Multimedia CD-ROM Single User License Agreement

1. NOTICE. WE ARE WILLING TO LICENSE THE MULTI-MEDIA PROGRAM PRODUCT TITLED **Clinical Immunology: Principles and Practice 2e** ("MULTIMEDIA PROGRAM") TO YOU ONLY ON THE CONDITION THAT YOU ACCEPT ALL OF THE TERMS CONTAINED IN THIS LICENSE AGREEMENT. PLEASE READ THIS LICENSE AGREEMENT CAREFULLY BEFORE OPENING THE SEALED DISK PACKAGE. BY OPENING THAT PACKAGE YOU AGREE TO BE BOUND BY THE TERMS OF THIS AGREEMENT. IF YOU DO NOT AGREE TO THESE TERMS WE ARE UNWILLING TO LICENSE THE MULTIMEDIA PROGRAME TO YOU, AND YOU SHOULD NOT OPEN THE DISK PACKAGE. IN SUCH CASE, PROMPTLY RETURN THE UNOPENED DISK PACKAGE AND ALL OTHER MATERIAL IN THIS PACKAGE, ALONG WITH PROOF OF PAYMENT, TO THE ATHORISED DEALER FROM WHOM YOU OBTAINED IT FOR A FULL REFUND OF THE PRICE YOU PAID.

2. **Ownership and License.** This is a license agreement and NOT an agreement for sale. It permits you to use one copy of the MULTIMEDIA PROGRAM on a single computer. The MULTIMEDIA PROGRAM and its contents are owned by us or our licensors, and are protected by U.S. and international copyright laws. Your rights to use the MULTIMEDIA PROGRAM are specified in this Agreement, and we retain all rights not expressly granted to you in this Agreement.

- You may use one copy of the MULTIMEDIA PROGRAM on a single computer
- After you have installed the MULTIMEDIA PROGRAM on your computer, you may use the MULTIMEDIA PROGRAM on a different computer only if you first delete the files installed by the installation program from the first computer.
- You may not copy any portion of the MULTIMEDIA PROGRAM to your computer hard disk or any other media other than printing out or downloading non- substantial portions of the text and images in the MULITMEDIA PROGRAM for your own internal informational use.
- Your may not copy any of the documentation or other printed materials accompanying the MULTIMEDIA PROGRAM.

Neither concurrent use on two or more computers nor use in a local area network or other network is permitted without separate authorisation and the payment of additional license fees.

1. **Transfer and Other Restrictions.** You may not rent, lend, or lease this MULTIMEDIA PROGRAM. Save as permitted by law, you may not and you may not permit others to (a) disassemble, decompile, or otherwise derive source code from the software included in the MULTIMEDIA PROGRAM (the "Software"), (b) reverse engineer the Software, (c) modify or prepare derivative works of the MULTIMEDIA PROGRAM (d) use the Software in an on-line system, or (e) use the MULITIMEDIA PROGRAM in any manner that infringes on the intellectual property or other rights of another party.

However, you may transfer this license to use the MULTIMEDIA ROGRAM to another party on a permanent basis by transferring this copy of the License Agreement, the MULTIMEDIA PROGRAM, and all documentation. Such transfer of possession terminates your license from us. Such other party shall be licensed under the terms of this Agreement upon its acceptance of this Agreement by its initial use of the MULTIMEDIA PROGRAM. If you transfer the MULTIMEDIA PROGRAM, you must remove the installation files from your hard disk and you may not retain any copies of those files for your own use.

2. **Limited Warranty and Limitation of Liability.** For a period of sixty (60) days from the date your acquired the MULTIMEDIA PROGRAM from us or our authorised dealer, we warrant that the media containing the MULTIMEDIA PROGRAM will be free from defects that prevent you from installing the MULTIMEDIA PROGRAM on your computer. If the disk fails to conform to this warranty you may as your sole and exclusive remedy, obtain a replacement free of charge if you return the defective disk to us with a dated proof of purchase. Otherwise the MULTIMEDIA PROGRAM is licensed to you on an "AS IS" basis without any warranty of any nature.

WE DO NOT WARRANT THAT THE MULTIMEDIA PROGRAM WILL MEET YOUR REQUREMENTS OR THAT ITS OPERATION WILL BE UNINTERRUPTED OR ERROR-FREE. THE EXPRESS TERMS OF THIS AGREEMENT ARE IN LIEU OF ALL WARRANTIES, CONDITIONS, UNDERTAKINGS, TERMS AND OBLIGATIONS IMPLIED BY STATUTE, COMMON LAW, TRADE USAGE, COURSE OF DEALING OR OTHERWISE ALL OF WHICH ARE HEREBY EXCLUDED TO THE FULLEST EXTENT PERMITTED BY LAW, INCLUDING THE IMPLIED WARRANTIES OF SATISFACTORY QUALITY AND FITNESS FOR A PARTICULAR PURPOSE.

WE SHALL NOT BE LIABLE FOR ANY DAMAGE OR LOSS OF ANY KIND (EXCEPT PERSONAL INJURY OR DEATH RESULTING FROM OUR NEGLIGENCE) ARISING OUT OF OR RESULTING FROM YOUR POSSESSION OR USE OF THE MULTIMEDIA PROGRAM (INCLUDING DATA LOSS OR CORRUPTION), REGARDLESS OF WHETHER SUCH LIABILITY IS BASED IN TORT, CONTRACT OR OTHERWISE AND INCLUDING, BUT NOT LIMITED TO, ACUTAL, SPECIAL, INDIRECT, INCIDENTIAL OR CONSEQUENTIAL DAMAGES. IF THE FOREGOING LIMITATION IS HELD TO BE UNENFORCEABLE OUR MAXIMUM LIABILITY TO YOU SHALL NOT EXCEED THE AMOUNT OF THE LICENSE FEE PAID BY YOU FOR THE MULTIMEDIA PROGRAM. THE REMEDIES AVAILABLE TO YOU AGAINST US AND THE LICENSORS OF MATERIALS INCLUDED IN THE MULTIMEDIA PROGRAM ARE EXCLUSIVE.

3. **Termination.** This license and your right to use this MULTIMEDIA PROGRAM automatically terminate if you fail to comply with any provisions of this Agreement, destroy the copy of the MULTIMEDIA PROGRAM in your possession, or voluntarily return the MULTIMEDIA PROGRAM to us. Upon termination you will destroy all copies of the MULTIMEDIA PROGRAM and documentation.

6. **Miscellaneous Provisions.** This Agreement will be governed by and construed in accordance with English law and you hereby submit to the non-exclusive jurisdiction of the English Courts. This is the entire agreement between us relating to the MULTMEDIA PROGRAM, and supersedes any prior purchase order, communications, advertising or representations concerning the contents of this package, No change or modification of this Agreement will be valid unless it is in writing and is signed by us

Second Edition

CLINICAL IMMUNOLOGY

PRINCIPLES AND PRACTICE

Edited by

Robert R Rich

Thomas A Fleisher

William T Shearer

Brian L Kotzin

Harry W Schroeder Jr

Volume Two

Mosby

London • Edinburgh • New York • Philadelphia • St Louis • Sydney • Toronto 2001

MOSBY
An imprint of Elsevier Science Limited

Dr. Fleisher edited this book in his private capacity and no official endorsement of support by the National Institutes of Health is intended or should be inferred.

First edition 1996
Second edition published 2001
Reprinted 2002, 2003

ISBN 0 7234 3161 2

British Library Cataloguing in Publication Data
A catalogue record for this book is available from the British Library

Library of Congress Cataloging in Publication Data
A catalog record for this book is available from the Library of Congress

Note
Medical knowledge is constantly changing. As new information becomes available, changes in treatment, procedures, equipment and the use of drugs become necessary.
The editors, contributors and the publishers have taken care to ensure that the information given in this text is accurate and up to date. However, readers are strongly advised to confirm that the information, especially with regard to drug usage, complies with the latest legislation and standards of practice.

Printed in China by RDC Group Limited
B/03

Commissioning Editor: Miranda Bromage
Project Development Manager: Louise Cook
Project Manager: Hilary Hewitt
Designer: Jayne Jones
Illustrations Manager: Mick Ruddy
Illustrators: Robin Dean, Jenni Miller

Contents

Contributors

Ronald T Acton PHD HCLD DIP ABMLI
Professor of Microbiology
Immunogenetics and DNA Diagnostic Laboratory
University of Alabama at Birmingham
Birmingham, AL
USA

Rafi Ahmed PHD
Director, GRA Chair in Vaccine Research
Emory Vaccine Center
Emory University School of Medicine
Atlanta, GA
USA

John Altman PHD
Assistant Professor
Department of Microbiology and Immunology
Vaccine Research Center
Emory University
Atlanta, GA
USA

Jintanat Ananworanich MD
Clinical Trials Co-ordinator/Pediatrician
HIV-NAT, The Thai Red Cross
AIDS Research Center
Bangkok
Thailand

Aftab Ansari PHD
Professor, Department of Pathology and Laboratory Medicine
Winship Cancer Center
Emory University School of Medicine
Atlanta, GA
USA

Gregory M Anstead MD PHD
Assistant Professor
Department of Medicine
Division of Infectious Diseases
University of Texas Health Sciences Center
San Antonio, TX
USA

William P Arend MD
Head, Division of Rheumatology
Professor of Medicine and Immunology
Division of Rheumatology
University of Colorado Health Sciences Center
Denver, CO
USA

Frank C Arnett MD
Professor of Internal Medicine, Pathology and Laboratory Medicine
Elizabeth Bidgood Chair in Rheumatology
University of Texas-Houston Medical School
Houston, TX
USA

Jonathan D Ashwell MD
Chief, Laboratory of Immune Cell Biology
Centre for Cancer Research
National Cancer Institute
National Institutes of Health
Bethesda, MD
USA

Howard A Austin III MD
Senior Clinical Investigator
National Institute of Diabetes and Digestive and Kidney Diseases
National Institutes of Health
Bethesda, MD
USA

Elia M Ayoub MD
Distinguished Service Professor
Vice Chairman for Academic Affairs
Department of Pediatrics
Pediatric Immunology and Infectious Diseases
University of Florida College of Medicine
Gainesville, FL
USA

James R Baker Jr. MD
Professor of Medicine
Chief, Division of Allergy and Immunology
Director, Center for Biologic Nanotechnology
University of Michigan Medical School
Ann Arbor, MI
USA

Mark A Ballow MD
Professor of Pediatrics
State University of New York at Buffalo
School of Medicine and Biomedical Sciences
Chief of Allergy/Clinical Immunology and Pediatric Rheumatology Division
Children's Hospital of Buffalo
Buffalo, NY
USA

James E Balow MD
Clinical Director
National Institute of Diabetes and Digestive and Kidney Diseases
National Institutes of Health
Bethesda, MD
USA

Emil J Bardana Jr. MD
Professor of Medicine
Head, Division of Allergy and Clinical Immunology
The Oregon Health Sciences University
Portland, OR
USA

Fuad M Baroody MD
Pediatric Otolaryngologist
Department of Surgery
Section of Otolaryngology
Head and Neck Surgery
The Pritzker School of Medicine
University of Chicago
Chicago, IL
USA

Robert E Baughn PHD
Professor
Veterans Affairs Medical Center
Department of Microbiology and Immunology
Baylor College of Medicine
Houston, TX
USA

Matthias D Becker MD
Casey Eye Institute
Oregon Health Science University
Portland, OR
USA

John W Belmont MD PHD
Associate Professor
Department of Molecular and Human Genetics
Baylor College of Medicine
Houston, TX
USA

Claudia Berek PHD
Senior Scientist
Deutsches Rheuma-Forschungszentrum Berlin
Berlin
Germany

Kishor Bhatia PHD
Head, Research Centre at King Fahad National Cancer Centre for Children's Cancer and Research
Riyadh, Saudi Arabia
Adjunct Professor
Department of Pathology and Microbiology
University of Nebraska Medical Center
USA

Leonard Bielory MD
Associate Professor of Medicine, Pediatrics and Ophthalmology
Asthma and Allergy Research Center
New Jersey Medical School
Newark, NJ
USA

Barbara E Bierer MD
Chief, Laboratory of Lymphocyte Biology
National Heart, Lung and Blood Institute
Senior Investigator
National Institutes of Health
Bethesda, MD
USA

Jack JH Bleesing MD
Immunology Fellow
Department of Laboratory Medicine
Warren G Magnuson Clinical Center
National Institutes of Health
Bethesda, MD
USA

Mark Boguniewicz MD
Senior Faculty Member
National Jewish Medical and Research Center;
Professor, Department of Pediatrics
University of Colorado School of Medicine
Denver, CO
USA

Dimitrios T Boumpas MD FACP
Division of Rheumatology
Clinical Immunology and Allergy
University of Crete Medical School
Heraklion
Greece

Prosper N Boyaka PHD
Assistant Research Professor
Department of Microbiology
The Immunology Vaccine Center
University of Alabama at Birmingham
Birmingham, AL
USA

Mary L Brandt MD
Associate Professor of Surgery
Michael E DeBakey Department of Surgery
Baylor College of Medicine
Texas Children's Hospital
Houston, TX
USA

Malcom K Brenner MB PHD FRCP FRCPATH
Professor of Medicine and Pediatrics
Director, Center for Cell and Gene Therapy
Baylor College of Medicine
Texas Children's Hospital
Houston, TX
USA

Knut Brockow MD
Visiting Fellow
Laboratory of Allergic Diseases
National Institute of Allergy and Infectious Diseases
National Institutes of Health
Bethesda, MD
USA

Rebecca H Buckley MD
J Buren Sidbury Professor of Pediatrics
Professor of Immunology
Department of Pediatrics
Duke University Medical Center
Durham, NC
USA

Ralph C Budd MD
Professor of Medicine
Director, Immunobiology Program
Department of Medicine
University of Vermont College of Medicine
Given College of Medicine
Burlington, VT
USA

Dario Campana MD PHD
Member, Hematology, Oncology and Pathology
St. Jude Children's Research Hospital;
Professor of Pediatrics
University of Tennesse College of Medicine
Memphis, TN
USA

James J Campbell MD
Assistant Professor of Pathology
Childrens Hospital
Harvard Medical School
Boston, MA
USA

Charles B Carpenter MD
Professor of Medicine
Harvard Medical School
Laboratory of Immunogenetics and Transplantation
Brigham and Women's Hospital
Boston, MA
USA

Melody C Carter MD
Clinical Fellow
Allergy and Immunology
National Institute of Allergy and Infectious Disease
National Institutes of Health
Bethesda, MD
USA

Alan S Cohen MD
Distinguished Professor of Medicine in Rheumatology
Amyloid Program
Boston University School of Medicine
Boston, MA
USA

Helen L Collins PHD
Post-doctoral Fellow
Department of Immunology
Max Planck Institute for Infection Biology
Berlin
Germany

Anthony D Cristillo PHD
Visiting Fellow
Laboratory of Lymphocyte Biology
National Institutes of Health
Bethesda, MD
USA

Ponciano D Cruz Jr. MD
Vice-Chairman and Professor
Department of Dermatology
University of Texas Southwestern Medical Center
Dallas, TX
USA

Charlotte Cunningham-Rundles MD
Professor, Department of Medicine and Pediatrics
Mount Sinai Medical Center
New York, NY
USA

Marinos C Dalakas MD
Professor of Neurology
Chief, Neuromuscular Diseases Section
National Institutes of Health
Bethesda, MD
USA

Richard D deShazo MD
Professor of Medicine and Pediatrics
Director, Division of Allergy and Immunology
Department of Medicine
University of Mississippi School of Medicine
Jackson, MS
USA

David Diaz-Sanchez PHD
Assistant Professor
Department of Medicine
Division of Immunology and Allergy
University of California at Los Angeles
Los Angeles, CA
USA

Angela Dispenzieri MD
Senior Associate Consultant
Division of Hematology and Internal Medicine
Mayo Clinic and Mayo Foundation
Rochester, MN
USA

Colin S Duckett PHD
Tenure Track Investigator
Metabolism Branch
Division of Clinical Sciences
National Cancer Institute
National Institutes of Health
Bethesda, MD
USA

Todd N Eager PHD
Research Assistant
Department of Microbiology–Immunology
Northwestern University Medical School
Chicago, IL
USA

George S Eisenbarth MD PHD
Professor of Medicine and Pediatrics
Barbara Davis Center for Childhood Diabetes
University of Colorado Health Sciences Center
Denver, CO
USA

Keith B Elkon MD
Professor of Medicine and Immunology
University of Washington
Seattle, WA
USA

B Keith English MD
Professor of Pediatrics
Chief, Division of Pediatric Infectious Diseases
University of Tennessee Health Science Center
Crippled Children's Foundation Research Center
Le Bonheur Children's Medical Center
Memphis, TN
USA

C Garrison Fathman MD
Professor of Medicine and Rheumatology
Chief of Division of Immunology
Stanford University School of Medicine
Stanford, CA
USA

Susetta Finotto PHD
Assistant Professor of Immunology
Laboratory of Immunology
University of Mainz
Mainz
Germany

Alain Fischer MD PHD
Professor of Medicine
Necker University Hospital
Paris
France

Thomas A Fleisher, MD
Chief, Department of Laboratory Medicine
Warren G Magnuson Clinical Center
National Institutes of Health
Bethesda, MD
USA

Andrew P Fontenot MD
Assistant Professor of Medicine
Division of Pulmonary Sciences and Critical Care Medicine
University of Colorado Health Sciences Center
Denver, CO
USA

Karen A Fortner PHD
Research Associate
Immunbiology Program
University of Vermont College of Medicine
Burlington, VT
USA

Robert I Fox MD PHD
Allergy and Immunology Clinic
Scripps Medical Foundation
La Jolla, CA
USA

Christopher E Freise MD
Assistant Professor of Surgery and Transplant Services
University of California
San Francisco, CA
USA

Anthony J Frew MD FRCP
Professor of Allergy and Respiratory Medicine
Department of Medical Specialties
Southampton General Hospital
Southampton
UK

David M Frucht BA MD
Clinical Associate
National Institutes of Health
Bethesda, MD
USA

Kohtaro Fujihashi DDS PHD
Associate Professor
Department of Oral Biology
The Immunology Vaccine Center
University of Alabama at Birmingham
Birmingham, AL
USA

Gianluca Gaidano MD PHD
Associate Professor of Internal Medicine
Centre for the Study and Treatment of Blood Disorders
Division of Internal Medicine
Amedeo Avogadro University of Eastern Piedmont
Novara
Italy

Stephen J Galli MD
Mary Hewitt Loveless MD Professor
Professor of Pathology and Microbiology and Immunology
Chair, Department of Pathology
Stanford University School of Medicine
Stanford University Medical Center
Stanford, CA
USA

Paul Gatenby MB BS PHD FRACP FRCPA MRACMA
Professor of Medicine and Pathology
Canberra Clinical School
The Canberra Hospital
Canberra ACT
Australia

M Eric Gershwin MD
The Jack and Donald Chia Professor of Medicine
Chief, Division of Rheumatology, Allergy and Clinical Immunology
University of California
Davis, CA
USA

Dennis O Gor PHD
Postdoctoral Fellow
Institute of Pathology
Case Western Reserve University
Cleveland, OH
USA

Neil S Greenspan MD PHD
Professor of Pathology
Institute of Pathology
Case Western Reserve University
Cleveland, OH
USA

Linda M Griffith MD PHD
Senior Staff Fellow
Department of Transfusion Medicine
Warren G Magnuson Clinical Center
National Institutes of Health
Bethesda, MD
USA

Russell P Hall III MD
Professor and Chief
Department of Medicine
Division of Dermatology
Duke VA Medical Center
Durham, NC
USA

Teal S Hallstrand MD MPH
Acting Instructor
Division of Pulmonary and Critical Care Medicine
University of Washington
Seattle, WA
USA

Robert G Hamilton PHD
Associate Professor of Medicine and Pathology
DACI Reference Laboratory
Allergy and Clinical Immunology Division
Johns Hopkins University School of Medicine
Baltimore, MD
USA

I Celine Hanson MD
Adjunct Professor of Pediatrics
Bureau Chief
Bureau of Communicable Disease Control
Texas Department of Health
Austin, TX
USA

Gregory R Harriman MD
Vice-President
Research and Clinical Development
Therakos
Exto, PA
USA

David B Hellman MD FACP
Mary Betty Stevens Professor of Medicine
Executive Vice Chairman
Department of Medicine
John Hopkins University School of Medicine
Baltimore, MD
USA

William R Henderson Jr. MD
Professor of Medicine
Department of Medicine
Division of Allergy and Infectious Disease
University of Washington
Seattle, WA
USA

V Michael Holers MD
Smyth Professor of Rheumatology
Chief, Division of Rheumatology and Professor of Medicine
University of Colorado Health Sciences Center
Denver , CO
USA

Stephen T Holgate BSC MD DSC FRCP FMEDSCI
Medical Research Council Clinical Professor of Immunopharmacology
Respiratory Cell and Molecular Biology Division
School of Medicine
University of Southampton
Southampton General Hospital
Southampton, Hants
UK

Steven M Holland, MD
Senior Clinical Investigator
Head, Immunopathogenesis Unit
Clinical Pathophysiology Section
Laboratory of Host Defenses
National Institute of Allergy and Infectious Disease
National Institutes of Health
Bethesda, MD
USA

Henry A Homburger MD
Professor of Laboratory Medicine
Department of Laboratory Medicine and Pathology
Mayo Medical School and Mayo Graduate School of Medicine
Mayo Clinic
Rochester, MN
USA

Marek Honczarenko MD PHD
Fellow
Department of Pathology and Lab Medicine
University of Pennsylvania Medical Center
Philadelphia, PA
USA

Keith M Hull MD PHD
Clinical Associate
Arthritis and Rheumatism Branch
National Institute of Arthritis and Musculoskeletal and Skin Diseases
National Institutes of Health
Bethesda, MD
USA

Gene G Hunder MD
Department of Internal Medicine/Rheumatology
Mayo Clinic
Rochester, MN
USA

Shai Izraeli MD
Associate Professor
Tel Aviv University Faculty of Medicine
Research Section
Department of Pediatric Hematology/ Oncology
Chaim Sheba Medical Center
Tel Hashomer
Israel

Heidi Jacobe MD
Chief Resident
Department of Dermatology
University of Texas Southwestern Medical Center
Dallas, TX
USA

Elaine S Jaffe MD
Chief, Hematopathology Section
Laboratory of Pathology
National Cancer Institute
National Institutes of Health
Bethesda, MD
USA

Sirpa Jalkanen MD PHD
Professor of the Finnish Academy
MediCity Research Laboratory
University of Turku
National Public Health Institute
Turku
Finland

Peter M Johnson PHD DSC FRCPATH
Professor of Immunology
Department of Immunology
University of Liverpool
Liverpool
UK

Barry D Kahan PHD MD
Professor of Surgery
Department of Surgery
Division of Immunology and Organ Transplantation
University of Texas Medical School at Houston
Houston, TX
USA

Allen P Kaplan MD
Professor
Division of Pulmonary and Critical Care Medicine
Allergy and Clinical Immunology
Medical University of South Carolina
Charleston, SC
USA

Arnon Karni MD
Research Fellow in Neurology
Department of Neurology
Center for Neurologic Disease
Brigham and Women's Hospital
Harvard Medical School
Boston, MA
USA

Stefan HE Kaufmann PHD
Professor and Director
Department of Immunology
Max-Planck Institute for Infection Biology
Berlin
Germany

Arthur F Kavanaugh MD
Associate Professor of Medicine
Director, Center for Innovative Therapies
University of California, San Diego
Division of Rheumatology/Allergy and Immunology
Thornton Hospital
La Jolla, CA
USA

Ilan R Kirsch MD
Chair, Genetics Department
Medicine Branch
Center for Cancer Research
Division of Clinical Sciences
National Cancer Institute
Bethesda, MD
USA

Harvey G Klein MD
Chief, Department of Transfusion Medicine
Warren G Magnuson Clinical Center
National Institutes of Health
Bethesda, MD
USA

Gary A Koretzky MD PHD
Professor, Pathology and Laboratory Medicine
Investigator and Director
Signal Transduction Program
Leonard and Madlyn Abramson Family Cancer Research Institute at University of Pennsylvania Cancer Center
University of Pennsylvania School of Medicine
Philadelphia, PA
USA

Brian L Kotzin MD
Professor of Medicine and Immunology
Chief, Division of Clinical Immunology
Department of Medicine
University of Colorado Health Sciences Center
Denver, CO
USA

M T Krishna PhD PHD MRCP
Specialist Registrar in Allergy and Clinical Immunology and Honorary Clinical Lecturer
Medical Specialities
Southampton General Hospital
Southampton, Hants
UK

Douglas B Kuhns PHD
Head, Neutrophil Monitoring Laboratory
SAIC Frederick
National Cancer Institute -FCRDC
Frederick, MD
USA

Roger Kurlander MD
Senior Staff for Hematology
Department of Health and Human Services
National Institutes of Health
Bethesda, MD
USA

Robert A Kyle MD
Professor of Medicine and Laboratory Medicine
Mayo Medical School
Mayo Clinic
Rochester, MN
USA

H Clifford Lane MD
Clinical Director
National Institute of Allergy and Infectious Disease
Immunologic Diseases Section
Laboratory of Immunoregulation
National Institutes of Health
Bethesda, MD
USA

Thomas J Lawley MD
Dean
School of Medicine
Emory University
Atlanta, GA
USA

Ellen F Lazarus MD FCAP
Reviewing Medical Officer
Division of Hematology
Food and Drug Administration CBER
Bethesda, MD
USA

Howard M Lederman MD PHD
Associate Professor of Pediatrics
Division of Pediatric Immunology
John Hopkins Hospital
Baltimore, MD
USA

Françoise Le Diest MD PHD
Associate Professor
Laboratory of Pediatric Immunology
Hôpital Necker-Enfants Malades
Paris
France

Richard L Leff MD
Senior Medical Director
DuPont Parmaceuticals
Wilmington, DE
USA

Philip Lieberman MD
Clinical Professor of Medicine and Pediatrics
University of Tennessee College of Medicine
Memphis, TN
USA

Donald YM Leung MD PHD
Professor and Head
Division of Pediatric Allergy/Immunology
National Jewish Medical and Research Center;
Professor of Pediatrics
University of Colorado Health Sciences Center
Denver, CO
USA

Patrick SC Leung PHD
Associate Adjunct Professor of Medicine
Division of Rheumatology, Allergy and Clinical Immunology
School of Medicine
University of California
Davis, CA
USA

Arnold I Levinson MD
Professor of Medicine and Neurology
Chief, Section of Allergy and Immunology
University of Pennsylvania School of Medicine
Philadelphia Veterans Administration Medical Center
Philadelphia, PA
USA

Stuart M Levitz MD
Professor of Medicine and Microbiology
The Evans Memorial Department of Clinical Research and the Department of Medicine
Boston University School of Medicine
Boston, MA
USA

Dorothy E Lewis PHD
Professor of Immunology
Department of Immunology
Baylor College of Medicine
Houston, TX
USA

John D Lippolis PHD
Technical Director
NIAID MHC Tetramer Core Facility
Vaccine Research Center
Emery University
Atlanta, GA
USA

Peter Lipsky MD
National Institute of Arthritis and Musculoskeletal and Skin Diseases
National Institutes of Health
Bethesda, MD
Adjunct Professor
University of Texas Southwestern Medical Center
Dallas, TX
USA

Douglas L Mann MD
Professor of Medicine
Baylor College of Medicine
Houston, TX
USA

Michael P Manns MD
Professor and Chairman
Department of Gastroenterology and Hepatology
Medizinische Hochschule
Hannover
Germany

Mariarosaria Marinaro PHD
Senior Researcher
Laboratorio di Batteriologia e Micologia Medica
Istituto Superiore di Sanita
Rome
Italy

Gerald Marti MD PHD
Laboratory of Medical and Molecular Genetics
Center for Biologics Evaluation and Research
Food and Drug Administration
Bethesda, MD
USA

Mehrdad Mazlumzadeh MD
Instructor, Mayo Medical School
Mayo Clinic
Rheumatology
Rochester, MN
USA

Peter C Melby MD
Associate Professor
Department of Medicine
Division of Infectious Diseases
University of Texas Health Sciences Center
San Antonio, TX
USA

Elizabeth D Mellins MD
Associate Professor
Department of Pediatrics
Division of Immunology and Transplantation Biology
Stanford University Medical School
Stanford, CA
USA

Laurel J Mengle-Gaw MD PHD
President and Co-Founder
The Camden Group
St Louis, MO
USA

Dean D Metcalfe MD
Chief, Laboratory of Allergic Diseases
National Institute of Allergy and Infectious Diseases
National Institutes of Health
Bethesda, MD
USA

JoAnn M Mican MD
Staff Physician
Division of Intramural Research
National Institutes of Allergy and Infectious Diseases
Bethesda, MD
USA

Ted R Mikuls MD
Clinical Fellow
Division of Clinical Immunology and Rheumatology
University of Alabama at Birmingham
Birmingham, AL
USA

Stephen D Miller PHD
Congressman John E Porter Professor
Director, Interdepartmental Immunobiological Center
Department of Microbiology–Immunology
DeNorthwestern University Medical School
Chicago, IL
USA

John E Moffitt MD
Professor of Pediatrics
Associate Professor of Medicine
Associate Dean for Graduate Medical Education
University of Mississippi School of Medicine
Jackson, MS
USA

David R Moller MD
Associate Professor of Medicine
Division of Pulmonary and Critical Care Medicine
The John Hopkins University School of Medicine
Baltimore, MD
USA

Anthony Montanaro MD
Professor of Medicine
Division of Allergy and Clinical Immunology
Oregon Health Sciences University
Portland, OR
USA

Malcolm AS Moore DPHIL
Enid A Haupt Professor of Cell Biology
Memorial Sloan Kettering Cancer Center
New York, NY
USA

Larry W Moreland MD
Professor of Medicine and Vice-Chairman for Clinical Research
Division of Clinical Immunology and Rheumatology
University of Alabama at Birmingham
Birmingham, AL
USA

Edina H Moylett MD
Pediatric Allergy and Immunology Fellow
Department of Allergy and Immunology
Texas Children's Hospital
Baylor College of Medicine
Houston, TX
USA

Jerry R McGhee PHD
Professor of Microbiology and Director
Department of Microbiology
The Immunobiology Vaccine Center
University of Alabama at Birmingham
Birmingham, AL
USA

Peter A McSweeney MD
Associate Professor of Medicine
Director of Allogeneic Transplantation
University of Colorado Health Sciences Centre
Denver, CO
USA

Ted R Mikuls MD
Fellow, Division of Clinical Immunology and Rheumatology
University of Alabama at Birmingham
Birmingham, AL
USA

Robert M Naclerio MD
Professor and Chief
Section of Otolaryngology
Head and Neck Surgery
The Pritzker School of Medicine
University of Chicago
Chicago, IL
USA

Karen A Nelson PHD DIPABHI
Director, Immunogenetics Laboratory
Puget Sound Blood Center
Seattle, WA
USA

Barbara S Nepom MD
Associate Member
Immunology Program
Virginia Mason Research Institute
Department of Pediatrics
University of Washington
Seattle, WA
USA

Markus F Neurath MD
Associate Professor of Medicine
Laboratory of Medicine
University of Mainz
Mainz
Germany

Anna Nowak-Wegrzyn MD
Assistant Professor Department of Pediatrics
Division of Allergy and Immunology
Mount Sinai School of Medicine
New York, NY
USA

Thomas B Nutman MD
Head, Helminth Immunology Section
Laboratory of Parasitic Diseases
National Institute of Allergy and Infectious Diseases
National Institutes of Health
Bethesda, MD
USA

Petra Obermayer-Straub MD
Professor, Department of Gastroenterology and Hepatology
Medizinische Hochschule
Hannover
Germany

John O'Shea MD
Chief, Lymphocyte Cell Biology Section
National Institute of Arthritis and Musculoskeletal and Skin Diseases
National Institutes of Health
Bethesda, MD
USA

Robert I Parker MD
Associate Professor and Vice Chairman for Academic Affairs
Department of Pediatrics
Stony Brook
New York, NY
USA

Mary E Paul MD
Assistant Professor of Pediatrics
Department of Pediatrics
Section of Allergy and Immunology
Baylor College of Medicine
Texas Children's Hospital
Houston, TX
USA

Erik J Peterson MD
Instructor, Department of Medicine
Abramson Family Cancer Research Institute
University of Pennsylvania School of Medicine
Philadelphia, PA
USA

Stefania Pittaluga MD PHD
Staff Physician
Hematopathology Section
Laboratory of Pathology
National Cancer Institute
National Institutes of Health
Bethesda, MD
USA

Paul Plotz MD
Chief, National Arthritis and Rheumatism Branch
National Institute of Arthritis and Musculoskeletal and Skin Diseases
National Institutes of Health
Bethesda, MD
USA

Calman Prussin MD FAAAAI
Head, Clinical Allergy and Immunology Unit
Laboratory of Allergic Diseases
National Institute of Allergy and Infectious Diseases
National Institutes of Health
Bethesda, MD
USA

Ching-Hon Pui MD
Director, Leukemia-Lymphoma Division
St. Jude Children's Research Hospital;
Professor of Pediatrics
University of Tennessee
College of Medicine
Memphis, TN
USA

Andreas Radbruch PHD
Professor of Experimental Rheumatology
Scientific Director
Deutsches Rheuma-Forschungszentrum Berlin
Berlin
Germany

John Renz MD PHD
Surgical Fellow
Department of Surgery
University of California at San Francisco
San Francisco, CA
USA

Robert R Rich MD
Executive Associate Dean
Professor of Medicine, Microbiology and Immunology
Emory University
School of Medicine
Atlanta, GA
USA

David T Robles BS
Medical Scientist Training Program
Department of Immunology
Barbara Davis Center for Childhood Diabetes
University of Colorado Health Sciences Center
Denver, CO
USA

John R Rodgers PHD
Assistant Professor
Department of Immunology
Baylor College of Medicine
Houston, TX
USA

James T Rosenbaum MD
Professor of Opthalmology, Medicine and Cell Biology
School of Medicine
Casey Eye Institute
Oregan Health Science University
Portland, OR
USA

Roger D Rossen MD
Professor, Immunology and Medicine
Baylor College of Medicine;
Chief, Allergy and Immunology Section
Director, Research Center for AIDS and HIV Infections
Houston Veterans Affairs Medical Center
Houston, TX
USA

Barry T Rouse DVM DSC
Lindsay Young Distinguished Professor of Microbiology
Department of Microbiology
College of Veterinary Medicine
University of Tennessee
Knoxville, TN
USA

Shimon Sakaguchi MD PHD
Professor and Chair
Department of Experimental Pathology
Institute for Frontier Medical Sciences
Kyoto University
Kyoto
Japan

Marko Salmi MD PHD
Special Investigator
Medicity Research Laboratory
University of Turku
National Public Health Institute
Turku
Finland

S S Salvi MD PHD
Clinical Research Fellow
School of Medicine
Division of Infection, Inflammation and Repair
University of Southampton
Southampton General Hospital
Southampton, Hants
UK

Christy Sandborg MD
Associate Professor of Pediatrics
Department of Pediatrics
Stanford University Medical Center
Stanford, CA
USA

Andrew Saxon MD
Chief, Professor of Medicine
Department of Medicine
Division of Clinical Immunology
University of California at Los Angeles
Los Angeles, CA
USA

Mohamed H Sayegh MD
Associate Professor of Medicine
Harvard Medical School
Laboratory of Immunogenetics and Transplantation
Brigham and Women's Hospital
Boston, MA
USA

Geraldine P Schechter MD
Professor, Department of Medicine
Chief, Hematology Section
George Washington University
Hematology and Oncology Division
VA Medical Center
Washington, DC
USA

Ronald F Schell PHD
Professor of Medical Microbiology and Immunology
Wisconsin State Laboratory of Hygiene
University of Wisconsin
Madison, WI
USA

Harry W Schroeder Jr. MD PHD
Professor of Medicine and Microbiology
Division of Developmental and Clinical Immunology
University of Alabama at Birmingham
Birmingham, AL
USA

Marvin I Schwarz MD
James C Campbell Professor of Pulmonary Medicine
Head, Division of Pulmonary Sciences and Critical Care Medicine
University of Colorado Health Sciences Center
Denver, CO
USA

Benjamin D Schwartz MD PHD
CEO and Co-Founder
The Camden Group
St Louis, MO
USA

William E Seaman MD
Professor of Medicine and of Microbiology/Immunology
Department of Medicine
Immunology/Arthritis Section
Veterans Administration Medical Center
University of California, San Francisco
School of Medicine
San Francisco, CA
USA

William M Shafer PHD
Professor Microbiology and Immunology
Emory University School of Medicine and Medical Research
VA Medical Center
Atlanta, GA
USA

William T Shearer MD PHD
Professor of Pediatrics and Immunology
Baylor College of Medicine
Chief, Allergy and Immunology Service
Texas Children's Hospital
Houston, TX
USA

Jeffrey Sherman MD
Assistant Clinical Professor of Medicine
George Washington University Hospital
Washington, DC
USA

Shmuel Shoham MD
Fellow in Infectious Disease
Professor of Medicine and Microbiology
Department of Medicine
Division of Infectious Diseases
Boston University School of Medicine
Boston, MA
USA

Leslie E Silberstein MD
Professor of Pathology (Pediatrics)
Department of Pathology
Children's Hospital
Boston, MA
USA

Jean D Sipe PHD
Scientific Review Administrator
Center for Scientific Review
National Institutes of Health
Bethesda, MD
USA

C Wayne Smith MD
Professor and Head
Section of Leukocyte Biology
Department of Pediatrics
Baylor College of Medicine
Houston , TX
USA

Justine R Smith MD PHD FRACO FRACS
Post-doctoral Clinical Research Fellow
Casey Eye Institute
Oregon Health Sciences University
Portland, OR
USA

Phillip D Smith MD
Professor of Medicine and Microbiology
Department of Medicine
University of Alabama at Birmingham
Birmingham, AL
USA

Lesley E Smythies PHD BSC (hons) AKC
Research Associate
Department of Medicine
University of Alabama at Birmingham
Veterans Administration Medical Center
Birmingham, AL
USA

Michael C Sneller, MD
Chief, Immunologic Diseases Section
Laboratory of Immunoregulation
National Institute for Allergy and Infectious Diseases
National Institutes of Health
Bethesda, MD
USA

Joseph D Spahn MD
Director of Immunopharmacology Laboratory
Division of Clinical Pharmacology
Associate Professor of Pediatrics
University of Colorado School of Medicine
National Jewish Medical and Research Center
Denver, CO
USA

Allen C Steere MD
Natalie V and Milton O Zucker Professor of Rheumatology and Immunology
New England Medical Center
Boston, MA
USA

Lawrence Steinman MD
Professor of Neurology and Neurological Sciences
Department of Neurology and Neurological Sciences and Department of Medicine
Beckman Center for Molecular Medicine
Stanford University School of Medicine
Stanford, CA
USA

David S Stephens MD
Professor of Medicine and Microbiology and Immunology
Emory University School of Medicine
Atlanta, GA
USA

John H Stone MD MPH
Assistant Professor of Medicine
Co-Director, John Hopkins Vasculitis Center
John Hopkins University School of Medicine
Baltimore, MD
USA

Rainer Storb MD
Head and Member
Transplantation Program
Fred Hutchinson Cancer Research Center;
Professor of Medicine
University of Washington
Seattle, WA
USA

Warren Strober MD
Chief, Mucosal Immunity Section
NIH/LCI/NIAID/MIS
National Institutes of Health
Bethesda, MD
USA

Frank J Strobl MD PHD
Assistant Professor
Pathology and Laboratory Medicine
Transfusion Medicine Section
Hospital of University of Pennsylvania
Philadelphia, PA
USA

Richard E Sutton MD PHD
Assistant Professor
Department of Molecular Virology and Microbiology
Baylor College of Medicine
Texas Medical Center
Houston TX
USA

Paul Szabo MD
Associate Research Professor
Division of Geriatrics and Gerontology
Department of Medicine
Weill Medical College of Cornell Unoversity
New York, NY
USA

Stanley J Szefler MD
Helen Wohlberg and Herman Lambert Chair in Pharmacokinetics
Co-Director, Clinical Research Unit
National Jewish Medical and Research Center
Professor of Pediatrics and Pharmacology
University of Colorado Health Sciences Center
Denver, CO
USA

Russell H Tomar MD FCAP
Chair, Department of Pathology
Cook County Hospital
Professor of Pathology
Rush Medical College
Professor of Preventive Medicine
University of Wisconsin School of Medicine
Chicago, IL
USA

Stephen M Tompkins BS PHD
Post-doctoral Fellow
Department of Microbiology-Immunology
Northwestern University Medical School
Chicago, IL
USA

Raul M Torres PHD
Assistant Professor
Department of Immunology
University of Colorado Health Science Center
National Jewish Medical and Reasearch Center
Denver, CO
USA
and Scientific Member
Basel Institute for Immunology
Basel
Switzerland

Takashi Uchiyama MD PHD
Professor
Department of Hematology/Oncology
Graduate School of Medicine
Kyoto University
Kyoto
Japan

Gülbû Uzel MD
Clinical Associate
National Institute of Allergy and Infectious Diseases
National Institutes of Health
Bethesda, MD
USA

Gill S Vince BSC PHD
Lecturer in Reproductive Immunology
Department of Immunology
University of Liverpool
Liverpool
UK

Sharon M Wahl PHD
Chief, Oral Infection and Immunity Branch
National Institute of Dental and Craniofacial Research
National Institutes of Health
Bethesda, MD
USA

Bruce Walker MD
Professor of Medicine
Department of Infectious Disease
Harvard Medical School
Director of AIDS Research Center
Massachusetts General Hospital
Boston, MA
USA

Su He Wang MD PHD
Research Investigator of Medicine
Department of Internal Medicine
University of Michigan
Ann Arbor, MI
USA

Russell E Ware MD PHD
Professor of Pediatrics
Department of Pediatrics
Duke University Medical Center
Durham, NC
USA

Stephen I Wasserman MD
Professor
Department of Medicine
University of California San Diego Medical Center
San Diego, CA
USA

Jochen Wedemeyer MD
Medical Resident
Department of Gastroenterology and Hepatology
Medizenische Hochscule Hannover
Hannover
Germany

Bih-Rong Wei PHD
Research Associate
Institute of Pathology
Case Western Reserve University
Cleveland, OH
USA

Howard Weiner MD
Partners Multiple Sclerosis Center
Center for Neurologic Diseases
Brigham and Women's Hospital
Boston, MA
USA

Allan M Weissman MD
Senior Investigator
Laboratory of Immune Cell Biology
Center for Cancer Research
National Cancer Institute
National Institutes of Health
Bethesda, MD
USA

Marc E Weksler MD
Wright Professor of Medicine
Department of Medicine
Division of Geriatrics and Gerontology
Weill Medical College of Cornell University
New York, NY
USA

Peter F Weller MD FACP
Professor of Medicine
Harvard Medical School
Chief, Allergy and Inflammation Division
Co-Chief, Infectious Diseases Division
Beth Israel Deaconess Medical Center
Boston, MA
USA

Sally E Wenzel MD
Associate Professor
National Jewish Medical Research Center
Denver, CO
USA

Sterling G West MD
Professor of Medicine
Division of Rheumatology
University of Colorado Health Sciences Center
Denver, CO
USA

Barbara White MD
Fellow Member
University of Maryland
Department of Medicine
Division of Rheumatology and Clinical Immunology
The Baltimore Veterans Administration Medical Center
Baltimore, MD
USA

Cara C Wilson MD
Assistant Professor of Medicine and Immunology
Division of Medicine, Clinical Immunology and Infectious diseases
University of Colorado Health Sciences Center
Denver, CO
USA

Christopher B Wilson MD
Professor and Chair
Department of Pediatrics and Immunology
University of Washington
Seattle, WA
USA

Kim B Yancey MD
Professor and Chair
Department of Dermatology
Medical College of Wisconsin
Milwaukee, WI
USA

James C Yang MD
Senior Investigator
Surgery Branch
National Cancer Institute
Assistant Professor of Surgery
Uniformed Services University of the Health Sciences
Bethesda, MD
USA

Anne B Yates MD
Assistant Professor of Pediatrics and Medicine
Department of Pediatrics
University of Mississippi Medical School
Jackson, MS
USA

James B Young MD
Medical Director
Head, Section of Heart Failure and Cardiac Transplant Medicine
Department of Cardiology
Kaufman Center for Heart Failure
Cleveland, OH
USA

Ke Zhang MD PHD
Assistant Professor
Department of Medicine
Division of Clinical Immunology/Allergy
University of California at Los Angeles
Los Angeles, CA
USA

Preface to the First Edition

Clinical immunology is a discipline with a distinguished history, rooted in the prevention and treatment of infectious diseases in the late nineteenth and early twentieth centuries. The conquest of historical scourges such as smallpox and (substantially) polio and the relegation of several other diseases to the category of medical curiosities is often regarded as the most important achievement of medical science of the past fifty years. Nevertheless, the challenges facing immunologists in the efforts to control infectious diseases remain formidable; HIV infection, malaria and tuberculosis are but three examples of diseases of global import that elude control despite major commitments of monetary and intellectual resources.

Although firmly grounded in the study and application of defenses to microbial infection, since the 1960s clinical immunology has emerged as a far broader discipline. Dysfunction of the immune system has been increasingly recognized as a pathogenic mechanism that can lead to an array of specific diseases and failure of virtually every organ system. Paradoxically, although the importance of the immune system in disease pathogenesis is generally appreciated, the place of clinical immunology as a practice discipline has been less clear. As most of the noninfectious diseases of the immune system lead eventually to failure of other organs, it has been organ-specific subspecialists who have usually dealt with their consequences. Recently, however, the outlook has begun to change as new diagnostic tools increasingly allow the theoretical possibility of intervention much earlier in disease processes, often before irreversible target organ destruction occurs. More importantly, this theoretical possibility is increasingly realized as clinical immunologists find themselves in the vanguard of translating molecular medicine from laboratory bench to patient bedside.

In many settings, clinical immunologists today function as primary care physicians in the management of patients with inmune-deficiency, allergic, and autoimmune diseases. Indeed many influential voices in the clinical disciplines of allergy and rheumatology support increasing coalescence of these traditional subspecialities around their intellectual core of immunology. In addition to his or her role as a primary care physician, the clinical immunologist is increasingly being looked to as a consultant, as scientific and clinical advances enhance his or her expertise. The immunologist with a *'generalist'* perspective can be particularly helpful in the application of unifying principles of diagnosis and treatment across the broad spectrum of immunologic diseases.

Clinical Immunology: Principles and Practice has emerged from this concept of the clinical immunologist as both primary care physician and expert consultant in the management of patients with immunologic diseases. It opens in full appreciation of the critical role of fundamental immunology in this rapidly evolving clinical discipline. Authors of basic science chapters were asked, however, to cast their subjects in a context of clinical relevance. We believe the result is a well-balanced exposition of basic immunology for the clinician.

The initial two sections on basic principles of immunology are followed by two sections that focus in detail on the role of the immune system in defenses against infectious organisms. The approach is two-pronged. It begins first with a systemic survey of immune responses to pathogenic agents followed by a detailed treatment of immunologic deficiency syndromes. Pathogenic mechanisms of both congenital and acquired immune deficiency diseases are discussed, as are the infectious complications that characterize these diseases. Befitting its importance, the subject of HIV infection and AIDS receives particular attention, with separate chapters on the problem of infection in the immunocompromised host, HIV infection in children, anti-retroviral therapy and current progress in the development of HIV vaccines.

The classic allergic diseases are the most common immunologic diseases in the population, ranging from atopic disease to drug allergy to organ-specific allergic disease (e.g., of the lungs, eye and skin). They constitute a foundation for the practice of clinical immunology, particularly for those physicians with a practice orientation defined by formal subspecialty training in allergy and immunology. A major section is consequently devoted to these diseases, with an emphasis on pathophysiology as the basis for rational management.

The next two sections deal separately with systemic and organ-specific immunologic diseases. The diseases considered in the first of these sections are generally regarded as the core practice of the clinical immunologist with subdisciplinary emphasis in rheumatology. The second section considers diseases of specific organ failure as consequences of immunologically mediated processes that may involve virtually any organ system. These diseases include as typical examples the demyelinating diseases, insulin-dependent diabetes mellitus, the glomerulonephritides and inflammatory bowel diseases. It is in management of such diseases that the discipline of clinical immunology will have an increasing role as efforts focus on intervention early in the pathogenic process and involve diagnostic and therapeutic tools of ever-increasing sophistication.

One of the major clinical areas in which the expertise of a clinical immunologist is most frequently sought is that of allogeneic organ transplantation. A full section is devoted to the issue of transplantation of solid organs, with an introductory chapter on general principles of transplantation and management of transplant rejection followed by separate chapters dealing with the special problems of transplantation of specific organs or organ systems.

Appreciation of both the molecular and clinical features of lymphoid malignancies is important to the clinical immunologist regardless of subspecialty background, notwithstanding the fact that primary responsibility for management of such patients will generally fall to the hematologist/oncologist. A separate section is consequently devoted to the lymphocytic leukemias and lymphomas that constitute the majority of malignancies seen in the context of a clinical immunology practice. The separate issues of immune responses to tumors and immunologicial strategies to treatment of malignant diseases are subjects of additional chapters.

Another important feature is the attention to therapy of immunologic diseases. This theme is constant throughout the chapters on the allergic and immunologic diseases, and because of the importance the editors attach to clinical immunology as a therapeutic discipline, an extensive section is also devoted specifically to this subject. Subsections are devoted to issues of immunologic reconstitution, with three chapters on treatment of immunodeficiencies, malignancies and metabolic diseases by bone marrow transplantation. Also included is a series of chapters on pharmaceutical agents currently available to clinical immunologists, both as anti-allergic and anti-inflammatory drugs, as well as newer agents with greater specificity for T cell-mediated immune responses. The section concludes with a series of chapters that address established and potential applications of therapeutic agents and approaches that are largely based on the new techniques of molecular medicine. In addition to pharmaceutical agents the section deals in detail with such subjects as apheresis, cytokines, monoclonal antibodies and immunotoxins, gene therapy and new experimental approaches to the treatment of autoimmunity.

The book concludes with a section devoted to approaches and specific techniques involved in the diagnosis of immunologic diseases. Use of the diagnostic laboratory in evaluation of complex problems of immunopathogenesis has been a hallmark of the clinical immunologist since inception of the discipline and many clinical immunologists serve as directors of diagnostic immunology laboratories. Critical assessment of the utilization of techniques ranging from lymphocyte cloning to flow cytometric phenotyping to molecular diagnostics are certain to continue as an important function of the clinical immunologist, particularly in his or her role as expert consultant.

In summary, we have intended to provide the reader with a comprehensive and authoritative treatise on the broad subject of clinical immunology, with particular emphasis on the diagnosis and treatment of immunological diseases. It is anticipated that the book will be used most frequently by the physician specialist practicing clinical immunology, both in his or her role as a primary physician and as a subspecialty consultant. It is hoped, however, that the book will also be of considerable utility to the non-immunologist. Many of the diseases discussed authoritatively in the book are diseases commonly encountered by the generalist physician. Indeed, as noted, because clinical immunology involves diseases of virtually all organ systems, competence in the diagnosis and management of immunological diseases is important to virtually all clinicians. The editors would be particularly pleased to see the book among the references readily available to the practicing internist, pediatrician and family physician.

Robert R. Rich
Thomas A. Fleisher
Benjamin D. Schwartz
William T. Shearer
Warren Strober

Preface to the Second Edition

The rapid progress in biomedical research noted in the preface to the first edition of *Clinical Immunology: Principles and Practice* continues, and at a continuously accelerating rate. Understanding the genetic basis of disease is proceeding rapidly, and will be further enhanced by the complete sequencing of the human genome. With development of new gene-deletion mice announced virtually daily, experimental models of human disease are becoming increasingly sophisticated. Advances in molecular understanding of leukocyte function offer many new targets for therapeutic intervention.

Important changes in the practice of clinical immunology reflect this progress in fundamental research. In developed countries, AIDS is no longer regarded as the virtual 'death sentence' of a few years ago. However, the constant vigilance and adherence of patients to therapeutic regimens to maintain an equilibrium with their disease still stresses the need for a better understanding of the mechanisms of T-cell control of infection. Research with recombinant cytokines and 'designer' monoclonal antibodies is bringing new therapeutic approaches to the treatment of allergic, autoimmune and other inflammatory diseases. New immunosuppressive regimens of increased efficacy and reduced toxicity improve the treatment of organ transplant recipients and patients with autoimmune diseases. and the introduction of the 'blockbuster' cyclooxygenase-2 inhibitors has transformed the treatment of arthritis.

Meanwhile, formidable challenges remain. AIDS in developing countries continues on a devastating pathway of disability and death. Malaria and tuberculosis remain worldwide scourges. Definitive identification of the etiologic agents in autoimmune diseases remains frustratingly elusive. In each of these cases the development of a preventative or therapeutic vaccine seems most likely to lead to fundamental advances in treatment. But in each instance this is likely to come from further progress in basic science. In that respect, by providing a basic science context for the current and future practice of clinical immunology, this edition should prepare today's practitioners for tomorrow's 'break-throughs'.

The editors have been gratified by responses to the first edition of *Clinical Immunology*, with feedback from many readers indicating that it served an important need. Advances in the areas above, and many others, therefore mandate a second edition. The editors thus renew their commitment to the treatment of patients with immunologic diseases with this thoroughly updated and comprehensive reference text for the practitioner treating such patients.

Because of the ubiquity of immunologic diseases, involving virtually every organ system, we continue to believe that every generalist physician must, at some level, practice clinical immunology, and every subspecialist must approach the patient with immunologic disease from the perspective of a generalist. Reflecting this premise of the first edition, we hope to have again developed a comprehensive overview of immunology and immunologic diseases of usefulness to generalists and subspecialists alike. Basic precepts of immune function and of the etiologies and pathogenetic mechanisms of immunologic diseases are described in considerable detail. But in every chapter, a popular feature from the first edition, the highlighting of Key Concepts, assures that the busy generalist (or house officer) can quickly grasp the essence of an author's message. To enhance this presentation of essential material, in the second edition Key Concepts boxes are joined in basic science chapters by summary boxes on Clinical Relevance and in clinical chapters by boxes entitled Therapeutic Principles and Clinical Pearls.

In addition to a systematic description of immunologic diseases, in which the various chapters include approaches to disease management, this edition again provides the reader with separate sections on therapeutic modalities and diagnostic tools. Venerable drugs and diagnostics, such as antihistamines and skin tests, are treated in balanced approach with newer and less familiar drugs such as immunophilin-binding drugs and leukotriene inhibitors and diagnostic tests such as fluorescence *in situ* hybridization and heteroduplex DNA analysis for detection of mutations. Our intent has been to introduce new and promising approaches to disease management, while never ignoring the 'tried and true.'

With the strong support of the Publisher, this edition is enhanced over the first edition in several respects that we believe will facilitate its use. Line drawings have been prepared to a common style and the number of color plates has been substantially increased. The CD-ROM that accompanies the written text provides illustrative material in color which we believe will be especially useful to individuals involved in the teaching of clinical immunology.

As always, an undertaking of this magnitude represents the dedicated efforts of many individuals. We thank first the many chapter authors who worked with us, enduring an editorial 'heavy-hand' intended to provide a book that was up-to-date and accurate in content, and with consistency of organization and style. We are grateful for their indulgence. We hope the reader will be well served, for example, by those cases where we have asked for reductions from a list of hundreds of references, appropriate to a scholarly review, to a selected bibliography that we thought more useful to readers of a textbook.

We also thank the dedicated team from Mosby in London who saw this edition from first concept to completed product with frequent trans-Atlantic conference calls, occasional trans-Atlantic travel and unremitting cheerfulness. Our appreciation, then, to Miranda Bromage, Serena Bureau, and especially to Francesca Lumkin and Ian Stoneham. Their determination to meet deadlines without ever compromising quality was very much appreciated. Finally, Mary Middleton at Emory University School of Medicine deserves the special thanks of the editor-in-chief for helping to maintain focus on the task, coordinating the efforts of all the editors and assuring the flow of a mountain of paper, and trillions of electrons, around the globe.

Robert R. Rich
Thomas A. Fleisher
William T. Shearer
Brian L. Kotzin
Harry W. Schroeder, Jr.

Dedication

To the special persons in our lives who have inspired and supported our work . . .

Susan and Margaret Rich

Mary, Gisela and Gerard Fleisher

Lynn Des Prez, and Christine, Mark, Christopher, Martin, John, and Jesse Shearer

Kathryn Comick and Margaret and Ezra Kotzin

Dixie Lee Schroeder, Maria de los Angeles Melendez Vda. de Schroeder and Elena de la Garza Vda. de Melendez

Chapter 64

Systemic Sclerosis

Barbara White

DESCRIPTION/NATURAL HISTORY

In 1753 a new malady was reported by Curzio, who was the physician of a 17-year-old girl with 'excessive tension and hardness of her skin over all her body', who could 'scarce open her mouth', and who sensed 'an uneasy constriction round the belly' after eating.[1] One century later, Gintrac coined the term 'sclerodermie' (Greek: *skleros* hard, *derma* skin) to designate this illness. Medical literature through the 1920s emphasized the dermatologic manifestations of scleroderma. Over the subsequent decades, the systemic nature and heterogeneity of clinical expression of the disease have become obvious. Scleroderma can range from a mild, indolent ailment that blurs the border between illness and health to an abrupt, aggressive, ischemic and fibrotic process that destroys organs and causes death.

Precise incidence and prevalence figures for systemic sclerosis are not available. Although early prevalence estimates placed systemic sclerosis among the relatively rare diseases, more inclusive studies estimate the incidence of this disease at 19 cases per million per year[2] and the prevalence as high as 67–265 cases per 100 000 people.[3] Thus, 150 000 to 500 000 people in the USA are estimated to have systemic sclerosis. Systemic sclerosis occurs in all geographic locations and ethnic groups.[4] It strikes adults principally, especially women aged 35–65 years, with an overall female to male ratio of approximately 3:1.[4]

Scleroderma is a generic term used to describe both disease restricted to the skin (localized scleroderma) and disease with internal organ involvement (systemic sclerosis). There are two major categories of systemic sclerosis, limited cutaneous systemic sclerosis (lSSc) and diffuse cutaneous systemic sclerosis (dSSc).[5] Limited cutaneous systemic sclerosis is skin thickening confined to the extremities distal to the elbows and knees, without truncal involvement (facial involvement is allowed). Diffuse cutaneous systemic sclerosis is skin involvement that, at one time, includes the proximal extremities or trunk. Scleroderma sine scleroderma describes about 5% of systemic sclerosis patients who have no skin involvement but do have characteristic gut or other internal organ damage. Scleroderma overlap syndromes include illnesses with concomitant features of systemic sclerosis and polymyositis, rheumatoid arthritis, systemic lupus erythematosus, Sjögren syndrome, or biliary cirrhosis.

Limited cutaneous systemic sclerosis (lSSc) is more common than the diffuse version of disease, but exact ratios are unknown because of a bias towards under-diagnosis.[3] Patients with the CREST syndrome of *c*alcinosis, *R*aynaud's phenomenon, *e*sophageal dysmotility, *s*clerodactyly, and *t*elangiectasia are a subset of lSSc patients. Other patients with lSSc or dSSc may have calcinosis, Raynaud's phenomenon, esophageal dysmotility, or telangiectasia, and systemic sclerosis patients should not be given the diagnosis of CREST just because they have one or more of these later manifestations. The discriminating clinical feature of CREST is sclerodactyly, with skin fibrosis confined to the fingers (with or without facial involvement). The CREST patients usually have anticentromere antibodies. Classification of the patients into lSSc and dSSc categories helps the physician prognosticate the general clinical course (Table 64.1), although variability exists even within these subsets. Patients with lSSc may present with bothersome Raynaud's phenomenon, digital ulcers, esophageal reflux, or dysphagia. Less frequently, they present with symptoms related to interstitial lung disease or pulmonary hypertension. Those lSSc patients with anticentromere antibodies are at lower risk of developing interstitial lung disease than other lSSc patients, but are at higher risk for developing pulmonary hypertension. In general, patients with lSSc are at less risk of developing significant heart involvement, renal crisis, and pseudo-obstruction than patients with dSSc. The natural history of lSSc is that these patients often do well in the long-term, although they may have chronic or recurrent problems with digital ulcers and esophageal dysmotility. The lSSc patients who do poorly are those who develop significant interstitial lung disease, pulmonary hypertension, or other major internal organ impairment.

In contract to lSSc, patients with dSSc usually present with obvious, progressive skin thickening and constitutional symptoms of fatigue, anorexia, and weight loss. Many of these patients

> **KEY CONCEPTS**
>
> **Clinical features of systemic sclerosis**
> - Two major subsets of patients with different clinical courses:
>   - Limited cutaneous systemic sclerosis. Skin involvement limited to the face, neck, and extremities distal to the elbows and knees.
>   - Diffuse cutaneous systemic sclerosis. Skin involvement on the trunk or on the extremities proximal to the elbows or knees.
> - Symptoms and signs of the disease are caused by tissue fibrosis and ischemia.
> - The diagnosis is usually straightforward in patients with characteristic skin thickening of the hands.
> - Morbidity and mortality are related to extent and severity of internal organ involvement, which usually is worse in diffuse cutaneous systemic sclerosis.

Table 64.1 Major clinical subsets of systemic sclerosis.

Major clinical subsets of systemic sclerosis		
Sign or symptom	**Diffuse cutaneous systemic sclerosis**	**Limited cutaneous systemic sclerosis**
Fatigue, anorexia, weight loss	Common in early disease	Uncommon
Skin involvement	Proximal extremities or trunk	Distal extremities, face, neck
Rate of skin progression	Fast	Slow
Raynaud's phenomenon	Occurs with or after skin involvement	Precedes skin involvement
Arthralgias	May be pronounced, associated with contractures	Usually absent
Tendon friction rubs	May be present	Absent
Other organ involvement	Interstitial fibrosis Cardiac hypertrophy or dilatation Renal crisis Severe GI dysmotility	Interstitial fibrosis Pulmonary hypertension Biliary cirrhosis Sicca symptoms
Organ failure	Often within 3–4 years	If it occurs, usually later
Associated antibodies	Antitopoisomerase I, RNA polymerase III	Anticentromere
Two-year survival	60–80% 95–98%	

have arthralgias and develop joint contractures from involvement of tendons and joint capsules. Tendon friction rubs, dry leathery rubbing sensations that are palpable over tendons as they are moved, are characteristic of dSSc. The disease is most active during the first several years of illness, when the risk of developing significant internal organ involvement appears greatest. The dSSc patients are at greater risk of developing significant heart disease, renal crisis, and pseudo-obstruction than patients with lSSc. After the first 2–4 years of illness, the skin may soften spontaneously, the constitutional symptoms may abate, arthralgias may resolve, and the patients simply feel better. At this later stage of illness, symptoms result from whatever tissue damage is left over from the earlier period of more active disease. Again, as with lSSc, interstitial lung disease and pulmonary hypertension, alone or in some combination, are the main causes of death in these patients.[6]

The course of scleroderma is variable among individual patients, and the long-term outcome depends upon the severity of internal organ damage. Widespread or severe skin involvement is a poor prognostic indicator, because it correlates with development of severe internal organ involvement.[7] Mortality is greatest for patients with dSSc, with severe renal, heart, lung, and gut disease accounting for deaths within the first several years.[4,7,8] Two-year survival with dSSc is 60–80%, but nearly normal (95–98%) in patients with lSSc.[7,8] Overall 10-year survival is 40–50%.[4]

GENETIC AND ENVIRONMENTAL FACTORS

Genetic factors influence the development of systemic sclerosis, as well as disease manifestations. Choctaw Native Americans in southeastern Oklahoma have the highest prevalence of scleroderma or systemic sclerosis yet found (469/100 000), with disease prevalence significantly higher than that among non-full-blooded Choctaws.[9] Among the Oklahoma Choctaw cases, there is striking homogeneity of disease expression. The majority of patients have dSSc, pulmonary fibrosis, and autoantibodies to topoisomerase I.[9] No environmental exposures have been found to be in excess in these patients.[9] A 2-cM region on chromosome 15q that contains the gene encoding fibrillin-1 is associated with scleroderma in these Choctaws.[10] This chromosomal locus may have been inherited from common founders about 10 generations ago.[10] Autoantibodies to fibrillin-1 that correlate with disease can be detected in the sera from these patients.[11] An extended HLA-DR2 (DRB1*1602, DQA1*0501, DQB1*0301, DPB1*1301) haplotype also is significantly associated with scleroderma in the Oklahoma Choctaw, with no other significant associations with microsatellite marker alleles immediately flanking the HLA region.[12]

In other studies of scleroderma, associations with HLA genes were weak, but improved when clinical subsets of patients were analyzed. As prominent examples, production of anticentromere antibodies is associated with HLA-DQB1 proteins with a glycine or tyrosine at position 26,[13] and production of antitopoisomerase I antibodies is associated with DRB1*1101–*1104 in Whites and Blacks, DRB1*1502 in Japanese, and DRB1*1602 in Choctaws.[14] Of relevance to the discussion later in this chapter about microchimerism in scleroderma, HLA Class II compatibility of a child from the mother's perspective is more common among scleroderma patients than among controls.[15,16]

Scleroderma is not associated with alleles of the T-cell antigen receptor (TCR) α and β chain constant region gene complexes, although a weak association has been reported with an allele of the Cγ2 TCR gene.[17] There are conflicting reports of associations of scleroderma with the null phenotype of C4, and no associations have been reported for C3 or immunoglobulin gene complex polymorphisms. Other genetic studies have attempted to associate scleroderma with factors unrelated to the immune system. Weak associations of scleroderma with low activity of P450 enzymes involved in hydroxylation of dapsone and

S-mephenytoin have been noted. No associations of scleroderma with mutants of the fibronectin gene, alleles of proα_1(I), proα_2(II), or proα_1(III) collagen genes, or allotypes of α_1 antitrypsin have been reported.

Clinical and serologic features in systemic sclerosis patients are strongly influenced by ethnic background. Clinical manifestations, disease course, and autoantibody status are all modulated by ethnicity among North American White, North American Black, Japanese, and Choctaw Native American patients.[14] It is noteworthy that ethnic background is an independent determinant affecting development of severe lung disease as well as survival.[14]

Fibrosing illnesses with some clinical similarities to scleroderma can be induced by exposures to drugs or toxins, including vinyl chloride, bleomycin, silica, tainted rape seed oil, and L-tryptophan. Several studies have failed to find an association of silicone breast implants with systemic sclerosis in women. Occupational exposures are not associated with systemic sclerosis,[18] with the possible exception of long-term silica dust exposure.[19] Clinical and laboratory data indicate that silica-induced and idiopathic systemic sclerosis show similar pathophysiology and similar markers of the disease including vascular involvement, immunological abnormalities, and dysregulation of extracellular matrix metabolism.[19] Silica dust is able to activate microvascular endothelial cells, mononuclear cells from peripheral blood, and dermal fibroblasts in vitro.[19]

There is no direct evidence for a viral etiology of systemic sclerosis, although human parvovirus B19 infection has been detected in the bone marrow[20] and antibodies to human cytomegalovirus are increased[21] in systemic sclerosis patients. Some B-cell epitopes on the scleroderma-specific autoantigens topoisomerase I and PM/Scl include areas of homology to viruses.[22–24] Antitopoisomerase I antibodies bind regions of the molecule that have homology with cytomegalovirus or p30^{gag} proteins encoded by retroviruses that cause leukemia in felines and rodents.[22,23] Anti-PM-Scl antibodies bind an antigenic fragment with homology to the nuclear localization signal of SV-40 large T antigen and a molecular signal found in the HIV tat protein.[24]

KEY CONCEPTS

Pathogenesis of systemic sclerosis

- The etiology of systemic sclerosis is unknown.
- Early events in the pathogenesis of systemic sclerosis include:
  - — Endothelial cell activation and damage
  - — Fibroblast activation.
  - — Immune system activation, with perivascular infiltration principally with T cells.
- Later events include:
  - — Vasculopathy of small arteries, arterioles, and capillaries with endothelial cell loss, intimal proliferation, luminal narrowing, and thrombosis.
  - — Tissue fibrosis.
- Cytokines and other soluble mediators secreted by cells of the immune system probably contribute to the disease process through activation/damage of endothelial cells and stimulation of fibroblast chemotaxis, proliferation, and extracellular matrix production.

IMMUNOLOGY/PATHOGENESIS

The cause of systemic sclerosis is unknown. Examination of tissues from systemic sclerosis patients indicates that early disease is characterized by activation of endothelial cells and fibroblasts, and tissue infiltration with activated cells of the immune system, especially in perivascular areas.[25,26] As disease progresses, endothelial cell damage becomes apparent, with endothelial cell loss, intimal proliferation, luminal narrowing and thrombosis, and periadventitial fibrosis of small arteries and capillaries.[26] Similarly, fibroblast activation progresses to tissue fibrosis, with the deposition of excessive extracellular matrix.[26] Late in the disease, mononuclear cell infiltration may resolve and fibrosis may lessen. Pronounced small vessel vasculopathy and fibrosis set systemic sclerosis apart from other connective tissue diseases.

Activation of the immune system may be a pivotal event in the initiation or perpetuation of the small vessel vasculopathy and fibrosis seen in systemic sclerosis. Activated mononuclear cells invade tissues early in the course of the disease[26] and are capable of secreting cytokines and other factors that can activate or damage endothelial cells and fibroblasts. Interactions among cells found in small blood vessels, fibroblasts, and the immune system are undoubtedly complex and ultimately lead to vasculopathy and fibrosis in systemic sclerosis patients. One of many possible models of the pathogenesis of systemic sclerosis is presented in Figure 64.1.

Recent data suggest that fetal–maternal microchimerism, with a graft-versus-host reaction, may be one of multiple factors involved in the development of systemic sclerosis. Fetal CD34$^+$ CD38$^+$ cells have recently been found to persist in maternal peripheral blood for many years after pregnancy. CD34$^+$ CD38$^+$ cells are progenitor cells that can differentiate into mature immune-competent cells. This finding suggests that fetal cells persisting in the maternal circulation or tissues could initiate a graft-versus-host reaction, and graft-versus- host disease in bone marrow transplanted patients has been associated with a syndrome similar to systemic sclerosis. To detect microchimerism, polymerase chain reaction techniques can be used to identify Y-chromosome DNA in female patients who have had male children. Microchimerism is found more frequently and with higher numbers of allogeneic cells in peripheral blood mononuclear cells

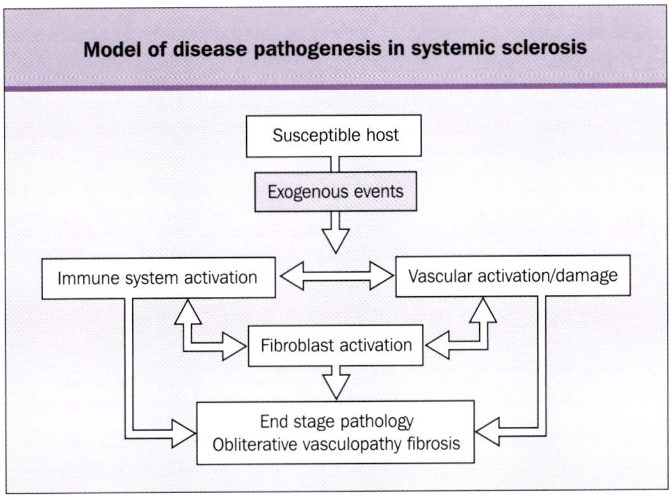

Figure 64.1 Model of disease pathogenesis in systemic sclerosis.

from women with scleroderma than controls.[27–29] Microchimerism can be detected in T-lymphocyte populations and can be identified in skin-biopsy specimens from women with systemic sclerosis.[29] HLA compatibility (i.e. matches of maternal and paternal HLA alleles) is not a requirement for persistent microchimerism in peripheral blood mononuclear cell subsets, but does occur more commonly in systemic sclerosis patients than controls.[27,29] These results raise the possibility that systemic sclerosis may be a form of chronic graft-versus-host disease.

T cells may be pivotal in the pathogenesis of systemic sclerosis. They are the predominant infiltrating cell in the perivascular areas.[26] Different T-cell subsets may contribute to the disease process in different organs and at different stages of systemic sclerosis. CD4 T cells are more common than CD8 T cells in the skin of patients with systemic sclerosis at all stages of disease.[26] Molecular analyses of T-cell receptor (TCR) genes expressed in the skin of systemic sclerosis patients reveal no differences in the dominant α and β genes used, when compared to controls.

CD8 T cells are more oligoclonal than normal in the blood and lungs of systemic sclerosis patients, as assessed by diversity of TCR expression.[30] Moreover, patients with active lung inflammation have increased numbers and percentages of CD8 T cells in their bronchoalveolar lavage (BAL).[30] These CD8 T cells produce type 2 cytokines, including interleukin (IL)-4.[31] The production of type 2 cytokines in the lungs of these patients is associated with greater subsequent decline in forced vital capacity, suggesting that CD8 T cells may be causally associated with the development of restrictive lung disease in these patients.[31]

The γδ T-cell repertoire is skewed in both the peripheral blood and BAL of patients with systemic sclerosis, with evidence for an oligoclonal expansion of the $V\delta1^+$ subset.[32] It is notable that, among unfractionated T cells, $CD8^+$ and γδ T cells, especially the $V\delta1^+$ subset, preferentially adhere to fibroblasts.[33] It has been suggested that γδ T cells may play a role in the vascular disease in systemic sclerosis.[34] The γδ T cells from systemic sclerosis patients adhere to cultured endothelial cells and proliferate at higher rates than control cells. Furthermore, significant endothelial cell cytotoxicity by systemic sclerosis γδ T cells is seen, which depends in part on granzyme A.[34]

T cells are responsible for the development of scleroderma-like disease in two animal models. In hereditary avian scleroderma, a particular subline of chickens have a defect in thymic maturation of T cells and develop severe perivascular T-cell infiltration of the skin and internal organs.[35] Subsequently, fibrosis and vascular occlusion develop. Lymphocytes in the papillary dermis are enriched for γδ T cells, 20% of which express CD8. Lymphocytes in the deeper dermis and subcutaneous tissues are enriched for αβ, CD4 T cells. The T cells are activated and express major histocompatibility complex (MHC) Class II molecules, and B-cell infiltration is sparse. In a second animal model of scleroderma, chronic graft-versus-host disease is induced in mice by CD8 T-cell allorecognition of MHC-encoded molecules.[36]

Although T cells may contribute to the disease process in systemic sclerosis, there is no evidence of any global abnormality of T cells in these patients. To the contrary, in vivo T-cell responses in systemic sclerosis patients are normal.[37] Scleroderma patients have normal cutaneous delayed-type hypersensitivity and antibody production in response to primary immunization and recall antigens with T-dependent antigens. It is likely that the activated T cells found in the tissues of patients are responding specifically to initiating antigens or antigens exposed secondary to the disease process itself. T cells from systemic sclerosis patients can be activated by skin extracts and purified collagen, including type I and type IV collagen. Cellular antigens on fibroblasts, epithelial cells, and muscle cells are reported to stimulate cytotoxic T-cell responses, although this is not consistently observed.

Abnormalities of humoral immunity in systemic sclerosis patients include hypergammaglobulinemia, with increases in IgG, IgA, IgM, and IgE, autoantibody production, and immune complex formation. Antinuclear antibodies (ANA) occur early and uniformly in patients with systemic sclerosis. The isotype of the ANA is usually IgG, especially the IgG3 subclass. Multiple autoantigens are recognized by autoantibodies from systemic sclerosis patients. Some autoantibodies are quite specific for this disease, including those directed to topoisomerase I, centromere, RNA polymerase I, RNA polymerase III, and U3 RNP antigens. Autoantibodies against centromeres recognize four centromeric proteins, CENP-A, -B, -C, and -D. Many of the systemic sclerosis-specific autoantigens share the ability to be uniquely cleaved into novel fragments by metal-dependent, nonenzymatic mechanisms[38] or by granzyme B.[39] Repeated episodes of ischemia reperfusion might lead to generation of oxygen radicals and thus facilitate the metal-dependent non-enzymatic cleavage of these autoantigens, promoting autoimmuno responses and autoantibody formation.[38] Alternatively, tissue damage caused by activated cytolytic CD8 T cells might initiate autoantibody formation in systemic sclerosis.[39]

Many other more nonspecific targets of autoantibodies in systemic sclerosis patients have been identified, including IgG, smooth muscle, endothelial cells, fibroblasts, thyroid tissue, salivary gland tissue, heat-shock proteins, single-stranded RNA, nuclear ribonucleoproteins, Th ribonucleoproteins, mitochondria, cardiolipin, types I, III and IV collagen, laminin, interleukin-6, Fcγ receptors, and fibrillin-1.

Evidence that autoantibodies cause tissue damage in scleroderma patients is largely limited to the demonstration that patient sera contain antibodies that bind to endothelial cells and fibroblasts and promote antibody-dependent cellular cytotoxicity. In patients with dSSc, a significant positive correlation is found between anti-endothelial cell antibodies and diffusing capacity, pulmonary artery pressures, digital ulcers, and capillaroscopic abnormalities, but not heart involvement, skin score, or pulmonary interstitial fibrosis.[40] These data suggest that in systemic sclerosis the anti-endothelial cell antibodies are linked to vascular injury and could reflect endothelial damage.[40] Anti-endothelial cell antibodies from systemic sclerosis patients can also induce endothelial cell apoptosis in vitro, through Fas-independent mechanisms.[41]

Many autoantibodies in systemic sclerosis sera do not activate the complement cascade, and serum complement levels are normal. Immune complexes may be present in the sera or bronchoalveolar lavage of patients, but there is no evidence that they are deposited in tissues or cause tissue damage.

Mast cells have also been implicated as possible contributors to pathology in systemic sclerosis patients. The best evidence for mast cell activation is the presence in the skin of mast cells containing tryptase, which are normally found in the gastrointestinal mucosa and alveolar walls of the lung.[42] It remains unresolved whether the numbers of mast cells are increased or whether the degranulation of mast cells is abnormally increased beyond that which might accompany increased numbers in involved skin. Mast cell degranulation is noted in chronic murine graft-versus-host disease and in the tight skin mouse model of systemic sclerosis.

It remains to be elucidated which of many different candidate cytokines or mediators actually contribute to the sclerodermatous process. TGF-β stimulates fibrosis and angiogenesis. Increased levels of TGF-β_2 mRNA and proα_1 (I) collagen mRNA co-localize within inflammatory infiltrates in skin from systemic sclerosis patients in the early phase of disease.[43] However, data for increased production of TGF-β in involved tissue are controversial and some investigators find no difference. Macrophage chemotactic protein-1 is strongly expressed in the epidermis, inflammatory mononuclear cells, and vascular endothelial cells in the sclerotic skin of systemic sclerosis patients, but not in control skin. Endothelial cell proliferation and fibroblast proliferation and chemotaxis can be stimulated by platelet-derived growth factor. Platelet-derived growth factor is found in increased amounts in the skin of systemic sclerosis patients, along with increased expression of type β receptors for this cytokine. Interleukin-4 stimulates fibroblast chemotaxis, proliferation, extracellular matrix production, and ICAM-1 expression. IL-4 mRNA is increased in bronchoalveolar lavage cells from systemic sclerosis patients with lung inflammation.[31] IL-8 mRNA and protein are increased in bronchoalveolar lavage fluids from systemic sclerosis patients with pulmonary fibrosis, where IL-8 may be responsible for influx of neutrophils. IL-1α, IL-1β, IL-2, IL-4, IL-6, IL-10, MCP-1, MIP-1α, MIP-1β, and tumor necrosis factor-α (TNF-α) have all been proposed as contributors to the pathogenesis of systemic sclerosis, based upon their more frequent presence in the sera of patients or their increased production by peripheral blood mononuclear cells. In contrast, IFN-γ protein has not been detected in blood of systemic sclerosis patients, and secretion of IFN-γ by systemic sclerosis peripheral blood mononuclear cells after mitogen stimulation is lower than that from controls.

CLINICAL MANIFESTATIONS AND PATIENT MANAGEMENT

The medical management of patients with systemic sclerosis is guided by the extent and severity of organ involvement. Organ involvement that causes little or no functional impairment requires a different therapeutic approach than that which is rapidly progressing or associated with significant functional impairment. Therapy often used to manage common problems in systemic sclerosis is outlined in Table 64.2.

THERAPEUTIC PRINCIPLES

Treatment of systemic sclerosis

- No therapy has been shown in controlled, double-blinded trials to modify the overall course of systemic sclerosis.
- The treatment of systemic sclerosis is determined by the severity of involvement of individual organs and is organ-based.
- Many organ-based therapies in systemic sclerosis are effective in reducing symptoms, and some may prevent further decline in organ function.

Organ-based therapies for systemic sclerosis

Problem	Therapies
Raynaud's phenomenon	Conservative measures, such as cold avoidance Ca^{++} channel blockers Nitrates
Skin involvement	Moisturizers for dryness Antihistamines for pruritis Cosmetics to mask pigmentary changes Laser ablation of telangiectasia
Digital ulcers	Local or systemic antibiotics, if infected Ca^{++} channel blockers Nitrates Prostaglandin E_2 infusions
Esophageal reflux	Avoid smoking, alcohol, and large meals H_2-blockers Proton pump inhibitors
Pseudo-obstruction	Prokinetic agents such as metaclopramide, erythromycin, or octreotide Total parenteral nutrition
Malabsorption	Prokinetic agents Antibiotics Dietary manipulations
Renal	Antihypertensives Angiotension-converting enzyme inhibitors

Table 64.2 Organ-based therapies for systemic sclerosis.

Over 95% of patients have Raynaud's phenomenon, which is caused by transient, reversible vasospasm of the small vessels of the hand. Episodes of vasospasm are usually precipitated by a decrease in environmental temperature or strong emotion. Raynaud's phenomenon usually precedes other symptoms in patients with lSSc, but may coincide with or follow disease onset in patients with dSSc. Systemic sclerosis patients have hyperresponsiveness of the $\alpha 2_c$-adrenergic receptors on the smooth muscle of their small blood vessels and, as a result, are more susceptible to cold-induced vasospasm. Moreover, they have significant narrowing of the lumen of their small blood vessels, as a result of intimal proliferation and endothelial cell apoptosis. Finally, systemic sclerosis patients appear to have reduced angiogenesis, with reduced growth of new blood vessels in what can become avascular tissue in their digits.

As a result of these functional and structural changes in small blood vessels, Raynaud's phenomenon may be particularly refractory to treatment in systemic sclerosis patients, and patients are prone to develop digital ulcers and infarctions (Fig. 64.2). Amputation of digits because of nonhealing ulcers or infarctions is occasionally necessary, especially in patients with lSSc. Conservative measures, with avoidance of cold, and calcium channel blockers are the mainstays of treatment of Raynaud's phenomenon in systemic sclerosis. A multicenter, randomized, parallel-group comparison of oral iloprost and placebo to treat Raynaud's phenomenon in systemic sclerosis showed significant treatment differences in the total daily duration of attacks and in the severity of attacks.[44] There was no difference in the frequency of attacks or percentages of patients improved at the end of treatment as assessed by the physician.[44] In contrast, another

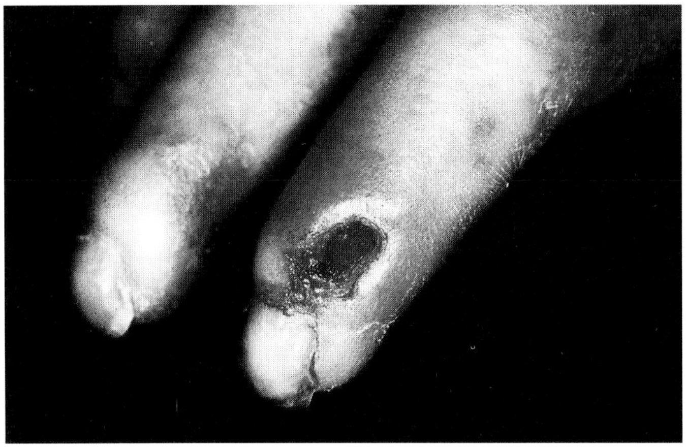

Figure 64.2 Digital ulcer in a man with limited cutaneous systemic sclerosis. Terminal digital reabsorption is present. (Photograph courtesy of Dr. Fredrick M. Wigley, The Johns Hopkins and University of Maryland Scleroderma Center.)

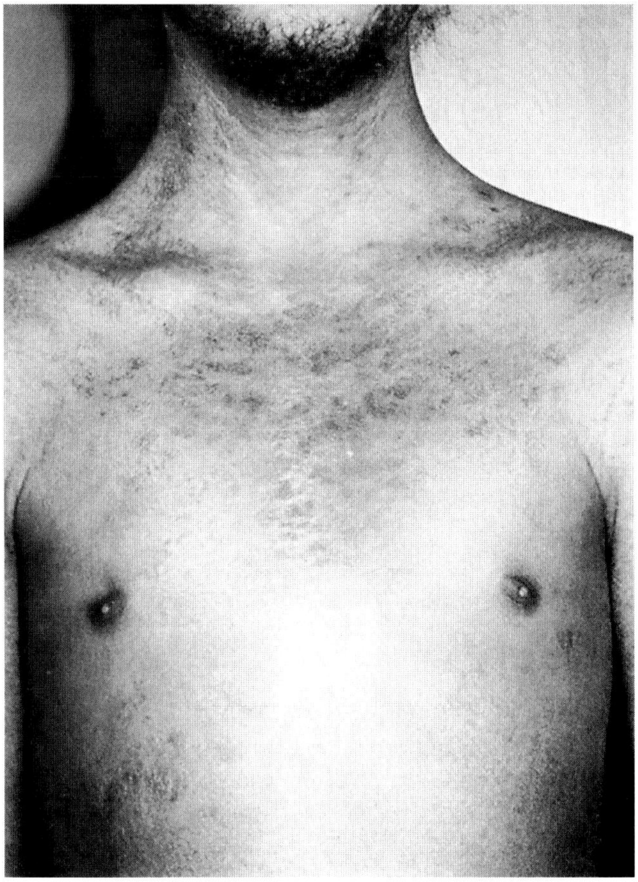

Figure 64.4 Tight, thickened skin on the trunk of a man with diffuse systemic sclerosis of 12 months duration. (Photograph courtesy of Dr. Fredrick M. Wigley, The Johns Hopkins and University of Maryland Scleroderma Center.) (See also color plate 64.4.)

similarly designed trial showed no benefit of oral iloprost over placebo.[45] Small clinical trials have suggested that angiotension II receptor antagonists and prostaglandin E1 infusions may be helpful in the management of severe Raynaud's phenomenon in systemic sclerosis.

Skin fibrosis affects all systemic sclerosis patients, except those with scleroderma sine scleroderma. Skin fibrosis develops more slowly and in a more restricted distribution in lSSc than in dSSc. Skin involvement progresses through three stages, with variable periods of time in each stage and with different stages present in different sites in the same individual. An edematous phase occurs first; the skin is swollen, shiny, and often erythematous and pruritic (Fig. 64.3). During the fibrotic phase, edema becomes less noticeable, and the skin is thickened (Fig. 64.4) and sometimes tethered if the fibrosis extends deep in the subcutaneous tissue to the fascia. Dryness and hair loss may be pronounced, and salt and pepper changes of hypo- and hyper-pigmentation may be a source of embarrassment for the patient. During the atrophic stage, the skin softens as fibrosis recedes, hair may return, and the only clinical indication of previous disease may be an atrophic epidermis and residual pigmentary changes. Regression of skin involvement occurs to a lesser extent on the fingers than elsewhere.

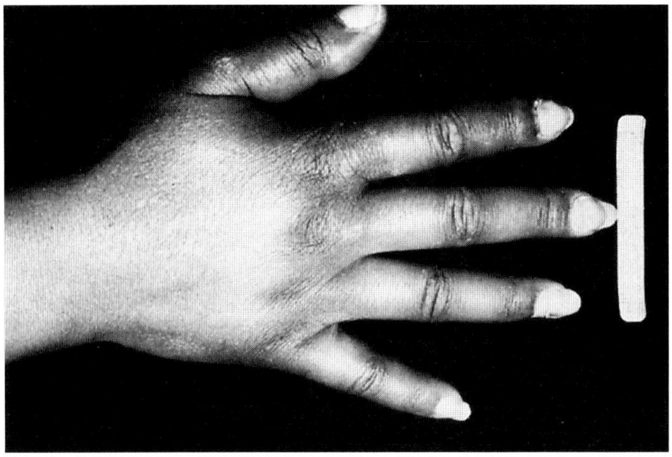

Figure 64.3 Hand swelling in a woman with diffuse systemic sclerosis of 6 months duration. Hyperpigmentation of the dorsum of the hand and hypopigmentation around the nails are noted. (Photograph courtesy of Dr. Fredrick M. Wigley, The Johns Hopkins and University of Maryland Scleroderma Center.) (See also color plate 64.3.)

The spontaneous improvement in skin thickening in systemic sclerosis patients points out the need, at this time, for controlled trials to demonstrate improvement in skin score. In placebo-controlled trials, photopheresis[46] and interferon-α[47] were ineffective in treating skin thickening. In a placebo-controlled trial, testing small numbers of patients, low-dose methotrexate injections were associated with improvement of total skin score, diffusion capacity, and a visual analog score. There have been several small trials, including placebo-controlled trials of interferon-γ in systemic sclerosis. Benefits of interferon-γ have been mild, if any, and side-effects frequent. When compared to low-dose D-penicillamine (125 mg every other day), high-dose D-penicillamine (1000 mg per day) did not provide improvement in skin score, pulmonary function, renal crisis, or survival.[48] In uncontrolled studies of small groups of patients, cyclosporin A, but not antithymocyte globulin, has been associated with improvement in skin score. A recently published preliminary (phase II) double-blind, placebo-controlled trial of recombinant human relaxin has reported that continuous subcutaneous infusion of relaxin over 24 weeks resulted in modest but significant reductions in skin scores, as well as improvement in other outcome measures.[49] Unfortunately, these promising findings did not hold true in a large phase III trial, which showed lack of efficacy of relaxin therapy in skin thickening.[50] Also in progress is a trial of the effects of induction of oral tolerance to bovine collagen in treating skin thickening.

Gut involvement is also nearly universal in systemic sclerosis patients, with sphincter dysfunction and dysmotility from smooth muscle fibrosis and atrophy. Esophageal reflux secondary to reduced lower esophageal sphincter pressure is the most common gut manifestation. Refractory cases of reflux may lead to esophageal erosions, strictures, and Barrett's esophagus. Agents that block gastric acidity, especially proton pump inhibitors, and prokinetic agents are effective in relieving symptoms of reflux and may prevent the development of erosions and other significant consequences. Dysphagia is caused by dysmotility in the distal two thirds of the esophagus, whereas postprandial bloating, early satiety, abdominal cramps, and pseudo-obstruction are manifestations of more distal gut dysmotility. Pseudo-obstruction can present as an acute abdominal process with anorexia, nausea, vomiting, obstipation, abdominal pain, and air–fluid levels on abdominal upright radiogram. Alternatively, it can have a more chronic presentation with intermittent abdominal distention, cramping, and diarrhea or constipation. As a result of reduced bowel motility, bacterial overgrowth and malabsorption may occur, with involuntary weight loss. Gut dysmotility is treated with prokinetic agents, antibiotics for malabsorption, attention to nutritional status, and, if needed, total parenteral nutrition. Fecal incontinence is a potential consequence of reduced anorectal sphincter function and may be improved with biofeedback.

Pulmonary and cardiac disease may remain largely silent in systemic sclerosis patients until organ damage is severe. Thirty to sixty per cent of systemic sclerosis patients have restrictive lung disease from interstitial fibrosis, which occurs with nearly equal frequency in patients with lSSc and dSSc. The presence of anti-DNA topoisomerase I antibodies (anti-Scl-70 antibodies) and African-American race are risk factors for interstitial lung disease. The fibrosis is thought to follow an inflammatory alveolitis, in which increased numbers of macrophages, neutrophils, lymphocytes, and eosinophils invade the lungs. This lung inflammation can be detected by an increased percentage of neutrophils in BAL fluids and is suggested by a ground-glass appearance on high-resolution computerized tomography of the lungs (Fig. 64.5). The presence of lung inflammation, as identified by bronchoalveolar lavage or lung biopsy, identifies patients at greater risk for subsequent decline in lung function or death.[51] Data from several uncontrolled trials and a large retrospective cohort study suggest that cyclophosphamide improves lung function outcome and perhaps even survival, with stabilization or improvement in lung function in treated patients.[51] Lung transplantation may be considered in patients with severe restrictive lung disease from scleroderma.

A severely reduced diffusing capacity for carbon monoxide, especially one out of proportion to the extent of restrictive lung disease, is a clue to the presence of pulmonary hypertension. Pulmonary hypertension occurs in approximately 15% of scleroderma patients (Fig. 64.6). It can be a devastating consequence of severe interstitial fibrosis or can occur in isolation, especially in patients with lSSc. Unfortunately, the diagnosis of systemic sclerosis may not be considered in some patients until they present with symptoma of right-sided heart failure. Diuretics, calcium channel blockers, and angiotension-converting enzyme

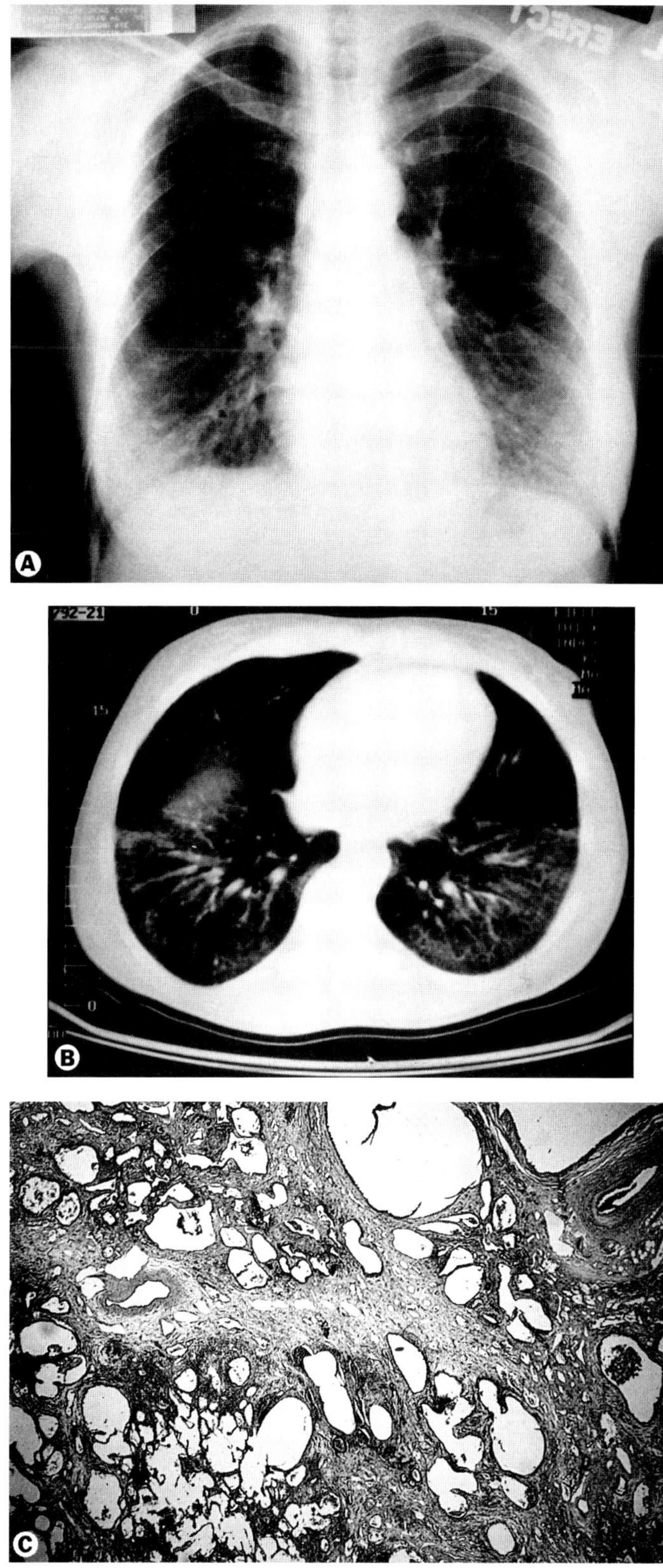

Figure 64.5 Interstitial fibrosis in a woman with diffuse systemic sclerosis of 16 months duration. (**A**) Bilateral basilar interstitial fibrosis is seen on chest radiograph. (**B**) A characteristic ground-glass appearance, which correlates with the presence of lung inflammation, is seen on high-resolution computerized axial tomography of the lung. (**C**) Interstitial fibrosis is present on lung biopsy. (See also color plate 64.5C.) (Photographs courtesy of Dr. Fredrick M. Wigley, The Johns Hopkins and University of Maryland Scleroderma Center.)

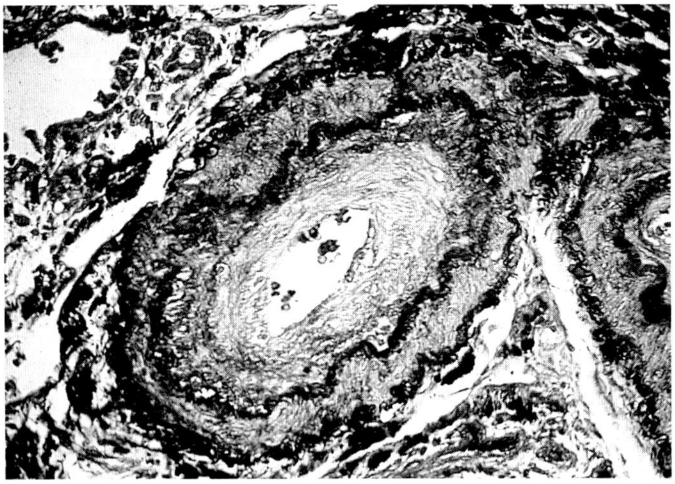

Figure 64.6 Pulmonary artery from a woman with limited cutaneous systemic sclerosis and pulmonary hypertension. Note the thickened intima, duplication of the basal lamina, and luminal narrowing. (Photograph courtesy of Dr. Fredrick M. Wigley, The Johns Hopkins and University of Maryland Scleroderma Center.) (See also color plate 64.6.)

inhibitors may be useful for symptomatic relief. A randomized, multicenter, placebo-controlled trial has demonstrated efficacy of continuous intravenous epoprostenol for pulmonary hypertension due to the scleroderma.[52] Lung transplantion may also be considered for patients with severe disease.

Cardiac pathology that is unique to systemic sclerosis is contraction band necrosis, which is small linear streaks of fibrosis caused by ischemia from small vessel vasculopathy. Thallium perfusion studies can show diffuse or patchy reduction in blood flow not in the distribution of any coronary artery, suggesting damage of the small cardiac vessels. Consequences of this small vessel disease can include cardiomegaly, reduced right or left ventricular ejection fraction, congestive heart failure, conduction defects, and arrhythmias. Asymptomatic pericardial effusions are common in systemic sclerosis, and moderate to large effusions are a poor prognostic indicator.

Hematuria, proteinuria, and mild progressive azotemia occur in systemic sclerosis patients, but processes independent of this disease (e.g. hypertension, diabetes, drug therapy) may independently account for most of these abnormalities. Two forms of renal damage clearly caused by the sclerodermatous disease process are scleroderma renal crisis and normotensive, rapidly progressive renal failure. Renal crisis is a dreaded complication caused by activation of the renin–angiotensin system. This severe complication generally presents within the first four years of dSSc as new diastolic hypertension and an abrupt decline in glomerular filtration associated with microangiopathic hemolytic anemia, hypertensive retinopathy, proteinuria, or hematuria. Prompt, aggressive antihypertensive therapy with angiotensin-converting enzyme inhibitors is the mainstay of therapy for scleroderma renal crisis. Even in patients with renal crisis who require dialysis, continuation of angiotensin-converting enzyme inhibitors may result in restoration of renal function adequate to discontinue dialysis, even as long as one year after dialysis began.

Joint and tendon involvement tends to be confined to patients with dSSc. Disabling arthralgias of large and small joints may be present, infrequently associated with joint warmth, swelling, and effusions. Tendon friction rubs, which are scratchy leathery sensations palpated over tendons during joint motion, are caused by fibrous encasement of the tendon sheath. Joint contractures, especially of the fingers, wrists, elbows, and knees, result from variable contributions of skin, tendon, and true joint involvement. Uncontrolled observations suggest that methotrexate therapy may be helpful in lessening pain and reducing the risk of contractures. When the skin softens over large joints such as the elbows and knees, contractures may also improve. Contractures in the fingers are usually permanent.

Two types of myositis occur in systemic sclerosis patients. More frequently, a bland fibrosis is seen. Patients with this process have no or minimal weakness, a several-fold increase in serum levels of creatinine phosphokinase (CPK), and a nonprogressive course which is steroid resistant. In contrast, a smaller subset of patients have disease that overlaps with polymyositis, with active muscle inflammation on biopsy, symptomatic progressive weakness, significantly elevated muscle enzymes, and steroid-responsiveness. Steroid therapy must be used with careful attention to blood pressure and renal function in dSSc patients. Case reports suggest that institution of steroid therapy can be temporally associated with the development of renal crisis in some patients.

Sicca symptoms frequently accompany systemic sclerosis, especially lSSc. As with joint and muscle involvement, two types of salivary gland involvement occur – a noninflammatory fibrosis and an inflammatory process that overlaps with another connective tissue disease. In most cases, salivary gland biopsies show a bland fibrosis, symptoms are mild, and antibodies to SSA and SSB are absent. Other patients have an overlap with Sjögren syndrome, with these autoantibodies present and lymphocytic infiltration on biopsy. Artificial tears and saliva may provide relief.

PATIENT EVALUATION AND DIFFERENTIAL DIAGNOSIS

The differential diagnosis of skin thickening includes localized cutaneous forms of scleroderma (morphea or linear scleroderma) and scleroderma-like illnesses such as eosinophilic fasciitis. Infrequently, under special clinical situations, it may also include scleredema of Buschke, scleromyxedema, lichen sclerosus et atrophicus, porphyria cutanea tarda, carcinoid syndrome, amyloidosis, phenylketonuria, Werner syndrome, progeria, acrogeria, congenital poikiloderma, localized lipoatrophy, acrodermatitis atrophicans, vinyl chloride disease, pentazocine-induced disease, bleomycin-induced disease, trichloroethylene-induced disease, and graft-versus-host disease. Despite this lengthy differential diagnosis, the presence of characteristic skin thickening proximal to the fingers is so specific for scleroderma that the diagnosis is usually straightforward. Thus, the diagnosis is usually not difficult in patients with dSSc, and skin biopsy is not generally needed to make the diagnosis.

Difficulty in making the diagnosis of scleroderma arises most frequently when skin changes are minimal or nonexistent, as may happen in lSSc and scleroderma sine scleroderma. Nailfold microscopy may be helpful in suggesting scleroderma in problematic cases. Typical nailfold capillary changes include dilated nailfold capillaries and capillary dropout. The presence of scleroderma-specific antibodies, typically anticentromere antibodies, also supports the diagnosis in difficult cases of lSSc.

The physician should be concerned that the diagnosis of scleroderma is incorrect in patients without Raynaud's phenomenon or without fibrosis of the skin of the fingers. Similarly, if the patient has puckering of the sucutaneous tissues, the physician should be concerned that the patient has fasciitis rather than systemic sclerosis.

The initial evaluation of a patient with systemic sclerosis should yield information about whether that patient has lSSc or dSSc, disease duration, what internal organs are likely to be involved, and the severity of internal organ involvement. Initial laboratory testing may include a complete blood count, tests of renal function, urinalysis, tests for antinuclear antibodies anti-Scl-70 antibodies, and anticentromere antibodies, thyroid function tests, chest radiographs, pulmonary function tests including spirometry, lung volumes, and diffusion capacity for carbon monoxide, and 2-dimensional echocardiogram to estimate baseline pulmonary artery pressures and evaluate ventricular function and pericardial effusion. Systemic sclerosis patients with significant dysphagia should have endoscopic evaluation to rule out esophageal stricture.

PITFALLS/CONTROVERSIES

The relationship of localized scleroderma to systemic sclerosis remains unclear. Increasingly, immunologic abnormalities are being identified in patients with localized scleroderma. Some of these abnormalities are similar to ones seen in patients with systemic sclerosis, suggesting that these diseases may have similar immune-mediated mechanisms of skin damage. It is not clear whether differences in the clinical course of these two types of scleroderma arise because of different initiating events or different hosts.

The data showing increased frequency and levels of fetal–maternal microchimerism in systemic sclerosis patients are exciting, because they suggest a novel mechanism for the development of this autoimmune process. Fetal or maternal cells can cross the placenta during pregnancy and remain unrecognized by the host for long periods of time due to Class II HLA compatibility. Later activation of these cells by an as yet unknown stimulus may result in the development of systemic sclerosis.[28] However, additional studies will be necessary to determine whether the increase in detectable microchimerism in systemic sclerosis patients actually plays a role in the pathogenesis of this disease. It is possible that it is merely an epiphenomenon that reflects overall activation of the immune system, making these cells easier to detect.

Similarly, the role of autoantibodies in the development of tissue damage in systemic sclerosis is unclear. Data suggest that anti-endothelial cell antibodies, which are not specific for systemic sclerosis, may cause endothelial cell apoptosis. If these antibodies cause vasculopathy in scleroderma, why is similar vascular pathology not seen in other patients with these same antibodies? Although certain autoantibodies are relatively specific for systemic sclerosis, there is little direct evidence to date that these antibodies are involved in tissue damage. If not, are these autoantibodies also just an epiphenomenon in systemic sclerosis patients?

Finally, it remains unclear whether vascular damage (or activation) is the initial pathologic event, or whether activation of the immune system is a more proximal event in disease initiation. The answer to this fundamental question would provide major insight into the etiology and pathogenesis of systemic sclerosis and may provide additional targets for therapeutic intervention.

REFERENCES

1. Rodnan G, Benedek T. An historical account of the study of progressive systemic sclerosis. Ann Intern Med 1962;57:305.
2. Steen VD, Conte C, Medsger TA Jr, et al. Twenty-year incidence survey of systemic sclerosis (scleroderma). Arthritis Rheum 1988;31:S57.
3. Maricq HR, Weinrich MC, Keil JE, et al. Prevalence of scleroderma spectrum disorders in the general population of South Carolina. Arthritis Rheum 1989;32:998.
4. Medsger TA J. Epidemiology of progressive systemic sclerosis. In: Black CM, Myers AR (eds) Systemic sclerosis (scleroderma). New York, Grover Medical Publishing, 1985, P. 53.
5. LeRoy EC, Black C, Fleishmajer R, et al. Scleroderma (systemic sclerosis): classification, subsets, and pathogenesis. J Rheumatol 1988;15:202.
6. Medsger TA Jr, Steen VD. Classification, prognosis. In: Clements PJ, Furst DE (eds) Systemic sclerosis. Baltimore, Williams & Wilkins, 1996, P51.
7. Clements PJ, Lachenbruch PA, Ng SC, et al. Skin score. A semiquantitative measure of cutaneous involvement that improves prediction of prognosis in systemic sclerosis. Arthritis Rheum 1990;33:1256.
8. Bulpitt KJ, Clements PJ, Lachenbruch PA, et al. Early undifferentiated connective tissue disease. III. Outcome and prognostic indicators in early scleroderma (systemic sclerosis). Ann Intern Med 1993;118:602.
9. Arnett FC, Howard RF, Tan F, et al. Increased prevalence of systemic sclerosis in a Native American tribe in Oklahoma. Association with an Amerindian HLA haplotype. Arthritis Rheum 1996;39:1362.
10. Tan FK, Stivers DN, Foster MW, et al. Association of microsatellite markers near the fibrillin 1 gene on human chromosome 15q with scleroderma in a Native American population. Arthritis Rheum 1998;41:1729.
11. Tan FK, Arnett FC, Antohi S, et al. Autoantibodies to the extracellular matrix microfibrillar protein, fibrillin-1, in patients with scleroderma and other connective tissue diseases. J Immunol 1999;163:1066.
12. Tan FK, Stivers DN, Arnett FC, Chakraborty R, Howard R, Reveille JD. HLA haplotypes and microsatellite polymorphisms in and around the major histocompatibility complex region in a Native American population with a high prevalence of scleroderma (systemic sclerosis). Tissue Antigens 1999;53:74.
13. Reveille JR, Owerbach D, Goldstein R, et al. Association of polar amino acids at position 26 of the HLA-DQB1 first domain with the anticentromere autoantibody response in systemic sclerosis (scleroderma). J Clin Invest 1992;89:1208.
14. Kuwana M, Kaburaki J, Arnett FC, Howard RF, Medsger TA Jr, Wright TM. Influence of ethnic background on clinical and serologic features in patients with systemic sclerosis and anti-DNA topoisomerase I antibody. Arthritis Rheum 1999;42:465.
15. Nelson JL, Furst DE, Maloney S, et al. Microchimerism and HLA-compatible relationships of pregnancy in scleroderma. Lancet 1998;351:559.
16. Artlett CM, Welsh KI, Black CM, Jimenez SA. Fetal-maternal HLA compatibility confers susceptibility to systemic sclerosis. Lancet 1998;351:559.
17. Kratz LE, Boughman JA, Cohen D, et al. Association of a T cell antigen receptor gamma gene restriction fragment length polymorphism with scleroderma. Arthritis Rheum 1990;33:569.
18. Conte C, Steen V. An epidemiologic study of occupational exposures in systemic sclerosis. Arthritis Rheum 1992;35:S150.
19. Haustein UF, Anderegg U. Silica induced scleroderma – clinical and experimental aspects. J Rheumatol 1998;25:1917.

20. Ferri C, Zakrzewska K, Longombardo G, et al. Parvovirus B19 infection of bone marrow in systemic sclerosis patients. Clin Exp Rheumatol 1999;17:718.
21. Neidhart M, Kuchen S, Distler O, et al. Increased serum levels of antibodies against human cytomegalovirus and prevalence of autoantibodies in systemic sclerosis. Arthritis Rheum 1999;42:389.
22. Maul GG, Jimenez SA, Riggs E, et al. Determination of an epitope of the diffuse systemic sclerosis marker antigen DNA topoisomerase 1: sequence similarity with retroviral $p30^{gag}$ protein suggests a possible cause for autoimmunity in systemic sclerosis. Proc Natl Acad Sci USA 1989;86:8492.
23. Muryoi T, Kasturi KN, Kafina MJ, et al. Antitopoisomerase I monoclonal autoantibodies from scleroderma patients and tight skin mouse interact with similar epitopes. J Exp Med 1992;175:1103.
24. Alderuccio F, Chan EKL, Tan EM. Molecular characterization of an autoantigen of PM-Scl in the polymyositis/scleroderma overlap syndrome: a unique and complete human cDNA encoding an apparent 75-kD acidic protein of the nucleolar complex. J Exp Med 1991;173:941.
25. Claman HN, Giorno RC, Seibold JR. Endothelial and fibroblast activation in scleroderma: the myth of the 'uninvolved skin'. Arthritis Rheum 1991;34:1495.
26. Prescott RJ, Freemont AJ, Jones CJP, et al. Sequential dermal microvascular and perivascular changes in the development of scleroderma. J Pathol 1992;166:255.
27. Nelson JL, Furst DE, Maloney S, et al. Microchimerism and HLA-compatible relationships of pregnancy in scleroderma. Lancet 1998;351:559.
28. Evans PC, Lambert N, Maloney S, Furst DE, Moore JM, Nelson JL. Long-term fetal microchimerism in peripheral blood mononuclear cell subsets in healthy women and women with scleroderma. Blood 1999;93:2033.
29. Artlett CM, Smith JB, Jimenez SA. Identification of fetal DNA and cells in skin lesions from women with systemic sclerosis. N Engl J Med 1998;338:1186.
30. Yurovsky VV, Wigley FM, Wise RA, White B. Skewing of the $CD8^+$ T cell repertoire in the lungs of systemic sclerosis patients. Human Immunol 1996;48:84.
31. Atamas SP, Yurovsky VY, Wise R, et al. Type 2 cytokines made by CD8+ lung cells predict decline in pulmonary function in patients with systemic sclerosis. Arthritis Rheum 1999;142:1168.
32. Yurovsky VV, Sutton PA, Schulze DH, Wigley FM, Wise RA, White B. Expansion of selected $V\delta1^+$ γ/δ T cells in systemic sclerosis patients. J Immunol 1994;153:881.
33. White BW, Korn JH, Piela-Smith TH. Preferential adherence of human γ/δ, CD8+ and memory T cells to fibroblasts. J Immunol 1994;152:4912.
34. Kahaleh MB, Fan PS, Otsuka T. Gammadelta receptor bearing T cells in scleroderma: enhanced interaction with vascular endothelial cells in vitro. Clin Immunol 1999;91:188.
35. Gruschwitz MS, Moormann S, Kromer G, et al. Phenotypic analysis of skin infiltrates in comparison with peripheral blood lymphocytes, spleen cells and thymocytes in early avian scleroderma. J Autoimmun 1991;4:577.
36. Jaffee BD, Claman HN. Chronic graft-versus-host disease (GVHD) as a model for scleroderma. 1. Description of model system. Cell Immunol 1983;77:1.
37. Lupoli S, Amlot P, Black C. Normal immune responses in systemic sclerosis. J Rheumatol 1990;17:323.
38. Casciola-Rosen L, Wigley F, Rosen A. Scleroderma autoantigens are uniquely fragmented by metal-catalyzed oxidation reactions: implications for pathogenesis. J Exp Med 1997;185:71.
39. Casciola-Rosen L, Andrade F, Ulanet D, Wong WB, Rosen A. Cleavage by granzyme B is strongly predictive of autoantigen status: implications for initiation of autoimmunity. J Exp Med 1999;190:815.
40. Pignone A, Scaletti C, Matucci-Cerinic M, et al. Anti-endothelial cell antibodies in systemic sclerosis: significant association with vascular involvement and alveolo-capillary impairment. Clin Exp Rheumatol 1998;16:527.
41. Bordron A, Dueymes M, Levy Y, et al. The binding of some human antiendothelial cell antibodies induces endothelial cell apoptosis. J Clin Invest 1998;101:2029.
42. Irani A-MA, Gruber BL, Kaufman LD, et al. Mast cell changes in scleroderma. Presence of MC_T cells in the skin and evidence of mast cell activation. Arthritis Rheum 1992;35:933.
43. Peltonen J, Kahari L, Jaakola S, et al. Evaluation of transforming growth factor β and type 1 procollagen gene expression in fibrotic skin diseases by in situ hybridization. J Invest Dermatol 1990;94:365.
44. Black CM, Halkier-Sorensen L, Belch JJ, et al. Oral iloprost in Raynaud's phenomenon secondary to systemic sclerosis: a multicentre, placebo-controlled, dose-comparison study. Br J Rheumatol 1998;37:952.
45. Wigley FM, Korn JH, Csuka ME, et al. Oral iloprost treatment in patients with Raynaud's phenomenon secondary to systemic sclerosis: a multicenter, placebo-controlled, double-blind study. Arthritis Rheum 1998;41:670.
46. Enomoto DN, Mekkes JR, Bossuyt PM, et al. Treatment of patients with systemic sclerosis with extracorporeal photochemotherapy (photopheresis). J Am Acad Dermatol 1999;41:915.
47. Black CM, Silman AJ, Herrick AI, et al. Interferon-alpha does not improve outcome at one year in patients with diffuse cutaneous scleroderma: results of a randomized, double-blind, placebo-controlled trial. Arthritis Rheum 1999;42:299.
48. Clements PJ, Furst DE, Wong WK, et al. High-dose versus low-dose D-penicillamine in early diffuse systemic sclerosis: analysis of a two-year, double-blind, randomized, controlled clinical trial. Arthritis Rheum 1999;42:1194.
49. Seibold JR, Korn JH, Simms R, et al. Recombinant human relaxin in the treatment of scleroderma. A randomized, double-blind, placebo-controlled trial. Ann Intern Med 2000;132:871.
50. Seibold JR, Korn JH, Simms R, et al. Recombinant human relaxin in the treatment of scleroderma. A randomized, double-blind, placebo-controlled trial. Ann Intern Med 2000, 132:871.
51. White B, Moore WC, Wigley FM, Xiao HQ, Wise RA. Cyclophosphamide is associated with pulmonary function and survival benefit in patients with sclerodema and alveolitis. Ann Intern Med 2000;132:947.
52. Badesch DB, Tapson VF, McGoon MD, et al. Continuous intravenous epoprostenol for pulmonary hypertension due to the scleroderma spectrum of disease. A randomized, controlled trial. Ann Intern Med 2000;132:425.

Section 6 Systemic Immune Diseases

Chapter 65 Inflammatory Muscle Diseases

Richard Leff, Jeffrey Sherman and Paul Plotz

Polymyositis, dermatomyositis, and related inflammatory muscle diseases, called collectively the idiopathic inflammatory myopathies (IIM), are among the least common immunologic illnesses. However, they are closely related to major immune diseases, since the IIM share many clinical features and laboratory abnormalities, particularly overlapping sets of autoantibodies. In addition, because their presentation and major clinical manifestations are weakness and rash, the differential diagnosis necessarily includes many more common diseases familiar to neurologists and dermatologists. Neurologists, dermatologists, rheumatologists, and clinical immunologists have all contributed to the understanding of IIM.

CLINICAL FEATURES

Symmetric proximal weakness is the most characteristic feature of inflammatory myositis. In some cases, muscle pain is the first or most troublesome symptom, but more often the patient is seen by a physician for the physical limitations imposed by weakness: difficulty arising from a chair or from a bed or getting into or out of a car; difficulty carrying packages, placing things on shelves, or combing and brushing hair. Rash is the first feature in a considerable proportion of patients who have dermatomyositis, but muscle weakness usually follows within a few months. Arthritis, Raynaud's phenomenon, fever, or lung disease presenting as cough or dyspnea may dominate the clinical picture. Heart and gastrointestinal symptoms other than dysphagia in severe cases are rarely early manifestations. Renal and central nervous system (CNS) involvement are almost never a part of the IIM.

Some of the rashes of dermatomyositis are virtually diagnostic; others are not disease specific (Fig. 65.1). The heliotrope rash, a purplish discoloration of the eyelids, is sometimes no more than a line along the margin of the upper lid but sometimes affects both upper and lower lids completely, and may be the only skin involvement in dermatomyositis. A reddish, sometimes raised and/or scaly eruption over the knuckles is Gottron's rash. In more advanced cases the knuckles of the toes, elbows, knees, and malleoli show a similar rash. Both heliotrope and Gottron's rashes can occur rarely in cases of frank systemic lupus erythematosus (SLE) without muscle involvement. Another common rash is a quite nondescript flat red blanching eruption of the face, the forehead, the upper chest (often in a V distribution), the upper back (where a shawl would touch), and sometimes the extensor surfaces of the upper arms and thighs. This rash looks quite lupus-like on the face, but, in contrast to lupus, the nasolabial folds are often affected. In some patients this rash is quite pruritic, and in some it is brought on by exposure to the sun. Less commonly, it may cover most of the body and break down or become infected. As in other connective tissue diseases, nailfold capillary dilatation and infarcts and cuticular overgrowth occur. A roughening and cracking of the sides of the fingers, resembling a condition found in many people

KEY CONCEPTS

Definition and incidence of idiopathic inflammatory myopathies (IIM)

- Polymyositis, dermatomyositis, and related inflammatory muscle diseases are called IIM.
- Indistinguishable muscle inflammation may accompany other autoimmune connective tissue diseases.
- The annual incidence in the USA is 5–10 cases per million. IIM are more common in women than men in all age groups.

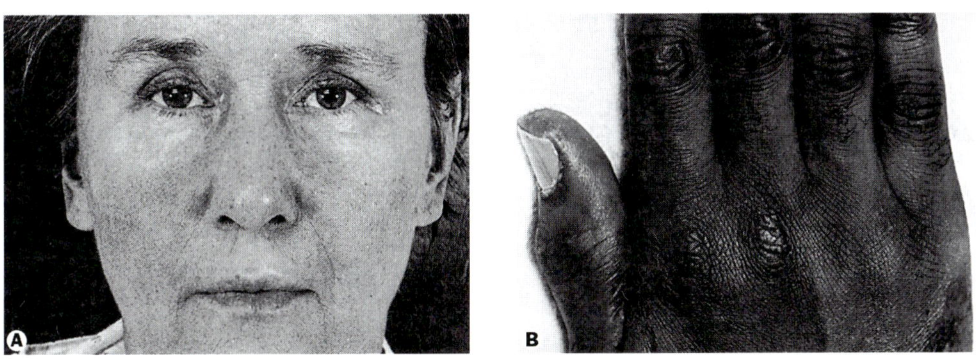

Figure 65.1 Dermatomyositis rash. (**A**) A flat red rash covers much of the lower face of this woman with dermatomyositis. Note particularly that the rash does not spare the nasolabial folds, as it often does in lupus erythematosus. (**B**) A raised shiny red rash – Gottron's rash – is apparent on the interphalangeal and the second and third metacarpo-phalangeal joints of this man with dermatomyositis (see also color plate 65.1).

Proposed revised criteria for the diagnosis of idiopathic inflammatory myopathies	
1	Symmetric[a] proximal muscle weakness
2	Elevation of the serum levels of enzymes including not only CK level but also aldolase, AST, ALT, and lactate dehydrogenase levels
3	Abnormal electromyogram with myopathic motor unit potentials, fibrillations, positive sharp waves, and increased insertional irritability
4	Muscle biopsy features of inflammatory infiltration and either degeneration/regeneration or perifascicular atrophy
5	Any one of the myositis-specific autoantibodies (an antisynthetase, anti-Mi-2, or anti-SRP)
6	Typical skin rash of DM that includes Gottron's sign, Gottron's papules, or heliotrope rash

[a] Symmetry is intended to denote bilateral but not necessarily equal involvement.
ALT = alanine aminotransferase; AST = aspartate aminotransferase; CK = creatine kinase.

Table 65.1 Possible idiopathic inflammatory myopathy (IIM) = any two criteria; probable IIM = any three criteria; definite IIM = any four criteria. Results of magnetic resonance imaging that are consistent with muscle inflammation may be substituted for either criterion 1 or 2. Patients with IIM who satisfy criterion 6 may be subclassified as having dermatomyositis. Those who satisfy the proposed criteria for inclusion body myositis (6) may be subclassified as having inclusion body myositis. The application of these criteria assumes that known infectious, toxic, metabolic, dystrophic, or endocrine myopathies have been excluded by appropriate evaluations. Criteria 1, 2, 3, 4 and 6 are the original Bohan and Peter criteria in similar form. Reproduced with permission from Targoff IN, Miller FW, Medsger TA Jr, Oddis CV. Classification criteria for the idiopathic inflammatory myopathies. *Curr Opin Rheumatol* 1997;9:527.[2]

KEY CONCEPTS

Characteristic hallmarks of inflammatory myositis

- The clinical hallmark is proximal limb and neck weakness, sometimes associated with muscle pain.
- The laboratory hallmarks are elevated serum levels of creatine kinase (CK), aldolase, lactic dehydrogenase, and the transaminases, and a characteristic pattern on electromyography (EMG). Elevated serum levels of autoantibodies are common.
- The pathologic hallmarks are focal muscle necrosis, regeneration, and inflammation.

who labor with their hands (mechanic's hands), is characteristic of one group of myositis patients.

Criteria proposed several decades ago have proved very useful in demarcating IIM from other muscle diseases.[1] Recent advances in immunologic tests and in imaging have led to an even more useful contemporary version[2] (Table 65.1).

CLASSIFICATION

It has been useful for some purposes to divide cases into several groups: polymyositis, dermatomyositis, juvenile myositis, myositis associated with another connective tissue disease (usually systemic sclerosis, SLE, or Sjögren syndrome), cancer-associated myositis (usually cases in which the diagnoses are made within 6–12 months of one another), inclusion body myositis, and a miscellaneous group that includes such rare entities as eosinophilic myositis (Table 65.2). This classification has allowed recognition of unique clinical and pathogenetic features and response to therapy. In the case of cancer-associated myositis, a more rational approach to workup based on recognition of groups at risk is now possible.[3]

Autoantibodies unique to myositis, the so-called 'myositis-specific autoantibodies', have allowed a useful alternative classification (Table 65.3). For example, patients with antibodies to one or another of a group of enzymes – the aminoacyl-tRNA (transfer RNA) synthetases, of which Jo-1 is the best known – have a characteristic syndrome that usually includes interstitial lung disease, arthritis, fevers, and Raynaud's phenomenon in addition to myositis. Those with antibodies to the signal recognition particle (anti-SRP) have severe disease of abrupt onset, often in the autumn, unaccompanied by rash. Those with antibodies to the nuclear antigen Mi-2 almost always have the V and shawl rashes and cuticular overgrowth in addition to myositis. Each of the different autoantibody-associated groups also has a predominant histocompatibility type and clinical course (Table 65.3).[4]

Traditional classification of idiopathic inflammatory myopathies	
Type I	Primary idiopathic polymyositis
Type II	Primary idiopathic dermatomyositis
Type III	Dermatomyositis or polymyositis associated with malignancy
Type IV	Childhood dermatomyositis or polymyositis
Type V	Myositis associated with another connective tissue disease
Type VI	Inclusion body myositis
Type VII	Miscellaneous: eosinophilic myositis, localized nodular myositis, etc.

Table 65.2 Traditional classification of idiopathic inflammatory myopathies.

Clinical features associated with myositis-specific autoantibodies

Autoantibodies	Characteristic clinical features
Anti-Jo-I and other antisynthetases	Relatively acute onset of myositis, frequent interstitial lung disease, fever, Raynaud's phenomenon, arthritis, mechanic's hands, moderate response to therapy, persistent disease. Patients sometimes meet criteria for SLE or RA, but muscle disease or lung disease dominate the clinical picture and prognosis
Anti-SRP	Very acute onset of myositis, often in autumn, severe weakness, no rash, palpitations, females predominate, poor response to therapy
Anti-Mi-2	Relatively acute onset of myositis, classic dermatomyositis rashes with V sign and shawl sign, cuticular overgrowth, good response to therapy

SRP = signal recognition particle.

Table 65.3 Clinical features associated with myositis-specific autoantibodies.

Inclusion body myositis (IBM) resembles an extremely chronic form of polymyositis. The diagnosis of IBM is important because, in contrast to patients with other inflammatory myopathies, those with IBM rarely improve in strength with immunosuppressive therapy.[5,6] Patients with IBM tend to be older than other patients with myositis; they are commonly men. They have gradual, painless, progressive weakness and focal atrophy that develop over years. There are few signs of disease outside of the skeletal musculature. Difficulties with swallowing can be a complaint of patients with any inflammatory myopathy and are frequently a major problem in patients with IBM.[5,7,8] The creatine kinase (CK) and other skeletal muscle-associated serum enzymes are normal in about one fourth of patients with IBM and only moderately elevated in the remainder. EMG in IBM frequently demonstrates both myogenic and neurogenic features secondary to the effective denervation of some muscle cells by inflammation and necrosis.

Proposed criteria for the diagnosis of IBM rely on both pathologic and clinical features. In the clinical setting of an inflammatory myopathy, the presence by light microscopy (with confirmation by electron microscopy) of the characteristic inclusions or rimmed vacuoles is diagnostic of IBM. The origin of the vacuoles in IBM has been the focus of investigation and remains a source of speculation. Among the inflammatory myopathies, IBM is distinguished by substantial numbers of rimmed cytoplasmic vacuoles with tubulofilamentous material within myofibers. A variety of proteins have been found by immunohistochemistry in the muscle cells in IBM, including ubiquitin, β-amyloid precursor protein, phosphorylated tau, and the transcription factor NF-κB, but it is not yet possible to tie them to the pathogenesis of the illness.[9] The infiltrates in the muscle of patients with IBM are composed predominantly of CD8 lymphocytes, closely resembling those found in the inflammatory infiltrate in the muscles of patients with polymyositis.[10] There is increased expression of human leukocyte antigen (HLA) in the muscle of patients with IBM.

IBM must be distinguished from other myopathies because of its chronic nature. These others include acquired myopathies, such as those caused by chloroquine, colchicine, and other toxins, and genetically-determined myopathies, such as some muscular dystrophies and the distal myopathies. There are several important differences between IBM and these other myopathies. The separation, however, is not as sharp as might be hoped. Although some of the familial forms of IBM have a distinctive clinical presentation, often early in life, there have been several families with the typical late onset and inflammatory picture of the presumed sporadic cases.[11] Several genetic loci have been identified in familial IBM, so it will be important to assess any identified mutations in familial IBM-associated genes in sporadic cases.[12] A further complexity is that IBM has now been described decades after typical dermatomyositis.[13]

ETIOLOGY

Immunologic clues to origin

The implications of myositis-specific autoantibodies that bind to and inhibit the function of native human enzymes involved with the formation of newly formed proteins are tantalizing and probably significant. These autoantibodies appear to develop before symptomatic weakness or serum creatine kinase (CK) elevation, suggesting a close link to an initiating factor.[14] Some of the clinical features, such as fever, arthritis, and lung disease, and the apparent seasonality in onset of disease in patients with anti-SRP are reminiscent of some viral infections.[15] In patients with autoantibodies against one of the aminoacyl-tRNA synthetases such as Jo-1 (histidyl-tRNA synthetase), the possible connection to a viral inciting agent appeared compelling since certain picornaviruses, which are closely related to viruses long suspected of causing myositis, such as coxsackieviruses, can mimic tRNA in acting as a substrate for an aminoacyl-tRNA synthetase.[16] Direct proof connecting picornaviruses to human myositis, however, has not been obtained.[17] Viral infections clearly associated with myositis include HIV, HTLV-I, influenza, and, in immunodeficient children, ECHO virus. A variety of other nonspecific immunologic abnormalities occur in the IIM.

Drugs and toxins

A large number of environmental agents have been associated with myopathies. Sometimes, the illness may strikingly resemble the spontaneous disease.[18] D-penicillamine, for example, can induce a variety of autoimmune phenomena, including an inflammatory myopathy closely resembling polymyositis. A number of drugs can also produce myopathies that are clinically confused with IIM but are histologically distinct. This large group includes corticosteroids, zidovudine (AZT), and 3-hydroxy-3-methylglutaryl-coenzyme A (HMG-CoA) reductase inhibitors. In corticosteroid-induced myopathy, type II muscle fiber atrophy is prominent on muscle biopsy and weakness improves when the dose is lowered. AZT produces a characteristic mitochondrial myopathy. The myopathy associated with HIV infection can be distinguished from that caused by AZT by examination of a muscle biopsy since, in the latter, characteristic mitochondrial abnormalities are found.[19] The HMG-CoA reductase inhibitors produce elevated CK and myalgias in some patients. Rhabdomyolysis has been reported but is rare. The antimalarial drugs chloroquine and hydroxychloroquine produce a vacuolar myopathy by raising the intralysosomal pH so that the acid cathepsins that digest waste products in the lysosome are inoperable, and waste products accumulate in vacuoles. For most other drugs, the mechanism of toxicity is unknown. The claims that injections of type I collagen or silicone breast implants can cause inflammatory myositis remain unsupported by epidemiological data.

Bacterial and parasitic diseases

Certain parasitic diseases can produce an illness by direct invasion of muscle. Weakness, fever, and eosinophilia are usually present. Bacterial pyomyositis is uncommon in North America but occurs more commonly in other parts of the world. It is attended by the signs of local infection and is difficult to confuse with an IIM.

PATHOGENESIS

The precise mechanisms of cell damage and death in the IIM are unknown. Apoptosis is absent in IIM biopsies,[20] but infiltrating CD8 T cells in polymyositis do appear to release perforin and granzyme into targeted muscle cells. After damage, a muscle fiber, which is a syncytium, can regenerate. Initially, on light microscopy one can appreciate loss of striations leading to a homogeneous appearance, fiber size variation, atrophy, and centralization of the nuclei. In the inflammatory myopathies, mononuclear cell invasion is a primary method of destruction. Macrophages and cytotoxic T cells invade the myofibers. The myocyte cytoplasm in the region of the invaginated cells appears vacuolated and swollen. Other regions of the same cell may show intense regeneration, as seen histologically by aggregates of nuclei with prominent nucleoli and fiber splitting. Thus, degeneration and regeneration may be present in the same fiber at the same time.

The inflammatory milieu in inflamed muscle has been studied. Pro-inflammatory cytokines were not always detectable, though the chemokines MIP-1α and RANTES were present in most biopsies,[21,22] and IL-1β was also usually present.[23] TGF-β is constitutively present in muscle. The muscle cells and inflammatory cells present in IIM often have costimulatory molecules on their surfaces, reinforcing the picture of a direct interaction between them.[24] Tissue culture observations of muscle cells have demonstrated that they can both produce and respond to a considerable range of cytokines.[25]

Engel and his colleagues have demonstrated several important pathologic distinctions between dermatomyositis and polymyositis,[10] and have suggested that, in dermatomyositis, the initial point of injury may be the capillaries. A model of disease has been proposed in which capillaries are primarily damaged and myocytes are secondarily involved. Complement and immunoglobulins may be found in the walls of the capillaries even where the remainder of the muscle is normal. The membrane attack complex of complement deposits there, and endothelial cells are swollen and pale. Even in unaffected regions of muscle, special staining reveals a marked decrease in capillary number.[26] More advanced changes include microtubular endothelial inclusions and microvacuoles. Evaluation of lymphocyte populations in dermatomyositis shows a high percentage of B cells in the perivascular regions and an increasing frequency of T cells toward the perimysium and endomysium. T cells found within the muscle are relatively rich in CD4 T cells. In dermatomyositis, especially the juvenile-onset form, inflammation and necrosis followed by atrophy appear in a perifascicular pattern. Perivascular lymphocytic infiltrates, typical of later disease, have not been described as an early change. Dermatomyositis thus may be the result of an immune complex deposition or a primary attack on endothelial cells. Consistent with the importance of immune complexes, histological abnormalities in the skin in dermatomyositis are indistinguishable from the changes in lupus.

In contrast to dermatomyositis, polymyositis and IBM do not demonstrate marked capillary changes, perivascular infiltrates are less pronounced, and T-cell infiltrates in the perimysial and endomysial regions are more pronounced. Non-necrotic fibers may be surrounded by T lymphocytes and macrophages. The T cells are enriched for the CD8 type. Attempts to culture these cells and look for lysis of autologous myocytes have met with limited success. There is negligible evidence of NK cell-like activity. Should cytotoxic T cells prove to be the major effector cells, it will be necessary to clone T cells to identify the antigenic targets.

Most cytotoxic T cells are of the CD8 phenotype and therefore recognize their antigenic peptide in association with major histocompatibility complex (MHC) Class I molecules. Although resting normal muscle has very low Class I expression, it is up-regulated in regenerating and degenerating fibers found in both

KEY CONCEPTS

Differential features of myositis

- In dermatomyositis the earliest changes involve vessel walls, and B cells and CD4 T cells dominate in the muscle biopsy.
- In polymyositis and inclusion-body myositis the dominant pathologic feature is attack on and invasion of muscle cells by CD8 cytotoxic cells.

inflammatory and noninflammatory myopathies.[27] Interestingly, in dermatomyositis, Class I is up-regulated predominantly in the perifascicular regions, around sites of atrophy, and near sites of cellular invasion. In contrast, in polymyositis, Class I may be diffusely up-regulated even where there is no cellular infiltrate.[28] IBM shows a more focal Class I distribution in regions of T-cell invasion. The presence of focal regions of MHC Class I expression in non-necrotic fibers at the site of activated CD8 T cells is compatible with cytotoxicity as a prime mechanism of myocyte necrosis in IBM and polymyositis.

The role of MHC Class II molecules remains to be clarified. Myoblasts in culture constitutively express high levels of Class I, and they are negative for Class II. Class II has been found to be up-regulated in the endothelial cells of patients with dermatomyositis, while its expression on T cells, a marker of activation, is more prominent in polymyositis.

Finally, γδ TCR T lymphocytes have been cloned from the muscle biopsy of one patient with polymyositis. Subsequent evaluation of his biopsy demonstrated γδ T cells and a 65 kDa heat shock protein in the endomysial region.[29] The relative importance of γδ T cells in the spectrum of IIM is unknown.

The role of the B cells within affected muscles is not understood. It is not yet known whether they produce any autoantibodies, particularly the myositis-specific antibodies, or whether they play a role in antigen presentation for the T cells.

The pathogenic role of the autoantibodies found in patients with IIM remains uncertain. Myositis-specific antibodies are found in 30–40% of patients, appear to delineate specific clinical entities, and each group has a strong but not absolute HLA association.[4] In a patient with myositis and antihistidyl-tRNA synthetase (Jo-1) autoantibodies, sera available from long before the onset of symptoms or biochemical damage to muscle tissue contained the autoantibodies, suggesting that the autoantibodies were not merely a response to release of tissue antigens.[31] The extraordinary specificity of myositis-specific antibodies for IIM and the lack of evidence for strong polyclonal stimulation in these diseases suggest that MSA are related to the fundamental causative process in IIM. Although 80–90% of patients with IIM are found to have antibodies to myosin or myoglobin, these antibodies are also found in patients with noninflammatory myopathies.[31]

The structures bound by myosin-specific antibodies are mostly intracellular ribonucleoproteins involved in protein synthesis such as the aminoacyl-tRNA synthetases and the signal recognition particle (SRP). These autoantigens are found in every nucleated cell.[31] The antibodies in general bind to conformational epitopes and, at least in the case of the antisynthetases, block enzymatic activity. It is possible that a structural property of muscle allows these particular proteins to be presented to the immune system when the cells are damaged, or, alternatively, the capacity of muscle fibers to degenerate alongside intense regeneration within the same fiber may allow these proteins to be efficiently displayed.[32] Recent experiments have suggested that some aminoacyl-tRNA synthetases have a direct pro-inflammatory role through a subsidiary chemokine-like action.[33]

Genetics

The IIM do not exhibit a simple mode of inheritance, and the rare familial cases mostly reflect IBM of early onset.[34] As noted above, there are HLA associations for particular myositis-specific autoantibodies. Specifically, HLA-DR52 has a strong association (90%) with antisynthetase-positive myositis in both Caucasians and African-Americans.[35] Even in drug-induced myositis there may be a predominance of a particular HLA type, implying immune specificity of drug-related myopathy. D-penicillamine-induced myositis is associated with DR4 in Caucasians.[36]

NATURAL HISTORY

The prognosis for patients with IIM varies greatly with clinical type, autoantibodies, extraskeletal muscle involvement, and the interval between diagnosis and the start of treatment.

Patients with dermatomyositis or myositis accompanying another connective tissue disease are likely to recover most of their strength with prompt and adequate therapy. Although recurrences are common, persistent profound weakness does not usually occur. Most patients with anti-Mi-2 autoantibodies also usually respond well to therapy. Strength usually recovers well in patients whose myositis is cancer related, but overall mortality due to the tumor is high. Indeed, death from an accompanying tumor remains the most frequent cause of death in patients with an IIM.

Patients with polymyositis fare less well, even when those with IBM are rigorously excluded. A return to normal strength is very unusual, and each recurrence is likely to be followed by greater residual weakness, even if inflammation is fully controlled. IBM has a poorer prognosis, but it is possible that the gradual decline in strength can be halted for long periods by corticosteroid and/or cytotoxic therapy if continuing inflammation is present. Patients with anti-SRP autoantibodies have the worst prognosis, since there is rampant muscle destruction at the very outset. Those with anti-Jo-1 autoantibodies or antibodies to another synthetase are likely to respond to therapy initially but to require continuing immunosuppression to treat frequent recurrences. In this group morbidity and mortality are heavily influenced by the progress of lung involvement.

PATIENT MANAGEMENT

The treatment of myositis is based on controlling skeletal muscle inflammation and damage. Immunosuppressive therapy and rest are used in the initial stages of the disease to decrease inflammation and muscle damage. After the inflammation is controlled, strengthening exercises are clearly useful in improving functional capabilities.

Corticosteroids

Corticosteroids are the main immunosuppressive agents used in the treatment of myositis. Patients generally require high doses (such as prednisone at 1 mg/kg/d) for at least 2–3 months before maximum clinical benefit occurs.[37–39] An initial course of pulses of methylprednisolone may be helpful, particularly in disease of acute onset. It is also helpful in managing flare-ups. Disease in about three quarters of myositis patients will be controlled initially with corticosteroids. If active muscle inflammation persists or the side-effects of corticosteroids are severe, other immunosuppressive treatments are employed. Alternate-day steroids are often not effective in these diseases.

Second-line immunosuppressive therapies

The most frequently used second-line agents in the treatment of myositis are azathioprine and methotrexate. Azathioprine has been shown to decrease long-term disability in polymyositis.[40] Methotrexate is useful in patients with little or no response to corticosteroid therapy.[41,42] Combination therapies, such as the combination of methotrexate with azathioprine, are useful even if patients have failed to respond to one of the agents alone.[43] High-dose intravenous immunoglobulin is of proven benefit in dermatomyositis.[44] Its usefulness in polymyositis is less predictable. Apheresis proved ineffective in a controlled blinded study.[45] Both cyclosporine and tacrolimus have been effective in some cases, as have cyclophosphamide and chlorambucil. There have not yet been careful trials of any biological agents.

Monitoring disease activity

Improvement in strength and normalization of serum CK activity are the best indirect measures of disease activity. A decrease in the serum CK activity may herald clinical improvement, but corticosteroid treatment alone may decrease the CK activity without associated clinical improvement. A lack of improvement in strength in a corticosteroid-treated patient may be due to the resistance of the inflammatory process, the presence of a corticosteroid-induced myopathy, or both. A diagnostic and therapeutic taper of the corticosteroids may then be warranted. If inflammation is present concurrently, other immunosuppressive agents are useful as the dosage of corticosteroids is lowered. If the CK value begins to rise, even if it is still within the normal range, and the symptoms of myositis are worsening in a patient whose disease has previously been controlled with corticosteroids, an increase in the dose may be warranted.[46]

Treatment-resistant myositis

Some treatment-resistant polymyositis patients have another disease. IBM or hereditary myopathy should be suspected in such patients. Unlike other myositis patients, those with IBM rarely, if ever, improve in strength with immunosuppressive therapy, but stabilization of strength may be achieved in some IBM patients with immunosuppressive agents.[6,47]

Nonskeletal muscle involvement

Other organs frequently involved in myositis include the skin, lungs, and joints. Such organ involvement and the systemic features of myositis (fever and weight loss) usually improve with immunosuppressive therapy that controls inflammation in the skeletal muscle. Hydroxychloroquine and other antimalarials are useful in controlling the rashes associated with myositis.[48]

Supportive therapy

Supportive therapies for skeletal muscle, for involved organs, and for the activities of daily life are important in the treatment of patients with myositis. These include bed rest during the acute illness followed by strengthening exercises, precautions to prevent falls and aspiration, supplemental oxygen for severe lung disease, vasodilator therapy for Raynaud's phenomenon, and counseling for a severe or chronic illness.

DIAGNOSTIC TOOLS, EVALUATION, AND DIFFERENTIAL DIAGNOSIS

Clinical, laboratory, pathologic, and electrodiagnostic findings contribute to the proper diagnosis of IIM. Even in individuals with typical clinical features of IIM, it is essential to exclude other diseases that may have similar symptoms and signs (Table 65.4). Certain clinical features should suggest a different diagnosis. These include: family history of a similar illness; sensory, reflex, or other neurologic changes; fasciculations; a relationship of the weakness to exercise, food intake, or fasting; major muscle cramping, myotonia (difficulty relaxing a contracted muscle), or myasthenia (increasing weakness with repeated contractions); significant early muscle atrophy or hypertrophy; marked asymmetry; weakness in the distribution of the cranial nerves; and dyspnea due to diaphragmatic weakness rather than lung fibrosis. All the above are findings that should lead away from a diagnosis of IIM.

CLINICAL PEARLS

Clinical features that suggest a non-IIM diagnosis

- Family history of a similar illness
- Weakness related to exercise, eating, or fasting
- Sensory, reflex, or other neurologic signs
- Cranial nerve involvement
- Fasciculations
- Muscle cramping (severe)
- Myasthenia (increasing weakness with repeated contractions)
- Myotonia (difficulty relaxing a contracted muscle)
- Significant atrophy or hypertrophy early in the illness
- Marked asymmetry
- Dyspnea due to diaphragmatic weakness with normal chest x-ray film

Differential diagnosis of IIM

Neuromuscular disorders
- Genetic muscular dystrophies
- Metabolic myopathies
  - Disorders of carbohydrate metabolism: McArdle disease, phosphofructokinase deficiency, adult acid maltase deficiency, and others
  - Disorders of lipid metabolism: carnitine deficiency, carnitine palmitoyl transferase deficiency
  - Disorders of purine metabolism: myoadenylate deaminase deficiency
- Mitochondrial myopathies
- Spinal muscular atrophies
- Neuropathies: Guillain–Barré and other autoimmune polyneuropathies, diabetes mellitus, porphyria
- Myasthenia gravis and Eaton–Lambert syndrome
- Amyotrophic lateral sclerosis
- Myotonic dystrophy and other myotonias
- Familial periodic paralysis

Endocrine and electrolyte disorders
- Hypokalemia, hypercalcemia, hypocalcemia, hypomagnesemia
- Hypothyroidism, hyperthyroidism
- Cushing syndrome, Addison's disease

Toxic myopathies (partial list)
- Alcohol
- Chloroquine and hydroxychloroquine
- Cocaine
- Colchicine
- Corticosteroids
- D-penicillamine
- Ipecac
- Statins and other lipid-lowering agents
- Zidovudine (AZT)

Infections
- Viral: HIV, HTLV-1, influenza
- Bacterial: staphylococcus, streptococcus, clostridia
- Parasitic: toxoplasmosis, trichinosis, schistosomiasis, cysticercosis

Miscellaneous
- Polymyalgia rheumatica
- Vasculitis
- Eosinophilia myalgia syndrome
- Paraneoplastic syndromes

Table 65.4 Differential diagnosis of IIM.

The single most useful laboratory feature of muscle destruction is an elevation of the serum CK, although a small proportion of patients – probably fewer than 5% – have a bona fide inflammatory muscle disease without ever having an elevated CK. Elevations of the serum levels of aldolase, serum glutamic-oxaloacetic transaminase (SGOT), serum glutamate pyruvate transaminase (SGPT), and lactate dehydrogenase (LDH) are as frequent but less specific for muscle disease. Hematologic abnormalities and elevation of the sedimentation rate are unreliable guides; if a significant abnormality is found, a physician should be alert to another cause for it.

Electromyographic (EMG) abnormalities are frequently present. Although the test is useful to exclude some neurologic diseases that resemble IIM, it is uncomfortable and not useful for following the course of the illness.

Magnetic resonance imaging, especially a combination of the T1 and the fat-suppressed T2 (STIR) sequences, is remarkably useful in defining the extent of involvement and planning a biopsy (Fig. 65.2).[49] Although not specific, the changes of inflammatory myopathy can provide considerable help in confusing cases as well as help in choosing a place to biopsy.

A muscle biopsy should be performed in every suspected case of myositis (Fig. 65.3). Although the spotty involvement means that the biopsy may occasionally miss inflammation, confounding diagnoses, for example amyloidosis, eosinophilic myositis, dystrophy, or some metabolic myopathies as well as the important variant IBM, can only be diagnosed definitively by biopsy. The identification of autoantibodies, particularly the myositis-specific autoantibodies, has distinct clinical and prognostic usefulness. At present, of these autoantibodies only anti-Jo-1 is commercially available, but tests for the others are carried out in research centers, and some will eventually become more widely available.

PITFALLS

It is increasingly apparent that the boundary between, on the one hand, polymyositis and inclusion body myositis and, on the

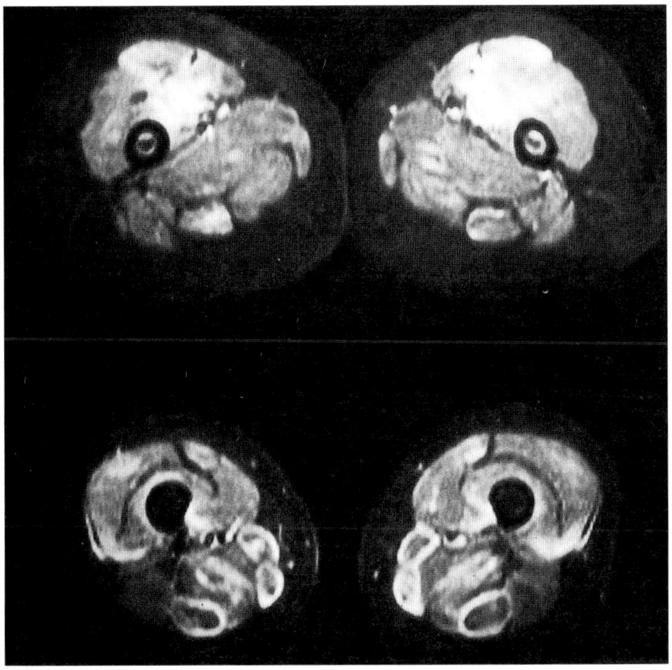

Figure 65.2 Magnetic resonance images of the upper and lower thighs of a patient with dermatomyositis done with the fat-suppressed T2 (STIR) technique. With this technique inflammation appears as a bright signal; normal muscle is gray; and bone, fat, fascia, and normal skin are dark. Blood vessels may appear as bright spots. Note the remarkable symmetry of the inflammation. In this patient most of the involvement is in the quadriceps in the upper thighs and around the periphery of the hamstring muscles in the lower thighs.

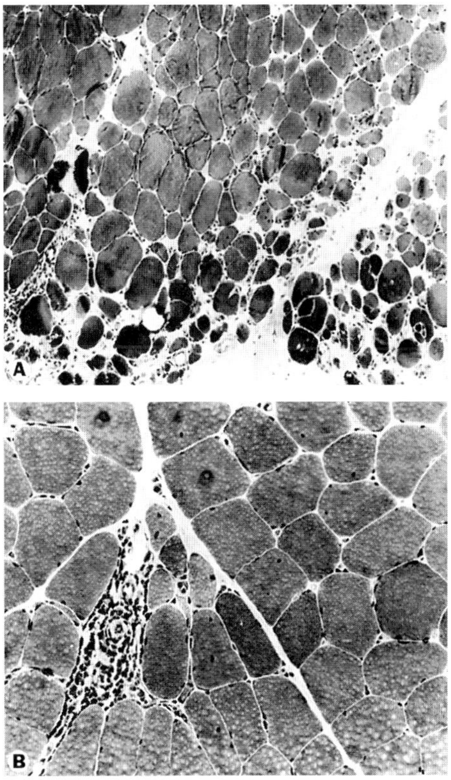

Figure 65.3 Biopsy in dermatomyositis. (**A**) Low-power (original magnification × 100) view of a muscle biopsy from a patient with dermatomyositis. Note the marked fiber size variation and the large number of atrophic myocytes, particularly at the periphery of the fascicles. (**B**) High-power (original magnification × 200) view of inflammation around the vessels in the muscle biopsy of a patient with dermatomyositis. There are nearby atrophic cells and cells whose nuclei have moved away from the periphery of the cell (centralized nuclei) (see also color plate 65.3).

other hand, some genetically determined myopathies cannot be cleanly drawn. In the last several years, dystrophies with an extraordinary variety of clinical manifestations (in regard to age and distribution of weakness) have also been described.[50] Not only can inflammation be seen on biopsy in some patients, but a partial clinical response to corticosteroids can occur. Furthermore, it is increasingly recognized that mitochondrial abnormalities can be limited to groups of skeletal muscles, leading to confusion with IIM. Toxic myopathies, of course, will continue to occur with the release of new drugs, and well continue to be a possible source of diagnostic confusion.

Thus, not only must the history, physical examination, and biopsy be performed and interpreted with compulsiveness and care, but molecular diagnostic techniques must be employed by clinicians in pursuit of accurate diagnosis and appropriate therapy. The correct response to disease that persists in the face of powerful immunosuppressive therapy is a careful re-thinking of the diagnosis, including, on occasion, re biopsy and molecular consultation.

REFERENCES

1. Bohan A, Peter JB, Bowman RL, Pearson CM. Computer-assisted analysis of 153 patients with polymyositis and dermatomyositis. Medicine (Baltimore) 1977;56:255.
2. Targoff IN, Miller FW, Medsger TA Jr, Oddis CV. Classification criteria for the idiopathic inflammatory myopathies. Curr Opin Rheumatol 1997;9:527.
3. Sigurgeirsson B, Lindelof B, Edhag O, Allander E. Risk of cancer in patients with dermatomyositis or polymyositis. A population-based study. N Engl J Med 1992;326:363.
4. Love LA, Leff RL, Fraser DD, et al. A new approach to the classification of idiopathic inflammatory myopathy: Myositis-specific autoantibodies define useful homogeneous patient groups. Medicine (Baltimore) 1991;70:360.
5. Lotz BP, Engel AG, Nishino H, Stevens JC, Litchy WJ. Inclusion body myositis. Observations in 40 patients. Brain 1989;112:727.
6. Leff R, Miller F, Hicks J, Fraser D, Plotz P. The treatment of inclusion body myositis (IBM): A retrospective review and a randomized, prospective trial of immunosuppressive therapy. Medicine (Baltimore) 1993;72:225.
7. Carpenter S, Karpati G, Heller I, Eisen A. Inclusion body myositis: a distinct variety of idiopathic inflammatory myopathy. Neurology 1978;28:8.
8. Wintzen AR, Bots GT, de Bakker HM, Hulshof JH, Padberg GW. Dysphagia in inclusion body myositis. J Neurol Neurosurg Psychiatry 1988;51:1542.
9. Yang CC, Askanas V, Engel WK, Alvarez RB. Immunolocalization of transcription factor NF-kappa B in inclusion-body myositis muscle and at normal human neuromuscular junctions. Neurosci Lett 1998;254:77.
10. Engel AG, Arahata K, Emslie-Smith A. Immune effector mechanisms in inflammatory myopathies. Res Publ Assoc Res Nerv Ment Dis 1990;68:141.

11. Amato AA, Robert RT. Inclusion body myositis in twins. Neurology 1998;51:598.
12. Argov Z, Eisenberg I, Mitrani-Rosenbaum S. Genetics of inclusion body myopathies. Curr Opin Rheumatol 1998;10:543.
13. McCoy AL, Bubb MR, Plotz PH, Davis JC. Inclusion body myositis long after dermatomyositis: A report of two cases. Clin Exp Rheum 1999;17:235.
14. Miller FW, Waite KA, Biswas T, Plotz PH. The role of an autoantigen, histidyl-tRNA synthetase, in the induction and maintenance of autoimmunity. Proc Natl Acad Sci USA 1990;87:9933.
15. Leff RL, Burgess SH, Miller FW, et al. Distinct seasonal patterns in the onset of adult idiopathic inflammatory myopathy in patients with anti-Jo-1 and anti-signal recognition particle autoantibodies. Arthritis Rheum 1991;34:1391.
16. Mathews MB, Bernstein RM. Myositis autoantibody inhibits histidyl-tRNA synthetase: a model for autoimmunity. Nature 1983;304:177.
17. Leff RL, Love LA, Miller FW, et al. Viruses in idiopathic inflammatory myopathies: absence of candidate viral genomes in muscle. Lancet 1992;339:1192.
18. Love LA, Miller FW. Noninfectious environmental agents associated with myopathies. Curr Opin Rheumatol 1993;5:712.
19. Miller RG. Neuropathies and myopathies complicating HIV infection. J Clin Apheresis 1991;6:110.
20. Schneider C, Gold R, Dalakas MC, et al. MHC Class I-mediated cytotoxicity does not induce apoptosis in muscle fibers nor in inflammatory T cells: studies in patients with polymyositis, dermatomyositis, and inclusion body myositis. J Neuropathol Exp Neurol 1996;55:1205.
21. Adams EM, Kirkley J, Eidelman G, Dohlman J, Plotz PH. The predominance of beta (CC) chemokine transcripts in idiopathic inflammatory muscle diseases. Proc Assoc Am Physicians 1997;109:275.
22. Lundberg I, Brengman JM, Engel AG. Analysis of cytokine expression in muscle in inflammatory myopathies, Duchenne dystrophy, and non-weak controls. J Neuroimmunol 1995;63:9.
23. Lundberg I, Ulfgren AK, Nyberg P, Andersson U, Klareskog L. Cytokine production in muscle tissue of patients with idiopathic inflammatory myopathies. Arthritis Rheum 1997;40:865.
24. Nagaraju K, Raben N, Villalba ML, et al. Costimulatory markers in muscle of patients with idiopathic inflammatory myopathies and in cultured muscle cells. Clin Immunol 1999;92:161.
25. Nagaraju K, Raben N, Merritt G, Loeffler L, Kirk K, Plotz P. A variety of cytokines and immunologically relevant surface molecules are expressed by normal human skeletal muscle cells under proinflammatory stimuli. Clin Exp Immunol 1998;113:407.
26. Estruch R, Grau JM, Fernandez-Sola J, Casademont J, Monforte R, Urbano-Marquez A. Microvascular changes in skeletal muscle in idiopathic inflammatory myopathy. Hum Pathol 1992;23:888.
27. Emslie-Smith AM, Arahata K, Engel AG. Major histocompatibility complex Class I antigen expression, immunolocalization of interferon subtypes, and T cell-mediated cytotoxicity in myopathies. Hum Pathol 1989;20:224.
28. Karpati G, Pouliot Y, Carpenter S. Expression of immunoreactive major histocompatibility complex products in human skeletal muscles. Ann Neurol 1988;23:64.
29. Hohlfeld R, Engel AG. The role of gamma-delta T lymphocytes in inflammatory muscle disease. Chem Immunol 1992;53:75.
30. Miller FW, Twitty SA, Biswas T, Plotz PH. Origin and regulation of a disease-specific autoantibody response: antigenic epitopes, spectrotype stability, and isotype restriction of anti-Jo-1 autoantibodies. J Clin Invest 1990;85:468.
31. Targoff IN. Autoantibodies in polymyositis. Rheum Dis Clin North Am 1992;18:455.
32. Rosen A, Casciola-Rosen L, Ahearn J. Novel packages of viral and self-antigens are generated during apoptosis. J Exp Med 1995;181:1557.
33. Wakasugi K, Schimmel P. Two distinct cytokines released from a human aminoacyl-tRNA synthetase. Science 1999;284:147.
34. Rider LG, Gurley RC, Pandey JP, et al. Clinical, serologic, and immunogenetic features of familial idiopathic inflammatory myopathy. Arthritis Rheum 1998;41:710.
35. Goldstein R, Duvic M, Targoff IN, et al. HLA-D region genes associated with autoantibody responses to histidyl-transfer RNA synthetase (Jo-1) and other translation-related factors in myositis. Arthritis Rheum 1990;33:1240.
36. Garlepp MJ, Dawkins RL, Christiansen FT. HLA antigens and acetylcholine receptor antibodies in penicillamine induced myasthenia gravis. Br Med J (Clin Res Ed) 1983;286:338.
37. Mulder DW, Winkelmann RK, Lambert EH, Diessner GR, Howard FM. Steroid therapy in patients with polymyositis and dermatomyositis. Ann Intern Med 1984;58:969.
38. Oddis CV, Medsger TA Jr. Relationship between serum creatine kinase level and corticosteroid therapy in polymyositis-dermatomyositis. J Rheumatol 1988;15:807.
39. Winkelmann RK, Mulder DW, Lambert EH, Howard FM, Diessner GR. Course of dermatomyositis-polymyositis: comparison of untreated and cortisone-treated patients. Mayo Clin Proc 1968;43:545.
40. Bunch TW. Prednisone and azathioprine for polymyositis: long-term followup. Arthritis Rheum 1981;24:45.
41. Metzger AL, Bohan A, Goldberg LS, Bluestone R, Pearson CM. Polymyositis and dermatomyositis: combined methotrexate and corticosteroid therapy. Ann Intern Med 1974;81:182.
42. Joffe MM, Love LA, Leff RL, et al. Drug therapy of the idiopathic inflammatory myopathies: predictors of response to prednisone, azathioprine, and methotrexate and a comparison of their efficacy. Am J Med 1993;94:379.
43. Villalba L, Hicks JE, Adams EM, et al. Treatment of refractory myositis: a randomized crossover study of two new cytotoxic regimens. Arthritis Rheum 1998;41:392.
44. Dalakas MC, Illa I, Dambrosia JM, et al. A controlled trial of high-dose intravenous immune globulin infusions as treatment for dermatomyositis. N Engl J Med 1993;329:1993.
45. Miller FW, Leitman SF, Cronin ME, et al. Controlled trial of plasma exchange and leukapheresis in polymyositis and dermatomyositis. N Engl J Med 1992;326:1380.
46. Oddis CV, Medsger TA. Current management of polymyositis and dermatomyositis. Drugs 1989;37:382.
47. Sayers ME, Chou SM, Calabrese LH. Inclusion body myositis: analysis of 32 cases. J Rheumatol 1992;19:1385.
48. Woo TY, Callen JP, Voorhees JJ, Bickers DR, Hanno R, Hawkins C. Cutaneous lesions of dermatomyositis are improved by hydroxychloroquine. J Am Acad Dermatol 1984;10:592.
49. Adams EM, Chow CK, Premkumar A, Plotz PH. The idiopathic inflammatory myopathies: spectrum of MR imaging findings. Radiographics 1995;15:563.
50. Emery AE. The muscular dystrophies. BMJ 1998;317:991.

Chapter 66 Spondyloarthropathies

Frank C. Arnett

INTRODUCTION

The term *spondyloarthropathies* encompasses a family of chronic inflammatory diseases characterized primarily by spinal and/or peripheral arthritis.[1,2] A variety of extra-articular manifestations also may occur and help to discriminate one disorder from another. Those entities classified as spondyloarthropathies include: (1) *ankylosing spondylitis*, primarily an ascending spinal arthritis resulting in bony fusion and deformity; (2) *juvenile spondyloarthropathy*, typically a peripheral arthritis beginning in childhood which eventually progresses to ankylosing spondylitis; (3) *Reiter syndrome* or *reactive arthritis*, a predominantly peripheral arthritis, with or without several distinctive mucocutaneous features, especially urethritis and conjunctivitis, following certain enteric and venereally acquired infections; (4) *psoriatic arthritis*, a peripheral and/or spinal arthritis occurring in individuals with cutaneous psoriasis; and (5) *enteropathic arthritis*, either peripheral or spinal arthritis occurring in the setting of one of the idiopathic inflammatory bowel diseases, either ulcerative colitis or Crohn's disease (Table 66.1). A variety of *atypical*,

KEY CONCEPTS

Important unifying features of the spondyloarthropathies

- A tendency for involvement of sacroiliac joints (sacroiliitis) and other axial structures (spondylitis)
- A pattern of peripheral arthritis which is typically oligoarticular and asymmetrical
- Inflammation of tendon and fascial insertions on bone (enthesitis) at both peripheral and axial sites
- Inflammatory lesions of the anterior uveal tract of the eye (uveitis or iritis) and/or cardiac tissues (aortic valvular disease and/or heart block)
- Onset of symptoms in young adults, especially men
- Absence of serum rheumatoid factor and other autoantibodies (i.e. seronegative)
- Strong but variable associations with the MHC class I allele, HLA-B27

Contrasting clinical and radiographic features of the spondyloarthropathies

Feature	Ankylosing spondylitis	Reiter syndrome	Psoriatic arthritis	Enteropathic arthritis
Male/female ratio	3:1	9:1	1:1	1:1
Usual onset	Insidious, low back or hip/buttock pain	Acute urethritis, conjunctivitis, and arthritis	Insidious, usually peripheral arthritis	Acute peripheral arthritis with active bowel symptoms or insidious low back pain or asymptomatic spinal fusion
Peripheral arthritis	Infrequent, except hips and shoulders; occasionally knees, ankles, and feet	100%; asymmetric, oligoarticular, lower extremities, sausage digits, heel pain	95%, asymmetric or symmetric, oligo- or polyarticular, esp. hands and feet, distal joints, sausage digits	20%, symmetric knees, ankles, wrists
Spinal arthritis	100%	20%	20%	10%
Sacroiliitis	Bilateral	Unilateral or bilateral	Unilateral or bilateral	Bilateral
Syndesmophytes	Symmetric	Asymmetric	Asymmetric	Symmetric
	Marginal	Nonmarginal	Nonmarginal	Marginal
Extra-articular features				
Fever	Rare	Frequent	Rare	Frequent
Uveitis	25%	20%	Rare	Occasional
Cardiac	5%	5%	Rare	Rare
Mucocutaneous	Rare	Keratoderma, circinate balanitis, painless oral ulcers, nail dystrophy	Psoriasis, nail pitting and/or dystrophy	Erythema nodosum with Crohn's disease Pyoderma gangrenosum with ulcerative colitis Painful oral ulcers

Table 66.1 Contrasting clinical and radiographic features of the spondyloarthropathies.

incomplete, or undifferentiated spondyloarthropathies also have been described.

Clinical, epidemiological and genetic studies have established important interrelationships among these disorders, as well as the fact that they are not variants of rheumatoid arthritis.

Although the causes of these diseases are unknown, there is substantial evidence that they arise as a consequence of abnormal immune responses to specific bacteria in which genetically determined HLA Class I molecules, especially HLA-B27, and several other as yet unidentified genetic loci play pivotal roles.

PREVALENCES AND EPIDEMIOLOGY

Prevalences for each of the spondyloarthropathies tend to parallel the frequencies of HLA-B27 in different racial and ethnic populations[3–5] (Table 66.2). High frequencies of exposure to endemic causative microorganisms in certain human populations also appear to influence the prevalence of Reiter syndrome or reactive arthritis.[6] The overall prevalence of spondyloarthropathies has been estimated to be 0.2–1.9% in US and European Caucasians.[5,7]

Ankylosing spondylitis occurs in 0.1–0.9% of American and European Caucasians, thus affecting approximately 2% of HLA-B27 carriers.[5,7] Within white families with ankylosing spondylitis, however, 20–30% of HLA-B27 positive relatives may develop disease, while there is almost no disease risk for HLA-B27 negative relatives.[5,8] Men appear to be affected more often than women (3:1), and the mean age of onset is approximately 28 years in American and European populations. The disease rarely begins after age 40. Younger mean ages of onset have been reported from developing countries such as Mexico.[9]

HLA-B27 frequencies in spondyloarthropathies and in selected normal populations

Disease	Frequency of HLA-B27[a]
Ankylosing spondylitis	90%
Reiters' syndrome (reactive arthritis)	63–75%
Psoriasis	Not increased[b]
With peripheral arthritis	Not increased[b]
With sacroiliitis/spondylitis	50%
Inflammatory bowel disease	Not increased[c]
With peripheral arthritis	Not increased[c]
With sacroiliitis/spondylitis	30–50%
Normal populations	**Frequency of HLA-B27**
American and European Caucasoids	6–14%
American and African Blacks	2–3%
Japanese	<1%
Chinese	7–8%
Middle Easterners	1–4%
Mexican Mestizos	3–5.5%
Eskimos/Inuits	30–40%
Navajo Native Americans	36%
Haida Native Americans	50%
Chippewa Native Americans	23%

[a] Based on studies primarily in Caucasian populations.
[b] Other Class I HLA antigens increased, including HLA-Cw6, B17(B57), B13, B37 and B16 (B38 and B39).
[c] Other non-HLA genes presumed but not identified.

Table 66.2 HLA-B27 frequencies in spondyloarthropathies and in selected normal populations.

Ankylosing spondylitis is less common in American and African Blacks, in whom the normal frequency of HLA-B27 is low (2–3%) and the disease association with HLA-B27 is weaker (only 50–70% of affected cases are positive).[4] Similarly, ankylosing spondylitis is rare in Japanese, in whom HLA-B27 is found in less than 1% of the normal population, but other Asian groups studied show disease and HLA-B27 frequencies similar to Caucasians.[4] The Haida indians of British Columbia have strikingly high frequencies of both HLA-B27 (50%) and ankylosing spondylitis (10%).[4]

The true prevalence of *Reiter syndrome* or *reactive arthritis* is unknown, although one study estimated it at 0.05% of men aged 20–29 years in Rochester, Minnesota.[6] It was once the most common cause of inflammatory peripheral arthritis in young white men in the US military, however, a decline in this prevalence has now been documented since the advent of the HIV epidemic and the practice of safer sexual behavior.[6] Men are affected disproportionately to women (9:1) in most studies, however, both genders appear to develop reactive arthritis with equal frequency following epidemics involving the causative enteric bacteria. The disease is rare in American and African Blacks. Reactive arthritis (Reiter syndrome) is common among Eskimos and Navajo indians who have high frequencies of HLA-B27 and who inhabit areas endemic for venereal infections and shigellosis, respectively.[4,6] Reiter syndrome was earlier reported to occur frequently (5–10%) in patients with AIDS, and HLA-B27 was found in approximately 75% of such cases. More recently, several large cohorts of homosexual men have been studied and only 0.1–0.5% had Reiter syndrome, regardless of HIV status, probably as a consequence of venereal exposure to the usual causative venereal or enteric infections.[10]

Cutaneous *psoriasis* is estimated to affect 1–2% of most Caucasian populations of Europe and the Americas.[11] It also appears to be common in the Indian subcontinent but rare in Africans and Japanese. *Psoriatic arthritis* affects males and females equally, and recent studies suggest that it develops in 20–34% of individuals with psoriasis. Psoriasis and psoriatic arthritis also have been associated with HIV infection. It appears that neither occurs in greater than expected frequencies in patients with HIV;[10] however, a clear relationship exists between exacerbations of pre-existing psoriasis and the profound immunodeficiency caused by AIDS.

The *inflammatory bowel diseases, ulcerative colitis and Crohn's disease*, are found worldwide with a prevalence approaching 0.1% for each disease, and arthritis is the most common extraintestinal manifestation. Peripheral arthritis develops in up to 20% of cases and spondylitis in 10%.[12]

ETIOLOGY AND PATHOGENESIS

Mechanisms underlying the various spondyloarthropathies are as yet unclear but interacting infectious and genetic factors seem likely. More information concerning infectious causes comes from reactive arthritis, while more genetic data are available in ankylosing spondylitis.

Infections

Reiter syndrome has been conceptualized as a '*reactive*' or sterile arthritis arising as a consequence of a distant infection in the bowel or genitourinary tract.[6,13] A variety of pathogenic bacteria

Microorganisms associated with reactive arthritis (Reiter syndrome) in HLA-B27 positive individuals	
	Certainty of association
Shigella flexneri	Definite
Shigella sonnei	Definite (rarely)
Salmonella (many species)	Definite
Yersinia enterocolitica 03	Definite
Yersinia pseudotuberculosis	Definite
Campylobacter jejuni (fetus)	Definite
Chlamydia trachomatis	Definite
Chlamydia psittaci	Possible
Chlamydia pneumoniae	Possible
Ureaplasma urealyticum	Possible
Giardia lamblia	Possible
Brucella	Possible
Others	

Table 66.3 Microorganisms associated with reactive arthritis (Reiter syndrome) in HLA-B27 positive individuals.

which trigger the disease have been implicated by clinical and epidemiologic studies (Table 66.3). In various epidemics of gastroenteritis caused by one of these pathogens, approximately 20% of the HLA-B27 positive individuals exposed develop a reactive arthritis. Similarly, studies from venereal disease clinics have reported that approximately 20% of HLA-B27 positive men develop Reiter syndrome after contracting *Chlamydia* urethritis.[13] Approximately one third of those developing arthritis are negative for HLA-B27. The male to female ratio of affected individuals appears to be equal following gastroenteritis; however, postvenereal Reiter syndrome appears to affect men disproportionately to women (9:1). The articular and extra-articular manifestations of Reiter syndrome appear to be the same regardless of whether the disease is triggered by enteric or venereal pathogens.

Recent evidence has challenged the concept that the joints in reactive arthritis are 'sterile'. *Chlamydia*-specific antigens have been demonstrated in phagocytic cells from synovial fluid and tissue. Furthermore, intracellular inclusions morphologically compatible with intact *Chlamydia* organisms have been seen.[2,14–17] While joint cultures for *Chlamydia* are consistently negative, several studies of synovial material using molecular probes have reported finding *Chlamydia* RNA or DNA, thus suggesting the presence of viable organisms. Similarly, specific *Yersinia*, *Salmonella* and *Shigella* lipopolysaccharide antigens also have been demonstrated in synovial fluid phagocytes from patients with reactive arthritis triggered by each of these organisms. Several attempts to detect *Yersinia* or *Salmonella* DNA by PCR in synovial fluids or tissues have been negative.[18,19] Nonetheless, it is clear that bacterial antigens, if not intact microorganisms, play an important role in the pathogenesis of reactive arthritis. Several studies have demonstrated bacterial antigens in joints many months to years after the initial infection, thus suggesting the following possibilities: (1) that in some individuals there is an inherent failure of bacterial degradation in the joints; (2) intact organisms may persist for long periods in synovial tissue and continue to elicit an inflammatory response; and/or (3) there may be chronic or recurrent dissemination of intact microorganisms and/or their antigens from the gut or genitourinary tract to joints, and possibly also to extra-articular sites of inflammation (eye, heart, skin, etc.).

Evidence for the microbial pathogenesis of reactive arthritis

- Initiation of arthritis 2–4 weeks following gastrointestinal or genitourinary infection with specific pathogens
- Foci of chronic asymptomatic inflammation in gut
- Persistent serum IgA antibodies specific for the triggering microorganism
- Bacterial-specific antigens in synovial phagocytes
- HLA-B27 transgenic rat does not develop arthritis in germfree environment

Table 66.4 Evidence for the microbial pathogenesis of reactive arthritis.

Chronic persistence of the triggering microorganisms also is suggested by many studies showing elevated serum levels of bacteria-specific IgA antibodies.[2,20] Moreover, chronic inflammatory lesions in the terminal ileum and proximal colon have been demonstrated by ileocolonoscopy in patients with reactive arthritis, especially those whose disease was triggered by enteric pathogens, in contrast to those with venereal infections.[12] Similar studies are not yet available for the genitourinary tract, but *Chlamydia trachomatis* is an organism known to potentially persist for long periods. Finally, several successful trials of chronic antibiotic therapy in *Chlamydia* reactive arthritis patients further support the likelihood that microbial persistence is a major pathogenetic mechanism underlying this disease[21,22] (Table 66.4).

A causative organism has not been established for *ankylosing spondylitis* although bowel flora are strongly suspected. One candidate, *Klebsiella pneumoniae*, has been the focus of much controversy, but a definite association with the disease has not been established.[23] Increased frequencies of serum IgA antibodies to *Klebsiella pneumoniae*, *E. coli*, and other enteric bacteria have been reported. Studies of spinal structures and entheses affected by this disease are difficult, but recent studies using PCR for detecting DNA from several bacteria in sacroiliac joint biopsies were negative.[24] Occult inflammatory lesions have been found in high frequency in the bowels of patients with ankylosing spondylitis,[12] and therapy with sulfasalazine appears to be effective,[25–28] thus suggesting that one or more enteric organisms may play a role in the pathogenesis of this disease.

Psoriasis, especially the guttate form, has been observed to begin with, or be exacerbated by, streptococcal infections.[11] Data supporting other candidate infections are few.

Genetic factors

Ankylosing spondylitis shows a strong familial tendency, with a 15% recurrence rate in families.[29] Other spondyloarthropathies, uveitis, psoriasis, and inflammatory bowel diseases also occur in higher than expected frequencies in relatives of individuals affected with ankylosing spondylitis. The concordance rate for ankylosing spondylitis in monozygotic twins is 63% compared to 12.5% in dizygotic twins.[30] Genetic modeling based on these findings in twins suggests that 97% of the population liability to ankylosing spondylitis results from additive genetic effects, while the environmental contribution is small and probably ubiquitous. Although ankylosing spondylitis shows linkage to HLA-B27 in families, its contribution is now estimated to be from 16–50% of the total genetic contribution.[31] Thus, other genes besides HLA-B27 are clearly necessary and help to explain the differential disease susceptibility of HLA-B27 positive relatives (20–30%)

compared to random HLA-B27 positive persons (2%). Other genes within the MHC have been implicated, including HLA-B40 (now designated B60 and B61) which increases disease risk 3-fold in both HLA-B27 positive and negative individuals, as well as HLA-B39 which is associated with disease in HLA-B27 negatives, especially in the Japanese population.[31] The HLA Class II alleles, DR1 and perhaps DR8, also appear to increase risk. Some evidence supporting additional roles for TNF-α alleles,[32] TAP, LMP, and MICA alleles, which also map within the MHC, has been presented but is controversial. A recent genome-wide linkage screen using 254 highly polymorphic microsatellite markers in 121 British sib pairs found evidence of disease linkage in 7 chromosomal regions, including the MHC.[33] Estimated susceptibility from the MHC was 31% of the total genetic risk. Other potentially linked chromosomal regions included several which have been linked to psoriasis and/or Crohn's disease (16q, 4q, 17q). There does not appear to be linkage of ankylosing spondylitis to T-cell receptor germline genes.[34]

Recent studies have relegated HLA-B27 to less than a predominant role; nonetheless, this gene confers a relative risk of approximately 100 for ankylosing spondylitis and shows linkage in families as a dominant genetic effect. Much research has been conducted on HLA-B27 over the last several decades. Until recently it was not clear whether HLA-B27 itself was directly involved or whether it was only a marker for another tightly linked disease-susceptibility gene within the MHC. The engineering of transgenic rats and mice expressing the human HLA-B27 and β2-microglobulin genes has now provided animal models that appear to recapitulate human spondyloarthropathies.[35,36] At 10–20 weeks of age, both male and female transgenic rats spontaneously develop diarrhea with inflammatory gut lesions, peripheral and spinal arthritis, enthesitis, psoriasis-like skin and nail lesions, genitourinary inflammation in males, and possibly uveitis. Only transgenic animals with 50–150 copies of the HLA-B27 gene develop disease, but control transgenes with high copy numbers of other human Class I HLA alleles (A2 and B7) do not develop disease. Cultures from diseased animals have been negative for the microbial pathogens known to incite disease in man; however, HLA-B27 transgenic rats raised in germfree environments do not develop the bowel or joint lesions, although the skin, nail, and genital lesions still appear.[35] The disease can be transferred into disease-susceptible non-transgenic rat strains using bone marrow-derived cells from HLA-B27 transgenics. Backcross of the B27 transgenic rat onto athymic and euthymic nude backgrounds has shown that T cells are necessary for disease; however, T-cell contact with B27 in the thymus is not required for rat spondyloarthropathy.[35] That the HLA-B27 molecule itself plays a direct role in disease now seems incontrovertible.

Another recent advance is the elucidation of the crystalline structure of HLA-B27 and the characterization of nonamer (or octamer) peptides that may bind within its 'peptide-binding' groove[37,38] (Chapters 6,7). Fifteen molecular subtypes of HLA-B27 have been discovered (Table 66.5) all differing from one another by one or more amino acid substitutions, most within the antigen-binding cleft in the C/F pocket[39–41] (Fig. 66.1). The various HLA-B27 subtypes in general are as different from one another in the peptide-binding groove as they are from most other HLA Class I alleles. There are only two characteristics that they all apparently share and that are unique from other Class I alleles: (1) a *lysine* in position 70; and (2) the same 'B' pocket around position 45 (Fig. 66.1).[38,39,41] HLA-B*2705 appears to be the primordial B27 allele from which the other subtypes evolved and is widely distributed among most racial groups, although in variable frequency[40,41] (Table 66.5). Most of the HLA-B27 subtypes have been associated with ankylosing spondylitis[40] (Table 66.5). The two major exceptions are HLA-B*2706 in southern Asians[42] and HLA-B*2709 in Sardinians. These two B27 alleles differ from the others at position 116, and can only bind aliphatic or aromatic amino acids rather than *tyrosine*.[43] It has been suggested, based on peptide-binding studies, that arthritogenic peptides binding to susceptibility B27 subtypes must carry a C-terminal *tyrosine*.[44] HLA-B27 subtypes have not been found to discriminate between the different spondyloarthropathies.

Association of molecular subtypes of HLA-B27 with spondyloarthropathies

Subtype	Racial groups	Associated with disease
B*2705	Primordial; 90% of Caucasians, Siberian and Alaska Eskimos, and Native Americans	Yes
B*2701	Unknown (rare)	Yes
B*2702	Caucasian 10%	Yes
B*2703	Africans 70%	Yes
B*2704	Chinese 90%	Yes
B*2706	Thais, Indonesians (60–80%)	No
B*2707	Indian, Chinese, Thais (7%)	Yes
B*2708	Azores, English (rare)	Yes
B*2709	Sardinians (30%)	No
B*2710	Japanese	Yes
B*2711	Japanese	Unknown
B*2712	Caucasian (Spanish, English)	Unknown
B*2713	Unknown	Unknown
B*2714	Unknown	Unknown
B*2715	Unknown	Unknown

Table 66.5 Molecular subtypes of HLA-B27, their distribution among different racial populations, and their associations with spondyloarthropathies

Although much is now known about the molecular structure and function of HLA-B27, it remains unclear why it causes the spondyloarthropathies. Moreover, whether the function of HLA-B27 in peptide binding and presentation to T cells plays a role in its propensity to cause disease also is unknown. If the HLA-B*2706 and B*2709 subtypes do not cause disease, then a role involving peptide binding is likely. Similarly, the sharing of the same 'B' pocket by all of the HLA-B27 subtypes may provide the appropriate peptide-binding motif for an arthritogenic bacterial and/or self peptide.

Molecular mimicry between HLA alleles and infectious agents has been a popular hypothesis to explain disease associations for

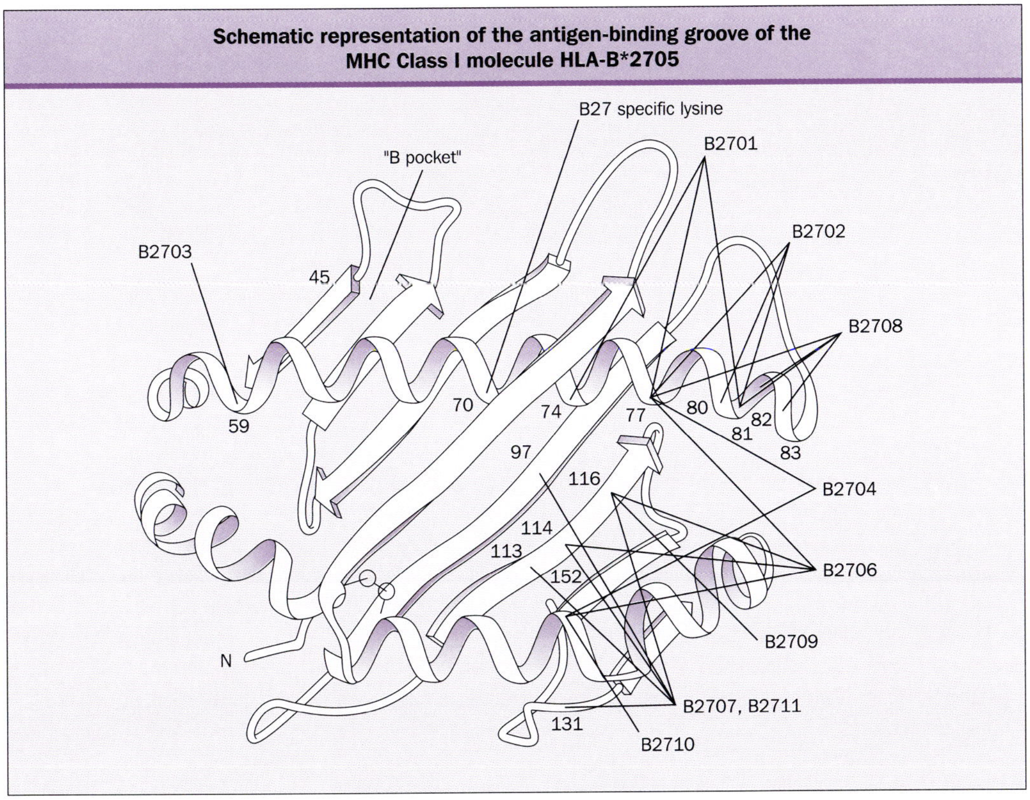

Figure 66.1 Schematic representation of the antigen-binding groove of the MHC Class I molecule, HLA-B*2705. Polymorphic amino acid changes which represent each of the other HLA-B27 subtypes are indicated. Also shown is the *lysine* in position 70 and the 'B' or '45 pocket' which are shared by all HLA-B27 subtypes. (Modified and adapted from Reveille JD. HLA-B27 and the seronegative spondyloarthropathies. *Am J Med Sci* 1998;316:239.[41])

many years.[45,46] Indeed, cross-reactivity between HLA-B27 and many of the arthritogenic bacteria has been demonstrated in many studies, and linear homologies in amino acid sequence have been defined. Computer searches have suggested that HLA-B27 shares more homologies with gram-negative enteric bacteria than any other HLA-B locus alleles.[47] In none of these examples, however, have antibodies to the shared sequence been reproducibly demonstrated.[48] Recently, T-cell repertoires in synovial fluids from patients with different types of reactive arthritis have shown a high degree of conservation in T-cell responses, as well as a CD8$^+$ T-cell clone reactive against HLA-B27.[49] Thus, mimicry between HLA-B27 and an antigen, perhaps a superantigen, shared among the causative bacteria could result in either a failure of immune recognition or a breakdown in tolerance and the elicitation of an autoimmune response, most likely of the cytotoxic T-cell arm of the immune system. The peptide-presenting function of HLA-B27 might or might not be involved in either of these scenarios. At this time, however, it remains unclear whether molecular mimicry has any disease role.

Finally, HLA-B27 may act through a nontraditional function in promoting bacterial persistence. Recent studies of several B27-transfected cell lines have shown that B27 modulates the survival of *Salmonella enteritidis*, perhaps via a pathway that impairs nitric oxide.[50]

Immunologic factors

Although much is now known about the molecular biology of HLA-B27, the immunologic consequences of the likely interaction between this Class I HLA molecule, other as yet unidentified genes, and the causative bacteria are largely unknown. Patients with spondyloarthropathies have elevated serum IgA levels, which now appear to represent antibodies to causative microbes, at least in reactive arthritis. It appears likely that persisting bacteria in gut and/or genitourinary mucosa are driving IgA antibodies.

In reactive arthritis, T-cell proliferative responses in the peripheral blood to causative organisms are not impressive. One study found that patients with post-*Salmonella* induced reactive arthritis showed a lack of proliferative response to the offending organisms compared to individuals infected with the same organism who did not have reactive arthritis.[51] The defect appeared to be in IL-2 production. More recently, significantly reduced blood levels of TNF-α (but not other cytokines), despite high levels of TNF-α in joints, have been reported in patients with reactive arthritis compared to patients with rheumatoid arthritis and normal controls.[52] Low blood TNF-α levels, probably genetically determined, correlated with disease chronicity.

Synovial fluid T cells appear to selectively recognize and proliferate to the microorganism that initiated the disease.[18] This proliferative response, however, appears to involve mostly CD4$^+$ lymphocytes and MHC Class II restricted responses, rather than the CD8$^+$ cytotoxic response expected from a Class I HLA associated disease. Nonetheless, cytotoxic T-cell responses to causal organisms as well as B27 itself have been detected.[18,53]

In summary, recent evidence suggests that reactive arthritis occurs as a result of an abnormal host response to selected bacterial pathogens, mediated in some way by HLA-B27 and other genes, which results in bacterial persistence and the dissemination of antigens (if not intact organisms) to articular, and perhaps extra-articular, structures. The immunologic events occurring as a result of such bacteria at mucosal surfaces and in the joints, as well as in extra-articular lesions, are largely unexplained. Whether reactive arthritis is a model for the other spondyloarthropathies also is unknown. HLA-B27 is so strongly associated with ankylosing spondylitis that it is not unreasonable to suspect that bacterial products might be gaining access to spinal joints and producing the inflammation characteristic of this disease; however, a link to definite causative organisms has yet to be established. It is now clear that several other as yet unidentified genes are also probably essential for disease, and their mechanisms cannot even be speculated. Psoriatic arthritis is less strongly associated with HLA-B27; however, genetic predisposition marked by other HLA Class I associations and linkage to non-MHC loci has been shown. The enteropathic arthropathies of Crohn's disease and ulcerative colitis require further genetic, immunologic, and microbiologic investigations.

CLINICAL FEATURES AND NATURAL HISTORY

Ankylosing spondylitis

History

The first pathological description of ankylosing spondylitis was provided by the Irish physician Bernard Connor in 1693 after uncovering an ankylosed skeleton in a French graveyard.[54] Classical clinical descriptions by Marie and Strumpel followed nearly 200 years later. Forestier and colleagues first described the characteristic roentgenographic findings of *sacroiliitis* and *syndesmophytes* in the early 20th century and suggested the designation 'ankylosing spondylitis'. Clinical, epidemiologic, and family studies by Moll, Wright, Haslock, and others in the 1960s established the interrelationships of ankylosing spondylitis, Reiter syndrome, psoriasis, and inflammatory bowel disease, and these investigators suggested the term *seronegative spondyloarthropathies*.[55] In 1973, the association of ankylosing spondylitis with the genetic marker HLA-B27 was established, and subsequent studies demonstrated similar correlations of HLA-B27 with the other spondyloarthropathies (Table 66.2). Subsequently, the application of HLA-B27 typing in clinical and epidemiologic studies has further broadened the clinical spectrum of this family of diseases.[54]

Symptoms

The usual first symptom of ankylosing spondylitis is low back pain with the typical 'inflammatory' characteristics.[29,56]

> **CLINICAL PEARLS**
>
> **Clinical features of 'inflammatory' back pain**
> - Insidious in onset
> - Present for 3 months or longer
> - Stiffness and worsening of pain with rest
> - Improvement of pain and stiffness with activity

Adapted from Calin A, Porta J, Fries JF, Schurman DJ. Clinical history as a screening test for ankylosing spondylitis. *JAMA* 1977;237:261.[56]

Alternating pain in the buttocks, indicative of sacroiliitis, is frequently interpreted as hip disease, and/or sciatic-like radiation down the posterior thigh as a herniated disc with nerve root compression. With time, usually over several years, similar symptoms of inflammatory pain and stiffness ascend into the lumbar, thoracic, and cervical regions. Chest wall pain may mimic pleurisy, and chest expansion is compromised by fusion of costovertebral joints. Gradually, spinal mobility is lost in affected regions and flexion deformity ensues (Fig. 66.2). In some patients, more often children and women than adult men, a peripheral arthritis, usually a monoarthritis of a knee or hip, heralds disease onset.

Physical examination

In early disease, there may be no objective abnormalities on spinal examination. Pain is usually elicited by compressing or stressing the sacroiliac joints, but higher spinal levels retain normal mobility. Later, as the disease progresses, the normal lumbar lordosis is lost and spinal flexion, extension, and lateral motion become restricted. The thoracic spine becomes fixed in an accentuated kyphosis. Chest expansion, measured at the 4th intercostal space as change in circumference from full expiration to full inspiration, is decreased to less than 3 cm (normal 6–10 cm). The cervical spine is usually affected last but eventually may lose all range of motion and assume a fixed position in flexion. Hips and/or shoulders also are frequently involved.

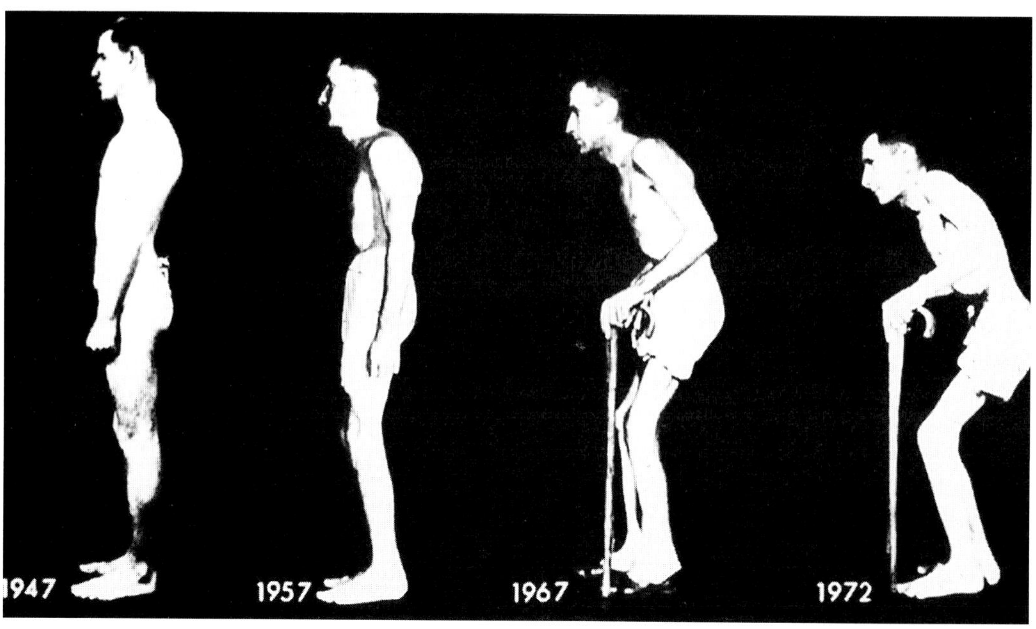

Figure 66.2 Severe progression of spinal deformity over a 25-year period in a patient with ankylosing spondylitis. (Reproduced from Little H, Swinson DR, Cruickshank G. *Am J Med* 1976;60:279 with permission.)

Pathological features

The inflammatory joint lesions of ankylosing spondylitis, as well as those of the other spondyloarthropathies, are comprised primarily of mononuclear inflammatory cells infiltrating synovium, cartilage, subchondral bone, joint capsule, and bony periosteum, especially at sites of tendon insertion (enthesitis).[57,58] $CD4^+$ T cells predominate in peripheral joint tissues, including $CD45RO^+$ memory T cells, along with lesser numbers of $CD8^+$ T cells, B cells ($CD19^+$), and macrophages ($CD14^+$ and $CD68^+$). Cytokine profiles in sacroiliac biopsies show high TNF-α mRNA, and perhaps decreased amounts of TGF-β.[59] Fibrosis and ossification also are prominent features. These lead to bony, ligamentous, and periarticular fusion which gives rise to the characteristic radiographic findings.

Roentgenographic features

Bilateral *sacroiliitis* is the radiographic hallmark of this disease, and a confident diagnosis cannot be established without it[1,60,61] (Fig. 66.3). *Bony sclerosis* on both sides of the sacroiliac joints is usually the first sign (grade 2), and it may be confused with the benign anomaly *osteitis condensens ilii* in postpartum women. The presence of sclerosis *and* erosions of the sacroiliac joints (grade 3) is a more definitive sign of sacroiliitis. Bony fusion across the joint (grade 4) with eventual disappearance of the sclerosis and the joints themselves is incontrovertible evidence of disease involvement and frequently represents the end result of disease progression. An anterior–posterior (AP) radiograph of the pelvis may not be adequate to assess the presence or absence of sacroiliitis. Instead, special sacroiliac radiographs may be necessary, i.e. either oblique-angled views of each joint and/or a Ferguson view (an AP pelvis view angled 30° cephalad).

Radiographs of vertebral bodies at lumbar, thoracic, and/or cervical levels may show 'squaring' of their normal configuration due to inflammatory erosion of anterior margins.[60] Ossified ligaments bridging intervertebral spaces give rise to the characteristic 'syndesmophytes' which, when numerous, lead to the appearance of a 'bamboo spine' (Fig. 66.4). Apophyseal and facet joints also may become fused into solid bone. Spinal osteoporosis is another common radiographic finding.[62]

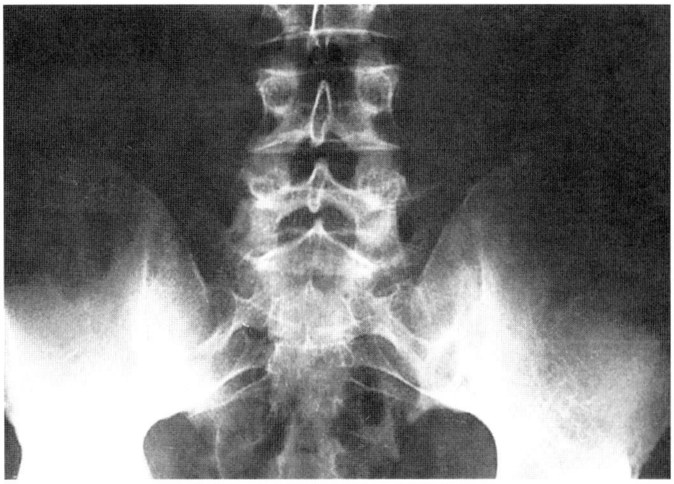

Figure 66.3 Anterior–posterior radiograph of the pelvis showing bilateral grade 3–4 sacroiliitis. Note sclerosis on both sides of each sacroiliac joint and nearly complete bony fusion across these joints.

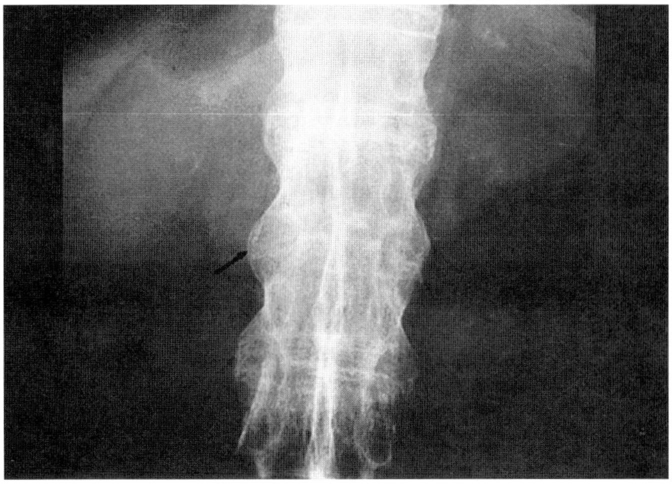

Figure 66.4 Anterior–posterior radiograph of the lumbar spine showing non-marginal syndesmophytes bridging intervertebral disc spaces.

Laboratory features

An elevated erythrocyte sedimentation rate (ESR) is the most consistent laboratory abnormality, especially during symptomatic phases of the disease. Some patients also will have a mild normocytic, normochromic anemia and/or thrombocytosis and/or polyclonal hyperglobulinemia (often high levels of IgA) secondary to the chronic inflammation.[20] Serum rheumatoid factor and antinuclear antibodies are typically negative. HLA-B27 is positive in over 90% of patients but is rarely required for diagnosis in typical cases.

Extra-articular features

Acute anterior uveitis (iritis), usually affecting one eye at a time, occurs episodically in 25% of patients without regard to activity of the arthritis.[63] Monocular pain, injection, and, especially photophobia, are the clinical hallmarks of uveitis, and the finding by slit-lamp examination of inflammatory cells in the anterior eye chamber confirms the diagnosis. Chronic uveitis with ensuing blindness may occur rarely.

Cardiac involvement occurs in approximately 5% of patients, usually after many years of active arthritis, but occasionally early in disease.[64] Inflammation and fibrotic thickening of the proximal aortic root and valve leaflets leads to progressive *aortic regurgitation*. Occasionally, *mitral regurgitation* may accompany the aortic valve disease. Moreover, the same inflammatory process may affect the adjacent atrioventricular node and lead to first-degree or complete *heart block*. Recent studies suggest that up to 13% of men requiring permanent cardiac pacemakers have underlying, often undiagnosed, spondyloarthropathies.

Renal involvement. *Amyloidosis* develops in approximately 1% of patients, usually after longstanding inflammatory disease, and typically presents as proteinuria and nephrotic syndrome.[65] *IgA nephropathy* may present similarly, and a definite relationship with spondyloarthropathies now appears likely.[20]

Pulmonary fibrosis, at times with cavitation of the lung apices, occurs rarely and must be discriminated from tuberculosis.[66]

Neurologic manifestations, although infrequent, most often involve the spinal cord. As the spine is brittle and osteoporotic, *fractures*, especially of the cervical region, may occur with relatively minor trauma, causing spinal cord damage and resulting in paralysis or sudden death.[67] Similarly, subluxation of the cervical C1 and C2 vertebrae also may cause cord compression. A *cauda equina syndrome* due to an arachnoiditis involving sacral nerves may produce lower extremity pain, weakness, and/or spasticity.[68]

Disease course

The clinical course of ankylosing spondylitis is highly variable. Approximately 10% of patients are asymptomatic or have negligible spinal symptoms despite radiographically obvious sacroiliitis or spondylitis. A predictable pattern of disease usually emerges in the first 10 years, with approximately 40% of patients stabilizing with mild to moderate spinal restriction and/or deformity, and another 40% progressing to severe spinal disease, often with hip and/or other peripheral joint involvement.[29,69,70] The majority of patients with ankylosing spondylitis function reasonably well, however, and significant disability occurs in less than 10%. Death from disease complications occurs in less than 5%, usually from cervical spinal fracture or dislocation, cardiac involvement, or amyloidosis.

Juvenile spondyloarthropathies

Ankylosing spondylitis commonly presents in late childhood and is termed juvenile ankylosing spondylitis or JAS.[9] Ten to twenty per cent of cases in adult Americans and Europeans have had onset of disease before age 16. Even higher frequencies (approximately 50%) of childhood-onset disease have been reported from Mexico and other developing countries. Adolescent boys are more frequently affected than girls.

The clinical presentation of JAS contrasts strikingly with that of adult-onset disease.[9] Peripheral arthritis and/or enthesopathy, usually mono- or pauciarticular and involving the lower extremities, are the most common initial symptoms, and axial involvement may not become apparent for many years. In fact, the term *SEA (seronegative enthesopathy and arthritis) syndrome* has been proposed to describe these patients. Other modes of onset include: (1) polyarticular arthritis, especially in girls, involving hands and wrists and mimicking rheumatoid arthritis;[71] (2) predominantly cervical spine arthritis leading to loss of neck movement and micrognathia;[71] and (3) an ankylosing tarsitis of the feet.[9] Less than 25% of JAS patients have clinical evidence of sacroiliac or spinal joint involvement at onset, and sacroiliac X-rays are difficult to interpret in children and adolescents. The same extra-articular complications described in adult ankylosing spondylitis may occur in JAS. JAS may be confused with any of the subgroups of juvenile rheumatoid arthritis (JRA), including pauciarticular, polyarticular and systemic (Still's disease) onsets. Typing for HLA-B27 may prove to be the most useful test in determining a correct diagnosis.[72] Because of its low frequency in most populations (<10%) and its high prevalence in patients with JAS, HLA-B27 typing may demonstrate both high sensitivity and specificity as a clinical test for this disease.

The natural history of JAS has not been well studied.[9] Some patients have a self-limited illness lasting months to years which spontaneously remits with or without residual joint or extra-articular damage. In other patients, peripheral joint involvement resolves but the typical axial picture of ankylosing spondylitis emerges, and in others peripheral joint disease with or without spinal involvement continues to progress into adulthood. Early hip involvement in JAS, as in adult ankylosing spondylitis, is a poor prognostic sign which portends future disability.

The other spondyloarthropathies, i.e. Reiter syndrome, psoriatic arthritis, and enteropathic arthritis, also may begin in childhood.

Reiter syndrome (reactive arthritis)

History

The classical triad of urethritis, conjunctivitis, and arthritis (Reiter syndrome) was first clearly described by Brodie in 1818, and it is impossible to discriminate possible earlier descriptions from gonococcal arthritis.[6,13,54] The eponym, Reiter syndrome, comes from the case report by Hans Reiter in 1916 who described the disease in a young German army officer following bacillary dysentery. Feisinger and Leroy also described several similar cases among French troops at the same time. Additional cases were reported during the Second World War, including an 'epidemic' of Reiter syndrome among Finnish soldiers following a large outbreak of shigella dysentery. Another similar but smaller epidemic occurred aboard the American naval vessel, USS Little Rock, in the early 1960s. These reports established that Reiter syndrome was a 'reactive arthritis', and this term was first used by Ahvohnen and colleagues to describe post-*Yersinia* induced arthritis in 1969. Over the same interval, it was found that venereal infections could also trigger Reiter syndrome. Genetic susceptibility to Reiter syndrome was reported in 1974 with the discovery that HLA-B27 occurred in 63–75% of cases. Shortly thereafter, the application of HLA-B27 testing demonstrated that incomplete forms of the disease were common, especially among young men.

Symptoms and physical examination

The first symptoms of typical Reiters syndrome are those of *urethritis* (cervicitis and/or vaginitis in women), *conjunctivitis*, and then *arthritis/enthesitis* beginning 2–4 weeks following venereal exposure or gastroenteritis.[6] Typically, symptoms of the inciting enteric infection have resolved completely prior to the onset of Reiter syndrome, and many patients cannot recall any gastrointestinal problems and will deny any extramarital sexual exposure. Approximately 40% of patients will have symptoms of arthritis and/or enthesopathy but can recall no dysuria, urethral discharge, or ocular irritation. Genitourinary involvement may occur in both postvenereal and postdysenteric Reiter syndrome and is thus an inherent feature of the disease and not necessarily a marker of venereal acquisition. In some patients, disease onset is acute and severe with high fever, prostration, and weight loss, while in others the symptoms begin insidiously and are not associated with systemic toxicity.

The urethral discharge is typically scant and mucopurulent and results in only mild dysuria. A first void morning urine examination may be necessary to document pyuria in asymptomatic individuals. Similarly, conjunctival injection and/or discharge is usually mild and transient, although some patients will develop frank acute anterior uveitis.

The *arthritis* of Reiter syndrome is typically oligoarticular and asymmetrical and affects lower extremity joints, especially the knees, ankles, and feet (Table 66.1). Upper extremity joints may be affected but hip and shoulder joints rarely so. Involvement of individual toes and/or fingers results in diffuse swelling, usually of the entire digit, resulting in a *sausage-like* appearance (or *dactylitis*). On examination, the joints are swollen, warm, tender, and often erythematous or dusky in coloration. Low back pain, with or without sacroiliac or lumbar tenderness, is a complaint in approximately 60% of cases, but radiographically apparent sacroiliitis develops in only 20% and is often unilateral (Fig. 66.3). Frank ankylosing spondylitis develops in approximately 10% of patients.

The *enthesopathy* of Reiter syndrome often gives rise to the most chronic and disabling complaints.[58] Heel pain due to enthesitis at the insertions of plantar and/or Achilles tendons is common and highly discriminating clinically for the diagnosis (Fig. 66.5). Pain may also occur at other sites of tendon or fascial insertion, such as the tibial tuberosity, various areas of the pelvis, or over the ribs.

A variety of *mucocutaneous lesions* may appear, usually early in disease, and one or more may be found in over 50% of cases.[1] *Keratoderma blennorrhagica* is a papulosquamous rash, most often appearing on soles and/or palms but also in other locations including the scalp (Fig. 66.6). The lesions initially appear as waxy maculopapular or pustular eruptions and then progress to marked hyperkeratosis and scaling. They are clinically and histopathologically indistinguishable from *pustular psoriasis*. At times, keratoderma may spread widely and result in an exfoliative erythroderma. *Circinate balanitis* appears as keratoderma-like scaling lesions on the glans penis in circumsized men (Fig. 66.7), or as moist, shallow, and painless ulcers in the uncircumcised.

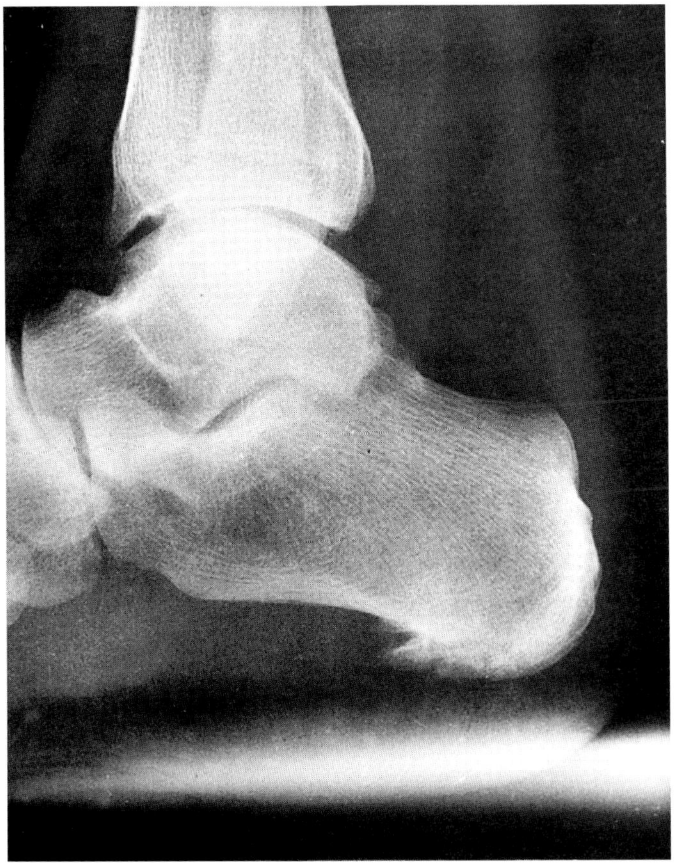

Figure 66.5 Lateral radiograph of the calcaneus showing periosteal reaction and spur formation at the insertion of the plantar aponeurosis (enthesitis) in a patient with Reiter syndrome.

CLINICAL PEARLS

Clues to the diagnosis of Reiter syndrome or reactive arthritis

- A young man (less often a woman) with arthritis
- Symptoms and physical findings:
  - acute diarrhea, urethritis (cervicitis), and/or conjunctivitis in the month preceding arthritis
  - lower extremity asymmetric oligoarthritis
  - heel pain and/or sausaging of digits
  - rash on soles or penis; painless oral ulcers; dystrophic nails
  - fever, weight loss, leukocytosis
- HLA-B27
- Pathognomonic changes of periostitis of calcaneus on heel radiograph (lover's heel)

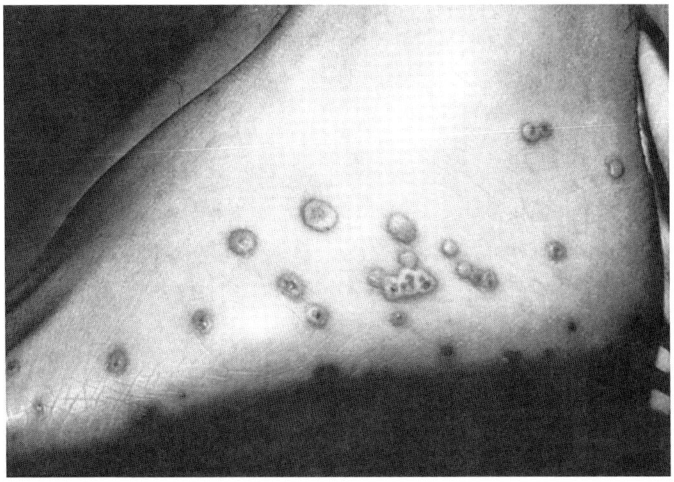

Figure 66.6 Keratoderma blennorrhagica (also termed 'pustular psoriasis') in a patient with Reiter syndrome.

Similarly, shallow and painless *oral ulcers* may occur on the tongue or palate. *Nail changes* include thickening, opacification, crumbling, and lifting-off of the nail from the nail bed but the characteristic pitting seen in psoriasis vulgaris is not present. Involved nails may resemble infected paronychia.

Other extra-articular features are similar to those of ankylosing spondylitis and include acute anterior uveitis in 20%, aortic regurgitation and/or heart block in 5%, and rarely amyloidosis or IgA nephropathy.[6,20,63,64]

Pathological features

Histopathological joint findings include microvascular injury, mild synovial cell hyperplasia, and synovial infiltration with chronic inflammatory cells but not granuloma formation. Inflammatory lesions also appear to involve cartilage, subchondral bone, joint capsule, and bony periosteum. Infiltrating T cells mostly express CD4, but $CD8^+$ cells are also present.[18] As in the spinal lesions of ankylosing spondylitis, prominent fibrosis and new bone formation are characteristic of the inflammatory process in peripheral joints and sites of enthesopathy.

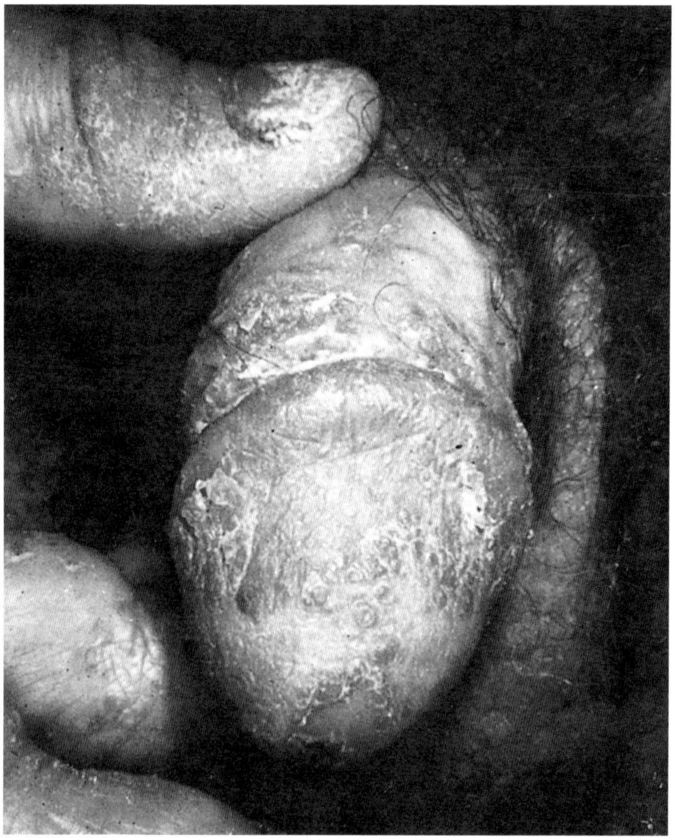

Figure 66.7 Circinate balanitis and onychodystrophy in a patient with Reiter syndrome.

Radiographic features

Abnormalities detectable on standard X-rays occur only after many months or years of active disease.[58,60] Most characteristic of the joint findings are loss of articular cartilage, periosteal reaction, and bony fusion across joints. New bone formation also may be found around joint capsules, marking sites of enthesopathy. Periostitis with bony erosions and/or the formation of 'fluffy' spurs on the calcaneus (so-called 'lover's heel') are virtually pathognomonic (Fig. 66.5).

Laboratory features

Most patients develop a mild normocytic, normochromic anemia due to chronic inflammation. A modest leukocytosis and thrombocytosis occurs in the majority, especially early in disease and in relation to systemic symptoms. The erythrocyte sedimentation rate is almost invariably elevated. Tests for rheumatoid factor and antinuclear antibodies are negative. HLA-B27 occurs in 63–75% of cases, but its frequency increases to over 90% in patients with uveitis, radiographic sacroiliitis, or longstanding disease.

Synovial fluid findings are those of an inflammatory process with high white blood cell counts (5000–50 000/mm^3) and elevated proteins. Unlike in infectious arthritis, the synovial fluid glucose is normal rather than low, and, in contrast to rheumatoid arthritis, complement levels are high rather than low. Occasionally, large mononuclear cells are seen which contain several ingested polymorphonuclear leukocytes (Reiter's cells).[14] By conventional culturing techniques, the fluid is negative for any microorganisms; however, recent studies have shown bacterial antigens to be present (see Etiology and pathogenesis).

Disease course

The clinical course of Reiter syndrome or reactive arthritis is usually that of a self-limited disease.[6,73] The majority of patients have near or complete resolution of symptoms in 3–12 months. Disease relapses are not uncommon, and it is unclear whether these relate to reinfection with causative microorganisms. Approximately 15% of patients continue to have persistent arthritis, enthesitis, and/or skin disease resulting in permanent joint deformities and disabilities. The most common causes of permanent disability are foot pain and deformity, or visual loss from uveitis. Approximately 10% develop ankylosing spondylitis but it is unclear whether this is an independent disease occurring in the same genetically predisposed host. There are also well-documented cases of ankylosing spondylitis in which Reiter syndrome has developed after an enteric infection. Death from the disease is rare and most commonly results from cardiac involvement or amyloidosis.

Psoriatic arthritis

History

Psoriasis and rheumatoid arthritis are both common diseases (prevalences of 1–2% for each), and the occurrence of arthritis and psoriasis together was once thought to be fortuitous. After the discovery of rheumatoid factor, it became apparent that most cases of arthritis developing in association with psoriasis were seronegative. The pioneering clinical, epidemiologic, and genetic studies of Wright and Moll, however, clearly demonstrated that psoriatic arthritis was an entity distinct from rheumatoid arthritis and one allied with the spondyloarthropathies.[55,60]

Symptoms and physical examination

Cutaneous psoriasis precedes or appears concomitantly with the arthritis in approximately 80% of adults. In children, the onset of arthritis is more likely to occur before the skin disease, and in some series 40% of children present with arthritis first, thus creating diagnostic confusion with JRA and JAS until psoriasis appears. There is a poor correlation between the extent and severity of psoriasis and the presence and/or severity of arthritis.

The onset of arthritis is typically insidious and not associated with systemic symptoms (Table 66.1). There is a predilection for involvement of the distal interphalangeal (DIP) joints of the fingers and toes, especially those joints adjacent to nails involved by psoriatic pitting or onychodystrophy. Any other joint may also become involved with swelling, erythema, pain, and stiffness. Diffuse swelling of fingers and/or toes commonly results in 'sausage-like' digits (dactylitis).

Several patterns of psoriatic arthritis have been described;[74] however, a great deal of overlap between these clinical types is observed. Arthritis mutilans is the most severe form of peripheral arthritis, in which nearly complete joint and bony resorption of the fingers (telescoping) results in the so-called 'opera glass hand' (Fig. 66.8). Spinal involvement occurs in approximately 20% of cases but rarely occurs in the absence of peripheral arthritis. Except for skin and nail involvement, extra-articular complications are uncommon.

Pathological features

There are few studies of joint histopathology in this disease. Chronic inflammatory mononuclear cells infiltrate synovium, cartilage, bone and joint capsule, and fibrosis with new bone formation is prominent.[74]

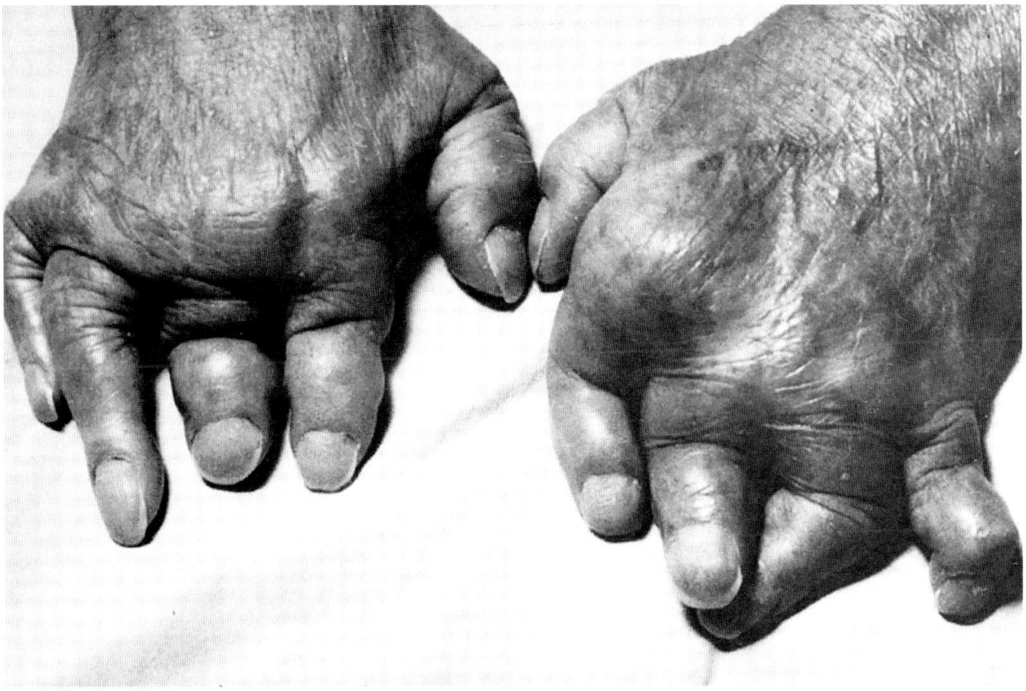

Figure 66.8 Hands of a patient with severe psoriatic arthritis with arthritis mutilans, also referred to as 'opera glass' hands.

> **KEY CONCEPTS**
>
> **Clinical patterns of psoriatic arthritis**
> - Distal interphalangeal joint involvement
> - Asymmetric oligoarticular
> - Symmetric polyarticular or 'rheumatoid-like'
> - Arthritis mutilans
> - Sacroiliitis and/or spondylitis.

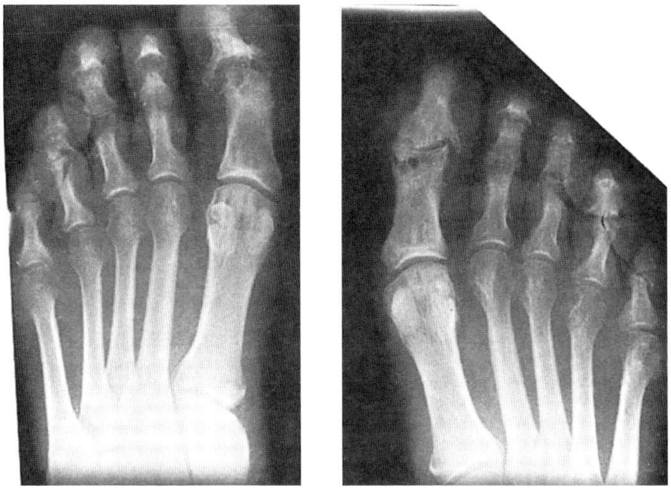

Figure 66.9 Radiographs of the feet in psoriatic arthritis. Note destruction primarily of most distal joints with periosteal reaction (whiskering), bony fusion of several small joints, and lack of osteopenia.

Radiographic features

The most characteristic X-ray changes occur in the fingers and toes, especially at the distal and/or proximal interphalangeal joints.[60] Bony hypertrophy and resorption with 'whiskering' at joint margins, loss of joint space (cartilage), and eventual bony fusion of joints, in the absence of osteopenia, are typical findings (Fig. 66.9). The development of a 'pencil-in-cup' deformity is pathognomonic.

Laboratory features

There are few laboratory abnormalities. A mildly elevated erythrocyte sedimentation rate is most common. Occasionally there is a mild anemia. Tests for rheumatoid factor and antinuclear antibodies are negative. Serum uric acid is elevated in approximately 40% of patients with psoriasis. Synovial fluid is inflammatory with white blood cell counts in the 5000–25 000/mm^3 range. Total protein and complement levels tend to be high and glucose levels in synovial fluid are normal. HLA-B27 occurs less frequently in psoriatic arthritis than in ankylosing spondylitis or Reiter syndrome (Table 66.2). Only 8–20% of cases overall are positive for HLA-B27; however, it occurs in approximately half of patients with spinal involvement.[11] Other Class I HLA antigens are found in increased frequencies in psoriasis and psoriatic arthritis, including HLA-Cw6, B17 (B57), B13, B37 and B16 (B38 and B39).[11]

Disease course

Psoriatic arthritis is a chronic and slowly progressive disease with exacerbations and periods of relative quiescence, or even remission. Overall, psoriatic arthritis tends to be less deforming and disabling than rheumatoid arthritis. Patients with initial oligoarticular disease tend to develop polyarticular involvement eventually. The worst disability occurs in the proportion of patients (approximately 5%) who progress to arthritis mutilans.

Enteropathic arthritis

Symptoms and physical examination

An inflammatory arthritis may complicate the course of either ulcerative colitis or Crohn's disease and occasionally may be the first symptom.[75] Peripheral joint involvement is most common, occurring in approximately 20% of patients. The appearance of arthritis indicates that the inflammatory bowel disease is active, regardless of whether or not gastrointestinal symptoms are present, and treatment should be directed to the bowel disease. Moreover, colectomy for ulcerative colitis, but not Crohn's disease, eliminates peripheral arthritis complications. Large joints are most often affected, usually knees, ankles, and wrists. Large warm effusions are typical. Joint damage and deformities are rare.

Sacroiliitis and/or spondylitis occur in approximately 10% of patients, independently of peripheral arthritis. Moreover, in contrast to peripheral arthritis, the spondylitis may progress regardless of the activity of the bowel disease, and colonic resection does not stop or slow progression of axial involvement. Many patients have asymptomatic spinal disease. Those with symptoms have complaints and physical findings similar to those described for ankylosing spondylitis.

Extra-articular features

Peripheral arthritis is only one of several extraintestinal manifestations of inflammatory bowel disease which may flare up together during periods of disease activity. Erythema nodosum is a characteristic skin complication of Crohn's disease, while pyoderma gangrenosum is associated with ulcerative colitis. Fever, acute anterior uveitis, painful oral ulcers, or ascending cholangitis may complicate either bowel disease. Cardiac complications are exceedingly rare.

Radiographic features

Spinal abnormalities in the axial skeleton are similar to those described in ankylosing spondylitis. Peripheral joints rarely show destructive changes.

Laboratory features

Active inflammatory bowel disease is usually accompanied by anemia, often severe, as a result of chronic inflammation, gastrointestinal blood loss, or both. Leukocytosis, thrombocytosis (often extreme), and marked elevation of the erythrocyte sedimentation rate are common findings. Serum rheumatoid factor and antinuclear antibodies are typically negative. Synovial effusions are mildly to moderately inflammatory but bacteriologically sterile. HLA-B27 is not increased in frequency in patients with inflammatory bowel diseases overall or in those with peripheral arthritis. However, it is positive in 30–50% of patients with associated sacroiliitis or spondylitis (Table 66.2).[76]

Disease course

The peripheral arthritis tends to exacerbate and remit in concert with the activity of bowel disease and usually leaves no permanent sequelae. Spondylitis, on the other hand, pursues a course independent of bowel inflammation which is comparable to that of ankylosing spondylitis.

Undifferentiated spondyloarthropathies

Many patients have combinations of peripheral and/or spinal arthritis, with or without extra-articular manifestations, which do not permit them to be confidently classified into any of the discrete disease categories described above.[77] Recently, criteria for 'spondylarthropathies' have been developed and validated for the accurate classification of such patients[78] (discussed below). In addition, even more limited presentations or *forme frustes* of these diseases have been identified, largely through the clinical and epidemiological use of HLA-B27 testing (Table 66.6).

Atypical spondyloarthropathies and forme frustes of HLA-B27 associated disease

	Reference
Inflammatory back pain without radiographic spondylitis	29
Inflammatory chest wall pain without radiographic spondylitis	29
Juvenile spondyloarthropathies	9
Pauciarticular arthritis (boys > girls)	71
Polyarticular arthritis (girls > boys)	
Seronegative enthesopathy and arthritis (SEA)	9
Ankylosing tarsitis	
Dominant cervical spine arthritis and fusion with micrognathia	71
Late-onset spondyloarthropathy	29
Incomplete Reiter syndrome	6
Characteristic peripheral arthritis alone	
Pustular psoriasis alone (keratoderma)	
Circinate balanitis alone	
Chronic dactyliitis alone	
Chronic heel pain (enthesitis) alone	
Acute anterior uveitis (with or without arthritis)	63
Lone aortic regurgitation and/or complete heart block (with or without arthritis)	64

Table 66.6 Atypical spondyloarthropathies and forme frustes of HLA-B27 associated disease.

SAPHO syndrome and acne-associated arthritis

Clinical features

SAPHO syndrome (Synovitis, Acne, Pustulosis, Hyperostosis, Osteomyelitis) is an acronym recently coined to encompass patients with a rare disorder that may be related to the spondyloarthropathies.[79,80] Children and young adults are most commonly affected.

Hyperostotic and/or osteomyelitis-like bone and joint lesions, most commonly of the chest wall (sternum, ribs, and clavicles) but also the mandible, long bones and vertebrae, have been described. Sacroiliitis, usually unilateral, and/or vertebral changes suggesting spondylitis, including syndesmophytes, appear to occur in approximately one third of cases. Dramatic skin lesions almost invariably accompany the musculoskeletal manifestations and include palmoplantar pustulosis resembling psoriasis, acne conglobata or fulminans, hidradenitis suppurativa, or dissecting cellulitis of the scalp. Thus, the term *acne arthritis* has been applied to some small series. The disease has variable exacerbations and remissions, often paralleled by the activity of skin disease. Therapy with antibiotics appears not to be very beneficial, and that with nonsteroidal anti-inflammatory drugs is also disappointing. Corticosteroids have most consistently been reported to be useful. Bacteriologic studies have been largely negative; however, *Propionibacterium acnes* has been reportedly grown from several bone biopsies, and is often found in the acneiform skin lesions.

HLA-B27 is present in approximately one third of cases.

Diagnosis and classification criteria

A definite diagnosis of idiopathic *ankylosing spondylitis* requires the radiographic demonstration of sacroiliitis along with clinical and/or radiographic evidence of higher spinal involvement.[81] In addition, other causes of spondylitis, i.e. Reiter syndrome, psoriasis and inflammatory bowel disease, should be excluded. Low back pain is a common complaint in the general population, and sacroiliitis/ankylosing spondylitis is the underlying cause in the minority of patients. The characteristic 'inflammatory spinal symptoms', especially in a young man or woman, should raise clinical suspicion.[56] Early in the disease, however, radiographic changes may be absent and may require many years to evolve. Computed tomography (CT) and magnetic resonance imaging (MRI) are more sensitive techniques for detecting sacroiliitis but are costly, and bone scans yield findings that are insufficiently specific.[60] Typing for HLA-B27, while not diagnostic for disease, may prove clinically useful.[72] As a test for ankylosing spondylitis, HLA-B27 has a sensitivity of 90% and specificity of 92% (based upon its 90% frequency in spondylitis patients and 8% prevalence in normal Whites, respectively). HLA-B27 is even more specific in patients of African or Japanese origin, in whom the gene frequency in the normal population is low (<1–3%). HLA-B27 is not at all specific in certain Native Americans and Eskimo groups with high gene frequencies (25–40%). Moreover, its predictive value as a test is optimal when there is a strong clinical likelihood of disease.

The diagnosis of *juvenile ankylosing spondylitis* is based upon the clinical picture, usually a chronic peripheral oligoarthritis with or without enthesopathy, the absence of serum rheumatoid factor and antinuclear antibodies, and the presence of HLA-B27. Spinal X-rays are usually of no diagnostic value early in this disease.[9]

Reiter syndrome or reactive arthritis is diagnosed clinically based upon its typical articular pattern and extra-articular manifestations, especially when they follow a recent gastroenteritis or genitourinary infection. Reiter syndrome should be considered in any young man with a peripheral arthritis. Infectious arthritis, especially due to gonococci, must always be excluded from the differential diagnosis and concomitant HIV infection also considered. Occasionally, in incomplete or atypical cases of Reiter syndrome, determination of HLA-B27 may be clinically useful; however, it is a less sensitive test for this disease than in ankylosing spondylitis, since it occurs in only 63–75% of cases.[72]

Psoriatic arthritis is a seronegative inflammatory arthritis occurring in a patient with cutaneous psoriasis, usually with concomitant nail pitting or other dystrophic changes.[74] Involvement of distal interphalangeal joints, sausaging of fingers and/or toes, and radiographic evidence of spinal involvement (sacroiliitis and/or syndesmophytes) are all features which strengthen the diagnosis. The similarity of cutaneous and nail changes leads to psoriatic arthritis often being confused with Reiter syndrome, and, in some patients, the two diseases cannot be discriminated from one another. HLA typing has no clinical role in diagnosis, since the association with HLA-B27 is weak and the other HLA alleles increased in psoriasis patients are multiple and occur in high frequencies in the normal population.

Enteropathic arthritis is diagnosed on clinical grounds on the basis of a seronegative peripheral and/or spinal arthritis in a patient with histopathologically and/or radiographically proven Crohn's disease or ulcerative colitis.

Recently, criteria have been developed for *spondyloarthropathies*, regardless of specific diagnosis[78] (Table 66.7). In fact, these criteria appear to perform well, with excellent sensitivity (82–90%) and specificity (80–94%).

Classification of spondyloarthropathy

Inflammatory spinal pain	***or***	**synovitis** Asymmetric or predominantly in the lower limbs
	and	

One or more of the following:
- *Positive family history* of AS, psoriasis, acute uveitis, reactive arthritis, or IBD
- *Psoriasis* – past or present diagnosis
- *Inflammatory bowel disease* – past or present diagnosis
- *Urethritis, cervicitis, or acute diarrhea* occurring within 1 month before arthritis
- *Buttock pain* alternating between right and left sides
- *Enthesopathy* – past or present pain and/or tenderness at insertion of Achilles tendon or plantar fascia
- *Sacroilitis* – X-ray finding of bilateral grade 2–4 or unilateral grade 3–4

Table 66.7 Classification of spondyloarthropathy. Proposed by Dougados M, van der Linden S, Juhlin R, et al. The European Spondyloarthropathy Study Group preliminary criteria for the classification of spondyloarthropathy. *Arthritis Rheum* 1991;34:1218.[78]

TREATMENT

The aims of treatment for each of the spondyloarthropathies should include the following considerations:

1. The suppression of inflammation in axial and/or peripheral joints and entheses so as to relieve pain and stiffness and to improve mobility. Nonsteroidal anti-inflammatory drugs (NSAIDs) are effective in the majority of patients. Agents most useful in these diseases include indomethacin, tolmetin, sulindac, and piroxicam. Aspirin and phenylacetic acid derivatives (profens) appear to be less effective in most patients. In severe cases of ankylosing spondylitis or Reiter syndrome (reactive arthritis) which have failed the usual first-line NSAIDs, phenylbutazone may prove to be effective; however, close monitoring for hematologic toxicity and interactions with other drugs is required. Low doses of corticosteroids may be beneficial at times but should not be used long term.

2. The use of drugs that can modify the natural history of the disease. It is not presently clear that such agents are available. A rationale for specific *antibiotic therapy* has been established for *Chlamydia*-induced reactive arthritis based upon the likelihood of persisting infections (see Etiology and pathogenesis). One double-blind controlled study of a tetracycline given for 3 months to

THERAPEUTIC PRINCIPLES

Treatment of spondyloarthropathies
- Relieve pain and stiffness with nonsteroidal anti-inflammatory drugs
- Sulfasalazine (2–3 g daily) proven effective as long-term agent
- Tetracycline or macrolide antibiotic for proven or suspected *Chlamydia*-induced reactive arthritis
- Methotrexate (or azathioprine) for refractory cases
- Physical therapy or self exercises and education about natural disease history and goals of treatment modalities

patients with *Chlamydia*-induced reactive arthritis has shown a significant reduction in disease duration. No improvement was seen in patients with enteric pathogen-induced reactive arthritis.[21] Similarly, early treatment of venereal infections with antibiotics in patients with prior or established Reiter syndrome appears to prevent recurrences and exacerbations.[22] The enteric antibiotic sulfasalazine also has been demonstrated in blinded, placebo-controlled trials to be effective in reactive arthritis, ankylosing spondylitis, and psoriatic arthritis.[25–28] Improvement in symptoms and inflammatory signs has been associated with lowering of serum acute-phase reactants. The active moiety responsible for sulfasalazine's efficacy has been shown to be sulfapyridine rather than the salicylate.[82] Recent clinical trials of quinolone antibiotics in reactive arthritis have not demonstrated effectiveness.[83] At the present time, it seems most logical in reactive arthritis to attempt to identify the causative bacteria, most importantly *Chlamydia*, perhaps by serologic surveys for antibodies to the known pathogens, and then to give appropriate antibiotic therapy. In most spondyloarthropathies, a trial of sulfasalazine should be considered, unless there is evidence of *Chlamydia*-induced disease where a trial of tetracycline first would be more appropriate.

Immunosuppressive agents such as methotrexate and azathioprine, have been used for patients with severe spondyloarthropathies unresponsive to conventional therapy; however, controlled clinical trials have not been reported. Newer tumor recresis factor-α (TNF-α) antagonists may be effective in severe disease.

3. The prevention of joint deformities and disabilities. The use of physical therapy to maintain both axial and peripheral joint function and a good range of motion remains an important aspect of treatment.[84] The spondyloarthropathies are characterized by prominent fibrous and bony fusion in both axial and peripheral joints which leads to contracture and loss of motion. A regular program of exercises and/or recreational activities, such as swimming, as well as instruction about maintenance of a good posture, may prevent disability.

4. Treatment of the extra-articular manifestations usually requires specialist consultation and management. Acute anterior uveitis must be treated and followed by an ophthalmologist and usually responds to topical mydriatics and corticosteroids, although some patients require brief courses of high-dose systemic corticosteroids. Sulfasalazine orally may reduce the number of recurrences. The cardiac complications of aortic valvular regurgitation and heart block usually require surgical replacement of the aortic valve and/or insertion of a cardiac pacemaker. Skin care for psoriatic lesions usually consists of local dermatologic creams and lotions, often corticosteroid based. Treatment of inflammatory bowel disease is multifaceted and best accomplished by a gastroenterologist.

REFERENCES

1. Arnett FC. Seronegative spondyloarthropathies. Sci Am 1998;Sect 15:1.
2. Khan MA (ed.) Spondyloarthropathies. Rheum Dis Clin North Am 1992;18:1.
3. al-Khonizy W, Reveille JD. The immunogenetics of the seronegative spondyloarthropathies. Baillières Clin Rheumatol 1998;12:567.
4. Lau CS, Burgos-Vargas R, Louthrenoo W, Mok MY, Wordsworth P, Zeng QY. Features of spondyloarthritis around the world. Rheum Dis Clin North Am 1998;24:753.
5. Braun J, Bollow M, Remlinger G, et al. Prevalence of spondyloarthropathies in HLA-B27 positive and negative blood donors. Arthritis Rheum 1998;41:58.
6. Amor B. Reiter's syndrome. Diagnosis and clinical features. Rheum Dis Clin North Am 1998;24:677.
7. Lawrence RC, Helmick CG, Arnett FC, et al. Estimates of the prevalence of arthritis and selected musculoskeletal disorders in the USA. Arthritis Rheum 1998;41:778.
8. van der Linden SM, Valkenburg HA, deJongh BM, Cats A. The risk of developing ankylosing spondylitis in HLA-B27 positive individuals. A comparison of relatives of spondylitis patients with the general population. Arthritis Rheum 1984;27:241.
9. Burgos-Vargas R, Petty RE. Juvenile ankylosing spondylitis. Rheum Dis Clin North Am 1992;18:123.
10. Clark MR, Solinger AM, Hochberg MC. Human immunodeficiency virus infection is not associated with Reiter's syndrome. Data from three large cohort studies. Rheum Dis Clin North Am 1992;18:267.
11. Gladman DD. Psoriatic arthritis: recent advances in pathogenesis and treatment. Rheum Dis Clin North Am 1992;18:247.
12. De Keyser F, Elewaut D, DeVos M, et al. Bowel inflammation and the spondyloarthropathies. Rheum Dis Clin North Am 1998;24:785.
13. Keat A. Reiter's syndrome and reactive arthritis in perspective. N Engl J Med 1983;309:1606.
14. Granfors K, Jalkanen S, VonEssen R, et al. Yersinia antigens in synovial fluid cells from patients with reactive arthritis. N Engl J Med 1989;320:216.
15. Granfors K, Jalkanen S, Lindberg AA, et al. Salmonella lipopolysaccharide in synovial cells from patients with reactive arthritis. Lancet 1990;335:685.
16. Nanagara R, Li F, Beutler A, Hudson A, Schumacher Jr HR. Alteration of chlamydia trachomatis biologic behavior in synovial membranes. Arthritis Rheum 1995;38:1410.
17. Gerard HC, Branigan PJ, Schumacher HR, Hudson AP. Synovial chlamydia trachomatis in patients with reactive arthritis/Reiter's syndrome are viable but show aberrant gene expression. J Rheumatol 1998;25:734.
18. Marker-Hermann E, Hohler T. Pathogenesis of human leukocyte antigen B27-positive arthritis. Information from clinical materials. Rheum Dis Clin North Am 1998;24:865.
19. Nikkari S, Rantakokko K, Edman P, et al. Salmonella-triggered reactive arthritis. Arthritis Rheum 1999;42:84.
20. Montenegro V, Monteiro RC. Elevation of serum IgA in spondyloarthropathies and IgA nephropathy and its pathogenic role. Curr Opin Rheumatol 1999;11:265.
21. Lauhio A, Leirisalo-Repo M, Lahdevirta J, Saikku P, Repo H. Double-blind, placebo-controlled study of three-month treatment with lymecycline in reactive arthritis, with special reference to chlamydia arthritis. Arthritis Rheum 1991;34:6.
22. Bardin T, Enel C, Cornelis F, et al. Antibiotic treatment of venereal disease and Reiter's syndrome in a Greenland population. Arthritis Rheum 1992;35:190.
23. Keat A. Is spondylitis caused by Klebsiella? Immunol Today 1986;7:144.
24. Braun J, Tuszewski M, Ehlers S, et al. Nested polymerase chain reaction strategy simultaneously targeting DNA sequences of multiple bacterial species in inflammatory joint diseases. Examination of sacroiliac and knee joint biopsies of patients with spondyloarthropathies and other arthritides. J Rheumatol 1997;24:1101.
25. Dougados M, van der Linden S, Leirisalo-Repo M, et al. Sulfasalazine in the treatment of spondyloarthropathy. Arthritis Rheum 1995;38:618.
26. Clegg DO, Reda DJ, Weisman MH, et al. Comparison of sulfasalazine and placebo in the treatment of ankylosing spondylitis. Arthritis Rheum 1996;39:2004.
27. Clegg DO, Reda DJ, Weisman MH, et al. Comparison of sulfasalazine and placebo in the treatment of reactive arthritis (Reiter's syndrome). A Department of Veterans Affairs Cooperative Study. Arthritis Rheum 1996;39:2021.

28. Clegg DO, Reda DJ, Mejias E, et al. Comparison of sulfasalazine and placebo in the treatment of psoriatic arthritis. Arthritis Rheum 1996;39:2013.
29. van der Linden S; van der Heijde D. Ankylosing spondylitis. Clinical features. Rheum Dis Clin North Am 1998;24:663.
30. Brown MA, Kennedy GL, MacGregor AJ, et al. Susceptibility to ankylosing spondylitis in twins – the role of genes, HLA, and the environment. Arthritis Rheum 1997;40:1823.
31. Wordsworth P. Genes in the spondyloarthropathies. Rheum Dis Clin North Am 1998;24:845.
32. Hohler T, Schaper T, Schneider PM, zum Buschenfelde KHM, Marker-Hermann E. Association of different tumor necrosis factor alpha promoter allele frequencies with ankylosing spondylitis in HLA-B27 positive individuals. Arthritis Rheum 1998;41:1489.
33. Brown MA, Pile KD, Kennedy LG, et al. A genome-wide screen for susceptibility loci in ankylosing spondylitis. Arthritis and Rheum 1998;41:588.
34. Brown MA, Rudwaleit M, Pile KD, et al. The role of germline polymorphisms in the T-cell receptor in susceptibility to ankylosing spondylitis. Brit J Rheumatol 1998;37:454.
35. Taurog JD, Maika SD, Satumtira N, et al. Inflammatory disease in HLA-B27 transgenic rats. Immunol Rev 1999;169:209.
36. Khare SD, Luthra HS, David CS. Animal models of human leukocyte antigen B27-linked arthritides. Rheum Dis Clin North Am 1998;24:883.
37. Madden DR, Gorga JC, Strominger JL, Wiley DC. The structure of HLA-B27 reveals nonamer self-peptides bound in an extended conformation. Nature 1991;353:321.
38. Buxton SE, Benjamin RJ, Clayberger C, Parham P, Krensky AM. Anchoring pockets in human histocompatibility complex leukocyte antigen (HLA) Class I molecules: Analysis of the conserved B ('45') pocket of HLA-B27. J Exp Med 1992;175:809.
39. Rojo S, Garcia F, Villadangos JA, Lopez de Castro JA. Changes in the repertoire of peptides bound to HLA-B27 subtypes and to site-specific mutants inside and outside pocket B. J Exp Med 1993;177:613.
40. Gonzalez-Roces S, Alvarez MV, Gonzalez S, et al. HLA-B27 polymorphism and worldwide susceptibility to ankylosing spondylitis. Tissue Antigens 1997;49:116.
41. Reveille JD. HLA-B27 and the seronegative spondyloarthropathies. Am J Med Sci 1998;316:239.
42. Ren EC, Koh WH, Sim D, Boey ML, Wee GB, Chan SH. Possible protective role of HLA-B*2706 for ankylosing spondylitis. Tissue Antigens 1997;49:67.
43. Garcia F, Marina A, Lopez de Castro JA. Lack of carboxyl-terminal tyrosine distinguishes the B*2706-bound peptide repertoire from those of B*2704 and other HLA-B27 subtypes associated with ankylosing spondylitis. Tissue Antigens 1997;49:215.
44. Fiorillo MT, Meadows L, D'Amato M, et al. Susceptibility to ankylosing spondylitis correlates with the C-terminal residue of peptides presented by various HLA-B27 subtypes. Eur J Immunol 1997;27:368.
45. Lahesmaa R, Skurnik M, Granfors K, et al. Molecular mimicry in the pathogenesis of spondylarthropathies: a critical appraisal of cross-reactivity between microbial antigens and HLA-B27. Brit J Rheumatol 1992;31:221.
46. Lopez-Larrea C, Gonzelez S, Martinez-Borra J. The role of HLA-B27 polymorphism and molecular mimicry in spondylarthropathy. Mol Med Today 1998;4:540.
47. Scofield RH, Warren WL, Koelsch G, Harley JB. A hypothesis for the HLA-B27 immune dysregulation in spondyloarthropathy: contributions from enteric organisms, B27 structure, peptides bound by B27, and convergent evolution. Proc Natl Acad Sci 1993;90:9330.
48. DeVries DD, Dekker-Saeys AJ, Gyodi E, Bohn U, Ivanyi P. Absence of autoantibodies to peptides shared by HLA-B27.5 and *Klebsiella pneumoniae* nitrogenase in serum samples from HLA-B27 positive patients with ankylosing spondylitis and Reiter's syndrome. Ann Rheum Dis 1992;51:783.
49. Dulphy N, Peyrat MA, Tieng V, et al. Common intra-articular T cell expansions in patients with reactive arthritis: identical beta-chain junctional sequences and cytotoxicity toward HLA-B27. J Immunol 1999;162:3830.
50. Virtala M, Kirkveskari J, Ganfors K. HLA-B27 modulates the survival of salmonella enteritidis in transfected L cells, possibly by impaired nitric oxide production. Infect Immun 1997;65:4236.
51. Inman RD, Chiu B, Johnston MEA, Vas S, Falk J. HLA-Class I-related impairment of IL-2 production and lymphocyte response to microbial antigens in reactive arthritis. J Immunol 1989;142:4256.
52. Braun J, Yin Z, Spiller I, et al. Low secretion of tumor necrosis factor alpha, but no other Th1 or Th2 cytokines, by peripheral blood mononuclear cells correlates with chronicity in reactive arthritis. Arthritis Rheum 1999;42:2039.
53. Ugrinovic S, Mertz A, Wu P, Braun J, Sieper J. A single nonamer from the Yersinia 60-kD heat shock protein is the target of HLA-B27-restricted CTL response in Yersinia-induced reactive arthritis. J Immunol 1997;159:5715.
54. Arnett FC. Ankylosing spondylitis 1992: From Connor to transgenes. J Irish Coll Phys Surg 1993;22:207.
55. Moll JMH, Haslock I, MacRae I, Wright V. Associations between ankylosing spondylitis, psoriatic arthritis, Reiter's disease, the intestinal arthropathies, and Behçet's syndrome. Medicine (Baltimore) 1974;53:343.
56. Calin A, Porta J, Fries JF, Schurman DJ. Clinical history as a screening test for ankylosing spondylitis. JAMA 1977;237:261.
57. Cunnane G, Bresnihan B, Fitzgerald O. Immunohistologic analysis of peripheral joint disease in ankylosing spondylitis. Arthritis Rheum 1998;41:180.
58. McGonagle D, Khan MA, Marzo-Ortega H, O'connor P, Gibbon W, Emery P. Enthesitis in spondyloarthropathy. Curr Opin Rheumatol 1999;11:244.
59. Braun J, Bollow M, Neure L, et al. Use of immunohistologic and *in situ* hybridization techniques in the examination of sacroiliac joint biopsy specimens from patients with ankylosing spondylitis. Arthritis Rheum 1995;38:499.
60. Braun J, Bollow M, Sieper J. Radiologic diagnosis and pathology of the spondyloarthropathies. Rheum Dis Clin North Am 1998;24:697.
61. Yu W, Feng F, Dion E, Yang H, Jiang M, Genant HK. Comparison of radiography, computed tomography and magnetic resonance imaging in the detection of sacroiliitis accompanying ankylosing spondylitis. Skeletal Radiol 1998;27:311.
62. Bronson WD, Walker SE, Hillman LS, Keisler D, Hoyt T, Allen SH. Bone mineral density and biochemical markers of bone metabolism in ankylosing spondylitis. J Rheumatol 1998;25:929.
63. Banares A, Hernandez-Garcia C, Fernandez-Gutierrez B, Jover JA. Eye involvement in the spondyloarthropathies. Rheum Dis Clin North Am 1998;24:771.
64. Bergfeldt L. HLA-B27-associated cardiac disease. Ann Intern Med 1997;127:621.
65. Gratacos J, Orellana C, Sanmarti R, et al. Secondary amyloidosis in ankylosing spondylitis. A systematic survey of 137 patients using abdominal fat aspiration. J Rheumatol 1997;24:912.
66. Casserly IP, Fenlon HM, Breatnach E, Sant SM. Lung findings on high-resolution computed tomography in idiopathic ankylosing spondylitis – correlation with clinical findings, pulmonary function testing and plain radiography. Brit J Rheumatol 1997;36:677.
67. Hunter T, Dubo HI. Spinal fractures complicating ankylosing spondylitis. Arthritis Rheum 1983;26:751.
68. Charlesworth CH, Savy LE, Stevens J, Twomey B, Mitchell R. MRI demonstration of arachnoiditis in cauda equina syndrome of ankylosing spondylitis. Neuroradiology 1996;38:462.
69. Carette S, Graham D, Little H, Rubenstein J, Rosen P. The natural disease course of ankylosing spondylitis. Arthritis Rheum 1983;266:186.
70. Gran JT, Skomsvoll JF. The outcome of ankylosing spondylitis: a study of 100 patients. Brit J Rheumatol 1997;36:766.
71. Arnett FC, Bias WB, Stevens MB. Juvenile-onset chronic arthritis: clinical and roentgenographic features of a unique HLA-B27 subset. Am J Med 1980;69:369.
72. Khan MA, Khan MK. Diagnostic value of HLA-B27 testing in ankylosing spondylitis and Reiter's syndrome. Ann Int Med 1982;96:70.
73. Leirisalo-Repo M. Prognosis, course of disease, and treatment of the spondyloarthropathies. Rheum Dis Clin North Am 1998;24:737.

74. Gladman DD. Psoriatic arthritis. Rheum Dis Clin North Am 1998;24:829.
75. Gravallese EM, Kantrowitz FG. Arthritis manifestations of inflammatory bowel disease: clinical review. Am J Gastroenterol 1988;83:703.
76. Enlow R, Bias WB, Arnett FC. The spondylitis of inflammatory bowel disease. Evidence for a non-HLA linked axial arthropathy. Arthritis Rheum 1980;23:1359.
77. Zeidler H, Mau W, Khan MA. Undifferentiated spondyloarthropathies. Rheum Dis Clin Am 1992;18:187.
78. Dougados M, van der Linden S, Juhlin R, et al. The European Spondyloarthropathy Study Group preliminary criteria for the classification of spondyloarthropathy. Arthritis Rheum 1991;34:1218.
79. Khan M-F, Chamot A-M. SAPHO syndrome. Rheum Dis Clin North Am 1992;18:225.
80. Winchester R. Psoriatic arthritis and the spectrum of syndromes related to the SAPHO (synovitis, acne, pustulosis, hyperostosis, and osteitis) syndrome. Curr Opin Rheumatol 1999;11:251.
81. van der Linden S, Valkenburg HA, Cats A. Evaluation of diagnostic criteria for ankylosing spondylitis: a proposal for modification of the New York criteria. Arthritis Rheum 1984;27:361.
82. Taggart A, Gardiner P, McEvoy F, Hopkins R, Bird H. Which is the active moiety of sulfasalazine in ankylosing spondylitis. Arthritis Rheum 1996;39:1400.
83. Sieper J, Fendler C, Laitko S, et al. No benefit of long-term ciprofloxacin treatment in patients with reactive arthritis and undifferentiated oligoarthritis. Arthritis Rheum 1999;42:1386.
84. Santos H, Brophy S, Calin A. Exercise in ankylosing spondylitis: how much is optimum? J Rheumatol 1998;25:2156.

Section 6 Systemic Immune Diseases

Chapter 67 Small and Medium Vessel Primary Vasculitis

David B. Hellmann and John H. Stone

Vasculitis is defined as inflammation within blood vessel walls. Inflamed blood vessels are liable to narrow, thrombose, or rupture, and thereby cause tissues served by those vessels to undergo ischemic damage. The many different forms of vasculitis offer several exciting challenges. First, these diseases often begin with nonspecific symptoms and signs, unfolding in an enigmatic fashion. Thus, vasculitis is one of the great diagnostic challenges in medicine. Knowledge of the clinical disguises worn by vasculitis often permits the physician to suspect or diagnose the condition at the bedside. Second, with therapy, most patients improve, some enter disease remissions, and a substantial portion are cured. Treating patients with vasculitis is therefore often as rewarding as making the diagnosis. Finally, rapidly expanding knowledge of the pathophysiology of vasculitides promises more specific and more effective therapies for these diseases in the near future.

CLASSIFICATION OF VASCULITIS

Over 20 different forms of vasculitis are recognized; because the causes of most forms are not known, the vasculitides are distinguished by their clinicopathologic differences.[1–3] One popular classification scheme separates the different forms of vasculitis according to the size of blood vessels affected (Table 67.1). Beyond vessel size, the vasculitides can also be distinguished by such considerations as the typical host, the organs most commonly affected, and the presence of certain pathologic features. For example, within the small-vessel vasculitides, Henoch–Schönlein purpura most commonly occurs in children, typically affects the gut, skin, joints, and kidneys, and produces vasculitis characterized by deposition of IgA. In contrast, Wegener's granulomatosis usually strikes adults, has a predilection for the upper airways, lungs, and kidneys, and causes granulomatous inflammation.

Finally, one additional basis for distinguishing the vasculitides is worth mentioning. Disorders in which vasculitis is the central cause of the symptoms and signs are designated 'primary'. 'Secondary' forms of vasculitides are those in which vasculitis complicates another type of disease, such as systemic lupus erythematosus (SLE) or rheumatoid arthritis (RA). This chapter focuses on primary vasculitides. Secondary forms of vasculitis are covered in other chapters.

Major categories of primary vasculitis
Large-vessel vasculitis
Giant-cell arteritis
Takayasu's arteritis
Medium-vessel vasculitis
Polyarteritis nodosa
Kawasaki's disease
Primary central nervous system vasculitis
Buerger's disease
Small-vessel vasculitis
ANCA-associated small-vessel vasculitis:
• microscopic polyangiitis
• Wegener's granulomatosis
• Churg–Strauss syndrome
• drug-induced ANCA-associated vasculitis
Immune-complex small-vessel vasculitis:
• hypersensitivity vasculitis
• cryoglobulinemic vasculitis
• connective tissue disorders
• urticarial vasculitis
• Behçet's disease
• Goodpasture's syndrome
• serum sickness
• infection-induced vasculitis
Paraneoplastic small-vessel vasculitis
Inflammatory bowel disease vasculitis

Table 67.1 Major categories of primary vasculitis. (Adapted from Jennette J, Falk R. Small vessel vasculitis. *N Engl J Med* 1997;337:1512.)

PATHOGENESIS

The pathogenesis of the vasculitides remains obscure. With few exceptions, the etiologies of these diseases are not known, and precise knowledge of how the immune system, endothelial cells, and cytokines interact to cause vascular inflammation is lacking. Still, enough is known about a few forms of vasculitis and discussion of their pathogenesis provides a framework for considering how perturbations of the immune system might cause others. The mechanisms described below are models of disease pathophysiology that have been proposed to explain some forms of vasculitis. Most remain of hypothetical importance, and it is conceivable that substantial overlap in disease models exists for some forms of vasculitis.[4]

Immune complex model

One established mechanism for causing vasculitis is the deposition of circulating immune complexes (ICs). After the formation of soluble ICs, the complexes are deposited in the subendothelium, an event facilitated by the release of vasoactive amines (e.g. histamine) from platelets and basophils. Once trapped in the subendothelial space, ICs fix complement and generate chemotactic factors for the recruitment and activation of neutrophils. Degranulation of these neutrophils leads to the release of oxygen radicals and lysosomal enzymes, which in turn damage the blood vessel walls.

The IC model of vasculitis, developed and studied in experimental animal models, accounts for several forms of vasculitis in humans. For example, it explains the transient vasculitis known as serum sickness that develops following exposure to some foreign antigens. Antigens as varied as the horse serum formerly used in immunizations, antibiotics (e.g. penicillin), virus-associated antigens (e.g. hepatitis B or C) or self-antigens (e.g. double-stranded DNA) are capable of causing immune complex-mediated vasculitis in humans.[3] In cases involving a 'one-shot' antigen exposure, the vasculitis resolves as the antigen is cleared. However, when the antigen persists – e.g. in chronic viral hepatitis, SLE, or RA – the vasculitis can be chronic (albeit the precise antigen is not always known).

It should be noted that the formation of ICs is common, even in healthy individuals, but the occurrence of vasculitis is relatively rare. Several factors determine the pathogenicity of ICs. Antigen load is one determinant, as only amounts of antigen large enough to overwhelm the reticuloendothelial system (RES) provoke a pathologic IC response. Another important factor is solubility of the immune complex, which changes with the ratio of antigen to antibody (Chapter 59). When the antigen:antibody ratio is very high, for example, complexes of antibody and antigen do not form. Conversely, when antibody is present in large excess compared to the antigen, the RES clears the antigen rapidly. ICs formed in slight antigen excess are most likely to be pathogenic, because they are both soluble and of sufficient size to deposit in blood vessel walls.[3] Finally, physical forces such as pressure within the blood vessel (which can damage vessels), temperature (certain ICs such as cryoglobulin form at colder temperatures), or locations of vascular branch points (where turbulence favors immune complex deposition) can influence the development of vasculitis.[3]

ANCA model

The inability to identify ICs in many forms of vasculitis prompted the search for other pathogenic mechanisms. One such mechanism may involve a novel group of autoantibodies, discovered in 1982, called antineutrophil cytoplasmic antibodies (ANCA).[2,4–7] ANCA are directed against different enzymes contained within primary granules of neutrophils and macrophages. These antibodies are usually detected by adding a patient's serum to a preparation of neutrophils, followed by the addition of an antibody tagged with a fluorescent label. In vasculitis, two main patterns of immunofluorescence (IF) are seen: a cytoplasmic pattern (C-ANCA) (Fig. 67.1) or a perinuclear pattern (P-ANCA). The C-ANCA pattern, usually caused by antibodies to serine proteinase 3 (PR-3), is highly specific for Wegener's granulomatosis.[7] The P-ANCA pattern, typically caused by antibodies to myeloperoxidase (MPO), is much less specific, being found in some patients with Wegener's granulomatosis, patients with microscopic polyarteritis, and in other conditions.

KEY CONCEPTS

ANCA patterns and associations with antigens and diseases

Pattern	Antigen	Disease association
C-ANCA	Proteinase-3	Wegener's granulomatosis
P-ANCA	Myeloperoxidase	Wegener's granulomatosis Microscopic polyarteritis Churg–Strauss syndrome

The P-ANCA pattern is an artifact of the tissue preparation. All of the antigens are located in the cytoplasm in vivo. However, alcohol fixation of neutrophils results in the translocation of MPO toward the nucleus, causing the P-ANCA pattern of immunofluorescence. 'Atypical' immunofluorescence patterns, caused by antibodies to lactoferrin and other proteins, are found in patients with diverse conditions, especially inflammatory bowel disease and SLE.[8] ELISA assays are used to verify the types of ANCA found by immunofluorescence.

Experiments have suggested that ANCA are not only markers for certain forms of vasculitis, but also may contribute to the pathogenesis of these conditions.[7] For example, certain inflammatory cytokines such as tumor necrosis factor (TNF) cause neutrophils to express PR-3 and MPO on their cell membranes.[9] The expressed antigens may then interact with the immune system, leading to the ANCA response. The combination of certain cytokines and ANCA leads to increased neutrophil degranulation and oxygen free radical production and, potentially, heightened vascular injury.[9] This model incorporates the accumulating evidence that endothelial cells and inflammatory cells communicate with each other through a large number of messengers and cytokines (Chapters 12, 22).

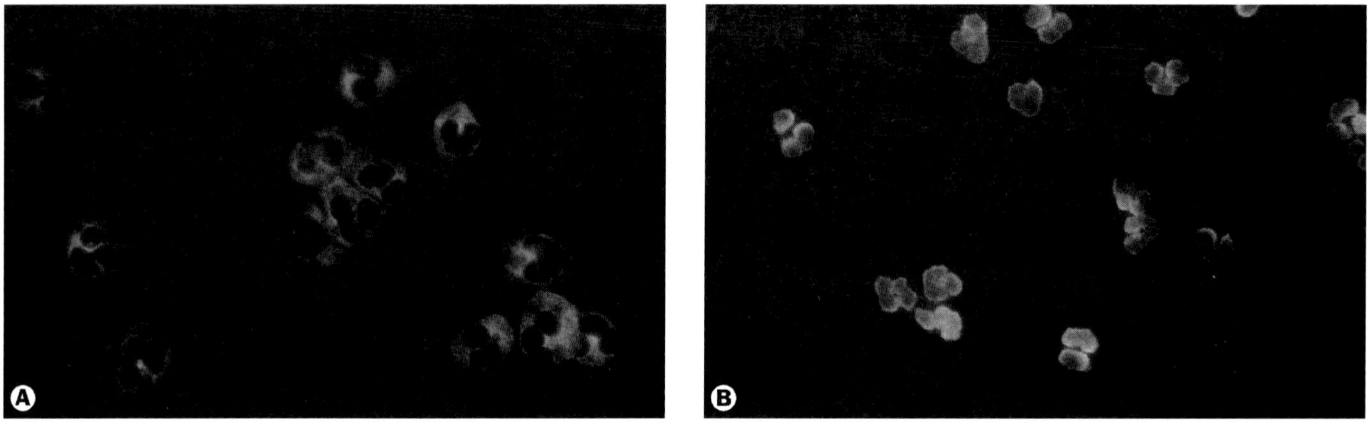

Figure 67.1 ANCA patterns. (**A**) Immunofluorescence study of serum on the substrate of human neutrophils, demonstrating cytoplasmic immunofluorescence (a positive ANCA assay, C-ANCA pattern). (**B**) Perinuclear immunofluorescence (P-ANCA pattern). (See also color plate 67.1.)

Granulomatous inflammation

Granulomatous inflammation is a central feature of several primary vasculitides, including Takayasu's arteritis, temporal arteritis, primary angiitis of the central nervous system, and Wegener's granulomatosis. Some forms of granulomatous vasculitis are associated with a Th1 response, possibly directed against antigens in the vessel wall.[3–4] Cells involved in the Th1 response produce a characteristic cytokine array, including interferon-gamma, IL–12, and TNF. These cytokines recruit and activate macrophages, which in turn release lysosomal enzymes that damage or destroy the vessel wall.[10]

Other possible mechanisms

There are many other potential ways in which the immune system could cause vasculitis.[4] Anti-endothelial cell antibodies have been described in several forms of vasculitis, but their full role requires further investigation.[4] Preliminary studies also suggest that some vasculitides result from antibody-dependent cytotoxicity. Cytotoxic T cells kill target cells either by the induction of target cell apoptosis (e.g. via the Fas/Fas ligand pathway) or by the release of two classes of secretory granules – performin or granzymes – which in turn destroy the target cell.[11] The relevance of these and other putative inflammatory mechanisms of vascular injury is under active investigation.

GENERAL CLUES TO DETECTING VASCULITIS

Inflamed vessels produce clinical symptoms and signs either by being associated with the release of inflammatory cytokines that cause malaise, fever, and weight loss, or by causing direct ischemic damage to specific tissues, such as the induction of digital gangrene. Since the vasculitides demonstrate predilections for certain tissues and organs, their presenting manifestations vary greatly. However, most of the vasculitides share four general features: first, they unfold in a subacute fashion, over weeks or months; second, pain is often a prominent feature of a vasculitis, be it from mononeuritis multiplex, myalgia, testicular infarction, or another consequence of vascular ischemia; third, signs of inflammation, such as fever, rashes, and arthritis are also prominent; fourth, evidence of multiorgan system dysfunction is common. Although not every case of vasculitis adheres strictly to all four of these guidelines, bearing these clues in mind helps clinicians to identify patients whose symptoms and signs may be caused by vasculitis.

CLINICAL PEARLS

General clues to detecting vasculitis

- Clinical symptoms and signs in vasculitis relate to:
  - the release of inflammatory cytokines that cause malaise, fever, and weight loss.
  - direct ischemic damage to specific tissues.
- Most of the vasculitides share four general features:
  - Disease manifestations usually unfold in a subacute fashion, over weeks to months.
  - Pain is often a prominent feature.
  - Signs of inflammation, such as fever, rashes, and arthritis are prominent.
  - Evidence of multiorgan system dysfunction is common.

POLYARTERITIS NODOSA

Polyarteritis nodosa (PAN), the grandfather of all the vasculitides, was described in 1866 by Kussmaul and Maier.[12] The patient was a 27-year-old journeyman tailor who died from a multisystem illness characterized by fever, weight loss, polyneuropathy, and abdominal pain. The nodular swellings found along the course of muscular arteries at autopsy prompted Kussmaul and Maier to term the disease 'periarteritis nodosa'. The term was unfortunate because in fact the inflammatory process consists of a panarteritis that involves the entire thickness of the vessel wall. Subsequent authors have adopted the more accurate name 'polyarteritis nodosa'.

In 1948, Davson et al.[13] suggested the division of PAN patients into two groups based on the presence or absence of glomerulonephritis. One group of patients, Davson noted, demonstrated renal vasculitis only in medium-sized vessels of the kidneys (sparing the glomerulus). In contrast, patients in the other group had glomerular inflammation (i.e. small-vessel vasculitis, with or without medium-sized vessel involvement). This subset of patients with small-vessel vasculitis of the kidney was designated as having 'microscopic PAN'. More recently, microscopic PAN has been renamed 'microscopic polyangiitis' (MPA), in recognition of the tendency of MPA to involve not only arteries but also capillaries and veins as well. The frequent occurrence of ANCA in patients with MPA argues that MPA and classic PAN differ not only pathologically, but also perhaps in terms of etiology. MPA is discussed further in the section on ANCA-associated vasculitis.

Epidemiology

PAN can begin in childhood or in the eighth decade of life, but the average age of onset is about 40–45 years.[3,14] Series vary in the proportion of men and women, afflicted (average male predominance is about two-fold). Ten to thirty percent of patients develop the disease related to infection with hepatitis B or C or both, probably as a result of deposition of ICs containing viral antigens.[15,16] In the remainder of the cases, the etiology remains unknown. Case reports suggest that PAN can rarely develop following vaccinations or other infections.[17] No genetic susceptibility to PAN has been identified, and familial PAN is rare.[18]

Clinical features

The initial symptoms of PAN are usually nonspecific, such as malaise, fatigue, fever, and extremity pain from myalgia or arthralgia (Table 67.2). Typically it is not until weeks or months later that patients develop signs of vasculitis (Table 67.2). The most helpful clinical clues often come from the skin and peripheral nerves because these areas are affected relatively early, and their manifestations of vasculitis are distinctive.[14] Skin lesions of PAN include livedo reticularis, subcutaneous nodules, leg ulcers, palpable purpura, and digital gangrene.[14]

Mononeuritis multiplex, a peripheral neuropathy characterized by the segmental infarction of named nerves, is one of the most specific clues to vasculitis.[19] In the absence of diabetes or multiple compression injuries, mononeuritis multiplex almost always indicates the presence of vasculitis. Mononeuritis multiplex affects the peroneal, tibial, ulnar, median, and radial nerves most often, leading to foot or hand symptoms (e.g. foot or wrist drop).[20] Cranial neuropathies are uncommon, and thoracic neuropathies very rare. Mononeuritis multiplex almost always causes

Clinical feature	Finding (percentage with finding)
General	
Fever	71
Weight loss	54
Organ system involvement	
Kidney	70
Musculoskeletal system:	64
• arthritis/arthralgia	53
• myalgias	31
Hypertension	54
Peripheral neuropathy	51
Gastrointestinal tract:	44
• abdominal pain	43
• nausea/vomiting	40
• cholecystitis	17
• bleeding	6
• bowel perforation	5
• bowel infarction	1
Skin:	43
• rash/purpura	30
• nodules	15
• livedo reticularis	4
Cardiac:	36
• congestive heart failure	12
• myocardial infarction	6
• pericarditis	4
Central nervous system:	23
• cerebral vascular accident	11
• altered mental status	10
• seizure	4

Table 67.2 Clinical features in patients with PAN. (From Cupps T, Fauci A. Systemic necrotizing vasculitis of the polyarteritis nodosa group. In: Smith LH (ed.) *The vaseulitides. Major problems in internal medicine, Vol 21*. Philadelphia, WB Saunders, 1981, p 26.)

sensory abnormalities, particularly painful dysesthesias. Motor involvement occurs in one third of patients. Sometimes patients with PAN appear to have a (nonspecific) symmetrical polyneuropathy. In such cases, electrodiagnostic testing may unmask greater asymmetry to the process than is evident clinically, and also confirm that the pattern of nerve injury is one of axonal degeneration (as seen in vasculitis) rather than demyelination.

The gastrointestinal tract is also frequently involved in PAN. The classic manifestation is 'intestinal angina' – periumbilical pain starting 30–60 min after eating. The pain results from intestinal ischemia occurring because the increased metabolic demands of the bowel after eating cannot be met by the limited blood flow in inflamed mesenteric vessels. Gangrenous bowel can be difficult to recognize, especially in patients receiving glucocorticoids, which blunt the signs of impending abdominal catastrophes. Perforation of ischemic bowel or rupture of a mesenteric microaneurysm can cause acute abdominal pain, shock, and death.[21] Vasculitis of the gallbladder may mimic cholecystitis, and vasculitis of the appendix may present as appendicitis.

Renal involvement is nearly universal at autopsy in PAN, but tends to produce few clinical symptoms. Nocturia may be the earliest manifestation, albeit a nonspecific one. The new onset of hypertension, hematuria, and rising serum creatinine are the most common signs. Renin-mediated hypertension, a hallmark of PAN, is rare in microscopic polyangiitis (MPA) and Wegener's granulomatosis, which tend to involve smaller vessels and glomeruli rather than the medium-sized interlobar renal arteries affected in PAN.[22]

Cardiac involvement, often striking at autopsy, is usually inconspicuous during life.[14] Pericardial effusions, cardiomyopathy, and myocardial infarctions are the most common manifestations. CNS disease usually results from hypertension rather than intracranial vasculitis, but involvement of cerebral blood vessels sometimes occurs. Scleritis is the most common ocular manifestation. Testicular infarction can occur early in the course, causing acute pain and swelling that mimics torsion of the testicle. Inexplicably, PAN usually spares the lungs.

Although PAN typically involves multiple organs, 'limited' forms have been described. 'Cutaneous PAN' is a medium-vessel vasculitis limited to the skin, causing nodules or ulcers. Over time, some of these patients develop systemic disease.

The laboratory features of PAN, though frequently strikingly abnormal, are nonspecific. Anemia, mild thrombocytosis (except in perforation of the gut, which is associated with thrombocytopenia), elevation of the erythrocyte sedimentation rate (ESR), and microscopic hematuria are common.[14]

The pathologic changes in PAN involve small and medium-sized arteries and may be macroscopic and microscopic. As observed by Kussmaul and Maier, involved arteries may show readily visible aneurysmal bulges of the vessel wall.[12] Infarctions, ruptured aneurysms, and gangrenous tissue may be easily visible. Histological sections show inflammatory cells infiltrating the vessel wall (Fig. 67.2), leading to fibrinoid necrosis.[3,12]

Varying degrees of intimal proliferation and thrombosis occur. Lesions tend to be segmental and to favor branch points. In the acute phase of the illness, the inflammatory infiltrate consists chiefly of neutrophils, whereas mononuclear cells predominate in the chronic phase. Granulomas are absent in PAN, and eosinophils rarely prominent.

Diagnosis

Criteria for the classification of PAN have been developed by the American College of Rheumatology (ACR) (Table 67.3).[23] The diagnosis requires a positive biopsy or an angiogram demonstrating

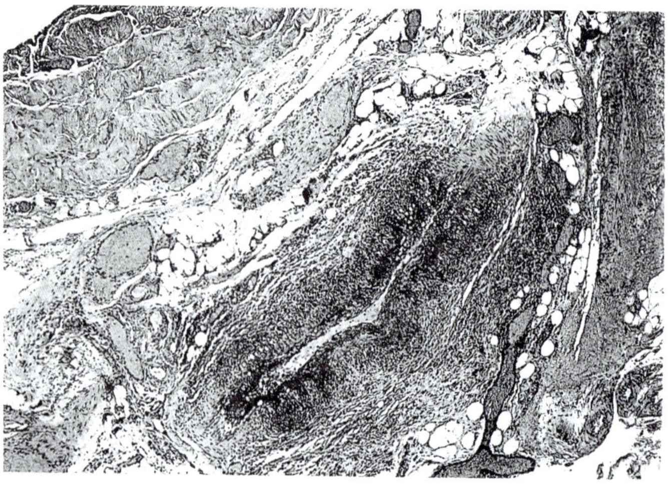

Figure 67.2 Polyarteritis nodosa histopathology. Medium-sized artery in the pericardium of a patient with polyarteritis nodosa showing acute vasculitis. (Reproduced with permission from Hu PJ, Shih I-M, Hutchins GM, et al. Polyarteritis nodosa diagnosed by pericardial biopsy. *J Rheumatol* 1997;24:2042.)

Criteria for classification of polyarteritis nodosa
1. Weight loss ≥ 4 kg
2. Livedo reticularis
3. Testicular pain or tenderness
4. Myalgias, weakness, or leg tenderness
5. Mononeuropathy or polyneuropathy
6. Diastolic BP >90 mmHg
7. Elevated BUN or creatinine
8. Hepatitis B virus
9. Arteriographic abnormalities
10. Biopsy of small or medium-sized artery containing polymorphonuclear cells in the vessel wall.
For classification purposes, a patient shall be said to have polyarteritis nodosa if at least 3 of these 10 criteria are present.

Table 67.3 Criteria for classification of polyarteritis nodosa. (From Lightfoot R, Michel B, Bloch D, et al. The American College of Rheumatology 1990 criteria for the classification of polyarteritis nodosa. *Arthritis Rheum* 1990;33:1088.)

characteristic microaneurysms (Fig. 67.3).[23,24] Biopsies of symptomatic sites such as nerve, muscle, or testicle are often useful (sensitivity, 60–70%; specificity ~97%), whereas biopsies of asymptomatic organs are of much lower yield (sensitivity ~20–30%) and frequently not helpful.[25,26] In contrast, in the absence of a symptomatic site to biopsy, mesenteric angiography may demonstrate telltale microaneurysms (sensitivity ~60%; specificity, 99%).

Treatment and prognosis

For patients with PAN unrelated to hepatitis B or C, treatment usually consists of prednisone and cyclophosphamide.[27,28] In the precorticosteroid era, only 13% of patients survived 5 years.[27] When corticosteroids became available, about half of the patients lived 5 years.[27] In uncontrolled trials, the addition of immunosuppressive drugs to corticosteroid treatment appeared to improve the 5-year survival to 80% or higher.[29] Especially good results in one small series of patients treated with daily cyclophosphamide (2 mg/kg per day) and prednisone (1 mg/kg per day)[27] prompted many physicians to adopt this as the standard initial treatment. However, the only randomized controlled trial comparing prednisone alone with prednisone and cyclophosphamide showed no difference in 10-year survival: about 70% in both treatment groups.[30] Patients treated with cyclophosphamide experienced fewer relapses than those treated with prednisone alone (9% vs. 38% patients).

During the 1990s, French investigators suggested that a 'five-factor score' correlated with prognosis and could be used to guide the choice of treatment.[31] The five factors are: proteinuria >1 g/d, renal insufficiency (i.e. creatinine > 140 moles/liter), cardiomyopathy, gastrointestinal manifestations, and central nervous system involvement. When none of these was present, survival at 5 years was 88%; when one was present, survival was 74%; and when two or more were present, survival fell to 54%.[31] These

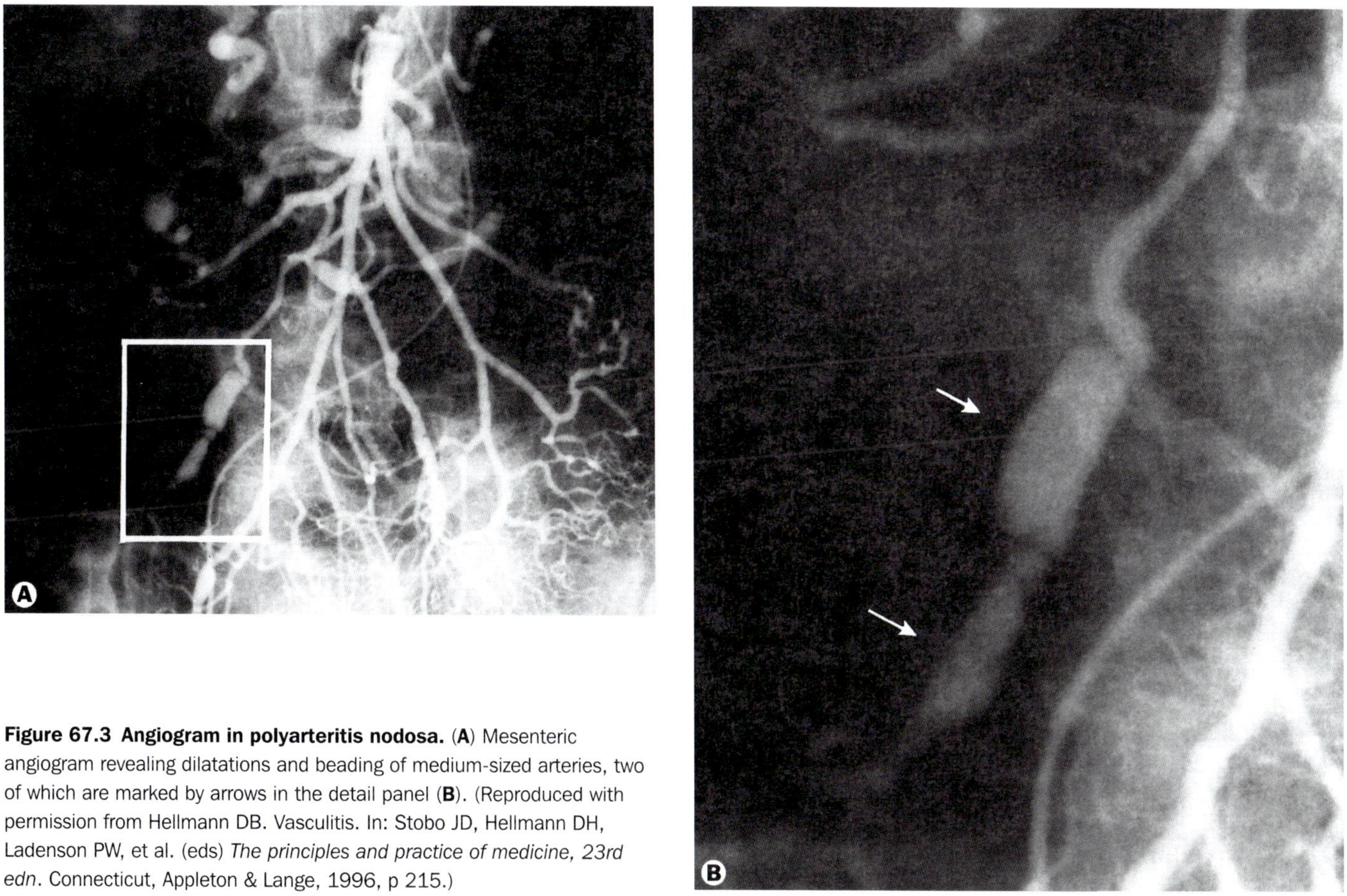

Figure 67.3 Angiogram in polyarteritis nodosa. (**A**) Mesenteric angiogram revealing dilatations and beading of medium-sized arteries, two of which are marked by arrows in the detail panel (**B**). (Reproduced with permission from Hellmann DB. Vasculitis. In: Stobo JD, Hellmann DH, Ladenson PW, et al. (eds) *The principles and practice of medicine, 23rd edn*. Connecticut, Appleton & Lange, 1996, p 215.)

data suggest that prednisone alone may be reasonable initial therapy for patients with low five-factor scores, and that cyclophosphamide should be used for those with high scores.[28,32,33] Controlled trials are needed to validate this approach.

It is controversial whether cyclophosphamide for PAN should be administered on a daily or intermittent (e.g. monthly) basis.[28] Intravenous pulse cyclophosphamide causes fewer opportunistic infections, a lower incidence of hemorrhagic cystitis, and probably fewer malignancies. When using cyclophosphamide to treat PAN, achieving leukopenia is neither required nor desirable.[27] Indeed, frequent monitoring of the white blood cell count (e.g. every 2 weeks) is advisable so that leukopenia can be detected early and cyclophosphamide reduced or stopped as needed.

Most patients begin to improve within 2–4 weeks of starting treatment. Tapering of prednisone may begin after the first month and is continued slowly until the drug is stopped after 6–18 months, depending on the patient's response.[27] Cyclophosphamide is continued for 6–18 months depending on response.[28]

Antiviral agents have revolutionized the treatment of PAN associated with hepatitis B. Before the availability of antiviral agents, all survivors of PAN treated with immunosuppression alone became chronic carriers of hepatitis B and assumed the risks of cirrhosis and hepatoma.[15] The availability of antiviral agents permitted a treatment strategy based on an understanding of disease pathogenesis.[28,32,34] Initially patients are treated with prednisone (1 mg/kg per day) to suppress the inflammation. After the first week, prednisone is rapidly tapered and then discontinued over 3–7 days, and antiviral therapy (e.g. lamivudine 100 mg/d) is started. For several weeks throughout this period, plasma exchange is carried out 2–3 times a week for an average of about 20 exchanges per patient, depending on clinical response. With this regimen, 80% of patients survive the vasculitis and 56% no longer demonstrate serologic evidence of hepatitis B replication.[15]

Treatment for PAN associated with hepatitis C

The treatment of hepatitis C-associated PAN is discussed in the section on cryoglobulinemia.

ESSENTIAL CRYOGLOBULINEMIA

Wintrobe discovered cryoglobulins in 1931 when, in the course of evaluating a 56-year-old woman with anemia, Raynaud's phenomenon, and symptoms of hyperviscosity, he refrigerated a tube of the patient's blood and noted the formation of a precipitate in her plasma.[35] To share his discovery with colleagues, he placed the tube in his coat pocket and walked to the wards. Pulling the tube from his warm pocket he was startled to see that his discovery had vanished. This experience helped to define the hallmark of cryoglobulins – antibodies that precipitate under conditions of cold and solubilize on re-warming (see below).[36]

Cryoglobulins are classified into three types (I, II, or III) (Table 67.4) based on whether or not they (a) are monoclonal, and (b) demonstrate rheumatoid factor activity.[36–38] Type I is monoclonal but does not have rheumatoid factor activity. Cryoglobulin types II and III are designated 'mixed' cryoglobulins, because they consist of both IgG and IgM. The IgM component in type II and type III cryoglobulinemia has rheumatoid factor activity. In type II cryoglobulinemia, the IgM is monoclonal, whereas in type III it is polyclonal. Not all patients with cryoglobulins have symptoms. Indeed, half of all patients with

Classification of cryoglobulins

Type	Monoclonal	Rheumatoid factor activity present	Clinical syndrome	Disease association
I	Yes (usually IgG)	No	Hyperviscosity	Malignancy
II	Yes (IgM)	Yes	Vasculitis	Hepatitis C Rheumatic diseases Malignancy Idiopathic
III	No	Yes	Vasculitis	Hepatitis C Rheumatic diseases Idiopathic

Table 67.4 Classification of cryoglobulins and their immunochemical features and clinical associations.

hepatitis C have demonstrable cryoglobulins, yet vasculitis occurs in only a minority. Symptoms induced by cryoglobulins depend on a number of factors, including their concentrations and thermal properties. The name 'cryoglobulinemia' is usually applied only to those patients who have developed symptoms of hyperviscosity or vasculitis. Vasculitis results when ICs containing cryoglobulins and antigenic components deposit in blood vessel walls and activate complement.

The clinical syndrome and underlying disease can be predicted from the type of cryoglobulin present. For example, monoclonal cryoglobulins without rheumatoid factor activity (type I) do not activate complement effectively and are more likely – as in Wintrobe's patient – to cause hyperviscosity than vasculitis.[36–38] In contrast, the mixed cryoglobulins (types II and III) often activate complement efficiently, and are prone to cause vasculitis. Monoclonal cryoglobulins (types I and II) are associated with B-cell malignancies (e.g. myeloma, Waldenström's macroglobulinemia, and chronic lymphocytic leukemia). Monoclonal cryoglobulins with rheumatoid factor activity (type II) also occur with some chronic infections (especially hepatitis C) and rheumatic diseases (e.g. Sjögren's syndrome, RA, and SLE). Polyclonal cryoglobulins (type III) are associated with rheumatic diseases or chronic infections, but not malignancies.

Until the last decade, 20–50% of patients with type II or III cryoglobulinemia had no identifiable underlying disease. These patients were said to have 'essential' mixed cryoglobulinemia (EMC).[36] After the discovery of hepatitis C virus (HCV) in 1989, it quickly became evident that this infection accounted for more than 80% of the cases of EMC vasculitis.[39–41] Several lines of evidence indicate that HCV-associated EMC is caused by the virus.[39] First, the concentrations of antibody to HCV and HCV-RNA are much higher in the cryoglobulin precipitate than in the serum. Second, antiviral therapy may lead to a reduction in the cryocrit and dramatic improvement in the symptoms of EMC. Third, among patients treated with antiviral agents, only those who clear the virus demonstrate improvement. Fourth, in treated EMC patients who relapse, rising titers of HCV-RNA herald the relapse of symptoms.[36,39]

Only a small subset of patients with HCV develop EMC. The prevalence of HCV in the American population is 1.8%.[42] In one series of 127 HCV patients, 54% demonstrated cryoglobulins but only 14% had symptoms of EMC.[43] Of the patients with symptoms, about one third had type II cryoglobulins and two thirds had type III. Type II EMC developed a mean of 7.6 years after infection, and type III EMC after a mean of 13.7 years following infection.[43] The genetic susceptibility of individual patients to EMC, the duration of HCV infection, and the genotype of particular HCV subspecies may explain why only some patients with HCV develop EMC.[36]

EMC causes small-vessel vasculitis with a predilection for the skin, peripheral nerves, and kidney. The most common manifestation is recurrent crops of palpable purpura on the legs (Fig. 67.4). These lesions may coalesce to form large, painful ulcerations. Other common manifestations are dysesthesias and mononeuritis multiplex caused by vasculitic neuropathy, glomerulonephritis, arthralgias, malaise, and fatigue.[36,38] Some patients develop mesenteric vasculitis, Raynaud's phenomenon, livedo reticularis, or secondary Sjögren's syndrome. Lung and heart disease are uncommon. Some patients with EMC develop a severe medium-vessel vasculitis that is clinically indistinguishable from PAN. Although the clinical pictures of type II and III cryoglobulinemia overlap considerably, only type II is associated with glomerulonephritis.[36]

Most patients with EMC have anemia, an elevated ESR, and liver transaminase elevations.[36] Those with type II usually show an IgM-kappa monoclonal spike. Ninety per cent of patients with EMC vasculitis are hypocomplementemic, with C4 levels characteristically more depressed than C3.[36] Biopsies of petechial lesions in the skin or gastrointestinal tract show leukocytoclastic vasculitis. Patients whose clinical picture resembles PAN have pathology mimicking that disease, i.e. medium-vessel arteritis. Renal biopsies in patients with type II EMC typically show membranoproliferative glomerulonephritis[36,44] (Chapter 79).

The only other 'common' form of vasculitis that causes recurrent palpable purpura of the lower extremities is Henoch–Schönlein purpura, which is principally a disease of children. The diagnosis of cryoglobulinemic vasculitis is established by isolating type II or type III cryoglobulins following refrigeration at 4° for several days and by demonstrating vasculitis pathologically (usually by skin biopsy). EMC is diagnosed if no underlying disease (except hepatitis C) is found.

The treatment of EMC is often unsatisfactory.[36] No form of EMC responds consistently to immunosuppressive drugs, and less than 30% of patients with HCV-associated EMC respond to antiviral therapy. For patients with mild symptoms such as infrequent crops of purpura, no therapy is required. For those with HCV-associated EMC, frequent purpura, and a mild vasculitic neuropathy, alpha-interferon (3×10^6 units 3 times per week) and ribavirin (1000–1200 mg/d) may be effective.[36,45,46] Patients below the age of 60 who do not have HCV genotype 1 (the most common in Americans) are more likely to respond.[36] This regimen eliminates purpura, reduces the cryocrit, normalizes complement levels, and eliminates HCV-RNA in 30–60% of patients. Unfortunately, up to 90% of patients relapse (clinically or serologically) if the therapy is discontinued. For this reason, antiviral therapy is sometimes continued indefinitely (albeit at lower doses). For those with life-threatening vasculities, high-dose prednisone, cyclophosphamide (in doses identical to those used in PAN), and plasmapheresis are recommended. If the vasculitis improves and the immunosuppression can be tapered, then antiviral therapy is added.[36]

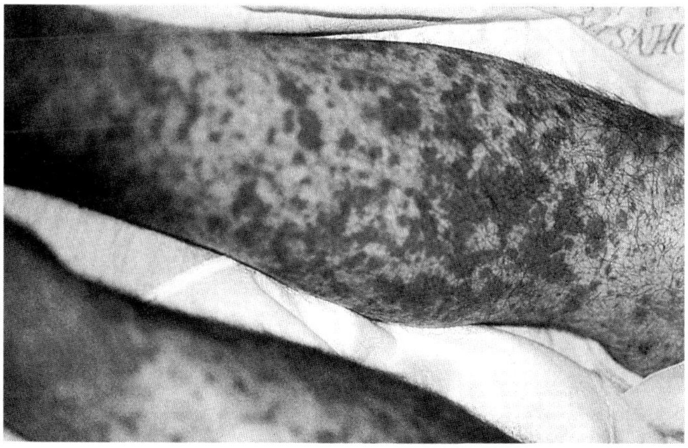

Figure 67.4 Purpura in vasculitis. Palpable purpura in a patient with cryoglobulinemic vasculitis. (See also color plate 67.4.)

THE 'ANCA-ASSOCIATED' VASCULITIDES

In a landmark 1954 paper, Godman and Churg[47] noted similar pathological features among three clinically distinct disease entities: Wegener's granulomatosis (WG), microscopic polyangiitis (MPA), and the Churg–Strauss syndrome (CSS). These diseases, Godman and Churg noted, 'group themselves into a compass, (ranging from) necrotizing and granulomatous processes with angiitis, through mixed forms, to vasculitis without granulomata'. The connections between these three diseases remain incompletely defined, but over the past 15 years WG, MPA, and CSS have become recognized as the cardinal forms of vasculitis associated with antineutrophil cytoplasmic antibodies (ANCA). They are commonly termed ANCA-associated vasculitides (AAV), although several shortcomings of reliance upon serological tests to define this complex group of diseases are now apparent.

The hallmarks of WG, MPA, and CSS are displayed in Table 67.5. Two additional conditions classified as ANCA-associated disorders – necrotizing crescentic glomerulonephritis

CLINICAL PEARLS

Vasculitides associated with antineutrophil cytoplasmic antibodies (ANCA)

- Wegener's granulomatosis (WG), microscopic polyangiitis (MPA), and the Churg–Strauss syndrome (CSS) have become recognized as the types of vasculitis associated with ANCA.
- Shortcomings of reliance upon ANCA to define this group of complex diseases:
  - The role (if any) of ANCA in the pathogenesis of these conditions is not understood.
  - Not all patients with these diseases have a positive test for ANCA.
  - A variety of systemic illnesses, including infections, malignancies and other conditions may be associated with a positive ANCA test, particularly when positive immunofluorescence tests are not confirmed by enzyme immunoassay.
  - Even when ANCA are present, they are unreliable indicators of disease activity.

Hallmarks of Wegener's granulomatosis (WG), microscopic polyangiitis (MPA), and Churg–Strauss syndrome (CSS)			
	WG	MPA	CSS
ANCA positive (%)	80–90%	75%	50%
Typical immunofluorescence/ EIA results	C-ANCA/PR-3	P-ANCA/MPO	P-ANCA/MPO
Upper respiratory tract	Nasal septal perforation Saddle-nose deformity Subglottic stenosis	Mild	Nasal polyps Allergic rhinitis
Lung	Nodules Cavitary lesions	Alveolar hemorrhage	Asthma Fleeting infiltrates
Kidney	NCGN, occasional granulomatous features	NCGN	NCGN (severe renal disease unusual)
Distinguishing feature	Destructive upper airway disease	No granulomatous inflammation	Allergy Eosinophilia

Table 67.5 Hallmarks of Wegener's granulomatosis (WG), microscopic polyangiitis (MPA), and Churg–Strauss syndrome (CSS). (Adapted from Rao JY, Weinberger M, Oddone EZ, et al. The role of antineutrophil cytoplasmic antibody (C-ANCA) testing in the diagnosis of Wegener's granulomatosis. *Ann Intern Med* 1995;123:425.)

(NCGN) and drug-induced AAV – are mentioned only briefly in this chapter. NCGN or 'renal-limited' vasculitis, is often considered a subset of WG, MPA, and CSS because of its similarities to the renal manifestations of those diseases. Drug-induced AAV has been described in association with a variety of medications, particularly propylthiouracil and hydralazine.[48] This disorder is generally self-limited, resolving upon cessation of the offending agent. In many cases of drug-induced AAV, vasculitis is limited to the skin.

Serologic testing for ANCA

Two types of ANCA tests, immunofluorescence (IF) and enzyme immunoassay (EIA), are now in common use. Proper use of the two different ANCA assays requires knowledge of the tests' trade-offs. IF tests are highly operator-dependent, require a high degree of experience for proper interpretation, and are not antigen-specific. On the other hand, IF assays are generally superior to EIA in terms of sensitivity. In contrast to IF assays, EIAs are antigen-specific and demonstrate substantially higher positive predictive values for AAV. One useful strategy for optimizing the utility of ANCA tests, therefore, is to screen patients with potential AAV by IF testing, and then to perform EIAs on patients who test positively.[49]

WG, MPA, and CSS have variable strengths of association with ANCA (Table 67.5). The strength of association for each disease is affected by several factors, including disease activity, disease extent, and intensity of therapy.[50] Even in WG, the disease for which the association with ANCA is the strongest, most series indicate that 10–20% of patients with active, 'disseminated', and untreated disease are ANCA negative.[7] For WG patients with 'limited' WG,[51] defined as the absence of an immediate threat to either the function of a vital organ or the patient's life, 30% or more of patients lack ANCA. In MPA, estimates of ANCA positivity generally approximate 75%.[28] This contrasts with classic PAN, which is generally not considered to be an ANCA-associated condition.[1] Finally, although relatively few data exist regarding the prevalence of ANCA in CSS, several studies have indicated that approximately 50% of such patients are positive for ANCA.[52]

Despite advances in ANCA testing techniques, histopathology remains the cornerstone of diagnosis in AAV (as in other forms of vasculitis). When the diagnosis is unconfirmed, all reasonable attempts to obtain a 'tissue diagnosis' should be pursued. On the other hand, appropriate sites for tissue biopsy are not always evident or readily accessible. Furthermore, even when performed, tissue biopsies are not always diagnostic. When carefully employed and properly interpreted, ANCA assays constitute an important, albeit imperfect, adjunct to diagnosis.

In the following sections, each of the three major forms of AAV is discussed. Treatment strategies for these disorders are discussed together in the final part of this section.

Wegener's granulomatosis

In 1936 a German pathologist, Friedrich Wegener, reported 3 patients in their mid 30s, whose innocuous presentations were those of a 'common cold'.[53] Within 7 months, all had succumbed to systemic inflammatory illnesses that culminated in uremia. Three years later, Wegener provided a more detailed description of this disease, which he referred to as 'a peculiar rhinogenic granuloma with particular involvement of the arterial system and the kidney'.[54]

Godman and Churg introduced the term 'Wegener's granulomatosis' to the English-language literature,[47] and recognized the three pathologic hallmarks: (1) necrotizing granulomas in the upper and/or lower respiratory tract; (2) necrotizing vasculitis affecting arteries or veins; and (3) segmental glomerulonephritis, associated with necrosis and thrombosis of capillary loops, with or without granulomatous lesions. Today, WG is regarded as one of the most common forms of systemic necrotizing vasculitis, with an annual incidence of 8.5 cases/million.[55] Although the disease has a predilection for Caucasians in the USA, WG occurs in all ethnic groups. Pathologic diversity in WG results in a remarkable array of clinical presentations.[56] 'Classic' WG involves the upper respiratory tract, the lungs, and the kidneys, but distinctive (if not diagnostic) features of this disease may also occur in the eye, ear, and other organs. Involvement of tissues as diverse as the prostate gland and meninges has been reported.

The numerous disease manifestations of WG throughout the respiratory tract have long engendered suspicion that the disease results from interactions between an inhaled microbial patho-allergen(s) and a susceptible host. Approximately 90% of patients with WG have nasal involvement.[56] The nasal manifestations of WG include crusting, bleeding, and obstruction. Cartilaginous inflammation may lead to nasal septal perforation and even to collapse of the nasal bridge, a condition known as a 'saddle-nose' deformity (Fig. 67.5). Most patients with nasal (or sinus) disease eventually develop secondary infections of these tissues. Nasal carriage of *S. aureus* has been associated with an increased risk of disease relapse.[57]

Erosive sinus disease is highly characteristic of WG. Among the AAV, only WG is likely to cause destructive lesions of the bony sinuses. Because destructive lesions in WG require time to develop, however, they are not present invariably at the time of diagnosis. The sinus destruction of WG may be mimicked by nonvasculitic disorders such as 'midline granuloma', a T-cell lymphoma, as well as granulomatous infections by acid-fast bacilli and fungi.

Subglottic stenosis, resulting from a peculiar predilection of WG to cause scarring inflammation in the region of the trachea inferior to the vocal cords, is a potentially disabling disease feature. Subglottic involvement is often asymptomatic and may manifest itself only as a subtle hoarseness. However, some patients present with the subacute onset of respiratory stridor. With time, airway scarring occurs, sometimes accompanied by profound tracheal narrowing. Severe cases require tracheostomy. Subglottic stenosis, particularly when associated with scarring and fibrosis, often responds poorly to immunosuppressive therapy. The most effective therapeutic approach to subglottic stenosis in these cases is usually mechanical, i.e. surgical dilatations and laser procedures to enlarge the obstructed airway.[58] Local glucocorticoid injections may also be useful. Pulmonary function tests, particularly flow-volume loops, provide a useful noninvasive means of quantifying both progression of the disease and its response to treatment.

Two principal forms of ear disease, conductive and sensorineural hearing loss, are typical of WG. 'Mixed' hearing loss, the conjoint occurrence of both auditory lesions, is also common. Conductive hearing loss results from granulomatous involvement of the middle ear cavity, most often leading to serous otitis media. In contrast, the mechanism of inner ear disease in WG is poorly understood.[59] WG patients frequently endure multiple courses of antibiotics, myringotomies, and other largely ineffectual interventions before the correct diagnosis is made. Granulomatous inflammation in the middle ear may compress the seventh cranial nerve (which courses through the middle ear cavity), leading to a peripheral facial nerve palsy. Less commonly, vasculitic neuropathy infarcts the nerve at some point during its path through the temporal bone.

WG has two signature ocular lesions: the retro-orbital mass and necrotizing scleritis (Fig. 67.6). Retro-orbital masses, among the most treatment-refractory WG lesions, may lead to proptosis and visual loss through ischemia of the optic nerve. Scleritis, which causes eye pain and an angry, purplish scleral hue, may lead to scleromalacia perforans and visual loss (Chapter 86). Other ocular manifestations of WG include episcleritis, keratitis, uveitis, conjunctivitis, nasolacrimal duct obstruction, and, occasionally, occlusion of the retinal arteries or veins.

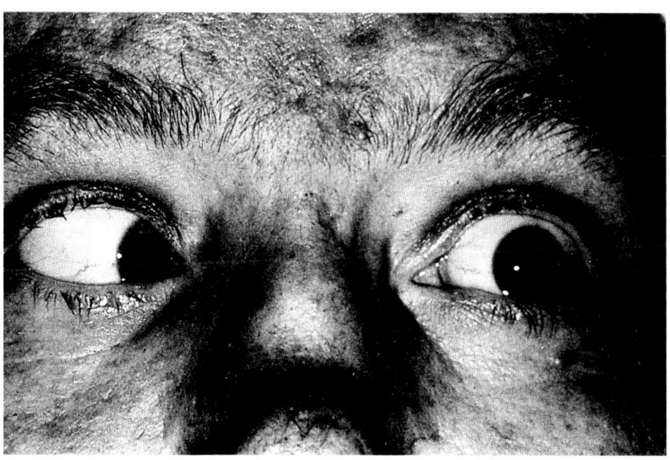

Figure 67.5 Saddle-nose deformity in Wegener's granulomatosis. Saddle-nose deformity and a left sixth cranial nerve lesion (the latter caused by meningeal inflammation) in a patient with Wegener's granulomatosis. (Reproduced with permission from Jinnah H, Dixon A, Brat D, Hellmann D. Chronic meningitis with cranial neuropathies in Wegener's granulomatosis: Case report and review of the literature. *Arthritis Rheum* 1997;40:573.)

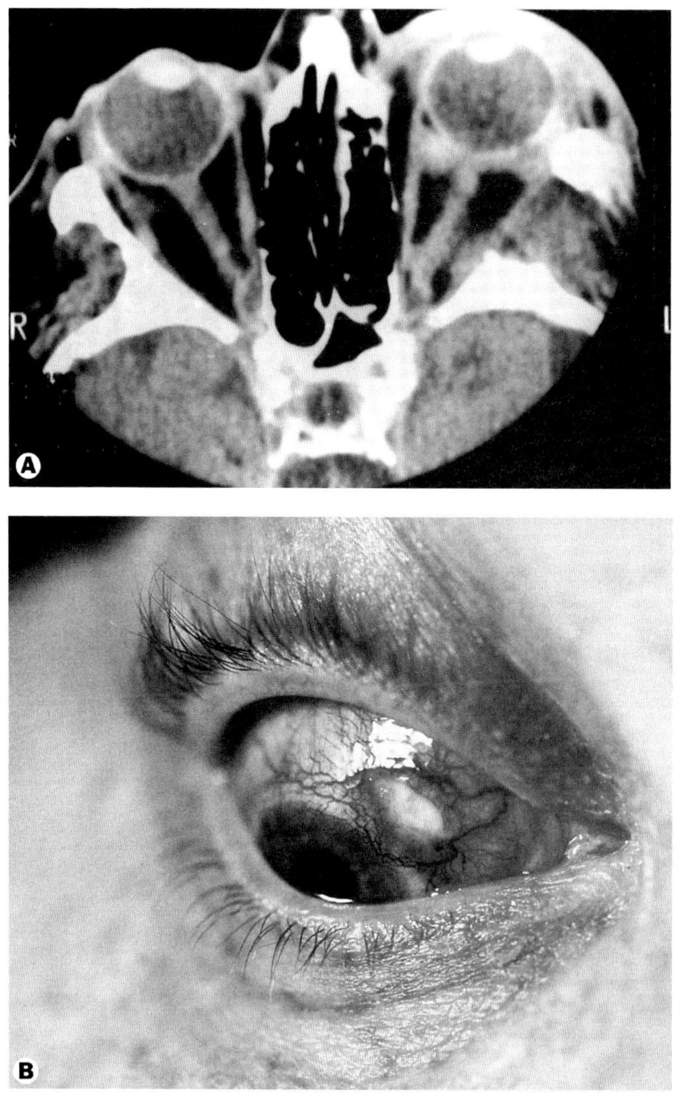

Figure 67.6 Ocular manifestations of Wegener's granulomatosis. The cardinal ocular manifestations of Wegener's granulomatosis: (**A**) bilateral retro-orbital masses, causing proptosis of the left eye; (**B**) necrotizing scleritis. (See also color plate 67.6.)

Although the histological features of pulmonary WG are similar to those found in specimens from other tissues, the full pathologic spectrum may be more apparent in lung biopsy specimens (Fig. 67.7). Both vasculitic and necrotizing granulomatous features, which do not invariably coexist, may be confirmed in lung biopsy specimens. In addition to these two processes, pulmonary WG frequently demonstrates an extensive, nonspecific inflammatory background. The leukocytoclastic vasculitis in the lung may involve arteries, veins, and capillaries, with or without granulomatous features. Vascular necrosis begins as clusters of neutrophils within the blood vessel wall (microabscesses) that degenerate and become surrounded by palisading histiocytes. Coalescence of such neutrophilic microabscesses leads to extensive regions of 'geographic' necrosis. The range of granulomatous inflammation found in WG may include palisading granulomas, scattered giant cells, and poorly-formed granulomas.

The clinical manifestations of pulmonary WG are equally diverse, ranging from asymptomatic lung nodules to fulminant alveolar hemorrhage. The most common radiographic findings are pulmonary infiltrates and nodules. The infiltrates, which may wax and wane, are often misdiagnosed initially as pneumonia. Nodules are usually multiple and bilateral, and often result in cavitation (Fig. 67.8). Hilar and/or mediastinal adenopathy is rare in WG; its presence suggests other diagnoses. Computed tomography is superior to chest radiography in demonstrating the extent of pulmonary disease. The substantial morbidity resulting from opportunistic infections in WG necessitates aggressive measures to exclude infections when WG patients present with new pulmonary lesions, while especially receiving treatment.

Renal involvement is the most ominous clinical manifestation of WG. The typical lesion of WG (indeed, of all forms of AAV) is segmental necrotizing glomerulonephritis, usually associated with the formation of glomerular crescents (Chapter 79). Thrombotic changes in the glomerular capillary loops are among the earliest histologic changes evident in WG. Immunofluorescence studies of renal biopsies indicate few immunoreactants (i.e. scant immunoglobulin or complement deposition). Consequently, WG and the other AAV are classified as 'pauci-immune' glomerulonephritis. Granulomatous changes, although frequently present, are identified only rarely in renal biopsies. The clinical presentation of renal disease in WG is that of rapidly progressive glomerulonephritis: hematuria, red blood cell casts, proteinuria (usually non-nephrotic), and progressive renal insufficiency. Without appropriate therapy, end-stage renal disease ensues within days to weeks. A commonly observed clinical occurrence is acceleration of the overall disease process once renal involvement is evident.

Less classic but nevertheless common features in WG are involvement of the musculoskeletal system, skin, and nervous system. Approximately half of all patients with WG are rheuma-

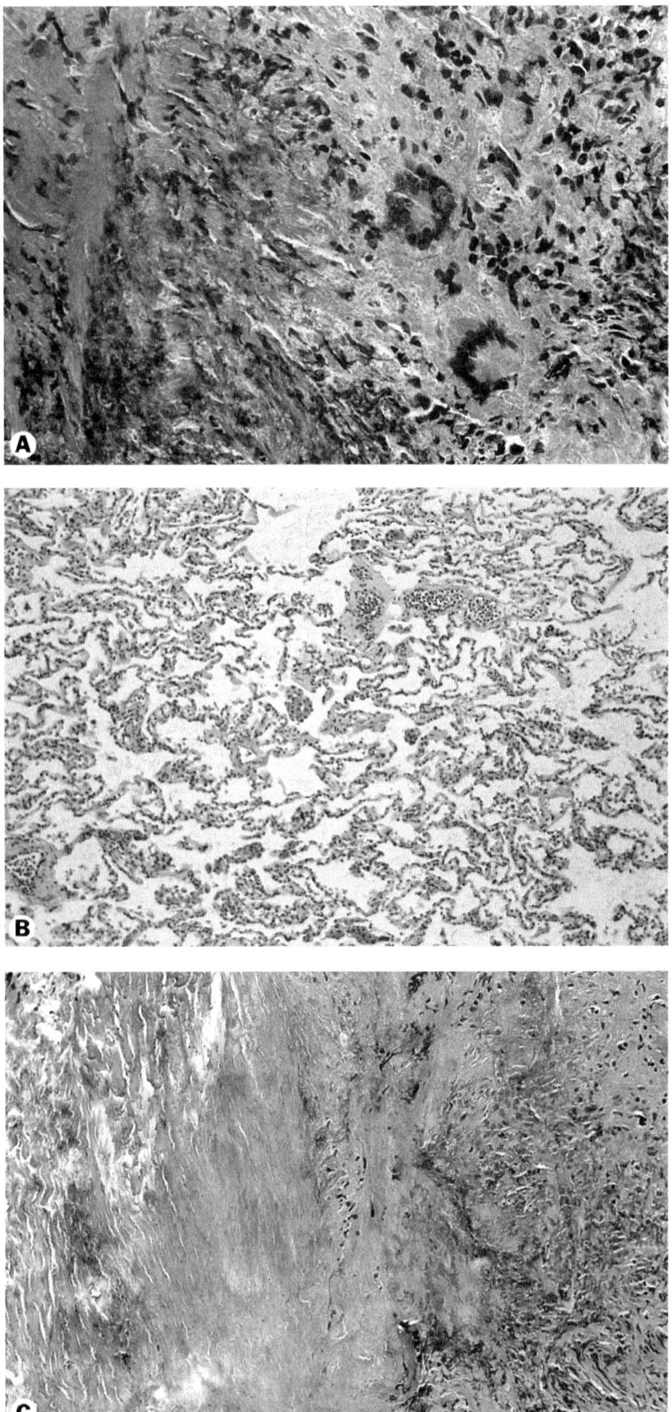

Figure 67.7 Histopathology of Wegener's granulomatosis. The pathologic features of Wegener's granulomatosis: (**A**) Langerhans giant cells and palisading granulomatous inflammation; (**B**) small-vessel vasculitis and fibrinoid necrosis of the lung; (**C**) 'geographic' necrosis. (See also color plate 67.7.)

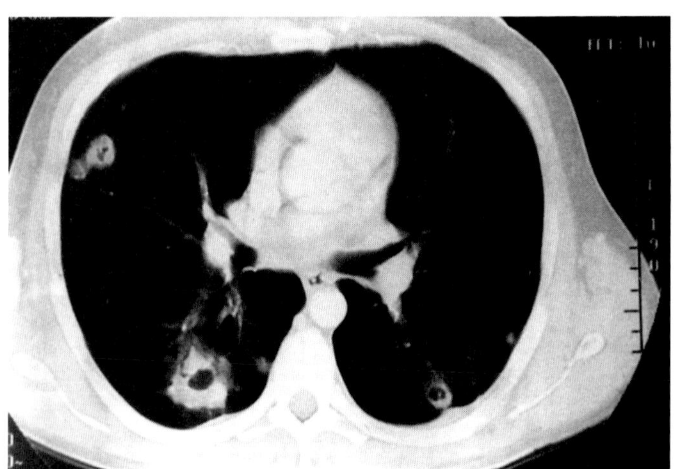

Figure 67.8 Chest CT abnormalities in Wegener's granulomatosis. Multiple, bilateral pulmonary nodules, several of which have cavitated.

toid factor positive, and rheumatoid arthritis (RA) is a common misdiagnosis early in the disease course when nonspecific arthralgias and arthritis may occur. Unlike RA, however, the arthritis of WG tends to involve large joints and to spare the small joints of the hands. Splinter hemorrhages, digital ischemia, and digital gangrene resulting from inflammation in large digital arteries are under-appreciated as manifestations of WG. Skin lesions in WG include the full panoply of lesions associated with cutaneous vasculitis (see Hypersensitivity vasculitis). Although involvement of the brain parenchyma with WG has been reported, meningeal inflammation presenting as excruciating headaches and cranial neuropathies are more common central nervous system manifestations of this disease. Finally, devastating mononeuritis multiplex may accompany WG, but this feature is less characteristic of WG than of the other major forms of AAV – MPA and CSS.

The clinical course of WG is marked by a tendency to recur following tapering or cessation of treatment. In a series from the National Institutes of Health, fewer than 40% of the patients achieved durable remissions following their initial courses of therapy with daily cyclophosphamide and corticosteroids.[56] The requirement for repeated administration of the potentially toxic treatments in WG (discussed below) leads to substantial long-term morbidity.[56,60] The greatest current challenge in the management of WG is the absence of a well-tolerated, effective medication for the maintenance of disease remission.

Microscopic polyangiitis

As noted earlier in this chapter, Davson[13] and colleagues drew the first distinction between classic PAN described by Kussmaul and Maier[12] and the disorder known today as MPA. This distinction was re-emphasized by the 1994 Chapel Hill Consensus Conference on the nomenclature of vasculitides,[1] which defined MPA as a process: (1) involving necrotizing vasculitis with few or no immune deposits; (2) affecting small blood vessels (capillaries, venules, or arterioles) as well as (perhaps) medium-sized arteries; and (3) demonstrating a tropism for the kidneys (glomerulonephritis) and lungs (pulmonary capillaritis). Microscopic poly*angiitis* (as opposed to poly*arteritis*) is the preferred term for this disorder, because the disease may affect arterioles, capillaries, venules, veins, and arteries in addition to arteries. Table 67.6 compares the principal features of MPA to those of classic PAN.

Distinguishing between two forms of vasculitis primarily on the basis of size of the involved blood vessels inevitably creates 'exceptions', because nature rarely acknowledges the artificial boundaries imposed by such schemes.[61] In the case of MPA and PAN, however, the distinction may be more than semantic: whereas approximately half of all patients with PAN respond well to corticosteroids alone, patients with MPA generally require treatment with a cytotoxic agent in addition to corticosteroids to control their disease.[28]

As with WG, a dominant feature of MPA is necrotizing glomerulonephritis with crescent formation (Fig. 67.9), which occurs in nearly 80% of patients.[67] In one study of 34 MPA patients with glomerulonephritis, the percentage of patients with functioning kidneys was only 55% and the actuarial survival only 65% at 5 years of follow-up, despite the use of corticosteroids, cytotoxic agents, and plasma exchange in various combinations.[63] Successful treatment of glomerulonephritis associated with AAV depends upon early recognition. Consequently, scrutiny of the urine sediment for red blood cells and casts is an essential early step in the evaluation of patients with possible MPA.

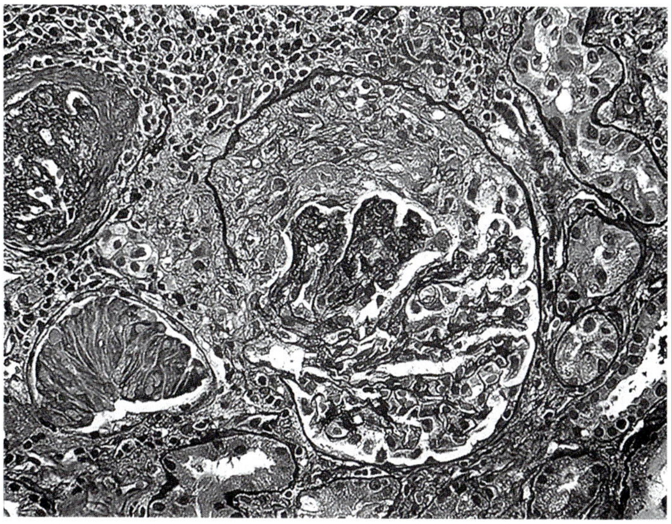

Figure 67.9 Crescentic glomerulonephritis in microscopic polyangiitis. Glomerular crescent in a patient with rapidly progressive glomerulonephritis secondary to microscopic polyangiitis. (See also color plate 67.9.)

Table 67.6 Features of MPA versus classic PAN.

Features of MPA versus classic PAN

Feature	Microscopic polyangiitis	Classic polyarteritis nodosa
Granulomas	No	No
Vessel size	Small (and medium)	Medium
Renovascular hypertension	No	Yes
Rapidly progressive glomerulonephritis	Yes	No
Lung involvement	Alveolar hemorrhage	No
Mononeuritis multiplex	Yes	Yes
ANCA positive	pANCA (anti-myeloperoxidase)	Rare
Hepatitis B association	No	Sometimes (10%)
Vascular aneurysms	Occasionally	Commonly

MPA is also commonly implicated in pulmonary–renal syndromes. Although Goodpasture syndrome (or, more precisely, anti-glomerular basement membrane disease) is the prototype of alveolar hemorrhage/glomerulonephritis syndromes (see Chapter 84), the AAV in aggregate constitute a far more common cause of this presentation.[64] Pulmonary capillaritis, most typical of MPA, may lead rapidly to life-threatening hemorrhage from the lungs, requiring prompt, aggressive treatment. Approximately 12% of patients with MPA develop alveolar hemorrhage.[62]

In the MPA series of Guillevin et al,[62] renal manifestations (79%), weight loss (73%), mononeuritis multiplex (58%), and fever (55%) were the most common disease manifestations. Upper respiratory tract symptoms in MPA are much milder than those associated with WG. MPA is not associated with erosion of the bony sinuses, scarring of the subglottic region, or saddle-nose deformities. Many experts regard the occurrence of any significant upper respiratory tract involvement (aside from the allergic rhinitis and nasal polyps that occur in CSS; see below) as an indication of WG. The essential difference between MPA and WG, however, is the absence of granulomatous inflammation in MPA.

The Churg–Strauss syndrome

In 1951, Churg and Strauss reported a series of 13 patients with 'periarteritis nodosa' who demonstrated, in addition to severe asthma, an unusual constellation of symptoms: 'fever ... hypereosinophilia, symptoms of cardiac failure, renal damage, and peripheral neuropathy, resulting from vascular embarrassment in various systems of organs'.[65] The investigators believed the syndrome to represent a new disease entity, which they termed 'allergic angiitis and allergic granulomatosis'. Three histologic criteria for this disorder, subsequently known as the Churg–Strauss syndrome (CSS), were specified: (1) presence of necrotizing vasculitis; (2) tissue infiltration by eosinophils; and (3) extravascular granulomas.[65] Finding all three criteria in one patient (autopsy series excepted) is often difficult.

The 1990 American College of Rheumatology criteria for the classification of CSS[66] are intended to distinguish patients with CSS from those with other vasculitic disorders (Table 67.7). The presence of four or more of the six disease criteria yielded a sensitivity and specificity of 85% and 99.7% for CSS, respectively. The Chapel Hill Consensus Conference defined CSS as the presence of eosinophil-rich, granulomatous inflammation involving the respiratory tract, with necrotizing vasculitis of small to medium-sized vessels, associated with asthma and eosinophilia.[1]

In addition to the other vasculitides, CSS must be distinguished from a group of hypereosinophilic disorders: Löffler syndrome, eosinophilic gastroenteritis, chronic eosinophilic pneumonia, the hypereosinophilic syndrome (HES), and eosinophilic leukemia.[67] Differentiating CSS from HES may be the biggest challenge. HES may cause even higher elevations of the peripheral eosinophil count than CSS (counts in excess of 100×10^9/l are not unusual in HES). In addition, whereas the eosinophilia of CSS responds dramatically to treatment with corticosteroids, HES is characteristically refractory to this measure.

Greater than 90% of CSS patients have histories of asthma. Typically the asthma is either of new onset or constitutes a significant exacerbation of long-standing disease. Upon encroachment of the vasculitis phase of CSS, patients' asthma may improve substantially, even before therapy for vasculitis is begun. Following successful treatment of the vasculitic phase, however, glucocorticoid-dependent asthma persists in many patients.

Chest radiographs are normal in the majority of CSS patients. Radiographic abnormalities are usually limited to fleeting pulmonary infiltrates, detected in one third of patients. Pulmonary hemorrhage is unusual, and cavitary lesions should suggest the alternative diagnosis of WG. The pathological features of lung disease in CSS vary according to the disease phase: in the pro-

CLINICAL PEARLS

Three phases of the Churg–Strauss syndrome (CSS)

- Prodromal phase, characterized by the presence of allergic disease (typically asthma or allergic rhinitis), which may last from months to many years.
- Eosinophilia/tissue infiltration phase, in which remarkably high peripheral eosinophilia may occur and tissue infiltration by eosinophils is observed in the lung, gastrointestinal tract, and other tissues.
- Vasculitic phase, in which systemic necrotizing vasculitis afflicts a wide range of organs, ranging from the heart and lungs to peripheral nerves and skin.

American College of Rheumatology classification criteria for Churg–Strauss syndrome

Criterion	Definition
Asthma	History of wheezing or diffuse high-pitched rales on expiration
Eosinophilia	Eosinophilia >10% on white blood cell differential count
Mononeuropathy or polyneuropathy	Development of mononeuropathy, multiple mononeuropathies, or polyneuropathy (i.e. stocking/glove distribution)
Pulmonary infiltrates, nonfixed	Migratory or transitory pulmonary infiltrates on radiographs
Paranasal sinus abnormality	History of acute or chronic paranasal sinus pain or tenderness, or radiographic opacification of the paranasal sinuses
Extravascular eosinophils	Biopsy including artery, arteriole, or venule, showing accumulations of eosinophils in extravascular areas

Table 67.7 American College of Rheumatology classification criteria for Churg–Strauss syndrome. (From Masi A, Hunder G, Lie J, et al. The American College of Rheumatology 1990 criteria for the classification of Churg–Strauss syndrome (allergic granulomatosis and angiitis). *Arthritis Rheum* 1990;33:1094.)

dromal phase, there is extensive eosinophilic infiltration of the alveoli and interstitium; during the vasculitic phase, necrotizing vasculitis and granulomas are evident. Upper airway disease in CSS usually takes the form of nasal polyps or allergic rhinitis. A high percentage of patients have histories of nasal polypectomies, often long before the diagnosis is considered. Although pansinusitis occurs frequently, destructive upper airway disease is not characteristic of CSS.

In contrast to WG, mononeuritis multiplex occurs with a remarkable frequency in CSS. This potentially disabling complication was evident in 74 of the 96 patients (77%) in one series.[52] Cardiac involvement (usually congestive heart failure) also occurs with a disproportionate frequency in CSS,[52] and cardiac complications are a common mode of death in CSS. Renal disease in CSS has been described as less common and less malignant compared to that associated with other AAV. When it occurs, histopathological findings are often indistinguishable from those of WG, MPA, and NCGN.[68]

In recent years, associations between the use of leukotriene antagonists and CSS have been reported.[69,70] It is possible, however, that the reduction in glucocorticoid dose afforded by these effective therapies for asthma 'unmasked' forme frustes of CSS. The true relationship between these medications and CSS requires further investigation.

Although clinical remissions may be obtained in more than 90% of patients with CSS,[52] disease recurrences are common upon cessation of therapy (as with other AAVs). In the largest series reported to date, flares were detected in more than 25% of the patients.[52] In most cases, relapses were heralded by the return of eosinophilia.

Treatment of the ANCA-associated vasculitides

Patients with WG, MPA, or CSS whose symptoms constitute immediate threats to either the function of vital organs or to the patient's life urgently require treatment with both a cytotoxic agent (usually cyclophosphamide) and high doses of glucocorticoids. 'Limited' forms of WG may respond to the combination of glucocorticoids and methotrexate, thus sparing patients the potential side-effects of cyclophosphamide. Increasing experience with methotrexate and prednisone has demonstrated, however, that durable remissions of WG with this regimen are rare, and smoldering or recurrent disease that reactivates upon taper of the medications is the rule.[71] A substantial number of patients with CSS achieve satisfactory responses with glucocorticoids alone, and monotherapy is a reasonable first approach for many of these patients. However, patients with evidence of rapidly progressive glomerulonephritis or symptoms of mononeuritis multiplex should be treated promptly with both cyclophosphamide and glucocorticoids to halt these devastating disease manifestations.

Practice regarding the use of either daily or intermittent (e.g. monthly intravenous) cyclophosphamide varies from center to center. In WG, daily cyclophosphamide is more likely to result in durable remissions,[72] but is also associated with a greater number of side-effects. Regardless of the route by which cyclophosphamide is administered, the treatment has potential hazards; careful monitoring, particularly of the white cell count, is essential. The induction of neutropenia is not required to achieve a therapeutic effect in AAV, and avoidance of this side-effect is highly desirable as a strategy to prevent opportunistic infections. Cyclophosphamide should be withheld temporarily if the WBC count falls below $4.0 \times 10^6/\mu l$. The multitude of side-effects associated with long-term use of cyclophosphamide has inspired the use of shorter courses of induction treatment (e.g. 3–6 months), followed by longer-term maintenance of remission with either azathioprine[73] or methotrexate.[74]

A wide array of other therapies, e.g. plasmapheresis or intravenous immunoglobulin, has been employed in small numbers of patients, but insufficient data exist to judge their efficacy. The use of alpha-interferon in the treatment of CSS appears promising,[75] but larger studies are required. The era of anticytokine therapy in AAV has begun.[71] For example, a multicenter trial of etanercept, a soluble tumor necrosis factor inhibitor, is under way in the USA.

THERAPEUTIC PRINCIPLES

Treatment of the ANCA-associated vasculitides

- The presence of symptoms that constitute immediate threats to either function of vital organs or to survival requires urgent treatment with both a cytotoxic agent and high doses of glucocorticoids.
- In patients with severe disease, cyclophosphamide is the cytotoxic drug of choice.
- Limited forms of WG may respond to a combination of glucocorticoids and methotrexate, but durable remissions with this regimen are rare.
- In CSS patients without serious organ involvement, treatment with glucocorticoids is a reasonable first approach. However, the presence of glomerulonephritis or mononeuritis multiplex requires immediate treatment with cyclophosphamide and glucocorticoids.

HYPERSENSITIVITY VASCULITIS

The complexity of vasculitis nomenclature is nowhere more evident than in discussions of vasculitis involving the skin. The proliferation of names for this clinical entity is principally due to the fact that, compared to the relatively limited number of disorders that cause large- or medium-vessel arteritis, a host of disorders may be associated with small-vessel vasculitis of the skin. These disorders include both primary vasculitides and secondary causes of vasculitic inflammation. Whereas some of these conditions cause only cutaneous vasculitis, others may also cause organ- or life-threatening involvement of vital organs, such as the lungs or kidney. This section focuses on types of small-vessel vasculitis confined to the skin. Other prominent causes of cutaneous vasculitis, e.g. cryoglobulinemia, Henoch–Schönlein purpura, urticarial vasculitis, the ANCA-associated disorders, and cutaneous polyarteritis nodosa (PAN), are discussed separately in other sections of this chapter.

In 1952, in the first classification scheme ever devised for the vasculitides, Zeek[76] coined the term 'hypersensitivity vasculitis'. The purpose of this term was to distinguish a form of necrotizing arteritis that involved only small blood vessels from PAN, which has a predilection for larger vessels. The word 'hypersensitivity' stemmed from animal models of vasculitis induced by the administration of horse serum, sulfonamides, and other drugs.

These vasculitis models – attempts to develop an animal model of PAN – differed from PAN in their prominent cutaneous involvement, their involvement of the venous as well as the arteriel circulation, and their involvement of 'small' blood vessels, i.e. arterioles, venules, and capillaries. Moreover, in contrast to PAN, all of the lesions in hypersensitivity vasculitis tended to occur in 'crops', and thus were approximately the same age. Finally, in contrast to the characteristically unrelenting nature of PAN, hypersensitivity vasculitis was self-limited.

Since Zeek's first description of hypersensitivity vasculitis, the term has been narrowed to denote small-vessel vasculitis confined principally to the skin and not associated with any other primary vasculitis (e.g. Henoch–Schönlein purpura, Wegener's granulomatosis, or cryoglobulinemia). The identification of an inciting antigen for the vasculitis is not a prerequisite to the diagnosis, because no such provocation is found in many patients who fit the clinical and pathological picture of the disease.[77]

The ACR formulated criteria for the classification of hypersensitivity vasculitis included: (1) age of onset greater than 16 years; (2) medication at disease onset; (3) palpable purpura; (4) maculopapular rash; and (5) biopsy of arteriole or venule showing granulocytes in a perivascular or extravascular location[78]. The presence of three of five criteria resulted in sensitivity of 71% and specificity of 84%.[78]

The 1994 Chapel Hill Consensus Conference on nomenclature of the vasculitides proposed an alternative term for hypersensitivity vasculitis – 'cutaneous leukocytoclastic angiitis' – because of the frequent failure to identify a precipitant (no manifest cause of 'hypersensitivity'). This designation is also problematical, however, because although most lesional skin biopsies demonstrate a neutrophil predominance, others show a primarily lymphocytic infiltration. Moreover, these two histopathological patterns do not appear to represent different evolutionary stages of the same process, but rather (at a minimum) two distinct processes, underscoring the difficulty of using a single term to define all patients with this clinical phenotype.

Regardless of the name, certain similarities exist among patients who present with symptoms and signs of cutaneous vasculitis. First, the lesions typically occur first in dependent regions, i.e. the lower extremities or buttocks. Second, the lesions may be asymptomatic, but are usually accompanied by a burning or tingling sensation. A wide array of skin lesions may occur, including palpable purpura, papules, urticaria/angioedema, erythema multiforme, vesicles, pustules, ulcers, and necrosis. The simultaneous occurrence of livedo reticularis usually indicates the involvement of medium-sized arteries as well. Most cases with a clearly identified precipitant resolve over a period over 1–4 weeks, often with some residual hyperpigmentation or (in the case of ulcerated lesions) scars. A subset of patients, however, have recurrent disease that remains confined to the skin and requires prolonged therapy.

The pleiomorphic lesions of cutaneous vasculitis and the large number of mimics of vasculitis make confirmation of the diagnosis by skin biopsy essential. Biopsy of an active lesion (<48 hours old, if possible) usually demonstrates leukocytoclastic vasculitis of the postcapillary venules (Fig. 67.10). Immunofluorescence shows variable quantities of immunoglobulin and complement deposition, with a diagnostic pattern. The performance of immunofluorescence studies, however, is an important (and often neglected) part of the workup, critical for the exclusion of Henoch–Schönlein purpura, urticarial vasculitis, and cryoglobulinemia. The workup for a patient with possible HSV includes a number of other laboratory studies to exclude internal organ involvement and to differentiate from other diseases (Table 67.8).

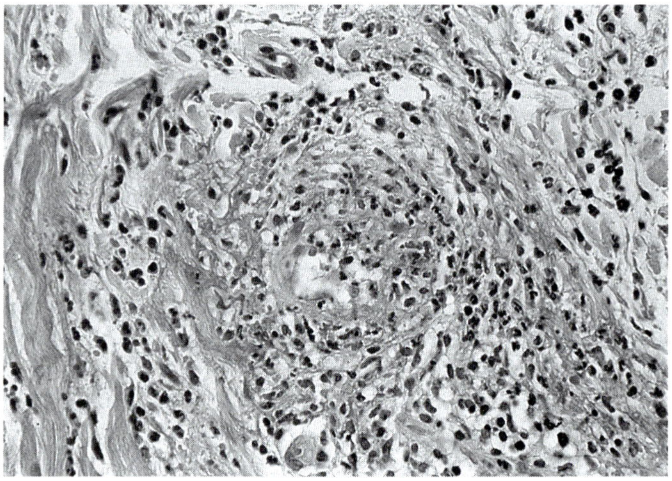

Figure 67.10 Histopathology of hypersensitivity vasculitis. Necrotizing vasculitis of a small cutaneous vessel, with fibrinoid necrosis. (See also color plate 67.10.)

Treatment strategies for hypersensitivity vasculitis are largely empiric. The type, intensity, and duration of therapy are based on the degree of disease severity in an individual patient. For cases in which a precipitant can be identified, removal of the offending agent usually leads to resolution of hypersensitivity vasculitis within days to weeks. Mild cases may be treated simply with leg elevation and the administration of nonsteroidal anti-inflammatory drugs (and/or H_1 antihistamines). Colchicine, hydroxychloroquine, or dapsone may be tried for persistent disease that does not lead to cutaneous gangrene. For refractory or more severe disease, immunosuppressive agents may be indicated, generally beginning with glucocorticoids. Failure of the

Workup for patient with possible cutaneous vasculitis
Skin biopsy with immunofluorescence
Complete blood count
Serum creatinine
Liver transaminases
Serum and urine electrolytes
Urinalysis with microscopy
Chest radiograph
Antinuclear antibody assay
Serum complement levels
Antineutrophil cytoplasmic antibodies
Cryoglobulins
Hepatitis C antibody
ESR

Table 67.8 Workup for patient with possible cutaneous vasculitis.

patient to tolerate a steroid taper over some weeks or the requirement for excessive glucocorticoids dictates the use of an additional immunosuppressive agent. Azathioprine is commonly used for this purpose.[79]

HENOCH–SCHÖNLEIN PURPURA

Henoch–Schönlein purpura (HSP) is a distinct form of small-vessel vasculitis characterized by nonthrombocytopenic purpura, arthritis, abdominal pain, and renal disease.[80–82] The histopathologic findings are those of a leukocytoclastic vasculitis with IgA deposition. HSP can develop at any age, but occurs most frequently in children. Indeed, HSP is the most common form of vasculitis in children.[81] The mean age of children with HSP is 5.9 years, and 93% of affected children are less than 9 years old.[81] The disease often remits spontaneously but sometimes causes life-threatening or chronic complications, most notably gastrointestinal hemorrhage (especially in children) and nephritis (especially in adults). Although the cause is unknown, an infectious trigger is suggested by the fact that two thirds of patients experience an acute, virus-like, upper respiratory illness an average of 10 days before the onset of HSP, and by the seasonal variation of the disease.[81] The central role of IgA in the pathogenesis of HSP is emphasized by the demonstration that most patients have increased serum IgA levels, IgA-containing circulating immune complexes, and IgA deposition in inflamed blood vessels.[81]

Typically, patients present with the acute onset of fever, palpable purpura on the lower extremities and buttocks, abdominal pain, arthritis, and hematuria (Table 67.9). The purpura tends to be extensive, producing lesions too numerous to count. Although the purpura is most extensive on the legs and buttocks, it may involve the arms and, very infrequently, the trunk. In some patients, the cutaneous involvement takes the form of maculopapular lesions, blisters, and ulcers.[81] The abdominal pain is often colicky and may worsen after eating (i.e. intestinal angina). Some patients experience nausea, vomiting, and upper or lower gastrointestinal bleeding. Joint disease manifests as arthralgias or arthritis in large joints, especially the knees and ankles, and to a lesser degree, the wrists and elbows. Migratory patterns can be seen.

The clinical hallmark of nephritis in HSP is hematuria, which is usually microscopic. Proteinuria almost never occurs in the absence of hematuria. Unlike gastrointestinal disease and arthritis, which occasionally precede the onset of purpura, nephritis almost always follows the appearance of skin disease. Other organs are rarely involved, but pulmonary involvement can be manifested by hemoptysis, and central nervous system involvement can result in subarachnoid or intracerebral bleeding. With the exception of renal disease, HSP is self-limited, lasting an average of 4 weeks (range, 3 days – 2 years).[81]

The manifestations of HSP vary with age.[81] Among children with HSP, infants have milder disease. Children under the age of 2 are less likely than older children to develop nephritis or abdominal complications. As a group, children differ from adults with HSP in having more frequent gastrointestinal symptoms and less frequent renal disease.[81,83] Gastrointestinal involvement in children can cause intussusception, which rarely occurs in adults. Renal disease in adults (affecting 50–85%) is also more likely to lead to renal insufficiency compared to children.[81]

Routine blood tests show few abnormalities other than a mild leukocytosis. The ESR is elevated only in about a third of patients. Urinalysis reveals hematuria, proteinuria, and red cell casts, but the serum creatinine is usually normal. Approximately 60% of patients have an elevated serum IgA.[81] Although there are two subclasses of IgA, HSP is associated with increases only in IgA_1.[81] Serum complement levels are usually normal. Assays for IgG ANCA are negative, but a few patients have positive tests for IgA ANCA.[81]

Leukocytoclastic vasculitis is the dominant finding in most affected organs, including the skin and gut. Deposition of IgA can be demonstrated in most lesional skin biopsies. Renal lesions range from minimal change disease to focal or diffuse proliferative glomerulonephritis with crescents. Immunofluorescence studies characteristically demonstrate IgA deposition in the mesangium.

Classification criteria for HSP have been established by the ACR to help differentiate this disease from other vasculitides.[84] The differential diagnosis of HSP includes other disorders that cause leukocytoclastic vasculitis. Cryoglobulinemia shares the predilection of HSP for producing purpura, hematuria, and abdominal pain. Cryoglobulinemia is more likely than HSP to recur chronically. Tests for cryoglobulin and HCV help to distinguish the two conditions, and the finding of IgA deposition within lesional biopsies strongly favors HSP. Hypersensitivity vasculitis is less likely than HSP to cause hematuria or gastrointestinal findings.[82] Unlike the ANCA-associated vasculitides (AAV), which can also produce purpura, hematuria, and arthritis, HSP seldom affects the lungs. Patients with AAV also differ from those with HSP in that the ANCA associated with those diseases are typically IgG and the glomerulonephritis is pauci-immune, not associated with substantial IgA deposition. Infrequently, bacterial endocarditis and other infections can produce purpura and hematuria that resemble HSP. The purpura associated with thrombocytopenia is usually not palpable.

Treatment of HSP has not been studied extensively. Most patients, especially children, have a self-limited disease course.

Clinical features in 100 children with HSP

Feature	Percentage
Purpura	100
Arthritis	82
Abdominal pain	63
Gastrointestinal bleeding:	33
• occult bleeding	23
• gross bleeding	10
Nephritis:	
• hematuria	40
• gross hematuria	7
• proteinuria	25
• nephrotic syndrome	3
Miscellaneous:	
• orchitis	5 (9% of boys)
• duodenal obstructions	1
Recurrence of symptoms	33

Table 67.9 Clinical features in 100 children with HSP. (From Saulsbury F. Henoch–Schonlein purpura in children. *Medicine* 1999;78:395.)

Nonsteroidal anti-inflammatory drugs may alleviate arthralgias but can aggravate gastrointestinal symptoms and should be avoided in any patient with renal disease. Although glucocorticoids have not been evaluated rigorously in HSP, they appear to ameliorate joint and gastrointestinal symptoms.[81] Glucocorticoids do not appear to improve the rash, however, and their effectiveness in renal disease is controversial.[81] Uncontrolled trials suggest that high-dose methylprednisolone followed by oral prednisone or high-dose prednisone combined with azathioprine or cyclophosphamide may help patients with severe nephritis (i.e. nephrotic syndrome and >50% crescents).[81] Chronic renal failure is rare except in adults with more than 50% crescents on renal biopsy.

BEHÇET'S DISEASE

The triad of recurrent mouth ulcers, genital ulcers, and eye inflammation was first recognized as a distinct syndrome in 1937 by the Turkish dermatologist, Dr Hulusi Behçet.[85] In addition to these manifestations Behçet's disease also affects different organ systems.[86,87] Most of the tissue damage in Behçet's disease results from vasculitis. Although Behçet's disease most commonly affects small and medium arteries, it may involve larger arteries and has a proclivity – unusual among the vasculitides – to involve veins as well as arteries. The cause is unknown. Most patients are in their 20s or 30s at disease onset. Behçet's disease is rare in North America, where it affects only 1 out of 500 000 people, but is 100 times more common along the ancient Silk Route, which includes Greece, Turkey, Saudi Arabia, Iran, Korea, China, and Japan.[86] Genetic factors also affect susceptibility to the disease, especially in Asia where up to 80% of patients have the HLA-B51 allele.[88]

The diagnosis of Behçet's disease rests upon a set of established criteria (Table 67.10): no single clinical or laboratory feature is pathognomonic.[86] The diagnosis is untenable in the absence of recurrent aphthous ulcers of the mouth (Fig. 67.11). The mouth ulcers usually number 2–10 and can affect the tongue, buccal mucosa, gums, and pharynx.[86,87] The oral ulcers can cause such severe odynophagia that some patients lose weight and become dehydrated. Most patients also experience intermittent, painful genital ulcers. Ocular disease most commonly presents as anterior or posterior uveitis. The anterior uveitis of Behçet's disease may be so intense that pus in the anterior chamber produces a white meniscus visible to the naked eye (called hypopyon). Visual loss commonly causes disability in Behçet's disease. Skin lesions are variable (Table 67.10): erythema nodosum is most typical. The phenomenon of pathergy – the development of pustules at the sites of sterile needle pricks – occurs rarely except in Turks.[86]

Manifestations of Behçet's disease are not limited to those encompassed by the diagnostic criteria. For example, meningoencephalitis, which produces recurrent 'sterile meningitis' with fever and encephalopathy, rivals uveitis as the most common cause of permanent disability. Strokes may also complicate Behçet's disease. Additional features seen in some patients include peripheral arthritis (usually nondeforming, oligoarticular, involving large joints in an asymmetrical pattern), sacroiliitis,

Criteria for the diagnosis of Behçet's disease

Finding	Definition
Recurrent oral ulceration	Minor aphthous, major aphthous, or herpetiform ulcers observed by the physician or patient, which have recurred at least three times over a 12-month period
Recurrent genital ulceration	Aphthous ulceration or scarring observed by the physician or patient
Eye lesions	Anterior uveitis, posterior uveitis, or cells in the vitreous on slit-lamp examination; or retinal vasculitis detected by an ophthalmologist
Skin lesions	Erythema nodosum observed by the physician or patient, pseudofolliculitis, or papulopustular lesions; or acneiform nodules observed by the physician in a postadolescent patient who is not receiving corticosteroids
Positive pathergy test	Test interpreted as positive by the physician at 24–48 hours

The criteria were drawn up by the International Study Group for Behçet's disease.[86] For the diagnosis to be made, a patient must have recurrent oral ulceration plus at least two of the other findings in the absence of other clinical explanations.

Table 67.10 Criteria for the diagnosis of Behçet's disease.

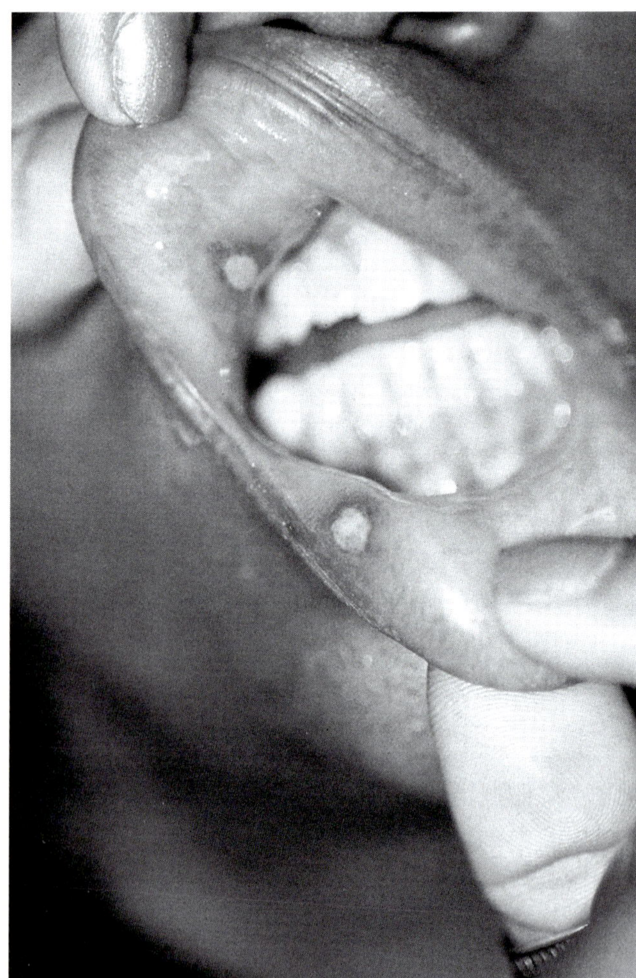

Figure 67.11 Aphthous oral ulcers in a patient with Behçet's disease. (See also color plate 67.11.)

thrombophlebitis (often migratory), gastrointestinal disease (mimicking Crohn's disease), epididymitis, and large artery vasculitis.[86,87,89]

Laboratory tests during active disease usually show mild leukocytosis, thrombocytosis, and an elevated erythrocyte sedimentation rate.[86] The cerebrospinal fluid (CSF) of patients with meningoencephalitis shows a lymphocytosis and elevated protein. Biopsies of the ulcers in the mouth, genital area, or colon show ulcerations and infiltration with mononuclear cells.[86] Granulomas are not seen, a feature that helps to distinguish Behçet's disease of the bowel from Crohn's disease. Biopsies in other affected organs usually reveal vasculitis.

Treatment depends on the type and severity of the disease.[86] Colchicine is sometimes effective for mild oral and genital ulcers. Severe disease in any organ system almost always requires high doses of prednisone (e.g. 1 mg/kg per day). Chlorambucil is useful for the most severe forms of uveitis or meningoencephalitis. Azathioprine, cyclosporine, methotrexate, alpha-interferon, and pentoxifylline have been reported to be effective in some patients.[86,89–92] Of these latter agents, only azathioprine has been studied in large clinical trials. Since disease activity in Behçet's disease tends to remit and relapse, drug therapy is slowly tapered once the patient improves.

BUERGER'S DISEASE

In 1908, Dr Leo Buerger reported pathological studies on the blood vessels obtained from 11 amputated lower extremities of patients with a disorder he termed 'thrombo-angiitis obliterans'.[93] Buerger wrote that the disorder usually occurred in young adults between the ages of 25 and 40, and was characterized by a thrombotic process in the arteries and veins, followed by organization and re-canalization. Portions above and below the diseased segment appear normal.

Buerger proceeded to describe the typical presentation and evolution of this disorder, from the onset of 'indefinite pains in the foot, in the calf of the leg, or in the toes, and particularly of a sense of numbness or coldness whenever the weather is unfavorable'. The initially nonspecific symptoms of Buerger's disease sometimes suggest a primary neuropathic process. Buerger observed that 'Some of these cases give the typical symptoms of intermittent claudication ...'. Upon the development of critical limb ischemia by the patient, Buerger described the development of a 'blister, hemorrhagic bleb, or ulcer ... near the tip of one of the toes ..., and when this condition ensues the local pain becomes intense'. Finally, Buerger reported, the condition resulted in dry gangrene and often in amputation because of unbearable pain.

Except for the remarkably strong association of Buerger's disease with the use of tobacco (see below), relatively little has been learned of this peculiar condition since the time of Buerger's original description. The classic patient with Buerger's disease is a young male who smokes cigarettes heavily. However, in populations where smoking is highly prevalent among females, Buerger's disease may afflict women as well. Although Buerger's disease has a predilection for the distal lower extremities, the distal upper extremities may also be involved severely.

Angiography of the extremities may suggest the diagnosis, but the findings are not pathognomonic (Fig. 67.12). The vessels most commonly involved are the digital arteries of the fingers and toes, as well as the palmar, plantar, tibial peroneal, radial, and ulnar arteries. Obliteration of these vessels leads to the development of collaterals that frequently have a 'corkscrew' appearance. Examination of the proximal vasculature by aortography is essential to exclude embolic sources and to demonstrate normality of the proximal vessels, which is characteristic of Buerger's disease.

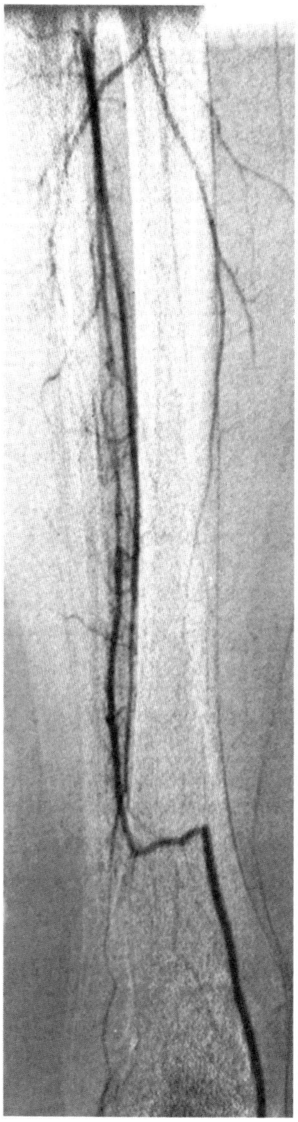

Figure 67.12 Angiogram in Buerger's disease. Lower extremity arteriogram in a 20 year-old woman with Buerger's disease. The anterior tibial artery attenuates in the mid-calf. The posterior tibial artery is occluded proximally, but is reconstituted above the ankle by collateral circulation from the peroneal artery. Distal to its reconstitution, the posterior tibial artery appears normal, consistent with the segmental nature of Buerger's disease.

Buerger's disease is unusual among the vasculitides in several respects: (1) the disease involves veins as well as arteries (even though the most striking symptoms are secondary to arterial involvement); (2) despite the intense involvement of medium-sized arteries, there is virtually no involvement of internal organs or any tissues besides the extremities; (3) although associated with the formation of a highly inflammatory thrombus, compared to other vasculitides there are fewer inflammatory changes within blood vessel walls and fibrinoid necrosis is absent; and

(4) Buerger's disease is less responsive than other forms of vasculitis to immunosuppression.

Buerger's disease does not occur in the absence of exposure to tobacco, usually large accounts of cigarette smoking. Once established, the disease may be maintained by even small exposures to tobacco (even smokeless tobacco or second-hand smoke), so cessation of smoking is essential in the treatment of this disease. Failure to stop smoking is associated with a dramatic increase in the risk of limb loss by amputation.[94] Although smoking is necessary, it is clearly not sufficient on its own to cause Buerger's disease. Other factors, including genetic factors and abnormalities of cellular and humoral immunity are currently under investigation.

In addition to encouraging cessation of smoking in the strongest possible terms, the therapy of Buerger's disease requires meticulous local wound care, avoidance of trauma to the involved areas, and ample use of narcotic analgesia. A variety of empiric therapies may be employed, including calcium channel blockers, pentoxifylline, iloprost, and sympathectomy, but this is currently little evidence to support their efficacy. In the authors' experience, glucocorticoids may be useful in the acute setting. The roles of anticoagulation and thrombolytic therapy require further investigation.[95]

COGAN SYNDROME

In 1945, Cogan reported 4 young patients (aged 20–35) who presented with either nonsyphilitic interstitial keratitis (bilateral eye pain, erythema, and photophobia) or symptoms of severe inner ear dysfunction (disabling vertigo, tinnitus, and progressive bilateral deafness). Regardless of which organ (eye or ear) became involved first, the onset of symptoms in one was followed within days to weeks by the development of symptoms in the other. Interstitial keratitis in the patients reported by Cogan waxed and waned, with only mild long-term ocular morbidity. In contrast, 3 of the 4 patients reported by Cogan suffered inexorable declines in auditory function, leading to deafness.

The combination of inflammatory eye disease and vestibulo/auditory dysfunction is the sine qua non of Cogan syndrome. The classic presentation is that of interstitial keratitis and sensorineural hearing loss. This disorder afflicts young adults, with no gender predominance. In approximately 10% of cases, eye and ear inflammation is associated with arthritis of medium- and large-sized vessels (including aortitis).[96,97] Consequently, the disorder is classified as a vasculitis. However, the true nature of the ocular and auditory inflammation, though clearly immune-mediated, remains obscure.[98]

Interstitial keratitis leads to the sensation of ocular irritation, excessive lacrimation, and photophobia, and is accompanied by moderate reductions (generally reversible) in visual acuity. The eye findings may be evanescent, and often require repeated examination for detection. Examination of the cornea by slit lamp (Fig. 67.13) reveals stromal clouding in the anterior and middle cornea. Pathologically, the cornea shows lymphocyte and plasma cell infiltration into the deep layers of the cornea, with varying degrees of neovascularization. Although vasculitis has been reported in other tissues in such patients, including cranial nerves II and VIII, vasculitis within the cornea has not been documented. Other forms of inflammatory eye disease occur in association with this disorder, including conjunctivitis, uveitis, episcleritis, scleritis, exophthalmos, papilledema, retinal vasculitis, and inflammation of the optic papilla suggesting optic neuritis.[96,97]

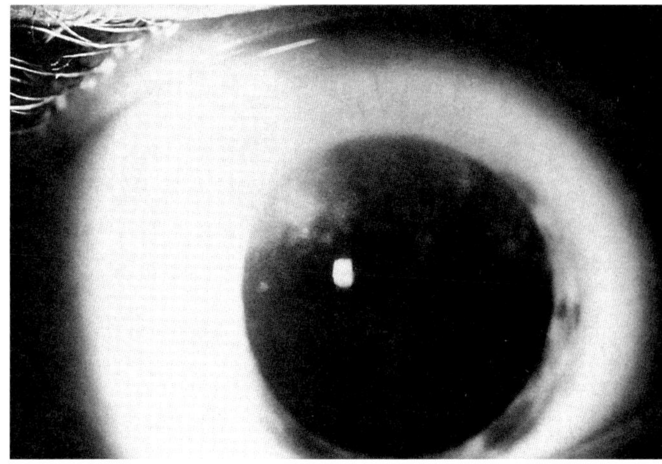

Figure 67.13 Interstitial keratitis in Cogan syndrome. Nonsyphilitic interstitial keratitis, demonstrated by slit-lamp examination in a patient with Cogan syndrome. (See also color plate 67.13.)

The greater cause of long-term morbidity in Cogan syndrome is the ear manifestations. Failure to recognize the nature of the problem promptly and institute appropriate therapy leads to more than half of the patients with Cogan syndrome suffering some degree of irreversible hearing loss.[96–98] A substantial percentage become profoundly deaf in at least one if not both ears, and become candidates for cochlear implantation. Audiologic testing reveals sensorineural hearing loss. The vestibular manifestations may also be severe, and usually present with the abrupt onset of vertigo, ataxia, tinnitus, and nausea and vomiting. The severity of these symptoms is often sufficiently great to confine patients to bed. Vestibular dysfunction may lead to the disabling visual complaint of oscillopsia, in which patients perceive objects to jiggle back and forth.

Access to tissue at any stage of ear involvement in Cogan syndrome is rare. Consequently, knowledge of the pathology of this disorder stems mostly from temporal bone specimens from patients with long-standing, intensively treated disease. These findings include endolymphatic hydrops, acute labyrinthitis resulting in atrophy of the hair cells and their supporting structures, focal or diffuse proliferation of fibrous tissue and bone ('neo-osteogenesis'), and neuronal degeneration. Once again, definitive evidence of vasculitis in these tissues is absent.

Medium- and large-vessel arteritis may lead to a host of complications in patients with Cogan syndrome, including aortitis, aortic regurgitation, coronary artery inflammation, mesenteric vasculitis, and limb claudication. In many respects the vascular disease of Cogan syndrome must be distinguished from that of Takayasu's arteritis (Chapter 68).

Interstitial keratitis generally responds well to topical steroid therapy, which often must be administered chronically. In contrast, sensorineural hearing loss must be treated early and aggressively, with high doses of systemic glucocorticoids. Failure to institute such therapy within the first 2 weeks of symptoms frequently results in irreversible hearing loss. Most patients who will respond generally do so within 2 weeks, and total courses lasting 2–3 months are usually sufficient.

PRIMARY ANGIITIS OF THE CENTRAL NERVOUS SYSTEM

Primary angiitis of the central nervous system (PACNS) is a rare disease of unknown etiology characterized by small- and medium-sized vessel vasculitis limited to the brain or spinal cord.[99] Some authors prefer the term 'isolated angiitis of the central nervous system'.[100] The once commonly used label – 'granulomatous angiitis' – has dropped out of favor because not all patients with vasculitis limited to the central nervous system demonstrate granulomatous inflammation, and other forms of vasculitis, including systemic diseases such as sarcoidosis and WG, can cause granulomatous vasculitis in the brain. Vasculitis limited to the central nervous system is the most difficult form of vasculitis to diagnose accurately. The protean manifestations of the disease, the unreliability of noninvasive diagnostic tests, and the difficulty of obtaining adequate brain biopsies all contribute to the diagnostic conundrum of PACNS.

Classically, patients with PACNS manifest the triad of headache, encephalopathy, and multifocal strokes.[99–102] However, only a minority of patients present with all three features, and many develop a wide range of other neurological manifestations (Table 67.11). Most patients present in the fourth or fifth decade of life, but may range in age from 3 to 74. The disease affects women and men equally often. The disease can begin suddenly or develop slowly. The first symptom is usually headache, often severe and sometimes associated with nausea and vomiting. Almost all patients eventually develop encephalopathy with lethargy, confusion, and memory loss. Some develop multifocal strokes, seizures, evidence of increased intracranial pressure, or myclopathy. Constitutional symptoms, a hallmark of most forms of vasculitis, are notably absent in patients with PACNS.

In keeping with the isolated nature of the inflammation of PACNS, routine laboratory tests are usually normal.[99–103] The majority of patients do not have anemia or an elevated erythrocyte sedimentation rate. The lumbar puncture yields abnormal cerebrospinal fluid (CSF) in approximately 80% of cases.[99,104] The most common abnormalities are a modest CSF monocytosis and an increased CSF protein.[99] The frequency of oligoclonal bands and elevated IgG indices in the CSF has not been studied in detail, but neither appears sensitive or specific for PACNS.[99]

The clinical and laboratory features described above apply to patients who are diagnosed by brain biopsy. Over the last 30 years, an increasing number of cases have been reported in which the diagnosis is based on CNS angiography alone, without the performance of a brain biopsy.[99,105] These patients differ from those with biopsy-confirmed cases in that the majority are women, the onset tends to be more abrupt, the neurological signs less severe, and the lumbar puncture normal.[99]

Of the noninvasive imaging tests, magnetic resonance (MR) imaging is more sensitive than computed tomography (CT).[104,106] The false negative rate of MR appears to be less than 10% in most series.[99,100,104–106] Most commonly the MR shows multiple, bilateral, bland infarctions, distributed in the subcortical white matter, cortical gray matter, deep gray matter, deep white matter, or cerebellum.[106] Hemorrhagic lesions and mass lesions also occur.[100] No MR pattern is specific for PACNS.

The classic abnormality on angiography is the 'string of beads' pattern produced by segmented arterial narrowing alternating with dilatations[99,107] (Fig. 67.14). Vascular occlusions, collateral formation, and prolonged circulation time may also be seen. Microaneurysms, so frequently seen on visceral angiograms in patients with PAN, rarely occur in PACNS. Unfortunately, no angiographic pattern is pathognomonic, and other disorders, including intravascular lymphoma, systemic infections, and vasospasm can produce similar angiographic abnormalities (see below). Angiograms are falsely negative in about 35% of patients with PACNS.[99,107]

The diagnosis of PACNS is definite if the patient: (1) presents with multifocal strokes or encephalopathy accompanied by

Presenting features of primary angiitis of the central nervous system

Feature	%
Encephalopathy	95
Headache	68
Focal cerebral dysfunction	50
Evidence of increased intracranial pressure	43
Brainstem or cranial nerve disease	40
Seizures	25
Spinal cord disease	20
Anorexia or weight loss	20

Table 67.11 Presenting features of primary angiitis of the central nervous system. (From Vollmer T, Guamaccia J, Harrington W, et al. Idiopathic granulomatous angiitis of the central nervous system. *Arch Neurol* 1993;50:925.)

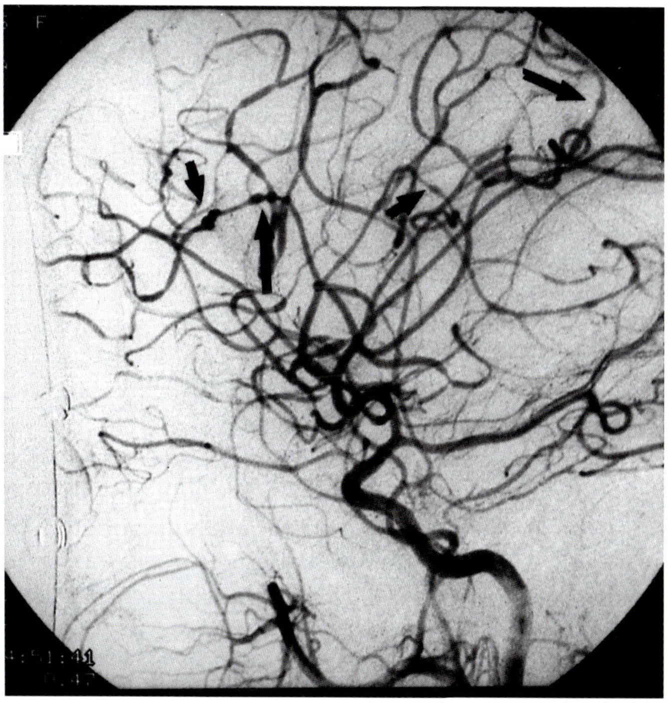

Figure 67.14 Cerebral angiogram in primary angiitis of the central nervous system. The angiogram illustrates the dilatations and narrowing of arteries typical of PACNS.

headache; (2) has a cerebral angiogram showing changes consistent with vasculitis; (3) has no evidence of systemic infection, neoplasm, or toxic exposure; and (4) has a biopsy of the leptomeninges or brain cortex demonstrating vasculitis in the absence of other causes.[100] The diagnosis of PACNS should be considered probable when the patient meets all criteria except that of a positive brain biopsy. In patients not having a positive biopsy, systemic vasculitides and other diseases that can mimic vasculitis must be excluded.

Histological specimens in PACNS show vasculitis of small and medium-sized leptomeningeal and cortical arteries. Veins and venules are involved less often.[99] The inflammatory infiltrate varies, but consists predominantly of lymphocytes admixed with histiocytes. Langerhans and foreign body giant cells occur in about half of the cases.[108] The inflammation usually targets the intima and media and produces variable degrees of necrosis.

The rarity of PACNS has prevented prospective treatment trials. Prednisone and cyclophosphamide are recommended for patients who have severe neurological deficits and a positive brain biopsy.[99,100] Prednisone alone (beginning at 1 mg/kg per day) appears to be adequate therapy for some patients, especially those who experience a sudden onset of mild to moderate abnormalities that are not progressive, have a normal CSF, and whose diagnosis is supported by an angiogram in the absence of a brain biopsy.[99] Mortality rates, once as high as 95% in untreated patients, have plummeted to less than 10% for treated patients.[99] Most patients improve with treatment; the degree of recovery correlates inversely with the severity of deficits at diagnosis and the age of the patient.

URTICARIAL VASCULITIS

In 1973, Mayo Clinic investigators described 4 patients with recurrent attacks of urticarial lesions and combinations of synovitis, abdominal symptoms, and glomerulonephritis.[109] Although transient, urticaria in these patients generally persisted for at least 24 hours (longer than the 6–8 hours typically associated with chronic idiopathic urticaria) and sometimes left traces of hyperpigmentation, indicative of red blood cell extravasation through damaged capillaries. Low complement levels were present in all of the patients during periods of active disease, and skin biopsies demonstrated evidence of an immune complex-mediated disease process. Investigations excluded systemic lupus erythematosus (SLE) and mixed cryoglobulinemia, leading to the report of a previously underscribed disorder now known as the hypocomplementemic urticarial vasculitis syndrome (HUVS).

HUVS is now recognized as one of a group of disorders known as urticarial vasculitis. At least three subtypes of urticarial vasculitis are known:[110] (1) a normocomplementemic form, which is generally idiopathic and benign; (2) a hypocomplementemic form, which is often associated with a systemic inflammatory disease; and (3) HUVS, a potentially severe condition usually associated with autoantibodies to the collagen-like region of C1q. Most patients with urticarial vasculitis have the hypocomplementemic subtype and demonstrate low C3, C4, and CH50. Patients with urticarial vasculitis who show evidence of complement activation are much more likely to manifest signs of a systemic disorder than those with normal complement levels. The majority of urticarial vasculitis patients (80–90%) have an underlying systemic disorder, usually SLE, Sjögren's syndrome, or cryoglobulinemia.

The lesions of urticarial vasculitis must be distinguished from chronic idiopathic urticaria, which is encountered far more commonly in clinical practice. Only about 10% of patients with chronic urticaria have urticarial vasculitis. In contrast to chronic idiopathic urticaria (the principal symptom of which is pruritus), urticarial lesions associated with vasculitis are often accompanied by stinging or burning. Urticarial vasculitis affects the capillaries and postcapillary venules, and the classic features of leukocytoclastic vasculitis may be evident on light microscopy. Immunofluorescence reveals both immunoglobulin and complement deposition in or around blood vessels of the upper dermis and/or the dermal – epidermal junction (Fig. 67.15).

HUVS frequently mimics SLE.[111] Like SLE, HUVS has a striking female predominance, with a female:male ratio of 8:1. However, SLE-specific antibodies (e.g. those to dsDNA and the Sm antigen) do not occur in HUVS, and there are several distinguishing clinical features. For example, HUVS may be associated with angioedema, ocular inflammation, and chronic obstructive pulmonary disease (COPD), all of which are highly atypical of SLE. Although exacerbated by tobacco use, COPD may occur in the absence of any history of cigarette smoking, and may be severe. The few cases of lung biopsies in patients with this complication have not demonstrated vasculitis, but rather shown panacinar emphysema. As in SLE, kidney biopsies in HUVS patients may reveal mesangial inflammation or membranoproliferative glomerulonephritis, but progression to end-stage renal disease in HUVS is unusual. Severe cardiac valve disease and Jaccoud's arthropathy have also been associated with HUVS.[112]

Most patients with HUVS make C1q 'precipitins', i.e. IgG autoantibodies to the collagen-like region of C1q.[111] Whether or not anti-C1q antibodies contribute to the pathogenesis of HUVS remains unclear. Anti-C1q antibodies are also detected in up to one third of patients with SLE, and in more than 80% of SLE patients with glomerulonephritis.[113] Despite the prevalence of these antibodies in SLE, few patients who are seropositive for anti-C1q antibodies develop urticarial lesions. Glomeruli from patients with lupus nephritis may contain large quantities of anti-C1q antibodies.[113]

The natural history of urticarial vasculitis is difficult to predict. Some cases, particularly those with normal complement levels

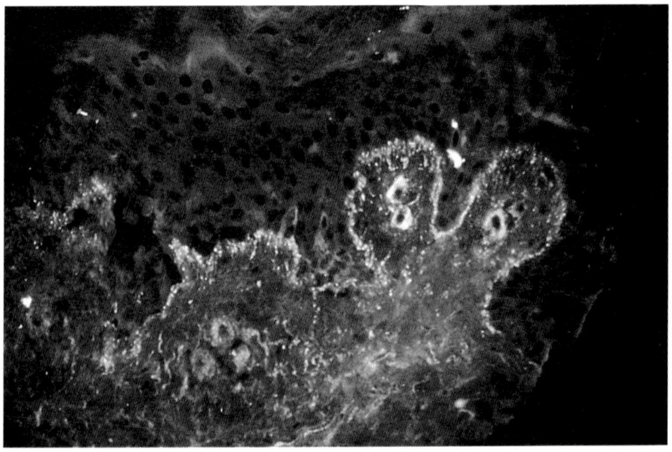

Figure 67.15 Immunofluorescence study of a skin biopsy from a patient with hypocomplementemic urticarial vasculitis syndrome (HUVS). There is positive staining for IgG along the basement membrane zone and around small arteries in the dermal papillae. (See also color plate 67.15.)

during attacks, are self-limited and require little therapy. Other cases, especially HUVS, may cause life-threatening involvement of the lungs or other organs, and require periods of intensive immunosuppression. The rarity of HUVS means that there exists little consensus regarding the optimal therapeutic strategy, and treatment decisions must be individualized according to each patient's clinical status. For hypocomplementemic urticarial vasculitis limited to the skin, antimalarial agents, dapsone, and low doses of glucocorticoids may be useful.

KAWASAKI'S DISEASE

The first case of the disease now known as Kawasaki's disease was described initially in 1939[114,115] and involved a 5-year-old girl who presented with high fever, sore throat, and nash and subsequently died from rupture of a coronary artery aneurysm. In 1961, Tomisaku Kawasaki evaluated a Japanese child with similar disease features, and also noted prominent cervical adenopathy. Over the next 6 years he performed a careful clinical and epidemiological study of the new disorder, and eventually reported the disease in the Japanese literature as 'mucocutaneous lymph node syndrome' in 50 patients.[114,116] The striking clinical features of this disease are summarized in Table 67.12. Formal diagnostic criteria for Kawasaki's disease have been developed.[117] The disease has a predilection for Asian children, but occurs in all races. Eighty per cent of all cases occur in children younger than 5 years of age. The annual attack rate in Japan is approximately 80–90 cases per 100 000 children under the age of 5, compared to roughly 10 per 100 000 among Caucasian children in the USA.[118]

In all of the patients described initially by Kawasaki, the symptoms resolved without sequelae within one month. In subsequent years, however, mortality from cardiac complications (usually coronary artery thrombosis) was reported. Cardiac complications of Kawasaki's disease result from a severe panvasculitis, leading to narrowing of the coronary lumina by the migration of myointimal cells from the media through the fragmented internal elastic lamina.[119] Although catastrophic heart complications occur in only a small minority of patients, evidence suggests that the preponderance of patients with Kawasaki's disease have at least some cardiac involvement. Heart lesions may include myocarditis, pericarditis, aneurysmal dilatation and thrombosis of the coronary arteries, and myocardial infarction. The tropism of the vascular inflammation for coronary arteries and its unusual propensity to cause aneurysm formation remain unexplained. The prompt institution of high-dose intravenous immunoglobulin (IVIG) may prevent this complication (see treatment, below).

Certain clinical features of Kawasaki's disease (fever, conjunctivitis, stomatitis, erythema multiforme-like rash, and the overwhelming predominance of the disease in young children) bear strong resemblance to a number of childhood exanthems. Moreover, the disease epidemiology of Japanese outbreaks is reminiscent of the classic spread of infectious agents.[118] The profound disturbances of immunoregulation in Kawasaki's disease,

Clinical features of Kawasaki's disease

Symptom	Frequency
Fever	95%
Conjunctival congestion	88%
Buccal/oral lesions:	
• dryness, erythema, fissuring of lips	90%
• protuberant tongue papillae	77%
• mucosal erythema	90%
Cutaneous findings:	
• erythema of palms/soles	88%
• edema/induration of acral regions	76%
• desquamation of skin from fingertips	94%
• polymorphous truncal rash	92%
Cervical adenopathy	75%
Sudden death due to coronary thrombosis	1–2%

Table 67.12 Clinical features of Kawasaki's disease. (Adapted from Kawasaki T, Kosaki F, Okawa S, et al. A new infantile acute febrile mucocutaneous lymph node syndrome (MLNS) prevailing in Japan. *Pediatrics* 1974;54:271.)

e.g. the unusual degree of T-cell and monocyte activation, far exceed the abnormalities accompanying most other febrile childhood illnesses, however. Skewing of the T-cell receptor Vβ distribution has been reported by some investigators,[120] but not confirmed by others.[121] The degree of immune activation in Kawasaki's disease and the acute but generally self-limited nature of the illness have implicated superantigens in the disease pathogenesis[120,122] (Chapter 7). Substantial attention has focused on toxic shock syndrome toxin-1 (TSST-1),[122,123] an exotoxin produced by *S. aureus*, but the true relationship of this and other potential superantigens to the etiology of Kawasaki's disease remains unclear.

Before the availability of effective therapy, at least 20% of patients with Kawasaki's disease developed coronary aneurysms and 2% succumbed to the disease.[124] To confirm earlier reports of efficacy of IVIG in Kawasaki's disease, seven pediatric centers in the USA enrolled 168 children with acute disease into a randomized trial. Half of the patients received IVIG 400 mg/kg/day on four consecutive days plus high-dose aspirin (100 mg/kg/day), and the other half received aspirin alone.[125] IVIG reduced the incidence of coronary aneurysms by 78% and relieved the symptoms of Kawasaki's disease with dramatic swiftness, establishing the combination of IVIG and aspirin as the standard for therapy of Kawasaki's disease. The mechanism of action of IVIG in this disorder remains unknown, but the rapidity of its benefit has implicated an anticytokine effect. The optimal dose of IVIG in Kawasaki's disease has not been defined: meta-analyzes suggest a lower rate of coronary aneurysms in patients who receive higher IVIG doses.[126]

REFERENCES

1. Jennette J, Falk R, Andrassy K, et al. Nomenclature of systemic vasculitides. Proposal of an international consensus conference. Arthritis Rheum 1994;37:187.
2. Jennette J, Falk R. Small vessel vasculitis. N Engl J Med 1997;337:1512.
3. Fauci A, Haynes B, Katz P. The spectrum of vasculitis. Clinical, pathologic, immunologic, and therapeutic considerations. Ann Intern Med 1978;89:660.
4. Robertson C, McCallum R. Changing concepts in pathophysiology of the vasculitides. Curr Opin Rheumatol 1994;6:3.
5. Davies D, Moran J, Niall J, Ryan G. Segmental necrotising glomerulonephritis with antineutrophil antibody: possible arbovirus aetiology. BMJ 1982;285:606.
6. Jennette J, Falk R. Disease associations and pathogenic role of antineutrophil cytoplasmic autoantibodies in vasculitis. Curr Opin Rheumatol 1992;4:9.
7. Hoffman G, Specks U. Antineutrophil cytoplasmic antibodies. Arthritis Rheum 1998;41:1521.
8. Rump JA, Schoelmerich J, Gross V, et al. A new type of perinuclear antineutrophil cytoplasmic antibody in ulcerative colitis but not in Crohn's disease, Immunobiology 1990;181:406.
9. Falk R, Terrell R, Charles L, et al. Anti-neutrophil cytoplasmic autoantibodies induce neutrophils to degranulate and produce oxygen radicals in vitro. Proc Natl Acad Sci USA 1990;87:4115.
10. Ludviksson B, Sneller M, Chua K, et al. Active Wegener's granulomatosis is associated with HLA-DR^{+} CD4^{+} T cells exhibiting an unbalanced Th1-Type T cell cytokine pattern: Reversal with IL-10. J Immunol 1998;160:3602.
11. Greidinger EL, Rosen A. Inflammatory rheumatic diseases. In: McPhee SJ, Lingappa VR, Ganong WF, et al. (eds) Pathophysiology of disease: an introduction to clinical medicine, 3rd edn. New York, McGraw-Hill, 2000, p. 576.
12. Kussmaul A, Maier R. Ueber eine bisher nicht beschriebene eigenthumliche arterienerkrankung (periarteritis nodosa), die mit morbus brightii und rapid fortschreitender allgemeiner muskellahmung einhergeht. Dtsch Arch Klin Med 1866;1:484.
13. Davson J, Ball J, Platt R. The kidney in periarteritis nodosa. QJM 1948;17:175.
14. Cupps T, Fauci A. Systemic necrotizing vasculitis of the polyarteritis nodosa group. In: Smith LH (ed.) The vaseulitides. Major problems in internal medicine, Vol 21. Philadelphia, WB Saunders, 1981, p 26.
15. Guillevin L, Lhote F, Cohen P, et al. Polyarteritis nodosa related to hepatitis B virus. A prospective study with long-term observation of 41 patients. Medicine 1995;74:238.
16. Carson C, Conn D, Czaja A, et al. Frequency and significance of antibodies to hepatitis C virus in polyarteritis nodosa. J Rheumatol 1993;20:304.
17. Libman B, Quismorio F, Stimmler M. Polyarteritis nodosa-like vasculitis in human immunodeficiency virus infection. J Rheumatol 1995;22:351.
18. Mason J, Cowie M, Davies K, et al. Familial polyarteritis nodosa. Arthritis Rheum 1994;37:1249.
19. Hellmann DB. Mononeuritis multiplex. In: Klippel JH, Dieppe UK (eds) Rheumatology. Baltimore, Mosby, 1994, p 6.
20. Hellmann DB, Laing TJ, Petri M, et al. Mononeuritis multiplex: The yield of the evaluation for occult rheumatic diseases. Medicine 1988;67:145.
21. Zizic T, Classen J, Stevens M. Acute abdominal complications of systemic lupus erythematosus and polyarteritis nodosa. Am J Med 1982;73:525.
22. Heptinstall R. Polyarteritis (periarteritis) nodosa, Wegener's syndrome, and other forms of vasculitis. Pathology of the kidney, 4th edn. 1992;16:1097.
23. Lightfoot R, Michel B, Bloch D, et al. The American College of Rheumatology 1990 criteria for the classification of polyarteritis nodosa. Arthritis Rheum 1990;33:1088.
24. Ewald E, Griffin D, McCune W. Correlation of angiographic abnormalities with disease manifestations and disease severity in polyarteritis nodosa. J Rheumatol 1987;14:952.
25. Albert D, Rimon D, Silverstein M. The diagnosis of polyarteritis nodosa. Arthritis Rheum 1988;31:1117.
26. Dahlberg P, Lockhart J, Overholt E. Diagnostic studies for systemic necrotizing vasculitis. Sensitivity, specificity, and predictive value in patients with multisystem disease. Arch Intern Med 1989;149:161.
27. Fauci A, Katz P, Haynes B, et al. Cyclophosphamide therapy of severe systemic necrotizing vasculitis. N Engl J Med 1979;301:235.
28. Guillevin L, Lhote F. Treatment of polyarteritis nodosa and microscopic polyangiitis. Arthritis Rheum 1998;41:2100.
29. Leib E, Restivo C, Paulus H. Immunosuppressive and corticosteroid therapy of polyarteritis nodosa. Am J Med 1979;67:941.
30. Guillevin L, Jarrousse B, Lok C. Longterm followup after treatment of polyarteritis nodosa and Churg–Strauss angiitis with comparison of steroids, plasma exchange and cyclophosphamide to steroids and plasma exchange. A prospective randomized trial of 71 patients. J Rheumatol 1991;18:567.
31. Guillevin L, Lhote F, Gayraud M, et al. Prognostic factors in polyarteritis nodosa and Churg–Strauss syndrome. A prospective study in 342 patients. Medicine 1996;75:17.
32. Guillevin L, Fain O, Lhote F, et al. Lack of superiority of steroids plus plasma exchange to steroids alone in the treatment of polyarteritis nodosa and Churg–Strauss syndrome. Arthritis Rheum 1992;35:208.
33. Fortin P, Larson M, Watters A, et al. Prognostic factors in systemic necrotizing vasculitis of the polyarteritis nodosa group – a review of 45 cases. J Rheumatol 1995;22:78.
34. Guillevin L, Lhote F, Cohen P, et al. Corticosteroids plus pulse cyclophosphamide and plasma exchanges versus corticosteroids plus pulse cyclophosphamide alone in the treatment of polyarteritis nodosa and Churg–Strauss syndrome patients with factors predicting poor prognosis. A prospective, randomized trial in sixty-two patients. Arthritis Rheum 1995;38:1638.
35. Wintrobe M, Buell M. Hyperproteinemia associated with multiple myeloma. Bull Johns Hopkins Hospital 1933;52:156.
36. Lamprecht P, Gause A, Gross W. Cryoglobulinemic vasculitis. Arthritis Rheum 1999;42:2507.
37. Meltzer M, Franklin E. Cryoglobulinemia – a study of twenty-nine patients. I. IgG and IgM cryoglobulins and factors affecting cryoprecipitability. Am J Med 1966;40:828.
38. Brouet J, Clauvel J, Danon F, et al. Biologic and clinical significance of cryoglobulins. A report of 86 cases. Am J Med 1974;57:775.
39. Agnello V, Chung R, Kaplan L. A role for hepatitis C virus infection in patients with Type II cryoglobulinemia. N Engl J Med 1992;327:1490.
40. Wener M, Johnson R, Sasso E. Hepatitis C virus and rheumatic disease. J Rheumatol 1996;23:953.
41. Marcellin P, Descamps V, Martinot-Peignoux M, et al. Cryoglobulinemia with vasculitis associated with hepatitis C virus infection. Gastroenterology 1993;104:272.
42. Gumber SC, Chopra S. Hepatitis C: A multifaceted disease. Review of extrahepatic manifestations. Ann Intern Med 1994;123:615.
43. Lunel F, Musset L, Cacoub P, et al. Cryoglobulinemia in chronic liver diseases: role of hepatitis C virus and liver damage. Gastroenterology 1994;106:1291.
44. Johnson R, Gretch D, Yamabe H, et al. Membranoproliferative glomerulonephritis associated with hepatitis C virus infection. N Engl J Med 1993;328:465.
45. Di Bisceglie A, Conjeevaram H, Fried M, et al. Ribavirin as therapy for chronic hepatitis C. A randomized, double-blind, placebo-controlled trial. Ann Intern Med 1995;123:897.
46. Poynard T, Bedossa P, Chevallier M, et al. A comparison of three interferon Alfa-2b regimens for the long-term treatment of chronic non-A, non-B hepatitis. N Engl J Med 1995;332:1457.
47. Godman G, Churg J. Wegener's granulomatosis: Pathology and review of the literature. Arch Pathol Lab Med 1954;58:533.
48. Merkel P. Drugs associated with vasculitis. Curr Opin Rheumatol 1998;10:45.

49. Hagen E, Daha M, Hermans J, et al. Diagnostic value of standardized assays for anti-neutrophil cytoplasmic antibodies in idiopathic systemic vasculitis. Kidney Int 1998;53:743.
50. Rao JY, Weinberger M, Oddone EZ, et al. The role of antineutrophil cytoplasmic antibody (C-ANCA) testing in the diagnosis of Wegener's granulomatosis. Ann Intern Med 1995;123:425.
51. Hoffman GS, Leavitt RY, Kerr GS, Fauci AS. The treatment of Wegener's granulomatosis with glucocorticoids and methotrexate. Arthritis Rheum 1992;35:1322.
52. Guillevin L, Cohen P, Gayraud M, et al. Churg–Strauss syndrome: Clinical study and long-term follow-up of 96 patients. Medicine 1999;78:26.
53. Wegener F. Uber generalisierte, septisehe Gefasserkrankungen. Verh Dtsch Ges Pathol 1936;29:202.
54. Wegener F. Uber eine eigenartige rhinogene Granulomatose mit besonderer Beteiligung des Arteriensystems und der Nieren. Beitr Pathol Anat Allg Pathol 1939;36:36.
55. Watts R, Carruthers D, Scott D. Epidemiology of systemic vasculitis: changing incidence or definition? Semin Arthritis Rheum 1995;25:28.
56. Hoffman G, Kerr G, Leavitt R, et al. Wegener's granulomatosis: An analysis of 158 patients. Ann Intern Med 1992;116:488.
57. Stegeman C, Tervaert J, Sluiter W, et al. Association of chronic nasal carriage of *Staphylococcus aureus* and higher relapse rates in Wegener granulomatosis. Ann Intern Med 1994;120:12.
58. Lebovics R, Hoffman G, Leavitt R, et al. The management of subglottic stenosis in patients with Wegener's granulomatosis. Laryngoscope 1992;102:1341.
59. Stone J, Francis H. Immune-mediated inner ear disease. Curr Opin Rheumatol 2000;12:32.
60. Talar-Williams C, Hijazi Y, Walther M, et al. Cyclophosphamide-induced cystitis and bladder cancer in patients with Wegener's granulomatosis. Ann Intern Med 1996;124:477.
61. Lie J. Nomenclature and classification of vasculitis: Plus ça change, plus c'est la même chose. Arthritis Rheum 1994;37:181.
62. Guillevin L, Durand-Gasselin B, Cevallos R, et al. Microscopic polyangiitis. Arthritis Rheum 1999;42:421.
63. Savage C, Winearls C, Evans D, et al. Microscopic polyarteritis: presentation, pathology, and prognosis. QJM 1985;56:467.
64. Niles J, Bottinger E, Saurina G, et al. The syndrome of lung hemorrhage and nephritis is usually an ANCA-associated condition. Arch Intern Med 1996;156:440.
65. Churg J, Strauss L. Allergic granulomatosis, allergic angiitis, and periarteritis nodosa. Am J Pathol 1951;27:277.
66. Masi A, Hunder G, Lie J, et al. The American College of Rheumatology 1990 criteria for the classification of Churg–Strauss syndrome (allergic granulomatosis and angiitis). Arthritis Rheum 1990;33:1094.
67. Lanham J, Elkon K, Pusey C, et al. Systemic vasculitis with asthma and eosinophilia: a clinical approach to the Churg–Strauss syndrome. Medicine 1984;63:65.
68. Clutterbuck E, Evans D, Pusey C. Renal involvement in Churg–Strauss syndrome. Nephrol Dial Transplant 1990;5:161.
69. Wechsler M, Pauwels R, Drazen J. Leukotriene modifiers and Churg–Strauss syndrome: adverse effect or response to corticosteroid withdrawal? Drug Saf 1999;21:241.
70. Stirling R, Chung K. Leukotriene antagonists and Churg–Strauss syndrome: the smoking gun? Thorax 1999;54:865.
71. Stone J, Tun W, Hellmann D. Treatment of non-life threatening Wegener's granulomatosis with methotrexate and daily prednisone as the initial therapy of choice. J Rheumatol 1999;26:1134.
72. Guillevin L, Cordier J-F, Lhote F, et al. A prospective, multicenter, randomized trial comparing steroids and pulse cyclophosphamide versus steroids and oral cyclophosphamide in the treatment of generalized Wegener's granulomatosis. Arthritis Rheum 1997;40:2187.
73. Jayne D, Rasmussen N. Treatment of antineutrophil cytoplasm autoantibody-associated systemic vasculitis: Initiatives of the European Community Systemic Vasculitis Clinical Trials Study Group. Mayo Clin Proc 1997;72:737.
74. Langford C, Talar-Williams C, Barron K, et al. A staged approach to the treatment of Wegener's granulomatosis: Induction of remission with glucocorticoids and daily cyclophosphamide switching to methotrexate for remission maintenance. Arthritis Rheum 1999;42:2666.
75. Tatsis E, Schnabel M, Gross W. Interferon-alpha treatment of four patients with the Churg–Strauss syndrome. Ann Intern Med 1998;129:370.
76. Zeek P. Periarteritis nodosa: A critical review. Am J Clin Path 1952;221:777.
77. Ekenstam E, Callen J. Cutaneous leukocytoclastic vasculitis: clinical and laboratory features of 82 patients seen in private practice. Arch Dermatol 1982;120:484.
78. Calabrese L, Michel B, Bloch D, et al. The American College of Rheumatology 1990 criteria for the classification of hypersensitivity vasculitis. Arthritis Rheum 1990;33:1108.
79. Callen J, Spencer L, Burruss J, et al. Azathioprine: An effective corticosteroid-sparing therapy for patients with recalcitrant cutaneous leukocytoclastic vasculitis. Arch Dermatol 1991;127:515.
80. Gairdner D. The Schönlein–Henoch syndrome (anaphylactoid purpura). Q J Med 1948;17:95.
81. Saulsbury F. Henoch–Schonlein purpura in children. Medicine 1999;78:395.
82. Michel B, Hunder G, Bloch D, et al. Hypersensitivity vasculitis and Henoch–Schönlein purpura: A comparison between the 2 disorders, J Rheumatol 1992;19:721.
83. Illan Y, Naparstek Y. Schönlein–Henoch syndrome in adults and children. Semin Arthritis Rheum 1991;21:103.
84. Mills J, Michel B, Bloch D, et al. The American College of Rheumatology 1990 criteria for classification of Henoch–Schonlein purpura. Arthritis Rheum 1990;33:1114.
85. Behçet H. Veber rezidivierende Aphthose, durch ein Virus verursachte Gerschwure am Mund, am Auge und de Genitalie. Dermat Wochenschr 1937;105:1552.
86. Sakane T, Tekeno M, Suzuki N, et al. Behçet's disease. N Engl J Med 1999;341:1284.
87. Kaklamani V, Variopoulos G, Kaklamanis P. Behçet's disease. Semin Arthritis Rheum 1998;27:197.
88. Mizuki N, Ota M, Katsuyama Y, et al. Association analysis between the MIC-A and HLA-B alleles in Japanese patients with Behçet's disease. Arthritis Rheum 1999;42:1961.
89. Zouboulis CC, Orfanos CE. Treatment of Adamantiades-Behçet's disease with systemic interferon-alpha. Arch Dermatol 1998;134:1010.
90. Hamuryudan V, Ozyazgan Y, Hizli N, et al. Azathioprine in Behçet's syndrome: effects on long-term prognosis. Arthritis Rheum 1997;40:769.
91. O'Duffy J, Calamia K, Cohen S, et al. Interferon-alpha treatment of Behçet's disease. J Rheumatol 1998;25:1938.
92. Yasui K, Ohta K, Kobayashi M, et al. Successful treatment of Behçet's disease with pentoxifylline. Ann Intern Med 1996;124:891.
93. Buerger L. Thromboangiitis obliterans: a study of the vascular lesions leading to presenile spontaneous gangrene. Am J Med Sci 1908;136:567.
94. Olin J, Young J, Graor R, et al. The changing clinical spectrum of thromboangiitis obliterans (Buerger's disease). Circulation 1990;(Suppl 4):3.
95. Hussein E, El Dorri A. Intra-arterial streptokinase as adjuvant therapy for complicated Buerger's disease: Early trials. Int Surg 1993;78:54.
96. Haynes B, Kaiser-Kupfer M, Mason P, Fauci A. Cogan syndrome: Studies in thirteen patients, long-term follow-up, and a review of the literature. Medicine 1980;59:426.
97. Vollertsen R, McDonald T, Younge B, Banks P, Stanson A, Ilstrup D. Cogan's syndrome: 18 cases and a review of the literature. Mayo Clin Proc 1986;61:344.
98. St. Clair E, McCallum R. Cogan's syndrome. Curr Opin Rheumatol 1999;11:47.
99. Calabrese L, Duna G, Lie J. Vasculitis in the central nervous system. Arthritis Rheum 1997;7:1189.
100. Moore P. Vasculitis of the central nervous system. Semin Neurol 1994;14:307.
101. Calabrese L, Furlan A, Gragg L, et al. Primary angiitis of the central nervous system: diagnostic criteria and clinical approach. Cleve Clin J Med 1992;59:293.
102. Vollmer T, Guamaccia J, Harrington W, et al. Idiopathic granulomatous angiitis of the central nervous system. Arch Neurol 1993;50:925.

103. Hellmann D, Roubenoff R, Healy R, et al. Central nervous system angiography: safety and predictors of a positive result in 125 consecutive patients evaluated for possible vasculitis. J Rheumatol 1992;19:568.
104. Stone J, Pomper M, Roubenoff R, et al. Sensitivities of non-invasive tests for CNS vasculitis: A comparison of LP, CT, and MRI. J Rheumatol 1994;21:1277.
105. Calabrese L, Gragg L, Furlan A. Benign angiopathy: A distinct subset of angiographically defined primary angiitis of the central nervous system. J Rheumatol 1993;20:2046.
106. Pomper M, Miller T, Stone J, et al. Central nervous system vasculitis: MR imaging and correlation with angiography. Am J Neuroradiol 1999;20:75.
107. Alhalabi M, Moore P. Serial angiography in isolated angiitis of the central nervous system. Neurology 1994;44:1221.
108. Parisi J, Moore P. The role of biopsy in vasculitis of the central nervous system. Semin Neurol 1994;14:341.
109. McDuffie F, Sams W Jr, Maldonado J, et al. Hypocomplementemia with cutaneous vasculitis and arthritis. Mayo Clin Proc 1973;48:430.
110. Wisnieski J. Urticarial vasculitis. Curr Opin Rheum 2000;12:24.
111. Wisnieski J, Baer A, Christensen J, et al. Hypocomplementemic urticarial vasculitis syndrome: Clinical and serological findings in 18 patients. Medicine 1995;74:24.
112. Palazzo E, Bourgeois P, Meyer O, et al. Hypocomplementemic urticarial vasculitis syndrome, Jaccoud's syndrome, valvulopathy: a new syndromic combination. J Rheumatol 1993;20:1236.
113. Mannik M, Wener M. Deposition of antibodies to the collagen-like region of Clq in renal glomeruli of patients with proliferative lupus glomerulonephritis. Arthritis Rheum 1997;40:1504.
114. Kawasaki T, Kosaki F, Okawa S, et al. A new infantile acute febrile mucocutaneous lymph node syndrome (MLNS) prevailing in Japan. Pediatrics 1974;54:271.
115. Spector S. Scarlet fever, periarteritis nodosa, aneurysm of the coronary artery with spontaneous rupture, hemopericardium. Arch Pediat 1939;25:319.
116. Kawasaki T. Acute febrile mucocutaneous syndrome with lymphoid involvement with specific desquamation of the fingers and toes in children [in Japanese]. Jpn J Allerg 1967;178.
117. Centers for Disease Control. Kawasaki disease. MMWR 1980;29:61.
118. Yanagawa H, Yashiro M, Nakamura Y, et al. Epidemiologic pictures of Kawasaki disease in Japan: from the nationwide incidence survey in 1991 and 1992. Pediatrics 1995;95:475.
119. Naoe S, Shibuya K, Takahashi K, et al. Pathologic observations concerning the cardiovascular lesions in Kawasaki disease. Cardiol Young 1991;1:212.
120. Abe J, Kotzin B, Meissner C, et al. Characterization of T cell repertoire changes in acute Kawasaki disease. J Exp Med 1993;177:791.
121. Pietra B, De Inocencio J, Giannini E, et al. T cell receptor Vβ family repertoire and T cell activation markers in Kawasaki disease. J Immunol 1994;153:1881.
122. Leung D, Meissner H, Fulton D, et al. Toxic shock syndrome toxin-secreting *Staphylococcus aureus* in Kawasaki syndrome. Lancet 1993;342:1385.
123. Terai M, Miwa K, Williams T, et al. The absence of evidence of staphylococcal toxin involvement in the pathogenesis of Kawasaki disease. J Infect Dis 1995;172:558.
124. Barron K, Shulman S, Rowley A, et al. Report of the National Institutes of Health workshop on Kawasaki disease. J Rheumatol 1999;26:170.
125. Newburger J, Takahashi M, Burns J, et al. The treatment of Kawasaki syndrome with intravenous gamma globulin. N Engl J Med 1986;315:341.
126. Terai M, Shulman S. Prevalence of coronary artery abnormalities in Kawasaki disease is highly dependent on gamma globulin dose but independent of salicylate dose. J Pediatr 1997;131:888.
127. Hu PJ, Shih I-M, Hutchins GM, et al. Polyarteritis nodosa diagnosed by pericardial biopsy. J Rheumatol 1997;24:2042.
128. Hellmann DB. Vasculitis. In: Stobo JD, Hellmann DH, Ladenson PW, et al. (eds) The principles and practice of medicine, 23rd edn. Connecticut, Appleton & Lange, 1996, p 215.
129. Jinnah H, Dixon A, Brat D, Hellmann D. Chronic meningitis with cranial neuropathies in Wegener's granulomatosis: Case report and review of the literature. Arthritis Rheum 1997;40:573.

Section 6 Systemic Immune Diseases

Chapter 68

Large Vessel Vasculitides

Gene G. Hunder and Mehrdad Mazlumzadeh

A number of forms of vasculitis can involve large arteries such as the aorta and its branches. Aside from Takayasu arteritis and giant cell (temporal) arteritis (GCA), however, such involvement is uncommon. Occasionally, patients with connective tissue disorders including rheumatoid arthritis, ankylosing spondylitis, Behçet disease, and Reiter syndrome develop aortitis. In addition, infectious aortitis may occur in tuberculosis and syphilis. However, in all these conditions, involvement of the large arteries is uncommon. In contrast, these arteries are the primary sites of involvement in Takayasu arteritis and giant cell (temporal) arteritis.

TAKAYASU ARTERITIS

Takayasu arteritis is a chronic inflammatory vasculitis of unknown etiology that occurs primarily in young women. It has a worldwide distribution, with greatest prevalence in Asians. It affects mainly the aorta and its primary branches. Several other names have also been used for this condition, including *aortic arch arteritis, aortitis syndrome, pulseless disease, brachiocephalic arteritis*, and *occlusive thromboarteropathy*. Narrowing, occlusion, and dilatation in varying degrees develop in involved portions of arteries, resulting in a wide variety of symptoms.

Clinical features

Over 90% of Takayasu arteritis patients are female.[1] The age at onset in the majority is between 10 and 40 years. In the early phase of the disease, systemic symptoms including fatigue, weight loss, and low-grade fever are common (Table 68.1). Arthralgias or myalgias occur in about half of the patients,[1–3] but clinically evident synovitis is less common. Articular symptoms may be transient or continuous over several months or more. Occasionally, early in the course of the disease before vascular findings become obvious, patients with prominent arthritis are mistakenly considered to have juvenile rheumatoid arthritis. In a minority of cases, skin lesions resembling erythema nodosum are found over the legs; on biopsy these lesions show vasculitis involving small vessels.[4] As the disease continues, evidence of vascular involvement and insufficiency becomes apparent as a result of narrowing or occlusion of proximal and/or distal branches of the aorta. The extremities become cool, and pain develops with use (arm or leg claudication). In advanced cases, occlusions of the vessels to the extremities may result in ischemic ulcerations or gangrene.[5] Because of the chronic nature of the disease, collateral circulation frequently develops in the affected areas.[3,6]

KEY CONCEPTS

Takayasu arteritis and giant cell arteritis compared

Finding	Takayasu arteritis	Giant cell arteritis
Sex ratio (M : F)	1 : 7	2: 3
Age at onset	<40 years	>50 years
Ethnic ancestry	Asian	European
Histopathology	Granulomatous inflammation	Granulomatous inflammation
Vessels most commonly involved	Aorta and branches	External carotid artery branches
Renovascular hypertension	Common	Rare
HLA association	HLA-B52	HLA-DR4
Course	Chronic	Self-limited
Response to corticosteroids	Excellent	Excellent
Surgical intervention needed	Common	Rare

Clinical features in patients with Takayasu arteritis

Finding	Percentage of patients
Malaise	33
Weight loss	20
Fever	27
Myalgias/arthralgias	50
Headache	50
Asymmetric or absent pulses of arms/legs	53/15
Claudication of arms/legs	62/32
Arterial bruits	80
Aortic valve insufficiency	20
Hypertension	33
Postural dizziness	33
Ischemic chest pain	10
Visual aberration/loss	20
Stroke/TIA	16

Table 68.1 Clinical features in patients with Takayasu arteritis.

Pulmonary arteries have been reported to be involved in up to 50% of cases.[7,8] However, symptoms related to the pulmonary arteries are less common. They include dyspnea, hemoptysis, and pulmonary hypertension.

Involvement of the carotid and vertebral arteries produces decreased cerebral blood flow and may cause vertigo, syncope, orthostasis, headaches, convulsions, and dementia. Visual impairment is a late manifestation and is due to severe cerebral ischemia.[1,9]

Abdominal pain, diarrhea, and hemorrhage may result from mesenteric artery ischemia. Angina pectoris may develop secondary to coronary artery ostial narrowing related to aortitis.[10]

On physical examination, the patient often looks chronically ill. Prior to treatment, fever may be present. As noted, reduced blood pressure in one or both arms is common, and a differential of over 10 mmHg between the arms is frequent. Arterial pulses in the arms and legs are diminished, often to an asymmetrical degree. Bruits are often audible over the subclavian arteries, brachial arteries, carotids, and abdominal vessels. Aortic valve insufficiency develops in some cases due to dilatation of the aortic root.[1,3,7] Early in the disease, synovitis may be palpable over larger joints.

Hypertension develops in more than half of patients secondary to narrowing of the renal artery or narrowing and decreased elasticity of the aorta and branches.[1,2] However, narrowing or occlusion of the arteries in the arms can make it difficult to assess the blood pressure. Blood pressure also can be measured by using a wide cuff on an uninvolved thigh or by direct measurements of the proximal aorta. It can also be estimated by ophthalmodynamometry.

Laboratory tests

In most patients with active disease, normochromic normocytic anemia is present.[3] The leukocyte count is usually normal. Other changes reflecting the underlying inflammatory process include an elevated erythrocyte sedimentation rate, reduced albumin concentration, increased quantity of α_2-globulins, and elevated levels of C-reactive protein.[3] Although not always precise or invariably reliable indicators, these tests usually reflect the state of activity of the disease.

Etiology

The cause of Takayasu arteritis is unknown. Although Takayasu arteritis occurs in all populations, it appears to be more frequent in persons of Asian ethnic background. In Japan, an autopsy survey suggested a frequency of 1 in 3000 persons.[5] In an American study, the incidence of Takayasu arteritis in Whites was found to be 2.6 new cases per million persons per year.[3] HLA-B52 has been increased in frequency in several studies, suggesting an immunogenetic association.[11] Elevated immunoglobulin levels seen in some patients have suggested a role for immune complexes. Anti-aorta antibodies have been reported, suggesting an autoimmune process.[12,13] However, these studies need further definition.

Pathogenesis

The disease may be localized to a portion of the thoracic or abdominal aorta and its branches, or involve the entire aorta. Pulmonary arteries are also affected in up to more than half of cases. Angiography and autopsy examinations of patients with Takayasu arteritis have usually shown patchy or continuous involvement of portions of the aorta, innominate, common carotid, and subclavian arteries. Additionally, coronary, celiac, mesenteric, renal, and iliac arteries are frequently affected.[1,14]

Inflammatory processes cause thickening of the walls of affected arteries.[15] The proximal aorta may become dilated secondary to the inflammatory injury and result in aortic valve insufficiency. The abdominal aorta and its branches are also frequently affected. Involvement of the proximal hepatic, celiac, or mesenteric artery may cause ischemic changes in these organs. Renal artery stenosis frequently results in renal hypertension.[3]

Anatomically, Takayasu arteritis has been classified into four types: type IA is the most typical, with involvement of the ascending aorta, aortic arch, and branches. Type IB is similar in location but with aneurysmal dilatation of the proximal thoracic aorta. Type II refers to involvement of the descending thoracic and abdominal aorta. Type III is a combination of types I and II. Type IV indicates pulmonary artery involvement, usually accompanied by aortitis.[2,14]

Histologically, a diffuse or patchy granulomatous inflammatory reaction is present in the arterial media. Lymphocytes, macrophages, and multinucleated giant cells are the predominant cells seen on histologic examination. Elastic fibers are disrupted, causing weakening of the vessel wall (Fig. 68.1). Variable, but often marked, intimal thickening is present. Few if any inflammatory cells are seen in the intima. As the lesions evolve, fibrosis and scarring cause narrowing or occlusion of the arterial lumen, and collateral circulation develops. Little is known about the molecular and cellular mechanisms that initiate and perpetuate the inflammatory processes in Takayasu arteritis.

Natural history

Takayasu arteritis tends to be a chronic disease. The degree of activity varies with apparent exacerbation, reduction, or remission in the intensity of the inflammatory processes. The disease may burn out eventually.[1,3] Although there is considerable variability, the initial vascular lesions frequently occur in the left middle or proximal subclavian artery. As the process progresses, the left common carotid, vertebral, brachiocephalic, right middle or proximal subclavian artery, right common carotid and vertebral arteries, and aorta are also affected. The abdominal aorta and pulmonary arteries are affected in approximately 50% of patients.

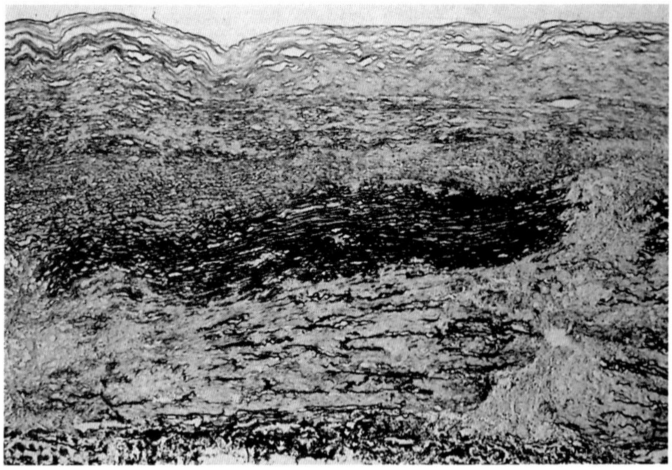

Figure 68.1 Takayasu arteritis specimen from ascending aorta. Low-power magnification with elastic tissue stain. Adventitia is at the bottom and thickened intima at the top. Extensive disruption of elastic tissue fibers in media can be seen.

Although vascular involvement tends to be progressive, the short-term outlook is good. In one follow-up study of 54 patients, an 83% 5-year survival was observed.[9] In another study of 32 patients, the 5-year survival was 94%.[3] A recent study of 120 patients revealed an overall 15-year survival rate of 83%. Major complications such as severe hypertension and cardiac involvement, a progressive course, and a younger age of onset indicate a poor prognosis.[16]

Diagnosis

The early diagnosis of Takayasu arteritis can be difficult. In the initial stages of the disease, the symptoms are often nonspecific. Typically, the patient complains of fatigue, malaise, and joint aches. Low-grade fever may also be present. In this period, sometimes called the *prepulseless phase*, vascular changes may not be marked enough to cause obvious extremity ischemia or arm claudication. However, a careful examination of the arteries may lead to the detection of a reduction in one or more pulses, differences in blood pressure between the arms, or bruits over the neck, supraclavicular areas, axillae, or abdomen. The detection of bruits or decreased pulses in a young woman narrows the focus of the differential diagnosis. Anemia of chronic disease and an elevated erythrocyte sedimentation rate (ESR) or C-reactive protein (CRP) support the diagnosis.

Arteriography is usually necessary to confirm the diagnosis (Fig. 68.2). The arteriographic changes tend to be most pronounced in the region of the aortic arch and its primary branches as noted, but in some cases involvement is most prominent in, or limited to, the more distal aorta and its branches. Arteriograms characteristically show smooth-walled, tapered, focal, or prolonged narrowed areas with some areas of dilatation. Collateral circulation is usually prominent because of the chronic nature of the disease.

Ultrasound examinations can help to detect alterations in the aorta or its branches.[17] Computed tomography (CT), CT angiography, or magnetic resonance (MR) imaging scans of the chest, abdomen, or other areas can also be helpful in detecting and evaluating the arterial tree (Fig. 68.3).[18,19]

The differential diagnosis includes fibromuscular dysplasia, which is usually more focal in its involvement. Excess ergotamine intake may cause reversible spasm of the large blood vessels. Ehlers–Danlos syndrome may cause vascular abnormalities. However, Ehlers–Danlos syndrome results in the development of aneurysms, which may rupture, and few, if any, stenoses. The American College of Rheumatology has established classification criteria for Takayasu arteritis (Table 68.2).[6] These criteria have a high sensitivity and specificity and should be used consistently.

Treatment

Glucocorticoids are effective in suppressing the systemic symptoms and usually arrest the progression of the disease. Normochromic anemia and elevated ESR and CRP also return to normal. A possible role for inflammatory cytokines such as IL-6 in the evaluation and management of Takayasu arteritis has been suggested.[20] In early cases, arterial stenosis may be reversed and ischemic symptoms improve. However, after fibrous tissue has formed in the involved vessels or thrombosis has occurred, the response to therapy is diminished.

An initial dose of 40–60 mg of prednisone or an equivalent dose of a similar glucocorticoid may be started in an adult of average size. A single morning dose is generally effective and convenient. When the symptoms and laboratory tests related to the inflammatory processes have improved to a maximum, the dose may be gradually reduced by a maximum of 10% of the daily amount per week. Long-term lower-dose prednisone therapy may be necessary to prevent progressive arterial stenosis. If the

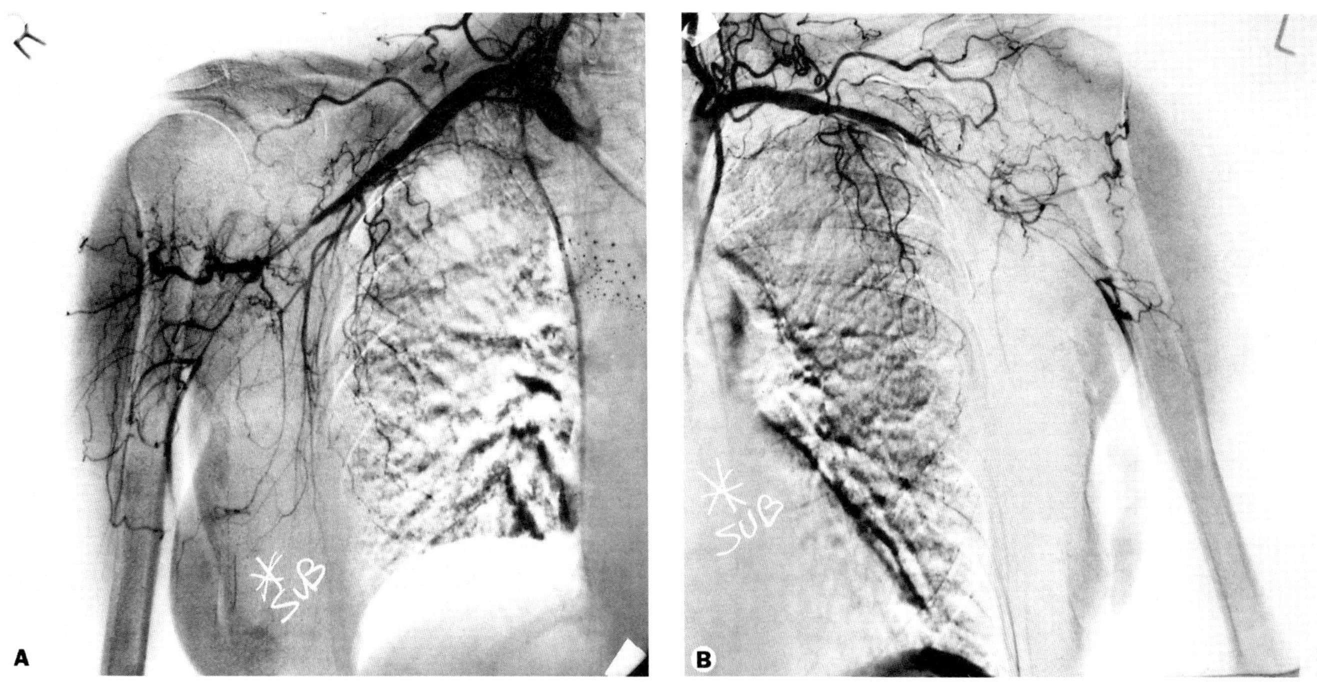

Figure 68.2 Selective arteriograms of right (**A**) and left (**B**) subclavian and more distal arteries in a patient with Takayasu arteritis. Irregularity of subclavian arteries is present and also marked tapered narrowing of axillary arteries (distal to clavicles). Brachial artery lumina are reconstituted at the level of proximal humerus (partially filled). Extensive collateral circulation has developed.

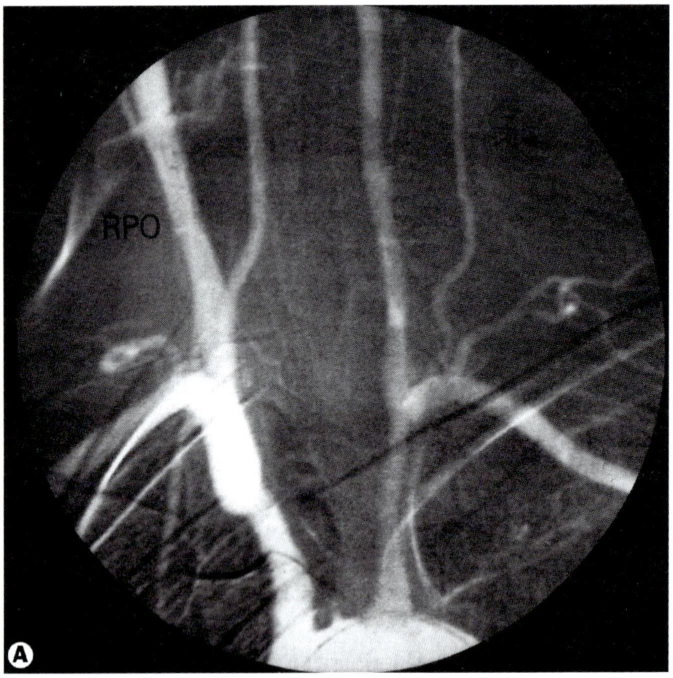

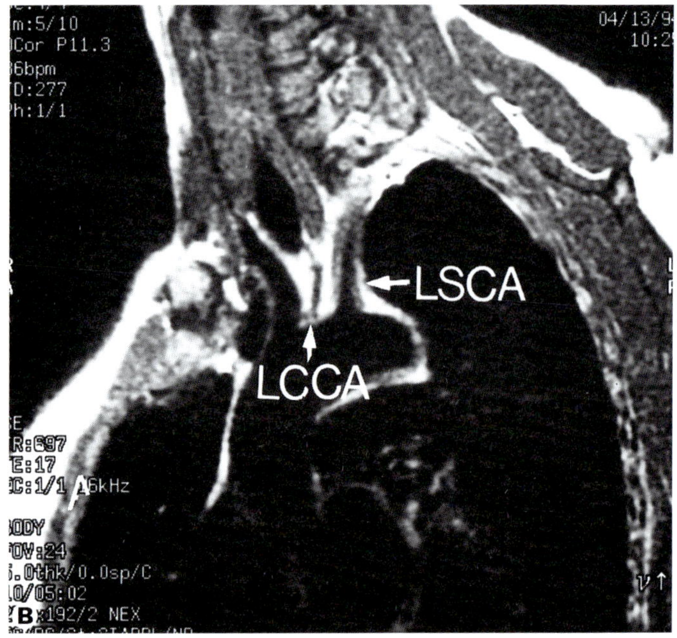

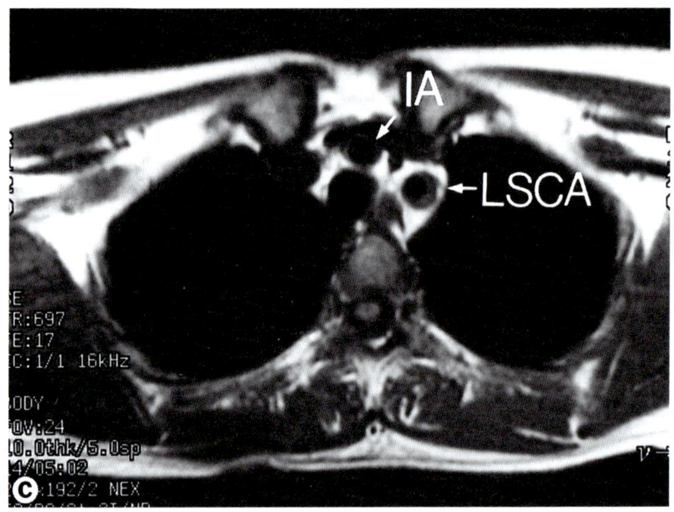

Figure 68.3 Takayasu arteritis. (**A**) Aortic arch arteriogram shows mild to moderate narrowing of great vessels. Changes are most prominent in proximal left subclavian artery. (**B**) T1 weighted, cardiac gated MRI, same patient. Oblique sagittal MRI shows thickened walls of left common carotid artery (LCCA) and left subclavian artery (LSCA). (**C**) Axial MRI, same patient, shows thickened walls of innominate artery (IA) and left subclavian artery (LSCA).

1990 Criteria for the classification of Takayasu arteritis (traditional format)

Criterion	Definition
Age at disease onset ≤ 40 years	Development of symptoms or findings related to Takayasu arteritis at age ≤ 40 years
Claudication of extremities	Development and worsening of fatigue and discomfort in muscles of one or more extremity while in use, especially the upper extremities
Decreased brachial artery pressure	Decreased pulsation of one or both brachial arteries
Blood pressure difference >10 mmHg	Difference of >10 mmHg in systolic blood pressure between arms
Bruit over subclavian arteries or aorta	Bruit audible on auscultation over one or both subclavian arteries or abdominal aorta
Arteriogram abnormality	Arteriographic narrowing or occlusion of the entire aorta, its primary branches, or large arteries in the proximal upper or lower extremities, not due to arteriosclerosis, fibromuscular dysplasia, or similar causes; changes usually focal or segmental

For purposes of classification, a patient shall be said to have Takayasu arteritis if at least three of these six criteria are present. The presence of any three or more criteria yields a sensitivity of 90.5% and a specificity of 97.8%.

Table 68.2 1990 Criteria for the classification of Takayasu arteritis (traditional format). (From Arend WP, Michel BA, Block DA, et al. The American College of Rheumatology 1990 Criteria for the Classification of Takayasu Arteritis. Arthritis Rheum 1990;33:1129. with permission.)

disease goes into remission, glucocorticoids may be discontinued. If exacerbations occur, the dosage may need to be increased once more. Alternate-day glucocorticoid therapy may be tried, but it is generally not as effectives as daily therapy. The efficacy of cytotoxic drugs is uncertain; however, a preliminary report suggested a favorable response to mycophenolate mofetil in three cases.[21] Methotrexate may help in some glucocorticoid-resistant or relapsing cases.[22] Antihypertensive drugs are useful if hypertension is present, and heart failure should be treated as in other diseases. Angioplasty or bypass grafts may be considered in late cases in which irreversible artery stenosis has occurred and significant ischemic symptoms are present. Angioplasty in some ways is a simpler procedure than surgery. However, stenoses or occlusions may affect a lengthy portion of the artery, making dilatation of the involved segment technically difficult. Furthermore, continued inflammation in a treated segment may result in restenosis, a problem that is avoided by bypass grafting.

GIANT CELL (TEMPORAL) ARTERITIS

Giant cell arteritis (GCA) is a vasculitis of unknown etiology that involves medium-sized and large arteries, particularly the arteries originating from the thoracic aorta and especially the external carotid artery. It is also referred to as *temporal arteritis*, *cranial arteritis*, and *granulomatous arteritis*.[23,24]

Clinical features

Giant cell arteritis nearly always begins after the age of 50 years, and 80% of the patients are 60 years of age or older at onset. The age at peak incidence is about 70 years. Two thirds of cases occur in women.[25]

The onset is usually gradual but may be abrupt. In most cases, symptoms have been present for weeks or months before the diagnosis is established. Constitutional symptoms including fatigue, malaise, fever, and weight loss are common and are often the initial manifestations. Fever is present in approximately one half of patients. It is usually low grade but occasionally reaches a level of 40°C (104°F) or more, accompanied by shaking chills resembling a septic process.[24,26]

The initial symptoms vary widely. The earliest manifestations in 100 consecutive biopsy-proven cases with giant cell arteritis in one series are shown in Table 68.3. Initial manifestations have also been described that were not seen in this group of patients, such as unexplained high ESR, anemia, cough, myocardial infarction, thrombocytosis of unknown cause, and stroke.[23,26–29]

Table 68.4 shows the overall clinical findings in the same 100 consecutive patients. Most patients with GCA have symptoms related to the vascular involvement at some time during the course of the illness. Headache is the most frequent symptom and is present in two thirds or more patients. It is often present early in the course of the disease and frequently is the initial manifestation. Headache may be mild or severe; it is often localized to the temporal, occipital, or periorbital areas but may be generalized. It may be present even when the temporal arteries are normal to palpation and may vary or improve even before the disease is treated. Scalp tenderness is common and most frequently is localized to the temporal or occipital arteries, but it also may be more generalized. Intermittent claudication of the muscles of mastication occurs in 40% or more of cases. This symptom is most frequently noted over the mandibular area in the region of the masseter and pterygoid muscles. Characteristically, it develops when the patient chews food, such as meat, that requires jaw muscles to exert extra effort. There is a progressive fatiguing discomfort that usually forces the patient to stop chewing for a short period of time. It is of varying severity and is usually bilateral. It may be more marked on one side

Initial manifestations of giant cell arteritis in 100 patients

Manifestation	Percentage of patients
Headache	32
Polymyalgia rheumatica (PMR)	25
Fever	15
Visual symptoms without loss	7
Weakness/malaise/fatigue	5
Tenderness over arteries	3
Myalgias	4
Weight loss/anorexia	2
Jaw claudication	2
Permanent loss of vision	1
Tongue claudication	1
Sore throat	1
Vasculitis on angiogram	1
Stiffness of hands and wrists	1
Total	*100*

Table 68.3 Initial manifestations of giant cell arteritis in 100 patients. (From Calamia KT, Hunder GG. Clinical manifestations of giant cell (temporal) arteritis. Clin Rheum Dis 1980;6:389 with permission.)

CLINICAL PEARLS

Important points when considering the diagnosis of giant cell arteritis

- Giant cell arteritis develops in older individuals; 80% of patients are over 60 years old.
- Systemic inflammation in giant cell arteritis causes constitutional symptoms and laboratory abnormalities (elevated ESR or increased CRP levels) in most patients.
- Giant cell arteritis should be considered when an older patient complains of a new type of headache, develops sudden vision changes or visual loss, or has unexplained evidence of systemic inflammation.
- Polymyalgia rheumatica (PMR), a syndrome characterized by proximal musculoskeletal pain and stiffness, is closely linked with giant cell arteritis.
- A temporal artery biopsy should be considered when the diagnosis of giant cell arteritis is strongly suspected.

Clinical findings in 100 patients with giant cell arteritis	
Finding	**Percentage of patients**
Onset: gradual/sudden	64/36
Weight loss, anorexia	50
Malaise/fatigue/weakness	40
Fever	42
Polymyalgia rheumatica	39
Other musculoskeletal pains	30
Synovitis	15
Symptoms related to arteries	83
Jaw claudication	45
Headache	68
Visual symptoms: transient/fixed	16/14
Swallowing claudication, dysphagia	8
Tongue claudication	6
Limb claudication	4
Signs related to arteries	66
Artery tenderness	27
Erythematous/nodular/swollen scalp arteries	23
Large artery: bruits/decreased pulses	21/7
Extraocular muscle weakness	2
Raynaud phenomenon	3
Central nervous system abnormalities	25
Sore throat	9

Table 68.4 Clinical findings in 100 patients with giant cell arteritis. (From Calamia KT, Hunder GG. Clinical manifestations of giant cell (temporal) arteritis. Clin Rheum Dis 1980;6:389 with permission.)

Visual manifestations in 34 of 245 patients with giant cell arteritis	
Symptoms	**Number of patients**
Amaurosis fugax	4
Diplopia	2
Permanent partial visual loss	22
Unilateral	15
Bilateral	7
Permanent complete visual loss	12
Unilateral	11
Bilateral	1

Table 68.5 Visual manifestations in 34 of 245 patients with giant cell arteritis. (Modified from Aiello PD, Trautmann JC, McPhee TJ, et al. Visual prognosis in giant cell arteritis. Ophthalmology 1993;100:550 with permission.)

than the other and, like other symptoms, may improve even before treatment has been started. It is caused by narrowing of the branches of the facial artery supplying the muscles involved in chewing. Similar symptoms may occur in the tongue muscles, those involved in deglutition, and in the extremities, particularly the arms. Occasionally, pain in the mandibular area is more continuous, and the discomfort is worse when the mouth is opened.

Visual complications are common in GCA. In most series, 15–20% of patients developed some permanent visual loss,[30,31] including partial or complete unilateral or bilateral blindness. Transient visual blurring or visual loss, diplopia, and ptosis may also be seen. Permanent visual loss occurs somewhat more frequently in patients who have antecedent amaurosis fugax. Visual loss is generally the result of narrowing or occlusion of the branches of the ophthalmic or posterior ciliary arteries, which produces ischemia of the optic nerve or tracts. Less commonly, visual loss is secondary to occlusion of the retinal arterioles. Occasionally, arteritis of vessels supplying the occipital lobes causes infarction of the visual cortex. The ophthalmoscopic examination usually shows findings of ischemic optic neuritis, with papilledema and scattered punctate hemorrhages. These changes generally develop simultaneously with or immediately after visual loss.

Table 68.5 shows the ophthalmic manifestations in a survey of 245 patients with giant cell arteritis who were studied over a 5-year period after the diagnosis.[30] Thirty-four patients (14%) permanently lost some vision. In nearly all of these patients, the visual deficit occurred before glucocorticoid therapy was started. In 2 others, the visual loss occurred after the diagnosis was made and therapy started. In 3 patients, visual loss progressed after the initiation of glucocorticoids, and in 5 others vision improved after treatment was started but did not return to normal. The probability of new visual loss developing over a 5-year period after initial glucocorticoid therapy was started was 1% (Kaplan–Meier technique), and the probability of additional loss after therapy was started in patients who had some loss of vision before therapy was initiated was 13%. Thus, development or progression of visual loss in giant cell arteritis after the initiation of glucocorticoid therapy is uncommon, and occasionally visual loss improves following therapy.[30,31]

Neurologic manifestations, which occur in about 30% of patients, are diverse. They include mononeuropathies and peripheral neuropathies. The symptoms are ischemic in nature, but pathologic documentation of vasculitis has rarely been obtained. Strokes or brainstem ischemic episodes occur in about 10% of patients and are mainly secondary to narrowing or occlusion of the carotid or vertebral arteries or branches.[27,32]

Large artery manifestations are present in 10–15% of patients.[29,32,33] Findings include decreased pulses in the arms or diminished blood pressure that has developed during the illness; new bruits over the cervical, subclavian, axillary, or brachial arteries; central nervous system events such as those described previously; and arm claudication. In some instances, aortic aneurysms develop that result in dissection and rupture.[33] Aneurysms or dissection can occur early in the course of disease and rarely may be the initial manifestation. However, it has become apparent that aortic aneurysm is most commonly a late complication that is found several years after other symptoms of the disease have resolved and when the patient is on low-dose glucocorticoids or the drugs have been discontinued.[33,34] Angiograms of involved large blood vessels show smooth-walled, tapered arterial stenoses or occlusions alternating with areas of normal caliber or aneurysms.[35] The findings tend to be most marked in the subclavian arteries and are often more marked on the left. The carotid, vertebral, axillary, and brachial arteries may also be involved extensively. Occasionally, the iliac or femoral arteries become narrowed and produce leg claudication. Recent preliminary studies have suggested a possible role for imaging modalities such as gallium scan, MRI angiography, or positron emission tomography (PET) in the diagnosis and therapeutic management of these patients.[36–38]

Polymyalgia rheumatica (PMR) is closely linked to GCA. It is a syndrome characterized by aching and morning stiffness (lasting longer than 30 minutes) in the proximal portions of the extremities and torso. Diagnostic criteria commonly include the presence of symptoms in two of the three commonly affected areas (shoulder girdle, hip girdle, and neck or torso) lasting 1 month or longer, accompanied by evidence of systemic inflammation, usually an erythrocyte sedimentation rate elevated to 40 or 50 mm in 1 hour or more (Westergren method). Some authors have also included a rapid response to a small dose of glucocorticoids (e.g. 10 mg prednisone daily) as a diagnostic criterion.[24,39,40]

PMR is found in approximately half of the patients with giant cell arteritis and is the initial symptom in about one fourth. It may also be a late manifestation and can appear initially as the glucocorticoid dose has been reduced after several weeks or more of treatment of GCA.[24] In patients with mild aching, the discomfort may resolve during the day but return again after prolonged sitting or the following morning. Those with more severe symptoms may be incapacitated by the pain and stiffness, which is accentuated by any movement.

The cause of aching and stiffness in patients with PMR is not completely understood. PMR appears to be due in large part to synovitis of proximal joints and periarticular tissues. The fact that many patients with GCA do not have PMR, even when large arteries in the shoulder girdle are affected, suggests that inflammation in the arteries is not the primary cause of the aching. Synovitis of the proximal joints and tenosynovial membranes and mild to moderate synovitis of the knees, shoulders, and elsewhere has been demonstrated in many patients by physical examination, MRI, and biopsies.[41–43] However, the degree of discomfort often seems out of proportion to the occlusion of the swollen joints.

When the relationship between GCA and PMR is analyzed from the perspective of PMR, numerous investigators have noted that about 15% of patients who have no clinical findings related to the arteries at the time of the diagnosis may nonetheless be found to have positive temporal artery biopsies when a 'blind' biopsy is performed.

Etiology

A number of causes have been considered for GCA, but the etiology remains unknown.[44] The increased incidence of GCA after the age of 50 years indicates a possible relationship to aging, but the significance of this finding is not currently understood. Several reports of familial cases and the observed increased frequency of GCA in Europe and in populations in the USA with mixed European backgrounds suggest a genetic predisposition.[44–46] Environmental factors, particularly infectious agents, have been proposed as additional associated etiological factors.[47–49]

In several studies, an increased frequency of HLA-DR4 in patients with giant cell arteritis has suggested a possible role for particular major histocompatibility complex (MHC) Class II alleles. In recent studies, genetic polymorphisms of the HLA-DRB1 gene were analyzed.[50] The B1*0401 or *0404/8 alleles were found in 60% of the patients in comparison to 19% of normal controls.[50] In addition, patients who did not have these HLA-DR4 alleles had other alleles that shared an amino acid sequence with HLA-DR4 alleles. The region of shared amino acid sequence forms part of the floor of the antigen-binding groove of the HLA-DR molecule. The sequence may therefore play a critical role in the selection and presentation of antigens to CD4 T lymphocytes in the immunopathogenesis of GCA.[50]

Pathogenesis

The inflammatory processes involve medium-sized and large arteries in an intermittent, apparently random distribution. However, longer segments may also be involved in some instances. The factors initiating the inflammatory reactions and the sequence of cellular events that result in the arteritis are poorly understood. GCA appears to be a T-cell-dependent disease which leads to an inflammatory reaction of the vessel walls in addition to a systemic activation of monocytes.[51,52] As noted, there appears to be a predilection for the thoracic aorta and its branches. The branches of the external carotid artery are the most commonly affected vessels from a clinical standpoint. The narrowing or occlusion of these vessels as a result of the inflammation produces many of the characteristic manifestations. As a result of the inflammation, the structures of the affected arteries are disrupted. Dilatation or occlusion may occur in the carotid, subclavian, and smaller arteries, but aortic aneurysm with dissection and rupture develops in about 10% of patients.

The inflammatory reaction may involve all layers of the blood vessels but is often most marked near the internal elastic lamina. Lymphocytes (mostly helper T cells), macrophages, and multinucleated giant cells are clustered together, forming a granulomatous inflammatory reaction (Fig. 68.4). Giant cells may be seen to contain particles of elastin. The intima becomes thickened, but generally there are few cells infiltrating this region. Clinical and autopsy studies have shown that the vascular inflammation stops as the cervical vessels penetrate the dura of the skull, coincident with a reduction of arterial wall elastin. These observations suggest a possible autoimmune response to age-altered elastin or possibly some material deposited near the elastic tissue. In some instances in GCA, immunoglobulins may be demonstrated along the internal elastic lamina in areas involved by the inflammatory process. An immune response to elastin in GCA has not been demonstrated, however.

Natural history

Giant cell arteritis may begin abruptly but usually develops insidiously. The symptoms increase in severity over weeks or longer, during which time new manifestations develop and some may resolve. In a minority, the initial manifestation may be a major vascular manifestation such as sudden loss of eyesight or rupture of the aorta. The degree of activity varies, and in most cases the disease appears to resolve gradually with occasional exacerbations, some of which become manifest as the glucocorticoid dose is being lowered. The disease tends to run a self-limited course over several months to several years. Occasionally, however, the activity continues at a lower level for a number of years. A small proportion of patients have recurrence after several years, but eventually the disease seems to resolve completely. The prognosis is usually good, life expectancy being similar to that of the general population.[53]

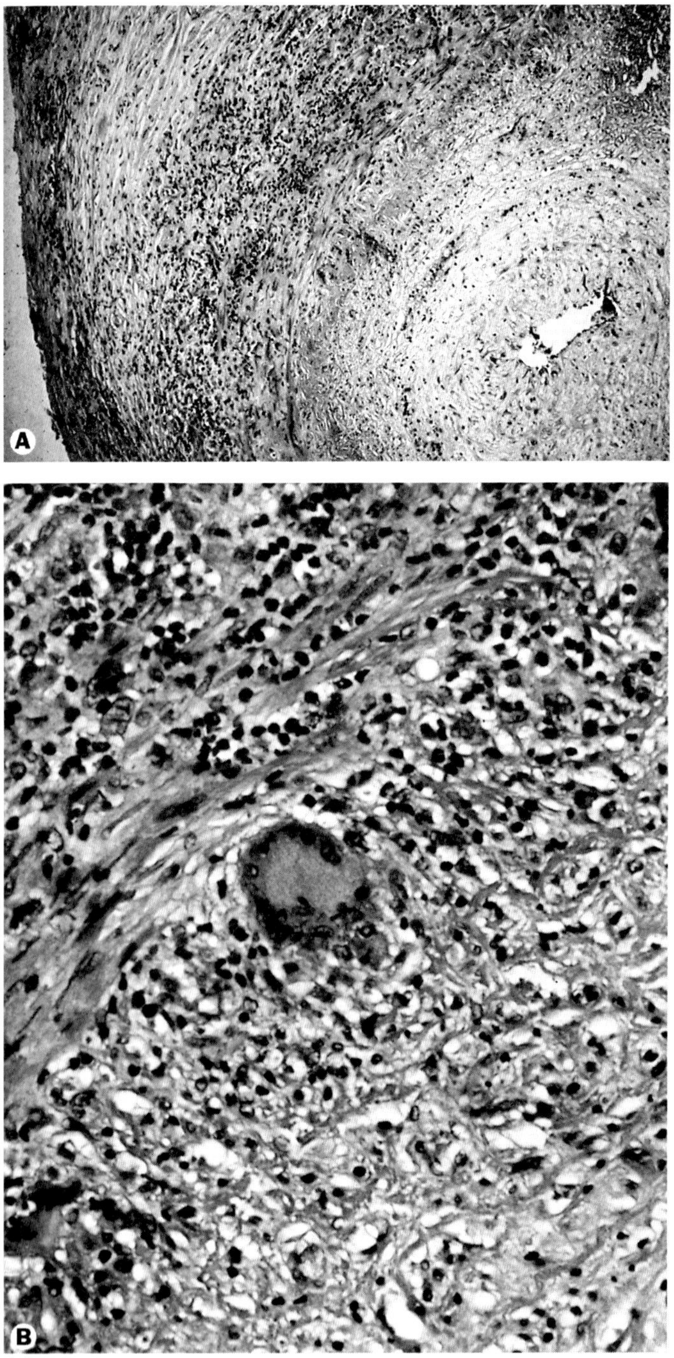

Figure 68.4 Giant cell arteritis. Temporal artery biopsy showing a chronic inflammatory reaction (**A**) most extensive in the media. The narrowed lumen at lower right is surrounded by a thickened intima (original magnification ×100). Higher-power magnification (**B**) shows multinucleated giant cell (original magnification ×250).

Diagnosis

Giant cell arteritis should be considered when a patient older than 50 years of age complains of a new form of headache, transient or sudden loss of vision, PMR, or unexpected fever, or develops unexplained anemia or a high erythrocyte sedimentation rate. A careful history may elicit the presence of more specific manifestations as described previously. The arteries of the head, neck, upper torso, and extremities should be examined for enlargement, tenderness, and the presence of pulsations.

A temporal artery biopsy for diagnosis is recommended for all patients suspected of having GCA. If the occipital artery is most abnormal, it can be biopsied. A clinically abnormal segment, if present, should be chosen for the biopsy because involvement may be focal. If the artery is obviously abnormal, only a small portion of the vessel needs to be removed, but when the temporal arteries feel normal and giant cell arteritis is being considered, a specimen 3–5 cm in length should be taken. It should be examined histologically at several different levels. If the first side is normal, biopsy of the second side also should be considered. Giant cells may not be seen in all biopsy sections. However, the presence of a lymphocytic infiltration in the media, along with interruption of the internal elastic lamina plus the clinical picture, is sufficient to make the diagnosis in most cases. Color duplex ultrasonography of the affected arteries may detect luminal abnormalities or periarterial hypoechogenic halos.[54,55] Although such findings may not discriminate between GCA and other inflammatory arteritides, the abnormalities may provide an additional guide to the site of biopsy. Arteriograms of the aortic arch and branches should be obtained in patients with symptoms or findings suggesting large artery abnormalities (Fig. 68.5). The subclavian, axillary, brachial, carotid, and vertebral arteries should be carefully evaluated.

Occasionally, other forms of vasculitis involve the temporal arteries, including polyarteritis nodosa, Wegener's granulomatosis, and hypersensitivity vasculitis. However, in these other forms of vasculitis, the different clinical findings and presence of polymorphonuclear leukocytes in the inflammatory infiltrate help to separate these cases from GCA. Occasionally, jaw or arm claudication may be present in patients with amyloidosis who have vascular involvement; in these cases, Congo red stains of artery biopsies or other tissues show birefringent deposits.

Giant cell arteritis may be distinguished from Takayasu arteritis by the age at onset and ethnic distribution, and separated from isolated vasculitis of the central nervous system in which the intracranial arteries are affected. Criteria for the classification of giant cell arteritis have been formulated (Table 68.6).[56]

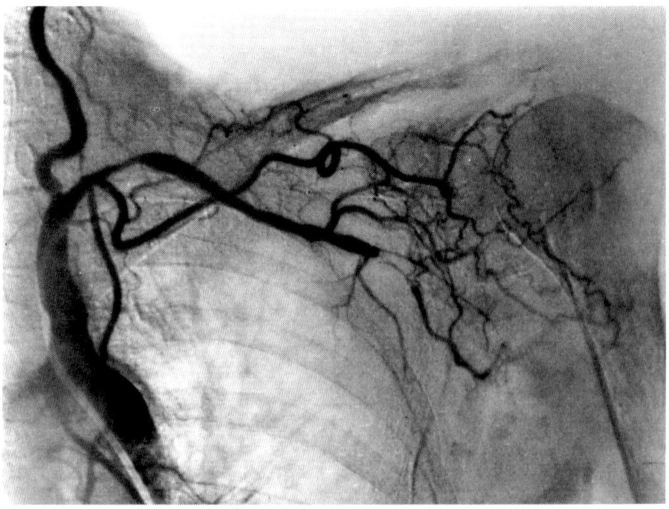

Figure 68.5 Giant cell arteritis. Angiogram showing a smooth-walled tapered stenosis of left subclavian artery and occlusion at level of the left axillary artery in a patient with an aortic arch syndrome. Numerous collateral vessels have formed.

Criterion	Definition
1. Age at disease onset ≥ 50 years	Development of symptoms or findings beginning at age 50 or older
2. New headache	New onset of or new type of localized pain in the head
3. Temporal artery abnormality	Temporal artery tenderness to palpation or decreased pulsation, unrelated to arteriosclerosis of cervical arteries
4. Elevated erythrocyte sedimentation rate	Erythrocyte sedimentation rate ≥ 50 mm/h by the Westergren method
5. Abnormal artery biopsy	Biopsy specimen with artery showing vasculitis characterized by a predominance of mononuclear cell infiltration or granulomatous inflammation, usually with multinucleated giant cells

1990 American College of Rheumatology criteria for the classification of giant cell (temporal) arteritis (traditional format)

For purpose of classification, a patient shall be said to have giant cell (temporal) arteritis if at least three of these five criteria are present. The presence of any three or more criteria yields a sensitivity of 93.5% and a specificity of 91.2%.

Table 68.6 1990 American College of Rheumatology criteria for the classification of giant cell (temporal) arteritis (traditional format). (From Hunder GG, Bloch DA, Michel B, et al. The American College of Rheumatology 1990 Criteria for the Classification of Giant Cell Arteritis. Arthritis Rheum 1990;33:1122 with permission.)

Treatment

Treatment with glucocorticoids should be started when the diagnosis is established. Patients in whom the diagnosis is strongly suspected may be started on glucocorticoids immediately or after blood tests have been obtained only for basic evaluations such as the hemoglobin and erythrocyte sedimentation rate. This immediate initiation of therapy is particularly necessary for those patients with a rapidly progressive course and those who appear to have impending complications such as blindness. Glucocorticoid treatment changes the histologic picture but does not completely abolish the vascular infiltrations for one or more weeks.[57] If temporal artery biopsy or biopsy of other arteries shows no vasculitis, but other clinical findings strongly favor the diagnosis, a trial of glucocorticoids may still be appropriate.

An initial dose of 40–60 mg of prednisone or the equivalent of a similar glucocorticoid in a single morning daily dose is adequate in nearly all cases. Patients with impending or recent vascular complications may be started on parenteral glucocorticoids. A pulse dose of 500–1000 mg of methylprednisolone for 1–3 days has been advocated by some as the initial treatment in those with blindness. If the initial oral dose does not result in rapid improvement, then it may need to be increased.

Increased secretion of inflammatory cytokines, especially interleukin-6 (IL-6), has been detected in GCA.[58] Although glucocorticoid therapy usually results in rapid normalization of symptoms and erythrocyte sedimentation rate, this may not correspond to suppression of IL-6 levels.[59] In fact, animal studies have shown that for complete suppression of inflammatory cytokines to occur there may be a need for higher glucocorticoid doses than conventional therapy in GCA.[60]

The effective initial prednisone dose should be maintained until all reversible symptoms and findings have resolved. Response usually occurs within 4 weeks. Subsequently, the dose can be reduced gradually by a maximum of 10% of the total daily amount each 1–2 weeks. The reduction program is determined by the continued suppression of symptoms and maintenance of a normal or near-normal erythrocyte sedimentation rate. Levels of C-reactive protein and hemoglobin are also helpful guides to therapy. If erythrocyte sedimentation rate or levels of C-reactive protein rise, further glucocorticoid reductions may need to be withheld for 2–4 weeks and subsequent reductions made by smaller amounts and at wider intervals. In some cases it may be necessary to continue doses of 15–25 mg of prednisone for several months. Gradual dose reduction allows a safer identification of the minimal suppressive dose needed and helps to avoid exacerbations that may result from too rapid withdrawal of glucocorticoids. Spontaneous exacerbations or recurrences occur in some patients. These are usually seen within the first 2 years of the disease but have been observed after several years. Alternate-day glucocorticoid therapy generally is not effective for giant cell arteritis.[61] Dapsone, antimalarials, penicillamine, cyclosporine, azathioprine, and methotrexate have been suggested as alternate therapies, but have neither been studied adequately nor proven to be efficacious.[62–66] However, these could be considered in patients who develop severe glucocorticoid side-effects and have not responded to treatment. The average length of treatment needed is 1–2 years but varies considerably. Due to the length of required glucocorticoid treatment, measures to prevent osteoporosis should be considered at the initiation of therapy.

THERAPEUTIC PRINCIPLES

Considerations in the treatment of giant cell arteritis

- Glucocorticoids are the mainstay of treatment.
- Treatment should be initiated in patients with an established diagnosis or in whom the diagnosis is strongly suspected, especially if visual or other vascular complications are suspected.
- Initial treatment in most patients should be oral prednisone at approximately 60 mg per day (or equivalent).
- The initial dose of prednisone should be maintained until all reversible signs and symptoms have resolved and inflammation has been suppressed.
- Prednisone tapering should be gradual, based on suppression of signs and symptoms and maintenance of a normal or near-normal erythrocyte sedimentation rate.
- Most patients need daily low doses of prednisone for at least 2 years.
- Other immunosuppressive medications, such as methotrexate, azathioprine, and cyclosporine have been suggested as alternative or additional therapies to glucocorticoids, but none has been proven to be efficacious.

REFERENCES

1. Kerr GS, Hallahan CW, Giordano J, Leavitt RY, Fauci AS, Rottem M, Hoffman GS. Takayasu arteritis. Ann Intern Med 1994;120:919.
2. Lupi-Herrera E, Sanchez-Torres G, Marcushamer J, et al. Takayasu's arteritis. Clinical study of 107 cases. Am Heart J 1977;93:94.
3. Hall S, Barr W, Lie JT, et al. Takayasu arteritis: A study of 32 North American patients. Medicine 1985;64:89.
4. Perniciaro CV, Winkelmann RK, Hunder GG. Cutaneous manifestations of Takayasu's arteritis: A clinicopathologic correlation. J Am Acad Dermatol 1987;17:998.
5. Nasu T. Takayasu's truncoarteritis in Japan: A statistical observation of 76 autopsy cases. Pathol Microbiol 1975;43:56.
6. Arend WP, Michel BA, Block DA, et al. The American College of Rheumatology 1990 Criteria for the Classification of Takayasu Arteritis. Arthritis Rheum 1990;33:1129.
7. Matsubara O, Yoshimura N, Tamura A, et al. Pathological features of the pulmonary artery in Takayasu arteritis. Heart Vessels 1992;7(suppl):18.
8. Sharma S, Kamalakar T, Rajani M, et al. The incidence and patterns of pulmonary artery involvement in Takayasu's arteritis. Clin Radiol 1990;42:177.
9. Subramanyan R, Joy J, Balakrishnan K. Natural history of aortoarteritis (Takayasu's disease). Circulation 1989;80:429.
10. Matsubara O, Kuwata T, Nemoto T, et al. Coronary artery lesions in Takayasu's arteritis: Pathological considerations. Heart Vessels 1992;7(suppl):26.
11. Dong R-P, Kimura P, Numano F, et al. HLA-linked susceptibility and resistance to Takayasu arteritis. Heart Vessels 1992;7(suppl):73.
12. Eichhorn J, Sima D, Thiele B, et al. Anti-endothelial cell antibodies in Takayasu arteritis. Circulation 1996;94:2396.
13. Blank M, Krause I, Goldkorn T, et al. Monoclonal anti-endothelial cell antibodies from a patient with Takayasu arteritis activate endothelial cells from large vessels. Arthritis Rheum 1999;42:1421.
14. Ishikawa K. Patterns of symptoms and prognosis in occlusive thromboaortopathy (Takayasu's disease). J Am Coll Cardiol 1986;8:1041.
15. Lie JT and members and consultants of the American College of Rheumatology Subcommittee on Classification of Vasculitis. Illustrated histopathologic classification criteria for selected vasculitis syndromes. Arthritis Rheum 1990;33:1074.
16. Ishikawa K, Maetani S. Peripheral arterial and aortic diseases: Long-term outcome for 120 Japanese patients with Takayasu's disease: clinical and statistical analyses of related prognostic factors. Circulation 1994;90:1855.
17. Sun Y, Yip PK, Jeng JS, Hwang BS, Lin WH. Ultrasonographic study and long-term follow-up of Takayasu's arteritis. Stroke 1996;27:2178.
18. Yamada I, Nakagawa T, Himeno Y, Numano F, Shibuya H. Takayasu arteritis: Evaluation of the thoracic aorta with CT angiography. Radiology 1998;209:103.
19. Hata A, Numano F. Magnetic resonance imaging of vascular changes in Takayasu arteritis. Int J Cardiol 1995;52:45.
20. Noris M, Daina E, Gamba S, Bonazzola S, Remuzzi G. Interleukin-6 and RANTES in Takayasu arteritis: A guide for therapeutic decisions? Circulation 1999;100:55.
21. Daina E, Schieppati A, Remuzzi G. Mycophenolate mofetil for the treatment of Takayasu arteritis: Report of three cases. Ann Intern Med 1999;130:422.
22. Hoffman GS, Leavitt RY, Kerr GS, Rottem M, Sneller MC, Fauci AS. Treatment of glucocorticoid-resistant or relapsing Takayasu arteritis with methotrexate. Arthritis Rheum 1994;37:578.
23. Calamia KT, Hunder GG. Clinical manifestations of giant cell (temporal) arteritis. Clin Rheum Dis 1980;6:389.
24. Hunder GG. Giant cell arteritis and polymyalgia rheumatica. Med Clin North Am 1997;81:195.
25. Salvarani C, Macchoni P, Ziggi F, et al. Epidemiologic and immunogenetic aspects of polymyalgia rheumatica and giant cell arteritis in Northern Italy. Arthritis Rheum 1991;34:351.
26. Calamia KT, Hunder GG. Giant cell arteritis (temporal arteritis) presenting as fever of undetermined origin. Arthritis Rheum 1981;24:1414.
27. Caselli RJ, Hunder GG. Neurologic aspects of giant cell (temporal) arteritis. Rheum Dis Clin North Am 1993;19:941.
28. Larson TS, Hall S, Hepper NGG, et al. Respiratory tract symptoms as a clue to giant cell arteritis. Ann Intern Med 1984;101:594.
29. Lie JT, Failoni D, Davis DC Jr. Temporal arteritis with giant cell aortitis, coronary arteritis, and myocardial infarction. Arch Pathol Lab Med 1986;110:857.
30. Aiello PD, Trautmann JC, McPhee TJ, et al. Visual prognosis in giant cell arteritis. Ophthalmology 1993;100:550.
31. Gonzalez-Gay MA, Blanco R, Rodriguez-Valverde V, Martinez-Taboada VM, Delgado-Rodriguez M, Figueroa M, Uriarte E. Permanent visual loss and cerebrovascular accidents in giant cell arteritis: Predictors and response to treatment. Arthritis Rheum 1998;41:1497.
32. Klein RG, Hunder GG, Stanson SW, et al. Large artery involvement in giant cell (temporal) arteritis. Ann Intern Med 1975;83:806.
33. Evans JM, Bowles CA, Bjornsson J, et al. Thoracic aortic aneurysm and rupture in giant cell arteritis. A descriptive study of 41 cases. Arthritis Rheum 1994;37:1539.
34. Evans JM, O'Fallon WM, Hunder GG. Increased incidence of aortic aneurysm and dissection in giant cell (temporal) arteritis: A population-based study. Ann Intern Med 1995;122:502.
35. Stanson AW, Klein RG, Hunder GG. Extracranial angiographic findings in giant cell (temporal) arteritis. Am J Roentgenol 1976;127:957.
36. Genereau T, Lortholary O, Guillevin L, et al. Temporal 67 gallium uptake is increased in temporal arteritis. Rheumatology 1999;38:709.
37. Mitomo T, Funyu T, Takahashi Y, Murakami K, Koyama K, Kamio K. Giant cell arteritis and magnetic resonance angiography. Arthritis Rheum 1998;41:1702.
38. Blockmans D, Maes A, Stroobants S, et al. New arguments for a vasculitic nature of polymyalgia rheumatica using positron emission tomography. Rheumatology 1999;38:444.
39. Salvarani C, Gabriel SE, O'Fallon WM, Hunder GG. Epidemiology of polymyalgia rheumatica in Olmsted County, Minnesota, 1970–1991. Arthritis Rheum 1995;38:369.
40. Lawrence RC, Helmick CG, Arnett FC, et al. Estimates of the prevalence of arthritis and selected musculoskeletal disorders in the United States. Arthritis Rheum 1998;41:778.
41. Salvarani C, Hunder GG. Musculoskeletal manifestations in a population-based cohort of patients with giant cell arteritis. Arthritis Rheum 1999;42:1259.
42. Salvarani C, Cantini F, Olivieri I, et al. Proximal bursitis in active polymyalgia rheumatica. Ann Intern Med 1997;127:27.
43. Salvarani C, Gabriel S, Hunder GG. Distal extremity swelling with pitting edema in polymyalgia rheumatica. Report of 19 cases. Arthritis Rheum 1996;39:73.
44. Hunder GG, Lie JT, Goronzy JJ, et al. Pathogenesis of giant cell arteritis. Arthritis Rheumatism 1993;36:757.
45. Boesen P, Sorensen SF. Giant cell arteritis, temporal arteritis, and polymyalgia rheumatica in a Danish County. Arthritis Rheum 1987;30:294.
46. Mathewson JA, Hunder GG. Giant cell arteritis in two brothers. A case report. J Rheumatol 1986;13:190.
47. Salvarani C, Gabriel SE, O'Fallon WM, Hunder GG. The incidence of giant cell arteritis in Olmsted County, Minnesota: Apparent fluctuations in cyclic pattern. Ann Intern Med 1995;123:192.
48. Gabriel S, Espy M, Erdman DD, Bjornsson J, Smith TF, Hunder GG. The role of parvovirus B19 in the pathogenesis of giant cell arteritis. Arthritis Rheum 1999;42:1255.
49. Russo MG, Waxman J, Abdoh AA, Serebro LH. Correlation between infection and the onset of the giant cell (temporal) arteritis syndrome: A trigger mechanism? Arthritis Rheum 1995;38:374.
50. Weyand CM, Hicok KC, Hunder GG, et al. The HLA-DRB1 locus as a genetic component in giant cell arteritis. J Clin Invest 1992;90:2355.
51. Brack A, Geisler A, Martinez-Taboada VM, Younge BR, Goronzy JJ, Weyand CM. Giant cell vasculitis is a T cell-dependent disease. Mol Med 1997;3:530.

52. Wagner AD, Goronzy JJ, Weyand CW. Functional profile of tissue-infiltrating and circulating CD68+ cells in giant cell arteritis. J Clin Invest 1994;94:1134.
53. Matteson EL, Gold KN, Bloch DA, Hunder GG. Long-term survival of patients with giant cell arteritis in the American College of Rheumatology Giant Cell Arteritis Classification Criteria Cohort. Am J Med 1996;100:193.
54. Schmidt WA, Kraft HE, Vorpahl K, Volker L, Gromnica-Ihle EJ. Color duplex ultrasonography in the diagnosis of temporal arteritis. N Engl J Med 1997;337:1336.
55. Hunder GG, Weyand CM. Sonography in giant cell arteritis. N Engl J Med 1997;337:1385.
56. Hunder GG, Bloch DA, Michel B, et al. The American College of Rheumatology 1990 Criteria for the Classification of Giant Cell Arteritis. Arthritis Rheum 1990;33:1122.
57. Achkar AA, Lie JT, Hunder GG, et al. How does previous corticosteroid treatment affect the biopsy findings in giant cell (temporal) arteritis? Ann Intern Med 1994;120:987.
58. Roche NE, Fulbright JW, Wagner AD, Hunder GG, Goronzy JJ, Wegard. Correlation of interleukin-6 production and disease activity in polymyalgia rheumatica and giant cell arteritis. Arthritis Rheum 1993;36:1286.
59. Weyand CM, Fulbright JW, Evans JM, Hunder GG, Goronzy JJ. Corticosteroid requirements in polymyalgia rheumatica. Arch Intern Med 1999;159:577.
60. Brack A, Rittner HL, Younge BR, Kaltschmidt C, Weyand CM, Goronzy JJ. Glucocorticoid-mediated repression of cytokine gene transplantation in human arteritis-SCID chimeras. J Clin Invest 1997;99:2842.
61. Hunder GG, Sheps SG, Allen GL, Joyce JW. Daily and alternate-day corticosteroid regimens in treatment of giant cell arteritis. Ann Intern Med 1975;82:613.
62. Schaufelberger C, Andersson R, Nordborg E. No additive effect of cyclosporin A compared with glucocorticoid treatment alone in giant cell arteritis: Results of an open, controlled, randomized study. Br J Rheumatol 1998;37:464.
63. De Silva M, Hazleman BL. Azathioprine in giant cell arteritis/polymyalgia rheumatica: A double-blind study. Ann Rheum Dis 1986;45:136.
64. Nesher G, Sonnenblick M. Steroid-sparing medications in temporal arteritis – report of three cases and review of 174 reported patients. Clin Rheumatol 1994;13:289.
65. Feinberg HL, Sherman JD, Schrepferman CG, Dietzen CJ, Feinberg GD. The use of methotrexate in polymyalgia rheumatica. J Rheumatol 1996;23:1550.
66. van der Veen MJ, Dinant HJ, van Booma-Frankfort C, van Albada-Kuipers GA, Bijlsma JW. Can methotrexate be used as a steroid sparing agent in the treatment of polymyalgia rheumatica and giant cell arteritis? Ann Rheum Dis 1996;55:218.

Section 6 Systemic Immune Diseases

Chapter 69

Rheumatic Fever

Elia M. Ayoub

INTRODUCTION

Acute rheumatic fever is a nonpurulent complication of group A streptococcal infection. A period of latency of about 3 weeks, during which the patient is asymptomatic, intervenes between the streptococcal infection and the onset of the clinical manifestations of acute rheumatic fever. Rheumatic fever is unique among collagen-vascular diseases in that the inciting cause is well defined. Despite the definition of the event that triggers the disease, the exact mechanism that leads to the evolution of the diffuse inflammatory process remains at issue.

Acute rheumatic fever is characterized by variable inflammation of several organs. These include the joints, the heart, and the brain. Underlying this inflammatory process is a vasculitis that involves these organs and, to a lesser extent, other organs such as the skin and tendons. Cardiac inflammation is potentially the most serious manifestation of acute rheumatic fever. Rheumatic fever is still the most common cause of acquired heart disease in children and young adults worldwide, particularly in developing countries.

EPIDEMIOLOGY

Infection of the upper respiratory tract by group A streptococci is the usual event that induces acute rheumatic fever. Only 2–3% of normal individuals will succumb to this complication following an untreated streptococcal pharyngitis. Localized infection of the skin, impetigo, does not lead to rheumatic fever.[1]

The incidence of rheumatic fever follows closely that of streptococcal pharyngitis, which peaks between the age of 5 and 15 years. Although rheumatic fever commonly affects young children in developing countries, it is rarely seen in children under the age of 5 years in the USA. There is no difference in the incidence of the disease between males and females, but racial and ethnic differences have been described.[2,3]

The annual incidence of rheumatic fever in developing countries is estimated at 100–150 cases per 100 000 population.[4] This incidence is similar to that seen in North America and Western Europe during the first quarter of this century and contrasts with the current incidence of 0.5–3 per 100 000 population in this part of the world. The decline in the incidence of rheumatic fever in the USA was reversed in 1985, when a significant increase in the number of patients with rheumatic fever was noted in several areas of the USA.[5,6] The resurgence of rheumatic fever had several noteworthy characteristics. In some locations, most of the children involved were of high- to middle-income families with established access to health care. A substantial number of these children had no history of a preceding respiratory infection or documented streptococcal pharyngitis prior to the onset of rheumatic fever.

The decline in the incidence of rheumatic fever in western countries has been attributed to improved living conditions, the advent of antibiotics, better access to medical care, and enhanced education regarding the treatment of streptococcal pharyngitis. However, observations derived from the recent resurgence of rheumatic fever suggest that changes in the virulence of the group A streptococcus may play a more pivotal role in influencing the incidence of this disease.

PATHOGENESIS

Acute rheumatic fever is the product of an interaction between a specific microorganism (the group A streptococcus) and a specific host (the individual susceptible to rheumatic fever) (Fig. 69.1). The interaction appears to involve an immune reaction that is peculiar to the microorganism and the host.

Microbial factors

The group A streptococcus, also known as *Streptococcus pyogenes*, is a member of the family of β-hemolytic streptococci that includes 20 separate groups identified serologically by Lancefield as group A to H and K to V. Group A streptococci are unique among the other serogroups for their capacity to induce rheumatic fever.

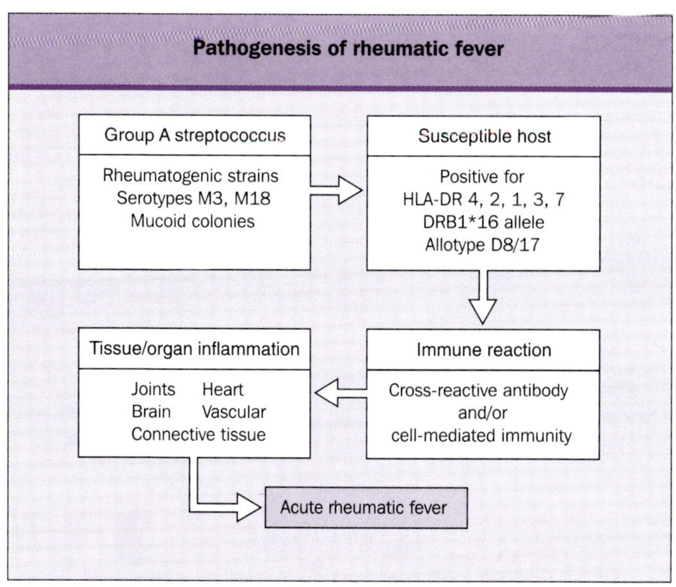

Figure 69.1 Steps in the interaction between bacterial and host factors that are involved in the pathogenesis of rheumatic fever.

Cellular components

The streptococcal cell consists of an inner protoplasm surrounded by a cell wall comprising three primary components: the cell wall peptidoglycan, the group-specific polysaccharide, and the cell wall protein(s) (Fig. 69.2). The peptidoglycan imparts rigidity to the cell wall. It has adjuvant properties. Injection of a peptidoglycan–polysaccharide complex derived from the cell wall of the group A streptococcus into the skin and joints of laboratory animals induces a chronic, recurrent, nodular dermal inflammation and arthritis.[7]

The cell wall polysaccharide is also designated as the group-specific carbohydrate, because its structure determines the serologic group specificity of the β-hemolytic streptococci. The group-specific carbohydrate of the group A streptococcus has been reported to share antigenic similarity with a glycoprotein isolated from human mitral valve tissue.[8] Some streptococcal strains are encapsulated. The presence of large amounts of hyaluronate capsular material imparts a mucoid characteristic to the colonies of these strains when grown on blood agar. Recovery of these highly mucoid strains has been associated with past and recent outbreaks of rheumatic fever.

A mosaic of proteins present in the cell wall consists of the M, R, and T proteins. The M protein is the type-specific antigen of the group A streptococci; its composition varies with each of the 100 or more known serotypes. This protein is of particular importance because it is a virulence factor of group A streptococci. When present on the surface of the cell, it inhibits phagocytosis of the organism. It is a coiled protein with an α-helical configuration. It has a hypervariable distal amino terminus and a proximal carboxy terminus that is anchored to the cell membrane. Type specificity resides in the hypervariable region. Antibody against the hypervariable region of an M protein abrogates its antiphagocytic activity and imparts immunity to the host against infection by a homologous serotype.[9]

The M protein has attracted attention because it carries several epitopes that impart antigenic cross-reactivity with tissues of the human heart, brain, and kidney. The presence of certain M proteins appears to be associated with specific biologic characteristics of the streptococcus. The M1 serotype has been associated with severe disease and with toxic shock.[10] Serotypes M3 and M18 have been associated with the recent outbreaks of acute rheumatic fever.[11] Epidemiologic data suggest that rheumatogenic capacity appears to reside more within strains of certain serotypes and not with the serotype itself.

Other proteins present in the cell wall include the T and R proteins, the SOR proteins, the fibronectin-binding proteins and Fc-binding proteins, and the recently identified peptidase that cleaves C5a. The T and R proteins have been utilized in subtyping of group A streptococci. The SOR proteins are α-lipoproteinases that are also type specific. The Fc-binding proteins, like protein A of *Staphylococcus aureus*, react with the Fc protein of IgG.

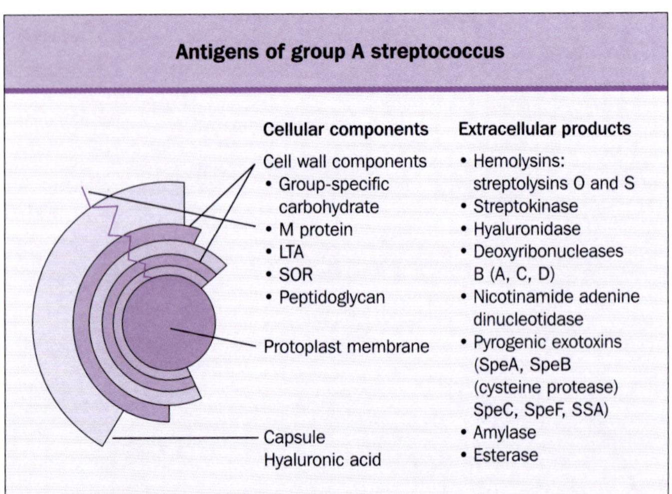

Figure 69.2 Cellular components and extracellular products of the group A streptococcus. LTA = leipoteichoic acid; SOR = serum opacity factor (α-lipoproteinase).

Extracellular products

The extracellular products of the group A streptococcus include the two streptolysins, O and S, that are responsible for the characteristic hemolysis that surrounds colonies of the organism when grown on blood agar. Streptolysin S exerts its activity under aerobic and anaerobic conditions, while streptolysin O requires an anaerobic environment for its action. Other products include hyaluronidase, streptokinase (which activates the fibrinolytic system), nicotinamide adenine dinucleotidase (NADase), a proteinase and proteinase precursor, an esterase, and an amylase. Four deoxyribonuclease (DNase) isozymes A, B, C, and D, are produced by streptococci; of these the DNase B is produced most commonly by group A streptococci.[12] A family of exotoxins have been identified as products of group A streptococci: streptococcal pyrogenic exotoxins A (SpeA), B (SpeB), C (SpeC), F (SpeF – previously known as mitogenic factor, MF), G (SpeG), H (SpeH), J (SpeJ), streptococcal mitogenic exotoxin Z (SMEZ), and streptococcal superantigen (SSA). These toxins act as superantigens, inducing massive T-cell stimulation and elaboration of lymphokines, including TNF-α, IL-1β, and IL-6.[13,14] Spe-A has been implicated in the pathogenesis of the streptococcal toxic shock syndrome and other members of the family may also be involved, etiologically in some cases of this disease (Chapter 7).[10,15] Except for streptolysin S, all of the above products are immunogenic in man.

Streptococcal antibody tests

A number of tests have been established for the assay of antibodies to some of the group A streptococcal antigens (Table 69.1). These antibody tests are used to provide evidence for antecedent streptococcal infection primarily in patients suspected of having acute rheumatic fever. The antistreptolysin O test (ASO), first described by Todd,[16] is still the most commonly used and best standardized of the streptococcal antibody tests. Most of the other tests that were developed subsequently are of limited use because of difficulties in standardization and reproducibility. The anti-DNase B test, which was developed more recently,[17] has proved to be quite reproducible and is now available in several laboratories.

The streptozyme test is an agglutination test that lacks specificity and reproducibility and should not be used as a primary test.

The streptococcal antigenic products are enzymes, and streptococcal antibody tests assay the serum neutralizing activity to these enzymes. Titers are determined by diluting the serum serially, and determining the highest dilution that neutralizes the enzymatic activity. The reciprocal of that dilution is the serum

Streptococcal antigen	Antibody test
Extracellular product	
Streptolysin O	Antistreptolysin O (ASO)
Streptokinase	Antistreptokinase (ASK)
Hyaluronidase	Antistreptococcal hyaluronidase (ASH)
Deoxyribonuclease B	Anti-DNase B
Nicotinamide adenine dinucleotidase	Anti-NADase
Multiple	Streptozyme[a]
Cellular component	
Type-specific M protein	Type-specific antibody
Group-specific polysaccharide	Anti-A-carbohydrate

[a]Not recommended because this test lacks specificity and reproducibility.

Table 69.1 Group A streptococcal antigens and corresponding antibody tests. From Ayoub EM. Streptococcal antibody tests in rheumatic fever. *Clin Immunol Newsletter* 1982;3:107, with permission.[17]

antibody titer for that antigen. The upper limit of normal for each test is usually determined by assaying sera from a normal population and determining the highest titer present in 80–85% of that population. Titers exceeding the upper limit of normal by two tube dilutions or 0.2 log, or paired sera that show a rise of 0.2 log, are indicative of an antecedent group A streptococcal infection.

The antibody response to these antigens generally peaks about 3 weeks after the acute streptococcal infection, stays at the peak level for 3–4 months, and then declines gradually to normal levels. Because patients with rheumatic fever present with their disease 2–4 weeks after the inciting infection, assay of antibody titers on a sample obtained then is usually sufficient.

Antibody tests to streptococcal cellular antigens include assays for antibody to the M protein (type-specific antigen) or antibody to the group A carbohydrate (the group-specific antigen). The former test helps determine immunity to a specific serotype. Antibody to the streptococcal group A carbohydrate has been found to persist at elevated levels for several years in patients with rheumatic mitral valve disease.[17]

Host factors

Evidence indicating that susceptibility to rheumatic fever is limited to certain individuals was suggested by a number of epidemiologic observations. These included the observation that only 2–3% of previously normal individuals who acquire a streptococcal pharyngitis will succumb to acute rheumatic fever. In contrast, 30–70% of individuals who have rheumatic fever will have recurrence of rheumatic fever manifestations if they have a subsequent episode of streptococcal pharyngitis. Several investigators have documented the familial incidence of rheumatic fever.[18,19] Studies by Zabriskie and associates have documented the presence of a B-cell alloantigen recognized by a specific monoclonal antibody, D8/17, that can be detected in high frequency on B cells of patients with rheumatic fever.[20] Other studies have documented a significant association of rheumatic fever with the inheritance of certain HLA class II alleles.[21] These findings provide strong support for the premise that susceptibility to rheumatic fever is genetically determined.

The documentation of an association between susceptibility to rheumatic fever with class II HLA is of particular importance in view of current knowledge regarding the role of HLA in antigen presentation and the immune response (Chapter 6).[22] Earlier theories on the pathogenesis of rheumatic fever had proposed that a peculiar state of immune hyperreactivity to streptococcal antigens might be an underlying cause for the disease. Subsequently, a number of investigators attempted to procure evidence for an abnormal response to group A streptococcal antigen(s). The most compelling of these observations was the finding of a hyperresponse to the group A streptococcal cell wall carbohydrate, the group-specific antigen, in patients with rheumatic mitral valve disease.[17,23] The hyperresponsiveness of these patients to this streptococcal antigen was associated with inheritance of HLA-DR2 or -DR4.[24] This finding is particularly relevant because the immune response to the group A carbohydrate has been documented to be under genetic control in experimental animals and in man.[25–27]

Mechanism of tissue injury

The current hypothesis regarding the mechanism of tissue injury in rheumatic fever and for cardiac involvement is that the inflammation seen in acute rheumatic fever is mediated by an autoimmune process. Evidence for an autoimmune reaction was provided by several investigators who described the presence of antibody to cardiac tissue in the serum of patients with rheumatic heart disease and of immune deposits in cardiac tissue of such patients.[28] These findings prompted a search for antigenic mimicry between the group A streptococcus and mammalian tissues (Chapter 58). The description of antigenic similarity between the streptococcus and human tissues has provided a potential explanation for the inflammation encountered in various organs in acute rheumatic fever.

Recent studies analyzing autoantibody-mediated cardiac injury in mice have provided possible insight into the pathogenic role of heart cross-reactive antibodies and genetic susceptibility to rheumatic heart disease.[29,30] These studies showed that injection of monoclonal antibodies to myosin induced myocarditis in certain murine strains (e.g. DBA/2) but not others (e.g. BALB/c). This susceptibility to autoimmune myocarditis was determined by genetic loci in the susceptible strain and appeared to be controlled by the expression of myosin in the myocardial extracellular matrix. These studies suggest that genetic susceptibility to rheumatic heart disease in humans could be associated with the genetic control of antigen display in the human heart.

Although formation of cross-reactive antibodies to common streptococcal and cardiac antigens may provide a potential explanation for the pathogenesis of rheumatic fever, other studies in experimental animals have supported the role of T-cell-mediated cardiac injury. In some studies, antibodies to myosin did not react with intact heart tissue and passive transfer of these antibodies did not induce myocarditis,[31] despite the development of disease after immunization or infection with Coxsackie virus. Additional evidence indicating that cross-reactive antibodies may not play a role in the pathogenesis of rheumatic carditis was reported in a study on the role of cell-mediated immunity in the pathogenesis of this disease.[32,33] In one of these studies, peripheral blood lymphocytes from patients with acute rheumatic carditis exerted a cytotoxic effect on myocardial cells cultured in vitro. Homologous serum from the patient abrogated the cytotoxic activity of the lymphocytes, suggesting that the antibody may protect against cardiac cytotoxicity in these patients. Thus, current information does not provide concrete evidence to support the role of antigenic mimicry and autoantibodies in the pathogenesis of rheumatic fever.

A major reason for our inability to assess the role of these antibodies and of other factors in the pathogenesis of rheumatic fever is the absence of an experimental animal model in which streptococcal infection leads to cardiac injury.

CLINICAL MANIFESTATIONS

The manifestations of acute rheumatic fever can be divided into major or minor manifestations. *Major manifestations* include arthritis, carditis, Sydenham's chorea, erythema marginatum, and subcutaneous nodules. These manifestations are quite specific for rheumatic fever. The *minor manifestations*, which include arthralgia, fever, and abnormal acute-phase reactants, are fairly nonspecific. A patient with acute rheumatic fever may present with one or more of the major and minor manifestations. These manifestations form the basis for the Jones' criteria that are used to establish the diagnosis of acute rheumatic fever.

Arthritis is the most common but the least specific of the major manifestations of acute rheumatic fever. It is seen in about 70% of the patients. Rheumatic fever arthritis affects mostly the large joints and is rarely symmetrical. Affected joints are painful, swollen, red, and warm. The arthritis is fleeting and migratory. The arthritis of rheumatic fever is self-limited, lasts for a few days, rarely leads to chronic changes, and is exquisitely responsive to salicylate therapy.

Carditis is the major cause of morbidity and mortality in rheumatic fever. It occurs in about 50% of patients. Clinical findings of carditis may be delayed for about a week after the onset of arthritis. Myocarditis and endocarditis are the primary lesions seen in patients with acute rheumatic carditis. Isolated pericarditis is uncommon as a primary manifestation of acute rheumatic carditis. It is usually encountered in association with pancarditis, a complication that is associated with high mortality. The presence of tachycardia at rest in a patient who is afebrile is reliable clinical evidence for myocarditis. Myocarditis may be associated with arrhythmias and varying degrees of heart block; these abnormalities are confirmed by the presence of abnormal rhythms and prolonged P–R interval on electrocardiogram.

Endocardial inflammation primarily affects valvular tissue. Valvulitis is the most common cardiac lesion seen in rheumatic fever. In our experience, the mitral valve is affected, either alone or in conjunction with the aortic valve, in 94% of patients with rheumatic carditis; isolated mitral disease is present in 65%, isolated aortic disease is found in 6%, and simultaneous involvement of both mitral and aortic valves is present in 29% of patients. Acute valvulitis is manifested clinically by signs of insufficiency or regurgitation. Auscultatory findings in mitral insufficiency include the presence of a high-frequency, smooth, apical holosystolic murmur that radiates to the left axilla. With marked mitral insufficiency, a low-frequency, mid-to-late diastolic murmur of relative mitral stenosis (Carey Coombs murmur) may be heard. Aortic insufficiency is characterized by an early diastolic murmur that starts with the aortic component of the second heart sound. This high-frequency decrescendo murmur is heard best in the third left intercostal space at the sternal edge. Murmurs of mitral or aortic stenosis usually reflect chronic valvular disease.

Sydenham's chorea is a manifestation of inflammation of the central nervous system involving the caudate nucleus in the basal ganglia. Chorea is seen in about 15% of patients. In some of the recent outbreaks, chorea was encountered in 30% of patients.[6] The onset of chorea usually follows the inciting streptococcal pharyngitis by a period of latency of 3–6 months, which may extend to 12 months. Choreiform manifestations include involuntary, purposeless movements and muscular incoordination of the upper and lower extremities. Characteristic signs include the presence of 'wormian' fasciculations in the tongue, 'spooning' of the hands on extension of the arms, pronation of the hands when the arms are raised vertically above the head, the 'milkmaid's grip', irregular contractions of the muscles of the hand when the patient grips the fingers of the examiner, inability to sustain phonation, and wavering of the upstroke when a patient draws vertical lines. Patients may show emotional lability associated with easy frustration and crying. These manifestations vary in severity and duration; they are usually self-limited and resolve in 2–4 weeks but may persist for months.

Auscultatory evidence of carditis in patients with Sydenham's chorea is often subtle and can be missed.

Erythema marginatum is a rash that is characteristic of acute rheumatic fever. It is seen in about 5% of patients. The rash is nonpruritic. Lesions appear as irregular circles of erythematous lines with a pale center. They are commonly found on the trunk and upper extremities, usually in the areas of limb juxtaposition. Warmth enhances the appearance of the rash.

Subcutaneous nodules, usually seen in patients with chronic rheumatic heart disease, occur in about 2–3% of patients. The nodules are located on the extensor tendons, mainly in elbows, knuckles, and ankles and over the spine. They are freely moveable, nontender, and about 1 cm in diameter.

A number of *minor manifestations* are associated with acute rheumatic fever. These nonspecific findings, commonly encoun-

KEY CONCEPTS

Guidelines for the diagnosis of initial attack of rheumatic fever

The presence of two major manifestations or of one major and two minor manifestations indicates a high probability of acute rheumatic fever, if supported by evidence of preceding group A streptococcal infection (Jones' criteria)

Major manifestations	**Minor manifestations**
Carditis	Clinical
Polyarthritis	Arthralgia
Chorea	Fever
Erythema marginatum	Laboratory
Subcutaneous nodules	Elevated acute-phase reactants
	Erythrocyte sedimentation rate
	C-reactive protein
	Prolonged P–R interval

Supporting evidence of antecedent group A streptococcal infection

Elevated or rising streptococcal antibody titer(s)

Positive throat culture or rapid streptococcal antigen test

Adapted from Dajani AS, Ayoub EM, Bierman FZ, et al. *JAMA* 1992;87:302, with permission.

tered in a variety of diseases, include fever, arthralgia (joint aches), abnormal acute-phase reactants (elevated ESR and C-reactive protein) and prolonged P–R interval on ECG.

DIAGNOSIS

The diagnosis of acute rheumatic fever is established by fulfilling the Jones' criteria. The use of the Jones' criteria is necessary because there is as yet no single clinical finding or laboratory test that allows a definitive diagnosis of acute rheumatic fever. Adherence to these guidelines will minimize the overdiagnosis of this disease.

Documentation of an antecedent group A streptococcal infection is a sine qua non in confirming the diagnosis of acute rheumatic fever. A positive throat culture or a 'rapid strep test', while acceptable as evidence for such an infection, is unreliable because the majority of patients with acute rheumatic fever have a negative throat culture. The use of streptococcal antibody tests provides a far more reliable means of confirmation of an antecedent group A streptococcal infection. It is recommended that an ASO be performed initially. About 15% of patients with acute rheumatic fever may have a normal ASO (Table 69.2), and one of the ancillary antibody tests such as the anti-DNase B should be performed if the ASO is normal in a patient whose clinical criteria support the diagnosis of acute rheumatic fever. Should evidence for an antecedent group A streptococcal infection be lacking, the diagnosis of acute rheumatic fever should be questioned.

TREATMENT

Management of a patient with acute rheumatic fever should address the treatment of the clinical manifestations and should include the administration of a streptococcus-eradicating course of antibiotic. This should be followed by the initiation of prophylactic measures for the prevention of recurrences of rheumatic fever and, in patients with carditis, the prevention of bacterial endocarditis. Patients with acute disease should be hospitalized and evaluated for the presence of carditis. Laboratory tests at the time of hospitalization include a complete blood count with an ESR, throat culture, and streptococcal antibody test(s) and, if needed, a chest roentgenogram, electrocardiogram, and echocardiogram. Treatment of heart failure is the most critical aspect of acute management. Bed rest is recommended during the acute disease for patients with acute arthritis and/or carditis. However, return to normal physical activity should be encouraged once the acute manifestations have subsided. While strenuous activity should be avoided initially, prolonged confinement should also be discouraged.

Percentage of patients with acute rheumatic fever showing an elevated antibody with ASO, anti-DNase B, or both tests

	ASO	Anti-DNase B	ASO and anti-DNase B
Normal controls	19	19	30
Acute rheumatic fever	83	82	92
Sydenham's chorea (isolated)	67	40	80

ASO = antistreptolysin O. DNase = deoxyribonuclease.

Table 69.2 Percentage of patients with acute rheumatic fever showing an elevated antibody with ASO, anti-DNase B, or both tests. Adapted from Ayoub EM, Wannamaker LW. *Pediatrics* 1962;29:527, and Ayoub EM, Wannamaker LW. *Pediatrics* 1966;38:946, with permission.

Treatment of acute manifestations

Treatment of acute **carditis** requires the use of anti-inflammatory agents. Salicylates at a dose of 80–100 mg/kg/day in 4 divided doses constitute adequate therapy for mild to moderate carditis. Salicylate therapy should be maintained for 4–8 weeks, depending on the response, then reduced gradually and terminated over the following 4 weeks. Patients with severe carditis and heart failure, particularly patients with pancarditis, are preferably treated with steroids.[34] Prednisone is administered orally in a dose of 2 mg/kg once daily. This dose should rarely be administered for longer than 2 weeks; it should then be tapered over the following 2–3 weeks. One week prior to termination of steroid therapy, salicylate therapy should be initiated in the above dosage so as to avert the clinical and laboratory rebound associated with rapid steroid withdrawal. Monitoring of acute-phase reactants is useful in gauging the duration of treatment with anti-inflammatory drugs. Adjunctive therapy for carditis and cardiac failure includes the use of digitalis, parenteral inotropic agents (dobutamine, dopamine, or amrinone) or vasodilators (captopril or enalapril), and diuretics.

Treatment of **arthritis**, in the absence of carditis, requires salicylates only. A characteristic of the arthritis of rheumatic fever is its extreme sensitivity to salicylates; if the arthritis does not respond promptly to salicylates, one should question the diagnosis of acute rheumatic fever. Patients can be started on 50–75 mg/kg/day of aspirin, divided in 4 daily doses. The aspirin dose may be increased to a maximum of 100 mg/kg/day if a response is not elicited. Treatment is continued for 2 weeks then tapered over the following 2–3 weeks.

The manifestations of **Sydenham's chorea** can be controlled with anticonvulsant therapy. Phenobarbital, haloperidol, and valproate have shown variable effectiveness in controlling choreiform activity. Anti-inflammatory agents are not needed if the patient presents with isolated chorea.

Antibiotic therapy

All patients should receive a streptococcus-eradicating course of antibiotics at the time of diagnosis (Table 69.3), even though the throat culture or rapid antigen test may be negative for group A streptococci. Penicillin is the primary agent to be used, with erythromycin reserved for patients who are allergic to penicillin. Intramuscular long-acting penicillin is preferred for patients with cardiac involvement. Sulfonamides, trimethoprim, and tetracyclines should not be used for streptococcal eradication.

Secondary prophylaxis is recommended for the prevention of streptococcal pharyngitis and recurrences of rheumatic fever. The regimens recommended by the American Heart Association are outlined in Table 69.3. Of these regimens, monthly injections of long-acting benzathine penicillin have been shown to be most effective and should be used for at least 5 years in patients with residual cardiac disease. Sulfonamides, though ineffective in streptococcal eradication and primary prevention, are quite effective in secondary prophylaxis. Other antibiotics such as ampicillin, semi-synthetic penicillins, and cephalosporins are effective in eradicating the streptococcus from the throat of patients with

Antibiotic	Dose	Route	Duration
Primary eradication			
Benzathine penicillin G	600 000–1 200 000 U[a]	Intramuscular	Single dose
Penicillin V	250 mg q 8 h	Oral	10 days
Erythromycin (eoslate or ethylsuccinate)	20–40 mg/kg/d (maximum 1.0 g/d) In 2–4 divided doses	Oral	10 days
Secondary prevention			
Benzathine penicillin G	600 000–1 200 000 U	Intramuscular	Every 4 weeks[b]
Penicillin V	250 mg q 12 h	Oral	
Sulfadiazine	1.0 g once daily	Oral	
Erythromycin ethylsuccinate	250 mg q 12 h	Oral	

Antibiotic regimens for primary prevention (streptococcus-eradicating) and secondary prevention of rheumatic fever

[a]See text for details.
[b]May be given every 3 weeks in a high-risk situation.

Table 69.3 Antibiotic regimens for primary prevention (streptococcus-eradicating) and secondary prevention of rheumatic fever. Adapted with permission from Dajani A, Taubert K, Ferrieri P, Peter G, Shulman S, and other Committee Members and the Committee on Rheumatic Fever, Endocarditis, and Kawasaki Disease of the Council on Cardiovascular Disease in the Young, the American Heart Association. Treatment of acute streptococcal pharyngitis and prevention of rheumatic fever: A statement for health professionals. *Pediatrics* 1995;96:758.[35]

pharyngitis. However, these antibiotics have not been tested as yet for efficacy in the primary or secondary prevention of rheumatic fever.

Present recommendations regarding the duration of prophylaxis are predicated on the presence of carditis and the risk for acquiring streptococcal infection.[35] Patients with cardiac involvement should be maintained on prophylaxis well into adulthood and preferably for life, even after valvular surgery. In addition, patients who had valvular disease should at all times follow the recommendations of the American Heart Association regarding prophylaxis against subacute bacterial endocarditis.[36] Patients who do not have cardiac involvement may have their prophylaxis discontinued after 5 years or once they reach the age of 21 years, if they have received at least 5 years of continuous prophylaxis. The pivotal role and effectiveness of prophylaxis in allowing resolution of valvular disease has been well documented[37] and should be emphasized to the patient in order to encourage compliance.

CLINICAL PEARLS

Evidence of carditis in rheumatic fever

Myocarditis

Tachycardia at rest in afebrile patient
Arrhythmias
Varying degrees of heart block on ECG

Endocarditis

Murmurs of valvular insufficiency in acute disease
- Mitral valve involvement in 94%
  - mitral valve alone in 65%
  - mitral and aortic valve in 29%
- Aortic valve involvement alone in 6%

Murmurs of mitral or aortic stenosis reflect chronic desease

REFERENCES

1. Wannamaker LW. Differences between streptococcal infections of the throat and of the skin. N Engl J Med 1970;282:23.
2. Caughey DE, Douglas R, Wilson W, Hassall IB. HLA antigens in Europeans and Maoris with rheumatic fever and rheumatic heart disease. J Rheumatol 1975;2:319.
3. Chun LT, Reddy DV, Yamamoto LG. Rheumatic fever in children and adolescents in Hawaii. Pediatrics 1987;79:549.
4. Markowitz M. The decline of rheumatic fever: Role of medical intervention. The Lewis W. Wannamaker Memorial Lecture. J Pediatr 1985;106:545.
5. Veasy LG, Wiedmeier SE, Orsmond GS, et al. Resurgence of acute rheumatic fever in the intermountain area of the United States. N Engl J Med 1987;316:421.
6. Ayoub EM. Resurgence of rheumatic fever in the United States. The changing picture of a preventable disease. Postgrad Med 1992;92:133.
7. Cromartie WJ, Craddock JG, Schwab JH, Anderle SK, Yang CH. Arthritis in rats after systemic injection of streptococcal cells or cell walls. J Exp Med 1977;146:1585.
8. Goldstein I, Halpern B, Robert L. Immunologic relation between streptococcus A polysaccharide and the structural glycoproteins of heart valve. Nature 1967;213:44.
9. Lancefield RC. Current knowledge of type specific M antigens of group A streptococci. J Immunol 1962;89:307.
10. Stevens DL. Invasive group A streptococcus infections. Clin Infect Dis 1992;14:2.
11. Johnson DR, Stevens DL, Kaplan EL. Epidemiologic analysis of group A streptococcal serotypes associated with severe systemic infections, rheumatic fever or uncomplicated pharyngitis. J Infect Dis 1992;166:374.
12. Gray ED. Nucleases of group A streptococci diseases. New York, Academic Press, 1971, p 143.
13. Braun MA, Gerlach D, Hartwig UF, et al. Stimulation of human T cells by streptococcal 'superantigen' erythrogenic toxins (scarlet fever toxins). J Immunol 1993;150:2457.
14. Proft T, Moffatt SL, Berkahn CJ, Fraser JD. Identification and characterization of novel superantigens from *Streptococcus pyogenes*. J Exp Med 1999;189:89.
15. Reiksson BKG, Andersson J, Holm SE. Invasive group A streptococcal infections: T1M1 isolates expressing pyrogenic exotoxins A and B in combination with selective lack of toxin-neutralizing antibodies are associated with increased risk of streptococcal toxic shock syndrome. J Infect Dis 1999;180:410.
16. Todd EW. Antihaemolysin titers in haemolytic streptococcal infections and their significance in rheumatic fever. Br J Exp Pathol 1932;13:248.
17. Ayoub EM. Streptococcal antibody tests in rheumatic fever. Clin Immunol Newsletter 1982;3:107.

18. Read SE, Reid H, Poon-King T. HLAs and predisposition to the non-suppurative sequelae of group A streptococcal infections. Transplant Proc 1977;9:543.
19. Wilson MG, Schweitzer M. Pattern of hereditary susceptibility in rheumatic fever. Circulation 1954;10:699.
20. Khanna AK, Buskirk DR, Williams RC, et al. Presence of a non-HLA B cell antigen in rheumatic fever patients and their families as defined by a monoclonal antibody. J Clin Invest 1989;83:1710.
21. Ayoub EM. Susceptibility to rheumatic fever: Host factors. In: Narula J, Virmani R, Reddy KS, Tandon R (eds) Rheumatic fever, 1st edn. Washington, DC, American Registry of Pathology, Armed Forces Institute of Pathology, 1999, p 181.
22. Braciale TJ, Morrison LA, Sweetser MT, Sambrook J, Gething M-J, Braciale VL. Antigen presentation pathways to class I and class II MHV-restricted T lymphocytes. Immunol Rev 1987;98:95.
23. Dudding BA, Ayoub EM. Persistence of streptococcal Group A antibody in patients with rheumatic valvular disease. J Exp Med 1968;128:1081.
24. Ayoub EM, Barrett DJ, Maclaren NK, Krischer JP. Association of class II human histocompatibility leukocyte antigens with rheumatic fever. J Clin Invest 1986;77:2019.
25. Eichman K, Kindt TJ. The inheritance of individual antigenic specificities of rabbit antibodies to streptococcal carbohydrate. J Exp Med 1971;134:532.
26. Klapper DG, Kindt TJ. Idiotypic cross-reactions among anti-streptococcal antibodies in an inbred rabbit population. Scand J Immunol 1974;3:483.
27. Saszuki T, Kaneoka H, Nishimura Y, Kaneoka R, Hayama M, Ohkuni H. An HLA-linked immune suppression gene in man. J Exp Med 1980;152:297S.
28. Kaplan MH, Meyeserian M. An immunological cross reaction between group A streptococcal cells and human heart tissue. Lancet 1962;1:706.
29. Liao L, Sindwani R, Rojkind M, Factor S, Leinwand L, Diamond B. Antibody-mediated autoimmune myocarditis depends on genetically determined target organ sensitivity. J Exp Med 1995;181:1123.
30. Kuan AP, Chamberlain W, Malkiel S, Lieu HD, Factor S, Diamond B, Kotzin BL. Genetic control of autoimmune myocarditis mediated by myosin-specific antibodies. Immunogenetics 1999;49:79.
31. Neu N, Ploier B, Ofner C. Cardiac myosin-induced myocarditis. J Immunol 1990;145:4094.
32. Yang LC, Soprey PR, Wittner MK, et al. Streptococcal induced cell mediated immune destruction of cardiac myofibers *in vitro*. J Exp Med 1977;146:344.
33. Hutto J, Ayoub EM. Cytotoxicity of lymphocytes from patients with rheumatic carditis to cardiac cells *in vitro*: Streptococcal disease and immune response. New York, Academic Press, 1980, p 733.
34. Combined Rheumatic Fever Study Group. A comparison of short-term intensive prednisone and acetylsalicylic acid therapy in the treatment of acute rheumatic fever. N Engl J Med 1965;272:63.
35. Dajani A, Taubert K, Ferrieri P, Peter G, Shulman S, and other Committee Members and the Committee on Rheumatic Fever, Endocarditis, and Kawasaki Disease of the Council on Cardiovascular Disease in the Young, the American Heart Association. Treatment of acute streptococcal pharyngitis and prevention of rheumatic fever: A statement for health professionals. Pediatrics 1995;96:758.
36. Dajani AS, Bisno AL, Chung KJ, et al. Prevention of bacterial endocarditis. Recommendations by the American Heart Association. Circulation 1990;264:2929.
37. Tompkins DG, Boxerbaum B, Liebman J. Long-term prognosis of rheumatic fever patients receiving regular intramuscular benzathine penicillin. Circulation 1972;45:543.

Section 6 Systemic Immune Diseases

Chapter 70 Lyme Disease

Allen C. Steere

DESCRIPTION/NATURAL HISTORY

Lyme disease, or Lyme borreliosis, which was first described in residents of Lyme, Connecticut,[1] is caused by the tick-borne spirochete *Borrelia burgdorferi* sensu lato (Fig. 70.1).[2] The illness usually begins in summer (stage 1) with a characteristic expanding skin lesion, erythema migrans, that occurs at the site of the tick bite. Within several days to weeks (stage 2), the spirochete may spread to many other sites, particularly to other skin sites, or the nervous system, heart, or joints. After months to years (stage 3), sometimes following long periods of latent infection, the spirochete may cause persistent disease, most commonly affecting the joints, nervous system, or skin.

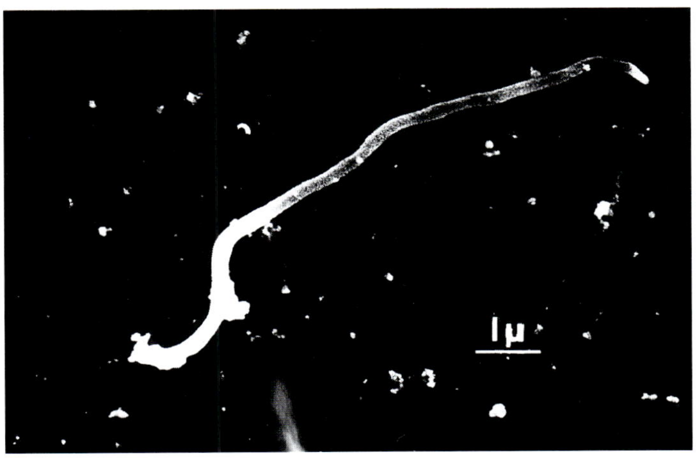

Figure 70.1 Scanning electron micrograph of *Borrelia burgdorferi*. The *Borrelia* spp. are longer and more loosely coiled than the other spirochetes. Of the *Borrelia* spp., *B. burgdorferi* is the longest (20–30 μm) and the narrowest (0.2–0.3 μm).

KEY CONCEPTS

Stages of infection in Lyme disease

Early infection

- Stage 1, localized skin infection – erythema migrans
- Stage 2, disseminated infection – particularly to other skin sites, or the nervous system, heart or joints

Late infection

- Stage 3, persistent infection – intermittent or chronic arthritis, chronic encephalopathy or polyneuropathy, or acrodermatitis chronica atrophicans

Three pathogenic groups of the *B. burgdorferi* sensu lato complex have been identified.[3] To date, all North American isolates have belonged to the first group, *B. burgdorferi* sensu stricto. All three groups have been found in Europe, but most isolates there have been group 2 (*Borrelia garinii*) and 3 (*Borrelia afzelii*) strains. Only group 2 and 3 strains have been found in Asia. Although the basic outlines of the disease are similar worldwide, there are regional variations. *B. burgdorferi* sensu stricto in the USA often disseminates widely early in the infection, and later, arthritis is a prominent manifestation of the illness. *B. garinii* seems to be particularly neurotropic, whereas *B. afzelii* may cause a chronic skin infection called acrodermatitis chronica atrophicans. The following clinical description is of *B. burgdorferi* sensu stricto infection in the USA.

Clinical manifestations: early infection

After an incubation period of 3–32 days, erythema migrans usually begins as a red macule or papule that expands slowly to form a large annular lesion, often with a bright red outer border and partial central clearing (stage 1: localized infection) (Fig. 70.2).[2] Within days to weeks, the spirochete often spreads hematogenously to many different sites (stage 2: disseminated infection). Such patients may develop secondary annular skin lesions, severe headache, mild neck stiffness, fever, chills, migratory musculoskeletal pain, or profound malaise and fatigue. Except for fatigue and lethargy, which are often constant, the early signs and symptoms of Lyme disease are typically intermittent and changing. Even in untreated patients, the early symptoms usually improve within several weeks.

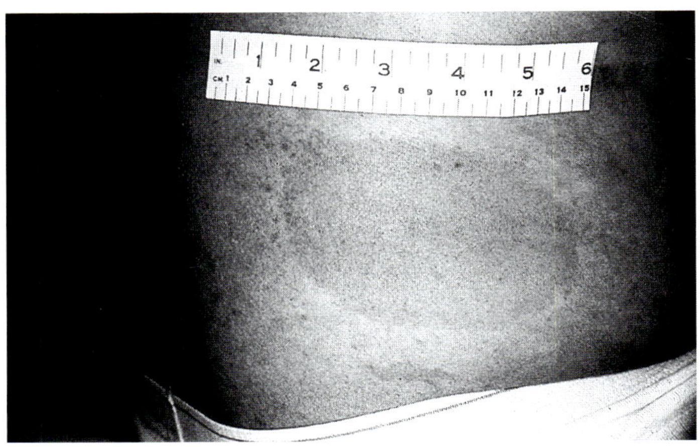

Figure 70.2 A 10-day-old erythema migrans skin lesion. The lesion expanded gradually and is beginning to have a redder outer border with partial central clearing. (See also colour plate 70.2.) (Reproduced with permission from Steere et al. The early clinical manifestations of Lyme disease. *Ann Intern Med* 1983;99:22.)

KEY CONCEPTS

Pathogenesis of Lyme arthritis

- Early in the infection, the spirochete disseminates hematogenously to joints, sometimes accompanied by migratory arthralgias.
- Months later, patients have onset of marked joint swelling, especially in knees, accompanied by a pro-inflammatory response to outer membrane lipoproteins of *B. burgdorferi*, often including outer-surface protein A (OspA).
- In genetically susceptible individuals, such as those with the HLA-DRB1*0401 allele, the T-cell response to the dominant epitope of OspA may cross react with human LFA-1, an adhesion molecule that is up-regulated on activated T cells.
- A cross-reactive T-cell response to LFA-1 may cause persistent joint inflammation after the apparent killing of *B. burgdorferi* with antibiotic therapy.

After several weeks to months, about 15% of untreated patients develop frank neurologic abnormalities, including meningitis, subtle encephalitic signs, cranial neuritis (including bilateral facial palsy), motor or sensory radiculoneuropathy, mononeuritis multiplex, or myelitis, alone or in various combinations. The usual pattern consists of fluctuating symptoms of meningitis accompanied by facial palsy or peripheral radiculoneuropathy, lasting weeks to months. In addition, about 8% of patients develop cardiac involvement. The most common abnormality is fluctuating degrees of atrioventricular block (first-degree, Wenckebach, or complete heart block), lasting weeks. Some patients have more diffuse cardiac involvement, including electrocardiographic changes of acute myopericarditis, left ventricular dysfunction on radionuclide scans, or, rarely, cardiomegaly or pancarditis.

Late infection

Months after the onset of infection, about 60% of untreated patients develop frank arthritis (stage 3: persistent infection) (Fig. 70.3).[4] The typical pattern is intermittent attacks of oligo-articular arthritis in large joints, especially knees, lasting weeks to months in a given joint. About 10% of patients develop chronic arthritis in the knees, defined as one year or more of continuous joint inflammation.

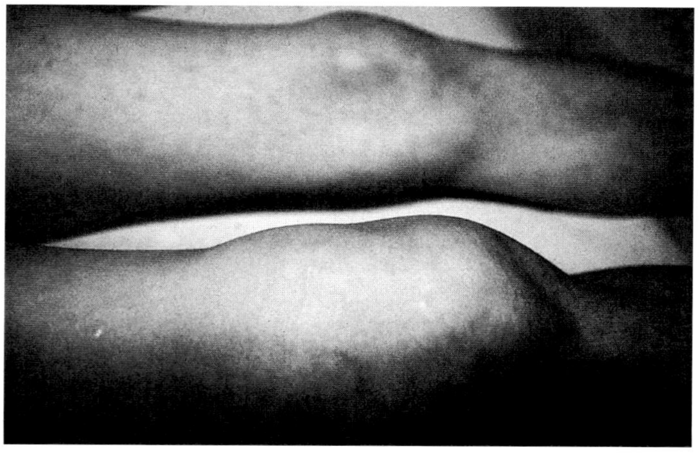

Figure 70.3 A 9-year-old boy with a markedly swollen knee caused by Lyme arthritis. Affected knees are commonly more swollen than painful and are often hot. (See also colour plate 70.3.)

Chronic neurologic involvement develops in approximately 5% of untreated patients months to years after the onset of infection, sometimes following long periods of latent infection.[5] The most common form of chronic central nervous system involvement is a subtle encephalopathy affecting memory, mood, or sleep. These patients frequently have evidence of memory impairment on neuropsychological tests and abnormal CSF analyses. Lyme encephalopathy is often accompanied by an axonal polyneuropathy manifested as either distal paresthesias or spinal radicular pain. Electromyography in these patients generally shows extensive abnormalities of proximal and distal nerve segments.

LIFE CYCLE OF SPIROCHETE

Lyme disease occurs in temperate regions of North America, Europe, and Asia. Throughout these regions, Lyme disease spirochetes have an enzootic cycle that involves ticks of the *Ixodes ricinus* complex and specific vertebrate hosts.[6] *I. scapularis* is the vector in the northeastern and midwestern USA from Maine to Maryland, and *I. pacificus* is the vector in the western states of California and Oregon. In Europe the vector is *I. ricinus*, and in Asia it is *I. persulcatus*. These ticks have different hosts in different locations. In the northeastern USA, immature larval and nymphal stages of *I. scapularis* prefer to feed on the white-footed mouse (*Peromyscus leucopus*), and the adult stage prefers to feed on white-tailed deer (*Odocoileus virginianus*). The lifecycle of the spirochete depends on horizontal transmission: from infected nymphs to mice in early summer, and in late summer from infected mice to larvae, which then molt to infected nymphs to begin the cycle again the following year. Deer are critical for the lifecycle of the tick, but are not involved in the lifecycle of the spirochete.

GENETIC FACTORS

The severity of disease is influenced by the genetics of both the spirochete and the vertebrate host (Chapter 27). The total genome of *B. burgdorferi* is small; it includes a linear chromosome of 950 kilobases along with 9 circular and 12 linear plasmids, which make up 40% of the genome.[7] The remarkable aspect of the *B. burgdorferi* genome is the large number of sequences for predicted or known lipoproteins, including outer-surface proteins (Osp) A through F. Some of these proteins are differentially expressed, and presumably help the spirochete to survive in markedly different arthropod and mammalian environments. For example, the spirochete expresses the highly related lipoproteins, OspA and OspB, in the mid-gut of the tick.[8] When the blood meal is taken, OspC is up-regulated as the organism traverses from the tick salivary gland to the vertebrate host. The sequences of OspC, which vary greatly among strains, have been divided into 21 major groups; these differences correlate with virulence. Certain groups do not appear to cause human disease, some strains seem only to cause local infection of the skin, and 4 groups (A, B, I, and K) are associated with disseminated infection.[9] There are surely other as yet unidentified genetic factors that influence spirochetal virulence.

Multiple host genetic factors are also likely to influence the severity of infection. For example, major histocompatibility complex (MHC) Class II alleles have been associated with severe and prolonged Lyme arthritis. In an initial study, an increased frequency of HLA-DR4 specificity, determined by serologic typing methods, was found in patients with chronic Lyme arthritis.[10] More recently, using contemporary molecular HLA typing techniques, HLA-DRB1*0401, 0404, 0101, 0102, and 0701 alleles have been associated with antibiotic treatment-resistant Lyme arthritis. These alleles, with the exception of 0701, are also associated with rheumatoid arthritis.

In inbred strains of mice, genetically determined differences in cytokine responses have been shown to influence the severity and duration of Lyme arthritis.[11,12] C3H/HeJ mice, which carry *H-2*^{k} alleles, develop severe arthritis when infected with *B. burgdorferi*, whereas BALB/c mice, which carry *H-2*^{d} alleles, develop only mild arthritis. C3H/HeJ mice produce IFN-γ (Th1 response) when infected with the spirochete,[11] but still have a large burden of spirochetes in joints. In comparison, *B. burgdorferi*-infected BALB/c mice initially produce even higher levels of IFN-γ, but the switch to IL-4 production (Th2 response).[12] Thus, BALB/c mice appear to reduce the numbers of spirochetes initially with a Th1 response, and then dampen the inflammatory response of the arthritis with a Th2 response.

IMMUNOLOGY/PATHOGENESIS

After injection into the skin, *B. burgdorferi* may migrate outward in the skin, resulting in erythema migrans, and may spread hematogenously to other organs. Spread within the host is probably facilitated by the binding of human plasminogen and urokinase-type plasminogen activator to the surface of the spirochete.[13] The spirochete can adhere to many different types of mammalian cells; it binds specifically to certain ubiquitous host integrin receptors in the extracellular matrix, vitronectin and fibronectin,[14] and to matrix glycoaminoglycans.[15] The organism seems to be particularly tropic for tissues of the skin, nervous system, and joint, but the specific reasons for these tropisms are not yet known. Histologically, all affected tissues show an infiltration of lymphocytes and plasma cells with some degree of vascular damage, including mild vasculitis or hypervascular occlusion, suggesting that the spirochete may have been in or around blood vessels.

Patients with untreated Lyme disease have a complex immune response to an increasing array of spirochetal proteins over a period of months to years.[16] After the first several weeks of infection, peripheral blood mononuclear cells (PBMC) generally have heightened responsiveness to *B. burgdorferi* antigens, and evidence of B-cell hyperactivity – elevated total serum IgM levels, cryoprecipitates, and circulating immune complexes. Specific IgM antibody titers to *B. burgdorferi* peak between the third and sixth week after disease onset. The specific IgG response develops gradually over months to an increasing array of 12 or more spirochetal polypeptides and reaches maximal expansion during the period of arthritis.

When arthritis is present, antigen-specific T cells from peripheral blood or synovial fluid secrete primarily the pro-inflammatory Th1 cytokine, IFN-γ,[17] and a Th1 response is dominant in the synovial tissue of such patients.[18] In a study of 10 patients with Lyme arthritis, the severity of joint swelling correlated directly with the ratio of Th1 to Th2 cells in synovial fluid, such that the larger the effusion, the higher the ratio.[17] Joint fluid samples from patients with Lyme arthritis also contain a large number of T cells that express γδ T-cell receptors and that proliferate upon stimulation with *B. burgdorferi*. Synovial fluid Vδ1$^+$ T cells may mediate an innate immune response to common lipoprotein products of spirochetes.[19]

Lyme arthritis typically occurs in intermittent attacks, but approximately 10% of patients have more persistent joint swelling, primarily in the knees.[20] Moreover, the arthritis often persists in these patients despite apparent killing of the spirochete with antibiotic therapy. These findings have suggested that treatment-resistant arthritis may result from the triggering of autoimmune responses within the joint in genetically susceptible individuals, such as those with DRB1*0401 alleles. Immune responses to specific spirochetal antigens may play a pathogenetic role in this process. In initial studies, the severity and duration of Lyme arthritis correlated with IgG antibody responses to outer-surface proteins A and B (OspA and OspB) of *B. burgdorferi*,[21] and among HLA-DR4-positive patients, those with antibodies to these proteins had arthritis for significantly longer after treatment than those who lacked such reactivity.[22] Similarly, comparisons of T-cell responses in treatment-responsive or treatment-resistant patients also implicated OspA reactivity in treatment-resistant arthritis. In a recent study, epitope mapping showed that 14 of the 16 patients with treatment-resistant arthritis had responses to OspA peptides (usually 4 or 5 epitopes), whereas only 5 of the 16 patients with treatment-responsive arthritis had reactivity with these peptides (usually 1 or 2 epitopes) ($P = 0.003$).[23] Moreover, the major difference was that 15 of the 16 patients with treatment-resistant arthritis had reactivity with an OspA peptide containing amino acids (aa) 154–173 compared with 1 of 5 patients with treatment-responsive arthritis ($P = 0.004$).

Using an algorithm by Hammer et al, which predicts epitopes presented by the DRB1*0401 molecule, the immunodominant epitope of OspA was predicted to be located at aa 165–173 with a secondary epitope at aa 237–245.[24] This is consistent with the data from human patients with Lyme arthritis. These dominant epitopes were verified using transgenic mice that were deficient in their own Class II molecules and expressed only a chimeric, human HLA-DRB1*0401 molecule. In a search of the Genetics Computer Group gene bank, a peptide from only one human protein, lymphocyte function associated antigen-1 (hLFA-1), showed sequence homology with $\text{OspA}_{165-173}$ and predicted binding to the DRB1*0401 molecule (Fig. 70.4).[24] Synovial fluid T cells from most patients with treatment-resistant arthritis responded to both OspA and hLFA-1, whereas those from patients with other forms of chronic inflammatory arthritis did not respond to either protein (Fig. 70.5). Molecular mimicry between the dominant T-cell epitope of OspA and hLFA-1 would provide a possible explanation for persistent joint inflammation after the apparent eradication of the spirochete from the joint with antibiotic therapy (Chapter 58).

Several caveats should be stressed regarding the OspA/hLFA-1 hypothesis. First, some patients, even those with the appropriate genetic susceptibility, may not develop treatment-resistant arthritis because the spirochete may not up-regulate OspA expression in the joint or because not enough time elapses prior

Molecular mimicry between *B. burgdorferi* and hLFA1α

B. burgdorferi OspA$_{165\text{-}173}$	Y	V	L	E	G	T	L	T	A
Human LFA-1α$_{L332\text{-}340}$	Y	V	I	E	G	T	S	K	Q
	↑ P1			↑ P4		↑ P6			

Figure 70.4 Molecular mimicry is shown between the dominant epitope of outer-surface protein A (OspA$_{165\text{–}173}$) of *B. burgdorferi* presented by the DRB1*0401 molecule and human lymphocyte function associated antigen-1 (hLFA-1α$_{L332\text{–}340}$). The LFA-1 peptide is located extracellularly in the region of LFA-1α$_L$ called the 'interactive' or 'I-domain', which mediates the binding of LFA-1 to its ligand, intracellular adhesion molecule-1 (ICAM-1). The spirochetal and human sequences have the same P1, 4, and 6 anchor sites. (Reproduced with permission from Steere A, et al. The early clinical manifestations of Lyme disease. *Ann Intern Med* 1983;99:22.)

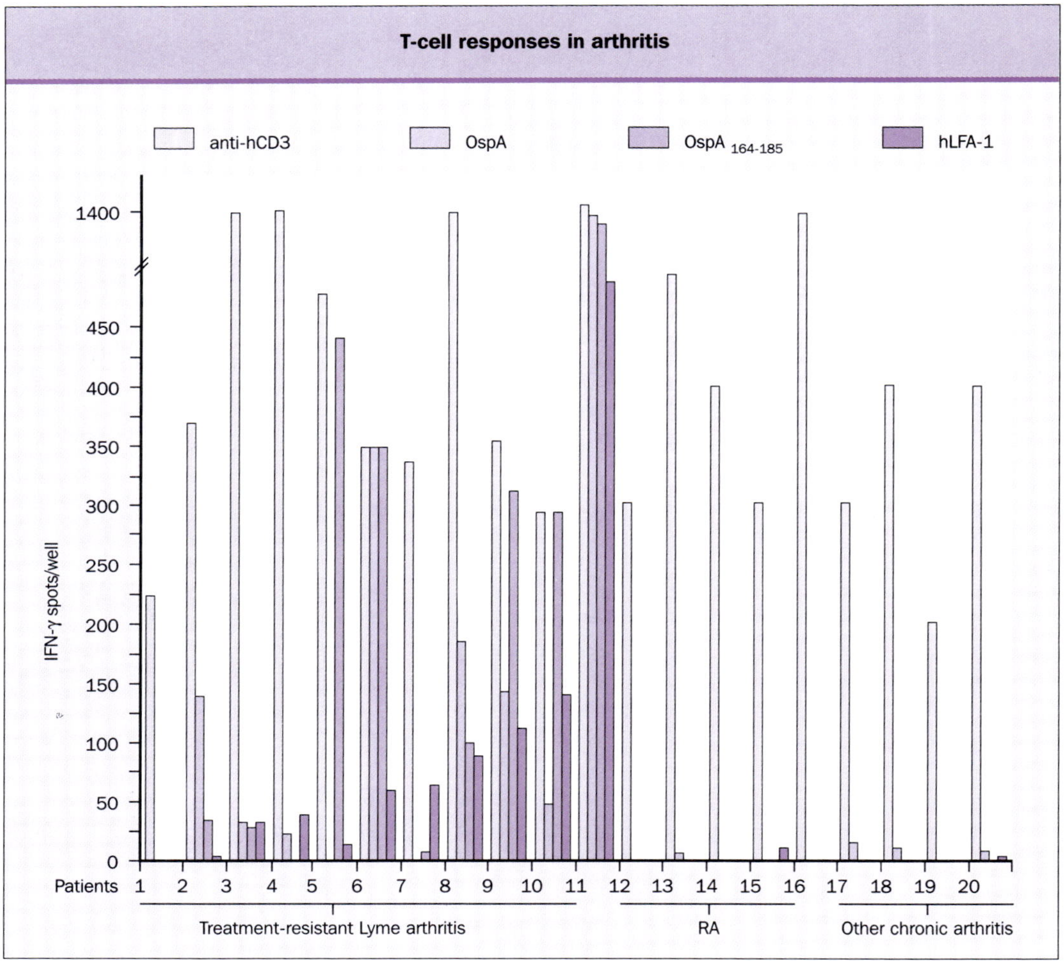

Figure 70.5 Responses of synovial fluid T cells to OspA or hLFA-1 in patients with treatment-resistant Lyme arthritis or other chronic inflammatory arthritides.[24] 3×10^5 SF cells were cultured with anti-CD3 monodonal antibody, OspA (10 μg/ml), OspA$_{164\text{–}173}$ (10 μg/ml), or hLFA-1 (70 ng/ml), or medium alone for 24 h, and reactivity was determined using an ElisaSpot assay. Values from medium alone were subtracted from those in wells containing antigen. Of the 11 patients with treatment-resistant Lyme arthritis, 10 had synovial fluid T-cell reactivity to OspA or hLFA-1, or in most instances, to both, whereas patients with other chronic inflammatory arthritides did not demonstrate responses to these proteins. (Reproduced with permission from Gross DM, et al. Identification of LFA-1 as a candidate autoantigen in treatment-resistant Lyme arthritis. *Science* 1998;281:703.)

to treatment for the development of this pathogenic response. Second, within this pro-inflammatory milieu, it is possible that other self peptides with less sequence homology than OspA and hLFA-1 may be stimulatory, even more stimulatory than hLFA-1. Third, other factors, such as genetically determined differences in cytokine responses, surely play a role. For example, patients who produce a sustained, pro-inflammatory response in the joint may be more likely to break tolerance. Finally, the DRB1*0401 molecule is predicted to bind the OspA$_{165\text{–}173}$ epitope of *B. garinii* or *B. afzelii* significantly less well than that of *B. burgdorferi* sensu stricto, which may explain why treatment-resistant Lyme arthritis has only been reported with *B. burgdorferi* sensu stricto infection in the USA.

PREVENTION

The risk of tick bites in high-risk areas can be reduced by simple measures, particularly by wearing long trousers tucked into socks and by checking for ticks after exposure in wooded areas. Prophylactic antibiotics for tick bites are not generally recommended. In a large, double-blind, placebo-controlled trial in the Lyme, Connecticut, region, the risk of Lyme disease in placebo-treated subjects with recognized tick bites was only 1.2%,[25] perhaps because 24–48 hours of tick attachment is often required for transmission of the spirochete. Thus, the simple act of removing an attached tick is often all that is required for appropriate prevention.

A vaccine is now available for the prevention of Lyme disease in the USA. In a pivotal efficacy and safety study, 10 936 subjects who lived in endemic areas for this infection received an injection of either recombinant OspA with adjuvant or placebo at enrollment and at 1 and 12 months later.[26] In the first year, after two injections, vaccine efficacy was 49%. In the second year, after the third injection, it was 76%. Injection of the vaccine was associated with mild to moderate, local or systemic reactions lasting a median duration of 3 days. High-titered antibody to OspA is necessary for protection, and yearly or every other year booster injections may be necessary to maintain adequate immunity. The American Committee on Immunization Practices of the Centers for Disease Control and Prevention states that vaccination should be considered for people who live in high-risk areas who have frequent exposure to ticks. Vaccination is not recommended for people who live in regions of low endemicity for the infection.

PATIENT MANAGEMENT

The various manifestations of Lyme disease can usually be treated successfully with oral antibiotic therapy, except for objective neurologic abnormalities, for which intravenous therapy is recommended (Table 70.1).[2,27] For early localized or disseminated Lyme disease, doxycycline is recommended in adult men and in nonpregnant women. Amoxicillin, cefuroxime axetil, or erythromyin are second-, third-, or fourth-choice alternatives. In children, amoxicillin should be prescribed; in cases of penicillin allergy, cefuroxime axetil or erythromycin may be used. For early Lyme disease, 20–30 days of therapy is recommended.

These oral antibiotic regimens, when given for 30–60 days, are usually effective for the treatment of Lyme arthritis. However, a small percentage of patients with arthritis, particularly those with the HLA-DRB1*0401, 0404, 0101, 0102, or 0701 alleles and an immune response to OspA, may have persistent joint

THERAPEUTIC PRINCIPLES

- Patients with early Lyme disease or Lyme arthritis can usually be treated successfully with oral antibiotic therapy.
- Patients with objective neurologic abnormalities usually require treatment with intravenous antibiotics.
- After 2 months of oral antibiotics or 1 month of intravenous therapy, patients with persistent Lyme arthritis who have negative PCR results for *B. burgdorferi* DNA in joint fluid are best treated with NSAIDs and disease-modifying antirheumatic drugs (DMARDs).
- Patients with post-Lyme disease syndrome should receive symptomatic treatment.

Table 70.1 Treatment regimens for Lyme disease.[a]

Treatment regimens for Lyme disease[a]	
Early infection (local or disseminated)	
Adults	Doxycycline, 100 mg orally 2 times/d for 20–30 d Amoxicillin, 500 mg orally 3 times/d for 20–30 d Alternatives in case of doxycycline or amoxicillin allergy: Cefuroxime axetil, 500 mg orally twice daily for 20–30 d Erythromycin, 150 mg orally 4 times a day for 20–30 d
Children (age 8 or less)	Amoxicillin, 250 mg orally 3 times a day or 20 mg/kg/d in divided doses for 20–30 d Alternatives in case of penicillin allergy: Cefuroxime axetil, 125 mg orally twice daily for 20–30 d Erythromycin, 250 mg orally 3 times a day or 30 mg/kg/d in divided doses for 20–30 d
Arthritis (intermittent or chronic)	Doxycycline 100 mg orally 2 times/d for 30–60 d Amoxicillin 500 mg orally 4 times/d for 30–60 d or Ceftriaxone 2 g IV once a day for 14–30 d Pen G, 20 million U IV in 4 divided doses daily for 30 d
Neurologic abnormalities (early or late)	Ceftriaxone 2 g IV once a day for 14–30 d Pen G, 20 million U IV in 4 divided doses daily for 30 d Alternative in case of ceftriaxone or penicillin allergy: Doxycycline, 100 mg orally 3 times a day for 30 d[b]
Facial palsy alone	Oral regimens may be adequate
Cardiac abnormalities	
First-degree AV block (P–R interval >0.3 s)	Oral regimens, as for early infection
High-degree AV block	Ceftriaxone, 2 g IV once a day for 30 d,[c] Pen G, 20 million U IV in 4 divided doses daily for 30 d[c]

[a] Treatment failures have occurred with any of the regimens given, and a second course of therapy may be necessary.
[b] In the author's experience, this regimen may be ineffective for the treatment of late neurologic abnormalities of Lyme disease.
[c] Once the patient has stabilized, the course may be completed with oral therapy.

inflammation for months or even several years despite either oral or intravenous antibiotic therapy. If there is persistent arthritis despite 2 months of oral therapy or 1 month of intravenous therapy, and if the results of PCR testing for *B. burgdorferi* DNA in joint fluid are negative the author treats such patients with anti-inflammatory agents, usually including both nonsteroidal anti-inflammatory agents (NSAIDS) and disease-modifying antirheumatic drugs (DMARDs) used in the treatment of rheumatoid arthritis. Arthroscopic synovectomy has also been used successfully for the treatment of such patients.

For objective neurologic abnormalities, with the possible exception of facial palsy alone, parenteral antibiotic therapy is generally recommended. A 2- or 4-week course of intravenous ceftriaxone is most commonly used, but IV cefotaxime or IV penicillin G for the same duration may also be effective. The symptoms of acute neuroborreliosis often improve rapidly, but those of chronic neurologic involvement subside slowly over a period of months. In patients with high-degree atrioventricular block or a P–R interval greater than 0.3 seconds, intravenous therapy for at least a part of the course and cardiac monitoring are recommended.

Despite recommended courses of antibiotic therapy, a small percentage of patients develop pain or fatigue syndromes along with or soon after Lyme disease.[28] The symptoms may include debilitating fatigue, severe headache, diffuse musculoskeletal pain, diffuse paresthesias, difficulty with concentration, sleep disturbance, or tender points in characteristic locations. This post-Lyme disease syndrome is the same or similar to chronic fatigue syndrome or fibromyalgia. Symptomatic treatment is recommended for these patients rather than repeated courses of antibiotic therapy.

PATIENT EVALUATION AND DIAGNOSIS

The diagnosis of Lyme disease is based primarily on the recognition of a characteristic clinical picture, exposure in an endemic area, and an elevated antibody response to *B. burgdorferi*. Culture of the spirochete from patient specimens permits definitive diagnosis, but, with few exceptions, the procedure has yielded positive results only from biopsies of erythema migrans skin lesions. Therefore, serologic testing is the most practical laboratory test for support of the diagnosis.

For serodiagnosis, the Centers for Disease Control and Prevention (CDC) recommend a two-step approach in which samples are tested first by ELISA and those yielding equivocal or positive results are tested by Western blotting.[29] During the first month of infection, both IgM and IgG responses to the spirochete should be determined, preferably in acute and convalescent serum samples. Approximately 20–30% of patients have a positive response in acute samples whereas, even after antibiotic treatment, about 70–80% have a positive response during convalescence 2–4 weeks later. After that time, the great majority of patients with active infection have a positive IgG antibody response, and a single test is usually sufficient. In persons with illness for longer than one month, a positive test for IgM antibodies alone is likely to be a false-positive result and, therefore, a positive IgM response should not be used to support the diagnosis after the first month of infection. According to current criteria adopted by the Centers for Disease Control and Prevention, a Western blot for IgM responses is considered positive if 2 of the following 3 bands are present: 23, 39, or 41 kDa, but the combination of the 23 and 41 kDa bands may still be a false-positive result. A Western blot for IgG responses is considered positive if 5 of the following 10 bands are present: 18, 23, 28, 30, 39, 41, 45, 58, 66, or 93 kDa. Patients with *B. garinii* or *B. afzelii* infection in Europe and Asia usually have less expansion of the antibody response than in observed with *B. burgdorferi* sensu stricto infection in the USA. Therefore, the CDC criteria cannot be used effectively in Europe or Asia.

The major limitation of serologic tests is that they do not distinguish clearly between active or inactive infection. IgG, and even IgM responses, may persist for years after antibiotic treatment. Since cultures are usually negative in Lyme disease, it had been hoped that PCR testing might serve as a substitute for culture in this infection. However, this test has been readily positive only in joint fluid samples from patients with Lyme arthritis prior to antibiotic treatment. In one study, 70 of 73 joint fluid samples (96%) had positive PCR results using primer-probe sets that detect OspA gene segments.[30] PCR testing is much less sensitive in detecting spirochetal DNA in CSF samples in patients with neuroborreliosis, and there seems to be little, if any role, for PCR in the detection of *B. burgdorferi* DNA from blood or urine samples.

CLINICAL PEARLS

Interpretation of serologic tests in Lyme disease

- IgM responses to *B. burgdor feri* are only helpful for diagnosis during the first several weeks of infection (when most patients have erythema migrans).
- In persons with illness for longer than one month, a positive test for IgM antibodies alone is likely to be a false-positive result.
- In persons with early infection, seroconversion between acute and convalescent samples provides more convincing support for diagnosis.
- After the first month of infection, the great majority of patients have a positive IgG antibody response.
- IgG, and even IgM responses, may persist for years after antibiotic treatment for active infection.
- Positive serologic tests do not clearly distinguish between active and inactive infection.
- Once a patient has seroconverted, subsequent antibody testing is of little help in determining the success of therapy.
- Although vaccinated individuals may have positive results by ELISA, a vaccine-induced antibody response can usually be distinguished from that of natural infection by Western blot analysis.

Differential diagnosis

One of the most common mistakes has been the failure to distinguish Lyme arthritis or chronic neuroborreliosis from chronic fatigue syndrome or fibromyalgia. This is compounded by the fact that a small percentage of patients develop fibromyalgia in association with or soon after Lyme disease. Compared to patients with Lyme disease, patients with chronic fatigue syndrome or fibromyalgia tend to have more generalized and disabling symptoms. In addition, patients with these conditions lack evidence of joint inflammation, have normal neurologic test results, and usually have more anxiety and depression.

Pitfalls/controversies

A common pitfall is the misinterpretation of serologic results in Lyme disease. In particular, IgM responses to *B. burgdorferi* are only helpful in supporting the diagnosis of Lyme disease during the first several weeks of infection when most patients have erythema migrans. Even then, serologic support for the diagnosis is more convincing if seroconversion is demonstrated between acute and convalescent samples. Once a patient has seroconverted, subsequent antibody testing is of little help in decisions about the adequacy of antibiotic therapy. After treatment, antibody responses typically remain positive for years, particularly if the disease had progressed to its late stages prior to treatment. In addition, there is considerable day-to-day variation in serologic test results, and therefore one cannot be certain that a given value is increasing or decreasing unless serial samples are tested in the same assay. Another problem is that about 10% of patients infected with *B. burgdorferi* in the USA and a higher percentage in Europe have asymptomatic infection. If these individuals or those with past infection subsequently develop another illness, the positive serologic test for Lyme disease may cause diagnostic confusion. Finally, with serologic tests that employ sonicated *B. burgdorferi* proteins, vaccinated individuals may have false-positive results by ELISA, but a vaccine-induced immune response can usually be distinguished from that of the natural infection by Western blot analysis.

The most controversial aspect of Lyme disease concerns the all too common practice of diagnosing pain or fatigue syndromes as Lyme disease, even in patients with little or no evidence of that infection. Although Lyme disease has many possible manifestations, it is usually associated with characteristic clinical findings and positive test results on standard laboratory tests.

REFERENCES

1. Steere AC, Malawista SE, Snydman DR, et al. Lyme arthritis: an epidemic of oligoarticular arthritis in children and adults in three Connecticut communities. Arthritis Rheum 1977;20:7.
2. Steere AC. Lyme disease. N Engl J Med 1989;321:586.
3. Baranton G, Postic D, Saint-Girons I, et al. Delineation of *Borrelia bugdorferi* sensu stricto: *Borrelia garinii* sp. nov., and group VS461 associated with Lyme borreliosis. Int J Syst Bacteriol 1992;42:378.
4. Steere AC, Schoen RT, Taylor E. The clinical evolution of Lyme arthritis. Ann Intern Med 1987;107:725.
5. Logigian EL, Kaplan RF, Steere AC. Chronic neurologic manifestations of Lyme disease. N Engl J Med 1990;323:1438.
6. Matuschka FR, Spielman A. The emergence of Lyme disease in a changing environment in North America and central Europe. Exp Appl Acarol 1986;2:337.
7. Fraser CM, Casjens S, Huang WM, et al. Genomic sequence of a Lyme disease spirochete: *Borrelia burgdorferi*. Nature 1997;390:580.
8. Montgomery RR, Malawista SE, Feen KJM, Bockenstedt LK. Direct demonstration of antigenic substitution of *Borrelia burgdorferi* ex vivo: exploration of the paradox of the early immune response to outer surface proteins A and C in Lyme disease. J Exp Med 1996;183:261.
9. Seinost G, Dykhuizen DE, Dattwyler RJ, et al. Four clones of *Borrelia burgdorferi* sensu stricto cause invasive infection in humans. Infect Immun 1999;67:3518.
10. Steere AC, Dwyer E, Winchester R. Association of chronic Lyme arthritis with HLA-DR4 and HLA-DR2 alleles. N Engl J Med 1990;323:219.
11. Keane-Myers A, Nickell SP. T cell subset-dependent modulation of immunity to *Borrelia burgdorferi* in mice. J Immunol 1995;154:1770.
12. Kang I, Barthold SW, Persing DH, Bockenstedt LK. T-helper-cell cytokines in the early evolution of murine Lyme arthritis. Infect Immun 1997;65:3107.
13. Klempner MS, Noring R, Epstein MP, et al. Binding of human plasminogen and urokinase-type plasminogen activator to the Lyme disease spirochete *Borrelia burgdorferi*. J Infect Dis 1995;171:1258.
14. Coburn J, Magoun L, Bodary SC, Leong JM. Integrins $\alpha v\beta 3$ and $\alpha 5\beta 1$ mediate attachment of Lyme disease spirochetes to human cells. Infect Immun 1998;66:1946.
15. Leong JM, Wang H, Magoun L, et al. Different classes of proteoglycans contribute to the attachment of *Borrelia burgdorferi* to cultured endothelial and brain cells. Infect Immun 1998;66:994.
16. Dressler F, Whalen JA, Reinhardt BN, Steere AC. Western blotting in the serodiagnosis of Lyme disease. J Infect Dis 1993;167:392.
17. Gross DM, Steere AC, Huber BT. Dominent T helper 1 response is antigen specific and localized to synovial fluid in patients with Lyme arthritis. J Immunol 1998;160:1022.
18. Yin Z, Braun Jurgen, Neure L, et al. T cell cytokine pattern in the joints of patients with Lyme arthritis and its regulation by cytokines and anticytokines. Arthritis Rheum 1997;40:69.
19. Vincent MS, Roessner K, Sellati T, et al. Lyme arthritis synovial $\gamma\delta$ T cells respond to *Borrelia burgdorferi* lipoproteins and lipidated hexapeptides. J Immunol 1998;161:5762.
20. Steere AC, Levin RE, Molloy PJ, et al. Treatment of Lyme arthritis. Arthritis Rheum 1994;37:878.
21. Akin E, McHugh GL, Flavell RA, Fikrig E, Steere AC. The immunoglobin (IgG) antibody response to OspA and OspB correlates with severe and prolonged Lyme arthritis and the IgG response to P35 correlates with mild and brief arthritis. Infect Immun 1999;67:173.
22. Kalish RA, Leong JM, Steere AC. Association of treatment resistant chronic Lyme arthritis with HLA-DR4 and antibody reactivity to OspA and OspB of *Borrelia burgdorferi*. Infect Immun 1993;61:2774.
23. Chen J, Field JA, Glickstein L, Molloy PJ, Huber BT, Steere AC. Association of antibiotic treatment-resistant Lyme arthritis with T cell responses to dominant epitopes of outer-surface protein A (OspA) of *Borrelia burgdorferi*. Arthritis Rheum 1999;42:1813.
24. Gross DM, Forsthuber T, Tary-Lehman M, et al. Identification of LFA-1 as a candidate autoantigen in treatment-resistant Lyme arthritis. Science 1998;281:703.
25. Shapiro ED, Gerber MA, Holabird NB, et al. A controlled trial of antimicrobial prophylaxis for Lyme disease after deer-tick bites. N Engl J Med 1992;327:1769.
26. Steere AC, Sikand VK, Meurice F, et al. Vaccination against Lyme disease with recombinant *Borrelia burgdorferi* outer-surface lipoprotein A with adjuvant. N Engl J Med 1998;339:209.
27. Wormser GP, Nadelman RB, Datturyler RJ, et al. Guidelines from the Infectious Diseases Society of America: practice guidelines for the treatment of Lyme disease. *Clin Infect Dis* 2000;31(Suppl I)51.
28. Dinerman H, Steere AC. Lyme disease associated with fibromyalgia. Ann Intern Med 1992;117:281.
29. Recommendations for test performance and interpretation from the Second International Conference on serologic diagnosis of Lyme disease. MMWR Morb Mortal Wkly Rep 1995;44:590.
30. Nocton JJ, Dressler F, Rutledge BJ, Rys PN, Persing DH, Steere AC. Detection of *Borrelia burgdorferi* DNA by polymerase chain reaction in synovial fluid in Lyme arthritis. N Engl J Med 1994;330:229.

Chapter 71

Amyloidosis

Jean D. Sipe* and Alan S. Cohen

NATURE AND CLASSIFICATION OF FIBRILS

Amyloidosis is a heterogeneous group of disorders in which normally soluble proteins assemble as insoluble amyloid fibrils with a β-pleated sheet conformation and are deposited in one or more organs of the body.[1] Amyloid fibrils are rigid, fine, and nonbranching, 8–10 nm in width, and indeterminate in length. Approximately 20 proteins, nonpathogenic when soluble, have been identified as insoluble amyloid fibrils in tissues. Each distinct fibril protein exhibits a unique anatomic pattern of deposition and is associated with characteristic clinical manifestations (Table 71.1).[2,3]

Amyloid fibril-forming monomers are small molecules, usually polyanionic proteins with a high content of glutamic and aspartic acids and serine. Amyloidosis occurs when this intact or partially catabolized precursor peptide undergoes changes in conformation to assume the cross β-pleated sheet conformation. This conformation favors hydrogen bonding between neighboring polypeptide chains rather than within one chain, as occurs with α-helical structure. It is thought that amyloid deposits in tissues become increasingly large because the fibrils associate with each other and bind extracellular matrix components such as glycosaminoglycans, apolipoprotein E, and amyloid P (AP) component. The avidity of amyloid fibrils for AP is actually used

Amyloid fibril proteins and clinical syndromes

Amyloid protein	Protein precursor	Clinical syndrome
Immunity/inflammation		
AL	Igλ Igκ	Idiopathic (primary); multiple myeloma; local nodular
AH	γ1 heavy chain	Idiopathic (primary); multiple myeloma
AA	Serum amyloid A	Reactive (secondary)
Aβ2M	β2-microglobulin	Chronic hemodialysis arthropathy
ACys	Cystatin C	Hereditary cerebral angiopathy with bleeding (Iceland)
ALys	Lysozyme	Nonneuropathic hereditary amyloid with renal disease
AFibA	Fibrinogen Aα	Nonneuropathic hereditary amyloid with renal disease
Endocrine hormones		
AIAPP	Islet amyloid polypeptide	Diabetes mellitus type II Insulinoma
AANF	Atrial natriuretic factor	Senile cardiac amyloid
ACal	Procalcitonin	Medullary carcinoma of the thyroid
APro	Prolactin	
AIns	Insulin, porcine	Iatrogenic
Transport molecules		
ATTR	Transthyretin	Familial amyloid polyneuropathy Senile cardiac amyloid
AApoAI	Apolipoprotein AI	Familial amyloid polyneuropathy
ALac	Lactoferrin	Familial subepithelial corneal amyloidosis; seminal vesicle amyloidosis
Nervous system		
Aβ	Aβ-protein precursor	Alzheimer's disease
APrP	Prion protein	Spongiform encephalopathies
Cell motility		
AGel	Gelsolin	Familial amyloid polyneuropathy

Table 71.1 Amyloid fibril proteins and clinical syndromes. Modified from Westermark P, Araki S, Benson MD, et al. Amyloid. *Int J Exp Clin Invest* 1999;6:63.

* The opinions contained herein do not necessarily reflect those of the Department of Health and Human Services or the National Institutes of Health.

diagnostically. In current clinical practice, the total body mass of amyloid is measured by a scintigraphic method using ^{123}I-labeled AP or, more recently, ^{131}I-labeled AP.[4]

The genesis of amyloid is multifactorial and not completely understood. Predisposition to disease may relate to genetic (germline or somatic mutation), infectious, inflammatory, or iatrogenic factors (Table 71.1).[2–6] The propensity with which a polypeptide forms amyloid fbrils is influenced by its primary structure and concentration. Additional effects may come from the local environment, susceptibility to conformational changes brought about by extracellular matrix components and/or nucleating agents, and any aberrations in proteolysis that may influence catabolism of precursor proteins, fibril-forming fragments, or nascent amyloid fibrils. The mononuclear phagocyte system plays a central role in many of the amyloidoses. Cytokines may stimulate expression of some amyloid precursors, the proteolytic enzymes that convert precursors to fibril proteins, and the phagocytic capacity for degradation and resorption of fibrils from amyloid deposits.

Amyloid is clinically heterogeneous. Depending upon the biochemical nature of the fibril protein, amyloid deposition may be limited to a single organ such as the brain or pancreas. Alternatively, amyloid deposition may be systemic and involve the cardiovascular system, gastrointestinal system, lymph nodes, spleen, liver, kidneys, and adrenals.[5–8]

The 1998 guidelines for nomenclature and classification of amyloid and amyloidosis, recommended by the Nomenclature Committee of the International Society for Amyloidosis, state that amyloid deposits should be classified using the capital letter A as the first letter of designation followed by the protein designation without any open space, for example, AL for amyloidosis involving immunoglobulin light chains (Table 71.1).[2]

SYSTEMIC AMYLOIDOSES

AL, AH (primary idiopathic amyloidosis; amyloidosis associated with multiple myeloma)

Pathogenesis

AL amyloid deposits consist of either intact or amino-terminal fibrillar fragments of monoclonal immunoglobulin light (L) chains. Deposits predominantly occur in heart, kidneys, liver, and spleen.[9,10] There have been a few reports of immunoglobulin heavy (H) chains deposited as amyloid fibrils (AH). The λ subclass of light chains is found in AL deposits more frequently than κ by a ratio of 2:1. This ratio is the inverse of that seen in multiple myeloma without amyloidosis and other monoclonal gammopathies. Certain light chain subsets (i.e. λ VI) have been reported exclusively in association with amyloidosis.

AL amyloidosis can be viewed as a subset of the immunoglobulin deposition diseases, related to, but distinct from, other forms in which light and heavy chains are deposited in tissues. However, in the nonamyloid deposition diseases, the deposited immunoglobulin protein is usually not fibrillar and is not stained by Congo red dye, nor is it associated with serum amyloid P component (SAP). Both fibrillar and nonfibrillar deposits of light chains exhibiting the same antigenic determinants have also been described as light chain deposition disease.[7]

The light chains that form amyloid fibrils in different individuals have been distinct and heterogeneous in amino acid sequence. Thus, it has been difficult to relate primary structure to fibril formation, as is easily done in some of the other forms of amyloidosis. Recent studies indicate that the variable domains of amyloidogenic light chains are thermodynamically less stable than the corresponding domains of those light chains that do not form amyloid fibrils. It has been postulated that there are no structural or sequence-specific features of the light chains that are associated with fibril formation, other than instability of light chain domain(s).[11]

Clinical features

Primary AL amyloidosis should be suspected in patients with hepatosplenomegaly or nephropathy of unknown origin.[10] It should be considered in patients with unexplained cardiomyopathy, congestive heart failure, carpal tunnel syndrome, peripheral neuropathy, and macroglossia. Individuals with a monoclonal immunoglobulin (M component) in the serum or with Bence-Jones proteinuria are also suspect. Primary idiopathic AL is differentiated from the AL of myeloma by the presence of immature plasma cells on bone marrow examination of the latter.

The renal, hepatic, and gastrointestinal manifestations of AL may be similar to those of AA amyloidosis (discussed later in this chapter), but the cardiovascular manifestations are far more severe. The latter include cardiomegaly and congestive heart failure. Intractable heart failure may be the presenting complication and is a major cause of death in AL disease. The myocardium is usually diffusely infiltrated with amyloid and presents a typical echocardiographic symmetric wall thickening with a granular sparkling appearance. Heart valves, endocardium, and pericardium also can be involved. Common abnormalities on electrocardiography include low voltage in QRS complex and atrioventricular and intraventricular conduction abnormalities.

AL deposits are common in other organ systems. In the skin the lesions can appear as waxy papules, plaques, nodules, purpura, or bullous lesions. Amyloid in the musculoskeletal system can cause a symmetric small-joint enlargement or an unusual shoulder pad sign. Synovial fluid may contain loose amyloid fragments. In rare instances, significant amyloid deposits occur in the respiratory system. Peripheral neuropathy or a carpal tunnel syndrome can be the presenting manifestation of primary AL amyloidosis. Adsorption of certain clotting factors, especially factors IX and X by large deposits in spleen, can cause selective factor deficiencies and bleeding to occur.

CLINICAL PEARLS

Consider the diagnosis of primary AL amyloidosis in patients with unexplained:

- Hepatosplenomegaly
- Nephropathy
- Cardiomyopathy or congestive heart failure
- Carpal tunnel syndrome
- Peripheral neuropathy
- Macroglossia
- Monoclonal immunoglobulin in serum or urine and unexplained clinical manifestations

Diagnosis

The diagnosis of any form of amyloidosis depends upon an appropriate tissue biopsy. Biopsy of a subcutaneous abdominal fat pad is the screening technique most frequently used. When stained with Congo red dye, lesions exhibit a classical green birefringence on polarization microscopy.[12] Electron microscopy of tissue lesions shows fine fibrils 9–10 nm in width in tissue sections. In the case of AL amyloid, laboratory studies reveal the presence of serum M components or Bence-Jones proteinuria in 70–80% of patients. This finding, however, is not specific for AL amyloidosis.

Treatment

The fact that immunoglobulin light chains are made by plasma cells has led to the use of alkylating agents, which are toxic and not very effective. A recent advance, which is far more effective, is the use of intravenous melphalan and autologous stem cell transplantation.[13] While long-term remissions are reported, serious complications, and even death, can occur, particularly if patients have inadequate cardiac function and status. Otherwise, treatment is supportive, with the use of dialysis or transplantation for renal lesions and, in selected cases, cardiac transplantation for those with primarily cardiac AL.

AA (secondary, reactive, or acquired amyloidosis)

Pathogenesis

A protein of unusual structure termed amyloid A (AA) is associated with reactive systemic amyloidosis.[14] AA proteins are 45–83 amino acid N-terminal fragments of serum amyloid A (SAA), a family of proteins identified through the study of AA amyloidosis.[8] SAA is now recognized to be a multigene family and, in human and mouse, allelic variants of active genes have been described (see references 8, 15 and 16 for reviews). The pathogenesis of AA amyloidosis has been significantly elucidated using well characterized animal models, particularly the mouse.[15] Revised SAA nomenclature was recently adopted by investigator(s) in whose laboratories AA and SAA proteins are currently being studied (see reference 16 for review), and has been recommended by the Amyloid Nomenclature Committee.[2] In both human and mouse, *SAA1* gene products are the major precursor of amyloid fibrils. The relevant SAA proteins are major acute-phase reactants and their production in liver is regulated by a cascade of cytokines, and especially tumor necrosis factor-α (TNF-α) and interleukins IL-1 and IL-6. It is likely that TNF-α plays a role early in the cascade, as blockage of TNF-α action leads to a reduction of SAA concentration in plasma of rheumatoid arthritis patients.[17] The complex network by which hepatic and extrahepatic expression of SAA genes is regulated involves positive and negative *cis*- and *trans*-acting promoter elements to ensure tissue-specific expression. Production of SAA proteins is also regulated by message stabilization (see reference 16 for review). At the peak of an acute-phase response, SAA can constitute as much as 80% of the total protein of plasma high-density lipoprotein. Normally, SAA is cleared rapidly in the peripheral microvasculature.[18] Although SAA production and structure are critical factors in AA amyloidogeneis, impaired clearance is probably the most important factor in fibril formation.[16]

Clinical features

Predisposing diseases include rheumatoid arthritis, ankylosing spondylitis and other rheumatic disorders, chronic granulomatous ileitis, and infections such as chronic tuberculosis, osteomyelitis, and bronchiectasis. AA amyloid can occur secondary to diseases in which the underlying disease is recessively inherited, as in familial Mediterranean fever[19] or autosomal dominant, as in TNF receptor-associated periodic fever syndromes (TRAPs).[20] FMF is caused by mutations in the *MEFV* gene encoding the transcription factor pyrin. There is a strong correlation between the M694V *MEFV* variant and development of AA amyloidosis. TRAPs are associated with missense mutations in the TNF receptor. One should suspect the presence of AA when there is an element of inflammation and patients develop unexplained hepatomegaly, splenomegaly, and especially proteinuria or other manifestations of renal disease.[21] Gastrointestinal lesions may also be significant in AA, but neuropathy and respiratory, cardiac, and musculoskeletal amyloid are very uncommon. The kidney disease is unusually slowly progressive, leading to azotemia. Hypertension is uncommon except in very long-standing disease. The kidney is classically described as large, but may be normal or small, depending upon the stage of the disease. Renal thrombosis or renal tubular acidosis may develop.

KEY CONCEPTS

Histological diagnosis of amyloidosis

Biopsy of appropriate site

- *Screening biopsy*
  — Subcutaneous abdominal fat aspirate
  — Rectum, gingiva
- *Directed to involved organ*
  Skin, heart, peripheral nerve, liver, kidney, synovium, small intestine, muscle

Analysis by:

- Staining with Congo red and polarizing microscopy
- Electron microscopy
- Immunohistochemical staining with antibodies specific for suspected amyloid protein

CLINICAL PEARLS

Consider the diagnosis of AA amyloidosis in patients with unexplained:

- Proteinuria and/or progressive renal unsufficiency
- Hepatomegaly
- Splenomegaly
- Gastrointestinal lesions

and chronic inflammation caused by another disease such as:

- Rheumatoid arthritis, other chronic arthritides, Crohn's disease, Behçet syndrome
- Chronic infections
- Familial Mediterranean fever or other familial periodic fever syndromes

Diagnosis

Diagnosis is similar to that described in the section on amyloid AL.

Treatment

The primary mode of treatment for AA amyloidosis is aggressive treatment of the inciting primary disease. Suppression of rheumatoid arthritis or removal of an osteomyelitic or tuberculous lesion can eventually result in regression of amyloidosis. As mentioned earlier, the hereditary recessive disorder familial Mediterranean fever (FMF) and the autosomal dominant periodic fever syndromes TRAPs[21] can be complicated by AA amyloid, particularly renal amyloid and azotemia in untreated cases. When colchicine was introduced as a form of therapy for the periodic attacks of FMF, the acute attacks decreased.[19] With the passage of time, it became clear that renal amyloid was prevented and, in some cases when it was already present, regressed on colchicine therapy. In a subset of FMF in which amyloid is the first presenting symptom, colchicine prophylaxis prevented AA amyloidosis. Treatment with soluble tumor necrosis factor receptors (sTNFRs), which act as natural inhibitors of TNF activity, also shows promise of preventing AA secondary to TRAPs.[22]

Renal disease remains a major cause of mortality in AA amyloidosis, but intervention has significantly improved the prognosis. Peritoneal dialysis, hemodialysis, and kidney transplantation are very useful.

ATTR and other hereditary amyloidoses

ATTR, in which the fibrils are variants of transthyretin (TTR), is the prototype form of hereditary amyloidosis, with nephropathy and cardiopathy. Familial amyloid polyneuropathy can be subclassified according to clinical symptoms; these subsets are associated with a specific amyloid fibril protein (Table 71.2). The heredofamilial forms of amyloid are characterized by deposition of fibrils of TTR, apolipoprotein AI, gelsolin, cystatin C, the α chain of fibrinogen A or lysozyme. The pathogenesis of ATTR and the other heredofamilial amyloidoses is distinct from that of AL and AA amyloidosis, in that, although the fibril precursor proteins are constitutive proteins present from birth, disease symptoms have a delayed onset of 3–7 decades.

In some unusual instances, reported for TTR and apolipoprotein AI, the wild-type protein can be the cause of the disease, indicating that a mutation in the protein product may not be the sole determinant for the appearance of amyloid deposits in those hereditary amyloidoses.

Pathogenesis and clinical features

ATTR

TTR is a tetrameric 55 kDa nonglycosylated plasma protein of 4 identical 127 amino acid subunits. Originally described as prealbumin, TTR was renamed because of its function as a carrier protein for thyroxine and for the retinal (vitamin A alcohol)-retinol binding protein (RBP) complex.[23] To date, more than 70 TTR variants have been identified by protein and DNA screening studies[24] (Table 71.2). Variant *TTR* gene carriers exhibit clinically heterogeneous amyloidoses according to the position and nature of the amino acid substitution. For example, the L55P mutation results in an early onset of disease manifestations and pronounced involvement of the heart, whereas the T119M mutation appears to protect against amyloid fibril formation. In Denmark, patients with the L111M mutation have severe

Heredofamilial amyloidoses		
Mutation	Geographic distribution	Clinical pattern
Transthyretin (ATTR)		
C10A	USA	E, H, PN
L12P	UK	L, LM
D18G	Hungary	LM
D18E	South America	PN
V20I	Germany, USA	CTS, H
S23N	Portugal, USA	E, H, PN
P24S	USA	CTS, H, PN
V30 M (prototype)	*Portugal, Japan, Sweden, China, Turkey, Germany, USA*	*PN, AN, GI, H, K, V, LM*
V30A	Germany, USA	AN, H
V30G	USA	E, LM
V30L	Japan, USA	PN, AN
F33I	Israel	E, PN
F33L	USA	PN
F33V	UK	PN
R34T	Italy	H, PN
K35N	France	AN, H, PN
A36P	USA	CTS, E
D38A	Japan	H
E42G	Japan, USA	AN, H, PN
E42O	France	H
F44S	USA	AN, H, PN
A45D	USA	H, PN
A45S		H
A45T	USA	H
G47R	Japan	AN, PN
G47A	Italy, Germany	AN, H
G47V	Sri Lanka	AN, CTS, PN
G47E		
T49A	France, Italy	AN, PN
T49I	Japan	H, PN
S50R	France, Italy, Japan	AN, PN
S50I	Japan	AN, H, PN, H
S52P	England	AN, H, K, PN
G53E	France	H, LM, N
E54G	England	AN, E, PN
E54Q		
E54K		PN
L55P	Taiwan, USA	AN, E, H
L55R		
L58H	Germany, USA	CTS, H
L58R	Japan	AN, CTS, E, H
T59K	Italy	AN, H, PN
T60A	Germany, UK, USA	CTS, H
E61K	Japan	PN
F64L	Italy, USA	CTS, PN
F64S	Canada, England	E, LM, PN
I68L	Germany, USA	H
Y69H	USA	E
K70N	USA	CTS, E, PN
V71A	France, Spain	CTS, E, PN
I73V	Bangladesh	AN, PN
S77Y	France, USA	H, K
S77F	France	PN
I84S	Hungary, USA	CTS, E, H, LM
I84N	USA	CTS, E, H
I84T	Germany, UK	H, PN
E89Q	Italy	CTS, H, PN
E89K	USA	H, PN
A91S	France	CTS, H, PN
A97G	Japan	H, PN
A97S		
R104H		
I107V	USA	CTS, H, PN
A109S	Japan	
L111M	Denmark	H
S112I	Italy	H, PN
Y114C	Japan	AN, E, H, LM, PN

Table 71.2 Heredofamilial amyloidoses.

Heredofamilial amyloidoses		
Mutation	**Geographic distribution**	**Clinical pattern**
Y114H	Japan	CTS
Y116S	France	PN
A120S		H
V122I	Africa, USA	H
V122A	USA	E, H, PN
dV122	Equador (USA)	H, PN
Non-amyloid TTR mutations		
G6S		
D74H		
H90N		
G101S		
P102R		
R104C		
A109T		
A109V		
T119M		
P125S		
Apolipoprotein A1 (Apo A1)		
Wild type	UK	K, S, SP
G26R	USA, Canada	K, L, LLN, peptic ulcer
L60R	England	K
W50R	Ashkenazi Jewish	K
d61–70VTinsertion	Spain	L
L90P		H, S
Gelsolin		
D187N	Finland, Japan, Netherlands, USA	Cranial neuropathy, lattice corneal dystrophy, LLN, S
D187Y	Denmark, Czechoslovakia	LLN
Fibrinogen A α		
R524L	USA	K
E526V	USA	K
R554L	Mexico	K, SP
Lysozyme		
I56T	England	K, S
D67H	England	K

AN = autonomic neuropathy; CTS = carpal tunnel syndrome; E = eye; GI = gastrointestinal tract; H = heart; K = kidney; L = liver; LLN = lower limb neuropathy; LM = leptomeninges; PN = polyneuropathy; S = skin; SP = spleen; V = vitreous.

Table 71.2 Heredofamilial amyloidoses. (*contd*) Modified in part from Connors LH, Richardson AM, Theberge R et al. Amyloid. *Int J Exp Clin Invest* 2000;7:54.[24]

cardiopathy. Several patients with homozygous methionine (M) residues at position 30 and compound heterozygotes with two mutant alleles have been described (Table 71.2). Fibrils are made up of both full-length TTR and fragments of TTR monomers and of variable quantities of both mutant and normal TTRs. In addition to the familial form of ATTR, normal TTR can be deposited in the heart of aged individuals.

In the case of ATTR, it is becoming apparent that the thermodynamic stability of TTR monomers is important, as a partially unfolded monomer appears to be required for fibril formation. To a certain extent, there is an inverse correlation between monomer stability and age of disease onset. Some TTR variants are stabilized by amino acid mutation or by its ligand thyroxine or other small molecules that stabilize the tetrameric protein, thereby preventing dissociation to monomers and the unfolding that is requisite to fibril formation.[23,25]

The clinical manifestations of the hereditary amyloidoses are protean. The prototype familial amyloid polyneuropathy, *V30M* mutation in ATTR, was extensively described in a Portuguese kinship (Andrade, Costa), but has also been found in defined areas of Japan and Sweden and in patients of Italian, Greek, French, German, Turkish and other ethnicities. Affected family members have neuropathy associated with nephropathy, cardiopathy, gastrointestinal disease, carpal tunnel syndrome, or vitreous opacities. Since so many single-point mutations in transthyretin and other proteins associated with the heredofamilial amyloidoses have been described, it is not surprising that there are differing clinical manifestations. Most patients, however, have an early lower limb peripheral neuropathy characterized by sensorimotor deficits. They may also have autonomic nervous system involvement with alternating constipation and diarrhea and severe malnutrition. Postural hypotension and impotence often develop. Clinically apparent cardiac involvement is sometimes part of the overall syndrome.

AGel

In patients with Finnish hereditary systemic amyloidosis (AGel), amyloid fibrils composed of gelsolin fragments are found in nerves and other tissues.[26] The 71 amino acid fragment contains the actin-binding domain residues 173–243 of secreted plasma gelsolin. Clinical manifestations include lattice corneal dystrophy, cranial neuropathy followed by peripheral neuropathy, dystrophic skin changes, and other organ involvement. A gelsolin mutation, A187D, has been associated with the development of disease in affected Finnish families. This mutation was also found in a similar familial amyloid polyneuropathy in patients of Japanese and Dutch background. The mutation A187Y has been found in patients of Danish and Czech background.

ACys

Several large families in Iceland are afflicted with hereditary cystatin C amyloid angiopathy (ACys) in which amyloid fibrils derived from the protease inhibitor cystatin C are deposited in the central nervous system and other tissues.[27] The disorder, which has also been described in familial and sporadic cases of cerebral hemorrhage afflicting elderly persons in Japan, is characterized by spontaneous cerebral bleeding and often death before age 30. A point mutation, N68L, is associated with the disease. Monocytes from these individuals demonstrate reduced cytstatin C secretion, raising the possibility that amyloid fibrils may form because of a secretory defect.

AFibA

Variant fibrinogen A chains have been identified in patients with hereditary nonneuropathic renal amyloidosis AFibA.[28] Three families have been identified with point mutations R24L, E526V, or R554L in the fibrinogen gene.

ALys

Lysozyme has been identified as the amyloid fibril protein in several English families afflicted with hereditary nonneuropathic systemic amyloidosis.[29] Two mutations have been described, I56T and D67H.

AApoAI

One apolipoprotein-AI variant, G26R, has been associated with an autosomal dominant hereditary amyloidosis that is characterized by peripheral neuropathy (clinically similar to ATTR) or by renal failure. Amyloid deposition in the kidney is the predominant clinical manifestation in patients with other mutations, such as L60R and W50R. The deletion of amino acids 61–70 with a VT insertion results in hepatic AApoAI, whereas the mutation L90P results in predominant skin and heart involvement.[30] ApoAI has been localized to atherosclerotic plaques, and wild-type apoAI amyloid deposits in skin, kidney, and spleen have been reported in a family in Great Britain.

Diagnosis

Demonstration of the presence of mutant TTR (or apoAI, gelsolin, etc.) in the presence of amyloidosis by either protein or DNA testing generally establishes the specific diagnosis of the disease. Isoelectric focusing is used as a simple screening test for variant TTRs associated with familial TTR amyloidosis.[12] Tissue sections also can be stained with anti-TTR, anti-AA or anti-light chain antibodies to determine the nature of the amyloid fibril.

Treatment

Genetic counseling is an important aspect of treatment in hereditary amyloidosis. Supportive measures for the autonomic neuropathy, renal, and cardiac disease can prolong life. Liver transplantation, to remove the site of synthesis of the mutant protein, has been carried out since 1990 for ATTR patients with familial amyloid polyneuropathy in Sweden, the USA, Portugal, Spain, and other countries. Disease progression is halted, to an extent that varies according to the particular mutation in the amyloid fibril protein, and there is generally some improvement in autonomic nervous system function.

IATROGENIC AMYLOIDOSIS

Aβ2M

Pathogenesis

β2-Microglobulin amyloid (Aβ2M) deposition in the musculoskeletal system is a serious and frequent complication for patients with renal failure who have received long-term hemodialysis using cuprophane membranes.[31] Aβ2M, which has been described only in the presence of renal problems usually requiring dialysis, is associated with the deposition of intact β2M, 11.8 kDa, often deposited with ectopic calcification in kidneys, heart, and synovium.

Clinical features

Aβ2M is a frequent rheumatologic complication of chronic hemodialysis, affecting almost 80% of patients who have been dialyzed for longer than 15 years. The manifestations are diverse, including carpal tunnel syndrome, chronic synovial involvement, extensive bone lesions with pathologic fractures, and a severe spondyloarthropathy, usually involving the upper spine. Visceral lesions with Aβ2M are being increasingly reported, but usually do not lead to organ failure. Lesions have also been reported in the tongue, intestines, and Achilles and quadriceps tendons. Histological examination of skin and internal organs shows predominantly small perivascular deposits.

Treatment

New dialysis membranes have been devised to filter out larger quantities of β2M. Renal transplantation in these patients has eased pain and improved function in the joints and has decreased the β2M blood levels. After kidney transplantation, long-term follow-up has shown neither progression nor regression of the radiologic lesions (bone cysts).

AIns

Insulin can also be readily converted to amyloid fibrils in vitro. Porcine insulin-derived amyloid fibrils have been isolated from insulin injection sites and have been shown to be a cause of failure of insulin implant devices.[32]

LOCALIZED AMYLOIDOSES

Aβ

Brain lesions in Alzheimer's disease are characterized by amyloid deposition in the brain. A novel protein, β-amyloid protein (Aβ), is the major fibril protein in the amyloid deposits of the cerebrovascular walls and in the cores of neuritic plaques in these individuals. Similar plaques can be found in patients with Down syndrome. The intracellular neurofibrillary tangles in Alzheimer's disease are distinct from deposits of Aβ. The lesions are composed of paired helical filaments arranged in a twisted β-pleated conformation characteristic of amyloid fibrils, and have as their major component an abnormally phosphorylated tau protein, a microtubule-associated protein. Aβ varies in length from 39 to 43 amino acids, and is derived from a large transmembrane glycoprotein, amyloid β precursor protein (AβPP).[33,34] Mutations in the *AβPP* gene on chromosome 21 are linked with familial Alzheimer's disease in about 5% of cases, and are also linked to another type of amyloidosis, hereditary cerebral hemorrhage with amyloidosis (Dutch type).[35] Other forms of familial Alzheimer's disease are associated with mutations in genes that encode presenilin.

APrP

Pathogenesis and clinical features

Prion diseases are transmissible neurodegenerative diseases, the spongiform encephalopathies, including scrapie and bovine spongiform encephalopathy (mad cow disease) in animals, and kuru, Creutzfeldt–Jakob disease (CJD) and Gerstmann–Straussler–Scheinker syndrome in man.[37] Cerebral amyloidosis is associated with these prion diseases. Like Alzheimer's disease, approximately 90% of the human cases occur sporadically throughout the world, while 10–15% are dominantly inherited.[36] It is the unique properties of the prion protein (PrP) molecule that give rise to sporadic, inherited, and transmissible forms of the disease. Wild-type PrP is glycolipid (GPI) anchored and localized to caveolae-like domains of the plasma membrane. In its protease-sensitive (designated PrP^c) conformation, the carboxyl portion of the molecule is comprised of 40% α helix and 3% β-pleated sheet, whereas the N-terminal half of the molecule is relatively unstructured and contains the copper-binding domain. PrP can also assume an abnormal protease-resistant conformation that is comprised of about 45% β sheet and about 30% α helix (designated PrP^{Sc}). It is thought that the β sheet region is localized to the formerly unstructured amino-terminal portion of the PrP molecule.

Two main categories of prion disease have been identified: the CJD/scrapie and the Gerstmann–Straussler–Scheinker (GSS) groups.[36] CJD/scrapie accounts for about 90% of the human and animal prion disease. In general, only a few mature amyloid plaques are associated with this group of disorders in 5–10% of cases; primitive plaque deposits that do not bind Congo red dye occur in a larger fraction of cases. However, new variant CJD that is epidemiologically linked to the bovine spongiform encephalopathy epidemic in Great Britain is associated with abundant PrP amyloid in brain and cerebellum.[38] The GSS group of dominantly inherited prion diseases has been described only in humans. GSS syndromes are transmitted by an autosomal dominant mode of inheritance and are accompanied by abundant and widespread PrP amyloid plaque formation.

Multiple disease-associated mutations within the PrP gene have been identified.[37] It is thought that the normal PrP molecule is near a threshold for transition to amyloidogenic conformation and that this transition for wild-type PrP is very slow, but irreversible. Amyloidogenic PrP can seed the conversion of normal molecules into the amyloidogenic form. Mutations in PrP can increase the tendency of PrP to become amyloidogenic. In this respect, APrP is similar to Aβ and to several forms of systemic amyloid. Familial amyloid results from accelerated fibril formation by mutant precursors, whereas, in sporadic cases, fibrils form from normal amyloid precursor molecules.

AIAPP

A novel polypeptide, islet amyloid polypeptide (IAPP), also known as amylin, is associated with amyloid deposits in the islets of Langerhans in more than 90% of individuals with type II (adult-onset) diabetes mellitus and in insulinoma endocrine tumors.[39] IAPP is derived from a prepropeptide and is produced by beta cells in the pancreas; it is stored and released together with insulin into plasma. The amyloidogenic region has been localized to residues 20–30 of the 37 amino acid IAPP molecule. This portion is the least conserved region of IAPP, and interspecies variation may explain why amyloid occurs in humans and some other species such as cat and monkey, but not others.

AANF

Isolated amyloid fibrils of atrial natriuretic factor occur in almost 80% of persons over 80 years of age.[39]

ACal

Medullary carcinoma of the thyroid (MCT) is frequently accompanied by amyloid deposition of a fragment of procalcitonin, thus the fibril is designated ACal.[39]

ALac

Lactoferrin, a product of lacrimal glands, has been identified as the amyloid fibril protein associated with familial subepithelial corneal amyloidosis.[40] Lactoferrin has also been associated with a localized form of seminal vesicle amyloidosis that is distinct from systemic amyloidosis with seminal vesicle involvement.[41]

REFERENCES

1. Cohen AS, Calkins E. Electron microscopic observations on a fibrous component in amyloid of diverse origins. Nature 1959;183:1202.
2. Westermark P and committee. Nomenclature of amyloid fibril proteins. Report from the meeting of the international nomenclature committee on amyloidosis. Amyloid Int J Exp Clin Invest 1999;6:64.
3. Sipe JD. Amyloidosis. Annu Rev Biochem 1992;61:947.
4. Hawkins PN, Aprile C, Capria G, et al. Scintigraphic imaging and turnover studies with iodine-131 labeled serum amyloid P component in systemic amyloidosis. Eur J Nuclear Med 1998;25:701.
5. Cohen AS. Amyloidosis. N Engl J Med 1967;277:522.
6. Glenner GG. Amyloid deposits and amyloidosis. The beta fibrilloses. N Engl J Med 1980;302:1283.
7. Buxbaum J, Chuba JV, Hellman GC, et al. Monoclonal immunoglobulin deposition disease: light chain and light and heavy chain deposition diseases and their relation to light chain amyloidosis. Ann Intern Med 1990;112:455.
8. Husby G, Marhaug G, Dowton B, Sletten K, Sipe JD. Serum amyloid A (SAA): Biochemistry, genetics and the pathogenesis of AA amyloidosis. Amyloid Int J Clin Exp Invest 1994;1:119.
9. Glenner GG, Harbaugh J, Ohms JI, et al. An amyloid protein: the amino-terminal variable fragment of an immunoglobulin light chain, Biochem Biophys Res Commun 1970;41:1287.
10. Kyle RA. Clinical aspects of multiple myeloma and related disorders including amyloidosis. Pathol Biol 1999;47:148.
11. Raffen R, Dieckman LJ, Szpunar M, et al. Physicochemical consequences of amino acid variations that contribute to fibril formation by immunoglobulin light chains. Protein Sci 1999;8:509.
12. Falk RH, Comenzo RL, Skinner M. The systemic amyloidoses. New Engl J Med 1997;337:898.
13. Skinner M. AL amyloidosis. Amyloid Int J Exp Clin Invest 2000;7:13.
14. Benditt EP, Eriksen N, Hermodson MA, et al. The major proteins of human and monkey amyloid substance: common properties including unusual N-terminal amino acid sequences. FEBS Lett 1971;19:169.
15. Sipe JD, Rokita H, de Beer FC. Cytokine regulation of the mouse SAA gene family. In: Baumann H, Gauldie J (eds) Acute phase proteins, molecular biology, biochemistry, and clinical applications. Boca Raton, CRC Press, 1993.
16. Sipe JD. Serum amyloid A: from fibril to function. Current status. Amyloid Int J Exp Clin Invest 2000;7:10.
17. Charles P, Elliott MJ, Davis D, et al. Regulation of cytokines, cytokine inhibitors, and acute-phase proteins following anti-TNF-alpha therapy in rheumatoid arthritis. J Immunol 1999;163:1521.
18. Bausserman LL. SAA kinetics in animals. In: Marrink EJ, van Rijswijk MH (eds) Amyloidosis. Dordrecht, M Nijhof, 1986.
19. Zemer D, Pras M, Sohar E, et al. Colchicine in the prevention and treatment of the amyloidosis of familial Mediterranean fever. N Engl J Med 1986;314:1001.
20. McDermott MF, Aksentijevich I, Galon J, et al. Germline mutations in the extracellular domains of the 55 kDa TNF receptor, TNFR1, define a family of dominantly inherited autoinflammatory syndromes. Cell 1999;97:133.
21. Cohen AS. Amyloidosis. In: McCarty DJ, Koopman WJ (eds) Arthritis and allied conditions, 12th edn. Philadelphia, Lea & Febiger, 1993.
22. Aksentijevich I, Galon J, McDermott MF, et al. TNF receptor associated periodic fever syndromes (TRAPS): novel TNFR1 mutations and early experience with etanercept therapy. Am J Hum Genet 1999;65:A281.
23. Kelly JW, Colon W, Lai ZH, et al. Transthyretin quaternary and tertiary structural changes facilitate misassembly into amyloid. Adv Protein Chem 1997;50:161.
24. Connors LH, Richardson AM, Theberge R, Costello CE. Tabulation of transthyretin (TTR) variants as of 1/1/2000. Amyloid Int J Exp Clin Invest 2000;7:54.
25. Kelly JW. The environmental dependency of protein folding best explains prion and amyloid diseases. Proc Natl Acad Sci USA 1998;95:930.
26. Kiuru S. Gelsolin-related familial amyloidosis, Finnish type (FAF), and its variants found worldwide. Amyloid Int J Exp Clin invest 1998;5:55.

27. Bjarnadottir M, Wulff BS, Sameni M, et al. Intracellular accumulation of the amyloidogenic L68Q variant of human cystatin C in NIH/3T3 cells. J Clin Pathol 1998;51:317.
28. Uemichi T, Liepnieks JJ, Alexander F, et al. The molecular basis of renal amyloidosis in Irish-American and Polish-Canadian kindreds. QJM 1996;89:745.
29. Gillmore JD, Booth DR, Madhoo S, et al. Hereditary renal amyloidosis associated with variant lysozyme in a large English family. Nephrol Dial Transplant 1999;14:2639.
30. Walsh MT. A novel amyloidogenic variant of apolipoprotein AI – Implications for a conformational change leading to cardiomyopathy. Am J Pathol 1999;154:11.
31. Hashimoto N, Naiki H, Gejyo F. Modification of beta(2)-microglobulin with D-glucose or 3-deoxyglucosone inhibits A beta 2M amyloid fibril extension in vitro. Amyloid Int J Exp Clin Invest 1999;6:256.
32. Renard E, Baldet P, Picot MC, et al. Catheter complications associated with implantable systems for peritoneal insulin delivery – An analysis of frequency, predisposing factors, and obstructing materials. Diabetes Care 1995;18:300.
33. Selkoe D. Cell biology of the amyloid β-protein precursor and the mechanism of Alzheimer's disease. Ann Rev Cell Biol 1994;10:373.
34. Abraham C. Amyloid β peptide: a century of discoveries. Amyloid Int J Exp Clin Invest 2000;7:7.
35. Bornebroek M, Haan J, Roos RAC. Hereditary cerebral hemorrhage with amyloidosis – Dutch type (HCHWA-D): a review of the variety in phenotypic expression. Amyloid Int J Exp Clin Invest 1999;6:215.
36. DeArmond SJ. Cerebral amyloidosis in prion diseases. Amyloid Int J Exp Clin Invest 2000;7:3.
37. Prusiner SB. Prions. Proc Natl Acad Sci USA 1998;95:13363.
38. Ironside JW. Review: Creutzfeldt–Jakob disease. Brain Pathol 1996;6:379.
39. Westermark P. Amyloid and polypeptide hormones – what is their interrelationship? Amyloid Int J Exp Clin Invest 1994;1:47.
40. Klintworth GK, Valnickova Z, Kielar RA, et al. Familial subepithelial corneal amyloidosis – A lactoferrin-related amyloidosis. Invest Ophthalmol Vis Sci 1997;38:2756.
41. Suess K, Moch H, Epper R, et al. Heterogeneity of amyloid in the seminal vesicles. Immunohistochemical evidence of lactoferrin and amyloid of the prealbumin-transthyretin type. Pathologe 1998;19:115.

Section 7 Organ-specific Inflammatory Disease

Chapter 72

Immune-mediated Anemia

Frank J. Strobl and Leslie Silberstein

INTRODUCTION

Immune-mediated anemia encompasses several disorders that result in the accelerated destruction of otherwise normal erythrocytes. The immunologically mediated injury most frequently involves antierythrocytic autoantibodies (autoimmune hemolytic anemia and drug-induced hemolytic anemia). The majority of cases of autoimmune hemolytic anemia are mediated by warm-reactive autoantibodies that optimally bind to red blood cells (RBC) at temperatures very close to 37°C. The remaining cases of autoimmune hemolytic anemia are induced by cold-reactive autoantibodies that preferentially bind to RBC at temperatures below 37°C. Cold-reactive autoantibodies include cold agglutinins and Donath–Landsteiner antibodies. In rare cases, a patient with autoimmune hemolytic anemia will exhibit both warm-reactive and cold-reactive autoantibodies. Immune hemolysis and anemia can also result from alloantibodies produced by the patient in response to foreign RBC (acute and delayed hemolytic transfusion reactions) or by alloantibodies produced by foreign lymphocytes against host RBC (post-transplant hemolysis and hemolytic disease of the newborn (HDN)).

MODES OF RBC DESTRUCTION

Whether facilitated by autoantibodies or alloantibodies, the accelerated erythrocyte destruction of immune-mediated anemia occurs via either or both of two mechanisms: extravascular hemolysis and intravascular hemolysis. In extravascular hemolysis splenic and hepatic macrophages trap and phagocytose either entire erythrocytes or portions of the erythrocyte membrane coated with antibody and/or complement. The specific opsonins responsible for extravascular hemolysis include IgG (rarely IgM and IgA), which binds to macrophage Fc receptors, and complement fragments C3b and C3bi, which bind to the macrophage complement receptors CR1 and CR3. Extravascular hemolysis predominates in warm-autoimmune hemolytic anemia (WAHA), drug-induced hemolytic anemia, HDN, and delayed hemolysis following transfusion or organ transplant. Extravascular hemolysis, however, can also occur to a variable degree in many patients with cold autoimmune disorders. In intravascular hemolysis the RBC are destroyed within the circulation. Antibody-induced (IgM or IgA, rarely IgG) complement fixation and the formation of C5b-9 membrane attack complexes on the RBC surface leads to phagocyte-independent lysis. Intravascular hemolysis is most frequently encountered in cold-autoimmune hemolytic anemia (CAHA) and acute hemolytic transfusion reactions.

KEY CONCEPTS

Major mechanisms of red cell destruction

Opson-mediated extravascular hemolysis

- Splenic and hepatic macrophages trap and phagocytose fragments of the plasma membrane from IgG- and/or C3b-coated RBC.
- Predominates in WAIHA, drug-induced hemolytic anemia, HDN and delayed hemolysis following transfusion or transplantation.
- Variable contribution to RBC destruction in CAHA.

Complement-mediated intravascular hemolysis

- Dependent on antibody fixation of complement with the formation of C5b-9 membrane attack complex.
- Frequently encountered in CAHA, the immune complex form of drug-induced hemolytic anemia, and acute hemolytic transfusion reactions.
- Rare contribution to RBC destruction in WAIHA.

THE CLINICAL CONSEQUENCES OF HEMOLYSIS

The clinical and laboratory changes associated with hemolysis reflect the physiologic mechanisms responsible for maintaining adequate tissue oxygenation, removing free hemoglobin from the plasma and restoring RBC mass. Patients with hemolytic anemia often develop fatigue, dyspnea, tachycardia, pallor, jaundice, congestive heart failure and splenomegaly. Within days of the onset of hemolysis and the development of anemia, increased erythropoiesis results in erythroid hyperplasia (decreased myeloid/erythroid ratio) in the bone marrow and reticulocytosis (polychromasia and macrocytosis) in the peripheral blood. The peripheral blood smear will often also demonstrate microspherocytes, fragmented RBC, nucleated RBC and leukocytosis. If the hemolysis and anemia become chronic, extramedullary erythropoiesis may develop in the spleen, liver and lymph nodes. Patients with chronic anemia and increased erythropoiesis may also develop folate deficiency and megaloblastosis. Intravascular hemolysis results in hemoglobinemia. Free plasma hemoglobin is excreted in the kidneys or bound to the plasma protein haptoglobin. At low levels much of the excreted hemoglobin is reabsorbed in the proximal renal tubules. The renal tubular cells catabolize the hemoglobin, converting iron into hemosiderin that is eventually shed along with renal tubular cells into the urine, resulting in hemosiderinuria. This is a reliable indicator of chronic intravascular hemolysis. At higher plasma levels, free hemoglobin is found in the urine (hemoglobinuria). Haptoglobin–hemoglobin complexes are cleared from the intravascular space by the reticuloendothelial system, resulting in reduced haptoglobin levels. Other common laboratory findings associated with hemolysis include elevated levels of serum unconjugated bilirubin, serum lactate dehydrogenase (LDH) and urinary urobilinogen. Within the reticuloendothelial system, hemoglobin is metabolized and released into the serum as unconjugated bilirubin. This is then conjugated in the liver, excreted in the gut, converted to fecal urobilinogen, partially reabsorbed, and excreted by the kidneys as urinary urobilinogen. The ubiquitous cellular enzyme LDH is released from lysed RBC into the plasma.

SEROLOGIC PRINCIPLES

Immune hemolysis may occur when either antibody (IgG, IgM or IgA) and/or complement binds to the erythrocyte surface. The distinction between immune-mediated hemolysis and other forms of hemolytic anemia rests on the direct antiglobulin test (DAT) or direct Coombs' test. The DAT detects the presence of IgG antibody or complement on the RBC surface (Fig. 72.1). In a positive DAT, IgG- or complement-coated RBC are agglutinated when incubated with antiserum to human IgG or human complement proteins, primarily C3d. C3d is the final complement fragment generated during normal C3b inactivation. C3d is not opsonically active and cannot induce lysis. IgM and IgA antibodies are not directly detectable with standard antiglobulin testing methods; rather, their presence is indirectly demonstrated by the detection of C3d on the erythrocyte. In rare cases the hemolytic anemia is due to noncomplement-fixing IgM or IgA antibodies, in which case the DAT will be falsely negative. Eluates containing the bound antibody can be obtained by washing the antibody-coated RBC. Alternatively, the antibody may also be free in the serum. Antibody specificity can be determined by the indirect antiglobulin test (IAT) or indirect Coombs' test (Fig. 72.2). In this test, the eluate or serum is screened against a panel of type O RBC which collectively possess all of the common blood group antigens. The pentavalent structure of IgM antibodies allows these immunoglobulins to agglutinate the test RBC directly. Binding of IgG to the test RBC is demonstrated by agglutination following the addition of antiserum to IgG. The antibodies detected by the DAT and IAT may be alloantibodies or autoantibodies. Alloantibodies have specificity for RBC antigen(s) not present on the patient's own erythrocytes. Thus, the DAT is positive in alloimmunization only when the patient has been recently transfused with RBC that possess the antigen against which the alloantibody is directed. Whereas alloantibodies have definable specificities, autoantibodies usually react with all RBC except those lacking rhesus (Rh) antigens.[1]

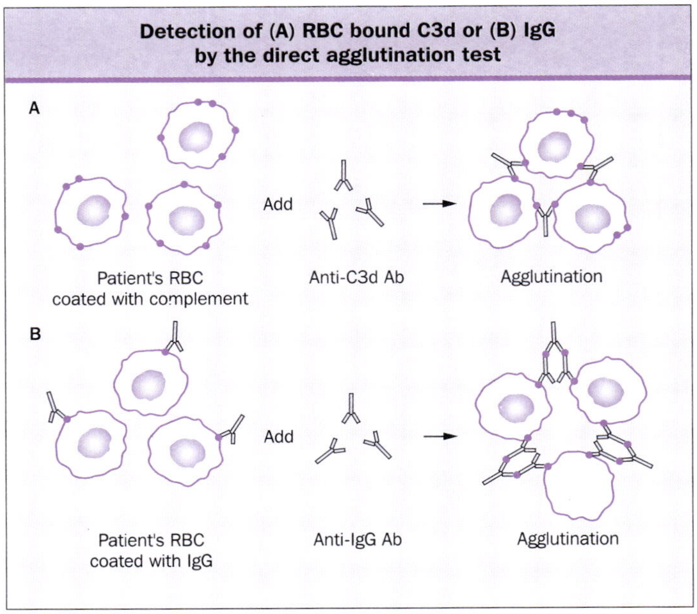

Figure 72.1 Detection of (A) RBC bound C3d or (B) IgG by the DAT. Agglutination results from bridging of sensitized RBC by anti-C3d or anti-IgG.

The presence of antibody or complement on the RBC, however, may not reflect ongoing hemolysis. Rather, the diagnosis of hemolytic anemia rests on the clinical findings and laboratory changes described earlier, such as RBC morphology, hemoglobin, bilirubin, haptoglobin and LDH levels, reticulocyte count, and the presence or absence of hemoglobinemia, hemoglobinuria or hemosiderinuria. The serologic findings provide information as to whether an immune basis exists and what type of immune hemolytic anemia may be present. The pathogenicity of RBC antibodies depends on the titer of the antibody, its avidity for the RBC antigen, and its ability to fix complement.[2]

AUTOIMMUNE HEMOLYTIC ANEMIA

Hemolytic antibodies directed against the individual's own RBC may arise as a primary/idiopathic event or be secondary to lym-

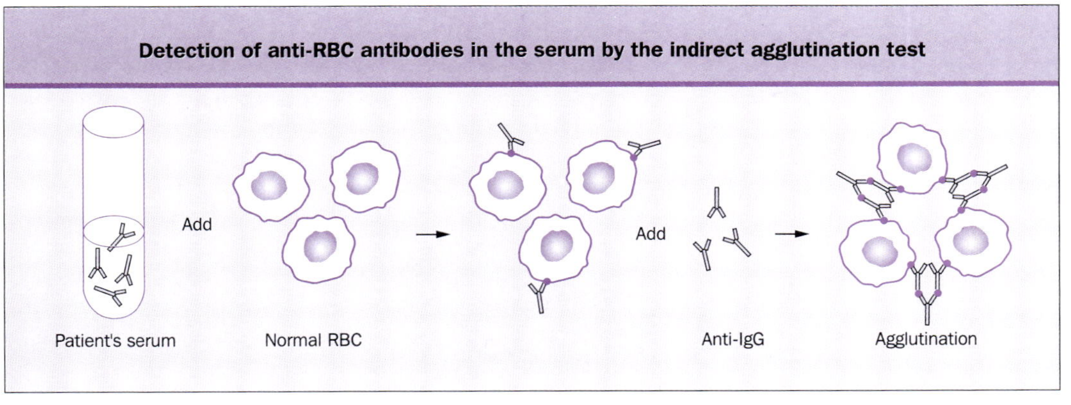

Figure 72.2 Detection of anti-RBC antibodies in the serum by the IAT. The patient's serum is mixed with normal RBC, some of which express the antigen(s) recognized by the serum antibodies. Agglutination results from bridging of antibody bound RBC by anti-IgG.

Classification of WAIHA
Warm autoimmune hemolytic anemia (WAIHA)
Primary (idiopathic)
Secondary
Lymphoproliferative diseases
Connective tissue diseases
Miscellaneous diseases
Drugs
Cold autoimmune hemolytic anemia (CAHA)
Primary (idiopathic)
Secondary
Lymphoproliferative disease
Infectious diseases
Mycoplasma pneumoniae
Infectious mononucleosis
Other
Miscellaneous disorders
Paroxysmal cold hemoglobinuria (PCH)
Tertiary syphilis
Viral infection

Table 72.1 Classification of autoimmune hemolytic anemia.

Diseases infrequently associated with WAIHA
Malignancy
Acute leukemia
Hodgkin's disease
Multiple myeloma
Mycosis fungoides
Solid-organ carcinoma
Thymoma
Waldenstrom's macroglobulinemia
Collagen vascular
Polyarteritis nodosa
Rheumatoid arthritis
Scleroderma
Serum sickness
Sjögren's syndrome
Miscellaneous
Congenital immunodeficiencies
Evans syndrome
Guillain–Barré syndrome
Kawasaki disease
Myelofibrosis
Pernicious anemia
Primary biliary cirrhosis
Ulcerative colitis

Table 72.2 Diseases infrequently associated with WAIHA.

phoid malignancies (chronic lymphocytic leukemia (CLL); non-Hodgkin lymphoma), connective tissue disorders (systemic lupus erythematosus (SLE)) or certain infections (*Mycoplasma* pneumonia; infectious mononucleosis; tertiary syphilis) (Table 72.1). Autoimmune hemolytic anemia is best classified according to the temperature at which the antibody optimally binds to the erythrocyte. The four major types of autoimmune hemolytic anemia are warm autoimmune hemolytic anemia, cold agglutinin syndrome, paroxysmal cold hemoglobinuria, and mixed-type autoimmune hemolytic anemia.

Warm autoimmune hemolytic anemia (WAIHA)

Etiology

The offending antibody in WAIHA is typically IgG (IgG_1 and IgG_3 subclasses) and can be found on the RBC, in the serum, or both. Rare cases involving warm-reactive IgM or IgA autoantibodies have been reported.[3–6] The exact specificity of the antibody is often difficult to determine. Most warm-reactive autoantibodies bind to all RBC tested. The nonspecific reactivity most likely reflects specificity for public epitopes shared by many membrane proteins. In approximately 50% of cases, proteins within the Rh system act as targets for the warm autoantibodies. In other rare cases the autoantibodies appear to possess specificities for non-Rh blood groups, including Wr^b,[7,8] En^a,[8] Lw,[9] U,[10] Ge,[11] Scl,[12] Kell,[13] N,[14] Jk^b,[15] S,[16] and Vel.[17] About half of all cases of WAIHA are idiopathic. The remainder are associated with lymphoma, CLL and SLE. WAIHA has also been infrequently associated with a variety of other disorders (Table 72.2).

Clinical features

The estimated incidence of WAIHA is one to two cases per 100 000 population. WAIHA can arise at any age but is more common in older individuals, with its peak incidence in the seventh decade. The tendency toward a late onset is probably the result of its association with lymphoid malignancies. However, the origin of the RBC antibodies involved in WAIHA appears distinct from the disorders with which it is often associated (i.e. lymphoma and SLE). Warm-reactive autoantibodies are polyclonal in nature, and most evidence indicates that they are not derived from the same B-cell clones responsible for the lymphoma or systemic autoimmune disease. Females are affected slightly more often than males, and there is no racial predisposition. The severity of WAIHA ranges from indolent to life-threatening. In its mildest form the DAT is positive but RBC survival is not significantly affected. In more aggressive forms symptomatic patients present with anemia, jaundice and splenomegaly. Most of these have a chronic stable anemia (Hgb < 8 g/dl). In its severest form, patients present with fulminant intravascular hemolysis, progressive anemia, congestive heart failure, respiratory distress and neurologic abnormalities. As with other hemolytic anemias, the peripheral smear often demonstrates anisocytosis and reticulocytosis, with spherocytes, macrocytes and polychromatophilia. The platelet count is usually normal except in patients with Evan's syndrome, where the autoantibody destroys both RBC and platelets.

CLINICAL PEARLS

Warm autoimmune hemolytic anemia (WAIHA)

- Most common (>80%) immune hemolytic anemia in adults.
- Occurs at any age, with peak incidence in the seventh decade.
- Warm autoantibodies are typically IgG.
- Hemolysis is primarily extravascular in the spleen or liver.
- Warm autoantibody specificity is predominantly against uncharacterized public antigens, including the Rh system (approximately 50% of cases).
- Primary therapy is corticosteroids; alternative therapies include splenectomy, IVIG, cyclophosphamide, azathioprine, danazol and plasma exchange.

Laboratory features

The DAT is positive for IgG and/or complement (C3d). A negative DAT, however, does not rule out WAIHA. Explanations for a negative DAT in a patient suspected of having WAIHA include rare warm-reactive IgA and IgM autoantibodies, low-affinity IgG autoantibodies,[18] and small numbers of RBC-bound IgG autoantibodies (<200 molecules of IgG bound per RBC). A positive DAT also does not definitively confirm the diagnosis of WAIHA. Approximately 1 in 10 000 blood donors[19] and up to 15% of hospitalized patients[20] have a positive DAT (IgG or C3d) without anemia or evidence of hemolysis. Explanations for a false positive DAT include tests performed on clotted samples,[21] the use of silicone gel tubes,[22] and medications that cause nonspecific binding of plasma proteins to the RBC surface.

Treatment

Corticosteroids

Corticosteroids are the primary therapy for WAIHA. The primary mechanism by which corticosteroids ameliorate the rate of hemolysis is their ability to cause Fc receptor blockade of macrophages and thus diminish immune clearance of RBC.[23,24] Corticosteroids can also inhibit antibody production, but this effect usually requires several weeks of therapy. Prednisone at a dose of approximately 1–2 mg/kg body weight is effective in most patients. In critically ill patients, intravenous methylprednisolone should be administered in divided doses ranging from 2 to 4 mg/kg/day. Higher doses rarely provide additional benefit, but rather increase the number and severity of side-effects. Treatment continues until the hemoglobin levels stabilize or improve. This may require up to 3 weeks. The initial dose of prednisone can then be tapered at a rate of 5–10 mg/week. Once a dose of 10 mg/day is reached, the steroid taper should progress more slowly in order to determine the minimum controlling dose. The side-effects of chronic steroid administration may be reduced by using an alternate-day schedule. After several months without relapse, attempts should be made to discontinue the prednisone. Approximately 25% of patients treated with corticosteroids experience complete remission; the remainder have either a partial response or no response at all.

Splenectomy

Splenectomy should be performed only in steroid-refractory patients or patients requiring unacceptably high (>15 mg/day) doses of prednisone to maintain remission. Splenectomy results in partial or complete remission in more than 50% of cases. The risk of sepsis following splenectomy can be lessened by immunization with pneumococcal and meningococcal vaccines.

Azathioprine and cyclophosphamide

More aggressive immunosuppressive therapy with drugs such as azathioprine (1.5 mg/kg/day) or cyclophosphamide (2 mg/kg/day) should be reserved for patients unfit for splenectomy or who have failed to respond to steroids and surgery. The potential acute and long-term side-effects of these drugs must be carefully considered when deciding to initiate therapy. Both azathioprine and cyclophosphamide can cause bone marrow suppression. In addition, the sustained use of cyclophosphamide has been associated with decreased fertility,[25,26] an increased risk of developing acute myelogenous leukemia and cancer of the bladder.

THERAPEUTIC PRINCIPLES

Therapy for WAIHA

- Prednisone (1–2 mg/kg) is the mainstay of therapy for WAIHA; prednisone reduces immune clearance of RBC by blocking macrophage Fc receptors and inhibiting antibody synthesis; approximately 25% of WAIHA patients treated with steroids experience complete remission.
- Splenectomy is performed in steroid-refractory or steroid-intolerant patients; it produces partial or complete remission in 50% of cases.
- More aggressive immunosuppressive therapy such as azathioprine (1.5 mg/kg/day) or cyclophosphamide (2 mg/kg/day) is reserved for steroid-refractory patients unfit for surgery.
- Alternative therapies with limited efficacy include IVIG (400 mg/kg/day for 5 days), danazol (400–600 mg/day) or plasma exchange.
- Experimental approaches include anti-B-cell monoclonal antibodies and costimulatory blockade (i.e. CTLA4-Ig and anti-CD40 ligand).

Intravenous immunoglobulin (IVIG)

IVIG is sometimes used in combination with steroids. IVIG probably competitively inhibits IgG-coated RBC interactions with macrophage Fc receptors, leading to an increase in erythrocyte survival. Soluble Ig in this product may also feed back to inhibit autoantibody synthesis. Selected patients have been reported to respond to IVIG alone at a dose of 400 mg/kg/day for 5 days. In the majority of cases, however, IVIG administration by itself has been of no benefit in WAIHA.

Danazol

Danazol, a synthetic androgen, has proved beneficial in a small number of patients with refractory WAIHA. The recommended dose is 400–600 mg/day orally.

Plasma exchange

Occasionally, plasma exchange has been used successfully as a temporizing measure in patients starting immunosuppressive therapy.[27,28] A typical 1–1.5 plasma volume exchange is expected to lower serum IgG levels by more than 50%. Unfortunately, continued antibody production, the large extravascular distribution of IgG, and plasma exchange's inability to effect a significant removal of IgG from circulating RBC limit the efficacy of plasma exchange in WAIHA.

Future directions

Experimental approaches for the treatment of WAIHA include the use of anti-B-cell monoclonal antibody therapy or approaches to modulate the uncontrolled B-cell immune responses via costimulatory blockade (i.e. CTLA4-Ig or anti-CD40 ligand).

Transfusion

Transfusion with ABO and Rh-compatible cross-match least-incompatible RBC should be performed in WAIHA patients with symptomatic anemia. Transfusion should not be withheld because of serologic incompatibility due to autoantibodies. Active serum autoantibodies, however, can mask the presence of clinically significant alloantibodies. Therefore, the most important consideration prior to transfusion is to confirm the presence or absence of alloantibodies in the patient's serum. Various autologous and allogeneic RBC absorption techniques exist to remove the autoantibody from a sample of the patient's serum and allow identification of any existing alloantibodies.[29] If clinically significant alloantibodies are present, RBC lacking the corresponding antigen(s) should be selected for transfusion. If the autoantibody has a definite specificity, RBC lacking that antigen should be selected.[30] In the absence of underlying alloantibodies, the survival of transfused cross-match incompatible RBC should be considered equivalent to circulating autologous RBC. Transfusions in life-threatening situations (severe anemia (<5 g/dl) with high-output cardiac failure or cerebral compromise) should never be delayed if the above tests are not readily available or completed. In all cases of transfusion in WAIHA the clinician must closely supervise and carefully monitor the patient for signs of hemolysis and volume overload.

Cold autoimmune hemolytic anemia (CAHA)

Cold agglutinin syndrome

Etiology

Cold agglutinin syndrome accounts for approximately one-quarter of all cases of autoimmune hemolytic anemia. No racial predisposition has been reported, but women appear to be affected more frequently than men. The disorder occurs as an acute or chronic condition. In cold autoimmune disorders the signs and symptoms of disease result either from the agglutination of RBC or from hemolysis. The autoantibodies are typically IgM and are most active at low temperatures (4°C). IgG cold autoantibodies are normally not associated with cold agglutinin disease, probably because of their reduced ability to fix complement. Rare examples of IgG and IgA, as well as mixed-type IgG/IgM and IgA/IgM cold agglutinins, however, have been reported.[31–41] In the lower temperatures of the peripheral circulation the IgM autoantibodies bind to RBC and induce the early steps of complement activation (C3b).[42,43] In warmer areas of the circulation the IgM dissociates from the erythrocyte, leaving activated complement fixed to the RBC surface. The late steps of complement activation leading to the formation of C5b-9 attack complexes can proceed in the absence of antibody. The severity of the disorder depends on both the titer of the antibody and the thermal range at which it is most active. Patients with high cold agglutinin titers (>1:1000) and high thermal amplitudes (closer to 37°C) have continuous RBC agglutination and destruction, whereas those with lower agglutinin titers and thermal amplitudes tend to have episodic hemolysis triggered by exposure to cold ambient temperatures. However, the thermal amplitude is a more accurate predictor of the severity of disease. The autoantibody specificity in cold agglutinin syndrome is usually against oligosaccharide RBC antigens of the I/i system.[44] The I and i antigens are precursors of the ABH blood group antigens. The expression of I and i is developmentally regulated so that the i antigen is strongly expressed on umbilical cord RBC, but weakly expressed on adult RBC. The converse is true for the I antigen. The antigenic specificity of cold agglutinins is usually determined by observing the degree of reactivity of patient serum with umbilical cord or adult RBC. Infrequently, the cold agglutinin specificity is for RBC antigens outside the I/i system, including the Pr,[45,46] Gd,[47] Sa,[48] Lud,[49] Fl,[50,51] M[52] and P[53] blood group antigens. The sera from such patients react similarly with both cord and adult RBC.

Clinical features

In CAHA, intravascular complement activation and RBC agglutination induced by the IgM autoantibody leads to hemolysis and acrocyanosis in the cool distal areas of the fingers, toes, ears and nose. Acute CAHA is most commonly seen in adolescents and young adults following infection with *Mycoplasma pneumoniae* or infectious mononucleosis. Hemolysis occurs approximately 1–2 weeks following infection and is associated with a rise in polyclonal anti-I IgM antibody with *Mycoplasma pneumoniae* or polyclonal anti-i IgM antibody with infectious mononucleosis. Postinfectious CAHA is self-limited, with full recovery occurring in approximately 1 month. Chronic CAHA occurs most commonly in the elderly, either idiopathically or associated with lymphoma, chronic lymphocytic leukemia or Waldenström's macroglobulinemia. Patients experience chronic intravascular hemolysis and anemia, with acute exacerbations induced by exposure to cold ambient temperatures. They are often also plagued by episodes of Raynaud's phenomenon. Monoclonal IgM antibodies with κ light chains and anti-I specificity usually cause the RBC agglutination and hemolysis in chronic CAHA.

> **CLINICAL PEARLS**
>
> **Cold autoimmune hemolytic anemia (CAHA)**
>
> **Cold agglutinin syndrome**
>
> - Acute form is a self-limited hemolytic anemia associated with *Mycoplasma* pneumonia or infectious mononucleosis; chronic form is idiopathic or associated with lymphoproliferative disorders.
> - Clinical presentation varies from chronic hemolytic anemia and acrocyanosis to episodic intravascular hemolysis following exposure to cold temperatures.
> - Antibodies typically IgM with specificity for oligosaccharide RBC antigens, most commonly of the I/i system; pathogenicity is dependent upon antibody titer, thermal amplitude and ability to fix complement.
> - Treatment involves keeping the patient warm; severe chronic cold agglutinin disease is treated with alkylating drugs or α-interferon; consider plasma exchange in critically ill patients.
>
> **Paroxysmal cold hemoglobinuria (PCH)**
>
> - The rarest form of CAHA in adults; more common in children as a self-limited, non recurring, postviral disorder.
> - Clinical presentation characterized by muscle aches, abdominal pain, fever, chills and hemoglobinuria following exposure to cold ambient temperatures.
> - The Donath–Landsteiner antibody is IgG with the ability to fix complement and a specificity for a glycosphingolipid within the P-antigen blood group system.
> - Treatment in the adult form consists primarily of avoidance of cold temperatures; in children, most cases require only supportive care.

Laboratory features

Examination of the peripheral smear shows RBC agglutination. The DAT is positive for complement. The IAT performed at 37°C is negative.

Treatment

A warm environment (>37°C) is often all that is required in patients with mild chronic and postinfectious CAHA. Severe CAHA secondary to a B-cell neoplasm can be treated with chlorambucil, cyclophosphamide or α-interferon.[54–56] Steroids and splenectomy are rarely beneficial, although prednisone may help in cases in which an IgG cold agglutinin is produced. Splenectomy has provided benefit in cases with splenomegaly secondary to lymphoid hyperplasia or localized splenic lymphoma. Blood transfusion should be avoided. In situations of life-threatening anemia the blood should be given slowly through a blood warmer. Hypothermia must be avoided during surgery in patients with CAHA, particularly surgical procedures involving extracorporeal circuits. Plasma exchange is often helpful in critically ill patients.

Paroxysmal cold hemoglobinuria (PCH)

Etiology

PCH is the rarest form of autoimmune hemolytic anemia. The disorder is caused by the nonagglutinating complement-fixing Donath–Landsteiner IgG antibody. In the colder temperatures of the peripheral microvasculature this antibody binds to and irreversibly fixes complement to the RBC membrane. Upon its return to warmer temperatures in the central circulation the antibody dissociates from the RBC, leaving activated complement to lyse the cell. In most cases the Donath–Landsteiner antibody appears to have specificity for the P blood group antigen, a glycosphingolipid found on practically all RBC.[57,58]

Clinical features

Adult patients with PCH experience recurrent episodes of acute intravascular hemolysis which occur following exposure to cold ambient temperatures. In children, PCH is a more common self-limited and nonrecurring disorder which develops following various viral infections.[59,60] Both children and adults develop muscle aches, abdominal pain, fever, chills, cold urticaria, hemoglobinemia and hemoglobinuria within minutes to hours following cold exposure. Soon after these initial symptoms, anemia and jaundice appear. In the past, PCH was commonly associated with congenital or tertiary syphilis, but now most cases in adults are idiopathic.

Laboratory features

During or shortly after a hemolytic episode the DAT is positive for complement but negative for IgG. Between attacks the DAT is negative for both complement and IgG. The IAT is usually negative.

Treatment

Most postinfectious cases of PCH are self-limited (2–3 weeks) and usually require only supportive care. Avoidance of cold temperatures can help to prevent recurrent attacks in patients with the chronic form of PCH. On occasion, however, severe anemia and renal failure can occur. No specific therapy for PCH exists; prednisone is not useful. Transfusion is indicated only for severe hemolysis and life-threatening anemia. As the Donath–Landsteiner antibody rarely causes agglutination, most random donor RBC units will be compatible with patient sera. Transfusions with extremely rare P-antigen-negative RBC should be reserved only for those who do not respond to random donor RBC. The use of a blood warmer should be considered.

Mixed-type autoimmune hemolytic anemia

Etiology

Approximately 8% of all autoimmune hemolytic anemias are of the mixed type.[61–63] Both IgG and complement are present on the RBC and both warm-reactive IgG autoantibodies and cold-reactive agglutinating IgM autoantibodies focused in the serum. The warm-reactive IgG autoantibodies are indistinguishable from autoantibodies encountered in WAIHA. The IgM autoantibodies usually have low titers (<1:64) at 4°C and have high thermal amplitudes reacting at 30°C or above. These IgM autoantibodies usually have no distinguishable specificity, although on occasion I or i specificities are observed.

Clinical features

Mixed-type autoimmune hemolytic anemia may be idiopathic or secondary, most commonly associated with systemic lupus erythematosus or lymphoma. The hemolytic anemia is often severe and chronic, with intermittent exacerbations. Exposure to cold does not increase the hemolysis.

Laboratory features

The DAT is positive for IgG and complement. Warm-reactive IgG panagglutinins will be demonstrated by the IAT.

Treatment

Steroids, splenectomy and cytotoxic agents often provide therapeutic benefit in mixed-type autoimmune hemolytic anemia. If blood transfusions are necessary the selection of blood should adhere to transfusion guidelines outlined earlier for WAIHA. The use of a blood warmer should be considered.

Drug-induced hemolytic anemia

Drugs may induce antibodies to bind to the erythrocyte surface, resulting in a positive DAT and/or hemolysis. There are four mechanisms by which drugs can cause a positive DAT: hapten; immune complex formation; autoantibody production; and [4]nonspecific absorption. Only the first three are associated with hemolysis and some drugs cause immune hemolysis by more

CLINICAL PEARLS

Mixed-type autoimmune hemolytic anemia

- Uncommon (8%) form of autoimmune hemolytic anemia; idiopathic or associated with SLE or lymphoma.
- Clinical presentation often severe; chronic hemolysis with intermittent exacerbations; degree of hemolysis unaffected by exposure to cold.
- Both IgG and complement are present on RBC; IgG and IgM autoantibodies are present in the serum; IgG-specificity typical of WAIHA; IgM specificity unidentifiable, rarely anti-I or anti-i.
- Therapeutic benefit seen with steroid administration, splenectomy or cytotoxic agents.

than one mechanism. Treatment and prevention are as straightforward as drug avoidance.

Hapten

Certain drugs bind to the RBC membrane with high affinity. Association of the drug with RBC membrane constituents allows the drug to act as a hapten. The antibodies produced are commonly IgG and are directed predominantly against the drug. Extravascular hemolysis develops gradually, but may be life-threatening if left untreated. After the offending drug is identified and withdrawn, the positive DAT and the hemolysis may persist for several weeks. Serum from these patients will not react with other RBC unless the drug is also present. β-Lactam antibiotics, including penicillin[64] and the cephalosporins,[65] are the most notorious examples of this phenomenon. Several other drugs,[66–68] listed in Table 72.3 have also been reported to cause immune hemolysis via the drug hapten mechanism. Approximately 3% of patients receiving large doses of penicillin G (millions of units per day) intravenously will develop a positive DAT for IgG. However, only the rare patient receiving >20 million units of penicillin per day develops hemolytic anemia. Patients with renal failure receiving more moderate doses of penicillin are also susceptible. The IgG-coated RBC are cleared by extravascular trapping, primarily in the spleen. Using the IAT, it can be demonstrated that antibodies in the patient's serum or in a RBC eluate do not react with untreated RBC, but do react with RBC preincubated in vitro with the suspected drug. The diagnosis is confirmed when the hemolysis ceases shortly after discontinuation of the suspected drug.

Drugs associated with hemolytic anemia

Mechanism	Absorption	Immune complex	Autoantibody
Drugs	Penicillins	Quinine	α-Methyldopa
	Cephalosporins	Quinidine	Mefenamic acid
	Tetracycline	Phenacetin	L-Dopa
	Streptomycin	Stibophen	Procainamide
	Tolbutamide	Hydrochlorothiazide	Ibuprofen
	Cianidanol	Rifampin	Diclofenac
		p-Aminosalicylic acid	Thioridazine
		Antihistamines	Interferon-α
		Sulfonamides	Latamoxef
		Isoniazid	Cianidanol
		Chlorpropramide	Nomifensine
		Chlorpromazine	Teniposide
		Pyramidan	Glafenine
		Dipyrane	
		Melphalan	
		Insulin	
		Tetracycline	
		Acetominophen	
		Streptomycin	
		Hydralazine	
		Probenecid	
		Carbimazole	
		Sulfonylureas	
		Anatazoline	
		Thiopental	
		Diclofenac	
		Cianidanol	
		Cephalosporins	
		Nomifensine	
		5-Fluorouracil	
		Tolmentin	
		Fenoprofen	
		Sulindac	
		Doxepin	
		Amphotericin B	

Table 72.3 Drugs associated with immune-mediated hemolytic anemia.

Immune complex

Other drugs bind to the RBC membrane with weak binding affinity (Table 72.3). These drugs induce the binding of IgM or IgG antibodies that activate complement and cause intravascular hemolysis. The antibodies appear to recognize both the drug and a component of the RBC cell membrane which together form a neoantigen. The DAT is often positive for complement but not antibody. The anemia tends to be acute and more severe than that associated with other mechanisms of drug-induced immune hemolysis. Hemoglobinemia and hemoglobinuria are common and renal failure occurs in about half of the cases. Once the offending drug is withdrawn the hemolysis stops. The drug, the antibody-containing serum and RBC must be incubated concurrently to demonstrate antibody binding by the IAT. Quinine,[69] phenacetin,[69] quinidine,[70] chlorpropramide[71] and sulfonylureas[72] are examples of drugs that can cause immune-mediated hemolysis via the immune complex mechanism.

Autoantibody induction

A number of drugs directly stimulate the synthesis of RBC autoantibodies (Table 72.3). Patient serum and RBC eluates react with normal autologous or donor RBC in the absence of the drug. The autoantibodies are indistinguishable from those found in WAIHA. In many cases the autoantibodies appear to have specificities within

CLINICAL PEARLS

Drug-induced immune hemolytic anemia

Hapten mechanism

- Clinical presentation and serology similar to WAIHA.
- The antibodies recognize RBC-bound drug, not RBC membrane constituents.
- Antibodies are typically IgG and induce extravascular hemolysis
- Treatment in most cases is simply withdrawing the offending drug; corticosteroids may be helpful.

Immune complex mechanism

- Clinical presentation and serology resemble CAHA.
- The antibodies recognize a complex consisting of both drug and RBC membrane constituents.
- IgM or IgG antibodies bind with low affinity, but are capable of fixing complement and inducing intravascular hemolysis.
- Treatment is simply withdrawing the offending drug: corticosteroids are ineffective.

Autoantibody induction mechanism

- Clinical presentation and serology similar to WAIHA.
- The antibodies recognize RBC membrane constituents.
- Antibodies are typically IgG and induce extravascular hemolysis.
- Treatment is stopping the offending drug; corticosteroids may be helpful.

the Rh system. The DAT usually becomes positive after 3–6 months of drug administration. The production of anti-RBC autoantibodies is reversible upon discontinuation of the drug. The hemolysis typically ceases within 2 weeks after withdrawal of the drug, but the DAT can remain positive for up to 2 years. α-Methyldopa,[73] L-dopa,[74] procainamide,[75] diclofenac[76] and mefenamic acid[77] are example of drugs that can stimulate the production of RBC autoantibodies. In the past, α-methyldopa was commonly used to treat hypertension and up to 20% of patients taking it developed a positive DAT. Higher doses of α-methyldopa were associated with an increased frequency of positive DAT. However, less than 1% of these patients developed significant hemolysis.[73] Interestingly, patients with drug-induced RBC autoantibodies often also have antinuclear antibodies, rheumatoid factor and antibodies to gastric parietal cells. The mechanism by which drugs induce autoantibodies is unknown.

Nonspecific protein adsorption

Often a drug-induced positive DAT reflects nonimmunologic adsorption of protein, including immunoglobulins. First-generation cephalosporins were originally associated with this phenomenon. More recently other drugs, including suramin, cisplatin and sulbactam, have also been implicated. This mechanism is not associated with reduced RBC survival.

ALLOIMMUNE HEMOLYTIC ANEMIAS

Acute hemolytic transfusion reactions

Etiology

The most catastrophic cases of alloimmune hemolysis occur following the transfusion of ABO-incompatible RBC.[78] Naturally occurring IgM anti-A and anti-B antibodies bind to the incompatible RBC and activate complement, resulting in intravascular hemolysis. Human error leading to the misidentification of patients, their blood samples or the units of RBC to be transfused, is responsible for virtually all cases of ABO incompatibility. Only rarely do other non-ABO IgG alloantibodies cause acute severe hemolysis.

Clinical features

Symptoms of an acute hemolytic transfusion reaction may begin after the infusion of as little as 10 ml of incompatible blood. The signs and symptoms include fever, chills, nausea, vomiting, hypotension, respiratory distress, hemoglobinuria, and chest or flank pain. The conscious patient will often express a feeling of 'impending doom'. Despite treatment, acute hemolytic transfusions reactions can result in renal failure, disseminated intravascular coagulation and even death. The incidence of ABO-incompatible RBC transfusions has been estimated to be 1:10 000–1:30 000,[79] with a fatality rate of approximately 5%.

Treatment

Once an acute hemolytic transfusion reaction is suspected the transfusion should be stopped immediately. Aggressive treatment of the hypotension with intravenous fluids and pressor agents (i.e., low-dose dopamine, 5 μg/kg/min) is recommended.[80] Other critical measures include monitoring the urine output and promoting renal blood flow with diuretics (furosemide 40–80 mg, or mannitol). Either heparin or the administration of platelets, plasma and cryoprecipitate can be used to treat organ or life-threatening bleeding secondary to disseminated intravascular coagulation.

Delayed hemolytic transfusion reactions

Etiology

Approximately 2–3% of transfusion recipients become alloimmunized to non-ABO RBC antigens.[81] Hemolysis is not generally seen during the primary immune response, as the transfused RBC often disappear from the circulation before antibody titers reach clinically significant levels. In the absence of further antigenic stimuli antibody titers can diminish to undetectable levels.[82] Subsequent transfusion of RBC possessing the offending antigen, however, will induce an anamnestic response, with reappearance of the IgG antibodies within hours to days. Binding of the IgG antibody to the transfused antigen-positive RBC results in a positive DAT and possibly mild to moderate extravascular hemolysis.

Clinical features

Most patients experiencing a delayed hemolytic transfusion reaction present with fever, jaundice and decreasing hemoglobin levels. Delayed hemolytic transfusion reactions are often discovered during evaluation for fever of unknown origin, or when the hemoglobin level fails to increase following transfusion.

Treatment

Treatment is rarely necessary, as acute renal failure or disseminated intravascular coagulation are uncommon. If a delayed hemolytic transfusion reaction is suspected, both the patient's serum and an eluate from the circulating RBC should be tested for alloantibodies. If alloantibodies are present, their specificities should be determined. Donor RBC units lacking the offending antigen should be selected for subsequent transfusions.

CLINICAL PEARLS

Hemolytic transfusion reactions (HTR)

Acute HTR

- Naturally occurring IgM anti-A and anti-B antibodies bind to transfused ABO-incompatible RBC.
- Intravascular hemolysis can lead to fever, chills, nausea, vomiting, chest/flank pain, hypotension, respiratory distress, hemoglobinuria, renal failure, DIC and death.
- **Stop transfusion immediately**; administer IV fluids and pressor agents for hypotension; promote diuresis to prevent renal failure; treat DIC if present.
- Due to human error, including misidentification of patient, patient's blood sample for type and cross-match, or RBC unit transfused.

Delayed HTR

- IgG alloantibodies to non-ABO RBC antigens (e.g. Rh, Kell, Kidd, Duffy antigen systems) bind to transfused antigen-positive RBC.
- Extravascular hemolysis leads to fever, jaundice and decreasing hemoglobin levels.
- Treatment rarely necessary; renal failure or DIC uncommon: identify antibody specificity; transfuse antigen-negative RBC.
- Initial alloimmunization occurs during prior pregnancy or transfusion.

Passenger lymphocyte hemolysis

Etiology

Recipients of a hematopoietic[83] or a solid organ transplant[84,85] may experience delayed extravascular hemolysis. In this circumstance, lymphocytes of donor origin produce hemolytic antibodies against ABO or other RBC antigens possessed by the recipient.

Clinical features

Hemolysis due to passenger lymphocytes is most commonly seen in out-of-group yet ABO-compatible liver and bone marrow transplants (group A or group B recipients of group O tissue), but can also occur in recipients of lung, heart and kidney transplants. This hemolysis can begin within several days after the transplant and continue for several months.

Treatment

If significant ABO hemolysis occurs, patients should be transfused with group O RBC. If non-ABO hemolysis is present, elution of the patient's RBC may help to identify the antibody specificity and allow the transfusion of antigen-negative RBC.

HEMOLYTIC DISEASE OF THE NEWBORN (HDN)

Hemolytic disease of the newborn occurs when maternal IgG antibodies cross the placenta and bind to fetal RBC, resulting in extravascular hemolysis. Usually these antibodies possess specificities within the Rh or ABO blood group systems, but occasionally they are directed against other RBC antigens, such as the Kell antigen. In the mildest cases, anemia develops several weeks after birth and is of little clinical consequence. In more severe cases the neonate develops progressive anemia and jaundice within the first week of life. If left untreated, bilirubin levels may reach levels associated with kernicterus, causing brain damage and death. In the severest cases the fetus develops profound anemia as early as the fifth month of gestation, and eventually is stillborn or delivered grossly edematous (hydrops fetalis). An infant with hydrops fetalis also has ascites, hepatosplenomegaly and erythroblastosis, and usually dies shortly after birth.

RhD incompatibility

HDN occurs most commonly and in its severest forms in RhD-negative women carrying a RhD-positive fetus. The mother has developed anti-D IgG antibodies following exposure to the D antigen either during a previous pregnancy or as a result of an inadvertent blood transfusion of D-antigen-positive cells. One half of all cases of RhD alloimmunization are due to transplacental hemorrhage from the fetus at the time of delivery. Spontaneous transplacental hemorrhage can also occur during gestation, particularly during the third trimester. The risk of transplacental hemorrhage increases with ectopic pregnancy, spontaneous or therapeutic abortion, chorionic villus sampling, cesarean section and trauma. Approximately 8% of untreated D-negative women who deliver a D-positive child will become alloimmunized to the D antigen.

It is essential to identify pregnant women at risk for RhD HDN and to prevent sensitization. All pregnant women should have their ABO and Rh types identified as early as possible, and their serum screened for alloantibodies against the D antigen and other RBC antigens.[86] Pregnant women who are D-antigen negative and have an initial negative antibody screen should have their serum retested for alloantibodies at 28 weeks of gestation. If an antibody screen is found to be positive, antibody titers should be followed at 2–4 week-intervals to determine whether further sensitization is occurring. The presence of an antibody, however, does not indicate ongoing hemolysis in all cases. Naturally occurring IgM antibodies such as anti-Lewis and anti-I are common during pregnancy, but do not cross the placenta. Furthermore, the fetal RBC may lack the antigen corresponding to the mother's antibody. Molecular typing of the father's DNA or even fetal DNA is available for several RBC antigens, including D, E/e,[87] C/c,[88] Jka/Jkb[89] and K1/K2.[90] A rising titer of anti-D antibody or other clinically significant RBC alloantibodies indicates ongoing sensitization and possible hemolytic disease of the newborn. From 18 weeks' gestation and onward, ultrasonography and fetal blood sampling can be used to assess the severity of hemolysis. After 28 weeks amniocentesis can be performed. If the fetus is experiencing significant hemolysis and anemia clinical intervention must be prompt. Prior to 34 weeks' gestation intrauterine transfusion with blood lacking the offending antigen should be performed. After 36 weeks induced labor should be considered. Upon the birth of an 'at-risk' fetus a sample of cord blood should be sent for DAT and measurements of hemoglobin and bilirubin. If the DAT is positive and the mother's antibody screen remains negative, hemolytic disease secondary to ABO incompatibility or antibodies against low-incidence RBC antigens should be considered. Infants with severe anemia (hemoglobin <12 g/dl) or severe jaundice (bilirubin >14 mg/dl) should undergo exchange transfusion. Phototherapy can also be used to assist in decreasing bilirubin levels. A D-antigen-negative mother's blood should also be tested to determine the amount

> **CLINICAL PEARLS**
>
> **Hemolytic disease of the newborn (HDN)**
> - Maternal IgG antibodies cross the placenta and bind to fetal RBC, causing extravascular hemolysis.
> - Antibody specificities include ABO, Rh and other RBC antigens (i.e. Kell, Kidd, Duffy etc.).
> - In the postpartum period cases of HDN range from mild, clinically insignificant anemia to sever hemolysis, anemia and jaundice associated with brain damage and death.
> - In the severest cases the fetus develops anemia during the second trimester and is born grossly edematous (hydrops fetalis) or dead.
> - HDN occurs most commonly and severely in RhD-negative women carrying an RhD-positive fetus; first pregnancies are unaffected.
> - HDN is rarely due to ABO incompatibility; group A or B infants of group O mothers are at greatest risk; ABO HDN can occur during the first and subsequent pregnancies; hydrops fetalis never occurs.
> - Infants and fetuses experiencing significant hemolysis and anemia should undergo exchange transfusion.
> - Prophylactic administration of Rh immunoglobulin at 28 weeks of gestation, following invasive procedures or traumatic events during pregnancy, and at delivery will essentially eliminate the risk of alloimmunization to RhD.

of fetomaternal hemorrhage at delivery. Administration of 300 μg of IgG anti-D (Rhogam) within 72 hours of delivery will protect 99% of D-antigen-negative mothers from developing anti-D antibodies. Prophylactic administration of Rhogam at 28 weeks' gestation and following invasive procedures or traumatic events will virtually eliminate the chance of alloimmunization.[91] Patients with large transplacental hemorrhages quantitated by the Kleihauer–Betke acid-elution technique should receive additional Rhogam at a dose equivalent to 300 μg for every 15 ml of fetal RBC.

ABO incompatibility

Although 15% of pregnancies are ABO incompatible, HDN due to ABO incompatibility is rare. Mild to moderate hemolysis and hyperbilirubinemia due to ABO incompatibility occurs in about 1.5 per 1000 pregnancies. Group A and group B infants of group O mothers are at the greatest risk. Unlike with RhD antigen, ABO-hemolytic disease of the newborn occurs during the first pregnancy as often as in subsequent pregnancies. Exchange transfusion with group O RBC is rarely required. Hydrops fetalis never occurs.

REFERENCES

1. Weiner W, Vos GH. Serology of acquired hemolytic anemias. Blood 1963;22:606.
2. Boros T, Rapp HJ. Complement fixation on cell surfaces by 19S and 7S antibodies. Science 1965;150:505.
3. Stratton F, Rawlinson VI, Chapman SA. Acquired hemolytic anemia associated with IgA anti-e. Transfusion 1972;12:157.
4. Reusser P, Osterwald B, Burri H, et al. Autoimmune hemolytic anemia associated with IgA: diagnostic and therapeutic aspects in a case with long term follow-up. Acta Haematol 1987;77:53.
5. Shirey RS, Kickler TS, Bell W, et al. Fatal immune hemolytic anemia and hepatic failure associated with a warm-reacting IgM autoantibody. Vox Sang 1987;52:219.
6. Freedman J, Wright J, Lim FC, et al. Hemolytic warm IgM autoagglutinins in autoimmune hemolytic anemia. Transfusion 1987;27:46.
7. Issit PD, Pavone BG, Goldfinger D, et al. Anti-Wr[b], and other antibodies responsible for positive direct antiglobulin test in 150 individuals. Br J Haematol 1976;34:5.
8. Bell CA, Zwicker H. Further studies on the relationship of anti-En[a] and antiWr[b] in warm autoimmune hemolytic anemia. Transfusion 1978;18:572.
9. Celano MJ, Levine P. Anti-LW specificity in autoimmune acquired hemolytic anemia. Transfusion 1967;7:265.
10. Marsh WL, Reid ME, Scott EP. Autoantibodies of U blood group specificity in autoimmune haemolytic anaemia. Br J Haematol 1972;22:625.
11. Shulman IA, Vengelen-Tyler V, Thompson JC, et al. Autoanti-Ge associated with severe autoimmune hemolytic anemia. Vox Sang 1990;59:232.
12. Owen I, Chowdhury V, Reid ME, et al. Autoimmune hemolytic anemia associated with anti-Scl. Transfusion 1992;32:173.
13. Marsh WL, Oyen R, Alicea E, et al. Autoimmune hemolytic anemia and the Kell blood groups. Am J Hematol 1979;7:155.
14. Dube VE, House RF, Moulds J, et al. Hemolytic anemia caused by auto-anti-N. Am J Clin Pathol 1975;63:828.
15. Ellisor SS, Reid ME, O'Day T, et al. Autoantibodies mimicking anti Jkb plus anti-JK3 associated with autoimmune hemolytic anemia in a primipara who delivered an unaffected infant. Vox Sang 1983;45:53.
16. Alessandrino EP, Costamanga L, Pagani A, et al. Late appearance of autoantibody anti-S in autoimmune hemolytic anemia. Transfusion 1984;24:369.
17. Becton DL, Kinney TR. An infant girl with severe autoimmune hemolytic anemia: apparent anti-Vel specificity. Vox Sang 1986;51:108.
18. Unger LJ. A method for detecting Rho antibodies in extremely low titer. J Lab Clin Med 1951;37:825.
19. Gorst DW, Rawlinson VI, Merry AH, et al. Positive direct antiglobulin test in normal individuals. Vox Sang 1980;38:99.
20. Judd WJ, Butch SH, Oberman HA, et al. The evaluation of a positive direct antiglobulin test in pretransfusion testing. Transfusion 1980;20:17.
21. Merry AH, Thomson EE, Rawlinson VI, et al. The quantification of C3 fragments on erythrocytes: estimation of C3 fragments on normal cells, acquired haemolytic anaemia cases and correlation with agglutination of sensitized cells. Clin Lab Haematol 1983;5:387.
22. Geisland JR, Milam JD. Spuriously positive direct antiglobulin tests caused by silicone gel. Transfusion 1980;20:711.
23. Atkinson JP, Schreiber AD, Frank MM. Effects of corticosteroids and splenectomy on the immune clearance and destruction of erythrocytes. J Clin Invest 1973;52:1509.
24. Atkinson JP, Frank MM. Complement independent clearance of IgG sensitized erythrocytes: inhibition by cortisone. Blood 1974;44:629.
25. Miller JJ, Williams GF, Leissring JC. Multiple late complications of therapy with cyclophosphamide, including ovarian destruction. Am J Med 1971;50:530.
26. Qureshi MSA, Goldsmith HJ, Pennington JH, et al. Cyclophosphamide therapy and sterility. Lancet 1972;2:1290.
27. Silberstein LE, Berkman EM. Plasma exchange in autoimmune hemolytic anemia (AIHA). J Clin Apheresis 1983;1:238.
28. Kutti J, Wadenvik H, Safai-Kutti S, et al. Successful treatment of refractory autoimmune hemolytic anemia by plasmapheresis. Scand J Haematol 1984;32:149.
29. Branch DR, Petz LD. A new reagent (ZZAP) having multiple applications in immunohematology. Am J Clin Pathol 1982;78:161.
30. Mollison PL. Measurement of survival and destruction of red cells in haemolytic syndromes. Br Med Bull 1959:15:59.
31. Hidajat M, Van Hoff A, Van Besien K, et al. Acute hemolysis due to IgG cold reactive anti-Pr antibodies in three patients. Transfusion 1992;32 (suppl):24S.
32. Silberstein LE, Berkman EM, Schreiber AD. Cold hemagglutinin disease associated with IgG cold-reactive antibody. Ann Intern Med 1987;106:238.
33. Garraty G, Petz LD, Brodsky I, et al. An IgA high-titer cold agglutinin with an unusual blood group specificity within the Pr complex. Vox Sang 1973;25:32.
34. Tonthat H, Rochant H, Henry A, et al. A new case of monoclonal IgA kappa cold agglutinin with anti Prld specificity in a patient with persistent antigen cirrhosis. Vox Sang 1976;30:464.
35. Angevine CD, Andersen BR, Barnett EV. A cold agglutinin of the IgA class. J Immunol 1966;96:578.
36. Dellagi K, Brouet JC, Schenmetzler C, et al. Chronic hemolytic anemia due to monoclonal IgG cold agglutinin with anti-Pr specificity. Blood 1981;57:189.
37. Moore JA, Chaplin H. Autoimmune hemolytic anemia associated with an IgG cold incomplete antibody. Vox Sang 1973;24:236.
38. Ambrus M, Bajtain G. A case of an IgG-type cold agglutinin disease. Haematologia 1969;3:225.
39. Szymanski IO, Teno R, Rybak ME. Hemolytic anemia due to a mixture of low-titer IgG lambda and IgM lambda agglutinins reacting optimally at 22°C. Vox Sang 1986;51:112.
40. Silberstein LE, Shoenfeld Y, Schwartz RS, et al. A combination of IgG and IgM autoantibodies in chronic cold agglutinin disease: immunologic studies and response to splenectomy. Vox Sang 1985;48:105.
41. Tschirhart DL, Kunkel L, Shulman IA. Immune hemolytic anemia associated with biclonal cold agglutinins. Vox Sang 1990;59:222.

42. Sokol RJ, Booker DJ, Stamps R, et al. Autoimmune haemolysis and red cell autoantibodies with ABO blood group specificity. Haematologia 1995;26:121.
43. Pruzanski W, Shumack KH. Biologic activity of cold-reacting autoantibodies. N Engl J Med 1977;297:538.
44. Hakomori S. Blood group ABH and Ii antigens of human erythrocytes: chemistry, polymorphisms, and their developmental change. Semin Hematol 1981;18:39.
45. Roelcke D, Anstee DJ, Jungfer H, et al. IgG-type cold agglutinins in children and corresponding antigens: detection of a new Pr antigen: Pra. Vox Sang 1971;20:218.
46. Roelcke D, Ebert W, Geisen HP. Anti-Pr3: serological and immunochemical identification of a new anti-Pr subspecificity. Vox Sang 1976;30:122.
47. Roelcke D, Riesen W, Geisen HP, et al. Serological identification of the new cold agglutinin specificity anti-Gd. Vox Sang 1977;33:304.
48. Roelcke D, Pruzanski W, Ebert W, et al. A new human monoclonal cold agglutinin Sa recognizing terminal *N*-acetylneuraminyl groups on the cell surface. Blood 1980;55:677.
49. Roelcke D. The Lud cold agglutinin: a further antibody recognizing *N*-acetylneuraminic acid-determined antigens not fully expressed at birth. Vox Sang 1981;41:316.
50. Roelcke D, Weber MT. Simultaneous occurrence of anti-F1 and anti-I cold agglutinins in a patient's serum. Vox Sang 1984;47:122.
51. Konig AL, Kather H, Roelcke D. Autoimmune hemolytic anemia by coexisting anti-I and anti-F1 cold agglutinins. Blut 1984;49:363.
52. Chapman J, Murphy MF, Waters AH. Chronic cold hemagglutinin disease due to an anti-M-like autoantibody. Vox Sang 1982;42:272.
53. Von dem Borne AEG, Mol JJ, Joustra-Mass N, et al. Autoimmune hemolytic anemia with monoclonal IgM (K) anti-P cold autohemolysins. Br J Haematol 1982;50:345.
54. Hippe E, Jensen KB, Olesen H, et al. Chlorambucil treatment of patients with cold agglutinin syndrome. Blood 1970;35:68.
55. Evans RS, Baxter E, Gilliland BC. Chronic hemolytic anemia due to cold agglutinins: a 20 year history of benign gammopathy with response to chlorambucil. Blood 1973;42:463.
56. O'Connor BM, Clifford JS, Lawrence WD, et al. Alpha-interferon for severe cold agglutinin disease. Ann Intern Med 1989;111:225.
57. Levine P, Celano MJ, Falkowski F. The specificity of the antibody in paroxysmal cold hemoglobinuria (PCH). Transfusion 1963;3:278.
58. Worlledge SM, Rousso C. Studies on the serology of paroxysmal cold haemoglobinuria (PCH) with special reference to its relationship with the P blood group system. Vox Sang 1965;10:293.
59. Nordhagen R, Stensvold K, Winsnes A, et al. Paroxysmal cold hemoglobinuria: the most frequent autoimmune hemolytic anemia in children? Acta Paediatr Scand 1984;73:258.
60. Gottsche B, Salama A, Mueller-Eckhardt C. Donath–Landsteiner autoimmune hemolytic anemia in children: a study of 22 cases. Vox Sang 1990;58:281.
61. Sokol RJ, Hewitt S, Stamps BK. Autoimmune haemolysis: an 18 year study of 865 cases referred to a regional transfusion centre. Br Med J 1981;282:2023.
62. Shulman IA, Branch DR, Nelson JM, et al. Autoimmune haemolytic anemia with both cold and warm autoantibodies. JAMA 1985;253:1746.
63. Sokol RJ, Hewitt S, Stamps BK. Autoimmune haemolysis. Mixed warm and cold antibody type. Acta Haematol 1983;69:266.
64. Petz LD, Fundenberg HH. Coombs-positive hemolytic anemia caused by penicillin administration. N Engl J Med 1966;274:171.
65. Gralnick HR, McGinnis MH, Elton W, et al. Hemolytic anemia associated with cephalothin. JAMA 1971;217:1193.
66. Simpson MB, Pryzbylik J, Innis B, et al. Hemolytic anemia after tetracycline therapy. N Engl J Med 1985;312:840.
67. Letona JML, Barbolla L, Frieyro E, et al. Immune haemolytic anaemia and renal failure induced by streptomycin. Br J Haematol 1977;35:561.
68. Malacarne P, Castaldi G, Bertusi M, et al. Tolbutamide-induced hemolytic anemia. Diabetes 1977;26:156.
69. Muirhead EE, Halden ER, Granes M. Drug dependen Coombs (antiglobulin) test and anemia: observations on quinidine and acetophenetide (phenacetin). Arch Intern Med 1958;101:827.
70. Freedman AL, Barr PS, Brody E. Hemolytic anaemia due to quinidine: observations on its mechanism. Am J Med 1956;20:806.
71. Logue GL, Boyd AE, Rosse WF. Chlorpropamide-induced immune hemolytic anemia. N Engl J Med 1970;283:900.
72. Kopicky JA, Packman CH. The mechanisms of sulfonyurea-induced immune hemolysis: case report and review of the literature. Am J Hematol 1986;23:283.
73. Worlledge SM, Carstairs KC, Dacie JV. Autoimmune haemolytic anaemia associated with alpha-methyldopa therapy. Lancet 1966;2:135.
74. Territo MC, Peters RW, Tanaka KR. Autoimmune hemolytic anemia due to levodopa therapy. JAMA 1973;226:1347.
75. Kleinman S, Nelson R, Smith L, et al. Positive direct antiglobulin tests and immune hemolytic anemia in patients receiving procainamide. N Engl J Med 1984;311:809.
76. Kramer MR, Levene C, Hershko C. Severe reversible autoimmune haemolytic anaemia and thrombocytopenia associated with diclofenac therapy. Scand J Haematol 1986;36:118.
77. Scott GL, Myles AB, Bacon PA. Autoimmune haemolytic anaemia and mefenamic acid therapy. Br Med J 1968;3:543.
78. Sazama K. Report of 355 transfusion-associated deaths: 1975–1985. Transfusion 1990;30:583.
79. Linden JV, Paul B, Dressler KP. A report of 104 transfusion errors in New York State. Transfusion 1992;32:601.
80. Capon SM, Goldfinger D. Acute hemolytic transfusion reaction, a paradigm of the systemic inflammatory response: new insights into pathophysiology and treatment. Transfusion 1995;35:513.
81. Heddle NM, Soutar RL, O'Hoski PL, et al. A prospective study to determine the frequency and clinical significance of alloimmunization post-transfusion. Br J Haematol 1995;91:1000.
82. Ramsey G, Smietana SJ. Long-term follow-up testing of red cell alloantibodies. Transfusion 1994;43:122.
83. Hows J. Donor-derived red blood cell antibodies and immune hemolysis after allogeneic bone marrow transplantation. Blood 1986;67:177.
84. Ramsey G. Red cell antibodies arising from solid organ transplants. Transfusion 1991;31:76.
85. Mangal AK, Growe GH, Sinclair M, et al. Acquired hemolytic anemia due to 'auto'-anti-a or 'auto'-anti-b induced by group O homograft in renal transplant recipients. Transfusion 1984;24:201.
86. Judd WJ, Luban NLC, Ness PM, et al. Prenatal and perinatal immunohematology: recommendations for serologic management of the fetus, newborn infant, and obstetric patient. Transfusion 1990;30:175.
87. Spence WC, Potter P, Maddalena A, et al. DNA-based prenatal determination of the RhEe genotype. Obstet Gynecol 1995;86:670.
88. Le Van Kim C. Mouro I, Brossard Y, et al. PCR-based determination of the Rhc and RhE status of the fetus at risk for Rhc and RhE hemolytic disease. Br J Haematol 1994;88:193.
89. Hessner MJ, Pircon RA, Luhm RA. Development of an allele specific polymerase chain reaction assay of prenatal genotyping of Jka and Jkb of the Kidd blood group system. Am J Obstet Gynecol 1998;178:52S.
90. Lee S, Bennett PR, Overton T, et al. Prenatal diagnosis of Kell blood group genotypes: KEL1 and KEL2. Am J Obstet Gynecol 1996;175:445.
91. Hartwell EA. Use of Rh immune globulin ASCP Practice Parameter. Am J Clin Pathol 1998;110:281.

Section 7 Organ-specific Inflammatory Disease

Chapter 73

Immune Neutropenia

Roger Kurlander

INTRODUCTION

Immune neutropenia is a term used to describe a heterogeneous population of patients who selectively destroy neutrophils and/or suppress neutrophil production on an immune basis. Usually antibodies directed against neutrophil-specific antigens play an important role in this process. Because immune destruction itself is clinically silent, these patients typically seek medical attention in response to infectious complications, particularly bacterial infections involving the skin, upper respiratory tract or middle ear. More serious systemic infections, such as sepsis or meningitis, also occur, but much less frequently. Patients with secondary neutropenia, i.e. associated with another underlying autoimmune disorder, can also present in this manner, or neutropenia might be noted incidentally during routine clinical monitoring of their coexistent illness.

By definition, all patients with active immune neutropenia have a circulating blood neutrophil count below the lower limit of normal (1800/mm^3 in adults and 1500/mm^3 in children). Reactive monocytosis is sometimes present. Typically, serious infections are uncommon until the patient develops more severe neutropenia, with counts of less than 500 neutrophils/mm^3. Generalized leukopenia should suggest the diagnosis of systemic lupus erythematosus or another systemic autoimmune illness. Additional abnormalities in red cell and platelet numbers or morphology should suggest the possibility of coexisting autoimmune hemolytic anemia (AIHA) or idiopathic thrombocytopenic purpura (ITP).

Abnormal increases in the absolute lymphocyte count should suggest the presence of a lymphoproliferative abnormality, such as chronic lymphocytic leukemia, or T-cell large granular lymphocyte (LGL) leukemia. The latter deserves special consideration because it is commonly associated with immune neutropenia, and the abnormality in peripheral blood can be quite subtle. In normal individuals LGL cells are large lymphocytes with pale cytoplasm and azurophilic granules (Fig. 73.1) that comprise 10–15% of peripheral blood mononuclear cells. The number of these cells circulating in the blood can increase in response to a variety of stresses, but the persistent presence of >2000 LGL/mm^3 strongly suggests the presence of LGL leukemia. Indeed, symptomatic neutropenia can sometimes be seen in patients with fewer circulating abnormal LGL.[1] Repeated blood counts, flow cytometric studies and molecular tests of T-cell receptor clonality are all important in making a definitive diagnosis.

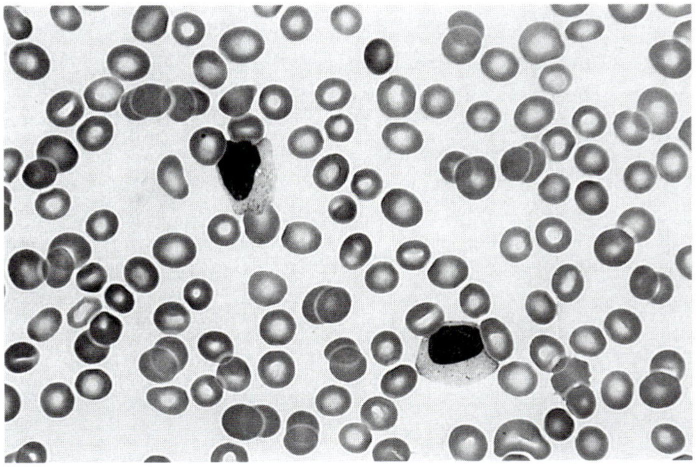

Figure 73.1 Representative large granular lymphocyte (LGL). LGL are moderate to large cells with round nuclei, abundant clear cytoplasm and distinctive azurophilic granules. Immunophenotyping is necessary to distinguish T-LGL from NK cells. (See also color plate 73.1.)

BONE MARROW MORPHOLOGY

In other immune cytopenias, such as AIHA or ITP, compensatory marrow hyperplasia in the affected cell line is common. A comparable pattern is often seen in patients with immune neutropenia. Patients typically have normocellular or slightly hypercellular marrows, with an increased proportion of myeloid precursors. In addition to an increase in the density of myeloid cells, however, there is usually a qualitative change in the pattern of maturation. The numbers of mature forms (neutrophils, stabs and metamyelocytes) are reduced, whereas the numbers of earlier precursor (particularly myelocytes and promyelocytes) increase. This loss of the most mature forms is termed 'maturation arrest'. Although maturation arrest can also be seen in a number of other diseases, in the setting of immune neutropenia this finding suggests (1) an expansion in the number of immature precursors; (2) the early release of mature components from the marrow; and (3) the in situ immune destruction of more mature cells as they begin to express higher levels of neutrophil-specific antigens. Although many patients with immune neutropenia have myeloid hyperplasia, others present with hypoplastic marrow and profound maturation arrest with the disappearance of myeloid cells differentiated beyond the level of the promyelocyte.

The interpretation of marrow findings in patients with secondary immune neutropenia can be difficult because marrow cellularity and maturation are often also affected by the underlying primary disease and the drugs used in its treatment. None the less, similar qualitative trends are usually discernible.

NATURAL HISTORY

There are several distinct subsets of patients who develop immune neutropenia (Table 73.1) and the clinical picture in these groups differs.

Immune neutropenia in childhood

Isoimmune neutropenia

Isoimmune neonatal neutropenia, analogous to neonatal immune hemolysis and thrombocytopenia, results when a pregnant woman develops an IgG antibody directed against neutrophil-specific alloantigens present on fetal cells. In most cases the disease is not severe and neutrophil counts return to normal as maternal antibodies disappear during the first 1–2 months of life.[2] Isoantibodies against neutrophils also develop in multiply transfused patients, and in rare patients after bone marrow transplantation.

Primary autoimmune neutropenia during childhood

This is the most homogeneous of the autoimmune neutropenia syndromes. Lyall et al reported an incidence of one case per 100 000 children per year in Scotland.[3] Patients with this entity have normal blood counts at birth and usually develop neutropenia between 3 and 36 months later.[4–6] Children presenting under 2 years of age have a very good prognosis for spontaneous recovery within 2–3 years of diagnosis, leading some to call this syndrome 'the benign neutropenia of childhood'. Nevertheless, a subset of children, particularly those manifesting other autoimmune findings, do develop a chronic neutropenia disorder, with a natural history more similar to secondary autoimmune neutropenia in adults.

> **KEY CONCEPTS**
>
> - Antibodies directed against surface antigens on neutrophils can cause clincally significant neutropenia
> - Primary autoimmune neutropenia is usually a self-limited disease of young children.
> - Immune neutropenia in adults more commonly is a chronic illness seen in association with other autoimmune or lymphoproliferative disease.

Classification of immune neutropenia
Isoimmune neutropenia
Isoimmune neonatal neutropenia
Isoimmune neutropenia after bone marrow transplanation
Primary immune neutropenia
Autoimmune neutropenia of childhood – self-limited
Autoimmune neutropenia in adulthood
Secondary autoimmune neutropenia associated with:
Other autoimmune disease
Rheumatoid arthritis, i.e. Felty syndrome
Systemic lupus erythematosus
Sjögren syndrome
Immune thrombocytopenic purpura
Autoimmune hemolytic anemia
Primary biliary cirrhosis
Lymphoproliferative malignancy
T-cell large granular lymphocyte (LGL) leukemia
Chronic lymphocytic leukemia
NonHodgkins lymphoma
Hodgkin lymphoma
Angioimmunoblastic lymphadenopathy with dysproteinemia

Table 73.1 Classification of immune neutropenia.

Immune neutropenia during adulthood

Primary neutropenia

Self-limited primary autoimmune neutropenia comparable to the disease noted in young children is uncommon. More often, adults develop the syndrome in the setting of other disease (Table 73.1). Rigorous data are not available concerning the incidence of immune neutropenia in adults, or about the natural history of disease. A small retrospective study in Sheboygan County, Wisconsin, found an overall annual incidence of 5–10 cases of primary or secondary neutropenia per 100 000 people.[7]

Felty syndrome

Immune neutropenia develops in perhaps 1% of patients with rheumatoid arthritis, most commonly in association with splenomegaly, a pattern designated Felty syndrome. Patients typically present with a history of long-standing seropositive rheumatoid arthritis complicated by erosive joint disease and extra-articular findings, such as subcutaneous nodules or leg ulcers, at the time neutropenia first develops. The natural history is often marked by repeated infection and increased mortality, with a 5-year mortality rate of approximately 30%.[8,9]

Neutropenia with other systemic autoimmune diseases

Most patients with active systemic lupus erythematosus (SLE) develop neutropenia in association with a more generalized leukopenia. Although the latter may have an immune etiology, it is distinct from the specific entity discussed here. A much smaller subset of SLE patients develops a disproportionate degree of neutropenia, which is presumably mediated by antineutrophil antibodies. Sjögren syndrome and other systemic autoimmune diseases also sometimes coexist with immune neutropenia.

Neutropenia associated with T-LGL leukemia

As noted above, some patients with immune neutropenia have an abnormal population of circulating LGL. There are at least two phenotypically distinct subsets of LGL found in the blood. One set, designated T-LGL, expresses CD2, CD3, CD8 and CD57. These cells often also express CD16, but usually do not express CD56. In T-LGL leukemia, the cells usually express $\alpha\beta$ T-cell receptors, but $\gamma\delta$ T-cell receptor-positive populations have also been reported. As would be expected in a 'leukemic' disorder, the abnormal cells are monoclonal and bear a single set of T-cell receptor rearrangements. The other class of LGL expresses CD2, CD16 and CD56, but lacks CD3, CD8, CD57 or surface T-cell receptors, a phenotype characteristic of natural killer cells.

Immune neutropenia and other autoimmune complications are seen almost exclusively in individuals with monoclonal T-LGL disease.[10] Furthermore, neutropenia is a surprisingly common complication in this disorder. Over 80% of these patients present with a neutrophil count of $<2000/mm^3$, and 30–40% have severe neutropenia with <500 neutrophils/mm^3. Although most patients show some evidence of bone marrow infiltration with abnormal cells that could influence production, neutropenia is usually out of proportion to marrow involvement, suggesting that immune mechanisms may also play a part. In fact, affected patients often show other evidence of autoimmunity. More than half the patients in one series had evidence of circulating rheumatoid factor, antinuclear antibodies or immune complexes. Over 30% of patients in some series develop clinical arthritis, 20–40% acquire thrombocytopenia, and 90% of patients in one series had neutrophil-reactive IgG.[11,12]

For patients with aggressive T-LGL these complications are easily recognized as manifestations of their primary disease. Others, however, have a stable or very slowly progressive condition which may be unrecognized for long periods. When these patients develop arthritis, splenomegaly and neutropenia, they may receive the diagnosis of Felty syndrome. Others without overt arthritis may be classified as having other 'idiopathic' autoimmune disorders.[13] Indolent monoclonal T-LGL disease deserves consideration whenever an adult presents with increased circulating LGL and autoimmune neutropenia.

Neutropenia associated with other lymphoproliferative diseases

Immune neutropenia, like other immune cytopenias, is also occasionally seen in association with CLL (chronic lymphoid leukemia) and other chronic B-cell malignancies.[14]

IMMUNOPATHOGENESIS

Regulation of antineutrophil antibody production

Isoimmune antibody production in pregnant women, which is responsible for immune neonatal neutropenia, represents a physiologic response to exposure to foreign antigens. By contrast, the production of autoimmune antineutrophil antibodies reflects a defect in immune regulation. Explaining autoantibody production remains a central goal in immunology, and there is little disease-specific insight into the causes for antineutrophil antibody production in adults.

Autoimmune neutropenia of early childhood, however, does represent a special case. Unlike most autoimmune disorders, this disease is age-dependent and self-limited. In older studies, several authors suggest that primary immune neutropenia of childhood may result from inadequate T-cell-mediated 'suppression' of B-cell activity.[4,6] In fact, newborn infants have a significantly increased ratio of CD4/CD8 cells in their peripheral blood compared to adults, and this ratio does not decrease to adult levels until the child is 2–3 years of age.[15] In addition to this quantitative abnormality, circulating CD8 cells isolated from neonates are qualitatively less effective than adult cells in suppressing B-cell immunoglobulin synthesis in vitro. It has been suggested that the spontaneous recovery often observed as children age may reflect the maturation of suppressor T cells. This general model is credible, but there has been little progress in defining at a molecular level why this disorder develops in only some children.

Clinically relevant neutrophil-specific antigens

The most important single target for antibody responses is the Fcγ receptor IIIb (FcγRIIIb), a low-avidity granulocyte-specific Fc receptor that binds IgG immune complexes. This product, one of two variant forms of CD16, is a glycosyl phosphatidylinositol-linked membrane protein selectively expressed on polymorphonuclear phagocytes. Unlike the other closely related variant of CD16, FcγRIIIa, which is expressed most prominently on macrophages and NK cells, FcγRIIIb has several significant polymorphisms.

NA1/NA2 is the most clinically important polymorphism associated with immune neutropenia. The two phenotypes, NA1 and NA2, can be explained by a set of five closely linked base substitutions within exon 3 of FcγRIIIb. The resulting products can be readily distinguished by SDS gel electrophoresis because two of the base substitutions in NA1 disrupt sites of *N*-linked glycosylation. Consequently, the less heavily glycosylated NA1 allelle migrates more rapidly than do NA2. The gene frequency of NA1 varies from 0.3 to 0.55 in different ethnic groups.[16]

SH is another common neutrophil antigen linked to a polymorphism in FcγRIIIb. This antigen, expressed in 5% of northern Europeans, is attributable to a single amino acid change at position 266 in a reduplicated copy of the NA2 allele of FcγRIIIb.[17]

FcγRIIIb-null is the most 'dramatic' of the FcγRIIIb-related variants. About 0.1% of the northern European population is homozygous for an extensive chromosomal deletion which includes all of FcγRIIIb.[18] Because affected individuals lack tolerance to endogenous FcγRIIIb, they often develop a broad antibody response after exposure through transfusion or pregnancy.

Neutrophil antigens unlinked to FcγRIIIb have also been identified. Perhaps most clinically relevant is NB1, which is expressed on an incompletely characterized 58–64 kDa neutrophil protein.[19] Antibodies against this target have been seen in patients with isoimmune and autoimmune neutropenia. A variety of other antigenic alleles have also been identified, such as 5b, NB2 and MART, but these are seen primarily in heavily transfused individuals and not with isoimmune neonatal or autoimmune neutropenia.[20] As described below, individuals with chronic immune neutropenia often develop antibodies against other surface antigens, including CD11b/CD18 and CD35.

Antineutrophil cytoplasmic antibodies (ANCA)

Antibodies directed against several intracellular products, including proteinase 3, actin and myeloperoxidase, have been noted in patients with vasculitis, biliary cirrhosis and other autoimmune conditions. Because these are located predominantly intracellularly, ANCA do not bind extensively to the surface of 'naive' circulating neutrophils and probably do not grossly influence neutrophil survival. Although they do not have a significant role in immune neutropenia, they may play a more important role in modulating the function of activated neutrophils at sites of vasculitis and other inflammation.[21]

Patterns of antibody reactivity in patients with immune neutropenia

Isoimmune neonatal neutropenia

Because many of the polymorphisms discussed above are common, maternal isoantibodies directed against alloantigens are fairly common. NA1 is the most common target,[2] but several other specificities have been observed.[20]

Primary immune neutropenia of childhood

Although patients with primary immune neutropenia of childhood have not been exposed to incompatible neutrophils, they frequently develop allospecific antineutrophil antibodies, most commonly directed against NA1 or NA2 epitopes on FcγRIIIb. The incidence of antibodies with this specificity has varied from 10 to 20% in Lalezari's early studies[4] to 34% in a recent large series from Germany,[22] and 85% in one smaller Dutch series studying a selected population of young children with uncomplicated self-limited autoimmune neutropenia.[23]

Although specificity for NA1 or NA2 is common, more refined techniques such as monoclonal antibody immobilization of granulocyte antigens (MAIGA) (Fig. 73.2) often detect a more complex pattern.[22] Sera from affected patients often also bind (albeit more weakly) to neutrophils expressing the alternative allele, and in some series more than half the patients with this entity produce antibodies capable of binding to nonpolymorphic elements within FcγRIIIb. Patient sera may also bind to other surface antigens. The best recent study addressing this pattern, studying antibodies from 125 patients, noted autoantibodies against CD11b/CD18 (CR3) in 21%, CD35 (CR1) in 14%, and FcRII in 2% of patients.[22]

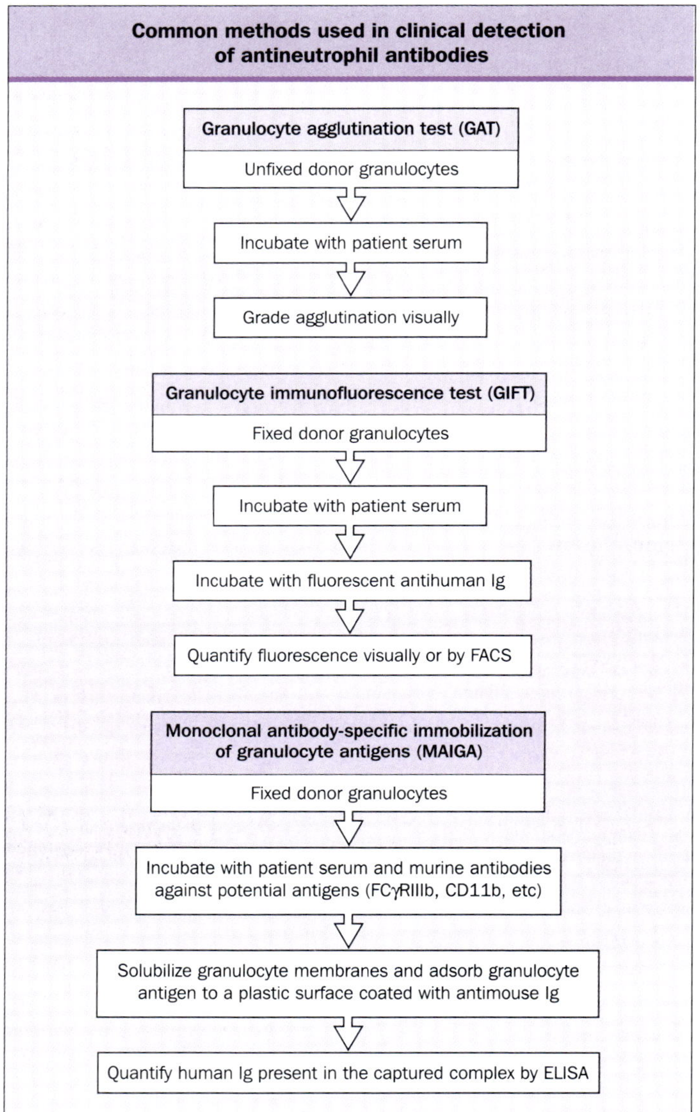

Fig. 73.2 Common methods used in clinical detection of antineutrophil antibodies. Schematic diagrams illustrate the sequence of steps required for antibody detection by granulocyte agglutination test (GAT), upper panel; granulocyte immunofluorescence test (GIFT), middle panel; and monoclonal antibody-specific immobilization of granulocyte antigens (MAIGA), lower panel.

CLINICAL PEARLS

- Congenital neutropenic disorders, primary bone marrow disease, drug-mediated neutropenia and idiosyncratic reactions to acute viral diseases should be ruled out in patients with suspected immune neutropenia.
- Laboratory studies to detect antineutrophil antibodies can be helpful, but a positive test is not diagnostic for antibody-mediated neutropenia. The results must be interpreted in the context of other clinical data.
- As drug-related neutropenia is common and difficult to prove, nonessential drugs should be discontinued in patients with a new onset of granulocytopenia.

The clinical value of delineating antibody specificity remains uncertain. Bruin et al, in one of the series cited above,[23] found that most young patients (18 of 21) with uncomplicated self-limited autoimmune neutropenia had antibodies with some degree of specificity for NA1 and/or NA2, and seven of seven children with evidence of chronic neutropenia and other generalized immune disorders had antibodies against nonpolymorphic determinants on the FcγRIIIb molecule. It remains to be determined in a larger prospective study whether this degree of concordance between antibody specificity and clinical course is common.

Autoimmune neutropenia in adults

There are no systematic large series addressing antibody specificity in adults; however, some points are clear. Specific autoantibodies directed against NA1 or NA2 are less common and autoantibodies against surface receptors such as CD11b/CD18, CR1 and FcγRII are more frequent.

The specificity of antineutrophil antibodies in adults with Felty syndrome and other systemic autoimmune diseases is even less certain. Evaluation is greatly complicated by the presence of immune complexes which can bind nonspecifically to neutrophils.[24,25] Although antineutrophil autoantibodies may be present in these patients, no systematic prospective evaluation of specificity is available.

Effects of antineutrophil antibodies on neutrophil survival in vivo

Reductions in the blood neutrophil count in patients with immune neutropenia are often assumed to reflect antibody-mediated destruction of circulating cells, but the pathophysiology is more complex than this. Sera from patients with immune- and drug-related neutropenia can cause transient neutropenia in normal volunteers;[26] however, subsequent studies using radiolabeled neutrophils to study cell survival in adult patients with autoimmune neutropenia have yielded variable results. In some patients neutrophil survival was markedly decreased,[27] whereas in others the most prominent abnormality was increased margination.[28] As many of these studies were performed on patients with Felty syndrome, who have high concentrations of circulating immune complexes and a large spleen, the general applicability of these results is unclear.

Perhaps the best controlled studies of the effects of antineutrophil antibodies on neutrophil survival were reported by McCullough et al who monitored the survival of donor neutrophils after therapeutic transfusion into allogeneic donors with known amounts of alloimmune antineutrophil antibodies.[29] These studies demonstrated an association between neutrophil agglutinating antibodies and accelerated neutrophil destruction in vivo.[29] On the other hand, in vitro lymphocytotoxic or granulocytotoxic activity correlated poorly with bioactivity in vivo. These results emphasize the importance of qualitative factors and the amount of antibody bound per cell in determining whether a given antibody can accelerate target cell destruction.

Effects of immune complexes on neutrophils

Because immune neutropenia often develops in a setting where immune complexes are present, there has been continuing speculation about their role in disease. Clearly, circulating immune complexes containing IgG and complement components can bind to Fc and complement receptors on the neutrophil surface. Indeed, this can cause false positive results in in vitro assays of antineutrophil antibodies.

Because immune complexes can also stimulate a variety of neutrophil functions and increase neutrophil adherence to endothelial cells in vitro, such complexes may also accelerate neutrophil clearance in vivo. Exploiting the capacity of IgG Fc and complement receptors on rodent leukocytes to recognize human ligands, Breedveld et al demonstrated that human immune complexes from neutropenic patients can induce significant neutropenia in animals.[30] On the other hand, clinical studies of adults with immune neutropenia do not show a close correlation between the immune complex levels and the severity of clinical neutropenia.[31] On balance, it is quite likely that some immune complexes (particularly those capable of 'targeting' neutrophils) may accelerate the margination and/or destruction of neutrophils in vivo. Circulating immune complexes alone, however, probably do not cause extensive granulocyte destruction.

Role of T-LGL in neutropenia

As noted above, patients with monoclonal T-LGL populations commonly manifest a range of autoimmune manifestations, including immune neutropenia. The mechanistic basis for this association remains uncertain. There are no data suggesting that T-LGL kill neutrophils directly, by either T-cell receptor-mediated or NK-like mechanisms. These cells, however, may influence myelopoiesis by suppressing myeloid colony formation.[32,33] This effect is mediated, at least in vitro, by humoral factors.[32,34]

As patients with T-LGL abnormalities and neutropenia often have other autoantibodies, it has been suggested that T-LGL cells can also stimulate B-cell hyperactivity, perhaps by overproducing IL-6 or other B-cell-stimulating factors.

In light of these hypotheses it is significant that cyclosporin A can partially reverse neutropenia in patients with T-LGL leukemia,[13,35,36] and in some cases these responses are seen without gross alteration in the number of circulating T-LGL cells.[35] Cyclosporin A is a potent inhibitor of cytokine production by stimulated T cells, and so this pattern of response circumstantially supports the hypothesis that soluble factors released from T-LGL, and not the cells themselves, play the critical role in mediating neutropenia in vivo.

THERAPY

Infection is a major concern in patients with immune neutropenia. All patients with neutrophil counts below 1000/mm^3 have at least a minimally increased risk of infection, yet some (particularly adults) remain asymptomatic with absolute neutrophil counts of 500/mm^3 or less. Given this variability in clinical course, the pattern of susceptibility in the individual patient should be considered in developing a therapeutic approach. As granulocyte counts drop progressively below 500/mm^3, concerted attempts to reverse granulocytopenia become increasingly justifiable. Where recurrent infection is a problem prophylactic antibiotics may be useful, particularly in children.[22]

Steroids and splenectomy

In patients with underlying diseases, such as rheumatoid arthritis or lymphoma, secondary immune neutropenia often improves as the primary disease is treated with anti-inflammatory agents or cytotoxic drugs. In severely symptomatic patients with primary or secondary disease, however, splenectomy and steroids have often been used to reverse neutropenia. Acutely, each modality reduces immune destruction by suppressing the body's capacity to clear IgG- and complement-coated cells. Over a longer time frame these treatments can also suppress antibody production, in the first case by removing a major site of production, and in the second by suppressing the cellular processes required for antibody production. Steroids can also prevent T-cell-mediated suppression of myelopoiesis, at least in patients with Felty syndrome.[37]

In retrospective analyses, steroids and splenectomy can each reverse neutropenia in some patients. Because these manipulations themselves may compromise immune clearance and/or cellular immunity, it is less clear how often they really improve patient outcome. One group noted persistent infections in splenectomized patients despite the correction of peripheral neutropenia.[38] With the availability of newer agents such as recombinant granulocyte colony-stimulating factor (G-CSF) and granulocyte–macrophage colony-stimulating factor (GM-CSF) and, to a lesser extent, intravenous immunoglobulin (IVIG), splenectomy and steroids should probably be considered only in severely or persistently granulocytopenic patients resistant to other forms of therapy.

Colony-stimulating factors (CSF)

The CSFs can be quite effective in enhancing neutrophil counts in children with autoimmune neutropenia[39] and adults with Felty syndrome or other autoimmune disease.[40,41] Clearly, these agents

THERAPEUTIC PRINCIPLES

- Asymptomatic patients with granulocyte counts higher than 1000/mm^3 usually require no therapy.
- Antibiotics are often life-saving in containing acute infection, and have been used prophylactically in selected high-risk patients to reduce the frequency of recurrent events.
- Patients with recurrent infections, especially with granulocyte counts below 500/mm^3, may benefit from specific therapy to correct granulocytopenia.
- G-CSF is probably the safest and most effective single agent for rapid symptomatic correction of neutropenia.
- Splenectomy and steroids should be reserved for use as a second line of therapy in patients with very persistent or refractory disease.

increase the rate of new neutrophil production. In addition, at least in some cases, CSFs stimulate the production of soluble antigen, which competitively inhibits antibody binding to neutrophils.[42] Because these agents are relatively safe, at least for short-term use, they may be used continuously or intermittently as needed, particularly in children. However, they are expensive and neutropenia recurs when they are stopped. Therefore judgment must be used in deciding when their use is warranted.

Intravenous immunoglobulin (IVIG)

This agent can transiently reverse immune neutropenia. Although it is reasonably effective in primary immune neutropenia of childhood,[43] it has not been as useful in adults, particularly in the setting of Felty syndrome.[44] Its mechanism of action has not been studied, but presumably it reduces Fc receptor-mediated clearance of antibody-coated neutrophils in vivo, without altering antibody production. Despite its moderate efficacy, its expense, short duration of action and inconvenience of administration have limited the usefulness of IVIG in chronic treatment plans.

Other immunosuppressive agents

Various drugs have been used in small numbers of steroid and splenectomy-resistant patients, with varying success. As noted above, cyclosporin A is particularly effective in the treatment of patients with neutropenia in the setting of T-LGL leukemia,[35,36] and also can be effective in some patients with Felty syndrome. The response rate to other drugs, such as cyclophosphamide and methotrexate, is less clear. Their use is more easily justified in a setting where they are also being used to treat some other primary condition.

PATIENT EVALUATION

The initial evaluation of selective neutropenia should include a history and physical examination, with evaluation of the blood counts and blood film. There are a number of alternative possibilities in the differential diagnosis of chronic neutropenia (Table 73.2). It is essential to note recent medication use, to uncover any family history of blood disorders, and to identify clinical symptoms or signs suggestive of underlying autoimmune or lymphoproliferative disease. The physical examination should include a careful evaluation for splenomegaly, lymphadenopathy, or evidence of systemic autoimmune disease. Review of blood counts and morphology is essential in identifying patients with increased numbers of large granular lymphocytes, other autoimmune cytopenias, or hematologic disorders that are associated with neutropenia. Absolute lymphocytosis on routine blood counts or a suggestion of increased LGL in a peripheral smear suggest the need for flow-cytometric studies. In cases of moderate to severe neutropenia, particularly in adults, a bone marrow examination is indicated to rule out myelodysplasia, lymphoproliferation or other hematologic disorders.

Antineutrophil antibody assays (discussed below) are the most disease-specific laboratory tool for confirming diagnosis. Neutrophil turnover and survival have been studied experimentally in the past, but have not proved practical for use in routine clinical practice.

Alternative etiologies for chronic neutropenia
Hereditary disorders
Kostmann syndrome
Cyclic neutropenia
Granulocytopenia associated with immunoglobulin abnormalities
Other less well defined syndromes of varying etiology
Hematologic disorders
Myelodysplastic syndromes
Hypersplenism
Drug-associated neutropenia[a]
Analgesics, especially aminopyrine
Sulfonamides
Antithyroid drugs, especially propylthiouracil
Penicillin and cephalosporin antibiotics
Cinchona alkaloids, especially quinidine and quinine
Phenothiazines
Diuretics especially thiazides
Many others reported with varying documentation of an immune etiology

[a] Some of these drugs may mediate neutropenia by immune mechanisms.

Table 73.2 Alternative etiologies for chronic neutropenia.

Detection of antineutrophil antibodies

With 10–20 years of published experience in detecting neutrophil-specific antibodies, some methodologic generalizations are possible:

1. Direct assays, measuring immunoglobulin on the surface of patient neutrophils, demonstrate increased cell-bound antibody more commonly than do indirect assays.[31] There are several disadvantages to this method, however. It is logistically difficult to perform these studies on freshly collected cells. Equally importantly, the specificity and significance of the results are unclear, partly because it is difficult to distinguish clinically significant cell-bound antibody from absorbed immunoglobulin or immune complexes. Consequently, direct assays are now less commonly used.

2. Indirect assays measuring the binding of antibodies from patient sera to donor granulocytes have become the standard approach for detecting antineutrophil antibodies. The most common assays are illustrated in Figure 73.2, and functional comparisons are summarized in Table 73.3. In practice, variants of the granulocyte immunofluorescent test (GIFT) are most commonly used. Granulocyte agglutination tests (GAT) can be useful in conjunction with GIFT, particularly in detecting antibodies against 5b or NA2, but they are too insensitive for use alone. Unfortunately, all these tests require freshly fixed donor granulocytes. As cell panels of defined antigen phenotype cannot be stored, defining antibody specificity is a burdensome process which is only practical in highly specialized centers.

At the second international granulocyte serology workshop, 12 centers independently tested a series of unknown sera.[20] Many laboratories could detect strong anti-NA1 antibodies, but the success rate was much lower in defining anti-NA2 or anti-NB1 antibodies. More disconcertingly, there was great variability in the proficiency of these laboratories. Whereas one correctly identified 12 of 12 unknowns, another identified none of 12 and several others did only slightly better. Clearly, technical problems in antibody characterization persist.[20]

3. Monoclonal antibody-specific immobilization of granulocyte antigens (MAIGA), described in Figure 73.2, is a useful research tool for characterizing the specificity of antineutrophil antibodies. However, the assay only detects antibodies directed

Comparison of indirect antineutrophil antibody detection assays	
Advantages	**Disadvantages**
Granulocyte agglutination test	
Simple to perform Sensitive to antibodies against unusual neutrophil antigens such as '5b'	Interpretation of endpoint is subjective Low sensitivity for most antibodies
Granulocyte immunofluorescence test (GIFT)	
Relatively simple to perform and interpret Sensitive for antibodies against most common antigens	False positive results with circulating immune complexes
Monoclonal antibody-specific immobilization of granulocyte antigens (MAIGA)	
Provides information about antibody specificity Few false positive results relatively insensitive to immune complexes	Relatively complex methodology Only detects antibodies against preselected target antigens

Table 73.3 Comparison of indirect antineutrophil antibody detection assays.

against selected immobilized antigens. Consequently, a positive result in a MAIGA provides useful information, but a negative study is of limited use.

4. Using recombinant techniques it may ultimately be possible to produce more stable, specific reagents, but development is still in its early stages.[45]

Role of antineutrophil assays in immune neutropenia of childhood

Using GIFT, with or without GAT, antineutrophil antibodies can be detected in more than 70% of patients with primary immune neutropenia. When two or more assay methods are used in tandem (usually one immunochemical and one agglutination based) the yield increases further.[4,6]

Role of antineutrophil assays in immune neutropenia in adults

Chronic neutropenia, even in adults, may arise through either immune or nonimmune mechanisms (Tables 73.1 and 73.2), and differentiation of these syndromes on clinical grounds can be difficult.[46] Van der Veen et al[31] detected serum antineutrophil antibodies in 15% of patients referred with chronic neutropenia. In a similar study, Logue[47] noted indirect antibodies in 36% of patients. As the true incidence of immune destruction is unknown, these frequencies may indicate either a low overall frequency of immune disorders in neutropenic adults, or low assay sensitivity.

Indirect assays yield far more positive results in studies of patients with Felty syndrome or other inflammatory conditions.[24,48] Although these positive results are reassuring to the clinician managing a neutropenic patient, there must be genuine concern about their significance. Circulating immune complexes, or even aggregated IgG, can cause strong false positive studies,[25] and so positive results must be considered of uncertain significance if they can not be confirmed using MAIGA or immunoprecipitation techniques.

DIFFERENTIAL DIAGNOSIS

Special considerations in children

Alloimmune neonatal neutropenia can cause severe immune neutropenia during the first month of life, but this usually corrects within 1–2 months. Ongoing neutropenia in a child 2 months of age or older is more consistent with primary autoimmune neutropenia. Apart from the infectious complications of neutropenia, affected infants are usually healthy, and so the main task in differential diagnosis is to rule out hereditary disorders, such as Kostman syndrome or drug-induced neutropenia, that might mimic primary autoimmune disease (Table 73.2). The demonstration of antineutrophil antibodies, either in the neonatal period or later, supports an immune etiology.

Special considerations in adults

Evaluation of the etiology of neutropenia in an otherwise healthy adult requires that drug-related neutropenia, undiagnosed autoimmune disease, lymphoproliferative disorder and myelodysplasia be ruled out. Even when these are excluded there remain a substantial subpopulation who have 'idiopathic', presumably nonimmune, neutropenia. The latter heterogeneous group[46,49] cannot be readily distinguished based on clinical picture, peripheral blood or bone marrow findings from patients with immune-mediated neutropenia. Because indirect assays are not absolutely reliable, in some cases the diagnosis remains uncertain and an empirical approach to management is warranted.

Felty syndrome

This clinical syndrome is defined by the triad of rheumatoid arthritis, splenomegaly and neutropenia. Although the pathophysiologic significance of a positive result remains controversial, an antineutrophil antibody assay is often performed to confirm the diagnosis, and it is usually positive.[41] Some authors suggest that patients with rheumatoid arthritis, granulocytopenia and an elevated antineutrophil antibody titer should be considered to have a variant of Felty syndrome, even if splenomegaly is absent.[48]

Patients with presumed Felty syndrome should be screened for evidence of abnormal circulating LGL on a peripheral blood smear, and if LGL abnormalities are suspected, lymphocyte immunophenotyping and T-cell clonality studies should also be obtained. Based on published estimates, some form of T-LGL abnormality may be seen in as many as one-third of patients with arthritis and neutropenia.[50]

Although Felty syndrome is pathophysiologically distinct from the immune neutropenia, splenomegaly and arthritis sometimes seen in patients with circulating monoclonal T-LGL, there is clinical overlap. Rheumatoid complications of T-LGL are preferentially seen in patients expressing HLA-DR4, the same MHC marker associated with severe symptoms in the classic rheumatoid arthritis population.

Drug-related neutropenia is also an important consideration in rheumatoid arthritis. Patients frequently receive gold, penicillamine, methotrexate or nonsteroidal anti-inflammatory agents, and each of these can cause neutropenia (Table 73.2). On occasion it is necessary to test for drug-related neutropenia by withdrawing one or more of these agents before concluding that neutropenia is attributable to Felty syndrome.

Other secondary immune neutropenic conditions

Diagnosis in this diverse population is sometimes difficult because the underlying disease and its therapy may confuse the clinical picture and contribute directly to the observed neutropenia. Circulating immune complexes in patients with systemic autoimmune disorders also present a problem, as they can cause false positive results in antineutrophil antibody assays. Often clinical judgment must be exercised in distinguishing immune neutropenia from underlying disease or complications of its treatment.

PITFALLS AND CONTROVERSIES

Diagnostic limitations

As noted above, currently available antineutrophil antibody assays have major limitations. In practice, a positive antineutrophil antibody assay in an otherwise healthy child or adult with neutropenia strongly supports the diagnosis of immune neutropenia, and a negative result points away from (but does not rule out) the diagnosis. The specificity of these tests, however, decreases when they are used in patients who may have other autoantibodies, e.g. those with rheumatologic disease, HIV etc. Until better tests are available, the clinician dealing with a complex patient must use clinical judgment as well as laboratory tools to establishing a diagnosis.

Management

Most of the available therapies are palliative to temporarily reverse neutropenia, or to contain infection without untoward complication. In practice, the early use of antibiotics during infection is probably the most important single intervention in improving clinical outcome. The value of antibiotics in prophylaxis is less clearly established, but this may be a reasonable approach. Among agents designed to correct neutropenia, G-CSF is the fastest and most reliable and its side effects are usually minimal. The main disadvantages are its cost, particularly when it must be used continuously, and the inconvenience.

Of the immunosuppressive agents, cyclosporin A clearly has a role in the therapy of neutropenia in T-LGL leukemia. Further studies should clarify whether this agent can also be effective in other forms of secondary disease. The efficacy of steroids, other potent cytotoxic drugs and splenectomy is limited, and clearly there is a need for more selective agents to suppress autoantibody production. Given the current pace of basic research and drug development, there is reason for optimism about future developments.

REFERENCES

1. Semenzato G, Zambello R, Starkebaum G, Oshimi K, Loughran TP Jr. The lymphoproliferative disease of granular lymphocytes: updated criteria for diagnosis. Blood 1997;89:256.
2. Cartron J, Tchernia G, Celton JL, et al. Alloimmune neonatal neutropenia. Am J Pediatr Hematol Oncol 1991;13:21.
3. Lyall EG, Lucas GF, Eden OB. Autoimmune neutropenia of infancy. J Clin Pathol 1992;45:431.
4. Lalezari P, Khorshidi M, Petrosova M. Autoimmune neutropenia of infancy. J Pediatr 1986;109:764.
5. Bussel JB, Abboud MR. Autoimmune neutropenia of infancy. CRC Crit Rev Oncol Hematol 1987;7:37.
6. Bux J, Mueller-Eckhardt C. Autoimmune neutropenia. Semin Hematol 1992;29:45.
7. Beatty PA, Stroncek DF. Autoimmune neutropenia in Sheboygan County, Wisconsin. J Lab Clin Med 1992;119:718.
8. Campion G, Maddison PJ, Goulding N, et al. The Felty syndrome: a case-matched study of clinical manifestations and outcome, serologic features, and immunogenetic associations. Medicine (Baltimore) 1990;69:69.
9. Thorne C, Urowitz MB. Long-term outcome in Felty's syndrome. Ann Rheum Dis 1982;41:486.
10. Loughran TPJ. Clonal diseases of large granular lymphocytes. Blood 1993;82:1.
11. Snowden N, Bhavnani M, Swinson DR, et al. Large granular T lymphocytes, neutropenia, and polyarthropathy: an underdiagnosed syndrome. Q J Med 1991;78:65.
12. Gentile TC, Wener MH, Starkebaum G, Loughran TP Jr. Humoral immune abnormalities in T-cell large granular lymphocyte leukemia. Leuk Lymphoma 1996;23:365.
13. Akashi K, Shibuya T, Taniguchi S, et al. Multiple autoimmune haemopoietic disorders and insidious clonal proliferation of large granular lymphocytes. Br J Haematol 1999;107:670.
14. Rustagi PK, Han T, Ziolkowski L, et al. Granulocyte antibodies in leukaemic chronic lymphoproliferative disorders. Br J Haematol 1987;66:461.
15. Yachie A, Miyawaki T, Nagaoki T, et al. Regulation of B cell differentiation by T cell subsets defined with monoclonal OKT4 and OKT8 antibodies in human cord blood. J Immunol 1981;127:1314.
16. Hessner MJ, Curtis BR, Endean DJ, Aster RH. Determination of neutrophil antigen gene frequencies in five ethnic groups by polymerase chain reaction with sequence-specific primers. Transfusion 1996;36:895.
17. Bux J, Stein EL, Bierling P, et al. Characterization of a new alloantigen (SH) on the human neutrophil Fc gamma receptor IIIb. Blood 1997;89:1027.
18. Fromont P, Bettaieb A, Skouri H, et al. Frequency of the polymorphonuclear neutrophil Fc gamma receptor III deficiency in the French population and its involvement in the development of neonatal alloimmune neutropenia. Blood 1992;79:2131.
19. Stroncek DF, Skubitz KM, Shankar RA, Mendiola JR, McCullough JJ. Biochemical characterization of the neutrophil-specific antigen NB1. Blood 1990;75:744.
20. Bux J, Chapman J. Report on the second international granulocyte serology workshop. Transfusion 1997;37:977.
21. Kallenberg CG, Tervaert JW. What is new with anti-neutrophil cytoplasmic antibodies: diagnostic, pathogenetic and therapeutic implications. Curr Opin Nephrol Hypertens 1999;8:307.
22. Bux J, Behrens G, Jaeger G, Welte K. Diagnosis and clinical course of autoimmune neutropenia in infancy: analysis of 240 cases. Blood 1998;91:181.
23. Bruin MC, von dem Borne AE, Tamminga RY, et al. Neutrophil antibody specificity in different types of childhood autoimmune neutropenia. Blood 1999;94:1797.
24. Starkebaum G, Arend WP, Nardella FA, et al. Characterization of immune complexes and immunoglobulin G antibodies reactive with neutrophils in the sera of patients with Felty's syndrome. J Lab Clin Med 1980;96:238.
25. Goldschmeding R, Breedveld FC, Engelfiet CP, et al. Lack of evidence for the presence of neutrophil-bound antibodies in the serum of patients with Felty's syndrome. Br J Haematol 1988;68:37.
26. Kissmeyer-Nielsen F. Demonstration of a thrombocytopenic and a leukopenic factor in the blood of patients with thrombocytopenia and leukopenia. Acta Haematol 1953;9:337.
27. Joyce RA, Boggs DR, Chervenick PA, et al. Neutrophil kinetics in Felty's syndrome. Am J Med 1980;69:695.
28. Vincent PC, Levi JA, MacQueen A. The mechanism of neutropenia in Felty's syndrome. Br J Haematol 1974;27:463.

29. McCullough J, Weibler BJ, Clay M, Richards K, et al. Effect of leukocyte antibodies on the fate in vivo of indium-111-labelled granulocytes. Blood 1981;58:164.
30. Breedveld FC, Lafeber GJM, De Vries E, et al. Immune complexes and the pathogenesis of neutropenia in Felty's syndrome. Ann Rheum Dis 1986;45:696.
31. van der Veen JPW, Hack CE, Engelfriet CP. Chronic idiopathic and secondary neutropenia: clinical and serological investigations. Br J Haematol 1986;63:161.
32. Nagler A, Greenberg PL. Bone marrow cell modulation and inhibition of myelopoiesis by large granular lymphocytes and natural killer cells. Int J Cell Cloning 1990;8:171.
33. Platanias L, Raefsky E, Young N. Neutropenia associated with large granular lymphocytes responsive to corticosteroids in vitro and in vivo. Eur J Haematol 1987;38:89.
34. Papadaki HA, Giouremou K, Eliopoulos GD. Low frequency of myeloid progenitor cells in chronic idiopathic neutropenia of adults may be related to increased production of TGF-beta1 by bone marrow stromal cells. Eur J Haematol 1999;63:154.
35. Sood R, Stewart CC, Aplan PD, et al. Neutropenia associated with T-cell large granular lymphocyte leukemia: long-term response to cyclosporine therapy despite persistence of abnormal cells. Blood 1998;91:3372.
36. Brinkman K, van Dongen JJ, van Lom K, et al. Induction of clinical remission in T-large granular lymphocyte leukemia with cyclosporin A, monitored by use of immunophenotyping with Vbeta antibodies. Leukemia 1998;12:150.
37. Bagby GC, Gabourel JD. Neutropenia in three patients with rheumatic disorders. J Clin Invest 1979;64:72.
38. Sienknecht CW, Urowitz MB, Pruzanski W, Stein HB. Felty's syndrome. Clinical and serological analysis of 34 cases. Ann Rheum Dis 1977;36:500.
39. Bauduer F. G-CSF: a very efficient therapy in chronic autoimmun neutropenia. A brief review of the literature. Hematol Cell Ther 1998;40:189.
40. Hellmich B, Schnabel A, Gross WL. Treatment of severe neutropenia due to Felty's syndrome or systemic lupus erythematosus with granulocyte colony-stimulating factor. Semin Arthritis Rheum 1999;29:82.
41. Shastri KA, Logue GL. Autoimmune neutropenia. Blood 1993;81:1984.
42. Kuijpers TW, de Haas M, de Groot CJ, von dem Borne AE, Weening RS. The use of rhG-CSF in chronic autoimmune neutropenia: reversal of autoimmune phenomena, a case history. Br J Haematol 1996;94:464.
43. Bussel J, Lalezari P, Hilgartner M, et al. Reversal of neutropenia with intravenous gammaglobulin in autoimmune neutropenia of infancy. Blood 1983;62:398.
44. Breedveld FC, Brand A, Van Aken WG. High dose intravenous gammaglobulin for Felty's syndrome. J Rheumatol 1985;12:700.
45. Bux J, Kissel K, Hofmann C, Santoso S. The use of allele-specific recombinant Fc gamma receptor IIIb antigens for the detection of granulocyte antibodies. Blood 1999;93:357.
46. Dale D, Guerry D, Wewerka J, Bull J, Chusid M. Chronic neutropenia. Medicine (Baltimore) 1979;58:128.
47. Logue GL, Shastri KA, Laughlin M, et al. Idiopathic neutropenia: antineutrophil antibodies and clinical correlations. Am J Med. 1991;90:211.
48. Logue GL, Shimm DS. Autoimmune granulocytopenia. Annu Rev Med 1980;31:191.
49. Kyle R. Natural history of chronic idiopathic neutropenia. N Engl J Med 1980;302:908.
50. Saway PA, Prasthofer EF, Barton JC. Prevalence of large granular lymphocyte proliferation in patients with rheumatoid arthritis and neutropenia. Am J Med 1989;86:303.

Chapter 74 Immune-mediated Platelet and Coagulation Disorders

Robert I. Parker

INTRODUCTION

Immune disorders may produce quantitative or qualitative platelet abnormalities or a decrease in coagulation factor activity. Frequently, these abnormalities result from the production of antibodies against platelets or clotting factors. This chapter reviews the pathophysiology and therapy of the more common immune-mediated platelet and coagulation disorders.

IMMUNE-MEDIATED PLATELET DEFECTS

Both platelet function and number can be affected in immune-mediated diseases; by far the more common finding, however, is thrombocytopenia. Abnormalities of platelet number and function can occur via any of several humoral or cell-mediated immune mechanisms.[1–7] The most commonly considered immune mechanism for thrombocytopenia is the formation of specific antiplatelet autoantibodies (Fig. 74.1). Platelets have a large number of immunogenic structures on their surface, the glycoprotein IIb/IIIa (GP IIb/IIIa) complex being the most numerous. Consequently, autoantibodies directed against epitopes on the GP IIb/IIIa complex are the most frequent when the specificity of the antibodies has been determined.[1] Platelet autoantibodies are usually IgG, although IgA, IgD and IgM autoantibodies have occasionally been demonstrated. Complement has also been found on the surface of platelets in clinical syndromes consistent with increased immune-mediated platelet destruction. However, most autoantibodies are not complement fixing, and removal of the immunoglobulin-coated platelets occurs in the spleen and other sites of reticuloendothelial tissue. Other platelet glycoproteins implicated in immune platelet destruction have been the GP Ib-IX complex and GP V (see next section).[1] Drugs can result in the production of 'antiplatelet' antibodies by several different mechanisms. These include antibodies generated against a neoantigen, Fc-mediated immune complex binding, and the hapten or 'innocent bystander' mechanism (Figs 74.2–74.4).

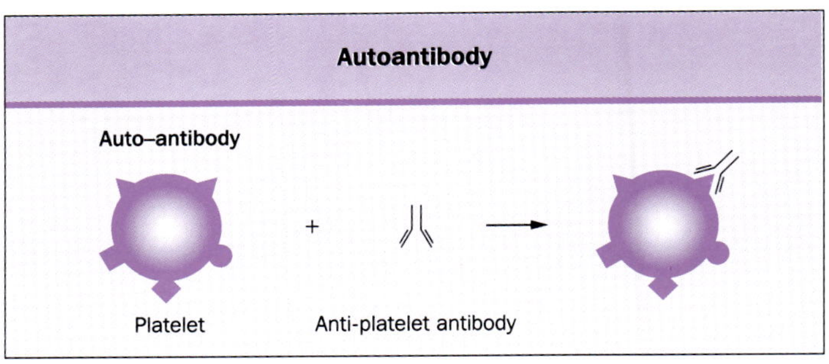

Fig. 74.1 Interaction of autoantibody with platelet.

KEY CONCEPTS

Mechanisms of immune-mediated thrombocytopenia
- Humoral
- Fab-mediated
  - Autoantibody directed against intrinsic platelet antigen
  - Antibody directed against neoantigen, e.g. platelet–drug complex
  - Innocent bystander or hapten mechanism
- Fc-mediated
  - Immune complex binding
- Cell-mediated
- Hemophagocytosis; monocyte or histiocyte activation
- Marrow suppression

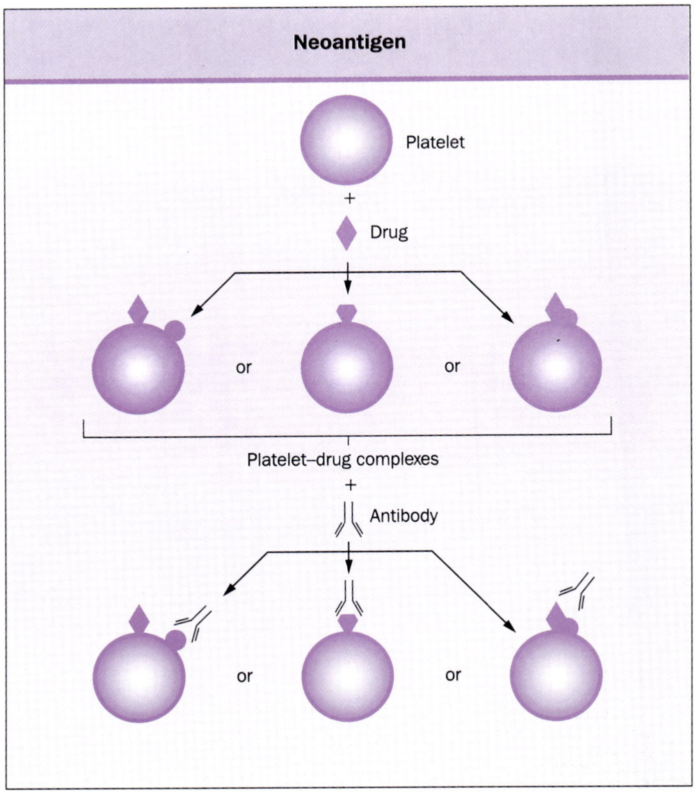

Fig. 74.2 Interaction of an autoantibody with a neoantigen on the platelet surface resulting from the interaction of a drug with the platelet membrane.

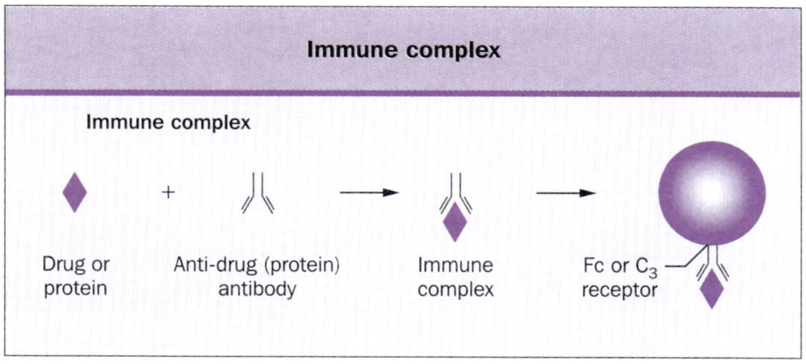

Fig. 74.3 Immune complex binding to the surface of a platelet via Fc or complement receptor.

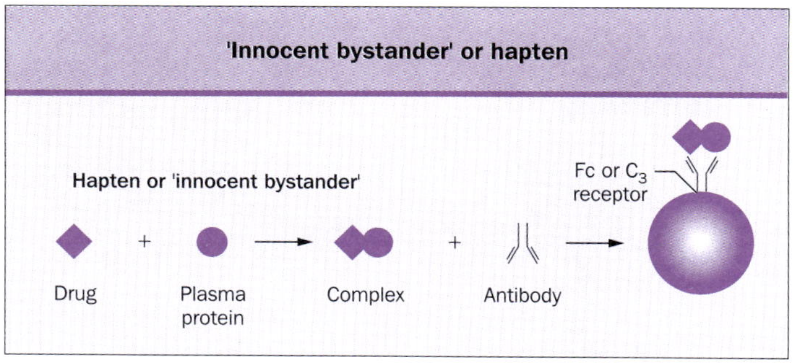

Fig. 74.4 Innocent bystander, or hapten, mechanism of antibody binding to platelets.

Cell-mediated events can also play a role in thrombocytopenia. Monocytes recognize and phagocytize antibody-coated platelets,[2] and in some cases monocyte activation may be a primary event in acute idiopathic thrombocytopenic purpura (ITP), as evidenced by the finding of increased levels of macrophage–colony-stimulating factor (M-CSF) in patients with acute ITP.[3] Expansion of NK and T-cell subsets has also been documented in ITP.[4–6] Thrombocytopenia can also be the result of decreased platelet production from generalized marrow suppression in immune disorders. This can be either cell- or antibody-mediated suppression of megakaryocyte proliferation.[7,8]

Idiopathic thrombocytopenia purpura

The clearest example of immune-mediated thrombocytopenia is idiopathic thrombocytopenic purpura (ITP), or autoimmune thrombocytopenia purpura (ATP). ITP is a syndrome rather than a single disease entity. Three major findings are necessary for the diagnosis of ITP, which may be accompanied by additional features. The three absolute findings for ITP are: thrombocytopenia; normal or increased megakaryocytes on bone marrow aspiration and/or biopsy, with other marrow elements being normal in number and morphology; and the absence of underlying disease or drug therapy that can result in thrombocytopenia. Some investigators have demonstrated a soluble cleavage product of the GP Ib-IX complex to be present in increased amounts in the sera of individuals with immune platelet destruction.[9]

The immune nature of ITP was shown by Harrington and coworkers[10] in 1951, in a study in which plasma from individuals with ITP was infused into normal laboratory volunteers. In these experiments a consistent and reproducible drop in platelet count occurred within hours and lasted for up to 5 days before recovery (Fig. 74.5). This experimental finding has been corroborated in vivo by generally finding a significantly shortened platelet survival in individuals considered to have ITP. However, platelet survival itself has not been useful in predicting the magnitude of the thrombocytopenia or the response to therapy. More recent studies, in which both platelet survival and platelet turnover were determined, have demonstrated a better correlation of platelet turnover with both thrombocytopenia and response to splenectomy.[11,12] Patients with shortened survival and increased

CLINICAL PEARLS

ITP: diagnostic criteria

- Required
  - Thrombocytopenia
  - Normal or increased marrow megakaryocytes
  - Absence of underlying condition associated with thrombocytopenia
- Supportive
  - Increased platelet-associated immunoglobulin
  - Large and/or bizarre platelets on peripheral smear
  - Shortened platelet survival
  - Increased platelet turnover

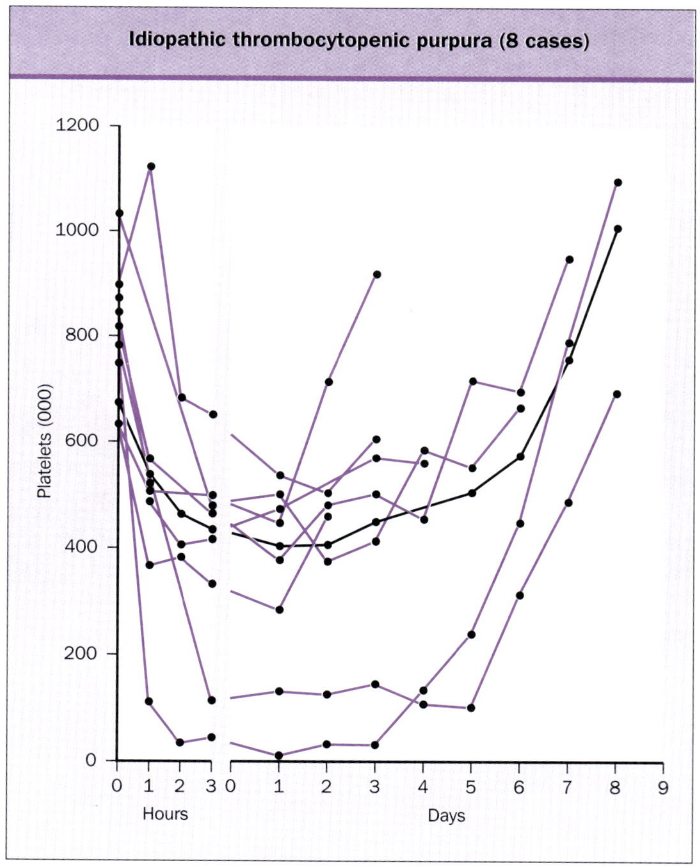

Fig. 74.5 Time course of thrombocytopenia following infusion of plasma from patients with immune thrombocytopenia. (From Harrington WJ, Minnich V, Hollingsworth JW, Moore CV. *J Lab Clin Med* 1951, 38:1 with permission.)

platelet turnover were much more likely to respond to splenectomy than those who had shortened survival and normal or decreased platelet turnover. It is believed that patients exhibiting an inappropriately low platelet turnover have a largely productive thrombocytopenia.[12]

Although 70–90% of patients with ITP demonstrate elevated platelet-associated IgG at some time during their disease, the significance of antiplatelet antibody testing in ITP is unclear because of the general lack of correlation with clinical course, degree of thrombocytopenia and response to therapy. Likewise, measurements of serum ('free') antiplatelet antibodies have not been useful in diagnosing ITP. Less than 50% of patients with ITP have measurable serum antiplatelet antibodies. In addition, there is generally little, if any, correlation between the titer of serum antiplatelet antibodies and clinical parameters.[1,13]

When the specificity of antiplatelet autoantibodies has been determined, a large number are directed against epitopes of platelet GP IIb/IIIa. The prospective determination of antibody specificity has not allowed early identification of individuals likely to progress to a chronic form of the disorder. Antibodies against GP V are noted in the postvaricella ITP syndrome. Antibodies directed against GP IIb/IIIa or GP Ib-IX complex may result in platelet dysfunction, as both of these glycoproteins contain functionally significant platelet receptors. GP IIb/IIIa contains the receptor for fibrinogen, von Willebrand factor and fibronectin; and the platelet GP Ib-IX complex contains the ristocetin-dependent receptor for von Willebrand factor. Binding of an antibody on or near these functionally active receptors has, in a small number of patients, resulted in both thrombocytopenia and significant platelet dysfunction.[14] The binding of immune complexes to platelets via the platelet Fc receptor or the binding of specific antiplatelet antibodies can result in the in vivo activation of platelets, with subsequent thrombocytopenia and paradoxical thrombosis.[15] This process can play a significant role in the microvascular thrombosis that has been demonstrated both in heparin-induced thrombocytopenia and in some patients with lupus anticoagulants and/or antiphospholipid antibodies. Although not yet confirmed in larger series, early studies suggest specific HLA profiles that may be predictive for the development of ITP and response to therapy.[16]

Children and adults with ITP display very different natural histories, clinical courses and responses to therapy. Because of this, many investigators feel that the immunologic mechanisms at play in these two patient groups must be different; this has yet to be clearly demonstrated.

Childhood ITP

In children, ITP is generally self-limited. The peak age of occurrence is between 2 and 6 years, although it can be seen in infants. The male:female ratio is roughly 1:1. ITP is generally noted 1–2 weeks following a viral illness, and has been observed following varicella, rubella, rubeola, Epstein–Barr virus (EBV) and cytomegalovirus (CMV) infections.[17] The syndrome is characterized by an acute onset of bruising. Eighty per cent of children exhibit a spontaneous remission within 6 months, and over 90% within 2 years. Only 4–5% of patients develop a chronic syndrome requiring long-term steroids or other drug therapies. In contrast to adult patients, spontaneous remissions have been documented up to and beyond 2 years after initial diagnosis. In general, the bleeding manifestations are relatively mild for the degree of thrombocytopenia. The most serious bleeding is intracranial hemorrhage: whereas initial series suggested an incidence of up to 5–10% for intracranial hemorrhage, more recent series have shown the incidence to be significantly less than 1%.[18]

> **CLINICAL PEARLS**
>
> **ITP: clinical parameters**
> - Children
>   - M:F ratio 1:1
>   - Peak incidence 2–6 years of age
>   - 80–90% exhibit a spontaneous remission, with relapses uncommon
>   - May spontaneously remit more than 2 years after presentation
> - Adults
>   - M:F ratio 1:3
>   - Peak incidence 20–50 years of age
>   - 10–20% spontaneous remission, with relapses common
>   - Spontaneous remission rare beyond 6 months after presentation

Adult ITP

Unlike children, adults exhibit a very broad incidence peak, occurring between 20 and 50 years of age, with a 3:1 female to male ratio. Spontaneous remissions are infrequent, with most series reporting a spontaneous remission rate of only 10–20%. Onset is usually indolent. Those patients who manifest a more acute onset are more likely to have a spontaneous or drug-assisted remission.[13] In contrast to children, treatment failures and relapses are quite common, and spontaneous remissions 6 months beyond presentation are rare. Most series report a high probability of associated immunologic disorders; all adults who present with isolated thrombocytopenia should be evaluated for immunologically mediated diseases such as systemic lupus erythematosus (SLE) or lymphoreticular neoplasia.

Therapy of ITP

Several therapies have been shown to be effective in ITP, but the current therapy of choice for acute ITP is the infusion of intravenous immunoglobulin (IVIG) (Chapter 104). The mechanism of action of IVIG may be one or more of the following: decreased reticuloendothelial (RE) clearance of immunoglobulin-coated platelets because of the nonspecific occupancy of splenic macrophage Fc receptors by the infused immunoglobulin; decreased synthesis of specific immunoglobulin; and, rarely, anti-idiotypic antibody present in the IgG preparation.[19,20]

The standard dose has been a total of 2 g/kg given in two to five doses. However, recent data in children and adults suggest that a single infusion of 0.8–1.0 g/kg produces responses equivalent to those seen with higher total doses, with less toxicity.[21,22] Commonly noted side-effects include flushing and hypertension during the infusion. Up to 20% of children treated with 2 g/kg will develop fever, headache, nausea, vomiting and meningismus thought to be secondary to immune complex deposition in the meninges.[21] The likelihood of developing this syndrome increases with higher single and total dose infused, but may be reduced by the concomitant administration of corticosteroids.[23]

THERAPEUTIC PRINCIPLES

ITP therapy

- First-line
  - IVIG
  - Corticosteroids (oral or intravenous)
  - Anti-D (WinRho)
  - Splenectomy (adults)
- Second-line
  - Immunosuppression (e.g. cyclosporine)
  - Alkylating agents
  - Splenectomy (children)
  - Immunoabsorption, plasmapheresis
  - Vincristine and related drugs
  - Danazol
  - Vitamin C
  - Colchicine
  - Interferon-α_{2b}

Prior to the use of IVIG, IV or oral corticosteroids were the mainstay of treatment. The usual oral regimen is 2–4 mg/kg/day (children) or 1–2 mg/kg/day (adults) in two or three divided doses given for 2 weeks, with a rapid taper thereafter. The overall response rate is similar to that of IVIG, but the lag time to response appears to be somewhat longer (2–3 days for corticosteroids vs. 1–2 days for IVIG).[21] The weight gain associated with corticosteroid therapy may be particularly troublesome, with most patients experiencing a 5–10% weight gain after 3 weeks of therapy. High-dose pulse intravenous methylprednisolone has been used by some investigators as a less expensive alternative to IVIG. The intravenous regimens usually call for 30 mg/kg/day for 3 days, followed by a slow taper over the next several weeks. Responses are comparable to those with IVIG; the toxicities include acute hypertension, flushing and transient carbohydrate intolerance.[24]

In individuals refractory to treatment with conventional IVIG preparations or corticosteroids, the use of an anti RhD antibody is beneficial.[21,25,26] The mechanism of action for this preparation is thought to be through the induction of a hemolytic anemia with secondary reticuloendothelial (RE) system blockade by red cell stroma. However, this therapy is also felt to produce some degree of immunosuppression by a mechanism that is as yet unidentified.[25] Limitations of this therapy are that it is only useful in Rh-positive individuals and is not beneficial post splenectomy. The usual dose is 25–50 μg/kg given as a single intravenous infusion, although single doses as high as 150 μg/kg have been used in patients not responsive to lower doses. The major toxicity is the expected hemolytic anemia, with up to 25% of treated patients developing a hemoglobin of less than or equal to 10 g/dl. Therapy with anti-RhD immunoglobulin is now advocated by many hematologists for the initial therapy of ITP.

Splenectomy is generally recommended for adults with chronic ITP refractory to or dependent on corticosteroids, but it is much less commonly utilized in children. This reluctance to use splenectomy as a therapy in childhood ITP is a product of the high spontaneous remission rate of ITP in children and concerns regarding postsplenectomy immune dysfunction (Chapter 42). Questions that remain for the treatment of splenectomized individuals are, for how long is penicillin prophylaxis required, and how frequently should these patients be reimmunized with pneumococcal vaccine? An additional problem in deciding when to perform splenectomy is the difficulty in identifying patients who will respond to this procedure. The determination of platelet turnover pre-splenectomy appears to be predictive of response.[12] Numerous other therapeutic measures have been tried, with a lower efficacy.

Immune complex-mediated thrombocytopenia

Immune complex-mediated thrombocytopenia can be seen in SLE as well as other autoimmune diseases, sepsis, malignancy and HIV infection. Thrombocytopenia can precede other clinical and serologic manifestations of lupus by several years; therefore, this diagnosis should be considered in any individual (particularly female) who presents with chronic, isolated thrombocytopenia without apparent cause. In some cases of SLE and related diseases, true antiplatelet antibodies have been demonstrated.[27] In addition, some investigators have demonstrated a component of myelosuppression contributing to the thrombocytopenia in SLE. Thrombocytopenia generally parallels the course of the disease, with relapses occurring during disease exacerbations.

Therapy of immune complex-mediated thrombocytopenia is generally directed toward treating the underlying immune disorder. Many of the modalities used to treat ITP have been used in the thrombocytopenia associated with lupus and related diseases, but are generally less effective unless the underlying autoimmune disorder is under control. Consequently, splenectomy should be considered only for patients in whom thrombocytopenia persists despite adequate control of their underlying disease, or unless optimal control of the underlying disease is not possible with medical management.

Thrombocytopenia of HIV infection

Thrombocytopenia is noted in up to 10% of asymptomatic and up to 40% of symptomatic HIV-positive adults, and up to 30% of symptomatic HIV-positive children.[28] AIDS patients with advanced disease and those who are IV drug abusers have a somewhat higher incidence of thrombocytopenia. Several studies have indicated that thrombocytopenia can be the initial manifestation of HIV infection, particularly in children, and thrombocytopenia is frequently an important contributor to the morbidity and mortality in children and hemophiliacs.[28] Both immune complexes and true antiplatelet antibodies have been demonstrated in HIV-associated thrombocytopenia; it appears that different subgroups of patients can have different mechanisms for their thrombocytopenia. Immune complex deposition on platelets is the primary cause of thrombocytopenia in HIV-positive homosexual men, and both immune complexes and autoantibodies have been implicated in the thrombocytopenia noted in HIV-positive IV drug abusers. HIV-positive hemophiliacs appear to have a largely autoantibody-mediated thrombocytopenia.[29] A cell-mediated thrombocytopenia has also been demonstrated in patients with advanced HIV infection. Anecdotal reports have demonstrated hemophagocytosis with monocyte–macrophage ingestion of platelets contributing to thrombocytopenia. HIV infection of bone marrow megakaryocytes, with resultant decreased platelet production, may affect some patients.[30]

Although the treatments for classic ITP have been useful in HIV-positive individuals, the thrombocytopenia associated with

HIV infection has been shown to respond to antiretroviral therapy with zidovudine (AZT) in up to 50% of patients.[31] The responses of HIV-positive individuals to IVIG, steroids and splenectomy are similar to those seen in HIV-negative adult ITP patients.[31] In addition, anti-D antibody preparations (WinRho) produce a good response in HIV-positive individuals when either the peak rise in platelet count or the interval between treatments is assessed.[25] Although anti-D has been useful in individuals who are refractory to treatment with IVIG, such individuals are less likely to respond to anti-D therapy than those who do respond to IVIG.

Drug-induced immune thrombocytopenia

Many drugs have the potential to induce an immune thrombocytopenia or immune-mediated platelet dysfunction; the ones most commonly implicated are listed in Table 74.1. Drugs that bind to the platelet surface, resulting in neoantigen formation, or that are highly immunogenic themselves, are more likely to be associated with a clinically significant effect on platelet number or function. The binding of an antibody or immune complex to or near a functionally significant platelet receptor (such as GPIIb/IIIa or GPIb-IX) can result in both thrombocytopenia and platelet dysfunction. As with ITP, the bleeding manifestations in thrombocytopenic states in which intrinsic platelet function is also compromised are significantly greater than in situations associated with thrombocytopenia alone.

Compounds associated with immune thrombocytopenia

Immunologic nature definite	
gold salts	acetazolamide
heparin	carbamazepine
quinine, quinidine	chlorpropamide
hydroxychloroquine, chloroquine	desipramine
methyldopa	digitoxin (digoxin, digitalis)
sulfonamides	*P*-aminosalicylic acid (PAS)
sulfa-trimethoprim	phenytoin
antithymocyte globulin	rifampin
chlorothiazides	stibophen
hydralazine	
Immunologic nature probable	
acetominophen	mercurial diuretics
aminopyrine	organic hair dyes
aspirin, sodium-salicylate	nitroglycerin
barbiturates	penicillins
bismuth	phenacetin
carbutamide	phenylbutazone
cephalosporins	potassium iodide
chlorpheniramine maleate	prednisone
chlorpromazine	prochlorperazine
codeine	propylthiouracil
dextroamphetamine sulfate	pyrazinamide
diazoxide	reserpine
disulfiram (Antabuse)	spironolactone
ergot	streptomycin
erythromycin	tetracycline
furosemide	tetraethylammoniun (TEA)
insecticides	thiourea
iopanoic acid (Telepaque)	trimethadione
isoniazid	turpentine
meperidine	
meprobamate	

Table 74.1 Compounds associated with immune thrombocytopenia.

The mechanisms by which drugs can induce immune platelet destruction are shown in Figures 74.2–74.4. Quinidine and quinine produce thrombocytopenia by the hapten mechanism.[32] In some cases of quinidine- or quinine-induced thrombocytopenia the immune complex reacts with elements of the platelet GP IIb/IIIa or Ib-IX complex.[32] Gold salts are associated with a relatively high incidence of drug-induced immune thrombocytopenia, occurring in 1–5% of all patients treated with these agents. The process appears to be idiosyncratic. The therapy of choice is to discontinue the drug. Typically, this is followed by rebound of the platelet count within 48 hours. Steroids and/or other immunosuppressive agents may be of benefit if the gold salt therapy must be continued.

Heparin is another drug commonly associated with thrombocytopenia. Because of its widespread use in medical practice, heparin-induced thrombocytopenia is an important clinical syndrome. There are at least two mechanisms responsible for this phenomenon. Type I, nonimmunologic thrombocytopenia, reflects the direct binding of heparin to the platelet membrane in a specific, saturable fashion. This binding is dependent on molecular size and charge and is not limited to heparin, as other glycosaminoglycans exhibit the same property. Larger glycosaminoglycans bind more avidly than do small ones, this being a function of charge density.[33] This type I thrombocytopenia is mild and generally resolves after 3–5 days, despite continued heparin exposure. Type II immune-mediated thrombocytopenia is more severe. This is an antibody-mediated process in which a heparin–antibody complex binds to the platelet surface, or alternatively, an antibody binds to a platelet–heparin complex neoantigen. Laboratory studies have demonstrated the involvement of both immunoglobulin and complement in the syndrome of severe immune-mediated heparin-induced thrombocytopenia.[34] Individuals who develop an immune-mediated (type II) heparin-induced thrombocytopenia exhibit a progressive and severe decrease in platelet count following heparin exposure. This is generally observed after rechallenge with heparin or after prolonged (more than 2 weeks) exposure to the drug. Up to 10–20% of individuals with severe immune-mediated thrombocytopenia develop thromboembolic manifestations as a result of in vivo platelet aggregate-induced microvascular obstruction. These patients may present with cutaneous (distal digital), renal, cerebral or pulmonary findings. The thrombocytopenia is persistent and progressive, and only resolves following complete cessation of heparin exposure, with platelet count recovery within 2–5 days.[34,35]

Type I, or nonimmunologic, heparin-induced thrombocytopenia is estimated to occur in up to one-third of patients receiving heparin, and type II is found in no more than 5–10% of exposed patients.[34,35] Low molecular weight heparin appears to cause a lower incidence of both type I and type II thrombocytopenia. The treatment of choice for heparin-induced thrombocytopenia is the cessation of all parenteral heparin. In a limited number of cases low molecular weight heparin has been successfully substituted to provide continued systemic anticoagulation when needed. Aspirin, prostacycline, IVIG and streptokinase have all been used in a small number of patients to treat microthrombotic manifestations of severe heparin-induced thrombocytopenia. Because of the risk of microvascular thrombosis, platelet transfusions are contraindicated unless all heparin exposure has ceased for at least 24–48 hours.

Sepsis and various malignancies have also been associated with immune-mediated thrombocytopenia. In most of these cases immune complex deposition on platelets is thought to result in increased platelet destruction, although true autoantibodies have been demonstrated in anecdotal reports.[36]

Other immune thrombocytopenias

Platelet-specific antigens have been shown to play a role in two unique syndromes of immunologic thrombocytopenia: post-transfusion purpura (PTP) and neonatal alloimmune thrombocytopenia (NAITP). The platelet antigens of interest in these syndromes are listed in Table 74.2. Post-transfusion purpura is a rare disorder (fewer than 200 cases described) characterized by the destruction of autologous platelets after the transfusion of a platelet-containing blood product.[37,38] Thrombocytopenia occurs 5–10 days after the transfusion and persists for up to 120 days. Most patients are women in their fifth or later decade, who have been exposed to blood by transfusion or pregnancy and are PL^{A1} (Zw^a) negative. Other platelet-specific antigens besides PL^{A1} have also been implicated.[39,40] The incidence of severe bleeding manifestations with this syndrome appears to be relatively high (at least 10%). The exact mechanism by which autologous platelets are destroyed as a consequence of exposure to heterologous platelet antigens is unknown. Schulman hypothesized an innocent bystander mechanism, in which the antibody induced by the transfused platelets combines to form soluble immune complexes which then secondarily attach to and destroy autologous platelets.[32] Morrison and Mollison[39] suggested that the anti-PL^{A1} antibody cross-reacts with autologous platelets. Muller-Eckardt and co-workers[40] suggested a third possibility, in which alloantibodies that bind to allogeneic and autologous platelets are induced by the transfused platelets. Steroids, plasmapheresis and plasma exchange have all been used with some benefit in PTP. More recently, high-dose IVIG has been shown to be beneficial in a limited number of patients with PTP, and this now is the treatment of choice.[40]

NAITP results from the transplacental passage of maternal IgG directed against fetal platelet antigens not present on maternal platelets. This syndrome is most commonly noted with PL^{A1}-negative mothers delivering PL^{A1}-positive infants. However, the PL^E, Bak (Lek), Pen (Yuk), Br (Zv) and K antigen systems can also be involved, with Bak^a (Lek^a) being the second most common antigen implicated in NAITP. Many of these antigens are located on functionally important platelet membrane glycoproteins (Table 74.2). Whereas this syndrome is the platelet analog of red cell Rh immunization, unlike Rh disease, thrombocytopenia frequently occurs during the first pregnancy owing to early transfer of fetal platelets into the maternal circulation. The degree of thrombocytopenia generally increases with each succeeding pregnancy. The risk of significant hemorrhage is quite high in this syndrome, with as many as 25% of affected infants suffering prenatal or perinatal intracranial hemorrhage.[41] Recent studies have demonstrated the efficacy of prenatal treatment of mothers with IVIG and corticosteroids.[43] Elective cesarean section is generally advocated in this syndrome because of the high incidence of severe perinatal bleeding. For severely affected infants postnatal treatment with IVIG has been advocated and – anecdotally – has been beneficial. Large controlled trials, however, have not been performed.

Neonatal passive immune thrombocytopenia occurs in infants of mothers with ITP, SLE and related diseases in which a maternal antiplatelet antibody (IgG) is transported transplacentally into the fetal circulation. These infants can be born significantly thrombocytopenic, although profound thrombocytopenia (<50 000) is unusual. Generally, these infants are at low risk for hemorrhage, and vaginal delivery is not contraindicated. The thrombocytopenia may persist for several weeks and is responsive to IVIG.[42] As the antiplatelet immunoglobulin is derived from the maternal circulation, using corticosteroids to suppress antiplatelet antibody production is ineffective.

Platelet alloimmunization is an increasing problem, particularly in cancer chemotherapy patients who are aggressively treated with platelet transfusions. Alloimmunization occurs upon exposure to allogeneic platelets following a blood product transfusion. Exposure of pregnant mothers to fetal platelets also appears to play a role in alloimmunization as multiparous women have a higher incidence of platelet alloimmunization than do nulliparous women. The antigens of interest in this process are HLA Class I antigens (HLA-A and HLA-B; HLA-C locus antigens are rarely implicated). Lymphocytotoxic, anti-HLA-A or HLA-B antibodies can be detected in 30–70% of alloimmunized individuals.[43] However, up to 30% of platelet alloimmunization will be the result of non-HLA antibodies, and the transfusion of HLA-A and HLA-B identical platelets is of limited benefit in these patients. Depletion of platelet concentrates of contaminating leukocytes significantly reduces the incidence of platelet alloimmunization.[44]

Platelet antigen systems

Antigen	Location
PL^{A1} (Zw^a)	GP IIa
PL^E	GP Ib
Bak (Lek)	GP IIb
Pen (Yuk)	GP IIIa
Br (Zv)	GP Ia–IIa
K_o	Undetermined

Table 74.2 Platelet antigen systems.

COAGULATION DEFECTS

Factor VIII inhibitors

Acquired inhibitors to factor VIII are the most common clinically significant inhibitors of coagulation.[45] These inhibitors most frequently occur in hemophiliac patients following exposure to factor VIII; however, they are also noted in nonhemophiliac patients in a variety of clinical settings. These inhibitory antibodies are generally IgG (particularly IgG_4), and can be of either light chain class, although κ chains dominate somewhat. They are generally not complement fixing and do not precipitate; hence the absence of immune complex disease in individuals with factor VIII inhibitors. The antibodies are most often directed against the AII and CII regions of the factor VIII molecule.[46] The inhibitors directed against the light-chain region (CII domain) appear to function by inhibiting factor VIII binding to phosphatidylserine.[46]

CLINICAL PEARLS

Factor VIII antibodies
- IgG (especially IgG_4)
- $\kappa > \lambda$ light-chain use
- Not complement fixing; nonprecipitating
- Most frequently directed against AII and CII domains
- Time- and temperature-dependent reactivity
- Type I
  - Simple kinetics, complete inhibitors
- Type II
  - Complex kinetics, incomplete inhibitors
  - Bind at or near von Willebrand factor-binding site

Factor VIII antibodies are both time and temperature dependent, with the inactivation of factor VIII increasing over time at 37°C. Two types of inactivation kinetics have been described. Type I (simple kinetics or complete) inhibitors are those that exhibit second-order kinetics; the amount of residual factor VIII or antibody is linearly related to the relative concentrations of each. Infusion of factor VIII results in a linear increase in the measured factor VIII activity once all antibody is neutralized. In general, these antibodies recognize sites on the factor VIII molecule near the active site and are not inhibited by the binding of von Willebrand factor (vWf) to the factor VIII molecule. This pattern is typical of inhibitors present in hemophiliacs but is occasionally noted in non-hemophiliac patients.[47] Type II inhibitors (complex kinetics, 'incomplete' inhibitors) are those in which the reaction kinetics with factor VIII is not linear. Incubation of antibody with factor VIII results initially in a rapid inactivation of factor VIII, followed by a slow rate of inactivation that fails to reach an endpoint. With this type of antibody, residual factor VIII activity is generally present, and the measured factor VIII activity does not predictably increase when additional factor VIII is added, indicating continued inactivation of factor VIII. The amount of residual factor VIII activity noted in these patients is not predictive of hemostatic function. These antibodies appear to react near the vWf binding site, and if vWf is removed from factor VIII the antibodies appear to react as type I inhibitors. This type of inhibitor is most typical of those found in nonhemophiliac patients, but is occasionally noted in hemophiliacs also.[47]

Population studies estimate an overall incidence of factor VIII inhibitors in hemophiliacs of 5–20%, with 15% generally being accepted.[48] Inhibitors are noted in severe, moderate and mild hemophilia, although the incidence is greater in the more severe forms. In a large survey of hemophiliacs with inhibitors, 80% had severe, 15% moderate and 4% had mild disease.[48] Inhibitors have been noted in patients who are cross-reacting material (CRM) positive as well as those who are CRM negative. The likelihood of developing an inhibitor is not strictly related to exposure. Most clinically significant inhibitors develop after relatively few exposures, with the majority occurring by the age of 20 years. The risk of developing an inhibitor has been estimated to be 24% by age 20.[48] New inhibitors have been noted to occur after hundreds of exposures late in life; these may be transient and most often are clinically insignificant. Previously untreated patients with hemophilia treated with recombinant human factor VIII have had as high as a 25% incidence of inhibitors developing early in the course of treatment.[49] Most of these are clinically insignificant, and some have been transient. However, the overall incidence of inhibitors in this population appears to be significantly increased over historical controls. The reasons for this are not clear, and may be partly due to closer surveillance.

Sibling studies of hemophiliacs have shown inhibitors to occur six times more frequently in patients whose brothers have inhibitors as in the general hemophiliac population.[50] Concordance is not complete, with only half of the brother pairs studied being concordant for inhibitors. In addition, two pairs of monozygotic twins have also been shown to be discordant for inhibitors despite similar clinical disease parameters.[50] A genetic linkage determining the risk of inhibitor development has been suspected. In one large study[51] the incidence of inhibitors in African-American hemophiliacs was noted to be 20.9% vs. 13.9% for white patients. A clear HLA linkage has not yet been documented, although a possible relationship to HLA-DR genotype as determined by restriction fragment length polymorphism (RFLP) mapping has been suggested.[52]

In the United States the Bethesda Unit assay is generally used to measure factor VIII inhibitor strength, whereas the New Oxford unit assay is generally used in the UK and parts of Europe. One Bethesda Unit equals approximately 1.21 New Oxford inhibitor units. Both types of assay are very reliable for measuring the magnitude of type I inhibitors, but are less useful when quantifying type II inhibitors owing to the residual factor VIII activity present with this type. Characteristically, the more the patient's plasma is diluted, the higher the measured inhibitor titer. For this reason, in the Bethesda Unit assay the inhibitor titer is the lowest dilution of patient plasma (i.e. the most concentrated patient specimen) that inactivates 50% of the normal plasma factor VIII activity, and is expressed as the reciprocal of the dilution producing a 50% inactivation of factor VIII.

Patients with factor VIII antibodies can generally be classified as either 'high responders' or 'low responders'. The distinction is based on the height of the inhibitor rise after rechallenge with factor VIII. High responders develop Bethesda Unit titers of at least 5, and low responders have BU titers below 5. Nonhemophiliac patients typically do not exhibit an anamnestic response to rechallenge with factor VIII, even though most have BU titers above 5 and are classified as high responders.

The survival of hemophiliac patients with inhibitors is increasing because of better methods for managing their acute hemorrhagic complications.[47] Generally, the presence of an inhibitor does not change the type or frequency of bleeding, the one exception being patients with mild hemophilia who develop high-titer inhibitors.[47,48] In contrast, patients with spontaneous factor VIII inhibitors have significant morbidity and mortality. These inhibitors are characterized by the sudden onset of marked bruising and bleeding, with gross hematuria and retroperitoneal, retropharyngeal and intracranial hemorrhage. The mortality rate for these patients is as high as 22% in some series.[53] Most spontaneous inhibitors exhibit complex kinetics (type II) with measurable residual factor VIII activity. The measured factor VIII activity does not correlate well with the severity of the coagulopathy, and in general the Bethesda Unit (or New Oxford) assay underestimates the potency of these inhibitors. The diseases and clinical syndromes in which spontaneous factor VIII inhibitors have been documented are listed in Table 74.3. Some 46% of patients developing a spontaneous factor VIII inhibitor have no

Condition	All cases (%)	Non-idiopathic cases (%)
Idiopathic	46.0	
Periparitum	7.6	14.0
Malignancy	7.5	12.0
Drug	5.4	10.0
SLE	5.4	10.0
Other autoimmune	4.3	8.0
Dermatologic	4.3	8.0
Respiratory	3.8	7.0
Multiple transfusions	2.7	5.0
Other	6.9	11.0

Table 74.3 Conditions associated with spontaneous factor VIII inhibitors.

underlying disease or drug exposure to explain the presence of the inhibitor, and typically are older individuals.[53] Spontaneous factor VIII inhibitors have been demonstrated in both hematologic and nonhematologic malignancies. A causal relationship between the inhibitor and the malignancy has not been determined; current data do not allow the determination of whether the factor VIII antibody is a tumor marker protein.

Particular mention should be made of the factor VIII inhibitors that occur in the peripartum period.[54] These represent 7% of spontaneous inhibitors and differ from other spontaneous factor VIII inhibitors in several ways. These inhibitors usually appear at or near parturition, suggesting a relationship to the immunosuppression of pregnancy. Spontaneous disappearance of these inhibitors is quite common and return with subsequent pregnancies is distinctly uncommon. As with other spontaneous factor VIII inhibitors, there is no anamnestic response to transfused factor VIII.

Autoimmune disorders, as a group, are the most common underlying diseases associated with spontaneous factor VIII inhibitors. Among these are several dermatologic diseases, including psoriasis, pemphigus vulgaris, exfoliative dermatitis, erythema multiforme and erythema annulare centrifugum. Some of these may be related to an unrecognized drug reaction, but in the case of pemphigus at least an underlying autoimmune disorder is thought to be present. The drugs that have been associated with spontaneous factor VIII inhibitors are:

Penicillin
Phenytoin
Chloramphenicol
Sulfonamides
Nitrofurazone
Pheylbutazone

Penicillins are the most commonly implicated.

Many different modalities exist to treat patients with factor VIII inhibitors, whether spontaneous or hemophilia-associated.[47] Factor VIII concentrate has been used in both bolus and continuous-infusion regimens. Bolus infusion is most useful in low-titer low-responder patients with simple kinetics. Continuous-infusion therapy has been equally beneficial in these patients, and the overall amount of factor VIII concentrate required has generally been less than with bolus therapy. The use of factor VIII concentrate is less successful in inhibitors with complex kinetics, although bolus therapy is often used in emergencies to treat these patients. Porcine factor VIII is immunologically different from human factor VIII, and many antifactor-VIII antibodies do not cross-react to a significant degree with the porcine protein. Therapy with this agent is beneficial for high-titer inhibitors with simple kinetics and for inhibitors with complex kinetics. FEIBA (factor VIII inhibitor bypassing activity), prothrombin complex concentrates and activated prothrombin complex concentrates are a family of products that contain, in various amounts, factors IX, X and VII. These products, along with purified factor VIIa, have been used as an alternative to factor VIII concentrate in patients with inhibitors, and appear equally efficacious with either type of inhibitor. Immune tolerance induction was initially utilized in Europe and continues to be more commonly used in Europe. This therapy requires infusions of large amounts of human factor VIII concentrate over a prolonged period of time, and is variably successful. Patients who have type I inhibitors are likely to benefit. Plasmapheresis has been useful in emergencies for acute reduction of the antibody titer. However, as most inhibitors are IgG, the reduction in inhibitor titer is transient and sustained reduction requires aggressive plasmapheresis. Immunoabsorption with ex vivo immunoperfusion over a staphylococcal protein A column to remove IgG has been beneficial acutely but, as with plasmapheresis, responses are generally transient and require several courses to effect a sustained response. Immunosuppression is the cornerstone of the treatment of spontaneous inhibitors and is generally not used in hemophiliac patients unless the inhibitor significantly interferes with clinical management. Several immunosuppressive agents have been used, including alkylating agents and antimetabolites. In addition, IVIG has been used with some success. The mechanism of action of IVIG remains to be fully elucidated, although cases have been reported in which the infused immunoglobulin preparation contained a high-titer antibody specific for the idiotype of the antifactor-VIII antibody.[20,55] When effective, this therapy results in a significant fall of the antifactor-VIII antibody within 24–48 hours, and in some patients antibody titers have remained low for long periods. The synthetic analog of argenine vasopressin, DDAVP (Desmopressin) is useful for the treatment of patients with low-titer type I or type II inhibitors. Infusion of DDAVP stimulates the secretion of factor VIII and vWf from intracellular storage sites and may result in a significant transient increase in circulating factor VIII clotting levels.[56]

Other factor inhibitors

Inhibitors to factor IX occur in up to 3% of hemophilia B patients. These antibodies are generally IgG subclasses 1, 2 and 4, and are not complement fixing or precipitating. Approximately 60% of hemophilia B patients who develop inhibitors have large gene deletions on genetic analysis. Spontaneous factor IX inhibitors occur much less commonly than do inhibitors to factor VIII. The principles of treatment for patients with factor IX inhibitors is similar to those for patients with factor VIII inhibitors. Inhibitors to vWf have been seen in both von Willebrand disease patients and as a spontaneous event. Over 100 patients have been reported, and these inhibitors may be associated with malignancy or autoimmune diseases. Fewer than 50 cases each of inhibitors to factors V, VII, X, XI, XII and XIII have been reported. Although some of these occur in congenitally deficient individuals, many are spontaneous and are associated with underlying autoimmune disorders, malignancy, infection or drug therapy (e.g. factor V deficiency with streptomycin, factor XIII deficiency with isoniazid or practalol). The response to immunosuppressive therapy is variable. The treatment of choice for drug-induced inhibitors is discontinuation of the drug, which generally results in remission.[54] Inhibitors to factor II (prothrombin) have generally been associated with lupus and the so-called lupus inhibitors.

Lupus inhibitors

Lupus inhibitors were first described in patients with SLE in 1953 by Conley and Hartman,[57] and subsequently in many other conditions. Lupus inhibitors are a heterogeneous group of IgG and IgM antibodies directed against negatively charged phospholipids. The anticardiolipin antibody was the first of this type described. More recent studies have demonstrated that the lupus inhibitor antibodies are directed against a complex involving phospholipid-binding proteins (e.g. β_2 GP-1), and not simply the phospholipids themselves.[58] The lupus inhibitor interferes with the prothrombin time (PT) and/or activated partial thromboplastin time (aPTT) in vitro, but does not produce a hemorrhagic diathesis. However, in the presence of another underlying coagulation or hemostasis defect (e.g. platelet dysfunction, thrombocytopenia, hypoprothrombinemia, etc.) bleeding can occur. Although lupus anticoagulants and/or anticardiolipin antibodies have been documented in 6–65% of patients with SLE,[59] only 50% of patients with lupus anticoagulants and/or anticardiolipin antibodies have been shown to have lupus.[60] In general, lupus anticoagulants and/or anticardiolipin antibodies usually remit with effective treatment of the underlying disorder. In several studies the presence of lupus anticoagulants and/or anticardiolipin antibodies (in patients with SLE) have been associated with an increased risk of thrombotic episodes (30–70% vs. 15% in those patients without lupus anticoagulants and/or anticardiolipin antibodies).[61] Whether lupus anticoagulants and anticardiolipin antibodies are identical is unclear, with conflicting reports in the literature.[62,63] It is likely that in most circumstances they are not. Of interest is the finding that patients with drug-induced lupus anticoagulants and/or anticardiolipin antibodies do not appear to be at risk for thrombosis.[60,64]

A well described clinical syndrome of thrombosis in the presence of lupus anticoagulants and/or anticardiolipin antibodies has been described and is referred to as the lupus inhibitor or the anticardiolipin antibody syndrome.[61,65] The risk of fetal wastage in young women with the lupus anticoagulant and/or anticardiolipin antibody syndrome appears to correlate with anticardiolipin antibody titers.[65] Although no clear relationship between antibody specificity and clinical manifestations has been identified, there is a growing body of experimental and epidemiological data suggesting that individuals with antibodies directed against phosphatidylethanolamine (PE) have an increased risk of thrombotic events.[66,67] It is thought that the antibody interaction with PE on the endothelial cell surface creates an environment that inhibits protein C activation and is conducive to thrombin generation.[68,69] In addition, the thrombotic risk of patients with the lupus anticoagulant syndrome may be further enhanced by the increased generation of tissue factor by blood mononuclear cells.[70]

Some patients with lupus anticoagulants will develop concomitant factor II (prothrombin) deficiency as a result of antibodies directed against prothrombin.[71] This antibody forms a complex with circulating prothrombin, resulting in enhanced clearance of this complex. Unlike lupus anticoagulants, only approximately 50% of prothrombin antibodies will remit with effective treatment of the underlying disease. All patients who present with a lupus anticoagulant and prolongation of both PT and aPTT should be evaluated for hypoprothrombinemia, as patients with hypoprothrombinemia are at risk for bleeding with invasive procedures. Inhibition of proteins C and S, as well as the contact-phase complex (prekallikrein, factor XII, factor XI), has also been demonstrated to occur in conjunction with lupus anticoagulants.[72–74] Thrombocytopenia and altered platelet aggregation have also been noted to occur in the presence of anticardiolipin antibodies.[75]

Lupus anticoagulants and/or anticardiolipin antibodies have been noted in up to 90% of HIV-positive individuals.[76,77] They have also been noted in hemophiliacs, although this is probably a result of HIV infection.[78] Other clinical settings in which lupus anticoagulants have been noted include acute inflammation, especially in children with acute or chronic tonsillitis,[79] monoclonal gammopathies[80] and chlorpromazine therapy.[81]

Most patients who manifest a lupus anticoagulant and/or anticardiolipin antibody require no specific therapy, the management of choice being to treat the underlying disorder causing aberrant antibody production. For patients who manifest thrombotic consequences associated with lupus anticoagulant or antiphospholipid antibody, anticoagulation, antiplatelet therapy and aggressive immunosuppression have all been used with some success. In a limited number of patients immunoabsorption and plasmapheresis have been attempted, with mixed results. Several clinical studies have shown the benefit of low-dose aspirin (75 mg daily) plus low-dose subcutaneous heparin (5000 U every 12 h) in reducing the risk of miscarriage in pregnant women with the lupus anticoagulant syndrome.[82] However, because of the increased risk of vertebral fractures, corticosteroids should not be given with heparin.[83]

CLINICAL PEARLS

Lupus anticoagulant anticardiolipin syndrome

- Common findings
  - Thrombosis (arterial or venous)
  - Thrombocytosis
  - Recurrent fetal loss
  - Livido reticularis
  - Pulmonary hypertension
  - False-positive VDRL
- Associated findings
  - Hemolytic anemia
  - Leg ulcers, peripheral vascular insufficiency
  - Labile hypertension
  - Migraine headaches
  - Seizures
  - Cardiac valve disease

REFERENCES

1. Hegde UM. Platelet antibodies in immune thrombocytopenia. Blood Rev 1992;6:340.
2. Court WS, Christensen AK, Sacks RW, LoBuglio AF. Human monocyte interaction with antibody-coated platelets I. General characteristics. Am J Hematol 1984;17:225.
3. Zeigler ZR, Rosenfeld CS, Nemunatis JJ, Vesa EC, Shadduck RK. Increased macrophage colony-stimulating factor levels in immune thrombocytopenia purpura. Blood 1993;81:1251.
4. Semple JW, Freedman S. Increased antiplatelet T helper lymphocyte reactivity in patients with autoimmune thrombocytopenia. Blood 1991;78:2619.
5. Mylvaganam R, Ahn YS, Harrington WJ, Kim CI, Gratzner HG. Differences in T cell subsets between men and women with idiopathic thrombocytopenic purpura. Blood 1985;66:967.
6. Garcia-Suarez J, Prieto A, Reyes E, Manzano L, Merino JL, Alvarez-Mon. Severe chronic autoimmune thrombocytopenic purpura is associated with an expression of CD 56+ CD3– natural killer cells subset. Blood 1993;82:1538.
7. Ballem PJ, Segal GM, Stratton JR, Gernsheimer T, Adamson JW, Slichter SJ. Mechanisms of thrombocytopenia in chronic autoimmune thrombocytopenic purpura, evidence of both impaired platelet production and increased platelet clearance. J Clin Invest 1987;80:33.
8. Parker RI, Siegel RS, Ratajczak MZ, Gewirtz AM. Deficient in vitro megakaryocytopoiesis and decreased in vivo platelet turnover in children and young adults with chronic thrombocytopenia. J Pediatr Hematol/Oncol 1998;20:196.
9. Steinberg MH, Kelton JG, Coller BS. Plasma glycocalicin: an aid in the classification of thrombocytopenic disorders. N Engl J Med 1987;317:1037.
10. Harrington WJ, Minnich V, Hollingsworth JW, Moore CV. Demonstration of a thrombocytopenia factor in the blood of patients with thrombocytopenic purpura. J Lab Clin Med 1951;38:1.
11. Tomer A, Hanson SR, Harker LA. Autologous platelet kinetics in patients with severe thrombocytopenia: discrimination between disorders of production and destruction. J Lab Clin Med 1991;118:546.
12. Siegel RS, Rae JL, Bart S, Coleman RE, Reba RC, Kurlander R, Rosse WF. Platelet survival and turnover: important factors in predicting response to splenectomy in immune thrombocytopenic purpura. Am J Hematol 1989;30:206.
13. Waters AH. Autoimmune thrombocytopenia: clinical aspects. Semin Hematol 1992;29:18.
14. Yanabu M, Suziki M, Soga T, et al. Influences of antiplatelet antibodies on platelet function in immune thrombocytopenic purpura. Eur J Haematol 1991;46:101.
15. Pfueller SL, David R, Firkin BG, Bilston RA, Cortizo WF, Raines G. Platelet aggregating IgG antibody to platelet surface glycoproteins associated with thrombosis and thrombocytopenia. Br J Haematol 1990;74:336.
16. Gratama JW, D'Amaro J, DeKoenig J, denOttolander GJ. The HLA system in immune thrombocytopenic purpura: its relation to the outcome of therapy. Br J Haematol 1984;56:287.
17. McWilliams NB, Maurer HM. Acute idiopathic thrombocytopenic purpura in children. Am J Hematol 1979;7:27.
18. Lusher JM, Emami A, Ravindranath Y, Warrier AI. Idiopathic thrombocytopenic purpura in children. A case for management without corticosteroids. Am J Pediatr Hematol/Oncol 1984;2:149.
19. Gernsheimer T, Stratton J, Ballem PJ, Slichter SJ. Mechanisms of response to treatment in autoimmune thrombocytopenic purpura. N Engl J Med 1989;320:974.
20. Berchold P, Dale G, Tani P, McMillian R. Inhibition of autoantibody binding to platelet glycoprotein IIb/IIIa by anti-idiopathic antibodies in intravenous gammaglobulin. Blood 1989;74:2414.
21. Blanchette V, Adams M, MacMillan L, Wang E. Initial therapy of childhood acute ITP: results of a randomized study comparing IV-IgG, oral prednisone and IV anti-D. Blood 1991;78(Suppl 1):345a, Abstract 1372.
22. Godeau V, Lesage S, Divine M, Wirquin V, Farcet JP, Bierling P. Treatment of adult chronic autoimmune thrombocytopenic purpura with repeated high-dose intravenous immunoglobulin. Blood 1993;82:1415.
23. Jayabose S, Mahmoud M, Levendoglu-Tugal O, et al. Corticosteroid prophylaxis for neurologic complications of intravenous immunoglobulin G therapy in childhood immune thrombocytopenic purpura. J Pediatr Hematol/Oncol 1999;21:514.
24. Ancona K, Prakash D, Mahan R, Gingliano DM, Parker RI. A randomized trial of high dose methylprednisolone vs. IVIG in the treatment of acute ITP in children. J Ped Hematol/oncol 22:373, Abstract 612,2000.
25. Bussel JB, Graziano JN, Kimberly RP, Pahwa S, Aledort LM. Intravenous anti-D treatment of immune thrombocytopenic purpura: analysis of efficacy, toxicity, and mechanism of effect. Blood 1991;77:1884.
26. Andrew M, Blancette V, Adams M, et al. A multi-center study of the treatment of childhood chronic idiopathic thrombocytopenic purpura with anti-D. J Pediatr 1992;120:522.
27. Berchtold P, Harris JP, Tani P, Piro L, McMillan R. Autoantibodies to platelet glycoproteins in patients with disease-related immune thrombocytopenia. Br J Haematol 1989;73:365.
28. Ratner L. Human immunodeficiency virus-associated autoimmune thrombocytopenic purpura: a review. Am J Med 1989;86:194.
29. Karpatkin S, Nardi MA. Immunologic thrombocytopenic purpura in human immunodeficiency virus-seropositive patients with hemophilia. Comparison with patients with classic autoimmune thrombocytopenic purpura, homosexuals with thrombocytopenia, and narcotic addicts with thrombocytopenia. J Lab Clin Med 1988;111:441.
30. Stella CC, Ganser A, Hoezler D. Defective in vitro growth of the hematopoetic progenitor cells in the acquired immunodeficiency syndrome. J Clin Invest 1987;80:286.
31. Oksenhendler E, Bierling P, Farset J-P, Rabian C, Seligmann M, Cauvel J-P. Response to therapy in 37 patients with HIV-related thrombocytopenic purpura. Br J Haematol 1987;66:491.
32. Shulman NR, Jordon JV. Platelet immunology. In: Coleman RW, Hirsh J, Marden VJ, Saltzman VW (eds) Hemostasis and thrombosis. Philadelphia, JB Lippincott, 1982.
33. Horne MK III, Chao ES. Heparin binding to resting and activated platelets. Blood 1989;74:238.
34. Cines DB, Kaywin P, Bina M, Tomaski A, Schreiber AD. Heparin-associated thrombocytopenia. N Engl J Med 1980;303:788.
35. Bell WR. Heparin-associated thrombocytopenia and thrombosis. J Lab Clin Med 1988;111:600.
36. Poskitt TR, Poskitt PKF. Thrombocytopenia of sepsis: the role of circulating IgG-containing immune complexes. Arch Intern Med 1985;45:891.
37. Shulman NR, Aster RH, Leitner A, Hiller MC. Immuno-reactions involving platelets. V. Post-transfusion purpura due to a complement-fixing antibody against a genetically controlled platelet antigen. J Clin Invest 1961;40:1597.
38. van Loghem JJ, Dorfeijer H, Hurt M van der, Sohrender F. Serological and genetic studies on a platelet antigen (Zw). Vox Sang 1959;4:161.
39. Morrison FS, Mollison PL. Post-transfusion purpura. N Engl J Med 1966;275:243.
40. Mueller-Eckhardt C. Post-transfusion purpura. Br J Haematol 1986;64:419.
41. Bussel JB, Berkowitz RL, McFarland JG, Lynch L, Chitkara U. Antenatal treatment of neonatal alloimmune thrombocytopenia. N Engl J Med 1988;319:1374.
42. Samuels P, Bussel JB, Braitman LE, et al. Estimation of the risk of thrombocytopenia in the offspring of pregnant women with presumed immune thrombocytopenic purpura. N Engl J Med 1990;323:229.
43. Lee EJ, Schiffer CA. Serial measurement of lymphocytotoxic antibody in response to non-matched platelet transfusions in alloimmunized patients. Blood 1987;70:1727.
44. van Marwijk Kooy M, van Prooijen HC, Moes M, Bosma-Stants I, Akkerman JW. Use of leukocyte-depleted platelet concentrates for the prevention of refractoriness and primary HLA-alloimmunization: a prospective, randomized trial. Blood 1991;77:201.
45. Shapiro SS, Siegel JE. Hemorrhagic disorders associated with circulating inhibitors. In: Ratinoff OD, Forbes CD (eds) Disorders of hemostasis, 2nd edn. Philadelphia, WB Saunders, 1984, p 245.

46. Arai M, Scandella D, Hoyer LW. Molecular basis for factor VIII inhibition by human antibodies: 1b. Antibodies that bind to the factor VIII light chain prevent the interaction of factor VIII with phospholipids. J Clin Invest 1989;83:1978.
47. Kasper CK. Treatment of factor VIII inhibitors. In: Coller BS (ed) Progress in hemostasis and thrombosis. WB Saunders, 1989, p 57.
48. Schwarzinger I, Pabinger I, Korninger C, et al. Incidence of inhibitors in patients with severe and moderate hemophilia A treated with factor VIII concentrates. Am J Hematol 1987;24:241.
49. Schwartz RS, Abildgaard CF, Aledort LM, et al. Human recombinant NA-derived anti-hemophilic factor (factor VIII) in the treatment of hemophilia A. N Engl J Med 1990;323:1800.
50. Bloom AL. The treatment of factor VIII inhibitors. In: Verstrate M, Vermylen J, Lijnen HR, Arnout J (eds) Thrombosis and haemostatis. Leuven, The Netherlands, Leuven University Press, 1987, p 447.
51. Gill FM. The natural history of factor VIII inhibitors of patients with hemophilia A. Prog Clin Biol Res 1984;150:19.
52. Lippert LE, Fisher LMcA, Schook LB. Relationship of major histocompatability complex Class II genes to inhibitor antibody formation in hemophilia A. Thromb Haemost 1990;64:564.
53. Greene D, Lechner K. A survey of 215 non-hemophilia patients with inhibitors to factor VIII. Thromb Haemost 1981;45:200.
54. Hultin MB. Acquired inhibitors in malignant and non-malignant disease states. Am J Med 91 1991;(Suppl 5A):95.
55. Sultan Y, Rossi F, Kazatchkine MD. Recovery from anti-VIII:C (anti-hemophilic factor) autoimmune disease is dependent on generation of anti-idiotypes against anti-VIII:C autoantibodies. Proc Natl Acad Sci USA 1987;84:828.
56. Naorose-Abidi SM, Bond LR, Chitolie A, Beuan DH. Desmopressin therapy in patients with acquired factor VIII inhibitors. Lancet 1988;i:366.
57. Conley CL, Hartman CA. A hemorrhagic disorder caused by circulating anticoagulants in patients with disseminated lupus erythematosus. J Clin Invest 1953;31:621.
58. Roubey RAS. Autoantibodies to phospholipid binding plasma protein: A new view of lupus anticoagulants and other antiphospholipid antibodies. Blood 1994;84:2854.
59. Petri M, Rheinschmidt M, Whiting-O'Keefe Q, Hellmann D, Corash L. The frequency of lupus anticoagulant in systemic lupus erythematosus. Ann Intern Med 1987;106:524.
60. Gastineau DA, Kazmier FJ, Nichols WL, Bowie EJW. Lupus anticoagulant: an analysis of the clinical and laboratory features of 219 cases. Am J Hematol 1985;19:265.
61. Glueck HI, Kant KS, Weiss MA, Pollak BE, Miller MA, Coots M. Thrombosis in systemic lupus erythematosus. Relation to the presence of circulating anticoagulants. Arch Intern Med 1985;145:1389.
62. Alving BM, Barr CF, Tang DB. Correlation between lupus anticoagulants and anticardiolipin antibodies in patients with prolonged activated partial thromboplastin times. Am J Med 1990;88:112.
63. McNeil HP, Chesterman CN, Krilis SA. Anticardiolipin antibodies and lupus anticoagulants comprise separate antibodies subgroups with different phospholipid binding characteristics. Br J Haematol 1989;73:506.
64. Love PE, Santoro SA. Antiphospholipid antibodies: antiocardiolipin and the lupus anticoagulant in systemic lupus erythematosis (SLE) and in non-SLE disorders. Prevalence and clinical significance. Ann Intern Med 1990;112:682.
65. Hughes GRV. The antiphospholipid syndrome: ten years on. Lancet 1993;342:342.
66. Drouvalakis KA, Buchanan RR. Phospholipid specificity of autoimmune and drug induced lupus anticoagulants; association of phosphatidylethanolamine reactivity with thrombosis in autoimmune disease. J Rheumatol 1998;25:290.
67. Esmon NL, Smirnov MD, Safa O, Esmon CT. Lupus anticoagulants, thrombosis and the protein C system. Haematologica 1999;84:446.
68. Field SL, Hogg PJ, Daly EB, et al. Lupus anticoagulants form immune complexes with prothrombin and phospholipid that can augment thrombin production in flow. Blood 1999;94:3421.
69. Zhao Y, Rumold R, Zhu D, et al. An IgG antiprothrombin antibody enhances prothrombin binding to damaged endothelial cells and shortens plasma coagulation times. Arthritis Rheum 1999;42:2132.
70. Dobado-Berrios P, Lopez-Pedrera C, Velasco F, et al. Increased levels of tissue factor mRNA in mononuclear blood cells of patients with primary antiphospholipid syndrome. Thromb Haemost 1999;82:1578.
71. Bajaj SP, Rapaport SI, Fierer DS, Herbst KD, Schwartz DB. A mechanism or the hypoprothrombinemia of the acquired hypoprothrombinemia–lupus anticoagulant syndrome. Blood 1983;61:684.
72. Malia RG, Kitchen S, Greaves M, Preston FE. Inhibition of activated protein C and its cofactor protein S by antiphospholipid antibodies. Br J Haematol 1990;76:101.
73. Sanfelippo MJ, Drayna CJ. Prekallikrein inhibition associated with the lupus anticoagulant. A mechanism of thrombosis. Am J Clin Pathol 1982;77:275.
74. Cariou R, Tobelem G, Bellucci S, et al. Effects of lupus anticoagulants on anti-thrombogenic properties of endothelial cells inhibition of thrombomodulin-dependent protein C activation. Thromb Haemost 1988;60:54.
75. Hasselaar P, Derksen RHWM, Blokzijl L, de Groot PG. Cross-reactivity of antibodies directed against cardiolipin, DNA, endothelial cells and blood platelets. Thromb Haemost 1990;63:169.
76. Bloom EJ, Abrams DI, Rodgers G. Lupus anticoagulant in the acquired immunodeficiency syndrome. JAMA 1986;256:491.
77. Stimmler MM, Quismorio FP Jr, McGehee WG, Boylen T, Sharma OP. Anticardiolipin antibodies in acquired immunodeficiency syndrome. Arch Intern Med 1989;149:1833.
78. Cohen H, Mackie IJ, Anagnostopoulos N, Savage GF, Machin SJ. Lupus anticoagulant, anticardiolipin antibodies, and human immunodeficiency virus in hemophilia. J Clin Pathol 1989;42:629.
79. Singh AK, Rao KPP, Kaizer J, Lazarchick J. Lupus anticoagulants in children. Ann Clin Lab Sci 1988;18:384.
80. Gleicher N, Friberg J. IgM gammopathy and a lupus anticoagulant syndrome in habitual aborters. JAMA 1985;253:3278.
81. Canoso RT, Size HS. Chloropromazine-induced lupus anticoagulant and associated immunologic abnormalities. Am J Hematol 1982;13:121.
82. Backos M, Rai R, Baxter N, et al. Pregnancy complications in women with recurrent miscarriage associated with antiphospholipid antibodies treated with low dose aspirin and heparin. Br J Obstet Gynaecol 1999;106:102.
83. Cowchock S. Treatment of antiphospholipid syndrome in pregnancy. Lupus 1998;7(Suppl 2):S95.

Chapter 75 Bullous Diseases of the Skin and Mucous Membranes

Russell P. Hall

Over the last four decades a number of skin diseases previously characterized only by their clinical presentations have been demonstrated to be organ-specific and autoimmune in nature. In most cases they have been associated with antibodies directed against specific proteins found in human skin. The discovery of these antibodies, followed by the subsequent characterization of the specific antigens, has led to a better understanding of the pathogenesis of these diseases and an increased understanding of the role these molecules play in the normal function of stratified squamous epithelium. This chapter focuses on the pathophysiology of the major autoimmune blistering skin diseases. These diseases not only increase our understanding of basic mechanisms of autoimmunity, but also provide insight into the structure–function relationship of these antigenic targets in the function of normal human skin.

PEMPHIGUS

Pemphigus is the term used to describe a group of diseases that have in common superficial blistering of the skin and mucous membranes.[1–3] Pemphigus can now be separated into four distinct groups: pemphigus vulgaris, pemphigus foliaceus, paraneoplastic pemphigus, and intraepidermal IgA neutrophilic dermatosis.

Pemphigus vulgaris

Pemphigus vulgaris (PV) is the most severe form of pemphigus. PV presents most often in the fourth to sixth decades, but has been reported to occur at any age.[1–3] Clinically, patients with PV are characterized by the presence of flaccid blisters and erosions of the skin and mucous membranes. Essentially all patients with PV will develop oral erosions at some point during the course of their disease. Most present with oral erosions and many have oral erosions as their only disease manifestation for months to years.[1–3] These lesions are often persistent, shaggy erosions that can involve all areas of the oral mucosa, extending into the esophagus.[1–3] In addition, in severe cases other mucous membranes, such as the conjunctiva, nasal, anal, cervical or urethral mucosa, can also be affected.

The blisters seen in patients with PV are flaccid, easily ruptured, and can occur on either inflamed or noninflamed skin.[1–3] The ease with which these blisters rupture is the origin of the Nikolsky sign, which is elicited when lateral traction on the skin results in desquamation of the superficial aspect of the skin. This sign, although helpful, is not unique to PV. The ease with which these blisters are broken results in large, nonhealing erosions. Blisters can occur on any area of the skin, most often beginning on the head and neck and trunk. Generalized blistering is not uncommon, especially if diagnosis and/or treatment has been delayed.

> **KEY CONCEPTS**
>
> **Pemphigus vulgaris**
> - Flaccid blisters with denuded epidermis
> - Oral mucous membrane lesions common
> - Suprabasilar blister with 'row of tombstones'
> - IgG deposits on keratinocyte cell surface (antigenic target = desmoglein-3)

Pemphigus vegetans is thought to represent an unusual variant of PV in which lesions develop that are localized primarily to the axilla, groin and other flexural areas. The lesions are characterized as hypertrophic granulation tissue with occasional pustules. This presentation can occur de novo or after healing of PV lesions. The etiology of this unusual clinical presentation is not known.

PV was almost uniformly fatal before the advent of systemic glucocorticoid therapy, with patients developing large areas of denuded skin and dying from overwhelming sepsis.[3] Since the advent of systemic glucocorticoids, however, the mortality rate has fallen to approximately 10%,[4] associated with the high doses required to treat the disease, particularly in debilitated or elderly patients.

Histologically, PV is characterized by the presence of an intraepithelial blister, with acantholysis or breaking apart of the suprabasilar portion of the epidermis.[1–3] Biopsy of an early lesion of PV reveals that the basal cells of the epidermis remain attached to the dermis, forming a 'row of tombstones', with a loss of attachment of individual keratinocytes to each other, resulting in the formation of an intraepidermal blister.

A major advancement in the understanding of PV occurred in the early 1960s, when Beutner and co-workers described IgG antibodies directed against the epithelial keratinocyte cell surface in the skin of patients with PV.[5,6] They also demonstrated that the serum of patients with PV had IgG antibodies that bound identically to normal human skin in vitro. These findings demonstrated that PV represented an autoimmune disease directed against a normal component of stratified squamous epithelium.[5]

Pemphigus foliaceus

Pemphigus foliaceus (PF) is the second major variant of the pemphigus group of diseases. It is characterized by blisters within the epidermis, resulting in the development of superficial erosions with scaling and crusting[1,2,7] (Fig. 75.1). Unlike patients with PV, those with PF rarely develop mucous membrane lesions. Because of the superficial nature of the blister many patients present with only erythematous, scaling and crusted plaques on the head, neck

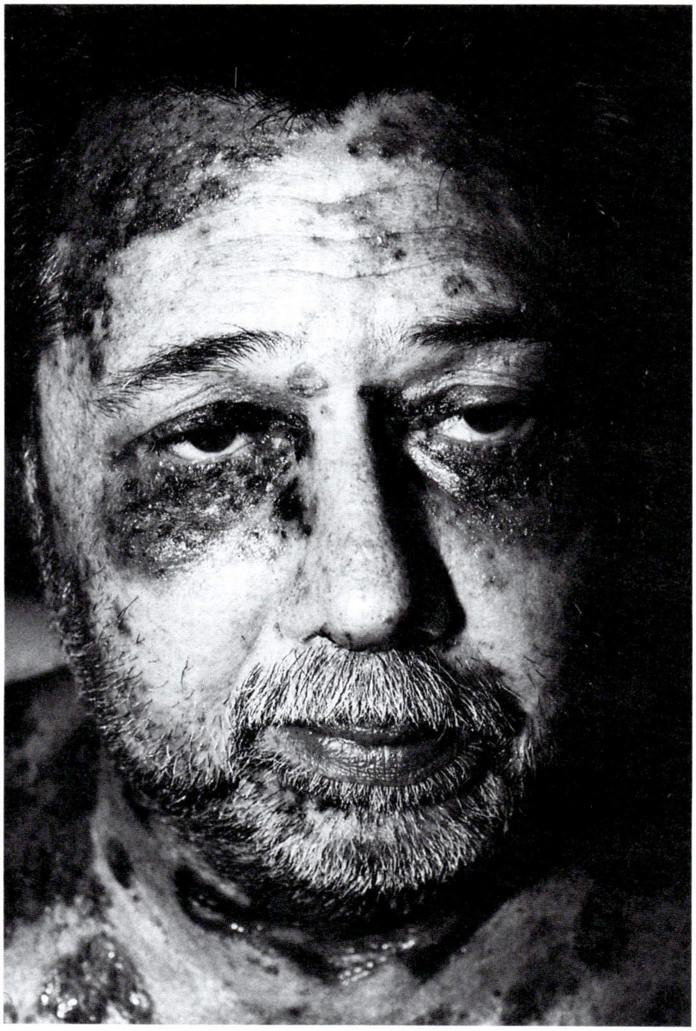

Figure 75.1 Patient with pemphigus foliaceus showing superficial erosions and crust formation on the head and neck.

and trunk. The prognosis for patients with PF is markedly better than for those with PV, although occasionally patients with severe disease can die, usually as a result of infectious complications of the disease and/or therapy. The improved prognosis is most likely secondary to the more superficial nature of the blistering process.

An unusual variant of PF is the endemic form of the disease, 'fogo selvagem' (Portuguese for wild fire).[7] This is identical to the sporadic form of PF but is endemic to certain rural areas of South America. The epidemiology suggests an infectious etiology, and preliminary data suggest that an arthropod vector may be relevant in the spread of the disease.[7–9]

Another variant of PF is pemphigus erythematosus, or Senear–Usher Syndrome.[10] These patients have typical features of PF with additional characteristics suggestive of systemic lupus erythematosus. The clinical course tends to parallel that of PF, and most patients do not develop systemic lupus erythematosus. The pathogenesis of this form of PF is poorly understood.

PF can also be associated with the use of drugs. The most common agents that induce pemphigus are D-penicillamine and captopril, or other angiotensin-converting enzyme inhibitors.[11] Although these drugs may induce a PV-like picture, the clinical manifestations are usually similar to those seen in patients with PF. The pathogenetic mechanism is not known, but it has been postulated that a reactive sulfhydryl or amide group common to these drugs plays an important part.

KEY CONCEPTS

Pemphigus foliaceus
- Flaccid blisters with scale and crust
- Oral mucous membrane lesions rare
- Intraepidermal blister, granular cell layer
- IgG deposits on keratinocyte cell surface (antigenic target = desmoglein-1)

The histology of a PF blister reveals a superficial, intraepidermal blister with acantholysis of only the most superficial portion of the skin.[3] This blistering occurs in the region of the granular cell layer of the skin, with the result that blisters have a base of epithelium and not the single basal cell layer as is seen in patients with PV.

The immunologic features of PF observed using direct or indirect immunofluorescence are indistinguishable from those seen in patients with PV (Fig. 75.2). Cell surface deposits of IgG are seen in the skin of patients with PF, and circulating IgG, which binds to normal stratified squamous epithelium, is present in patients with PF.[1,2] Although the immunofluorescence patterns are virtually identical between PF and PV, the antigenic targets of these autoantibodies are different, as discussed later in this chapter.

Paraneoplastic pemphigus

Anhalt and co-workers described occasional patients who presented with a heterogeneous picture of severe oral erosions and polymorphic skin lesions suggestive of both PV and erythema multiforme.[12,13] In each of these cases the patients had an associated malignancy, generally lymphoreticular and including lymphoma, chronic lymphocytic leukemia or thymomas. The

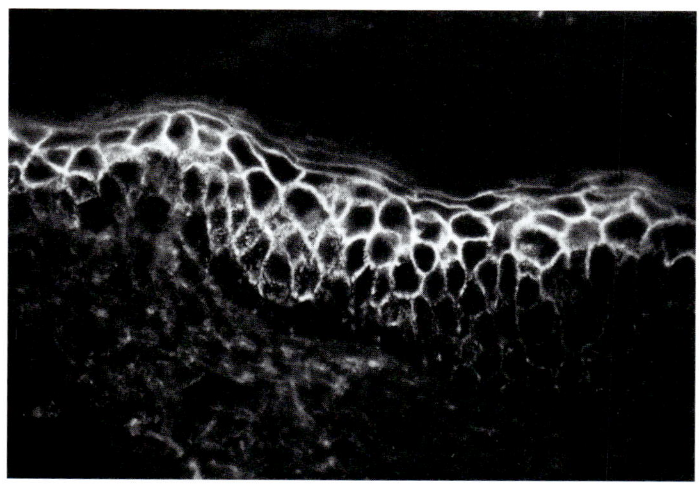

Figure 75.2 Direct immunofluorescence of perilesional normal-appearing skin from a patient with pemphigus foliaceus using antibodies directed against human IgG. Cell surface IgG deposits are seen on the epidermal keratinocytes.

histologic features of the skin lesions in these patients resembled that seen in patients with PV, with suprabasilar blister formation but with the additional finding of keratinocyte cell necrosis, as seen in erythema multiforme. The immunopathology of skin biopsies from these patients revealed IgG bound to keratinocyte cell surfaces, and granular–linear deposits of IgG and C3 at the basement membrane. In addition, circulating IgG was present in the serum of these patients, which bound to normal keratinocyte cell surfaces of squamous epithelium.[13] Although initial reports suggested that this antibody bound to both nonstratified and stratified squamous epithelium, this has not proved to be the case in all instances. The antigenic targets of these antibodies are also distinct from both PV and PF, as discussed later.

Intraepidermal neutrophilic IgA dermatosis

In 1985, a patient with an annular, vesiculopustular eruption characterized by intraepidermal blisters with numerous polymorphonuclear leukocytes (PMN) and intercellular deposits of IgA on direct immunofluorescence staining was described by Huff et al.,[14] who proposed the name intraepidermal neutrophilic IgA dermatosis. This entity has subsequently been described by other investigators and has been referred to by several different names, including IgA pemphigus, intercellular IgA vesiculopustular dermatosis and intercellular IgA dermatosis.

Patients with this disorder present with a heterogeneous clinical picture. Some present with tense blisters that enlarge peripherally to form a 'flower-like' grouping, whereas others present with superficial pustules, erosions and crusts. Sites of involvement include the trunk, abdomen, face, scalp and extremities, but mucosal involvement has not been reported. Routine histology of lesional skin reveals the presence of either a subcorneal or an intraepidermal blister, with acantholytic cells and a polymorphous infiltrate marked by the predominance of polymorphonuclear leukocytes.[14]

The immunopathology of these patients has proved distinctive. Direct immunofluorescence of perilesional skin biopsies from all patients shows keratinocyte cell surface deposits of IgA. These deposits have been localized to the lower two-thirds of the epidermis in a subset of patients with a superficial pustular dermatitis-like disease. Approximately half of these patients with intraepidermal neutrophilic IgA dermatosis have detectable but low-titer circulating IgA antibodies specific for epithelium.[14]

Pathogenesis

The discovery by Beutner and co-workers that IgG antibodies directed against normal human skin were present in the skin and serum of patients with pemphigus provided the first suggestion that these diseases may be the result of antibodies reacting with autoantigens.[5,6] Over the last decade the specific nature of the antigenic targets in these diseases has been defined (Table 75.1). Sera from patients with different forms of pemphigus bind to different components of desmosomes, a key structure involved in the adhesion of keratinocytes.[15–18] IgG from patients with PF binds to a 160 kDa glycoprotein, desmoglein-1.[19,20] Immunoprecipitation studies by Korman and co-workers demonstrated that desmoglein-1 is complexed with an 85 kDa protein, plakoglobin, which is found in the cytoplasmic plaque of both types of intercellular junctions (adherens junctions and desmosomes).[16,19] In contrast, IgG from patients with PV binds to a distinct 130 kDa glycoprotein, desmoglein-3, a unique epithelial cadherin with significant homology to desmoglein-1.[15,20] This 130 kDa protein is also complexed to plakoglobin.

Immunopathology of autoimmune blistering diseases

Disease	Direct IF (patient's skin)	Indirect IF (patient's serum)	Antigen(s)
Pemphigus vulgaris	IgG keratinocyte cell surface	IgG binds keratinocyte cell surface (normal stratified squamous epithelium)	Desmoglein-3, DG3
Pemphigus foliaceus	IgG keratinocyte cell surface	IgG binds keratinocyte cell surface (normal stratified squamous epithelium)	Desmoglein-1, DG1
Paraneoplastic pemphigus	IgG keratinocyte cell surface; C3, granular/linear at epidermal basement membrane	IgG binds keratinocyte cell surface (normal stratified and nonstratified squamous epithelium)	Desmoplakin I, II envoplakin, periplakin 230 kDa, BPAg1 190 kDa, antigen
Herpes gestationis	Linear C3 at epidermal basement membrane (in 30–50% of patients linear IgG also seen)	IgG binds in linear pattern normal stratified squamous epithelium basement membrane (epithelial side)	180 kDa, BPAg2
Bullous pemphigoid	Linear IgG, C3 at epidermal basement membrane	IgG binds in linear pattern normal stratified squamous epithelium basement membrane (epithelial side)	180 kDa, BPAg2 230 kDa, BPAg1
Epidermolysis bullosa acquisita	Linear IgG epidermal basement membrane (IgA rarely)	IgG binds in linear pattern normal stratified squamous epithelium basement membrane (dermal side)	Type VII collagen (noncollagenous domain)
Dermatitis herpetiformis	Granular IgA dermal papillary tips	Negative	Unknown
Linear IgA bullous dermatosis	Linear IgA at epidermal basement membrane	IgA binds linear pattern normal stratified squamous epithelium basement membrane (epithelial side)	97 kDa protein (portion of BPAg2)

Table 75.1 Immunopathology of autoimmune blistering diseases.

In paraneoplastic pemphigus IgG antibodies have immunoprecipitated a complex of 250 000, 230 000, 210 000 and 190 000 kDa proteins,[13,17] which are members of the plakin family of desmosomal/hemidesmosomal proteins.

Sera from patients with intraepidermal IgA neutrophilic dermatosis have also been used to determine the antigenic targets relevant for this disease. Serum from a patient with the intraepidermal neutrophilic variant recognized a 120 kDa protein from extracts of normal human skin and bovine desmosomes.[21,22] In contrast, sera from patients with subcorneal pustular dermatosis-like disease recognized proteins in a bovine desmosomal extract that were identified as the desmosomal proteins desmocollin I and II.[21,22]

In addition to the identification of the specific antigens against which the IgG from patients with pemphigus react, it has been clearly demonstrated that these antibodies are pathogenic. Anhalt and co-workers developed an animal model that demonstrated the pathogenicity of the autoantibodies found in many forms of pemphigus.[23] In this model neonatal mice were injected with IgG from patients with pemphigus. Cutaneous blisters and erosions, histologic changes and immunofluorescence findings consistent with pemphigus were present in the animals injected with pemphigus IgG, but not those with normal IgG. This has been shown to be true for sera from patients with PV, PF and paraneoplastic pemphigus.[13,23,24] This animal model has also been used to further define an antigenic epitope of the PV antigen to the amino-terminal cadherin-binding domain of desmoglein-3.[25] Similar studies demonstrated that specific antibodies against desmoglein-1 are responsible for blister formation in pemphigus foliaceus.[26] Together, studies demonstrate that the IgG directed against desmogleins-1 and -3, found in the sera of patients with PV and PF, respectively, can induce the clinical, histologic and immunologic manifestations of the diseases.

Despite the clearly demonstrated importance of these autoantibodies in disease pathogenesis, the exact mechanism by which they cause acantholysis is not known. The finding of complement components (C3, C1q) in the lesional skin of patients with pemphigus, as well as the findings of low levels of complement in blister fluid, initially suggested that complement may play a crucial role in blister formation. It has been shown that IgG from patients with pemphigus can fix complement, and that complement fixation in vitro can lead to keratinocyte cell membrane damage in vitro.[27] There is, however, evidence that autoantibodies can induce acantholysis both in vitro and in the neonatal mouse model without complement activation.[28] In total, these data suggest that although complement may play a role in acantholysis, especially in an additive fashion, pemphigus IgG alone is capable of attaching to the keratinocyte and inducing the characteristic loss of cell–cell adhesion.

A new mouse model has recently been developed that may help define the regulation of the immune response in patients with pemphigus and other autoimmune skin diseases.[29] This model involves the immunization of desmoglein-3 knockout mice with native desmoglein-3, leading to an immune response against this antigen. Lymphocytes from these mice are then transferred into Rag-2 immunodeficient recipients which lack their own T and B cells but express desmoglein-3. Studies showed that the immune reconstituted Rag-2$^{-/-}$ desmoglein-3-expressing mice developed circulating antibody directed against desmoglein-3 along with clinical and histologic evidence of pemphigus vulgaris-like disease.[29] Although this model does not address the events that lead to the development of autoantibodies, it may prove useful for studying factors critical in regulating and maintaining disease.

Although it is clear that serum IgG autoantibodies are of primary importance in the development of pemphigus, the factors that lead to the development of the autoimmune response are not known. A possible role of genetics in pemphigus was first postulated because of the increased incidence of this disease in Askenazi Jews, and early work focused on the possible contribution of the HLA system to the development of pemphigus. A number of investigators have demonstrated an increased frequency of HLA-DR4 and HLA-DR6 in patients with PV.[30,31] Healthy relatives of patients with PV were also shown to have low levels of autoantibodies directed against an epidermal antigen similar to the PV antigen, and the presence of these antibodies was associated with HLA-DR4 or -DR6.[32] Additional studies have shown that a specific HLA-DR4 subtype (DRB1*0402) is associated with pemphigus vulgaris.[33] This DR4 subtype is distinct from those DR4 molecules associated with rheumatoid arthritis (Chapters 58 and 61). Studies also showed that T cells from patients with PV secreted high levels of IL-4 and IL-10 in response to specific desmoglein-3 peptides when presented by DRB1* 0402.[33] Other workers have also shown that T cells reactive against desmoglein-3 are present in patients with PV, and that T cells from some normal HLA DRB1*0402 subjects also responded to desmoglein-3.[34] It is still not clear what additional factors are required for HLA-susceptible individuals to develop clinical disease, but it seems that additional susceptibility genes and environmental factors are probably needed for the disease to develop (Chapter 58).

Fogo selvagem, a form of pemphigus foliaceus that is endemic in certain regions of Brazil, is associated with particular HLA-DRB1 alleles (DRB1*1042, *1406 and *0404).[8,35] The prevalence of antibodies against desmoglein-1 is high among normal subjects living in areas where fogo selvagem is endemic, and the onset of desease is preceded by a sustained antibody response.[9] These findings support the concept that the production of antibodies against desmoglein-1 is initiated by an environmental agent in these areas. In this regard, fogo selvagem has been associated with exposure to the hematophagous black flies found in the endemic areas of Brazil.[36] It has been suggested that the development of fogo selvagem may be related to an immune response to the bite of this fly in the HLA-susceptible individuals who develop cross-reactive antibodies against desmoglein-1. Further investigation of this phenomenon holds promise for developing a new understanding of the initial events that may occur in patients with PF, PV, and potentially other organ-specific autoimmune diseases.

Therapy

Before the advent of systemic glucocorticoids, pemphigus, especially PV, was uniformly fatal.[2,3] Since that time, the use of high-dose systemic glucocorticoids and improvements in wound care have markedly reduced the mortality. Most blistering in patients can be controlled with doses of 1–2 mg/kg/day of prednisone, often in divided doses,[1,2] and the dose can be tapered slowly toward alternate-day therapy. Although the majority of patients are controlled by this method, occasional patients may flare during the taper. These patients must be managed on an individual basis, taking into account the adverse effects of continuing high-dose systemic glucocorticoid therapy.

The chronic nature of this disease makes long-term follow-up of all patients mandatory. Often the addition of immunosuppressive agents, such as azathioprine, cyclophosphamide, mycophenolate mofetil, methotrexate or cyclosporin A, is needed.[4] However, no prospective, controlled trials have demonstrated the efficacy of these agents in the treatment of PV.[4] The relatively low toxicity of azathioprine (1–3 mg/kg/day) may make this drug a more frequent first-line immunosuppressive agent. Other agents, including parenteral gold compounds, plasmapheresis, high-dose intravenous immunoglobulin, and extra corporeal photochemotherapy, have been suggested as adjunctive therapy. However, none have been shown in controlled studies to improve results compared to glucocorticoids alone.

Treatment for patients with PF follows many of the same guidelines as for those with PV; however, it should be noted that this disease is in general less severe and rarely fatal, and therapy should be designed with this in mind. Indeed, many patients with limited disease can be treated with high-potency topical glucocorticoids. Dapsone has proved to be the mainstay of therapy for patients with intraepidermal IgA neutrophilic dermatosis, most probably owing to the presence of a neutrophilic infiltrate in their skin.[14] Occasionally systemic glucocorticoid therapy may be needed, either alone or in conjunction with dapsone, to control the eruption in some patients. Therapy for paraneoplastic pemphigus has been disappointing and in general unsuccessful.

BULLOUS PEMPHIGOID

Clinical features

Bullous pemphigoid (BP) is characterized clinically by the presence of extremely pruritic, tense blisters that can occur on either inflamed or noninflamed skin[1,37] (Fig. 75.3). These can range in size from small (1–5 mm) vesicles to large bullous lesions several centimeters in diameter. Because the blister is subepidermal its roof comprises the entire epidermis and, as such, often remains intact. In addition to the characteristic tense blisters, patients with BP can also present with a variety of other skin manifestations, including urticarial lesions, vesicular lesions or, rarely, eczematous dermatitis. Blisters can occur on any part of the skin, but often localize to the extremities, groin and axilla. Oral and ocular mucosal lesions occur infrequently in patients with BP and, when seen, are often of minor importance. This is in contrast to patients with cicatricial pemphigoid, who have predominantly mucosal lesions.

KEY CONCEPTS

Bullous pemphigoid

- Tense subepidermal blisters
- Oral mucous membrane lesions rare
- Subepidermal blister, most often with inflammatory infiltrate with eosinophils
- Linear deposits of IgG and C3 at the dermal–epidermal junction (antigenic target 230 and 180 kDa hemidesmosomal proteins)

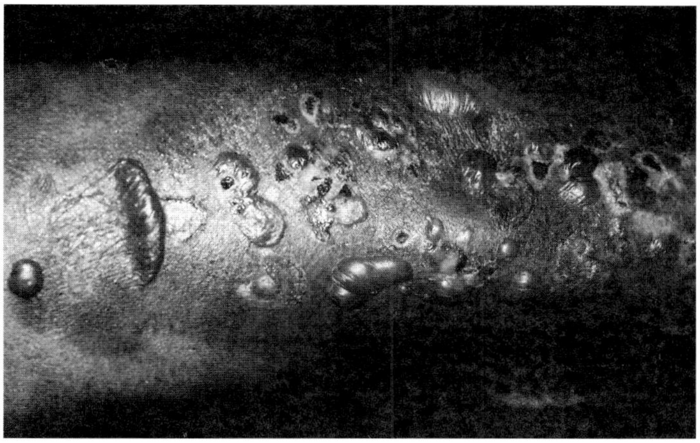

Figure 75.3 Patient with bullous pemphigoid showing erythematosus plaques with tense subepidermal blisters.

Although BP is primarily a disease of the elderly, with most patients being over the age of 60, BP can develop at any age. It has also been reported to be associated with other diseases, including diabetes mellitus, psoriasis, other autoimmune diseases and malignancy.[37] The association with malignancy has been noted in case reports and retrospective studies for many years. However, when age- and sex-matched control studies were performed, no statistically increased incidence of malignancy was documented in patients with BP.[38] BP has also been associated with the ingestion of drugs, with furosemide and phenacetin being the most commonly noted. Finally, environmental factors such as ultraviolet light and therapeutic radiation have been reported to precipitate BP.

Biopsy of an early lesion of BP can reveal a number of different patterns, consistent with the polymorphic appearance of the eruption. The classic finding is a subepidermal blister with an inflammatory infiltrate in the dermis, comprised predominantly of eosinophils with an admixture of lymphocytes, histiocytes and neutrophils.[37] The epidermis over this blister is often intact with minimal abnormality, whereas the blister cavity is filled with inflammatory cells. Variants of this presentation can be seen, including a neutrophil-predominant inflammatory infiltrate, or a 'cell-poor' variant with few inflammatory cells. Occasionally an early lesion of BP may not show a subepidermal blister but rather only edema of the epidermis, with an infiltrate of eosinophils. Because of the polymorphic histology of BP, it is important to realize that the diagnosis of this disease cannot rely solely on the histologic and clinical findings.

Patients with BP usually have IgG present in a linear pattern at the dermal–epidermal junction (DEJ),[6] as well as circulating IgG antibodies that bind in a similar linear pattern at the DEJ of normal human skin.[39] Direct and indirect immunofluorescence studies are currently the mainstay of the diagnosis of BP. Whereas 70–90% of patients have linear deposits of IgG at the DEJ, 90–100% of patients with BP have linear deposits of C3 at the DEJ[37] (Fig 75.4). C3 may be the only immunoreactant seen in the skin of patients with BP.[6] By indirect immunofluorescence analysis, 70–90% of patients with BP have a circulating IgG that binds in a linear pattern at the DEJ of normal human skin. Although these antibodies are often present at high levels, no consistent relationship has been demonstrated between the presence or

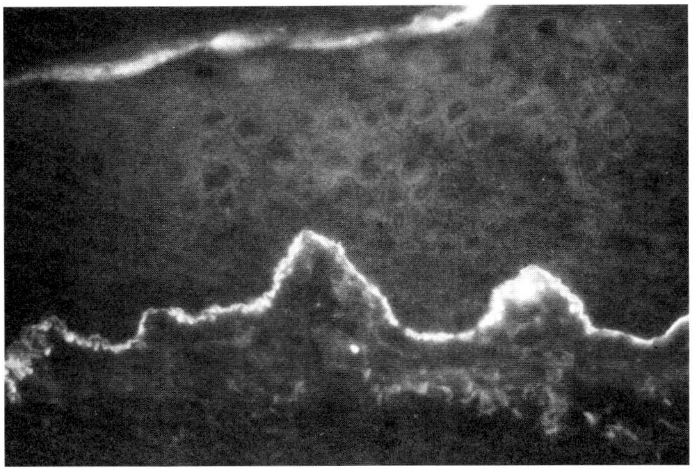

Figure 75.4 Direct immunofluorescence of perilesional normal-appearing skin from a patient with bullous pemphigoid using antibodies directed against human C3. A linear band of C3 is present at the basement membrane.

level of antibodies directed against the DEJ and clinical disease activity or prognosis.[37,40]

Although the immunofluorescent findings in patients with BP are characteristic, they are not diagnostic. Other immunologically mediated blistering diseases, such as the bullous eruption of systemic lupus erythematosus, herpes gestationis and epidermolysis bullosa acquisita (EBA), can have similar patterns of immunoreactivity.[41,42] Gammon and co-workers reported that the use of normal human skin split with 1 M NaCl can help in distinguishing antibodies directed against the BP antigen and the EBA antigen.[43] NaCl treatment splits the skin within the lamina lucida, and IgG from patients with BP binds to the epidermal side only or to the epidermal and dermal sides, whereas antibodies from patients with EBA bind only to the dermal side (Fig. 75.5). Similar studies with NaCl-treated skin of BP patients demonstrated that IgG deposited in vivo is also localized to the epidermal side of the split skin.[44]

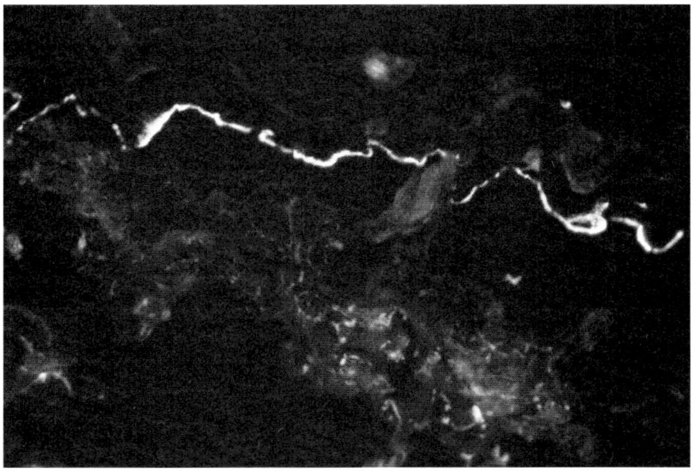

Figure 75.5 Indirect immunofluorescence using serum from a patient with bullous pemphigoid. Serum was incubated with frozen sections of normal human skin which had been incubated with 1 M NaCl. IgG deposits are present on the epithelial basement membrane associated with the epidermis and not on the dermal side of the split skin.

Pathogenesis

The presence of IgG and C3 at the DEJ has suggested that the interaction of an IgG autoantibody with a component of normal stratified squamous epithelium is the underlying pathogenetic event involved in BP. Initial steps to better understand the pathogenesis of BP have therefore focused on the antigenic target(s) of the IgG antibody.

Immunoelectron microscopic studies have demonstrated that the in vivo deposits of IgG are localized to the lamina lucida of the basement membrane, and that the target antigen is a component of hemidesmosomes,[45] which are the major attachment site of epidermal basal cells. Hemidesmosomes also serve as the site of linkage for cytoskeletal proteins, the keratins, through the plasma membrane to the dermis.[46] Further characterization of the antigen–antibody interaction in patients with BP revealed that a major bullous pemphigoid antigen is a 230 kDa protein present in epidermal cell extracts.[47,48a] Sera from 97% of BP patients with antibodies to the basement membrane zone immunoprecipitate this protein.[46–47]. Sera from 30–50% of patients with BP also react with other proteins, including a 166 kDa band on immunoblot (180 kDa band on immunoprecipitation).[48b] The 230 and 180 kDa BP antigens are distinct proteins, associated as a complex within the hemidesmosome in the native state.[49] Using a sensitive and specific ELISA assay it has been shown that essentially all patients with BP have antibodies to the 180 kDa BP antigen.[50]

The 230 kDa and the 180 kDa BP antigens have both been cloned and sequenced, confirming that the 230 kDa (BPAg1) and the 180 kDa BP (BPAg2) antigens are distinct proteins.[51,52] The 230 kDa BP antigen (BPAg1) contains sequence homology with desmoplakin I, a protein found in desmosomes, suggesting that 230 kDa BPAg and desmoplakin I are members of an adhesion junction plaque protein family.[52] In addition, it is important to note that no extracellular regions of the 230 kDa BP antigen have been identified. Epitope mapping studies have been performed using the cDNA of the 230 kDa BP antigen to characterize the immunorelevant regions of the antigen, and have demonstrated that antibodies in the sera of patients with BP are directed against multiple epitopes on the native protein, most consistent with an antigen-driven immune response. The 180 kDa BP antigen (BPAg2) contains both intra- and extracellular domains joined by a transmembrane region. The extracellular portion of this protein is remarkable for the presence of alternating collagen and noncollagen domains with identity to a chick corneal protein.[51] Epitope mapping studies of the 180 kDa protein have identified an immunodominant epitope that maps to an extracellular domain adjacent to the transmembrane region.[53] This same region of the 180 kDa protein is a target for circulating antibodies in the sera of patients with herpes gestationis.[53]

Although patients with BP have antibody reactivity against both the 230 kDa and the 180 kDa antigens, the role of these autoantibodies in the pathogenesis of BP has not been clearly established. The 230 kDa BPAg1 is located inside the cell, and it is unclear how the autoantibodies may have access to the antigen. Attempts to develop an animal model of BP by passively transferring IgG from patients to animals have been unsuccessful.

Hall and co-workers[54] developed an animal model using rabbits that had been immunized with peptides derived from the 230 kDa BP antigen cDNA. Immunized animals developed high-titer antibody against the 230 kDa BP antigen, but there was no evidence of blistering or immunoglobulin deposition in skin. When the rabbits were irradiated with ultraviolet light, producing a minimal erythema, the animals with circulating antibody against the 230 kDa BP antigen developed a marked inflammatory response. Histology showed loss of the epidermis and a linear band of C3 and IgG at the DEJ. Target disruption of the gene encoding BPAg1 did not result in blister formation or epidermal–dermal adhesion abnormalities.[54a] These studies suggest that antibodies to BPAg1 do not directly inhibit BPAg1 its function. They may, however, play an important role in maintaining or enhancing the inflammatory response in patients with BP.

Patients with both BP and herpes gestationis develop antibodies against a noncollagenous, extracellular portion of the BPAg2 molecule.[53] In order to develop an animal model of BP, rabbits were immunized to produce antibodies directed against the region of the mouse 180 kDa BP antigen which corresponds to the immunodominant region of the human 180 kDa BP antigen.[55] Passive transfer of this rabbit IgG to newborn mice resulted in the development of clinical blisters, an inflammatory infiltrate and the deposition of immunoreactants. These experiments therefore document the ability of antibodies against the 180 kDa BP antigen to directly induce disease. Serum levels of autoantibodies directed against the BP 180 kDa antigen have also been correlated with disease activity in patients with BP.[56] Further evidence for the important role for BPAg2 in BP is provided by the observation that patients with a form of inherited skin blistering and generalized atrophic benign epidermolysis bullosa, have a mutation in BPAg2 that results in a dysfunctional or missing protein [57]

Complement activation and other extracellular mediators also appear to be involved in the pathogenesis of skin lesions in BP. IgG from patients with BP binds to normal human skin and activates the complement cascade, resulting in the accumulation of neutrophils at the cutaneous basement membrane.[58] Complement and the terminal components of the complement cascade are also present in the skin of patients with BP. Early lesions in patients with BP have eosinophil granule proteins, suggesting that eosinophils play an important role in the early development of the lesions. A 92 kDa gelatinase produced by eosinophils present in the skin of patients with BP is capable of cleaving BPAg2.[59] Together, these findings support the hypothesis that the IgG autoantibody binds to the BP antigen, initially most likely BPAg2, activates the complement cascade and the local production of cytokines, resulting in an accumulation of eosinophils and neutrophils that release enzymes, including gelatinases, leading to blister formation. Recent studies in the animal models of BP have confirmed that the BP-like lesions do not develop in complement-deficient or gelatinase-deficient mice, and that the inhibition of neutrophils also prevents lesion development.

The factors that induce the development of autoantibodies in patients with BP are unknown. Budinger and co-workers demonstrated that T cells from patients with BP respond in vitro to the extracellular region of the BPAg2.[60] In addition, they reported that this reactivity was restricted by HLA-DQB1*0301 and that normal HLA-DQB1*0301 showed similar T-cell reactivity. Interestingly, T cells from the patients with BP produced both Th1- and Th2-type cytokines, whereas normal subjects only produced Th1-type cytokines. These results suggest that the ability to mount a Th2 T-cell response to the BP antigen(s) may play a critical role in the development of the disease.

Therapy

The mainstay of therapy for patients with bullous pemphigoid is systemic glucocorticoids.[37] The majority respond rapidly to 0.5–2.0 mg/kg/day of oral prednisone. Mild or localized disease can sometimes be managed by the use of potent topical corticosteroids; however, this form of the disease often progresses to more severe involvement, necessitating systemic therapy. When new blister formation has stopped and healing has begun, a slow taper of the systemic steroids can be instituted. The speed at which the taper is undertaken is often dictated by the severity of the patient's initial disease and the minor flares that may occur during the taper. The majority of patients can be totally tapered off systemic steroids within 6–18 months. Recurrence of active disease is not uncommon. These episodes should be managed with the minimal amount of systemic steroids possible and can occasionally be treated using topical corticosteroid therapy alone. In general, BP is a self-limited process, often lasting 1.5–5 years, which responds promptly to systemic glucocorticoids.

A minority of patients require prolonged high-dose systemic glucocorticoids. In these individuals the addition of cytotoxic agents such as azathioprine, cyclophosphamide or methotrexate will often allow tapering or discontinuation of systemic steroid therapy.[4,37,40] However, few prospective controlled studies have been done to determine which of these drugs, if any, is superior as a steroid-sparing agent. One controlled study failed to demonstrate a substantial benefit from the use of either plasmapheresis or azathioprine in addition to systemic glucocorticoids in the treatment of patients with BP.[61] It is important to note, however, that this study did not address the utility of these agents in patients who had initially been unable to discontinue therapy with systemic glucocorticoids. Other unproven adjunctive therapies suggested to be possibly beneficial in some patients include mycophenolate mofetil, dapsone, cyclosporin A, and tetracycline with niacinamide. When additional therapy is needed, we favor the use of azathioprine at doses of 1–2 mg/kg/day. Although few patients die of BP, the need for systemic glucocorticoids and/or immunosuppressive drugs makes it mandatory that patients be carefully followed and that the least possible amount of medication be used to control the disease.

EPIDERMOLYSIS BULLOSA ACQUISITA (EBA)

Epidermolysis bullosa acquisita (EBA) is a chronic subepidermal blistering disease that typically presents in the fourth to sixth decades. The original description of patients with EBA emphasized the similarity with patients who have dystrophic forms of hereditary epidermolysis bullosa.[62,63] Patients with the 'classic' form of EBA present with acrally distributed blisters that heal with scarring and milia formation.[42,62] The skin of these patients is extremely fragile, often resulting in numerous erosions in areas of mechanical trauma, such as the hands, feet, elbows and knees. Oral mucous membrane lesions, including esophageal involvement, are often seen. In addition, patients with 'classic' EBA may develop lesions in the ocular, vaginal, urethral and rectal mucosae.

> **KEY CONCEPTS**
>
> **Epidermolysis bullosa acquisita**
> - 'Classic EBA' with subepidermal blisters, extreme fragility of acral skin
> - 'Inflammatory EBA' subepidermal blisters similar to BP
> - Oral, conjunctival and other mucous membrane lesions frequent
> - Linear deposits of IgG at the dermal–epidermal junction, localize to the dermis (antigenic target = type VII collagen)

Ocular changes are common and many of these patients may clinically resemble those with cicatricial pemphigoid. Other cutaneous manifestations include scarring alopecia and variable degrees of nail dystrophy. EBA has been associated with a variety of other diseases, particularly inflammatory bowel disease and systemic lupus erythematosus. Part of the explanation for these associations may be the result of the association of EBA with the specific HLA type, DR-2.[42,64] Over the last two decades it has become apparent that the clinical spectrum of EBA is broader than originally appreciated. Patients also present with a 'nonclassic' or 'inflammatory' type of EBA,[65] the clinical presentation of which is essentially identical to that seen in BP, with widespread tense blisters on an erythematous base, which heal without scarring.

Skin biopsies of early lesions from patients with EBA reveal a subepidermal blister with variable degrees of an inflammatory response. In patients with 'classic' EBA lesional skin biopsies often have a minimal inflammatory cell infiltrate.[62] In contrast, patients with the 'inflammatory' variant may have substantial collections of inflammatory cells in the superficial dermis, usually consisting of an admixture of mononuclear cells, polymorphonuclear leukocytes and eosinophils.[65]

An important advance in our understanding of EBA was the demonstration that patients with EBA had deposition of immunoreactants, most often IgG and complement, on direct immunofluorescence at the DEJ. Direct immunofluorescence of perilesional skin biopsies from patients with EBA displays a pattern of immunoreactants similar to that seen in patients with BP, with linear deposits of IgG and C3 at the DEJ.[63] Linear deposits of other immunoreactants, including IgM, IgA and fibrinogen, have also been reported in patients with EBA. The immunoreactants in the skin of patients with EBA have, however, a different localization from those present in the skin of patients with BP. In EBA, immunoelectron microscopy has demonstrated that the immunoreactants are localized exclusively below the lamina lucida.[63,66] One method that distinguishes between patients with EBA and those with BP, by DIF, is to incubate the patient's biopsy specimen in 1 M NaCl skin-splitting buffer, as discussed earlier.[44] With this technique, the in vivo deposited immunoreactants, both IgG and C3, can be demonstrated to be localized to the floor of the in vitro generated blister, whereas in BP the IgG localizes to the blister roof.

Indirect immunofluorescence using stratified squamous epithelia such as normal human skin as a substrate, detects circulating anti-basement membrane zone antibodies in 30–50% of patients with EBA.[42] Indirect immunofluorescence using NaCl-treated split skin as a substrate results in positive antibody detection in up to 85% of patients, making it a more sensitive and specific substrate for clinical testing.[67] As would be expected based on the in vivo deposition pattern, the IgG from patients with EBA localizes to the blister floor.[67] With the improved immunologic characterization of patients with EBA it has become apparent that those with a number of other clinical presentations also have antibodies in sera and skin identical to those seen in patients with EBA. One such group are patients with the bullous eruption of systemic lupus erythematosus.[42,68] These patients have a vesiculobullous eruption clinically and histologically similar to the findings in patients with dermatitis herpetiformis. However, many of these patients have a linear band of IgG at the DEJ which localizes to the floor of 1 M NaCl split skin. Another clinical presentation with EBA-like antibodies against the DEJ of skin is cicatricial pemphigoid. These patients have a limited blistering eruption of the skin with marked mucosal involvement, including oral and ocular inflammation and scarring. The inclusion of these phenotypes in the spectrum of EBA has been made possible by the immunologic studies described above, as well as the discovery that antibodies against type VII collagen are demonstrable in each of them.

Pathogenesis

Immunoelectron microscopy has shown immunoglobulin deposits in patients with EBA localized to the lamina densa zone of the basement membrane, below the lamina lucida.[63] Routine electron microscopy of lesional skin of patients with EBA has revealed that the anchoring fibrils are decreased or absent.[69] These findings may be relevant in the development of the clinical feature of skin fragility, as anchoring fibrils are postulated to play a role in epidermal–dermal adherence via the linkage of the hemidesmosome through the basement membrane. The lack of an inflammatory infiltrate in many patients with EBA suggests that these autoantibodies may disrupt the interaction between anchoring fibrils and dermal matrix proteins.

The target antigen for the IgG autoantibodies present in the sera of patients with EBA is type VII collagen, a 290 kDa glycoprotein composed of a 145 kDa collagenase-insensitive carbohydrate-rich domain and a 145 kDa collagenase-sensitive domain.[70,71] IgG antibodies from patients with EBA appear to be specific for the carbohydrate-rich noncollagenous carboxyl domain of the protein.[71,72] Type VII collagen is the major structural component of anchoring fibrils and is produced by both epithelial keratinocytes and dermal fibroblasts. In vitro, type VII collagen interacts specifically with other extracellular matrix proteins, particularly fibronectin, and its expression is influenced by cell–mesenchymal interactions. In addition, wound healing and embryo development experiments have demonstrated that hemidesmosomes and type VII collagen appear synchronously, again suggesting a coordinate expression of these important basement membrane proteins. Using recombinant fusion proteins of type VII collagen, the IgG from patients with EBA has been shown to bind to four immunodominant epitopes within the noncollagenous amino-terminal domain of the type VII molecule.[73] The identification of these epitopes, however, will allow investigators to begin to address how these autoantibodies can cause disruption of the normal interaction of anchoring fibrils with dermal matrix proteins.

Treatment

Spontaneous resolution is infrequent in patients with EBA, and management is difficult. Goals are to minimize blistering and scar formation, with particular concern for ocular and oral mucosal lesions. Systemic glucocorticoids are the mainstay of therapy, especially for patients with the inflammatory variant of EBA.[42] Unfortunately, even high-dose systemic steroids usually do not affect fragility and trauma-induced blister formation. Mucosal lesions often respond to systemic steroids in doses of 0.5–1.5 mg/kg/day, but recur with tapering and/or discontinuation of the drug. Several agents have been proposed as adjunctive agents, including azathioprine, cyclophosphamide, dapsone, hydroxychloroquine and plasmapheresis. However, none has been consistently demonstrated to be effective.[42] Cyclosporin A has been used to treat patients with EBA with some success, although toxicity has limited therapy in some cases. Photophoresis and intravenous immunoglobulin have also been reported to be effective in some patients with refractory EBA.[74]

Mucous membrane lesions can prove particularly difficult to manage and may necessitate the use of systemic therapy. Ocular lesions should be followed with an ophthalmologist and may require the use of systemic glucocorticoids to prevent conjunctival scarring. Oral mucous membrane lesions can be managed with the frequent application of potent topical steroid ointments or gels (0.05% clobetasol propionate, 0.05% fluocinonide). If this fails and the degree of oral erosions is inhibiting the maintenance of appropriate nutrition, systemic glucocorticoid therapy may be required.

The management of chronic skin wounds in remains of prime importance in the care of EBA patients. Protection of the skin from trauma and the use of topical and systemic antibiotics when infections develop are critical to improving the rate of healing. The recent development of new biological dressings for chronic ulcers has also proved helpful in the management of these wounds.

HERPES GESTATIONIS

Herpes gestationis (HG) is a rare, itchy blistering disease of pregnancy and the puerperium that is characterized in part by the presence of linear deposits of IgG and C3 at the DEJ.[75,76] The name herpes gestations was initially chosen because of the frequent appearance of groups of vesicular lesions; however, this disease has no relationship to herpesvirus infections. Recently some workers have proposed renaming this eruption pemphigoid gestationis, emphasizing its close association with bullous pemphigoid.

HG is rare, occurring in less than 1 per 50 000 pregnancies in North America. It often presents in the third trimester or in the immediate postpartum period.[75,76] Although it may recur in subsequent pregnancies, such recurrence is not absolute. Disease flares in the immediate postpartum period do occur, and patients have been reported to develop blisters when menses return or when oral contraceptives are used.

HG presents as tense blisters, often on an urticarial base, ranging in size from small (3–5 mm) vesicles to large (1–2 cm) bullae. The blisters often begin on the abdomen, although the entire body can be involved. Pruritus is a common feature and can be quite severe.

HG is associated with morbidity for the mother and an increased morbidity and mortality for the fetus.[75–77] The morbidity for the mother is related mainly to the skin disease, with extensive itching and blister formation. Fetal morbidity and mortality were previously estimated to range as high as 30%, but a number of studies have suggested that this figure is too high. These studies have suggested that prematurity and low birthweight may be associated with HG, and that there may be a small but significant risk of fetal morbidity. Infants born to mothers with HG may also develop skin lesions similar to those seen in the mother, probably partly related to the transplacental passage of maternal autoantibodies, as the lesions resolve spontaneously with the clearance of maternal immunoglobulin.

The histopathology of HG lesions is not diagnostic. Subepidermal blisters are seen with a perivascular infiltrate containing eosinophils, neutrophils, lymphocytes and monocytes.[76] Necrotic basal keratinocytes can also be seen. None of these findings is sufficiently distinct, however, to separate HG from other subepidermal blistering diseases on the basis of histologic appearance alone.

Direct immunofluorescence studies of the skin of patients with HG reveals a linear pattern of C3 at the DEJ.[79–81] In addition, 30–50% of patients have linear deposits of IgG in a similar pattern. Occasionally other immunoreactants, including IgA, IgM, C1q, C4, properidin, Factor B and C5, may be present, localized to the lamina lucida region of the DEJ. Indirect immunofluorescence reveals the presence of a circulating IgG antibody directed against the epidermal basement membrane in only approximately 30% of patients. If, however, a complement fixation technique is used, 50–75% of patients will have evidence of an IgG antibody directed against epithelial basement membrane.[79,80] This is detected by its ability to fix complement in vitro, but owing to its low concentration cannot be detected by routine indirect immunofluorescence. This autoantibody can cross the placenta, and infants born to mothers with HG will often have C3 deposits at the DEJ, even in the absence of clinical skin disease. The use of 1 M NaCl split skin as the substrate for indirect immunofluorescence has revealed that the IgG antibody present in the serum of patients with HG binds to the epithelial side of the split skin,[74] a pattern identical to that seen in patients with BP.

Pathogenesis

Sera from a majority of patients with HG bind a 180 kDa protein present in human stratified squamous epithelial extracts.[81] In contrast, sera from patients with HG do not react with the 230 kDa BP antigen. The 180 kDa antigen has been cloned and sequenced and is identical to the 180 kDa antigen to which sera from patients with BP bind.[53,82,83] This antibody reacts with the noncollagenous extracellular region of the 180 kDa BP antigen, similar to what is seen in patients with BP. In addition, T cells from patients with HG react to peptides from this region of the 180 kDa BP antigen.[84] The critical role of pregnancy and other hormonal factors in the development of HG is not understood.

An increased frequency of the HLA-DR3 haplotype has been demonstrated in patients with HG, and the greatest relative risk is associated with the presence of both HLA-DR3 and -DR4.[85] It has also been reported that patients with HG have an increased frequency of anti-HLA antibodies compared to multiparous control subjects. Although some data suggest that the paternal haplotype is important in the pathogenesis of HG, further prospective studies are indicated. Patients with HG are also reported to have an increased frequency of the C4 null allele, although this has been postulated to be secondary to the increased frequency of HLA-DR3 in this patient population (Chapter 58).

Treatment

Therapy of patients with HG is directed at relieving the significant pruritus and preventing the development of new blisters. If the extent of disease is limited, patients can be managed with topical glucocorticoids and antihistamines.[75,76] Most patients, however, have more significant disease and require the use of systemic glucocorticoids. Treatment with 20–60 mg/day of prednisone is sufficient to control both the pruritus and new blister formation in the vast majority of cases. Every attempt should be made to reduce the prednisone to the lowest possible effective dose. Occasionally it may be possible to stop prednisone before delivery. However, the physician should be aware that flares of HG are often seen in the immediate postpartum period. Only rarely will patients require therapy beyond that time. In patients who require prolonged therapy postpartum, immunosuppressive agents such as those used in the other blistering diseases should be considered. Patients being treated with either systemic steroids or immunosuppressive drugs should be counseled with regard to breast-feeding restrictions.

Occasionally infants born to mothers with HG will have skin lesions.[75,77,81] These are limited in extent and resolve spontaneously with the disappearance of maternal IgG from the infant's circulation.

CICATRICIAL PEMPHIGOID (CP)

Cicatricial pemphigoid is a rare, chronic, scarring blistering disease that affects predominantly the oral and conjunctival mucosae.[86,87] Involvement of the conjunctiva can range from a mild conjunctivitis to severe conjunctival inflammation leading to symblepharon formation, entropion, trichiasis, corneal scarring and, eventually, blindness in some patients. Oral mucosal lesions include gingivitis, often with erosions and desquamation, and erosions and ulcerations on the buccal mucosa and the hard and soft palates. Rarely esophageal and laryngeal involvement is seen with resultant scarring and stenosis. Other mucosal sites that can be involved include the genitalia, rectum and nasopharynx. Cutaneous involvement occurs in approximately 10–25% of patients, often on the scalp, back or face. The skin lesions are often indistinguishable from those seen in BP or EBA.

Mucosal biopsys reveals a subepidermal blister with a cellular infiltrate that is usually composed of lymphocytes and plasma cells. Increased numbers of neutrophils or eosinophils have also been reported. Skin biopsies of lesions in patients with CP are essentially indistinguishable from those seen in patients with BP.

Direct immunofluorescence of perilesional skin or mucosal samples reveals a linear deposit of immunoreactants at the basement membrane zone.[88] The majority of patients with CP have IgG and C3 deposit at the basement membrane, although the presence of other immunoreactants, including IgA, IgM and fibrin, has also been reported. The presence of more than two immunoreactants on direct immunofluorescence is highly suggestive of either EBA or CP. The immunoreactants in CP have been described as thick and discontinuous, in contrast to those in BP, which occur as a fine linear band within the lamina lucida. Significant variance from this observation has been noted, however, limiting its utility in the diagnosis of CP.[89] It is important to note that in patients with CP who do not have skin lesions, an undirected skin biopsy for immunofluorescence offers little diagnostic utility. Similarly, biopsy of the conjunctiva can sometimes yield negative immunofluorescence results in patients with otherwise typical CP. This may be due to the inflammation present in the conjunctiva. In such patients a careful evaluation for mucosal lesions and biopsy of the perilesional mucosa is often diagnostic. On immunoelectron microscopy, immunoreactants have been localized both within the lamina lucida and the lamina densa.

Circulating anti-basement membrane zone antibodies are usually absent, or present in low titer, in patients with CP. Attempts to improve the yield of indirect immunofluorescence by using a variety of tissue substrates, including oral and conjunctival mucosa, normal human skin and normal human split skin, have for the most part been unsuccessful. Sarret et al[90] reported 100% positive indirect immunofluorescence in patients with CP who had a positive DIF, using undiluted sera and salt-split skin as a substrate.[90] These authors observed both epidermal and dermal staining, with a linear band of IgA on the epidermal side of the blister being most commonly seen.

Pathogenesis

Both the heterogeneous clinical presentation and the lack of high-titer antibodies in the circulation have hampered a better understanding of the pathogenesis of CP. The presence of different immunoglobulin classes at the basement membrane using immunofluorescence, and the different localization of those immunoglobulins in the basement membrane as detected by immunoelectron microscopy, support the hypothesis that CP may be a heterogenous disease, with a variety of basement membrane zone proteins serving as relevant targets. Chan and coworkers[88] correlated the clinical presentation, immunopathology and target antigens in a group of patients with immune-mediated subepithelial blistering disorders of the mucous membranes. Patients with skin and mucous membrane lesions or mucous membrane lesions alone had immunoreactants present on direct immunofluorescence about 90% of the time. In contrast, patients with ocular disease only had C3 and/or IgG deposits present in approximately 40% of cases. This finding may reflect the difficulty encountered in biopsies of the inflamed conjunctiva. Of more interest, however, were the results of indirect immunofluorescence: 11 of 14 (81%) patients with skin and mucous membrane disease had circulating IgG anti-basement membrane zone antibodies, of which nine identified the 180 kDa and 230 kDa antigens associated with BP by immunoblot and/or immunoprecipitation. In contrast only three of 24 patients with oral mucosal lesions or ocular lesions alone had positive indirect immunofluorescence, one of which reacted with the BP antigens.

Other investigators have reported antibody reactivity in patients with CP to a variety of epidermal and dermal proteins. Sera from patients with CP have been shown to react with the 180 kDa BP antigen.[91,92] A 120 kDa protein has also been identified by immunoblot using sera from patients with CP.[93] Sera from ocular cicatricial pemphigoid patients has been reported to react with a 205 kDa protein that has homology with the cytoplasmic domain of β_4-integrin[94] and a 45 kDa protein.[95] Some patients with a clinical phenotype suggestive of CP have autoantibodies directed against epiligrin, a ligand for a major keratinocyte integrins ($\alpha_3\beta_1$ and $\alpha_6\beta_4$).[96] These data suggest that the clinical presentation of CP is associated with a heterogenous group of autoantibodies that react with multiple antigens of the skin basement membrane zone. The different clinical presentations may therefore result from not only different target antigens, but also perhaps different antibody-binding sites on antigens such as the BP antigen.

DQB1*0301 has been found to occur in Caucasian patients with ocular cicatricial pemphigoid and with cicatricial pemphigoid with ocular and oral mucosal lesions.[97,98] Chan and coworkers reported that this association was not noted in patients with oral mucosal disease without ocular disease, and suggested that the increased frequency of the DQB1*0301 allele may play a role in the development of ocular disease.[98] These results need to be confirmed in larger populations.

Therapy

Treatment of CP is difficult and directed at minimizing the scarring and resultant complications that can occur in the eye. Dapsone in doses of 100–200 mg/day has been found by many investigators to be effective at controlling the early inflammatory response in patients with CP.[99] Some investigators have also found that tetracyclines, often in combination with nicotinamide, can control the inflammatory process seen in patients with cicatricial pemphigoid.[100] If this therapy is unsuccessful, treatment with systemic glucocorticoids (1–2 mg/kg/day), often with adjunctive immunosuppressive therapy such as azathioprine or cylophosphamide, may be needed.[101] Isolated case reports also suggest that therapy with mycophenolate mofetil, intravenous immunoglobulin or plasmapheresis may be of benefit in some patients with cicatricial pemphigoid; however, no control studies or large series using these therapies have been reported. It is important to note that the course of cicatricial pemphigoid is difficult to predict and that the response to treatment in some patients is often less than optimal. Some patients are able to achieve long-lasting remissions, but active disease frequently recurs and patients in remission should be followed closely.

Oral mucosal lesions can often be managed with potent topical corticosteriods (0.05% clobetasol propionate ointment, 0.05% fluocinonide gel) applied frequently to lesions. In severe cases dapsone or systemic glucocorticoids may be needed. Patients with limited amounts of skin disease can often be managed with topical therapy alone. If this fails, management techniques such as those discussed for patients with BP are usually successful.

LINEAR IgA BULLOUS DISEASES

Linear IgA bullous disease (LABD) is a clinically heterogeneous blistering disease in which direct immunofluorescence of perilesional skin biopsies reveals the presence of a linear band of IgA at the basement membrane zone.[102–104] The majority of patients with LABD present with pruritic vesicles and papules, localized primarily to the extensor surfaces similar to those in patients with dermatitis herpetiformis (DH). They do not, however, have an associated gluten-sensitive enteropathy, are not able to control their disease by a gluten-free diet, and do not have HLA associations that are characteristic of patients with DH.

Other patients with linear IgA deposits may present with a clinical picture more suggestive of bullous pemphigoid, with pruritic tense blisters on an erythematous base. Other clinical presentations have been described with clinical as well as histologic and immunopathologic overlap between patients with LABD and cicatricial pemphigoid or epidermolysis bullosa acquisita.[102–104] Finally, children can develop a subepidermal blistering disease with linear IgA deposits, which was previously termed chronic bullous disease of childhood.[103,104] In these cases the blisters occur mainly in flexural areas, with pruritus that is more variable in degree than that which is present in many other blistering diseases.

Routine histopathology of lesional skin of patients with LABD reflects the clinical heterogeneity seen in these patients.[102–104] Biopsy usually reveals collections of neutrophils in the dermal papillary tips in a pattern virtually identical to that seen in biopsies from patients with dermatitis herpetiformis (DH). However, subepidermal blisters with eosinophils, as observed in patients with BP, may also be seen.

Direct immunofluorescence of perilesional skin in patients with LABD reveals a linear band of IgA at the basement membrane zone, which has been characterized on isotyping experiments to be almost exclusively IgA_1.[103,104] Other immunoreactants, especially IgG and C3, have been found in 30–40% of these patients. Further characterization of these IgA deposits in the skin has revealed that both κ and λ light chains are present, indicating that the antibodies are polyclonal. In addition, J chain has not been detected, suggesting that the IgA is monomeric and may not be of gut origin. Immunoelectron microscopic localization of the immunoreactants has most often revealed IgA deposits in the lamina lucida; however, sublamina densa IgA deposits have also been noted. Circulating IgA antibodies against the basement membrane zone of stratified squamous epithelium have been detected in only 10–30% of patients (children and adults) with linear IgA deposits.

Pathogenesis

The absence of circulating antibody has made it difficult to determine the antigenic target in linear IgA dermatosis. Zone et al[104] reported that sera from both adults and children with linear IgA deposits within the lamina lucida reacted with a 97 kDa protein from dermal extracts on immunoblot. Further characterization of this 97 kDa protein revealed that it is identical to a portion of the 180 kDa bullous pemphigoid antigen BPAg2.[105] In patients with LABD or linear IgA disease of childhood that have sublamina densa deposits IgA deposits, investigators have identified reactivity to type VII collagen, and to an unknown 285 kDa dermal protein.[106] These findings support the hypothesis that the target antigens in LABD, including linear IgA disease of childhood, are heterogeneous. The mechanism of lesion formation in patients with LABD regardless of the location of the IgA deposits or the specific antigenic target, is not known.

Therapy

The mainstay of therapy of patients with all forms of the linear IgA-bullous dermatosis is dapsone.[107] The exact mechanism of its action is not known but, as discussed above, this drug seems most useful in diseases with marked neutrophil infiltrates in lesional skin.[108] The dosage needed to control the cutaneous eruption can range from 25 to 200 mg/day. Most patients can be controlled with 100 mg/day, with minimal side-effects. Although dapsone is well tolerated by most patients, it does have significant pharmacologic and idiosyncratic adverse effects and should only be used by physicians experienced in its use.[107] Occasionally patients may not response to dapsone alone. In these cases the addition of low doses of systemic glucocorticoids (prednisone 10–20 mg/day) may result in a significant improvement. If patients cannot tolerate dapsone, systemic glucocorticoids in doses of 40–60 mg/day are usually effective. As most adult patients with linear IgA dermatosis require long term therapy, however, treatment with prednisone should be avoided whenever possible.

DERMATITIS HERPETIFORMIS

Clinical features

Dermatitis herpetiformis (DH) is an intensely pruritic blistering disease that classically presents in the second or third decade with erythematous papules and/or vesicles localized over the extensor surfaces[109–111] (Fig. 75.6). However, patients often present with a broad spectrum of lesions. Because of the severe pruritus, patients will often present with multiple erosions, with and without crusts. Patients also can present with urticarial plaques or, more rarely, frank bullae. Lesions are most often symmetrically distributed over the extensor surfaces, especially the elbows, knees, buttocks, back and posterior hairline.[109–111] Symptomatic mucous membrane lesions are rarely present. One clinical hallmark of DH is the extreme pruritus that patients experience: they characteristically report feeling a severe burning or stinging 12–24 hours before the appearance of a lesion, which persists until the vesicle is broken and the crust forms. Although clinical manifestations of DH may wax and wane, in general DH is a lifelong dermatosis. The wide variety of clinical presentations of DH often suggests a long differential diagnosis, including erythema multiforme, herpes gestationis, bullous pemphigoid, transient acantholytic dermatitis, papular urticaria, scabies, bug bites and neurotic excoriations.[109]

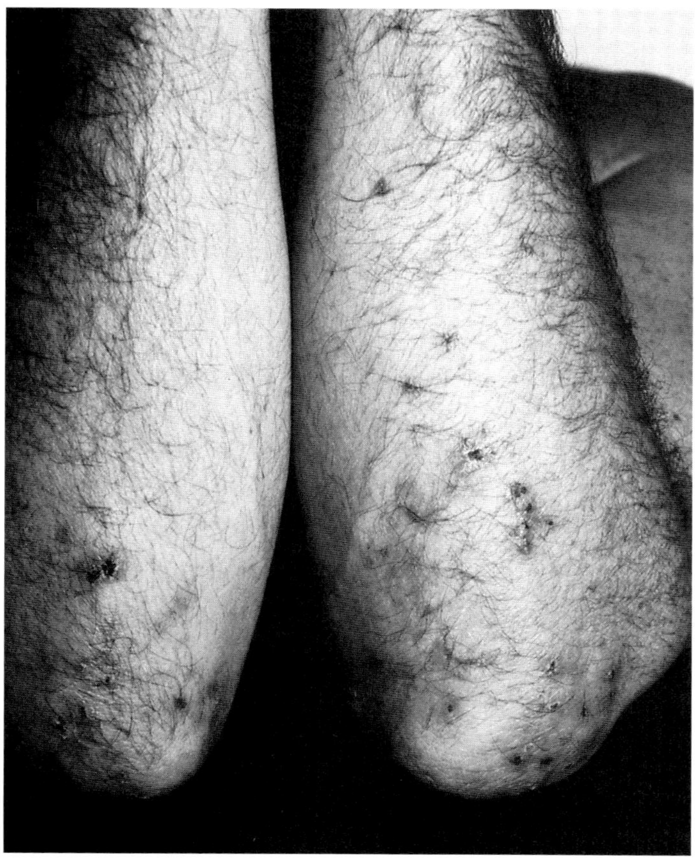

Figure 75.6 Patient with dermatitis herpetiformis showing erythematosus papules with crusts on the elbows. Rare intact vesicles are present.

KEY CONCEPTS

Dermatitis herpetiformis
- Extremely itchy, small blisters on extensor surfaces
- Associated with asymptomatic/gluten-sensitive enteropathy
- Increased frequency HLA-B8, -DR3, -DQ2 haplotype
- Granular deposits of IgA at the dermal–epidermal junction (antigenic target unknown)
- Skin disease controlled by gluten-free diet

The frequency of DH differs with the ethnicity of the population. In Anglo-Saxon and Scandinavian populations it has been estimated to be between 10 and 39 per 100 000 persons, whereas other populations, such as African-Americans and Asians, DH occurs much less frequently. This relates in part to the different frequency of the HLA antigens associated with DH in different ethnic populations.

In addition to the striking association of DH with gluten-sensitive enteropathy, a number of other diseases associations have also been noted. For example, patients with DH have an increased frequency of gastric atrophy and gastric hypochlorhydria.[110] Thyroid abnormalities, including hypothyroidism, hyperthyroidism, thyroid nodules and thyroid cancer, have also been reported to occur more frequently in patients with DH.[113] A number of other autoimmune diseases, including systemic lupus erythematosus, dermatomyositis, myasthenia gravis, Sjögren's syndrome and rheumatoid arthritis, have also been reported in patients with DH. It is thought that many of these associations are related to the high frequency of the HLA-B8, -DR3, DQ-2 haplotype in patients with DH. Another important clinical association in patients with DH is an increased frequency of malignancy, specifically gastrointestinal lymphomas. An overall incidence of malignancy of about 6.4% has been reported, which represents an increased relative risk for malignancy of 2.38.[114]

Biopsy of an early lesion of DH reveals a characteristic neutrophilic infiltrate in the dermal papillae with the presence of fibrin, neutrophilic fragments, edema and variable numbers of eosinophils.[109] This histologic pattern is not specific; it has been reported in patients with bullous pemphigoid, linear IgA disease, the bullous eruption of systemic lupus erythematosus and leukocytoclastic vasculitis. When older bullous lesions are biopsied in patients with DH, the histologic features are often indistinguishable from those seen with other blistering disorders.

IgA is present at the DEJ of the skin of patients with DH (Fig. 75.7). Two patterns of IgA deposition were initially described in patients with identical clinical findings: 85–90% of patients had granular deposits of IgA at the DEJ, and 10–15% had a linear band of IgA at the DEJ.[115,116] These patterns, consistent within a given individual, have now been shown to distinguish between two different diseases. Patients with linear IgA deposits have linear IgA bullous dermatosis (see previous section), whereas patients with granular deposits of IgA are considered to have

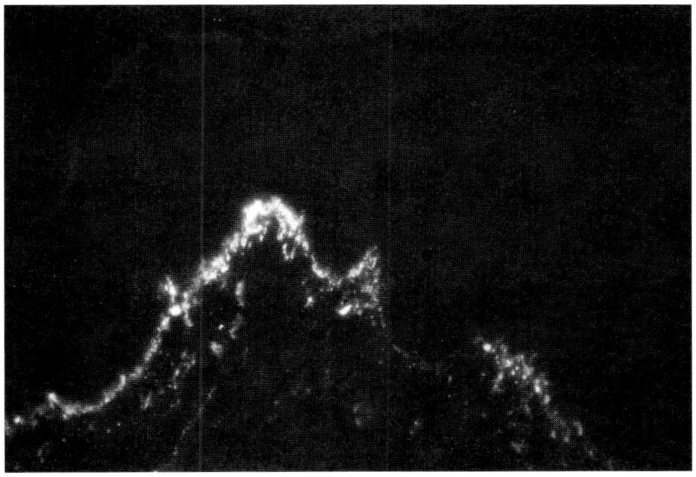

Figure 75.7 Direct immunofluorescence of normal appearing perilesional skin of a patient with dermatitis herpetiformis using antibodies against human IgA. Granular deposits of IgA are present at the dermal–epidermal junction.

dermatitis herpetiformis. The granular deposits of IgA at the DEJ are specific for patients with DH and have not been found in those with isolated gluten-sensitive enteropathy (GSE) or asymptomatic relatives of patients with DH.

Granular deposits of IgA are found in both involved and uninvolved skin of patients with DH, including the oral mucosa.[117] Consistent regional variations in the amount of IgA in the skin of patients with DH have not been reported. However, Zone and co-workers[118] reported that IgA was either markedly decreased or absent in skin in which the patient reported never having had any lesions. These observations suggest that biopsies taken for direct immunofluorescence studies should be obtained from normal-appearing perilesional skin in order to maximize the diagnostic yield.

IgG, IgM and IgE are not usually found in the skin of patients with DH. Complement component, C3, along with early components of the alternative complement pathway, may be present.[119] The neoantigens of the C5–C9 membrane attack complex have also been reported to be present in normal-appearing skin of patients with DH.[119] The colocalization of vitronectin with the C9 neoantigen, however, suggests that the C5–C9 neoantigen that is present in DH skin is deposited as part of the nonlytic C5–C9 complex, and that the lytic membrane attack complex of complement may not play a primary role in the development of skin lesions in patients with DH.[120]

Characterization of IgA in DH skin has shown that it contains both κ and λ light chains, indicating that the IgA is polyclonal. Secretory component, a transport protein bound to secretory IgA, has not been found in these IgA deposits. Attempts to determine whether the IgA in the skin of patients with DH is of mucosal origin have focused on determining whether the IgA contains joining (J) chain. Although Unsworth and co-workers reported that J chain is present in DH skin, others have been unable to detect it.[121–123] The detection of J chain in intact IgA molecules is difficult, however, presumably because of the masking of the antigenic site on the J chain by the IgA molecules, and this may account for the discrepancy between these investigators.

Additional attempts to characterize the origin of the IgA have included examination of the IgA subclass of the cutaneous deposits. Secretory IgA, in addition to being primarily polymeric, also is composed of relatively equal amounts of IgA_1 and IgA_2 compared to serum IgA, which is comprised of approximately 90% IgA_1. Using monoclonal antibodies directed against the IgA subclasses a number of investigators have found that IgA_1 is the predominant subclass found in the skin of patients with either minimal or no deposits of IgA_2 detected.[122,124,125] Although this would seem to suggest that the IgA in DH skin may not be mucosal in origin, IgA_1 is also the predominant subclass in the gastrointestinal secretions of patients with DH.[126] Thus, the IgA immune response to wheat protein found in the gut secretions of patients with DH may be similar to the IgA in DH skin.

Immunoelectron microscopic studies have demonstrated that the IgA deposits in the skin of patients with DH are present as large, amorphous collections in the dermis, sometimes adjacent to the basement membrane or the extended anchoring plaque network.[127] These deposits are not localized to the microfibrillar bundles, suggesting that they may be bound to degraded basement membrane or represent IgA that is deposited in the dermis owing to physical characteristics, such as altered solubility or carbohydrate composition.[127] The mechanism by which IgA binds and/or deposits in the skin of patients with DH is not known.

In 1966 Marks and co-workers[128] noted a gastrointestinal abnormality in 60–70% of patients with DH, which was histologically similar to that seen in isolated gluten-sensitive enteropathy (GSE). This abnormality was reversible with the avoidance of dietary gluten, confirming that this was a gluten-sensitive disease. The histologic changes seen in the small bowel of patients with DH are characterized by a flattening of the normal villous architecture of the jejunal epithelium, with elongation of the intestinal crypts and a mononuclear cell infiltrate both within the lamina propria and in an intraepithelial location. This disease is often patchy in character in both DH and isolated GSE, and in general the findings in patients with DH are less severe than those seen in isolated GSE. Essentially all patients with the clinical features of DH and granular IgA deposits have an associated GSE.[108]

Despite the morphological similarity of the intestinal abnormality seen in patients with DH and those with isolated GSE, most patients with DH have no gastrointestinal symptoms. Only 10% of patients with DH have the typical symptoms of isolated GSE, including bloating, diarrhea and malabsorption, whereas 20–30% may have mild steatorrhea.[108] However many patients with DH do have abnormal intestinal function, as documented by abnormal D-xylose, iron, folate, glucose, water and bicarbonate absorption.

Despite the asymptomatic nature of the GSE associated with DH, it is clear that it plays a critical role in the pathogenesis of DH. The ability of patients with DH to control their skin disease, to normalize the morphologic changes of the small intestine, as well as to decrease or eliminate IgA deposits by years of gluten avoidance, is strong evidence that the GSE associated with DH plays a fundamental role in the pathogenesis of DH. However, the mechanism of the interaction of the skin disease, the cutaneous IgA deposits and the associated GSE, remains unknown.

With the discovery of the association of GSE with DH, a number of investigators began studies to determine whether HLA associations were present in patients with DH, as they were in patients with isolated GSE. Initial studies of HLA associations in patients with DH and granular deposits of IgA revealed that 70–90% of those with DH express the HLA Class I antigen B8, compared to only 20–30% of control subjects.[108,129,130] Subsequent studies showed that 90–95% of patients with DH express HLA-DR3, compared to about 23% of controls.[130–133] In addition, 95–100% of DH patients express HLA-DQ2 (which is in linkage disequilibrium with HLA-DR3), compared to 40% of controls.[130] The HLA-DR and HLA-DQ alleles involved in the pathogenesis of DH are DQB1*0201, DQA1*0501 and DRB1*0301.[131–133] These associations are essentially identical to those that have been described for patients with isolated GSE.[131–133] The vast majority of individuals who express these HLA molecules, however, do not develop DH or isolated GSE. In addition, family studies have demonstrated the presence of normal individuals who are HLA identical with siblings who have developed DH, although a strong familial component to both DH and isolated GSE has been documented.[134] Together, these observations strongly suggest that multiple genes and additional environmental factors are important in the pathogenesis of DH.

Pathogenesis

The pathogenesis of DH rests on three distinct associations: (1) skin biopsies from patients with DH reveal granular deposits of IgA at the DEJ; (2) patients with DH have an associated gluten-sensitive enteropathy; and (3) the increased frequency of the HLA-DR3/DQ2 haplotype. Attempts to understand DH must integrate each of these three distinct factors.

The mechanism by which IgA binds to DH skin is not known. Indirect immunofluorescence, using normal human skin or 1 M NaCl split skin as substrates, has not detected IgA antibodies that bind to skin in a granular pattern. This suggests that the structures to which the IgA bind are not present in normal human skin, or that the mechanism of binding cannot be reproduced in vitro. The IgA deposits also do not appear to be the result of the presence of IgA-containing circulating immune complexes (IgA-CIC). These complexes have been found in 25–35% of patients with DH, but have also been detected in the serum of patients with isolated GSE, who do not have cutaneous IgA deposits.[135] Although these data suggest that circulating IgA immune complete are not responsible for the IgA found in DH skin, it is possible that pathogenic immune complex have escaped detection by the available techniques.

A third mechanism by which IgA might bind to DH skin is that IgA produced in the gut as a response to wheat or other dietary antigens reaches the circulation, and IgA antibodies directed against dietary antigens such as wheat proteins could either bind to wheat protein deposited in skin or cross-react with normal-appearing antigens in the skin. Wheat or other dietary protein antigens, however, have not been detected in the skin of DH patients, and no specific interaction of DH skin with either serum or secretory IgA has been documented in such patients.[108] Finally, IgA deposits in the skin of DH patients may occur as a result of the unique properties of IgA of mucosal origin that persist in the circulation of patients with DH and may slowly accumulate in skin via a nonantigen–antibody-binding mechanism.

IgA antibodies against a connective tissue element surrounding smooth muscle, endomysium, have been found in the serum of patients with DH.[136] These antibodies have also been found in patients with isolated gluten-sensitive enteropathy and are thought to be related to the degree of underlying intestinal disease.[137] Although these antibodies may prove important in the diagnosis of isolated GSE, their role in the pathogenesis of DH is not clear. Only 70% of patients with DH have IgA antiendomysial antibodies compared to essentially all patients with active GSE. Recently IgA antiendomysial antibodies have been determined to be directed against tissue transglutaminase.[138] Furthermore, the gliadin component of wheat has been identified as a preferred substrate for the tissue transglutaminase.[138] In vitro studies have demonstrated that treatment of gliadin with tissue transglutaminase modifies gliadin peptides to allow recognition by T cells from the gut of patients with isolated GSE.[138,139] These observations suggest that modification of the wheat protein by tissue transglutaminase may play a role in the development of immunity to wheat seen in patients with isolated GSE and DH. It is not known whether differences exist in tissue transglutaminase or in the specificity of the T cells against wheat protein in patients with DH versus those with isolated GSE. Smith and coworkers[140] have recently demonstrated that the cytokine profile in the gut of patients with DH differs from that in those with symptomatic isolated GSE.[140] Gut biopsies from patients with isolated GSE expressed significantly more IFN-γ than those with DH, whereas DH patients' gut biopsies expressed more IL-4. It remains to be determined whether different antigenic specificities play a role in these observations.

Patients with DH and those with isolated GSE have elevated levels of soluble IL-2 receptor in their serum.[141,143] Elevated levels of IL-2 receptors in the circulation are thought to occur as the result of shedding of IL-2 receptor during T-cell activation. These results provide indirect evidence for the presence of activated T cells in patients with both isolated GSE and DH. In patients with DH this elevation in soluble IL-2R was noted in the absence of any active cutaneous disease and correlated with the presence of serum IgA antibodies against dietary antigens, suggesting that elevated IL-2R levels were the result of an ongoing T-cell mediated immune response in the gastrointestinal mucosa.

Therapy

Dermatitis herpetiformis can be treated either with dapsone or by adherence to a gluten-free diet, and the choice of therapy must be individualized to the patient.[109] The treatment of choice for most patients with DH is dapsone or sulfapyridine, owing to both the lack of gastrointestinal symptoms in most cases, as well as the difficulty of adhering to a strict gluten-free diet. Dapsone 100–200 mg/day is sufficient to control the cutaneous eruption in the majority of cases, with minimal side-effects.[109] Dapsone results in an almost immediate cessation of symptoms of the skin disease. It does not, however, affect the gastrointestinal mucosal defect or the gastrointestinal symptoms. Patients with DH on dapsone therefore have an ongoing (albeit low-grade) gluten-sensitive enteropathy. Dapsone appears to function at the level of the effector cells in the skin lesions, most likely the polymorphonuclear leukocyte, rather than affecting the mucosal immune response to wheat protein. The exact mechanism of action of dapsone, however, is not known. Dapsone is a potentially toxic drug[107] and patients must avoid increasing the dose when disease flares occur without first consulting their physician.

The second mechanism of controlling the cutaneous eruption of DH is by strict adherence to a gluten-free diet. Studies have shown that nearly 80% of patients with DH who follow such a diet are able to stop or substantially reduce the dose of dapsone required to control their skin disease.[108] Patients may require at least 5 months on a gluten-free diet before being able to reduce their dose of dapsone, and 8–48 months of such a diet are necessary before they can discontinue their dapsone. Gluten-reduced diets, in which gluten content is not totally eliminated, appear to be less effective in controlling the cutaneous manifestations of DH, but may provide some relief. Patients on a reduced gluten diet are able to decrease their dapsone dosage by approximately 50% compared to a 75% or greater reduction in patients on a gluten-free diet.

Although strict adherence to a gluten-free diet controls the cutaneous manifestations of DH and reverses the morphological changes in the small intestine, decreases in the cutaneous IgA deposits of patients on the diet are less well documented. Different investigators have mostly reported either no significant change or a decrease in cutaneous IgA deposits after the institution of a gluten-free diet.[142] The disappearance of IgA deposits appears to be uncommon.[142]

Rarely patients with DH do not respond to a gluten-free diet despite what appears to be total dietary compliance. This has also been reported in patients with isolated GSE, and other dietary factors have been postulated to play a role. In support of this concept is the observation that the skin lesions and gastrointestinal changes seen in patients with DH may also respond to an elemental diet, often within only 2–3 weeks of starting the diet.[144] These results may be due to other proteins besides gluten playing a role in the pathogenesis of DH or, alternatively, that small amounts of gluten are ingested by patients on even the most strict gluten-free diet. Although a gluten-free diet is an attractive alternative to medication for many patients, such a diet is difficult to maintain. Gluten is present in most common grains (wheat, rye, barley, oats) but not in rice and corn. It is often helpful for a dietitian to assist the patient. The patient must also be informed that the success or failure of the diet cannot generally be assessed until at least a year of therapy has been completed.

REFERENCES

1. Nousari HC, Anhalt GJ. Pemphigus and bullous pemphigoid. Lancet 1999;354:667.
2. Udey MC, Stanley JR. Pemphigus – diseases of antidesmosomal autoimmunity. JAMA 1999;282:572.
3. Lever WF. Pemphigus. Medicine 1953;32:1.
4. Bystryn JC, Steinman NM. The adjuvant therapy of pemphigus. An update. Arch Dermatol 1996;132:203.
5. Beutner EH, Jordon RE. Demonstration of skin antibodies in the sera of pemphigus vulgaris patients by indirect immunofluorescent staining. Proc Soc Exp Biol Med 1964;117:505.
6. Beutner EH, Jordon RE, Chorzelski T. The immunopathology of pemphigus and bullous pemphigoid. J Invest Dermatol 1968;51:63.
7. Sampaio SA, Rivitti EA, Aoki V, Diaz LA. Brazilian pemphigus foliaceus, endemic pemphigus foliaceus, or fogo selvagem (wild fire). Dermatol Clin 1994;12:765.
8. Hans-Filho G, Aoki V, Rivitti E, Eaton DP, Lin MS, Diaz LA. Endemic pemphigus foliaceus (fogo selvagem) – 1998. The Cooperative Group on Fogo Selvagem Research. Clin Dermatol 1999;17:225.
9. Warren SJP, Lin M-SL, Giudice GJ, et al. The prevalance of antibodies against desmoglein 1 in endemic pemphigus foliaceus in Brazil. N Engl J Med 2000;343:23.
10. Chorzelski T, Jablonska S, Blaszczyk M. Immunopathological investigations in the Sener–Usher syndrome (co-existence of pemphigus and lupus erythematosus). Br J Dermatol 1968;80:211.
11. Mutasim DF, Pelc NJ, Anhalt GJ. Drug-induced pemphigus. Dermatol Clin 1993;11:463.
12. Anhalt GJ. Paraneoplastic pemphigus. Adv Dermatol 1997;12:77.
13. Anhalt GJ, Kim SC, Stanley JR. Paraneoplastic pemphigus. An autoimmune mucocutaneous disease associated with neoplasia. N Engl J Med 1990;323:1729.
14. Huff JC, Golitz LE, Kunke KS. Intraepidermal neutrophilic IgA dermatosis. N Engl J Med 1985;313:1643.
15. Eyre RW, Stanley JR. Identification of pemphigus vulgaris antigen extracted from normal human epidermis and comparison with pemphigus foliaceus antigen. J Clin Invest 1988;81:807.
16. Korman NJ, Eyre RW, Klaus-Kovtun V, Stanley JR. Demonstration of an adhering-junction molecule (plakoglobin) in the autoantigens of pemphigus foliaceus and pemphigus vulgaris. N Engl J Med 1989;321:631.
17. Mahoney MG, Aho S, Uitto J, Stanley JR. The members of the plakin family of proteins recognized by paraneoplastic pemphigus antibodies include periplakin. J Invest Dermatol 1998;111:308.
18. Stanley JR. Pemphigus and pemphigoid as paradigms of organ-specific, autoantibody-mediated diseases. J Clin Invest 1989;83:1443.
19. Koulu L, Kusumi A, Steinberg MS, Klaus-Kovtun V, Stanley JR. Human autoantibodies against a desmosomal core protein in pemphigus foliaceus. J Exp Med 1984;160:1509.
20. Stanley JR, Koulu L, Thivolet C. Distinction between epidermal antigens binding pemphigus vulgaris and pemphigus foliaceus autoantibodies. J Clin Invest 1984;74:313.
21. Ebihara T, Hashimoto T, Iwatsuki K, Takigawa M, Ando M, Ohkawara A. Autoantigens for IgA anti-intercellular antibodies of intercellular antibodies of intercellular IgA vesiculopustular dermatosis. J Invest Dermatol 1991;97:742.
22. Hashimoto T, Kiyokawa C, Mori O, et al. Human desmocollin 1 (Dsc 1) is an autoantigen for the subcorneal pustular dermatosis type of IgA pemphigus. J Invest Dermatol 1997;109:127.
23. Anhalt GJ, Labib RS, Voorhees JJ, Beals TF, Diaz LA. Induction of pemphigus in neonatal mice by passive transfer of IgG from patients with the disease. N Engl J Med 1982;306:1189.
24. Rock B, Martins CR, Theofilopoulos AN, et al. The pathogenic effect of IgG_4 autoantibodies in endemic pemphigus foliaceus (fogo selvagem). N Engl J Med 1989;320:1463.
25. Amagai M, Karpati S, Prussick R, Klaus-Kovtun V, Stanley JR. Autoantibodies against the amino-terminal cadherin-like binding domain of pemphigus vulgaris antigen are pathogenic. J Clin Invest 1992;90:919.
26. Amagai M, Hashimoto T, Green KJ, Shimizu N, Nishikawa T. Antigen-specific immunoadsorption of pathogenic autoantibodies in pemphigus foliaceus. J Invest Dermatol 1995;104:895.
27. Kawana S, Geoghegan WD, Jordon RE. Complement fixation by pemphigus antibody. III Altered epidermal cell membrane integrity mediated by pemphigus antibody and complement. J Invest Dermatol 1986;86:29.
28. Rock B, Labib RS, Diaz LA. Monovalent Fab′ immunoglobulin fragments from endemic pemphigus foliaceus autoantibodies reproduce the human disease in neonatal Balb/c mice. J Clin Invest 1990;85:296.
29. Amagai M, Tsunoda K, Suzuki H, Nishifuji K, Koyasu S, Nishikawa T. Use of autoantigen-knockout mice in developing an active autoimmune disease model for pemphigus. J Clin Invest 2000;105:635.
30. Scharf SJ, Friedman A, Brautbar C, et al. HLA Class II allelic variation and susceptibility to pemphigus vulgaris. Proc Natl Acad Sci USA 1988;85:3504.
31. Ahmed AR, Yunis EJ, Khatri K, et al. Major histocompatibility complex haplotype studies in Ashkenazi Jewish patients with pemphigus vulgaris. Proc Natl Acad Sci USA 1990;87:7658.
32. Ahmed AR, Mohimen A, Yunis EJ, et al. Linkage of pemphigus vulgaris antibody to the major histocompatibility complex in healthy relatives of patients. J Exp Med 1993;177:419.

33. Wucherpfennig KW, Yu B, Bhol K, et al. Structural basis for major histocompatibility complex (MHC)-linked susceptibility to autoimmunity: charged residues of a single MHC binding pocket confer selective presentation of self-peptides in pemphigus vulgaris. Proc Natl Acad Sci USA 1995;92:11935.
34. Hertl M, Amagai M, Sundaram H, Stanley J, Ishii K, Katz SI. Recognition of desmoglein 3 by autoreactive T cells in pemphigus vulgaris patients and normals. J Invest Dermatol 1998;110:62.
35. Moraes ME, Fernandez-Vina M, Lazaro A, et al. An epitope in the third hypervariable region of the DRB1 gene is involved in the susceptibility to endemic pemphigus foliaceus (fogo selvagem) in three different Brazilian populations. Tissue Antigens 1997;49:35.
36. Eaton DP, Diaz LA, Hans-Filho G, et al. Comparison of black fly species (Diptera: Simuliidae) on an Amerindian reservation with a high prevalence of fogo selvagem to neigboring disease-free sites in the State of Mato Grosso do Sul, Brazil. The Cooperative Group on Fogo Selvagem Research. J Med Entomol 1998;35:120.
37. Stanley JR. Bullous pemphigoid. In: Freedberg IM, Eisen AZ, Wolff K, et al. (eds) Fitzpatrick's dermatology in general medicine. New York, McGraw-Hill, 1999;666.
38. Venning VA, Wojnarowska F. The association of bullous pemphigoid and malignant disease: a case control study. Br J Dermatol 1990;123:439.
39. Jordon RE, Beutner EH, Witebsky E, Blumenthal G, Hale WL, Lever WF. Basement zone antibodies in bullous pemphigoid. JAMA 1967;200:91.
40. Venning VA, Wojnarowska F. Lack of predictive factors for the clinical course of bullous pemphigoid. J Am Acad Dermatol 1992;26:585.
41. Jenkins RE, Hern S, Black MM. Clinical features and management of 87 patients with pemphigoid gestationis. Clin Exp Dermatol 1999;24:255.
42. Gammon WR, Briggaman RA. Epidermolysis bullosa acquisita and bullous systemic lupus erythematosus. Diseases of autoimmunity to type VII collagen. Dermatol Clin 1993;11:535.
43. Gammon WR, Fine JD, Briggaman RA. Immunofluorescence on split skin for the detection and differentiation of basement membrane zone autoantibodies. J Am Acad Dermatol 1992;27:79.
44. Domloge-Hultsch N, Bisalbutra P, Gammon WR, Yancey KB. Direct immunofluorescence microscopy of 1 mol/L sodium chloride-treated patient skin. J Am Acad Dermatol 1991;24:946.
45. Mutasim D, Takahashi Y, Labib RS, Anhalt GJ, Patel H, Diaz LA. A pool of bullous pemphigoid antigen(s) is intracellular and associated with the basal cell cytoskeleton hemidesmosome complex. J Invest Dermatol 1985;84:47.
46. Stanley JR. Cell adhesion molecules as targets of autoantibodies in pemphigus and pemphigoid, bullous diseases due to defective epidermal cell adhesion. Adv Immunol 1993;53:291.
47. Stanley JR, Hawley-Nelson P, Yuspa SH, Shevach EM, Katz SI. Characterization of bullous pemphigoid antigen: a unique basement membrane protein of stratified squamous epithelia. Cell 1981;24:897.
48a. Mueller S, Klaus-Kovtun V, Stanley JR. A 230-kDa basic protein is the major bullous pemphigoid antigen. J Invest Dermatol 1989;92:33.
48b. Mutasim DF, Morrison LH, Takahashi Y, et al. Definition of bullous pemphigoid antibody binding to intracellular and extracellular antigen associated with hemidesmosomes. J Invest Dermatol 1989;92:225.
49. Robledo MA, Kim SC, Korman NJ, et al. Studies of the relationship of the 230-kD and 180-kD bullous pemphigoid antigens. J Invest Dermatol 1990;94:793.
50. Zillikens D, Mascaro JM, Rose PA, et al. A highly sensitive enzyme-linked immunosorbent assay for the detection of circulating anti-BP180 autoantibodies in patients with bullous pemphigoid. J Invest Dermatol 1997;109:679.
51. Li KH, Sawamura D, Giudice GJ, et al. Genomic organization of collagenous domains and chromosomal assignment of human 180-kDa bullous pemphigoid antigen-2, a novel collagen of stratified squamous epithelium. J Biol Chem 1991;266:24064.
52. Tanaka T, Parry DA, Klaus-Kovtun V, Steinert PM, Stanley JR. Comparison of molecularly cloned bullous pemphigoid antigen to desmoplakin I confirms that they define a new family of cell adhesion junction plaque proteins. J Biol Chem 1991;266:12555.
53. Giudice GJ, Emery DJ, Zelickson BD, Anhalt GJ, Liu Z, Diaz LA. Bullous pemphigoid and herpes gestationis autoantibodies recognize a common non-collagenous site on the BP180 ectodomain. J Immunol 1993;151:5742.
54. Hall RP, Murray JC, McCord MM, Rico MJ, Streilein RD. Rabbits immunized with a peptide encoded for by the 230-kD bullous pemphigoid antigen cDNA develop an enhanced inflammatory response to UVB irradiation: a potential animal model for bullous pemphigoid. J Invest Dermatol 1993;101:9.
55. Liu Z, Diaz LA, Troy JL, et al. A passive transfer model of the organ-specific autoimmune disease, bullous pemphigoid, using antibodies generated against the hemidesmosomal antigen, BP180. J Clin Invest 1993;92:2480.
56. Schmidt E, Obe K, Brocker EB, Zillikens D. Serum levels of autoantibodies to BP180 correlate with disease activity in patients with bullous pemphigoid. Arch Dermatol 2000;136:174.
57. McGrath JA, Darling T, Gatalica B, et al. A homozygous deletion mutation in the gene encoding the 180-kDa bullous pemphigoid antigen (BPAG2) in a family with generalized atrophic benign epidermolysis bullosa. J Invest Dermatol 1996;106:771.
58. Gammon WR, Merritt CC, Lewis DM, Sams WM, Wheeler CE, Carlo J. Leukocyte chemotaxis to the dermal epidermal junction of human skin mediated by pemphigoid antibody and complement: mechanism of cell attachment in in vitro leukocyte attachment method. J Invest Dermatol 1981;76:514.
59. Stahle-Backdahl M, Inoue M, Guidice GJ, Parks WC. 92-kD gelatinase is produced by eosinophils at the site of blister formation in bullous pemphigoid and cleaves the extracellular domain of recombinant 180-kD bullous pemphigoid autoantigen. J Clin Invest 1994;93:2022.
60. Budinger L, Borradori L, Yee C, et al. Identification and characterization of autoreactive T cell responses to bullous pemphigoid antigen 2 in patients and healthy controls. J Clin Invest 1998;102:2082.
61. Guillaume JC, Vaillant L, Bernard P. Controlled trial of azathioprine and plasma exchange in addition to prednisolone in the treatment of bullous pemphigoid. Arch Dermatol 1993;129:49.
62. Roenigk HH-Jr, Ryan JG, Bergfield WF. Epidermolysis bullosa acquisita: Report of 3 cases and a review of all published cases. Arch Dermatol 1971;103:1.
63. Yaoita H, Briggaman RA, Lawley TJ, Provost TT, Katz SI. Epidermolysis bullosa acquisita: ultrastructural and immunological studies. J Invest Dermatol 1981;76:288.
64. Gammon WR, Heise ER, Burke WA, Fine JD, Woodley DT, Briggaman RA. Increased frequency of HLA-DR2 in patients with autoantibodies to epidermolysis bullosa acquisita antigen: evidence that the expression of autoimmunity to type VII collagen is HLA Class II allele associated. J Invest Dermatol 1988;91:228.
65. Gammon WR, Briggaman RA, Wheeler CE Jr. Epidermolysis bullosa acquisita presenting as an inflammatory bullous disease. J Am Acad Dermatol 1982;7:382.
66. Domloge-Hultsch N, Anhalt GJ, Gammon WR, et al. Antiepiligrin cicatricial pemphigoid. A subepithelial bullous disorder. Arch Dermatol 1994;130:1521.
67. Gammon WR, Fine JD, Forbes M, Briggaman RA. Immunofluorescence on split skin for the detection and differentiation of basement membrane zone autoantibodies. J Am Acad Dermatol 1992;27:79.
68. Gammon WR, Briggaman RA. Bullous SLE: a phenotypically distinctive but immunologically heterogeneous bullous disorder. J Invest Dermatol 1993;100:28S.
69. Nieboer C, Boorsma DM, Woerdeman MJ, Kalsbeek GL. Epidermolysis bullosa acquisita. Immunofluorescence, electron microscopic and immunoelectron microscopic studies in four patients. Brit J. Dermatol 1980;102:383.
70. Woodley DT, Briggaman RA, O'Keefe EJ, Inman AO, Queen LL, Gammon WR. Identification of the skin basement-membrane autoantigen in epidermolysis bullosa acquisita. N Engl J Med 1984;310:1007.
71. Woodley DT, Burgeson RE, Lunstrum G, Bruckner-Tuderman L, Reese MJ, Briggaman RA. Epidermolysis bullosa acquisita antigen is the globular carboxyl terminus of type VII procollagen. J. Clin Invest 1988;81:683.

72. Gammon WR, Murrell DF, Jenison MW, et al. Autoantibodies to type VII collagen recognize epitopes in a fibronectin-like region of the non-collagenous (NCI) domain. J Invest Dermatol 1993;100:618.
73. Lapiere JC, Woodley DT, Parente MG, et al. Epitope mapping of type VII collagen. Identification of discrete peptide sequences recognized by sera from patients with acquired epidermolysis bullosa. J Clin Invest 1993;92:1831.
74. Mohr C, Sunderkotter C, Hildebrand A, et al. Successful treatment of epidermolysis bullosa acquisita using intravenous immunoglobulins. Br J Dermatol 1995;132:824.
75. Yancey KB. Herpes gestationis. Dermatol Clin 1990;8:727.
76. Shornick JK. Herpes gestationis. Dermatol Clin 1993;11:527.
77. Lawley TJ, Stingl G, Katz SI. Fetal and maternal risk factors in herpes gestationis. Archives 1978;114:552.
78. Shornick JK, Black MM. Fetal risks in herpes gestationis. J Am Acad Dermatol 1992;26:63.
79. Jordon RE, Heine KG, Tappeiner G, Bushkell LL, Provost TT. The immunopathology of herpes gestationis. Immunofluorescence studies and characterization of 'HG factor'. J Clin Invest 1976;57:1426.
80. Katz SI, Hertz KC, Yaoita H. Herpes gestationis. Immunopathology and characterization of the HG factor. J Clin Invest 1976;57:1434.
81. Shornick JK, Bangert JL, Freeman RG, Gilliam JN. Herpes gestationis: clinical and histologic features of twenty-eight cases. J Am Acad Dermatol 1983;8:214.
82. Morrison LH, Labib RS, Zone JJ, Diaz LA, Anhalt GJ. Herpes gestationis autoantibodies recognize a 180-kD human epidermal antigen. J Clin Invest 1988;81:2023.
83. Diaz LA, Ratrie H III, Saunders WS, et al. Isolation of a human epidermal cDNA corresponding to the 180-kD autoantigen recognized by bullous pemphigoid and herpes gestationis sera. Immunolocalization of this protein to the hemidesmosome. J Clin Invest 1990;86:1088.
84. Lin MS, Gharia MA, Swartz SJ, Diaz LA, Giudice GJ. Identification and characterization of epitopes recognized by T lymphocytes and autoantibodies from patients with herpes gestationis. J Clin Invest 1999;162:4991.
85. Shornick JK, Stastny P, Gilliam JN. High frequency of histocompatibility antigens HLA-DR3 and DR4 in herpes gestations. J Clin Invest 1981;68:553.
86. Mutasim DF, Pelc NJ, Anhalt GJ. Cicatricial pemphigoid. Dermatol Clin 1993;11:499.
87. Yancey KB. Cicatricial pemphigoid. In: Freedberg IM, Eisen AZ, Wolff K, et al. (eds) Fitzpatrick's dermatology in general medicine. New York, McGraw-Hill, 1999;674.
88. Chan LS, Yancey KB, Hammerberg C, et al. Immune-mediated subepithelial blistering diseases of mucous membranes. Pure ocular cicatricial pemphigoid is a unique clinical and immunopathological entity distinct from bullous pemphigoid and other subsets identified by antigenic specificity of autoantibodies. Arch Dermatol 1993;129:448.
89. Bedane C, Prost C, Bernard P, Catanzano G, Bonnetblanc JM, Dubertret L. Cicatricial pemphigoid antigen differs from bullous pemphigoid antigen by its exclusive extracellular localization: a study by indirect immunoelectronmicroscopy. J Invest Dermatol 1991;97:3.
90. Sarret Y, Hall R, Cobo LM, Thivolet J, Patton DL, Woodley DT. Salt-split human skin substrate for the immunofluorescent screening of serum from patients with cicatricial pemphigoid and a new method of immunoprecipitation with IgA antibodies. J Am Acad Dermatol 1991;24:t.
91. Balding SD, Prost C, Diaz LA, et al. Cicatricial pemphigoid autoantibodies react with multiple sites on the BP180 extracellular domain. J Invest Dermatol 1996;106:141.
92. Bedane C, McMillan JR, Balding SD, et al. Bullous pemphigoid and cicatricial pemphigoid autoantibodies react with ultrastructurally separable epitopes on the BP180 ectodomain: evidence that BP180 spans the lamina lucida. J Invest Dermatol 1997;108:901.
93. Sarret Y, Reano A, Nicolas JF, Su H, Thivolet J. Bullous pemphigoid and cicatricial pemphigoid: immunoblotting detection of involved autoantigens. Autoimmunity 1989;2:145.
94. Tyagi S, Bhol K, Natarajan K, Livir-Rallatos C, Foster CS, Ahmed AR. Ocular cicatricial pemphigoid antigen: partial sequence and biochemical characterization. Proc Natl Acad Sci USA 1996;93:14714.
95. Smith EP, Taylor TB, Meyer LJ, Zone JJ. Identification of a basement membrane zone antigen reactive with circulating IgA antibody in ocular cicatricial pemphigoid. J Invest Dermatol 1993;101:619.
96. Domloge-Hultsch N, Gammon WR, Briggaman RA, Gil SG, Carter WG, Yancey KB. Epiligrin, the major human keratinocyte integrin ligand, is a target in both an acquired autoimmune and an inherited subepidermal blistering skin disease. J Clin Invest 1992;90:1628.
97. Ahmed AR, Foster S, Zaltas M, et al. Association of DQw7 (DQB1*0301) with ocular cicatricial pemphigoid. Proc Natl Acad Sci USA 1991;88:11579.
98. Chan LS, Hammerberg C, Cooper KD. Significantly increased occurrence of HLA-DQB1*0301 allele in patients with ocular cicatricial pemphigoid. J Invest Dermatol 1997;108:129.
99. Ciarrocca KN, Greenberg MS. A retrospective study of the management of oral mucous membrane pemphigoid with dapsone. Oral Surg Oral Med Oral Pathol Oral Radiol Endod 1999;88:159.
100. Reiche L, Wojnarowska F, Mallon E. Combination therapy with nicotinamide and tetracyclines for cicatricial pemphigoid: further support for its efficacy. Clin Exp Dermatol 1998;23:254.
101. Neumann R, Tauber J, Foster CS. Remission and recurrence after withdrawal of therapy for ocular cicatricial pemphigoid. Ophthalmology 1991;98:858.
102. Peters MS, Rogers RS. Clinical correlations of linear IgA deposition at the cutaneous basement membrane zone. J Am Acad Dermatol 1989;20:761.
103. Wojnarowska F, Bhogal BS, Black MM. Chronic bullous disease of childhood and linear IgA disease of adults are IgA1-mediated diseases. J Dermatol 1994;131:201.
104. Hall RP III. Linear IgA dermatosis and chronic bullous disease of childhood. In: Freedberg IM, Eisen AZ, Wolff K, et al. (eds) Dermatology in general medicine. New York, McGraw-Hill, 1999; p 680.
105. Zone JJ, Taylor TB, Meyer LJ, Petersen MJ. The 97 kDa linear IgA bullous disease antigen is identical to a portion of the extracellular domain of the 180 kDa bullous pemphigoid antigen, BPAg2. J Invest Dermatol 1998;110:207.
106. Wojnarowska F, Whitehead P, Leigh IM, Bhogal BS, Black MM. Identification of the target antigen in chonic bullous disease of childhood and linear IgA disease of adults. Br J Dermatol 1991;124:157.
107. Coleman MD. Dapsone: modes of action, toxicity and possible strategies for increasing patient tolerance. Br J Dermatol 1993;129:507.
108. Thuong-Nguyen V, Kadunce DP, Hendrix JD, Gammon WR, Zone JJ. Inhibition of neutrophil adherence to antibody by dapsone: a possible therapeutic mechanism of dapsone in the treatment of IgA dermatoses. J Invest Dermatol 1993;100:349.
109. Katz SI (moderator). Dermatitis herpetiformis: the skin and the gut. Ann Intern Med 1980;93:857.
110. Gawkrodger DJ, Blackwell JN, Gilmour HM, Rifkind EA, Heading RC, Barnetson RS. Dermatitis herpetiformis: diagnosis, diet and demography. Gut 1984;25:151.
111. Buckley DB, English J, Molloy W, Doyle CT, Whelton MJ. Dermatitis herpetiformis: a review of 119 cases. Clin Exp Dermatol 1983;8:477.
112. Stockbrugger R, Andersson H, Gillberg R, Kastrup W, Lundquist G, Mobacken H. Autoimmune atrophic gastritis in patient with dermatitis herpetiformis. Acta Derm Venereol 1997;56:111.
113. Gaspari AA, Huang CM, Davey RJ, Bondy C, Lawley TJ, Katz SI. Prevalence of thyroid abnormalities in patients with dermatitis herpetiformis and in control subjects with HLA-B8/-DR3. Am J Med 1990;88:145.
114. Leonard JN, Tucker WF, Fry JS, et al. Increased incidence of malignancy in dermatitis herpetiformis. Br Med J 1983;286:16.
115. Yaoita H, Hertz KC, Katz SI. Dermatitis herpetiformis: immunoelectronmicroscopic and ultrastructural studies of a patient with linear deposition of IgA. J Invest Dermatol 1976;67:691.
116. Chorzelski TP, Beutner EH, Jablonska S, Blaszczyk M, Triftshauser C. Immunofluorescence studies in the diagnosis of dermatitis herpetiformis and its differentiation from bullous pemphigoid. J Invest Dermatol 1971;56:373.

117. Haffenden G, Wojnarowska F, Fry L. Comparison of immunoglobulin and complement deposition in multiple biopsies from the uninvolved skin in dermatitis herpetiformis. Br J Dermatol 1979;101:39.
118. Zone JJ, Meyer LJ, Petersen MJ. Deposition of granular IgA relative to clinical lesions in dermatitis herpetiformis. Arch Dermatol 1996;132:912.
119. Dahl MV, Falk RJ, Carpenter R, Michael AF. Membrane attack complex of complement in dermatitis herpetiformis. Arch Dermatol 1985;121:70.
120. Dahlback K, Lofberg H, Dahlback B. Vitronectin colocalizes with Ig deposits and C9 neoantigen in discoid lupus erythematosus and dermatitis herpetiformis, but not in bullous pemphigoid. Br J Dermatol 1989;120:725.
121. Unsworth DJ, Payne AW, Leonard JN, Fry L, Holborow EJ. IgA in dermatitis-herpetiformis skin is dimeric. Lancet 1982;1:478.
122. Barghuthy FS, Kumar V, Valeski E, Beutner EH, Chorzelski TP. Identification of IgA subclasses in skin of dermatitis herpetiformis patients. Int Arch Allergy Appl Immunol 1988;85:268.
123. Hall RP3: Dermatitis herpetiformis. J Invest Dermatol 1992;99:873.
124. Olbricht SM, Flotte TJ, Collins AB, Chapman CM, Harrist TJ. Dermatitis herpetiformis. Cutaneous deposition of polyclonal IgA1. Archives 1986;122:418.
125. Wojnarowska F, Delacroix D, Gengoux P. Cutaneous IgA subclasses in dermatitis herpetiformis and linear IgA disease. J Cutan Pathol 1988;15:272.
126. Hall RP, McKenzie KD. Comparison of the intestinal and serum antibody response in patients with dermatitis herpetiformis. Clin Immunol Immunopathol 1992;62:t.
127. Lightner VA, Sakai LY, Hall RP. IgA-binding structures in dermatitis herpetiformis skin are independent of elastic-microfibrillar bundles. J Invest Dermatol 1991;96:88.
128. Marks J, Shuster S, Watson AJ. Small bowel changes in dermatitis herpetiformis. Lancet 1966;1280.
129. Hall RP, Sanders ME, Duquesnoy RJ, Katz SI, Shaw S. Alterations in HLA-DP and HLA-DQ antigen frequency in patients with dermatitis herpetiformis. J Invest Dermatol 1989;93:501.
130. Sachs JA, Awad J, McCloskey D, et al. Different HLA associated gene combinations contribute to susceptibility for coeliac disease and dermatitis herpetiformis. Gut 1997;27:515.
131. Hall MA, Lanchbury JS, Bolsover WJ, Welsh KI, Ciclitira PJ. HLA association with dermatitis herpetiformis is accounted for by a cis or transassociated DQ heterodimer. Gut 1991;32:487.
132. Spurkland A, Ingvarsson G, Falk ES, Knutsen I, Sollid LM, Thorsby E. Dermatitis herpetiformis and celiac disease are both primarily associated with the HLA-DQ (alpha 1*0501, beta 1*02) or the HLA-DQ (alpha 1*03, beta 1*0302) heterodimers. Tissue Antigens 1997;49:29.
133. Balas A, Vicario JL, Zambrano A, Acuna D, Garcia-Novo D. Absolute linkage of celiac disease and dermatitis herpetiformis to HLA-DQ. Tissue Antigens 1997;50:52.
134. Reunala T. Incidence of familial dermatitis herpetiformis. Br J Dermatol 1996;134:394.
135. Hall RP, Lawley TJ, Heck JA, Katz SI. IgA-containing circulating immune complexes in dermatitis herpetiformis, Henoch–Schönlein purpura, systemic lupus erythematosus and other diseases. Clin Exp Immunol 1980;40:431.
136. Leonard JN, Chorzelski TP, Beutner EH, IgA anti-endomysial antibody detection in the serum of patients with dermatitis herpetiformis following gluten challenge. Arch Dermatol Res 1985;277:349.
137. Reunala T, Chorzelski TP, Viander M, et al. IgA anti-endomysial antibodies in dermatitis herpetiformis: correlation with jejunal morphology, gluten-free diet and anti-gliadin antibodies. Br J Dermatol 1987;117:185.
138. Dieterich W, Ehnis T, Bauer M, et al. Identification of tissue transglutaminase as the autoantigen of celiac disease. Nature Med 1997;3:797.
139. Molberg O, McAdam SN, Korner R, et al. Tissue transglutaminase selectively modifies gliadin peptides that are recognized by gut-derived T cells in celiac disease. Nature Med 1998;4:713.
140. Smith AD, Bagheri B, Streilein RD, Hall RP III. Expression of interleukin-4 and interferon-gamma in the small bowel of patients with dermatitis herpetiformis and isolated gluten-sensitive enteropathy. Dig Dis Sci 1999;44:2124.
141. Ward MM, Pisetsky DS, Hall RP. Soluble interleukin-2 receptor levels in patients with dermatitis herpetiformis. J Invest Dermatol 1991;97:568.
142. Leonard J, Haffenden G, Tucker W, et al.: Gluten challenge in dermatitis herpetiformis. N Engl J Med 1983;308:816.
143. Crabtree JE, Heatley RV, Juby LD, Howdle PD, Losowsky MS. Soluble interleukin-2 receptor in coeliac disease: response to treatment and gluten challenge. Clin Exp Immunol 1989;77:345.
144. Kadunce DP, McMurry MP, Avots-Avotins A, Chandler JP, Meyer LJ. The effect of an elemental diet with and without gluten on disease activity in dermatitis herpetiformis. J Invest Dermatol 1991;97:175.

Section 7 Organ-Specific Inflammatory Disease

Chapter 76

Myasthenia Gravis

Arnold I. Levinson

INTRODUCTION

Myasthenia gravis (MG) is a disease characterized by weakness of striated muscles. The weakness is due to impaired neuromuscular transmission resulting from a reduction in the number of receptors for the neurotransmitter acetylcholine (ACh) at the postsynaptic myoneural junction. This reduction is caused by the action of anti-acetylcholine receptor (anti-AChR) antibodies. MG is a prototypical autoimmune disease; the immune effector mechanisms and autoantigenic target have been delineated. The disease occurs with a reported prevalence of 0.5–5/100 000 and an incidence of 0.4/100 000/year. Although MG can occur at any age, it typically presents in the second and third decades of life, with a later peak occurring after age 50 (late-onset disease). A female preponderance (3:1–4:1) has been reported in the first 40 years of life; thereafter the incidence is comparable between the sexes.

CLASSIFICATION

MG patients have traditionally been divided into two categories: those with generalized disease and those presenting with disease limited to the ocular muscles.[1] Within these two groups patients can be further subdivided on the basis of age of onset. Neonatal MG affects 10–20% of offspring born to myasthenic mothers. Disease manifestations are those of generalized MG (see below) but are transient, dissipating with the metabolism of maternal anti-AChR antibodies that had been transmitted across the placenta during the third trimester of pregnancy. Several congenital myasthenic syndromes have been described. For the most part these manifest during the neonatal period, persist into adulthood, and are characterized by the absence of anti-AChR antibodies.[2]

A variety of pathophysiologic mechanisms have been delineated, whose unifying feature is their interference with the safety factor of neuromuscular transmission. Juvenile MG describes those patients who present with disease between 1 year of age and puberty. Apart from the age of onset, juvenile myasthenics behave like adult patients with MG.

Adults may present with ocular involvement or signs of more generalized disease. The ocular involvement is characterized by impaired ocular muscle motility and lid weakness, manifesting as diplopia and ptosis, respectively. The vast majority of patients will experience signs of ocular MG, with roughly 50% of patients presenting with ocular signs at the time of diagnosis. An important question that remains to be answered is which of the patients that present with ocular MG will go on to develop more generalized disease. Those at risk of disease progression fall into the following categories: (1) patients with evidence of subclinical disease on electrophysiological testing of limb muscles; and (2) patients who have markedly elevated titers of anti-AChR antibodies. However, these statements can only serve as rough guidelines. In general, patients with ocular symptoms for longer than 2 years will not progress to a more generalized form of disease.

In the generalized disease group patients can be classified into mild, moderate and severe on the basis of clinical activity. Any skeletal muscle group may be affected, but typically the palatal, pharyngeal and upper esophageal muscles are involved. This results in dysarthria, dysphagia and difficulty in handling secretions. Involvement of the diaphragm and intercostal muscles produces dyspnea and may lead to respiratory failure. Involvement of the muscles of the extremities and trunk occurs in 20–30% of patients at initial presentation and causes difficulties with activities of daily living. The hallmark of all of the muscle involvement in MG is its variability over time, with weakness usually exacerbated by repetitive use.

DIAGNOSIS

The differential diagnosis is extremely broad, encompassing neuropathies, primary and secondary myopathies, muscular dystrophy, demyelinating disorders, degenerative diseases, cerebrovascular accidents, mass lesions and infectious diseases. The clinical features that point to a diagnosis of MG include the variable nature of the muscle weakness, normal sensation, and normal deep tendon reflexes. The diagnosis can usually be confirmed by pharmocologic and electrophysiologic testing. A decremental pattern is characteristically seen following repetitive nerve stimulation (Fig. 76.1) and this pattern is normalized following treatment with the anticholinesterase agent tensilon. Further confirmation rests on detecting anti-AChR antibodies, which are found in 90% of patients with generalized disease. In the standard assay, sera are reacted with a nicotinic AChR preparation labeled with ^{125}I-α-bungarotoxin, a snake venom polypeptide that binds irreversibly to the receptor. Bound antibodies are immunoprecipitated by an anti-immunoglobulin reagent or staphylococcal protein A, and the quantity of antibodies detected is expressed in terms of the amount of α-bungarotoxin bound.

CLINICAL PEARLS

Telltale signs of myasthenia

- Variable muscle weakness
- Weakness in cranial nerve distribution
- Normal reflexes and sensation

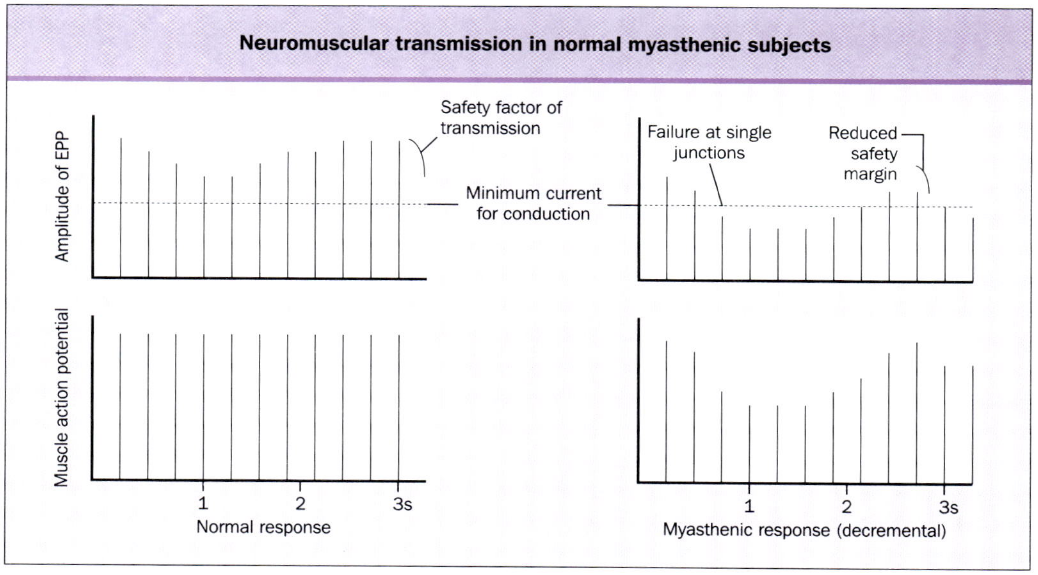

Figure 76.1 Neuromuscular transmission in normal and myasthenic subjects. With repetitive stimulation there is a reduction in the efficiency of ACh release, with a subsequent recovery in efficiency as the train of stimuli continues. Although the endplate potential (EPP) fluctuates at the normal junction, sufficient current is generated to stimulate an action potential of constant magnitude. At the myasthenic junction, however, the amplitude of the EPP in response to a given amount of ACh is reduced. Under conditions of inefficient ACh release, e.g. repetitive stimulation, the minimum current for conduction is not generated, resulting in a profile of action potentials that shows a progressive decline or 'decrement' with subsequent recovery.

AChR STRUCTURE

The nicotinic acetylcholine receptor (nAChR) is a member of a larger family of ligand-gated ion channels. The muscle-type receptor, which is involved in myasthenia, can be subclassified further into mature junctional receptors, and immature, extrajunctional or denervated receptors. The nAChR at a mature myoneural junction is composed of four subunits, labeled α, β, δ and ε (Fig. 76.2). The genes for the α, δ, and γ subunits are located on chromosome 2 in humans, and subunits β and ε on chromosome 17. There are two isoforms of the α subunit, which are generated by alternative splicing.[3] The larger, which includes an additional sequence of 25 amino acids between exons 3 and 4, is found only in humans and other primates. These subunits of the AChR are homologous to each other and to their counterparts across species, with the greatest conservation of sequence being in the α subunit. Two α subunits and one of each of the other subunits are assembled to form an asymmetric hourglass channel spanning the membrane. Each subunit has a large amino terminus located extracellularly, four transmembrane regions, and a short cytoplasmic tail formed by a loop between the third and fourth transmembrane domains. The receptor appears as a dimer owing to disulfide bonding between the δ subunits of two receptors. The two α subunits are not contiguous in each receptor but are separated by another subunit. One ACh-binding site is found on each of the α subunits around the pair of cysteines at amino

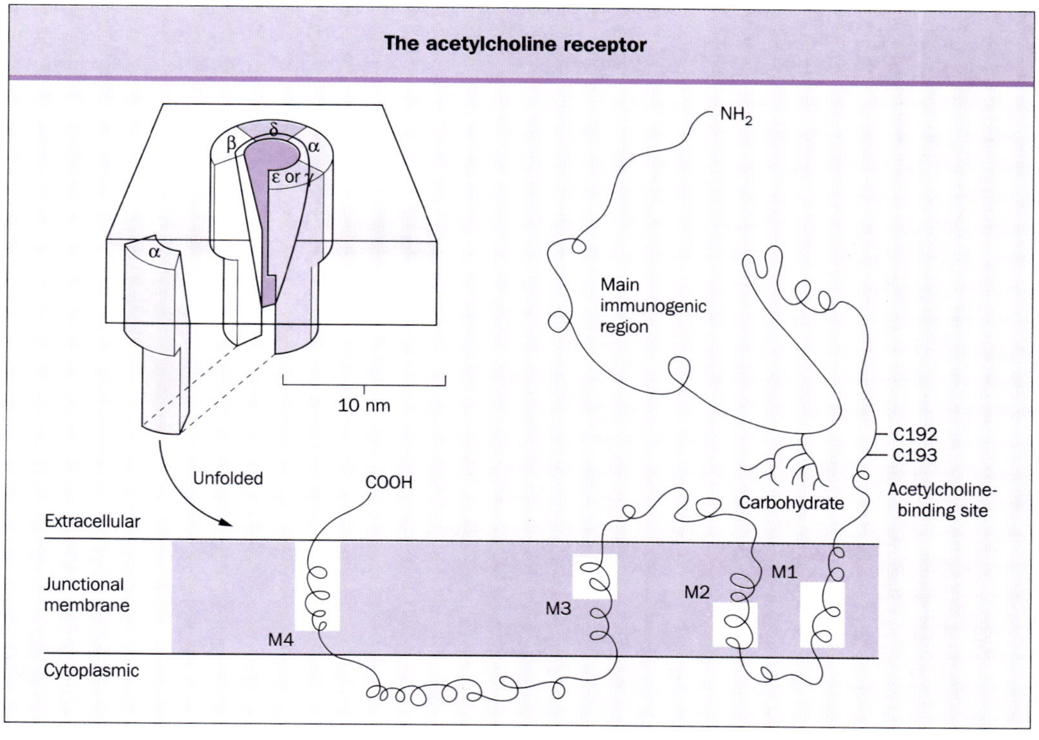

Figure 76.2 The acetylcholine receptor. The subunits of the acetylcholine receptor – α, β, δ, and γ or ε – are arranged like barrel staves around the central ion pore. Each subunit winds through the junctional membrane four times (sites M1, M2, M3 and M4). In the unfolded view of the α subunit, the amino-terminal end of the α subunit is extracellular, where it is accessible to acetylcholine, which binds at the site shown (amino acids 192 and 193). In myasthenia gravis, autoantibodies may bind to various epitopes of all subunits, but a high proportion of antibodies bind to the main immunogenic region of the α subunit.

acids 192 and 193. The binding of ACh to the α subunits is believed to engender a conformational change, possibly resulting in rearrangement of charged groups. The binding of ACh to both α subunits increases the probability of transition of the channel to an open conformation. Binding of curare or α-bungarotoxin to the α subunits blocks this channel.

In normal innervated neuromuscular junctions there are two forms of the AChR, the predominant form having a long half-life, and a small subset that is rapidly turned over.[4] The rapidly turned-over receptors are the precursors of the stable receptors. It is not clear how these two types differ, or how they are regulated. The receptors are concentrated at the top of the folds in the muscle endplate, adjacent to the nerve terminus, at a density of 10 000/μm^2. This localization reflects the action of agrin, a nerve-derived synaptic organizing molecule.[5] The AChRs are organized into clusters by rapsyn, a 43-kDa cytoplasmic protein.[5] The clustered AChRs are linked to the cytoskeleton by connections between rapsyn and a dystrophin–glycoprotein complex.

In fetal muscle, as in adult denervated muscle or nonjunctional membrane, a γ subunit replaces the ε subunit found in mature innervated muscle endplates. This form of the receptor differs from the mature junctional form by its lower density (500 receptors/μm^2) and its distribution over most of the surface of the sarcolemma. The immature receptor also has a lower conductance, a longer open time and a more rapid turnover. Denervation results in a decrease in the amount of AChR with an ε subunit, and an increase in AChR with a γ subunit. This change reverses with reinnervation. Denervation also results in a decrease in the half-life of the AChR that increases with reinnervation. The substitution of a γ for an ε subunit does not coincide exactly with the changes in receptor half-life.

NEUROMUSCULAR TRANSMISSION

When an impulse is transmitted along an axon terminal it results in the release of the neurotransmitter ACh across its presynaptic membrane (Fig. 76.3). ACh, stored in vehicles located throughout the cytoplasm, is concentrated at the points of release in areas called active zones. The release of ACh is dependent on the availability of intracellular calcium, which moves into the nerve terminal through voltage-gated channels. ACh diffuses across a 50 nm synaptic cleft, where it interacts with AChRs that are displayed in greatest density at the tops of the junctional folds of the postsynaptic muscle membrane or endplate. This interaction leads to a local depolarization or endplate potential caused by increased membrane permeability to sodium and potassium. The endplate potential is terminated by acetylcholinesterases, which are present in highest concentrations in the synaptic cleft around the junctional folds. If the summation of endplate potentials attains a prescribed threshold it produces an action potential which depolarizes the surrounding sarcolemma and causes muscle contraction. In a healthy individual the arrival of an impulse at the presynaptic membrane of a motor nerve releases considerably more ACh than is required to generate an action potential. This reserve, roughly four times the current needed for propagation of the impulse, is referred to as the safety factor of neuromuscular transmission.

Neuromuscular transmission is most efficient following the arrival of the initial impulse. The vesicles of ACh are lined up at the active zones and optimal amounts of ACh are available for release.

Schematic representation of the myoneural junction

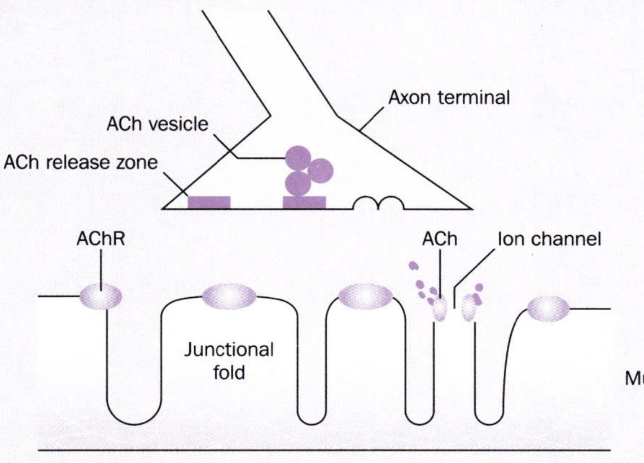

Figure 76.3 Schematic representation of the myoneural junction. Vesicles of ACh release their contents at active zones across from AChRs in response to impulses conducted down nerve axons. ACh diffuses across synaptic cleft and binds to AChRs, with opening of the ion channel and the generation of endplate potential. Action potential is propagated to muscle when sufficient amplitude of summated endplate potentials is attained.

Subsequent stimuli in a repetitive train will be associated with depletion of ACh vesicles. However, the repetitive stimuli cause a net increase in the concentration of presynaptic calcium, which tends to enhance the efficiency of ACh release. Consequently, the first several stimuli in a burst of five per second are associated with a decrease in the efficiency of conduction, but conduction efficiency recovers as the train of stimuli continues. These counteracting forces produce a fluctuation in the amplitude of endplate potentials, with an initial fall followed by a return towards normal values. In the normal state, owing to the safety factor of transmission, the reduced efficiency of vesicle release is clinically inconsequential. Because of the severe reduction in receptor number in MG, the electrical threshold for propagation of an action potential cannot be attained and muscle contraction is prevented. With a less severe reduction in receptor numbers neuromuscular transmission may proceed normally unless the efficiency of presynaptic vesicle release is compromised, as occurs with repetitive use of muscles. The combination of decreasing availability of ACh and the reduced number of receptors accounts for the characteristic decremental nerve conduction pattern seen on electromyograms of patients with MG following repetitive nerve stimulation (Fig. 76.1).

IMMUNOPATHOGENESIS OF MG

Anti-AChR antibodies are detected in 90% of MG patients and are responsible for the impaired neuromuscular transmission.[6] There are many lines of evidence to support this contention IgG, along with C3 and the terminal attack complex (C5–C9) is deposited at AChR-containing areas of the postsynaptic membrane, and anti-AChR/AChR complexes can be extracted from the muscles of patients with MG. Transfer of myasthenic serum from mother to fetus, or from human to mouse, results in symptoms or signs of myasthenia in the recipient. Plasmapheresis, which decreases anti-AChR antibody levels, is associated with clinical improvement (Chapter 118).

> **KEY CONCEPTS**
>
> **Involvement of anti-AChR antibodies in the pathogenesis of MG**
> - Anti-AChR antibodies found in serum of 90% of MG patients.
> - Infants born to myasthenic mothers sometimes develop MG.
> - IgG and complement deposited at the postsynaptic junction.
> - Transfer of IgG from MG patients to mice induces neuromuscular blockade.

Structural properties of anti-AChR and characterization of B-cell epitopes

Anti-AChR antibodies are produced by a small subset of B cells in affected people. The frequency of IgG-producing AChR-specific peripheral blood mononuclear cells is estimated to be 1 in 15 000–70 000.[7] IgG anti-AChR-secreting cells are also found in the peripheral blood of healthy volunteers, albeit to much lower numbers. The proportion of immunoglobulin producing AChR-specific B cells or plasma cells is greater in the germinal centers of hyperplastic thymuses, but still only 1 in 1000–10 000 antibodies produced is AChR specific. Anti-AChR antibodies are predominantly IgG_1 and IgG_3 but IgG_2 and IgG_4 isotypes have also been found. IgA and IgM anti-AChR antibodies are present in some patients, but never in the absence of IgG anti-AChR antibodies.[8] The IgA and IgM anti-AChR antibodies tend to appear in patients whose disease is of longer duration and greater severity, and in association with high IgG titers.

The pathogenic anti-AChR antibodies in MG are thought to be directed to conformationally dependent structures. Immunization of animals with irreversibly denatured AChR does lead to the formation of anti-AChR antibodies capable of binding to native AChR, but those antibodies are not capable of causing disease. This observation indicates that conformationally-dependent epitope(s) are important in the induction of disease. Many of the anti-AChR antibodies are directed against the α subunit, particularly to a small region on the extracellular portion referred to as the main immunogenic region (Fig. 76.2). Approximately 60% of the anti-AChR antibodies are directed against this region, which encompasses a set of overlapping epitopes clustered around amino acids 67–76 of the α subunit, with Asn 68 and Asp 71 being critical for antibody binding.[9] The reason for the predominant role of the α chain in the antibody response in myasthenia is not known. Not all disease-producing antibodies in man or rats appear to be directed to this region. Many patients also have antibodies recognizing the γ-containing embryonic form of AChR. This observation has spawned speculation about a nonmuscle source of sensitization.

The molecular diversity of the anti-AChR response has also been examined. When evaluated by in situ[10] and Southern[11] hybridization techniques, the B cells from the germinal centers of myasthenic hyperplastic thymuses exhibit a pattern of polyclonal activation with variable region gene usage similar to that of normal peripheral blood lymphocytes. The variable heavy- and light-chain regions of three monoclonal anti-AChR antibodies (two IgM and one IgG) derived from the peripheral blood lymphocytes of patients with myasthenia have been sequenced.[12] Based on their nucleotide sequences, the two IgM antibodies appeared to be direct copies of germline gene segments. The variable heavy-chain sequences utilized in these antibodies have been seen in antibodies with other autoimmune specificities. The IgG antibody appeared to have undergone antigenic selection, as evidenced by the appearance of somatic mutations in its variable region segments.

Anti-AChR antibody levels and relationship to disease activity

The relationship of anti-AChR antibody and disease activity in MG is complicated. In general, serum levels of anti-AChR antibody or anti-AChR/AChR complexes correlate poorly with disease severity. Among patients within one clinical grade, anti-AChR antibody levels can vary by several orders of magnitude. In addition, approximately 10% of patients with clinical MG have no anti-AChR antibody by standard assays, indicating that disease may not require antibody, or at least antibody of the specificity detected. Conversely, the finding of anti-AChR-producing B cells in normal subjects suggests that anti-AChR antibodies are not sufficient to cause disease.[7] However, anti-AChR antibody is more likely to be present if the disease is generalized or severe, and there is a tendency for higher levels of anti-AChR antibody to correlate with more severe disease. Also, in an individual patient an increase or decrease in anti-AChR antibody levels often accompanies deterioration or improvement, respectively, in clinical activity.

As the quantity of anti-AChR antibodies produced does not fully explain disease severity, studies have also focused on qualitative differences in these antibodies among different patients. These studies, however, have not been able to distinguish properties of anti-AChR antibodies that lead to grater pathogenicity. Differences in specificity and avidity of binding to AChR have not been associated with particular functional effects or disease severity. Anti-AChR antibodies that bind or compete for the same region of AChR can have different functional effects. Anti-AChR antibodies show extensive heterogeneity by isoelectric focusing, but this characteristic also does not correlate with pathogenic potential.

Ten per cent of MG patients are persistently antibody negative. There is some evidence that this may be a truly distinct subgroup of patients, as one study[14] found that 70% of this group had no thymic pathology (essentially the reverse of myasthenia as a whole), and other investigators found no germinal centers, typically seen in seropositive MG. Thymi in these antibody-negative patients were notable for expanded medullary T-cell areas.[15] Some studies suggest that seronegative patients have less severe disease. However, there is also evidence that some of these so-called antibody-negative patients have anti-AChR antibodies that are not being detected by the routine assay systems. For example, plasma from some of these patients can passively transfer a defect in neuromuscular transmission, and disease activity in a subset of seronegative patients improved with plasmapheresis. Anti-AChR antibodies have been demonstrated in some of these patients by rosetting assays using BC3H1 cells (a mouse tumor cell line that expresses AChR on its surface). Anti-AChR secreting B cells have also been identified in seronegative patients by immunospot assay. Consistent with this finding, human IgG was demonstrated at the neuromuscular synapse when peripheral blood mononuclear cells from seronegative patients were transferred to SCID mice. These findings are difficult to reconcile with those from mice administered plasma from seronegative patients. Although these mice had impaired neuromuscular transmission on electromyography, immunoglobulin was not detected at the myoneural junction.

There are several plausible explanations why antibodies in these patients might not be detected in the serum: the antibodies might be completely bound up by AChR in vivo; the conformational epitopes to which the antibodies bind might be lost or altered during the extraction of AChR from its tissue source; and finally, antibodies might be binding to some structure other than AChR and interfering with neuromuscular transmission by another mechanism. It might also be argued that the seronegative patients have some other, nonimmunoglobulin, factor in their plasma fraction that interferes with neuromuscular transmission.

Patients with purely ocular symptoms of myasthenia (OMG) have a distinctive antibody profile compared to patients with generalized disease. About half of ocular myasthenia patients are seronegative. When antibodies are present, they are more often directed against normal junctional nAChR than the extrajunctional form even though the extrajunctional γ subunit has been identified in extraocular muscles.[16] In contrast, the latter specificity usually predominates in generalized myasthenia. Perhaps most significantly, some patients with OMG have antibodies directed against AChR found in a clustered form on the motor endplate seen at neuromuscular synapses in extraocular muscle but not in limb muscle.[17] It is also interesting that whereas antinuclear antibodies are commonly found in generalized myasthenia, they are absent in ocular myasthenia. Antithyroid antibodies, which are absent in generalized myasthenia, are found in 40% of patients with ocular myasthenia and are particularly common in the anti-AChR subset without detectable antibodies.

Patients with myasthenia gravis associated with thymoma also show distinct patterns of antibody production. Almost all patients with thymoma are anti-AChR antibody positive and most produce antistriational antibodies.[18] These antibodies react with titin, a giant filamentous protein of striated muscle. Titin filaments are involved in muscle assembly and contribute to the muscle's ability to recoil following stimulation. Such antistriational antibodies are also found in approximately 50% of the sera of older, nonthymoma MG patients who have thymic atrophy, but are not frequently detected in patients with early-onset disease and thymic hyperplasia. The finding of antistriational antibodies in an MG patient less than 40 years old strongly suggests the presence of thymoma. There is no evidence that antistriational antibodies are involved in muscle weakness.

MG sera also contain antibodies reacting with the ryanodine receptor.[18] These receptors, which are critically involved in muscle contraction, are Ca^{2+} release channels located in the sarcoplasmic reticulum of striated muscles. Antibodies to ryanodine receptors are found in 50% of MG patients with thymoma, and patients with high levels have a worse prognosis than do antibody-negative MG patients with thymoma. In vitro studies have suggested a pathogenic role for these autoantibodies in MG.

Antirapsyn antibodies have been detected in a small subset of MG patients.[19] Seropositive patients with MG are indistinguishable from seronegative patients with regard to clinical and laboratory features of disease. The presence of this autoantibody specificity is not specific for MG, having been detected in the sera of an occasional MS patient and a majority of the lupus patients tested.

PATHOGENIC EFFECTS OF ANTI-AChR ANTIBODIES

Complement-mediated damage

The critical problem in MG is the anti-AChR antibody-mediated reduction in the number of nAChRs at the myoneural junction. There are several possible mechanisms by which the anti-AChR antibodies could lead to impaired neuromuscular transmission.[20] Ultramicroscopic studies show marked destructive changes in some endplates, particularly at the peaks of the postsynaptic folds, where AChR is usually present in the greatest concentration. The architecture of the muscle endplate is simplified, with loss of junctional folds and widening of the synaptic cleft that contains membrane debris. C3, C9 and the membrane attack complex are deposited at the muscle endplate, suggesting a role for complement in membrane destruction.[21] Indeed, the anti-AChR antibodies in many patients can fix complement in vitro when bound to skeletal muscle, and can damage cultured rat myotubes with a resultant decrease in AChR content.

Although antibody-directed complement-mediated destruction is important in the pathophysiology of MG, it is not the entire story. The rapid clinical improvement in MG following certain therapeutic interventions and the lack of destructive changes in many neuromuscular junctions of symptomatic areas despite prominent immunoglobulin deposition suggest that a more readily reversible process is also likely to be involved in the neuromuscular block.

Acceleration of AChR degradation

In vitro and in vivo studies have shown that anti-AChR antibodies can accelerate the rate of degradation of extrajunctional and junctional receptors, respectively.[22] This reaction is complement independent and is due to the endocytosis of AChRs via shallow depressions, presumably clathrin-coated pits. Other membrane receptors are not affected. Both stable and rapidly turned-over receptors appear to be affected, thereby explaining the greater than expected antibody-mediated loss of AChRs observed at neuromuscular junctions. The reaction requires cross-linking of adjacent AChRs, as it can be mediated by $F(ab')_2$ fragments, but not Fab fragments, of anti-AChR antibodies. The effect of antibody on the synthesis of new AChR is controversial.

Receptor blockade

The inhibition of ACh binding has been assessed by studying the effects of MG serum on the binding of the neurotoxin α-bungarotoxin to AChRs. Such blocking antibodies are found in a

> **KEY CONCEPTS**
>
> **Effects of anti-AChR antibodies in MG pathology**
> - Reduced number of receptors
> - Widening of the synaptic cleft
> - Distorted geometry of the synaptic membrane
>
> **Mechanisms of damage**
> - Complement dependent damage to muscle endplate
> - Enhanced rate of AChR degradation
> - Block cholinergic binding sites

variable number of MG sera. Blockade has been generally attributed to steric hindrance of the ligand-binding site, rather then direct binding to the ACh-binding site.[23] The importance of these antibodies in the pathophysiology of MG remains unclear. However, in one study the functional ability of an individual serum to accelerate degradation and cause blockade of AChRs paralleled most closely the clinical status of the patient. The in vivo significance of such antibodies has also been demonstrated by passive transfer of certain rat monoclonal anti-AChR antibodies into chicks. Complete paralysis was observed within 1 hour of the transfer, presumably before there was time for complement-mediated damage. In MG patients it has been reasoned that such blocking antibodies could further diminish synaptic function already decreased owing to complement-mediated damage or accelerated receptor degradation. This could result in acute clinical deterioration or a rapid clinical improvement after plasmapharesis, before the repair of damaged membrane and regeneration of new AChRs.

Role of T cells

An overwhelming body of data indicates that anti-AChR antibody production in MG patients and rodents with experimental autoimmune myasthenia gravis (EAMG) is dependent on the activity of CD4 T cells.[26] Researchers have used freshly isolated CD4 T cells, T-cell lines and T-cell clones stimulated with AChR purified from the electric organs of *Torpedo californica* (T-AChR), recombinant human AChR, human AChR concentrated on immunomagnetic beads, and synthetic AChR peptides. Most of the T cells derived from MG patients have responded to the complete AChR or the α subunit, but responses to the δ, ε and γ subunits have also been demonstrated.[24] Unlike experimental autoimmune myasthenia gravis (EAMG), a T-cell immunodominant epitope has not been found in humans. However, T cells from most patients recognize a limited number of AChR sequences. In an individual patient, T cells reactive with a particular AChR epitope can show limited TCR Vβ usage, but the same TCR VB usage has not been observed for different patients. A range of MHC class II molecules can present AChR epitopes. This is not surprising, given the degenerate binding capabilities of MHC molecules needed to present an extremely large and diverse group of peptides to the immune system. T cells from normal controls respond to some of the same epitopes to which MG patient's T cells respond, albeit in smaller numbers and less vigorously.

Experimental autoimmune myasthenia gravis (EAMG)

The serendipitous discovery that rabbits injected with purified AChR developed not only anti-AChR antibodies but signs of myasthenia gravis provided the evidence for the pivotal role of antibodies in this disease, and paved the way for the development of an experimental model of human MG.[25] Experimental autoimmune myasthenia gravis (EAMG) has been studied in a number of different animal species.[26] It is generally induced by immunizing animals with AChR purified from the electric organs of *Torpodo californica* and emulsified in adjuvant. Disease may also be passively transferred by immunoglobulin from affected animals or from patients with myasthenia. The induced disease is similar to the spontaneous human disease in a number of ways. Both humans and animals suffer from fatigue, hypoactivity, weight loss, paralysis, difficulty in breathing and dysphagia; these signs are reversible with anticholinesterases. There is a decremental response to repetitive nerve stimulation on electromyography in EAMG as well as in MG. Myasthenic animals share their human counterparts' hypersensitivity to curare. Anti-AChR antibodies are present and most are directed against the main immunogenic region (Fig. 76.2). They are deposited along with complement at the muscle endplate. Similar to the pathology in humans, there is simplification of the muscle endplate and a loss of AChR content of muscles in the experimental disease.

Despite these similarities between the human disease and animal models, there are some striking differences between the manifestations of EAMG in different species, and some notable differences between the model and the human disease. In rabbits and monkeys the disease is generally acute and fatal. It is generally mild and transient in rats, in which it is characterized by acute and chronic phases. In rats the acute phase is characterized by infiltration with macrophages, whereas infiltration of the muscle endplate by inflammatory cells is not a feature of human MG. In mice, EAMG varies from extremely mild to rapidly fatal. Notably, there is no thymic pathology in any of the animal models of EAMG. In spite of these caveats, the establishment of a murine model, where the genetics are well defined and the immunology well studied, has enhanced our understanding of the disease pathogenesis and has more clearly defined questions that remain to be answered.

In murine models there are disease-resistant and disease-susceptible strains. The major histocompatibility complex (MHC) determines this susceptibility in part, with specific H-2 alleles associated with susceptibility or resistance. However, even in the high-responder strains only 50–70% of immunized animals manifest disease. This lack of concordance remains to be fully explained. Differences in the level of complement activation and the physiologic safety factor of neuromuscular transmission may partly account for the variability in disease expression.

Most immunized animals demonstrate anti-AChR antibodies whether or not they develop EAMG. Induction of pathogenic antibody production requires the integrity of the three-dimensional structure of the receptor, as immunization with denatured AChR elicits antibody production but not disease, even in susceptible animals. Anti-AChR antibody levels correlate with anti-AChR/AChR complexes and with the AChR content of the muscle, but not with clinical disease severity. No characteristic feature distinguishing disease-producing and nonpathogenic autoantibodies has been defined. Antibodies in rats with and without disease are predominantly of the same immunoglobulin isotope and subclass, express similar clonotypic heterogeneity, and show similar acidities.[27] The percentage of antibodies that recognize the native receptor (as opposed to the foreign eel receptor immunogen) is low (0.2–2%), but similar between the symptomatic and the asymptomatic mice. The percentage of antibody directed against the main immunogenic region of AChR is also similar. The antibodies that develop in asymptomatic animals can bind and cause a decrease in receptor half-life, as well as those that develop in paralyzed animals. In fact, EMG abnormalities can be demonstrated in mice who appear disease free.[28] An analogous situation in humans may be the high frequency of single fiber EMG abnormalities in asymptomatic family members of patients with MG. Importantly, antibodies from affected animals will cause disease in resistant strains, indicating that disease differences between strains is not caused by differences in the AChR receptor itself.

Although EAMG is mediated by autoantibodies, it is a T-cell-dependent process. Examination of T-cell responses in rats and mice has shown that EAMG requires the action of CD4 T cells. These cells recognize immunodominant T-cell epitopes located on the α subunit.[26] The T-cell responses to the immunodominant epitope in rats involve a variety of TCRVβ and Jβ gene segments. However, in susceptible C57BL/6 mice there is a predominant use of the TCRVβ6 family in the CD4 T-cell response.[26] CD4 T cells in susceptible and resistant strains recognize different immunodominant AchR α-chain epitopes.[29]

Early reports suggested that AChR-reactive T-cell clones did not fit neatly into T-helper 1 (Th1) and Th2 subsets. However, recent studies suggest that interferon-γ production by Th1 cells is essential for the development of disease. Thus, disruption of the interferon-γ gene in disease-susceptible mice is associated with a marked reduction in the titer and affinity of IgG anti-AChR antibodies and decreased severity of EAMG following immunization with AChR and adjuvant.[26] In contrast, IL-4 knockout mice show little change in acute EAMG compared to wildtype counterparts and also go on to develop a chronic form of disease.[30] Further evidence of the importance of a Th1 response in the pathogenesis of EAMG comes from studies of IL-12. Coadministration of IL-12 with a sensitizing dose of AChR to susceptible mice results in increased IgG2a anti-AChR antibody titers, increased AChR-induced interferon-γ production by peripheral lymphocytes in vitro, and an earlier and more severe form of EAMG.[31] Relative to wild-type mice, IL-12 knockout mice demonstrate less IgG2a anti-AChR antibodies, less AChR-induced interferon-γ production by peripheral lymphocytes in vitro, and less severe EAMG following immunization with AChR. Collectively, these studies suggest that interferon-γ is required for the production of pathogenic anti-AChR antibodies and disease expression, whereas IL-4 may subserve a protective role.

The roles of CD28/B7 and CD40/CD40 ligand interactions have been investigated in EAMG.[26] Interactions between these respective receptor–ligand pairs appear to be required for the development of the primary immune response to AChR. However, they play a less important role in the secondary response or in the maintenance of the immune response to this autoantigen.

THE THYMUS IN MYASTHENIA GRAVIS

Several lines of evidence have implicated the thymus in the pathogenesis of MG.

Pathology

Early observations from autopsy material and later analyses of thymectomy specimens indicated that the thymus is pathologically abnormal in 80–90% of MG patients.[32] The majority of patients (65–75%) have thymic follicular hyperplasia. This histologic picture is seen most frequently in women with a relatively early disease onset and with HLA-B8 and DR3 haplotypes. The architecture of the hyperplastic thymi is generally preserved, with well demarcated cortical and medullary regions. However, the medulla is crowded by numerous germinal centers that display the architectural features and cellular constituents of germinal centers in the secondary follicles of peripheral lymph nodes from normal individuals. Although these germinal centers in patients are generally thought to occupy an intraparenchymal position, some observers feel that they may actually lie extraparenchymally in the perivascular space. The appearance of thymic germinal centers is not unique to MG. They have been observed in the thymi of healthy subjects who have died suddenly from traumatic injury, and in autopsy specimens of patients with SLE, thyrotoxicosis and multiple sclerosis. Nevertheless, they are widely regarded to be larger and more numerous in patients with MG.

Patients with MG and associated thymomas tend to be older and show no gender predominance or HLA associations. Histologic sections show neoplastic epithelial cells admixed with thymocytes and a loss of the normal corticomedullary definition. The affected epithelial cells belong to the cortical epithelial compartment, and the thymocytes have the immunophenotypic properties of normal immature cortical thymocytes.

> **KEY CONCEPTS**
>
> **Pathogenic role of the thymus in MG**
>
> *Clinical*
> - Improvement associated with thymectomy
>
> *Pathological*
> - 75% of patients have germinal hyperplasia, 10% have thymomas
>
> *Immunological*
> - nAChR-reactive T and B cells localized in thymus
> - nAChR expressed on cells within thymus

Clinical

The demonstration of thymic pathology prompted empiric trials of thymectomy in patients with MG. Although no controlled study has been performed, there is general agreement that removal of the thymus, particularly in young patients with follicular hyperplasia, leads to clinical improvement. This topic is considered in more detail in the discussion on therapy later in this chapter.

Intrathymic AChR

For some time there has been evidence that nAChR is expressed in the thymus.[32,33] This finding, in conjunction with the thymic pathology described above, has raised the hypothesis that thymic expression of AChR may be involved in the initiation or perpetuation of the autoimmune response in MG. At the protein level, the AChR α chain is expressed on thymic myoid cells and epithelial cells. Most of the current evidence is consistent with the expression of a fetal receptor on myoid cells and an adult receptor on thymic epithelial cells. In addition, an epitope localized to residues 373–380 of the AChR α-chain cytoplasmic domain has been detected on neoplastic epithelial cells of thymomas and thymic carcinomas, and is most often seen in thymomas associated with MG. This epitope is also found in smaller amounts on normal thymic medullary cells. The source of the epitope is not AChR but a cross-reactive protein with a molecular weight of 153 kDa.[34] The overexpression of this protein in thymomas may trigger an anti-AChR antibody response, leading to the development of MG.

Studies relying on molecular probes of AChR expression indicate that both major isoforms of the α subunit are expressed in human thymus.[33,35] The smaller P3A⁻ isoform is present in approximately a fivefold excess in both MG and control thymic tissue,[35] which differs from the aquivalent expression of these isoforms in control and MG muscle. These observations suggest that the expression of mRNAs encoding the $P3A^-$ and $P3A^+$ isoforms is regulated differently in human thymus compared to muscle. As the same disproportionate expression of $P3A^-$ was observed in control and MG thymus, the differential pattern of expression observed in thymus relative to muscle is probably not a manifestation of thymic pathology in MG. Rather, this pattern may reflect control processes that are unique to these two distinct tissue compartments. It is currently not known whether the disproportionate expression of $P3A^-$ and $P3A^+$ isoforms has pathogenic significance. Notably, the expression of both $P3A^+$ and $P3A^-$ mRNAs is increased in MG thymus relative to control thymus. This finding parallels that reported for skeletal muscle, where AChR mRNA expression is greater in MG muscle than in control muscle. The finding of increased AChRα mRNA expression in MG thymus may represent an attempt to compensate for the destructive action of locally secreted anti-AChR antibodies. The increased AChR mRNA expression may also reflect the antecedent action of other local environmental factors, e.g. cytokines.

Sequencing of $P3A^+$ and $P3A^-$ cDNA clones recovered from control and MG thymi indicates that they share the same nucleotide sequence as their respective counterparts at the myoneural junction.[33,36] Therefore, unless there are post-translational changes, the structure of the AchRα proteins expressed in the thymus and the periphery are likely to be identical. These results provide a structural basis for proposing that an immune response directed at thymic nAChRα is indeed responsible for initiating or perpetuating disease.

Immunologic

From an immunologic standpoint the MG thymus has unique features that could reflect pathogenic involvement and help explain some of the histologic abnormalities.[32] Although B cells and Ig-secreting cells are rare intramedullary inhabitants of normal thymi, they are increased in cell suspensions of MG thymus, particularly hyperplastic thymus (obtained from subjects undergoing elective cardiothoracic surgery). The B cells in suspension are largely surface IgG positive, even though the predominant B cells in hyperplastic thymus tissue sections are surface IgM positive. When stimulated in vitro with the polyclonal B-cell activator pokeweed mitogen, both MG and normal thymus cell suspensions produced surprisingly large amounts of immunoglobulin, with the IgG isotype greatly exceeding IgM.

There has been great interest in determining whether the heightened B-cell activity in MG thymus reflects local immune events. Single cell suspensions from thymi of MG patients with follicular hyperplasia secrete anti-AChR antibody.[32] However, the thymic B-cell repertoire also includes anti-influenza specificity and anti-tetanus toxoid specificity. The latter is only detected when patients are booster immunized to tetanus toxoid 3–4 weeks prior to thymectomy. Thus, the B-cell repertoire in the MG thymus may reflect systemic as well as local immune events.

AChR-reactive CD4 T cells have been detected and propagated as long-term lines and clones from MG thymus (both thymoma and hyperplasia), but not from normal thymus. These antigen-specific T cells seem to be enriched in the thymus relative to the blood of the same MG patient. Migration of T cells reactive to foreign antigen into the thymus is known to occur.[37] Therefore, it is not clear whether AChR-reactive T cells in MG thymus are sensitized in the periphery with subsequent intrathymic localization, or are sensitized in situ.

In addition, hyperplastic MG thymus shows increased numbers of IL-1- and IL-6-producing cells. These cells were found largely in the perifollicular areas and connective tissue adjacent to the septae of disrupted cortex. Cells producing IL-2 were less prominent and confined largely to perifollicular areas. This distribution of cytokine production was not seen in normal thymus or in hyperplastic lymph nodes.

Together, the above studies indicate that MG thymus contains all the cellular constituents necessary for an immune response directed against AChR. These include AChR-reactive B cells and helper T cells, as well as a local source of the autoantigen. Moreover, there appears to be an array of cytokines produced that may facilitate T- and B-cell activation. It is still not known whether autosensitization occurs in the thymus with spillover to the myoneural junction, or whether the thymic pathology is causally related to the pathogenesis of MG. Thymic pathologic changes are not typically seen in the thymi of rodents with actively or passively induced MG. These studies provide evidence that the pathologic changes seen in MG thymus are not secondary to the autoimmune response and may be linked to the etiopathogenesis of this disease. The trigger for the putative intrathymic sensitization remains to be determined.

ETIOLOGIC FACTORS

Genetic factors

Similar to most autoimmune diseases, the MHC represents an important genetic susceptibility locus for the development of MG. Studies indicate that the MHC haplotype with HLA-B8, DR3 and DQ2 is associated with early-onset MG and hyperplastic thymus in Caucasian individuals. An association with HLA-B7 and DR2, although weaker, has also been described for patients with onset of MG after the age of 40 years associated with atrophic thymic histology. In murine studies the MHC Class II molecules $I\text{-}A^b$ and $I\text{-}E^k$ have been associated with suceptibility to EAMG.[26] In EAMG the permissive MHC Class II molecules are capable of binding AChR peptides that are recognized by antigen-specific CD4 T cells.

Studies have also addressed the potential genetic contributions of other immune system-related genes in the pathogenesis of MG. An association has been reported for a particular IL-1β allele and MG.[38] This was most pronounced in patients who lacked disease-susceptible HLA genes. Several groups have reported an association between MG and the presence of particular TNF-α polymorphisms.[39–41] The expression of a high-transcription TNF-α allotype correlated with early-onset MG and the absence of anti-titin antibodies. In this regard, MG patients demonstrate increased serum levels of TNF-α and their peripheral blood mononuclear cells display increased expression of TNF-α mRNA.[41] Polymorphisms in the IL-10 promoter region have also been reported to be associated with distinct patterns of thymic histology.[42] No correlations have been made between IL-4 alleles and MG. Finally, allotypic markers on IgG and FcγRIIa receptors have been associated with the coexistence of MG and thymoma.[43]

Exogenous factors

Whether or not sensitization to AChR occurs in the thymus or the periphery, the stimulus for this autoimmune response remains a conundrum. As mentioned earlier in this chapter, analysis of anti-AChR antibody sequences suggests that these autoimmune responses are driven by antigen. However, it remains to be determined whether the stimulus is self-antigen (AChR) or a foreign antigen that mimics the receptor's molecular structure. In this regard, several examples of molecular mimicry between AChRα chain and other molecules have been reported. Studies carried out with certain monoclonal anti-AChR antibodies demonstrated epitope sharing between the receptor and several bacteria, including *Klebsiella pneumoniae*, *Eschericchia coli*, *Proteus vulgaris* and *Yersinia enterocolitica*.[44] However, for the most part no difference was observed in the binding of polypeptides from these organisms by either MG patient or control sera. A computer search of protein banks revealed a sequence homology between AChRα chain and a short peptide in herpes simplex glycoprotein D,[45] although the significance of this finding is unknown. Finally, similarities were reported between idiotypic determinants on anti-AChR antibodies and antibodies reactive with α1,3 dextran. Interestingly, antidextran antibodies were detected in approximately 13% of MG patients but rarely in normal controls.[46] α1,3 Dextran is found in the cell walls of several common enteric pathogens and thus represents a potential ubiquitous source of immunogen. This type of idiotypic network connectivity led the investigators to postulate that an unregulated anti-idiotypic response to anti-α1,3 dextran antibodies might lead, in certain individuals, to an anti-AChR antibody response. Unfortunately, there has been no follow-up to these observations.

A striking association has been reported between the development of MG and treatment with the drug penicillamine,[47,48] particularly in individuals with HLA DR1. MG developed in patients with rheumatoid arthritis and patients with Wilson's disease treated with this agent. After discontinuation of penicillamine, resolution of MG symptoms was reported in some patients but not others. Penicillamine treatment was associated with the development of anti-AChR antibodies that appeared to have the same type of specificity profile as found in idopathic myasthenia. Additional evidence suggests that penicillamine may directly interfere with neuromuscular transmission. Although penicillamine has been shown to have diverse effects on the immune response in the normal host, and has reactive sulfhydryl groups capable of modifying self-antigens, its role in the development of MG remains to be determined.

TREATMENT OF MYASTHENIA GRAVIS

Therapeutic intervention in MG usually proceeds in a stepwise manner, beginning with anticholinesterase agents.[49]

THERAPEUTIC PRINCIPLES

Therapeutic approaches
- Anticholinesterase agents
- Thymectomy
- Plasmapheresis
- Corticosteroids
- Immunosuppressive agents
- Intravenous γ-globulin

Anticholinesterases

Anticholinesterases are the mainstay of treatment. These agents protect acetylcholine from hydrolysis by cholinesterase, thereby increasing the amount of neutrotransmitter and the number of contacts with the reduced number of receptors at the postsynaptic junction. This in turn raises the probability of attaining the necessary threshold for neuromuscular transmission. In addition, some of the anticholinesterase agents have a direct agoinst effect at the postsynaptic junction. The three most popular agents in this group are neostigmin bromide (prostigmin), pyridostigmin bromide (mestinon) and ambenonium chloride (mytelase). Although there are only slight differences between these agents, mestinon remains the most commonly used. It has an onset of action of 30–60 minutes, peak action at about 2 hours, and loss of activity occurring after 4 hours. The drug is usually initiated at a dose of 60 mg every 3–4 hours and increased if necessary in 30–60 mg increments. Additional benefit is usually not seen at doses higher than 240 mg every 3–4 hours or 120 mg every 2 hours. It is important to individualize the dosing schedule for each patient according to their needs. For example, the patient with bulbar symptoms should be instructed to take anticholinesterase 30 minutes to 1 hour before meals. Adverse effects of these agents are due to excessive stimulation of nicotinic and muscarinic receptors. The nicotinic side-effects include fasciculations, muscle cramps and increased weakness. Muscarinic side-effects include diarrhea, abdominal cramps, palpitations, increased sweating, and nasal and bronchial secretions. Adding atropine or an atropine analog to the regimen can minimize the latter group of reactions. This provides a cushion for increasing the amount of drug, and hence, its effect at the postsynaptic junction. Auxiliary drugs that have been purported to have a salutary effect on neuromuscular transmission are ephedrine and xanthine derivatives (theophylline), which are thought to increase the presynaptic release of ACh. The minimal effect of their added benefit has not warranted their common usage.

Thymectomy

Another mainstay in the therapy of the adult with generalized MG is thymectomy.[49–52] The benefit is greatest in younger patients and those with thymic hyperplasia, although many centers include older patients as well. Although no controlled study has ever been carried out, the accumulated experience indicates that thymectomy is associated with an excellent outcome, measured as either remission or an improvement in clinical symptoms. In one study 90% of patients were asymptomatic or in complete remission within a few years of thymectomy, and 46% were off all medications. With improvements in preoperative care, anesthesia, surgical technique and postoperative care, thymectomy has become a very safe procedure, but its value and safety in children and older patients is less well established. There is still some controversy over what represents the best surgical procedure, although the trans-sternal approach is the choice in most centers. Unlike the transcervical approach, it is less likely to be complicated by residual thymic tissue. The mechanism responsible for the salutary effect of thymectomy remains to be elucidated. No obvious effects on immunoregulatory mechanisms have been demonstrated, although anti-AChR titers tend to fall months after the procedure. Thymectomy is also the recommended treatment for patients of all ages suspected of having thymoma.

Corticosteroids

Corticosteroids are used in patients with generalized MG who fail to respond to anticholinesterase agents or thymectomy, and in patients needing optimization of their clinical condition in preparation for thymectomy.[53] They are generally not used as a first-line agent to replace thymectomy. They are also used in patients with ocular myasthenia who fail to respond to anticholinesterases. Corticosteroids are initially given on a daily basis, with therapy begun in hospital. This cautious approach is followed because of the fear of clinical deterioration that occurs in some patients during the introduction of corticosteroids. Because of this concern, some groups advocate starting patients on alternate-day therapy, which is not typically associated with clinical deterioration and can be carried out on an outpatient basis. Daily corticosteroids are usually started in patients with generalized MG at a dose >1 mg/kg prednisone. Patients should be continued on this dose until clinical improvement is maintained for several days, and then gradually weaned on to alternate-day therapy. With improvement sustained over several months, an effort should be made to reduce the dose (usually in 5 mg decrements) administered on the alternate day. Although no controlled studies have ever been carried out, the improvement rate is estimated to be 60–90%. Complete remission is rare and most patients will require some dose of steroids indefinitely. The physician should be alert to the possibility that anticholinesterase requirements may decrease as the patient responds to corticosteroids.

Plasmapheresis

Plasmapheresis has enjoyed popularity since its introduction as an auxiliary treatment modality in 1976, particularly as a temporizing measure.[54] It appears to be most beneficial in patients in myasthenic crisis and in those experiencing progressive deterioration despite treatment with anticholinesterases and corticosteroids. Plasmapheresis has also proved to be useful in preparing patients for thymectomy whose course is complicated by involvement of the bulbar and respiratory musculature. Such patients may also require short-term plasmapheresis during the postoperative period. Although there are no hard and fast rules, the average exchange is 1–2 l/day for 7–14 days. Improvement is usually observed within a few days of concluding the treatment course, although patients in crisis often benefit more quickly. The mechanism of action most likely involves the removal of the pathogenic autoantibody, as a reduction in titer of anti-AChR antibody correlates with clinical improvement. However, it is also possible that the removal of other phlogistic humoral factors contributes to clinical efficacy.

Immunosuppressive agents

Immunosuppressive drugs have been tried primarily in patients who have failed treatment with anticholinesterases, thymectomy, plasmapheresis and corticosteroids.[55–57] Most of the experience has been obtained with azathioprine, which has strong anti-inflammatory effects as well as immunosuppressive activity. The dose of azathioprine has varied between 1 and 3 mg/kg/day, with improvement seen between 5 and 20 weeks. The drug is usually started at a lower dose and escalated weekly to achieve the maintenance dose. The patient should be followed with complete blood counts, particularly during the initiation of therapy, as azathioprine has a suppressive effect on the bone marrow. A white blood cell count below 2500 or a neutrophil count below 1500 should prompt a reduction or termination of the dosage. The results of a randomized double-blind placebo-controlled trial indicated that the addition of azathioprine (2.5 mg/kg) to alternate-day prednisolone was associated with a reduction of the prednisolone dose, fewer treatment failures, longer remissions and fewer side-effects.[57] There is considerably less experience with cyclophosphamide, another powerful immunosuppressive agent. In the hands of most clinicians, its use is associated with more adverse effects and does not appear to offer any significant advantage. Methotrexate has been used in some uncontrolled studies but there is no information to indicate that it is more efficacious or safer than azathioprine. As is true for corticosteroid therapy, it is the rare patient who enjoys a permanent remission following institution of immunosuppressive therapy, and those who show some improvement often require treatment indefinitely.

Cyclosporin A (Cy-A), a potent immunosuppressive agent, has been investigated because it interferes with IL-2-mediated T-cell proliferation and thus would be expected to interfere with the generation of T cells that would 'help' the anti-AChR antibody response. Treated patients showed greater improvement and a more impressive fall in anti-AChR antibody titer. However, a number of patients enrolled in the treatment group had to be withdrawn because of drug toxicity. In a subsequent 12-month European trial, Cy-A appeared to be as efficacious as azathioprine in producing clinical improvement.

Intravenous immunoglobulin

There have been several uncontrolled trials of intravenous immunoglobulin (IVIG) in MG. Interest in the use of this agent grew out of its demonstrated efficacy in other autoimmune diseases, most notably autoimmune thrombocytopenia. IVIG has generally been administered at a dose of 2 g/kg over 2–4 days. The results of these trials suggest that IVIG therapy can be associated with rapid clinical improvement in some patients, independent of whether they had undergone thymectomy or were being treated concurrently with corticosteroids or immunosuppressive agents. In some patients improvement was sustained over a period of several weeks. The mechanism(s) of this apparent salutary effect is unknown; improvement was not always accompanied by a consistent reduction in anti-AChR antibody titers. The efficacy of this agent in the treatment of MG can only be determined by controlled clinical trials, which are currently in progress.

POSSIBLE FUTURE THERAPEUTIC OPTIONS

There are a number of possible experimental avenues of approach. These are aimed at interrupting the sensitization process of helper CD4 T cells or interrupting their effector function. Such strategies include blocking the presentation of immunogenic AChR peptides by antigen presenting cells with nonimmunogenic forms of peptides, the induction of anergy or apoptosis of AChR-reactive T cells, or possibly suppressing AChR-specific Th1 responses. All of these approaches have achieved some degree of success in EAMG, where a limited number of immunodominant AChR T-cell epitopes are operative.[26] Delivery of synthetic AChR peptides via the mucosal route (i.e. oral tolerance) has been used in animals to prevent EAMG and, in some studies, to suppress ongoing disease. Nasal administration of AChR peptides prior to the induction of disease in susceptible mice and after the induction of disease in susceptible rats resulted in the prevention and suppression of EAMG, respectively. Notably, treated animals generally showed markedly depressed AChR-specific Th1 immune responses, with little effect on AChR-specific Th2 responses. At present it is not known whether such peptide-based approaches will work in human MG, particularly as the range of AChR peptides recognized by T cells is likely to be more diverse. In animal studies the costimulatory molecules CD28/B7 and CD40 ligand/CD40 are required for the primary AChR response, but may be less important in the maintenance of this autoimmune response. The possible effect of CTLA4-Ig or monoclonal antibody to CD40 ligand in the treatment of patients with ongoing disease is unclear. Interferon-α trials are in progress, based on the ability of this cytokine not only to prevent the development of EAMG but also to suppress established disease.[26] However, interferon-α may be a two-edged sword as its use in hepatitis C patients has been associated with the de novo appearance or accentuation of autoimmune disease.

ACKNOWLEDGMENT

This work was supported by National Institutes of Health (NIH) grant NS19546.

REFERENCES

1. Lisak RP, Barchi RL. Myasthenia gravis. In: Walton JN (ed) Major problems in neurology, vol 11. Philadelphia, WB Saunders; 1982: p5.
2. Engel A. The investigation of congenital myasthenic syndromes. Ann NY Acad Sci 1993;681:425.
3. Beeson D, Vincent A, Morris A, et al. cDNA and genomic clones encoding the muscle acetylcholine receptor. Ann NY Acad Sci 1993;681:165.
4. Karlin A. Explorations of the nicotinic acetylcholine receptor. The Harvey Lectures 1991;85:71.
5. Sanes JR, Apel ED, Gautam M, et al. Agrin receptors at the skeletal neuromuscular junction. Ann NY Acad Sci 1998;841:1.
6. Levinson AI, Zweiman B, Lisak RP. Immunopathogenesis and treatment of myasthenia gravis. J Clin Immunol 1987;7:187.
7. Yi Q, Pirskanen R, Lefvert AK. Human muscle acetylcholine receptor reactive T and B lymphocytes in the peripheral blood of patients with myasthenia gravis. J Neuroimmunol 1993;42:215.
8. Tindal RSA. Humoral immunity in myasthenia gravis: biochemical characterization of acquired anti-receptor antibodies and clinical correlations. Ann Neurol 1981;10:437.
9. Papadouli I, Sakarellos C, Tzartos SJ. High-resolution epitope mapping and fine antigenic characterization of the main immunogenic region of the acetylcholine receptor: Eur J Biochem 1993;211:227.
10. Guigou V, Emilie D, Berrih-Aknin S, et al. Individual germinal centres of myasthenia gravis human thymuses contain polyclonal activated B cells that express all the V_H and V_k families. Clin Exp Immunol 1991;83:262.
11. Tesch H, Hohfeld R, Toyka KV. Analysis of immunoglobulin and T cell receptor rearrangements in the thymus of myasthenia gravis patients. J Neuroimmunol 1989;21:169.
12. Killen JA, Hochschwender SM, Lindstrom JM. Human anti-acetylcholine receptor antibodies use variable gene segments analogous to those used in autoantibodies of various specificities. Mol Immunol 1992;29:1501.
13. Killen JA, Hochschwender SM, Lindstrom JM. The main immunogenic region of acetylcholine receptors does not provoke the formation of antibodies of a predominant idiotype. J Neuroimmunol 1985;9:229.
14. Oger JJ-F. Thymus histology and acetylcholine receptor antibodies in generalized myasthenia gravis. Ann NY Acad Sci 1993;681:110.
15. Willcox N, Schluep M, Ritter MA, Newsom-Davis J. The thymus in seronegative myasthenia gravis patients. J Neurol 1991;238:256.
16. Horton RM, Manfredi AA, Conti-Tronconi BM. The 'embryonic' gamma subunit of the nicotinic acetylcholine receptor is expressed in adult extraocular muscle. Neurology 1993;43:983.
17. Oda K. Differences in acetylcholine receptor-antibody interactions between extraocular and extremity muscle fibers. Ann NY Acad Sci 1993;681:238.
18. Aarli JA, Skeie GO, Mygland A, et al. Muscle striation antibodies in myasthenia gravis. Ann NY Acad Sci 1998;841:505.
19. Agius MA, Zhu S, Kirvan CA, et al. Rapsyn antibodies in myasthenia gravis. Ann NY Acad Sci 1998;841:516.
20. Drachman DB, Adams RN, Josifek LF, et al. Antibody-mediated mechanisms of ACh receptor loss in myasthenia gravis: clinical relevance. Ann NY Acad Sci 1981;377:175.
21. Engel AG, Sahashi K, Fumagalli G. The immunopathology of acquired myasthenia gravis. Ann NY Acad Sci 1981;377:158.
22. Drachman DB, Angus CW, Adams RN, Michelson JD, Hoffman GJ. Myasthenic antibodies cross-link acetylcholine receptors to accelerate degradation. N Engl J Med 1978;298:1116.
23. Richman DP, Wollmann RL, Maselli RA, et al. Effector mechanisms of myasthenic antibodies. Ann NY Acad Sci 1993;681:264.
24. Conti-Fine B, Navaneetham D, Karachunski PI, et al. T cell recognition of the acetylcholine receptor in myasthenia gravis. Ann NY Acad Sci 1998;841:283.
25. Patrick J, Lindstrom J. Autoimmune response to acetylcholine receptor. Science 1973;180:871.
26. Christadoss P, Poussin M, Deng C. Animal models of myasthenia gravis. Clin Immunol 2000;94:75.
27. Zoda T, Yeh T-M, Krolick KA. Clonotypic analysis of anti-acetylcholine receptor antibodies from experimental autoimmune myasthenia gravis-sensitive Lewis rats and experimental autoimmune myasthenia gravis-resistant Wistar Furth rats. J Immunol 1991;146:663.
28. Pachner AR, Kantor FS. The relation of clinical disease to antibody titre, proliferative response and neurophysiology in murine experimental autoimmune myasthenia gravis. Clin Exp Immunol 1983;51:543.
29. Bellone M, Ostile N, Lei S, Conti-Tronconi BM. Experimental myasthenia gravis in congenic mice. Sequence mapping and H-2 restriction of T helper epitopes on the α subunits of *Torpedo californica* and murine acetylcholine receptors. Eur J Immunol 1991;21:2303.
30. Karachunski PI, Ostlie NS, Okita DK, Conti-Fine BM. Interleukin-4 deficiency facilitates development of experimental myasthenia gravis and precludes its prevention by nasal administration of CD4+ epitope sequences of the acetylcholine receptor. J Neuroimmunol 1999;95:73.
31. Moiola L, Galbiati F, Martino G, et al. IL-12 is involved in the induction of experimental autoimmune myasthenia gravis, an antibody-mediated disease. Eur J Immunol 1998;28:2487.
32. Levinson AI, Wheatley LM. The thymus and the pathogenesis of myasthenia gravis. Clin Immunol Immunopathol 1995;78:1.
33. Wheatley LM, Urso D, Zheng Y, Loh E, Levinson AI. Molecular analysis of intrathymic nicotinic acetylcholine receptor Ann N Y Acad Sci 1993;681:74.
34. Schultz A, Hoffacker V, Wilisch A, et al. Neurofilament is an autoantigenic determinant in myasthenia gravis. Ann Neurol 1999;46:167.
35. Zheng Y, Wheatley LM, Liu T, Levinson AI. Acetylcholine receptor alpha subnit mRNA expression in human thymus: augmented expression in myasthenia gravis and upregulation by interferon-γ. Clin Immunol 1999;91:170.

36. Wheatley L, et al. Molecular characterization of the nicotinic acetylcholine receptor alpha chain in mouse thymus. J Immunol 1992;148:3105.
37. Naparstek Y, Ben-Nun A, et al. T lymphocyte lines producing or vaccinating against autoimmune encephalomyelitis (EAE). Functional activation induces peanut agglutinin receptors and accumulation in the the brain and thymus of line cells. Eur J Immunol 1983;13:418.
38. Huang D, Pirskanen R, Hjelmstrom P, Lefvert AK. Polymorphisms in IL-1beta and IL-1 receptor antagonist genes are associated with myasthenia gravis. J Neuroimmunol 1998;81:76.
39. Skeie GO, Pandey JP, Aarli JA, Gilhus NE. TNFA and TNFB polymorphisms in myasthenia gravis. Arch Neurol 1999;56:457.
40. Hjelmstrom P, Peacock CS, Giscombe R, et al. Polymorphism in tumor necrosis factor genes associated with myasthenia gravis. J Neuroimmunol 1998;88:137.
41. Huang DR, Pirskanen R, Matell G, Lafvert AK. Tumour necrosis factor-alpha polymorphism and secretion in myasthenia gravis. J Neuroimmunol 1999;94:165.
42. Huang DR, Zhou YH, XiaSQ, et al. Markers in the promoter region of interleukin-10 (IL-10) gene in myasthenia gravis: implications of diverse effects of IL-10 in the pathogenesis of the disease. J Neuroimmunol 1999;94:82.
43. Raknes G, Skeie GO, Gilhus NE, Aadland S, Vedeler C. FcgammaRIIa and FcgammaRIIIB polymorphisms in myasthenia gravis. J Neuroimmunol 1998;81:173.
44. Stefansson K, Dieperink ME, Richman DP, Marton LS. Sharing of epitopes by bacteria and the nicotinic acetylcholine receptor: a possible role in the pathogenesis of myasthenia gravis. Ann NY Acad Sci 1987;505:451.
45. Schwimmbeck PL, Dyrberg T, Drachman DB, Oldstone MB. Molecular mimicry and myasthenia gravis: an autoantigenic site of the acetylcholine receptor α-subunit that has biologic activity and reacts immunochemically with herpes simplex virus. J Clin Invest 1989;84:1174.
46. Dwyer DS, Vakil M, Bradleg RT, Ol SJ, Kearney JF. A possible cause of myasthenia gravis: Idiotypic networks involving bacterial antigens. Ann NY Acad Sci 1987;505:461.
47. Bever CT Jr, Chang HW, Penn AS, Jaffe IA, Bock E. Chemical alteration of acetylcholine receptor by penicillamine: a mechanism for induction of myasthenia gravis. Neurology 1982;32:1077.
48. Penn A, Jacques JJ. Cells from mice exposed chronically to D-penicillamine show proliferative responses to D-penicillamine-treated self (macrophage/dendritic cells): a graft-versus-host response? Ann NY Acad Sci 1993;681:319.
49. Genkins G, Sivar M, Tartte PI. Treatment strategies in myasthenia gravis. Ann NY Acad Sci 1993;681:603.
50. Grob D, Arsura EL, Brunner NG, Namba T. The course of myasthenia gravis and therapies affecting outcome. Ann NY Acad Sci 1987;505:472.
51. Genkins G, Kornfeld P, Papatestas AE, Bender AN, Matta RJ. Clinical experience in more than 2000 patients with myasthenia gravis. Ann NY Acad Sci 1987;505:500.
52. Olanow CW, Wechsler AS, Sirotkin-Roses M, Stajich J, Roses AD. Thymectomy as primary therapy in myasthenia gravis. Ann NY Acad Sci 1987;505:595.
53. Johns TR. Long-term corticosteroid treatment of myathenia gravis. Ann NY Acad Sci 1987;505:568.
54. Seybold M. Plasmapheresis in myasthenia gravis. Ann NY Acad Sci 1987;505:584–594.
55. Cornelio F, Antozzi C, Mantegazza R, et al. Immunosuppressive treatments, their efficacy on myasthenia gravis patients' outcome and on the natural course of the disease. Ann NY Acad Sci 1993;681:594.
56. Matell G. Immunosuppressive drugs: azathioprine in the treatment of myasthenia gravis. Ann NY Acad Sci 1987;505:588.
57. Palace J, Newsom-Davis J, Lecky B. A randomized double-blind trial of prednisolone alone or with azathioprine in myasthenia gravis. Myasthenia Gravis Study Group. Neurology 1998;50:1778.

Section 7 Organ-specific Inflammatory Disease

Chapter 77

Multiple Sclerosis

Arnon Karni and Howard L. Weiner

Multiple sclerosis (MS), an inflammatory demyelinating disorder of the human central nervous system (CNS), is the leading cause of nontraumatic neurological disability in young adults in North America and Europe, and affects nearly 1 million people worldwide. Neurologic disability generally increases over the course of the disease, which runs its course over a 10–20-year period. Thus, MS has a major personal and social impact on those afflicted with the illness. The description of MS as an isolated entity with an accurate clinicopathological correlation was made in the second half of the 19th century by the French neurologist Charcot.[1]

CLINICAL FEATURES

Multiple sclerosis can be broadly defined clinically into relapsing–remitting and progressive forms, although there are mixed patterns and two different classifications of progressive disease.[2] It is generally the progressive form that leads to disability. Different immunologic mechanisms may be linked to the different stages of the illness, and treatment may also differ depending on the stage of the disease. Most commonly, MS begins as a relapsing–remitting illness, with an average age of onset of 28–30 years.[3] In this stage the patient experiences discrete neurologic attacks, with full or partial recovery and lack of progression between relapses. The relapse rate tends to decline with time, with an average rate of 1.2–1.8 relapses per person-year at the first year from diagnosis, to 0.8–1.0 in the fifth year and 0.5–0.9 in the 10th year.

A large percentage (at least half) of patients with the relapsing–remitting form enter a stage in which the disease becomes progressive (secondary progressive stage). At this time the clinical course is continuously progressive, with no or only occasional relapses. Another progressive form is termed primary progressive, in which there is continuous progression from the onset. The primary progressive form is different pathologically and perhaps etiologically from the relapsing–remitting and secondary progressive forms. In approximately 10–15% of cases there is minimal accumulation of disability over a 10–15-year period, and the MS is classified as benign. In rare instances MS may be an acute fulminating illness or may present primarily as a cognitive disorder. The average time to accumulate disability that involves the use of a cane for at least 50% of patients is 15 years for those with a relapsing–remitting course, but only 5–6 years for those with a progressive course. Life expectancy is not significantly affected. It has been reported that MS patients may have lower incidence of some malignant diseases compared to the general population.

Certain factors have been associated with a better prognosis (Table 77.1). Most studies show that female gender, early age of onset, onset of a relapsing–remitting course as opposed to a primary progressive course, complete recovery from the first attack, low frequency of attacks in the early course, and long time to moderate disability are associated with a better outcome. In addition, the type of the signs or symptoms at onset may have some predictive value, as patients with optic neuritis or sensory symptoms at onset have a better prognosis.

CLINICAL PEARLS

Important clinical considerations in multiple sclerosis

- MS can be broadly defined clinically into relapsing–remitting and progressive forms of disease activity.
- The progressive form of disease leads to disability.
- Different immunologic mechanisms may be linked to the different stages of the illness, and treatment may be different depending on the stage of disease.
- A large percentage (at least half) of patients with the relapsing–remitting form enter a secondary progressive stage.
- Magnetic resonance imaging (MRI) has shown relapsing–remitting disease to be a much more chronically active process than can be discerned clinically.
- The initial clinical presentation in MS occurs when there is reversible disability and minimal chronic nervous system damage. Thus, the opportunity exists to prevent central nervous system damage and disability by early intervention.

Favorable predictive factors in multiple sclerosis
Female gender
Early age of onset
Onset of relapsing remitting rather than progressive course
Complete recovery after the first attack
Low frequency of attacks in the early course
Long time to moderate disability
Optic neuritis and sensory symptoms at onset

Table 77.1 Favorable predictive factors in multiple sclerosis.

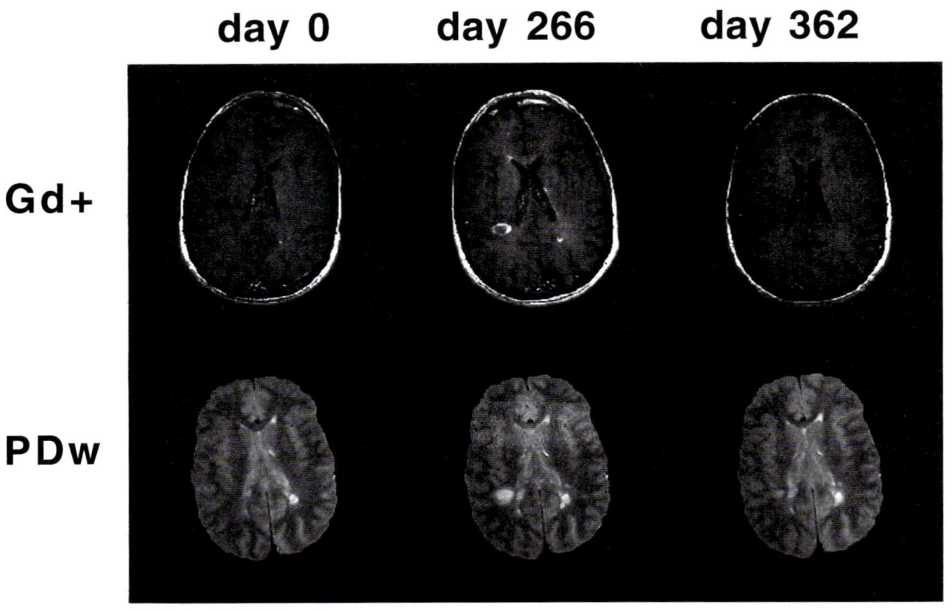

Figure 77.1 Serial MRI scans in multiple sclerosis. Proton density and gadolinium-enhanced MRI on a single patient carried out on days 0, 266 and 362, demonstrating periventricular lesions and the appearance and disappearance of a gadolinium-enhancing lesion over time.

DIAGNOSIS AND LABORATORY FINDINGS

Although there is no pathognomonic test for MS, diagnosis is generally based on the clinical presentation, magnetic resonance imaging (MRI), and cerebrospinal fluid (CSF) examination. The most valuable diagnostic aid is MRI, which shows multiple white matter lesions in more than 90% of patients (Fig. 77.1). A characteristic distribution and morphology of plaques on T_2-weighted MRI are associated with MS. MS plaques are found in the white matter in a periventricular distribution, the posterior poles of the lateral ventricles and the area of the centrum semiovale being most frequently involved. The most common appearance is of homogeneously hyperintense lesions; less commonly, ring or cystic lesions may occur. Nonspecific white matter abnormalities may be confused with MS, particularly in patients older than 50 years. Injection of gadolinium demonstrates intermittent breakdown of the blood–brain barrier, which occurs more frequently in the relapsing–remitting than the progressive stages and is correlated with clinical attacks. In addition, it has become clear that the disease is more chronically active as measured by MRI than as evidenced by clinical attacks. Thus, MS is a chronic, recurrent inflammatory process affecting the CNS. With progression of the disease there are fewer attacks and fewer gadolinium-enhancing lesions, but increased T_2 lesion burden and axonal loss (Fig. 77.2).

Examination of the CSF provides supportive information for diagnosis. There is increased CSF IgG that is produced locally in the CSF and the presence of oligoclonal IgG bands by electrophoretic analysis. This pattern is not seen in normal people, in whom the CSF IgGs are passively derived from the serum and appear as diffuse broad bands in electrophoretic gels. More than 90% of patients with clinically definite MS have oligoclonal bands, although they are also found in patients with other CNS inflammatory or infectious diseases.

Conditions that may be confused with MS include acute disseminated encephalomyelitis, Lyme disease, HIV- or HTLV-I associated myelopathy, CNS vasculitis, Sjögren's syndrome, Behçet's disease and sarcoidosis.

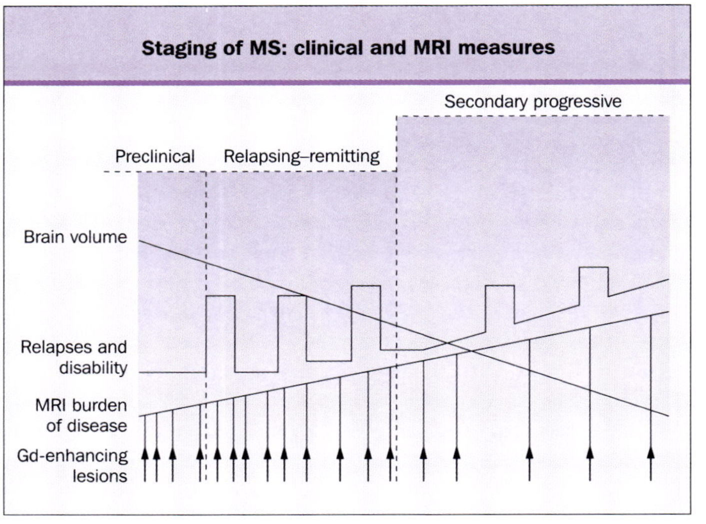

Figure 77.2 Staging of MS: clinical and MRI measures.

EPIDEMIOLOGY AND GENETICS

Multiple sclerosis is approximately twice as common in females as in males (Table 77.2), and prevalence, and incidence appear to increase with distance from the equator. The disease affects 1–1.8 people per 1000, resulting in a prevalence of 250 000– 350 000 cases in the United States. MS is unusual before adolescence, and then steadily rises in incidence from the teens to age 35, gradually declining thereafter. Epidemiologic studies support both genetic and environmental components of susceptibility. Reports of clusters, small 'epidemics', geographic variation in prevalence and alteration of MS susceptibility after migration support an environmental factor or factors.[4] The higher risk for MS in Europeans and in relatives of patients, especially in monozygotic versus dizygotic twins, adoption studies, and the existence of MS-resistant ethnic groups support a genetic predisposition.[1] In several population-based studies the concordance rate for monozygotic

Epidemiology of MS
Most frequent in Caucasians of European descent
Prevalence and incidence appear to increase with distance from the equator. In the USA there is a north–south gradient of decreasing risk
Twice as common in females as in males
Onset unusual before adolescence, then steadily rises in incidence from the teens to age 31–35, and declines gradually thereafter

Table 77.2 Epidemiology of MS.

Inheritance and genetics of MS
Familial aggregation
Concordance in monozygotic twins is 6–11 times higher than in dizygotic twins
Association with the HLA haplotype HLA-DRB1*1501-DQA1*0102-DQB1*0602
Linkage analysis through genomic screen studies of affected sibling pairs revealed possible susceptibility loci on chromosomes 2p53, 5q13, 6p21 and 19q13.

Table 77.3 Inheritance and genetics of MS.

twins varied from 5.9 to 25.9% (with average 17.8%) versus 0–3.6% (with average of 2.0%) for dizygotic twins (Table 77.3). Furthermore, in MS patients of European descent a strong association was found for HLA-DR2, that is, the extended haplotype HLA-DRB1*1501/DQA1*0102/DQB1*0602. In a recent series of studies microsatellite markers were used in genome screens to identify genomic regions potentially harboring MS susceptibility genes. Several regions had been identified as having a mild to moderate influence on genetic risk for MS, among them the major histocompatibility complex (MHC) region on chromosome 6. The results support a multifactorial etiology, including environmental factors and multiple genes of a moderate effect.

There is no evidence for a single or unique environmental agent in MS. An important question is how environmental factors trigger exacerbations or influence whether the course of disease will be severe or mild. Correlations have been found between upper respiratory tract viral infections and exacerbations of relapsing–remitting MS.[5,6] Infections could affect the course of MS in a variety of ways. One of the most popular theories is that of molecular mimicry[7] (Chapter 58). It could also be connected with antigen-nonspecific polyclonal activation of T cells, with increased T-cell traffic into the CNS or with a virus-induced burst of IFN-γ that has been associated with exacerbation of the disease.[8]

PATHOLOGY

The inflammatory infiltrate in the MS lesion is composed of T lymphocytes, small numbers of B lymphocytes and plasma cells, activated microglia, and macrophages (particularly in demyelinating active lesions) which interact with myelin sheaths and are actively engaged in the demyelinating process. There is local production or expression of immune-related molecules such as MHC, molecules, adhesion molecules, cytokines and chemokines.[9,10] These

> **KEY CONCEPTS**
>
> **Pathology**
> - Perivascular infiltration of macrophages, T and B lymphocytes, and plasma cells
> - Demyelination
> - Axonal damage
> - Loss of oligodendrocytes
> - Astrocytic hypertrophy
> - Increased expression of MHC Class I & II

patterns suggested that the basic immunopathology is a Th1-type T cell-mediated immune response.

The neuropathology of the MS lesion is heterogeneous. There is selective destruction of myelin sheath and relative sparing of axons. However, axonal destruction does occur from the beginning of MS, is more pronounced in progressive MS patients, and correlates with the permanent neurological deficit. In early stages of the disease there is partial remyelination after the inflammation subsides.

Apart from the inflammatory response, the other major pathologic feature of MS is demyelination. Of note, in experimental models, encephalitogenic T-cell infiltration of the brain does not always cause demyelination, and in humans acute demyelinating encephalomyelitis (ADEM), which is an extensive T-cell-mediated inflammation, does not result in MS-like demyelinating plaques. This has led investigators to postulate additional mechanisms besides T-cell infiltration as part of the pathologic process.

Lassmann and colleagues[11] have classified MS into different neuropathologic categories: (1) demyelination with no or minor oligodendrocyte loss; (2) demyelination with concomitant destruction of oligodendrocytes; (3) primary demyelination with secondary gradual loss of oligodendrocytes in inactive plaque areas; and (4) primary oligodendrocyte destruction with secondary demyelination (Table 77.4). These categories correspond to different mechanisms of demyelination. A particular pathologic profile may be highly conserved in different plaques of an individual patient, whereas there may be major differences in the pathological patterns between patients. Specific aspects of some of these mechanisms of demyelination are described below.

Inflammatory demyelination induced by a synergy of encephalitogenic T cells and demyelinating antibodies

This immunological mechanism was shown by transferring encephalitogenic T cells with or without antibodies to myelin

Mechanism of demyelination
Synergic effect of encephalitogenic T cells and demyelinating antibodies T-cell-mediated myelin and oligodendrocyte damage Macrophage-mediated demyelination Imbalance in oligodendrocyte metabolism.
Axonal damage Direct attack on axons of demyelinating fibers by immunological mediators Secondary effect of demyelination

Table 77.4 Mechanism of demyelination.

oligodendrocyte glycoprotein (MOG) into experimental animals.[12] Injection of encephalitogenic T cells alone induced acute inflammation without demyelination. This process was augmented by antibodies that caused widespread demyelination. Repeated co-transfer of these cells and antibodies resulted in a chronic relapsing disease with plaques of demyelination and impaired remyelination.[13] MOG has epitopes that can stimulate both encephalitogenic T cells and demyelinating antibodies.[14] Immunoglobulins precipitate at the active edge of the MS plaque, at sites where macrophages interact with the disintegrating myelin sheath. Also, complement activation has been demonstrated at these sites, and antibodies against MOG may be present.[15] Thus, in a subgroup of MS patients it is possible that demyelinating antibodies may amplify the pathologic damage on the background of the T cell-mediated inflammatory response.

T cell-mediated destruction of myelin and oligodendrocytes

It has been shown that T cells and their products, such as lymphotoxin or perforin, can mediate demyelination.[16,17] In addition, activation of the Fas-signaling pathway in oligodendrocytes by Fas ligand on T cells may destroy oligodendrocytes selectively.[18] It has been shown that Fas receptor is expressed on a variety of glial cells in MS patients, especially on oligodendrocytes, and that Fas ligand is found on activated T cells as well as on microglial cells.[18,19]

Toxic effects of macrophage products

Macrophage products, such as complement components, oxygen free radicals or cytokines (e.g. TNF-α) can destroy oligodendrocytes in vitro.[20–22] Thus, activated macrophages alone, in the course of T cell-mediated inflammation in the CNS, can cause demyelination. In MS there may be massive activation of macrophages in the plaques, and TNF-α has been detected in the plaques.[23,24] It also has been shown that in some cases of MS active demyelination occurs without the deposition of antibodies or complement components, but instead is caused by activated macrophages and microglia.[11]

Disturbance of the metabolism of oligodendrocytes, the myelin producing cells

This hypothesis of myelin damaging by aberrant metabolism is based on the fact that there is dysregulation of expression of mRNA myelin proteins in MS plaques. In addition, the pattern of demyelination in a subset of chronic progressive MS patients suggests primary oligodendrocyte damage, followed by demyelination.[25,26] The mechanism by which these putative metabolic changes to the oligodendrocytes are induced is not understood.

Axonal damage

Axonal pathologic changes in MS were initially described by Charcot. More recent studies have suggested that axonal injury in this disease may be closely related to the development of permanent neurological disabilities. Neurologic disability has been correlated with parenchymal atrophy.[27] Magnetic resonance spectroscopy studies have shown that the signal of the neuronal marker *N*-acetyl aspartate is decreased in the plaques of MS patients with a relapsing–remitting course. In these patients the decrease of the signal is confined to the area of the lesions, whereas chronic progressive patients have reduced *N*-acetyl aspartate even in normal-appearing white matter.[27,28] Another study reported axonal accumulation of the amyloid precursor protein in MS lesions and raised the possibility of irreversible axonal damage. In support of this mechanism of pathology, immunocytochemistry and confocal microscopy showed that transected axons were a consistent feature of the brain lesions in MS, and that their frequency was related to the degree of inflammation within a lesion.[29] Thus, axonal transection may be the pathologic correlate of the irreversible neurologic impairment in MS.

Remyelination

It is quite clear that a process of remyelination occurs in MS plaques, especially in lesions, that occur in the early years of the disease process. The production of the myelin layer that surrounds the nerve fibers is dependent on the availability of the oligodendrocyte progenitor cell and preservation of the neural axons. In chronic plaques there may be a lack of remyelination, probably due to repeated demyelination in the same lesion and therefore exhaustion of the progenitor cell fraction.

IMMUNOPATHOGENESIS

The putative immunological events that lead to the pathology of MS (Table 77.5; Fig. 77.3) are based on animal experiments in experimental autoimmune encephalomyelitis (EAE) and observations in human MS. Autoreactive T cells specific for myelin and other antigens of the CNS pre-exist in the normal immune system of animals and human (Chapter 58). These clones escaped deletion by thymic negative selection and they are normally controlled by one of the modes of peripheral tolerance, such as maintenance of immunological ignorance, clonal inactivation (anergy), or active suppression by regulatory cells. In MS these autoreactive clones undergo activation outside the CNS (Fig. 77.3). There are several possibilities for such activation, one being molecular mimicry with a viral or bacterial antigen and cross-stimulation of autoantigen-specific T cells. For example, in vitro activation of myelin basic protein (MBP) peptide autoreactive T cells was demonstrated with seven viral and one bacterial peptides that have the predictive molecular mimicry motif of this MBP peptide.[7] It should be stressed that the primary amino acid sequences of these peptides could be quite different from the relevant MBP peptide. Another possibility for cross-reactivity occurs when T cells carry a dual T-

Immunopathogenesis of MS
The normal immune system contains T cells capable of recognizing myelin autoantigens that escaped negative selection in the thymus
These autoimmune clones are normally controlled by peripheral mechanisms of tolerance, including maintenance of immunological ignorance, anergy/deletion, and regulatory T cells
In MS there is failure of tolerance mechanism; activation of autoreactive T cells occurs outside the central nervous system
Initial activation of antimyelin autoreactive T-cell clones may be secondary to infectious agents that act via molecular mimicry
Activated autoreactive Th1-type T cells traffic to the central nervous system after acquiring specific surface adhesion molecules and chemokine receptors

Table 77.5 Immunopathogenesis of MS.

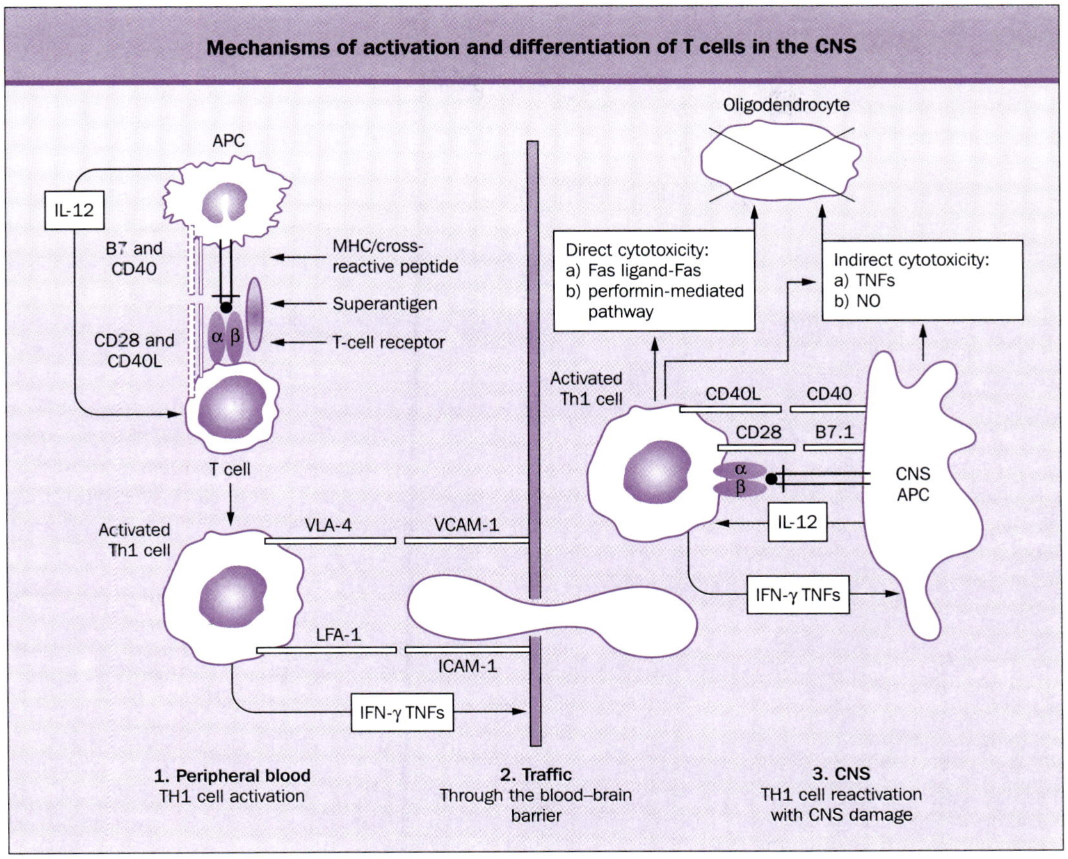

Figure 77.3 Mechanisms of activation and differentiation of T cells in the CNS. The minimal requirement to induce inflammatory autoimmune disease in the CNS white matter is the activation of CD4 T cells specific for a CNS-associated antigen. In one prevalent model of MS, an inducing event, such as a bacterial superantigen or viral peptide (via molecular mimicry), activates autoreactive T cells. A second costimulatory molecule, such as B7.1, is required for activation. The interaction of T cells with APCs via CD40 ligand–CD40 is important for induction of IL-12 synthesis by APC and consequent Th1-type cell generation in MS. Activated Th1-type cells then migrate into the CNS, where they recognize CNS antigens in the context of MHC and recruite effector cells which cause an inflammatory response. Oligodendrocytes can be lysed either directly via the cell–cell contact by cytotoxic T cells or via the production of soluble cytotoxic mediators, such as TNF-α or nitric oxide.

cell receptor (TCR) by expressing two TCR α-chains or two β-chains.[30] Thus, one could be specific for a viral or bacterial epitope, whereas the second is specific for autoantigen. In this case, activation of the T cell by the specific viral or bacterial epitope could activate an autoimmune reaction. Autoreactive T cells could also be activated in the periphery by microbial superantigens because the superantigen-binding site of the TCR β chain is probably shared by many T-cell clones specific for autoantigens. In EAE, it has been shown that exacerbation of disease can be induced by staphylococcal superantigen.

Upon activation, the autoreactive T cells express chemokine receptors and adhesion molecules that enable them to migrate into brain tissue (Fig. 77.3). Upon entering the brain, the autoantigen-specific T cells encounter autoantigen through its presentation by MHC Class II expressing microglia and macrophages. Cytokines such as interferon-γ, lymphotoxin and TNF-α that are produced by the entering CD4 T cells (Th1-type cells) as well as by activated local antigen-presenting cells induce up-regulation of MHC Class II expression. Once the inflammatory reaction begins, there is increased production of inflammatory mediators, leading to change in the blood–brain-barrier and thence to additional inflammatory cells entering the brain. These mediators also activate astrocytes, endothelium and pericytes, resulting in their increased expression of MHC Class II and therefore perpetuation of the autoimmune response.

In addition to MBP, other myelin and brain proteins have been found to be encephalitogenic in animal models (Table 77.6). Proteolipid protein (PLP) and MOG have been studied extensively in EAE, S100β is an example of a nonmyelin antigen expressed by astrocytes that can induce EAE.[31] Different autoantigens and different epitopes of a particular autoantigen can be targeted by the autoimmune response in different stages of the disease. Determinant spreading is a process by which the immune response to one epitope spreads to other epitopes on the same molecule (intramolecular spreading) as well as to other autoantigens (intermolecular spreading)[32,33] (see Chapter 58). Both processes have been demonstrated in the course of EAE.

The humoral immune system also participates in the pathogenesis, as there is overproduction of IgG in the CSF and antibodies are detected in the lesions. B cells are usually found in MS plaques, and their numbers relative to T cells increase as the lesion become chronic.[25] There is evidence that after binding to the myelin surface, demyelinating autoantibodies activate

KEY CONCEPTS

Multiple sclerosis as a Th1-type cell-mediated autoimmune disease

- Exacerbation of MS induced by administration of IFN-γ
- Increased production of INF-γ and TNF in the blood and CNS
- Increased production of IL-12 in progressive MS
- Increased expression of chemokine receptors CCR5 and CXCR3 on T cells
- Expression of MIP-1α and IL-10 in MS lesions
- Presence of IL-12 and B7.1 in MS lesions
- Similarities between MS and EAE, which is a Th1-type cell-mediated autoimmune disease

Potential autoantigens in multiple sclerosis
Myelin basic protein (MBP)
Proteolipid protein (PLP)
Myelin oligodendrocyte glycoprotein (MOG)
s100-β
AlphaB crystallin
Transaldolase
Oligodendrocyte myelin glycoprotein
2′,3′-cyclic nucleotide 3′-phosphodiesterase (CNP)

Table 77.6 Potential autoantigens in multiple sclerosis.

complement and attract macrophages/microglia.[34] Glia presumably also contribute to the myelin damage, as reactive astrocytes in the MS plaques contain NADH diaphorase activity that reflect the activity of inducible nitric oxide synthase (iNOS). High expression of iNOS has also been detected in macrophages in the region of active demyelination in MS.[35]

Autoantigens and autoreactive T cells

The identification of MBP, PLP and MOG as potential target autoantigens in the pathogenesis of human demyelinating disease have come primarily from studies of EAE (Table 77.6). EAE is an autoimmune inflammatory disease of the CNS characterized by perivascular and subpial inflammatory infiltrates and lesions of demyelination after immunization with autoantigens, together with adjuvant, or by transfer of autoreactive T lymphocytes.[36] The involvement of oligodendroglial transaldolse as a candidate antigen based on studies in animal models has also been suggested.[37] Other candidate autoantigens include 2′,3′-cyclic nucleotide 3′-phosphodiesterase (CNP) expressed by oligodendrocytes[29] and oligodendrocyte myelin glycoprotein (OMgp).[38] MS is predominantly, although not exclusively, a CNS disease and there are usually no lesions in the peripheral nervous system. The anatomic localization of the target autoantigens in MS is likely to influence the distribution of inflammatory lesions. PLP, the most abundant protein of CNS myelin, and MOG are found in the CNS and not in peripheral nervous system (PNS). In contrast, MBP and myelin-associated glycoprotein (MAG) are expressed in both the CNS and the PNS.[40] It is of interest that MBP induces only CNS lesions in EAE. In the past, it was thought that an immune response against a single autoantigen could be viewed as the cause of MS. It is now clear that there are reactivities against more than one myelin autoantigen in MS.[39] This is true of most inflammatory organ-specific autoimmune diseases, as inflammation in the organ releases antigens that lead to sensitization to additional antigens in the target organ.

Immune responses against nonmyelin antigens can also induce CNS disease in experimental animals and be involved in the autoimmune response in MS. For example, immunization with the protein s100-β, which is expressed in astrocytes, thymus and spleen, induces T-cell responses in rats, and transfer of s100-β-reactive T cells induces inflammation in the CNS of recipients.[31] Another family of proteins, heat-shock proteins (HSP), can function as immune targets during infection and inflammation and there is a possibility of cross-reactive responses to epitopes shared by host and microbial HSP. These responses, if not properly regulated, could also theoretically contribute to the patho genesis of multiple sclerosis. Increased immune responses to *Mycobacterium tuberculosis* HSP have been detected in T-cell lines and spinal fluid lymphocytes from MS patients compared to controls.[41] Also, altered expression of several HSP were observed in areas of active MS lesions on brain sections.[42] Furthermore, expression of the small HSP αB crystalline by both oligodendrocytes and astrocytes in MS lesions, and the capacity of this antigen to induce a specific T-cell response, suggests that this nonmyelin antigen could also be a potential autoantigen in MS.[43]

Although an inflammatory organ-specific autoimmune disease such as MS is presumably mediated by autoantigen-reactive T cells, such T cells are found at about the same frequency in normal individuals as in MS patients using conventional lymphocyte proliferation assays. However, an increase in MBP and PLP reactive cells was demonstrated in the peripheral blood and CSF of MS patients versus controls when IL-2 receptor positive (i.e. activated) T cells were studied.[44,45] Another approach to study relative MBP reactivity in MS involved estimation of the frequency of MBP-specific T-cell lines that carry mutations in the hypoxanthine-guanine phosphoribosyl transferase (HPRT) gene.[46] HPRT-mutated cells have been hypothesized to represent actively dividing T cells and an increased frequency of MBP-reactive T cells in the population of HPRT mutant cells in MS has been reported.[46]

In some susceptible strains of mice and rats, there is a limited usage of particular TCRs in the response to encephalitogenic epitopes of MBP.[36,47] Vaccination with synthetic peptides with sequence homology to the complementary-determining regions of the utilized TCRs was shown to prevent and even suppress disease. This approach has been applied to multiple sclerosis using T-cell or T-cell receptor vaccination with TCR Vβ peptides believed to be overutilized in the human disease.[48] Analysis of TCR Vβ usage in MBP-reactive T-cell clones, clones from patients (with undefined antigen specificity) isolated from MS brain and control clones was performed at an international workshop on TCR usage in human and experimental demyelinating diseases.[47] In separate studies, preferential expansion of T lymphocytes bearing αδ TCR in both MS lesions, CSF and peripheral blood was observed by different laboratories in MS patients.[48,49] In regard to these observations, human oligodendrocytes and human fetal astrocytes express HSP and stimulate the preferential expansion of cytotoxic γδ T cells.[50,51]

ALTERED PEPTIDE LIGANDS, MOLECULAR MIMICRY AND MYELIN-SPECIFIC T-CELL RESPONSES

The TCR on a particular T-cell clone is capable of being stimulated by a relatively large number of different peptides when complexed with the relevant MHC molecule.[52] Although an individual T-cell clone recognizes the 'original' peptide used to generate the clone, there are other peptides that are capable of stimulating the same clone. These 'variant' peptides can come from viral or bacterial proteins (molecular mimicry) or can be artificially synthesized by a simple substitution of one or another particular amino acid within the original peptide (altered peptide ligand, or APL).[53] Variant or altered peptides can induce variable types of responses in T cells compared to the original peptide. Furthermore, APL can induce different patterns of cytokine secretion in T-cell clones compared to the original peptide. As discussed above, molecular mimicry could allow an immune response to an infectious agent that might lead to a subsequent attack against an autoantigen in the target organ[54] (Chapter 58). Responses to a variant or altered peptide could change a Th1-type to Th2-type response (see below) or cause a decrease in the production of the Th1 proinflammatory cytokines. This concept has been exploited in a number EAE studies to stimulate protection from the disease[56–57] and is being tested as a possible treatment for MS patients (see below).

Th1-type vs. Th2-type cytokines in MS

Investigation of murine T cells has led to the broad division of CD4 T cells into Th1 and Th2 types based on cytokine profile: Th1-type cells secrete IL-2, IFN-γ and TNF-α whereas Th2-type cells secrete IL-4, IL-5, and IL-10 (see Chapters 15, 16 and 58). Th0-type cells have a mixed cytokine profile. Th1-type cytokines favor delayed-type hypersensitivity responses, whereas Th2-type cytokines favor antibody production and allergy-associated responses. Furthermore, Th1- and Th2-type cytokines cross-regulate the expression of each other. In a number of murine models of organ-specific autoimmune diseases, including EAE, Th1 cells contribute to the pathogenesis of the disease, whereas Th2 cells can prevent disease[58] (Chapter 58). However, there are differences regarding this division in murine and human systems. Based on results in EAE, investigators have searched for an inverse correlation between the development of MS (a putative Th1-type disease) and the expression of allergic reactions (a Th2-type responses). MS patients have been reported to have fewer allergic symptoms, a lower number of positive allergen-specific IgE test results and lower composite allergy indexes than control subjects.[59]

IFN-γ, a cytokine that is the hallmark of Th1-type immune responses, appears to play an important role in MS disease pathogenesis as increased production of IFN-γ precedes clinical attacks[60] and injection of MS patients with recombinant IFN-γ induced exacerbations of the disease.[8] Furthermore, within the nervous system the inflammatory process is characterized by increased IFN-γ expression.[61] IL-12, a cytokine produced by non-T cells, is the most potent inducer of IFN-γ and Th1-type immune responses.[62] In studies performed by the authors, anti-IL-12 antibodies reduced anti-CD3-induced IFN-γ production by cells from MS patients to normal levels. Investigation of the cellular basis for increased IL-12 expression demonstrated that T cells from MS patients induced increased IL-12 secretion from non-T cells, which was blocked by anti-CD40 ligand antibody. The CD40 ligand (CD40L; CD154)-dependent Th1-type immune activation was observed in the progressive but not in the relapsing–remitting form of MS, suggesting a link to the pathogenesis of progression in disease and providing a basis for immune intervention.[63] Elevated serum IL-12 p70 has also been detected in chronic progressive MS[64] and can be produced by activated microglial cells in vitro.[65] Increased expression of IL-12p40, CD40 and CD40-L can be detected in MS lesions.[66,67] In EAE, animals treated with IL-12 in vivo have a more severe and prolonged form of EAE and relapses, whereas anti IL-12 reduces the incidence and severity of adoptively transferred EAE.[68] In addition, treatment of animals with anti-CD40L antibody completely prevented development of the disease and CD40L-deficient mice failed to develop EAE.[69] Taken together, these studies provide a basis for future clinical trials in MS with agents that have anti-IL-12 or anti-CD40L activity.

Antigen-nonspecific immunologic abnormalities in MS

A variety of antigen-nonspecific abnormalities have been descriped in patients with MS. How they are involved in the pathogenesis of the disease is not understood, but they are consistent with MS being a Th1-type autoimmune disease. The abnormalities described include defects of T-cell suppressor function;[8,66] increased TNF-α receptor expression on peripheral T cells;[70] IFN-γ-induced influx of Ca^{2+} in T lymphocytes;[71] increased lymphocyte β-adrenergic receptor density in progressive MS;[72] abnormalities in the levels of soluble ICAM-1 (CD54) and VCAM-1;[73,74] increased numbers of B7.1 (CD80)-positive B cells in the peripheral blood, CSF and lesions of active MS patients.[66,75,77]

IMMUNE-MEDIATED MECHANISMS OF MYELIN DESTRUCTION

There are two predominant hypotheses to explain oligodendrocyte destruction in MS lesions: direct T-cytotoxic lymphocyte (CTL)-mediated lysis of oligodendrocytes, or an indirect mechanism in which activated T cells induce toxic cytokine production (e.g. nitric oxide or TNF-α) by accessory cells. T-cell-produced cytokines may be also involved in the damage to oligodendrocytes.[16,22] Studies have demonstrated that cytotoxicity mediated by CTLs may be secondary to the secretion of electron-dense cytoplasmic granules (perforin and serine esterase granzyme B) or a nonsecretory pathway based on the interaction of Fas ligand with Fas (CD95) on target cells and the induction of apoptosis.[16–19,22,24,77]

Fas–Fas ligand

During the course of demyelination in murine models of MS, such as EAE and Theiler's, murine encephalomyelitis virus infection oligodendroglial apoptosis is observed, suggesting that the demyelinating process may share a common terminal pathway and lead to a similar clinical and pathological picture.[78] Apoptosis of oligodendroglial cells has also been observed in MS lesions.[19,78,79] The role of Fas and Fas ligand, the molecules that are involved in one of the pathways of CTL-mediated lysis of target cells has been studied in EAE, but the results in have been mixed. For example, studies showing that Fas deficiency prevents or enhances EAE have been reported.[80–82] In humans, both Fas and Fas ligand-positive cells have been demonstrated in MS lesions.[18,19] However, dying oligodendrocytes did not exhibit evidence of apoptosis.[18,19]

Perforin

The role of a perforin-mediated pathway in the destruction of oligodendrocytes in MS has not been extensively studied. Oligodendrocytes are highly susceptible to attack by T-cell perforin, and respond similarly to sublethal attack by shedding membrane vesicles.[17] A higher number of CD4 T cells in the peripheral blood of active MS patients compared to controls express perforin and MBP-specific CD4 T-cell clones can mediate cytotoxicity via a perforin-mediated cytotoxic mechanism.[83] These findings suggest that perforin-mediated lysis of oligodendrocytes could be involved in the pathogenesis of MS.

Toxic cytokines and lymphotoxin-α

TNF-α has also been considered as a factor possibly causing the destruction of oligodendrocytes in vitro.[16] TNF-α can be produced by T cells, astrocytes and microglia cells and, together with lymphotoxin-α, can be found in MS lesions.[16] In addition, TNF-α and lymphotoxin-α are increased prior to and during MS exacerbations.[62,84,85] TNF-α has also been reported to be elevated in the serum and CSF in MS patients,[86] and, the number of TNF-α and lymphotoxin-α mRNA-expressing cells are increased in the CSF of MS patients.[87,88] Consistent with an important role for TNF-α in disease pathogensis, antibodies against TNF-α abrogated T-cell transfer of EAE in mice, whereas recombinant TNF-α augmented disease.[89,90]

Other molecules considered to be important in pathogenesis include IFN-α and nitric oxide (NO). IFN-γ is expressed in the lesions of MS brains and has been shown to be a potent inducer of apoptosis in oligodendrocytes. Nitric oxide (NO) synthesis is associated with nonspecific immune-mediated cellular cytotoxicity, and inducible NO synthase (iNOS) mRNA has been detected in MS lesions but not in control brains.[91] It has been suggested that NO may be a mechanism of death of oligodendrocytes, although further studies are needed to define the role of NO in the pathology of MS.[92]

THERAPY

Therapy of multiple sclerosis can be divided into three categories: (1) treatment to prevent the ongoing destruction of nervous system tissue by inflammatory cells; (2) symptomatic treatment to allow a damaged nervous system to function at a higher level; and (3) treatment designed to repair damaged CNS myelin. If the destructive inflammatory process in the CNS could be arrested at an early stage it would prevent the accumulation of neurologic disability. Symptomatic treatments are also available for MS patients, e.g. those that relieve spasticity, improve bladder function or help fatigue. Treatment to repair damaged myelin remains in the research stage. The clinical features of the disease make therapy difficult, as MS is a chronic, relapsing– progressive disease with an unpredictable clinical course that generally spans 10–20 years, during which time neurologic disability accumulates.

PRINCIPLES OF IMMUNOTHERAPIES USED IN THE TREATMENT OF MS

A number of immunotherapeutic approaches are being used to treat multiple sclerosis and are under active investigation. Interferon-β1a, interferon-β1b, and glutiramer acetate are approved specifically for use in multiple sclerosis in the treatment of relapsing–remitting disease. IFN-β is the most widely used drug and has been shown in clinical trials to decrease the frequency of relapses, favorably affect MRI lesions, and in some instances slow disease progression.[93,94] The mechanism of action of the β-interferon drugs is not clearly understood; however, they most likely function by decreasing IFN-γ-induced secretion of IL-4, IL-10 and TNF-α from lymphoid cells. They may also affect the trafficking of cells into the nervous system. IFN-β1b is given by subcutaneous injection every other day, and IFN-β1a by weekly intramuscular injection. Gluteramer acetate is a random copolymer of four amino acids given as daily injection.[95] This drug appears to work as an MBP analog that induces Th2 and Th3 regulatory cells.[96]

Drugs used for the treatment of inflammatory or malignant conditions have also been found useful in MS. Intravenous methylprednisolone can speed recovery from acute attacks, and patients with optic neuritis treated with intravenous methylprednisolone have a delay in onset of MS.[97] Other therapies reportedly beneficial in MS include cyclophosphamide, methotrexate, cladribine, mitoxantrone, intravenous immunoglobulin and total lymph node irradiation (reviewed in[98]). Over the past 15 years the authors have acquired extensive experience using pulse cyclophosphamide for the treatment of progressive and relapsing progressive types of MS using protocols analogous to those for lupus nephritis.[98] Although cyclophosphamide is a cytotoxic drug, recent work has suggested that it causes profound immune deviation to a Th2-type pattern, Specifically, patients treated with pulse cyclophosphamide have demonstrated eosinophilia and increased IL-4 and IL-10 secretion.[99] In addition, a marked decrease in IL-12 secretion by mononuclear cells in patients treated with cyclophosphamide was observed.[100]

Antigen-specific immune modulation of autoreactive cells in MS is being tested using a number of paradigms, including oral tolerance, T-cell receptor vaccination and altered peptide ligands. It appears that the mechanism of action for these therapeutic approaches is bystander suppression.[101] Because there is reactivity against multiple antigens in the target organ, the use of antigen-specific therapy is problematic if one is inducing anergy or deletion. However, these approaches induce regulatory T cells that secrete cytokines such as IL-4, IL-10 and TGF-β. They therefore suppress inflammation in an antigen-nonspecific fashion after arriving at the site of pathology. For oral tolerance the dose is important, as antigen-specific regulatory cells and bystander suppression are preferentially induced at lower doses.[102] A trial of single-dose bovine myelin in relapsing–remitting MS did not show differences in MS.[102] Future studies of oral tolerance will involve the administration of gluteramer acetate, which is now given by injection in MS and immune adjuvants.[103,104] Other therapies being studied include the use of the antiadhesion molecule anti-α_4-integrin, which has been shown to suppress EAE.[105] Paradoxically, a recent trial of anti-TNF antibody worsened MS, even though it has been of benefit in the EAE model and in rheumatoid arthritis.[106] This paradoxical affect may be explained by the burst of IFN-γ that may occur with anti-TNF therapy. Other future approaches to treatment may involve targeting factors related to the recruitment of cells to the nervous system (chemokines)[107] and antibodies directed against costimulatory molecules such as anti-CD40L and anti-CD80. Also, based on experimental data, anti-IL-12 compound would be expected to be of benefit in MS.

In summary, immunotherapy of MS involves (1) antigen-specific approaches that induce regulatory cells that act via bystander suppression; (2) antigen-nonspecific therapies that induce immune deviation or decrease IFN-γ secretion; and (3) drugs that affect lymphocyte trafficking or affect soluble products released by lymphocytes or mononuclear cells that cause CNS damage.

REMYELINATION

Studies in both humans and experimental models demonstrate that myelin repair occurs in the CNS and is a normal physiologic response to myelin injury.[108] Although remyelination in MS is often incomplete and limited, the extent of remyelination correlates well with the presence of oligodendrocytes in the lesions. The source and origin of the remyelinating cells is still unclear. They may be derived from either undifferentiated progenitor cells or, in part, from mature oligodendrocytes that have escaped destruction during lesion activity. Complete remyelination of plaques is possible, leading to the formation of 'shadow plaques'. No reliable data are available at present on the frequency of remyelination in different forms of MS. However, most studies agree that remyelination is especially prominent at the early stages of the disease, whereas it is sparse after several years of disease duration. Very little remyelination is found in cases of primary progressive MS.[108] Furthermore, given that axonal loss occurs in MS, when significant axonal loss accumulates irreversible damage to the nervous system has occurred and myelin repair is not possible.

SPECIFIC AGENTS USED IN THE TREATMENT OF MS

First-line, 'nontoxic' therapy for relapsing–remitting disease

Currently available treatments are interferon-β1b (Betaseron), interferon-β1a (Avonex), and glatiramer acetate (Copaxone).

Interferon-β

Two forms of recombinant IFN-β, 1a and 1b, are approved for the treatment of relapsing–remitting multiple sclerosis.[93,94] IFN-β1b (Betaseron) is a nonglycosylated recombinant bacterial cell product in which serine is substituted for cysteine at position 17. INF-β1a (Avonex) is a glycosylated recombinant mammalian-cell product with an amino acid sequence identical to that of natural interferon. IFN-β1b given subcutaneously in alternate-day injections was shown to decrease the relapse rate by 31%, increase the proportion of patients who were relapse free, and reduce the number of patients who had moderate and severe relapses. There was no difference in the proportions of patients whose disability increased, or in disability score changes between treatment groups. However, MRI progression, as measured by new MRI lesions and T_2-weighted area, was reduced in IFN-β1b-treated patients. IFN-β1a is given as a weekly intramuscular injection and demonstrated in a multicenter trial that the length of time to progression of disability was improved in treated patients compared to those given placebo.[93] In addition, IFN-β1a-treated patients had fewer gadolinium-enhancing lesions on MRI. Side-effects of IFN-β include injection-site reactions, influenza-like symptoms, and worsening of pre-existing depression. The choice between the different preparations depends on the patient and the individual physician. IFN-β1a is often prescribed, as it requires only weekly injections and appears to be better tolerated.

Glatiramer acetate (Copaxone)

This is a mixture of random synthetic peptides synthesized initially as a compound to mimic myelin basic protein, a long-studied autoantigen in multiple sclerosis. Glatiramer acetate was effective in the animal model of MS (EAE), and in a double-blind trial of relapsing–remitting MS its use decreased the relapse rate.[95] Treatment consists of daily subcutaneous injections of 20 mg. The most common side-effects are a mild reaction at the injection site and, in some patients, unexplained reactions involving episodes of flushing, chest tightness, shortness of breath and palpitations.

The choice of starting a relapsing–remitting patient as IFN-β verses glatiramer acetate has not been resolved. Patients with depression, those very early in their course, or those who cannot tolerate IFN-β are often preferentially treated with glatiramer acetate. Patients who do not respond to either IFN-β or glatiramer acetate may be treated with the other medication, depending on how active the disease has become (see below).

Intravenous steroids for relapses

Based on what is currently known about IFN-β and other relatively nontoxic drugs that could be given early in the disease course, it is expected that patients will continue to have relapses. Thus, short courses of intravenous methylprednisolone are given when a significant relapse occurs in order to speed recovery and, given what was reported in the optic neuritis study, perhaps to have a salutary effect on the disease course.[97] As part of the optic neuritis study it was found that treatment with a 3-day course of high-dose methylprednisolone reduced the rate of development of multiple sclerosis over a 2-year period.[97] The protective effect was most apparent in patients at highest risk for MS, i.e. those with multiple focal brain MRI abnormalities.

Second-line, immunotherapy to halt refractory or progressive disease

Although some patients may respond to first-line treatments it is expected that others will be refractory to therapy or enter the progressive stage. In these instances more potent immunotherapy or immunosuppression may be warranted, depending on the individual case. Options at this stage include drugs that are used for progressive disease, such as cyclophosphamide and mitoxantrone.[109] Treatment directed at the progressive phase is the most difficult as the disease may be harder to affect once the progressive stage has been initiated. Beta-interferon may benefit progressive MS patients in the secondary progressive phase (110) though patients may be less responsive to immunotherapy the longer they have been in the progressive phase (111).

THERAPEUTIC PRINCIPLES

Principles of therapy in multiple sclerosis

- Magnetic resonance imaging (MRI) has shown MS to be a much more chronically active process that can be discerned clinically. MRI is central to disease monitoring and has become an important outcome measure in clinical trials.
- First-line 'nontoxic' therapy for relapsing–remitting disease
  - interferon β
  - glatiramer acetate
- Intravenous steroids for relapses
- Plasmapheresis or intensive immunosuppression for refractory fulminant CNS demyelination
- Immunosuppression to halt refractory or progressive disease (cyclophosphamide, mitoxantrone, IVIG, methotrexate)
- Reinstitution of first-line therapy in patients who have achieved remission
- Combination and pulse therapy

Reinstitution of first-line therapy

One of the principles of second- or third-line therapy is to induce a remission, after which first-line nontoxic therapy can be instituted to maintain the remission. The degree to which subsequent first-line therapy will be effective is unknown.

Combination and pulse therapy

Until the pathogenesis of MS is precisely understood, it is unlikely that a single treatment will be effective in all patients. The principle of combination therapy has found utility in cancer treatment and is likely to be an important principle for the therapy of MS and other autoimmune diseases. Pulse steroids or relatively nontoxic immunosuppression may find utility in conjunction with antigen-specific forms of therapy. Furthermore, because MS appears to be more chronically active as viewed by MRI than can be evident clinically, and because some forms of therapy cannot be given chronically, intermittent pulse therapy with drugs that affect the immune system may become an important principle for MS therapy.

Disease monitoring

The major problem confronting the therapy of MS remains its unpredictable course and the length of time over which disability accumulates. Even for treatments that have proven efficacy it may be difficult to determine in an individual patient whether the treatment is having a therapeutic effect unless the disease becomes truly quiescent clinically, or the patient improves on therapy. In some instances it is clear that a patient is either a responder or a nonresponder to a particular treatment. Magnetic resonance imaging (MRI) has provided a surrogate marker of disease activity and was one of the major factors in the approval of IFN-β for the treatment of relapsing–remitting MS. Even though MRI is not a perfect correlate of disease activity, it may ultimately serve as the best objective measure of ongoing disease in the nervous system, given that it is now known that MS is chronically active even when clinical activity is not present. Because MS is felt to be an immune-mediated disease, ultimately an immune marker of disease activity will need to be found. We have found that IL-12 may be a marker of disease activity.[100]

CONCLUSION

Multiple sclerosis is a disease that affects young adults and generally runs its course over 10–20 years from onset. Unlike type I diabetes, which becomes clinically evident once the majority of islet cell damage has occurred, the initial presentation in MS occurs when there is reversible clinical disability and minimal nervous system damage. Thus, the opportunity exists to prevent CNS damage and disability by early intervention, followed by more aggressive immunotherapy if the disease continues to be active. Thus, the future of therapy for MS is to find compounds that can be given early in the course of the disease and to treat aggressively if the disease is active, either clinically or by MRI.

REFERENCES

1. Compston A, Ebers G, Lassmann H, et al. McAlpine's multiple sclerosis. London, Churchill Livingstone, 1998.
2. Lublin FD, Reingold SC. Defining the clinical course of multiple sclerosis: results of an international survey. National Multiple Sclerosis Society (USA) Advisory Committee on Clinical Trials of New Agents in Multiple Sclerosis. Neurology 1996;46:907.
3. Weinshenker BG, Bass B, Rice GP, et al. The natural history of multiple sclerosis: a geographically based study. I. Clinical course and disability. Brain 1989;112:133.
4. Hogancamp WE, Rodriguez M, Weinshenker BG. The epidemiology of multiple sclerosis. Mayo Clin Proc 1997;72:871.
5. Sibley WA, Bamford CR, Clark K. Clinical viral infections and multiple sclerosis. Lancet 1985;1:1313.
6. Andersen O, Lygner PE, Bergstrom T, Andersson M, Vahlne A. Viral infections trigger multiple sclerosis relapses: a prospective seroepidemiological study. J Neurol 1993;240:417.
7. Wucherpfennig KW, Strominger JL. Molecular mimicry in T cell-mediated autoimmunity: viral peptides activate human T cell clones specific for myelin basic protein. Cell 1995;80:695.
8. Panitch HS, Hirsch RL, Schindler J, Johnson KP. Treatment of multiple sclerosis with gamma interferon: exacerbations associated with activation of the immune system. Neurology 1987;37:1097.
9. Balashov KE, Rottman JB, Weiner HL, Hancock WW. CCR5(+) and CXCR3(+) T cells are increased in multiple sclerosis and their ligands MIP-1alpha and IP-10 are expressed in demyelinating brain lesions. Proc Natl Acad Sci USA 1999;96:6873.
10. Sorensen TL, Tani M, Jensen J, et al. Expression of specific chemokines and chemokine receptors in the central nervous system of multiple sclerosis patients. J Clin Invest 1999;103:807.
11. Lassmann H. Neuropathology in multiple sclerosis: new concepts. Mult Scler 1998;4:93.
12. Schluesener H, Sobel R, Linington C, Weiner HL. A monoclonal antibody against a myelin oligodendrocyte glycoprotein induces relapses and demyelination in CNS autoimmune disease. J Immunol 1987;139:4016.
13. Linington C, Engelhardt B, Kapocs G, Lassman H. Induction of persistently demyelinated lesions in the rat following the repeated adoptive transfer of encephalitogenic T cells and demyelinating antibody. J Neuroimmunol 1992;40:219.
14. Johns TG, Kerlero de Rosbo N, Menon KK, et al. Myelin oligodendrocyte glycoprotein induces a demyelinating encephalomyelitis resembling multiple sclerosis. J Immunol 1995;154:5536.
15. Raine CS, Cannella B, Hauser SL, Genain CP. Demyelination in primate autoimmune encephalomyelitis and acute multiple sclerosis lesions: a case for antigen-specific antibody mediation. Ann Neurol 1999;46:144.
16. Selmaj K, Raine CS, Farooq M, Norton WT, Brosnan CF. Cytokine cytotoxicity against oligodendrocytes. Apoptosis induced by lymphotoxin. J Immunol 1991;147:1522.
17. Scolding NJ, Jones J, Compston DA, Morgan BP. Oligodendrocyte susceptibility to injury by T-cell perforin. Immunology 1990;70:6.
18. D'Souza SD, Bonetti B, Balasingam V, et al. Multiple sclerosis: Fas signaling in oligodendrocyte cell death. J Exp Med 1996;184:2361.
19. Dowling P, Shang G, Raval S, et al. Involvement of the CD95 (APO-1/Fas) receptor/ligand system in multiple sclerosis brain. J Exp Med 1996;184:1513.
20. Scolding NJ, Morgan BP, Houston A, et al. Normal rat serum cytotoxicity against syngeneic oligodendrocytes. Complement activation and attack in the absence of anti-myelin antibodies. J Neurol Sci 1989;89:289.
21. Griot C, Vandevelde M, Richard A, Peterhans E, Stocker R. Selective degeneration of oligodendrocytes mediated by reactive oxygen species. Free Radical Res Commun 1990;11:181.
22. Selmaj KW, Raine CS. Tumor necrosis factor mediates myelin and oligodendrocyte damage in vitro. Ann Neurol 1988;23:339.
23. Bruck W, Porada P, Poser S, et al. Monocyte/macrophage differentiation in early multiple sclerosis lesions. Ann Neurol 1995;38:788.
24. Selmaj K, Raine CS, Cannella B, Brosnan CF. Identification of lymphotoxin and tumor necrosis factor in multiple sclerosis lesions. J Clin Invest 1991;87:949.

25. Ozawa K, Suchanek G, Breitschopf H, et al. Patterns of oligodendroglia pathology in multiple sclerosis. Brain 1994;117:1311.
26. Bruck W, Schmied M, Suchanek G, et al. Oligodendrocytes in the early course of multiple sclerosis. Ann Neurol 1994;35:65.
27. Losseff NA, Wang L, Lai HM, et al. Progressive cerebral atrophy in multiple sclerosis. A serial MRI study. Brain 1996;119:2009.
28. Matthews PM, Pioro E, Narayanan S, et al. Assessment of lesion pathology in multiple sclerosis using quantitative MRI morphometry and magnetic resonance spectroscopy. Brain 1996;119:715.
29. Trapp BD, Peterson J, Ransohoff RM, et al. Axonal transection in the lesions of multiple sclerosis. N Engl J Med 1998;338:278.
30. Davodeau F, Peyrat MA, Romagne F, et al. Dual T cell receptor beta chain expression on human T lymphocytes. J Exp Med 1995;181:1391.
31. Kojima K, Berger T, Lassmann H, et al. Experimental autoimmune panencephalitis and uveoretinitis transferred to the Lewis rat by T lymphocytes specific for the S100 beta molecule, a calcium binding protein of astroglia. J Exp Med 1994;180:817.
32. Sercarz EE, Lehmann PV, Ametani A, et al. Dominance and crypticity of T cell antigenic determinants. Annu Rev Immunol 1993;11:729.
33. Miller SD, McRae BL, Vanderlugt CL, et al. Evolution of the T-cell repertoire during the course of experimental immune-mediated demyelinating diseases. Immunol Rev 1995;144:225.
34. Brosnan CF, Raine CS. Mechanisms of immune injury in multiple sclerosis. Brain Pathol 1996;6:243.
35. De Groot CJ, Ruuls SR, Theeuwes JW, Dijkstra CD, Van der Valk P. Immunocytochemical characterization of the expression of inducible and constitutive isoforms of nitric oxide synthase in demyelinating multiple sclerosis lesions. J Neuropathol Exp Neurol 1997;56:10.
36. Martin R, McFarland HF, McFarlin DE. Immunological aspects of demyelinating diseases. Annu Rev Immunol 1992;10:153.
37. Colombo E, Banki K, Tatum AH, et al. Comparative analysis of antibody and cell-mediated autoimmunity to transaldolase and myelin basic protein in patients with multiple sclerosis. J Clin Invest 1997;99:1238.
38. Mikol DD, Stefansson K. A phosphatidylinositol-linked peanut agglutinin-binding glycoprotein in central nervous system myelin and on oligodendrocytes. J Cell Biol 1988;106:1273.
39. Zhang J, Markovic S, Raus J, et al. Increased frequency of IL-2 responsive T-cells specific for myelin basic protein and proteolipid protein in peripheral blood and cerebrospinal fluid of patients with multiple sclerosis. J Exp Med 1993;179:973.
40. Sobel RA. The pathology of multiple sclerosis. Neurol Clin 1995;13:1.
41. Birnbaum G, Kotilinek L, Albrecht L. Spinal fluid lymphocytes from a subgroup of multiple sclerosis patients respond to mycobacterial antigens. Ann Neurol 1993;34:18.
42. Aquino DA, Capello E, Weisstein J, et al. Multiple sclerosis: altered expression of 70- and 27-kDa heat shock proteins in lesions and myelin. J Neuropathol Exp Neurol 1997;56:664.
43. Bajramovic JJ, Lassmann H, van Noort JM. Expression of alphaB-crystallin in glia cells during lesional development in multiple sclerosis. J Neuroimmunol 1997;78:143.
44. Zhang J, Markovic-Plese S, Lacet B, et al. Increased frequency of interleukin 2-responsive T cells specific for myelin basic protein and proteolipid protein in peripheral blood and cerebrospinal fluid of patients with multiple sclerosis. J Exp Med 1994;179:973.
45. Hafler DA, Weiner HL. Immunologic mechanisms and therapy in multiple sclerosis. Immunol Rev 1995;144:75.
46. Allegretta M, Nicklas J, Sriram S, Albertini R. T-cells responsive to myelin basic protein in patients with multiple sclerosis. Science 1990;247:718.
47. Hafler DA, Saadeh MG, Kuchroo VK, Milford E, Steinman L. TCR usage in human and experimental demyelinating disease. Immunol Today 1996;17:152.
48. Shimonkevitz R, Colburn C, Burnham J, Murray RS, Kotzin BL. Clonal expansion of activated gamma/delta T-cells in recent onset multiple sclerosis. Proc Natl Acad Sci USA 1993;90:923.
49. Liedtke W, Meyer G, Faustmann PM, Warnatz H, and Raine CS. Clonal expansion and decreased occurrence of peripheral blood gamma delta T cells of the V delta 2J delta 3 lineage in multiple sclerosis patients. Int Immunol 1997;9:1031.
50. Freedman MS, D'Souza S, Antel JP. Gamma delta T-cell-human glial cell interactions. I. In vitro induction of gammadelta T-cell expansion by human glial cells. J Neuroimmunol 1997;74:135.
51. Freedman MS, Bitar R, Antel JP. gamma delta T-cell-human glial cell interactions. II. Relationship between heat shock protein expression and susceptibility to cytolysis. J Neuroimmunol 1997;74:143.
52. Nanda NK, Arzoo KK, Geysen HM, Sette A, Sercarz EE. Recognition of multiple peptide cores by a single T cell receptor. J Exp Med 1995;182:531.
53. Evavold BD, Sloan-Lancaster J, Wilson KJ, Rothbard JB, Allen PM. Specific T cell recognition of minimally homologous peptides: evidence for multiple endogenous ligands. Immunity 1995;2:655.
54. Hemmer B, Fleckenstein BT, Vergelli M, et al. Identification of high potency microbial and self ligands for a human autoreactive Class II-restricted T cell clone. J Exp Med 1997;185:1651.
55. Prabhu Das M, Nicholson LB, Greer JM, Kuchroo VK. Autopathogenic T helper cell type 1 (Th1) and protective Th2 clones differ in their recognition of the autoantigenic peptide of myelin proteolipid protein. J Exp Med 1997;186:867.
56. Nicholson L, Greer J, Sobel R, Lees M, Kuchroo V. An altered peptide ligand mediates immune deviation and prevents EAE. Immunity 1995;3:397.
57. Brocke S, Gijbels K, Allegretta M, et al. Treatment of experimental encephalomyelitis with a peptide analogue of myelin basic protein. Nature 1996;379:343.
58. Liblau RS, Singer SM, McDevitt HO. Th1 and Th2 $CD4^+$ T-cells in the pathogenesis of organ-specific atuoimmune diseases. Immunol Today 1995;16:34.
59. Oro AS, Guarino TJ, Driver R, Steinman L, Umetsu DT. Regulation of disease susceptibility: decreased prevalence of IgE- mediated allergic disease in patients with multiple sclerosis. J Allergy Clin Immunol 1996;97:1402.
60. Dettke M, Scheidt P, Prange H, Kirchner H. Correlation between interferon production and clinical disease activity in patients with multiple sclerosis. J Clin Immunol 1997;17:293.
61. Woodroofe MN, Cuzner ML. Cytokine mRNA expression in inflammatory multiple sclerosis lesions: detection by non-radiactive in situ hybridization. Cytokine 1993;5:583.
62. Trinchieri G. Interleukin-12: a proinflammatory cytokine with immunoregulatory functions that bridge innate resistance and antigen-specific adaptive immunity. Annu Rev Immunol 1995;13:251.
63. Balashov KE, Smith DR, Khoury SJ, Hafler DA, Weiner HL. Increased IL-12 production in progressive multiple sclerosis: Induction by activated CD4+ T-cells via CD40 ligand. Proc Natl Acad Sci USA 1997;94:599.
64. Nicoletti F, Patti F, Cocuzza C, et al. Elevated serum levels of interleukin-12 in chronic progressive multiple sclerosis. J Neuroimmunol 1996;70:87.
65. Becher B, Dodelet V, Fedorowicz V, Antel JP. Soluble tumor necrosis factor receptor inhibits IL-12 production by stimulated human adult microglial cells in vitro. J Clin Invest 1996;98:1539.
66. Windhagen A, Newcombe J, Dangond F, et al. Expression of costimulatory molecules B7-1 (CD80), B7-2 (CD86), and interleukin 12 cytokine in multiple sclerosis lesions. J Exp Med 1995;182:1985.
67. Gerritse K, Laman JD, Noelle RJ, et al. CD40–CD40 ligand interactions in experimental allergic encephalomyelitis and multiple sclerosis. Proc Natl Acad Sci USA 1996;93:2499.
68. Leonard JP, Waldburger KE, Goldman SJ. Prevention of experimental autoimmune encephalomyelitis by antibodies against interleukin 12. J Exp Med 1995;181:381.
69. Grewal IS, Foellmer HG, Grewal KD, et al. Requirement for CD40 ligand in constimulation induction, T cell activation, and experimental allergic encephalomyelitis. Science 1996;273:1864.
70. Bongioanni P, Meucci G. T-cell tumor necrosis factor-alpha receptor binding in patients with multiple sclerosis. Neurology 1997;48:826.
71. Martino G, Clementi E, Brambilla E, et al. Gamma interferon activates a previously undescribed Ca2+ influx in T lymphocytes from patients with multiple sclerosis. Proc Natl Acad Sci USA 1994;91:4825.

72. Karaszewski JW, Reder AT, Anlar B, Kim WC, Arnason BG. Increased lymphocyte beta-adrenergic receptor density in progressive multiple sclerosis is specific for the CD8+, CD28– suppressor cell. Ann Neurol 1991;30:42.
73. Droogan AG, McMillan SA, Douglas JP, Hawkins SA. Serum and cerebrospinal fluid levels of soluble adhesion molecules in multiple sclerosis: predominant intrathecal release of vascular cell adhesion molecule-1. J Neuroimmunol 1996;64:185.
74. Rieckmann P, Altenhofen B, Riegel A, Baudewig J, Felgenhauer K. Soluble adhesion molecules (sVCAM-1 and sICAM-1) in cerebrospinal fluid and serum correlate with MRI activity in multiple sclerosis. Ann Neurol 1997;41:326.
75. Genc K, Dona D, Reder AT. Increased CD80+ B cells in active multiple sclerosis and reversal by interferon β-1b therapy. J Clin Invest 1997;99:2664.
76. Svenningsson A, Dotevall L, Stemme S, Andersen O. Increased expression of B7–1 costimulatory molecule on cerebrospinal fluid cells of patients with multiple sclerosis and infectious central nervous system disease. J Neuroimmunol 1997;75:59.
77. Moretta A. Molecular mechanisms in cell-mediated cytotoxicity. Cell 1997;90:13.
78. Tsunoda I, Fujinami RS. Two models for multiple sclerosis: experimental allergic encephalomyelitis and Theiler's murine encephalomyelitis virus. J Neuropathol Exp Neurol 1996;55:673.
79. Dowling P, Husar W, Menonna J, et al. Cell death and birth in multiple sclerosis brain. J Neurol Sci 1997;149:1.
80. Tonegawa SMS. Tolerance induction and autoimmune encephalomyelitis amelioration after administration of myelin basic protein-derived peptide. J Exp Med 1997;186:507.
82. Waldner H, Sobel RA, Howard E, Kuchroo VK. Fas- and FasL-deficient mice are resistant to induction of autoimmune encephalomyelitis. J Immunol 1997;159:3100.
82. Sabelko KA, Kelly KA, Nahm MH, Cross AH, Russell JH. Fas and Fas ligand enhance the pathogenesis of experimental allergic encephalomyelitis, but are not essential for immune privilege in the central nervous system. J Immunol 1997;159:3096.
83. Rubesa G, Podack ER, Sepcic J, Rukavina D. Increased perforin expression in multiple sclerosis patients during exacerbation of disease in peripheral blood lymphocytes. J Neuroimmunol 1997;74:198.
84. Sharief MK, Hentges R. Association between tumor necrosis factor-α and disease progression in patients with multiple sclerosis. N Engl J Med 1991;325:467.
85. Rieckmann P, Albrecht M, Kitze B, et al. Tumor necrosis factor-alpha messenger RNA expression in patients with relapsing-remitting multiple sclerosis is associated with disease activity. Ann Neurol 1995;37:82.
86. Rentzos M, Nikolaou C, Rombos A, et al. Tumour necrosis factor alpha is elevated in serum and cerebrospinal fluid in multiple sclerosis and inflammatory neuropathies. J Neurol 1996;243:165.
87. Matusevicius D, Navikas V, Soderstrom M, et al. Multiple sclerosis: the proinflammatory cytokines lymphotoxin-alpha and tumour necrosis factor-alpha are upregulated in cerebrospinal fluid mononuclear cells. J Neuroimmunol 1996;66:115.
88. Navikas V, He B, Link J, et al. Augmented expression of tumour necrosis factor-alpha and lymphotoxin in mononuclear cells in multiple sclerosis and optic neuritis. Brain 1996;119:213.
89. Ruddle NH, Bergman CM, McGrath KM, et al. An antibody to lymphotoxin and tumor necrosis factor prevents transfer of experimental allergic encephalomyelitis. J Exp Med 1990;172:1193.
90. Kuroda Y, Shimamoto Y. Human tumor necrosis factor-α augments experimental allergic encephalomyelitis in rats. J Neuroimmunol 1991;34:159.
91. Bagasra O, Michaels FH, Zheng YM, et al. Activation of the inducible form of nitric oxide synthase in the brains of patients with multiple sclerosis. Proc Natl Acad Sci USA 1995;92:12041.
92. Parkinson JF, Mitrovic B, Merrill JE. The role of nitric oxide in multiple sclerosis. J Mol Med 1997;75:174.
93. Jacobs LD, Cookfair DL, Rudick RA, et al. Intramuscular interferon beta-1a for disease progression in relapsing multiple sclerosis. Ann Neurol 1996;39:285.
94. The IFNB Multiple Sclerosis Study Group and The University of British Columbia MS/MRI Analysis Group. Interferon beta-1b in the treatment of multiple sclerosis: final outcome of the randomized controlled trial. Neurology 1995;45:1277.
95. Johnson KP, Brooks BR, Cohen JA, et al. Copolymer 1 reduces relapse rate and improves disability in relapsing-remitting multiple sclerosis: results of a phase III multicenter, double-blind placebo-controlled trial. The Copolymer 1 Multiple Sclerosis Study Group. Neurology 1995;45:1268.
96. Miller A, Shapiro S, Gershrein R, et al. Treatment of multiple selerosis with copolymer-1 (Copaxone): implicating mechanisms of Th1 to Th2/Th3 immune-deviation. J Neurnimmunol. 1998 Dec 1:92(1–2):113–21.
97. Beck RW, Cleary PA, Trobe JD, et al. The effect of corticosteroids for acute optic neuritis on the subsequent development of multiple sclerosis. N Engl J Med 1993;239:1764.
98. Weiner H, Hohol M, Khoury S, Dawson D, Hafler D. Therapy for MS. Neurol Clin 1995;13:173.
99. Smith DR, Balashov KE, Hafler DA, Khoury SJ, Weiner HL. Immune deviation following pulse cyclophosphamide/methylprednisolone treatment of multiple selerosis: increased interleukin-4 production and associated eusinophilia. Ann. Neurol. 1997 Sep:42(3):313–8.
100. Comabella M, Balashov K, Issazadeh S, et al. Elevated interleukin-12 in progressive multiple sclerosis correlates with disease activity and is normalized by pulse cyclophosphamide therapy. J Clin Invest 1998;102:671.
101. Miller A, Lider O, Weiner HL. Antigen-driven bystander suppression following oral administration of antigens. J Exp Med 1991;174:791.
102. Faria AMC, Weiner HL. Oral tolerance: mechanisms and therapeutic applications. Adv Immunol 1999;73:153.
103. Weiner HL. Oral tolerance with copolymer 1 for the treatment of multiple sclerosis. Proc Natl Acad Sci USA 1999;96:3333.
104. Sun JB, Rask C, Olsson T, Holmgren J, Czerkinsky C. Treatment of experimental autoimmune encephalomyelitis by feeding myelin basic protein conjugated to cholera toxin B subunit. Proc Natl Acad Sci USA 1996;93:7196.
105. Yednock TA, Cannon C, Fritz LC, et al. Prevention of exprimental autoimmune encephalomyelitis by antibodies against alpha 4 beta 1 integrin. Nature 1992 Mar 5;536(6364):63–6.
106. Van Oosten BW, Barkhof F, Truyen L, et al. Increased MRI activity and immune activation in two multiple selerosis patients treated with the monoclonal anti-tumor necrosis factor antibody CA2. Neurology. 1996;47:1531.
107. Balashov KB, Rottman JB, Weiner HL, Hancock WW. CCR5(+) and CXR3(+) T cells are increased in multiple selerosis and their ligands. MIP-1 alpha and IP-10 are expressed in demyclinating brain lesions. Proc Natl Acad Sci USA. 1999;96:6873.
108. Lassmann H, Bruck W, Lucchinetti C, Rodriguez M. Remyelination in multiple sclerosis. Mult Scler 1997;3:133.
109. Edan G, Miller D, Clanet M, et al. Therapeutic effect of mitoxantrone combined with methylprednisolone in multiple sclerosis: a randomised multicentre study of active disease using MRI and clinical criteria. J Neurol Nerurosrg Psychiatry. 1997;62:112.
110. Placebo-controlled multicentre randomised trial of interferon beta-1b in treatment of secondary progressive MS. Lancet. 1998;352:1491.
111. Hohol MJ, Olek MJ, Orav EJ, et al. Treatment of progressive multiple selerosis with pulse cyctophosphamide/methylprednisolone: response to therapy is linked to the duration of progressive disease. Mult Scler. 1999;5:403.

Section 7 Organ-specific Inflammatory Disease

Chapter 78 Autoimmune Peripheral Neuropathies

Marinos C. Dalakas

Autoimmune peripheral neuropathies occur when immunologic tolerance to peripheral nerve components (myelin, Schwann cell, axon and motor or ganglionic neurons) is lost. In some of these neuropathies there is direct evidence for autoimmune reactivity mediated by specific antibodies or autoreactive T lymphocytes against peripheral nerve. In others, the underlying immune-mediated mechanism is secondary or indirect, and an autoimmune cause is suspected when the neuropathy coexists with another systemic autoimmune disease or viral infection.

Autoimmune peripheral neuropathies are potentially treatable or amenable to immunomodulating and immunosuppressive therapies, hence the need for early recognition and accurate diagnosis. Further, the study of these diseases provides the opportunity to investigate how sensitized T cells or antimyelin antibodies cause demyelination; what are the principal immunogenic epitopes of the peripheral nerve antigens; how the immune reaction can be suppressed; and finally, how best to design target-specific immunotherapies.

This chapter reviews the most common autoimmune neuropathies (Table 78.1), their clinical features and diagnostic criteria, the prevailing autoimmune phenomena that govern each neuropathy, and the most effective therapeutic approach.

Common autoimmune neuropathies
Guillain–Barré syndrome and clinical variants (C. Miller Fisher syndrome, pharyngeal–cervical branchial plexopathy, lumbar polyradiculopathy and plexopathy, pure sensory ataxic neuronopathy, acute axonal motor neuropathy)
Chronic inflammatory demyelinating polyneuropathy (CIDP) and its newly recognized variants
Polyneuropathy associated with paraproteinemias: IgG and IgA monoclonal gammopathy Polyneuropathy, organomegaly, endocrinopathy, myeloma and skin changes (POEMS) syndrome Polyneuropathy with IgM monoclonal gammopathies (demyelinating–anti-MAG, sensorimotor, ataxic, and pure motor with GM1 antibodies) Cryoglobulinemic polyneuropathy
Multifocal motor neuropathy with conduction block, often associated with GM1 antibodies
Paraneoplastic neuropathies associated with anti-Hu antibodies Vasculitic neuropathies
Human immunodeficiency virus (HIV) neuropathies and other neuropathies associated with viruses or bacteria (herpes, Lyme disease, leprosy, Chagas' disease, diphtheria)

Table 78.1 Common autoimmune neuropathies.

CLINICAL FEATURES, DIAGNOSIS, AND IMMUNOPATHOGENETIC MECHANISMS

Acute inflammatory demyelinating polyneuropathy (Guillain–Barré syndrome)

Guillain–Barré syndrome (GBS) is an acute demyelinating polyneuropathy characterized by acute (within 1 week) or subacute (within 4 weeks) ascending motor weakness, areflexia, and mild or moderate sensory abnormalities.[1,2] It is a disease of all ages and occurs sporadically, although occasional outbreaks have been noted. In typical cases of GBS the maximum deficit is reached by the fourth week, a sign conventionally used to separate GBS from chronic inflammatory demyelinating polyneuropathy (CIDP), in which the disease begins slowly and progresses over several months, as discussed later. Rare patients who progress beyond the fourth week, but not more than the eighth week, are better classified as having an intermediate form.[3,4] The intermediate form is probably a variant of both GBS and CIDP and a link between the two. Although these criteria are somewhat arbitrary, they are clinically helpful in determining prognosis and making therapeutic decisions in the early phase of the illness.

In patients with GBS the acute onset of weakness may be limited to one or two limbs or to cranial nerves.[2,3] In classic cases the weakness is ascending and symmetric, starting from the legs and spreading up to the arms, the intercostal and diaphragmatic muscles and the facial or bulbar muscles, causing dysphagia and dysarthria. The facial weakness, which can be unilateral or bilateral, occurs in more than half of patients. The oculomotor muscles can be also affected, resulting in diplopia, ptosis or pupillary dysfunction. Sphincter involvement is rare in classic cases except for transient urinary retention or overflow incontinence, which may be seen in up to 20% of patients.[2,3] Although respiratory failure in the absence of limb and trunk weakness is not a feature of GBS, diaphragmatic weakness and respiratory failure occur in parallel with the limb, neck, bulbar and trunk weakness. Patients with acute GBS need to be monitored very carefully for impending respiratory failure, hence the need for early admission to intensive care units (ICUs). Although sensory complaints, such as tingling paresthesias and pain in the calves, buttocks, legs or back, are not uncommon, objective sensory findings may be mild or even absent early in the disease. After the acute phase of the illness, however, a reduction or loss is often detected in vibratory and proprioceptive sensation owing to involvement of the large myelinated fibers or to an impaired pinprick and temperature sensation in a stocking-and-glove distribution as a result of involvement of the small unmyelinated axons.[3] The tendon reflexes are usually abolished early in the disease.

Autonomic dysfunction of varying degree occurs in up to 65% of patients.[2,3] If severe, autonomic dysregulation can be associated with sudden death due to cardiac arrhythmias, or with various hemodynamic changes such as hypertension, orthostatic hypotension and reduced peripheral vascular tone. Gastrointestinal involvement, with ileus, hiccoughs, salivary hypersecretion, oversweating or impaired sweating ability, and loss of thermal regulation or diabetes insipidus can be part of the autonomic dysfunction.[2,3] In respirator-bound patients other secondary complications, such as pulmonary emboli, GI bleeding, sepsis, electrolyte disturbances, depression, and poor motivation for aggressive respiratory therapy, can prolong recovery or contribute to a poor outcome.

Diagnosis

The classic laboratory abnormalities in GBS patients are elevated cerebrospinal fluid (CSF) protein and abnormal nerve conduction studies consistent with active demyelination.

The CSF protein may be normal in the early phase of the disease, but can be as high as 1000 mg/dL by the sixth week of the illness. The elevation of CSF protein may be due to involvement of the roots related to inflammation, but as the blood–nerve barrier becomes impaired serum albumin and IgG may enter freely into the CSF, contributing further to protein elevation. The CSF cell count is usually normal unless GBS occurs in a setting of HIV infection. Mild CSF lymphocytosis may also suggest another coexisting viral illness or a lymphomatous process. When the CSF protein is very high, papilledema may develop because of impaired reabsorption of CSF and raised intracranial pressure.[3] Oligoclonal IgG bands can be also seen.[5]

The abnormal electrophysiologic findings in the classic cases consist of slow nerve conduction velocity, prolonged F-wave latencies, conduction block, and temporal dispersion of the muscle action potentials. In the classic cases only mild signs of denervation are seen early in the disease. Revised criteria for the electrophysiologic diagnosis of GBS have been generally accepted.[1,6] An early sign suggestive of incomplete recovery is the reduction in amplitude of the mean distal compound muscle action potential *by the first week of the illness*, indicative of substantial loss of axons.[6,7] Early signs of denervation by needle electromyography are also consistent with extensive axonal loss and less favorable recovery.

Clinical variants

GBS is a spectrum or group of acute neuropathies with a varying degree of involvement of the motor or sensory axons in which the pathology may primarily involve the myelin sheath (most often); the axon; the motor or sensory roots; all of the above. The degree of involvement defines the clinical picture, the electrophysiological findings, certain serological abnormalities and the response to therapy.

The recognized GBS variants include the following.

Acute inflammatory demyelinating polyneuropathy (AIDP) is the most common form as described above, accounting for up to 75% of cases.

Acute motor axonal neuropathy (AMAN), often associated with *Campylobacter jejuni* infection and GM1 antibodies, as discussed later.[8–11] The primary axonal damage in this variant is due either to massive acute demyelination and inflammation, as occurs in experimental allergic neuritis when the animals are immunized with a high dose of myelin antigen,[12] or to a primary axonal event mediated by macrophages without associated demyelination. At times these patients have a fulminant clinical course, with severe paralysis, complete electrical inexcitability of motor nerves as early as 3–5 days after onset, and generally poor or incomplete recovery of motor function.[12] Infection with *Campylobacter* and at times with cytomegalovirus may be responsible for the majority of these cases,[8–11,13] as discussed later. In AMAN there is nodal and periaxonal deposition of immunoglobulin and complement, whereas macrophages invade the periaxonal space. This is in contrast to the classic demyelinating GBS (AIDP), in which the immunoglobulin deposits and macrophages are noticeable at the abaxonal side of the myelin sheath.[8,9]

Acute motor–sensory axonal neuropathy (AMSAN) is like AMAN but with concurrent involvement of the sensory axons, in which there is massive macrophage-mediated attack on the axonal membrane of motor and sensory nerves.[12]

C. *Miller-Fisher syndrome* is characterized by an acute onset of ophthalmoplegia, gait ataxia and areflexia.[14] The ataxia can occur in a setting of normal sensation, although 50% of patients complain of tingling paresthesias.[2,3] Muscle weakness may be absent at onset in two-thirds of cases, but in approximately a third of all patients weakness leading to paralysis, with pharyngeal, facial, trunk and respiratory muscle involvement, can occur.[3] Nerve conduction studies are consistent with proximal demyelination. The C. Miller-Fisher syndrome is a distinct variant characterized by the presence of a unique IgG antibody against GQ1b ganglioside,[15] as described later.

Pharyngeal–cervical branchial variant, with acute weakness of the pharyngeal and upper extremity muscles and electrophysiologic signs of demyelination.

Lumbar polyradiculopathy and plexopathy variant, with acute weakness of the lower extremities in the distribution of multiple roots or plexus and electrophysiologic signs of proximal demyelination.

Sensory ataxic GBS due to acute involvement of roots and ganglionic neurons. In these patients antibodies against GQ1b ganglioside were recently found, suggesting that ataxic GBS and Miller-Fisher variants share autoantibody with the same fine specificity that may form a continuous spectrum.[15]

Acute pandysautonomic neuropathy. In these cases there is no evidence of detectable demyelination, and the target antigen is probably components of the autonomic nervous system (sympathetic ganglia?).[16]

The differential diagnosis of GBS should include other forms of acute paralysis, such as botulism, tick paralysis, acute intermittent porphyria, acute paralytic poliomyelitis, acute myelopathy, acute myositis, or acute paralysis in patients treated with neuromuscular blocking agents and steroids, as seen in critically ill patients.

Antecedent illnesses or events

Two-thirds of patients with GBS give a history of a flu-like illness, with upper respiratory signs or acute dysenteric episodes that precede the development of GBS by 1–3 weeks.[2,3] Among the implicated viruses are cytomegalovirus, identified as the predominant viral cause in 10–15% of cases, Epstein–Barr virus, herpesviruses, outbreaks of hepatitis A and HIV.[17] Among bacteria, *Mycoplasma pneumoniae* may precede up to 8–10% of cases, but *Campylobacter jejuni* is the most frequent, having been implicated in up to 35% of cases worldwide; in Japan and China the incidence may be as high as 45–60%.[17] *Campylobacter jejuni* is of special interest because it contains glycoconjugates that share epitopes with the peripheral myelin. Cytomegalovirus may also directly infect the nerve and cross-react with GM2 glycolipid and Po protein of the peripheral nerve.[13] Two vaccines, one against rabies and the other against the swine flu A/New Jersey influenza strain that caused an outbreak of GBS in 1976,[2,3] have been convincingly connected with the development of GBS. Apart from these two vaccines, however, there is no convincing evidence that the incidence of GBS is increased in connection with other vaccines, in spite of anecdotal reports of patients who developed GBS 1–3 weeks after vaccinations.

Surgery can precede the development of GBS in up to 10% of patients.[2,3] Surgical stress, the release of nerve autoantigens, and infections have been proposed as possible explanations for this association.

There are also four drugs causally associated with acute demyelinating neuropathy: gold, perhexiline, suramin (used now for prostatic carcinoma) and chronassial (used in Europe to treat various neuropathic symptoms). Chronassial (now withdrawn) was of special interest because it contained a mixture of gangliosides, including GM1, and elicited a strong anti-GM1 antibody response along with a clinical picture identical to that of AMAN.[18]

GBS has occurred in patients who suffer from neoplasms, especially lymphoma, melanoma and Hodgkin disease. Melanoma is of special interest because it contains GM2 gangliosides and may cause disease through a molecular mimicry phenomenon (discussed later). In spite of the autoimmune nature of GBS, the disease is rarely seen as part of another connective tissue disorder.[2,3]

Immunopathology

GBS is an inflammatory demyelinating polyneuropathy in which the peripheral myelin, the Schwann cells and, at times, axonal components are target antigens of an immune attack, triggered by the various antecedent events discussed above. Both the cellular and the humoral components of the immune system have been implicated in the immunopathogenesis of GBS. In spite of newly identified myelin antigens, the exact target antigen is still unknown.

Cellular factors

The nerves of GBS patients possess two prominent histologic features: (1) perivascular and endoneurial inflammatory infiltrates consisting of lymphocytes and macrophages, found throughout the cranial nerves, ventral and dorsal roots, plexuses and peripheral nerves;[1–3] and (2) segmental demyelination in areas associated with the lymphoid infiltrates. Although CD4 cells appear to predominate over CD8 cells and macrophages in the infiltrates[3], if one takes into account that most tissue macrophages express CD4, the dominant cells are the macrophages. By electron microscopy, macrophages break through the basement membrane of healthy Schwann cells and make direct contact with the outermost myelin lamellae, leading finally to lysis of the superficial myelin sheath. Macrophages may exert their myelinolytic activity via lymphokines, especially interleukin (IL)-1. Interferon-γ released by the activated T cells and complement activation may increase capillary permeability and enhance recruitment of additional macrophages.[10] When the demyelination is extensive it is followed by axonal degeneration.[1–3] At sites of segmental demyelination there is proliferation of Schwann cells along the denuded axons, whereas in areas of axonal degeneration the Schwann cells proliferate in columns to guide the regenerating axons. The proliferating Schwann cells are responsible for remyelination and axonal regeneration, which may begin even during the phase of active myelin breakdown. The degree and effectiveness of remyelination and axonal regeneration dictate the degree of clinical recovery.

A number of studies indicate that activated T cells play a role in GBS.[3] Peripheral blood lymphocytes from GBS patients exert myelinotoxic activity when applied to cultures of myelinated axons. Further, levels of IL-2 and soluble IL-2 receptors are increased in the serum during the acute phase of GBS and decline during recovery, suggesting ongoing T-cell proliferation.[10] Inflammatory cytokines, such as tumor necrosis factor α (TNF-α), are increased during the acute phase whereas down-regulatory cytokines such as transforming growth factor-β (TGF-β) are decreased at presentation but increased after recovery.

A more convincing role for a T-cell-mediated process in GBS is derived by analogy from the animal model of experimental allergic neuritis (EAN), which resembles GBS in both its pathology and its clinical course.[3] Animals sensitized to whole human nerve, to various myelin proteins such as P0, P2, and to the neutral glycolipid galactocerebroside, develop segmental demyelination with mononuclear cell infiltrates consisting of macrophages and T cells. In EAN the T cells are sensitized against myelin, and T cells from EAN animals or cloned P2-specific T-cell lines can passively transfer the disease to healthy animals.[3]

Humoral factors

There is even stronger evidence that humoral factors are involved in the pathogenesis of GBS. On clinical grounds this is supported by the beneficial effect of plasmapheresis, presumably by removing pathogenic antibodies. On laboratory grounds it is supported by the variety of autoantibodies detected in the serum of acute GBS patients. Studies have also shown that sera taken from patients in the acute phase of GBS can demyelinate rodent dorsal root ganglionic extracts in a complement-dependent manner.[20] Further, GBS serum injected into rat sciatic nerves caused demyelination and conduction block.[21] Immunocytochemical studies of the peripheral nerves of GBS patients have demonstrated deposits of IgG, IgM and components of the complement membrane attack complex, implying complement-fixing antibody activity of the serum immunoglobulin.[3,8,9] Complement-fixing IgM antibodies against a human neutral glycolipid of peripheral nerve myelin that contains a carbohydrate epitope similar to the one found on the Forssman antigen have been found.[22] These antibodies, which are part of the heterophile response, are directed against a neutral glycolipid widely distributed on bacteria, viruses and parasites, but not in humans. They may be nonspecific and their presence has not been confirmed by others. In contrast, acidic glycolipids may be more specific targets. High titers of autoantibodies against sulfated and acidic glycolipids are found in the serum of acute GBS as well as CIDP patients.[23–24] In one study, IgG or IgM antibodies to acidic glycolipids were demonstrated in 36 of 53 (68%) GBS patients and in 8 of 16 (50%) CIDP patients and autoantibody levels correlated with clinical symptoms in 9 of 11 GBS patients.[24] The target glycolipids in these patients were LM1, GM1, GD1b and GT1a.[23–25] LMI is present only in the peripheral nerve, and antibodies to this antigen have been speculated to be of pathogenic significance. In contrast to other neuropathies or motor neuron syndromes in which anti-GM1 antibodies of the IgM class are seen, as in GBS patients, these antibodies are mostly of the IgG class.[10,18] These patients have a high incidence of C. *jejuni* infection,[26] implying a cross-reactivity between determinants on both C. *jejuni* and GM1.

The pathogenic significance of these antibodies with wide specificity for various ganglioside epitopes is poorly understood. They are associated with different clinical phenotypes and are not directed against a common 'GBS antigen'. It is conceivable that antibodies against different acidic glycolipids or sulfatides are related to different viral or bacterial antecedent factors. In one model, molecular mimicry between epitopes of viral proteins and myelin components might result in the sensitization of cross-reactive T cells that could initiate the autoimmune process. The activated T cells could then stimulate B cells to produce specific antibodies directed against myelin components and could recruit macrophages as effector cells.[10] Cytokines triggered by the initiating event (virus, bacteria) could also up-regulate intercellular adhesion cell molecule (ICAM)-1 expression on the endothelial cells and facilitate the entrance of activated T cells or antibodies to the endoneurial parenchyma. The mechanism by which these autoantibodies can cause conduction block is under study. They may access the peripheral nerve proximally at the root or distally at the end plate, and depress or block sodium channels at the nodes of Ranvier.[8,18] Figure 78.1 summarizes these immunopathogenic mechanisms

Among the autoantibodies to different gangliosides, the only one that correlates with a specific clinical syndrome is directed to GQ1b.[8] IgG anti-GQ1b antibodies are present in approximately 90–100% of patients with the C. Miller-Fisher variant of GBS. These autoantibodies are also found in post-infectious ophthalmoplegias, as well as in GBS patients with ophthalmoplegia,

KEY CONCEPTS

Characteristics of cellular autoimmune response in Guillain–Barré syndrome

- Peripheral myelin or Schwann cells express the target antigens.
- Activated macrophages are the dominant infiltrating endoneurial cells and lift the outermost myelin lamellae, lysing the superficial myelin sheaths.
- Peripheral blood lymphocytes from patients with GBS exert myelinotoxic activity in vitro.
- Levels of IL-2 and soluble IL-2 receptors are increased during the acute phase of the disease and decline during recovery.
- Adhesion molecules on endothelial cells are elevated during the acute phase of the disease.

but not in other subsets of GBS patients or in other autoimmune conditions. The recent finding of GQ1b in the ataxic GBS suggests a continuous spectrum with the C. Miller-Fisher variant.[15] Interestingly, anti-GQ1b antibodies immunostain the paranodal regions of oculomotor nerves III, IV and VI, suggesting that these autoantibodies may block impulse generation at the nodes of Ranvier, resulting in a conduction block that is characteristic of GBS. GQ1b is also found in high quantities in cranial nerve III.

Relationship between Campylobacter jejuni and GBS

GBS is associated with *Campylobactor jejuni* infection (Penner D:19 Serotype) in 15–60% of GBS patients, depending on the geographic area being studied.[11,13,17] Further, such patients also have a higher frequency of anti-GM1 antibodies, axonal damage

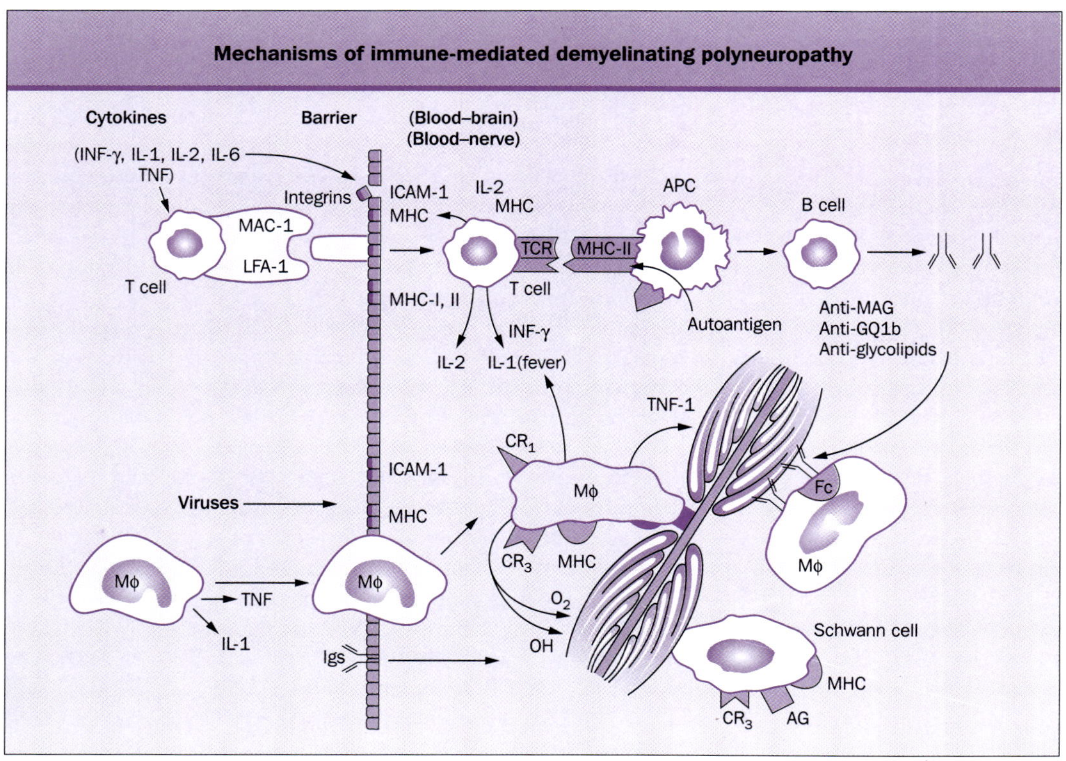

Figure 78.1 Mechanisms of immune-mediated demyelinating polyneuropathy. Cytokines lead to increased expression of major histocompatibility complex (MHC) molecules and intercellular adhesion molecules. The latter allow the sensitized T cells and macrophages to exit the endothelial cell wall and traffic to the peripheral nerve, where they recognize myelin antigen and induce a macrophage-mediated demyelination. The antigen-presenting cells (probably Schwann cells or macrophages), in concert with MHC Class II expression, interact with CD4+ T cells and lead to clonal expansion of B cells and the production of antibodies against various peripheral nerve antigens.

KEY CONCEPTS

Characteristics of humoral autoimmune response in Guillain–Barré syndrome

- Serum IgG from patients exerts a complement-dependent demyelination in vitro.
- Intraneural injections of serum from acute GBS patients cause demyelination and conduction block.
- IgG, IgM and membranolytic attack complex are detected immunocytochemically on the patients' nerves.
- High titers of IgG antibodies against peripheral nerve acidic glycolipids (GM1, LM1, GT1α and GQ1b) and sulfatides are detected in the serum and correlate with disease activity.
- IgG antibodies against GQ1b ganglioside are specific for the C. Miller-Fisher variant and cause blockade of neuromuscular transmission.
- High incidences of antibodies to *Campylobacter jejuni* and GM1 are seen in acute GBS, implying molecular mimicry (the enterotoxin of *Campylobacter* utilizes GM1 as its receptor).

and poorer recovery. Because these bacteria are a common cause of diarrheal illness worldwide, and diarrhea has been reported to be an antecedent event in up to 50% of GBS patients, infection with C. *jejuni* may trigger the disease in many cases. Isolation of C. *jejuni* from stools early in acute GBS varies from 44% to 88% of patients, and IgG or IgM antibodies to C. *jejuni* are found in 36% of GBS patients compared to 10% of controls.[11] The titers of anti-GM1 or anti-GD1b antibodies are also higher in GBS patients who have serologic evidence of C. *jejuni* infection.[27–29] This association has generated great interest because C. *jejuni* elaborates an enterotoxin of 68 kDa that utilizes GM1 as its receptor. Further, the monoclonal IgM anti-GM1 antibodies from patients with motor neuropathies bind to lipopolysaccharides from C. *jejuni*, suggesting that molecular mimicry may result in these lipopolysaccharides stimulating B cells to produce anti-GM1 antibodies. A similar mechanism of molecular mimicry may be also implicated in cytomegalovirus (CMV) associated GBS, for which IgM anti-GM2 antibodies have been found.[3] Even though the distribution of GM2 on human myelin sheath and peripheral nerve is unclear, antibodies to GM2 cross-react with CMV.[30]

Chronic inflammatory demyelinating polyneuropathy

Chronic inflammatory demyelinating polyneuropathy (CIDP) is the most common of the chronic autoimmune peripheral neuropathies. It is considered the chronic counterpart of GBS because of the clinical, electrophysiologic, histologic and laboratory similarities with GBS and its common autoimmune features. CIDP differs from GBS predominantly by its tempo, mode of evolution, prognosis and responsiveness to steroids.

Clinical features

CIDP presents with a slowly progressive weakness and paresthesias that evolve over several weeks (usually more than 4–6) or months. Maximum deficit is usually reached after 2 months from onset.[31,32] Although initially the weakness is predominantly distal, proximal muscle involvement can be prominent, especially late in the course of the disease. CIDP can be either monophasic or characterized by spontaneous remissions and relapses. Nowadays, with early initiation of therapy, it is difficult to distinguish spontaneous relapses from treatment-related relapses.[31]

Along with the muscle weakness there is areflexia and, in chronic cases when axonal loss has taken place, muscular atrophy. Cranial nerves can be affected, but not as often as in GBS. Optic neuritis can be seen rarely, implying coexisting central demyelination. Sensory symptoms are almost always present, and sensory findings (often due to large fiber loss) are very frequent. In rare cases, however, the disease can be purely motor, and when it is asymmetric the distinction from multifocal motor neuropathy is difficult, as discussed later. Pain and autonomic dysfunction in CIDP are unusual. A mild action tremor (neuropathic tremor) during the active phase of the disease has been seen in several patients.[32a]

Diagnosis

The diagnostic criteria include:[31,33]

1. Subacute onset of sensorimotor polyneuropathy, which is progressive over several weeks or months or has a relapsing–-remitting course;
2. Absence of another systemic disease that can cause neuropathy. Specifically, the patients should not have diabetes, thyroid disease, neoplasms, amyloidosis, paraproteinemia, myelomas, vasculitis, alcoholism, collagen vascular disease, systemic infections, exposures to neurotoxic agents or drugs, or a family history of neuropathy. Although CIDP can occur in a patient who is diabetic, alcoholic, or HIV-positive, or who has an IgG or IgA benign gammopathy, for a strict definition all these diseases should be excluded.
3. Elevated CSF protein (up to sixfold) without pleocytosis. No oligoclonal bands are found, but a single band is often seen on agarose gel electrophoresis, probably reflecting the high amount of protein.[5]
4. Demyelination of motor and sensory fibers by electrophysiologic testing and nerve biopsy.[32] Although a nerve biopsy is not essential when the electrophysiology is characteristic of CIDP,[34] it can be useful in confirming the diagnosis and studying the immunopathology of this disease. Characteristic electrophysiologic findings include slow nerve conduction velocity (at least below 60% of normal), prolonged F-wave latencies, prolonged distal motor and sensory latencies, and an associated conduction block in one or more nerves, with dispersion of the compound muscle or nerve action potentials.[31–35] An associated axonal loss is also common, with evidence of denervation detected by needle electromyography (EMG) in the majority of cases.

CIDP may mimic the following autoimmune peripheral neuropathies: (1) multifocal motor neuropathy with conduction block, when the sensory findings are not prominent (discussed later); (2) demyelinating neuropathies associated with IgA or IgG gammopathies (discussed later); (3) the intermediate form of GBS when the onset of GBS is not very acute and its maximum deficit is reached between 4 and 8 weeks[4] (discussed previously); and (4) the relapsing form of GBS. Up to 3% of GBS patients relapse;[3] however, in some cases the new relapse may not be as acute and typical as the original attack of GBS but slower, resembling the intermediate form.

Variants of CIDP have been recently recognized.[34] These include a multifocal sensorimotor but asymmetric form of

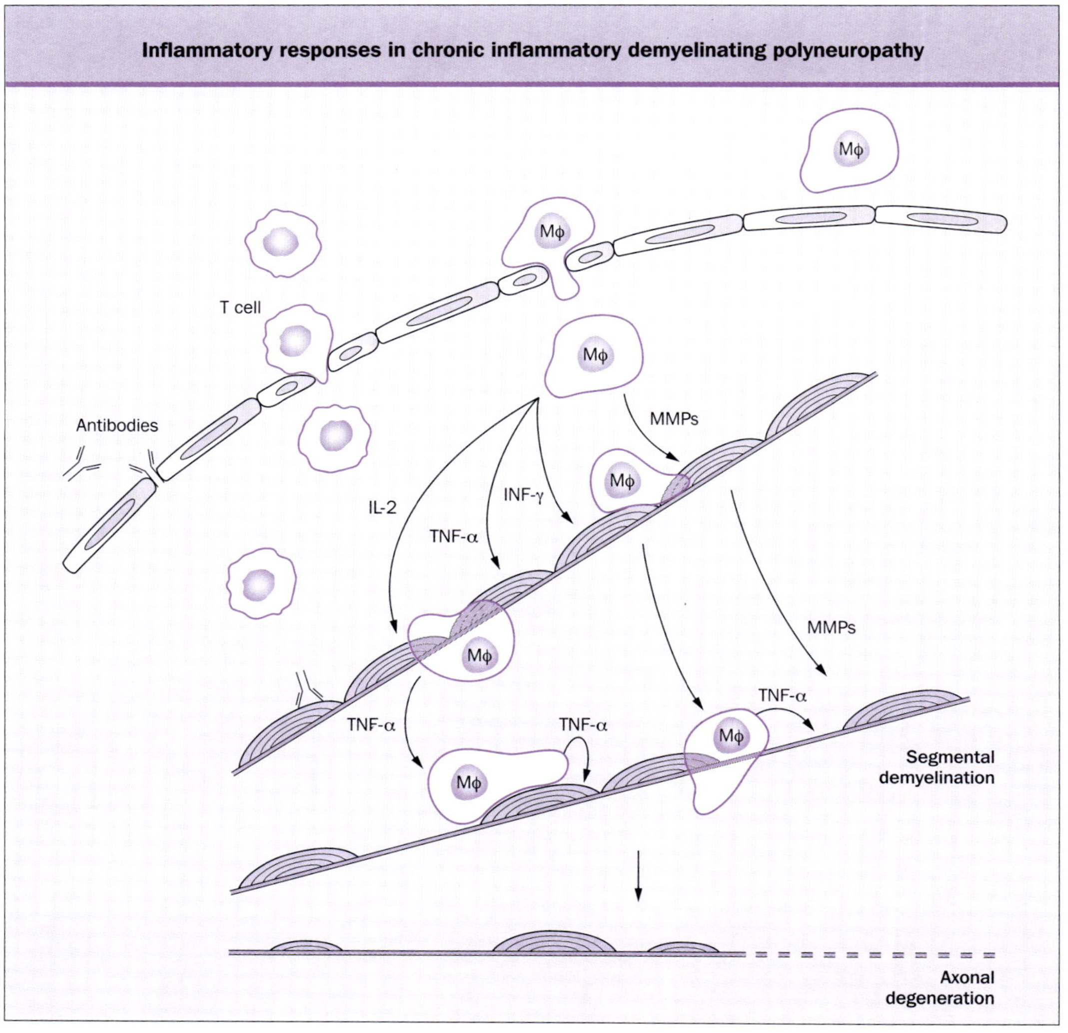

Figure 78.2 Inflammatory responses in chronic inflammatory demyelinating polyneuropathy (CIDP). Activated macrophages (Mφ) and T cells cross the endothelial cell wall of the blood–nerve barrier and reach the myelinated fibers. Activated, TNF-α producing Mφ invade the myelin sheath, causing Mφ-mediated segmental demyelination. Axonal loss secondary to demyelination, probably enhanced by production of TNF-α and metalloproteinases, may become prominent in the chronic phases of the disease. Other cytokines, T cells sensitized to unidentified antigens and putative antibodies may participate. IL, interleukin; INF, interferon; MMP, metalloproteinase; Mφ, activated macrophage; TNF, tumor necrosis factor.

CIDP[36,37] and a multifocal, regional form, with a predominantly upper or lower extremity involvement.[38] When CIDP occurs in children it presents like the disease in adults, but usually follows a stable course after the first few years.

In contrast to GBS, patients with CIDP do not have an increased incidence of infection, vaccination or trauma preceding the development of the neuropathy. The significance of a few isolated case reports that followed an infectious illness[31] is unclear. CIDP is a chronic disease and although it may respond to various therapies many patients have incomplete recovery and are left with residual weakness.[35]

Immunopathogenesis

Although CIDP is defined as an inflammatory polyneuropathy, there is usually only minimal evidence of inflammation visible with hematoxylin and eosin stains of sural nerve biopsies. A biopsy during a relapse may, however, show a mild perivascular or endoneurial inflammatory cellular infiltrate. The predominant endoneurial mononuclear cell is the macrophage and not the lymphocyte.[37] Electron microscopic studies demonstrate that the demyelinating process in CIDP is always associated with the presence of macrophages, which sequentially penetrate the basement membrane of the Schwann cell, displace the cytoplasm, and finally disrupt the myelin by focal lysis of the superficial myelin lamellae.[32] Similarities may exist between the immunopathology and GBS and the chronic or relapsing–remitting form of experimental allergic neuritis in which macrophages, activated T cells and components of the complement membrane attack complex C5b-9 are noted on the myelin sheath of the peripheral nerves.[10]

Evidence for autoimmunity in CIDP is mostly indirect, related to its resemblance to GBS. As in GBS, humoral factors may play an important role in CIDP. Complement-fixing IgG and IgM are deposited on the patient's myelin sheath, suggestive of antimyelin antibodies.[31] Antibodies to glycolipids LM1, GM1 or GD1b are found in some CIDP patients, but less frequently than in GBS patients.[24] The up-regulation of HLA-DR antigens on endothelial cells and Schwann cells,[39] ICAM-1 expression on the endothelial cells[40] and differentiation antigens on endoneurial macrophages[41] suggest that cytokines, such as interferon-γ (IFN-γ) and TNF-α may participate in the disease process. Up-regulation of mRNA for TNF-α, IFN-γ and IL-2 has been seen within the endoneurial macrophages and around the active demyelinating lesions.[34] In CIDP, Schwann cells express the molecules associated with antigen-presenting cells, such as the costimulatory molecule BB1. In addition, the counter-receptors CTLA-4 and CD28 are up-regulated on the endoneurial CD4 T cells.[39] The immunopathogenesis scheme illustrated in Figure 78.1, proposed for GBS, is also appropriately applied to CIDP with some modification

> **KEY CONCEPTS**
>
> **Autoimmunity in CIDP**
> - Activated macrophages are the predominant infiltrating endoneurial cell causing displacement of Schwann cell cytoplasm, disruption of myelin and lysis of superficial myelin lamellae.
> - Complement-fixing IgG and IgM antibodies are deposited on the myelin sheath.
> - IgG antibodies to acidic glycolipids LM1, GM1 or GD1b are found in the serum of some patients.
> - There is up-regulation of HLA-DR expression on Schwann cells and endothelial cells and of ICAM-1 on the endothelial cells of the peripheral nerves.
> - The Schwann cells express the costimulatory molecule BB-1, whereas surrounding T cells show up-regulated expression of the ligands CTLA-4 and CD28.

(Figure 78.2). In CIDP there may be prominent axonal loss, which becomes evident as the disease becomes more chronic. TNF-α secreted by the activated macrophages in the endoneurium may play a role in this axonal injury.

Molecular mimicry may be also implicated in patients with CIDP associated with melanoma.[42] Carbohydrate epitopes such as GM3, GM2, GD3 are expressed on melanoma cells, and antibodies raised against melanoma cell lines react with myelin glycoproteins. Cross-reactivity of antibodies to GM2 on melanoma cells and peripheral nerve myelin have been demonstrated in a patient with melanoma who developed CIDP and had circulating antibodies against GM2.[42]

Multifocal motor neuropathy with conduction block

Patients with multifocal motor neuropathy (MMN) present with progressive weakness, atrophy, and areflexia in muscle groups supplied by many individual peripheral nerves (multifocal).[43] It differs from vasculitic neuropathy because it is slow and painless and affects clinically only the motor nerve fibers. It also differs from a lower motor neuron disease because it progresses very slowly, over years rather than months, and the distribution of the weakness is not multisegmental but within distributions of peripheral nerves. Further, the weakness and atrophy do not always coexist as in lower motor neuron disease, and weak muscles may not be severely atrophic. In MMN, the cranial musculature is often spared; atrophy of the tongue or the face is the exception. As with motor neuron disease, however, patients with MMN can experience cramps and fasciculations. The weakness and atrophy begin in the hands and are more prominent distally and in the upper extremities, even in advanced chronic cases. There is no evidence of other systemic illness. The CSF protein is normal, an important finding that distinguishes MMN from CIDP.[34]

In spite of the term MMN, however, the disease is not strictly motor. For example, one of the author's patients had sensory complaints and very minimal sensory findings, and another had minor sensory abnormalities on examination. The mild sensory abnormalities reported have raised the question whether MMN is a distinct entity or a variant of CIDP.[34,44] Most investigators view MMN as a distinct disease that should be recognized early because it is treatable. It affects men more often than women, and is more common in people younger than 50 years. The identification of MMN has been important because of the hope that a small number of patients with amyotrophic lateral sclerosis (ALS) who present as a lower motor neuron disease may not have ALS but rather MMN, a potentially treatable and clearly nonfatal condition.[43]

MMN is characterized by the multifocal conduction block always seen in more than one motor nerve by electrophysiologic techniques. High IgG or IgM anti-GM1 antibody levels determined by ELISA are found in up to 60 or 70% of these patients. In contrast to CIDP, in which sensory conduction block is also present, the sensory conduction in MMN remains normal across those nerve segments that have a severe motor block.[43] This important distinction is not absolute, however, because CIDP occasionally exhibits a predominance of motor conduction block that spares sensory fibers. Further, sural nerve biopsies from patients with MMN show subtle changes of segmental demyelination and loss of myelinated axons, implying that MMN may have more similarities with CIDP than usually thought.[43] The reason for a selective motor conduction block is unclear. Differences in the antigenic specificities in the myelin components between the motor and sensory fibers are suspected because the ceramide composition of gangliosides differs between sensory and motor fibers.[43] Confusion has recently emerged with the suggestion that there is also a MMN without identifiable conduction block, when the block is too proximal to detect it. Such rare cases exist and should be sought because they are potentially treatable.

The role of GM1 antibodies in the pathogenesis of MMN, or as an aid in the diagnosis and distinction of MMN from CIDP or ALS, is unsettled because (1) high GM1 antibody titers can be seen in up to 25% of ALS patients who do not have conduction block,[45] (2) high GM1 antibody titers are also seen in some CIDP patients; and (3) not all patients with MMN have high GM1 antibodies.

The GM1 ganglioside has been implicated in the cause of MMN because it is present on the surface of motor neurons and at the nodes of Ranvier.[46] Consequently, IgM anti-GM1 antibodies, may interfere with saltatory conduction. Further, sera from MMN patients with GM1 antibody titers, when injected into the sciatic nerves of rats, produced conduction block and demyelination.[46] Although GM1 antibodies can be helpful in diagnosis, the author's approach is to treat aggressively all patients with bona fide MMN with conduction block regardless of their GM1 antibody titers.

PARAPROTEINEMIC POLYNEUROPATHIES

A distinct subset of acquired polyneuropathies has been associated with circulating monoclonal gammopathies.[47] Although neuropathy occurs in a setting of myeloma, plasmacytoma or Waldenström macroglobulinemia, the majority of paraproteinemic neuropathies occur in patients without an underlying lymphoproliferative disease. The gammopathy in such patients is of undetermined significance (monoclonal gammopathy of undetermined significance; MGUS),[48] even though the IgM monoclonal protein may recognize specific antigenic determinants of the human myelin, and many of these patients have a favorable response to immunotherapy.

The association of neuropathy with benign monoclonal gammopathy was originally thought to be rare and coincidental because a causal relationship between the neuropathy and the paraproteinemia had not been established. Further, benign gammopathies occur nonspecifically in many chronic inflammatory or infectious conditions, and their incidence increases with age, occurring in up to 2% of normal people older than 70 years.[48] In 1979, in the largest series reported to that date, it was hypothesized that the paraprotein may bind to peripheral nerve, and in a number of patients the neuropathy responded to immunosuppressive therapy.[47] The causal association between the paraprotein and the neuropathy was strengthened when it was shown that the monoclonal IgM of a patient with demyelinating polyneuropathy had specific antimyelin activity directed against myelin-associated glycoprotein (MAG).[49] Today, polyneuropathies with monoclonal gammopathy comprise 10% of patients with acquired neuropathy.[48,50] Importantly, the paraproteinemic polyneuropathies are considered to be a potentially treatable group of autoimmune peripheral neuropathies.

A monoclonal gammopathy is considered benign[48,50] when the patient has the following: (1) less than 3 g/dL of monoclonal protein in their serum and, rarely, the same monoclonal protein in the urine; (2) fewer than 5% plasma cells in the bone marrow aspirate; (3) no systemic signs of renal insufficiency, osteolytic or osteosclerotic lesions in the bone survey, or signs of anemia and hypercalcemia; (4) no suppression of the rest of the uninvolved polyclonal immunoglobulins (background immunoglobulins); (5) no signs of a lymphoproliferative disease; and (6) a stable amount of the monoclonal protein during follow-up examinations (Chapter 97). In contrast, ominous findings of malignant plasma cell dyscrasia are lytic bone lesions, Bence Jones proteinuria, a reduction of the uninvolved (background) immunoglobulin level, abnormal bone marrow examination, and a progressively increased amount of monoclonal protein in serial measurements. Even in patients with the benign gammopathies, however, long-term follow-up may reveal that up to 20% of the patients develop malignant plasma cell dyscrasia, especially macroglobulinemia; hence the need for periodic screening.[50]

Frequency of polyneuropathies in patients with monoclonal gammopathy

Based on routine blood bank screening, up to 1% of normal people over 50 years may have a monoclonal gammopathy. This incidence increases to 1.7% of the normal population above age 70 and up to 6% of normal people above the age of 90 (Chapter 97). Monoclonal gammopathies, however, are 10 times more frequent in patients with polyneuropathy than in an age-matched control population, and almost 10% of patients with acquired polyneuropathy have an associated monoclonal gammopathy.[48] If one categorizes these gammopathies into subclasses, the incidence of polyneuropathy among patients with IgM monoclonal proteins can be as high as 50%.[48,50,51]

Monoclonal gammopathy, polyneuropathy and amyloid

Some patients with paraproteins may have associated amyloidosis derived from the variable region of the immunoglobulin light chain (Chapters 71, 97). A λ light chain is more often associated with amyloidosis. If present in a patient with gammopathy and neuropathy, deposits of amyloid should be thoroughly sought. When amyloidosis is present, the neuropathy is often painful and has a strong autonomic component. In addition to painful paresthesias in the hands and feet, these patients have mild to moderate distal weakness, often with pedal edema, and autonomic symptoms consisting of orthostatic hypotension, dizziness, impotence, impaired gastric mobility or frequent diarrhea. The disease is difficult to treat; apart from symptomatic therapy (mostly opiates), immunosuppressive therapies have been largely unsuccessful. The diagnosis is frequently made via a muscle or nerve biopsy that demonstrates the amyloid in the connective tissue or around blood vessels. In the author's experience, muscle and skin biopsies have a higher yield than nerve biopsy for finding amyloid deposits. Overall, biopsy of the abdominal fat, along with skin, may give the highest yield in finding amyloid.

Polyneuropathies associated with IgG or IgA monoclonal gammopathies

Patients with polyneuropathy and benign IgG or IgA monoclonal gammopathy who do not have myeloma, plasmacytoma, cryoglobulinemia or amyloidosis usually have an axonal neuropathy. Their IgG or IgA generally cannot be demonstrated to recognize a specific neuronal or myelin protein although monoclonal IgA from one patient recognized certain glycoconjugates.[52] When the neuropathy is demyelinating it may behave like CIDP and respond to immunosuppressive therapies. The mechanism of the neuropathy in such patients is not understood, and the causal association between the monoclonal protein and the neuropathy has not been established.

Polyneuropathy, organomegaly, endocrinopathy, myeloma and skin changes

A subset of patients with malignant IgG or IgA gammopathy have polyneuropathy with osteosclerotic myeloma. Most of them comprise the POEMS syndrome (*p*olyneuropathy, *o*rganomegaly, *e*ndocrinopathy, *m*yeloma, and *s*kin changes).[53–55] More than 50% of patients with osteosclerotic myeloma of IgA or IgG type have a sensorimotor, symmetric polyneuropathy with mixed demyelinating and axonal features and high (usually 200 mg/dL) CSF protein.[53–55] Pure axonal neuropathies can be also seen. In POEMS the neuropathy tends to be associated with edema in the legs, with hyperpigmentation, sclerodermatous thickening or papular angiomas of the skin, and hypertrichosis with dark hair. Endocrinopathy most often includes gonadal failure, amenorrhea, impotence, gynecomastia, hypothyroidism, diabetes or elevated prolactin levels. The IgG class is slightly more common than the IgA class, but the λ light chain is present in the majority (up to 90%) of patients.[53–55] CT scans of the abdomen reveal an enlarged spleen and calcifications. The bone lesions can be sclerotic, solitary or multiple, sparing the skull and the extremities. The pathologic changes in the lymph nodes, which can be enlarged, may at times resemble those of Castleman disease, which can also be associated with polyneuropathy. Not all patients with POEMS, however, have all these features. Overproduction of various proinflammatory cytokines seem to play a fundamental role in POEMS.[55]

Polyneuropathies associated with IgM monoclonal gammopathies

This entity is composed of a clinically heterogeneous group of neuropathies in which the immunoglobulin appears to be an antibody to various glycoproteins or glycolipids of the peripheral nerve. These neuropathies can be best divided into the following subsets.

Demyelinating polyneuropathy with IgM anti-MAG antibodies

Sera from approximately 50% of patients with neuropathy and IgM monoclonal gammopathy react with myelin-associated glycoprotein (MAG), a 100 kDa glycoprotein of the central and peripheral nerve myelin, as well as other glycoproteins or glycolipids that share antigenic determinants with MAG. Most patients with anti-MAG antibodies present with a sensory, large-fiber demyelinating polyneuropathy manifested as a sensory ataxia.[56,57] Other patients have a sensorimotor polyneuropathy with mixed features of demyelination and axonal loss. A tremor of neurogenic origin is common.[32a,56]

The CSF protein is elevated, up to 250 mg/dL (normal ≤ 50 mg/dL). The monoclonal IgM may also enter the CSF compartment, in spite of its high molecular weight, probably via the dorsal root ganglia, which lack a blood–CSF barrier, or via a disrupted root–CSF barrier.[57a]

Nerve conduction studies are consistent with demyelination characterized by slow conduction velocity and by prolonged distal motor and sensory latencies. Conduction block, as seen in CIDP or GBS, is usually absent. The amplitude of the muscle action potential can be diminished, and the needle EMG often shows denervation potentials due to a concomitant axonal degeneration.

The sural nerve biopsy demonstrates a diminished number of myelinated axons (Fig. 78.3). Lymphocytic infiltrates are rarely seen within the endoneurial parenchyma. On electron microscopy there is splitting of the outer myelin lamellae, associated with the presence of IgM deposits.[58]

Antibodies to myelin-associated glycoprotein (MAG)

MAG, a 100 kDa glycoprotein of the central and peripheral nerve myelin, is the most extensively studied antigen recognized by IgM paraproteins. The antigenic determinant resides in the carbohydrate component of the MAG molecule, as demonstrated by the loss of reactivity following deglycosylation of purified human MAG.[59] The anti-MAG IgM paraproteins also react with an acidic glycolipid in the ganglioside fraction of the human peripheral nerve, which can be separated from the whole ganglioside fraction by ion-exchange chromatography.[60] This antigenic glycolipid, chromatographed between GM1 and GD1a, is a novel sulfoglucuronyl glycosphingolipid[61] (Fig. 78.4). In contrast to MAG, which is mostly present within the CNS, this sulfoglucuronyl glycosphingolipid is found only in the peripheral nerve and may be the most specific antigenic target in demyelinating polyneuropathy with IgM gammopathy.

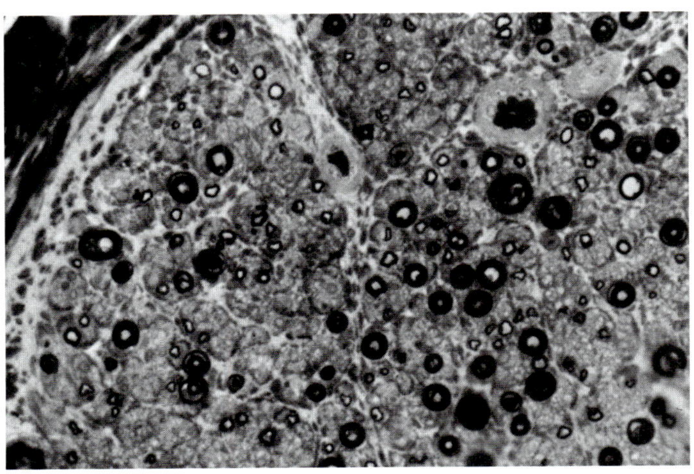

Figure 78.3 Cross-section of a sural nerve biopsy from a patient with sensorimotor demyelinating polyneuropathy, stained with toluidine blue. Note the reduction in the number of myelinated fibers and some signs of axonal degeneration.

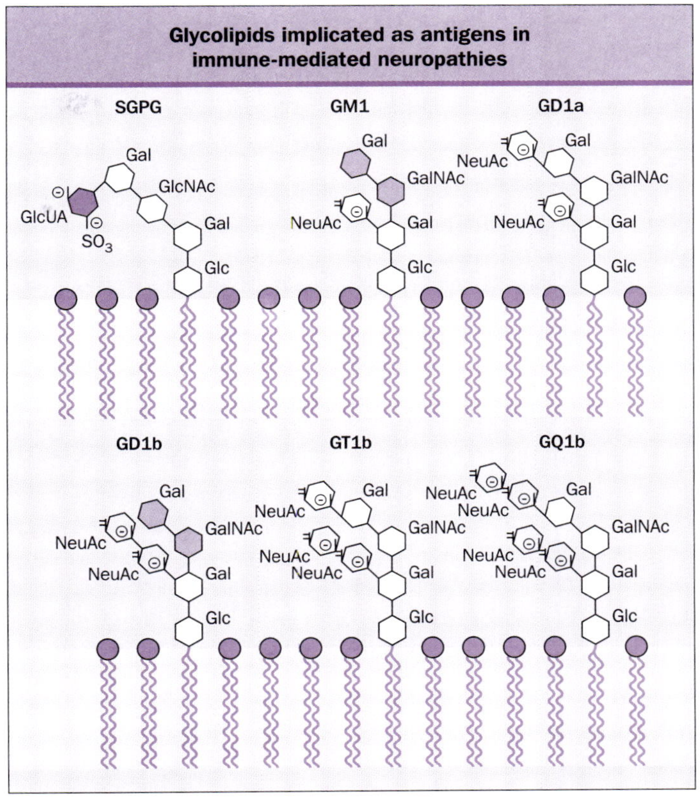

Figure 78.4 Glycolipids implicated as antigens in immune-mediated neuropathies. Sulfate-3-glucuronyl paragloboside (SGPG) is the glycolipid sharing a carbohydrate epitope with myelin-associated glycoprotein (MAG), and the terminal sulphated glucuronic acid is a key part of the epitope. GM1 is the ganglioside implicated in motor nerve disorders, and in most cases the terminal Gal (β1–3) GalNAc epitope, which is shared with GD1b, is involved. The disialosyl moiety implicated in sensory neuropathies consists of NeuAcα2–8NeuAc- and is present in GD1b and GT1b gangliosides, as well as the simpler GD2 and GD3 gangliosides (not shown). GQ1b ganglioside, which is the target antigen in C. Miller-Fisher syndrome, has two disialosyl moieties. Although GD1a ganglioside has two sialic acid residues, they are not linked to each other, so antibodies to GD1a do not cross-react with the anti-GD1b antibodies. The color-coded sugar moieties represent key aspects of the various epitopes, but carbohydrate sequences recognized by the antibodies may include additional sugar residues. GlcUA, glucuronic acid; Gal, galactose; G1cNAc, *N*-acetylglucosamine; Glc, glucose; GalNAc, *N*-acetylgalactosamine; NeuAc, *N*-acetylneuraminic acid (sialic acid).

Demyelinating polyneuropathies with monoclonal IgM antiganglioside antibodies (but not antibodies to MAG)

The sera of some patients with IgM monoclonal gammopathy and sensorimotor or pure sensory demyelinating polyneuropathy may not react with MAG, in spite of its clinical similarities with anti-MAG paraproteins. The IgM in several of these patients reacts with various gangliosides, such as those containing a disialosyl moiety, or with GalNAc-GM1b and GalNAc-GD1a, two gangliosides that share eptiopes with GM2 or with a combination of GM2 and GM1, or GM1 and GD1b[57,62] (Fig. 78.4).

Sensory ataxic neuropathies with monoclonal IgM anti-GD1b antibodies

Sera from patients with a chronic sensory large-fiber demyelinating ataxic neuropathy have been noted to react with GD1b glycolipids.[57,61,63] Patients with this combination of clinical and immunopathologic findings represent a distinct clinical entity. Antibodies to GD1b are believed to be pathogenic in these patients because immunization of rabbits with GD1b antigens caused an ataxic neuropathy with inflammatory infiltrates and destruction of the dorsal root ganglionic neurons, which express GD1b on their surface.[64] Although GD1b and GM1 both have the Gal (β1–3) Gal Nac epitope, the NeuNAc(a2–8) NeuNAc moiety is present only in GD1b (Fig. 78.4). The data suggest that when IgM binds to the Gal (β1–3) GalNAc moiety of GM1, which is found on the surface of motor neurons, a motor neuropathy results (as described earlier). In contrast, if the IgM binds to epitopes containing disialosyl groups of GD1b, which are present on the surface of the dorsal root ganglionic neurons, a sensory neuronopathy develops. Thus, the sugar structure of the reactive gangliosides may determine cellular specificity and the ensuing clinical manifestations.[57,65]

Sensory neuropathies with antisulfatide antibodies

Antisulfatide antibodies have also been associated with a sensory neuropathy and may bind to the surface of the dorsal root ganglionic neurons.[66] Antisulfatide antibodies may be also seen in some patients with IgM anti-MAG-associated polyneuropathy, Guillain–Barré syndrome and CIDP. The significance of antisulfatide antibodies in autoimmune peripheral neuropathies remains to be defined. Thus, antibodies are found in clinically and pathologically heterogeneous autoimmune neuropathies, but a cause and effect relationship has not been established.

Motor, axonal neuropathies with monoclonal IgM anti-GM1-antibodies

A small number of patients with IgM paraprotein have a predominantly motor neuropathy that resembles a lower motor neuron disease syndrome.[67] The IgM in some of these patients shows strong immunoreactivity with GM1 and asialoGM1 and, to a lesser degree, with GD1b.[52] Because GM1 is present on the surface of motor neurons and the nodes of Ranvier, these findings led to a search for polyclonal GM1 antibodies in patients with a variety of conditions, including those with motor neuron diseases, patients with multifocal motor neuropathy with conduction block, as well as in patients with Guillain–Barré syndrome and CIDP. The role of GM1, present in a small number of these patients and in up to 60% of patients with multifocal motor neuropathy with conduction block, remains unclear.

Cryoglobulinemic neuropathy

Cryoglobulins are proteins that precipitate in the cold and redissolve when heated. There are three types: type I, which is monoclonal, often of the IgM and IgG class; type II, which is mixed polyclonal with one monoclonal (often monoclonal IgM with polyclonal IgG); and type III, which is polyclonal (often IgM and IgG).

Polyneuropathy occurs most often with mixed cryoglobulinemias and presents as distal, sensory, symmetric polyneuropathy or as mononeuropathy multiplex. These patients also have purpura, polyarthralgias, cutaneous vasculitis, Raynaud phenomenon, renal involvement with proteinuria, and polyneuropathy. Type II cryoglobulinemia may be associated with an underlying lymphoproliferative process. However, most patients (up to 90%) have infection with hepatitis C virus, which appears to be the cause of the cryoglobulinemia.[68] This association is of more than theoretical interest because these patients can respond to treatment with interferon-α (IFN-α), especially in combination with ribavirin. This neuropathy is often axonal. The nerve biopsy shows perivascular inflammatory cuffing with axonal degeneration which, if focal, may suggest ischemia. Especially in patients in whom the virus cannot be eradicated, the neuropathy is treated with cyclophosphamide and prednisone.

Causal relationship between monoclonal IgM and neuropathy

MAG is present in small amounts in the peripheral nervous system (PNS) but abundant in the CNS, yet the CNS is spared in these patients. It was suggested that the reactivity of IgM to MAG may therefore represent nonspecific binding to carbohydrate antigens. However, the discovery of the PNS-specific glycolipid sulfate-3-glucuronyl paragloboside (SGPG; see Fig. 78.4), with which all the anti-MAG-reacting monoclonal IgMs react, has led to the hypothesis that the glycolipids, rather than the glycoproteins, may serve as primary antigenic targets in these patients. More than half of the IgM paraproteins in these patients recognize both MAG and SGPG, whereas two-thirds of those who are anti-MAG-negative and have demyelinating neuropathy recognize ganglioside antigens. Collectively, in more than 75% of these patients acidic glycolipids are the target antigens. Although the role of these antibodies in the pathogenesis of the neuropathy has been questioned, the author's view is that many of these antibodies are causally related to the neuropathy, as supported by the following:

1. IgM and complement are deposited on the homologous myelinated nerve fibers of patients' sural nerve biopsy (Fig. 78.5).[47,49]
2. In a double-immunolabeling technique of light and electron microscopy, the IgM has been demonstrated in the areas of the split myelin lamellae.[59] The separation of myelin is a unique feature of the IgM-associated demyelinating polyneuropathies, and the deposition of IgM in these areas of the myelin sheath may contribute to the separation of the myelin lamellae, disrupting normal function. It is relevant that the monoclonal IgM anti-MAG antibodies also react with high molecular weight glycoproteins of the neural cell adhesion molecules (N-CAM). Because N-CAM is an important molecule in cell–cell adhesion and interaction, such binding can cause myelin disadhesion.[70]
3. Injection of serum from patients with IgM anti-MAG/SGPG paraprotein supplemented with fresh complement into feline peripheral nerve causes complement-dependent demyelination and conduction block within 2–9 days after the injection.[71] The IgM injected intraneurally immunolocalizes to the outer layer of the myelin sheath. In addition, systemic transfusion of anti-MAG IgM paraproteins produced segmental demyelination in chickens.[72] In this experiment, the IgM immunolocalized to the outer lamellae of the myelin and resulted in widening of the intermediate line, similar to that observed in the human neuropathy. The reported failures to induce intraneural demyelination in other animals such as the rat or mouse probably relates to the fact that nerves from these animals express few or no glycoconjugates that cross-react with the human anti-MAG IgM paraproteins.
4. Reduction of IgM anti-MAG antibody levels with chemotherapy has led to clinical improvement of the neuropathy in some patients.[23]

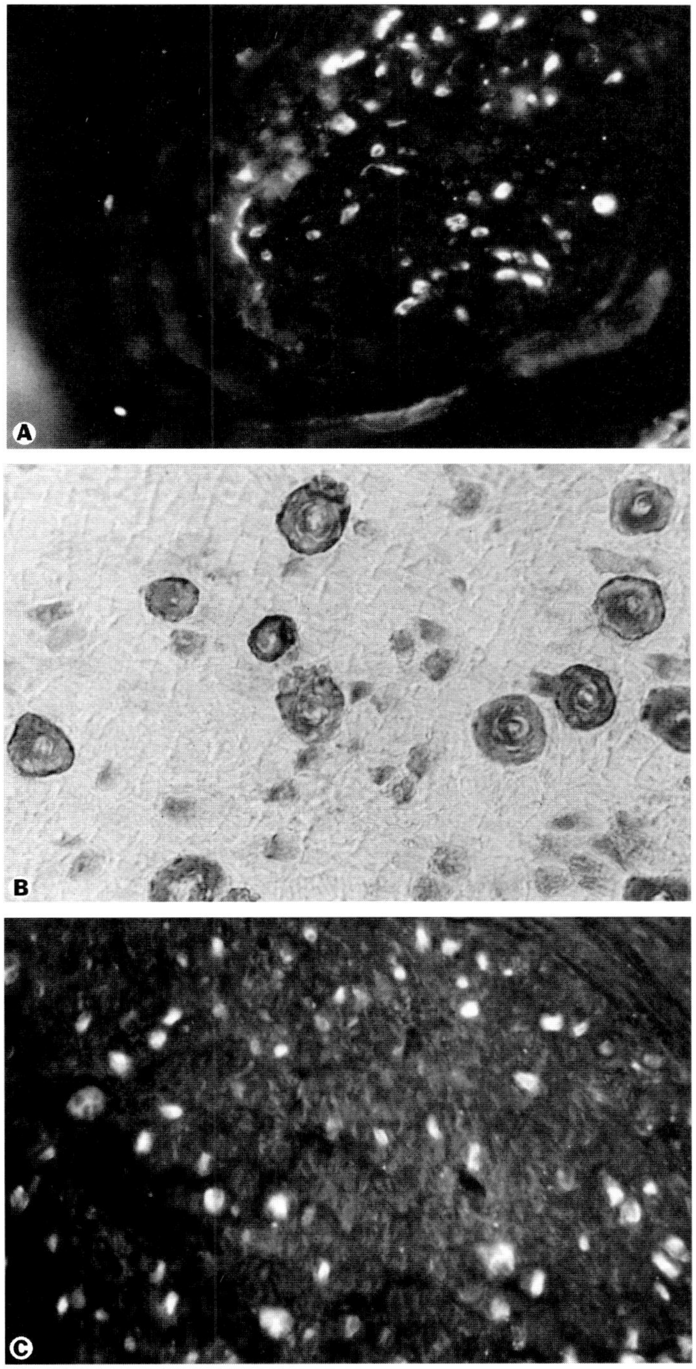

Figure 78.5 (A) Cross-section of a sural nerve from a patient with IgM paraproteinemia and demyelinating polyneuropathy. Fresh-frozen nerve specimen stained with FITC-conjugated antibodies to human IgM reveals IgM deposits in many myelinated fibers. (**B**) Same section immunostained with avidin-biotin immunoperoxidase shows the IgM deposited in the outer layer of the myelin sheath. (**C**) Cross-section of a normal human nerve incubated first with the serum from a patient with IgM demyelinating polyneuropathy and then with FITC-conjugated antihuman IgM. Note deposits of IgM in most of the normal myelinated fibers.

5. IgM anti-GD1b antibodies have been implicated in the sensory ataxia in humans. Injection of GD1b in rabbits reproduces the human disease, and anti-GD1b in phrenic nerve preparation induces impaired neural transmission.[57,64]

CLINICAL PEARLS

Autoimmunity in polyneuropathy associated with IgM monoclonal gammopathy

- In more than 50% of patients the IgM reacts with two antigens, the myelin-associated glycoprotein (MAG) and the glycosphingolipid SGPG.
- In many patients with non-MAG-reacting monoclonal IgM, the IgM recognizes (a) gangliosides containing disialosyl moieties including GM1, GM2, GD1b, GD1a and LM1 (see Fig. 78.4); (b) sulfatides; and (c), rarely, chondroitin sulfate.
- Overall, in at least 75% of the patients the IgM recognizes gangliosides that may be the primary antigenic targets.
- The IgM is deposited on the homologous myelin sheath and activates complement.
- The IgM, when deposited on the myelin sheath, results in disadhesion and separation of the myelin lamellae and disruption of normal myelin function.
- Intraneural injection of anti-MAG-reacting IgM or passive transfusion into experimental animals causes segmental demyelination, whereas complement-fixing IgM is immunolocalized to the myelin sheath, causing myelin separation.
- The GD1b-reacting monoclonal IgM causes sensory ataxia in humans and in an animal model and impairs neuronal transmission in vitro.

Paraneoplastic peripheral neuropathies with anti-Hu antibodies

Peripheral neuropathy is an occasional complication of systemic cancer, related either to the systemic effects of the tumor or, more often, to various neurotoxic chemotherapeutic agents. Cancer-associated peripheral neuropathy is usually mild, axonal and at times painful, and affects mostly the small nerve fibers. It is frequently difficult to distinguish from the coexisting toxic neuropathy of chemotherapeutic drugs. There is, however, a distinct sensory paraneoplastic neuropathy, the *paraneoplastic sensory neuronopathy (PSN)*, which has a unique clinical picture and an autoimmune pathogenesis.

PSN is most often associated with small cell lung cancer and, to a lesser degree, with breast cancer or other neoplasms.[74,75] It is frequently the presenting symptom, sometimes preceding the discovery of the tumor by months. PSN presents with a unique clinical picture characterized by (1) burning or aching paresthesias; (2) sensory loss of the large fibers, causing sensory gait ataxia and chorioathetotic movements related to loss of proprioception in the feet and hands; (3) normal strength; and (4) areflexia. Some patients may have a varying degree of other associated neurologic manifestations, including autonomic dysfunction, encephalopathic symptoms or cerebellar disturbances. Laboratory studies show increased CSF protein, an axonal sensory neuropathy by electrophysiologic testing, and an axonal degeneration with rare mononuclear cell infiltrates in the nerve biopsy. PSN is a ganglionopathy (sensory neuronopathy) caused by involvement of the dorsal root ganglionic neurons. Histologically there is a variable degree of inflammation in the dorsal root ganglia.

The autoimmune nature of PSN is supported by the presence of specific IgG autoantibodies to the antigen Hu.[74,75] These antibodies are present in almost all patients who have small cell lung carcinoma and, less often, in patients with other cancers. In sections of human brain, spinal cord or dorsal root ganglia the anti-Hu antibody-containing serum stains the nuclei, but not the nucleoli, of the neurons. Immunoblots of extracts from human neuronal nuclei show that the anti-Hu antibodies are directed against a closely spaced group of proteins with a 35–40 kDa molecular weight. Anti-Hu antibodies may also be found in higher titers in the CSF, suggesting intrathecal synthesis.

The antigens of the Hu protein are present not only in the tumors of patients with PSN but also in the small cell lung cancer from patients without anti-Hu antibodies or neurologic disease. Further, low titers of anti-Hu antibodies can be seen in up to 20% of patients with small cell lung cancer without neurologic symptoms. This observation suggests that PSN may be the result of an autoimmune reaction against antigens shared by both the tumor cells and the dorsal root ganglionic neurons. The Hu protein may also be an antigenic target of CD4 Th1-type T cells, which may be involved in cell-mediated injury of the peripheral nerve.[76] Although the pathogenic role of anti-Hu antibodies has not been clearly established and cellular immunity may be important, these antibodies appear to be highly specific as markers to detect an occult small cell lung cancer in patients who present with sensory ataxic neuropathy.

Localized, isolated vasculitis of the peripheral nerves

Polyneuropathy is a common manifestation of systemic vasculitis[77] (Chapter 67). It occurs in patients with (1) polyarteritis nodosa; (2) vasculitis associated with connective tissue diseases, such as rheumatoid arthritis, Sjögren syndrome or systemic lupus erythematosus; (3) hypersensitivity vasculitis; or (4) temporal arteritis, in which it may occur in up to 14% of cases. There is, however, a distinct vasculitic entity localized only to the peripheral nerve, the isolated peripheral nerve vasculitis (PNV).[78]

PNV involves the small and medium-sized arteries of the epineurium and perineurium and causes ischemic changes within the peripheral nerve. The presentation is similar to the vasculitic neuropathy seen in patients with systemic vasculitis, the only difference being the lack of systemic organ involvement. Fever, malaise or weight loss may occur, however. Patients with PNV present with a mononeuropathy multiplex with motor and sensory involvement of acute onset restricted to individual peripheral nerves. The diagnosis is confirmed by biopsy of the sural, superficial personeal or superficial radial nerve. When nerve biopsy is combined with a muscle biopsy, the diagnostic yield is higher. PNV has a better prognosis than the systemic vasculitides, and patients may respond to immunosuppressive therapy. Work-up for PNV should include all the tests needed to exclude systemic vasculitis, including hepatitis B and C and HIV. Vasculitis of the peripheral nerves is common in the vasculitis associated with these infections.

Neuropathy associated with HIV infection

Neuropathy can be seen in a setting of a variety of viral or bacterial infections. For example, in patients with Lyme disease (Chapter 70), various neuropathies, including GBS or mononeuritis (Bell's palsy), have been noted. Other infections, such as cytomegalovirus, hepatitis viruses, herpes, leprosy, Chagas' disease and diphtheria, can be associated with an autoimmune peripheral neuropathy. However, the most common neuropathy seen today in a setting of viral infection is the group of neuropathies associated with HIV infection (Chapter 38).

HIV-related peripheral neuropathies usually develop in a stage-specific fashion in infected adults.[79–81] Two immune neuropathies, GBS and CIDP, can occur early in the infection, or can be the presenting manifestation of unsuspected HIV infection. One distinguishing feature of HIV-associated GBS or CIDP is pleocytosis in the spinal fluid. The sural nerve biopsy shows segmental demyelination associated with a large number of macrophages within the endoneurial parenchyma. Perivascular inflammation can also be seen. Less common peripheral neuropathies that may develop in early-stage HIV infection include acute ganglioneuronitis coincident with seroconversion and mononeuritis multiplex.[81]

The most common neuropathy in AIDS patients occurs in the later stage of the infection and may affect up to 70% of adults with AIDS. This syndrome is characterized by a painful sensory axonal neuropathy.

Despite the relative lack of motor involvement, severe neuropathic pain in such patients can be disabling. Pain may be so uncomfortable that even contact with light stimuli (e.g. bed sheets) is intolerable. Clinical findings include distal pansensory loss or hypesthesia, areflexia and, in advanced cases, distal weakness. Pathologic studies at autopsy indicate that peripheral nerve pathology is ubiquitous in AIDS patients, whether or not they had clinical evidence of peripheral neuropathy.

Another neuropathy seen in later-stage HIV infection is a lumbosacral polyradiculoneuropathy affecting roots and sensory ganglia, which is often associated with cytomegalovirus (CMV) infection. CMV polyradiculoneuropathy presents with lower extremity muscle weakness, sacral and distal paresthesias, areflexia and atrophy, mostly of the legs, associated with sphincteric dysfunction resembling a cauda equina syndrome. The spinal fluid may show pleocytosis or harbor CMV detected by cultures or cytologic examinations. CMV inclusions are often found within the Schwann cells or the endothelial cells (Fig. 78.6). The disease is thought to represent reactivated CMV infection of the nerve root rather than primary infection. Recognition is important because anti-CMV therapy with ganciclovir or foscarnet can improve the quality of life and prolong patient's lives.

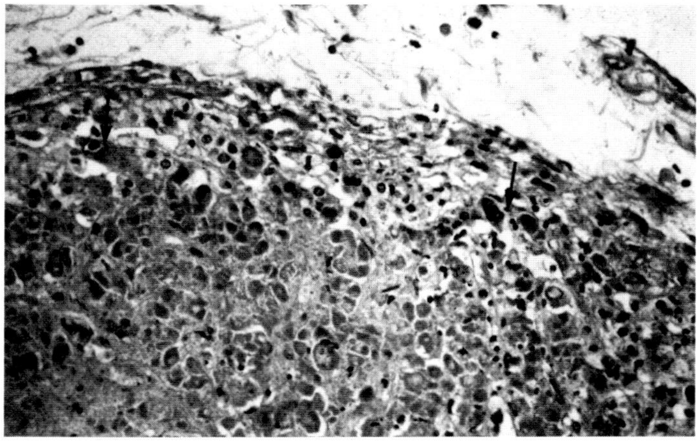

Figure 78.6 Cross-section of a root from a patient with HIV-associated Guillain–Barré syndrome shows cytomegalovirus inclusions within the Schwann cell (*arrow*).

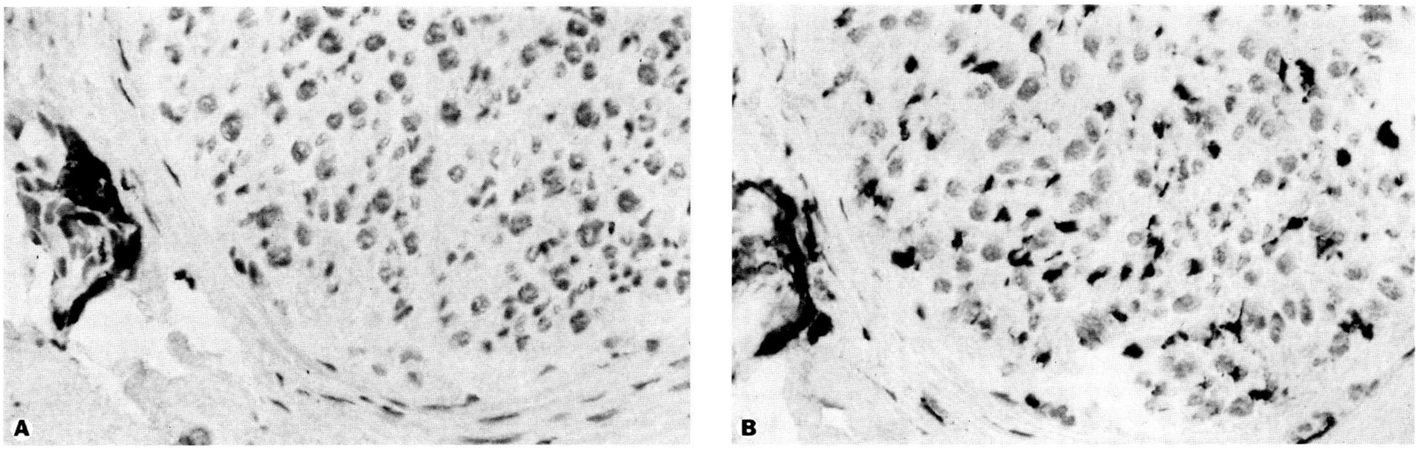

Figure 78.7 Serial sections of a new biopsy from a patient with HIV-associated chronic inflammatory demyelinating polyneuropathy stained for CD8 cells (**A**) and macrophages (**B**). This section shows that the majority of the endoneurial cells are macrophages. Only a few CD8 cells are noted in a perivascular area between the nerve fascicles.

Although zidovudine (AZT) is myotoxic,[82] the two other antiretroviral drugs, ddC and ddI, are neurotoxic, causing a dose-dependent reversible axonal painful sensory neuropathy.[83,84] The major feature that distinguishes a ddI- or ddC-related painful neuropathy from the painful sensory axonal neuropathy of AIDS is that the latter tends to be progressive, whereas the nucleoside-related peripheral neuropathies tend to improve when the drugs are discontinued. Another clinical feature of nucleoside neuropathy is 'coasting', or worsening of symptoms for a period after the drug is discontinued, followed by clinical improvement.[84]

Possible mechanisms for the peripheral neuropathy in HIV infection include direct viral infection; immune alterations triggered by the viral illness; complications of antiretroviral therapy; sequelae of chronic illness, and a combination of all these factors (Chapter 38).

HIV has been cultured from peripheral nerves and HIV viral RNA has been amplified from sural nerve biopsies. There is no convincing evidence, however, that the neuropathy results from direct infection of the peripheral nerve with the virus. The author's immunocytochemical studies of sural nerve biopsies have shown that HIV is present only in rare endoneurial macrophages, but not within the Schwann cells or the axons. With immunocytochemistry the endoneurial infiltrates in the sural nerve biopsies from such patients consist mostly of macrophages. CD8 T cells are sparse, and CD4 T lymphocytes absent (Fig. 78.7). There is also strong expression of HLA-DR antigens on Schwann cells, endothelial cells and macrophages, as well as up-regulation of costimulatory molecules on the Schwann cells.[39] The proliferating macrophages may play an important role as immune effector cells in the demyelination, similar to that described previously for the Guillain–Barré syndrome and CIDP in HIV-negative patients. The frequency of antimyelin, GM1-specific or antisulfatide autoantibodies in the serum of these patients is also similar to that described previously in HIV-negative patients with demyelinating polyneuropathies.

As HIV infection progresses, immune dysregulation gives way to frank immunosuppression, setting the stage for direct infection by opportunistic infections such as CMV that may be harbored by the Schwann cells. Furthermore, the peripheral nerve becomes susceptible to the effects of the systemic illness and the various neurotoxins, lymphokines or cytokines that contribute to the development of neuropathy. Antibiotics, particularly antimycobacterial and chemotherapeutic agents, are also known peripheral neurotoxins.

PATIENT MANAGEMENT

Autoimmune peripheral neuropathies are clinically important because they comprise potentially treatable disorders amenable to various immunosuppressive, immunomodulating or chemotherapeutic agents. The selection of an effective protocol is based on the results of experimental therapeutic trials, clinical experience and the risk–benefit ratio of the available therapies. The author's approach to the treatment of each one of these disorders is as follows.

Guillain–Barré syndrome

Supportive care

The dramatic reduction in mortality of GBS is mainly due to the availability of intensive care units for these patients as well as improvements in respiratory support, antibiotic therapy and control of autonomic cardiac dysregulation. A GBS patient is best monitored in the intensive care unit, even if respiratory compromise is not evident at the time of admission. When forced vital capacity drops or bulbar weakness is severe, intubation is in order. A team approach provides the best results.

Plasmapheresis

In double-blind studies[3,7] plasmapheresis (Chapter 118) has been shown to be effective, improving the degree and rate of recovery if performed early in the course of the illness. A continuous-flow machine is preferable and a central venous catheter may be required for some patients. To be effective, plasma exchanges should begin within the first week of disease onset. A series of five or six exchanges, with one exchange every other day, is sufficient. Early relapses can occur in up to 20% of patients, who may require a second series of plasma exchanges. Plasmapheresis is effective even in milder cases. Based on controlled studies, two exchanges are sufficient for mild GBS, and four exchanges are optimal for moderate cases or mild cases that continue to progress.[85]

High-dose intravenous immunoglobulin

On the basis of two controlled studies comparing intravenous immunoglobulin (IVIG) and plasmapheresis, IVIG (Chapter 104), given at 2 g/kg in 2–5 days, was equally as effective as plasmapheresis.[86,87] A trial of plasma exchange followed by IVIG added mild but not significant benefit.[87] The decision as to which treatment to use first (plasmapheresis or IVIG) is governed by individual circumstances, such as the availability of the treatment modality, experience of the treating physicians, the age of the patient and other associated or concurrent illnesses.[88] Early relapses can occur with IVIG as often as with plasmapheresis. Because IVIG is easier to use and more readily available, it has become the treatment of choice at many centers worldwide.

Glucocorticoids are contraindicated in GBS. In a multicenter trial it was convincingly shown that glucocorticoids are ineffective and increase the incidence of future relapses.

Chronic inflammatory demyelinating polyneuropathy

Prednisone

CIDP is a glucocorticoid-responsive polyneuropathy as demonstrated in a controlled study.[89] A high-dose regimen of 80–100 mg prednisone daily is the author's preference. After clinical response and stability, the dose can be tapered to an alternate day schedule.[31] The starting dose can be a little lower and the tapering faster in patients with coexisting cardiac disease or severe osteoporosis, or in the elderly. The goal of therapy is to increase muscle strength, and this is the single parameter to follow. Azathioprine, cyclosporine and mycophenolate have been used as steroid-sparing agents.

IVIG

In controlled studies, IVIG has been effective in the majority of patients with CIDP.[90] With more chronic disease and more severe axonal degeneration, the likelihood of complete or significant recovery is decreased, hence the need for early treatment. IVIG can be used effectively as a first-line therapy to avoid steroid-related side-effects. It is increasingly becoming the first treatment of choice

Plasmapheresis

Plasmapheresis has been shown to be effective in CIDP in controlled studies.[91] The improvement can be as dramatic as with IVIG. After a series of six plasma exchanges, maintenance therapy with one exchange at least every 8 weeks may be required. IVIG has mostly replaced plasmapheresis as the initial therapy of choice, although different patients may benefit more from steroids, IVIG, or plasmapheresis. Other therapies recently tried in patients resistant to the above treatments include IFN-α and cyclophosphamide.

Polyneuropathy with paraproteinemia

Patients with benign IgG or IgA demyelinating polyneuropathies respond similar to the CIDP patients. On the basis of a controlled study[92], plasmapheresis may be more effective for some patients, but the response is variable. Whether plasmapheresis is superior to IVIG is unclear, and the choice of which method to use first is empirical and, currently, dependent on clinical experience.

The patients with malignant paraproteinemias should be treated with chemotherapy as recommended for the underlying disease. Often, the neuropathy responds to chemotherapy.[93] However, when the neuropathy is axonal, treatments are, in general, disappointing.

The neuropathy in some patients with POEMS syndrome responds to steroids, tamoxifen or alkylating agents. In others the neuropathy responds to the removal or irradiation of the solitary sclerotic lesion, suggesting that the tumor may secrete neurotoxic factors, perhaps a neurotoxic IgG or IgA.

For the IgM demyelinating polyneuropathies treatments have included prednisone plus chlorambucil,[93] plasmapheresis,[94] IVIG[95] and chemotherapy with an anti-B-cell (Rituxan) monoclonal antibody.[96] Individual patients have responded to each of these therapies but the degree and rate of improvement may be quite variable. IFN-α in a controlled study was not effective.[97]

Multifocal motor neuropathy

This neuropathy responds very well to IVIG, which is the treatment of choice, based on controlled trials.[98,99] Cyclophosphamide is also effective.[100] Aggressive treatment with cyclophosphamide followed by plasmapheresis and then IVIG has also been shown to be of benefit in the author's experience.

Paraneoplastic neuropathy

Some of these patients have, anecdotally, improved with plasma exchange or IVIG, but overall this neuropathy is not generally responsive to available therapies.

Vasculitic neuropathies

Patients with isolated peripheral nerve vasculitis are treated less aggressively than those with systemic vasculitis (see Chapter 67). A combined treatment of prednisone 1.5 mg/kg/day, and oral cyclophosphamide 2 mg/kg/day, is currently recommended as the initial treatment of choice. Although treatment may vary between patients, the administration of cyclophosphamide may not be necessary for more than 12 months as in systemic vasculitis. Often, 6–12 months of treatment may suffice. Plasmapheresis has been tried with variable results in cryoglobulinemic neuropathies.

HIV-associated neuropathies

The demyelinating neuropathies, GBS and CIDP, in HIV-infected patients are treated with the same immunomodulatory therapies used in HIV-negative patients. In uncontrolled studies plasmapheresis and IVIG have each been effective. IVIG may be preferred because it does not suppress immune function and it is easier to administer.

Ganciclovir appears to be effective in CMV-related polyradiculoneuropathy.[101] The role of foscarnet (approved for CMV retinitis) in this disorder remains to be delineated. Painful sensory neuropathy can be quite disabling because of intractable pain, even though muscle weakness may be minimal. Tricyclic antidepressants, nonsteroidal anti-inflammatory drugs, anticonvulsants (carbamazepine and phenytoin), narcotic analgesics and topical capsaicin in various combinations may provide some relief from the neuropathic pain in these patients, but, symptomatic management of this condition is a difficult clinical problem.[101]

REFERENCES

1. Asbury AK, Cornblath DR. Assessment of current diagnostic criteria for Guillain–Barré syndrome. Ann Neurol 1990;27(suppl):21.
2. Ropper AH. The Guillain–Barré syndrome. N Engl J Med 1992;326:1130.
3. Arnason BGW, Soliven B. Acute inflammatory demeylinating polyradiculoneuropathy. In: Dyck PJ, Thomas PK, Griffin JW, et al., (eds) Peripheral neuropathy. Philadelphia, WB Saunders, 1993;1437.
4. Hughes R, Sanders E, Hall S, et al. Subacute idiopathic demyelinating polyradiculoneuropathy. Arch Neurol 1992;49:612.
5. Dalakas M, Houff SA, Engel WK, et al. CSF monoclonal bands in chronic relapsing polyneuropathy. Neurology 1980;30:864.
6. Cornblath DR. Electrophysiology in Guillain–Barré syndrome. Ann Neurol 1990;27(suppl):17.
7. McKhann GM, Griffin JW, Cornblath DR. The Guillain–Barré syndrome study group. Plasmapheresis and Guillain–Barré syndrome: analysis of prognostic factors and the effect of plasmapheresis. Ann Neurol 1988;23:347.
8. Griffin JW, Li CY, Ho TW, et al. Pathology of the motor–sensory axonal Guillain–Barré syndrome. Ann Neurol 1996;39:17.
9. Ho TW, Hsieh S-T, Nachamkin I, et al. Motor nerve terminal degeneration provides a potential mechanism for rapid recovery in acute motor axonal neuropathy after *Campylobacter* infection. Neurology 1997;48:717.
10. Hartung HP, van der Meche FGA, Pollard JD. Guillain–Barré syndrome, CIDP and other chronic immune-mediated neuropathies. Curr Opin Neurol 1998;11:497.
11. Rees JH, Soudain SE, Gregson NA, Hughes RAC. *Campylobacter jejuni* infection and Guillain–Barré syndrome. N Engl J Med 1995;333:1374.
12. Feasby TE, Hahn AF, Brown WF, et al. Severe axonal degeneration in acute Guillain–Barré syndrome: evidence of two different mechanisms? J Neurol Sci 1993;116:185.
13. Visser LH, van der Meche FG, Meulstee J, et al. Cytomegalovirus infection and Guillain–Barré syndrome: the clinical, electrophysiologic, and prognostic features. Dutch Guillain–Barré Group. Neurology 1996;47:668.
14. Fisher CM. An unusual variant of acute idiopathic polyneuritis (syndrome of ophthalmoplegia, ataxia and areflexia). N Engl J Med 1956;255:57.
15. Yuki N, Susuki K, Hirata K. Ataxic Guillain–Barré syndrome with anti-GQlb antibody: relation to Miller-Fisher syndrome. Neurology 2000;54:1851.
16. Feldman EL, Bromberg MB, Blaivas M, Junck L. Acute pandysautonomic neuropathy. Neurology 1991;41:746.
17. Hartung HP. Infections and the Guillain–Barré syndrome. J Neurol Neurosurg Psychiatr 1999;66:277.
18. Illa I, Ortiz N, Gallard E, Juarez C, Grau JM, Dalakas MC. Acute axonal Guillain–Barré syndrome with IgG antibodies against motor axons following parenteral injection of gangliosides. Ann Neurol 1995;38:218.
19. LaRocca RV, Meer J, Gilliatt R, et al. Suramin-induced polyneuropathy, Neurology 1990;40:954.
20. Cook SD, Dowling PC. The role of autoantibody and immune complexes in the pathogeneis of Guillain–Barré syndrome. Ann Neurol 1981;9(suppl):70.
21. Saida T, Saida K, Lisak RP, et al. In vivo demyelinating activity of sera from patients with Guillain–Barré syndrome. Ann Neurol 1982;11:69.
22. Koski CL, Chou DKH, Jungalwala FB. Anti-peripheral nerve myelin antibodies to Guillain–Barré syndrome bind a neutral glycolipid of peripheral myelin and cross-react with Forssman antigen. J Clin Invest 1989;84:280.
23. Ilyas AA, Mithen FA, Dalakas MC, et al. Antibodies to sulfated glycolipids in Guillain–Barré syndrome. J Neurol Sci 1991;105:108.
24. Ilyas AA, Mitchen FA, Dalakas MC, et al. Antibodies to acidic glycolipids in Guillain–Barré syndrome and chronic inflammatory demyelinating polyneuropathy. J Neurol Sci 1992;107:1111.
25. Ilyas AA, Cook SD, Mithen FA, et al. Antibodies to GT1a ganglioside in patients with Guillain–Barré syndrome. J Neuroimmunol 1998;82:160.
26. Yuki N, Tagawa Y, Irie F, Hirabayashi Y, Handa S. Close association of Guillain–Barré syndrome with antibodies to minor monosialogangliosides GM1b and GM1a. J Neuroimmunol 1997;74:30.
27. Kuroki S, Saida T, Nukina M, et al. *Campylobacter jejuni* strains from patients with Guillain–Barré syndrome belong mostly to Penner serogroup 19 and contain beta-*N*-acetylglucosamine residues. Ann Neurol 1993;33:243.
28. Enders U, Karch H, Toyka KV, et al. The spectrum of immune responses to *Campylobacter jejuni* and glycoconjugates in Guillain–Barré syndrome and in other neuroimmunologic disorders. Ann Neurol 1993;34:130.
29. Vriesendorp FJ, Mishu B, Blaser MK, Koski CL. Serum antibodies to GM1, GD1b, peripheral nerve myelin, and *Campylobacter jejuni* in patients with Guillain–Barré syndrome and controls: correlation and prognosis. Ann Neurol 1993;34:130.
30. Yuki N, Tagawa Y. Acute cytomegalovirus infection and IgM anti-GM2 antibody. J Neurol Sci 1998;154:14.
31. Dalakas MC, Engel WK. Chronic relapsing (dysimmune) polyneuropathy: pathogenesis and treatment. Ann Neurol 1981;10(suppl):134.
32. Dyck PJ, Prineas J, Pollard J. Chronic inflammatory demyelinating polyradiculoneuropathy. In: Dyck PJ, Thomas PK, Griffin JW, et al., eds. Peripheral neuropathy. Philadelphia, WB Saunders, 1993;1498.
32a. Dalakas MC, Teravinen H, Engel WK. Tremor as a feature of chronic relapsing and dysgammaglobulinemic polyneuropathies; Indence and management. Arch Neurol 1984;41:711–714.
33. Ad Hoc Subcommittee of the American Academy of Neurology AIDS Task Force. Research criteria for the diagnosis of chronic inflammatory demyelinating polyneuropathy (CIDP). Neurology 1991;41:617.
34. Dalakas MC. Advances in chronic inflammatory demyelinating polyneuropathy: disease variants and inflammatory response mediators and modifiers. Curr Opin Neurol 1999;12:403.
35. Barohn RK, Kissell JT, Warmolts JR, Mendell JR. Chronic inflammatory demyelinating polyradiculoneuropathy clinical characteristics, course, and recommendations for diagnostic criteria. Arch Neurol 1989;46:878.
36. Parry GJ. Are multifocal motor neuropathy and Lewis–Sumner syndrome distinct nosologic entities? Muscle Nerve 1999;22:557.
37. Saperstein DS, Amato AA, Wolfe GI, et al. Multifocal acquired demyelinating sensory and motor neuropathy: the Lewis–Sumner syndrome. Muscle Nerve 1999;22:560.
38. Gorson KC, Ropper AH, Weinberg DH. Upper limb predominant, multifocal chronic inflammatory demyelinating polyneuropathy. Muscle Nerve 1999;22:758.
39. Murata K, Dalakas MC. Expression of the costimulatory molecule BB-1, the ligands CTLA-4 and CD28, and their mRNA in chronic inflammatory demyelinating polyneuropathy. Brain 2000;123:1660.
40. Gold R, Archelos JJ, Hartung HP. Mechanisms of immune regulation in the peripheral nervous system. Brain Pathol 1999;9:343.
41. Kiefer R, Kiessier BC, Bruck W, Hartung HP, Toyka KV. Macrophage differentiation antigens in acute and chronic autoimmune polyneuropathies. Brain 1998;121:469.
42. Weiss MD, Luciano CA, Semino-Mora C, Dalakas MC, Quarles RH. Molecular mimicry in chronic inflammatory demyelinating polyneuropathy and melanoma. Neurology 1998;51:1738.
43. Parry GJ. Motor neuropathy with conduction block. Semin Neurol 1993;13:269.
44. Lange DJ, Trojaberg W, Latov N, et al. Multifocal motor neuropathy with conduction block: is it a distinct clinical entity? Neurology 1992;42:497.
45. Pestronk A. Motor neuropathies, motoneuron disorders and antiglycolipid antibodies. Muscle Nerve 1991;14:927.
46. Uncini A, Santoro M, Corbo M, et al. Conduction abnormalities induced by sera of patients with multifocal motor neuropathy and anti-GM1 antibodies. Muscle Nerve 1993;16:610.
47. Dalakas MC, Engel WK. Polyneuropathy and monoclonal gammopathy: studies of 11 patients. Ann Neurol 1981;10:45.
48. Gosselin S, Kyle RA, Dyck PJ. Neuropathy associated with monoclonal gammopathies of undetermined significance. Ann Neurol 1991;30:54.

49. Latov N, Sherman WH, Nemi R, et al. Plasma cell dyscrasia and peripheral neuropathy with a monoclonal antibody to peripheral nerve myelin. N Engl J Med 1980;303:618.
50. Kyle RA, Garton JP. The spectrum of IgM monoclonal gammopathy in 430 cases. Mayo Clin Proc 1987;62:719.
51. Latov N, Hays A, Sherman WH. Peripheral neuropathy and anti-MAG antibodies. Crit Rev Neurobiol 1988;3:301.
52. Farrer RG, Dalakas MC, Quarles RH. Multiple antibodies to nerve glycoconjugates in an unusual patient with neuropathy and monoclonal IgA gammopathy. J Neuroimmol 1996;66:71.
53. Diego Miralles G, O'Fallon JR, Talley NJ. Plasma cell dyscrasia with polyneuropathy. N Engl J Med 1992;327:1919.
54. Bardwick PA, Zvaifler WJ, Gill GN, et al. Plasma cell dyscrasia with polyneuropathy, organomegally, endocrinopathy, M-protein and skin changes. The POEMS syndrome. Medicine (Baltimore) 1980;59:311.
55. Gherardi RK, Belec L, Soubrier M, et al. Overproduction of proinflammatory cytokines imbalanced by their antagonists in POEMS syndrome. Blood 1996;87:1458.
56. Dalakas MC. Ataxia and paraproteinemic polyneuropathy. Ann Neurol 1987;22:94.
57. Dalakas MC, Quarles RH. Autoimmune ataxic neuropathies (sensory ganglionopathies): are glycolipids the responsible autoantigens? Ann Neurol 1996;39:419.
57a. Dalakas MC, Papadopouls NM. Paraproteins in the spinal fluid of patients with paraproteinemia polyneutropathies. Ann Neural 1984;15:590–593.
58. Vital A, Vital C, Julien J, et al. Polyneuropathy associated with IgM monoclonal gammopathy. Immunological and pathological study in 31 patients. Acta Neuropathol (Berlin) 1989;79:160.
59. Ilyas AA, Quarles RH, McIntosh TD, et al. IgM in a human neuropathy related to paraproteinemia binds to a carbohydrate determinant in the myelin-associated glycoprotein and to a ganglioside. Proc Natl Acad Sci USA 1984;81:1225.
60. Ilyas AA, Quarles RH, Dalakas MC, Brady RO. Polyneuropathy with monoclonal gammopathy: glycolipids are frequently antigens for IgM paraproteins. Proc Natl Acad Sci USA 1985;82:6697.
61. Ilyas AA, Dalakas MC, Brady RO, Quarles RH. Sulfated glucuronyl glycolipids reacting with anti-myelin-associated glycoprotein monoclonal antibodies including IgM paraproteins in neuropathy: species distribution and partial characterization of epitopes. Brain 1986;385:1.
62. Ilyas AA, Li SC, Chou DKH, et al. Gangliosides GM_2, IV^4Gal NaC GM_{1B}, and IV^4Gal NaC GD1a as antigens for monoclonal immunoglobulin M neuropathy associated with gammopathy. J Biol Chem 1988;263:4369.
63. Duane GC, Farrer RG, Dalakas MC, Quarles RH. Sensory neuropathy associated with monoclonal IgM to GD1b ganglioside. Ann Neurol 1992;31:683.
64. Kusunoki S, Shimizu T, Chiba A, et al. Experimental sensory neuropathy induced by sensitization with ganglioside GD1b. Ann Neurol 1996;39:424.
65. Quarles RH, Dalakas MC. Do antiganglioside antibodies cause human peripheral neuropathies? J Clin Invest 1996;97:1136.
66. Quattrini A, Corbo M, Dhaliwal SK, et al. Anti-sulfatide antibodies in neurological disease; binding to rat dorsal root ganglia neurons. J Neurol Sci 1992;112:152.
67. Latov N, Hays AP, Donofrio PD, et al. Monoclonal IgM with unique specificity to gangliosides GM1 and GD1b, and to lactop-*N*-tetraose, associated with human motor neuron disease. Neurology 1988;38:763.
68. Authier FJ, Ponvlotsky JM, Viard JP, et al. High incidence of hepatitis C virus infection in patients with cryoglobulinemic neuropathy. Ann Neurol 1993;34:749.
69. Monaco S, Bonetti B, Ferrari S, et al. Complement dependent demyelination in patients with IgM monoclonal gammopathy and polyneuropathy. N Engl J Med 1990;322:844.
70. Steck AJ, Murray N, Dellagi K, et al. Peripheral neuropathy associated with monoclonal IgM autoantibody. Ann Neurol 1987;22:764.
71. Trojaborg W, Galassi G, Hays AP, et al. Electrophysiological study of experimental demyelination induced by serum of patients with IgM M-proteins and neuropathy. Neurology 1989;39:1581.
72. Tatum AH. Experimental paraprotein neuropathy: demyelination by passive transfer of human IgM anti-MAG. Ann Neurol 1993;33:502.
73. Nobile-Orazio E, Baldini L, Barbieri S, et al. Treatment of patients with neuropathy and anti-MAG M-proteins. Ann Neurol 1988;34:93.
74. Dropcho EJ. Paraneoplastic peripheral neuropathies. Semin Neurol 1994;14:179.
75. Dalmau J, Furneaux HM, Gralla RJ, et al. Detection of the anti-Hu antibody in the serum of patients with small cell lung cancer. Ann Neurol 1990;27:544.
76. Benyahia B, Liblau R, Beral H. Cell mediated autoimmunity in paraneoplastic neurological syndromes with anti-Hu antibodies. Ann Neurol 1999;45:162.
77. Chalk CH, Dyck PJ, Conn DL. Vasculitis neuropathy. In: Dyck PJ, Thomas PK, Griffin JW, et al., eds. Peripheral neuropathy. Philadelphia, WB Saunders, 1993;1424.
78. Said G. Necrotizing peripheral nerve vasculitis. Neurol Clin 1997;15:835.
79. Dalakas MC, Wichman A, Sever JL. AIDS and the nervous system. JAMA 1989;261:2396.
80. Parry GJ. Peripheral neuropathies associated with human immunodeficiency virus infection. Ann Neurol 1988;23(suppl):49.
81. Dalakas MC, Cupler EJ. Polyneuropathies in HIV infection. Peripheral Neuropathies: Part II, Baillière's Clinical Neurology. London, WB Saunders, 1996;99.
82. Dalakas MC, Illa I, Pezeshkpour GH, et al. Mitochondrial myopathy caused by long-term zidovudine therapy. N Engl J Med 1990;332:1092.
83. Berger AR, Arezzo JC, Schaumberg HH, et al. 2′3′ dideoxycytidine (ddC) toxic neuropathy: a study of 52 patients. Neurology 1993;43:358.
84. Dalakas MC. Myopathies and neuropathies in HIV-infected adults and children. In: Pizzo PA, Wilfert CM (eds) Pediatric AIDS, 3rd edn. Baltimore, Williams & Wilkins, 1998;403.
85. French Cooperative Group on Plasma Exchange in Guillain–Barré Syndrome. Appropriate number of plasma exchanges in Guillain–Barré syndrome. Ann Neurol 1997;41:298.
86. Van der Meche FGA, Schmitz PIM. The Dutch Guillain–Barré syndrome. N Engl J Med 1992;326:1123.
87. Plasma exchange/sandoglobulin Guillain–Barré syndrome trial group. Randomized trial of plasma exchange, intravenous immunoglobulin, and combined treatments in Guillain–Barré syndrome. Lancet 1997;949:225.
88. Dalakas MC. Intravenous immunoglobulin in the treatment of Autoimmune neuromuscular diseases: present status and practical therapeutic guidelines. Muscle Nerve 1999;22:1479.
89. Dyck PJ, O'Brien PC, Oviatt KF, et al. Prednisone improves chronic inflammatory demyelinating polyradiculoneuropathy more than no treatment. Ann Neurol 1982;11:136.
90. Hahn AF, Bolton CF, Zochodne D, Feasby TE. Intravenous immunoglobulin treatment in chronic inflammatory demyelinating polyneuropathy. A double-blind, placebo-controlled, cross-over study. Brain 1996;119:1067.
91. Hahn AF, Bolton CF, Pillay N, et al. Plasma-exchange therapy in chronic inflammatory demyelinating polyneuropathy. A double-blind, sham-controlled, cross-over study. Brain 1996;119:1055.
92. Dyck PJ, Low PA, Windebank AJ. Plasma exchange in polyneuropathy associated with monoclonal gammopathy of undetermined significance. N Engl J Med 1991;325:1482.
93. Nobile-Orazio E, Baldini L, Barbieri S, et al. Treatment of patients with neuropathy and anti-MAG IgM M-proteins. Ann Neurol 1988;24:93.
94. Haas DC, Tatum AH. Plasmapheresis alleviates neuropathy accompanying IgM anti-myelin-associated glycoprotein paraproteinemia. Ann Neurol 1988;23:394.
95. Dalakas MC, Quarles RH, Farrer RG, et al. A controlled study of intravenous immunoglobulin in demyelinating neuropathy with IgM gammopathy. Ann Neurol 1996;40:792.
96. Levine TD, Pestronk A. IgM antibody-related polyneuropathies: B-cell depletion chemotherapy using Rituximab. Neurology 1999;52:1701.
97. Mariette X, Chastang C, Clavelou P, Louboutin JP, Leger JM, Brouet JC. A randomized clinical trial comparing interferon-alpha and intravenous immunoglobulin in polyneuropathy associated with monoclonal IgM.

The Igm-associated Polyneuropathy Study Group. J Neurol Neurosurg Psychiatry 1997;3:28.
98. Chaudhry V, Corse Am, Cornblath DR, et al. Multifocal motor neuropathy: response to human immune globulin. Ann Neurol 1993;33:237.
99. Nobile-Orazio E, Meucci N, Barbieri S, et al. High dose intravenous immunoglobulin therapy in multifocal motor neuropathy. Neurology 1993;43:537.
100. Meucci N, Cappellari A, Barbieri S, Scarlato G, Nobile-Orazio E. Long term effect of intravenous immunoglobulin and oral cyclophosphamide in multifocal motor neuropathy. J Neurol Neurosurg Psychiatry. 1997;63:765.
101. Jay C, Dalakas MC. Neuropathies myopathies in pediatric AIDS. In: Pizzo A, Wilfert CM (eds) Pediatric AIDS, 2nd edn. Baltimore, Williams & Wilkins, 1994, 559.

Chapter 79

Immunologic Renal Diseases

James E. Balow and Howard A. Austin III

Immunologically mediated kidney diseases represent the third most common cause of end-stage renal failure (after diabetic and hypertensive nephropathies). Disappointingly large numbers of patients first present for medical attention with advanced renal insufficiency. Several factors contribute to the often late diagnosis and treatment of immune-mediated kidney diseases. Patients with primary glomerular diseases tend to experience few symptoms that prompt them to seek medical evaluation. Shortcomings within the medical system also contribute to late diagnosis and treatment. Subtle abnormalities in urinary screening tests are too commonly missed or misattributed to inconsequential intercurrent conditions; moreover, definitive diagnostic tests are sometimes deferred because of a certain degree of nihilism about treatment, particularly the utility of immunomodulating drugs. Notwithstanding the notable deficiencies in evidence-based indications for treatment, it is clear from both experimental and clinical studies that early detection is one of the most important determinants of the success of treatment in both primary and secondary forms of immune-mediated renal disorders.

PRINCIPLES OF DIAGNOSIS

Appropriate evaluation of patients with immune-mediated kidney diseases requires a meticulous history and physical examination, with particular attention to the urinalysis,[1] tests of renal function[2] and often renal biopsy.[3] The urinalysis plays a pivotal role in the assessment of urinary disorders. The physician should be mindful of the many 'false negative' urinalyses reported by practice-oriented clinical pathology laboratories with high throughput. As a general rule, reports of positive findings are much more likely to be accurate than are negative reports. The thorough clinician should personally review microscopic urinalysis in any case in which there is a reasonable index of suspicion of immune-mediated renal disease.

Hematuria

Evaluation of hematuria should begin with the determination of whether the urinary bleeding is due to upper urinary tract (glomerular and/or tubulointerstitial) pathology or to lower urinary tract abnormalities. Urinary erythrocyte morphology helps to determine the cause of hematuria. Red blood cells that emanate from lesions of the calices, ureters, bladder or urethra tend to maintain their normal morphology; when nondysmorphic red blood cells are present it is usually appropriate to refer the patient to urology for further evaluation. Red blood cells that result from glomerular or tubulointerstitial pathology are more likely to appear dysmorphic (abnormal shapes and sizes, fragmented); when dysmorphic red blood cells are present it is usually appropriate to refer the patient to nephrology for further evaluation.

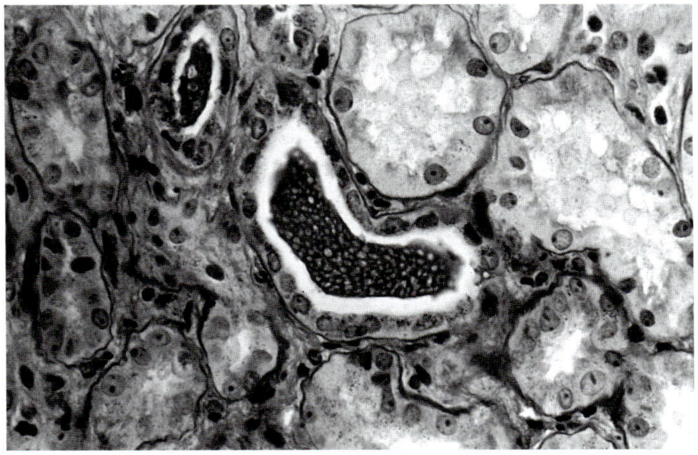

Figure 79.1 Red blood cell cast in situ within the lumen of a distal renal tubule. (PAS stain.)

Erythrocyte and/or leukocyte casts are indicative of glomerulonephritis (or interstitial nephritis). Cellular casts can be formed from erythrocytes and/or leukocytes that enter the tubular lumen because of glomerular or tubular inflammation (Fig. 79.1). To find cellular casts it is best to examine several freshly prepared urine sediments. The detection of any cellular casts is more important in diagnosis than is determining their exact frequency.

Proteinuria

Proteinuria is a cardinal feature of renal parenchymal disease and may indicate glomerular or tubular pathology. Glomerular proteinuria results from a loss of the size- and/or charge-selective properties of the glomerular capillary wall, allowing plasma proteins (especially albumin) to leak into the filtrate. Tubulointerstitial nephropathy often leads to impaired tubular absorption of other normally filtered low molecular weight proteins; this so-called ('tubular proteinuria' exhibits a characteristic pattern on urine protein electrophoresis, rarely exceeds 2 g/day, and often is associated with other manifestations of tubular dysfunction (e.g. Fanconi syndrome).

The completeness of 24-hour urine collections for quantitative proteinuria is often an issue. The accuracy of timed urine collection can be estimated from concurrent measurements of creatinine and protein excretion rates. Typically, females excrete 10–15 mg creatinine/kg/day, and males excrete 15–20 mg/kg/day. Problems associated with timed urine collections (especially in children) can be circumvented by determining the urinary protein-to-creatinine concentration ratio in random urine samples. Normally, this is less than 0.1. This random urine sample method has continued to gain favor as an efficient, cost-effective method to monitor proteinuria in both children and adults.

Filtration of abnormal plasma proteins may be responsible for proteinuria (e.g. multiple myeloma or light-chain disease). This type of proteinuria may be undetected or underestimated by the dipstick method of evaluating proteinuria. Abnormal light-chain excretion may be detected by urine protein electrophoresis, but immunofixation electrophoresis is particularly important for the detection and definitive diagnosis of paraproteinuria.[4]

Nephrotic syndrome

The nephrotic syndrome is characterized by substantial degrees of proteinuria (≥ 3.5 g/day), resulting in hypoalbuminemia, edema, hyperlipidemia and lipiduria. Nephrotic proteinuria usually results from global involvement of the glomerular capillaries. The degree of proteinuria may offer a helpful diagnostic clue because some immune-mediated conditions with typically diffuse glomerular disease (e.g. membranous nephropathy, systemic lupus, amyloidosis) are more likely than others with typically focal disease (e.g. IgA nephropathy, microscopic polyangiitis, Wegener's granulomatosis) to be associated with the nephrotic syndrome.

Acute nephritic syndrome

The acute nephritic syndrome is characterized by hematuria, erythrocyte casts, abnormal proteinuria, fluid retention, azotemia and hypertension. Histologically, this constellation of clinical findings is due to proliferative glomerulonephritis. A variant of this syndrome, called rapidly progressive glomerulonephritis, is defined by loss of 50% or more of glomerular filtration rate over 3 months and cellular crescents on renal biopsy. Rapidly progressive glomerulonephritis may present subtly as hematuria and/or proteinuria without oliguria, edema, hypertension or azotemia, and may be the premonitory sign of several immunologic renal diseases, particularly Wegener's granulomatosis, microscopic polyangiitis, Henoch–Schönlein nephritis, Goodpasture's syndrome and proliferative lupus nephritis.

Chronic glomerulonephritis

Chronic glomerulonephritis is not a diagnosis but is a stage in the evolution of immune-mediated renal disease. The urinalysis often provides valuable clues regarding the duration of glomerular disease. Broad granular casts and waxy casts are features of chronic renal disease that are not likely to be seen in recent-onset acute glomerulonephritis.

Renal biopsy

After extensive clinical and laboratory evaluations, a renal biopsy may be indicated to establish or confirm a tissue diagnosis, to clarify the precise type of renal involvement, to formulate a prognosis, and to help direct therapy.[5] To assist the reader in recognizing patterns of glomerular disease, a normal glomerulus is illustrated in Figure 79.2.

MINIMAL-CHANGE NEPHROPATHY (LIPOID NEPHROSIS)

Nephrotic syndrome of childhood is due to minimal-change nephropathy in over 90% of cases. There is a strong male predominance in preadolescent children. The frequency of minimal-change nephropathy in adult nephrotic syndrome is low, but this disease has been seen even into the ninth decade of life.

CLINICAL PEARLS

Indications for renal biopsy
- Active 'nephritic' urine sediment
  - Dysmorphic erythrocytes: >10 per high-power field
  - Cellular casts: erythrocyte or leukocyte.
- Proteinuria >2 g day.
- Abnormal renal function
  - Associated with the above features of active nephritis
  - Particularly important if the duration of renal disease and/or rate of change are unknown.
- Document indications for use of high-risk therapeutic interventions.

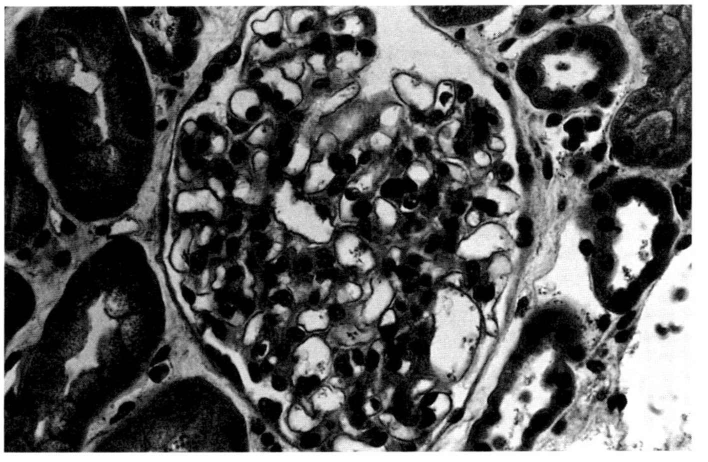

Figure 79.2 Normal glomerular architecture. Note the thin, delicate capillary walls. Neither cells nor matrix encroach upon the patency of the capillary lumina. (Hematoxylin and eosin.)

Clinical features

Minimal-change nephropathy characteristically presents with a rather precipitous onset of severe nephrotic syndrome in the absence of signs of a systemic disease. Massive generalized edema and ascites can be very debilitating; these features may be difficult to control with diuretics because of the typically extreme hypoalbuminemia.

Etiology

The cause of minimal-change nephropathy is largely unknown, hence the designation idiopathic nephrotic syndrome. Rare cases

KEY CONCEPTS

Minimal-change nephropathy
- Most common cause of nephrotic syndrome in children.
- High rate of response to glucocorticoids.
- Cyclophosphamide is useful for frequent relapsers.
- Renal prognosis is excellent.
- Subset may evolve to focal segmental glomerulosclerosis.

of recurrent minimal-change nephropathy are associated with precipitating events, such as allergic reactions or insect stings. Lymphomas, particularly Hodgkin lymphoma, have occasionally been associated with minimal-change nephropathy and should be considered in the differential diagnosis and comprehensive medical evaluation.

Pathogenesis

The basic lesion of minimal-change nephropathy is loss or neutralization of the normal high density of anionic proteoglycans in the glomerular capillary loops. Dissipation of the negative charge barrier allows anionically charged albumin to pass freely. Selective albuminuria is commonly seen in minimal-change disease because larger proteins are retained by the normal size-selective filtration barrier. The factor(s) responsible for loss of the glomerular charge-selective barrier are not known. The leading hypothesis is that it is a lymphokine or monokine because of the occasional association of minimal-change nephropathy with lymphoproliferative disorders, and because of its frequent response to glucocorticoids and cytotoxic drugs. Standard immunologic screening tests are usually normal in minimal-change nephropathy.

Diagnosis and treatment

Minimal-change nephropathy is typically exquisitely sensitive to glucocorticoids. The disease remits completely in over 90% of children within the first few weeks of therapy.[6] Because minimal-change nephropathy is the predominant cause of nephrotic syndrome in children, empiric glucocorticoid therapy is the standard practice without verification of the pathologic cause of the nephrotic syndrome. Thus, unless atypical clinical findings raise the suspicion of diagnoses other than minimal-change nephropathy, renal biopsy is not regularly performed for evaluation of nephrotic syndrome in children. On the other hand, renal biopsy is usually necessary in adults to make a diagnosis of the cause of the nephrotic syndrome. On light microscopy the biopsy shows normal glomerular cellularity and capillary wall thickness. The characteristic pathologic lesion is seen by electron microscopy, where there is fusion of the foot processes of the epithelial cells.

The response rate of minimal-change nephropathy to glucocorticoids in adults is somewhat lower and more delayed than in children; prednisone should be continued for up to 4 months in refractory cases. A substantial portion of patients with minimal-change nephropathy face long-term difficulties with the disease and its therapy: some are steroid resistant from the inception; others are steroid dependent for control of nephrotic syndrome; still others become frequent relapsers and suffer substantial steroid toxicity with repeated treatments.[7] Relapse is more common in adults than in children with minimal-change nephropathy. Controlled trials have shown that alkylating agents (cyclophosphamide or chlorambucil) increase response rates and/or decrease relapse rates for these groups of patients.[8] Cyclosporine has also been shown to be an effective alternative to prolonged steroid therapy.[9]

The risk of progression to end-stage renal failure is extremely low in true minimal-change nephropathy.[10] However, there is some apparent overlap between minimal-change nephropathy and focal segmental glomerulosclerosis, the latter being typically more refractory to therapy and having a much more adverse renal prognosis. There is debate about whether renal biopsy sampling error accounts for mistaken diagnoses of minimal-change disease in a certain portion of focal segmental glomerulosclerosis, and whether a subset of cases of minimal-change nephropathy can progress to focal segmental glomerulosclerosis.[11]

FOCAL SEGMENTAL GLOMERULOSCLEROSIS

Few features distinguish patients with new onset idiopathic nephrotic syndrome due to minimal-change nephropathy versus focal segmental glomerulosclerosis (FSGS). Hypertension, microscopic hematuria and azotemia are suggestive of the latter diagnosis. FSGS is distinguished from minimal-change nephropathy mainly by a more adverse renal prognosis, a higher frequency of persistent nephrotic syndrome and poorer response to immunosuppressive drug therapies. The incidence of FSGS is clearly increasing as a cause of nephrotic syndrome, particularly among black patients, in whom the search for genetic predisposing factors is under way.

The etiology and pathogenesis of FSGS are mostly unknown. The characteristic renal pathology includes segmental areas of podocyte damage and detachment, and collapse of glomerular capillaries associated with a marked local increase in matrix and collagen accumulation (Fig. 79.3). The areas of glomerular histology apart from the segmental sclerosing lesions resemble minimal-change nephropathy: indeed, some cases of FSGS may simply represent advanced forms of minimal-change nephropathy. Several distinctive pathologic subtypes of FSGS are recognized. Collapsing FSGS is one such form that has been associated with viral infections, notably HIV, and follows a particularly aggressive course.[12,13] Some forms of FSGS, such as those associated with morbid

KEY CONCEPTS

Focal segmental glomerulosclerosis

- Nephrotic syndrome with progressive renal insufficiency
- Glomerular permeability factor in plasma of some cases
- Unpredictable responses to glucocorticoids or cyclophosphamide
- Cyclosporine effective but relapses common
- Moderately high relapse rate in renal allografts

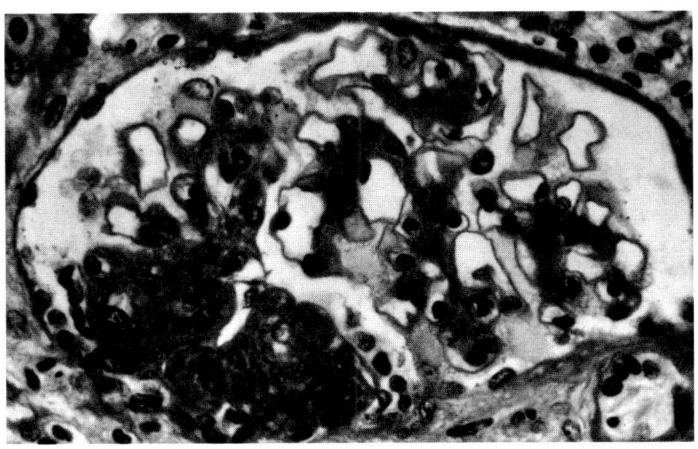

Figure 79.3 Focal segmental glomerulosclerosis. The glomerular capillary loops at the lower left are collapsed and obliterated by excessive matrix and connective tissue. (Masson trichrome.)

obesity, appear to result from nonimmunologic glomerular hyperfiltration injury. Potential new insights into the pathogenesis of FSGS emanate from the discovery of plasma factors which in vitro increase the permeability of normal glomerular capillaries to albumin.[14] Although this is controversial, some investigators have found permeability factors in a subset of cases of FSGS and claim that levels of these factors correlate with remissions and exacerbations of nephrotic syndrome.

The treatment of the common form of primary FSGS is basically similar to that of minimal-change nephropathy and includes prednisone, cyclophosphamide and cyclosporine. Recent controlled trials have shown that cyclosporine is much more effective than prednisone alone in inducing remission of nephrotic syndrome, and in preserving renal function in patients with steroid-resistant FSGS.[15,16] Prolonged courses up to several months of immunosuppressive drugs may be necessary to realize maximum benefit in FSGS. Long-term prognosis depends mainly on achievement of remission of nephrotic syndrome; the renal prognosis at 10 years is approximately 50–60%.[17,18] Angiotensin-converting enzyme inhibitors or angiotensin receptor antagonists are commonly used to counter the potential contribution of hyperfiltration injury. Preliminary studies have suggested a small benefit of plasma exchange therapy in patients with high plasma levels of permeability factors.[19] The rate of recurrence of FSGS in renal transplants is high, particularly in those with permeability factors.[20] Treatment is controversial and warrants further study under experimental protocols.

MEMBRANOUS NEPHROPATHY

Membranous nephropathy is identified in approximately 20% of adults who undergo renal biopsy for nephrotic syndrome. It is a less frequent cause of nephrotic syndrome in children. Secondary causes of membranous nephropathy can be identified in a substantial portion of cases; primary (idiopathic) membranous nephropathy should be considered a diagnosis of exclusion. Membranous nephropathy has been attributed to a large number of medications, infections, neoplasms and systemic illnesses. The etiologic association has been strengthened in some cases by a remission of the nephrotic syndrome following elimination of a medication, a malignancy or an infection.

Pathogenesis

Membranous nephropathy is characterized by subepithelial (epimembranous) immune deposits containing IgG and complement components. Two general hypotheses regarding the immune deposits have been considered:[21] immune complexes could be formed in the circulation and then trapped in the glomerulus; alternatively, they could be formed in situ by the interaction of a pathogenic antibody with an endogenous glomerular antigen, or with an antigen that had been planted in the glomerulus as a consequence of the physicochemical characteristics of the antigen and the glomerular capillary wall (e.g. charge–charge interaction). Extensive studies of animal models of membranous nephropathy have provided strong evidence for the hypothesis of in situ immune complex formation leading to the activation of complement and generation of the C5b-9 membrane attack complex. Monoclonal antibodies that potentially modulate the complement-mediated injury are under investigation as an approach to the treatment of membranous nephropathy.

Clinicopathologic features

The majority of patients with membranous nephropathy present with the nephrotic syndrome. Some are discovered by the detection of asymptomatic proteinuria on routine urinalysis. Renal biopsy is usually required to establish the diagnosis of membranous nephropathy. In the early stages of the disease glomeruli may appear normal by light microscopy. In most cases light microscopy shows uniform thickening of the glomerular capillary walls without endocapillary cell proliferation (Fig. 79.4). Characteristic subepithelial (epimembranous) and/or intramembranous deposits are seen an electron microscopy (Fig. 79.5). The diagnosis of secondary membranous nephropathy depends on ancillary clinical and laboratory data.

Natural history

The clinical course of idiopathic membranous nephropathy is highly variable. On average, about one-quarter of adult patients progress to end-stage renal failure within 10 years.[6] Another quarter of patients experience a spontaneous remission of proteinuria. The majority are likely to have persistent proteinuria and moderately impaired renal function over an extended period of observation. Patients with sustained hyperlipidemia are at risk for premature cardiovascular disease,[22] and reduction of cardiovascular risk may be an important part of therapy.

KEY CONCEPTS

Membranous nephropathy
- Common cause of idiopathic nephrotic syndrome in adults
- Several secondary causes: systemic lupus, drugs, chronic hepatitis, certain malignancies
- One-quarter of patients have spontaneous remission
- One-quarter of patients develop ESRD within a decade
- Protracted nephrotic syndrome confers risks of cardiovascular and thromboembolic events
- Therapy: steroids, alkylating agents, lipid-lowering drugs, angiotensin antagonists

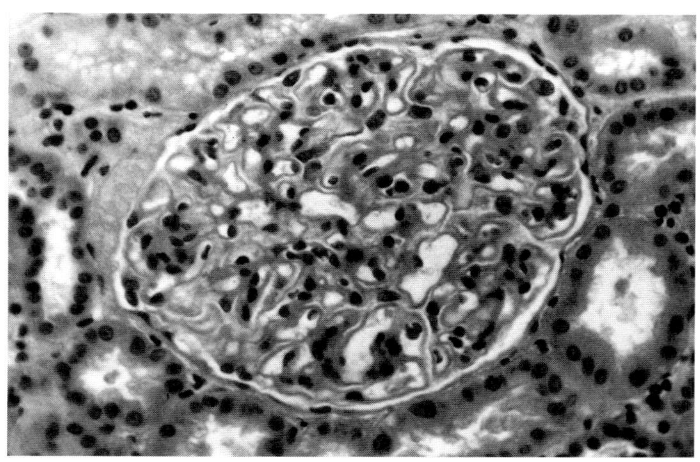

Figure 79.4 Membranous nephropathy. The capillary walls are nearly uniformly thickened but remain widely patent, and the cellularity of the glomerulus is normal. (Hematoxylin and eosin.)

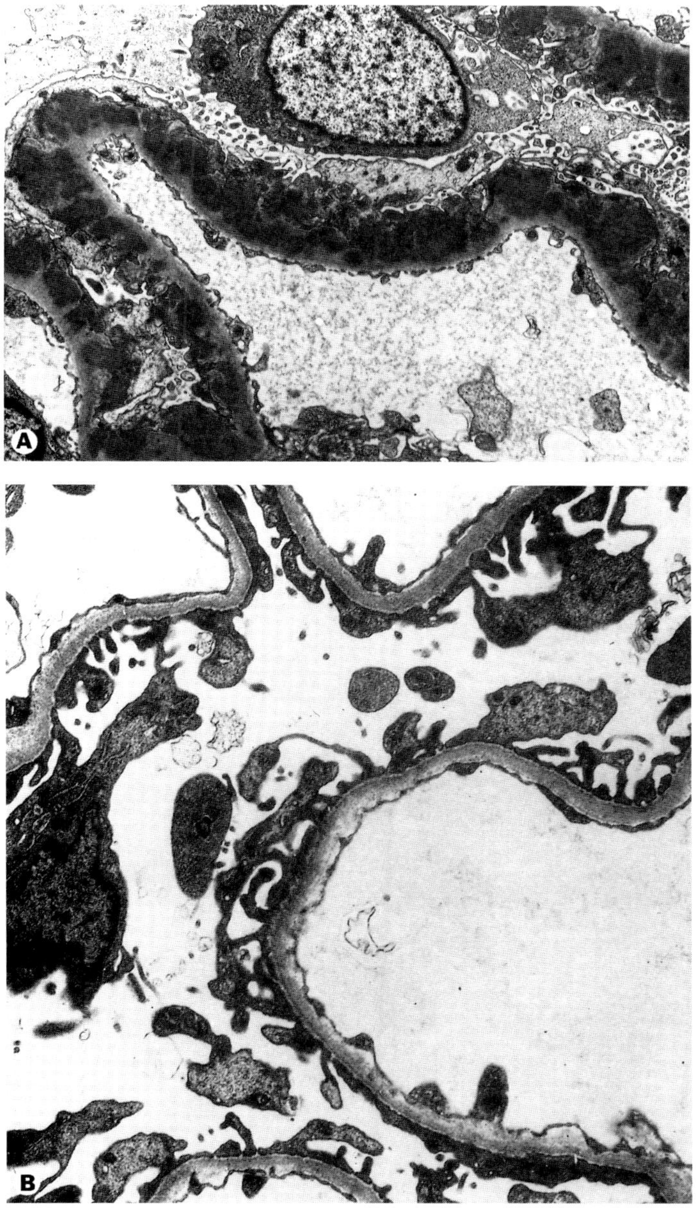

Figure 79.5 Membranous nephropathy. (**A**). This electron micrograph demonstrates heavy, dark-staining immune complex deposits along the outer surface of the glomerular basement membrane and beneath the epithelial foot processes (hence the terms subepithelial or epimembranous deposits). Note the thickening and projections of the gray-staining basement membrane between the electron-dense deposits. (**B**). The ultrastructure of a normal glomerular capillary wall for comparison. (Electron micrographs courtesy of Drs T. Antonovych and S. Sabnis, Armed Forces Institute of Pathology; Washington DC.)

It is difficult to predict the clinical course of individual patients with membranous nephropathy. Women, children and patients with low-grade proteinuria (<2 g/day) tend to have a favorable prognosis. In contrast, several studies have indicated that severe nephrotic syndrome, hypertension and azotemia on presentation are associated with a poor prognosis. Glomerular and/or interstitial scarring on renal biopsy also have an adverse effect on prognosis. Predictions of renal outcome can be enhanced by considering observations over a period of time.[23] Persistent high-grade nephrotic-range proteinuria for more than 6 months and declining renal function are relatively strong predictors of an adverse renal outcome. On the other hand, complete remission is associated with an excellent long-term prognosis.[24]

Treatment

The management of patients with membranous nephropathy usually includes diuretics to reduce edema, lipid-lowering drugs (for severe hyperlipidemia), anticoagulant therapy for thromboembolic complications, and antihypertensive agents.[25] Angiotensin-converting enzyme inhibition has been shown to have a substantial antiproteinuric effect in membranous nephropathy.[26] The remainder of this discussion will focus on the controversial role of immunosuppressive therapy in the treatment of idiopathic membranous nephropathy.

Patients with severe nephrotic syndrome due to membranous nephropathy are usually treated with high-dose alternate-day prednisone.[25] Proteinuria has been shown to be reduced in some, but not all, studies of alternate-day prednisone, but relapses of proteinuria after prednisone treatment are common. It also remains controversial whether prednisone treatment reduces the risk of progression to renal failure.

Studies have suggested that a combination of prednisone and cytotoxic drug therapy might provide more benefit than prednisone alone. Azathioprine does not appear to have a role in membranous nephropathy. However, a recent pilot study of the related drug mycophenolate mofetil, in patients resistant to other immunosuppressive therapies, showed encouraging evidence of benefit.[27] The most compelling results from controlled trials have shown that patients with membranous nephropathy treated with alternating monthly courses of pulse methylprednisolone and chlorambucil or cyclophosphamide[28] were more likely than controls to experience a remission of the nephrotic syndrome and achieve stable renal function. Some authors have reported stable or improved renal function and reduction of nephrotic-range proteinuria in patients with deteriorating renal function treated with prednisone and long-term daily oral cyclophosphamide.[29] Concerns regarding the potential adverse effects of daily cytotoxic drug therapy have led to studies of intermittent pulse cyclophosphamide analogous to that described for lupus nephritis. However, evidence to date indicates that intermittent pulse cyclophosphamide is not effective in the treatment of idiopathic membranous nephropathy.[30]

Several anecdotal series and one controlled trial of cyclosporine in membranous nephropathy have suggested a moderate benefit on proteinuria and renal function.[31] However, relapses of proteinuria are common, particularly after a short course of cyclosporine therapy. At the present time cyclosporine is usually relegated to the status of alternative therapy for patients with poor prognostic profiles who fail to respond or do not tolerate combination steroid and cytotoxic drug therapy.

MEMBRANOPROLIFERATIVE GLOMERULONEPHRITIS

Membranoproliferative glomerulonephritis (MPGN) is a rare condition sometimes called mesangiocapillary glomerulonephritis (Fig. 79.6).[32] Besides the presence of pathologic immunoreactants in glomerular sites, the immune-mediated nature of this disease is suggested by the high frequency of persistent hypocomplementemia. It is of interest that both congenital complement

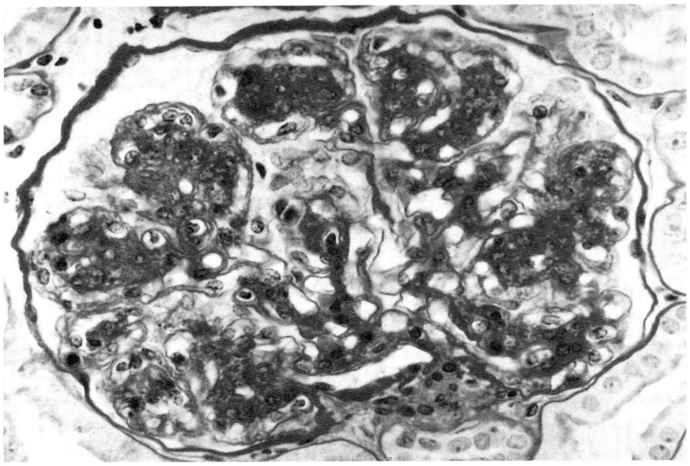

Figure 79.6 Membranoproliferative glomerulonephritis (MPGN). The glomerulus exhibits the typical lobulated appearance of this disease. Note the markedly increased mesangial cells and matrix in all of the lobules. The mesangium extends outward into the capillary loops and forms double contours with the glomerular basement membrane. (PAS stain.)

KEY CONCEPTS

Membranoproliferative glomerulonephritis (MPGN)

- Rare form of chronic nephritis, mostly discovered as asymptomatic hematuria, variable proteinuria and/or insidious chronic renal insufficiency
- Type I MPGN: subendothelial immune complex deposits
- Type II MPGN: dense intramembranous deposits (containing C3 complement)
- Hypocomplementemia associated with C3 nephritic factor, an autoantibody to C3 convertase of the alternative complement pathway
- Response to immunosuppressive drug treatment generally poor
- Both types MPGN tend to recur in renal allografts

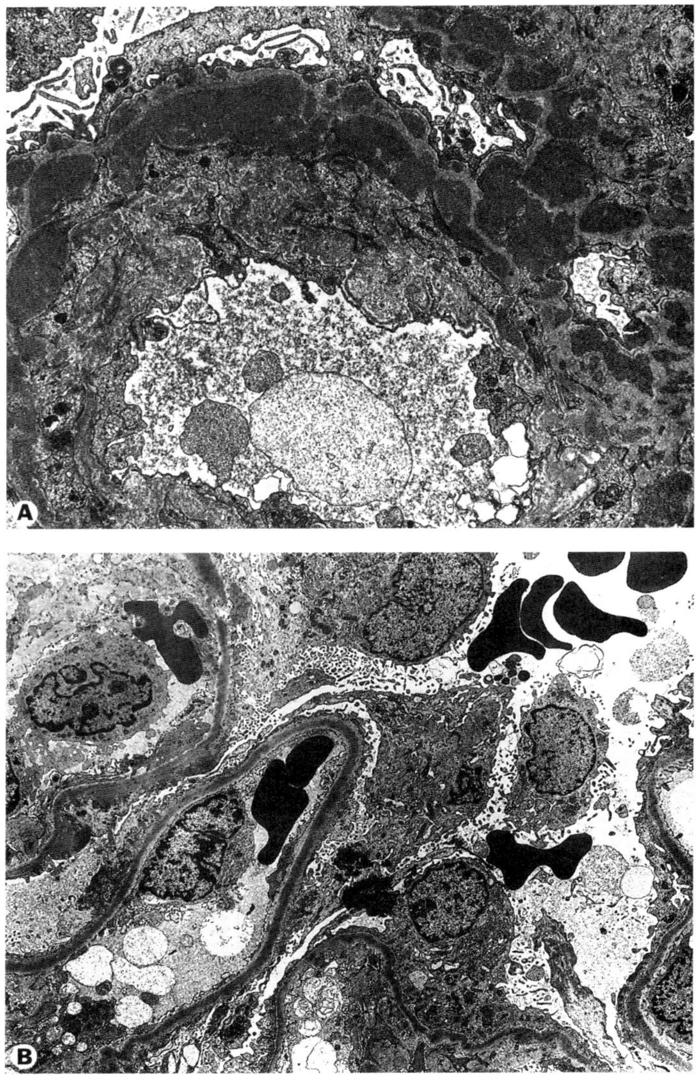

Figure 79.7 Membranoproliferative glomerulonephritis (MPGN). (**A**) Type I MPGN: the capillary wall is markedly thickened and contains heavy, dark-staining electron dense immune complexes in the subendothelial space. The mesangium (lighter material) extends into the capillary loop where it is interposed between the basement membrane and the endothelium. This interposition gives the appearance of a massively thickened capillary loop by hematoxylin and eosin stain and the split appearance by PAS and silver stain. (**B**) Type II MPGN (dense intramembranous deposit disease): the capillary loops contain smooth, continuous linear dense material within the basement membrane. (Electron micrographs courtesy of Drs. T. Antonovych and S. Sabnis; Armed Forces Institute of Pathology; Washington, DC.)

deficiencies (e.g. deficiency of complement component C3) and sustained hypocomplementemia induced by nephritic factor autoantibodies or circulating immune complexes have been associated with MPGN.[33]

Pathologic variants

The nomenclature of MPGN includes two main pathological subsets: type I, MPGN with subendothelial deposits (Fig. 79.7A), and type II, MPGN with dense intramembranous deposits (Fig. 79.7B); a third subset (type III) with mixed subendothelial and subepithelial deposits has been proposed. Some argue that this third subset is a variant of type I MPGN, although recent evidence of a difference in response to treatment indicates a true distinction between types I and III.[34] Although most cases of MPGN are of unknown etiology, studies over the past decade have shown that chronic hepatitis C infection, often with cryoglobulinemia, accounts for a substantial portion of cases of type I MPGN.[35]

Types I and II idiopathic MPGN are clinically indistinguishable. Typically, asymptomatic hematuria and proteinuria are discovered incidentally. Judging from the chronicity found on renal biopsy, MPGN probably goes undetected for long periods in most patients. Whereas in many cases it is a chronic low-grade nephropathy, other patients experience complicated nephrotic syndrome and even rapidly progressive and crescentic phases of the disease.

Nephritic factors

Patients with type II MPGN, and to a lesser extent type I, exhibit a complement-activating antibody called nephritic factor.[33] The typical nephritic factor is an IgG autoantibody that binds to the complement alternative pathway convertase C3b, Bb (Chapter 21). Nephritic factor stabilizes and prolongs the activity of the enzyme by interfering with normal factors controlling the convertase activity. This leads to sustained activation and severe depletion of serum C3 levels, which is a hallmark of MPGN. Whether or how C3 nephritic factor plays a role in the pathogenesis of either form of MPGN is unknown. Interestingly, in type II MPGN there are no immunoglobulin components in the dense intramembranous deposits, whereas there are heavy linear deposits of C3, possibly indicating an effect of the prolonged C3 activation.

Treatment

There is no consensus about the treatment of MPGN, and the preponderance of opinion is that no therapy is effective in inducing remission or in protecting against progressive renal failure. Overall, renal survival is approximately 50% at 10 years from diagnosis, although a subset of patients have a rapidly progressive course if they develop superimposed crescentic glomerulonephritis.[6] Alternate-day prednisone is commonly tried in children with MPGN, but no controlled trials are available and the long-term prognosis remains unfavorable. The efficacy of cytotoxic drug therapy, anticoagulants and antiplatelet drugs is similarly unproven. Both forms of MPGN tend to recur in renal allografts, although recurrence of type I MPGN has the greater detrimental effect on graft survival.[36]

POSTINFECTIOUS NEPHROPATHIES

An ever-expanding list of infectious agents has been implicated in the pathogenesis of immune-mediated nephropathies. Some are acute and self-limited, but many of the nephritogenic infections are protracted and are associated with circulating immune complexes, cryoglobulins, high-titer rheumatoid factor and hypocomplementemia.

KEY CONCEPTS

Infectious-related nephropathies

- *Viral*: hepatitis B – membranous nephropathy; hepatitis C – cryoglobulinemic membranoproliferative glomerulonephritis; HIV – focal segmental glomerulosclerosis (HIV nephropathy)
- *Bacterial (mainly gram-positive)*: nephritogenic streptococcal infections, prosthetic device (shunt) infections, subacute bacterial endocarditis, chronic deep tissue abscesses – mainly diffuse or focal proliferative glomerulonephritis; secondary syphilis – membranous nephropathy
- *Parasitic*: schistosomiasis mansoni (chronic hepatosplenic form) – focal segmental glomerulosclerosis and membranoproliferative glomerulonephritis
- Effective control of renal disease in most conditions (except perhaps schistosomiasis) depends on eradication of the organism; immunosuppressive or anti-inflammatory drug therapies are rarely indicated

VIRAL INFECTIONS

Hepatitis B

Chronic hepatitis B virus (HBV) has been associated with membranous nephropathy, membranoproliferative glomerulonephritis and polyarteritis nodosa.[37] Available evidence suggests that HBV-associated nephropathy is immune complex mediated. The deposition of circulating immune complexes containing HBV antigens is most likely involved in the pathogenesis of membranoproliferative glomerulonephritis. In HBV-associated membranous nephropathy, in situ immune complex formation or the induction of autoantibodies to intrinsic glomerular antigens are more likely to be involved. The possibility that viral replication within the kidney itself initiates the injury has also been hypothesized.

Hepatitis B-associated nephropathy most frequently presents as nephrotic syndrome accompanied by microscopic hematuria; only rarely is evidence of renal functional impairment or progressive liver disease apparent on presentation. Hepatic disease may be present for many years prior to the onset of nephropathy. Progressive nephritis with the development of chronic renal failure is common in adults. Nearly all patients with chronic HBV have HBsAg, anti-HBc antibodies and elevated serum aminotransferase levels. Serum C3 and C4 are decreased in some patients.

Renal biopsy most commonly shows membranous nephropathy; membranoproliferative glomerulonephritis is less common in HBV-associated renal disease. Immunofluorescence studies usually show immunoglobulin, C3 and viral antigens, particularly HBsAg and HBeAg. Electron microscopy shows subepithelial and intramembranous deposits but, unlike idiopathic membranous nephropathy, there may also be mesangial and even some subendothelial deposits. Glucocorticoids and cytotoxic agents may promote viral replication, whereas recombinant human interferon-α (IFN-α) has been shown to produce remission of both liver and kidney disease.[38]

Hepatitis C

Hepatitis C virus (HCV) is a major cause of both transfusion-associated and sporadic chronic hepatitis. Persistent infection occurs in approximately 50% of patients and may result in chronic active hepatitis, cirrhosis, mixed cryoglobulinemia and membranoproliferative glomerulonephritis.[39] The pathogenesis of the renal disease is unknown but may relate to deposition within glomeruli of immune complexes containing HCV, anti-HCV antibody and virus-related (or unrelated) cryoglobulins.[35] Treatment with IFN-α results in decreased viral replication and regression of renal and liver disease.[40] Ribavirin is currently under investigation as an alternative therapy and combination therapy with IFN-α for chronic hepatitis C and its systemic complications.

Human immunodeficiency virus (HIV)

Patients with the acquired immunodeficiency syndrome (AIDS) develop a wide variety of renal abnormalities, including focal segmental glomerulosclerosis, tubulointerstitial disease and drug-related interstitial nephritis.[41] Black patients and intravenous drug abusers are more likely to develop an aggressive form of glomerular disease, currently designated HIV-associated nephropathy (HIVAN).[42] HIVAN is characterized by focal segmental glomerulosclerosis (collapsing type) with extensive tubular ectasia and interstitial fibrosis. Treatment with highly active antiretroviral therapies appears to have partially improved the otherwise poor renal prognosis of HIVAN, although complications of drug therapy itself have been observed.[43] The use of standard immunosuppressive drug therapies for HIVAN is controversial.

BACTERIAL INFECTIONS

Post-streptococcal glomerulonephritis

Post-streptococcal glomerulonephritis is the result of skin or throat infection with nephritogenic strains of group A streptococci.[44] Nephritic syndrome usually occurs about 2 weeks after the appearance of infection. Whereas the role of streptococcal infection in causing the disease is widely accepted, the demonstration of streptococcal antigens and antibodies in glomeruli has been controversial.

Post-streptococcal glomerulonephritis is characterized by the nephritic syndrome, consisting of smoky or rust-colored urine, generalized edema, hypertension, and nephritic urine sediment. Proteinuria is typically mild. Although antistreptolysin titers usually rise, the emergence of this antibody may be blunted by effective antibiotic therapy. Patients have depressed C3 complement levels early in nephritis but normal or minimally depressed C4 levels, indicating activation of the alternative complement pathway.

Complete clinical resolution of nephritis is the rule and therefore in children renal biopsy is not usually indicated. In adults biopsy is often necessary for diagnosis. Proliferative glomerulonephritis with polymorphonuclear leukocyte and monocyte infiltration, granular immune deposits of IgG and C3, and dome-shaped electron-dense subepithelial deposits (humps) are characteristic. The prognosis is excellent: almost all children will recover with supportive care. Progressive renal failure accompanied by hypertension may be more common in adults.

Glomerulonephritis associated with focal infections

Renal disease has been associated with infective endocarditis, infection of artificial vascular devices, and localized abscesses.[45,46] A variety of organisms have been implicated in the pathogenesis of renal disease, which seems to be immune-complex mediated. Overlap with renal vasculitic diseases is common.[47] Renal biopsy findings in fulminant infections resemble those of acute post-streptococcal glomerulonephritis. In subacute forms (e.g., endocarditis), focal segmental proliferative glomerulonephritis is more common. The course and prognosis are variable. Antibiotic therapy in most cases is associated with improvement in the renal lesions.

Syphilis

Nephropathy may occur in both congenital and acquired syphilis. In acquired syphilis it usually becomes apparent during the secondary phase of the infection. Most patients present with nephrotic syndrome and have secondary membranous nephropathy on renal biopsy.[48] Patients with concurrently positive syphilis serologies and antinuclear antibodies may have lupus-related rather than syphilis-associated membranous nephropathy. Following the institution of antimicrobial therapy most, but not all, patients with syphilis-associated nephropathy recover.

PARASITIC DISEASES

Schistosomiasis

Schistosomal infections affect millions of patients in tropical countries. Nephropathy usually occurs after the development of the hepatosplenic form of *Schistosoma mansoni* and is characterized by proteinuria, hypertension and progressive renal failure.[49] Renal biopsy usually demonstrates focal segmental glomerulosclerosis or membranoproliferative glomerulonephritis. Long-standing schistosomiasis rarely produces secondary renal amyloidosis. Treatment of the underlying schistosomiasis or the nephropathy with corticosteroids and immunosuppressive therapy does not seem to affect the progression of the schistosomiasis-associated nephropathy.

IgA NEPHROPATHY

Idiopathic IgA nephropathy (also known as Berger's disease) is among the most common forms of glomerular disease in many parts of the world, especially southern Europe, Australia and Asia.[50,51] This appears to reflect, in part, the widespread routine screening of healthy schoolchildren and military recruits for urinary abnormalities, and the frequent use of renal biopsy to evaluate asymptomatic isolated hematuria. Renal histologic features and aspects of immunopathogenesis are comparable to those of Henoch–Schönlein nephritis.

Clinical features

IgA nephropathy can affect patients of all ages, especially children and young adults, with a male preponderance. Unexplained is the fact that IgA nephropathy is rare in Black patients. This observation and examples of familial clustering of IgA nephropathy support a role for genetic susceptibility in the immunopathogenesis of disease. IgA nephropathy is frequently discovered as asymptomatic microscopic hematuria. Alternatively, patients (especially children) may present with recurrent episodes of macroscopic hematuria that occur within 24–48 hours after an intercurrent infection, usually upper respiratory or gastrointestinal tract infections. A transient elevation in serum creatinine has been associated with macroscopic hematuria in about one-third of cases. This has been attributed to tubular injury and obstruction caused by intraluminal red blood cell casts. An episode of macroscopic hematuria is occasionally associated with extensive cellular crescent formation, rapidly deteriorating renal function, hypertension and nephrotic syndrome.

KEY CONCEPTS

IgA nephritis

- Common cause of asymptomatic microscopic hematuria, recurrent macroscopic hematuria and/or low-grade proteinuria.
- Spectrum of disease, including idiopathic IgA nephritis and Henoch–Schönlein purpura nephritis; IgA in skin and renal biopsies.
- Mostly benign prognosis, especially in children.
- Patients with progressive renal insufficiency and/or crescentic glomerulonephritis warrant trial of glucocorticoids and/or cytotoxic drug therapy.

Natural history

IgA nephropathy typically has a benign renal prognosis. However, it is recognized that at least one-third of patients with IgA nephropathy progress to end-stage kidney failure. Twenty years after apparent disease onset, the probability of renal failure is 25%, and about half of patients demonstrate some renal dysfunction. Hypertension occurs frequently as the disease progresses and forebodes a poor prognosis.[52]

Other clinical features that have been associated with a poor prognosis include older age at apparent disease onset, male gender, persistent proteinuria (> 0.5 g/day), and persistent azotemia. On renal biopsy evaluation extensive cellular crescents, endocapillary proliferation and extension of immune deposits to the peripheral glomerular capillary walls are indicative of severe immune-mediated glomerulonephritis and a poor prognosis. Evidence of irreversible renal parenchymal injury (glomerular sclerosis, interstitial fibrosis and tubular atrophy) also identifies high-risk patients.

Treatment

The treatment of progressive IgA nephropathy remains undefined. Control of hypertension is clearly important. Some controlled trials suggest that fish oil dietary supplements (eicosanoids) have a salutary effect on IgA nephropathy.[53] Investigators have not found convincing evidence that phenytoin (which decreases serum IgA levels), danazol or antiplatelet agents favorably affect the course of this disease. Conventional immunosuppression with steroids and cytotoxic drugs is indicated in the subset of patients with poor prognostic factors who are at risk for progressive renal failure.[54]

HENOCH–SCHÖNLEIN NEPHRITIS

Henoch–Schönlein purpura (HSP) is a generalized vasculitis that usually affects children and typically involves the skin, joints, kidneys and gastrointestinal tract (Chapter 67).[55,56] Classic HSP, manifested as palpable purpuric skin lesions with joint, kidney and/or gastrointestinal involvement, is readily recognized. Characteristic skin and renal biopsy findings may support the diagnosis. Skin biopsies reveal leukocytoclastic vasculitis with granular deposits of IgA along dermal vessels of purpuric and uninvolved skin.

Although in most patients the disease remits spontaneously, some develop serious renal and/or gastrointestinal complications. Evidence of immune complex causation has prompted recommendations for immunosuppressive treatment of severe HSP nephritis, but the data are uncontrolled and controversial.

Clinical features

Urinary abnormalities were seen in about one-third of a largely unselected sample of children with HSP.[57] Microscopic hematuria is detected in nearly all cases with nephritis and is accompanied by variable proteinuria in more than 90% of cases. Approximately 40% of patients with HSP nephritis reported from referral centers had nephrotic-range proteinuria, and in two-thirds of these there were complicating features, including various combinations of hypertension, azotemia and hypoproteinemia. Renal biopsy findings range from mild mesangial proliferation to crescentic glomerulonephritis. Immune deposits are predominantly mesangial and characteristically contain IgA.

KEY CONCEPTS

Renal involvement in systemic vasculitis

- Vasculitis with glomerular involvement includes microscopic polyangiitis, Wegener's granulomatosis and necrotizing crescentic glomerulonephritis (renal-limited vasculitis).
- Associated with anti-neutrophil cytoplasmic antibodies (ANCA).
- Rapidly progressive glomerulonephritis is common; early treatment includes pulse methylprednisolone, cyclophosphamide (possibly adjunctive plasma exchange).
- Maintenance therapy: azathioprine, mycophenolate, methotrexate.

Natural history

Most patients with HSP nephritis follow a relatively benign clinical course. The probability of maintaining life-supporting renal function is nearly 90% at 10 years. It is debated whether adults are at greater risk for renal failure than children. Patients who present with microscopic hematuria without proteinuria rarely progress to renal failure. Approximately 80% of patients who initially manifest hematuria and proteinuria have normal renal function with little or no urinary abnormality after extended observation; another 10% are likely to progress to renal failure.[58] Patients who present with complicated nephrotic syndrome are at substantial risk for end-stage kidney failure. The renal biopsy also provides useful prognostic information. The proportion of glomeruli exhibiting crescents is proportional to the risk of renal failure.

Therapy

Decisions regarding the treatment of HSP nephritis are made difficult by a lack of compelling data from prospective randomized therapeutic trials and by the highly unpredictable nature of this disease. Glucocorticoids and cytotoxic drugs should be reserved for high-risk patients as described above. Pulse intravenous methylprednisolone seems to offer additional benefit.[59] Renal transplantation is a reasonable option for patients who progress to terminal renal failure, provided that the disease has been in remission for several months preoperatively.

NEPHROPATHIES ASSOCIATED WITH ANTINEUTROPHIL CYTOPLASMIC ANTIBODIES (CLASSIC POLYARTERITIS, MICROSCOPIC POLYANGIITIS, WEGENER'S GRANULOMATOSIS AND IDIOPATHIC NECROTIZING CRESCENTIC GLOMERULONEPHRITIS)

Systemic vasculitis is covered in detail in Chapter 67. The present discussion is limited to the renal components of the major vasculitic syndromes.

Clinical and pathologic features

Renal involvement is common in the systemic vasculitides but varies in type and severity. In classic polyarteritis nodosa the vasculitis affects mainly arteries outside the glomerulus, producing ischemia, hypertension, segmental infarctions and renal failure. In microscopic polyangiitis, Wegener's granulomatosis and renal-limited necrotizing and crescentic glomerulonephritis, the vasculitis occurs mainly within the glomerulus.[60–62] The glomerular

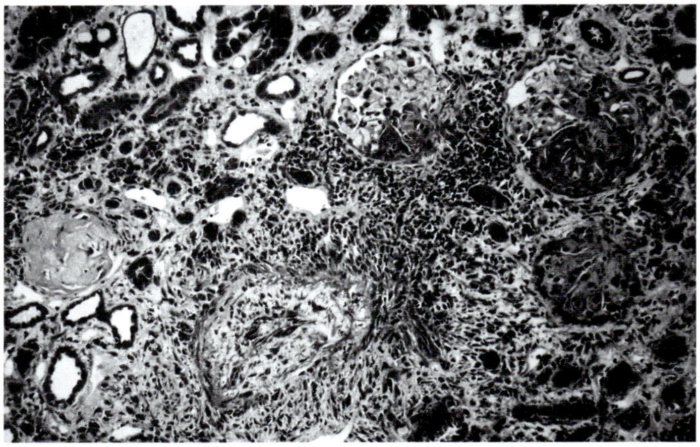

Figure 79.8 Vasculitis with both glomerular and arteriolar lesions. The small renal vessel shows healing arteritis with proliferation, edema, and fibrosis which severely compromise the lumen. Lesions in the four glomeruli include segmental fibrinoid necrosis (upper right), cellular crescent (lower right) and hyalinized glomerulus (middle left). Tubular atrophy and interstitial fibrosis are prominent. Masson stain. (Micrograph courtesy of Drs. T. Antonovych and S. Sabnis; Armed Forces Institute of Pathology; Washington, DC.)

abnormalities are similar among these groups (Fig. 79.8). The lesions are characteristically focal and segmental in distribution, with fibrinoid necrosis and crescent formation but few, if any, immune deposits (some use the term pauci-immune glomerulonephritis). Clinically, rapidly progressive glomerulonephritis is a common manifestation of these renal vasculitides, making the early detection of glomerulonephritis critically important in management.

Another common feature of the renal vasculitides is the presence of autoantibodies to neutrophil cytoplasmic antigens (anti-neutrophil cytoplasmic antibodies; ANCA).[63] As shown in Table 79.1, microscopic polyangiitis, Wegener's granulomatosis and idiopathic necrotizing crescentic glomerulonephritis are all associated with ANCA, but in somewhat different patterns. There is a strong correlation between the presence of ANCA and glomerular involvement in systemic vasculitis. However the precise mechanism(s) by which ANCA contribute to the pathogenesis of the vasculitic diseases is not understood. The value of ANCA titers for monitoring the activity of renal vasculitis is controversial.

Prevalence of ANCA in renal vasculitis

Type of renal vasculitis	ANCA test positivity (%) P-ANCA or Anti-MPO	ANCA test positivity (%) C-ANCA or Anti-PR3
Polyarteritis nodosa	10–20	10–20
Microscopic polyangiitis	50–80	10–20
Wegener's granulomatosis	10–20	80–90
Necrotizing and crescentic GN	50–80	10–20

MPO, myeloperoxidase; PR3, proteinase 3.

Table 79.1 Prevalence of ANCA in renal vasculitis.

Treatment and prognosis

Renal involvement in these vasculitides tends to be severe and fulminant. Even with early diagnosis, approximately one-third of patients will progress to renal failure within 5 years. Relapsing courses are common in patients with microscopic polyangiitis and Wegener's granulomatosis.[64–66] Glucocorticoids are important in the early treatment of renal vasculitis, but their long-term efficacy is limited, Maintenance should include alternate-day therapy whenever possible.

In patients with rapidly progressive glomerulonephritis, pulse methylprednisolone, followed by prednisone and daily cyclophosphamide, is commonly instituted. Plasma exchange has also been added in cases of aggressive pulmonary–renal syndrome,[67] but its value is not proven.

Although controversial, some recent experience indicates that intermittent pulse cyclophosphamide may be substituted for daily cyclophosphamide in order to reduce the toxicity of extended therapy in ANCA-associated glomerulonephritis.[65,68] Wegener's granulomatosis is generally considered an exception to this recommendation, in which case most investigators advocate daily cyclophosphamide for remission induction therapy, with conversion to azathioprine, mycophenolate or methotrexate for maintenance.[69,70] Cyclosporine has not proved to be an effective alternative to conventional cytotoxic drugs, either as primary therapy or in preventing renal relapse following kidney transplantation.[71]

ANTI-GBM ANTIBODY-MEDIATED NEPHRITIS: GOODPASTURE'S SYNDROME

Goodpasture's syndrome is a rare but classic cause of severe pulmonary–renal syndrome (Chapter 84).[72] Its essential components include pulmonary hemorrhage and rapidly progressive glomerulonephritis, both of which are characteristically (but not universally) fulminant. The cardinal pathogenic factor is autoantibody to a component of type IV collagen present in the capillary basement membranes of the lung and kidney. These autoantibodies are called antiglomerular basement membrane (anti-GBM) antibodies because glomerular antigens are normally used for their detection in immunoassays. The immunopathogenesis of Goodpasture's syndrome is unknown. Iatrogenic cases of anti-GBM disease have occurred when normal kidneys have been transplanted into patients with hereditary Alport's nephropathy who lack the normal GBM antigen and tolerance thereto. Such patients mount an anti-GBM antibody response to the neoantigen. Evidence suggests that anti-GBM antibodies are expressed for a limited duration (weeks to months) in Goodpasture's syndrome. This is of little consolation because of the devastating nature of the disease during the height of the pulmonary–renal syndrome. Hence, aggressive treatment with pulse methylprednisolone, cyclophosphamide and plasma exchange is indicated early in the course of Goodpasture's disease (Chapter 84).[73] Renal disease is unlikely to be reversible if renal function is substantially impaired or oliguria ensues before treatment is begun. Immunosuppressive treatment is normally continued until the patient has been in sustained clinical remission and anti-GBM titers are minimal or absent for at least 3 months.

RENAL INVOLVEMENT IN SELECTED SYSTEMIC CONNECTIVE TISSUE DISEASES

Lupus nephritis

Renal involvement affects most patients with systemic lupus erythematosus (SLE) (see Chapter 60). Lupus nephritis has a wide spectrum of disease expressions and outcomes in different patient populations; in particular, it generally exhibits a substantially more ominous prognosis and poorer response to treatment in Black patients than in Whites.[74,75] Nephritis is a major cause of morbidity and mortality, and accounts for a large proportion of all hospital admissions in the lupus population. The majority of patients experience chronic renal disease with remissions and exacerbations.

Pathogenesis

Several different mechanisms appear to be involved in the pathogenesis of lupus nephritis, resulting in a wide spectrum of renal lesions (see Chapter 60). DNA and anti-DNA antibodies are known to be concentrated in glomerular deposits in the subendothelial location and are likely to play a central role in the pathogenesis of proliferative lupus nephritis. Deposition of immune complexes from the circulation into the kidney and in situ complex formation may both be important in the pathogenesis of proliferative lupus nephritis; however, only a subset of immune complexes appears to be nephritogenic. Unfortunately, there are fewer insights into the pathogenesis of the lupus membranous nephropathy with its characteristic epimembranous immune deposits. Although T cells are almost certainly involved in autoantibody production, it is unknown whether they have a direct role in the pathogenesis of lupus nephritis.

Clinical features

Asymptomatic hematuria or proteinuria may be the presenting feature, but they often progress to nephritic and/or nephrotic syndromes. Nephrotic syndrome is seen in both severe proliferative and membranous forms of lupus nephritis. Hypertension, azotemia, nephritic urine sediment (with hematuria and cellular casts), hypocomplementemia and high anti-DNA titers are more commonly found in patients with proliferative lupus nephritis. Rapidly progressive glomerulonephritis is usually associated with the appearance of cellular crescents and may be superimposed on severe proliferative or membranous forms of lupus nephritis.[76]

Diagnosis

Proper evaluation of the urinary sediment is very helpful in assessing and monitoring renal disease activity. Active glomerulonephritis is indicated by hematuria (with dysmorphic erythrocytes) as well as cellular casts. Broad and/or waxy casts indicate long-standing or advanced glomerulonephritis. Serum complement levels (especially C3 and C4) have been found to correlate with glomerular disease activity on renal biopsy. Falling levels of complement components may indicate a flare of lupus nephritis; other tests (including anti-DNA antibodies) are less reliable. Therapeutic decisions should not be based on serologic tests alone because none of these have adequate sensitivity or specificity to justify treatment decisions. Renal biopsy is indicated only if the patient has laboratory evidence of urinary abnormalities.

The most widely used scheme for the classification of renal biopsy in lupus nephritis is that of the World Health Organization (WHO) (Figs. 79.9–79.12) (Chapter 60). In addition, scoring of

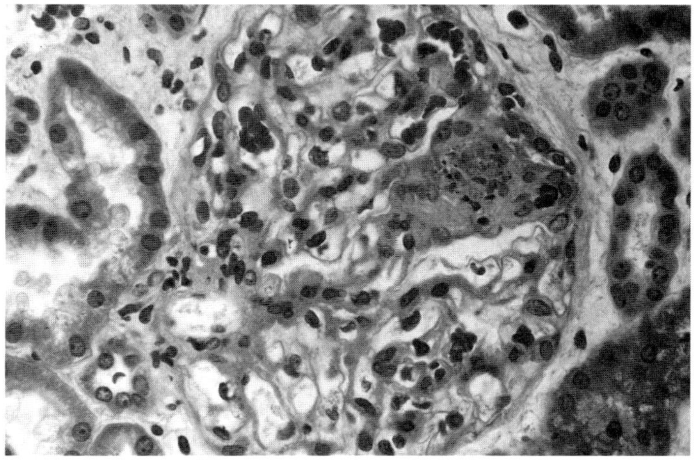

Figure 79.9 Focal proliferative lupus nephritis. The solid lesion at the right demonstrates segmental fibrinoid necrosis. Note the nuclear fragments (karyorrhexis) in the fibrinous exudate. Hematoxylin and eosin.

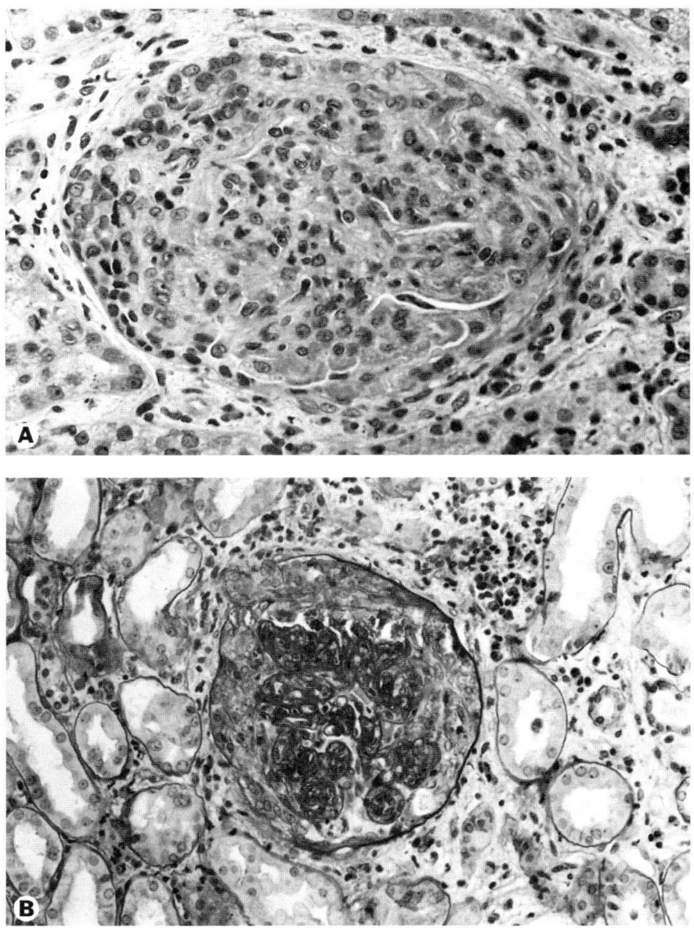

Figure 79.10 Diffuse proliferative lupus nephritis. (**A**) The glomerulus is globally affected with proliferating and swollen cells; these processes severely compromise the circulatory space of the glomerulus which also contains a cellular crescent. Hematoxylin and eosin. (**B**) The glomerulus exhibits a more advanced fibrocellular crescent. Its circumferential position has produced a global collapse of the glomerular tuft. This lesion is likely destined to 'heal' by sclerosis. PAS stain.

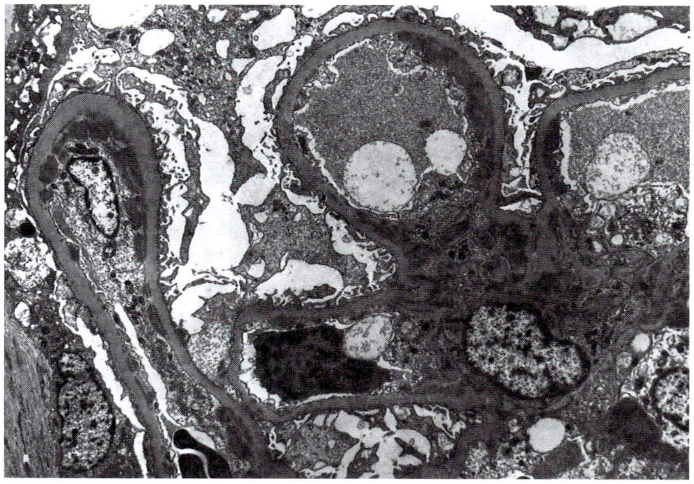

Figure 79.11 Proliferative lupus nephritis. This electron micrograph demonstrates the characteristic mesangial deposits (dark materials dispersed within the centrally located amorphous gray mesangial matrix) and subendothelial deposits (dark materials extending along the peripheral capillary loops).

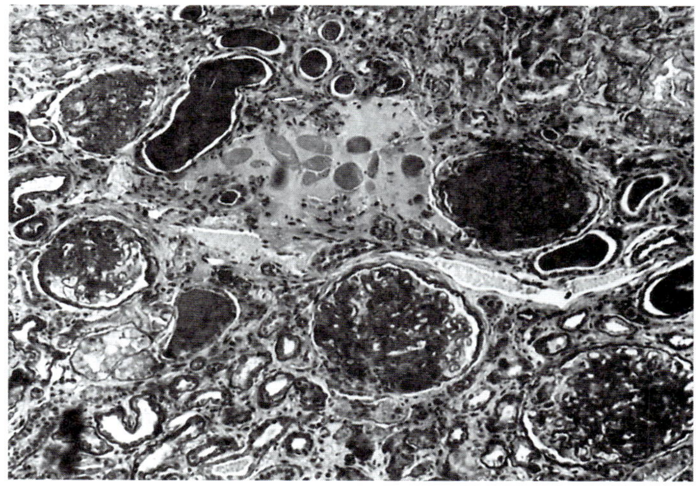

Figure 79.12 Advanced chronic lupus nephritis. This section demonstrates features of atrophy, sclerosis and fibrosis resulting from persistently active lupus nephritis. Two glomeruli are completely hyalinized and the others are compromised by marked mesangial expansion, which is a precursor to glomerulosclerosis. The tubules show loss of epithelial lining cells, broad waxy (renal failure) casts, and separation by bands of fibrous connective tissue. This patient entered chronic dialysis within 1 year of this biopsy. (Masson trichrome.)

the type and extent of individual lesions is widely accepted in evaluating renal biopsies in lupus patients. A composite score (Activity index) can be made for selected histologic features that represent active (potentially reversible) lesions. A different score (Chronicity index) attempts to quantity chronic, sclerosing, atrophic and/or fibrosing (i.e. irreversible) lesions. The combination of WHO classification with the Activity and Chronicity Indices provides useful information, both therapeutic and prognostic. A summary of the histologic features in each WHO class is presented in Table 79.2. Transitions between the different classes are common.

Treatment

Treatment of mesangial lupus nephritis is usually not indicated unless protein excretion exceeds 2 g/day.[77] However, distinguishing between early mesangial lesions that are in transition to more ominous classes from those that reflect mild and stable nephropathy is difficult. Patients with focal or diffuse proliferative glomerulonephritis with a relative paucity of activity and/or chronicity features on renal biopsy may benefit from oral glucocorticoids or monthly pulses of intravenous methylprednisolone.[77,78] A prolonged course of intravenous cyclophosphamide pulses is more efficacious than pulses of methylprednisolone in

Table 79.2 WHO classification of lupus nephritis.

WHO classification of lupus nephritis

WHO Class	Histologic features/comments
I Normal	No evidence of changes by light microscopy (LM), immunofluorescence (IF) or electron microscopy (EM)
II Mesangial	Abnormalities limited to the mesangium; mesangial disease represents the lowest common denominator of lupus nephritis LM: increased mesangial cellularity and/or matrix IF and EM: mesangial immune deposits
III Focal proliferative	Glomerular capillary obliteration in $<50\%$ of nephrons. LM: Increased numbers of mesangial, endothelial and/or hematogenous cells. Active inflammatory lesions (karyorrhexis, fibrinoid necrosis, adhesion to Bowman's capsule, cellular crescents, interstitial inflammatory infiltrates). Wire loop lesions. Hyaline thrombi IF and EM: Mesangial and peripheral capillary loop (subendothelial) immune complex deposits
IV Diffuse proliferative	Qualitatively similar histologic lesions as in Class III. Glomerular capillary obliteration involving more than 50% of nephrons
V Membranous	LM: Regular thickening of the peripheral capillary loops of the glomerulus. Mesangial expansion EM: Subepithelial, intramembranous, mesangial (but no or very rare subendothelial) immune complex deposits

patients with severe focal or diffuse proliferative nephritis.[77,79] Plasmapheresis offers no significant advantage over cytotoxic therapy.[80,81] Controlled studies have shown that intermittent pulse cyclophosphamide is more effective than either high-dose conventional prednisone or extended courses of pulse methylprednisolone therapy.[82,83] Indeed, pulse cyclophosphamide therapy has become the standard treatment for severe proliferative lupus nephritis. Studies suggest that treatment should continue for at least 1 year after the remission of renal disease to prevent exacerbations.[84]

Pulse cyclophosphamide is not universally effective and is associated with several undesirable side-effects, particularly gonadal failure. Hence, alternative treatment regimens, including mycophenolate,[85] immunoablation without[86] or with stem cell reconstitution,[87] and immunological costimulation inhibitors, continue to be explored for the treatment of severe lupus nephritis.[88]

Definitive therapeutic guidelines have not been established for lupus membranous nephropathy. High-dose alternate-day glucocorticoids, cyclophosphamide and cyclosporine have been used, with mixed results.[89,90] The preliminary results of a prospective controlled trial indicate that both cyclophosphamide and cyclosporine are more effective than steroids alone in inducing complete remission of proteinuria in lupus membranous nephropathy (Austin and Balow, unpublished observations).

Scleroderma (systemic sclerosis)

Renal disease occurs in the diffuse form of systemic sclerosis and is a major cause of morbidity and mortality in these patients. (Chapter 64). Patients with renal disease may experience rapidly progressive disease and early death.

Renal disease in scleroderma covers a spectrum of manifestations, with a slowly progressive form of chronic renal disease at the one extreme and acute scleroderma renal crisis at the other (Fig. 79.13).[91] Proteinuria, urine sediment abnormalities (hematuria or pyuria), hypertension and renal insufficiency are markers of impending renal disease and should alert the physician to this possibility. Rapid progression of skin disease has also been associated with an increased frequency of renal crisis. Renal disease is more likely to occur in the first 5 years of the disease. Plasma renin activity increases with the onset of renal injury but there is no convincing evidence that the rise precedes the onset of scleroderma renal crisis.

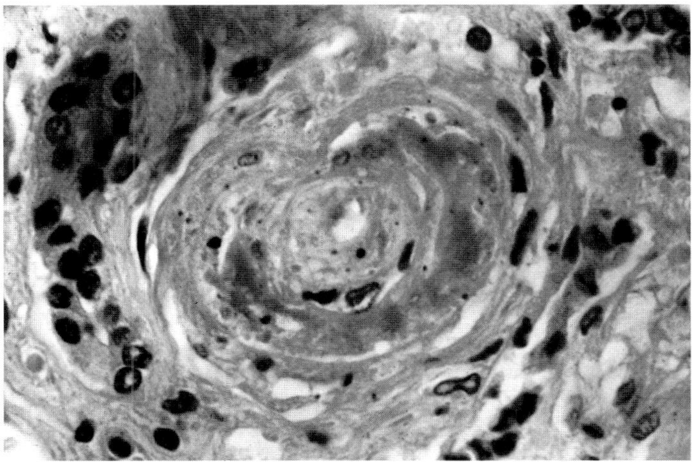

Figure 79.13 Scleroderma renal crisis. The renal arteriole demonstrates extensive fibrin deposition (dark material) within multiple layers of its wall. The lumen is further compromised by severe swelling and intimal hyperplasia.

Scleroderma renal crisis is characterized by malignant hypertension, rapid deterioration of renal function and proteinuria (usually nonnephrotic) (Chapter 64). Rapid deterioration of renal function alone in the absence of hypertension can occur in some patients with scleroderma renal crisis. The primary pathogenic process appears to be a renal vasculopathy involving predominantly the interlobular arteries and arterioles. Marked intimal thickening with an attendant 'mucoid' appearance, and fibrinoid necrosis in the absence of vasculitis, are common and characteristic of the disease. Adventitial fibrosis is often observed. Glomeruli typically exhibit ischemic changes but in severe cases may develop crescents. Immune deposits are rarely observed by fluorescence or electron microscopy studies. Hyperplasia of the juxtaglomerular apparatus may be common and correlates with the presence of hypereninemia. Renal cortical flow is markedly reduced, with an attendant reduction in glomerular filtration rate.

The most significant therapeutic advance in the treatment of renal involvement is the use of angiotensin-converting enzyme inhibitors and angiotensin receptor antagonists, which have dramatically increased the 1-year survival of patients with scleroderma renal crisis.[92] Despite this initial improvement, approximately half will subsequently progress to death or renal failure. Survival of patients undergoing any form of treatment for end-stage renal disease due to scleroderma (hemodialysis, peritoneal dialysis or transplantation) has been poor.[93]

Sjögren's syndrome

A variety of renal manifestations occur in approximately one-third of patients with primary Sjögren's syndrome (Chapter 63), including tubular dysfunction (distal or proximal tubular acidosis, nephrogenic diabetes insipidus), nephrocalcinosis, interstitial nephritis, pseudolymphoma, necrotizing vasculitis and glomerulopathy.[94] Mild, nonspecific glomerular changes are common, but overt glomerular disease is rare. Membranous nephropathy and proliferative glomerulonephritis (focal or diffuse, and membranoproliferative) have been reported in primary Sjögren's syndrome. In such cases the possibility of overlap with systemic lupus should be considered.

Rheumatoid arthritis

Although early studies described a condition called rheumatoid glomerulonephritis, several investigators have questioned whether a specific nephritis related to rheumatoid is arthritis does in fact exist.[95] From a clinical standpoint, renal disease from drugs used for its therapy or secondary amyloidosis developing as a result of the disease are more common.

Membranous nephropathy in the setting of rheumatoid arthritis may be a complication of gold or D-penicillamine therapy. Its pathogenesis is poorly understood. In most cases proteinuria resolves spontaneously after the cessation of therapy. Mesangial glomerulonephritis has been described in several patients with rheumatoid arthritis who had renal biopsy because of hematuria and/or proteinuria. Some of these patients were also receiving gold or penicillamine therapy, whereas in others the renal disease was classified as IgA glomerulonephritis. In a number of patients there is an association between high titers of rheumatoid factor and the occurrence of mesangial nephritis, leading to the hypothesis that the renal lesion represents a functional response of the mesangium to remove IgM rheumatoid factor–IgG complexes. Proliferative glomerulonephritis is extremely rare and may be found in patients with rheumatoid vasculitis. Rheumatoid arthritis can be a cause of secondary amyloidosis.[95]

RENAL DISEASES IN DYSPROTEINEMIAS AND PARAPROTEINEMIAS

Multiple myeloma

Multiple myeloma results from a neoplastic proliferation of plasma cells which produce one or more abnormal monoclonal proteins (M-proteins) (Chapter 97). Abnormal bands of immunoglobulin light or heavy chains are present in the urine of 50–70% of patients with myeloma. These paraproteins have a predilection to precipitate in the tubular lumina to produce the so-called cast nephropathy or myeloma kidney. Acute renal failure (precipitated by dehydration or contrast dyes) and chronic renal failure may result from the cast tubulopathy. Distal renal tubular acidosis may also occur as a manifestation of myeloma protein deposition in renal tubules. Myeloma paraproteins are not detected by urine protein dipstick methods. Urinary protein electrophoresis and immunofixation electrophoresis are therefore critically important for diagnosis.[4]

Light-chain deposition disease

In light-chain deposition disease monoclonal immunoglobulin light chains, usually κ type, are usually deposited in the vessel walls of multiple organs, especially the renal glomeruli.[96] Proteinuria (accompanied by nephrotic syndrome in about 30% of cases), microscopic hematuria, hypertension and progressive renal failure are common. Renal biopsy shows nodular sclerosing glomerulonephritis (Fig. 79.14) similar to diabetic glomerulosclerosis and amyloidosis. Up to one-third of these patients do not have abnormalities in the serum or urine immunofixation electrophoresis. In such cases the bone marrow may reveal monoclonal plasma cells when stained for κ or λ light chains. Diagnosis depends on finding monoclonal light chains by immunofluorescence studies of renal biopsy tissue. Treatment with prednisone and alkylating agents may halt or reverse the progression of renal failure.

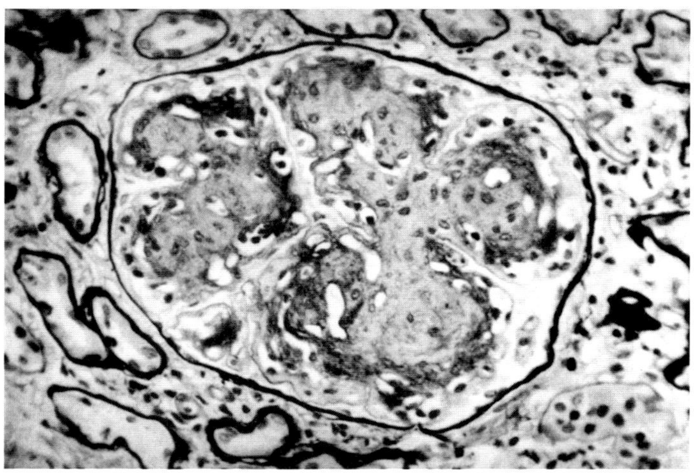

Figure 79.14 Light-chain nephropathy. The glomerulus has the characteristic appearance of an extrinsic deposition disease. The mesangial areas are filled with pale-staining material that produces a lobular pattern and severely compromises the capillary loops. Immunofluorescence studies are needed to distinguish the light-chain deposits from amyloid infiltration. (Silver stain.)

Amyloidosis

Deposition of amyloid fibrils in glomeruli and renal blood vessels is common[97,98] (Chapter 71). Both immunoglobulin-associated (primary, AL) and protein A-associated (secondary, AA) amyloid have been associated with renal involvement.

Proteinuria (often within the nephrotic range) is the most frequently noted presentation and is found in 35–50% of all patients. Hematuria and hypertension are uncommon. Longstanding amyloidosis is regularly accompanied by autonomic neuropathy and postural hypotension. Glomerular involvement is found in all cases of AA amyloidosis, whereas in AL amyloidosis glomerular disease is present in only half of patients.

Deposition of amyloid protein is recognized by the characteristic staining with metachromatic dyes such as Congo red, which exhibits birefringence on polarized light microscopy. Involvement is typically generalized and diffuse in distribution, and not associated with any significant cellular proliferation or glomerular inflammation (Fig. 79.15A). Amyloid deposits initially involve the mesangium, but with progression of the disease process they extend on to the glomerular capillary surfaces, which become markedly and irregularly thickened; this extension ultimately results in capillary luminal occlusion, glomerular obliteration and end-stage renal disease. Amyloid deposits are also found in the intrarenal vasculature, and resemble hyaline arteriosclerosis on hematoxylin and eosin-stained sections. Interstitial deposits of amyloid are associated with foci of tubular atrophy. Electron microscopic findings of fibrillar material with characteristic morphology confirms the diagnosis (Fig. 79.15B).

Treatment of primary AL amyloidosis with cytotoxic agents has generally not resulted in favorable long-term outcomes. However, there are some recent encouraging reports of salutary effects of aggressive cytotoxic drug therapy with stem cell reconstitution.[99] For patients with secondary amyloidosis control of the underlying diseases may prevent, stabilize or even reverse this process. Colchicine can prevent the deposition of amyloid in familial Mediterranean fever if started early.

Cryoglobulinemia

Cryoglobulins (immunoglobulins that reversibly precipitate on cooling) are present in the serum of patients with a wide variety of autoimmune, lymphoproliferative and infectious diseases. Cryoglobulinemia with membranoproliferative glomerulonephritis secondary to chronic hepatitis C is the most common variety and is discussed earlier. Essential mixed cryoglobulinemia (ECM) is an idiopathic clinical syndrome consisting of recurrent episodes of palpable purpura involving the lower extremities, constitutional symptoms, arthralgias, vasculitis, hepatosplenomegaly, lymphadenopathy and neuropathy.[100]

Renal complications are common with mixed cryoglobulinemia. A waxing and waning course is characteristic of this disease. Glomerular involvement may develop acutely, particularly after dehydration or exposure to cold, and may be associated with oliguric acute renal failure. Other clinical syndromes may also occur, including nephrotic syndrome, hematuria, renal insufficiency, and chronic or rapidly progressive glomerulonephritis. Deposition of cryoglobulins usually occurs in the glomerular subendothelial space, and these deposits exhibit a unique fibrillar appearance on electron microscopy (Fig. 79.16). The glomerulonephritis is typically membranoproliferative and/or crescentic in nature. Large eosinophilic, PAS-positive intraluminal deposits ('thrombi') are found in more than one-third of patients.

Treatment with combinations of glucocorticoids, cytotoxic drugs and plasma exchange has been successful in controlling cryoglobulinemic nephritis. Spontaneous remissions can occur. Patients with rapid deterioration of renal function may benefit from intravenous glucocorticoid pulses. Interferon-α has been shown to be efficacious in small nonrandomized studies, even in patients refractory to conventional therapy.

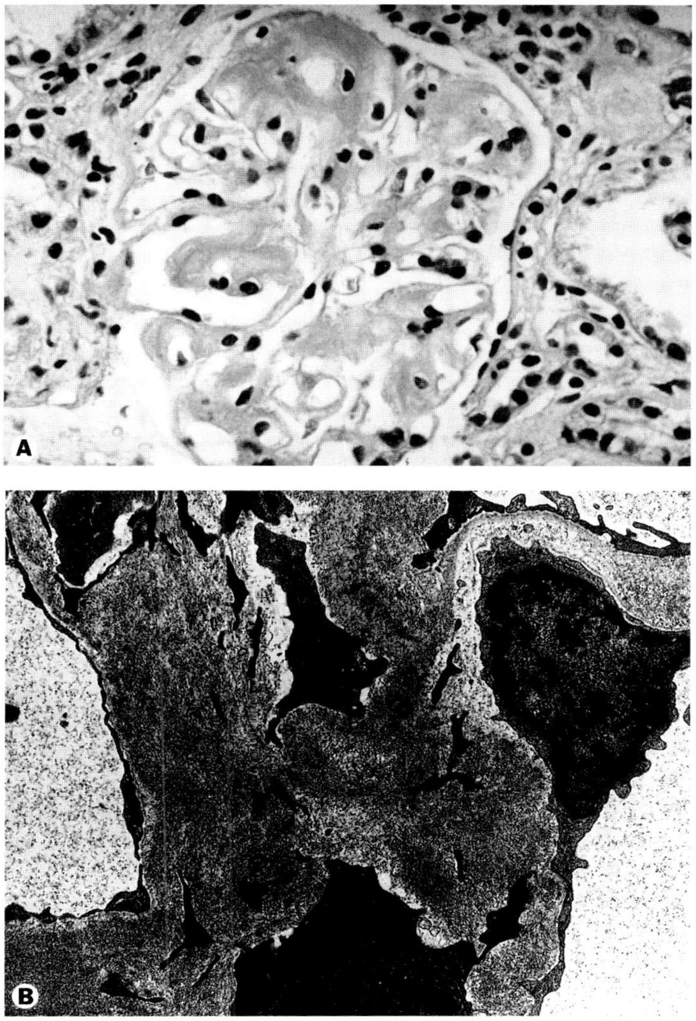

Figure 15 Amyloidosis of the kidney. (**A**) The glomerulus contains pale-staining amorphous material in and around several capillary loops. This material is birefringent when stained with Congo red and examined under polarized light. Hematoxylin and eosin. (**B**) This electron micrograph shows characteristic tangles of fibrillar amyloid within the glomerular capillary wall. (Electron micrographs courtesy of Drs. T. Antonovych and S. Sabnis, Armed Forces Institute of Pathology, Washington DC.)

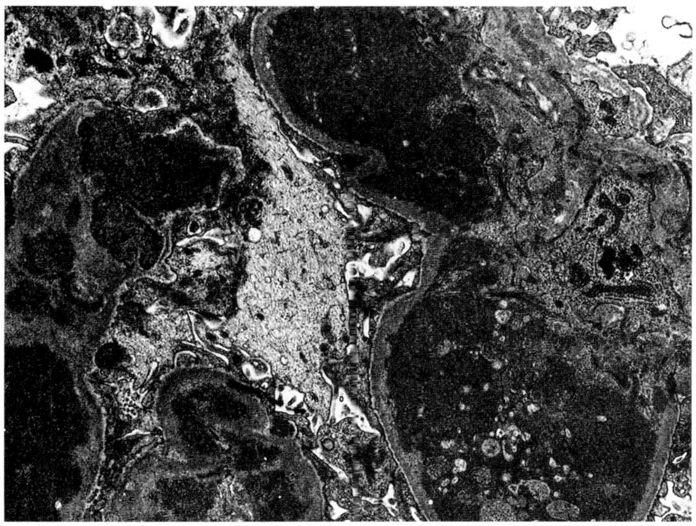

Figure 16 Cryoglobulinemic nephropathy. This electron micrograph demonstrates dense material completely filling the glomerular capillary lumina. By light microscopy these capillary 'plugs' have the appearance of microvascular thrombi, but ultrastructural studies show the crystalline structure of immune aggregates, not fibrin tactoids. (Electron micrographs courtesy of Drs T. Antonovych and S. Sabnis, Armed Forces Institute of Pathology; Washington DC.)

REFERENCES

1. Fogazzi GB, Ponticelli C, Ritz E. The urinary sediment: an integrated view, 2nd edn. Oxford, Oxford University Press, 1999;1.
2. Levy AS. Clinical evaluation of renal function. In: Greenberg A, ed. Primer on kidney diseases, 2nd edn. San Diego, Academic Press, 1998;20.
3. Churg J, Bernstein J, Glassock RJ. Renal disease: classification and atlas of glomerular diseases, 2nd edn. New York, Igaku-Shoin, 1995;1.
4. Levinson SS. Urine protein electrophoresis and immunofixation electrophoresis supplement one another in characterizing proteinuria. Ann Clin Lab Sci 2000; 30:79.
5. Shaw GA, Croker BP, Tisher CC. Renal biopsy as a guide to the treatment of glomerulonephritis. In: Brady HR, Wilcox CS, eds. Therapy in nephrology and hypertension. Philadelphia, WB Saunders, 1999,81.
6. Cameron JS. The long-term outcome of glomerular disease. In: Schrier RW, Gottschalk CW, eds. Diseases of the kidney, 6th edn. Boston, Little Brown, 1997;1919.
7. Dember LM, Salant DJ. Minimal change disease. In: Brady HR, Wilcox CS, eds. Therapy in nephrology and hypertension. Philadelphia, WB Saunders, 1999;165.
8. Niaudet P. Comparison of cyclosporine and chlorambucil in the treatment of steroid-dependent idiopathic nephrotic syndrome. Pediatr Nephrol 1992;6:1.
9. Klein M, Radhakrishnan J, Appel G. Cyclosporine treatment of glomerular diseases. Annu Rev Med 1999;50:1.
10. Mak SK, Short CD, Mallick NP. Long-term outcome of adult-onset minimal-change nephropathy. Nephrol Dial Transplant 1996;11:2192.
11. Fogo A, Hawkins EP, Berry PL, et al. Glomerular hypertrophy in minimal change disease predicts subsequent progression to focal segmental glomerular sclerosis. Kidney Int 1990;38:115.
12. Singh HK, Baldree LA, McKenney DW, et al. Idiopathic collapsing glomerulopathy in children. Pediatr Nephrol 2000;14:132.

13. Schwartz MM, Evans J, Bain R, Korbet SM. Focal segmental glomerulosclerosis: prognostic implications of the cellular lesion. J Am Soc Nephrol 1999;10:1900.
14. Sharma M, Sharma R, McCarthy ET, Savin VJ. 'The FSGS factor:' enrichment and in vivo effect of activity from focal segmental glomerulosclerosis plasma. J Am Soc Nephrol 1999;10:552.
15. Lieberman KV, Tejani A. A randomized double-blind placebo-controlled trial of cyclosporine in steroid-resistant idiopathic focal segmental glomerulosclerosis in children. J Am Soc Nephrol 1996;7:56.
16. Cattan DC, Appel GB, Hebert LA, et al. A randomized trial of cyclosporine in patients with steroid-resistant focal segmental glomerulosclerosis. Kidney Int 1999; 56:2220.
17. Cattran DC, Rao P. Long-term outcome in children and adults with classic focal segmental glomerulosclerosis. Am J Kidney Dis 1998;32:72.
18. Korbet SM. Clinical picture and outcome of primary focal segmental glomerulosclerosis. Nephrol Dial Transplant 1999;14 (Suppl 3):68.
19. Feld SM, Figueroa P, Savin V, et al. Plasmapheresis in the treatment of steroid-resistant focal segmental glomerulosclerosis in native kidneys. Am J Kidney Dis 1998;32:230.
20. Savin VJ, Sharma R, Sharma M, et al. Circulating factor associated with increased glomerular permeability to albumin in recurrent focal segmental glomerulosclerosis. N Engl J Med 1996;334:878.
21. Couser WG. Glomerulonephritis. Lancet 1999; 353:1509.
22. Ordonez JD, Hiatt RA, Killebrew EJ, et al. The increased risk of coronary heart disease associated with nephrotic syndrome. Kidney Int 1993;44:638.
23. Cattran DC, Pei Y, Greenwood CM, et al. Validation of a predictive model of idiopathic membranous nephropathy: its clinical and research implications. Kidney Int 1997;51:901.
24. Laluck BJ, Cattran DC. Prognosis after complete remission in adult patients with idiopathic membranous nephropathy. Am J Kidney Dis 1999;33:1026.
25. Austin HA, Falk RJ. Idiopathic membranous nephropathy. In: Brady HR, Wilcox CS, eds. Therapy in nephrology and hypertension. Philadelphia, WB Saunders, 1999,189.
26. Ruggenenti P, Mosconi L, Vendramin G, et al. ACE inhibition improves glomerular size selectivity in patients with idiopathic membranous nephropathy and persistent nephrotic syndrome. Am J Kidney Dis 2000;35:381.
27. Miller G, Zimmerman R, Radhakrishnan J, Appel G. Use of mycophenolate mofetil in resistant membranous nephropathy. Am J Kidney Dis 2000;36:250.
28. Ponticelli C, Altieri P, Scolari F, et al. A randomized study comparing methylprednisolone plus chlorambucil versus methylprednisolone plus cyclophosphamide in idiopathic membranous nephropathy. J Am Soc Nephrol 1998; 9:444.
29. Branten AJ, Reichert LJ, Koene RA, Wetzels JF. Oral cyclophosphamide versus chlorambucil in the treatment of patients with membranous nephropathy and renal insufficiency. Q J Med 1998;91:359.
30. Falk RJ, Hogan SL, Muller KE, Jennette JC. Treatment of progressive membranous glomerulopathy: a randomized trial comparing cyclophosphamide and corticosteroids with corticosteroids alone. Ann Intern Med 1992;116:438.
31. Cattran DC, Greenwood C, Ritchie S, et al. A controlled trial of cyclosporine in patients with progressive membranous nephropathy. Kidney Int 1995;47:1130.
32. Holley KE, Donadio JV. Membranoproliferative glomerulonephritis. In: Tisher CC, Brenner BM, eds. Renal pathology: with clinical and functional correlations, 2nd edn. Philadelphia, JB Lippincott, 1994,294.
33. West CD, McAdams AJ. The alternative pathway C3 convertase and glomerular deposits. Pediatr Nephrol 1999;13:448.
34. Braun MC, West CD, Strife CF. Differences between membranoproliferative glomerulonephritis types I and III in long-term response to an alternate-day prednisone regimen. Am J Kidney Dis 1999;34:1022.
35. D'Amico G. Renal involvement in hepatitis C infection: cryoglobulinemic glomerulonephritis. Kidney Int 1998;54:650.
36. Andresdottir MB, Assmann KJ, Hoitsma AJ, et al. Recurrence of type I membranoproliferative glomerulonephritis after renal transplantation: analysis of the incidence, risk factors, and impact on graft survival. Transplantation 1997; 63:1628.
37. Johnson RJ, Couser WG. Hepatitis B infection and renal disease: clinical, immunopathogenetic and therapeutic considerations. Kidney Int 1990;37:663.
38. Conjeevaram HS, Hoofnagle JH, Austin HA, et al. Long term outcome of hepatitis B virus related glomerulonephritis after therapy with interferon alfa. Gastroenterology 1995;109:540.
39. Daghestani L, Pomeroy C. Renal manifestations of hepatitis C infection. Am J Med 1999;106:347.
40. Jefferson JA, Johnson RJ. Treatment of hepatitis C associated glomerular disease. Semin Nephrol 2000;20:286.
41. Kopp JB, Balow JE. Renal complications. In: DeVita VT, Hellman S, Rosenberg SA, eds. AIDS: etiology, diagnosis, treatment and prevention, 4th edn. Philadelphia, Lippincott-Raven, 1997,423.
42. Klotman PE. HIV-associated nephropathy. Kidney Int 1999;56:1161.
43. Kopp JB, Miller KD, Mican JA, et al. Crystalluria and urinary tract abnormalities associated with indinavir. Ann Intern Med 1997;127:119.
44. Tejani A, Ingulli E. Poststreptococcal glomerulonephritis. Current clinical and pathologic concepts. Nephron 1990;55:1
45. Montseny JJ, Meyrier A, Kleinknecht D, Callard P. The current spectrum of infectious glomerulonephritis: experience with 76 patients and review of the literature. Medicine (Baltimore) 1995;74:63.
46. Jaffner D, Schindera F, Aschoff A, et al. The clinical spectrum of shunt nephritis. Nephrol Dial Transplant 1997;12:1143.
47. Choi HK, Lamprecht P, Niles JL, et al. Subacute bacterial endocarditis with positive cytoplasmic antineutrophil cytoplasmic antibodies and anti-proteinase 3 antibodies. Arthritis Rheum 2000;43:226.
48. Hunte W, al-Ghraoui F, Cohen RJ. Secondary syphilis and the nephrotic syndrome. Am J Kidney Dis 1993;3:1351.
49. Barsoum RS. Schistosomal glomerulopathies. Kidney Int 1993;44:1.
50. Schena FP. A retrospective analysis of the natural history of primary IgA nephropathy worldwide. Am J Med 1990;89:209.
51. Hunley TE, Kon V. IgA nephropathy. Curr Opin Pediatr 1999;11:152.
52. Alamartine E, Sabatire JC, Guerin C, et al. Prognostic factors in mesangial IgA glomerulonephritis: an extensive study with univariate and multivariate analysis. Am J Kidney Dis 1991;18:12.
53. Donadio JV, Grande JP, Bergstralh EJ, et al. The long-term outcome of patients with IgA nephropathy treated with fish oil in a controlled trial. J Am Soc Nephrol 1999; 10:1772.
54. Roccatello D, Ferro M, Cesano G, et al. Steroid and cyclophosphamide in IgA nephropathy. Nephrol Dial Transplant 2000;15:833.
55. Austin HA, Balow JE. Henoch–Schönlein nephritis: prognostic features and the challenge of therapy. Am J Kidney Dis 1983;2:512.
56. Rai A, Nast C, Adler S. Henoch–Schönlein purpura nephritis. J Am Soc Nephrol 1999;10:2637.
57. Goldstein AR, White RH, Akuse R, et al. Long-term follow-up of childhood Henoch–Schönlein nephritis. Lancet 1992;339:280.
58. Fogazzi GB, Pasquali S, Moriggi M, et al. Long-term outcome of Schönlein–Henoch nephritis in the adult. Clin Nephrol 1989;31:60.
59. Niaudet P, Habib R. Methylprednisolone pulse therapy in the treatment of severe forms of Schönlein–Henoch purpura nephritis. Pediatr Nephrol 1998;12:238.
60. Balow JE, Fauci AS. Vasculitic diseases of the kidney. In: Schrier RW, Gottschalk CW, eds. Diseases of the kidney, 6th edn. Boston, Little Brown, 1997, 1851.
61. Jennette JC, Falk RJ. Small vessel vasculitis. N Engl J Med 1997;337:1512.
62. Harris AA, Falk RJ, Jennette JC. Crescentic glomerulonephritis with a paucity of glomerular immunoglobulin localization. Am J Kidney Dis 1998; 32:179.
63. Savige J, Davies D, Falk RJ, et al. Antineutrophil cytoplasmic antibodies and associated diseases: a review of the clinical and laboratory features. Kidney Int 2000; 57:846.
64. Hoffman GS, Kerr GS, Leavitt RY, et al. Wegener granulomatosis: an analysis of 158 patients. Ann Intern Med 1992;116:488.
65. Nachman PH, Hogan SL, Jennette JC, Falk RJ. Treatment response and relapse in antineutrophil cytoplasmic autoantibody-associated microscopic polyangiitis and glomerulonephritis. J Am Soc Nephrol 1996;7:33.

66. Aasarod K, Iverson BM, Hammerstrom J, et al. Wegener's granulomatosis: clinical course in 108 patients with renal involvement. Nephrol Dial Transplant 2000;15:611.
67. Pusey C, Rees AJ, Evans D, et al. Plasma exchange in focal necrotizing glomerulonephritis without anti-GBM antibodies. Kidney Int 1991;40:757.
68. Kunis CL, Kiss B, Williams G, et al. Intravenous 'pulse' cyclophosphamide therapy of crescentic glomerulonephritis. Clin Nephrol 1992;37:1.
69. Langford CA, Talar-Williams C, Barron KS, Sneller MC. A staged approach to the treatment of Wegener's granulomatosis: induction of remission with glucocorticoids and daily cyclophosphamide switching to methotrexate for remission maintenance. Arthritis Rheum 1999;42:2666.
70. Nowack R, Gobel U, Klooker P, et al. Mycophenolate mofetil for maintenance therapy of Wegener's granulomatosis and microscopic polyangiitis: a pilot study in 11 patients with renal involvement. J Am Soc Nephrol 1999;10:1965.
71. Nachman PH, Segelmark M, Westman K, et al. Recurrent ANCA-associated small vessel vasculitis after transplantation: a pooled analysis. Kidney Int 1999; 56:1544.
72. Bolton WK. Goodpasture's syndrome. Kidney Int 1996; 50:1753.
73. Kluth DC, Rees AJ. Anti-glomerular basement membrane disease. J Am Soc Nephrol 1999;10:2446.
74. Austin HA, Boumpas DT, Vaughan EM. Balow JE. High-risk features of lupus nephritis: importance of race and clinical and histological factors in 166 patients. Nephrol Dial Transplant 1995;19:1670.
75. Dooley MA, Hogan S, Jennette JC, Falk RJ. Cyclophosphamide therapy for lupus nephritis: poor survival in black Americans. Kidney Int 1997;51:1188.
76. Balow JE, Boumpas DT, Austin HA. Systemic lupus erythematosus and the kidney. In: Lahita RG, ed. Systemic lupus erythematosus, third edition. San Diego, Academic Press, 1999; 657.
77. Balow JE, Boumpas DT, Austin HA. Lupus nephritis. In: Brady HR, Wilcox CS, eds. Therapy in nephrology and hypertension. Philadelphia, WB Saunders, 1999, 130.
78. Boumpas DT, Austin HA, Vaughan EM, et al. Controlled trial of pulse methylprednisolone versus two regimens of pulse cyclophosphamide in severe lupus nephritis. Lancet 1992;340:741.
79. Gourley MF, Austin HA, Scott D, et al. Methylprednisolone and cyclophosphamide, alone or in combination, in patients with lupus nephritis: a randomized, controlled trial. Ann Intern Med 1996;125:366.
80. Lewis EJ, Hunsicker LG, Lan S-P, et al. A controlled trial of plasmapheresis therapy in severe lupus nephritis. N Engl J Med 1992;326:1373.
81. Wallace DJ, Goldfinger D, Pepkowitz SH, et al. Randomized controlled trial of pulse/synchronization cyclophosphamide/apheresis for proliferative lupus nephritis. J Clin Apheresis 1998;13:163.
82. Austin HA, Klippel JH, Balow JE, et al. Therapy of lupus nephritis: controlled trial of prednisone and cytotoxic drugs. N Engl J Med 1986;314:614.
83. Balow JE, Austin HA, Muenz LR, et al. Effect of treatment on the evolution of renal abnormalities in lupus nephritis. N Engl J Med 1984;311:491.
84. Moroni G, Quaglini S, Maccario M, Banfi G, Ponticelli C. 'Nephritic flares' are predictors of bad long-term renal outcome in lupus nephritis. Kidney Int 1996; 50:2047
85. Dooley MA, Cosio FG, Nachman PH, et al. Mycophenolate mofetil therapy in lupus nephritis: clinical observations. J Am Soc Nephrol 1999;10:833.
86. Brodsky RA, Petri M, Smith BD, et al. Immunoablative high-dose cyclophosphamide without stem-cell rescue for refractory, severe autoimmune disease. Ann Intern Med 1998;129:1031.
87. Burt RK, Traynor AE, Pope R, et al. Treatment of autoimmune disease by intense immunosuppressive conditioning and autologous hematopoietic stem cell transplantation. Blood 1998;92:3505.
88. Balow JE, Austin HA. Progress in the treatment of proliferative lupus nephritis. Curr Opin Nephrol Hypertens 2000;9:107.
89. Hallegua D, Wallace DJ, Metzgar AL, et al. Cyclosporine for lupus membranous nephritis: experience with ten patients and review of the literature. Lupus 2000;9:241.
90. Austin HA, Balow JE. Treatment of lupus nephritis. Semin Nephrol 2000;20:265.
91. Donohoe JF. Scleroderma and the kidney. Kidney Int 1992;41:562.
92. Steen VD. Scleroderma renal crisis. Rheum Dis Clin North Am 1996;22:861.
93. Chang YJ, Spiera H. Renal transplantation in scleroderma. Medicine (Baltimore) 1999;78:382.
94. Aasarod K, Haga HJ, Berg KJ, et al. Renal involvement in primary Sjogren's syndrome. Q J Med 2000; 93:297.
95. Nakano M, Ueno M, Nishi S, et al. Analysis of renal pathology and drug history in 158 Japanese patients with rheumatoid arthritis. Clin Nephrol 1998;50:154.
96. Buxbaum J, Gallo G. Nonamyloidotic monoclonal immunoglobulin deposition disease. Hematol Oncol Clin North Am 1999;13:1235.
97. Falk RH, Skinner M. The systemic amyloidoses: an overview. Adv Intern Med 2000;45:107.
98. Kyle RA, Gertz MA, Greipp PR, et al. A trial of three regimens for primary amyloidosis: colchicine alone, melphalan and prednisone, and melphalan, prednisone and colchicine. N Engl J Med 1997;336:1202.
99. Comenzo RL, Vosburgh E, Falk RH, et al. Dose-intensive melphalan with blood stem-cell support for the treatment of AL (amyloid light-chain) amyloidosis: survival and responses in 25 patients. Blood 1998;91:3662.
100. Dispenzieri A, Gorevic PD. Cryoglobulinemia. Hematol Oncol Clin North Am 1999;13:1315.

Chapter 80

Myocardial Inflammation

Roger D. Rossen and Douglas L. Mann

A variety of external agents can cause focal or even generalized myocardial cell injury and the accumulation of leukocytes in heart tissues. These include allergic or anaphylactoid reactions, virtually any infectious agent, ischemia, and other traumas. Myocardial inflammation can also result from autoimmune and collagen vascular diseases, systemic vasculitides and neoplastic diseases. All elements of the heart, including the vasculature, connective tissue, myocytes and pericardium, may be involved. The heart is not a passive bystander to proinflammatory stimuli: its response to agents that generate inflammation within it is to produce a diverse array of neurohumoral substances, proteolytic enzymes and cytokines that can cause profound alterations in cardiac structure and function. In the short term these responses are probably compensatory, but in the long term they often cause progressive loss of muscle function and loss of cardiac myocytes. The result is a condition known as dilated cardiomyopathy. Heart failure usually follows and many patients die unless they receive cardiac transplants.

> **KEY CONCEPTS**
>
> **Presentation of myocarditis is highly variable**
> - Patients present:
>   - Without symptoms (most common)
>   - With slowly progressive cardiac insufficiency resulting in dilated cardiomyopathy
>   - With syncope caused by cardiac arrhythmias
>   - With thromboembolism caused by intraventricular clots
>   - With fulminant congestive heart failure

CLINICAL FEATURES OF MYOCARDIAL INFLAMMATION

Affected individuals are frequently asymptomatic at first. Much later they may develop evidence of left ventricular dilation and then signs and symptoms of heart failure. They may also experience systemic or pulmonary embolism as a first sign of this condition. Because of the frequently long asymptomatic interval it is rarely possible to assign an etiologic diagnosis for most of the 2 million patients under treatment for dilated cardiomyopathy in the USA.[1] Acute myocarditis may present at the outset with fulminant congestive heart failure, or with less dramatic evidence of cardiac insufficiency. Symptomatic patients can recover completely, or they may progress to severe, intractable heart failure within a matter of months. For the latter group, long-term survival prospects are not promising. According to a 1994 report, approximately 200 000–250 000 people die annually of congestive heart failure following the development of dilated cardiomyopathy.[2] A more recently published study of patients with biopsy-documented myocarditis showed, paradoxically, that 93% of the relatively small subset that had fulminant disease survived for 11 years, but only 45% of the majority who had acute or subacute manifestations of myocarditis survived for that interval.[3]

Initially, symptoms are often nonspecific and may include fatigue, dyspnea and, less frequently, palpitations; these symptoms may not call attention to the heart as the source of the problem. Some patients may have vague precordial discomfort and experience syncope. It is important to establish whether precordial discomfort varies with respiration or position, as may occur with pericarditis. Syncope may indicate atrioventricular (AV) conduction block and require urgent treatment, possibly pacemaker implantation.[4] Typically, only patients with fulminant myocarditis are febrile.[5] These patients also have extreme fatigue, orthopnea and dyspnea on exertion or at rest, together with rapidly developing peripheral edema.[3] Rapid onset of congestive heart failure in these cases often follows 2 weeks after an otherwise nondescript viral illness. Hemodynamic compromise may be sufficient to require immediate hospitalization, treatment with vasopressors or even a left ventricular assist device.

PHYSICAL EXAMINATION

Except in those who also have pericarditis and may have a friction rub, the physical examination is often unrevealing.[6] Tachycardia is generally present, however, even in the absence of fever. Heart size may be normal in clinically silent cases, or massively enlarged in patients with dilated cardiomyopathy and congestive heart failure. On auscultation the first heart sound may be muffled; the second heart sound is generally normal unless there is AV block or severe left ventricular dysfunction. In these cases there may be paradoxical splitting of the second heart sound. There may be a transient apical systolic murmur or, in cases with heart failure, a protodiastolic gallop. Diastolic murmurs are rare unless the inflammatory process includes the heart valves, as may occur in acute rheumatic fever or infective endocarditis. Evidence of heart failure includes rales, neck vein distention, and sometimes dependent peripheral edema.

LABORATORY EVALUATION

Rhythm disorders occur more frequently than symptoms or physical findings. These may include AV and intraventricular conduction defects and atrial and ventricular arrhythmias. Transient electocardiographic abnormalities include ST segment and T-wave abnormalities. Q-waves are rarely seen. Complete AV block, although rare, may cause sudden death; it has been specifically noted as a feature of carditis caused by *Borrelia burgdorferi*, the infectious agent that causes Lyme disease.[7]

Chest radiographs in asymptomatic patients show a generally unremarkable heart size and configuration. In patients with heart failure one sees the expected cardiac enlargement and pulmonary congestion characteristic of this condition. Echocardiography may demonstrate either regional or global left ventricular dysfunction. This test may also reveal left ventricular thrombi, thickening of the atrioventricular valves and, in some cases, pericardial effusions. Doppler echocardiography may show mild regurgitant valvular disease and demonstrate abnormal diastolic filling, even when the systolic function remains normal.

Radioisotopic imaging can be used to identify foci of inflammation within the heart. The inflammation avid isotope, gallium-67 (^{67}Ga) is reported to be quite sensitive in detecting active myocarditis.[8] 99m-Technetium (^{99m}Tc) pyrophosphate is not reported to be helpful in humans.[6] However ^{111}In-labeled antimyosin antibodies can be used to detect intracardiac inflammation and necrotic regions in the heart.[9] Recently EKG-triggered T_1-weighted images obtained by gadolinium-enhanced MRI has been used to investigate the hearts of patients with suspected myocarditis.[10] In Chagas' disease the images obtained by gadolinium-enhanced MRI have been used to guide myocardial biopsies.[11]

Theoretically, myocardial damage should result in elevated circulating levels of the MB fraction of creatine kinase (CK-MB). However, even in patients with biopsy-proven disease plasma CK-MB levels are infrequently abnormal. On the other hand, increased cardiac troponin I levels were noted in 15 of 25 of patients tested within the first month following the onset of heart failure. This test may also be useful, at least early in the course of the disease, for monitoring myocardial damage.[12] Other laboratory tests, such as an elevated sedimentation rate, or leukocytosis, only help to support the idea that these patients have an inflammatory process. A fourfold or greater increase in virus-specific antibody titers, as may be found in some patients with cryptic viral myocarditis, provides evidence that the patient has had a recent viral illness. Identification of leukocytic infiltrates in transvenous endomyocardial biopsies is considered to be the closest to a diagnostic gold standard, but this test is only helpful when positive.[6] In order to set up a large multi-institutional collaborative study to test the efficacy of immunosuppressive therapy for myocarditis (Myocardial Treatment Trial), a group of pathologists met in Dallas to develop uniform criteria for the evaluation of cardiac muscle biopsies. According to the 'Dallas criteria, active myocarditis is defined histologically as 'an inflammatory infiltrate of the myocardium with necrosis and/or degeneration of adjacent myocytes not typical of the damage associated with ischemic coronary artery disease'.[13] The character of the inflammatory infiltrates can also be distinctive. For example, myocardial biopsy is the only way to diagnose giant cell myocarditis (also known as granulomatous myocarditis), which is a rare, rapidly fatal disease that sometimes occurs in association with collagen vascular, infectious or hypersensitivity diseases.[14] Figure 80.1 shows the type of myocardial inflammation seen in Chagas' disease and is emblematic of the type of information that one can obtain from endomyocardial biopsy.

The sensitivity and specificity of myocardial biopsies cannot be determined because the only reference standard is provided by autopsy studies. Only 10% of the 2233 patients with recent-onset congestive heart failure screened for the Myocarditis Treatment Trial had endomyocardial evidence of myocarditis that satisfied the Dallas criteria.[15] Because foci of inflammation are often patchy and may come and go with time, it is possible to biopsy at the wrong time or to miss involved tissue. Multiple biopsies and a series of biopsies over time may be needed to make a diagnosis, but this sort of persistence may be justified only if the biopsy is necessary to allocate the patient to a specific treatment protocol. MRI-guided biopsy may be a real advance if it increases the frequency of positive findings.

Routine light microscopy of a myocardial biopsy provides little insight into the possible cause of myocarditis. To take advantage of new and emerging treatments, additional immunohistological studies have been recommended to search for deposits of autoantibodies, neurohumoral agents, and various cytokines that may be pathophysiologically important.[6] Tagged antibodies can be used to probe for viral antigens, and viral nucleic acids can be amplified by the polymerase chain reaction (PCR) to identify likely infectious causes of myocarditis.[16] The presence of viral DNA or RNA in myocardial samples is currently undergoing evaluation as a more sensitive means of diagnosing viral myocarditis. Indeed, enteroviral RNA has been detected in the myocardium of patients at all stages of the disease process, including acute myocarditis and chronic dilated cardiomyopathy. Persistence of viral RNA, particularly enteroviral RNA, has also been implicated in progression to dilated cardiomyopathy. Koide et al detected enteroviral RNA sequences in human endomyocardial biopsy samples in 32% of patients with clinical dilated cardiomyopathy and in 33% of patients with clinical myocarditis, using PCR technology.[17] In their study, patients who had histologic findings of myocarditis and clinical features resembling dilated cardiomyopathy had a high incidence (85%) of enteroviral RNA sequences detected by PCR. Importantly, approximately 25% of patients with dilated cardiomyopathy and no histologic findings of active myocarditis also had enteroviral RNA sequences detected by PCR. However, it bears emphasis that there is a significant variability in the frequency of detection of enteroviral RNA in endomyocardial tissue samples, with values ranging from 0 to 42%. Thus, the validation of PCR technology as a reliable means for diagnosing viral myocarditis will require further refinement and study. Considering the difficulties associated with obtaining endomyocardial biopsies and the resources needed to evaluate these tissue samples, properly this procedure is probably best undertaken in centers with special expertise and as part of a study designed to find qualified patients for new treatment modalities.[18]

DIAGNOSIS OF MYOCARDITIS

The clinical diagnosis of viral myocarditis should be suspected in a patient who presents with signs and symptoms suggestive of dilated cardiomyopathy with no apparent cause, and whose clinical history suggests an antecedent viral illness within the preceding weeks to months. The diagnosis of viral myocarditis is supported by the presence of myocarditis and/or the detection of viral genomic DNA on endomyocardial biopsy, or by the identification of virus in stool, throat washings, blood or pericardial fluid. A fourfold increase in virus neutralizing antibody, complement fixation or hemagglutination inhibition titers is also supportive, although not routinely performed in most clinical settings. As noted above, the examination of the endomyocardial

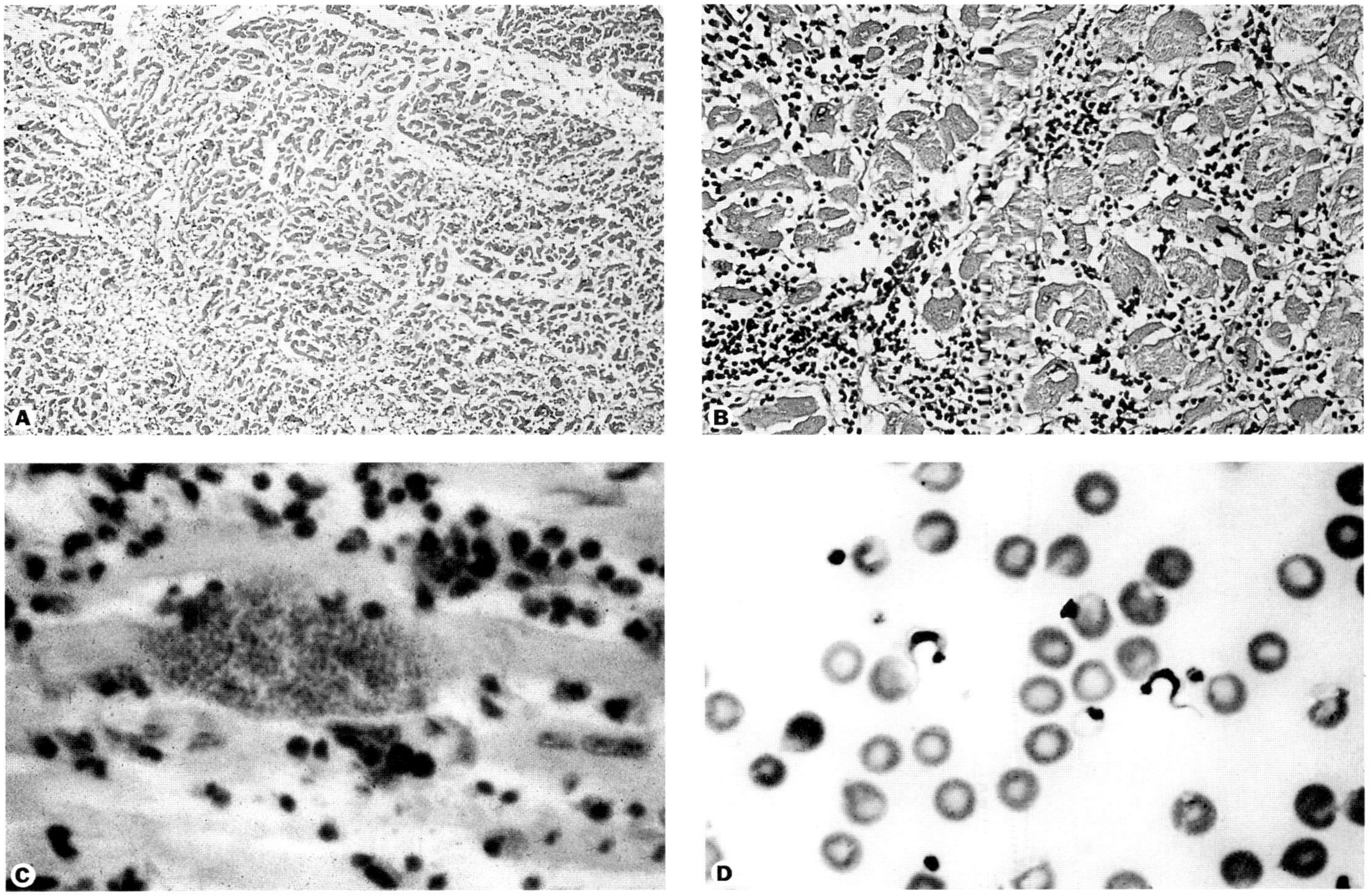

Figure 80.1 Infiltrates of leukocytes in between the muscle bundles is a characteristic feature of myocarditis, regardless of etiology. (**A**) Section of normal myocardium that is generally free of interstitial leukocytes. (**B**) Myocardium from a patient infected with *Trypanosoma cruzi*, the etiologic agent of Chagas' disease or American trypanosomias. Note the many interstitial leukocytes. (**C**) High-power (×1000) view of the predominantly mononuclear infiltrate seen in Chagas' disease. In the middle of this figure is a large pseudocyst containing *Trypanosoma cruzi* amastigotes. (**D**) Giemsa-stained blood smear that contains the characteristic sickle cell-shaped free-swimming trypomastigote form of *T. cruzi*. These trypomastigotes can be found in the peripheral blood of ~25% of infected patients. (Photomicrographs courtesy of Dr Robert M. Genta, Chief of Laboratory Services, the Houston Veterans Affairs Medical Center and Professor, Department of Pathology, Baylor College of Medicine.)

CLINICAL PEARLS

Diagnosis of myocarditis is suspected when there is:

- Dilated cardiomyopathy *not* readily explainable by documented
  - Coronary artery disease
  - Hypertension
  - Congenital cardiomyopathy
- A history of antecedent viral infection
- A history of unexplained cardiac arrhythmias
- Inflammatory cell infiltrates in endomyocardial biopsies

biopsy specimen may be particularly helpful in making a diagnosis of myocarditis. However, the sampling error and differences in interpretation of myocardial biopsies by pathologists who specialize in cardiovascular pathology decreases the overall specificity and sensitivity. The absence of classic findings on a myocardial biopsy does not exclude the diagnosis of myocarditis in a patient with a clinical presentation strongly suggestive of this diagnosis.

MANAGEMENT OF PATIENTS WITH INFLAMMATORY DISEASES OF THE MYOCARDIUM

In many cases myocarditis is a self-limited condition. The course of disease also cannot be predicted. Thus therapy for viral myocarditis is initially supportive and the first requirement is to optimize conventional treatment. In this regard there are two principal aims: 1) to reverse in so far as possible cardiac functional abnormalities, and 2) to control or prevent cardiac arrhythmias.[19] Supportive treatment involves the judicious use of diuretics, vasodilators, β-adrenergic receptor blocking drugs and angiotensin-converting enzyme (ACE) inhibitors. Warfarin is indicated if clots are identified by echocardiography on the ventricular or atrial walls. Stressful exercise should be avoided and patients should be at rest at least initially, based on evidence in murine coxsackie B3 virus myocarditis that exercise increases

THERAPEUTIC PRINCIPLES

Patients with myocarditis with or without dilated cardiomyopathy
- Optimize cardiac function by judicious use of β-blockers, vasodilators, diuretics and angiotensin-converting enzyme antagonists
- Control cardiac arrhythmias
- Encourage bed rest
- Avoid anti-inflammatory drugs and digitalis derivatives, especially in the first 2 weeks

Patients with fulminant myocarditis and congestive heart failure
- Often need aggressive inpatient management:
  - Optimize cardiac contractile function with a left ventricular assist device, if necessary
  - Control arrhythmias
  - Prevent thromboembolic complications
  - Use appropriate immunomodulatory and/or immunosuppressive therapy.
- Often have excellent recovery, if properly supported during acute phase of disease

intracardiac inflammation and necrosis.[6] The use of digoxin is contraindicated during the acute phase of the illness because this drug may aggravate potentially lethal ventricular arrhythmias.

If hemodynamic function is badly compromised the patient may need to be hospitalized for close observation, intravenous medications and mechanical circulatory assistance. Cardiac rhythm in such cases must be closely monitored and appropriate antiarrhythmic agents used to prevent life-threatening ventricular arrythmias or sudden death. Aggressive support for patients with fulminant myocarditis is worth undertaking, not only as a bridge to cardiac transplantation but also because these patients often recover sufficient cardiac function to provide a good quality of life thereafter.[3]

A key decision in patients with myocarditis is whether to begin treatment designed to reverse the inflammatory process and, if so, what type of treatment should be employed. Options include anti-inflammatory drugs, immunosuppressive agents or immunomodulatory therapies. Recently treatment with intravenous immunoglobulin or, paradoxically, removal of the majority of the circulating IgG by non-selective immunoadsorption, has been added to the list of alternatives.[20,21] Another option is treatment with cytokine inhibitors or antagonists.[22] Anti-viral drugs may also help patients who have evidence of a persistent intracardiac viral infection. The large and somewhat disparate array of agents previously used to treat myocarditis and its sequel, dilated cardiomyopathy, probably reflects uncertainty about the pathophysiology of this multifactorial disease process.

The hypothesis that stimulated the Myocardial Treatment Trial was that biopsy-proven lymphocytic myocarditis is driven by an autoimmune response to cardiac tissues that develops idiopathically or as the result of an antecedent viral infection. Previous uncontrolled studies in biopsy-documented myocarditis had suggested that treatment with glucocorticoids, azathioprine, antilymphocyte globulins, cyclosporine or other immunosuppressive agents benefited some patients. The controlled Myocarditis Treatment Trial found that treatment for 24 weeks with prednisone and either azathioprine or cyclosporine did not improve cardiac function or patient survival of 1 year and 4.3 years of follow-up.[23] Subsequently a composite review of all studies in the literature between 1980 and 1997 concurred that immunosuppressive therapy for biopsy-proven myocarditis is ineffective.[24] The Myocardial Treatment Trial was nevertheless criticized for rigidly restricting enrollment to patients with biopsy-proven lymphocytic myocarditis, thereby excluding those who did not fit the diagnostic criteria but who might still have had myocarditis by other criteria. It was also criticized because the treatment period was only 24 weeks, a period considered by some to be too short to see the benefits of immunosuppressive therapy. More importantly, perhaps, it was criticized for failing to identify and exclude patients with active viral myocarditis in whom suppression of the host immune response might increase virus-induced tissue injury, thereby offsetting any therapeutic successes achieved with immunosuppressive drugs in patients who only had cardiac-specific autoimmunity.

Regardless of these criticisms, on the basis of the results of the Myocardial Treatment trial, immunosuppressive therapy is no longer routinely recommended for myocarditis patients with a stable clinical course. However, many clinicians still recommend aggressive immunosuppressive therapy for patients with fulminant myocarditis and/or those who have a deteriorating clinical course. The results of a multicenter study of patients with giant cell myocarditis showed that in the 22 who were treated with glucocorticoids and cyclosporine, azathioprine or both survived for an average of 12.3 months, compared to an average of 3.0 months for the 30 patients who received no immunosuppressive therapy.[14] Of the 34 patients who underwent heart transplantation in this study, nine (26%) had a giant cell infiltrate in the transplanted heart but only one patient died of recurrent giant cell myocarditis. Thus, immunosuppressive therapy appears efficacious in a special subset of patients with myocarditis; the results of this study also suggest that cardiac transplantation may be successfully performed in many patients with fulminant myocarditis.

To address the perceived shortcomings of the Myocarditis Treatment Trial, a group of European clinical investigators has embarked on the 'European Study of the Epidemiology and Treatment of Cardiac Inflammatory Disease (ESETCID). Table 80.1 provides a plan for the evaluation and treatment of myocarditis that is founded on the expanded list of diagnostic measures and corresponding treatments put in place for the ESETCID.[18,25] Immunohistochemical studies of myocardial biopsies are used to evaluate (a) the likelihood that the myocarditis is caused by continued production of virus and/or virus-encoded antigenic subunits, and (b) whether the myocardial inflammation is the result of a humoral and/or cellular immune response against autologous cardiac antigens. The plan of this highly ambitious placebo-controlled trial is, for example, to treat patients with cytomegalovirus-induced myocarditis with immunoglobulin and ganciclovir. Patients with enterovirus-positive myocarditis will be treated with interferon-α. Immunosuppressive drugs will be given only to those with virus-negative inflammatory lesions in the heart. A battery of tests for autoimmune responses to cardiac tissue antigens will also be performed to shore up the rationale for treatment with immunosuppressive drugs. Although the ESETCID has not yet been completed, a preliminary report of

Plan for the evaluation and treatment of patients with myocarditis in the European study of the epidemiology and treatment of cardiac inflammatory disease*

Evaluation

1 Obtain medical history suggestive of cardiac dysfunction
2 Demonstrate cardiac dysfunction by EKG, stress test &/or echocardiography
3 Measure troponin I levels
4 Look for antibodies to the β_1 adrenoreceptor, to cardiac myosin, the adenine nucleotide transporter, and other heart cell-specific antigens.
5 Measure serum proinflammatory cytokines, especially TNF-α and IL-1
6 Obtain cardiac endomyocardial biopsy
- Routine histology: characterize leukocyte infiltrates in cardiac tissue, if present
- Immunocytochemistry and polymerase chain reaction technology to evaluate cardiac tissue for proteins and nucleic acids originating from infectious agents that commonly cause myocarditis

Treatment

1 Optimize medical management with diuretics, vasodilators, digoxin, antiarrhythmia agents, β-adrenoreceptor blocking agents and ACE inhibitors
2 Monitor effects of treatment on cardiac function and serum troponin I
3 Consider adjunctive therapy for special categories of patients with ejection fraction <45% and:
- Viral nucleic acids/proteins in heart: Treat with interferon-α, and/or broad-spectrum antiviral agents, appropriate for the infecting organism
- Circulating autoantibodies to cardiac tissue antigens and deposits of immunoglobulin in cardiac biopsy: Treat with IVIG. If no functional improvement, consider immunoadsorption therapy and/or immunosuppressive medications.
- Mononuclear cell infiltrate in cardiac tissue without evidence of viral proteins or nucleic acids: Treat with immunosuppressive drugs, especially if patients have autoantibodies reactive with cardiac tissue antigens
- High serum TNF-α levels. Treat with infusions of TNF-α scavenging agents

4 Treatments to avoid: Digitalis derivatives, corticosteroids and nonsteroidal anti-inflammatory drugs during the first 2 weeks of the illness
5 The special case of patients with fulminant myocarditis
- Hospitalize and monitor for heart failure and cardiac arrhythmias
- Treat with immunosuppressive drugs
- Provide aggressive functional support, including ventricular assist device, if needed

Table 80.1 Plan for the evaluation and treatment of patients with myocarditis in the European study of the epidemiology and treatment of cardiac inflammatory disease. (Based on the guidelines of the European Study of the Epidemiology and Treatment of Cardiac Inflammatory Disease. Maisch B, Hufnagel G, Schonian U, Hengstenberg C. The European Study of Epidemiology and Treatment of Cardiac Inflammatory Disease (ESETCID). *Eur Heart J* 1995;16:173.)

the endomyocardial biopsies obtained from the 3055 patients recruited so far suggests that 17.2% showed signs of inflammation by light microscopy and had evidence of virus infection.[16] Enterovirus, cytomegalovirus or adenovirus infections could be detected in 11.8% of the patients. Only 6%, however, had an ejection fraction less than 45%, the cut-off that qualified patients for enrollment in one of the treatment arms. Completion of this comprehensive study should greatly improve our understanding of the epidemiology of cardiac inflammation and the modalities available to treat it.

Caution is the watchword in treating intracardiac inflammatory responses. Many patients, even very sick patients, improve on their own or with aggressive supportive therapy. In addition there is the real risk that anti-inflammatory drugs may worsen the prognosis for patients with myocarditis, as they may in patients with ischemia–reperfusion injury. For example, treatment with NSAIDs, including indomethacin, salicylates and ibuprofen, increase tissue necrosis and viral replication in experimental models of acute myocarditis. Therefore, they are generally withheld during the first 2 weeks of viral myocarditis,[6] but they can be safely given in the later phases of the disease process.

ETIOLOGY OF CARDIAC INFLAMMATORY DISORDERS

A recent review lists 60 drugs or chemical agents, exemplified by sympathomimetic agents, anthracycline derivatives and IL-2, that can cause cardiac injury either by direct toxic effects or by their ability to invoke hypersensitivity responses in the heart.[6] Myocarditis can be a prominent feature of over 23 systemic diseases and be caused by more than 50 infectious diseases[6] including 21 viruses, 20 bacteria or spirochetes, four rickettsial species, nine fungal organisms and nine species of protozoa and helminths. The initial host response in almost all cases is directed against the infectious agent, but continued stimulation with the antigens associated with these agents can elicit cardiac-specific autoimmune responses that cause persistent intracardiac inflammation. It has been estimated that autoimmune responses to cardiac tissue antigens after viral myocarditis occur in approximately 10% of patients.[26] Because the interval between the time of the infection and the onset of heart failure is often very great and the patient is frequently asymptomatic during that time, these patients are often classified as having an 'idiopathic' dilated cardiomyopathy. Specific examples of disorders that cause myocardial inflammation are discussed below.

Reactions to drugs and chemicals

Cocaine, a sympathomimetic agent that magnifies the physiological effects of norepinephrine, is one of the more commonly encountered cardiotoxic agents. It increases blood pressure, heart rate and myocardial oxygen demand, and causes spasm of the small and medium arteries. Crack cocaine users may exhibit symptoms and signs of cardiac ischemia and show global cardiac hypokinesia an echocardiography.[27] Histologic examination of cardiac tissue in these patients may show myocarditis, contraction band necrosis (a feature indicative of myocardial cell necrosis) and thickening of the walls of the coronary arteries.

Doxorubicin, an example of the anthracycline class of cancer chemotherapeutic agents, is directly cardiotoxic.[28] It causes cardiac arrhythmias and a pericarditis–myocarditis syndrome characterized by intracardiac leukocyte infiltrates and myocyte necrosis. Although its mechanism of action is not clear, doxorubicin has a high affinity for cardiolipin, a phospholipid of the inner membrane of cardiac mitochondria.[29] Thus it may interfere with the energy metabolism of these cells.

Cardiomyopathy with or without myocarditis has also been seen after treatment with interferon-α chloroquine, emetine, antimony-containing drugs, lithium and many other agents. Interleukin-2 (IL-2) causes a capillary leak syndrome that may provoke cardiac ischemic injury and cause an eosinophilic myocarditis and arrhythmias.[30]

Infectious agents

In the United States viral infections, especially infections with strains of coxsackie B virus, adenoviruses and herpesviruses, are among the most common causes of myocarditis and its sequelae, dilated cardiomyopathy and heart failure.[6] However the link between viral myocarditis and the subsequent development of cardiomyopathy and heart failure is highly variable.

HIV-1 infection is emerging as an important and frequently overlooked cause of heart failure.[31] Approximately one-third of patients dying with HIV infections have evidence of myocarditis. In 80% of these patients no other cause besides HIV infection can explain the myocarditis. Cofactors, including infections with a number of opportunistic infectious agents and Kaposi sarcoma, are implicated in the remainder. Although cardiac failure is only rarely a cause of mortality, signs and symptoms of cardiac dysfunction are common in AIDS patients. Because they may respond symptomatically to conventional treatment for heart failure, this diagnosis should be considered when evaluating HIV-1 infected patients who complain of fatigue, shortness of breath or generalized weakness.

Epidemics of rheumatic fever have been extremely infrequent in North America and other parts of the developed world for more than two generations, but in many parts of the world the demographic and epidemiological factors that cause recurrent infections with 'rheumatogenic' strains of group A streptococci persist[32] (Chapter 63). In these areas, rheumatic fever and the related valvular heart disease are frequently found. For example, a 1980 World Health Organization survey in Peru and Pakistan suggested that up to 5% of school-aged children have evidence of rheumatic valve disease. Rheumatic fever is prototypical of diseases that may cause tissue injury because structural components of the microorganism cross-react immunologically with specific proteins or other tissue components of the host, a phenomenon called molecular mimicry (Chapter 58). A vigorous immune response to the infecting organism results in the expansion of clones of autoreactive T and B lymphocytes, and the production of autoantibodies. Molecular mimicry is not a unique feature of the host response to streptococcal antigens. Recent reports suggest that the immune response to a cysteine-rich outer membrane protein of chlamydia can cross-react with murine heart muscle myosin; similarly, a cross-reaction between myosin and a protein of coxsackie virus 3B has been reported.[33]

Chagas' disease, a result of chronic infection with *Trypanosoma cruzi*, continues to be a frequent cause of myocarditis and heart failure in South and Central America.[34,35] As many as 20 million people may harbor this parasite, and it is estimated that 10–30% of these will eventually develop symptomatic heart disease. Blood transfusion has been identified as a cause of transmission of this parasite in Brazil. Whereas Chagas' disease is still rarely diagnosed in the United States, there may be as many as 50 000–100 000 infected people among immigrants from South and Central America who now reside in the continental USA. In Los Angeles County, one report suggests that the prevalence of antibodies to *T. cruzi* among recent immigrants from endemic areas may be as high as 1:500–1:1000. A species of the reduviid bug, the insect vector for this infectious agent, is found in southern Texas and California.

It is important to consider Chagas' disease in young or middle-aged patients who have developed otherwise unexplained cardiac insufficiency, with or without gastrointestinal motility disorders involving either the esophagus or colon. Suspicion should increase if the patient originated from endemic areas, or has received blood transfusions from former residents of these areas. Serologic tests are available at the Centers for Disease Control and Prevention to confirm the diagnosis; specialized research laboratories offer other tests, including PCR amplification of blood samples, and xenodiagnosis, a technique in which blood suspected of containing very low numbers of parasites is fed to laboratory-raised reduviid bugs; these serve as a culture vessel for the trypanosomes, which are then identified in the gut of the insect. Although there is currently no treatment that can arrest established infections, early diagnosis is nevertheless important. Serial assessment of patients by electrocardiography and echocardiography to monitor for disorders of cardiac rhythm, ventricular dysfunction, and left or right ventricular or atrial wall clots that can be the source of systemic or pulmonary emboli, help to manage the complications of this disorder.[35] There are reports of successful cardiac transplants for end-stage Chagas' disease,[36] despite the problems of immunosuppression.

Anaphylaxis and anaphylactoid reactions

Cardiac arrhythmias and hypotension are well recognized features of anaphylaxis (Chapter 46). One of the reasons for this is that the heart muscle is well endowed with mast cells.[37] Their density appears to be increased in the hearts of patients with ischemic heart disease and idiopathic dilated cardiomyopathy.[38] Cardiac mast cells contain similar levels of histamine to lung and skin mast cells, and can be activated in vitro to release histamine, tryptase, chymase, prostaglandin D_2 and leukotriene C_4. In addition, their secretory granules contain tumor necrosis factor-α (TNF-α) and other cytokines. Thus, stimuli that provoke anaphylactic (IgE-mediated) or anaphylactoid (non-IgE-mediated) reactions can directly offer the heart. Although anaphylactoid reactions to radiographic contrast media are one of the risks of cardiac catheterization, there have also been rare reports of intracardiac anaphylactic reactions triggered by latex in the balloons of cardiac catheters. A careful medical history to identify patients who have had reason to be sensitized to latex should be part of the preliminary evaluation of anyone scheduled for cardiac catheterization.[39]

Radiographic contrast media activate the complement cascade and release of the complement dependent anaphylatoxins, C3a and C5a, may stimulate mast cells to release histamine, thromboxane A_2 and other mentioned arachidonic acid metabolites. The incidence of clinically significant reactions is approximately 0.23% in patients given intra-arterial injections of these agents in the cardiac catheterization laboratory.[40] In patients with a prior history of reactions to these agents, pretreatment with 0.5 mg/kg methylprednisolone 12 and 2 hours before a diagnostic procedure reduces the risk of such reactions.

Histamine increases the heart rate and, acting together with adenosine, an endogenous nucleoside released by mast cells and by ischemic myocardial cells, may cause defects in atrioventricular conduction.[41–42] Initially, histamine increases the force of cardiac contraction. Later, contractility and coronary artery flow are reduced, reflecting the combined effects of histamine acting upon H_1 and H_2 receptors in the heart and arachidonic acid metabolites acting directly on the myocardial cells. Depending on the severity, one may consider treating anaphylaxis with both H_1 and H_2 receptor antagonists and parenteral glucocorticoids in addition to epinephrine, particularly in patients who experience hypotension, even though the peak anti-inflammatory effects of glucocorticoids may be delayed for several hours. This delay in onset of action of glucocorticoids may actually be beneficial, as it may help to suppress the late-phase response (Chapter 46).

Thrombolytic therapy of acute coronary occlusions with either recombinant tissue plasminogen activators or streptokinase also activates the complement cascade acutely.[43] The frequency and severity of the resulting reactions are greater after streptokinase.[44] Patients are more likely to have circulating antistreptokinase antibodies as a result of prior streptococcal infections, and experience immune complex-mediated reactions following injection of this agent as well. Clinically evident serum sickness is a late complication of thrombolytic therapy with streptokinase, occurring in approximately 6% of patients.[45] Although treatment with glucocorticoids may help control this process it must be undertaken with extreme caution in patients who were given streptokinase to restore coronary artery flow, because treatment with glucocorticoids or even nonsteroidal antiinflammatory drugs adversely affects myocardial healing after ischemia–reperfusion injury. In short, although the cost of thrombolytic therapy with streptokinase may be lower, the risks of post-treatment complications are greater.

PATHOPHYSIOLOGY OF MYOCARDIAL INJURY AND INFLAMMATION

Cardiac muscle ischemia, blunt trauma or other injuries that rupture cardiac cells release intracellular organelles that activate the complement cascade and trigger leukocyte infiltration. Infectious agents can cause direct myocardial cell injury or induce the release and presentation of cardiac subcellular molecules that stimulate autoimmune responses to cardiac tissue components. Finally, heart failure, regardless of cause, often results in the production of agents such as norepinephrine, angiotensin II, TNF-α, IL-1 and IL-6, which can adversely affect cardiac structure and function.[46,47]

Inflammation and repair following ischemic injury

Experimental occlusion of a coronary artery that reduces microvascular flow by more than 50% and that lasts for more than 20–25 minutes causes irreversible myocardial injury, even when flow is eventually restored.[48] Because the time of onset is known and the extent and the location of the myocardial injury can be measured, myocardial ischemia–reperfusion injury provides an excellent model to study host responses to acute cardiac tissue injury. Following occlusion, osmotically active metabolites accumulate and cause cardiac muscles to swell; fluid-filled blebs develop under the myocardial cell membranes.[49] Mitochondria just beneath the cell membrane migrate into these blebs, and can escape when the blebs rupture. Their internal membranes unfold and expose integral membrane proteins that display the negatively charged phospholipid cardiolipin. Figures 80.2 and 80.3 show scanning and transmission electron micrographs of injured but intact cardiac myocytes undergoing such a process. The cardiolipin–protein complexes avidly bind C1q and activate the classic complement pathway.[50] Normal cardiac myocytes express decay-accelerating factor and other regulatory proteins that block assembly of the complement C3 convertase. However, ischemic cardiac myocytes do not express these regulatory proteins and the complement cascade can proceed to the membrane attack complex.[51] Complement activation is facilitated by amine groups in mitochondrial membranes that provide sites for the attachment and assembly of the C3- and C5-converting enzymes. The generation of C5a attracts leukocytes to the ischemic myocardium. *N*-formyl methionyl residues of proteins encoded by the mitochondrial genome also provide leukocyte chemotactic stimuli.[52] Complement-mediated ischemia–reperfusion injury may also be amplified and prolonged by complement proteins that are displayed by damaged cardiocytes.[53]

Reperfusion provides fresh complement and a relatively inexhaustible supply of leukocytes that greatly amplify the initial inflammatory response. Leukocytes that localize in the damaged heart muscle can cause considerable injury.[46] Thus without reperfusion myocardial injury is extensive and inevitable. Prompt reperfusion salvages myocardial cells but at the same time it triggers an intense inflammatory response that can damage living myocytes at the border of the infarct. Without this inflammatory response, healing is impaired. Research on the mechanisms that regulate the inflammatory response to myocardial injury continues in the expectation that a better understanding of these mechanisms will help to minimize loss of myocardial cells without compromising healing.

Activation of complement, the initial stimulus for leukocyte infiltration into damaged myocardium, is quickly followed by the release of bound stores of transforming growth factor-B1 (TGF-β1) and then by the biosynthesis of IL-8 and monocyte chemotactic protein-1 by vascular endothelial cells in the injured cardiac muscle.[54,55] Sequential release of these chemotactic agents causes both neutrophils and mononuclear leukocytes to enter the zone of injury. Proinflammatory cytokines, such as IL-1β and TNF-α, released by activated mononuclear phagocytes migrating into the myocardium and by cardiac mast cells, stimulate the production of IL-6.[46] This cytokine induces myocardial cells on the borders of the infarct to express intercellular adhesion molecule-1 (ICAM-1). Neutrophils that have been activated by C5a and express high levels of the ICAM-1 counterligand, CD11b/CD18 (MAC-1), adhere to these myocytes and kill myocytes by releasing oxidative radicals. Thus, the induction of ICAM-1 on the myocyte cell surface is a signaling event that targets damaged cells for killing. Three or more hours after they migrate into the heart, neutrophils lose cell surface staining for CD11b but continue to express CD11a.[46] Neutrophils lacking CD11b can no longer adhere to cardiocytes; presumably they also lose their ability to kill cardiac muscle cells.

Monocytes begin to migrate into damaged myocardium at the same time as neutrophils. Monocytes tend to localize in the epicenter of the ischemic tissue, where their numbers increase progressively with time. Tissue-infiltrating monocytes are a rich source of proinflammatory cytokines and other agents that help

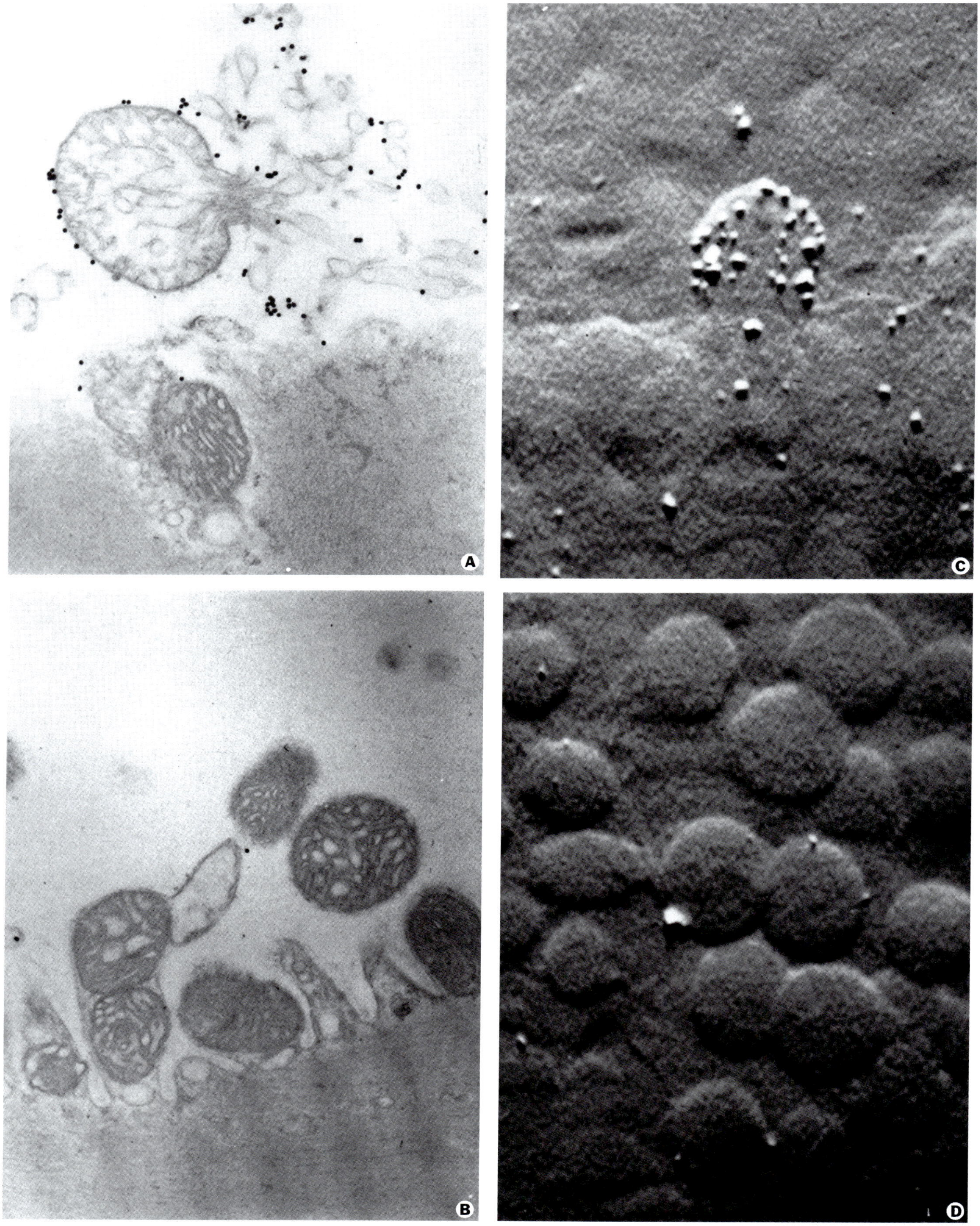
A
C
B
D

Figure 80.2 Cardiac mitochondria bind anticardiolipin antibody. To identify the very first events that result in activation of the complement cascade by subcellular components of injured cardiac tissue, single cardiac myocytes were isolated from adult canine hearts after extensive treatment of the muscle with collagenase. Although more than 80% of the cells isolated by these methods are viable by usual histologic criteria, some show small breaks in the outer cell membrane when examined with an electron microscope. Mitochondria, which are normally clustered between the sarcolemma and the myofibrils, push through these breaks in the cell membrane; some may escape altogether from the damaged myocytes. Because it is recognized that the cardiac subcellular constituent that activates C1 is cardiolipin, a phospholipid that is abundant in cardiac mitochondrial membranes, these damaged cardiac myocytes were evaluated to see if their cell surfaces display cardiolipin. The cells were incubated with affinity-purified highly specific rabbit anticardiolipin antibodies, washed, and then exposed to antibodies to rabbit IgG labeled with colloidal gold. The cells were then washed again, fixed, and prepared for scanning and transmission electron microscopy. (**A**) (× 30 000), (**C**) (× 35 000). Transmission and scanning electronmicrographs, respectively, stained sequentially with the anticardiolipin antibodies and gold–colloid-conjugated second antibody. Gold beads that have deposited on the membranes of mitochondria that protrude through the myocyte cell membrane may be seen in both (**A**) and (**C**), suggesting that immunoreactive cardiolipin is abundantly displayed on these mitochondrial membranes. (**B**) (×24 000) and (**D**) (×28 000) Controls that were treated only with the gold-labeled second antibody. Note in (**D**) that mitochondria protruding through the myocyte cell membrane may be visualized in this scanning electronmicrograph as round humps on the otherwise homogeneous cell surface. Gold beads are not seen. (From Rossen RD, Michael LH, Hawkins HK et al. *Circ Res* 1994; 75:546, with permission.)

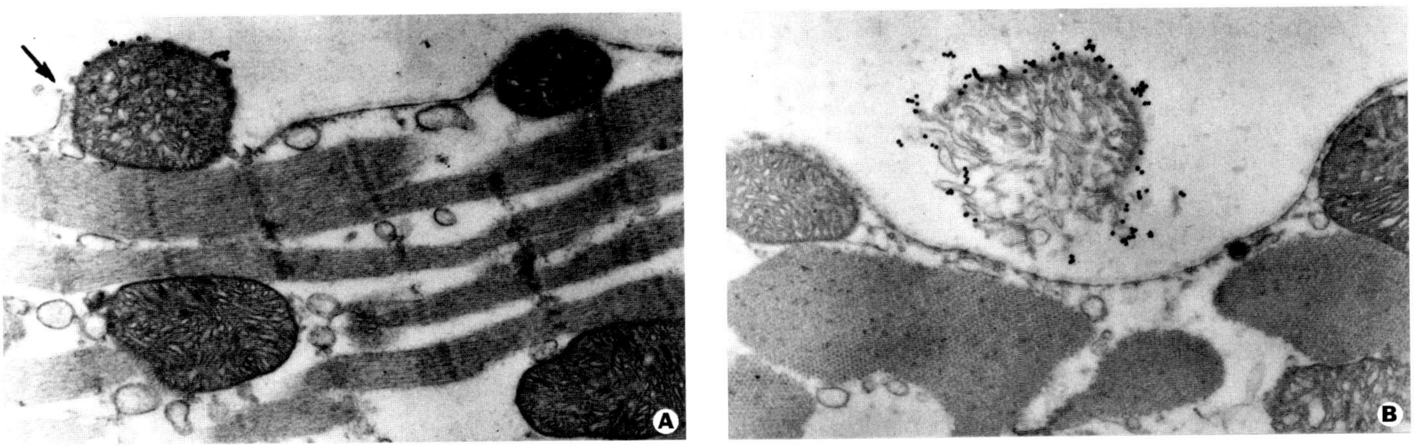

Figure 80.3 Cardiac mitochondria are released from injured myocytes. (**A**) A mitochondrion is caught in the act of protruding through a break in the cardiac muscle cell membrane. There are abundant deposits of gold beads only on the surface of the mitochondrion that has emerged through the myocyte membrane, indicating that this part of the mitochondrial surface was accessible to the anticardiolipin antibodies, but the mitochondrion on the right is still covered by an intact myocardial cell membrane. It does not bind anticardiolipin antibodies (×35 000). (**B**) A mitochondrion that has just been released from a cardiac myocyte. Once released, the cristae of the mitochondrion begin to unfold and the inner membranes display numerous sites that can react with and bind anticardiolipin antibodies. Note that, as in (**A**), mitochondria that are covered by an intact myocardial cell membrane do not react with the anticardiolipin antibodies (×37 000). (From Rossen RD, Michael LH, Hawkins HK et al. *Circ Res* 1994; 75:546, with permission.)

to protect cardiac myocytes near the zone of injury. Besides TNF-α, tissue-infiltrating monocytes release insulin-like growth factor-1, acidic fibroblast growth factor and IL-6, all agents that help to protect myocytes injured from hypoxia.[56] Tissue-infiltrating macrophages and their products may salvage myocardial cells that might otherwise succumb to the acute inflammatory response, and they also remove damaged myocardial cells. Activated macrophages also can damage myocardial cells after adhering to cells that have been induced to display high cell surface levels ICAM-1 and/or phosphatidyl serine,[57] by releasing oxygen free radicals, nitric oxide and TNF-α.

Myocardial cells in the ischemic zone can die either by necrosis or by apoptosis. Mechanisms that cause necrosis have been mentioned above. Programmed cell death (apoptosis) has only recently been recognized as a cause of myocardial cell death. One consequence of initiating the cell-death program is that phosphatidylserine, a phospholipid that normally resides on the inner leaf of the lipid bilayer, migrates to the outer side of the cell membrane. Apoptotic myocytes can be identified in patients experiencing acute myocardial infarctions by imaging myocardium with ^{99m}Tc-labeled annexin V.[58] Annexin V is an endogenous protein that binds with high affinity to membrane phosphatidylserine. A number of stressors may induce apoptosis in cardiac myocytes.[59] Apoptosis can be inhibited by β-adrenergic blocking drugs such as carvedilol and propanolol.[60] Acute cardiac ischemia–reperfusion experiments in mice that are double knockouts for both tumour necrosis factor receptor-1 (TNFR1) and TNFR2 suggest that TNF-α may also help to protect myocardial cells from apoptosis even though it does not protect against necrosis.[61] To remove dead and dying cardiocytes, killed either by apoptosis or by necrosis, the extracellular matrix (ECM) that ties them to their neighbors must be dissolved.

Proteolysis of connective tissue matrix attachments may be another key function of the tissue-infiltrating neutrophils and monocytes. The brisk inflammatory response that follows prompt reperfusion of ischemic myocardium may clear away damaged tissues relatively rapidly, so that repair can begin without prolonged exposure to proteolytic enzymes and other agents generated during ischemia.[62–64] Plasmin generated by microvascular thromboses and leukocyte granular enzymes such as elastase and metalloproteinases cause fragmentation of extracellular matrix (ECM) proteins. Fragments of ECM proteins often have distinct signaling properties that help regulate monocyte migration and differentiation. For example, cryptic binding sites for the β_1-integrin, $\alpha_5\beta_1$ (VLA-5), generated by proteolysis of fibronectin, enable the resulting fibronectin fragments to attract monocytes to the site of myocardial injury.[56] At the higher concentrations found in the center of myocardial infarcts these same fibronectin fragments stimulate monocytes to express serine proteases that cleave the α_5 chain of the monocytes' own VLA-5 molecules, significantly reducing the ability of these cells to migrate further in the ECM. This may explain why migrating monocytes seem to accumulate in the most damaged parts of the infarcted myocardium, where fibronectin fragment concentrations are very high. Fibronectin fragments and other stimuli also provide signals that stimulate monocytes to differentiate into macrophages, which remove necrotic and apoptotic cells and produce factors that stimulate angiogenesis, fibroblast proliferation and collagen production.

Matrix-bound cytokines such as TGF-β are also likely to be among the agents that stimulate repair of ischemic myocardium.[65] TGF-β is mobilized from tissue depots shortly after reperfusion. During the first 24 hours tissue stores decrease, but within 48 hours of the occlusion production is increased, particularly at the margins of the infarct.[66] This cytokine is not only a potent chemoattractant for monocytes: it also modulates monocyte production of reactive oxygen intermediates, specifically down-regulating the expression of cardiac muscle cell-inducible nitric oxide synthase. Nitric oxide-mediated cytotoxicity is thereby reduced. TGF-β also stimulates fibroblasts to produce collagen and fibronectin. Overproduction of this cytokine may cause excessive fibrosis.[65]

Some of the signals that influence monocyte/macrophage behavior may be derived from T lymphocytes that accumulate along with other leukocytes in reperfused myocardium. At present, there is no compelling evidence that these T cells localize in cardiac tissue by specific recognition of cardiac tissue antigens. Nevertheless, beginning 5–6 hours after reperfusion, and for 4–5 days or more thereafter, T cells infiltrating ischemic or formerly ischemic myocardium produce IL-10.[46] The production of this 'anti-inflammatory' cytokine may help to shut down synthesis of IL-6 in the damaged tissue and stimulate the production of inhibitors of metalloproteinases. Both IL-10 and monocyte colony-stimulating factor (M-CSF) stimulate monocytes to differentiate, and one can demonstrate mRNA for M-CSF in ischemic and reperfused myocardium by the third hour after reperfusion. Recent studies suggest that infiltrating lymphocytes also release activated metalloproteinases.[67] Adhesive interactions with fibronectin stimulate T cells to produce these collagenolytic enzymes. The same signals down-regulate T-cell production of the tissue inhibitor of metalloproteinases, TIMP-2.

In summary, all classes of leukocyte participate in the host response to ischemia–reperfusion injury. When limited in time and duration, as most commonly occurs with an acute coronary occlusion, the inflammatory response to this insult effectively removes dead cells and their surrounding connective tissue matrix proteins and causes a strong scar that can resist the deforming internal pressures of the heart and allow it to continue to function as an efficient pump. However, when stimuli that drive intracardiac inflammation are recurrent or persistent, the host response can become maladaptive.

CARDIAC INFLAMMATION ASSOCIATED WITH VIRAL INFECTIONS AND AUTOIMMUNITY

From clinical investigations it is difficult to ascertain why only some patients develop overt manifestations of myocarditis following infection with certain viruses. Why myocarditis in some individuals resolves without sequelae, whereas in others it progresses rapidly, or after a variable latent period, to end-stage dilated cardiomyopathy is also poorly understood. As viral myocarditis and its sequel dilated cardiomyopathy remains a major cause of mortality and morbidity this disease has been studied intensively in experimental animals. These studies have shown that dendritic cells are regularly found in the hearts of healthy experimental animals,[68] and that these cells can stimulate cloned cardiac myosin-specific CD4 T cells to proliferate. Thus, even in healthy animals, there is intracardiac presentation of myosin-derived peptides in the context of MHC Class II molecules.

Experimental studies in mice have demonstrated that viruses that infect the heart vary widely in their ability to provoke an acute myocarditis. They also vary in their ability to cause progressive intracardiac inflammation.[69] For example, there are strains of coxsackie B virus that invoke direct cardiac injury, strains that are not cardiotoxic, and strains that seem only to stimulate autoimmune responses directed against cardiac tissue. Infections with coxsackie B virus types 1 or 4 (CVB1 or CVB4) cause myocardial injury that parallels the recovery of virus from the heart. In contrast, coxsackie B type 3 virus (CVB3) strain variants, cause a myocarditis that begins well after peak virus titers are achieved and continues to progress after infectious virus has been eliminated from the host.

The persistence and the severity of the resulting myocardial disease also depend on the genetic background of the infected host. For example, that CVB3 causes a severe and persistent myocarditis in some mouse strains but not others.[69] The host response to these infections include T cells that recognize virus-encoded antigens, T cells that recognize self-antigens, and perhaps NK cells that become armed with antibodies directed against cardiac cell surface proteins that can mediate antibody-dependent cellular cytotoxicity (ADCC).

Cytolytic T cells kill myocardial cells either by membrane insertion of perforin or by Fas-Fas ligand-induced apoptosis. Cardiac myocyte death by apoptosis may occur because enterovirus infections induce expression of Fas (CD95).[70] These cells can then be targeted by cytotoxic lymphocytes that express Fas ligand (CD95L). Although both antigen-specific T cells expressing α/β T-cell receptors (TCR) and T cells expressing γ/δ TCR can kill cardiac myocyte target cells, recent studies suggest that γ/δ T cells infiltrating the heart in CVB3-induced myocarditis are particularly important effectors of myocardial cell injury.[71] T cells expressing the γ/δ TCR constitute up to 12% of the inflammatory cells in the heart.[71] In addition to their role as cytolytic effector cells, they also appear to have an immunoregulatory role. Specifically, they may help to perpetuate a Th1 phenotype among the cells infiltrating the heart by selectively destroying IL-4-producing CD4+ Th2-type cells. The ultimate effect of this is to prolong the host immune response to the cardiac tissue.

Depending on the genetic background of the host and the virus causing the myocarditis, different classes of effector cells are mobilized in response to the infection.[69] Treatment with anti-CD4, anti-CD8 or pan-T-cell antibodies prior to infection has been effective in eliminating effector T cells that cause myocardial cell injury, depending on the particular virus used to initiate the myocardial cell infection and the MHC phenotype of the murine host. Viral antigens, displayed in the context of Class II MHC, become a target of CD4 cells that recognize them. Viral proteins produced in the endoplasmic reticulum of infected host cells, on the other hand, will associate with Class I MHC antigens at the cell surface and be recognized by CD8 CTL. Antigenic targets of these CTL include virus-encoded peptides as well as self-antigen arising in infected host cells as a result of the virus infections.

Not all the antigens that stimulate autoimmune responses have been fully characterized. Considering the fact that dendritic cells from healthy normal hearts express cardiac myosin, it is not surprising that antibodies against myosin are found in myocarditis patients. The adenine nucleotide translocator, a cardiac mitochondrial protein involved in energy metabolism, has also been identified as a possible autoantigen in postviral myocarditis.[72] Immune responses to CVB3 have been shown to cross react with this cellular protein.

CHRONIC INTRACARDIAC INFLAMMATION, CARDIAC REMODELING AND HEART FAILURE

Large myocardial infarctions, immune responses to infectious agents that target cardiac tissues, and cardiac tissue-specific autoimmune responses are among the conditions that can engender a long-standing and deleterious inflammatory response in cardiac tissue and the development of congestive cardiomyopathy (Fig. 80.4). A common consequence of all of these conditions is the overproduction of specific peptides and cytokines, including norepinephrine, the angiotensins, endothelins and proinflammatory cytokines, most notably TNF-α, IL-1 and IL-6.[73,74] Myocardial cells themselves begin to produce these factors. These cytokines can also further amplify their own production in an autocrine and paracrine fashion. Some of them appear to be responsible for cardiac myocyte loss. For example, concentrations of norepinephrine in the myocardium and the blood of

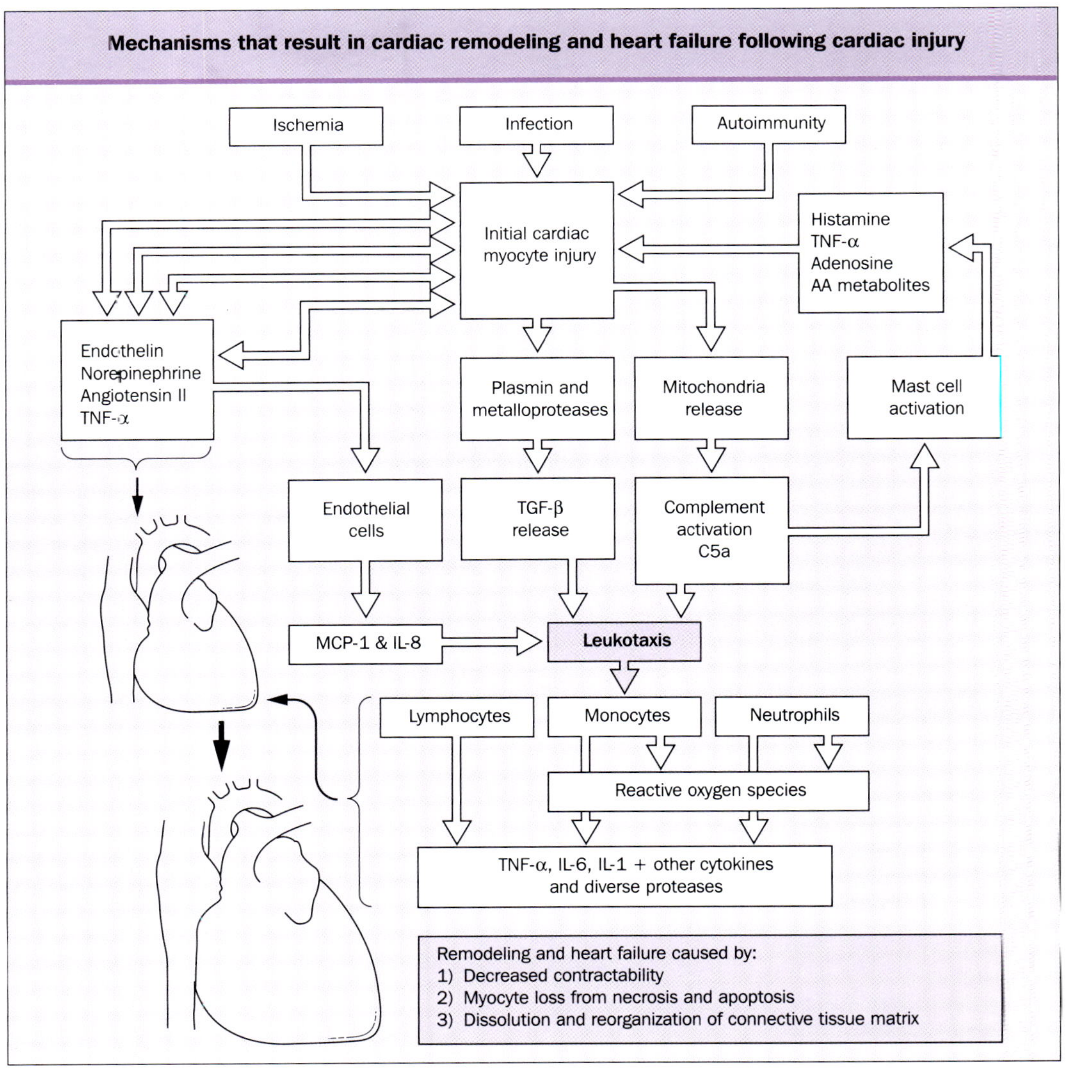

Figure 80.4 Mechanisms that result in cardiac remodeling and heart failure following cardiac injury. Remodeling results from (a) the production of various mediators such as endothelin, norepinepherine, angiotensin II and TNF-α by the heart muscle cells, as well as (b) the production and release of proteolytic enzymes, cytokines and chemokines by invading leukocytes attracted into the damaged myocardium by a cascade of chemotactic agents. Activation of cardiac mast cells in the course of the response to injury may facilitate both processes by producing histamine, TNF-α, adenosine and arachidonic acid (AA) metabolites.

patients with advanced heart failure are sufficient to cause myocyte necrosis in experimental model settings. Likewise, high concentrations of endothelin or angiotensin II kill cardiac myocytes in experimental model systems. The production of these agents often results in cardiac failure and a process known as 'cardiac remodeling'. Remodeling describes the changes in both the shape and the function of the left ventricular muscle, which dilates the left ventricular cavity.[74] Normally this cavity is bullet-shaped; in remodeling it balloons out and become almost spherical.[75] This results in increased wall stress, persistent endocardial ischemia, leakage of the atrioventricular valves and decreased left ventricular ejection. The increase in wall stress is a sufficient stimulus to cause cardiac muscle cells to produce TNF-α. The intracardiac release of this cytokine further depresses the contractile properties of the cardiac myocytes. Remodeling is ultimately caused by the death of myocardial cells and the attenuation of the connective tissue matrix that links the cardiac cells together. Figure 80.4 summarizes the reaction to cardiac injury that ultimately results in cardiac remodeling and heart failure.

The illumination of the role of TNF-α in heart failure provides a particularly clear example of the impact of inflammation on the pathophysiology of heart disease. Although TNF-α does not initiate heart failure, the toxic effects of this cytokine cause it to progress. Table 80.2 lists the documented adverse effects of TNF-α on the heart. A Kaplan–Meier analysis of the survival of heart failure patients categorized according to their plasma TNF-α levels suggests that those who have circulating TNF-α levels >6.5 pg/mL die sooner than those with lower TNF-α levels.[76] Administration of TNF-α in rats to levels found in the sera of heart failure patients is sufficient to cause left ventricular dilation and remodeling.[77] In addition, transgenic mice that overexpress TNF-α in the heart develop progressive left ventricular failure. Several hypotheses have been offered to explain why high levels of this cytokine are found in so many patients, regardless of the etiology of their heart failure. Surprisingly it is not due to overproduction of TNF-α by circulating leukocytes or by activated lymphoid tissues. Rather, as noted above, the cardiac myocytes themselves appear to produce this cytokine as part of a common pathway of response to cardiac injury of all types. This assertion is supported by measurements of TNF-α mRNA and protein in failing human hearts collected at the time of cardiac transplantation. These observations and others have stimulated attempts to treat this condition by controlling either the production or the effects of this cytokine.

Untoward effects of tumor necrosis factor-α in heart failure
In humans
Left ventricular dysfunction
Pulmonary edema
Cardiomyopathy
Reduced leg blood flow
In experimental animals
Left ventricular remodeling
Abnormalities in myocardial metabolism
Anorexia and cachexia
β-receptor uncoupling from adenylate cyclase
Abnormal mitochondrial energetics
Activation of the fetal gene program

Table 80.2 Untoward effects of tumor necrosis factor-α in heart failure. (Modified from Bozkurt B, Kribbs SB, Clubb FJ, et al. Pathophysiologically relevant concentrations of tumor necrosis factor-alpha promote progressive left ventricular dysfunction and remodeling in rats. *Circulation* 1998;97:1382.)

EMERGING TREATMENTS FOR MYOCARDIAL INFLAMMATION

Vaccine strategies

The difficult-to-treat cardiomyopathy of diphtheria is extremely rare in well-immunized populations such as the United States, and usually represents an isolated failure of immunization. Vaccines also have had a salutary effect on an endocardial fibroelastosis, formerly the most common form of dilated cardiomyopathy in children with an incidence of 1 in 5000 live births until the late 1960s. Studies of heart tissue from children with this condition showed that ~90% of samples contain mumps virus genomic RNA sequences, suggesting that this cardiomyopathy resulted from mumps virus infections acquired in utero.[2] Endocardial fibroelastosis has dramatically declined following the introduction of mumps vaccine. With these success stories in mind, it is important to consider vaccination as a means of preventing other cardiomyopathies, including those caused by coxsackie B viruses and certain strains of adenovirus. Recently, molecular biological techniques have been used in mice[78] to develop hybrid viruses or chimeras that induce protective immunity to coxsackie 3B and adenoviruses without inducing cardiac inflammation. An alternative approach, the development of attenuated strains of these viruses, has also been shown to protect against wild-type virus infection without infecting heart tissue and without eliciting cardiac-specific autoimmune responses.[79,80] Clearly, the information and the technology are available to develop vaccines likely to protect against infection with agents that commonly cause myocarditis.

MODULATING THE HOST RESPONSE TO CARDIAC INFLAMMATION

Despite optimal treatment with angiotensin-converting enzyme inhibitors and β-adrenergic blockers, heart failure continues its downhill course in a large proportion of patients who have progressed from myocarditis to dilated cardiomyopathy. This suggests the persistence of biologically active systems that are involved in creating the heart failure phenotype.[73] Left ventricular assist devices (LVADs) are mechanical pumps designed to supplement the actions of the failing heart and have served as a 'bridge to cardiac transplantation'. Clinical experience with LVADs has demonstrated that reducing the work of the heart substantially slows the progression of heart failure and may reverse many of its physiological consequences, at least temporarily.[73,81] Comparative studies performed before and after the implantation of LVADs showed that this treatment decreases the frequency of necrotic and apoptotic myocardial cells, improves myocardial cell contractility and reverses the changes in the connective tissue matrix associated with cardiac remodeling. In a few patients cardiac function improved so dramatically that the pumps could be removed and the patients continued to function without further support or need for transplantation.[82] In short, these studies suggest that in some cases irreversible end-stage heart failure is in fact neither end-stage nor irreversible.

A growing body of evidence suggests that one of the key molecules driving the progression of heart failure, regardless of etiology, is TNF-α. As discussed earlier, this cytokine is produced in the myocardium in response to volume overload. It is therefore not too surprising to note that mechanical circulatory support with an LVAD substantially reduces TNF-α production by the failing heart.[83] A short-term phase 1 trial suggested that a single dose of 4 or 10 mg/m^2 of the soluble p75 TNF receptor, etanercept, increased cardiac output, and improved the quality of life for up to 14 days in a small group of patients with advanced heart failure.[22] The potential benefit of TNF-α inhibition may be further supported by the favorable results of treatment trials with amrinone, adenosine, pentoxifylline and other agents that block TNF-α transcriptional activation by altering intracellular cyclic AMP levels.[47] While etanercept and infliximab are already available and approved for the treatment of patients with rheumatoid arthritis and other chronic inflammatory diseases, they must still be used with caution in inflammatory heart disease. For when it is produced as part of the acute response to injury, TNF-α may be beneficial in that it may protect against myocyte apoptosis. A large multicenter trial is under way to evaluate the effects of treatment with soluble TNF receptors in heart failure.

The decision to suppress TNF-α production or block its effects was based on a detailed elucidation of basic mechanisms responsible for the development of dilated cardiomyopathy and heart failure. The same cannot be said for the decision to use high-dose IVIG as therapy for myocarditis and dilated cardiomyopathy. Yet, three reports suggest that IVIG given over a relatively short time for a total dose of 2 g/kg caused sustained improvement in cardiac function in all treated subjects for as long as 1 year.[20,84,85] The results of these trials, despite being uncontrolled, were sufficiently encouraging to stimulate a randomized placebo-controlled trial of IVIG therapy in chronic heart failure, the results of which are still pending. Like the trials of immunosuppressive therapy for myocarditis, the use of IVIG treatment was based on the hypothesis that autoimmunity to cardiac tissue antigens contributes to the pathophysiology of disease, and that exogenous immunoglobulin may modulate these autoimmune responses. Studies of mice infected with coxsackie virus 3B support the notion that immunoglobulin therapy can reduce inflammation in the heart, decrease myocardial tissue injury and improve survival.[86] Additional evidence that the humoral immune response may contribute to the pathophysiology of heart failure has come from an interventional study in patients with idiopathic dilated cardiomyopathy, chosen because they had autoantibodies to the β_1-adrenoreceptors.[21] In this case-controlled trial the patients' immunoglobulin levels were reduced by immunoadsorption over columns that contained sheep anti-human immunoglobulin antibodies. Sequential immunoadsorptions reduced anti-β_1 autoantibody levels by more than 90% and was associated with a sustained and highly significant improvement in left ventricular ejection fraction and evidence for a reduction in remodeling. Illuminating the molecular basis for the apparent success for either IVIG or immunoadsorption therapy in the treatment of heart failure may significantly improve our understanding of and ability to manage this condition.

REFERENCES

1. Heart Failure: management of patients with left-ventricular systolic dysfunction. In: Quick reference guide for clinicians No. 11. 1994, Agency for Health Policy and Research, USPHS, DHHS: Rockville, MD.
2. Bowles NE, Towbin JA. Molecular aspects of myocarditis. Curr Opin Cardiol 1998;13:179.
3. McCarthy RE, Boehmer JP, Hruban RH, et al. Long-term outcome of fulminant myocarditis as compared with acute (nonfulminant) myocarditis. N Engl J Med 2000;342:690.
4. Marboe CC, Fenoglio JJ. Pathology and natural history of human myocarditis. Pathol Immunopathol Res 1988;7:226.
5. Reyes MP, Lerner AM. Coxsackie virus myocarditis – with special reference to acute and chronic effects. Prog Cardiovasc Dis 1985;27:373.
6. Pisani B, Taylor D, Mason JW. Inflammatory myocardial diseases and cardiomyopathies. Am J Med 1997;102:459.
7. Kimball SA, Janson PA, LaRaia PJ. Complete heart block as the sole presentation of lyme disease. Arch Intern Med 1989;149:1987.
8. O'Connell JB, Henkin RE, Robinson JA. Gallium-67 imaging in patients with dilated cardiomyopathy and biopsy-proven myocarditis. Circulation 1984;70:58.
9. Dec GW, Palacios I, Yasuda T, et al. Antimyosin antibody cardiac imaging: its role in the diagnosis of myocarditis. J Am Coll Cardiol 1990;16:97.
10. Friedrich MG, Strohm O, Schulz-Menger J, et al. Contrast media-enhanced magnetic resonance imaging visualizes myocardial changes in the course of viral myocarditis. Circulation 1998;97:1802.
11. Bellotti G, Bocchi EA, de Moraes AV, et al. In vivo detection of *Trypanosoma cruzi* antigens in hearts of patients with chronic Chagas' heart disease. Am Heart J 1996;131:301.
12. Smith SC, Ladenson JH, Mason JW, Jaffe AS. Elevations of cardiac troponin I associated with myocarditis: experimental and clinical correlates. Circulation 1997;95:163.
13. Aretz HT, Billingham ME, Edwards WD, et al. Myocarditis: a histopathologic definition and classification. Am J Cardiovasc Pathol 1987;1:3.
14. Cooper LT, Berry GJ, Shabetai R. Idiopathic giant-cell myocarditis-natural history and treatment. Multicenter Giant Cell Myocarditis Study Group Investigators. N Engl J Med 1997;336:1860.
15. Mason JW. Myocarditis. In: Advances in internal medicine. St. Louis, Mosby, 1999;293.
16. Hufnagel G, Pankuwelt S, Richter A, Schonian U, Maisch B. The European Study of Epidemiology and Treatment of Cardiac Inflammatory Diseases (ESETCID) First epidemiological results. Herz 2000;25:279.
17. Koide H, Kitaura Y, Deguchi H, et al. Genomic detection of enteroviruses in the myocardium – studies on animal hearts with coxsackievirus B3 myocarditis and endomyocardial biopsies from patients with myocarditis and dilated cardiomyopathy. Jpn Circ J 1992;56:1081.
18. Maisch B, Hufnagel G, Schonian U, Hengstenberg C. The European Study of Epidemiology and Treatment of Cardiac Inflammatory Disease (ESETCID). Eur Heart J 1995;16:173.
19. Parrillo JE. Myocarditis: how should we treat in 1998? J Heart Lung Transplant 1998;17:941.
20. McNamara D, Rosenblum WD, Janosko KM, et al. Intravenous immune globulin in the therapy of myocarditis and acute cardiomyopathy. Circulation 1997;95:2476.
21. Muller J, Wallukat G, Dandel M, et al. Immunoglobulin adsorption in patients with idiopathic dilated cardiomyopathy. Circulation 2000;101:385.
22. Deswal A, Bozkurt B, Seta Y, et al. Safety and efficacy of a soluble p75 tumor necrosis factor receptor (Enbrel, Etanercept) in patients with advanced heart failure. Circulation 1999;99:3224.
23. Mason JW, O'Connell JB, Herskowitz A, et al. A clinical trial of immunosuppressive therapy for myocarditis. N Engl J Med 1995;333:269.
24. Garg A, Shiau J, Guyatt G. The ineffectiveness of immunosuppressive therapy in lymphocytic myocarditis: an overview. Ann Intern Med 1998;129:31.

25. Maisch B, Herzum M, Hufnagel G, Schonian U. Immunosuppressive and immunomodulatory treatment for myocarditis. Curr Opin Cardiol 1996;11:310.
26. Lange LG, Schreiner GF. Immune mechanisms of cardiac disease. N Engl J Med 1994;330:1129.
27. Bunn WH, Giannini AJ. Cardiovascular complications of cocaine abuse. Am Fam Phys 1992;46:769.
28. Bristow MR, Mason JW, Billingham ME, Daniels JR. Dose–effect and structure–function relationships in doxorubicin cardiomyopathy. Am Heart J 1981;102:709.
29. Porumb H, Petrescu I. Interaction with mitochondria of the anthracycline cytostatics adriamycin and daunomycin. Prog Biophys Mol Biol 1986;48:103.
30. Samlowski WE, Ward JH, Craven CM, Freedman RA. Severe myocarditis following high-dose interleukin-2 administration. Arch Pathol Lab Med 1989;113:838.
31. Rerkpattanapipat P, Wongpraparut N, Jacobs LE. Cardiac manifestations of acquired immunodeficiency syndrome. Arch Intern Med 2000;160:602.
32. Hutchison SJ. Acute rheumatic fever. J Infect 1998;36:249.
33. Bachmaier K, Neu N, de la Maza LM, et al. Chlamydia infections and heart disease linked through antigenic mimicry. Science 1999;283:1335.
34. Kirchhoff LV. Chagas disease. American trypanosomiasis. Infect Dis Clin North Am 1993;7:487.
35. Hagar JM, Rahimtoola SH. Chagas' heart disease in the United States. N Engl J Med 1991;325:763.
36. de Carvalho VB, Sousa EF, Vila JH, et al. Heart transplantation in Chagas' disease. 10 years after the initial experience. Circulation 1996;94:1815.
37. Marone G, de Crescenzo G, Adt M, et al. Immunological characterization and functional importance of human heart mast cells. Immunopharmacology 1995;31:1.
38. Marone G, de Crescenzo G, Florio G, et al. Immunological modulation of human cardiac mast cells. Neurochem Res 1999;24:1195.
39. Myers GE, Crick WF, King SW, et al. Latex versus iodinated contrast media anaphylaxis in the cardiac cath lab. Cathet Cardiovasc Diagn 1995;35:228.
40. Goss JE, Chambers CE, Heupler FA Jr. Systemic anaphylactoid reactions to iodinated contrast media during cardiac catheterization procedures: guidelines for prevention, diagnosis, and treatment. Cathet Cardiovasc Diagn 1995;34:99.
41. del Balzo U, Polley MJ, Levi R. Activation of the third complement component (C3) and C3a generation in cardiac anaphylaxis: histamine release and associated inotropic and chronotropic effects. J Pharmacol Exp Ther 1988;246:911.
42. Belardinelli L, Linden J, Berne RM. The cardiac effects of adenosine. Prog Cardiovasc Dis 1989;32:73.
43. Bennett WR, Yawn DH, Migliore PJ, et al. Activation of the complement system by recombinant tissue plasminogen activator. J Am Coll Cardiol 1987;10:627.
44. Davidson JR, Bush RK, Grogan EW, Boh LA, Graziano FM. Immunology of a serum sickness/vasculitis reaction secondary to streptokinase used for acute myocardial infarction. Clin Exp Rheumatol 1988;6:381.
45. Siebert WJ, Ayres RW, Bulling MT, et al. Streptokinase morbidity – more common than previously recognised. Aust NZJ Med 1992;22:129.
46. Frangogiannis NG, Youker KA, Rossen RD, et al. Cytokines and the microcirculation in ischemia and reperfusion. J Mol Cell Cardiol 1998;30:2567.
47. Mann DL. Cytokines as mediators of disease progression in the failing heart. In: Hosenpud JD, Greenberg BH, Ed. Congestive heart failure. Philadelphia, Lippincott Williams & Wilkins, 2000, 213.
48. Rossen RD, Swain JL, Michael LH, et al. Selective accumulation of the first component of complement and leukocytes in ischemic canine heart muscle. Circ Res 1985;57:119.
49. Jennings RB, Reimer KA. The cell biology of acute myocardial ischemia. Annu Rev Med 1991;42:225.
50. Rossen RD, Michael LH, Hawkins HK, et al. Cardiolipin–protein complexes and initiation of complement activation after coronary artery occlusion. Circ Res 1994;75:546.
51. Zimmermann A, Gerber H, Nussenzweig V, Isliker H. Decay-accelerating factor in the cardiomyocytes of normal individuals and patients with myocardial infarction. Virchows Arch A Pathol Anat Histopathol 1990;417:299.
52. Carp H, Mitochondrial *N*-formylmethionyl proteins as chemoattractants for neutrophils. J Exp Med 1982;155:264.
53. Yasojima K, Kilgore KS, Washington RA, Lucchesi BR, McGeer PL. Complement gene expression by rabbit heart: upregulation by ischemia and reperfusion. Circ Res 1998;82:1224.
54. Birdsall HH, Green DM, Trial J, et al. Complement C5a, TGF-β1, and MCP-1, in sequence, induce migration of monocytes into ischemic myocardium within the first 1 to 5 hours following reperfusion. Circulation 1997;95:684.
55. Kumar AG, Ballantyne CM, Michael LH, et al. Induction of monocyte chemoattractant protein-1 in the small veins of the ischemic and reperfused canine myocardium. Circulation 1997;95:693.
56. Trial J, Baughn RE, Wygant JN, et al. Fibronectin fragments modulate monocyte VLA-5 expression and monocyte migration. J Clin Invest 1999;104:419.
57. Simms MG, Walley KR. Activated macrophages decrease rat cardiac myocyte contractility: importance of ICAM-1-dependent adhesion. Am J Physiol 1999;277:H253.
58. Hofstra L, Liem IH, Dumont EA, et al. Visualization of cell death in vivo in patients with acute myocardial infarction. Lancet 2000;356:209.
59. Sabbah HN, Sharov VG. Apoptosis in heart failure. Prog Cardiovasc Dis 1998;40:549.
60. Yue TL, Ma XL, Wang X, et al. Possible involvement of stress-activated protein kinase signaling pathway and Fas Receptor expression in prevention of ischemia/reperfusion-induced cardiomyocyte apoptosis by carvedilol. Circ Res 1998;82:166.
61. Kurrelmeyer KM, Michael LH, Baumgarten G, et al. Endogenous tumor necrosis factor protects the adult cardiac myocyte against ischemic-induced apoptosis in a murine model of myocardial infarction. Proc Natl Acad Sci USA 200;97:5456.
62. Lindsey MH, Wedin K, Brown MD, et al. Matrix-dependent mechanism of neutrophil-mediated release and activation of MMP-9 myocardial ischemia/reperfusion. Circulation 2001 (in press).
63. Peterson JT, Dillion L, Bryant JW. Evolution of matrix metalloprotease and tissue inhibitor expression during heart failure progress in the infarcted rat. Cardiovasc Res 2000;46:307.
64. Mann DL, Spinale FG. Activation of matrix metalloproteinases in the failing human heart breaking the tie that binds. Circulation 1998;98:1699.
65. Sporn MB, Roberts AB. Transforming growth factor-beta. Multiple actions and potential clinical applications: clinical conference. JAMA 1989;262:938.
66. Thompson NL, Bazoberry F, Speir EH, et al. Transforming growth factor beta-1 in acute myocardial infarction in rats. Growth Factors 1988;1:91.
67. Esparza J, Vilardell C, Calvo J, et al. Fibronectin upregulates gelatinase B (MMP-9) and induces coordinated expression of gelatinase A (MMP-2) and its activator MT1-MMP (MMP-14) by human T lymphocyte cell lines. A process repressed through RAS/MAP kinase signaling pathways. Blood 1999;94:2754.
68. Spencer SC, Fabre JW. Characterization of the tissue macrophage and the interstitial dendritic cell as distinct leukocytes normally resident in the connective tissue of rat heart. J Exp Med 1990;171(6):1841.
69. van Houten N, Huber SA. Role of cytotoxic T cells in experimental myocarditis. Springer Semin Immunopathol 1989;11:61.
70. Huber SA. T cells expressing the gamma delta T cell receptor induce apoptosis in cardiac myocytes. Cardiovasc Res 2000;45:579.
71. Huber SA, Budd RC, Rossner K, Newell MK. Apoptosis in coxsackievirus B3-induced myocarditis and dilated cardiomyopathy. Ann NY Acad Sci 1999;887:181.
72. Huber SA. Autoimmunity in myocarditis: relevance of animal models. Clin Immunol Immunopathol 1997;83:93.
73. Mann DL. Mechanisms and models in heart failure, a combinatorial approach. Circulation 1999;100:999.
74. Givertz MM, Colucci WS. New targets for heart-failure therapy: endothelin, inflammatory cytokines, and oxidative stress. Lancet 1998;352(Suppl I):34.

75. Mendes LA, Picard MH, Dec GW, et al. Ventricular remodeling in active myocarditis. Am Heart J 1999;138:303.
76. Torre-Amione G, Bozkurt B, Deswal A, Mann DL. An overview of tumor necrosis factor alpha and the failing human heart. Curr Opin Cardiol 1999;14:206.
77. Bozkurt B, Kribbs SB, Clubb FJ, et al. Pathophysiologically relevant concentrations of tumor necrosis factor-alpha promote progressive left ventricular dysfunction and remodeling in rats. Circulation 1998;97:1382.
78. Hofling K, Tracy S, Chapman N, Kim KS, Leser JS. Expression of an antigenic adenovirus epitope in a group B coxsackievirus. J Virol 2000;74:4570.
79. Chapman NM, Ragland A, Leser JS, et al. A group B coxsackievirus/poliovirus 5′ nontranslated region chimera can act as an attenuated vaccine strain in mice. J Virol 2000;74:4047.
80. Zhang H, Morgan-Capner P, Latif N, et al. Coxsackievirus B3-induced myocarditis. Characterization of stable attenuated variants that protect against infection with the cardiovirulent wild-type strain. Am J Pathol 1997;150:2197.
81. Mann DL, Willerson JT. Left ventricular assist devices and the failing heart, a bridge to recovery, a permanent assist device, or a bridge too far? Circulation 1998;98:2367.
82. Frazier OH, Myers TJ. Left ventricular assist system as a bridge to myocardial recovery. Ann Thorac Surg 1999;68:734.
83. Torre-Amione G, Stetson SJ, Youker KA, et al. Decreased expression of tumor necrosis factor-alpha in failing human myocardium after mechanical circulatory support: a potential mechanism for cardiac recovery. Circulation 1999;100:1189.
84. Drucker NA, Colan SD, Lewis AB, et al. Gamma-globulin treatment of acute myocarditis in the pediatric population. Circulation 1994;89:252.
85. Bozkurt B, Villaneuva FS, Holubkov R, et al. Intravenous immune globulin in the therapy of peripartum cardiomyopathy. J Am Coll Cardiol 1999;34:177.
86. Takada H, Kishimoto C, Hiraoka Y. Therapy with immunoglobulin suppresses myocarditis in a murine coxsackievirus B3 model. Antiviral and anti-inflammatory effects. Circulation 1995;92:1604.

Section 7 Organ-specific Inflammatory Disease

Chapter 81 Autoimmune Thyroid Disease

Su He Wang and James R. Baker

Autoimmune thyroid disease is a group of thyroid disorders in which autoimmune processes target various constituents of thyroid tissues, including cells, receptors and enzymes. The classification of autoimmune thyroid disease encompasses primarily two entities: autoimmune hyperthyroidism and autoimmune thyroiditis (Table 81.1).

The concept of a thyroid autoimmune process originated more than 50 years ago, when antithyroid antibodies were found in the serum of patients with Hashimoto's thyroiditis,[1] followed by the induction of experimental autoimmune thyroiditis in animals.[2] The long-acting thyroid stimulator (LATS) was then discovered as the cause of Graves' disease.[3] Since then, there has been continuing growth in both knowledge and concepts concerning the nature of immunologic molecules, the mechanisms of autoimmune processes, and their clinical and laboratory manifestations. This progress greatly increases our understanding of the pathogenesis of autoimmune thyroid disease, especially Graves' disease and Hashimoto's thyroiditis, which are the most common thyroid disorders. This chapter will discuss the basic and clinical aspects of each of these disorders.

GRAVES' DISEASE

Graves' disease accounts for most cases of hyperthyroidism. It is named after the Irish physician Robert J. Graves, who first gave a clinical description of the disease in 1835, although the symptoms of hyperthyroidism were noted in the early 1800s. It was nearly 50 years after Graves' description, however, that excessive production of thyroid hormones was proposed as the cause of the disease.[4] After several decades' active study of hyperthyroid-related hormones, in 1956 Adams and Purves[3] discovered an abnormal thyroid stimulator protein named LATS in the serum of patients with Graves' disease. The nature of LATS was later identified as an autoantibody against thyroid follicular cell thyrotropin (TSH) receptors, and since that time Graves' disease has been classified as an autoimmune disease.

The classification of autoimmune thyroid disease
Autoimmune hyperthyroidism
Graves' disease
Autoimmune thyroiditis
Hashimoto's (lymphocytic) thyroiditis
Postpartum thyroiditis

Table 81.1 The classification of autoimmune thyroid disease.

Genetic and environmental factors

Graves' disease is common in the general population, with an incidence of 1–1.5 cases per 1000 population. Its etiology is largely unknown, but it develops predominantly in genetically susceptible individuals. Family members of a patient with Graves' disease are more likely to have autoimmune thyroid disease or other organ-specific autoimmune disease than the general population. For example, autoimmune thyroid disease is more frequently associated with type 1 diabetes.[5] Studies of monozygotic twins have indicated that the disease has a concordance rate of 30–60%.[6] These studies also suggest that the expression of Graves' disease in genetically susceptible individuals is affected by environmental agents or perhaps endogenous factors in either permissive or protective ways.

One of the pathological features seen in Graves' disease is infiltration of the thyroid gland with activated lymphocytes. Increased expression of the major histocompatibility complex (MHC) Class II antigens has been noted on these lymphocytes, as well as on the thyroid cells. MHC genes and their products play a crucial role in determining the immune response, particularly in antigen presentation (Chapter 6). The HLA region on chromosome 6 is therefore an obvious candidate as a Graves' disease susceptibility gene. A number of studies have suggested that there is an association between Graves' disease and HLA-DR3 in Caucasian populations,[3] although this might not be the case in other races.[9,10] More recent studies indicate that HLA-DR3 is in strong linkage disequilibrium with DQB1*0201 and DQA1*0501, both of which are strongly associated with Graves' disease.[11,12] HLA-DQB1*0303 has been suggested to be a race-specific susceptibility allele for Graves' disease in Hong Kong Chinese.[10] Conversely, a few studies have implied that HLA-DQ alleles play a role in resistance to autoimmune thyroid disease.[13] A few studies have also found no evidence of associations between MHC genes and Graves' disease.[14]

Genetic studies also support the involvement of non-MHC genes in the pathogenesis of Graves' disease (Table 81.2). CTLA-4 (cytotoxic T-lymphocyte antigen-4) plays an important role in the down-regulation of T-cell activation. Genetic studies have provided evidence that particular alleles of the gene encoding CTLA-4 are linked and associated with various organ-specific autoimmune diseases in general, including Graves' disease.[15–18] These associations have been present in different races.[15–17] Because the presence of autoantibodies against the TSH receptor is the most important pathogenic feature of Graves' disease, the TSH receptor gene has also been an obvious candidate for disease contribution.[19] However, most studies have failed to show any significant association of TSH receptor alleles in the genetics of Graves' disease. GD-1, a locus on chromosome 14 at 14q31, has

Genes or locus	Reference
HLA-DR,DQ	7,8, 10–12
Cytotoxic T-lymphocyte antigen-4 (CTLA-4)	15–17
TSH receptor	19
Graves' disease-1 (GD-1, 14q31)	20
X-chromosome at Xq21.33–22	21
Interleukin-1 receptor antagonist (IL-1RA)	22
Glyoxalase I	23

Table 81.2 Genes or loci associated with Graves' disease.

KEY CONCEPTS

Environmental factors in the development of Graves' disease

Clinical/epidemiological phenomenon observed	*Pathogenic factors suggested*
• Increased incidence or recurrent rate in high iodine intake areas	Excess iodine
• Increased incidence in populations exposed to wars	Stress
• Female predominance	Female hormones
• Increased incidence after viral or bacterial infections	Infections

been linked with susceptibility to Graves' disease.[20] This locus colocalizes with the multinodular goiter-1 locus. A locus on the X-chromosome at Xq21.33–22 has also been linked with Graves' disease.[21] Considering that Graves' disease predominates in females, this preliminary result is very interesting as it may possibly relate to the female predisposition to the disease. Interleukin-1 is implicated in the pathogeneses of a number of inflammatory disorders and autoimmune diseases. One case-control study has shown that the frequency of an allele for the gene encoding the IL-1 receptor antagonist (IL-IRa) is significantly increased in patients with Graves' disease.[22] However, possible population stratification and genetic mismatching between cases and controls need to be excluded, and a family-based linkage study will prove or disprove the role of this gene in Graves' disease. A recent study has suggested that there is an association between the gene encoding the glyoxalase I and Graves' disease and Hashimoto's thyroiditis in the Chinese population.[23] Finally, although interferon-α is involved in the immunopathogenesis of Graves' disease, there is so far no evidence that its gene plays a role in genetic susceptibility to the disease.[24]

Together, the data suggest that Graves' disease, like other autoimmune diseases, is a complex genetic trait related to contributions from MHC and multiple non-MHC genes, most of which have yet to be identified. Although a number of genes have been associated with susceptibility to Graves' disease, their relative contributions to its pathogenesis have yet to be clearly defined. Moreover, as previously mentioned, additional non-genetic factors contribute significantly to the etiology of this disorder.

Both human and animal studies have indicated that chronic excess iodine supplementation may modulate the expression of autoimmune thyroid disease in genetically susceptible individuals. The mechanism for this is unknown and may be multiple. For example iodine is known to stimulate B lymphocytes to increase the production of immunoglobulins,[25] enhance T-lymphocyte activity,[26] and influence the expression of MHC antigens.[27] The incorporation of dietary iodine into thyroglobulin has also been reported to increase thyroglobulin immunogenicity in an animal study.[28] Although excess iodine is unlikely to cause Graves' disease in normal subjects, the recurrence of this disorder is clearly affected by iodine intake. Patients given iodine supplementation after discontinuing treatment with antithyroid drugs are more likely to have relapses than those who do not receive iodine.[29] Graves' disease is also more likely to recur following thyroidectomy in areas of high iodine intake than in areas of normal iodine intake.[30] Comparable doses of antithyroid drugs are more likely to cause hypothyroidism in patients with Graves' disease who reside in areas of iodine deficiency.[31]

It is well known that stress can affect the immune system and hormone secretion. Studies have shown that stress can change thyroid function by increasing iodine uptake and stimulating TSH and thyroid hormones secretion.[32] This may relate to studies showing that the incidence of Graves' disease increased significantly in populations exposed to a major war.[33] Although there is evidence that stress may affect the development of Graves' disease, it is unlikely that it can itself induce expression of the disease.

Graves' disease has a marked female predominance (M:F ratio 7:1), and sex hormones have been proposed to play a role in its development.[34] The basic reasons for this phenomenon are largely unknown; however, it has been noted that sex hormones have some significant effects on the immune system (see Postpartum thyroiditis, below).

There is increasing evidence for a connection between infectious agents and the development of Graves' disease. The frequency of antibodies to *Yersinia enterocolitica*, a gram-negative bacillus, is significantly increased in patients with Graves' disease.[35] Furthermore, *Yersinia enterocolitica* appears to have saturable TSH-binding sites;[36] this bacillus may contain antigenic determinants that cross-react with human thyroid autoantigens. Other organisms, including retroviruses, may also predispose to the development of Graves' disease, perhaps by breaking tolerance to autoantigens through molecular mimicry, stimulating the production of cytokines, or changing host cell components (Chapter 60).

Pathogenesis

An immune response can be initiated when $CD4^+$ T cells recognize foreign or self-antigenic peptides presented by MHC Class II molecules such as HLA-DR or HLA-DQ. Class II molecules are usually expressed only on antigen-presenting cells, such as dendritic cells, B cells and macrophages, and not on epithelial cells such as thyrocytes. As mentioned above, particular alleles of several Class II HLA molecules have been reported to be associated with Graves' disease. Abnormal or aberrant expression of these antigens on thyrocytes may possibly play a key role in the development of Graves' disease. It has been well established that TSH receptor antibodies (TRAb, previously named LATS), cause Graves' disease by binding to TSH receptors on thyroid follicular cells and inducing excess production of thyroid hormones. The mechanism by which TRAb are induced is still not fully known. It is likely that $CD4^+$ T cells drive this response by recognizing TSH peptides in conjunction with MHC Class II. Epitope mapping, made possible by the cloning of the TSH receptor gene,[41] has suggested that T-cell recognition of peptide 158–176 may be a relevant early event in the disease process.[42] A number of possible mechanisms have been suggested to explain how peripheral T-cell tolerance to thyroid antigens could be overcome in autoimmune thyroid disease (Chapter 60).

Graves' disease is characterized by T- and B-cell infiltration of the thyroid gland (Fig. 81.1). $CD4^+$ T cells predominate.[37] Studies of intrathyroidal T-cell receptor expression have demonstrated limited α region expression and these activated CD4 T cells may be providing help for antibody production by locally abundant B cells. Although $CD8^+$ cells are usually only a small fraction of infiltrating cells in early disease, it is interesting that this subset may increase after treatment with antithyroid drugs.[38]

Two types of TRAb exist in thyroid diseases.[42] In Graves' disease TRAb act as agonists and are named thyroid-stimulating antibodies (TSAb) The TSAb bind to the TSH receptor, stimulate the release of thyroid hormones, and ultimately lead to hyperthyroidism. In atrophic thyroiditis TRAb act as antagonists and are named thyroid-blocking antibody (TBAb). These also bind to the receptor but fail to stimulate. TSH is also prevented from binding to the receptor, and hypothyroidism occurs. It has been proposed that some patients with Graves' disease proceed to develop hypothyroidism, not because the thyroid gland itself is eventually destroyed by autoreactive cells, but because the TRAb switch from agonist to antagonist.[43] In healthy individuals thyroid hormone release is normally regulated by feedback inhibition from TSH, but the presence of TSAb disrupts this system, as the generation of TSAb is independent of thyroid hormones. As a result, the TSH receptor is under continuing stimulation by TSAb. Apart from the disease-specific TSAb, other autoantibodies against various components of the thyroid gland, including thyroid peroxidase (TPO) and thyroglobulin, may also be present in Graves' disease.

KEY CONCEPTS

Immunologic features of Graves' disease
- Presence of autoantibodies, particularly TSAb
- Predominant $CD4^+$ T cell infiltration of thyroid gland
- Increased local expression of MHC Class II molecules, especially HLA-DR
- Evidence for local stimulation of $CD4^+$ T cells and recognition of thyroid antigens.

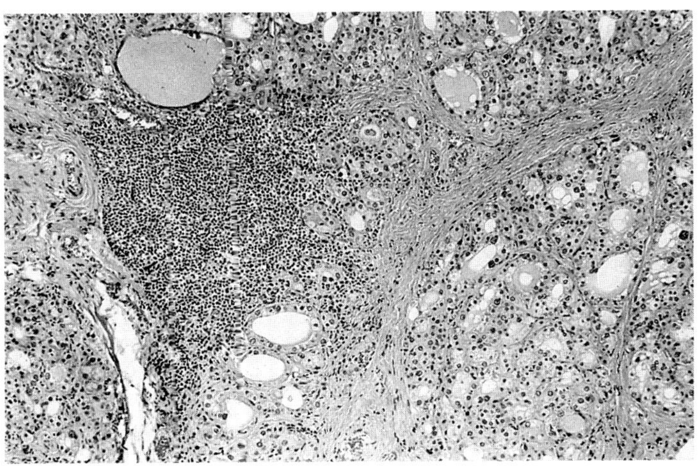

Figure 81.1 Graves' disease. Graves' disease showing epithelial hyperplasia, lymphocytic infiltration and fibrous bands. (Courtesy of Dr Thomas Giordano, Department of Pathology, University of Michigan.) (See also colour plate 81.1)

Prevention and patient management

There is no effective way to prevent the occurrence of Graves' disease. Prior to a confirmatory diagnosis, an effective means of controlling symptoms is the use of β-adrenergic receptor inhibitors such as propranolol. After diagnosis β-adrenergic blocking agents can also be used with other therapies. However, their use should be carefully considered when patients have contraindications such as congestive heart failure, bronchospastic disease and diabetes mellitus. A suitable antithyroid therapy should be given as soon as the diagnosis has been established. These regimens include thionamide antithyroid medicines, radioactive iodine and surgical thyroidectomy. Various medications are available for the treatment of Graves' disease. Propylthiouracil and methimazole are the two antithyroid drugs that are most frequently used by physicians. They not only inhibit the production of thyroid hormones, relieving hyperthyroidism, but also reduce the size and vascularity of the goiter, making it more amenable to a definitive therapy with surgery or radioactive iodine if necessary. Both radioactive iodine and surgical subtotal thyroidectomy are definitve ablative treatments. Destructive therapy with ^{131}I is beneficial because patients do not relapse, but it may increase the risk of developing or worsening ophthalmopathy. Corticosteroids, lithium, ipodate and amiodarone have also been reported to be used in the treatment of Graves' disease.

THERAPEUTIC PRINCIPLES

Therapies used in treatment of Graves' disease

β Blockers	Inhibition of peripheral T_4 conversion to the active hormone T_3
	Block of sympathetic action
Iodine	Inhibition of thyroid hormone release
	Inhibition of TSH action on thyroid
Ipodate	Inhibition of thyroid hormone synthesis
	Decrease in serum T_3 and increase of serum rT_3
Lithium	Inhibition of T_4 release
Steroids	Immunosuppressive actions
	Inhibition of peripheral monodeiodination, causing a decrease in serum T_3 and an increase in serum rT_3
Thionamides	Inhibition of thyroglobin synthesis
	Correction of abnormal immune responses

Treatment protocols vary and decisions are based on particular symptoms, physician experience, medical support services available, and patient preference.

One study[44] provides evidence that initial treatment with antithyroid drugs plus thyroxine, followed by suppressive doses of thyroxine alone, maintains a low level of TSAb and thus prevents the recurrence of hyperthyroidism.[44] However, other groups have been unable to obtain the same result.[45,46]

In order to determine the optimal dosage and length of maintenance therapy, some pathological markers should be monitored during the treatment. Thyroid hormone and TSH concentrations are perhaps the most useful. Measurement of TSAb levels has also been used to assess the response to treatment and to predict relapses.

Pregnant patients with Graves' disease require special attention. The aim of treatment in this situation is to control disease activity so that the potential deleterious effect of hyperthyroidism on the fetus can be avoided. The therapies employed must not interfere with the normal development of the fetus. Antithyroid drugs are considered the first line of therapy in pregnant patients. Surgical intervention is only selected for those who are either allergic to or respond poorly to antithyroid medicines. Radioactive iodine is contraindicated.

Most patients with thyroid-associated ophthalmopathy do not need special treatment for the eye problem because its pathology is self-limiting. However, patients with severe orbital involvement may require immunosuppressants and corticosteroids, orbital irradiation or surgical intervention.

Patient evaluation and differential diagnosis

Graves' disease typically presents with a diffuse enlargement of the thyroid gland (goiter) and thyrotoxicosis. The classic signs of hyperthyroidism are heat intolerance, hand tremor, nervousness, irritability, warm moist skin, weight loss, muscle reflex changes, hyperdynamic cardiovascular status with tachycardia, hyperdefecation, and changes in mental status.

Approximately 20–25% of patients present with clinical thyroid-associated ophthalmopathy, characterized by proptosis. However, subclinical thyroid-associated ophthalmopathy can be found in the majority of patients with Graves' disease when more sensitive imaging techniques (CT scan or MRI) are used. Surprisingly, clinically significant thyroid-associated ophthalmopathy can rarely occur without evidence of Graves' hyperthyroidism, although antithyroid autoantibodies are usually detected. TSH receptors are known to be expressed in connective tissues of the orbit in patients with ophthalmopathy, but a potential role for them in the immunopathogenesis of Graves' ophthalmopathy remains to be established. Thyroid-associated dermopathy usually presents as a swelling in the pretibial area (myxedema), but can also involve the feet, face or hands. Skin involvement rarely occurs on other parts of the body. Interestingly, dermopathy typically coexists with thyroid-associated ophthalmopathy.

Laboratory findings in patients with hyperthyroidism include elevated levels of total and free T_3 and T_4. TSH levels are low or undetectable because the stimulation of the thyroid gland is exogenous rather than from the pituitary axis, and the elevated thyroid hormone levels cause a feedback inhibition of the pituitary TSH secretion. The appearance of TSAb is regarded as a specific and pathogenic marker for Graves' disease. This autoantibody can be demonstrated in the serum of about 90% of patients. Insensitive assays may be responsible for the failure to detect TSAb in all patients with Graves' disease. The thyroid gland in patients with Graves' disease always shows an increased uptake of radioactive iodine, and a diffuse homogeneous uptake on a radioisotope scan of the thyroid is almost pathognomonic of Graves' disease.

The differential diagnosis of Graves' disease involves the exclusion of other thyroid disorders with hyperthyroidism, such as Hashimoto's thyroiditis, pituitary tumors or thyroid adenomas. Most of these can be ruled out by determining that the thyroid gland has a diffuse increase of iodine uptake. The presence of ophthalmopathy also strongly suggests the diagnosis. Sometimes it is difficult to differentiate Graves' disease from Hashimoto's thyroiditis, and fine-needle biopsy of the thyroid may be useful. In Hashimoto's thyroiditis the lymphocytic infiltrate is usually diffuse and considerably more intense than in Graves' disease. Oxyphilic cells, typical of Hashimoto's thyroiditis, are not usually seen in Graves' disease.

The hypermetabolic state of pregnancy can be confused with Graves' disease. Systemic symptoms such as fatigue, heat intolerance, emotional lability and hyperhidrosis often accompany normal pregnancy and cannot be used for diagnosis. Normal pregnancy may also be associated with a slight increase in the size of the thyroid gland. Laboratory confirmation of the clinical suspicion of hyperthyroidism is essential in the setting of pregnancy. Radioisotope tests should be avoided because of the risk to the fetus.

Pitfalls/controversies

Continuing advances have increased our understanding of Graves' disease. However, many key questions are still unanswered or remain controversial.

1. Which genes are involved in the susceptibility to Graves' disease? Can individuals with greatly increased risk be prospectively identified?
2. How does TRAb (TSAb or TBAb) react structurally and functionally with the TSH receptor? What is the molecular mechanism for its agonism (stimulation) and antagonism (blocking) of the TSH receptor?
3. What are the pathways of damage to the thyroid gland during the course of disease?
4. Can the thyroid antigen epitopes for T and B cells be fully characterized?
5. How can we develop a therapy directed at aberrant autoimmune response or abnormal apoptosis?
6. What is the role of female hormones in disease occurrence?

HASHIMOTO'S THYROIDITIS

Hashimoto's thyroiditis was first described by Hashimoto in 1912 as struma lymphomatosa. Autoantibodies present in this disorder were found in 1956 by Roitt et al.[1] Hashimoto's thyroiditis is characterized by lymphocytic infiltration of the thyroid parenchyma, causing thyroid enlargement, and by the presence of thyroid autoantibodies to thyroglobulin and to thyroid peroxidase. Hashimoto's thyroiditis is the most common underlying cause for hypothyroidism. It has been estimated that about 3–4% of the population suffers from Hashimoto's thyroiditis. It is found most commonly in middle-aged and elderly women, but also occurs in other age groups. Although it is distributed throughout the world without racial and ethnic restriction, it occurs more commonly in families where another member has an autoimmune thyroid disease or other autoimmune disease such as lupus erythematosus (SLE), chronic active hepatitis or scleroderma.

Genetic and environmental factors

The etiology of Hashimoto's thyroiditis is not known but, like Graves' disease, it is believed to involve both genetic and environmental factors. Thyroid antibodies are found with a high frequency among first-degree relatives, and there is a high degree of concordance among identical twins. Siblings of adult patients with Hashimoto's thyroiditis have about a 50% chance of developing thyroid autoantibodies.[47] As with Graves' disease, most genetic studies have focused on the HLA region. In Caucasians HLA-DR5 has been associated with a 3.4-fold increased risk of disease whereas HLA-DR3 was associated with a 5.7-fold increased risk of primary myxedema,[48] suggesting that these two diseases are distinct in cause. High frequencies of HLA-DRB4*0101 and HLA-A2 were demonstrated in Japanese patients and the presence of both alleles confers a great risk for Hashimoto's thyroiditis.[49] One study suggested that HLA-DQA1*0102 might have a protective role in the development of disease as its frequency is reduced in patients with Hashimoto's thyroiditis.[49] A summary of the different HLA types associated with Hashimoto's thyroiditis is given in Table. 81.3.

Hashimoto's thyroiditis has also been associated with particular alleles of CTLA-4.[15] As discussed above, the CTLA-4 gene has been known to be associated with Graves' disease and other autoimmune diseases.[20,21]

Although 95% of patients with Hashimoto's thyroiditis are women,[59] the basis for this gender effect remains unclear. Rodent studies have shown that testosterone suppresses and estrogen exacerbates experimental autoimmune thyroiditis induced by immunization or by thymectomy, and that castration of a male animal increases the severity of experimental autoimmune thyroiditis.[60,61] Furthermore, the expression of a functional estrogen receptor in thyroid cells suggests that thyrocytes may be directly affected by sex hormones.[62] Infection, iodine and irradiation might also increase the risk of developing Hashimoto's thyroiditis, but convincing epidemiological data have yet to be provided. It is interesting that the use of interferon-α (IFN-α) for the treatment of hepatitis has been associated with a significantly increased incidence of autoimmune thyroid disease.[63] A high frequency of HLA-A2 was observed in patients with hepatitis who developed autoimmune thyroid disease during or after IFN-α therapy.

> **KEY CONCEPTS**
>
> **Immunologic features in Hashimoto's thyroiditis**
> - Presence of antithyroid peroxidase (TPO) antibody and antithyroglobulin antibody
> - Imbalance of decreased suppressor T cells, with increased helper and cytotoxic T cells
> - Expression of MHC Class II antigens, especially HLA-DR antigen
> - Recognition of thyroid antigens by T cells
> - Presence of immune complexes

Pathogenesis

The pathogenesis of Hashimoto's thyroiditis is complex, with evidence of autoimmune cellular and humoral immune responses. The thyroid gland in Hashimoto's thyroiditis shows a dense accumulation of lymphocytes, plasma cells and macrophages with germinal center formation (Fig. 81.2). Thyroid follicles are damaged and their numbers are reduced. Traditionally it is thought that the thyroid follicles are injured by cytotoxicity, but there is recent evidence that apoptosis, or a combination of cytotoxicity and apoptosis, plays a key role in this pathogenic process.[64] A model for the immunopathogenesis of Hashimoto's thyroiditis is illustrated in Figure 81.3. A key immunologic event may relate to the increased HLA Class II antigen expression on infiltrating lymphocytes and thyrocytes in affected glands. Both CD4+ T cells and CD8+ cytotoxic T cells are increased. It is hypothesized that infiltrating T cells recognize processed peptides

Association of HLA types with Hashimoto's thyroiditis

Population studied	HLA associated	Reference
Caucasian (Canada)	DR4, DR5	50,53
Caucasian (Canada+UK)	DR4, DR5	54
Caucasian (Denmark)	Dw5	51
Caucasian (Hungary)	DR3	52
Caucasian (UK)	DR3	55
Oriental (China)	DR9, Bw46	56
Oriental (Japan)	DRB4*0101, A2	49
Oriental (Japan)	DR53	57
Oriental (Korea)	DR8, DQB1*0302	58

Table 81.3 Association of HLA types with Hashimoto's thyroiditis.

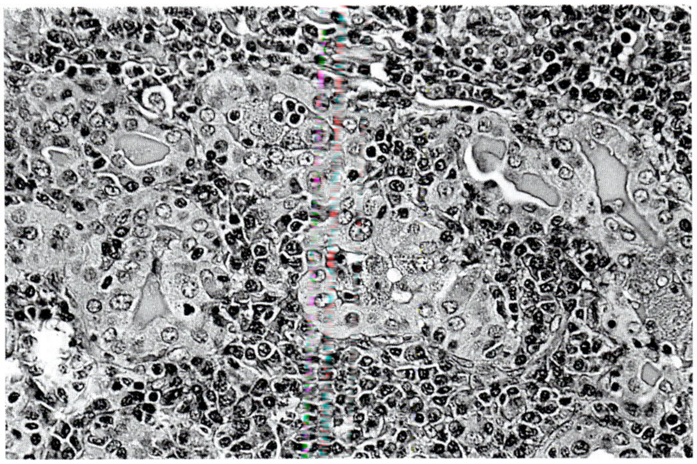

Figure 81.2 Hashimoto's thyroiditis, with prominent infiltration by lymphocytes, plasma cells and oncocytic metaplasia of residual follicular epithelium. (Courtesy of Dr Thomas Giordano, Department of Pathology, University of Michigan.) (See also colour plate 81.2)

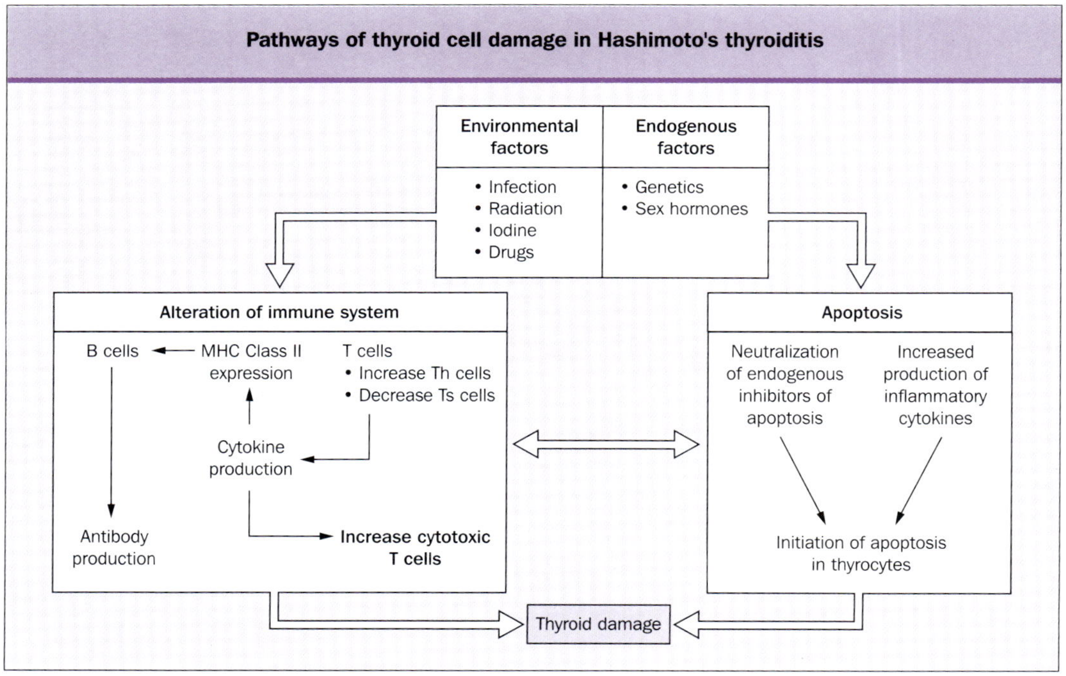

Figure 81.3 Pathways of thyroid cell damage in Hashimoto's thyroiditis. Under the influence of environmental factors the immune system in genetically susceptible individuals loses its surveillance function. Excess autoantibody is produced and the activity of cytotoxic T cells increases. On the other hand, the balance between proapoptotic and antiapoptotic factors shifts to the former and thyroid cell death occurs. Extensive thyroid damage is thus caused by both an overactive immune system and an overactive apoptotic system.

of thyroid peroxidase (TPO) and thyroglobulin. With assistance from T cells, B cells produce antibodies to thyroid antigens which are exposed or modified by the destructive process. Depending upon the methods of detection used, 55–90% of patients exhibit antithyroglobulin antibodies, and 82–91% exhibit anti-TPO antibodies.[65,66] In addition, intrathyroidal lymphocytes and surrounding lymphoid tissues may still be capable of producing thyroid antibodies in patients with negative serology.[65] TPO antigen can also be a central antigen for cytotoxic antibodies in Hashimoto's thyroiditis. The molecular nature of TPO antibodies has been characterized, and the variable-region genes involved are restricted mainly to V_H1, V_H3, $V_\kappa I$ and $V_\kappa III$ family members, which are among the most common V families.

Thyroid damage in Hashimoto's thyroiditis is associated with infiltrating cytotoxic T cells and evidence of increased apoptosis of follicular thyroid cells (Fig. 81.4). Thyroid cells have been shown to express molecules involved in apoptosis, such as TNF receptor and Fas.[67] Fas-mediated apoptosis of thyroid cells can be induced by CD8 cytotoxic T cells. The mechanism of apoptosis in thyroid cells is under active investigation. Although Fas is expressed constitutively on thyrocytes (Fig. 81.5), normally it does not cause apoptosis even in the presence of excess anti-Fas antibodies. The Fas–FasL pathway may therefore be regulated in thyrocytes, and certain combinations of inflammatory cytokines may reverse the inhibition.[69] In addition, the normal thyroid may utilize the Fas–FasL system to protect against invading lymphocytes. A recent study demonstrated that the process of lymphocytic infiltration in an inflamed thyroid was inhibited by direct injection of a FasL-expression vector,[68] suggesting that apoptosis was induced in the infiltrating lymphocytes by the expressed FasL on thyroid follicular cells.

In involved thyroid glands, thyroid cells show increased expression of intercellular adhesion molecules ICAM-1, VCAM-1 and LFA-3. Adhesion molecules are extensively involved in a network of cell–cell and cell–matrix interactions in the immune system. They are implicated not only in cell adhesion per se, but

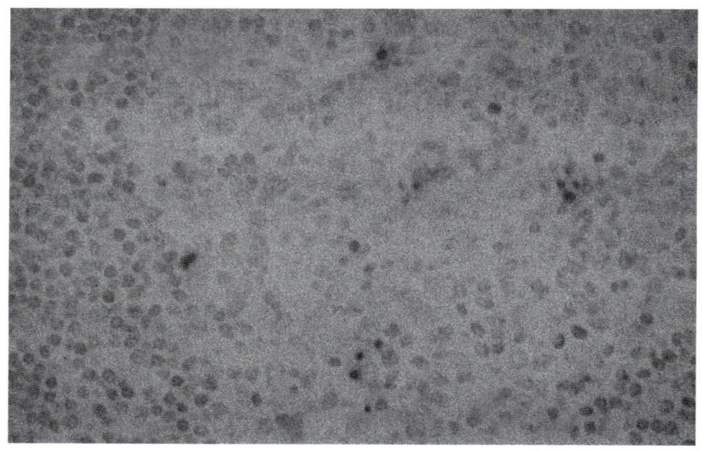

Figure 81.4 Apoptosis occurs in thyrocytes from Hashimoto's thyroiditis. The apoptotic cells were detected with ApopTag staining kit, where the nuclear fragmented DNA is demonstrated by the brown color. (See also colour plate 81.4)

also in signal transduction, leading to cellular events such as activation and proliferation. The presence of these adhesion molecules in patients with Hashimoto's thyroiditis may enhance the binding of lymphocytes to thyroid follicular cells and significantly increase thyroid cell damage. As mentioned earlier, one of the important characteristics of Hashimoto's thyroiditis is the formation of germinal centers within the thyroid gland. Germinal centers constitute a specialized microenvironment essential for the induction of antibody synthesis, affinity maturation of B cells, memory B-cell formation, and the maintenance of T-cell memory. The interactions between thyroid follicular cells, dendritic-like cells, infiltrating B cells and T cells in germinal centers may have a key role in the generation of autoantibodies, the production of cytokines, and the formation of memory B and T cells. Basement membranes on thyroid

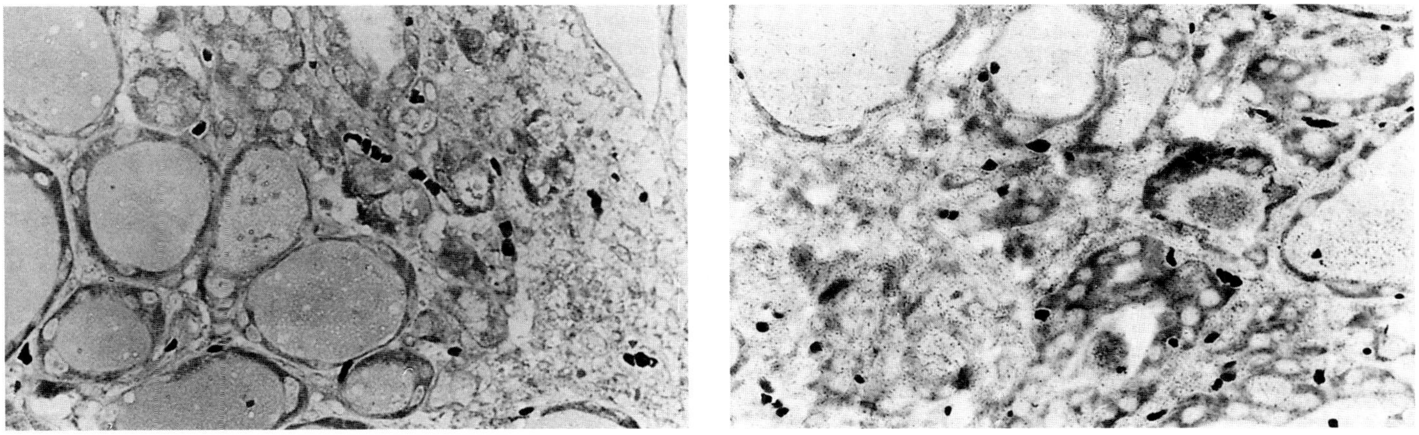

Figure 81.5 **Expression of Fas in Hashimoto's thyroiditis.** Fas is constitutively expressed on thyrocytes in Hashimoto's thyroiditis (left panel: control antibody; right panel: anti-Fas antibody). (See also colour plate 81.5)

follicular cells in Hashimoto's thyroiditis also demonstrate immune complex deposition and terminal complement complexes indicative of complement activation.[48]

Prevention and patient management

The cause of Hashimoto's thyroiditis is largely unknown, and no preventive medications are available. Treatment usually consists of thyroid hormone replacement for hypothyroidism, and this is generally required lifelong to prevent recurrence. A response to thyroid hormone therapy often includes a decrease in the levels of antithyroid antibodies. If the patient has a symptomatic goiter, a dose of thyroid hormones that suppresses TSH secretion may reduce the size of the gland. Although corticosteroids and immunosuppressive therapy may reduce thyroid enlargement, the high risk/benefit ratio does not support their use in the treatment of this disease. Patients with coexisting thyrotoxicosis should be treated with antithyroid drugs and levels of thyroid hormones carefully monitored. An appropriate therapy is not available for patients who are euthyroid but have enlarged glands. Thyroid hormone therapy may result in a decrease in the size of the gland in some cases, but an increase in others.

Occasionally Hashimoto's thyroiditis coexists with Graves' disease, and patients often present with typical symptoms of hyperthyroidism. Antithyroid treatment should be handled with extreme caution in such cases, because patients with both diseases are more likely to become hypothyroid after surgical or radioactive iodine therapy than are those with Graves' disease alone.[70]

Patient evaluation and differential diagnosis

Hashimoto's thyroiditis presents primarily with the symptoms of altered thyroid function. Early in the course of the disease the patient is usually euthyroid, but may experience clinical thyrotoxicosis owing to the breakdown of thyroid follicles, with the release of thyroid hormones. In contrast, later in the disease patients are often hypothyroid because of progressive destruction of the thyroid gland. The most common eventual outcome of Hashimoto's thyroiditis is hypothyroidism. Properly diagnosed and treated, Hashimoto's thyroiditis is not life-threatening.

A consistent physical sign seen in Hashimoto's thyroiditis is an enlarged thyroid gland. The goiter is often symmetrical, large, and feels very firm. Fine modularity is also often present. The size of an enlarged thyroid gland and the number of nodules are variable, depending on the amount of lymphocytic infiltration, the formation of fibrosis and the degree of compensatory hyperplasia. Lymph nodes surrounding the gland often become enlarged, and lymphoma must be excluded. Sometimes patients will show symptoms of other autoimmune diseases, such as generalized vasculitis with urticaria and nephritis, and these are believed to be caused by the cross-reaction of antithyroid autoantibodies with other organs, or the presence of circulating immune complexes containing thyroid antigens, predominantly thyroglobulin.

Other than tests of thyroid status, general laboratory findings are not very useful in making the diagnosis. In the early phase of the disease thyroid hormone levels may be normal, high or low. An increased TSH in the presence of normal thyroid hormones (T_4 and T_3) may presage clinical hypothyroidism. Patients with hyperthyroidism are differentiated from those with Graves' disease by the demonstration of patchy or decreased uptake on a radioiodine scan of the thyroid. Screening tests for specific autoantibodies against thyroid (antithyroglobulin and antithyroid TPO) may be helpful diagnostically in certain patients.

Sometimes it may be difficult to differentiate Hashimoto's thyroiditis from Graves' disease and other types of thyroiditis (focal lymphocytic, subacute, Riedel's). On occasion, the rapid enlargement of one lobe of the thyroid gland in Hashimoto's thyroiditis also needs to be differentiated from malignant lymphoma or thyroid carcinoma. The fibrous variant of Hashimoto's thyroiditis may also mimic carcinoma. In subacute thyroiditis the involvement of the gland is focal, whereas in Hashimoto's thyroiditis the gland is diffusely nodular and only rare nodules may be spared from the process. In some patients fine-needle biopsy will be necessary to provide a pathologic diagnosis. Cytologically, Hashimoto's thyroiditis is characterized by the presence of lymphoid infiltration of follicules, follicular cells with oxyphilic changes of varying degrees, polymorphous lymphocyte populations, and histiocytes.

POSTPARTUM THYROIDITIS

Postpartum thyroiditis is characterized by the development of transient thyrotoxicosis and/or hypothyroidism during the first 6 months of the postpartum period. A significant percentage of these patients (25–30%) suffer from chronic hypothyroidism. The symptoms of postpartum thyroiditis were first described by Robert in 1948, but the nature of the disease was not fully established until 1976.[71] The incidence of postpartum thyroiditis has been reported to range from 2% to 21% in different races and geographical locations. However, a much narrower range of 5–8% is generally accepted.[34]

Genetic and environmental factors

As with other autoimmune thyroid diseases, the development of postpartum thyroiditis is believed to involve genetic and environmental factors. A familial form has been reported.[72] A number of studies have indicated that HLA antigens, particularly DR antigens, are associated with the development of postpartum thyroiditis. A positive association of HLA-DR5 with disease has been reported.[77] A negative association with HLA-DR2 has also been observed,[78] suggesting that DR2 might confer a protective effect against the disease. Frequencies of DR3, DR4 and DR7 have also been reported to be increased in postpartum thyroiditis.[79,80]

Iodine consumption may affect the incidence or severity of postpartum thyroiditis, and this concept is in agreement with the fact that the administration of iodine exacerbates autoimmune thyroid disease.[25–31] One study[73] showed that the administration of 150 μg of iodine daily increased the severity of hypothyroidism in women with postpartum thyroiditis. A history of smoking more than 20 cigarettes per day may also be a risk factor of the development of postpartum thyroiditis.[74]

Pathogenesis

Complement-fixing anti-TPO antibodies are present in the majority of patients with postpartum thyroiditis, and the titer of this autoantibody is closely associated with the severity of the disease. Thus, the degree of hypothyroidism, determined by TSH levels, correlates with TPO antibody titers obtained both early in pregnancy and 5–7 months postpartum.[75] Although serum anti-TPO antibody levels are significantly elevated, the role they play in the pathogenesis of postpartum thyroiditis remains unclear. As the histomorphologic changes seen in postpartum thyroiditis are similar to those in Hashimoto's thyroiditis,[76,81] it is possible that the antibody only reflects the degree of thyroid damage and that the damage is executed by lymphocyte-, complement- and apoptosis-mediated mechanisms similar to those of Hashimoto's thyroiditis. However, there is evidence that the pathways leading to the final presentation of the disease appear somewhat different between these two types of thyroiditis. It is also likely that the alterations in humoral and cell-mediated immunity that accompany pregnancy (Chapter 83) are involved in the pathogenesis of this disorder.[76,81]

Patient management

Treatment is usually not recommended for the thyrotoxic phase unless symptoms are severe. As thyrotoxicosis in postpartum thyroiditis is caused by hormone release from the damaged gland, and is not secondary to increased synthesis and secretion of thyroid hormones, antithyroid medicines are not useful. In the hypothyroid phase the management of this disorder is similar to that of hypothyroidism caused by other diseases. Thyroid hormone therapy is not required unless hypothyroidism is clinically and biochemically significant. The administration of thyroxine prevents hypothyroid symptoms but does not alter the course of the disease.

Patient evaluation and differential diagnosis

The classic clinical course of postpartum thyroiditis consists of a hyperthyroid phase, followed by a hypothyroid phase and recovery. The hyperthyroidism is often mild and not recognized, or does not occur at all. During this phase irritability and lack of energy are prominent, even in autoantibody-positive women who do not develop thyroid dysfunction. In contrast, symptoms in the hypothyroid phase may be profound. Most patients recover, and about 80% are euthyroid within 12 months after delivery. However, many will have a recurrence of postpartum thyroiditis with subsequent pregnancies, and these individuals are also at a greater risk of becoming permanently hypothyroid. Patients are also more likely to become persistently hypothyroid if they have relatively high autoantibody titers or lack a hyperthyroid phase of their disease.

Results from laboratory tests need to be analyzed with consideration given to the two phases in the course of disease. TSH levels are usually a little lower or at the lower limit of detection in the hyperthyroid phase, but increased during the hypothyroid phase. Thyroid hormones are also consistent with the two-phase changes. Antithyroid autoantibodies, especially anti-TPO, are present in most patients. TRAb is usually not found unless there is coexisting Graves' disease.

The first phase (hyperthyroidism) of postpartum thyroiditis is sometimes difficult to distinguish from Graves' disease. If necessary, a thyroid radioactive iodine uptake (RAIU) test can be performed to differentiate between these two diseases. A low uptake suggests postpartum thyroiditis, whereas a high one is consistent with Graves' disease. In postpartum patients ^{123}I should be used rather than ^{131}I, and appropriate precautions should be taken to avoid exposure of the child.

A possible relationship between postpartum thyroiditis and the outcome of the infant has recently received increased attention. Infants of affected mothers demonstrated a decrease in their growth during the first 30 days, although Apgar scores, birthweight and length, and the levels of thyroid hormones were not significantly different from those of infants born to unaffected women.[83] Low IQ has also been associated with children born of women with postpartum thyroiditis.[84]

REFERENCES

1. Roitt IM, Doniach D, Campbell RN, Hudson RV. Autoantibodies in Hashimoto's thyroiditis (lymphadenoid goitre). Lancet 1956;2:820.
2. Rose NR, Witebsky E. Studies on organ-specificity. V. Changes in the thyroid gland of rabbits following active immunization with rabbit thyroid extract. J Immunol 1956;76:417.
3. Adams DD, Purves HD. Abnormal responses in the assay of thyrotropin. Proc Univ Otago Med Sch 1956;34:11.
4. Horsley V. Remarks on the function of the thyroid gland. A critical and historical review. Br Med J 1892;1:215.
5. Payami H, Joe S, Thomson G. Auntoimmune thyroid diseases in type I diabetic families. Genet Epidemiol 1989;7:83.
6. Tomer Y, Davies TF. The genetic susceptibility to Graves' disease. Baillières Clin Endocrinol Metab 1997;11:431.
7. Stenszky V, Kozma L, Balazs C, et al. The genetics of Graves' disease: HLA and disease susceptibility. J Clin Endocrinol Metab 1985;61:735.
8. Weetman AP, McGregor AM. Autoimmune thyroid disease: further developments in our understanding. Endocrinol Rev 1994;15:788.
9. Katsuren E, Awata T, Matsumoto C, Yamamoto K. HLA Class II alletes in Japanese patients with Graves' disease: weak associations of HLA-DR and -DQ. Endocrinol J 1994;41:599.
10. Wong GWK, Cheng SH, Dorman JS. The HLA-DQ associations with Graves' disease in Chinese children. Clin Endocrinol 1999;50:493.
11. Barlow ABT, Wheatcroft N, Waston P, Weetman AP. Association of HLA-DQA10501 with Graves' disease in English Caucasian men and women. Clin Endocrinol 1996;44:73.
12. Chuang L-M, Wu HP, Chang CC, et al. HLA DRB1/DQA1/DQB1 haplotype determines thyroid autoimmunity in patients with insulin dependent diabetes mellitus. Clin Endocrinol 1996;45:631.
13. Tamai H, Kimura A, Dong R-P, et al. Resistance to autoimmune thyroid disease is associated with HLA-DQ. J Clin Endocrinol Metab 1994;78:94.
14. Roman SH, Greenberg D, Rubinstein P, Wallenstein S, Davies TF. Genetics of autoimmune thyroid disease: lack of evidence for linkage to HLA within families. J Clin Endocrinol Metab 1992;74:496.
15. Yanagawa T, Taniyama M, Enomoto S, et al. CTLA4 gene polymorphism confers susceptibility to Graves' disease in Japanese. Thyroid 1997;7:843.
16. Vaidya B, Imrie H, Perros P, et al. The cytotoxic T lymphocyte antigen-4 is a major Graves' disease locus. Hum Molec Genet 1999;8:1195.
17. Donner H, Rau H, Walfish PG, et al. CTLA Alanine-17 confers genetic susceptibility to Graves' disease and to type I diabetes mellitus. J Clin Endocrinol Metab 1997;82:143.
18. Kemp EH, Ajjan RA, Husebye ES, et al. A cytotoxic T lymphocyte antigen-4 (CTLA-4) gene polymorphism is associated with autoimmune Addison's disease in English patients. Clin Endocrinol 1998;49:609.
19. De Roux N, Shields DC, Misrahi M, Ratanachaiyavong S, McGregor AM, Milgrom E. Analysis of the thyrotropin receptor as a candidate gene in familial Graves' disease. J Clin Endocrinol Metab 1996;81:3483.
20. Tomer Y, Barbesina G, Greenberg DA, Concepcion E, Davies TF. Linkage analysis of candidate genes in autoimmune thyroid disease. III. Detailed analysis of chromosome 14 localizes Grave's disease-1 close to multinodular goiter (MNG-1). J Clin Endocrinol Metab 1998;83:4321.
21. Barbesina G, Tomer Y, Concepcion E, Davies TF, Greenberg DA. Linkage analysis of candidate genes in antoimmune thyroid disease. II. Selected gender-related genes and the X-chromosome. J Clin Endocrinol Metab 1998;83:3290.
22. Blakemore AIF, Waston PF, Weetman AP, Duff GW. Association of Graves' disease with an allele of the interleukin-1 receptor antagonist gene. J Clin Endocrinol Metab 1995;80:111.
23. Yangwei W, Tian L. Association of GLO I with Graves' disease and Hashimoto's thyroiditis. J Xi'An Med Uni 1998;19:575.
24. Siegmund T, Usadel KH, Donner H, Braun J, Walfish PG, Badenhoop K. Interferon-gamma gene microsatellite polymorphisms in patients with Graves' disease. Thyroid 1988;8:1013.
25. Weetman AP, McGregor AM, Campbell H, et al. Iodide enhances IgG synthesis by human peripheral blood lymphocytes in vitro. Acta Endocrinol (Copenh) 1983;103:210.
26. Champion BR, Rayner DC, Byfield PGH, Page KR, Chan CTJ, Riott IM. Critical role of iodination for T cell recognition of thyroglobulin in experimental murine thyroid autoimmunity. J Immunol 1987;139:3665.
27. Schupper F, Tangiguchi S-I, Schroder S, Dralle H, von Zur Muhlen A, Kohn LD. In vivo and in vitro evidence for iodide regulation of MHC Class I and Class II expression in Graves' disease. J Clin Endocrinol Metab 1996;81:3622.
28. Sundick RS, Herdegen DM, Brown TR, Bagchi N. The incorporation of dietary iodine into thyroglobulin increases its immunogenicity. Endocrinology 1987;120:2078.
29. Alexander WD, Harden RMcG, Koutras DA, Wayne E. Influence of iodine intake after treatment with antithyroid drugs. Lancet 1965;2:866.
30. Thjodleifsson B, Hedley AJ, Donald D, et al. Outcome of sub-total thyroidectomy for thyrotoxicosis in Iceland and Northeast Scotland. Clin Endocrinol (Oxford) 1975;7:367.
31. Azizi F. Environmental iodine intake affects the response to methimazole in patients with diffuse toxic goiter. J Clin Endocrinol Metab 1985;61:374.
32. Winsa B, Adami H, Bergstrom R, et al. Stressful life events and Graves' disease. Lancet 1991;338:1475.
33. Gorman CA. A critical review of the role of stress in hyperthyroidism. In: Drexhage HA, de Vijlder JJM, Wiersinga WM (eds) The thyroid gland environment and autoimmunity. Amsterdam, Elsevier Science, 1990, p. 191.
34. Baker JR Jr Endocrine disease. In Stites DP, Terr AI, Parslow TG (eds) Basic and clinical immunology, 8th edn. Norwalk, Conn., Appleton & Lange, 1994, p. 412.
35. Bech K, Larsen JH, Hansen JM, Nerup J. *Yersinia enterocolitica* infection and thyroid disorders. Lancet 1974;2:951.
36. Weiss M, Inghar SH, Winbald S, Kaspar DL. Demonstration of a saturable binding site for thyrotropin in *Yersinia enterocolitica*. Science 1983;219:1331.
37. Weetman AP, McGregor AM. Autoimmune thyroid disease: further developments in our understanding. Endocrinol Rev 1994;15:788.
38. Volpe R, Karlsson A, Jansson R, Dahlberg PA. Edvidence that antithyroid drugs induce remissions in Graves' disease by modulating thyroid cellular activity. Clin Endocrinol (Oxford) 1986;25:453.
39. Libert F, Lefort A, Gerard C, et al. Cloning, sequencing and expression of the human thyrotropin (TSH) receptor: Evidence for binding of autoantibodies. Biochem Biophys Res Commun 1989;165:1250.
40. Soliman M, Kaplan E, Guimaraes V, Yanagawa T, DeGroot LJ. T cell recognition of residue 158–176 in TSH receptor confers risk for development of thyroid autoimmunity in siblings in a family with Graves' disease. Thyroid 1996;6:545.
41. Davies TF, Martin A, Concepcion ES, Graves P, Chen L, Ben-Nun A. Evidence of limited variability of antigen receptors on intrathyroidal T cells in autoimmune thyroid disease. N Engl J Med 1991;325:238.
42. Konishi J, Iida Y, Endo K, et al. Inhibition of thyrotropin-induced adenosine 3′,5′-monophosphate increase by immunoglobulins from patients with primary myxoedema. J Clin Endocrinol Metab 1983;57:544.
43. Drexhage HA, van der Gaag RD. Immunoglobulins affecting thyroid growth. In: McGregor AM (ed) Immunology of endocrine diseases. Lancaster, MTP Press, 1986, p. 51.
44. Hashizume K, Ichikawa K, Sakurai A, et al. Administration of thyroxine in treated Graves' disease: effects on the level of antibodies to thyroid-stimulating hormone receptors and on the risk of recurrence of hyperthyroidism. N Engl J Med 1991;324:947.
45. McIver B, Rae P, Beckett G, Wilkinson E, Gold A, Toft A. Lack of effect of thyroxine in patients with Graves' hyperthyroidism who are treated with an antithyroid drug. N Engl J Med 1996;334:220.

46. Rittmaster RS, Zwicker H, Abbott EC, et al. Effect of methimazole with or without exogenous L-thyroxine on serum concentrations of TSH receptor antibodies in patients with Graves' disease. J Clin Endocrinol Metab 1996;81:3283.
47. Hall R, Owen SG, Smart GS. Evidence for genetic predisposition to formation of thyroid autoantibodies. Lancet 1964;2:187.
48. Weetman AP. Autoimmune thyroiditis: predisposition and pathogenesis. Clin Endocrinol 1992;36:307.
49. Wan XL, Kimura A, Dong RP, Honda K, Tamai H, Sasazuki T. HLA-A and DRB4 genes in controlling the susceptibility to Hashimoto's thyroiditis. Hum Immunol 1995;42:131.
50. Thompson C, Farid NR. Post-partum thyroiditis and goitrous (Hashimoto's) thyroiditis are associated with HLA-DR4. Immunol Lett 1985;11:301.
51. Thompson M, Ryder LP, Beth K, et al. HLA-D in Hashimoto's thyroiditis. Tissue Antigens 1983;21:173.
52. Stenszky V, Balazs C, Kraszits E, et al. Association of goitrous autoimmune thyroiditis with HLA-DR3 in eastern Hungary. J Immunogenet 1987;14:143.
53. Vargas MT, Bropnes-Urbina R, Gladman D, Papsin FR, Walfish PG. Antithyroid microsomal autoantibodies and HLA-DR5 are associated with postpartum thyroid dysfunction: evidence supporting an endocrine pathogenesis. J Clin Endocrinol Metab 1988;67:327.
54. Badenhoop K, Schwarz G, Walfish PG, et al. Susceptibility to thyroid autoimmune disease: molecular analysis of HLA-D region genes identifies new markers for goitrous Hashimoto's thyroiditis. J Clin Endocrinol Metab 1990;71:1131.
55. Tandon N, Zhang L, Weetman AP. HLA association with Hashimoto's thyroiditis. Clin Endocrinol 1991;34:383.
56. Hawkins BR, Lam KSL, Ma JTC, Wang C, Yeung RTT. Strong association between HLA-DRw9 and Hashimoto's thyroiditis in southern Chinese. Acta Endocrinol 1987;114:543.
57. Onuma H, Ota M, Sugenoya A, Kasuga Y, Asanuma K, Inoko H, Iida F. Association between HLA and Hashimoto thyroiditis in Japanese. In: Nagataki S, Mori T, Torizuka K (eds) 80 years of Hashimoto disease. Amsterdam, Elsevier, 1993, p. 65.
58. Cho BY, Chung JH, Lee HK, Koh C-S. Immunogenetic heterogeneity of atrophic antoimmune thyroiditis according to thyrotropin receptor blocking antibody. In: Nagataki S, Mori T, Torizuka K (eds) 80 years of Hashimoto disease. Amsterdam, Elsevier, 1993, p. 45.
59. Levine SN. Current concepts of thyroiditis. Arch Intern Med 1983;143:1952.
60. Ansar Ahmed S, Young PR, Penhale WJ. The effects of female sex steroids on the development of autoimmune thyroiditis in thymectomized and irradiated rats. Clin Exp Immunol 1983;54:351.
61. Okayasu I, Kong YM, Rose NR. Effect of castration and sex hormones on experimental autoimmune thyroiditis. Clin Immunol Immunopathol 1981;20:240.
62. Clark OH, Gerend PL, Davus M, Goretzki PE, Hoffman PG Jr. Estrogen and thyroid-stimulating hormone (TSH) receptors in neoplastic and nonneoplastic human thyroid tissue. J Surg Res 1985;38:89.
63. Kakizaki S, Takagi H, Murakami M, Takayama H, Mori M. HLA antigens in patients with interferon-α-induced antoimmune thyroid disorders in chronic hepatitis C. J Hepatol 1999;30:794.
64. Baker JR Jr. Dying (apoptosing?) for a consensus on the Fas death pathway in the thyroid. J Clin Endocrinol Metab 1999;84:2593.
65. Baker JR Jr. Immunologic aspects of endocrine diseases. Ann Intern Med 1988;108:26.
66. Bonger U, Finke R, Hegedus L, Hanseb JM, Schleusener H. Cytotoxicity and antithyroid peroxidase antibodies in patients with autoimmune thyroiditis. In: Nagataki S, Mori T, Torizuka K (eds) 80 years of Hashimoto disease. Amsterdam, Elsevier, 1993, p. 383.
67. Arscott PL, Baker JR Jr. Apoptosis and thyroiditis. Clin Immunol Immunopathol 1998;87:207.
68. Batteux F, Tourneur L, Trebeden H, Charreire J, Chiocchia G. Gene therapy of experimental autoimmune thyroiditis by in vivo administration of plasmid DNA coding Fas ligand. J Immunol 1999;162:603.
69. Bretz JD, Arscott PL, Myc A, Baker JR Jr. Inflammatory cytokine regulation of Fas-mediated apoptosis in thyroid follicular cells. J Biol Chem 1999;274:25433.
70. Irvine WJ, McGregor AG, Stuart AE. The prognostic significance of thyroid antibodies in the management of thyrotoxicosis. Lancet 1962;2:843.
71. Amino N, Miyai KJ, Onishi T, et al. Transient hypothyroidism after delivery in autoimmune thyroiditis. J Clin Endocrinol Metab 1976;42:296.
72. Singer PA, Gorsky JE. Familial postpartum transient hypothyroidism. Arch Intern Med 1985;145:240.
73. Kampe O, Jansson R, Karlsson FA. Effects of L-thyroxine and iodide on the development of autoimmune postpartum thyroiditis. J Clin Endocrinol Metab 1990;70:1014.
74. Jansson R, Dahlberg PA, Karlsson FA. Postpartum thyroiditis. In: Baillieṙe's Clin Endocrinol Metab. 1988;2:619.
75. Jansson R, Bernander S, Karlsson A, Levin K, Nilsson G. Autoimmune thyroid dysfunction in the postpartum period. J Clin Endocrinol Metab 1984;58:681.
76. Stagnaro-Green A, Roman SH, Cobin RH, et al. A prospective study of lymphocyte-initiated immunosuppression in normal pregnancy: evidence of a T-cell etiology for postpartum thyroid dysfunction. J Clin Endocrinol Metab 1992;74:645.
77. Vargas MT, Briones-Urbina R, Gladman D, et al. Antithyroid microsomal autoantibodies and HLA-DR5 are associated with postpartum thyroid dysfunction: evidence supporting an autoimmune pathogenesis. J Clin Endcrinol Metab 1988;67:327.
78. Kologlu M, Fung H, Darke C, et al. Postpartum thyroid dysfunction and HLA status. Eur J Clin Invest 1990;20:56.
79. Thompson P, Farid NR. Post-partum thyroiditis and goitrous (Hashimoto's) thyroiditis are associated with HLA-DR4. Immunol Lett 1985;11:301.
80. Parkes AB, Darke C, Othman S, et al. MHC Class II and complement polymorphism in postpartum thyroiditis. Eur J Endocrinol 1996;134:449.
81. Mizukami Y, Michigishi T, Nonomura A, et al. Postpartum thyroiditis a clinical, histological, and immunopathologic study of 15 cases. Am J Clin Pathol 1993;100:200.
82. Davies TF. The thyroid immunology of the postpartum period. Thyroid 1999;9:675.
83. Beth K, Hertel J, Rasmussen NG, et al. Effect of maternal thyroid autoantibodies and post-partum thyroiditis on the fetus and neonate. Acta Endocrinol 1991;125:146.
84. Pop VJ, de Vries E, van Baar AL, et al. Maternal thyroid proxidase antibodies during pregnancy: a marker of impaired child development. J Clin Endocrinol Metab 1995;80:3561.

Section 7 Organ-specific Inflammatory Disease

Chapter 82

Diabetes and Related Autoimmune Diseases

David T. Robles and George S. Eisenbarth

INTRODUCTION

Diabetes mellitus is a heterogeneous group of disorders characterized by glucose intolerance and hyperglycemia. The clinical manifestations of this disease are the result of either an absolute or a relative deficiency of insulin secretion. Recently, an expert committee of the American Diabetes Association proposed four categories of diabetes, based on etiology rather than the age of disease onset (e.g. juvenile-onset versus adult-onset) or the requirement for insulin therapy (insulin-dependent versus non-insulin-dependent diabetes).[1] The categories are type 1 (formerly termed insulin-dependent diabetes – IDDM); type 2 (with a major component of insulin resistance); diabetes with known genetic mutations (e.g. the maturity-onset diabetes of youth syndromes with mutations in glucokinase, hepatic nuclear factor genes etc.); and gestational diabetes (Table 82.1). Type 1 diabetes is divided into type 1A (immune mediated) and type 1B (idiopathic loss of insulin secretion), depending primarily upon the presence or absence respectively of anti-islet autoantibodies.

The subject of this chapter is type 1A or immune-mediated diabetes, and there is now convincing evidence that this form of diabetes results from immune-mediated destruction of the cells that produce insulin. Despite older designations for this category, approximately the same number of adults develop type 1A diabetes as do children, and many individuals early in the course of type 1A diabetes are not 'insulin dependent' but can transiently be treated with oral hypoglycemic agents. The incidence of type 2 diabetes increases dramatically with age, whereas that of type 1A changes relatively little with age (less than threefold).[2] Thus, when a child develops diabetes they usually (>90% for non-Hispanic White children) have type 1A diabetes mellitus. There is, however, heterogeneity of diabetes even among children with the disorder. For example, almost half of African-American and Hispanic-American children who develop diabetes do not have type 1A, but have primarily type 2 or type 1B diabetes.[3] Given such heterogeneity, it is likely that the diagnostic classification of diabetes will in the future depend upon the immunologic parameters to be discussed and identification of specific genetic mutations associated with specific disorders of glucose metabolism.

The information indicating that type 1A diabetes is an immune-mediated autoimmune illness has greatly increased during the past two decades. The recognition that there might be a form of 'juvenile' or insulin-dependent diabetes of autoimmune origin came from the observation that diabetes was often associated with disorders thought to be of autoimmune origin, such as Addison's disease, Graves' disease and thyroiditis.[4,5] Nevertheless, considerable confusion existed because of the failure to separate diabetes into distinct disease categories (type 1 versus type 2). Although insulitis had been observed in a few children who had come to autopsy shortly after the development of diabetes, this was an extremely rare event for diabetes as a whole.[6,7]

Table 82.1 Classification of diabetes mellitus (DM).

Classification of diabetes

Diabetes mellitus	Previous designations	Etiologic distinctions	Clinical distinctions
Type 1		β-cell destruction	
A. Immune-mediated	Juvenile onset/IDDM	Immune	Both result in insulin dependence, with loss of β-cells
B. Idiopathic	Type 1.5/Flatbush DM	Unknown	
Type 2	NIDDM	Insulin resistance and relative insulin deficiency	Oral hypoglycemic agents are effective early in the disease
Other specific types	MODY Secondary diabetes	Specific genetic defects Pancreatic disease Endocrinopathies Chemical induced Infection related Immune-mediated forms Genetic syndromes	Specific mutations identified and defined clinical syndromes
Gestational	Unchanged		Onset during pregnancy

IDDM, insulin-dependent diabetes; MODY, maturity-onset diabetes of youth.

Studies of monozygotic twins with diabetes revealed very different patterns of inheritance for insulin-dependent and non-insulin-dependent diabetes mellitus, and two major forms of the disease were proposed. Specific HLA alleles were found to be associated with the insulin-dependent form,[8] and in 1974 cytoplasmic islet cell autoantibodies were found for diabetic patients with polyendocrine autoimmunity (e.g. Addison's disease).[9] Islet cell autoantibodies were then found to be present prior to the development of diabetes, and studies of monozygotic twins of patients with type 1 diabetes led to the observation that this was a chronically progressive autoimmune disorder.[10] In identical twins developing diabetes, islet cell autoantibodies and loss of insulin secretion preceded the development of diabetes by years.[11] As discussed below, the measurement of anti-islet autoantibodies has improved dramatically during the past two decades, and for many individuals the development of type 1A diabetes can now be predicted.

Despite the emphasis on anti-islet autoantibodies, most investigators believe that T cells and not autoantibodies mediate the immune destruction of insulin-producing cells.[12–14] Studies of T cells have benefited from the discovery of two remarkable animal models of type 1A diabetes, the NOD mouse and the BB rat.[13,14] In animal models diabetes can be transferred to nondiabetic animals by T-cell clones. In addition, a clinical observation by Sutherland and co-workers was particularly informative in terms of demonstrating the importance of T cells in this disease.[15] They transplanted the tail of the pancreas from monozygotic twins who had not developed diabetes into their respective twin pairs with more than a decade of diabetes. The transplanted islets were invaded by lymphocytes, and islet β cells (the cells that produce insulin) were specifically and rapidly destroyed.

KEY CONCEPTS

Type 1A diabetes is an autoimmune disease

- Genetic and familial clustering of diabetes and additional autoimmune disorders
- Presence of high-affinity autoantibodies and T cells reactive to islet cell autoantigens
- Strong HLA association (DR3/DR4)
- Ability to transfer the disease in animal models through adoptive transfer of islet cell-reactive T-cell clones
- Recurrence of disease in pancreas transplanted between identical twins

Key questions in type 1A diabetes

Basic questions
What genes determine type 1A diabetes susceptibility?
What triggers or suppresses the activation of autoimmunity?
What are the major target molecules and is there a primary autoantigen?
What are the effector mechanisms for islet destruction?

Clinical questions
Is type 1A diabetes predictable?
Is the rate of progression to overt diabetes predictable?
Is type 1A diabetes preventable?

Table 82.2 Key questions in type 1A diabetes.

Despite considerable progress in studies of type 1A diabetes, a series of basic and clinical questions remain unanswered or have only partial answers (Table 82.2). This chapter reviews current knowledge concerning many of these questions. Although the chapter cannot address all viewpoints on controversial issues, controversies are emphasized, as many issues concerning the pathogenesis of type 1A diabetes are not settled.

DIAGNOSIS

The demonstration of elevated plasma glucose is the *sine qua non* for diagnosis of diabetes mellitus. Recent recommendations by the American Diabetes Association have lowered the diagnostic level of fasting glucose from 140 mg/dl (7.8 mmol/l) to 126 mg/dl (7.0 mmol/l). Other diagnostic criteria include a random plasma glucose level >200 mg/dl (11.1 mmol/dl) or a plasma glucose level >200 mg/dl (11.1 mmol/dl) 2 hours following 75 g of oral glucose ingestion (the oral glucose tolerance test – OGTT). In children this is usually not necessary for diagnosis.

The clinical signs and symptoms associated with hyperglycemia and osmotic diuresis (e.g. polyuria and polydypsia) are recognized by clinicians and lay people alike, making the diagnosis relatively straightforward. Insulin deficiency, if untreated, leads to the utilization of fats for fuel, with subsequent metabolism of fatty acids and the production of ketoacids. Thus, the presentation of ketonuria, ketonemia and ketoacidosis, often associated with nausea or hyperventilation, is an important clinical feature. Unexplained weight loss, along with the classic signs and symptoms mentioned above, is highly suggestive for the diagnosis of diabetes. Despite the classic signs and symptoms, approximately 1 in 200 children die at the onset of type 1 diabetes. If the first healthcare provider to see the child fails to make a diagnosis of diabetes, the child may subsequently present with severe ketoacidosis and may develop cerebral edema, which is usually fatal.

Although not specifically recommended as a diagnostic criterion by the National Diabetes Data Group, an elevated glycosylated hemoglobin concentration (HbA1c) may also be useful for diagnosis. The HbA1c level correlates with mean glucose levels over several months and eventually with the development of diabetic complications, including diabetic retinopathy.

The diagnosis of specific diabetic syndromes, including type 1A diabetes, requires further information. Several clinical criteria increase or decrease the probability that an individual has type 1A diabetes (e.g. increase: onset at age <35, nonobese, presence of ketoacidosis, immediate therapy with insulin required, family or personal history of organ-specific autoimmunity; decrease: age of onset >35, effective therapy with oral hypoglycemic agents, African-American or Hispanic-American child, obesity). These clinical criteria are, however, imprecise guidelines to diagnosis at best. For example, as many as 10% of obese White adults presenting with diabetes have type 1A. The hallmark of type 1 versus type 2 diabetes is the early (several years post diagnosis) development of severe insulin deficiency. The connecting peptide (C-peptide) of the proinsulin molecule is secreted in equimolar quantity to insulin by pancreatic β cells. Within 3 years of the onset of type 1A diabetes, most children have a severe impairment of insulin secretion such that fasting C-peptide is not detectable. The range of C-peptide secretion, however, is large at the onset in both type 1 and type 2 diabetes. Secretion is influenced by metabolic control, such that determination of C-peptide at onset has limited diagnostic utility in distinguishing type 1 from type 2 diabetes. The maintenance of C-peptide secretion can also be used as a measure of effective immunotherapy in clinical trials.

It should be recognized that both type 1A and type 2 diabetes are relatively common disorders, and thus individuals might have both diseases. Type 2 diabetes would be manifested by resistance to insulin, such that overt hyperglycemia will present earlier in the course of the islet β-cell destruction associated with type 1A diabetes.

The best immunologic markers for distinguishing type 1A from other forms of diabetes is the presence of islet cell autoantibodies. Diagnostic accuracy depends upon the sensitivity and specificity of the autoantibody assays employed. Assays for autoantibodies reacting with insulin, glutamic acid decarboxylase (GAD65) and ICA512 (IA-2), when performed with fluid-phase assays (not ELISA), can be set such that fewer than 1 in 100 nondiabetic individuals are positive. One or another of these three autoantibodies is present in approximately 95% of children with recent-onset type 1A diabetes. However, approximately half of Hispanic-American children presenting with diabetes do not express any of the three anti-islet antibodies (compared to less than 10% of non-Hispanic white children). We believe that the majority of the antibody-negative population represents a type 2 diabetes variant.

CLINICAL PEARLS

- Type 1A diabetes can occur at any age. Testing of islet cell autoantibodies identifies 10% of adults (thought to have type 2 diabetes) as having type 1A diabetes.
- Half of African-American and Hispanic-American children are negative for anti-islet autoantibodies and have type 2 or type 1B diabetes.
- Organ-specific autoimmunity (in particular celiac disease, thyroid disease, Addison's disease and pernicious anemia) is greatly increased in patients with type 1A diabetes.
- The more common the organ-specific autoimmune disease in the general population the more common the disease in patients with type 1A diabetes. For example, thyroid autoimmunity is common and routine TSH testing is advised.
- In diabetic patients with decreasing insulin need or severe hypoglycemia, rule out Addison's disease.

EPIDEMIOLOGY/INCIDENCE

Type 1A diabetes is one of the most common chronic diseases of childhood and is the most common type of diabetes in persons under 40 years of age. Diabetes is the leading cause of blindness, amputations and end-stage renal disease, and is a major factor contributing to cardiovascular disease and premature death.[17] It typically presents in children (with a peak onset at 12–13 years of age), but it may occur at any age and can be found in all racial groups, with a similar prevalence in both females and males.

The annual incidence of type 1A diabetes varies dramatically. In children the incidence is approximately 15/100 000 in the United States, 35/100 000 in Finland, and fewer than 1/100 000 in Japan.[16] The prevalence of type 1A diabetes in the US is approximately 1/300, and 90% of children developing diabetes do not have a first-degree relative with the disorder. Approximately 1 in 20 first-degree relatives of patients develop the disease. The risk to offspring of a father with type 1A diabetes is approximately twice that of offspring of an affected mother. In the US, non-Hispanic White Americans are approximately one and a half times more likely to develop type 1A diabetes than are other groups.

The prevalence of type 1A diabetes is greatest in countries where the predominant population is Caucasian. For example, it is most prevalent in Finland and Sardinia and rare in Japan, Korea and China. A child in Finland has a 35 fold greater risk of developing diabetes than a child in Japan. In Japan, for example, monozygotic twins of patients with type 1A diabetes and their first-degree relatives have a risk of diabetes similar to that of twins and relatives in the United States.[18] This suggests that the bulk of differences between countries relates to genetic differences and not environmental factors. Studies of migrant populations from developed countries have failed to reveal major differences in diabetes incidence based on migration from a high-incidence to a lower-incidence country.[19] Nevertheless, there are less well characterized populations where diabetes incidence may have changed dramatically with migration, e.g. Yemenite Jews migrating to Israel.

Seasonal variation in the incidence of type 1A diabetes has been well documented, with more children presenting with the disease in the fall and winter months. This seasonal variation has been ascribed to potential viral infections causing β-cell destruction; however, with increased knowledge of the natural history of type 1A diabetes it is more likely that such seasonal variation may simply reflect factors (e.g. viral infections) that either bring children to medical attention or produce insulin resistance when limited islet β-cell mass remains.

The incidence of type 1A diabetes in Finland is among the highest in the world and has been increasing by 2–3% per year over the last three decades.[17,20] Furthermore, the age of onset of type 1A diabetes in Finland is becoming younger, with children <5 years of age showing an increase in incidence.[20] One hypothesis to explain these trends is that increases in the number or timing of vaccinations may be related to changes in incidence.[21] Classen and Classen[22] suggested that immunization with *Haemophilus influenzae* type B (HiB) after the age of 2 months is associated with an increased risk of type 1A diabetes in humans. However, one study[23] reported that there was no statistically significant difference in the incidence of type 1A diabetes between three cohorts of Finnish children who either were not vaccinated or who were vaccinated at 3 months or at 24 months. In 1998, a workshop reviewing type 1A diabetes and immunization, held at the Johns Hopkins School of Public Health, found no evidence that vaccines increase the risk of type 1A diabetes in humans.[24] In a cohort study in Denver, Colorado, no association was found between β-cell autoimmunity and hepatitis B, HiB, polio or DTP vaccinations given either at birth or at 9 months of age.[25] Despite the conclusions of these studies, public concern over this matter is still high and there will probably be further studies.

KEY CONCEPTS

Epidemiology and incidence of type 1A diabetes

- One of the most common chronic diseases of childhood and the most common type of diabetes in persons under 40 years of age.
- The leading cause of blindness, amputations, and end-stage renal disease, and contributes to premature death.
- Peak age of onset is 12–13 years, but may occur at any age, in all racial groups, with equal prevalence between males and females.
- More children are diagnosed in the fall and winter months, but it is likely that this reflects factors that bring children to medical attention.
- The incidence of type 1A diabetes has been increasing in many countries.
- No conclusive evidence exists for an association between vaccination and incidence of type 1A diabetes.

Stages in the development of type 1A diabetes

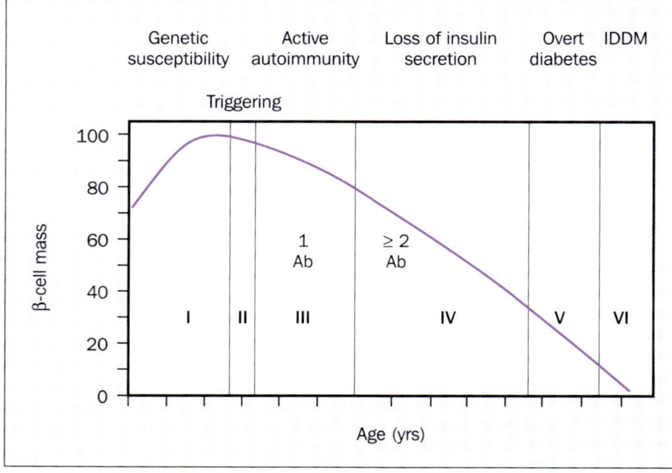

Figure 82.1 Stages in the development of type 1A diabetes. Eisenbarth GS. Type I diabetes mellitus. A chronic autoimmune disease. *N Engl J Med* 1986;314:1360.

NATURAL HISTORY

Studies over the past decade in humans are defining details of the chronology of development of type 1A diabetes. In addition, studies in animal models have contributed to a greater understanding of the pathogenesis of the disease. At present, there are three major hypotheses (described below) concerning the natural history of type 1A diabetes, with a fourth hypothesis having almost no supporters. The fourth hypothesis, which was prominent two decades ago, was that type 1A diabetes was an acute disorder induced by viral infection.[26] If the acute development of diabetes occurs, it is likely to be extremely rare, given studies of both relatives and the general population. Anti-islet autoantibodies almost always precede diabetes by years, as does the loss of first-phase insulin secretion.[27,28]

Hypothesis 1 Type 1A diabetes is a chronic and progressive disorder resulting from immune-mediated destruction of islet β cells.[10,29] A corollary of this hypothesis is that as immunologic and immunogenetic assays are refined, one would be able to predict both the risk of diabetes and the approximate time of progression to diabetes, with different individuals progressing at different rates. This hypothesis is encapsulated in the division of type 1A diabetes into a series of stages (I, genetic susceptibility; II, triggering of autoimmunity; III, active immunity; IV, loss of insulin secretion; and V, overt diabetes) (Fig. 82.1).[10,30]

Hypothesis 2 Type 1A diabetes is preceded by a long prodromal phase of autoimmunity, but actual islet β-cell destruction is acute and occurs at the end of the process.[31]

Hypothesis 3 Type 1A diabetes results from 'multiple' hits, perhaps viral, and thus develops slowly, but would be difficult to predict as the 'hits' are not predictable.[32]

It is possible that a combination of all three hypotheses will eventually be found to apply to different individuals developing diabetes. For example, a diabetic identical twin who receives half of the pancreas from their nondiabetic twin rapidly develops recurrent diabetes within several weeks.[15] Thus, the immune system has the potential to rapidly destroy human β cells. Nevertheless, there is considerable evidence that the first hypothesis is generally applicable. It reflects the progressive loss of first-phase insulin secretion which precedes diabetes, and the chronic loss of C-peptide secretion (over years) after the diagnosis of diabetes. This hypothesis is also consistent with recent detailed analysis of β-cell loss and regeneration in NOD mice prior to diabetes.[33]

Despite evidence for progressive loss of β cells in the NOD mouse,[33] there is evidence for important changes in the immune system at the onset of diabetes. In the NOD mouse, splenocytes from recently diabetic – but not nondiabetic – mice transfer diabetes. Close to the time of diabetes, but not at early ages, NOD mice destroy islet transplants.[34] Finally, anti-CD3 therapy produces long-term improvement of blood sugar if given at diabetes onset, but not with early treatment.[35]

TWIN STUDIES

Monozygotic twins of patients with type 1A diabetes have approximately a 50% concordance rate for type 1A diabetes. This concordance is markedly different from that of dizygotic twins (5%), who have a risk similar to a sibling of a patient with type 1A diabetes. This difference reflects a significant role for genetic factors but suggests that environmental and possibly somatic mutations or other stochastic events may also play a significant role in the pathogenesis. Although the risk of a discordant twin progressing to type 1A diabetes decreases proportionately with the duration of discordance, twins can become concordant after many years.[36] In a prospective study involving 187 monozygotic twins from the UK and the US who were discordant at the time of enrolment, 47 became concordant with a range of time of onset of 0.4–39 years. The median discordance time of the twin pairs was 4.2 years, and 25% became concordant after 14 years of discordance.[37]

HLA genes

A major determinant of genetic susceptibility resides in the MHC Class II region (*IDDM1*). HLA Class II molecules, particularly DR and DQ, account for approximately 50% of the genetic risk

High-risk and protective HLA haplotypes			
High risk			
DR3	DRB1*0301	DQA1*0501	DQB1*0201
DR4	DRB1*0401	DQA1*0301	DQB1*0302
	DRB1*0402	DQA1*0301	DQB1*0302
	DRB1*0405	DQA1*0301	DQB1*0302
Moderate risk			
DR1	DRB1*01	DQA1*0101	DQB1*0501
DR8	DRB1*0801	DQA1*0401	DQB1*0402
DR9	DRB1*0901	DQA1*0301	DQB1*0303
Protective			
Strong protection			
DR2	DRB1*1501	DQA1*0102	DQB1*0602
DR6	DRB1*1401	DQA1*0101	DQB1*0503
DR7	DRB1*0701	DQA1*0201	DQB1*0303
Moderate protection			
DR5	DRB1*1101	DQA1*0501	DQB1*0301
Weak protection			
DR4	DRB1*0401	DQA1*0301	DQB1*0301
	DRB1*0403	DQA1*0301	DQB1*0302
DR7	DRB1*0701	DQA1*0201	DQB1*0201

Table 82.3 High-risk and protective HLA haplotypes.

for type 1A diabetes development.[38] As the MHC region displays a significant degree of linkage disequilibrium (e.g. specific DQ and DR alleles are nonrandomly associated with each other) associations of HLA with disease must be thought of as haplotype specific and not allele specific. Class I HLA alleles can also influence disease, and it is possible that unknown genes linked to the HLA region are important. Nevertheless, the identification of HLA Class II alleles associated with high, moderate, low risk and even 'protection' is useful in disease prediction (Table 82.3).

Individuals with the highest risk for type 1A diabetes in the US express both DQA1*0501-DQB1*0201 (DQ2), which is almost always inherited with DRB1*0301, and DQA1*0301-DQB1*0302 (DQ8), inherited with DRB1*0401 or *0402. These individuals have been referred to as DR3/DR4 or DQ2/DQ8 heterozygotes. The genotype, DQ2/DQ8 (DR3/DR4) is commonly observed in type 1A diabetics. Although only 2% of children in the US have this genotype, they constitute approximately 40% of those developing diabetes.[39] Observations of transmission frequencies of particular haplotypes have helped illustrate the importance of certain haplotypes in contributing to diabetes susceptibility. For example, analysis of the Human Biological Data Interchange (HBDI) family collection has revealed that DQA1*0501-DQB*0201 and DQA1*0301-DQB1*0302 are transmitted to more than 80% of diabetic children. DQB1 alleles without an aspartic acid at position 57 of the β chain have been proposed to determine diabetes risk. No simple amino acid rule, however, adequately describes the risk associated with DQ allelles, and with current technology it is possible to define all polymorphic residues.

HLA DQ alleles have also been associated with dominant protection from type 1A diabetes. Approximately 20% of the general population have DQA1*0102-DQB1*0602, the HLA haplotype that provides dominant protection from type 1A diabetes.[40] Interestingly, autoantibody-positive relatives of affected individuals who express the HLA haplotype DQA1 0102, DQB1*0602 are protected (though not completely) from progression to diabetes.[41]

HLA Class I and DP alleles are also associated with diabetes risk. For example, the A24 allele is associated with early age of onset of type 1A diabetes.[42] There are probably additional loci linked to HLA, such as loci near microsatellite D6S2223, also conferring risk.

NON-HLA GENES

Genome-wide screens for loci linked with diabetes (using microsatellite markers from all of the chromosomes) have led to the identification of 18 genetic loci contributing to diabetes susceptibility in the NOD mouse and over 15 in humans, with variable statistical significance (Table 82.4). However, actual genes have not been identified for the great majority of these putative loci.

Because the autoimmune response against the β-cell-specific molecule insulin is a major component of type 1A diabetes, the insulin gene would be an ideal candidate locus. In fact, polymorphisms in the 5′ flanking sequence (promoter region) of the insulin gene have been associated with diabetes risk, and account for about 10% of the familial aggregation of type 1A diabetes.[43] The insulin gene is located on the short arm of chromosome 11 and has been termed *IDDM2*. Polymorphisms in the 5′ sequence leading to alterations in insulin gene expression could be envisaged as potentially modulating the development of tolerance in the thymus or yolk sac.[44,45] A low level of insulin gene expression in the thymus may allow insulin-reactive T cells to escape negative

Locus	Chromosome	Comment
– IDDM1	6p21.31	Major histocompatibility locus
– IDDM2	11p15.5	Insulin gene 5′ VNTR
IDDM3?	15q26	
IDDM4?	11q13	
– IDDM5	6q25	
IDDM6?	18q21	
IDDM7	2q31-33	
IDDM8	6q27	
IDDM9	3q21	
IDDM10?	10p11-q11	
IDDM11?	14q24.3-14q31	
IDDM12	2q33	CTLA4
IDDM13	2q34	
– IDDM15	6q21	Confirmed multiple studies
IDDM17	10q25.1	Single Bedouin Arab family

?, negative evidence for linkage in two or more large linkage studies.
–, evidence for linkage found in more than one major study.
Underlined, definitive evidence for linkage or association.

Table 82.4 IDDM loci in humans.

Three genetic models of type 1A diabetes inheritance

Monogenic model
Susceptibility to type 1A diabetes and other endocrine and nonendocrine autoimmune diseases can be determined by a mutation in a single gene. An example is the autoimmune polyendocrine syndrome type I (APS-I) with a mutation in the autoimmune regulator (AIRE) gene.[48]

Polygenic model
A major role for Class II molecules (DQ, DR) in determining susceptibility for type 1A diabetes is well recognized. In the NOD mouse model more than 15 non-MHC loci have been found to contribute to diabetes risk. The idea that multiple genetic polymorphisms, each contributing a small component to disease susceptibility, is a popular model.

Oligogenic model
Diabetes risk may be determined by HLA alleles in conjunction with one or two non-MHC disease genes in each family. For different families the specific major 'diabetogenes' would differ. This model is supported by studies of a large Bedouin Arab family[49] and the finding of a risk of 40% for DQ2/DQ8 siblings of patients with type 1A diabetes.[39]

Table 82.5 Three genetic models of type 1A diabetes inheritance.

selection. The insulin gene polymorphism (larger repeat region), which results in greater thymic expression of proinsulin, is associated with protection.[46,47]

Some of the loci identified through genome-wide screens for linkage have not been replicated by different groups. The reasons for this lack of reproducibility may include the following: genetic heterogeneity in different populations; heterogeneity of disease phenotypes; ethnic differences; statistical 'artifacts'; and differences in the markers utilized. It is possible that genetic heterogeneity between different families having different non-MHC genes may underlie the inability of sibling-pair studies to identify loci accounting for a major proportion of the familial aggregation of type 1A diabetes. Three potential patterns of inheritance for diabetes will be addressed: monogenic, polygenic and oligogenic models (Table 82.5).

In 1989, Pnini Vardi identified a unique family with a high frequency of type 1A diabetes. This Bedouin Arab family consisted of over 250 members, with 18 affected (Fig. 82.2). A genome-wide scan for linkage in this family revealed that the risk for diabetes was associated with a susceptibility locus on chromosome 10 which is termed *IDDM17*. In family members expressing the DR3 or DR4 haplotypes, the risk for diabetes was 30%, as opposed to <2% for those members who do not have a DR3 or DR4 haplotype.[49] Linkage analysis and association studies revealed that in this family a pattern of oligogenic inheritance may underlie disease susceptibility.

RODENT MODELS

Studies in animal models have contributed greatly to our understanding of the pathogenesis of type 1A diabetes. Numerous models exist, with both induced (e.g. with alloxan, streptozotocin

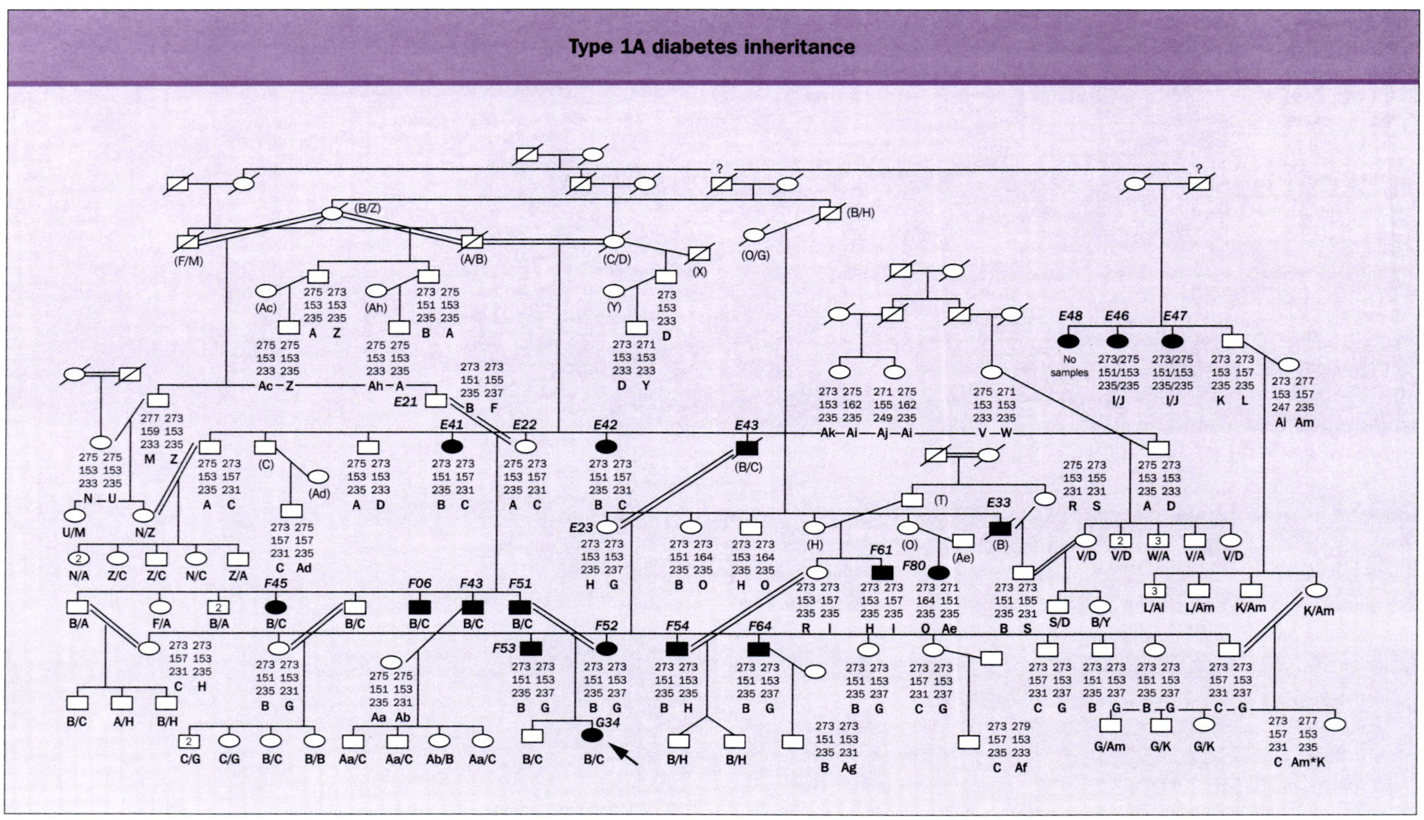

Figure 82.2 Type 1A diabetes inheritance. Family tree in which 18 members have developed type 1 diabetes and diabetes appears to be inherited as an autosomal recessive mutation at a locus on chromosome 10 plus typical type 1 HLA alleles. The B haplotype on chromosome 10 occurs in the majority of patients with diabetes (numbers refer to chromosome 10q25.1 microsatellite alleles) and diabetics have homologous B like 10q25.1 regions for other diabetic haplotypes (e.g. haplotypes, Ae, O, I, J, C, G, and H).

Spontaneous animal models of type 1A diabetes
BB rat (oligogenic inheritance)
Homozygosity lymphopenia gene
RT1-U MHC Class II alleles
Additional loci
NOD mouse (polygenic inheritance of diabetes)
I-A^{g7}; I-Eα deletion; Class I allele
IL-2 polymorphism
More than 15 additional IDDM loci
Tokushima rat (oligogenic inheritance)
RT1-U MHC alleles
Homozygosity chromosome 11

Table 82.6 Spontaneous animal models of type 1A diabetes.

treatment) and spontaneous (e.g. NOD mouse, BB rat) forms being available (Table 82.6). Some important advantages of an autoimmune model include: access to the pancreas at various stages in the immunopathology; ability to breed and genetically manipulate the animals; and intervention strategies that can be employed at various disease stages (e.g. preinsulitis, insulitis/presymptomatic stage etc.).

NOD MOUSE

The best-studied animal model for type 1A diabetes is the nonobese diabetic (NOD) mouse, which develops diabetes spontaneously. In the NOD mouse, cellular and humoral immune responses specific for β cells are present, anti-insulin autoantibodies precede overt diabetes, and disease is associated with MHC alleles.[13] Pancreatic insulitis in the NOD mouse can be detected as early as 2 weeks with electron microscopy, and becomes detectable by light microscopy at 4–5 weeks of age. Approximately 80% of female mice and 20% of male mice progress to diabetes by 30 weeks of age. The reason for the excess of female cases is unknown, but may be related to the effects of sex hormones.

Multiple genetic loci in this mouse determine disease susceptibility, with the MHC (termed *Idd1*) being necessary but not sufficient for disease. The Class II region in NOD mice encodes the I-A^{g7} molecule, the homolog of the human Class II DQ8 and DQ2. I-A^{g7} is unique among the known I-A molecules in that it has a serine instead of an aspartic acid at position 57 of the β chain. Like a number of normal strains, NOD mice do not express I-E (the murine homolog of HLA-DR) because of a mutation in the Eα promoter. The introduction of a normal I-Eα gene inhibits diabetes development in the NOD mouse, implying that its absence is important.[50] Transgenic NOD mice expressing a 'normal' I-A, or with amino acid substitutions of position 56 and 57 of the NOD I-A^{g7}, are protected from disease.

BB RAT

The BB rat also spontaneously develops diabetes, with equal frequency among males and females.[14] Ninety per cent of both sexes developing insulitis progress to overt diabetes between 50 and 90 days of age. Selective breeding of BB rats resulted in the production of diabetes-prone (DP) and a diabetes-resistant (DR) BB strains.

Genetic susceptibility for type 1A diabetes in the BB rat is also determined in part by the MHC genes. In the BB rat, diabetes is independent of Class I alleles but requires the MHC Class II haplotype RT-1U (*Iddm2*) in which at least one allele must be present for diabetes development. A second locus (*Iddm1*) is inherited in an autosomal recessive manner and is responsible for T-cell lymphopenia in these animals. The DP-BB rat is deficient in T cells expressing the surface antigen RT6. RT6 is a surface marker that appears to distinguish a subset of T cells capable of immunoregulation, as adoptive transfer of these cells into a DP-BB rat abrogates diabetes. In addition, monoclonal antibodies targeting RT6 can induce β-cell destruction in the nonlymphopenic, diabetes-resistant BB rats.

The DR-BB rats are nonlymphopenic and diabetes can be induced with either the administration of RT6 monoclonal antibodies or infection with the Kilham rat virus. The Kilham rat virus does not infect β cells but is believed to alter immune regulation. Table 82.6 lists several animal models of type 1A diabetes.

TRANSGENIC MODELS

The use of transgenic and knockout technology has allowed investigators to begin to determine the role of various immune factors in the etiology and pathology of type 1A diabetes. In these models, the breakdown of organ specific tolerance can be examined by creating DNA constructs that allow tissue-specific expression of the transgene under the control of tissue-specific promoters (e.g. insulin promoter). Most of the transgenic models of type 1A diabetes involve the NOD mouse, and a brief summary of some of these studies is provided (Table 82.7).

NOD mice that have been crossed with mice with a target mutation of the μ chain in the IgM heavy chain do not develop diabetes,[51] suggesting that B lymphocytes play an important role in the disease process. As autoantibodies do not appear to be directly pathogenic to β cells, the role of B cells in the pathogenesis of type 1A diabetes appears to be that of antigen presentation.[52] When B-cell-deficient (MT–/–) mice were crossed with NOD mice expressing a B7.1 transgene in the pancreatic β cells, progression to diabetes was accelerated, suggesting that B-cell presentation can be bypassed.

The perhaps overly simplistic hypothesis that Th1 cells are destructive and Th2 protective is the basis for efforts to skew the cytokine environment towards Th2 cytokines. In support of this idea, the administration of IL-4[53] or IL-10[54] has been associated with disease protection in NOD mice, whereas systemic administration of Th1-type cytokines, IL-12[55] and TNF-α[56] can precipitate disease. However, studies of transgenic and knockout NOD models involving cytokines have suggested that the Th1/Th2 paradigm is an oversimplification. For example, NOD mice expressing an IL-4 transgene specifically in the islet β cells show protection from diabetes, whereas IL-4 knockout NOD mice do not show accelerated diabetes. In addition, anti-IFN-γ treatment prevents diabetes development in the NOD mouse,[57] but IFN-γ-deficient NOD mice continue to develop diabetes, albeit at a reduced rate.[58] Furthermore, whereas NOD mice administered IL-10 are protected from diabetes,[54] mice expressing an IL-10 transgene specifically in the islet β cells develop accelerated diabetes.[59] Although the reasons for these differences remain to be clarified, it suggests that the ability to dissect

Transgenic and knockout studies on NOD mice

Transgene	Observation	Conclusion
I-Eα	Diabetes prevented	I-E prevents diabetes
I-A_{β} proline 56, Asp57	Diabetes prevented	I-A sequence is important
Proinsulin with Class II promoter	Diabetes prevented	Insulin 'key' autoantigen
Heat-shock protein with Class II promoter	Small decrease in diabetes	Potential importance of HSP
GAD65 with Class II promoter	No decrease in diabetes	'Tolerance' to GAD65 not induced
GAD65/67 antisense transgene	Two strains with decreased diabetes	GAD important, not necessary[a]
IL-2 B6 variant	Diabetes decreased	IL-2 polymorphisms contribute to diabetes
Expression in β cells		
TNF-α	Accelerated diabetes	
IL-10	Accelerated diabetes	
FasL	Accelerated diabetes	Neutrophil infiltration induced
B7.1	Accelerated diabetes	B7.1 Costimulation is important
TGF-β	Decreased incidence of diabetes	TGF-β may induce suppression of islet-reactive CD4 T cells and/or induce regulatory T-cell subsets
IL-4	Abrogates insulitis and development of diabetes	IL-4 may induce a 'protective' Th2 response
Expression in T cells		
IL-10	Protection with limited diabetes	
Expression in α cells (paracrine effect)		
TGF-β	Protected against spontaneous and cyclophosphamide-induced diabetes	Paracrine TGF-β is important for suppressing autoimmunity, perhaps through induction of regulatory T cells
In vitro		
Bcl-2 transgenic islet cells	Protected from IL-1β, TNF-α, IFN-γ-induced destruction	Bcl-2 antiapoptotic factor blocks cytokine-induced apoptosis
Knockout/inactivating mutation		
Rag, SCID	Diabetes prevented	T-cell receptors or Igs are essential
Mu chain of immunoglobulin	Diabetes prevented	B cells important
Class II deficient B lymphocytes	Diabetes prevented	B-cell expression of Class II important
β_2-microglobulin ('Class I knockout')	Diabetes prevented	Class I and CD8 T cells are important
CIITA 'Class II transactivator' (deficient in MHC II and peripheral CD4 T cells)	Pancreatic infiltration/seldom insulitis/diabetes prevented	CD4 T cells needed for progression to insulitis and diabetes
Perforin	Insulitis severity unchanged Incidence/onset of diabetes is reduced and delayed	Perforin-dependent cytotoxicity is important in the late effector phase of disease
Fas	Fas–/– prevents diabetes	Fas is important for autoimmune β-cell destruction
GAD65	Diabetes rate/incidence unchanged	GAD65 is not required
GAD67	Normal islet development but perinatal death unrelated to diabetes (respiratory distress)	GAD67 not tested
IFNγ	Develop diabetes at a slower rate	
TNF Receptor 1	Insulitis but no diabetes	TNFR1 signaling is important for progression to diabetes
IL-12	Diabetes unchanged	Other cytokines may substitute
IL-4	Diabetes unchanged	Other cytokines may substitute

Table 82.7 Summary of transgenic and knockout studies on the NOD background.

out the role of individual cytokines may be complicated by a variety of factors, which may include functional redundancy in cytokine action; the fact that individual cytokines may modulate the expression of other cytokines and/or chemokines; cytokine influence may vary at different periods during the course of disease development; and the microenvironment of cytokine production; can all serve to muddy the waters of the cytokine regulation of the disease process.

Several caveats should be considered when evaluating animal models. First, no single model exactly replicates the disease process in humans, and genus-specific differences may contribute to this variance. In addition, the highly inbred nature of these models (owing to multiple brother–sister matings) and the controlled housing environment of these animals implies that the model is not directly analogous to humans, in that inbred mice are monoallelic at all loci. Despite these disadvantages, animal models remain an invaluable tool to research immunopathology.

STAGE II: TRIGGERING OF AUTOIMMUNITY (POTENTIAL ENVIRONMENTAL FACTORS)

Environmental factors suggested to influence the development of type 1A diabetes include viral infections, bacterial and/or viral superantigens, dietary components and environmental toxins. Many investigators support a viral etiology for type 1A diabetes. However, so far there has been no formal demonstration that viral infections directly cause type 1A diabetes in humans. Congenital rubella, but only congenital infection, is associated with diabetes risk, but such infection increases the risk of a series of autoimmune disorders.

The mechanism by which microbial infections might influence the autoimmune process of type 1A diabetes is poorly defined. Hypotheses include: (1) microbial-specific T and B cells, may cross-react with self-antigens (molecular mimicry); (2) virally-infected β cells may be directly destroyed by cytotoxic T lymphocytes reacting to viral epitopes displayed on MHC Class I; (3) indirect or 'bystander' activation of autoreactive lymphocytes may occur owing to a local increase in inflammatory cytokines associated with viral infection;[60] and (4) the effects of congenital infection (e.g. rubella) on the developing immune system may contribute to disease susceptibility. Without convincing epidemiological evidence for relevant environmental factors it is difficult to test these hypotheses.

Rubella virus

Congenital rubella infection is a well defined environmental factor contributing to the development of type 1A diabetes in humans. Approximately 12–20% of individuals infected in utero with rubella develop diabetes in 5–20 years,[61] in what appears to be an autoimmune process. One hypothesis to explain this association involves a molecular mimicry mechanism, supported by the fact that there is a shared epitope between a rubella viral noncapsid protein and a 52 kDa islet autoantigen.[62] Alternatively, the rubella virus may alter β-cell antigens as it buds from the membrane, resulting in the formation of a novel antigenic determinant. A separate hypothesis would be that rubella infection might modulate T-cell development and result in abnormal immunologic tolerance to islet and thyroid tissues.[63]

Coxsackie B viruses

Coxsackie viruses are RNA-containing picornaviruses that have been implicated in the etiology of type 1A diabetes. The coxsackie viruses are members of the enterovirus class and have six B serotypes (B1–B6). The precise role these viruses play in the etiology of type 1A diabetes has yet to be defined.

Sequence similarity exists between the coxsackie viral protein 2C (P2-C) and the glutamic acid decarboxylase (GAD65) autoantigen that is expressed in the pancreas. This amino acid sequence homology is highly conserved in coxsackie B4 isolates, and the relevant peptide has been found to bind to HLA-DR3 but not DR4, giving rise to speculation that the molecular mimicry may be limited to the HLA DR3 subpopulation of type 1A diabetics.[64] In another study, a GAD-peptide AA 247–279 similar to the coxsackie B virus was shown to stimulate Th1-like lymphocytes derived from children with recent-onset type 1A diabetes. Lymphocytes from these patients were found to have increased IFN-γ mRNA expression, which was not seen in lymphocytes derived from HLA-matched controls.[65]

Attempts to relate antibodies to coxsackie viruses in the development of type 1A diabetes revealed both positive and negative results.[66–68] Because these viruses are ubiquitous in the environment and thus not unique to individuals with type 1A diabetes, it has been difficult to definitively associate viral infection with the disease. One alternative hypothesis is that a coxsackie B viral infection may act as a final insult and induce hyperglycemia in individuals who have already lost a substantial amount of β cell mass.[7,69]

In addition to the coxsackie and rubella viruses, numerous other viruses have been implicated in the etiology of type 1A diabetes, including cytomegalovirus herpesviruses, mumps, retroviruses, rotaviruses, Epstein–Barr viruses and echoviruses.[2,70]

Superantigens

Superantigens are nonconventional antigens derived from microbes that bind outside the MHC binding groove and crosslink the MHC molecule with the Vβ portion of the T-cell receptor (TCR)[71] (Chapter 7). By the very nature of this interaction, a large fraction of T cells (5–20%) bearing the appropriate Vβ region (each with their own unique specificity) can become activated. In one study, splenic and pancreatic tissue from patients with new-onset type 1A diabetes revealed a high expression of TCRVβ7 (30%) compared to healthy controls (8–11%).[72] Subsequently, Conrad et al[73] described the isolation of an endogenous HERV-K10-like retroviral genome, $IDDM_{1,2}22$. $IDDM_{1,2}22$ is related to a mouse mammary tumor virus in which a superantigen is encoded by the *env* gene. Using RT-PCR for transcripts related to the $IDDM_{1,2}22$ genome, Conrad reported that 10 of 10 new-onset type 1A diabetics, but not 10 age-matched controls, were positive for the transcripts. However, other groups have been unable to replicate these results and have concluded that these transcripts are not specific for diabetic patients but can be found in control individuals with the same frequency.[74,75]

Milk proteins

Milk proteins, namely bovine serum albumin (BSA) and casein, have received the most attention as possible dietary components important for the development of type 1A diabetes. Studies from Scandinavia show a correlation between the reduction in breast feeding and an increase in the incidence of type 1A diabetes.[76] Antibodies against BSA have been found in humans, NOD mice and BB rats. One proposed hypothesis is that a peptide of BSA,[77] homologous to the islet antigen ICA-69,[78] results in the activation of autoimmunity through molecular mimicry. Most of the studies associating the ingestion of milk with the development of diabetes are retrospective and with relatively small effects (odds ratio of 1.6). Importantly, several prospective studies examining the possible association between the expression of anti-islet autoimmunity and early infant exposure to cow milk in high-risk first-degree relatives failed to find an association.[79,80] Furthermore, in at least one prospective study the duration of breast feeding did not appear to modulate the development of anti-islet autoimmunity in children at high risk.[79,86]

STAGE III ACTIVE IMMUNITY

Islet-cell autoantibodies can be detected in the sera prior to the development of type 1A diabetes and in new-onset patients prior to insulin therapy.[81] For three of the autoantigens (glutamic acid decarboxylase (GAD65), insulin and ICA512/IA2) the frequency of positive autoantibody tests is high, and the assays are in a form that allow the testing of thousands of samples (Table 82.8). However, there is no evidence that autoantibodies play a direct role in the immunopathogenesis of type 1A diabetes. Evidence against autoantibodies contributing directly to β-cell damage come from studies of infants born to mothers with type 1A diabetes. Anti-islet autoantibodies of mothers are transplacentally transferred to the infant, yet these infants do not develop disease. If anything, the offspring of diabetic mothers develop diabetes less often than do the offspring of diabetic fathers. Furthermore, adoptive transfer studies in the NOD mouse have clearly shown that β-cell destruction can be mediated by T cells in the absence of antibodies. As discussed above, the lack of an influence exerted by autoantibodies does not rule out an important role for B lymphocytes in the pathogenesis of diabetes. Studies from B-cell-deficient NOD mice indicate that the development of diabetes is markedly suppressed in such animals.

AUTOANTIGENS/AUTOANTIBODIES

Insulin

The insulin molecule is the only β-cell-specific autoantigen so far associated with type 1A diabetes, and antibodies against insulin are one of the earliest clinical markers of prediabetes. Insulin autoantibodies (IAA) can be detected in the sera of approximately 60% of newly diagnosed type 1A patients prior to insulin therapy. The presence of IAA is inversely correlated with age of diabetes onset, with almost 100% of newly diagnosed children less than 5 years of age expressing IAA, compared to less than 20% of those diagnosed after 15 years of age. Moreover, the levels of IAA are associated with the rate of the autoimmune destruction of the β cells, making their detection an important aspect of diagnosis and prevention.[82]

GAD65

Glutamic acid decarboxylase (GAD) is an enzyme that converts glutamate to γ-amino butyric acid (GABA). Two isoforms, GAD65 and GAD67, named for their molecular weights in kilodaltons, have been identified and their expression is not limited to the central nervous system. GAD65 is expressed in human β cells (but is also expressed by α and δ cells of islets) and is a major target autoantigen in type 1A diabetes. Although antibodies to GAD65 can be detected in the sera of 70% of new-onset type 1A patients, only 20% of GAD antibody-positive relatives progress to type 1A diabetes (with long-term follow-up) if no other islet antibodies are expressed.[83,84]

ICA512 (IA-2)

ICA512 was identified by screening an islet cDNA library with sera from new-onset type 1A diabetics.[85] The gene encodes a putative tyrosine phosphatase-related molecule expressed in the pancreas (associated with the β-cell secretory granules) and the brain. Despite its homology with tyrosine phosphatase, no enzymatic activity has been demonstrated. The molecule appears to be produced in two alternative splice variants, with the variant lacking the transmembrane exon 13 domain usually termed ICA512 bdc. Autoantibodies usually react with both variants although approximately 10% of sera from new-onset patients react with one or the other.

The above-mentioned autoantibodies appear in a sequential manner rather than simultaneously, with insulin and GAD65 usually appearing first. This appearance reflects the progression of humoral autoimmunity to β cells, which develops chronically, with early responses often directed against insulin.

STAGE IV LOSS OF INSULIN SECRETION

Given the presence of anti-islet autoantibodies, the loss of first-phase insulin secretion following the administration of intravenous glucose is a parameter that aids in defining the time to development of overt diabetes. Most adults have lost first-phase secretion (below the first percentile of normal individuals) years before the development of diabetes, whereas most children developing diabetes lose first-phase secretion 1–3 years prior to the onset of disease. The measurement of insulin autoantibodies can be combined with first-phase insulin secretion to develop a linear regression model for predicting diabetes onset.[82]

STAGE V OVERT DIABETES

By the time overt diabetes develops in humans, most (80–90%) of the β cells are apparently destroyed. In patients who die shortly after the onset of type 1A diabetes, insulitis can be found within the islets that still contain β cells. After β-cell destruction has occurred in humans and in the various animal models, islets with no β cells remain and the insulitis resolves. The decrease in β-cell mass accompanying the onset of overt diabetes is associated with a lack of first-phase insulin secretion, which is not restored

Assays for anti-islet autoantibodies using recombinant antigens

Antigen	Sensitivity (%)	(Specificity) (%)	Comment
Insulin	40–95	(99)	Prevalence inversely correlated with the age of onset
GAD	70	(99)	Prevalence increases with age
ICA512 (IA-2)	60	(99)	Islet tyrosine phosphatase homolog
IA2β (Phogrin)	55	(99)	These autoantibodies are predominantly a subset of ICA512/IA2/autoantibodies

Table 82.8 Assays for anti-islet autoantibodies using recombinant antigens.

even if patients are treated with cyclosporin. At the time of diagnosis anti-islet autoantibodies can still be detected in the sera of these patients, and probably reflects the insulitis and β-cell destruction that is still on-going. Newly diagnosed type 1A diabetes is often associated with a brief metabolic remission, termed the 'honeymoon phase', in which low doses of insulin are required or, in some cases, patients may be transiently insulin independent. This brief metabolic remission usually lasts for less than 1 year. It is likely that this period reflects decreased insulin resistance after treatment of severe hyperglycemia. The ability to induce this temporary remission makes the search for an agent that can maintain long-term remission an important goal.

EFFECTOR MECHANISMS OF β-CELL DESTRUCTION

An important feature supporting the conclusion that type 1A diabetes is an autoimmune disorder is the finding of a lymphocytic infiltrate in the islets. The mechanism by which these cells gain access to the islets and mediate the selective destruction of the insulin-secreting β cells, while leaving other islet cells intact, is still unclear. It is believed by many investigators that the destruction of β-cells occurs through apoptosis in a process that requires B lymphocytes and CD4 and CD8 T lymphocytes. Studies in which B cells[65] or macrophages[86] are depleted in the NOD model show that these antigen-presenting cells are important in the disease process.

Although some studies have shown that either CD4 or CD8 T cells may, under certain experimental conditions, be sufficient to cause β cell destruction alone, it would be difficult to imagine that these cells are acting in isolation. It is more likely that there is a complex interaction between antigen-presenting cells (dendritic cells, macrophages and B cells), T lymphocytes and numerous cytokines that bring about the destruction of the β cells. Studies have supported the role of proinflammatory cytokines, including TNF-α, IL-1, IL-6 and IFN-γ, as well as Fas–FasL interactions, perforin and granzymes and reactive oxygen intermediates (for example nitric oxide). Despite numerous reports describing the involvement of many of these molecules, the extent to which each of them participates in β-cell destruction is still controversial.

CD4 T cells

CD4 T cells appear to be critical in the pathogenesis of type 1A diabetes. In NOD mice depleted of CD4 T cells using anti-CD4 antibodies, or engineered to be genetically deficient in CD4, diabetes does not develop. Islet-specific T-cell clones have been isolated from the spleen, lymph nodes and islets of Langerhans of NOD mice, and such islet-specific T cells are capable of inducing diabetes after adoptive transfer. Nearly all of these T-cell clones are CD4$^+$ and require peptide presentation in the context of the NOD Class II I-A^{g7} molecule. Of the CD4$^+$ T-cell clones isolated from NOD islets, 55% have been found to be insulin reactive and the remainder reactive with unknown antigens. More than 95% of the insulin-reactive clones recognize a single peptide of insulin which spans the amino acid residues 9–23 of the insulin B chain. This epitope has been termed B9-23, or the B2 peptide. Molecular characterization of the known B9-23 reactive CD4$^+$ T-cell clones derived from the NOD islet reveals that the TCR α chain is highly restricted to Vα13 and Jα45 or Jα34.[87] This TCR motif is expressed in up to 60% of insulin-reactive T-cell clones.

CD8 T cells

Studies of knockout mice have confirmed the importance of CD8 T cells in islet cell pathology. In the β_2-microglobulin-null NOD mice, which are deficient in CD8 T cells, neither diabetes nor insulitis occurs. A similar finding is observed when NOD mice are treated with a monoclonal antibody against CD8. Recently, Wong and colleagues[88] identified insulin as the autoantigen recognized by a NOD-derived pathogenic CD8 T cell. Interestingly, the region recognized by the CD8 T cells overlapped with the portion of the insulin B chain recognized by the majority of the insulin-reactive CD4 T cells.

Despite the importance of T lymphocytes for the development of type 1A diabetes, both in humans and in animal models, T-cell assays useful for the prediction or follow-up of the diabetes process are essentially nonexistent. In humans an international workshop with multiple laboratories participating indicated that none had an antigen-specific T-cell assay that could reliably distinguish a group of controls from patients with diabetes. Most of the assays evaluated depended upon in vitro proliferation of T lymphocytes to autoantigens such as GAD, insulin or heat-shock proteins. It is hoped that with improved knowledge of T-cell autoimmunity better assays will be developed, but a major limitation is likely to be the frequency of autoreactive T cells outside the islets that are available for study.

Histopathology

Studies in the NOD model have provided the opportunity to examine the islets at various stages of the natural history of the disease. Through these studies it has become clear that intra-islet infiltration evolves from a stage of peri-insulitis and MHC Class I hyperexpression in the NOD islet β cells. The perivascular and periductal T-cell infiltration, termed peri-insulitis, is usually observed at 4–6 weeks of age. Animals at this stage have been described by some authors as being in a state of 'benign autoimmunity', in which case the peri-insulitis is thought to be nondestructive.[89] The conversion to invasive insulitis and β-cell destruction ('malignant autoimmunity') in these mice was reported to occur abruptly and in an unpredictable fashion as the mice aged. However, O'Brien and colleagues[90] reported that apoptosis in the NOD islets was detectable throughout the period of peri-insulitis. Apoptotic death of the islets preceded lymphocytic infiltration and then declined when progression to overt diabetes occurred. In another study, NOD mice were observed to have an early increased 'compensatory' β-cell proliferation. This was unable to keep pace with the progressive β-cell destruction and resulted in a reduction in β-cell mass that became worse with time and correlated with a decrease in the insulin secretory response.[33]

Histological analyses of the islets in humans have been limited for several reasons, which include the relative inaccessibility of the pancreas for biopsy; the fact that the islets make up only 2–3% of the pancreatic tissue; and the fact that histologic examination of the islets at the time of disease initiation (which precedes clinical presentation) has not been possible. Histological evaluation of pancreata from children who have died at disease onset also suggests a slowly evolving autoimmune process in type 1A diabetes.[6] Foulis and colleagues[91] have described three histologically distinguishable types of islets in patients with new-onset diabetes:

(1) insulin-deficient islets, which make up the largest fraction (approximately 70%); (2) insulin-containing islets with a chronic inflammatory cell infiltrate; and (3) insulin-containing islets that appear normal. T cells make up most of the infiltrate, with CD8 T cells comprising a larger fraction than CD4 in some studies.

In contrast to the characteristic peri-insulitis associated with the early stages of immunopathology in the NOD mouse, peri-insulitis does not appear to be a common feature in humans. Another distinction is that insulitis in the NOD mouse is associated with massive mononuclear cell infiltrates not typically seen in man. The mechanisms that underlie these differences remain unclear. It is, however, a good reminder that the NOD mouse, although an excellent model, is clearly not identical to humans.

TYPE 1A DIABETES PREDICTION

By the time the diagnosis of type 1A diabetes is made, approximately 80–90% of the β cells may have been destroyed. Therefore, the ability to predict who will develop type 1A diabetes among high-risk individuals (siblings of type 1A diabetics) has become an important goal. With studies of disease prevention it has become increasingly important to identify individuals at high risk. Using HLA haplotype analysis and 'combinatorial' autoantibody analyses, clinicians should be able to identify high-risk individuals. Because the initiation of the autoimmune process in type 1A diabetes occurs years before the progression to overt symptoms, the chance of early intervention is feasible. Furthermore, if a definable environmental trigger exists for type 1A diabetes, as it does for celiac disease (wheat gliadin), preventing exposure may be important.

Over the past decade the prediction of type 1A diabetes has improved substantially. The most important risk factor for disease development is the expression of multiple anti-islet autoantibodies,[92] particularly, two or more of GAD65, ICA512 (IA-2) or insulin autoantibodies (Fig. 82.3). However, there is a subset of relatives who express a single autoantibody, and an even smaller subset expressing multiple autoantibodies, who have the 'protective' HLA alleles DQA1*0102, DQB1*0602. In individuals with DQB1*0602 the risk of progressing to diabetes is low, but still present. Approximately 1% (versus 20% of the general population) of patients with type 1A diabetes has this allele.

PREVENTION

Immunosuppression

The first major trial of general immunosuppressive therapy for newly diagnosed subjects involved the administration of cyclosporin A (CyA).[93,94] CyA was effective in prolonging insulin secretion when treatment lasted 1 year and was initiated during the first 6 weeks of insulin therapy. Long-term benefit was limited, however, with relapse of hyperglycemia occurring within 3 years despite continued CyA therapy, and despite continued maintenance of improved insulin secretion as measured with C-peptide. When CyA was discontinued, insulin secretion was rapidly lost. Because of the potential for nephrotoxicity and the risk of malignancy associated with long-term CyA treatment, such therapy has not been adopted. Other immunosuppressive agents have been studied, including prednisone, anti-CD5, anti-CD25, antithymocyte globulin and anti-T12, but so far they have had little success in providing long-term protection.

Progression to diabetes vs number of autoantibodies (GAD65, insulin, ICA512,)

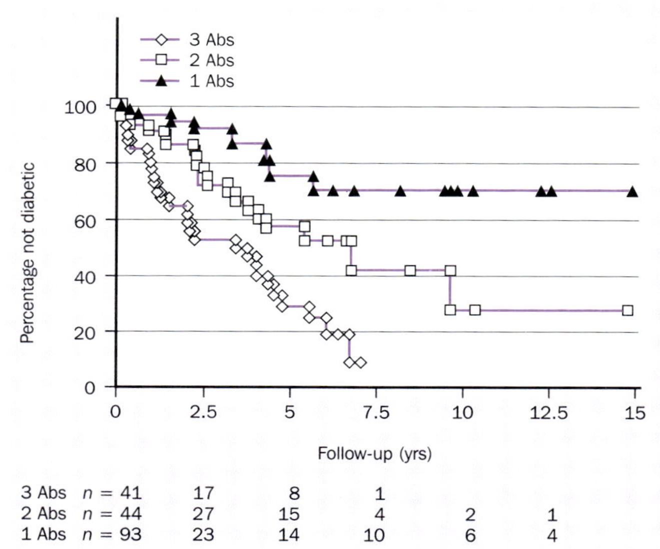

Figure 82.3 Life table analysis of progression to type 1A diabetes in relatives of affected patients sub-divided by the number of autoantibodies (GAD65, insulin, ICA512) expressed.

Autoantigen administration

The administration of certain islet cell autoantigens, such as insulin and GAD, and derivatives of these autoantigens can prevent diabetes in animal models.[94] For example, in the NOD mouse long-term (up to 1 year) oral ingestion of these autoantigens has been reported to delay the onset and/or reduce the incidence of disease.[95,96] Subcutaneous and intranasal administration of the insulin B chain, B9-23, can prevent diabetes in the NOD mouse.[97] Although the precise mechanism by which subcutaneous administration of the insulin peptide mediates immunoprotection is unknown, the isolation of B9-23-reactive CD4 T-cell clones[98] expressing TGF-β suggests that protection may be mediated by regulatory T cells. Much evidence exists that in type 1A diabetes a Th1-dominant response enhances β-cell destruction, whereas a Th2 response is protective. Autoantigen administration appears to dampen the autoimmune response via bystander suppression through the generation of regulatory T cells secreting a Th2 cytokine profile.[99]

In the US individuals at moderate risk for type 1A diabetes are being randomized to receive either oral insulin or placebo in the Diabetes Prevention Trial-1 (DPT-1). In this same study, individuals at high risk are being randomized to parenteral insulin therapy. Relatives of patients with type 1A diabetes are eligible for this trial if they express anti-islet autoantibodies and have additional (HLA, low insulin secretion) high-risk factors. To date over 60 000 relatives have been screened and results from the oral trial should be available within 4 years and within 1 year for the parenteral trial. Screening is available for the DPT-1 trial at centers throughout the United States.

Adjuvants

In the NOD mouse a single injection of complete Freund's adjuvant prevents the development of diabetes[100] but not insulitis. A single injection of incomplete Freund's adjuvant (IFA) was unable to induce this effect. However, when combined with an injection of B chain of insulin or the B9-23 peptide, IFA was able to prevent diabetes in the NOD mouse.[97] Vaccination with the bacillus Calmette–Guérin (BCG) strain of *Mycobacterium bovis* has also been found to prevent diabetes in the NOD mouse.[101] Spurred by these results, several clinical trials were designed to test the efficacy of BCG vaccination for type 1A diabetes prevention in humans. In a small nonrandomized placebo-controlled trial involving intradermal BCG vaccination, the clinical remission rate of diabetes in new-onset type 1A diabetes was reported to be improved in those receiving vaccination. However, in several randomized double-blinded placebo-controlled trials intradermal BCG vaccination did not alter remission rate or protect β cells.

Nicotinamide

In the NOD mouse large doses of the vitamin nicotinamide delayed the development of diabetes, and preliminary non-controlled trials suggested that such therapy might also be successful in humans. In light of this, two randomized controlled trials of nicotinamide, the small German DENIS (Deutsche Nicotinamide Trial) trial and the larger ENDIT (European Nicotinamide Trial) trial in Europe, were initiated. Although the European ENDIT trial is still ongoing, the German DENIS trial has been discontinued with no evidence of benefit.

THERAPEUTIC PRINCIPLES

- Autoantibody testing in combination with HLA testing can be used to predict type 1A diabetes.
- Insulin therapy is mandatory in type 1A patients who are ketosis prone, and insulin therapy is recommended for adults who initially can be controlled with oral hypoglycemic agents. Testing of islet cell autoantibodies identifies 10% of adults (thought to have type 2 diabetes) as having type 1A diabetes.
- Prevention of diabetic complications is feasible; it requires routine screening for retinal lesions and microalbuminuria.

TREATMENT WITH INSULIN

Insulin is administered subcutaneously to millions of individuals with diabetes. Over the past three decades, not only has the purity of the insulin preparations improved, but in developed countries human insulin has essentially replaced the use of porcine or bovine insulin. Porcine insulin differs from human insulin by only one amino acid, whereas bovine insulin differs by three amino acids. Most recently, a recombinant form of human insulin, in which the lysine and proline of the B chain of insulin are reversed (LysPro insulin, or Humalogue insulin), has been introduced into clinical practice. This change in the insulin molecule disrupts the natural ability of insulin to form hexamers and greatly speeds subcutaneous absorption. Although the insulin is modified, it has not been associated with an increase in insulin antibodies or immunologic reactions to insulin.

Essentially all patients treated with insulin, even human insulin, develop a low level of antibodies that cross-react with native insulin. These antibodies are of relatively low affinity compared to the insulin autoantibodies of prediabetic patients, and do not usually interfere with insulin action. Insulin resistance due to induced insulin antibodies (defined as patients requiring more than 200 U of insulin per day, and insulin antibodies with a capacity that usually exceeds 50 U of insulin per liter of serum) was always rare and appears to be nearly disappearing as human insulin replaces animal insulins. Allergic or hypersensitivity reactions to insulin and (in the past) lipoatrophy or lipohypertrophy at the site of insulin injection, are also very rare at present. Such allergic reactions can be treated by changing the formulation of insulin used (e.g. NPH insulin to Lente insulin) or, for delayed hypersensitivity, adding small amounts of glucocorticoids to the insulin preparation.

ASSOCIATED AUTOIMMUNE DISORDERS

Type 1A diabetes is associated with several autoimmune diseases, including Addison's disease, thyroiditis, Graves' disease, pernicious anemia, celiac disease, myasthenia gravis and vitiligo. The association with other organ-specific autoimmune diseases points to the importance of screening for these diseases in type 1A patients. Several commonly associated diseases or unique syndromes are discussed in this section.

Autoimmune polyendocrine syndromes

Polyendocrine syndromes are characterized by multiple autoimmune disorders. Two distinct forms have been described: autoimmune polyendocrine syndrome I (APS-I) and II (APS-II).

Autoimmune polyendocrine syndrome type I (APS-I)

APS-I consists of a triad of chronic mucocutaneous candidiasis, hypoparathyroidism and Addison's disease, which often present in that order. Other endocrine and nonendocrine disorders can also be present or develop later in patients with this syndrome (Table 82.9). Eighteen per cent of patients develop type 1A diabetes. APS-I is also known as autoimmune polyendocrinopathy candidiasis ectodermal dystrophy (APECED), and is an autosomal recessive disorder in which males and females are equally affected. In contrast to APS-II, in which the manifestations of disease usually occur in middle age, APS-I usually manifests in infancy or early childhood. In both syndromes the detection of autoantibodies against endocrine and nonendocrine tissues precedes overt disease.

APS-I is of considerable importance in that it has a defined monogenic etiology. In addition, no association with HLA alleles is found. The gene underlying the pathogenesis of APS-I is localized to the long arm of chromosome 21 (21q22.3) and is termed autoimmune regulator (AIRE).[48] AIRE has two zinc-finger motifs and a DNA-binding domain, and is localized to the nucleus,[102] suggestive of a role in modulating transcription. Heino and colleagues[103] have recently demonstrated that AIRE is expressed in both thymic epithelial and nonepithelial cells, as well as cells in the lymph node, spleen and fetal liver, but not in the target organs. These results suggest that AIRE may regulate the expression of genes important for the development of immunologic tolerance.

Autoimmune polyendocrine syndrome type 2 (APS-II)

APS-II, or Schmidt's syndrome, is the most common of the polyendocrine syndromes and, in contrast to APS-I, the incidence is greater (2–3-fold) in females than in males, with onset typically

Table 82.9 Autoimmune polyendocrine syndrome types I and II.

APS I and II		
	APS-I[a]	APS-II[b]
Inheritance	Autosomal recessive AIRE gene 21q22.3	Autosomal dominant polygenic/oligogenic
HLA association	None	HLA DR3 and DR4
Immunodeficiency	Mucocutaneous candidiasis, asplenism	Not well defined
Age of onset	Infancy or early childhood	Adulthood (peak 20–60)
Sexual prevalence	Equal among males and females	Greater in females (by 2–3-fold)
[a]Mucocutaneous candidiasis	73–100%	Not associated
[a]Hypoparathyroidism	80–89%	Not associated
[a,b]Addison's disease	60–72%	70%
[b]Type 1 diabetes	4–15%	52%
[b]Autoimmune thyroid disease	10–40%	70%
Gonadal failure	38–60% of females 7–14% of males	3.5–10% of females 5–50% of males
Vitiligo	4–9%	4.5%
Hepatitis	10–15%	Rare
Pernicious anemia	12–15%	<1%
Malabsorption	18%	With celiac disease

[a]Classic triad for APS-I.
[b]Classic triad for APS-II.

in adulthood. The classic triad of APS-II involves Addison's disease, autoimmune thyroid disease and type 1A diabetes, but other endocrine and nonendocrine disorders can be seen in affected patients. Unlike APS-I, APS-II is strongly associated with HLA alleles and susceptibility is probably determined by an interaction between *multiple* genetic loci and environmental factors. The Class II HLA alleles associated with most of the component disorders of APS-II are DR3 (DQB*0201) and DR4 (DQB1*0302).

Addison's disease

Addison's disease, or primary adrenocortical insufficiency, is an autoimmune disease characterized by the presence (in 70% of patients) of autoantibodies that are directed predominantly against 21-hydroxylase, a key regulator of mineralocorticoid and glucocorticoid synthesis. The myriad clinical manifestations of Addison's disease, including muscle weakness and fatigue, hypotension and hyponatremia, and loss of axillary and pubic hair in women, are the result of cortisol, aldosterone and sex hormone deficiencies, respectively. Addison's disease is the principal component disorder of APS-II.

In 'DR4' patients with Addison's disease DRB1*0404 is the DR4 allele most often carried by the affected patient. Individuals with type 1A diabetes have a 100-fold greater risk of developing Addison's disease. This significant increase justifies anti-21 hydroxylase autoantibody screening in type 1A diabetics. The MICA-5.1 allele is an additional major independent determinant of Addison's disease.[104] This nontraditional Class I allele has an extra nucleotide that disrupts the transmembrane portion of the molecule.

Celiac disease

Celiac disease is a common autoimmune disease (incidence of 1:250 in the US)[105] characterized by immune-cell-induced intestinal lesions which may lead to malabsorption and growth failure. The highest incidence occurs in type 1A diabetics and their relatives, with most of these patients expressing DQA1*0501; DQB1*0201 (DR3, DR3/3 or DR5/7).[106] Of the autoimmune diseases, celiac disease is unique in that intestinal pathology is entirely dependent on the ingestion of cereal proteins, namely wheat, rye and barley. Remarkably, the removal of wheat gliadin from the diet resolves the intestinal lesions and also leads to the disappearance of autoantibodies associated with the disease.

Tissue transglutaminase (tTG), an enzyme that catalyzes the cross-linking of proteins via glutamyl–lysine bonds, has been shown to be the primary autoantigen of the autoantibodies directed to the intestinal tissues (antiendomysial antibodies).[107] Glutamine residues make up over 40% of the amino acid residues of the gliadin protein, making it a good substrate for transglutaminase. It is postulated that gliadin may become cross-linked to transglutaminase, creating a novel antigenic determinant that is then recognized by self-T cells.

Tissue transglutaminase IgA antibodies have been assessed using both an enzyme-linked immunoadsorbent assay (ELISA)[107] and a radioisotope-binding assay.[108] Ten per cent of all type 1A

diabetics are positive for tTG autoantibodies. Using the radioisotope-binding assay, 22/68 (32%) of type 1A diabetics homozygous for HLA-DQ2 express tTG autoantibodies, as opposed to <2% of those lacking DQ2 or DQ8.[108] Approximately 70% of antiglutaminase-positive patients have celiac disease on biopsy, and the finding of high serum levels of these antibodies revealed a 100% positive predictive value for biopsy evidence of intestinal lesions.[109]

PITFALLS/CONTROVERSIES

General population screening

Current trials that target individuals at increased risk for the development of type 1A diabetes, such as the large multicenter randomized trial headed by the National Institutes of Health (Diabetes Prevention Trial), are aimed at intervening in the prediabetic stage with the hope of either delaying or preventing disease onset. The success of such trials relies in part on our ability to reliably detect at-risk individuals (e.g. siblings of affected patients). However, 90% of patients with type 1A diabetes do not have an affected first-degree relative, making prediction in the general population an important goal.

General population screening depends on the development of an effective intervention that can be instituted prior to the development of diabetes, and potentially prior to autoimmunity. Given the natural history of type 1A diabetes (for many individuals), this will mean that treatment would need to be initiated in infancy. Further complicating this intervention is that only a subset of genetically susceptible individuals progress to diabetes. This subset is highest (40–50%) for DQ8/DQ2 heterozygous first-degree relatives of patients with type 1A diabetes. Trials can be designed that will determine whether autoantibodies, and subsequently disease, are preventable. Because only 10% of first-degree relatives of patients with type 1A diabetes are DQ8/DQ2 heterozygous, such trials will require the screening of more than 1000 neonates. This is obviously a logistical hindrance to such trials, but the major impediment is likely to be the consideration that antigen-based trials have some probability of activating disease. Thus, it is likely that therapies will initially be evaluated in patients with recent-onset type 1A diabetes, and in individuals expressing autoantibodies and progressing to diabetes, before instituting trials involving individuals with genetic susceptibility alone. Increased knowledge of the basic mechanisms of disease and mechanisms of immunotherapies and new assays that predict efficacy are a high priority, so that safe and effective preventive trials can be carried out.

Distinguishing various forms of diabetes

Not all children presenting with diabetes mellitus have type 1A diabetes. Whereas only 10% of non-Hispanic White children do not express GAD65, ICA512 or insulin autoantibodies, as many as 50% of Hispanic and African-American children do not express these antibodies. For patients with type 2 diabetes oral hypoglycemic agents may be the more appropriate therapy. In such cases, clinicians need to carefully monitor these patients for possible decompensation requiring insulin treatment.

In a fraction of adults presenting with what appears to be type 2 diabetes, anti-islet autoantibodies can be detected.[110] When these patients are followed, most eventually require exogenous insulin for glycemic control. It is likely that such patients, who represent approximately 5–10% of adults presenting with diabetes mellitus, actually have type 1A diabetes. One goal for clinicians is to identify both of the groups described above to ensure that they receive the appropriate therapy in a timely fashion.

Large quantities of antibodies to insulin can occur separately from treatment with insulin as part of the insulin autoimmune syndrome (also termed Hirata syndrome). The two forms of this syndrome, both very rare, are characterized by high-titer antiinsulin antibodies. In the rarest form, monoclonal insulin autoantibodies are produced. The form of the syndrome with polyclonal anti-insulin autoantibodies is frequently associated with ingestion of sulfhydryl-containing drugs such as methimizole (treatment for Graves' disease) in East Asian patients. For both syndromes, hypoglycemia and not insulin resistance is the usual presenting abnormality. The polyclonal syndrome is strongly associated with a specific DRB1 allele (DRB1*0406) and usually resolves with discontinuation of the inciting drug. Ninety-six per cent of Japanese patients (48/50) were found to have DR4, and 42 of these had DRB1*0406.[111]

Autoantibodies to the insulin receptor are present in a rare syndrome characterized by both hypoglycemia and hyperglycemia in the same patient at different times. It is thought that the anti-insulin receptor antibodies can act as agonists or antagonists. Patients with this syndrome frequently have systemic autoimmune disorders such as lupus erythematosus, rheumatoid arthritis and Sjögren syndrome. There are case reports of favorable response to immunosuppression (e.g. cyclosporine).

REFERENCES

1. Gavin JR, Alberti G, Davidson MB, et al. Report of the Expert Committee on the Diagnosis and Classification of Diabetes Mellitus. Diabetes Care 1997;20:1183.
2. Rewers M, Norris JM. Epidemiology of type I diabetes. In: Eisenbarth GS, Lafferty KJ (eds) Type I diabetes: molecular, cellular, and clinical immunology. New York, Oxford University Press, 1996;172.
3. Pinhas-Hamiel O, Dolan LM, Daniels SR, Standiford D, Khoury PR, Zeitler P. Increased incidence of non-insulin dependent diabetes mellitus among adolescents. J Pediatr 1996;128:608.
4. Nerup J. Addison's disease – clinical studies: a report of 108 cases. Acta Endocrinol 1974;76:127.
5. Irvine WJ. Autoimmunity in endocrine disease. Recent Prog Horm Res 1980;36:509.
6. Foulis AK, Liddle CN, Farquharson MA, Richmond JA, Weir RS. The histopathology of the pancreas in type I diabetes (insulin dependent) mellitus: a 25-year review of deaths in patients under 20 years of age in the United Kingdom. Diabetologia 1986;29:267.
7. Foulis AK, McGill M, Farquharson MA, Hilton DA. A search for evidence of viral infection in pancreases of newly diagnosed patients with IDDM. Diabetologia 1997;40:53.
8. Johnston C, Pyke DA, Cudworth AG, Wolf E. HLA-DR typing in identical twins with insulin-dependent diabetes: difference between concordant and discordant pairs. Br Med J 1983;286:253.
9. Bottazzo GF, Florin-Christensen A, Doniach D. Islet-cell antibodies in diabetes mellitus with autoimmune polyendocrine deficiencies. Lancet 1974;2:1279.

10. Eisenbarth GS. Type I diabetes mellitus. A chronic autoimmune disease. N Engl J Med 1986;314:1360.
11. Srikanta S, Ganda OP, Eisenbarth GS, Soeldner JS. Islet cell antibodies and beta cell function in monozygotic triplets and twins initially discordant for type I diabetes mellitus. N Engl J Med 1983;308:322.
12. Bach JF. Etiology and pathogenesis of human insulin-dependent diabetes mellitus. In: Volpe R (ed) Contemporary endocrinology: autoimmune endocrinopathies. Totowa, Humana Press, 1999,293.
13. Atkinson MA, Leiter EH. The NOD mouse model of type 1 diabetes: as good as it gets? Nature Med 1999;5:601.
14. Mordes JP, Bortell R, Doukas J, et al. The BB/Wor rat and the balance hypothesis of autoimmunity. Diabetes Metab Rev 1996;12:103.
15. Sutherland DE, Sibley R, Xu XA, et al. Twin-to-twin pancreas transplantation: reversal and reenactment of the pathogenesis of type I diabetes. Trans Assoc Am Phys 1984;97:80.
16. Karvonen M, Tuomilehto J, Libman I, LaPorte R, WHO DIAMOND Project Group. A review of the recent epidemiological data on the worldwide incidence of type 1 (insulin-dependent) diabetes mellitus. Diabetologia 1993;36:883.
17. WHO Study Group. Diabetes mellitus – Technical Report Series 727. Geneva, World Health Organization, 1985.
18. Ikegami H, Ogihara T. Genetics of insulin-dependent diabetes mellitus. Endocrinol J 1996;43:605.
19. Muntoni S, Fonte MT, Stoduto S, et al. Incidence of insulin-dependent diabetes mellitus among Sardinian-heritage children born in Lazio region, Italy. Lancet 1997;349:160.
20. Karvonen M, Pitkaniemi J, Tuomilehto J. The onset age of type 1 diabetes in Finnish children has become younger. The Finnish Childhood Diabetes Registry Group. Diabetes Care 1999;22:1066.
21. Classen DC, Classen JB. The timing of pediatric immunization and the risk of insulin-dependent diabetes mellitus. Infect Dis Clin Prac 1997;6:449.
22. Classen JB, Classen DC. Public should be told that vaccines may have long term adverse effects. Br Med J 1999;318:193.
23. Karvonen M, Cepaitis Z, Tuomilehto J. Association between type 1 diabetes and *Haemophilus influenzae* type b vaccination: birth cohort study. Br Med J 1999;318:1169.
24. Anonymous. Childhood immunizations and type 1 diabetes: summary of an Institute for Vaccine Safety Workshop. The Institute for Vaccine Safety Diabetes Workshop Panel. Pediatr Infect Dis J 1999;18:217.
25. Graves PM, Barriga KJ, Norris JM, et al. Lack of association between early childhood immunizations and beta-cell autoimmunity. Diabetes Care 1999;22:1694.
26. Yoon JW, Austin M, Onodera T, Notkins A. Isolation of a virus from the pancreas of a child with diabetic ketoacidosis. N Engl J Med 1979;300:1173.
27. Bingley PJ, Bonifacio E, Williams AJK, Genovese S, Bottazzo GF, Gale EAM. Prediction of IDDM in the general population: strategies based on combinations of autoantibody markers. Diabetes 1997;46:1701.
28. Rewers M, Norris JM, Eisenbarth GS, et al. Beta-cell autoantibodies in infants and toddlers without IDDM relatives: Diabetes Autoimmunity Study in the Young (Daisy). J Autoimmun 1996;9:405.
29. Verge CF, Eisenbarth GS. Prediction of type I diabetes: the natural history of the pre-diabetic period. In: Eisenbarth GS, Lafferty KJ (eds) Type I diabetes: molecular and cellular immunology. New York, Oxford University Press, 1996;230.
30. Verge CF, Eisenbarth GS. Natural history of autoimmunity in type I diabetes mellitus. In: LeRoith D, Taylor SI, Olefsky JM (eds) Diabetes mellitus: a fundamental and clinical text. Philadelphia, Lippincott-Raven, 1996;287.
31. Shimada A, Charlton B, Taylor-Edwards C, Fathman CG. β-cell destruction may be a late consequence of the autoimmune process in nonobese diabetic mice. Diabetes 1996;45:1063.
32. Greenbaum CJ, Sears KL, Kahn SE, Palmer JP. Relationship of B-cell function and autoantibodies to progression and nonprogression of subclinical type 1 diabetes. Diabetes 1999;48:170.
33. Sreenan S, Pick AJ, Levisetti M, Baldwin AC, Pugh W, Polonsky KS. Increased β-cell proliferation and reduced mass before diabetes onset in the nonobese diabetic mouse. Diabetes 1999;48:989.
34. Gazda LS, Charlton B, Lafferty KJ. Diabetes results from a late change in the autoimmune response of NOD mice. J Autoimmun 1997;10:261.
35. Chatenoud L, Thervet E, Primo J, Bach JF. Anti-CD3 antibody induces long-term remission of overt autoimmunity in nonobese diabetic mice. Proc Natl Acad Sci USA 1994;91:123.
36. Verge CF, Gianani R, Yu L, et al. Late progression to diabetes and evidence for chronic β-cell autoimmunity in identical twins of patients with type I diabetes. Diabetes 1995;44:1176.
37. Redondo MJ, Yu L, Hawa M, et al. Heterogeneity of type 1 diabetes: analysis of twins in the United Kingdom and United States. 1999; (Unpublished).
38. Pugliese A, Eisenbarth GS. Human type I diabetes mellitus: genetic susceptibility and resistance. In: Eisenbarth GS, Lafferty KJ (eds) Type I diabetes: molecular, cellular, and clinical immunology. New York, Oxford University Press, 1996;134.
39. Rewers M, Bugawan TL, Norris JM, et al. Newborn screening for HLA markers associated with IDDM: diabetes autoimmunity study in the young (DAISY). Diabetologia 1996;39:807.
40. Baisch JM, Weeks T, Giles R, Hoover M, Stastny P, Capra JD. Analysis of HLA-DQ genotypes and susceptibility in insulin-dependent diabetes mellitus. N Engl J Med 1990;322:1836.
41. Pugliese A, Gianani R, Moromisato R, et al. HLA-DQB1*0602 is associated with dominant protection from diabetes even among islet cell antibody-positive first-degree relatives of patients with IDDM. Diabetes 1995;44:608.
42. Nakanishi K, Kobayashi T, Murase T, Naruse T, Nose Y, Inoko H. Human leukocyte antigen-A24 and -DQA1*0301 in Japanese insulin-dependent diabetes mellitus: independent contributions to susceptibility to the disease and additive contributions to acceleration of beta-cell destruction. J Clin Endocrinol Metab 1999;84:3721.
43. Bennett ST, Lucassen AM, Gough SCL, et al. Susceptibility to human type I diabetes at IDDM2 is determined by tandem repeat variation at the insulin gene minisatellite locus. Nature Genet 1995;9:284.
44. Kennedy GC, German MS, Rutter WJ. The minisatellite in the diabetes susceptibility locus IDDM2 regulates insulin transcription. Nature Genet 1995;9:293.
45. Eisenbarth GS, Jackson RA, Pugliese A. Insulin autoimmunity: the rate limiting factor in pre-type I diabetes. J Autoimmun 1992;5:241.
46. Pugliese A, Zeller M, Fernandez A, et al. The insulin gene is transcribed in the human thymus and transcription levels correlate with allelic variation at the INS VNTR-IDDM2 susceptibility locus for type I diabetes. Nature Genet 1997;15:293.
47. Vafiadis P, Bennett ST, Todd JA, et al. Insulin expression in human thymus is modulated by INS VNTR alleles at the IDDM2 locus. Nature Genet 1997;15:289.
48. Nagamine K, Peterson P, Scott HS, et al. Positional cloning of the APECED gene. Nature Genet 1997;17:393.
49. Verge CF, Vardi P, Babu S, et al. Evidence for oligogenic inheritance of type 1A diabetes in a large Bedouin Arab family. J Clin Invest 1998;102:1569.
50. Nishimoto H, Kikutani H, Yamamura K, Kishimoto T. Prevention of autoimmune insulitis by expression of I-E molecules in NOD mice. Nature 1987;328:432.
51. Akashi T, Nagafuchi S, Anzai K, et al. Direct evidence for the contribution of B cells to the progression of insulitis and the development of diabetes in non-obese diabetic mice. Int Immunol 1997;9:1159.
52. Serreze DV, Fleming SA, Chapman HD, Richard SD, Leiter EH, Tisch RM. B lymphocytes are critical antigen-presenting cells for the initiation of T cell-mediated autoimmune diabetes in nonobese diabetic mice. J Immunol 1998;161:3912.
53. Rapoport MJ, Jaramillo A, Zipris D, et al. Interleukin 4 reverses T cell proliferative unresponsiveness and prevents the onset of diabetes in nonobese diabetic mice. J Exp Med 1993;178:87.
54. Pennline KJ, Rogue-Gaffney E, Monahan M. Recombinant human IL-10 prevents the onset of diabetes in the nonobese diabetic mouse. Clin Immunol Immunopathol 1994;71:169.
55. Trembleau S, Penna G, Bosi E, Mortara A, Gately MK, Adorini L. Interleukin 12 administration induces T helper type 1 cells and accelerates autoimmune diabetes in NOD mice. J Exp Med 1995;181:817.

56. Yang XD, Tisch R, Singer SM, et al. Effect of tumour necrosis factor alpha on insulin-dependent diabetes mellitus in NOD mice. I. The early development of autoimmunity and the diabetogenic process. J Exp Med 1994;180:995.
57. Campbell IL, Oxbrow L, Harrison LC. Reduction in insulitis following administration of IFN-gamma and TNF-alpha in the NOD mouse. J Autoimmun 1991;4:249.
58. Hultgren B, Huang X, Dybdal N, Stewart TA. Genetic absence of γ-interferon delays but does not prevent diabetes in NOD mice. Diabetes 1996;45:812.
59. Wogensen L, Lee M-S, Sarvetnick N. Production of interleukin 10 by islet cells accelerates immune-mediated destruction of β cells in nonobese diabetic mice. J Exp Med 1994;179:1379.
60. Tough DF, Borrow P, Sprent J. Induction of bystander T cell proliferation by viruses and type I interferon in vivo. Science 1996;272:1947.
61. Ginsberg-Fellner F, Witt ME, Franklin BH, et al. Triad of markers for identifying children at high risk of developing insulin-dependent diabetes mellitus. JAMA 1985;254:1469.
62. Karounos DG, Wolinsky JS, Thomas JW. Monoclonal antibody to rubella virus capsid protein recognizes a β-cell antigen. J Immunol 1993;150:3080.
63. Rabinowe SL, George KL, Loughlin R, Soeldner JS, Eisenbarth GS. Congenital rubella. Monoclonal antibody-defined T cell abnormalities in young adults. Am J Med 1986;81:779.
64. Vreugdenhil GR, Geluk A, Ottenhoff TH, Melchers WJ, Roep BO, Galama JM. Molecular mimicry in diabetes mellitus: the homologous domain in coxsackie B virus protein 2C and islet autoantigen GAD65 is highly conserved in the coxsackie B-like enteroviruses and binds to the diabetes associated HLA-DR3 molecule. Diabetologia 1998;41:40.
65. Karlsson MG, Ludvigsson J. Determination of mRNA expression for IFN-gamma and IL-4 in lymphocytes from children with IDDM by RT-PCR technique. Diabetes Res Clin Prac 1998;40:21.
66 Hyöty H, Hiltunen M, Knip M, et al. A prospective study of the role of coxsackie B and other enterovirus infections in the pathogenesis of IDDM. Diabetes 1995;44:652.
67. Clements GB, Galbraith DN, Taylor KW. Coxsackie B virus infection and onset of childhood diabetes. Lancet 1995;346:221.
68. D'Alessio DJ. A case-control study of group B Coxsackievirus immunoglobulin M antibody prevalence and HLA-DR antigens in newly diagnosed cases of insulin-dependent diabetes mellitus. Am J Epidemiol 1992;135:1331.
69. Graves PM, Rewers M. The role of enteroviral infections in the development of IDDM: limitations of current approaches. Diabetes 1997;46:161.
70. Dahlquist G. Environmental risk factors in human type 1 diabetes – an epidemiological perspective. Diabetes Metab Rev 1998;11:37.
71. Jardetzky TS, Brown JH, Gorga JC, et al. Three-dimensional structure of a human Class II histocompatibility molecule complexed with superantigen. Nature 1994;368:711.
72. Conrad B, Weidmann E, Trucco G, et al. Evidence for superantigen involvement in insulin-dependent diabetes mellitus aetiology. Nature 1994;371:351.
73. Conrad B, Weissmahr RN, Böni J, Arcari R, Schüpbach J, Mach B. A human endogenous retroviral superantigen as candidate autoimmune gene in type 1 diabetes. Cell 1997;90:303.
74. Jaeckel E, Heringlake S, Berger D, Brabant G, Hunsmann G, Manns MP. No evidence for association between $IDDMK_{1,2}22$, a novel isolated retrovirus, and IDDM. Diabetes 1999;48:209.
75. Kim A, Jun HS, Wong L, et al. Human endogenous retrovirus with a high genomic sequence homology with IDDMK (1,2)22 is not specific for type I (insulin-dependent) diabetic patients but ubiquitous. Diabetologia 1999;42:413.
76. Martin JM, Trink B, Daneman D, Dosch H-M, Robinson B. Milk proteins in the etiology of insulin-dependent diabetes mellitus (IDDM). Ann Med 1991;23:447.
77. Karjalainen J, Martin JM, Knip M, et al. A bovine albumin peptide as a possible trigger of insulin-dependent diabetes mellitus. N Engl J Med 1992;327:302.
78. Pietropaolo M, Castaño L, Babu S, et al. Islet cell autoantigen 69 kDa (ICA69): molecular cloning and characterization of a novel diabetes associated autoantigen. J Clin Invest 1993;92:359.
79. Norris JM, Beaty B, Klingensmith G, et al. Lack of association between early exposure to cow's milk protein and β-cell autoimmunity: Diabetes Autoimmunity Study in the Young (DAISY). JAMA 1996;276:609.
80. Couper JJ, Steele C, Beresford S, et al. Lack of association between duration of breast-feeding or introduction of cow's milk and development of islet autoimmunity. Diabetes 1999;48:2145.
81. Palmer JP, Asplin CM, Clemons P, et al. Insulin antibodies in insulin-dependent diabetics before insulin treatment. Science 1983;222:1337.
82. Eisenbarth GS, Gianani R, Yu L, et al. Dual parameter model for prediction of type 1 diabetes mellitus. Proc Assoc Am Phys 1998;110:126.
83. Yu L, Gianani R, Eisenbarth GS. Quantitation of glutamic acid decarboxylase autoantibody levels in prospectively evaluated relatives of patients with type I diabetes. Diabetes 1994;43:1229.
84. Ujihara N, Daw K, Gianani R, Boel E, Yu L, Powers AC. Identification of glutamic acid decarboxylase autoantibody heterogeneity and epitope regions in type I diabetes. Diabetes 1994;43:968.
85. Gianani R, Rabin DU, Verge CF, et al. ICA512 autoantibody radioassay. Diabetes 1995;44:1340.
86. Jun HS, Yoon CS, Zbytnuik L, van Rooijen N, Yoon JW. The role of macrophages in T cell-mediated autoimmune diabetes in nonobese diabetic mice. J Exp Med 1999;189:347.
87. Simone E, Daniel D, Schloot N, et al. T cell receptor restriction of diabetogenic autoimmune NOD T cells. Proc Natl Acad Sci USA 1997;94:2518.
88. Wong FS, Karttunen J, Dumont C, et al. Identification of an MHC Class I-restricted autoantigen in type 1 diabetes by screening an organ-specific cDNA library. Nature Med 1999;5:1026.
89. Dilts SM, Lafferty KJ. Autoimmune diabetes: the involvement of benign and malignant autoimmunity. J Autoimmun 1999;12:229.
90. O'Brien BA, Harmon BV, Cameron DP, Allan DJ. Apoptosis is the mode of β-cell death responsible for the development of IDDM in the nonobese diabetic (NOD) mouse. Diabetes 1997;46:750.
91. Itoh N, Hanafusa T, Miyazaki A, et al. Mononuclear cell infiltration and its relation to the expression of major histocompatibility complex antigens and adhesion molecules in pancreas biopsy specimens from newly diagnosed insulin-dependent diabetes mellitus patients. J Clin Invest 1993;92:2313.
92. Bingley PJ, Christie MR, Bonifacio E, et al. Combined analysis of autoantibodies improves prediction of IDDM in islet cell antibody-positive relatives. Diabetes 1994;43:1304.
93. Stiller CR, Dupre J, Gent M, et al. Effects of cyclosporine immunosuppression in insulin-dependent diabetes mellitus of recent onset. Science 1984;223:1362.
94. Tian J, Clare-Salzler M, Herschenfeld A, et al. Modulating autoimmune responses to GAD inhibits disease progression and prolongs islet graft survival in diabetes-prone mice. Nature Med 1996;2:1348.
95. Ramiya VK, Shang X, Pharis PG, et al. Antigen based therapies to prevent diabetes in NOD mice. J Autoimmun 1996;9:349.
96. Zhang ZJ, Davidson L, Eisenbarth G, Weiner HL. Suppression of diabetes in nonobese diabetic mice by oral administration of porcine insulin. Proc Natl Acad Sci USA 1991;88:10252.
97. Daniel D, Wegmann DR. Protection of nonobese diabetic mice from diabetes by intranasal or subcutaneous administration of insulin peptide B-(9–23). Proc Natl Acad Sci USA 1996;93:956.
98. Zekzer D, Wong FS, Wen L, et al. Inhibition of diabetes by an insulin-reactive CD4 T-cell clone in the nonobese diabetic mouse. Diabetes 1997;46:1124.
99. Maron R, Melican NS, Weiner HL. Regulatory Th2-type T cell lines against insulin and GAD peptides derived from orally- and nasally-treated NOD mice suppress diabetes. J Autoimmun 1999;12:251.
100. Sadelain MW, Qin H-Y, Lauzon J, Singh B. Prevention of type I diabetes in NOD mice by adjuvant immunotherapy. Diabetes 1990;39:583.
101. Harada M, Kishimoto Y, Makino S. Prevention of overt diabetes and insulitis in NOD mice by a single BCG vaccination. Diabetes 1990;8:85.

102. Bjorses P, Pelto-Huikko M, Kaukonen J, Aaltonen J, Peltonen L, Ulmanen I. Localization of the APECED protein in distinct nuclear structures. Hum Mol Genet 1999;8:259.
103. Heino M, Peterson P, Kudoh J, et al. Autoimmune regulator is expressed in the cells regulating immune tolerance in thymus medulla. Biochem Biophys Res Commun 1999;257:821.
104. Gambelunghe G, Falorni A, Ghaderi M, et al. Microsatellite polymorphism of the MHC Class I chain-related (MIC-A and MIC-B) genes marks the risk for autoimmune Addison's disease. J Clin Endocrinol Metab 1999;84:3701.
105. Not T, Horvath K, Hill ID, et al. Celiac disease risk in the USA: high prevalence of antiendomysium antibodies in healthy blood donors. Scand J Gastroenterol 1998;33:494.
106. Polvi A, Eland C, Koskimies S, Maki M, Partanen J. HLA DQ and DP in Finnish families with celiac disease. Eur J Immunogenet 1996;23:221.
107. Dietrich W, Ehnis T, Bauer M, et al. Identification of tissue transglutaminase as the autoantigen of celiac disease. Nature Med 1997;3:797.
108. Bao F, Yu L, Babu S, et al. One third of HLA DQ2 homozygous patients with type 1 diabetes express celiac disease associated transglutaminase autoantibodies. J Autoimmun 1999;13:143.
109. Hoffenberg EJ, Bao F, Eisenbarth GS, et al. Silent celiac disease in children with a genetic risk. 1999 (Unpublished).
110. Turner R, Stratton I, Horton V, et al. UKPDS 25: autoantibodies to islet-cell cytoplasm and glutamic acid decarboxylase for prediction of insulin requirement in type 2 diabetes. UK Prospective Diabetes Study Group. Lancet 1997;350:1288.
111. Uchigata Y, Hirata Y. Insulin autoimmune syndrome (IAS, Hirata disease). In: Eisenbarth G (ed) Molecular mechanisms of endocrine and organ specific autoimmunity. Austin, TX, R.G. Landes, 1999;133.

Chapter 83

Human Reproductive Immunology

Gill S. Vince, Peter M. Johnson and Paul Gatenby

Pregnancy has been held to present an immunological paradox: 'How does the pregnant mother continue to nourish within herself for many weeks or months a fetus that is an antigenically foreign body?'. This question, posed first by Peter Medawar almost 50 years ago,[1] provided a framework for research in reproductive immunology and, in particular, the immunology of pregnancy. In the intervening time, many of the cellular and molecular components contributing fundamentally to successful viviparity in genetically outbred pregnancy have been identified – even if not all the functional detail is yet known. This chapter focuses on human reproductive immunology, highlighting the specialized immunological features of both fetal trophoblast and maternal leukocytes within the decidualized endometrium (decidua) that contribute to the unique transplantation protection of the intrauterine fetal allograft. The topic of reproductive immunology has also broadened significantly and the latter part of this chapter covers clinical aspects of reproductive immunopathology.

BASIC CONCEPTS

Male reproductive tract

The male urogenital tract is part of the mucosal immune system that provides initial immune defense against potentially infectious organisms. The blood–testis barrier, provided by the Sertoli cell layer, excludes immune cells from human seminiferous tubules. T cells are usually absent from the testis, but are found in the rete testis, epididymis, and vas deferens. CD8 T cells are predominant within the epithelium, with CD4 T cells mainly in the stroma.[2] Macrophages comprise 20–40% of the interstitial cell population in the testis, where they are known to scavenge dead sperm, and are also present in the epididymis and penile urethra. Human prostate contains numerous lymphocytes and macrophages, but few plasma cells are detected even though levels of IgG, IgM, and IgA are approximately 10 times higher in prostatic fluid than in semen.[2]

The male reproductive tract is considered an immunosuppressive microenvironment and human seminal plasma also contains many immune mediators, such as prostaglandins, TGF-β, complement inhibitors, spermine and defensins, all indicative of the immunosuppressive action of semen.[3]

Although all spermatozoa and cellular precursors are HLA-negative, there are HLA-positive nonmotile cells present normally in the ejaculate – mainly epithelial cells and leukocytes. A concentration of $>1\times10^6$ nonspermatozoal cells/ml is the WHO definition of leukocytospermia; this is considered abnormal and indicative of genital tract infection, but is often asymptomatic and can occur in over 20% of men attending infertility clinics. Infection can compromise fertility, and there is an association between leukocytospermia and poor semen function.[4]

Female reproductive tract

The female reproductive tract is also part of the mucosal immune system. Plasma cells are located within the endocervix, ectocervix, vagina, and fallopian tube, and epithelial cells in the fallopian tube and endocervix constitutively express secretory component. Plasma cells and immunoglobulin-containing cells are only rarely detected in the human endometrium and thus there is little intrinsic endometrial production of IgA – the majority of IgA in the uterine lumen is synthesized in tissues higher up the reproductive tract.[2] Few T cells are present in the ectocervix and vaginal stroma, but numerous CD8–T cells occur within the ectocervical and vaginal epithelium. Cervicovaginal T cells express the β chemokine receptor CCR5, which functions as a coreceptor for HIV-1 and thus could provide a target for transmission of HIV-1 in women.[5] Macrophages are present in the endocervix, vagina, and ectocervix; the antigen-presenting cell population also includes dendritic (Langerhans) cells. The fallopian tube contains T cells as well as a population of granulocytes; indeed, the fallopian tube and uterus contain a higher proportion of leukocytes than the cervix and vagina.[2]

The interaction between the female immune system and spermatozoa is not fully understood. The presence of sperm in the female reproductive tract results in a leukocytic infiltrate, predominantly neutrophils, in the cervical mucus. The high concentration of prostaglandins in semen may effect a cytokine-mediated switch away from a cell-mediated immune response, inducing a state of nonresponsiveness to sperm antigens in the female reproductive tract. This would be of benefit to sperm, but responses to infectious agents may also be compromised.[3]

The endometrium contains significant numbers of leukocytes, both intraepithelial and within the stroma, where they can be individually scattered or in large aggregates mainly adjacent to glands. The absolute numbers and proportions of constituent cell populations vary during the menstrual cycle and early in pregnancy[6] (Table 83.1). A population of large granular lymphocytes (LGL) increases significantly in number in the late secretory phase, and increases further if pregnancy occurs, suggesting that LGL are under hormonal control. However, uterine leukocytes do not express progesterone or estrogen receptors and thus effects must be indirect, possibly via epithelial or stromal cells that do express progesterone receptors. In the latter half of the menstrual cycle, the most abundant leukocyte is a population of phenotypically distinctive $CD3^- CD16^- CD56^{bright}$ LGL. Around implantation, LGL comprise 70–80% of leukocytes in the endometrium.[6] These cells contain perforin and granzymes, indicating the potential for decidual LGL-mediated cytolytic function.

T-cell numbers remain relatively constant through the menstrual cycle although, in contrast to peripheral blood, more than

Leukocyte populations in the human endometrium and decidua				
	Endometrium		Decidua	
	Proliferative phase	Secretory phase	First trimester	Term
B cells and granulocytes	–	–	–	±
T cells	+	+	+	+
Macrophages	+	+/++	++	++
LGL (CD56^{bright})	+	++	+++	+

Table 83.1 Leukocyte populations in the human endometrium and decidua.

two thirds express CD8. The majority of endometrial T cells carry the αβ T-cell receptor. γδ T cells form only a small proportion of total T-cell numbers (around 5–10%) which is similar throughout the menstrual cycle and early pregnancy.[7]

Macrophages are present in the endometrium and increase in number premenstrually, although to a lesser extent than LGL. Macrophages are found in the placental bed throughout gestation, in contrast to decidual LGL which have essentially disappeared at term.[6] In the absence of a pronounced antigen-specific cellular immune system within human uteroplacental tissues, it is likely that decidual macrophages (along with fetal macrophages in the placenta) provide an immediate antigen-nonspecific host defense to infection that may be essential for maintaining the integrity of pregnancy.

Feto-maternal tissue contact

Direct tissue contact between maternal endometrium and the embryonic blastocyst is established at implantation, approximately 6–9 days after fertilization. The preimplantation embryo consists of a small inner cell mass encased within trophectoderm. Trophoblast is the first cell type to differentiate following fertilization and forms the entire continuous surrounding tissue interface with maternal blood and decidualized endometrium (Fig. 83.1). An additional feature of human pregnancy is invasion of decidualized endometrium, myometrium, and arteries by extravillous cytotrophoblast. During the first weeks of pregnancy, columns of cytotrophoblast cells proliferate from chorionic villi and spread laterally to form the cytotrophoblastic shell from which extravillous cytotrophoblast invades uterine tissues. Cytotrophoblast migrates up uterine spiral arteries in two waves, reaching the terminal segments of myometrial radial arteries at 16–20 weeks' gestation and mediating the physiological alterations required to accommodate a 10-fold increase in uterine blood supply to nourish the feto-placental unit. Interstitial cytotrophoblast also infiltrates through decidua and myometrium, where some cells fuse to form multinucleate syncytial giant cells. Extraembryonic trophoblast thus has direct contact with both maternal blood and cells within decidual tissue (Fig. 83.1).

Expression of HLA molecules

Neither syncytiotrophoblast nor extravillous cytotrophoblast express the classical Class I HLA molecules HLA-A or -B. However, fetal cells within the mesenchymal core of placental villi, e.g. macrophages, express HLA Class I (from 8–11 weeks) and HLA Class II molecules (from the end of the second trimester) but are sequestered from maternal leukocytes by the HLA-negative layer of syncytiotrophoblast (Fig. 83.1). In contrast, human extravillous cytotrophoblast selectively and strongly express the nonclassical Class I HLA-G molecule from early pregnancy.[8] HLA-G (molecular weight 39 kDa) is a transmembrane molecule with a truncated cytoplasmic tail, associated with β_2-microglobulin at the cell surface. It has a high degree of sequence similarity to HLA-A2 at both nucleotide and amino acid level. Unlike other Class I HLA molecules, HLA-G demonstrates very limited polymorphism but undergoes alternative splicing to produce different proteins (HLA-G1, G2, G3), two of which also have soluble forms (HLA-G1sol, HLA-G2sol).[9] These different HLA-G proteins could have multiple functions in pregnancy. HLA-G may have the ability to provoke a maternal allogeneic response since HLA-G1 is potentially capable of presenting 9 residue peptide antigens to T cells, and hence could play a role in defense to local infection.

Extravillous cytotrophoblast also expresses an additional Class I molecule (HLA-E) which, like HLA-G, shows limited polymorphism but also a low level of protein expression. HLA-E can bind other Class I HLA leader sequence peptides. HLA-C is also expressed by extravillous cytotrophoblast,[10] and HLA-G, -E and -C could all be involved in protection of trophoblast from NK cell killing by acting as killer inhibitory receptor (KIR) ligands (see below).

KEY CONCEPTS

Protection of the fetus from maternal cytotoxic effectors

- The interface of fetal tissue with the maternal host is the various differentiated forms of trophoblast throughout the uteroplacental site and extraembryonic membranes.
- Syncytiotrophoblast, in direct contact with maternal blood, does not express surface classical Class I MHC molecules HLA-A, -B – thus protecting the placenta from attack by cytotoxic T cells.
- Extravillous trophoblast, in direct contact with maternal decidua, express the Class I MHC molecules HLA-E and -G. Unlike HLA-A, -B and -C, HLA-E and -G show limited genetic polymorphism. Expression of HLA-E and -G protects trophoblast from attack from large granular lymphocytes (LGL) in maternal decidua, probably via interaction with killer inhibitory receptors (KIR).
- Passive immunity is provided to the fetus by the selective transfer of maternal IgG, occurring significantly from 20 weeks' gestation; however, maternal IgG antifetal HLA alloantibodies are trapped and retained within placental tissue.
- Trophoblast express high surface levels of complement regulatory proteins, thus providing protection from maternal complement-mediated damage at the maternal–fetal tissue interface.
- Other cellular mechanisms may also protect the fetal tissue interface from cellular cytotoxic attack – notably expression of Fas ligand and local catabolism of tryptophan by indoleamine 2,3-dioxygenase (IDO).

Trophoblast populations at the implantation site

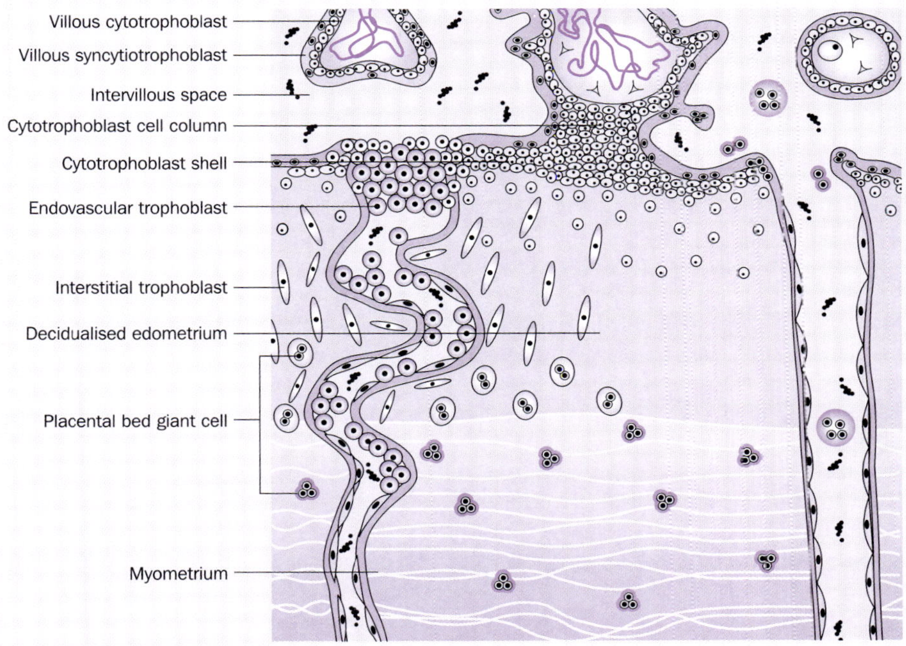

Figure 83.1 Trophoblast populations at the implanation site. The definitive villous placenta is at the top of the diagram surrounded by the intervillous space. Beneath the placenta is the decidua basalis with the myometrium at the bottom of the picture. A spiral artery is represented schematically on the left of the diagram with a vein on the right. The endothelium and media of the decidual portion of the spiral artery are replaced by trophoblast and fibrinoid material as a result of infiltration by endovascular and interstitial trophoblast. Placental bed giant cells are present in the myometrium. Syncytial sprouts originating from the villous syncytiotrophoblast are deported via uterine veins to the lungs. (Adapted from Loke YW, King A. *Human Implantation: Cell Biology and Immunology*. Cambridge, Cambridge University Press, 1995).

Expression of complement regulatory proteins

All fetal trophoblast populations throughout gestation, from the preimplantation embryo to the term placenta, express high levels of cell surface complement regulatory proteins – notably, membrane cofactor protein (MCP; CD46), decay accelerating factor (DAF; CD55) and membrane attack complex inhibitory factor (CD59)[11] (Chapter 21). CD46 and CD55 down-regulate the complement cascade at the level of component C3 convertase activity, whereas CD59 inhibits the formation of the terminal membrane attack complex. The unusually strong expression of complement regulatory proteins by trophoblast provides exceptional protection from maternal complement-mediated damage at the maternal–fetal interface, thus minimizing tissue damage at potential sites of complement activation, for example during trophoblast invasion and tissue remodeling.

Recent experiments have highlighted the potential importance of protection from complement activation at the maternal–fetal interface. Mice deficient in a murine complement regulator, *Crry*, were unable to reproduce successfully: embryos died in mid-gestation due to excessive complement deposition and consequent placental inflammation.[12]

CD46 is also expressed selectively on the surface of acrosome-reacted spermatozoa. In contrast, CD55 and CD59 are expressed on both acrosome-reacted and unreacted sperm. The expression of complement regulatory proteins on sperm could provide protection from complement-mediated cytolytic damage in the female tract. In addition, certain anti-CD46 antibodies inhibit human sperm binding and pronuclear formation in an autologous zona-free oocyte penetration assay, suggesting a role for CD46 in apposition or fusion of spermatozoa and oocyte.

Evasion of maternal cytotoxic effector cells: killer inhibitory receptors (KIR)

Both endometrial and decidual LGL have been shown to express natural killer (NK) cell type cytotoxicity against classical NK cell targets, although to a lesser extent than peripheral blood NK cells. However, cytotoxicity against cytotrophoblast is induced only after activation by IL-2 and, since decidual LGL express only the IL-2 receptor β chain, these cells are not readily activated by IL-2. HLA-G, -E or -C could protect cytotrophoblast from maternal NK cell attack – the 'missing self' hypothesis.[13] Indeed, expression of HLA-G by cell transfectants leads to decreased NK target cell killing. Basal HLA-nonrestricted cytolytic activity of decidual LGL would be prevented by expression of KIR molecules, including CD94 and the p58 molecules on the cell surface of decidual LGL.[14]

HLA-C alleles are ligands for p58 KIR molecules and thus HLA-C expression on extravillous trophoblast could act as an allotype-dependent KIR ligand. CD94 may be the more important ligand for protecting HLA-G-expressing target cells from lysis by NK cells, and HLA-E is also recognized by CD94 receptors. HLA-G and -E would therefore act as allotype-independent KIR ligands, and cytotrophoblast would be expected to be susceptible to lysis only by cells lacking all of these KIRs, a phenotype that has not been identified for decidual LGL. Differences in expression of KIRs in relation to HLA phenotype could be a mechanism for the unexplained association between certain HLA types and recurrent pregnancy loss.

Herpes simplex virus (HSV) blocks intracellular transport of HLA-G in a choriocarcinoma cell line, and hence could also provide a reason for the association of HSV infection and spontaneous fetal loss.[15] In addition, certain viral products (together with IL-15 and TGF-β) have been shown to enhance CD94 expression and therefore down-regulate lytic activity. Expression of HLA-G1 protein is not essential for fetal survival since, in a homozygous individual lacking HLA-G1, there was no expression of HLA-G1 protein in the placenta but the individual survived to adulthood.[16]

Indoleamine 2, 3-dioxygenase

Immunosuppression mediated by indoleamine 2,3-dioxygenase (IDO), an enzyme that catabolizes tryptophan, may prevent fetal rejection by the maternal immune system. Macrophages induced to express IDO inhibit T-cell proliferation in vitro by consuming tryptophan. In mice, inhibition of IDO leads to rejection of allogeneic conceptuses a few days after implantation.[17] A role for IDO in human pregnancy is unclear as yet, but cells producing IDO are present in term placenta, and maternal serum levels of tryptophan decline from the first to the third trimester of pregnancy coinciding with development and growth of the placenta. By metabolizing tryptophan, the mammalian conceptus could suppress T-cell activity and hence maternal IDO expression may prevent immune rejection of fetal allografts.[17]

Fas

The fetus can be considered a semi-allograft exposed to the host (mother's) immune system which should generate an immune rejection response. Normally, this does not take place (for reasons outlined above) and maternal tolerance to the fetus occurs. The basic mechanisms involved in tolerance are poorly understood.

Fas ligand (Fas-L) and its receptor Fas play an important role in regulation of the immune response. Fas is expressed constitutively by a number of tissues. In contrast, Fas-L is expressed as an inducible protein on activated T and NK cells, where it participates in effector function as well as programmed elimination of activated T cells. Fas-L is also expressed in various tissue sites where it can trigger apoptosis of infiltrating Fas-expressing T cells, thus enforcing immune privilege and mediating immune tolerance. Fas-L is expressed on syncytiotrophoblast and cytotrophoblast in the placenta and on extravillous cytotrophoblast, while Fas is expressed on leukocytes in decidua.[18] Apoptotic decidual leukocytes are found mainly in areas where trophoblast have invaded, suggesting that trophoblastic Fas-L may induce apoptosis in activated leukocytes, thus providing a mechanism for maternal immune tolerance to the fetus. Villous cytotrophoblast also express Fas, but the Fas response appears inactivated. In addition, the TNF-related apoptosis-inducing ligand (TRAIL) is expressed by syncytiotrophoblast, suggesting a similar role for TRAIL in the establishment of placental immune privilege.[19]

Cytokines

Recent attention has focused on possible immunobiological roles of cytokines in pregnancy following the accumulated evidence of extensive and complex cytokine activity within uteroplacental tissues. It has been suggested that Th1-type cytokine responses (e.g. IFN-γ, IL-2) are impaired in pregnancy and that this impairment is accompanied by local expression of Th2-type cytokines (e.g. IL-4, IL-6, IL-10) that are beneficial for placental growth and development.[20] Partial suppression of systemic Th1 responses in human pregnancy is compatible with clinical evidence that infectious diseases caused by intracellular pathogens, e.g. CMV and malaria, are sometimes exacerbated in pregnancy. It is important to remember, however, that both fetal and maternal leukocyte populations, as well as uterine epithelium and fetal trophoblast, have the potential to produce Th1- and Th2-type cytokines.

There is constitutive decidual expression of additional cytokines, such as TNF-α and GM-CSF, as well as expression on fetal trophoblast of specific receptors for these cytokines. Soluble factors, produced locally by implanting blastocysts, may therefore recruit and activate decidual macrophages and LGL at the implantation site. Cytokine production by these maternal cells then has the potential to affect trophoblast growth and invasion (termed immunotrophism).[20]

Although many cytokines are represented at high levels in uteroplacental tissue, IL-2 stands out by its marked local absence. This has implications for the activation of LGL, as well as relative T-cell anergy within uteroplacental tissues. However, high levels of IL-15 mRNA have been detected in placenta and decidua, and IL-2 and IL-15 share many effects on T and B cells, but IL-15 has unique activity on cells of nonhematopoietic lineage.

Antibody and cellular transfer from mother to fetus and from mother to neonate

Antibody transfer

Transplacental transport of maternal IgG to the developing fetus, and hence acquisition of passive immunity, is vitally important in protection of the subsequent newborn from infection. The placenta contains several known IgG Fc (Fcγ) receptors as well as other proteins that bind immunoglobulins, and maternal IgG is selectively transferred from maternal blood in the intervillous spaces into fetal circulation via Fcγ receptors expressed by trophoblast cells.[21] The precise mechanisms of selective IgG transfer across the placenta are not fully understood. The Class I MHC-related IgG receptor, FcRn, is expressed on human syncytiotrophoblast and, in rodents, has been shown to be involved in transcellular IgG transport. Protected cellular transport of IgG occurs within intracellular endocytic vesicles in syncytiotrophoblast prior to release and subsequent movement into the lumen of fetal stem vessels. IgG is internalized via fluid-phase endocytosis, and binding to the FcRn occurs in acidic endosomes, allowing preferential intracellular sorting into the transcytotic pathway such that the receptor prevents entry into the degradative pathway in lysosomes.[22]

Significant transplacental passage of IgG to the human fetus begins around the 20th week of gestation and all four IgG subclasses are transferred. In contrast to the beneficial transfer of immunity, deleterious maternal IgG antibodies might also be passively transferred into the fetal circulation. However, locally formed immune complexes would be trapped in the placental stroma by Fcγ receptors on fetal macrophages (FcγRI, FcγRII, FcγRIII) as well as on fetal capillary endothelial cells (FcγRII).[21] Thus, for example, maternal IgG alloantibodies directed towards a fetal HLA allele will be bound and retained within the placental villus and will not reach the fetal circulation. Potentially deleterious antibodies are therefore trapped by a mechanism termed the placental 'sink' or 'sponge'. This results in extensive IgG and complement deposition within term placental villous tissues. There are exceptions, and some maternal IgG autoantibodies escape placental trapping; these are considered later in this chapter.

Cellular transfer

It has been known for over 100 years that some fetal cells can pass into the maternal circulation.[23] Indeed, fetal cells can persist in the maternal circulation for up to 30 years such that, following pregnancy, a woman may effectively become a chimera.[24] Similarly, maternal cells are known to be able to engraft and persist in immunocompetent, as well as immunodeficient, children into adult life.[25] Cellular microchimerism has been suggested to have a role in the pathogenesis of systemic sclerosis by initiating a graft-versus-host-like response (Chapter 64). Persistent fetal microchimerism is more frequent in the peripheral blood of women with systemic sclerosis, and fetal cells have been detected in affected tissues.[26] Fetal cells may persist due to either maternal immune tolerance or HLA compatibility between mother and offspring.

Fetal cells in maternal circulation have been evaluated as a potential source of DNA for noninvasive prenatal diagnosis.[27] Indeed, both intact fetal cells and fetal DNA are increased in the maternal circulation in Down syndrome, possibly due to abnormalities in the placental microenvironment.[27]

Immunogenetics in pregnancy

Anti-HLA antibodies

Sera from pregnant individuals may contain pregnancy-induced anti-HLA alloantibodies (lymphocytotoxic antibodies) directed against paternal antigens expressed by fetal leukocytes. Fifteen per cent of primiparous and up to 60% of multiparous women may develop such cytotoxic antibodies in pregnancy. Cytotoxic T cells specific for paternally-inherited fetal HLA molecules occur only rarely in peripheral blood during pregnancy. The presence (or absence) of pregnancy-derived maternal anti-HLA antibodies is neither advantageous nor deleterious to pregnancy.

Maternal–fetal HLA compatibility

Marked genetic polymorphism within MHC contributes substantially to fetal–maternal genetic disparity. Since HLA molecules encoded within the MHC region are the focus of mechanisms of T-cell restriction and allograft rejection, they may play a central role in the immunogenetic enigma of reproduction. It has been suggested that maternal–fetal incompatibility is advantageous to mammalian pregnancy. HLA-matched couples could therefore have poorer reproductive outcomes. However, over 30 retrospective studies of HLA-matching in couples with recurrent miscarriage have yielded conflicting results and no clear relationship between HLA-matching and fetal loss can be extrapolated.[28]

Endogenous retroviruses

Human syncytiotrophoblast normally express intact endogenous retroviruses (ERV), leading to speculation about involvement in placental formation or function. The envelope (*env*) gene of the human ERV family, HERV-W, encodes a protein (syncytin) highly expressed in syncytiotrophoblast; it may mediate cytotrophoblast fusion in vivo (without the need for a receptor) and may therefore be important in placental morphogenesis.[29]

Endogenous retroviruses may also have had a role in the evolution of mammalian placentation and help to protect the fetus from rejection by local suppression of the maternal immune system. ERV3 is expressed in human fetal heart, and the presence of high levels of antibodies to ERV3 in mothers of babies with congenital heart block suggests a possible role for ERV3 in the pathogenesis of this condition[30] (see below).

CLINICAL ASPECTS OF REPRODUCTIVE IMMUNOLOGY

Immunological infertility

Antisperm antibodies occur in some women, as well as in men, and may contribute to infertility by inhibiting spermatogenesis, motility, or other functions of sperm.[31] There is a better correlation of these antibodies with clinical infertility in men compared with women. Their presence in genital secretions of the male or female reproductive tract is of greater significance than in serum, and IgA appears to be the primary mediator of immunological infertility at these sites. The choice of assay for antisperm antibodies is also important. Assays that detect only surface antigens (e.g. agglutination test, mixed antiglobin reaction, or immunobead binding) demonstrate a better clinical correlation than assays that also detect cytoplasmic antigens (e.g. ELISA).[31] Only about 5% of antibodies to sperm are donor-specific.

Endometriosis

Endometriosis, characterized by the presence of endometrial tissue outside the uterus, has an estimated prevalence of around 10% in women of reproductive age. Endometriosis may originate either by development in situ by metaplasia or, more likely, by dissemination of endometrium to the peritoneal cavity by retrograde menstruation. However, retrograde menstruation is believed to be a universal phenomenon and there has been speculation on the role of the immune system in determining susceptibility to endometriosis.[32] There is little evidence for defective immune surveillance in the etiology of endometriosis. In common with other inflammatory conditions, a number of nonorgan-specific autoantibodies can be detected in individuals with this problem. Immune alterations in endometriosis include increased number and activation of peritoneal macrophages, resulting in increased cytokine concentrations and decreased T-cell reactivity and NK-cell cytotoxicity.[32]

Autoimmune disease and pregnancy

Antiphospholipid autoantibodies (aPL)

Several prospective studies support the link between aPL (autoantibodies reactive with negatively charged phospholipids) and recurrent pregnancy loss (Chapter 60). Up to 20% of women with recurrent pregnancy loss have aPL.[33] Fetal loss can occur in the first and second trimesters, and term pregnancies are also associated with complications that could be secondary to placental ischaemia. Up to half of women with aPL suffer pre-eclampsia, and placental insufficiency occurs in 15–30% of women with aPL, leading to a preterm birth rate of 12–35%.[33] Most evidence suggests that a thrombophilic state is important and late pregnancy loss may be associated with a decidual vasculopathy. However, this mechanism alone does not appear sufficient. aPL may also bind directly to both the villous cytotrophoblast and syncytiotrophoblast which may contribute to defective placentation.

It is now recognized that the apolipoprotein, β_2 glycoprotein 1 (β_2 GP1), is an important plasma cofactor for binding of aPL to phospholipid and, increasingly, assays to β_2 GP1 are being employed in the context of aPL-related pregnancy pathology.[34] β_2 GP1 has a potential role as a natural anticoagulant and may be the 'true' target for the autoimmune response. The risk of complications in pregnancy is higher in women with medium to high titers of IgG aCL or LA, but complications may also occur in those with lower levels or with IgM antibodies.[33] The association of aPL with preimplantation failure is controversial, both with regard to unexplained infertility and failure of in vitro fertilization.

Systemic lupus erythematosus

Systemic lupus erythematosus (SLE; Chapter 60) is the most common systemic autoimmune disease in young women and hence has important implications for pregnancy. Indeed, early studies suggested that women with SLE placed themselves at high risk of morbidity or mortality if they became pregnant. Although the outcome is no longer so gloomy, about 15–60% of women with SLE will 'flare' during pregnancy or the postpartum period.[35] In general, predisposition to exacerbation is small and mostly treatable with medium to low glucocorticoid doses. The rate of SLE exacerbation in pregnancy may be lower for women in remission prior to conception, as is the rate of renal deterioration.

Pregnancy loss is more common in women with SLE and may be over 30%. Women with SLE also have a higher rate of late (second or third trimester) pregnancy losses. Most, if not all, fetal deaths in women with SLE are associated with maternal aPL activity. Many women with active lupus during pregnancy, particularly those requiring therapy with glucocorticoids, experience gestational diabetes, hypertension, intrauterine growth retardation, and pre-eclampsia. These individuals are also at risk for a syndrome characterized by hemolysis, elevated liver enzymas, and thrombocytopenia as well as at risk for exacerbations of diabetic retinopathy.[35] Preterm birth is also more common in women with flares of lupus activity during pregnancy (20–60%). In addition, patients with a degree of renal impairment may suffer further renal impairment during pregnancy because of an increased glomerular filtration rate imposing an extra workload on an already compromised kidney. The mortality rate in women with SLE-associated nephropathy may be as high as 2.5%.

Neonatal lupus erythematosus

Neonatal lupus erythematosus (NLE) is a relatively rare complication characterized by dermatologic, cardiac or hematologic abnormalities due to passive autoantibody transfer, particularly anti-Ro/SS-A, from mother to the fetus.[36] Maternal anti-Ro/SS-A antibodies are found in 75–95% of NLE cases, including those

THERAPEUTIC PRINCIPLES

Antiphospholipid autoantibodies (aPL)

- The most widely used laboratory measures of aPL activity are anticardiolipin aCL and the lupus anticoagulant CA.
- Women are only considered aPL-positive after two positive tests (not in pregnancy), six weeks apart.
- Treatment with low molecular weight heparin and low-dose aspirin achieves final pregnancy outcomes as good as prednisolone (with or without low-dose aspirin) and with fewer side-effects.
- Heparin interferes with thrombosis in the placental circulation, and low-dose aspirin (60–100 mg) improves placental flow by decreasing the thromboxane to prostacyclin ratio.
- Lower doses of heparin are probably as effective as full anticoagulant doses, although the latter are required if there is a previous history of thrombosis.
- Heparin and low-dose aspirin are superior to low-dose aspirin alone.
- Most studies have shown a live birth rate in aPL-positive women treated with heparin and low-dose aspirin to be around 70%, compared with 15% for untreated women.

CLINICAL PEARLS

Neonatal lupus erythematosus (NLE)

Neonatal skin disease

- Most common presentation.
- Notably a subacute cutaneous lupus erythematosus, which manifests after delivery and exacerbates after exposure to ultraviolet light.
- New lesions, typically on the face and scalp, can continue to develop for several months, with a resolution by 6–8 months.

Cardiac disease

- Less common.
- Onset coincides with the transfer of maternal IgG antibodies across the placenta.
- An inflammatory infiltrate can be detected around the cardiac conducting tissues which may extend to a myopericarditis.
- Typically, the fetus has a slow fixed heart rate (60–80 bpm) and, as gestation continues, this may be associated with cardiac failure and hydrops.
- Congenital complete heart block (CHB) is a significant problem – 65% of infants require a pacemaker and, in one large registry, 25% died within a few years of birth.
- At-risk pregnancies should be monitored serially from 16 to 20 weeks' gestation using high-quality fetal cardiac ultrasound.

with congenital complete heart block (CHB), and antibodies to La/SS-B are also found in association with congenital CHB. These autoantibodies are directed against intracellular antigens, and the mechanism by which they may actually mediate disease is still under investigation. Substantial indirect evidence suggests that after IgG autoantibodies have crossed the placenta, they bind to fetal antigens and cause immunological damage resulting in NLE. IgG has been demonstrated in the heart and skin of affected neonates.

Not all fetuses exposed to these autoantibodies are affected, and this can even result in discordance between twins. Thus, the risk of a mother with anti Ro/SS-A and/or anti La/SS-B having an NLE-affected fetus is uncertain and depends on factors other than autoantibodies alone. For women with SLE, the risk of NLE is probably less than 5%.[37] In women with SLE and anti Ro/SS-A, the risk of NLE skin disease is around 15%. Fortunately, the risk of congenital CHB is low (1–2%) among women with SLE, even if they have anti Ro/SS-A, although the risk may be higher (15%) in women with a previously affected fetus.[37]

Rheumatoid arthritis (RA)

It has been recognized for over 60 years that about 70% of RA patients improve during pregnancy[38] but there is a high incidence of relapse within 3 months of delivery. Sex hormones, particularly estrogen, were considered likely candidates for pregnancy-induced remission but, more recently, attention has focused on immunologic mechanisms. As discussed above, pregnancy may lead to down-regulation of Th1 cytokines which may in turn down-regulate RA activity (Chapter 61).[39]

The relationship of maternal–fetal HLA has also been examined in pregnancies characterized by remission compared to pregnancies in which the disease was active. The greater the degree of feto-maternal disparity in Class II HLA-DRB1, DQA and DQB alleles, the greater the likelihood of improvement during pregnancy – the strongest association is for HLA-DQA disparity.[40] Feto-maternal HLA differences may also influence the onset of RA in the mother. In general, the risk of developing RA during pregnancy is decreased but there is a five-fold increase in RA in the postpartum period. DQA1 and DQB1 allele disparities between mother and fetus during pregnancy are associated with an increased incidence of RA post partum.[40] In practical terms, the amelioration of RA that can occur during pregnancy is of benefit to patient management as many of the second-line antirheumatic drugs are potentially teratogenic and need to be stopped during pregnancy.

Passive autoimmune disease

Thrombocytopenia

Most forms of autoimmune (idiopathic) thrombocytopenic purpura (ITP) are antibody mediated. Women are not at greater risk of ITP during pregnancy, when control is readily achieved by measures acceptable to fetal well-being, but the fetus is at risk from effects of maternally-derived IgG autoantibody on fetal platelets and hemorrhagic complications.[41] Maternal immunosuppression does not reliably raise the fetus' platelet count, and management has tended towards cesarean section.

Alloimmune thrombocytopenia (AIT) is a far more serious fetal disorder. Neonatal platelet counts of $<20 \times 10^9/l$ are common and AIT is associated with an intracranial hemorrhage rate of up to 30%. Maternal and neonatal IVIG and fluorinated corticosteroids may help, but fetal platelet transfusions may also be indicated.[41]

Thyroid disease

In Graves disease, IgG autoantibodies to thyroid-stimulating hormone (TSH) receptor can cross the placenta and be associated with neonatal hyperthyroidism, often manifest by fetal tachycardia and a goiter. Less commonly, neonatal hypothyroidism can occur because of maternal IgG antibodies that bind and block the TSH receptor.

Myasthenia gravis

Myasthenia gravis can also be associated with a fetal syndrome due to passively acquired maternal IgG autoantibodies to the acetylcholine receptor. The syndrome can lead to respiratory failure in the neonate requiring treatment, on a temporary basis, with long-acting anticholinesterase preparations.

Pemphigoid gestationis

Pemphigoid gestationis (PG) previously called herpes gestationis, is a rare autoimmune bullous disorder of pregnancy (Chapter 75). The condition is characterized by linear deposition of C3 and sometimes IgG along the basement membrane of maternal perilesional skin.[42] Circulating IgG complement-binding autoantibodies are directed against the hemidesmosome of the basement membrane. Most cases present in the second and third trimester of pregnancy and recede within 6 months of birth. There is a low incidence (2–5%) of PG in the neonate, presumably due to passive IgG antibody transfer, that resolves in less than 3 months. The condition can recur in over 50% of subsequent pregnancies, a rate unaltered by a change in partner, fetal gender, or HLA-DR sharing with the fetus.

Mild disease appears to respond to systemic antihistamines and topical corticosteroids. However, most patients require systemic glucocorticoids, e.g. prednisolone. The subsequent use of oral contraceptives in women who have had PG is contentious since a small number (about 10%) experience a recrudescence of the condition.[42]

Fetal hemolytic disease (Rhesus disease)

Immune destruction of fetal red cells by passively acquired maternal IgG antibody was one of the first observations that maternal immune sensitization could adversely affect the fetus. The blood group system mostly associated with fetal hemolytic disease is the Rhesus (Rh)-D system, but other Rh products and over 20 minor red cell loci can be involved as well. ABO hemolytic disease is generally much milder, probably because AB expression is usually lower on fetal red cells and the antibodies are predominantly IgM and thus do not cross the placenta.[43]

Rh disease is observed primarily in parous D-negative women with at least one previous pregnancy. D-positive cells cross the placenta, particularly at the time of delivery, and invoke anti-D antibodies which are boosted by minor feto-maternal bleeds in subsequent pregnancies. The secondary response is more potent because it is predominantly IgG. Approximately 20% of women appear to be nonresponders; the reason for nonresponsiveness may often be ABO incompatibility, leading to early removal and destruction of red cells. These IgG antibodies are non-complement fixing and the spleen is the major site of removal of red cells.

In highly sensitive women, attempts are made to reduce the titer of anti-RhD antibodies by plasma exchange and intravenous immunoglobulin (IVIG). For the fetus, treatment includes early delivery. If the fetus is too immature, intrauterine blood transfusion is the standard approach. Treatment of the neonate includes exchange transfusion, which may need to be carried out several times under intensive care conditions. Exchange transfusion has little impact upon the bilirubin level, and phototherapy is used to try to reduce bilirubin levels.[43]

The incidence of Rh disease has been reduced greatly since the worldwide introduction of maternal prophylactic anti-D passive immunization in the perinatal period; this should be used whenever there is potential for RhD exposure in a RhD-negative woman.

Recurrent pregnancy loss

Recurrent pregnancy loss (RPL), defined by the occurrence of three or more consecutive, clinically detectable, pregnancy losses prior to the 20th week of gestation, is estimated to occur in around 1 in 300 pregnancies.[44] Causative or contributory factors can be identified in a proportion of these women, and include chromosomal abnormalities, endocrine problems, or the presence of antiphospholipid autoantibodies (see section earlier in this chapter and Chapter 60). However, the reason for miscarriage remains unknown in the majority of couples and an immunologic etiology has been proposed for many of these cases. It is important to remember that it is unlikely that a single mechanism will be responsible for all cases of 'unexplained' RPL.

Much research has focused on the pregnancy-related production of so-called 'blocking antibodies' which inhibit a wide variety of in vitro lymphocyte proliferation or other types of immune function assays, most noticeably the mixed lymphocyte reaction. It was suggested that these blocking antibodies may be absent from women with RPL, either during or after unsuccessful pregnancies.[45] However, doubt remains about these observations since other pregnancy-related immunoregulatory serum components (notably steroidal hormones), may be influential at relatively high concentrations, and blocking antibody may also be a consequence rather than a cause of successful pregnancy.[46] In addition, in vitro assays can be technically erratic and interpretation of results may vary according to the equation used to calculate the inhibitory effect. The broad hypothesis that a proportion of unexplained RPL cases can be ascribed to a failure of normal active maternal immune adaption to early pregnancy has provoked extensive debate of controversial concepts and introduced use of alloimmunization with paternal or third-party lymphocytes as a treatment for pregnancy failure (immunotherapy).

Initial successful immunotherapy for recurrent miscarriage stimulated interest in the concept of immune-mediated pregnancy loss.[47] However, to date, virtually no supportive data have emerged and a meta-analysis of a number of trials indicated a possible small positive treatment effect with the need to immunize 11 women to produce one additional successful pregnancy.[48] Furthermore, it is not possible to identify those women who would benefit from the treatment, and a Cochrane collaboration concluded that there is no firm evidence for the efficacy of this procedure.[49] Importantly, a recent large multicenter randomized trial showed no benefit of paternal lymphocyte immunization.[50] In fact, the miscarriage rate was higher in those women who had been immunized.

Intravenous immuneglobulin (IVIG) has also been used in the treatment of RPL and, although meta-analysis of four published randomized double-blind trials showed an increase in successful pregnancy outcome, this did not reach significance.

More recently, studies suggesting an abnormal Th1-type cellular immune response formed the basis of a hypothesis for a different type of immunological failure in pregnant women.[51] This theory states that conceptus may be a target of local cell-mediated immunity (probably acting via release soluble factors or cytokines), culminating in a spontaneous miscarriage. Cell mediated immune reactivity could be changed in some women with RPL. In some studies, peripheral blood mononuclear cells (PBMC) from women with RPL responded to trophoblast extracts in vitro by (1) releasing soluble factors that adversely affect embryo and trophoblast viability, (2) releasing Th1-type cytokines (TNF-β and IFN-γ), and (3) showing a reduction in Th2-type cytokine production (IL-4 and IL-10).[51] In contrast, PBMC from women with a history of successful pregnancy primarily produced Th2-type cytokines when exposed to trophoblast extracts. Circulating levels of TNF-α are high in patients with subsequent miscarriage compared to those with a successful pregnancy, suggesting that TNF-α could be a potentially relevant factor in RPL patients. Higher production of Th2-type cytokines from PBMC appears to be associated with successful pregnancy, whereas Th1-type cytokines are associated with RPL.[52] Decidual T cells from women with RPL also show decreased production of Th2-type cytokines.

Pre-eclampsia

An inadequate maternal vascular response to pregnancy, manifest as inadequate cytotrophoblast invasion of the spiral arteries in early pregnancy, leads later in pregnancy to the maternal syndrome of pre-eclampsia (PE) characterized by hypertension, edema, and proteinuria. This syndrome is thought to result from maternal endothelial cell dysfunction.[53] PE can occur severely in hydatidiform mole, demonstrating that the placenta is of central importance. There is a strong genetic component to disease susceptibility and daughters of women with PE have an increased relative risk of developing the disease. The incidence in first pregnancy is much higher than in subsequent pregnancies, and even a previous abortion may confer protection. However, a change of partner in women with at least one previous normal pregnancy significantly increases the risk of PE in a subsequent pregnancy. Prior blood transfusions and previous sexual exposure to sperm are also associated with a decreased risk of PE. These lines of evidence suggest an immunological mechanism, and it has been proposed that PE results from an inadequate maternal immune adaption to pregnancy. More recently, it has been suggested that excessive activation of the maternal innate immune system may lead to pre-eclampsia.[54]

Infection in the female reproductive tract

In the absence of a pronounced antigen-specific cellular immune defense system within human uteroplacental tissues, both placental and decidual macrophages provide an important immediate antigen-nonspecific host defense to infection. The elucidation of host immune functional capacity within the reproductive tracts is an area of much current activity, particularly in the context of sexually transmitted diseases and potential vaccine design and delivery.

Most cases of pediatric human immunodeficiency virus (HIV) infection are acquired by vertical transmission (Chapter 39), with the rate of transmission from noninfected mothers to infants varying from 17% to 30%. Precise mechanisms of intrauterine transmission are poorly defined, but viral antigens and nucleic acids have been clearly identified within placentas from some HIV-infected women. Placental macrophages (Hofbauer cells) can act as a reservoir of HIV, and as a vehicle for vertical transplacental transmission from mother to fetus in perinatal infection since placental macrophages express CD4.[55] The low level of HIV replication in placental macrophages, together with their apparently lower susceptibility to productive infection than blood monocytes, may contribute to the selective nature of transmission of HIV to the fetus.

The presence of maternal IgG anti-HIV antibodies could potentially also act to focus HIV to Fc receptors on the surface of CD4+ extraembryonic fetal macrophages. However, maternal IgG anti-HIV antibody may block HIV transmission in utero, possibly by denying intimate cellular contact through masking HIV binding sites to CD4 and other receptors.[56]

Immunocontraception

It is theoretically possible to use immune methods to interfere with fertility in both the male and female although, in practice, antigens considered as potential birth control vaccine candidates in humans are largely restricted to those capable of fertility control in women. This represents an entirely novel approach to develop a vaccine to a 'self' component with the aim of producing a safe, effective, readily applicable, relatively long-lasting but 'reversible' (ie. not boosted by repeated natural antigen exposure) method of fertility control. There are five potential stages in the reproductive process in which fertility-regulating vaccines could act: ovulation, sperm transport, fertilization, implantation, and blastocyst development. A number of potential targets have been considered, including sperm antigens in men and human chorionic gonadotrophin (hCG) in women, notably the unique C-terminal peptide of the β-subunit of hCG and zona pellucida antigens of varying types.[57,58] Vaccines against hCG have progressed to clinical trials, and early trials have also occurred with some sperm antigens but, despite much promise, the progress made with immunocontraceptive vaccines has been less than ideal; overall, this is an area in which much work remains to be done.

REFERENCES

1. Medawar PB. Some immunological and endocrinological problems raised by the evolution of viviparity in vertebrates. Symp Soc Exp Biol 1953;VII:320.
2. Anderson DJ. The importance of mucosal immunology to problems in human reproduction. J Reprod Immunol 1996;31:3.
3. Kelly RW, Critchley HO. Immunomodulation by human seminal plasma: a benefit for spermatozoa and pathogen? Hum Reprod 1997;12:2200.
4. Wolff H. The biologic significance of white blood cells in semen. Fertil Steril 1995;63:1143.
5. Hladik F, Lentz G, Delpit E, McElroy A, McElrath MJ. Coexpression of CCR5 and IL-2 in human genital but not blood T cells: implications for the ontogeny of the CCR5+ Th1 phenotype. J Immunol 1999;163:2306.
6. Bulmer JN. Cellular constituents of human endometrium in the menstrual cycle and early pregnancy. In: Bronson RA, Alexander NJ, Anderson D, Branch DW, Kutteh WH (eds) Reproductive immunology. Oxford, Blackwell Science, 1996, p. 212.
7. Vassiliadou N, Bulmer JN. Quantitative analysis of T lymphocyte subsets in pregnant and nonpregnant human endometrium. Biol Reprod 1996;55:1017.
8. Ellis SA, Palmer MS, McMichael AJ. Human trophoblast and choriocarcinoma cell line BeWo express a truncated HLA Class I molecule. J Immunol 1990;144:731.
9. Ober C, Aldrich CL. HLA-G polymorphisms: neutral evolution or novel function? J Reprod Immunol 1997;36:1.
10. King A, Burrows TD, Hiby SE, et al. Surface expression of HLA-C antigen by human extravillous trophoblast. Placenta 2000;21:376.
11. Holmes CH, Simpson KL, Okada H, et al. Complement regulatory proteins at the feto-maternal interface during human placental development: distribution of CD59 by comparison with membrane cofactor protein (CD46) and decay accelerating factor (CD55). Eur J Immunol 1992;137:1604.
12. Xu C, Mao D, Holers VM, Palanca B, Cheng AM, Molina H. A critical role for murine complement regulator Crry in fetomaternal tolerance. Science 2000;287:498.
13. Ljunggren G, Karre K. In search of the 'missing self' – MHC molecules and NK cell recognition. Immunol Today 1990;11:237.
14. Gudelj L, Deniz G, Rukavina D, et al. Expression of functional molecules by human CD3 decidual granular leucocyte clones. Immunology 1996;87:609.
15. Schust DJ, Hill AB, Ploegh HL. Herpes simplex virus blocks intracellular transport of HLA-G in placentally derived human cells. J Immunol 1996;157:3375.
16. Ober C, Aldrich C, Rosinsky B, et al. HLA-G1 protein expression is not essential for fetal survival. Placenta 1998;19:127.
17. Munn D, Zhou M, Attwood J, et al. Prevention of allogeneic fetal rejection by tryptophan catabolism. Science 1998;281:1191.
18. Kauma SW, Huff TF, Hayes N, Nilkaeo A. Placental Fas ligand expression is a mechanism for maternal immune tolerance to the fetus. J Clin Endocrinol Metab 1999;84:2188.
19. Phillips TA, Ni J, Pan G, et al. TRAIL (Apo-2L) and TRAIL receptors in human placentas: Implications for immune privilege. J Immunol 1999;162:6053.
20. Wegmann TG, Lin H, Guilbert L, Mosmann TR. Bidirectional cytokine interactions in the maternal-fetal relationship: is successful pregnancy a Th2 phenomenon? Immunol Today 1993;14:353.
21. Simister NE, Story CM. Human placental Fc receptors and the transmission of antibodies from mother to fetus. J Reprod Immunol 1997;37:1.
22. Ellinger I, Schwab M, Stefanescu A, Hunziker W, Fuchs R. IgG transport across trophoblast-derived BeWo cells: a model system to study IgG transport in the placenta. Eur J Immunol 1999;29:733.
23. Schmorl G. Pathologisch-anatomische Untersuchungen ueber Puerperal-Eklampsie. Leipzig, Verlag von F.C.W. Vogel, 1893.
24. Bianchi DW, Zickwolf GK, Weil GJ, Sylvester S, DeMaria MA. Male fetal progenitor cells persist in maternal blood for as long as 27 years postpartum. Proc Natl Acad Sci USA 1996;93:705.
25. Maloney S, Smith A, Furst DE, et al. Microchimerism of maternal origin persists into adult life. J Clin Invest 1999;104:41.
26. Nelson JL, Furst DE, Maloney S, et al. Microchimerism and HLA-compatible relationships of pregnancy in scleroderma. Lancet 1998;351:559.
27. Bianchi DW. Fetomaternal cell trafficking: A new cause of disease. Am J Med Genet 2000;91:22.
28. Ober C, van der Ven K. HLA and fertility. In: Hunt JB (ed.) HLA and the maternal–fetal relationship. Austin, RG Landes, 1996; p 133.
29. Mi S, Lee X, Li X-P, et al. Syncytin is a captive retroviral envelope protein involved in human placental morphogenesis. Nature 2000;403:785.
30. Li J-M, Fan WS, Horsfall AC, et al. The expression of human endogenous retrovirus-3 in fetal cardiac tissue and antibodies in congenital heart block. Clin Exp Immunol 1996;104:388.

31. Bronson RA. Antisperm antibodies: a critical evaluation and clinical guidelines. J Reprod Immunol 1999;45:159.
32. Hill JA. Immunology and endometriosis. Fact, artifact or epiphenomenon? Obstet Gynecol Clin North Am 1997;24:291.
33. Kutteh WH, Rote NS, Silver R. Antiphospholipid antibodies in reproduction: the antiphospholipid syndrome. Am J Reprod Immunol 1999;41:133.
34. Lee RM, Emblen W, Scott JR, Branch DW, Silver RM. Anti-β2 glycoprotein 1 antibodies in women with recurrent spontaneous abortion, unexplained fetal death, and antiphospholipid syndrome. Am J Obstet Gynecol 1999;181:642.
35. Petri M. Pregnancy in SLE. Baillières Clin Rheumatol 1998;12:449.
36. Tseng C, Buyon J. Neonatal lupus syndromes. Rheum Dis Clin North Am 1997;23:31.
37. Branch DW, Silver RM. Autoimmune disease and pregnancy: Maternal and fetal implications in systemic lupus erythematosus and antiphospholipid syndrome. In: Bronson RA, Alexander NJ, Anderson D, Branch DW, Kutteh WH (eds) Reproductive immunology. Oxford, Blackwell Science, 1996, p 443.
38. Hench PS. The ameliorating effect of pregnancy on chronic atrophic arthritis, fibrositis and intermittent hydrarthrosis. Mayo Clin Proc 1938;13:161.
39. Russell AS, Johnston C, Chew C, Maksymowych WP. Evidence for reduced Th1 function in normal pregnancy: A hypothesis for the remission of rheumatoid arthritis. J Rheumatol 1997;24:1045.
40. Hazes J. Fetomaternal HLA differences and the onset and course of rheumatoid arthritis. Rev Rheum 1998;65:611.
41. Bussel JB. Immune thrombocytopenia in pregnancy: autoimmune and alloimmune. J Reprod Immunol 1997;37:35.
42. Jenkins RE, Hern S, Black MM. Clinical features and management of 87 patients with pemphigoid gestationis. Clin Exp Dermatol 1999;24:255.
43. Bowmans JM. Alloimmune hemolytic disease of the fetus and newborn. In: Lee GR, Faerster J, Lukens J, Paraskevas F, Greer JP, Rodgers GM (eds) Wintrobe's Clinical hematology. Baltimore, Williams & Wilkins, 1998, p 210.
44. Alberman E. The epidemiology of repeated abortion. In: Early pregnancy loss, mechanisms and treatment. New York, Springer Verlag, 1988, p 9.
45. Beer AE, Semprini AE, Xiaoyn Z, Quebbeman JF. Pregnancy outcome in human couples with recurrent spontaneous abortion: HLA antigen profiles, HLA antigen sharing, female serum MLR blocking factors and paternal leucocyte immunization. Exp Clin Immunogenet 1985;2:137.
46. Sargent IL, Wilkins T, Redman CWG. Maternal immune responses to the fetus in early pregnancy and recurrent miscarriage. Lancet 1988;ii:1099.
47. Mowbray JF, Gibbings C, Liddell H, et al. Controlled trial of treatment of recurrent spontaneous abortion by immunisation with paternal cells. Lancet 1985;i:94.
48. The Recurrent Miscarriage Immunotherapy Triallists Group. Worldwide collaborative observational study and meta-analysis on allogenic leukocyte therapy for recurrent spontaneous abortion. Am J Reprod Immunol 1994;32:55.
49. Scott JR. Immunotherapy for recurrent miscarriage. The Cochrane database for systemic reviews. The Cochrane Library, 1998.
50. Ober C, Karrison T, Odem RR, et al. Mononuclear-cell immunisation in prevention of recurrent miscarriages, a randomised trial. Lancet 1999;354:365.
51. Hill JA, Polger K, Anderson DJ. T-helper 1-type immunity to trophoblast in women with recurrent spontaneous abortion. JAMA 1995;273:1933.
52. Raghupathy R, Makseed M, Azizieh F, et al. Cytokine production by maternal lymphocytes during normal pregnancy and in unexplained recurrent spontaneous abortion. Hum Reprod 2000;196:122.
53. Roberts JM, Taylor RN, Musci MD, Rodgers GM, Hubel C, McLaughlin MK. Pre-eclampsia: an endothelial cell disorder. Am J Obstet Gynecol 1989;161:1200.
54. Redman CWG, Sacks GP, Sargent IL. Preeclampsia: an excessive maternal inflammatory response to pregnancy. Am J Obstet Gynecol 1999;180:499.
55. Lairmore MD, Cuthbert PS, Utley LL, et al. Cellular localization of CD4 in the human placenta. Implications for maternal-to-fetal transmission of HIV. J Immunol 1993; 151:1673.
56. Schwartz DH, Sharma UK, Perlman EJ, Blakemore K. Adherence of human immunodeficiency virus-infected lymphocytes to fetal placental cells: a model of maternal fetal transmission. Proc Natl Acad Sci USA 1995;92:978.
57. Frayne J, Hall L. The potential use of sperm antigens as targets for immunocontraception; past, present and future. J Reprod Immunol 1999;43:1.
58. Talwar GP. Fertility regulating and immunotherapeutic vaccines reaching human trials stage. Hum Reprod Update 1997;3:301.

Chapter 84

Immunologic Lung Diseases

Andrew P. Fontenot and Marvin I. Schwarz

The lung serves as an interface between the environment and the sanctuary of the body. The defense systems of the upper airways clear the majority of inhaled particulates. Those that evade the upper airway defenses are combated by the innate and acquired immune responses. Macrophages and lymphocytes are the key cells involved in the initiation and perpetuation of the acquired immune response in the lung. In the normal host, the macrophage is the predominant cell type in the bronchoalveolar lavage (BAL).[1] Macrophages serve as scavenger cells, ingesting and degrading the inhaled antigenic load. In addition, these cells serve as antigen-presenting cells for T lymphocytes. Relatively few lymphocytes are present in the normal lung parenchyma. However, after stimulation by the relevant antigen in the surrounding lymphoid tissues, lymphocytes specific for that antigen migrate to the lung and participate in the inflammatory response.

Immunologic lung diseases develop when the normal mechanisms of immune self-tolerance fail. Essentially all autoimmune diseases appear to be dependent on the inappropriate activation of autoreactive CD4 T cells as well as autoreactive B cells responsible for the pathogenic autoantibodies. This chapter will deal with the pulmonary manifestations of these disorders.

KEY CONCEPTS

Classification of the idiopathic interstitial pneumonias

- The idiopathic interstitial pneumonias comprise a group of seven histologically distinct disorders. The distinction is important since response to treatment and prognosis differs.
  - Idiopathic pulmonary fibrosis (IPF) with histopathology labeled as usual interstitial pneumonitis (UIP). The pathology of UIP can occur in other diseases such as collagen vascular diseases.
  - Acute interstitial pneumonitis (AIP).
  - Desquamative interstitial pneumonitis (DIP).
  - Respiratory bronchiolitis associated interstitial lung disease (RB–ILD)
  - Nonspecific interstitial pneumonitis (NSIP).
  - Lymphocytic interstitial pneumonitis (LIP).
  - Cryptogenic organizing pneumonia (COP).
- In order to differentiate between these diseases, a thorascopic lung biopsy is often required.

IDIOPATHIC INTERSTITIAL PNEUMONIAS

The idiopathic interstitial pneumonias comprise a group of seven histologically distinct disorders, which previously had been included under the heading of idiopathic pulmonary fibrosis (IPF). These include IPF (usual interstitial pneumonitis – (UIP)) acute interstitial pneumonitis (AIP), desquamative interstitial pneumonitis (DIP), respiratory bronchiolitis-associated interstitial lung disease (RB–ILD), nonspecific interstitial pneumonitis (NSIP), lymphocytic interstitial pneumonitis (LIP), and cryptogenic organizing pneumonia (COP). In order to differentiate between these diseases, a thoracoscopic lung biopsy is often required. The distinction is important since response to treatment and outcome differs.

Idiopathic pulmonary fibrosis

IPF, also known as cryptogenic fibrosing alveolitis, represents one of the most common diffuse parenchymal lung diseases of unknown etiology.[2–4] It is characterized by progressive clinical deterioration despite available therapy. Although there are characteristic clinical, radiographic, and histologic appearances of IPF, other interstitial lung diseases including the collagen vascular diseases, drug toxicities, and environmental exposures can mimic these findings. The pathogenesis of IPF remains poorly understood, but current evidence suggests that the disease is mediated through an interplay between immunologic, genetic, and environmental factors.[5–9]

Clinical manifestations

The incidence and prevalence of IPF remains unknown although recent studies have reported prevalence rates for men and women as 20.2 per 100 000 and 13.2 per 100 000, respectively.[10] In addition, evidence suggests that both the incidence and prevalence of disease increase with age, with most patients presenting between 40 and 70 years of age.[11,12] Although the clinical features of IPF are variable, most patients present with the insidious onset of exertional dyspnea with an associated dry, nonproductive cough. The physical examination typically reveals dry, end-inspiratory crackles, and clubbing may be present in 25–50% of patients.[13,14]

CLINICAL PEARLS

Idiopathic pulmonary fibrosis

- IPF is one of the most common causes of diffuse parenchymal lung disease of unknown etiology and is characterized by the insidious onset of cough and dyspnea.
- The histopathologic pattern of IPF is usual interstitial pneumonitis.
- A confident diagnosis of IPF based on HRCT can only be made in two thirds of the cases.
- IPF is a fatal disorder characterized by relentless progression and a 5-year survival of 30–50%

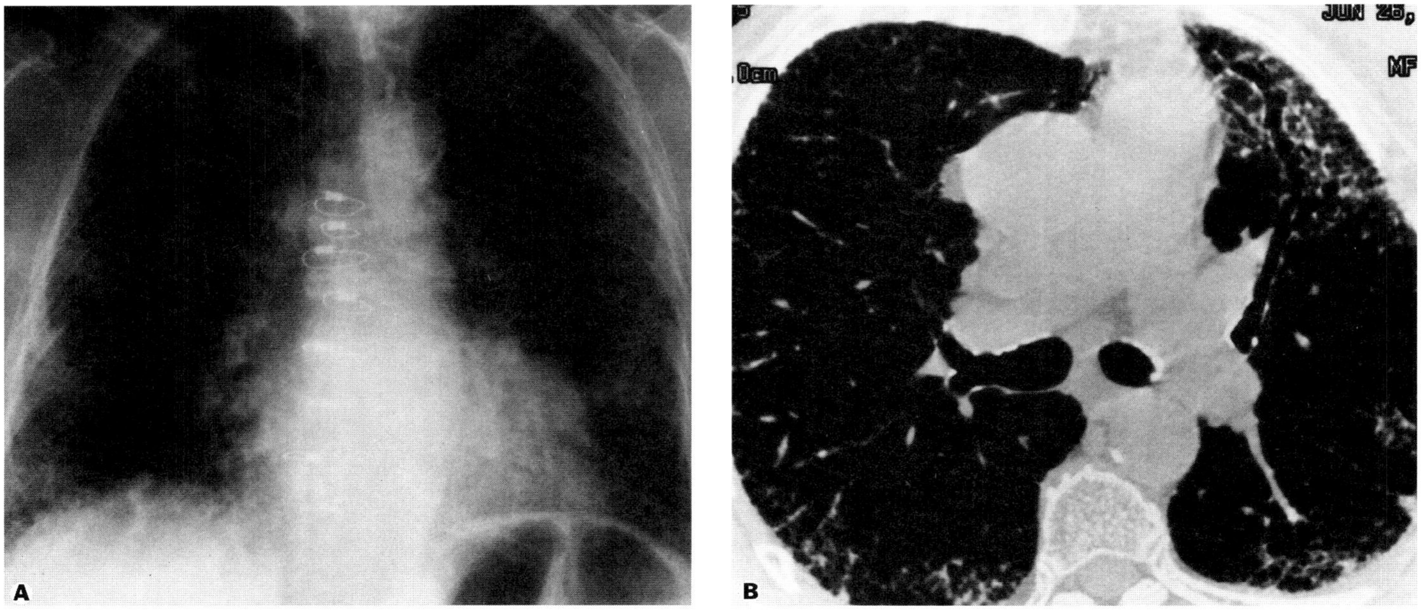

Figure 84.1 Radiographic manifestations of idiopathic pulmonary fibrosis. (**A**) Chest radiograph in a patient with IPF showing diffuse, coarse reticular opacities with a lower lung zone predominance. Cystic radiolucencies, consistent with honeycombing, are evident. (**B**) HRCT shows peripheral reticular opacities, honeycombing, and traction bronchiectasis.

The majority of patients with IPF have an abnormal chest radiograph on presentation.[13] The chest radiograph typically shows diffuse reticular opacities predominant in the lower zone and periphery of the lung.[15] Ground-glass opacities, small cysts (honeycombing), and reduced lung volumes may also be seen (Fig. 84.1A). These radiographic changes often precede the onset of symptoms, and serial chest radiographs usually reveal progression with associated volume loss. High-resolution computed tomography (HRCT) findings include bibasilar peripheral reticular opacities (Fig. 84.1B).[16,17] Honeycombing, traction bronchiectasis, and subpleural fibrosis may also be present. The finding of ground-glass opacities on the initial HRCT may be associated with alveolar inflammation and may identify patients with IPF who are more likely to respond to glucocorticoid therapy.[18,19]

The typical physiologic abnormalities in IPF are those of a restrictive lung disease with a low diffusing capacity for carbon monoxide and severe gas exchange abnormalities exacerbated by exercise.[20–22]

Histopathology

The gross appearance of the lungs in IPF shows a nodular pleural surface with the histopathologic pattern of IPF being usual interstitial pneumonitis (UIP). UIP is characterized by nonuniform and variable distribution of the interstitial changes. At low magnification, alternating zones of interstitial fibrosis, mild inflammation, honeycombing, and normal lung may be seen (Fig. 84.2A). At higher magnification, findings include derangement of alveolar walls with edema, fibrinous exudate, fibroblast proliferation, and fibrosis. Honeycomb change refers to enlarged airspaces lined by metaplastic bronchial epithelium and surrounded by walls thickened with collagen (Fig. 84.2B). These changes are irreversible and represent end-stage lung. Another distinct feature of UIP is the fibroblast focus (Fig. 84.2C). This is thought to represent the earliest finding in UIP and is characterized by distinct clusters of fibroblasts and myofibroblasts in a loose connective tissue matrix within the alveolar wall with minimal interstitial inflammation or intra-alveolar macrophage accumulation.[23,24] Findings of granulomatous inflammation, vasculitis, or evidence of pneumoconiosis exclude the diagnosis of IPF.

It was previously thought that DIP represented an earlier stage of IPF and that UIP was the more advanced phase of IPF. However, it is now clear that UIP, DIP, RB-ILD, and NSIP represent separate pathologic entities.[2,25] Tables 84.1 and 84.2 compare the clinical and pathologic features of these disorders.

Pathogenesis

The etiologic agent(s) responsible for the initiation of IPF remains unknown. Evidence suggests that an interaction between genetic, environmental, and viral factors may be involved[5–9] (Fig. 84.3). The presence of familial cases of IPF suggests the involvement of genetic factors. Familial IPF is inherited as an autosomal dominant trait with variable penetrance.[26] To date, there are no identified associations between IPF and HLA alleles. Environmental exposure to both wood and metal dust has been associated with the development of fibrosis independent of cigarette smoking.[11,27] Despite numerous viruses, including Epstein–Barr virus, being implicated in the pathogenesis of IPF, no definitive evidence exists to substantiate such a relationship.

At present, the mechanisms involved in the induction of the inflammatory events leading to the development of lung fibrosis remain poorly understood. However, little doubt exists regarding the immunologic nature of this disease. For example, an identical pathologic process can be seen in several immune-mediated diseases such as collagen vascular diseases, inflammatory bowel disease, and primary biliary cirrhosis. It is also clear that no single stimulus is responsible for all causes of pulmonary fibrosis. More likely, the fibrotic response represents a final common pathway following certain immune and inflammatory events.

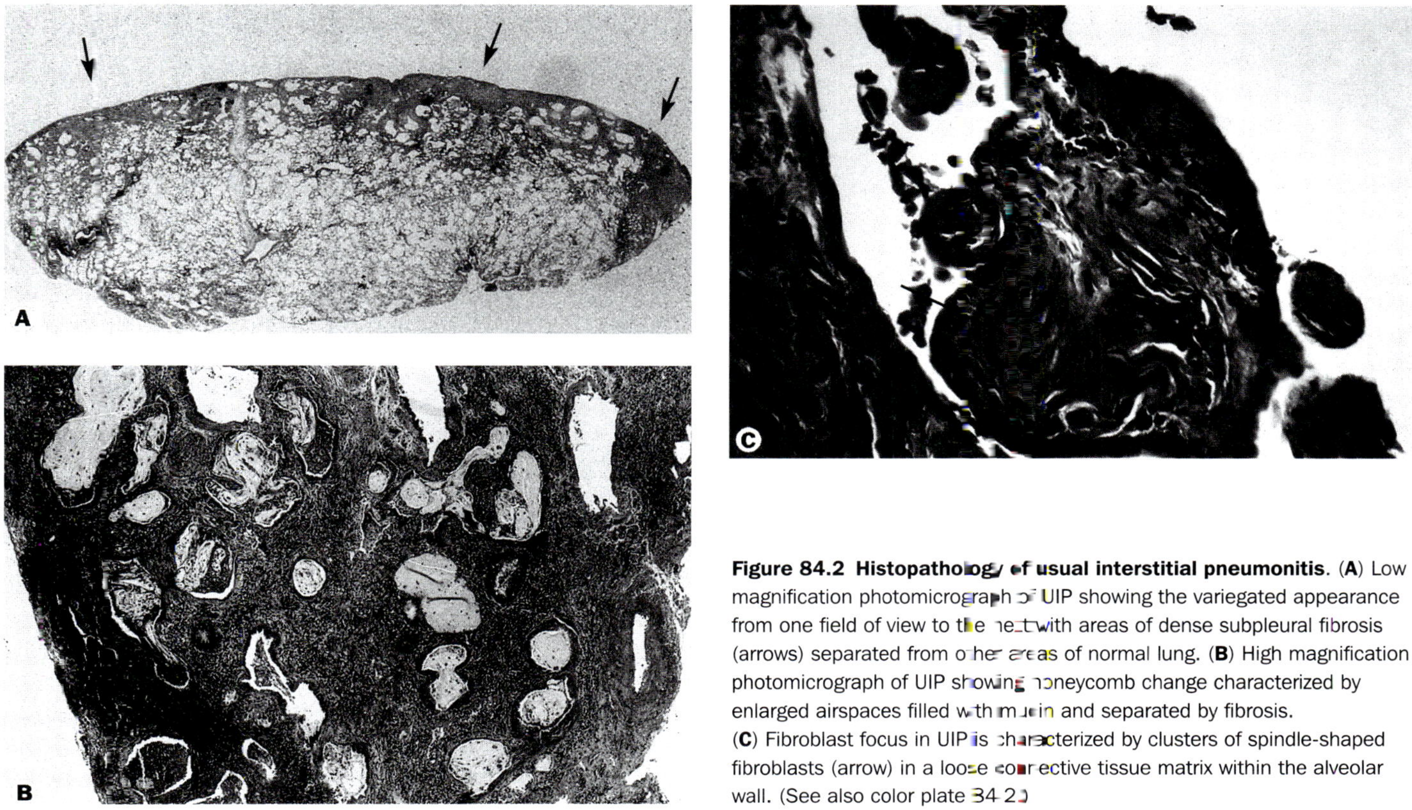

Figure 84.2 Histopathology of usual interstitial pneumonitis. (**A**) Low magnification photomicrograph of UIP showing the variegated appearance from one field of view to the next with areas of dense subpleural fibrosis (arrows) separated from other areas of normal lung. (**B**) High magnification photomicrograph of UIP showing honeycomb change characterized by enlarged airspaces filled with mucin and separated by fibrosis. (**C**) Fibroblast focus in UIP is characterized by clusters of spindle-shaped fibroblasts (arrow) in a loose connective tissue matrix within the alveolar wall. (See also color plate 84.2.)

Table 84.1 Clinical features of the idiopathic interstitial pneumonias. Adapted from Katzenstein AL, Myers JL. Idiopathic pulmonary fibrosis: clinical relevance of pathologic classification. *Am J Respir Crit Care Med* 1998;157:1301.

Clinical features of the idiopathic interstitial pneumonias

	UIP	DIP	RB–ILD	AIP	NSIP
Mean age, yrs	57	42	36	49	49
Childhood	No	Rare	No	Rare	Occasionally
Onset	Insidious	Insidious	Insidious	Acute	Subacute, insidious
Mortality (mean survival)	68% (5–6 yrs)	27% (12 yrs)	0%	62% (1–2 mos)	11% (17 mos)
Response to steroids	Poor	Good	Good	Poor	Good
Recovery possible	No	Yes	Yes	Yes	Yes

UIP = usual interstitial pneumonitis; DIP = desquamative interstitial pneumonitis; RB–ILD = respiratory bronchiolitis associated interstitial lung disease; AID = acute interstitial pneumonitis; NSIP = nonspecific interstitial pneumonitis.

In the normal lung, the interstitium is thin and delicate with few lymphoid cells and fibroblasts. Following the initiation of the inflammatory process, damage to the alveolar epithelium occurs, followed by the infiltration of the interstitium with activated immune cells. In addition, immune complexes have been identified in the serum and lungs of IPF patients.[5] Activated alveolar macrophages secrete IL-1, IL-8, tumor necrosis factor-α (TNF-α), platelet-derived growth factor (PDGF), and insulin-like growth factor-1 (IGF-1).[28,29] This cytokine milieu promotes the activation and recruitment of neutrophils and lymphocytes to the area of alveolitis.

T lymphocytes, which accumulate in the alveolar space and interstitium, express an activated phenotype, including the expression of HLA-DR and IL-2 receptor.[30] Following activation, CD4 T cells evolve into two major subsets distinguished by the cytokines produced[31] (Chapter 12). In IPF, T cells expressing a Th2-type phenotype predominate, producing IL-4, IL-5, IL-10, and IL-13.[32,33] Th2 cells are mainly involved in the development of humoral immunity by helping B cells through the promotion of class switching and enhancement of the production of certain IgG isotypes and production of IgE. Evidence suggests that a switch to Th2-type cells may be important in the development

Histopathologic features of the idiopathic interstitial pneumonias

	UIP	DIP/RB–ILD	AIP	NSIP
Temporal appearance	Variegated	Uniform	Uniform	Uniform
Interstitial inflammation	Scant	Scant	No	Prominent
Collagen/fibrosis	Patchy	Diffuse (DIP) Focal (RB–ILD)	No	Diffuse
Fibroblast proliferation	Fibroblast foci prominent	No	Diffuse	Rare
BOOP	No	No	No	Focal
Honeycomb change	Yes	No	No	Rare
Intra-alveolar macrophages	Focal	Diffuse (DIP) Focal (RB–ILD)	No	Patchy
Hyaline membranes	No	No	Focal	No

UIP = usual interstitial pneumonitis; DIP = desquamative interstitial pneumonitis; RB–ILD = respiratory bronchiolitis associated interstitial lung disease; AIP = acute interstitial pneumonitis; NSIP = nonspecific interstitial pneumonitis; BOOP = bronchiolitis obliterans organizing pneumonia.

Table 84.2 Histopathologic features of the idiopathic interstitial pneumonias. Adapted from Katzenstein AL, Myers JL. Idiopathic pulmonary fibrosis: clinical relevance of pathologic classification. *Am J Respir Crit Care Med* 1998;157:1301.

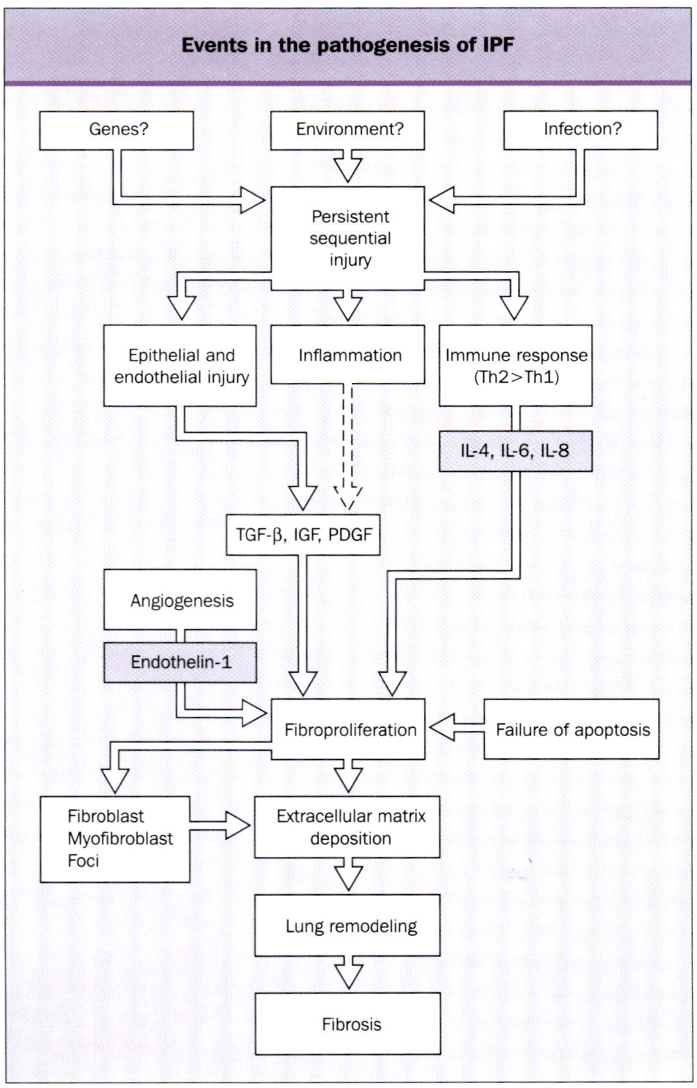

Figure 84.3 Events hypothesized to be involved in the pathogenesis of idiopathic pulmonary fibrosis. The initiating event(s) leading to persistent lung injury remains poorly understood. The interaction between genetic factors, environmental exposures, and infectious agents leads to epithelial and endothelial injury, resulting in the secretion of macrophage-derived growth factors, including transforming growth factor-β (TGF-β), insulin-like growth factor-1 (IGF-1), and platelet-derived growth factor (PDGF). This cytokine milieu stimulates fibroblast proliferation and collagen deposition. In addition, the resulting Th2 immune response stimulates extracellular matrix production and fibroblast proliferation, resulting in lung remodeling and, eventually, lung fibrosis.

KEY CONCEPTS

Pathogenesis of the idiopathic interstitial pneumonias

- Although the inciting event(s) is unknown in the different diseases, a common result is a dysregulated fibroproliferative response (similar to wound healing), which leads to excessive extracellular matrix production and lung remodeling.
- A genetically-determined inability to adequately repair and re-epithelialize the denuded basement membranes may be a contributing factor and may relate to the familial occurrence of some cases of idiopathic pulmonary fibrosis.
- The presence of a chronic stimulus (autoantigen), as is seen in the pneumoconioses, may result in a persistent inflammatory and immune response and lead to a failure in the normal healing process.
- The release of TGF-β following epithelial injury stimulates collagen synthesis and the prevention of apoptosis of proliferating fibroblasts in the lung and may impair collagen degradation by inhibiting the production of metalloproteases.
- A predominant Th2 response in the lung and the absence of interferon-gamma (IFN-γ) favor the development of a fibrotic response.

of fibrosis through the deposition of matrix components. Thus, a switch to Th2-type cells may occur in IPF followed by the release of Th2-type cytokines stimulating production of extracellular matrix as well as attracting the influx of fibroblasts.[30,34]

In addition to their role as scavengers, alveolar macrophages are vital in the reparative phase of the inflammatory process. However, the distinguishing feature between a self-resolving inflammatory process and a fibrotic response as seen in IPF is the accumulation of collagen. Current evidence suggests that the fibrotic process in IPF is a consequence of dysregulation of both collagen synthesis and degradation.[35] Macrophage-derived growth factors, including transforming growth factor-β (TGF-β), PDGF, and IGF-1, stimulate both fibroblast proliferation and collagen deposition. Adequate resolution of an inflammatory process requires matrix degradation. Metalloproteases produced by both macrophages and fibroblasts are involved in matrix degradation, and control of metalloprotease production involves substances known as tissue inhibitors of metalloproteases (TIMPs). TIMPs are elevated in the lungs of patients with IPF.[36] In addition, TGF-β can markedly augment TIMP production. Thus, there appears to be a loss of balance between the events mediating resolution and those mediating perpetuation of the inflammatory response, setting the stage for lung injury, tissue remodeling, and the development of irreversible pulmonary fibrosis.[34]

Diagnosis

The diagnostic evaluation of a patient with diffuse parenchymal lung disease includes a thorough history and physical examination with particular attention to symptoms and signs that could indicate collagen vascular diseases, occupational and environmental exposures, or medication and drug usage. A careful family history is also important.

The history and physical findings in IPF are nonspecific. However, extrapulmonary involvement does not occur, and fever, arthralgias, myalgias, and pleuritis should suggest a collagen vascular disorder. The presence of antinuclear antibodies and rheumatoid factor occurs in 10–20% of IPF patients, but titers greater than 1:160 should suggest the possibility of an alternative diagnosis.[5,37]

The majority of patients with IPF have an abnormal chest radiograph at the time of presentation.[13] Basilar, peripheral reticular opacities are the characteristic radiographic findings of IPF. The presence of confluent opacities, pleural involvement, or lymphadenopathy should suggest an alternative diagnosis. A 'confident' diagnosis of IPF can be made from the chest radiograph in 48–87% of the cases.[17,38,39]

A confident diagnosis of IPF from HRCT of the lung requires the presence of patchy, peripheral, bibasilar reticular abnormalities. The presence of extensive ground-glass opacities on HRCT should suggest an alternative diagnosis, such as DIP, hypersensitivity pneumonitis, BOOP, or NSIP.

The diagnostic accuracy of HRCT for the diagnosis of IPF is dependent on the experience of the observer.[38] With a trained observer, the accuracy of a confident diagnosis based on HRCT findings was shown to be approximately 90%.[38–40] However, a confident HRCT diagnosis can only be reached in two thirds of the cases with histologically proven UIP.[41]

A surgical lung biopsy is recommended in suspected IPF patients without a definitive HRCT appearance and who do not have contraindications to the procedure. This is especially important in patients with atypical clinical or radiographic findings, which could suggest the possibility of one of the other histologic patterns of the idiopathic interstitial pneumonias and an improved prognosis. The elderly (greater than 70 years of age), patients with cardiovascular disease, or those with evidence of extensive honeycomb change may forego biopsy confirmation of their disease. Video-assisted thoracoscopic (VATS) biopsy is the preferred surgical technique and has been associated with less morbidity and a decreased hospital stay compared with open lung biopsy.[42,43]

Treatment and outcome

The usual course of IPF is relentless progression without spontaneous remission, commonly with a fatal outcome. Recent studies in patients with biopsy-proven IPF indicate a shorter survival than previously thought (30–50% 5-year survival).[19,44,45] Currently available treatment options include glucocorticoids or immunosuppressant drugs either alone or in combination. However, despite the fact that the glucocorticoids are considered the mainstay of therapy for IPF, no prospective, randomized, double-blind, placebo-controlled trial has demonstrated their efficacy in the treatment of IPF.[25,46] Previous studies had reported that 10–30% of IPF patients initially responded to corticosteroids.[25,45,46] However, it is unclear if all of these patients had IPF based on current criteria since many did not have tissue confirmation. Recently, an International Consensus Conference on the diagnosis and treatment of IPF recommended the use of combined therapy (glucocorticoids and either cyclophosphamide or azathioprine).[25] Initiation of glucocorticoids (0.5 mg/kg/day) for 4 weeks followed by tapering to 0.125 mg/kg/day is recommended. The recommended dose of cyclophosphamide is 2 mg/kg/day, and a trial of at least 3–6 months is required to determine a clinical response. The recommended dose of azathioprine in the treatment of IPF is 2 mg/kg/day with a maximum dose of 150 mg/day. The combination of azathioprine and corticosteroids has been associated with both objective improvement and enhanced survival in some IPF patients.[47]

After 6 months of treatment, re-evaluation for an objective response to therapy is recommended. If an objective response is seen, maintenance prednisone and cytotoxic therapy at the same dosage is continued. Based on the likelihood of relapse, prolonged therapy of 1–2 years is recommended for individuals

THERAPEUTIC PRINCIPLES

Treatment of patients with idiopathic pulmonary fibrosis

- No data exist to show that any currently available therapy alters survival and improves quality of life.
- Therapy is not recommended in all IPF patients (e.g. age >70 years, end-stage honeycomb lung, and significant comorbid diseases, e.g. cardiac disease, diabetes mellitus).
- Until studies define the best therapeutic regimen in IPF, combined therapy including prednisone at 0.5 mg/kg/day for 4 weeks followed by a taper to 0.125 mg/kg/day plus azathioprine or cyclophosphamide at 2 mg/kg/day is recommended.
- At least 3 months are needed to determine an objective response to any intervention.

exhibiting an objective response to treatment. If continued disease progression is noted, therapy should be stopped or altered to include a different cytotoxic agent, alternative therapy, or consideration of lung transplantation.

Since current therapies have minimal beneficial effects on survival in patients with IPF, it is clear that improved survival will depend on the development of new therapeutic approaches based on an improved understanding of the immunopathogenesis of this disease.[48] Trials using interferon-gamma (IFN-γ),[49] relaxin, and pirfenidone[50] are being undertaken in the treatment of IPF.

Lung transplantation should be considered in patients with progressive clinical and physiologic deterioration who meet established criteria. Early listing is crucial since the waiting time may exceed two years.

The most common cause of death in patients with IPF is progression of the underlying disease. In one study, 39% of IPF patients died of respiratory failure with cardiovascular complications (ischemic heart disease, heart failure, stroke) accounting for 27% of the deaths.[51] Bronchogenic carcinoma accounted for 10% of the IPF deaths followed by infection (7%) and pulmonary embolism (3%). Whether the presence of IPF increases the risk of lung cancer remains a controversial issue. However, a recent study showed a seven-fold increased risk of lung cancer in the IPF group compared to control subjects.[52]

Acute interstitial pneumonia

In 1944, Hamman and Rich reported four cases of what they termed 'acute diffuse interstitial fibrosis'.[53] Acute interstitial pneumonia (AIP) is a fulminant form of idiopathic interstitial pneumonia. Although it was previously thought to represent an acute phase of UIP, recent studies indicate that it is a distinct entity.

Clinical manifestations

AIP usually presents with the acute onset of dyspnea followed by rapid progression to respiratory failure.[54,55] The clinical, radiographic, physiologic, and histologic features are identical to those of the adult respiratory distress syndrome (ARDS) but, in the case of AIP, no cause is identified. Most patients are previously healthy individuals greater than 40 years of age. There is no sex predilection. A viral prodrome lasting one to two weeks is common, and symptoms include fever, nonproductive cough, and dyspnea. Most patients require ventilatory support. Laboratory studies are nonspecific. Chest radiographs show diffuse, bilateral airspace opacities, and ground-glass attenuation is seen on chest CT examination. A similar presentation may complicate or represent the initial manifestation of a collagen vascular disease.

Histopathology

AIP is characterized by diffuse interstitial fibrosis that is temporally uniform (Fig. 84.4).[23] The changes are identical to the organizing phases of diffuse alveolar damage, as seen in ARDS. Within the thickened interstitial space, there is active, diffuse fibroblast proliferation similar to the focal fibroblast foci seen in UIP. If this is progressive, honeycomb change occurs. However, these airspaces are lined with alveolar epithelium as opposed to the bronchiolar epithelium lining honeycomb spaces. Another feature of acute lung injury, which is frequently seen in AIP, are intra-alveolar hyaline membranes.

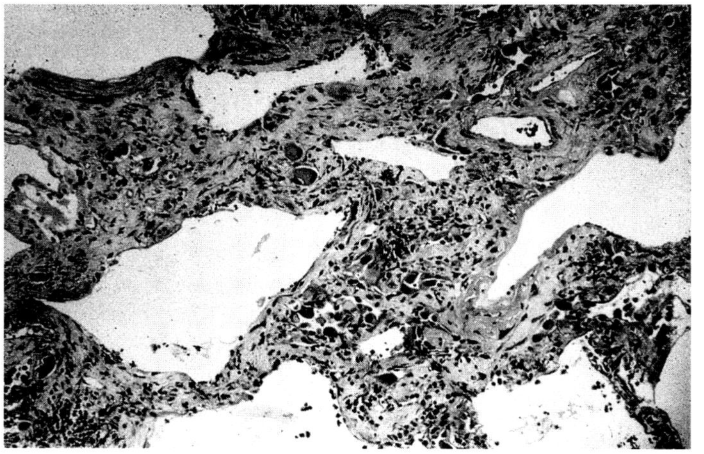

Figure 84.4 Histopathology of acute interstitial pneumonitis. Diffuse thickening of the alveolar septum with an infiltration of mononuclear cells is the characteristic abnormality. The temporal uniformity of this process is also apparent. (See also color plate 84.4.)

Diagnosis

The diagnosis of AIP requires a clinical syndrome of idiopathic ARDS and the presence of organizing diffuse alveolar damage on lung biopsy. Thus, an open lung biopsy or video-assisted thoracoscopic lung biopsy is suggested to secure the diagnosis and exclude other causes of acute interstitial lung disease.

Treatment and outcome

To date, no effective therapy exists for patients with AIP. Glucocorticoids are utilized in most cases; however, no survival benefit has been shown.[56] The prognosis of patients with AIP is poor, with mortality rates ranging from 50% to 88%.[54–56] Half of the patients die within 6 months of disease onset. The early mortality seen in AIP reflects the massive degree of lung injury present. However, those individuals who survive may have complete recovery of lung function. Recurrent injury is not thought to be a feature of AIP although recurrent episodes of AIP have been noted.

Desquamative interstitial pneumonitis

Desquamative interstitial pneumonitis (DIP) represents less than 3% of all cases of interestitial lung disease. However, it is a distinct clinicopathological entity that differs substantially from UIP. DIP was previously thought to represent an early cellular form of UIP. However, as discussed earlier in this chapter, the earliest change identified in UIP is the fibroblast focus, which is characterized by the cluster of fibroblasts and myofibroblasts in the alveolar septum. At this stage of UIP, there is minimal if any intra-alveolar macrophage accumulation.

Clinical manifestations

DIP affects individuals in their fourth to fifth decades of life; a male predominance is noted in most studies.[57,58] This disease occurs predominantly in cigarette smokers. Clinically, most individuals present with the subacute onset of a dry, nonproductive cough and dyspnea. Clubbing is present in approximately 50% of DIP patients. Laboratory evaluation is usually nonspecific.

The chest radiograph typically reveals bibasilar ground-glass opacities, which are not disease specific. Reticulonodular inter-

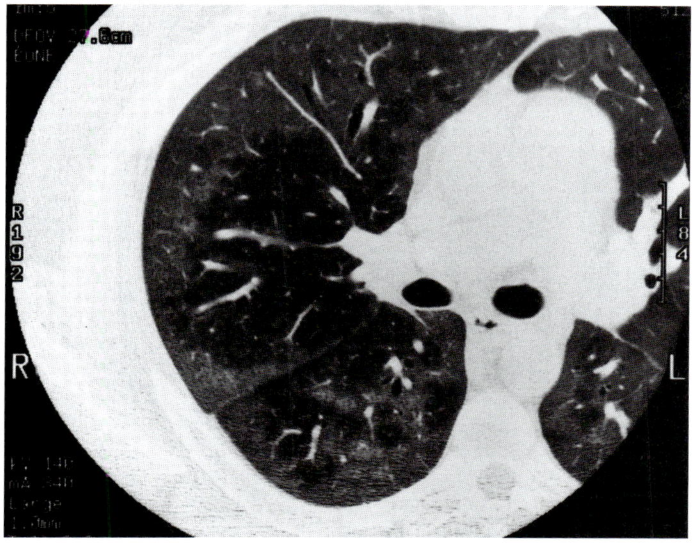

Figure 84.5 Radiographic manifestations in desquamative interstitial pneumonitis. HRCT in a patient with DIP shows ground-glass attenuation in the periphery of the upper and lower lung fields.

stitial infiltrates have also been reported. In addition, a normal chest radiograph may be seen in up to 20% of symptomatic individuals. HRCT confirms the chest radiograph findings, showing ground-glass attenuation in the periphery of the lower lung zones (Fig. 84.5).[59] Pulmonary function testing shows a restrictive defect with an associated decreased diffusing capacity and hypoxemia.

Histopathology

DIP is a misnomer. It was initially thought that the intra-alveolar cells represented sloughed or 'desquamated' alveolar epithelial cells. However, DIP is pathologically defined by a uniform, diffuse accumulation of macrophages in the alveolar space (Fig. 84.6).[23] At low magnification, the overall appearance is one of uniformity from one field of view to the next as opposed to the variegated

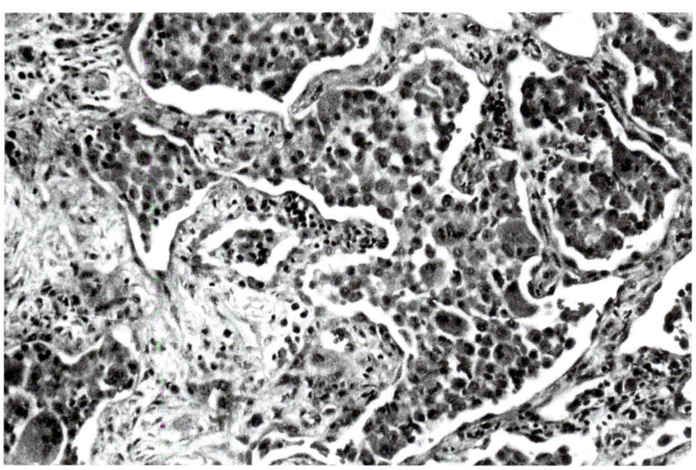

Figure 84.6 Histopathology of desquamative interstitial pneumonitis. A high magnification photomicrograph of DIP shows the uniform, diffuse accumulation of macrophages within the alveolar space with associated thickening of the alveolar septum. These aggregates of macrophages almost completely fill the alveolar spaces. (See also color plate 84.6.)

appearance of UIP. In addition, scant interstitial inflammation with varying degrees of fibrosis of the alveolar septum is present.

Diagnosis

The diagnosis of DIP requires tissue confirmation of the pathologic lesion. This is important since this process is associated with an improved prognosis and a response to therapeutic interventions compared to IPF. A DIP-like lesion is frequently seen in the other idiopathic interstitial pneumonias as well as in eosinophilic granuloma, drug reactions, and other unrelated conditions. Thus, the diagnosis of DIP requires correlation of pathologic findings with clinical and radiologic findings.

Treatment and outcome

The primary intervention in DIP is smoking cessation. Since there are a limited number of cases, it is unclear whether glucocorticoids alter the natural history of this disease. Carrington and associates reported a mortality of 23% with a mean survival of 12 years, compared to a 66% mortality and a mean survival of 5.6 years in UIP.[57] Of note, 22% of their patients spontaneously improved and 60% responded to glucocorticoid therapy. This improvement is dramatically different from IPF in which spontaneous improvement rarely if ever occurs and response to glucocorticoids is seen only in 10–15% of patients. There are, however, a number of patients with DIP who fail to respond to treatment and progress to respiratory failure, secondary to advanced fibrosis.

Respiratory bronchiolitis–interstitial lung disease

Respiratory bronchiolitis–interstitial lung disease (RB–ILD) is a distinct clinical entity that occurs in current or former cigarette smokers.[60] However, it remains unclear whether RB–ILD and DIP represent different diseases or different ends of the spectrum of the same disease process.[23] Both disorders occur predominantly (in the case of DIP) or exclusively (in RB–ILD) in cigarette smokers, suggesting a common pathogenesis related to cigarette smoke.

Clinical manifestations

In the two studies to date evaluating RB–ILD, the mean age at the time of presentation was 36 years.[58,60] A male predominance was noted, and all individuals with RB–ILD were cigarette smokers. The most common symptoms were a dry, nonproductive cough and dyspnea. Yousem et al.[59] noted the absence of clubbing in contrast to its frequent presence in patients with DIP. Laboratory evaluation is nonspecific.

The chest radiograph typically shows diffuse, fine reticular or nodular interstitial opacities with normal lung volumes. Additional findings include bronchial wall thickening and a prominent peribronchovascular interstitium. HRCT may reveal ground-glass opacification as well as emphysema.

Pulmonary function tests most commonly reveal a mixed restrictive-obstructive pattern with a reduced diffusing capacity and mild hypoxemia. An isolated elevation of the residual volume may also be observed.

Histopathology

The pathology of RB-ILD has similarities to DIP. However, in RB–ILD, the intra-alveolar macrophages accumulate primarily within the peribronchiolar airspaces and are associated with thickening of the alveolar septum in these areas (Fig. 84.7). The

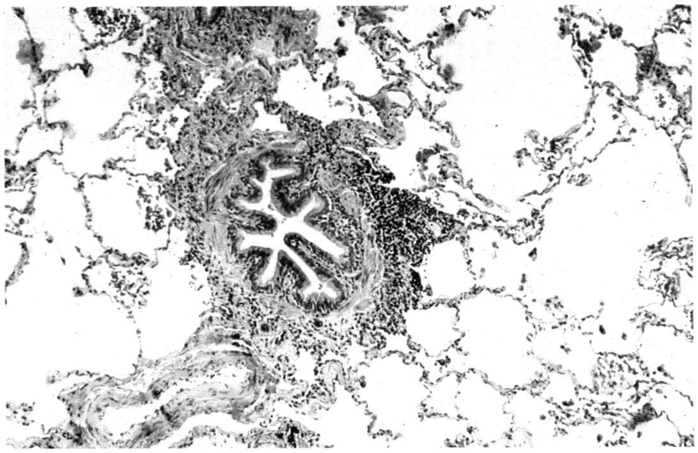

Figure 84.7 Histopathology of respiratory bronchiolitis–interstitial lung disease. An ectatic bronchiole with a thickened wall and a mononuclear infiltrate extending into the immediately surrounding alveoli is shown. (See also color plate 84.7.)

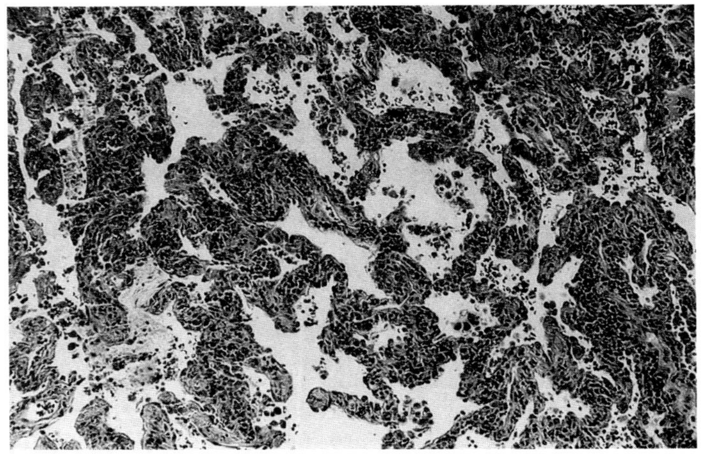

Figure 84.8 Histopathology of nonspecific interstitial pneumonitis. Low magnification photomicrograph of cellular NSIP shows diffuse, uniform thickening of the alveolar septum due to the presence of a lymphoplasmacytic infiltrate. (See also color plate 84.8.)

differentiation of this lesion from DIP requires sparing of distal airspaces with the lesion confined to the peribronchiolar airspaces in RB–ILD.

Diagnosis

RB–ILD should be suspected in young individuals with a history of cigarette use who complain of cough and dyspnea with a chest radiograph or HRCT showing nodular and/or reticular interstitial opacities. The diagnosis requires tissue confirmation of the pathologic findings noted above.

Treatment and outcome

The key therapeutic intervention in RB–ILD is cessation of smoking. The use of glucocorticoids has been associated with favorable results. At present, the clinical course and prognosis of patients with RB–ILD is unknown. All patients in the series by Myers[60] and Youchem[58] either improved or stabilized with no deaths reported.

Nonspecific interstitial pneumonitis

The term nonspecific interstitial pneumonitis (NSIP) was first used to describe cases of interstitial pneumonia that did not demonstrate a pattern of UIP, AIP, or DIP.[61] Currently, the term NSIP is applied to an idiopathic interstitial pneumonia or to a similar histologic pattern, which occurs in collagen vascular diseases, hypersensitivity pneumonitis, or drug-induced lung disease. In fact, 16% of the patients in the original description of NSIP had one of the collagen vascular diseases.[61] The following deals with idiopathic NSIP.

Clinical manifestations

NSIP is most often seen in middle-aged individuals, and a slight female predominance has been noted.[61–64] A dry, nonproductive cough and exertional dyspnea are the most common symptoms although fever is present in 25% of patients. Symptoms are usually present for 6–10 months prior to diagnosis. As in other interstitial pneumonias, the laboratory evaluation is nonspecific.

The chest radiograph usually shows bilateral interstitial infiltrates and sometimes can be normal in a symptomatic patient. The HRCT characteristically shows bilateral, patchy ground-glass attenuation indistinguishable from DIP or RB–ILD.[62]

Histopathology

NSIP is characterized by varying but temporally uniform degrees of fibrosis and inflammation of the alveolar septum without histopathologic features indicative of UIP, AIP, or DIP (Fig. 84.8). Katzenstein and Fiorelli[61] divided NSIP cases into three groups depending on the presence or absence of interstitial fibrosis: interstitial lymphoplasmacytic inflammation (48% of cases); inflammation and fibrosis (38%); and fibrosis (14%). Although the changes are temporally uniform, they may be patchy with intervening areas of normal lung.

This temporal uniformity is in contrast to the variegated pattern seen in UIP. Fibroblast foci, the earliest lesion seen in UIP, are found in 20% of patients with NSIP, making the differentiation of fibrotic NSIP from UIP difficult. The key feature in this circumstance is the temporal uniformity of the lesion in NSIP.

Treatment and outcome

Unlike the poor outcome of UIP, individuals with NSIP have a favorable prognosis. In the original paper, 45% of the subjects completely recovered while another 42% remained stable or improved.[61] Only 11% of the patients died, with a mean survival of 16 months. All of the individuals who suffered the aggressive course were in the fibrotic group. This was recently confirmed by another study that separated NSIP into a cellular and a fibrotic pattern.[65] A 90% 10-year survival occurred in the cellular group compared to 35% in patients with the fibrotic pattern. Despite the worse prognosis of NSIP with a fibrosing pattern, it was still significantly better than the 10-year survival of UIP patients (15% vs. 35%).[65]

Lymphocytic interstitial pneumonia

Although lymphocytic interstitial pneumonia (LIP) was originally thought to represent one of the idiopathic interstitial pneumonias, it is now considered one of the lymphoproliferative disorders of the lung.[66] It has a similar presentation to the aforementioned idiopathic interstitial pneumonias, however, and so will be discussed here.

LIP is an unusual cause of interstitial lung disease; it occurs either as an isolated entity or in association with an autoimmune process, such as Sjögren syndrome, pernicious anemia, rheumatoid arthritis, or chronic active hepatitis. In addition, an increased incidence of LIP has been seen in children infected with human immunodeficiency virus.[67] Approximately 50–77% of cases of LIP are associated with dysproteinemia, which is most often polyclonal.

Clinical manifestations

In adults, LIP occurs more commonly in women, and most patients present between the fourth and seventh decades.[68] The mean age at diagnosis is 56 years. Insidious onset of cough and dyspnea are the most common presenting symptoms. Other findings depend on the presence of associated disorders (e.g. Sjögren syndrome) and include keratoconjunctivitis sicca, hepatosplenomegaly, lymphadenopathy, parotid gland enlargement, and arthritis.

Bilateral mixed reticulonodular and alveolar infiltrates with a lower lung zone predominance are the characteristic chest radiographic changes. However, these findings as well as the HRCT findings are nonspecific. The presence of hilar and/or mediastinal adenopathy could suggest a complicating lymphoma. The physiologic impairment in LIP is similar to that seen in the other interstitial lung diseases and includes reduction of lung volumes with decreased diffusing capacity and hypoxemia.

Histopathology

LIP is characterized by the infiltration of the alveolar septum with monotonous sheets of lymphocytes and plasma cells, which expand the interstitium and compress alveolar space (Fig. 84.9).[68] These lymphoid aggregates may be either diffuse or focal, and immunofluorescent staining has shown these cells to be polyclonal in nature. Other features of LIP include well-formed germinal centers, noncaseating granulomatous inflammation with giant cells, and type II pneumocyte hyperplasia.

Pathogenesis

An autoimmune etiology of LIP is suggested by its frequent association with various autoimmune disorders. Rarely, immune complexes have been found in LIP patients.[5] Based on the increased incidence of LIP in individuals infected with HIV, a viral etiology is another attractive possibility. Improvement in the lung disease has been noted with initiation of antiretroviral therapy, suggesting that HIV may be responsible for the proliferation of lymphocytes in the lung in those cases associated with HIV. Although the role of Epstein–Barr virus (EBV) in the pathogenesis of LIP is unknown, the role of this virus in the generation of lymphoproliferative disorders in the immunocompromised host is well known. In situ hybridization of lung biopsies from LIP patients showed increased EBV genomic material compared to other chronic lung diseases.[69] In Japanese patients, an association between LIP and human T-cell lymphotropic virus type 1 (HTLV-1) has been reported.[70]

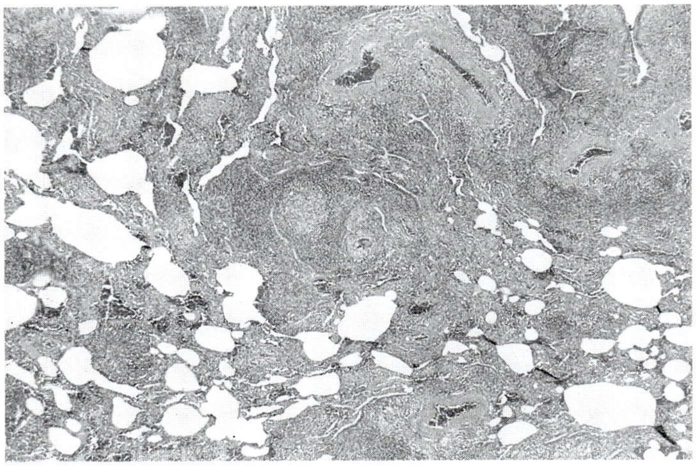

Figure 84.9 Histopathology of lymphocytic interstitial pneumonitis. Low magnification photomicrograph of LIP shows a dense lymphocytic infiltrate. In the center of the photomicrograph, noncaseating granulomatous inflammation with a multinucleated giant cell is seen. (See also color plate 84.9.)

Diagnosis

Based on the presence of nonspecific symptoms, signs, physiology, and radiology, the diagnosis of LIP depends on tissue confirmation of the pathologic findings. In the immunocompromised host, infection should be adequately excluded prior to the institution of therapy.

Treatment and outcome

Although glucocorticoids are the mainstay of therapy for LIP, no controlled trial has demonstrated their efficacy in the treatment of this disease. In addition, the optimal dose and duration of glucocorticoids remains unknown.

Possible outcomes of LIP include: (1) resolution following therapy, (2) progression to fibrosis and death, (3) development of a respiratory or systemic infection, or (4) progression to a lymphoma.[71] Although several series have indicated no evidence of progression of LIP to lymphoma, case reports document this progression. The lymphomas complicating LIP usually develop years after the diagnosis of LIP and are associated with slow growth and prolonged survival.

Cryptogenic organizing pneumonia

Cryptogenic organizing pneumonia (COP) or idiopathic bronchiolitis obliterans organizing pneumonia (BOOP) is a specific clinicopathologic disorder of unknown etiology characterized by excessive proliferation of granulation tissue within the lumen of the distal airspaces.[72–74] The term COP is reserved for cases demonstrating BOOP without an obvious cause, since this histologic appearance also occurs in a variety of inflammatory lung disorders including collagen vascular diseases, malignancy, infections, and those caused by medications.

Clinical manifestations

A prevalence of 6–7 per 100 000 has been suggested.[74] The onset of disease is usually in the fifth to sixth decades of life, men and women are affected equally. Most individuals have symptoms for less than 2 months prior to diagnosis. The initial presentation is characterized by a dry, nonproductive cough with flu-like symptoms including fever, sore throat, and malaise. This is followed by progressive dyspnea and cough. Routine laboratory evaluation is nonspecific.

The chest radiograph is characterized by diffuse, often patchy alveolar opacities in the setting of normal lung volumes (Fig. 84.10A).[72–74] These opacities can be migratory and can have a peripheral distribution similar to those seen in chronic eosinophilic pneumonia. Other rare radiographic manifestations include linear or nodular interstitial opacities and honeycombing. The presence of a pleural effusion or pleural thickening should suggest an associated collagen vascular disease.

HRCT of the chest shows patchy airspace consolidation more commonly located in the lung periphery with a lower lung zone predominance (Fig. 84.10B).[75] Other findings include ground-glass attenuation, small nodular opacities, and bronchial wall thickening.

As in other interstitial lung diseases a restrictive ventilatory defect is the most common pulmonary function abnormality. Gas exchange abnormalities are common and are accompanied by decreased diffusing capacity, widening of the alveolar–arterial gradient, and exercise-induced hypoxemia.[72,76]

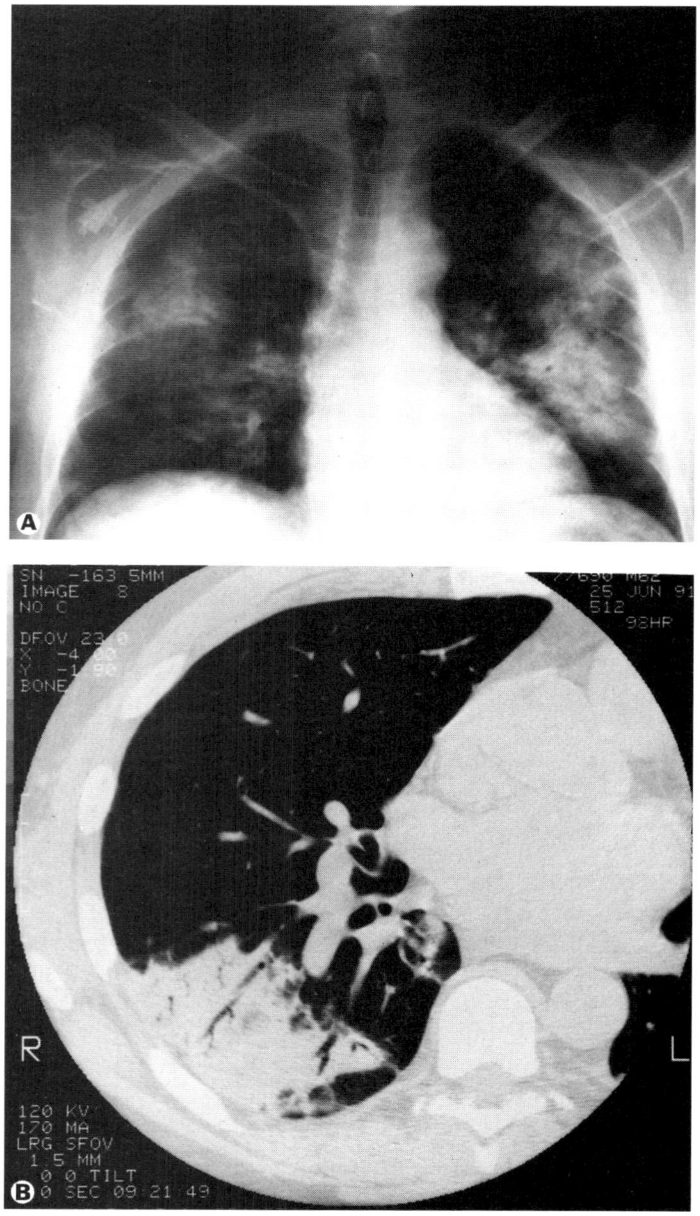

Figure 84.10 Radiographic findings in Cryptogenic organizing pneumonia. (**A**) Chest radiograph in a patient with COP shows bilateral, patchy alveolar opacites with a peripheral distribution in the setting of normal lung volumes. (**B**) Chest CT shows a dense right lower lung consolidation with the presence of air bronchograms.

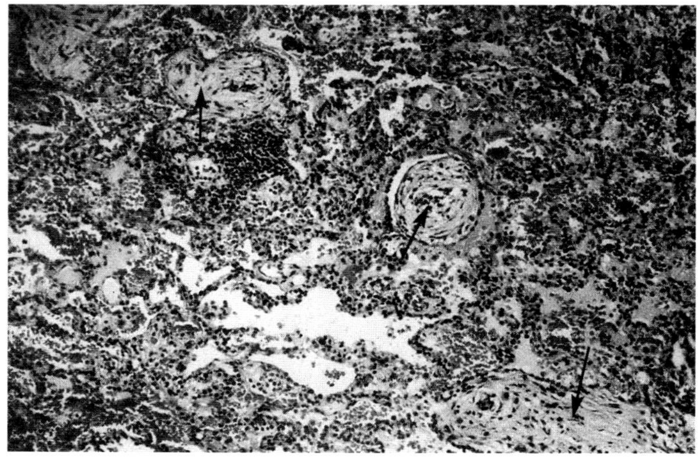

Figure 84.11 Histopathology of Cryptogenic organizing pneumonia. A photomicrograph of COP shows intra-alveolar fibroblast proliferation (arrows) and early collagen production. In addition, thickening of the alveolar septa with a lymphoplasmacytic infiltrate consistent with cellular NSIP is present. (See also color plate 84.11.)

Histopathology

The histopathology of COP is characterized by excessive proliferation of granulation tissue in the small airways and alveolar ducts with associated chronic inflammation in the alveolar walls (Fig. 84.11).[76] The intraluminal fibrotic buds (Masson bodies) consist of loose collagen-embedding fibroblasts and myofibroblasts and have a tendency to extend from one alveolus to the next, giving a characteristic 'butterfly' pattern.[73] The lesions are patchy in nature and have a uniform temporal appearance at low magnification with preservation of the underlying lung parenchyma.

Diagnosis

The presence of BOOP in a lung biopsy does not necessarily represent COP since this is a diagnosis of exclusion. Organizing pneumonia is a nonspecific response to many lung injuries and may be seen adjacent to another pathologic process or as a component of other primary pulmonary disorders such as infections, irradiation, collagen vascular diseases, Wegener's granulomatosis, or chronic eosinophilic pneumonia (Table 84.3).

Treatment and outcome

Treatment with glucocorticoids usually offers dramatic clinical and radiographic improvement within days to weeks. Complete clinical, physiologic, and radiographic recovery occurs in two thirds of the cases.[15,72,76] However, in the remainder, persistent disease with progression to fibrosis can be expected. It is common for relapses to occur with prednisone tapering, followed by improvement with retreatment; because of this, at least 6 months of therapy is recommended. The 5-year survival in COP is 73%, compared to a 44% 5-year survival of patients with BOOP due to other causes (e.g. collagen vascular diseases) or the 30% 5-year survival of IPF.[76]

VASCULITIS

The primary systemic vasculitides are a heterogeneous group of disorders of unknown etiology with a wide spectrum of clinical

Disorders associated with a BOOP pattern
Idiopathic BOOP (cryptogenic organizing pneumonia)
Collagen vascular diseases: • systemic lupus erythematosus • rheumatoid arthritis • polymyositis/dermatomyositis • Sjögren syndrome
Hypersensitivity pneumonitis
Chronic eosinophilic pneumonia
Drug-induced: • gold • penicillamine • amiodarone • bleomycin • sulfa drugs
Wegener's granulomatosis
Bone marrow transplantation
Lung transplantation/rejection
Inhalational injury
Neoplasms
Lung irradiation
Virus-associated: • HIV • influenza • adenovirus
BOOP = bronchiolitis obliterans organizing pneumonia; HIV = human immunodeficiency virus.

Table 84.3 Disorders associated with a BOOP pattern.

manifestations (Chapter 67). The complexity of the clinical and histopathologic features, as well as the potential for overlap, can make specific diagnosis difficult. The 1992 Chapel Hill International Consensus Conference was convened to reconcile definition and classification schemata.[77] This nomenclature is based on histopathologic criteria including size of vessels involved and the presence or absence of serum anti-neutrophil cytoplasmic antibody (ANCA).

Most of the pulmonary vasculitides are systemic in nature. Consequently, the lung is one of many organ systems involved in the disease process. The systemic vasculitides, which typically involve the small vessels of the lung, include Wegener's granulomatosis, Churg–Strauss syndrome, and microscopic polyangiitis. Involvement of alveolar capillaries (pulmonary capillaritis) in the inflammatory process results in intra-alveolar bleeding and the clinical syndrome known as diffuse alveolar hemorrhage (DAH).

Wegener's granulomatosis

Wegener's granulomatosis (WG) (Chapter 67) is a systemic vasculitis of small arteries and veins involving the upper and lower respiratory tract, often with associated glomerulonephritis. A limited form of WG involving only the upper and lower respiratory tract has been observed in 28% of patients.[78] Classically, the inflammatory lesions include necrosis, granulomatous inflammation, and vasculitis.[79,80]

Clinical manifestations

The incidence of WG is unknown. Men and women are affected equally; the mean age at presentation is 40 years, with approximately 15% of patients presenting prior to the age of 19 years.[79–81] The clinical presentation is characterized by upper respiratory tract signs and symptoms including recurrent epistaxis, mucosal ulcerations, and septal perforation.[79] At initial presentation, 90% of patients have evidence of upper and lower respiratory tract involvement. The most frequent lower respiratory symptoms are cough, dyspnea, and hemoptysis. Diffuse alveolar hemorrhage is an uncommon presenting manifestation of WG, occurring in 5% of patients.[82] Only 18% of patients have renal involvement at initial presentation, but 75% eventually develop signs of glomerulonephritis within two years of presentation. Other nonspecific findings include fever, malaise, and weight loss.

Laboratory findings in WG include elevated erythrocyte sedimentation rate, mild anemia, leukocytosis, and thrombocytosis. c-ANCA, an autoantibody directed against a neutrophil cytoplasmic serine protease, proteinase 3, is highly specific (>95%) for WG.[83] The sensitivity of c-ANCA parallels disease activity and may be as low as 65–70% in patients with inactive disease.[83] In limited WG, the sensitivity of the c-ANCA is only 65%. Thus, a negative c-ANCA in the setting of limited WG does not exclude the diagnosis.

The most common radiographic findings in WG are single or multiple pulmonary nodules with or without cavitation.[79,80,84] Less common findings include pleural effusions, bilateral alveolar opacities representing diffuse alveolar hemorrhage, hilar adenopathy, and the presence of an aspergilloma in a pre-existing cavity. Moreover, endobronchial involvement can cause lobar atelectasis.

Histopathology

The pulmonary histopathology of WG is characterized by the presence of vasculitis, parenchymal necrosis, and granulomatous inflammation accompanied by a mixed infiltrate of neutrophils, lymphocytes, histiocytes, and eosinophils.[78] The necrotizing granulomas vary from punctate microabscesses to large geographic zones of necrosis, and the vasculitis typically involves pulmonary arteries, veins, and capillaries.

The histopathologic correlate of diffuse alveolar hemorrhage in WG is pulmonary capillaritis. Even though the frequency of this manifestation of WG is low, capillaritis was observed in 35% of the granulomatous lesions, usually located adjacent to the granulomatous process.

> **CLINICAL PEARLS**
>
> **Lung involvement in Wegener's granulomatosis (WG)**
> - WG is a small-vessel vasculitis involving the upper and lower respiratory tracts and associated with glomerulonephritis.
> - Although 15% of patients are diagnosed prior to the age 19 years, the mean age at presentation is 40 years.
> - The sensitivity of c-ANCA in the setting of limited WG is only 65%.
> - The lung histopathology is characterized by the presence of vasculitis, necrosis, and granulomatous inflammation.
> - The histopathologic correlate of diffuse alveolar hemorrhage in WG is capillaritis.

The renal histopathology in WG shows a focal, segmental necrotizing glomerulonephritis with or without crescent formation[85] (Chapters 67 and 79). This lesion is not specific for WG as it occurs in other small-vessel vasculitidies and Goodpasture syndrome.

Treatment and outcome

The recommended therapy for WG consists of cyclophosphamide (2 mg/kg/day) and prednisone (1 mg/kg/day). The prednisone dosage is subsequently tapered once a remission is achieved; cyclophosphamide is continued for 6–12 months after the disappearance of symptoms and tapered gradually over the next several months.

With this regimen, a partial remission occurs in 90% of patients and a complete remission occurs in 75% of patients.[80] Approximately 50% of patients who experience a complete remission suffer one or more relapses. Although this regimen has converted a previously fatal disease into a treatable disorder with prolonged survival and often a cure, it is associated with significant toxicity. Treatment-related side-effects include infections, hemorrhagic cystitis, bladder cancer and myelodysplasia.[86] The increased incidence of *Pneumocystis carinii* pneumonia in patients with WG has led to the recommendation that all WG patients who are receiving daily glucocorticoids should be given chemoprophylaxis against *P. carinii*.[87]

Churg–Strauss syndrome

The Churg–Strauss syndrome (CSS), previously referred to as allergic angiitis and granulomatosis, is a rare disorder characterized by allergic rhinitis, asthma, eosinophilia, and a granulomatous vasculitis.[88–90] The lung is the most common organ involved. The diagnosis is sometimes unclear due to similarities with other vasculitides, such as WG. Of the 807 patients with vasculitis submitted to the American College of Rheumatology classification study, only 2.5% had CSS.[91]

Clinical manifestations

The incidence and prevalence of CSS are unknown. The mean age at diagnosis is 38 years; men and women are affected equally.[89] In most cases there are three phases of the disease. The prodromal phase is characterized by atopy (rhinitis and asthma) and occurs during the second and third decades of life. This is followed by the eosinophilic phase with peripheral blood eosinophilia and eosinophilic tissue infiltration including chronic eosinophilic pneumonia. Finally, the vasculitic phase is heralded by the onset of life-threatening medium and small-vessel vasculitis. This classic presentation is not always the case, and, in 20% of the cases, asthma, eosinophilia, and vasculitis develop simultaneously.[88–90]

Asthma and allergic rhinitis are the most consistent nonvasculitic findings in CSS. Complications related to the vasculitis include skin changes in two thirds of patients, manifesting as subcutaneous nodules and palpable purpura. The most common neurologic complication is a peripheral neuropathy due to mononeuritis multiplex. Cardiovascular involvement accounts for approximately 50% of the deaths due to CSS and includes pericarditis, coronary arteritis, and eosinophilic myocarditis. Renal involvement is more common than previously reported with one study showing some degree of renal involvement in approximately 90% of patients.[92]

Laboratory tests are nonspecific, but abnormalities include peripheral blood eosinophilia ($5–10 \times 10^9$/l), anemia, leukocytosis, and an elevated erythrocyte sedimentation rate. Approximately 50% of CSS patients are p-ANCA positive, usually related to autoantibodies to myeloperoxidase.[93] Bronchoalveolar lavage shows eosinophilia, but this is nonspecific.

The chest radiograph is abnormal in 72% of the cases, with the most common abnormality being transient, patchy alveolar opacities.[89] Pleural effusions are present in greater than 15% of cases, and eosinophils usually comprise more than 60% of the pleural fluid cells.[94]

In patients with steroid-dependent asthma treated with zafirlukast, a syndrome characterized by pulmonary infiltrates, eosinophilia, and cardiomyopathy has occurred following the withdrawal of corticosteroids.[95] Other cases of eosinophilia and CSS have been reported with other leukotriene antagonists including pranlukast and montelukast. At the present time, it is unclear if these manifestations represent a class-specific drug effect or the unmasking of a primary eosinophilic disorder due to steroid withdrawal.

Histopathology

The major histologic findings of CSS include eosinophil infiltration of vascular media and perivascular tissues accompanied by lymphocytes, plasma cells, and histiocytes. There is a necrotizing vasculitis of small arteries and veins and necrotizing extravascular granulomatosis.[88–91]

Diagnosis

Three criteria were proposed by Lanham et al.[89] to establish a diagnosis of CSS: (1) asthma (2) eosinophilia exceeding 1.5×10^9/l, and (3) systemic vasculitis of two or more extrapulmonary organs. Using the American College of Rheumatology criteria,[91] a sensitivity of 85% and a specificity of 99.7% are obtained if four or more of the following criteria are met: (1) asthma, (2) greater than 10% peripheral blood eosinophilia, (3) mononeuritis or polyneuropathy, (4) paranasal sinus abnormality, (5) transient alveolar opacities on chest radiograph, and (6) extravascular eosinophils on a vessel biopsy. The finding of a positive p-ANCA further strengthens the diagnosis.

Treatment and outcome

Glucocorticoids are the mainstay of therapy. Most patients respond favorably to prednisone administered at a dosage range of 0.5–1.5 mg/kg/day. Persistent ANCA positivity does not appear to correlate with underlying disease activity.[96] Without treatment, CSS is characterized by a 50% mortality at 3 months.[89] In contrast, a survival rate of 70% at 5 years with treatment has been recently reported.[97] The presence of cardiac involvement, gastrointestinal disease, renal insufficiency, proteinuria, or central nervous system involvement are poor prognostic factors.[97]

Microscopic polyangiitis

Microscopic polyangiitis is a necrotizing small-vessel vasculitis associated with focal, segmental, necrotizing glomerulonephritis, and is considered a microscopic variant of classic polyarteritis nodosa (PAN) (Chapter 67).

Clinical manifestations

Nearly all patients have a systemic illness characterized by fever, malaise, and weight loss. Other common findings include neuropathy, sinusitis, vasculitic skin lesions (i.e. palpable purpura), gastrointestinal bleeding, and muscle involvement. Pulmonary involvement is heralded by the onset of hemoptysis and dyspnea due to diffuse alveolar hemorrhage. In addition, all patients have focal, segmental glomerulonephritis (Chapter 79). Antibodies to either hepatitis B or C are seen in up to a third of patients.

Histopathology

Microscopic polyangiitis is characterized by necrotizing vasculitis affecting capillaries, arterioles, and venules (Fig. 84.12).[77]

Diagnosis

The differentiation of microscopic polyangiitis from WG and classic PAN is difficult. There is no granulomatous inflammation in microscopic polyangiitis. The differentiating feature between microscopic polyangiitis and PAN revolves around the size of the vessels predominantly involved. In classic PAN, medium- and small-sized muscular arteries are involved, resulting in hypertension, microaneurysms, and renal infarcts. The capillaritis of microscopic polyangiitis results in rapidly progressive glomerulonephritis, which is not a feature of PAN. In addition, involvement of pulmonary capillaries (capillaritis) in microscopic polyangiitis may result in diffuse alveolar hemorrhage. This severe complication is present in one third of patients with microscopic polyangiitis, whereas clinically apparent lung disease in classic PAN is rare. Approximately 80% of patients with microscopic polyangiitis have a positive p-ANCA, and the remainder are c-ANCA positive.[93]

Treatment and outcome

The treatment regimen is similar to that for other pulmonary vasculitides. With reduction or discontinuation of immunosuppressive therapy, recurrence of alveolar hemorrhage may occur. An early mortality of 25% is associated with the presence of diffuse alveolar hemorrhage in microscopic polyangiitis.[98] Overall, a 5-year survival rate of 65% has been reported. The presence of c-ANCA has been associated with a worse prognosis.

Isolated pauci-immune pulmonary capillaritis

Most pulmonary capillaritis occurs as part of a systemic vasculitis (e.g. WG or microscopic polyangiitis), a collagen vascular disease, or another autoimmune process (Table 84.4).

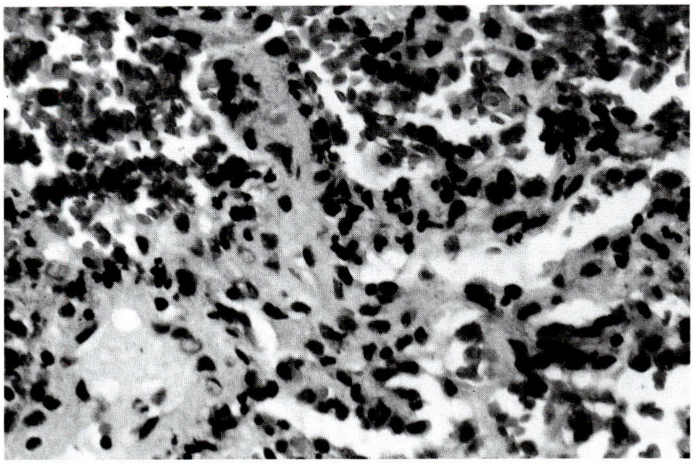

Figure 84.12 Histopathology of pulmonary capillaritis. A high magnification photomicrograph of pulmonary capillaritis shows marked thickening of the alveolar septa with the infiltration of neutrophils. The alveolar spaces are filled with red blood cells. (See also color plate 84.12.)

Isolated pauci-immune pulmonary capillaritis is a small-vessel vasculitis which is isolated to the lung, occurring with or without the presence of ANCA. Bosch and coworkers reported the occurrence of pulmonary capillaritis in p-ANCA-positive individuals without manifestations of extrapulmonary disease.[99] These cases could represent a limited form of microscopic polyangiitis. Studies have suggested that isolated pauci-immune pulmonary capillaritis (ANCA-negative) is the most common cause of pulmonary capillaritis, followed by WG and microscopic polyangiitis.[100]

Clinical manifestations

The incidence and prevalence of isolated pauci-immune pulmonary capillaritis is unknown. Men and women are equally affected, and the mean age at presentation is 30 years. The most common presenting symptoms are cough, dyspnea, chest pain, hemoptysis, and fever.[100] Rapid progression to respiratory failure occurred in 75% of the patients. Laboratory findings invariably show anemia, and the chest radiograph shows bilateral, diffuse, patchy alveolar infiltrates.

Histopathology

Capillaritis allows red blood cells and fibrin to escape through the damaged alveolar–capillary basement membrane into the alveolar space. The end result is diffuse alveolar hemorrhage. Histopathology in this entity is characterized by the presence of (1) fibrin thrombi occluding capillaries in the alveolar septum, (2) fibrin clots attached to the alveolar septum in a sessile fashion, (3) neutrophils and nuclear dust in the interstitium and adjacent blood vessels, and (4) interstitial red blood cells (Fig. 84.12).[101] Direct immunofluorescent studies of lung tissue have been negative for immune complexes.

Disease associations with pulmonary capillaritis
Isolated pauci-immune pulmonary capillaritis (ANCA-negative)
Isolated pulmonary capillaritis (ANCA-positive)
Wegener's granulomatosis
Microscopic polyangiitis
Systemic lupus erythematosus
Rheumatoid arthritis
Scleroderma
Mixed connective tissue disease
Henoch–Schönlein purpura
Primary antiphospholipid syndrome
Behçet's disease
Goodpasture syndrome
IgA nephropathy
Ulcerative colitis
Cryoglobulinemia

Table 84.4 Disease associations with pulmonary capillaritis.

Diagnosis

The diagnosis of isolated pauci-immune pulmonary capillaritis should be suspected in an individual who presents with DAH and without other clinical or laboratory evidence for a systemic disease. The diagnosis requires tissue confirmation. In addition, the absence of giant cells, eosinophils, and large- or small-vessel vasculitis is necessary for this diagnosis.

Treatment and outcome

The treatment regimen for isolated pulmonary capillaritis is similar to that of other pulmonary vasculitides. Jennings and colleagues[100] reported that five of their seven surviving subjects were in clinical remission after 43 months of follow-up, and none of these subjects had developed clinical or serologic evidence of an underlying vasculitis or collagen vascular disease.

Goodpasture syndrome

Goodpasture syndrome is a rare disorder characterized by diffuse alveolar hemorrhage and rapidly progressive glomerulonephritis, related to the production of autoantibodies reactive with glomerular and alveolar basement membranes.[102] This syndrome is part of a spectrum of diseases known as anti-basement membrane antibody (ABMA) diseases (also referred to as anti-glomerular basement membrane (AGBM) diseases). In the majority of cases, the lung and renal involvement occur simultaneously (Goodpasture syndrome). However, in approximately one third of cases, glomerulonephritis is the sole manifestation of disease and in less than 5% of patients, diffuse alveolar hemorrhage occurs without clinical evidence of renal involvement.

Clinical manifestations

The disease occurs two to three times more commonly in men than in women, with a peak incidence in the second and third decades of life. A genetic basis for ABMA production is suggested by its association in Caucasians with certain HLA antigens, including DRB1*1501 and DQB1*0602 alleles.[103,104]

The clinical presentation of Goodpasture syndrome is similar to other disorders associated with diffuse alveolar hemorrhage and glomerulonephritis. The most common symptoms include cough, dyspnea, and hemoptysis. Fatigue due to a combination of iron deficiency anemia and renal failure may be the presenting symptom in patients without diffuse alveolar hemorrhage. Evidence of microscopic hematuria, proteinuria, and red blood cell casts as well as an increase in the serum creatinine are common. Gross hematuria and hypertension are uncommon. The chest radiograph shows patchy or diffuse alveolar infiltrates, and pulmonary physiology reveals an increase in the diffusing capacity during periods of active bleeding.

The presence of serum or tissue ABMA in a patient with diffuse alveolar hemorrhage or glomerulonephritis, or both, establishes the diagnosis of ABMA disease. These antibodies are almost always IgG, and most commonly of the subclass IgG_1. The level of the ABMA in the serum correlates with the severity of the renal disease but not with that of the lung disease.

Histopathology

The diffuse alveolar hemorrhage in Goodpasture syndrome represents either bland pulmonary hemorrhage or pulmonary capillaritis (see Table 84.4). In those with capillaritis, alveolar wall necrosis is not seen. Similar to renal involvement in the systemic vasculitides (Chapters 67 and 79), the renal histology shows focal segmental necrotizing glomerulonephritis with crescent formation. Immunofluorescent staining of alveolar and glomerular basement membranes shows an uninterrupted linear deposition of immunoglobulin (Fig. 84.13).

Pathogenesis

Studies have demonstrated that the pathologic damage in Goodpasture syndrome is related to the binding of the autoantibodies directed against the noncollagenous domain (α3 chain) of type IV collagen in the basement membrane.[105–107] Despite the widespread distribution of type IV collagen in the body, disease expression is limited to the lungs and kidneys. This limited disease expression suggests the possibility that other factors allow exposure of this autoantigen selectively in alveolar or glomerular basement membranes. Since not all patients with ABMA develop diffuse pulmonary hemorrhage, it is possible that some additional injury is necessary to increase alveolar capillary permeability and permit the passage of the antibody. For example, the clinical onset of alveolar hemorrhage has been associated with influenza A2,[108] hydrocarbon exposure,[109] and cigarette smoking.[110] On the other hand, the glomerular basement membrane is directly exposed to the vascular compartment through endothelial fenestrations, explaining the positive association between the level of ABMA and the severity of the glomerulonephritis.

Molecular mimicry has been linked to the pathogenesis of several autoimmune disorders including multiple sclerosis and type I diabetes mellitus[111] (Chapter 58). This concept proposes that a susceptible host is exposed to an infectious agent that has antigens that are immunologically similar to the host but sufficiently different to induce an immune response. Subsequently, tolerance to the autoantigen breaks down, and the pathogen-specific immune response is generated that cross-reacts with host structures resulting in tissue damage. The possibility of molecular mimicry between antigens from infectious agents and basement membrane antigens is suggested by the finding of sequence homology between the α3 chain of type IV collagen in the basement membrane and a segment of influenza A hemagglutinin.[112]

Treatment and outcome

The establishment of a rapid diagnosis is essential since the severity of the renal lesion at the time of presentation correlates with the potential recovery of renal function. Prior to the introduction of plasmapheresis, the mortality of Goodpasture syndrome was between 75% and 90%. In patients with diffuse alveolar hemorrhage alone, glucocorticoids are effective; however, if glomerulonephritis is present with or without alveolar hemorrhage, monotherapy is usually unsuccessful. Cytotoxic therapy, usually azathioprine or cyclophosphamide, may reverse the renal dysfunction, but the main role of these medications is to control alveolar hemorrhage. However, the combination of plasmapheresis, glucocorticoids, and cytotoxic therapy may be the most efficacious regimen, particularly for patients with oliguria who do not require hemodialysis. Plasmapheresis (3–6 l/day) is generally continued for 2 weeks.

The 2-year survival of all patients with Goodpasture syndrome is approximately 50%, with the majority dying from alveolar hemorrhage, often precipitated by a concomitant infection. Severe renal failure reduces survival to 50% at 6 months. Renal biopsy provides both a diagnosis and prognostic information.[113]

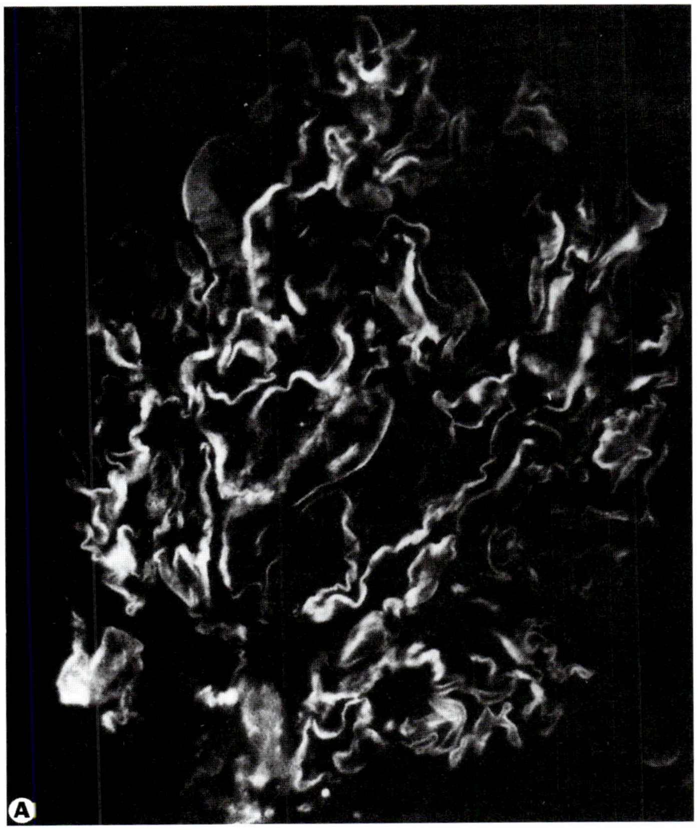

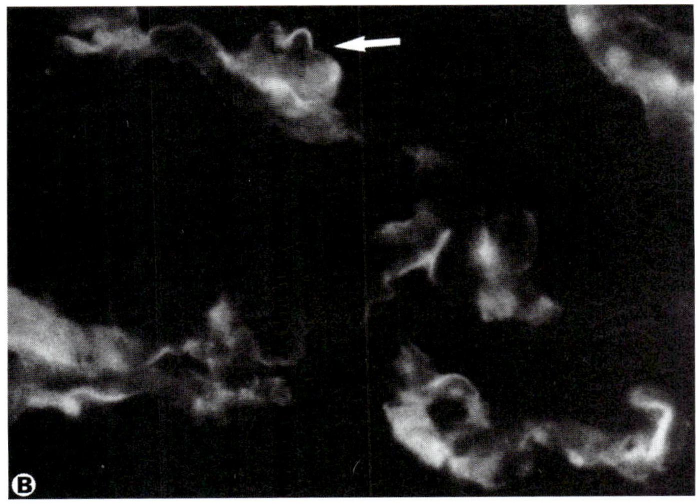

Figure 84.13 This figure demonstrates the typical immunofluorescence staining patterns of Goodpasture syndrome with IgG deposits on the basement membrane. The characteristic linear deposit of antibody reacting with the continuously distributed basement membrane antigen(s) of (**A**) glomerular basement membrane (GBM) in the kidney and (**B**) alveolar basement membrane in the lung can be appreciated; it easily separates this from the more common granular or interrupted patterns of staining seen with immune complex forms of immune renal injury.

Involvement of less than 30% of the glomeruli with crescent formation is associated with preserved renal function, significant response to therapy, and prologed survival. However, when greater than 70% of the glomeruli are involved with crescent formation, progressive renal dysfunction is expected, requiring hemodialysis and consideration of renal transplantation.

LUNG INVOLVEMENT IN COLLAGEN VASCULAR DISEASES

The collagen vascular diseases (CVD) are a heterogeneous group of systemic autoimmune diseases, which frequently involve the lungs. The pleuropulmonary manifestations of these diseases are diverse, affecting all anatomic locations of the respiratory tract (i.e. airways, alveoli, blood vessels, and pleura) (Table 84.5).[114,115] Although pulmonary complications generally occur in patients with well-established disease occasionally the lung involvement is the first manifestation of the autoimmune disorder. This section discusses the pleuropulmonary manifestations of systemic lupus erythematosus (SLE), rheumatoid arthritis (RA), systemic sclerosis (SS), and polymyositis/dermatomyositis (PM/DM) (for a discussion of other manifestations in these diseases, see Chapters 60–64).

Systemic lupus erythematosus

SLE is a disease of unknown etiology characterized by the presence of autoantibodies directed against various nuclear antigens. These autoantibodies and the resultant immune complexes mediate many of the manifestations of SLE (Chapter 60). This disease primarily affects young women (female to male ratio >8:1) and is characterized by possible involvement and

Pleuropulmonary manifestations of collagen vascular diseases

	SLE	RA	SS	PM/DM
Pulmonary hypertension	+	+	+++	±
Vasculitis	+	±	±	−
Pleural disease	+++	+++	+	−
Bronchiolitis obliterans	±	++	+	−
Aspiration pneumonia	−	−	++	+++
Diaphragmatic dysfunction	+−	−	−	±
Lung nodules	−	++	−	−
Diffuse alveolar damage	+	±	±	+
BOOP	±	+	±	+
UIP	+	++	+++	++
Capillaritis	++	+	±	±
LIP	−	+	+	±
NSIP	−	++	+	++

SLE = systemic lupus erythematosus; RA = rheumatoid arthritis; SS = systemic sclerosis; PM/DM = polymyositis/dermatomyositis

Table 84.5 Pleuropulmonary manifestations of collagen vascular diseases.

dysfunction of virtually every organ system. Pleuropulmonary involvement occurs at some point in the disease course in 38–89% of cases.[116] Thus, the respiratory system is affected more commonly in SLE than in any other CVD.[115] Although not a manifestation specific for SLE, infectious pneumonia is the most common cause of pulmonary disease in this patient population, and infection is one of the most common causes of death. Thus, in the presence of a febrile illness with accompanying pulmonary infiltrates, a community-acquired or an opportunistic infection must be promptly excluded.

Acute lupus pneumonitis

Acute lupus pneumonitis is an uncommon pulmonary manifestation of SLE, occurring in less than 5% of cases.[116,117] The clinical presentation mimics that of an infectious pneumonia with the abrupt onset of fever, cough, and dyspnea.[118] Serum complement levels are often low and the chest radiograph typically shows diffuse alveolar opacities. It may be accompanied by pericarditis and often pleuritis and pleural effusion.

It can be difficult to distinguish acute lupus pneumonitis from an infectious pneumonia, and BAL followed by thoracoscopic lung biopsy is often recommended prior to instituting corticosteroid therapy. The histopathology varies and includes diffuse alveolar damage, bronchiolitis obliterans organizing pneumonia (BOOP), nonspecific interstitial pneumonitis (NSIP), or a combination of these.

There are no controlled trials of therapy for acute lupus pneumonitis. Treatment includes high-dose glucocorticoids (1–2 mg/kg/day) with or without accompanying cytotoxic drugs, such as cyclophosphamide. Mortality rates as high as 50% have been reported.[118] In those patients who fail to respond to treatment, respiratory failure is the usual cause of death.

Diffuse alveolar hemorrhage

Diffuse alveolar hemorrhage occurs in less than 5% of patients with SLE, and it represents the initial manifestation of disease in 11–20% of those cases.[119] However, the majority of cases develop in individuals with well-established diagnoses of SLE, usually with pre-existing lupus nephritis.

The symptoms of diffuse alveolar hemorrhage mimic those of infectious pneumonia and acute lupus pneumonitis. Hemoptysis is present in 42–66% of patients at presentation.[119] Therefore, the absence of hemoptysis does not exclude the diagnosis, particularly in the setting of a falling hematocrit, diffuse pulmonary infiltrates, and a serosanguinous BAL. When possible to perform, which is often not the case due to respiratory failure, a diffusing capacity will be elevated because of the increased availability of hemoglobin to bind carbon monoxide. Diffuse alveolar hemorrhage in SLE is most often due to pulmonary capillaritis, but it can also be caused by diffuse alveolar damage. Immunofluorescence studies show granular deposits of IgG and C3 along alveolar walls, interstitium, and capillary endothelial cells.

There are no controlled trials for the treatment of alveolar hemorrhage in SLE. Glucocorticoids, cytotoxic drugs, and plasmapheresis have all been used in various combinations. The mortality rate associated with diffuse alveolar hemorrhage is approximately 50%.[119] Poor prognostic factors include the need for mechanical ventilation, presence of infection, and prior treatment with cyclophosphamide.

Lupus pleuritis

The pleura is the most common site of respiratory involvement in SLE, with pleurisy and pleural effusions occurring in 50–80% of patients.[116,117] Lupus pleuritis may be the presenting manifestation of disease, but, more commonly, develops in patients with established SLE. It is often recurrent. The clinical manifestations include chest pain, fever, and dyspnea, and the chest radiograph typically shows bilateral pleural effusions. The pleural fluid is serous or serosanguinous and exudative in nature. Compared to effusions in rheumatoid arthritis, the glucose is higher and the lactate dehydrogenase (LDH) level is lower. The most helpful measurement is a pleural fluid antinuclear antibody titer greater than 1:160.[115] Examination of the pleura reveals infiltration with plasma cells and lymphocytes accompanied by pleural thickening and fibrosis. Treatment with nonsteroidal anti-inflammatory drugs and/or glucocorticoids is usually effective for relief of pleural discomfort.

Interstitial lung disease

The presence of interstitial lung disease (ILD) in SLE was once thought to be uncommon, especially when compared to systemic sclerosis or rheumatoid arthritis. However, utilization of HRCT, as opposed to chest radiography and physiologic testing, indicates that interstitial abnormalities are present in approximately one third of SLE patients.[120] The significance and natural history of these subclinical findings are uncertain. The presence of anti-SSA (Ro) has been noted in approximately 80% of lupus patients with interstitial changes.[121] In addition, the prevalence of ILD is increased in a subset of SLE patients with sclerodermatous skin changes.

The diagnosis of SLE is usually well established in the group of patients who develop the insidious form of ILD. The disease course is characterized by progressive dyspnea and cough; the chest radiograph shows reduced lung volumes and reticular interstitial infiltrates. A restrictive pattern with a reduced diffusing capacity and exercise-induced hypoxemia are typically seen on pulmonary function testing. The histopathology of chronic interstitial disease in SLE resembles usual interstitial pneumonitis (UIP) although cases of brochiolitis obliterans organizing pneumonia (BOOP), lymphocystic interstitial pneumonitis (LIP), and nonspecific interstitial pneumonitis (NSIP) have been described. Response to therapy depends on the underlying histopathology, with the UIP-like form being least responsive as discussed earlier in this chapter.

Pulmonary vascular disease

In acutely ill SLE patients, a syndrome of acute reversible hypoxemia has been described.[122] These patients have hypoxemia and a widened alveolar–arterial oxygen gradient with a normal chest radiograph and ventilation–perfusion scan. The etiology of this syndrome is unknown, but complement-mediated intravascular neutrophil aggregation has been suggested. The hypoxemia usually resolves with glucocorticoid treatment and resolution of the acute exacerbation.

The development of pulmonary hypertension secondary to plexogenic arteriopathy in the setting of SLE, although previously thought to be unusual, has been increasingly noted, the incidence ranging from 5% to 14%.[123,124] Pulmonary hypertension in SLE has been associated with the presence of Raynaud syndrome, serositis, digital vasculitis, and antiphospholipid antibodies.

Dyspnea and fatigue in the face of a normal chest radiograph is the most common presentation. As the pulmonary hypertension advances, enlargement of the central pulmonary arteries occurs. Pulmonary function testing is characterized by an isolated decrease in the diffusing capacity for carbon monoxide. Ventilation–perfusion scanning and, occasionally, pulmonary angiography may be indicated in order to exclude thromboembolic disease. Treatment consists of oxygen and calcium-channel blockers. Whether the use of continuous intravenous epoprostenol in patients with secondary pulmonary hypertension due to SLE alters exercise capacity and cardiopulmonary hemodynamics is currently unknown.

Respiratory muscle dysfunction

The *shrinking or vanishing lung syndrome* is due to diaphragmatic weakness as well as weakness of other respiratory muscles.[124] This entity accounts for the findings of dyspnea without evidence of interstitial infiltrates or pulmonary vascular disease. It is estimated to occur in 25% of patients with SLE, and the chest radiograph typically shows elevated diaphragms and basilar atelectasis. The pathogenesis of respiratory muscle weakness is unknown, but it is not associated with generalized muscle weakness. Glucocorticoids are frequently ineffective in the treatment of this syndrome. Improvement has been noted with inhaled β-agonist and theophylline therapy. Despite a variable response to therapy, a progressive course of this manifestation of SLE is unusual.

Rheumatoid arthritis

Rheumatoid arthritis (RA) is characterized by the presence of a symmetric, inflammatory polyarthritis occurring more frequently in women, with a 2:1 female to male ratio (Chapter 61). Disease onset is most commonly in the fourth to fifth decades of life. The pleuropulmonary complications of RA occur more commonly in individuals with subcutaneous nodules, high titers of rheumatoid factor, and more severe chronic articular involvement. Although RA is more common in women, the pleuropulmonary manifestations have a higher incidence in men. The pleuropulmonary complications of RA are numerous. Moreover, treatment-related lung toxicity and pulmonary infections are at times difficult to differentiate from the primary pleuropulmonary manifestations of the disease.

> **CLINICAL PEARLS**
>
> **Lung involvement in rheumatoid arthritis**
> - Despite the increased prevalence of RA in women, pleuropulmonary complications occur more frequently in men.
> - The pleuropulmonary complications of RA occur most commonly in individuals with more severe articular involvement, subcutaneous nodules, and high levels of rheumatoid factor.
> - Similar to SLE, pleural effusions are the most common complication, characterized by an exudate and a low glucose and low pH.
> - The differentiation of rheumatoid nodules from malignant lesions can be difficult; however, the rapid growth of a nodule should prompt an aggressive search for a malignant cause.

Pleuritis and pleural effusions

As in SLE, pleural abnormalities are one of the most common pulmonary complications of RA. Pleural effusions are clinically evident in approximately 5% of patients, and these may occur prior to the development of arthritis. Often, pleural disease is discovered on a routine chest radiograph. However, the presence of nonspecific chest pain, dyspnea, and fever is not unusual. The effusion may be unilateral or bilateral and may coexist with interstitial lung disease.

Typically, the effusion is exudative in nature and is characterized by a glucose level less than 30 mg/ml in 70–80% of the cases.[125] The mechanism underlying the low pleural fluid glucose is impaired membrane transport of glucose. A low pleural fluid pH is thought to occur secondary to impaired carbon dioxide exit from the pleural space. If the effusion is chronic, the cholesterol concentration can be increased, and the pleural fluid may have a milky appearance (pseudochylothorax). Cytologic examination of the pleural fluid in RA typically reveals multinucleated giant cells, spindle-shaped macrophages, and necrotic debris.

Most rheumatoid effusions are small and asymptomatic, and therefore require no treatment. They resolve over several months without complications. Occasionally, fibrothorax can occur. The use of glucocorticoids for active articular disease will hasten the resolution of the pleural process.

Rheumatoid nodules

Rheumatoid or necrobiotic nodules are the only pleuropulmonary manifestation specific for RA.[115] These nodules most commonly are seen in men with active articular disease, high rheumatoid factors, and subcutaneous nodules. Most individuals are asymptomatic and are diagnosed on routine chest radiograph. Radiographically, these nodules may be singular or multiple with an upper to mid lung zone predominance. Cavitation occurs in approximately 50% of the cases. HRCT of the lung indicates a higher frequency of nodules than previously thought. Rarely, subpleural necrobiotic nodules can erode into the pleural space, resulting in a pneumothorax with a complicating bronchopleural fistula. The diagnostic dilemma arises in the differentiation of these nodules from malignant lesions, and frequently open lung biopsy is necessary. The presence of rapid growth should prompt an aggressive diagnostic evaluation. Typically, no treatment is necessary.

Caplan syndrome refers to the rapid development of pulmonary nodules with an upper lung zone predominance originally described in Welsh coal miners with rheumatoid arthritis.[125] Histologically, these nodules are identical to necrobiotic nodules. Other occupational dust exposures have also been associated with this syndrome.

Pulmonary vascular disease

Although systemic vasculitis with nailfold infarcts, cutaneous ulcers, mononeuritis multiplex, and digital ischemia can develop in RA, pulmonary vascular disease is the least common pleuropulmonary complication of RA. Rarely, pulmonary capillaritis can result in diffuse alveolar hemorrhage.[126] In addition, unlike SLE and SS, primary pulmonary vascular disease resulting in pulmonary hypertension is rare.

Airway disease

Airflow limitation is a common finding in patients with RA, being present in approximately one third of patients. The mechanism(s) responsible for airway disease is poorly understood. The interplay of cigarette smoking and RA may play a role.

A life-threatening complication of RA is upper airway obstruction, resulting from synovitis of the cricoarytenoid joint. Common presenting complaints include a sore throat, hoarseness, and a fullness in the throat. It can progress to inspiratory stridor and upper airway obstruction. This complication occurs more commonly in women, particularly in those with advanced RA. Seventy five per cent of patients were found to have cricoarytenoid abnormalities when screening with direct or indirect laryngoscopy and computed tomography was utilized.[127] The treatment of cricoarytenoid arthritis includes anti-inflammatory medications.

Bronchiolitis obliterans is a progressive form of obstructive lung disease that is being increasingly recognized as a complication of RA.[128,129] This entity was thought to develop secondary to the use of penicillamine for the treatment of RA, but most cases occur in the absence of this therapy. The histopathologic lesion of bronchiolitis obliterans is constrictive bronchiolitis, which is characterized by the presence of concentric submucosal and peribronchiolar fibrosis resulting in extrinsic compression and obliteration of the bronchiolar lumen. The insidious onset of cough and dyspnea with a normal or hyperinflated chest radiograph is the typical clinical presentation. This complication occurs more commonly in women than in men. Pulmonary function studies show airflow limitation with hyperinflation and a reduced diffusing capacity. Expiratory HRCT shows multiple areas of air trapping (mosaic pattern). Some individuals respond to high-dose glucocorticoids and cytotoxic drugs, but most patients with bronchiolitis obliterans progress to respiratory failure.

Bronchiectasis occurs at an increased frequency in RA, usually in individuals with long-standing articular disease. In most patients, bronchiectasis is not clinically significant. However, a productive cough and dyspnea are the most common respiratory symptoms. Recurrent pneumonia and respiratory failure are potentially fatal complications of this problem.

Interstitial lung disease

Although ILD is a common complication of RA, the incidence is difficult to determine, since different methods of detection have been employed and dissimilar populations of patients have been studied. Gabbay and colleagues identified clinically significant ILD in 14% of patients and findings compatible with ILD that were not clinically significant in 44% of patients.[130] The development of ILD in relation to the onset of arthritis is variable.[115] Most often, the ILD develops subsequent to arthritis, but, in approximately 20% of patients, the lung disease precedes the onset of arthritis.

The most common histopathologies identified in this patient population are usual interstitial pneumonitis (UIP), lymphocytic interstitial pneumonitis (LIP), nonspecific interstitial pneumonitis (NSIP), and bronchiolitis obliterans organizing pneumonia (BOOP) (see discussion of these types of ILD earlier in this chapter). The clinical manifestations of ILD in RA resemble those seen in idiopathic disease and include a dry, nonproductive cough and dyspnea on exertion. The chest radiograph and HRCT show increased reticular markings with a predilection for the periphery and lower lung zones. Often, pleural abnormalities accompany the interstitial changes. With advanced disease, progression to honeycomb lung occurs. LIP usually occurs in cases of RA complicated by Sjögren syndrome, and presence of keratoconjunctivitis sicca and xerostomia in a patient with RA and ILD should suggest this histologic type.

In general, ILD in RA appears more indolent than in idiopathic interstitial pneumonitis. Thus, due to uncertain treatment benefits and possible adverse effects, the decision to institute therapy should be based on clinical, radiographic, and physiologic deterioration.

Drug-induced lung disease

Methotrexate and gold used for the treatment of RA are capable of causing lung injury. Methotrexate administered weekly (10–20 mg/week) is associated with the development of interstitial changes in 1–5% of patients with RA.[131] No correlation with age, sex, disease duration, or cumulative dose has been identified. The clinical presentation is subacute in nature, characterized by the presence of fever, cough, and dyspnea occurring 1–5 months after the initiation of the drug. The chest radiograph shows mixed interstitial-alveolar infiltrates. Nonspecific laboratory abnormalities include a leukocytosis, sometimes with mild eosinophilia and an elevated erythrocyte sedimentation rate. In most cases, bronchoalveolar lavage reveals a lymphocytosis. Histologically, cellular nonspecific interstitial pneumonitis (NSIP) with areas of organizing pneumonia is seen. In addition, noncaseating, granulomatous inflammation similar to that seen in hypersensitivity pneumonitis may be present. The primary treatment of methotrexate-induced pneumonitis is withdrawal of the medication and supportive care.

Gold-induced pneumonitis occurs in less than 1% of RA patients treated with gold therapy.[132] Dyspnea and cough usually begin after 4–6 weeks of therapy, and eosinophilia may occur in a minority of patients. The chest radiograph typically reveals mixed alveolar-interstitial opacities with an upper lung zone predilection. The histology is similar to that seen in RA patients with complicating ILD. Thus, the differentiation of gold-induced pneumonitis from rheumatoid interstitial lung disease can be established only when discontinuation of the medication results in remission.

Systemic sclerosis (scleroderma)

Systemic sclerosis is characterized by an excessive deposition of extracellular matrix in the skin and internal organs and vascular involvement (Chapter 64). The degree of visceral organ involvement determines morbidity and mortality. Pulmonary involvement develops in 70–100% of patients with systemic sclerosis. There is no correlation with the degree of extrapulmonary disease.[114] Interstitial lung disease is the most common pulmonary manifestation of systemic sclerosis. Of note, with the improved mortality associated with renal involvement in systemic sclerosis, lung disease has become the most significant cause of morbidity and mortality.[133]

Interstitial lung disease

The incidence of interstitial lung disease in systemic sclerosis depends on the method of detection. Autopsy studies have reported an incidence in interstitial lung disease of 60–100% of cases,[133,134] whereas studies based on chest radiographs have noted interstitial changes in only 14–66% of cases.[115]

Similar to other interstitial lung diseases, cough and dyspnea on exertion are the most common symptoms. Physical examination reveals bibasilar rales. Clubbing is unusual due to capillary

destruction in the nail beds. The radiographic findings include basilar reticulonodular infiltrates, enlargement of pulmonary arteries, and progressive volume loss with associated honeycomb change. Pulmonary function testing reveals restrictive lung disease, preservation of flow rates, and a decreased diffusing capacity. A disproportionate decrease in diffusing capacity compared to lung volume changes should suggests pulmonary hypertension, especially in individuals with limited scleroderma (CREST syndrome). The predominant histopathologic abnormality is usual interstitial pneumonitis with honeycomb changes and is identical to that seen in idiopathic pulmonary fibrosis. Rarely, lymphocytic interstitial pneumonitis may complicate cases of systemic sclerosis that are associated with Sjögren syndrome. Although the 5-year survival for systemic sclerosis patients with interstial lung diseases is 38–45%, it is better than that of patients with idiopathic pulmonary fibrosis.[135]

Pulmonary vascular disease

Pulmonary hypertension is a frequent complication of systemic sclerosis. It occurs in approximately 30% of patients with diffuse scleroderma and in 10–50% of those with limited scleroderma[134,137] (Chapter 64). The pulmonary hypertension may either be associated with interstitial fibrosis or result from involvement of small- and medium-sized arteries and arterioles with smooth muscle hyperplasia, medial hypertrophy, and intimal proliferation (plexogenic). Direct involvement of the pulmonary circulation is more common with limited scleroderma while pulmonary hypertension in patients with diffuse scleroderma is more likely associated with interstitial lung disease.

The clinical presentation is characterized by the insidious onset of dyspnea on exertion and fatigue. Physical examination and chest radiographs show signs typical of pulmonary hypertension, and a decreased diffusing capacity is seen on pulmonary function testing.

The prognosis of isolated pulmonary hypertension is worse than that for pulmonary hypertension associated with interstitial fibrosis, with a 2-year survival rate of 40%.[138] A recent study using continuous intravenous epoprostenol in patients with hypertension associated with scleroderma showed improvement in exercise capacity and cardiopulmonary hemodynamics as compared to control subjects treated with conventional therapy alone.[139]

Pleural disease

Clinically significant pleural disease is uncommon in systemic sclerosis although pleural fibrosis and adhesions are frequent findings in postmortem studies.

Aspiration pneumonitis

Patients with systemic sclerosis have an increased incidence of esophageal dilatation and decreased peristalsis, and this esophageal dysmotility predisposes to aspiration pneumonitis. However, it is unclear if a relationship exists between the presence of gastroesophageal reflux and the development of lung disease. A study by Troshinsky and colleagues[140] showed that gastroesophageal reflux did not correlate with physiologic impairment of the lung in these patients.

Polymyositis/dermatomyositis

Polymyositis (PM) and dermatomyositis (DM) are idiopathic inflammatory myopathies characterized by proximal muscle weakness and, in the case of DM, a characteristic skin rash (Chapter 65). Pulmonary complications in PM/DM are important causes of morbidity and mortality and may overshadow the muscle involvement. Studies have indicated that approximately 40% of patients with PM/DM have pulmonary involvement.[141] As opposed to the other collagen vascular diseases, lung involvement in PM/DM does not primarily involve the airways or the pleura.

Aspiration pneumonia

Aspiration pneumonia is the most common pulmonary complication in patients with PM/DM. Protection of the upper airway is impaired secondary to a reduced cough reflex resulting from weakness of striated muscles of the soft palate, pharynx, and upper esophagus. This weakness results in dysphagia, and, as a consequence, aspiration pneumonitis occurs in 15–20% of PM/DM patients. A history of aspiration pneumonia portends a poor prognosis since these complications tend to occur in patients with more extensive muscle (and/or skin) involvement.[114,141]

Respiratory muscle dysfunction

Hypercapnic respiratory failure secondary to generalized respiratory muscle dysfunction occurs infrequently in patients with PM/DM. Mucous plugging with resultant atelectasis occurs secondary to the inadequate cough reflex. Chest radiograph may reveal reduced lung volumes with associated bibasilar atelectasis. The respiratory muscle weakness results in both inspiratory and expiratory dysfunction, and measurement of maximal inspiratory and expiratory pressures is useful in the determination of respiratory muscle dysfunction as the cause of restrictive lung disease in patients with PM/DM.[141] Sequential measurements are important in monitoring the clinical course and response to therapy.

Interstitial lung disease

Depending on the method of screening, 5–30% of patients with PM/DM have interstitial lung disease.[141] Usual interstitial pneumonitis (UIP) is the most common histopathologic lesion in PM/DM. However, nonspecific interstitial pneumonitis (NSIP), diffuse alveolar hemorrhage secondary to capillaritis, diffuse alveolar damage, and bronchiolitis obliterans organizing pneumonia (BOOP) may also occur.[142] No relationship exists between the interstitial changes and the degree of skin and/or muscle involvement.

Depending on the underlying lung pathology, several clinical syndromes may occur. The most common presentation is the insidious onset of cough and dyspnea due to the presence of UIP or NSIP. The laboratory findings include an elevation of creatine phosphokinase and the presence of anti-Jo-1 antibodies, which are directed against histidyl-tRNA-synthetase. This autoantibody specificity serves as a marker for the subset of PM/DM patients who have interstitial fibrosis, being present in 50% of these individuals[143] (Chapter 65). The chest radiograph in PM/DM is similar to that seen in IPF. Physiologic testing shows a restrictive pattern with a reduction in diffusing capacity. The natural history and optimal treatment of interstitial lung disease in PM/DM is unknown.

Some individuals present with the acute development of diffuse alveolar infiltrates and associated respiratory failure. The underlying histopathologic lesion in this situation may be either diffuse alveolar damage, capillaritis, or BOOP. The differentiation of diffuse alveolar damage from capillaritis and BOOP is critical since the response to treatment and survival are dramatically different. In diffuse alveolar damage, recovery is unusual despite aggressive anti-inflammatory and immunosuppressive treatment. On the other hand, both BOOP and capillaritis are responsive to available therapeutic options.

REFERENCES

1. Reynolds HY. Bronchoalveolar lavage. Am Rev Respir Dis 1987;135:250.
2. King TE Jr. Idiopathic pulmonary fibrosis. In: Schwarz MI, King TE Jr (eds) Interstitial lung disease. Hamilton, BC Decker, 1998, p 597.
3. Schwarz MI. Idiopathic pulmonary fibrosis [clinical conference]. West J Med 1988;149:199.
4. du Bois RM. Idiopathic pulmonary fibrosis. Annu Rev Med 1993;44:441.
5. Dreisin RB, Schwarz MI, Theofilopoulos AN, Stanford RE. Circulating immune complexes in the idiopathic interstitial pneumonias. N Engl J Med 1978;298:353.
6. Schwarz MI, Dreisin RB, Pratt DS, Stanford RE. Immunofluorescent patterns in the idiopathic interstitial pneumonias. J Lab Clin Med 1978;91:929.
7. Hogg JC. Epstein–Barr virus and cryptogenic fibrosing alveolitis. Thorax 1995;50:1232.
8. Iwai K, Mori T, Yamada N, Yamaguchi M, Hosoda Y. Idiopathic pulmonary fibrosis. Epidemiologic approaches to occupational exposure. Am J Respir Crit Care Med 1994;150:670.
9. Raghu G, Hert R. Interstitial lung diseases: genetic predisposition and inherited interstitial lung diseases. Semin Respir Med 1993;14:323.
10. Coultas DB, Zumwalt RE, Black WC, Sobonya RE. The epidemiology of interstitial lung diseases. Am J Respir Crit Care Med 1994;150:967.
11. Scott J, Johnston I, Britton J. What causes cryptogenic fibrosing alveolitis? A case-control study of environmental exposure to dust. BMJ 1990;301:1015.
12. Mannino DM, Etzel RA, Parrish RG. Pulmonary fibrosis deaths in the United States, 1979–1991. An analysis of multiple-cause mortality data. Am J Respir Crit Care Med 1996;153:1548.
13. Johnston ID, Prescott RJ, Chalmers JC, Rudd RM. British Thoracic Society study of cryptogenic fibrosing alveolitis: current presentation and initial management. Fibrosing Alveolitis Subcommittee of the Research Committee of the British Thoracic Society. Thorax 1997;52:38.
14. Crystal RG, Fulmer JD, Roberts WC, Moss ML, Line BR, Reynolds HY. Idiopathic pulmonary fibrosis. Clinical, histologic, radiographic, physiologic, scintigraphic, cytologic, and biochemical aspects. Ann Intern Med 1976;85:769.
15. Guerry-Force ML, Muller NL, Wright JL, et al. A comparison of bronchiolitis obliterans with organizing pneumonia, usual interstitial pneumonia, and small airways disease. Am Rev Respir Dis 1987;135:705.
16. Mathieson JR, Mayo JR, Staples CA, Muller NL. Chronic diffuse infiltrative lung disease: comparison of diagnostic accuracy of CT and chest radiography. Radiology 1989;171:111.
17. Muller NL, Miller RR, Webb WR, Evans KG, Ostrow DN. Fibrosing alveolitis: CT–pathologic correlation. Radiology 1986;160:585.
18. Muller NL, Staples CA, Miller RR, Vedal S, Thurlbeck WM, Ostrow DN. Disease activity in idiopathic pulmonary fibrosis: CT and pathologic correlation. Radiology 1987;165:731.
19. Gay SE, Kazerooni EA, Toews GB, et al. Idiopathic pulmonary fibrosis: predicting response to therapy and survival. Am J Respir Crit Care Med 1998;157:1063.
20. Chinet T, Jaubert F, Dusser D, Danel C, Chretien J, Huchon GJ. Effects of inflammation and fibrosis on pulmonary function in diffuse lung fibrosis. Thorax 1990;45:675.
21. Keogh BA, Lakatos E, Price D, Crystal RG. Importance of the lower respiratory tract in oxygen transfer. Exercise testing in patients with interstitial and destructive lung disease. Am Rev Respir Dis 1984;129:S76.
22. Nugent KM, Peterson MW, Jolles H, Monick MM, Hunninghake GW. Correlation of chest roentgenograms with pulmonary function and bronchoalveolar lavage in interstitial lung disease. Chest 1989;96:1224.
23. Katzenstein AL, Myers JL. Idiopathic pulmonary fibrosis: clinical relevance of pathologic classification. Am J Respir Crit Care Med 1998;157:1301.
24. Fukuda Y, Basset F, Ferrans VJ, Yamanaka N. Significance of early intra-alveolar fibrotic lesions and integrin expression in lung biopsy specimens from patients with idiopathic pulmonary fibrosis. Hum Pathol 1995;26:53.
25. Idiopathic Pulmonary Fibrosis: Diagnosis and Treatment. International consensus statement. Am J Respir Crit Care Med 2000;161:646.
26. Bitterman PB, Rennard SI, Keogh BA, Wewers MD, Adelberg S, Crystal RG. Familial idiopathic pulmonary fibrosis. Evidence of lung inflammation in unaffected family members. N Engl J Med 1986;314:1343.
27. Hubbard R, Lewis S, Richards K, Johnston I, Britton J. Occupational exposure to metal or wood dust and aetiology of cryptogenic fibrosing alveolitis. Lancet 1996;347:284.
28. Shaw RJ. The role of lung macrophages at the interface between chronic inflammation and fibrosis. Respir Med 1991;85:267.
29. Zhang Y, Lee TC, Guillemin B, Yu MC, Rom WN. Enhanced IL-1 beta and tumor necrosis factor-alpha release and messenger RNA expression in macrophages from idiopathic pulmonary fibrosis or after asbestos exposure. J Immunol 1993;150:4188.
30. Sheppard M, Harrison NK. Lung injury, inflammatory mediators, and fibroblast activation in fibrosing alveolitis. Thorax 1992;47:1064.
31. O'Garra A. Cytokines induce the development of functionally heterogeneous T helper cell subsets. Immunity 1998;8:275.
32. Furuie H, Yamasaki H, Suga M, Ando M. Altered accessory cell function of alveolar macrophages: a possible mechanism for induction of Th2 secretory profile in idiopathic pulmonary fibrosis. Eur Respir J 1997;10:787.
33. Wallace WA, Ramage EA, Lamb D, Howie SE. A type 2 (Th2-like) pattern of immune response predominates in the pulmonary interstitium of patients with cryptogenic fibrosing alveolitis (CFA). Clin Exp Immunol 1995;101:436.
34. Agostini C, Siviero M, Semenzato G. Immune effector cells in idiopathic pulmonary fibrosis. Curr Opin Pulm Med 1997;3:348.
35. Chan ED, Worthen GS, Augustin A, Lapadat R, Riches DWH. Inflammation in the pathogenesis of interstitial lung disease. In: Schwarz MI, King TE Jr (eds) Interstitial lung disease. Hamilton, BC Becker, 1998, p 135.
36. Pardo A, Selman M, Ramirez R, et al. Production of collagenase and tissue inhibitor of metalloproteinases by fibroblasts derived from normal and fibrotic human lungs. Chest 1992;102:1085.
37. Chapman JR, Charles PJ, Venables PJ, et al. Definition and clinical relevance of antibodies to nuclear ribonucleoprotein and other nuclear antigens in patients with cryptogenic fibrosing alveolitis. Am Rev Respir Dis 1984;130:439.
38. Grenier P, Valeyre D, Cluzel P, Brauner MW, Lenoir S, Chastang C. Chronic diffuse interstitial lung disease: diagnostic value of chest radiography and high-resolution CT. Radiology 1991;179:123.
39. Tung KT, Wells AU, Rubens MB, Kirk JM, du Bois RM, Hansell DM. Accuracy of the typical computed tomographic appearances of fibrosing alveolitis. Thorax 1993;48:334.
40. Lynch DA, Newell JD, Logan PM, King TE Jr, Muller NL. Can CT distinguish hypersensitivity pneumonitis from idiopathic pulmonary fibrosis? Am J Roentgenol 1995;165:807.
41. Swensen SJ, Aughenbaugh GL, Myers JL. Diffuse lung disease: diagnostic accuracy of CT in patients undergoing surgical biopsy of the lung. Radiology 1997;205:229.
42. Carnochan FM, Walker WS, Cameron EW. Efficacy of video assisted thoracoscopic lung biopsy: an historical comparison with open lung biopsy. Thorax 1994;49:361.
43. Bensard DD, McIntyre RC Jr, Waring BJ, Simon JS. Comparison of video thoracoscopic lung biopsy to open lung biopsy in the diagnosis of interstitial lung disease. Chest 1993;103:765.

44. Hubbard R, Johnston I, Britton J. Survival in patients with cryptogenic fibrosing alveolitis: a population-based cohort study. Chest 1998;113:396.
45. Mapel DW, Hunt WC, Utton R, Baumgartner KB, Samet JM, Coultas DB. Idiopathic pulmonary fibrosis: survival in population based and hospital based cohorts. Thorax 1998;53:469.
46. Mapel DW, Samet JM, Coultas DB. Corticosteroids and the treatment of idiopathic pulmonary fibrosis. Past, present, and future. Chest 1996;110:1058.
47. Raghu G, Depaso WJ, Cain K, et al. Azathioprine combined with prednisone in the treatment of idiopathic pulmonary fibrosis: a prospective double-blind, randomized, placebo-controlled clinical trial. Am Rev Respir Dis 1991;144:291.
48. Mason RJ, Schwarz MI, Hunninghake GW, Musson RA. NHLBI Workshop Summary. Pharmacological therapy for idiopathic pulmonary fibrosis. Past, present, and future. Am J Respir Crit Care Med 1999;160:1771.
49. Ziesche R, Hofbauer E, Wittmann K, Petkov V, Block LH. A preliminary study of long-term treatment with interferon gamma-1b and low-dose prednisolone in patients with idiopathic pulmonary fibrosis. N Engl J Med 1999;341:1264.
50. Raghu G, Johnson WC, Lockhart D, Mageto Y. Treatment of idiopathic pulmonary fibrosis with a new antifibrotic agent, pirfenidone: results of a prospective, open-label Phase II study. Am J Respir Crit Care Med 1999;159:1061.
51. Panos RJ, Mortenson RL, Niccoli SA, King TE Jr. Clinical deterioration in patients with idiopathic pulmonary fibrosis: causes and assessment. Am J Med 1990;88:396.
52. Hubbard R, Venn A, Lewis S, Britton J. Lung cancer and cryptogenic fibrosing alveolitis. A population-based cohort study. Am J Respir Crit Care Med 2000;161:5.
53. Hamman L, Rich A. Acute diffuse interstitial fibrosis of the lung. Bull Johns Hopkins Hosp 1944;74:177.
54. Olson J, Colby TV, Elliott CG. Hamman–Rich syndrome revisited. Mayo Clin Proc 1990;65:1538.
55. Primack SL, Hartman TE, Ikezoe J, Akira M, Sakatani M, Muller NL. Acute interstitial pneumonia: radiographic and CT findings in nine patients. Radiology 1993;188:817.
56. Katzenstein AL, Myers JL, Mazur MT. Acute interstitial pneumonia. A clinicopathologic, ultrastructural, and cell kinetic study. Am J Surg Pathol 1986;10:256.
57. Carrington CB, Gaensler EA, Coutu RE, FitzGerald MX, Gupta RG. Natural history and treated course of usual and desquamative interstitial pneumonia. N Engl J Med 1978;298:801.
58. Yousem SA, Colby TV, Gaensler EA. Respiratory bronchiolitis-associated interstitial lung disease and its relationship to desquamative interstitial pneumonia. Mayo Clin Proc 1989;64:1373.
59. Hartman TE, Primack SL, Swensen SJ, Hansell D, McGuinness G, Muller NL. Desquamative interstitial pneumonia: thin-section CT findings in 22 patients. Radiology 1993;187:787.
60. Myers JL, Veal CF Jr, Shin MS, Katzenstein AL. Respiratory bronchiolitis causing interstitial lung disease. A clinicopathologic study of six cases. Am Rev Respir Dis 1987;135:880.
61. Katzenstein AL, Fiorelli RF. Nonspecific interstitial pneumonia/fibrosis. Histologic features and clinical significance. Am J Surg Pathol 1994;18:136.
62. Park JS, Lee KS, Kim JS, et al. Nonspecific interstitial pneumonia with fibrosis: radiographic and CT findings in seven patients. Radiology 1995;195:645.
63. Bjoraker JA, Ryu JH, Edwin MK, et al. Prognostic significance of histopathologic subsets in idiopathic pulmonary fibrosis. Am J Respir Crit Care Med 1998;157:199.
64. Nagai S, Kitaichi M, Itoh H, Nishimura K, Izumi T, Colby TV. Idiopathic nonspecific interstitial pneumonia/fibrosis: comparison with idiopathic pulmonary fibrosis and BOOP. Eur Respir J 1998;12:1010.
65. Travis WD, Matsui K, Moss J, Ferrans VJ. Idiopathic nonspecific interstitial pneumonia: prognostic significance of cellular and fibrosing patterns: survival comparison with usual interstitial pneumonia and desquamative interstitial pneumonia. Am J Surg Pathol 2000;24:19.
66. Carrington BC, Liebow AA. Lymphocytic interstitial pneumonia. Am J Pathol 1966;48:36.
67. White DA, Matthay RA. Noninfectious pulmonary complications of infection with the human immunodeficiency virus. Am Rev Respir Dis 1989;140:1763.
68. Koss MN, Hochholzer L, Langloss JM, Wehunt WD, Lazarus AA. Lymphoid interstitial pneumonia: clinicopathological and immunopathological findings in 18 cases. Pathology 1987;19:178.
69. Barbera JA, Hayashi S, Hegele RG, Hogg JC. Detection of Epstein–Barr virus in lymphocytic interstitial pneumonia by in situ hybridization. Am Rev Respir Dis 1992;145:940.
70. Setoguchi Y, Takahashi S, Nakiwa T, Kira S. Detection of human T-cell lymphotropic virus type I-related antibodies in patients with lymphocytic interstitial pneumonia. Am Rev Respir Dis 1991;144:1361.
71. Schwarz MI. Lymphoplasmacytic infiltrations of the lung. In: Schwarz MI, King TE Jr (eds) Interstitial lung disease. Hamilton, BC Decker, 1998, p 685.
72. Epler GR, Colby TV, McLoud TC, Carrington CB, Gaensler EA. Bronchiolitis obliterans organizing pneumonia. N Engl J Med 1985;312:152.
73. Cordier JF. Cryptogenic organizing pneumonitis. Bronchiolitis obliterans organizing pneumonia. Clin Chest Med 1993;14:677.
74. Alasaly K, Muller N, Ostrow DN, Champion P, FitzGerald JM. Cryptogenic organizing pneumonia. A report of 25 cases and a review of the literature. Medicine (Baltimore) 1995;74:201.
75. Lee KS, Kullnig P, Hartman TE, Muller NL. Cryptogenic organizing pneumonia: CT findings in 43 patients. Am J Roentgenol 1994;162:543.
76. King TE Jr. Bronchiolitis. In: Schwarz MI, King TE Jr (eds) Interstitial lung disease. Hamilton; BC Decker, 1998, p 645.
77. Jennette JC, Falk RJ, Andrassy K, et al. Nomenclature of systemic vasculitides. Proposal of an international consensus conference. Arthritis Rheum 1994;37:187.
78. Travis WD, Hoffman GS, Leavitt RY, Pass HI, Fauci AS. Surgical pathology of the lung in Wegener's granulomatosis: review of 87 open lung biopsies from 67 patients. Am J Surg Pathol 1991;15:315.
79. Fauci AS, Haynes BF, Katz P, Wolff SM. Wegener's granulomatosis: prospective clinical and therapeutic experience with 85 patients for 21 years. Ann Intern Med 1983;98:76.
80. Hoffman GS, Kerr GS, Leavitt RY, et al. Wegener's granulomatosis: an analysis of 158 patients. Ann Intern Med 1992;116:488.
81. Fontenot A, Jennings C, King TE Jr. Pulmonary opacities and glomerulonephritis in a 15-year-old boy. Chest 1998;113:525.
82. Colby TV. Diffuse alveolar hemorrhage in Wegener's granulomatosis. Semin Respir Med 1989;10:136.
83. Rao JK, Weinberger M, Oddone EZ, Allen NB, Landsman P, Feussner JR. The role of antinuclear cytoplasmic antibody (c-ANCA) testing in the diagnosis of Wegener granulomatosis. Ann Intern Med 1995;123:925.
84. Cordier JF, Valeyre D, Guillevin L, Loire R, Brechot J-M. Pulmonary Wegener's granulomatosis. A clinical and imaging study of 77 cases. Chest 1990;97:906.
85. Jennette JC, Falk RJ. The pathology of vasculitis involving the kidney. Am J Kidney Dis 1994;24:130.
86. Talar-Williams C, Hijazi YM, Walther MM, et al. Cyclophosphamide-induced cystitis and bladder cancer in patients with Wegener granulomatosis. Ann Intern Med 1996;124:477.
87. Ognibene FP, Shelhamer JH, Hoffman GS, et al. *Pneumocystis carinii* pneumonia: a major complication of immunosuppressive therapy in patients with Wegener's granulomatosis. Am J Respir Crit Care Med 1995;151:795.
88. Churg JC, Strauss L. Allergic granulomatosis, allergic angiitis, and polyarteritis nodosa. Am J Pathol 1951;27:277.
89. Lanham JG, Elkon KB, Pusey CD, Hughes GR. Systemic vasculitis with asthma and eosinophilia: a clinical approach to the Churg–Strauss syndrome. Medicine (Baltimore) 1984;63:65.
90. Guillevin L, Lhote F, Gayraud M, et al. Prognostic factors in polyarteritis nodosa and Churg–Strauss syndrome. A prospective study in 342 patients. Medicine (Baltimore) 1996;75:17.
91. Masi AT, Hunder GG, Lie JT, et al. The American College of Rheumatology 1990 criteria for the classification of Churg–Strauss

syndrome (allergic granulomatosis and angiitis). Arthritis Rheum 1990;33:1094.
92. Clutterbuck EJ, Evans DJ, Pusey CD. Renal involvement in Churg–Strauss syndrome. Nephrol Dial Transplant 1990;5:161.
93. Cohen Tervaert JW, Goldschmeding R, Elema JD, et al. Association of autoantibodies to myeloperoxidase with different forms of vasculitis. Arthritis Rheum 1990;33:1264.
94. Erzurum SC, Underwood GA, Hamilos DL, Waldron JA. Pleural effusion in Churg–Strauss syndrome. Chest 1989;95:1357.
95. Wechsler ME, Garpestad E, Flier SR, et al. Pulmonary infiltrates, eosinophilia, and cardiomyopathy following corticosteroid withdrawal in patients with asthma receiving zafirlukast. JAMA 1998;279:455.
96. Cohen P, Guillevin L, Baril L, Lhote F, Noel LH, Lesavre P. Persistence of antineutrophil cytoplasmic antibodies (ANCA) in asymptomatic patients with systemic polyarteritis nodosa or Churg–Strauss syndrome: follow-up of 53 patients. Clin Exp Rheumatol 1995;13:193.
97. Guillevin L, Cohen P, Gayraud M, Lhote F, Jarrousse B, Casassus P. Churg–Strauss syndrome. Clinical study and long-term follow-up of 96 patients. Medicine (Baltimore) 1999;78:26.
98. Leatherman JW, Davies SF, Hoidal JR. Alveolar hemorrhage syndromes: diffuse microvascular lung hemorrhage in immune and idiopathic disorders. Medicine (Baltimore) 1984;63:343.
99. Bosch X, Lopez-Soto A, Mirapeix E, Font J, Ingelmo M, Urbano-Martinez A. Antineutrophil cytoplasmic autoantibody-associated alveolar capillaritis in patients presenting with alveolar hemorrhage. Arch Pathol Lab Med 1994;118:517.
100. Jennings CA, King TE Jr, Tuder R, Cherniack RM, Schwarz MI. Diffuse alveolar hemorrhage with underlying isolated, pauciimmune pulmonary capillaritis. Am J Respir Crit Care Med 1997;155:1101.
101. Travis WD, Colby TV, Lombard C, Carpenter HA. A clinicopathologic study of 34 cases of diffuse pulmonary hemorrhage with lung biopsy confirmation. Am J Surg Pathol 1990;14:1112.
102. Schwarz MI. Diffuse alveolar hemorrhage. In: Schwarz MI, King TE Jr (eds) Interstitial lung disease. Hamilton, BC Decker, 1998, p 535.
103. Perl SI, Pussell BA, Charlesworth JA, Macdonald GJ, Wolnizer M. Goodpasture's (anti-GBM) disease and HLA-DRw2 [letter]. N Engl J Med 1981;305:463.
104. Rees AJ, Peters DK, Amos N, Welsh KI, Batchelor JR. The influence of HLA-linked genes on the severity of anti-GBM antibody-mediated nephritis. Kidney Int 1984;26:445.
105. Wieslander J, Barr JF, Butkowski RJ, et al. Goodpasture antigen of the glomerular basement membrane: localization to noncollagenous regions of type IV collagen. Proc Natl Acad Sci U S A 1984;81:3838.
106. Kalluri R, Gunwar S, Reeders ST, et al. Goodpasture syndrome. Localization of the epitope for the autoantibodies to the carboxyl-terminal region of the alpha 3(IV) chain of basement membrane collagen. J Biol Chem 1991;266:24018.
107. Kalluri R, Gattone VH II, Noelken ME, Hudson BG. The alpha 3 chain of type IV collagen induces autoimmune Goodpasture syndrome. Proc Natl Acad Sci U S A 1994;91:6201.
108. Wilson CB, Smith RC. Goodpasture's syndrome associated with influenza A2 virus infection. Ann Intern Med 1972;76:91.
109. Keogh AM, Ibels LS, Allen DH, Isbister JP, Kennedy MC. Exacerbation of Goodpasture's syndrome after inadvertent exposure to hydrocarbon fumes. Br Med J 1984; 288:188.
110. Donaghy M, Rees AJ. Cigarette smoking and lung haemorrhage in glomerulonephritis caused by autoantibodies to glomerular basement membrane. Lancet 1983; 2:1390.
111. Albert LJ, Inman RD. Molecular mimicry and autoimmunity. N Engl J Med 1999; 341:2068.
112. Feng L, Xia Y, Wilson CB. Alternative splicing of the NCI domain of the human alpha 3(IV) collagen gene. Differential expression of mRNA transcripts that predict three protein variants with distinct carboxyl regions. J Biol Chem 1994; 269:2342.
113. Johnson JP, Moore J Jr, Austin HAD, Balow JE, Antonovych TT, Wilson CB. Therapy of anti-glomerular basement membrane antibody disease: ananlysis of prognostic significance of clinical, pathologic and treatment factors. Medicine (Baltimore) 1985; 64:219.
114. Schwarz MI. Pulmonary manifestations of the collagen vascular diseases. In: Fishman AP, Elias JA, Fishman J, Grippi MA, Kaiser LR, Senior RM (eds) Fishman's Pulmonary diseases and disorders, vol. 1. New York, McGraw-Hill, 1998, p 1115.
115. King TE Jr. Connective tissue disease. In: Schwarz MI, King TE Jr (eds) Interstitial lung disease. Hamilton, BC Decker, 1998, p 451.
116. Orens JB, Martinez FJ, Lynch JP III. Pleuropulmonary manifestations of systemic lupus erythematosus. Rheum Dis Clin North Am 1994;20:159.
117. Murin S, Wiedemann HP, Matthay RA. Pulmonary manifestations of systemic lupus erythematosus. Clin Chest Med 1998;19:641, viii.
118. Matthay RA, Schwarz MI, Petty TL, et al. Pulmonary manifestations of systemic lupus erythematosus: review of twelve cases of acute lupus pneumonitis. Medicine (Baltimore) 1975;54:397.
119. Zamora MR, Warner ML, Tuder R, Schwarz MI. Diffuse alveolar hemorrhage and systemic lupus erythematosus. Clinical presentation, histology, survival, and outcome. Medicine (Baltimore) 1997;76:192.
120. Bankier AA, Kiener HP, Wiesmayr MN, et al. Discrete lung involvement in systemic lupus erythematosus: CT assessment. Radiology 1995;196:835.
121. Boulware DW, Hedgpeth MT. Lupus pneumonitis and anti-SSA(Ro) antibodies. J Rheumatol 1989;16:479.
122. Abramson SB, Dobro J, Eberle MA, et al. Acute reversible hypoxemia in systemic lupus erythematosus. Ann Intern Med 1991;114:941.
123. Simonson JS, Schiller NB, Petri M, Hellmann DB. Pulmonary hypertension in systemic lupus erythematosus. J Rheumatol 1989;16:918.
124. Asherson RA, Higenbottam TW, Dinh Xuan AT, Khamashta MA, Hughes GR. Pulmonary hypertension in a lupus clinic: experience with twenty-four patients. J Rheumatol 1990;17:1292.
125. Caplan A. Certain unusual radiographic appearances in the chest of coal miners suffering from rheumatoid arthritis. Thorax 1953;8:19.
126. Torralbo A, Herrero JA, Portoles J, Barrientos A. Alveolar hemorrhage associated with antineutrophil cytoplasmic antibodies in rheumatoid arthritis. Chest 1994;105:1590.
127. Geterud A, Ejnell H, Mansson I, Sandberg N, Bake B, Bjelle A. Severe airway obstruction caused by laryngeal rheumatoid arthritis. J Rheumatol 1986;13:948.
128. Penny WJ, Knight RK, Rees AM, Thomas AL, Smith AP. Obliterative bronchiolitis in rheumatoid arthritis. Ann Rheum Dis 1982;41:469.
129. Schwarz MI, Lynch DA, Tuder R. Bronchiolitis obliterans: the lone manifestation of rheumatoid arthritis? Eur Respir J 1994;7:817.
130. Gabbay E, Tarala R, Will R, et al. Interstitial lung disease in recent onset rheumatoid arthritis. Am J Respir Crit Care Med 1997;156:528.
131. Barrera P, Laan RF, van Riel PL, Dekhuijzen PN, Boerbooms AM, van de Putte LB. Methotrexate-related pulmonary complications in rheumatoid arthritis. Ann Rheum Dis 1994;53:434.
132. Cooper JA Jr, White DA, Matthay RA. Drug-induced pulmonary disease. Part 2: Noncytotoxic drugs. Am Rev Respir Dis 1986;133:488.
133. Arroliga AC, Podell DN, Matthay RA. Pulmonary manifestations of scleroderma. J Thorac Imaging 1992;7:30.
134. Weaver AL, Divertie MB, Titus JL. Pulmonary scleroderma. Dis Chest 1968; 54:490.
135. Wells AU, Cullinan P, Hansell DM, et al. Fibrosing alveolitis associated with systemic sclerosis has a better prognosis than lone cryptogenic fibrosing alveolitis. Am J Respir Crit Care Med 1994;149:1583.
136. Ungerer RG, Tashkin DP, Furst D, et al. Prevalence and clinical correlates of pulmonary arterial hypertension in progressive systemic sclerosis. Am J Med 1983;75:65.
137. Thurm CA, Wigley FM, Dole WP, Wise RA. Failure of vasodilator infusion to alter pulmonary diffusing capacity in systemic sclerosis. Am J Med 1991;90:547.
138. Stupi AM, Steen VD, Owens GR, Barnes EL, Rodnan GP, Medsger TA Jr. Pulmonary hypertension in the CREST syndrome variant of systemic sclerosis. Arthritis Rheum 1986;29:515.
139. Badesch DB, Tapson VF, McGoon MD, et al. Continuous intravenous epoprostenol for pulmonary hypertension due to the scleroderma spectrum of disease. A randomized, controlled trial. Ann Intern Med 2000;132:425.

140. Troshinsky MB, Kane GC, Varga J, et al. Pulmonary function and gastroesophageal reflux in systemic sclerosis. Ann Intern Med 1994;121:6.
141. Schwarz MI. The lung in polymyositis. Clin Chest Med 1998;19:701, viii.
142. Schwarz MI, Sutarik JM, Nick JA, Leff JA, Emlen JW, Tuder RM. Pulmonary capillaritis and diffuse alveolar hemorrhage. A primary manifestation of polymyositis. Am J Respir Crit Care Med 1995;151:2037.
143. Wasicek CA, Reichlin M, Montes M, Raghu G. Polymyositis and interstitial lung disease in a patient with anti-Jo1 prototype. Am J Med 1984;76:538.

Chapter 85

Sarcoidosis

David R. Moller

INTRODUCTION

Sarcoidosis is a multisystem disorder of unknown etiology characterized by noncaseating epithelioid granulomas in affected organs.[1,2] The disease most commonly affects the lungs and intrathoracic lymph nodes, although granulomatous inflammation may be present in any organ system. Eye and skin involvement is seen in as many as 25% of patients; symptomatic involvement of other organs occurs less frequently.

The clinical presentation and course of sarcoidosis varies greatly.[3–5] Based on mass population screening with chest radiographs in some European countries, it is estimated that 30–60% of patients with sarcoidosis are asymptomatic, usually with isolated bilateral hilar adenopathy.[6] Symptomatic presentations most frequently involve the respiratory system, with symptoms of cough, dyspnea and chest discomfort.[7] Other clinical manifestations depend on the range and extent of extrapulmonary involvement, most commonly involving the eyes, skin, liver and peripheral lymph nodes (Table 85.1). Cardiac and neurologic sarcoidosis may have devastating consequences, but are seen in less than 10% of patients. Löfgren's syndrome is a well defined acute presentation characterized by erythema nodosum, bilateral hilar adenopathy, polyarthritis and often uveitis.[8] Fever, malaise, arthragias and other constitutional symptoms are common in Löfgren's syndrome, and in patients with significant hepatic and widespread lymph node involvement.

Sarcoidosis is found worldwide, though there are striking differences in the prevalence of the disease in different geographic areas and racial groups.[9] In Europe the prevalence ranges from 64 cases per 100 000 population in Sweden to 9 per 100 000 in Italy, with 10–60 cases per 100 000 in most other European countries. In North America the prevalence of sarcoidosis is estimated to range from 3 to 47 per 100 000, with the higher rates

KEY CONCEPTS

- Sarcoidosis is characterized by noncaseating epithelioid granulomas and mononuclear cell inflammation, usually in multiple organ systems.
- Genetic susceptibility to sarcoidosis and its various clinical presentations is suggested by family studies and associations with MHC haplotypes.
- Granulomatous inflammation in sarcoidosis is characterized by oligoclonal expansions of Th1 cells and activated mononuclear phagocytes producing TNF-α, IL-12 and IL-15.
- Pulmonary involvement with bilateral hilar adenopathy, restrictive or obstructive interstitial lung is seen in over 90% of patients.
- Symptomatic, extrapulmonary sarcoidosis is often chronic, requiring treatment to prevent serious permanent organ damage.
- Standard treatment for progressive, symptomatic sarcoidosis involves corticosteroid therapy, although the long-term benefits remain unproven.

Major clinical features of systemic sarcoidosis

Organ system (approx. % involvement)	Major clinical features
Pulmonary (90)	Bilateral hilar adenopathy, restrictive and obstructive disease, fibrocystic disease, bronchiectasis, mycetomas
Upper airway (5–10)	Hoarseness, laryngeal or tracheal obstruction, nasal congestion, sinusitis, saddle nose deformity
Ocular (25)	Anterior and posterior uveitis, chorioretinitis, conjunctivitis, optic neuritis, glaucoma, lacrimal gland enlargement
Skin (20)	Erythema nodosum, chronic nodules and plaques, lupus pernio, alopecia
Hepatic (10)	Hepatomegaly, pruritis, jaundice, cirrhosis
Cardiac (5–10)	Arrhythmias, heart block, cardiomyopathy, sudden death
Central nervous system (5–10)	Cranial neuropathy, e.g. Bell's palsy, aseptic meningitis, brain mass, seizures, obstructing hydrocephalus, myelopathy, polyneuropathy, mononeuritis multiplex
Salivary and parotid gland (10)	Salivary and parotid gland enlargement, sicca syndrome
Hematologic (30–50)	Lymphadenopathy, splenomegaly, hypersplenism anemia, lymphopenia, thrombocytopenia
Joints/musculoskeletal (10–20%)	Polyarthritis, bone cysts, Achilles' tendonitis, heel pain, myopathy
Endocrine (<10)	Hypercalciuria (more common), hypercalcemia, hypopituitarism, diabetes insipidus
Renal (<5)	Renal calculi, nephrocalcinosis, renal failure, epididymitis, testicular mass

Table 85.1 Major clinical features of systemic sarcoidosis

in African-American populations.[10,11] In countries where tuberculosis is common and healthcare uncertain, no reliable epidemiologic data are available because of the difficulty in distinguishing these diseases. Worldwide there is a slight female preponderance. Although all ages can be affected, more than 80% of cases present between the ages of 20 and 50 years.

The frequency of different clinical presentations and the severity of sarcoidosis vary between different groups.[4,5] Löfgren's syndrome has a particularly high frequency among Scandinavians, Irish female immigrants in Britain and Puerto Rican women in New York City, but occurs in less than 5% of African-American patients with sarcoidosis. Lupus pernio, a disfiguring nodular facial condition associated with chronic sarcoidosis, is more frequent in patients of African descent. Cardiac sarcoidosis is present in as many as 50% of Japanese patients with sarcoidosis, but less than 10% of European and North American patients.[9] Hospital statistics and anecdotal experience suggest that race is an important prognostic indicator, with black patients more likely to have chronic persistent disease and suffer from increased morbidity and mortality than white patients with sarcoidosis. In one recent study of mortality data from hospitals in the United States from 1979 to 1991, age-adjusted mortality was consistently higher among Blacks than Whites, and among women compared with men.[12] Overall, sarcoidosis accounted for 0.02% of total deaths in the United States. Other retrospective studies suggest that sarcoidosis is the direct cause of death in <1–6% of cases, with pulmonary insufficiency, massive hemoptysis and cardiac disease the most common causes.

GENETICS AND ENVIRONMENTAL FACTORS

Although the cause of sarcoidosis remains unknown, there is substantial evidence for a genetic predisposition.[13] Familial clustering occurs in approximately 5–16% of patients, with a greater frequency in Black than in White populations.[14] Within the same family sibling pairs are most common, followed by mother–daughter pairs and father–son pairs. A genetic predisposition is strongly supported by the fact that monozygotic twins appear two to four times more likely to develop sarcoidosis than do dizygotic twins. Studies from Germany estimate that the risk of siblings suffering from sarcoidosis is 8–20 times that of the general population.[15] The lack of a clear genetic pattern suggests that susceptibility to sarcoidosis is polygenic and interacts importantly with environmental factors.

HLA studies in sarcoidosis have shown inconsistent results from different ethnic and geographic regions.[13] In Sweden, HLA-DR17 (DR3) has been associated with bilateral hilar adenopathy or erythema nodosum and a good prognosis, whereas DR14 and DR15 were found to be associated with severe, chronic disease.[16] Other studies have reported associations with B27 and uveitis, B13 and chronic disease, DR5 and Italian patients, and DRw52 and Japanese patients. Although one study found that sarcoidosis was associated with MHC haplotypes containing glutamate at position 69 of the DPβ1-chain, the same alleles reported to be a risk factor for chronic beryllium disease, these findings have not been confirmed in other populations.[17–19]

Studies of non-HLA polymorphisms have yielded few clues to the genetic basis of sarcoidosis. Polymorphisms of the angiotensin-converting enzyme (ACE) gene, a protein up-regulated in many patients with sarcoidosis, have been associated with sarcoidosis in Japan, but not in US or European studies. In one study, specific tumor necrosis factor-α (TNF-α) gene polymorphisms were associated with patients with Löfgren's syndrome, although the overall disease frequency of the sarcoidosis cohort did not differ from that of a control group.[20]

Environmental factors may play a role in the etiology of sarcoidosis, given reports of a higher incidence of disease in the springtime months, with time–space clustering, and in certain occupations such as healthcare workers.[21] A noninfectious environmental cause is suggested by a comparison to chronic beryllium disease. This granulomatous lung disease, histologically identical to sarcoidosis, is caused by beryllium dust in a minor proportion of exposed workers. Whether beryllium or other metal dusts, pine pollen, organic dusts or molds that cause hypersensitivity pneumonitis are capable of causing the multisystem disorder recognized as sarcoidosis remains unproven.

Since the initial descriptions of sarcoidosis, investigators have postulated an infectious cause of the disease based on its clinical similarities to other infectious diseases, most notably tuberculosis. Reports of acid-fast organisms and cultivatable mycobacterial or cell wall-deficient organisms have not been confirmed in other centers. Recently, polymerase chain reaction (PCR) methods have been used to search for traces of genetic elements from microbial organisms in sarcoidosis.[22] Studies report mycobacterial DNA or RNA in 0–>50% of tissues from patients with sarcoidosis, but also in control tissues; the lack of consistent results among different investigators has led to skepticism regarding a role for these organisms in sarcoidosis.[22] Recently, Japanese investigators have found high numbers of *Proprionibacterium acnes* or *granulosum* genomes in lymph nodes from Japanese patients with sarcoidosis but not tuberculosis.[23] Given that these organisms are part of the normal skin and upper airway flora, it is not clear how these findings relate to the pathogenesis of the disease. The presence of high titers of antibodies against many viral agents (Epstein–Barr virus, human herpesvirus-8, cytomegalovirus, parainfluenzae, adenovirus) and bacterial antigens (*Proprionibacterium* spp., *Chlamydia* spp., *Borrelia burgdorferi*) in sarcoidosis sera may reflect generalized B-cell activation and not a direct causal relationship. In support of an infectious etiology of sarcoidosis, transmission of systemic granulomas by allogeneic bone marrow transplantation or from a cardiac transplant has been reported.[24]

In the 1940s, Ansgar Kveim reported that the intradermal inoculation of a suspension of sarcoid lymph node tissue resulted in a nodular skin reaction that contained sarcoid-like granulomas in patients with suspected sarcoidosis, but not in control individuals. In this reaction, well formed granulomas take 2–4 weeks to develop, similar to the Mitsuda reaction in patients with tuberculoid leprosy. The active component appears to be a heat-stable cell wall-associated microparticulate, but precise characterization has not been accomplished.[25] No evidence of microbial DNA has been found in this reagent.

Investigators in the 1970s suggested that sarcoidosis may be the result of autoimmunity, owing to the concurrence of sarcoidosis with other autoimmune diseases and the frequent presence of antinuclear antibodies, rheumatoid factor, hypergammaglobulinemia and immune complexes in sarcoidosis.[26] This hypothesis fell into disfavor when sarcoidosis was found to be dominated by activated CD4 T cells at sites of disease. Nonetheless, recent evidence of dysregulated cytokine production and oligoclonal expansions of T cells at sites of disease in sarcoidosis can be marshaled to support an autoimmune origin.[27,28]

IMMUNOLOGY/PATHOGENESIS

The histologic hallmark of sarcoidosis is the presence of discrete, compact noncaseating granulomas (Fig. 85.1). The dominant cell in the central core is the epithelioid cell, thought to be a differentiated form of a mononuclear phagocyte. CD4 lymphocytes and mature macrophages are interspersed throughout the epithelioid core, whereas both CD4 and CD8 lymphocytes are seen around the periphery of the granuloma. Multinucleated giant cells, often containing cytoplasmic inclusions such as Schaumann bodies or asteroid bodies, are scattered throughout the inflammatory locus. In the lung, granulomas tend to form along areas that are rich in lymphatic vessels, such as bronchovascular, bronchial submucosal, subpleural and interlobular septal regions, as well as alveolar and bronchial walls. Granulomas in sarcoidosis tend to vary from cellular forms to acellular, hyalinized ghosts of granulomas that probably reflect an evolution to an inactive or fibrotic form.

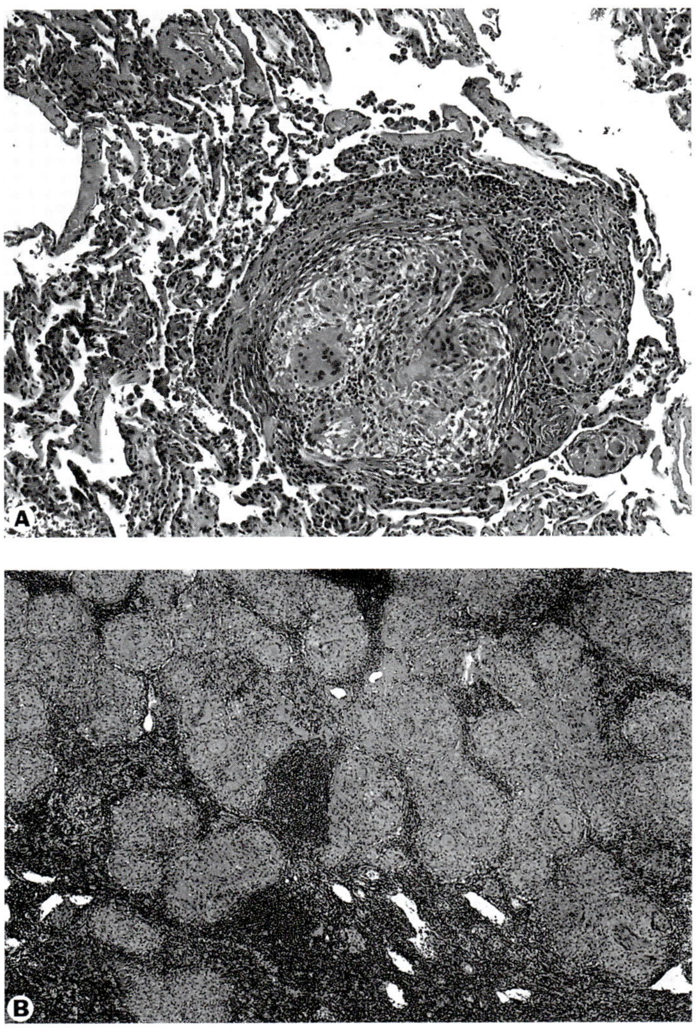

Figure 85.1. (A) Open lung biopsy showing typical noncaseating epithelioid granuloma, giant cells and lymphocytic infiltrates in lung parenchyma in sarcoidosis. **(B)** Lymph node biopsy showing extensive replacement with well-defined epithelioid granulomas in a patient with sarcoidosis. (See also colour plate 85.1B)

Current concepts of the immunopathogenesis of sarcoidosis have been based largely on studies using bronchoalveolar lavage (BAL) to recover cells and fluid from patients with active pulmonary disease.[29] Landmark studies in the early 1980s demonstrated that patients with pulmonary sarcoidosis are characterized by increased proportions and numbers of activated CD4 alveolar lymphocytes, reflective of enhanced cell-mediated immune processes at sites of granuloma formation.[30] Prior to this development, sarcoidosis was thought to be a disease of immune depression exemplified by circulating lymphopenia and cutaneous anergy.

Lung T cells in pulmonary sarcoidosis express a phenotype indicative of recent activation.[28] Approximately 5–10% of lung T cells are IL2R$^+$, 30–50% are class II MHC DR$^+$ and >50% express the late activation marker VLA-1 (very late activation antigen-1, CD49a). Importantly, sarcoid lung T cells demonstrate reduced surface density of the CD3:T-cell receptor complex, a hallmark of T cells activated through the T-cell antigen receptor (TCR) pathway.[31] Consistent with recent activation, greater numbers of lung T cells express the cell cycle-related nuclear antigen Ki67, and a small proportion of lung T cells are spontaneously proliferating. These activated cells produce greater amounts of IL-2, IFN-γ and IL-6 ex vivo than do BAL cells from healthy controls, findings that are also consistent with in situ mRNA cytokine analyses of sarcoid tissue.[32] In contrast to the lung, patients with sarcoidosis often demonstrate CD4 T-cell lymphopenia in their blood.

In order to define disease-specific T cells and potentially identify etiologically relevant antigens, investigators have analyzed TCR gene expression in sarcoidosis.[28] Results from these studies have shown that subgroups of patients are characterized by expanded oligoclonal populations of lung, blood or skin T cells expressing specific gene segments from the variable regions of the TCR.[33–35] The most compelling data involve studies demonstrating expanded numbers of Vα2.3$^+$ lung T cells in Swedish patients with DR17(3)/DQ2 haplotypes, suggesting T-cell responses to a specific peptide/MHC complex.[34] Sequence analyses demonstrate that expanded $\alpha\beta^+$ T-cell subsets are oligoclonal and sometimes contain shared amino acid motifs in the CDR3 region of their Vβ or Vα/Jα genes, consistent with a local antigen-driven T-cell response.[36,37] These studies provided the first direct evidence that granulomatous inflammation in sarcoidosis is an antigen-driven response to a conventional antigen(s). Despite intense efforts, the reactivities of these expanded T-cell clones have yet to be identified.

As many as 30% of sarcoidosis patients have greater proportions of $\gamma\delta^+$ T cells in their blood,[38,39] predominantly of the Vγ9$^+$Vδ2$^+$ subset. Other studies have found that the increase in $\gamma\delta^+$ T cells is secondary to a reduction in circulating $\alpha\beta^+$ T cells, or have found no difference from control populations.[40] As $\gamma\delta^+$ T cells are rarely found around granulomas in lymph nodes or skin, their role in the pathogenesis of sarcoidosis remains uncertain.[41]

Alveolar macrophages are thought to play a central role in the development of granulomatous inflammation in sarcoidosis by presenting disease-specific antigens and producing cytokines that regulate granuloma formation.[29,42] Investigators have reported that alveolar macrophages from patients with sarcoidosis express higher levels of surface class II MHC (DR, DQ, DP) molecules, leukocyte function associated-antigen-1 (LFA-1), intracellular adhesion molecule-1 (ICAM-1) and the accessory molecules CD86 (B7.2), CD80 (B7.1) and CD40 than do alveolar macrophages from healthy controls.[43] These characteristics probably contribute to the enhanced ability of sarcoid alveolar macrophages to present antigen to autologous T cells compared to normal alveolar macrophages.[44] These cells also produce increased amounts of lysozyme, angiotensin-converting enzyme and reactive oxygen species, and less than normal amounts of the counterinflammatory prostaglandin E_2. Importantly, sarcoid alveolar macrophages spontaneously produce TNF-α, IL-6, IL-12, IL-15 and IL-18, cytokines known to regulate granuloma formation.[45–47] Lung macrophages release increased amounts of fibronectin and insulin-like growth factor-1 (IGF-1), which are important in fibroblast recruitment and replication.

Several chemotactic cytokines (chemokines), including monocyte chemotactic protein (MCP)-1, RANTES, macrophage inflammatory protein (MIP)-1, MIG (monokine-induced by IFN-γ), IL-8 and osteopontin (early T-lymphocyte activation protein), are produced by BAL cells in sarcoidosis.[42,48] These chemokines probably assist in the recruitment of T cells, blood monocytes and granulocytes to inflammatory loci in sarcoidosis. NK cells, B cells and mast cells are also occasionally seen around granulomas; their contributions to the inflammatory response are uncertain.

Substantial evidence indicates that granulomatous inflammation in sarcoidosis is dominated by a Th1 cytokine profile (Fig. 85.2).[49] BAL studies demonstrate increased mRNA and protein levels of IFN-γ and IL-2, with low or undetectable levels of IL-4 and IL-5 in pulmonary sarcoidosis.[46,50] Consistent with a polarized type 1 process, IL-12 has been found to be markedly up-regulated in BAL fluid and in cells from the lungs and lymph nodes of patients with sarcoidosis.[32,46] Alveolar macrophages from some patients who had sarcoidosis for years were found to produce greater than normal amounts of IL-12 without stimulation or when stimulated with bacterial products, suggesting that dysregulated IL-12 production is a feature of chronic sarcoidosis.[46] As higher than normal proportions of lung T cells from patients with sarcoidosis express IL-12 receptor β_2 chains, a marker of Th1 cells, it is likely that locally produced IL-12 contributes to Th1 cell activation and development in sarcoidosis.[51] Because IFN-γ and IL-12 are potent costimulators of each other, Th1-driven granulomatous inflammation in sarcoidosis may be maintained by a positive feedback loop between IL-12 and IFN-γ, similar to processes documented in several experimental models of infectious and autoimmune diseases.[49] Consistent with this scenario, IFN-α therapy, a known inducer of type 1 cytokine expression, has been associated with the development of sarcoidosis during treatment of hepatitis C.[52]

Over 50% of all patients with sarcoidosis have remission of their disease. The determinants of this outcome are unknown. Importantly, a recent study found that patients with active sarcoidosis who underwent spontaneous remission within 6 months had significantly greater production of transforming growth factor-β (TGF-β) from their cultured BAL cells at the time of initial evaluation than did patients who later required therapy or who demonstrated progressive disease.[53] Because TGF-β is a potent endogenous inhibitor of IL-12 and $CD4^+$ Th1 development, these observations suggest that TGF-β may be important in the down-regulation of Th-1 driven granulomatous responses in sarcoidosis.

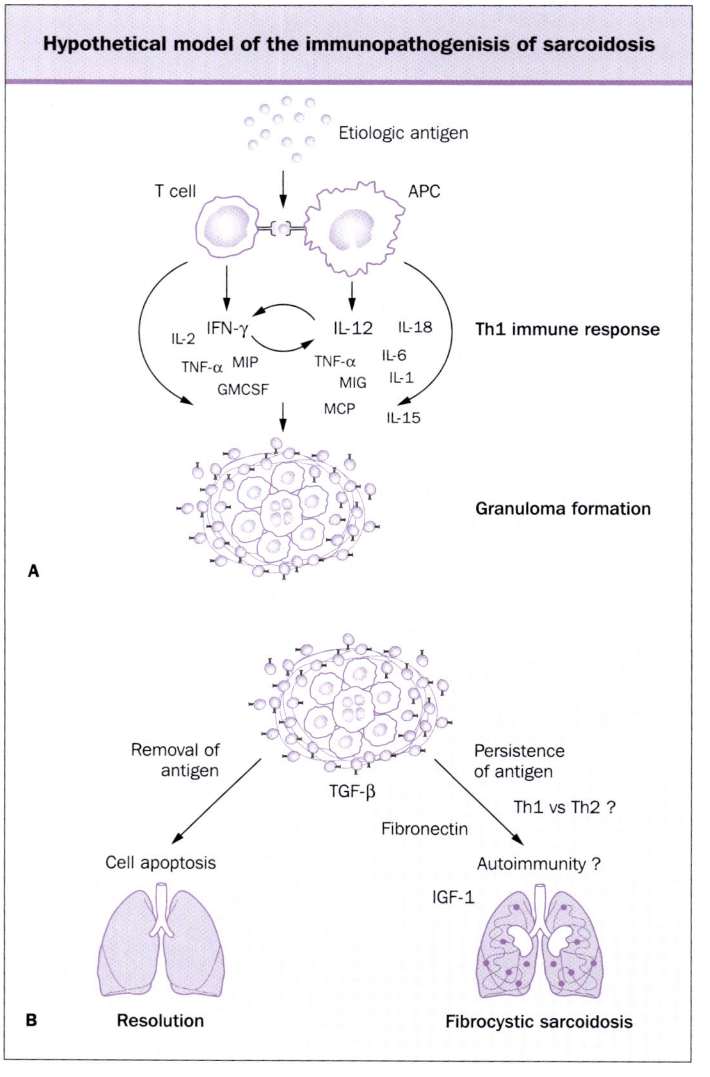

Figure 85.2. Hypothetical model of the immunopathogenesis of sarcoidosis. (A) Granuloma formation in sarcoidosis results from stimulation by an insoluble antigen that evokes an adaptive T-cell immune response and stimulates the production of IL-12 along with other cytokines from mononuclear phagocytes and dendritic cells. Granulomatous inflammation is maintained by a Th1 immune response driven by IFN-γ, IL-12 and IL-18. **(B)** Remission vs. chronic fibrotic sarcoidosis. After the removal of stimulating antigen(s), suppression of Th1-driven granuloma formation is mediated by TGF-β, IL-10 and other mediators, followed by granuloma resorption with cell apoptosis. Progressive fibrosis results from persistent, possibly autoimmune, antigenic stimulation in the presence of either Th1 or Th2 cytokines and TGF-β, IGF-1 and other profibrotic mediators.

Although fibrocystic lung disease occurs in 10–20% of patients with pulmonary sarcoidosis, the pathogenesis of fibrosis in these patients is largely unstudied. Rodent models of immune-mediated granulomatous processes indicate that the propensity to develop fibrosis is greater with type 2 than with type 1-dependent granulomatous responses.[54] Theoretically, fibrocystic sarcoidosis could develop in a subset of patients with Th2-driven granulomatous inflammation, or could result from unremitting Th1-mediated lung injury with subsequent reparative fibrosis. In either scenario, profibrotic cytokines such as TGF-β, insulin-like growth factor-1 and fibronectin, which are expressed in the lungs of patients with pulmonary sarcoidosis, probably contribute to a fibrotic outcome.[55]

PATIENT EVALUATION AND DIFFERENTIAL DIAGNOSIS

Pulmonary sarcoidosis

The most common symptoms of pulmonary sarcoidosis are a progressive shortness of breath, a nonproductive cough and ill-defined, variably severe chest discomfort (Table 85.1). Chronic sputum production and hemoptysis are more frequent in advanced fibrocystic disease. Typically, there are few physical findings in pulmonary sarcoidosis. Lung crackles are heard in less than 20% of patients and clubbing is rare. Findings of pulmonary hypertension or cor pulmonale are seen in 1–4% of patients, usually from severe fibrocystic sarcoidosis or, rarely, a granulomatous vasculitis of the pulmonary vessels.

Chest radiographs are abnormal in more than 90% of patients with sarcoidosis. By international convention, the chest radiograph is divided into the following stages or types:[4,5]

Stage 0: normal chest radiograph
I: bilateral hilar adenopathy
II: bilateral hilar adenopathy + interstitial infiltrates
III: interstitial infiltrates only (non-fibrotic)
IV: fibrocystic interstitial lung disease.

A normal chest X-ray is found in 5–10% of patients with sarcoidosis, frequently in those with extrathoracic manifestations. Stage I is seen in 40–50% of cases on initial presentation. Typically, the hilar adenopathy is discrete, symmetric, and often accompanied by right paratracheal adenopathy. A stage II chest radiograph, often with mid- or upper-zone infiltrates, is seen in 20–30% of cases on initial presentation (Fig. 85.3). A stage III radiograph is seen in 10–20% of cases on initial presentation. Chest radiographs with fibrocystic changes and scarring are frequently placed in a separate subgroup, stage IV, in recognition of the poor outcome of this group of patients (Fig. 85.4). Mycetomas are mobile fungus balls that colonize pre-existing cystic spaces in fibrocystic sarcoidosis. More unusual patterns of pulmonary sarcoidosis include large, well defined nodular infiltrates, miliary disease, or a pattern of patchy air-space consolidation with air bronchograms, termed 'alveolar sarcoidosis'. Differential diagnoses often include mycobacterial or fungal infection, malignancy or Wegener's granulomatosis. Pleural effusions and pneumothorax are rare.

Computed tomography (CT) of the chest is more sensitive than plain radiography in demonstrating enlarged lymph nodes and pulmonary infiltrates.[56] Chest CT typically demonstrates nodular infiltrates that follow central bronchovascular structures (Fig. 85.5). Lymphangitic carcinomatosis also follows a bronchovascular distribution and must be considered in the differential diagnosis.

Pulmonary function tests do not correlate well with chest radiographs.[56] In patients with stage I chest radiographs pulmonary function tests are normal in about 80% of cases, or have only an isolated reduction in diffusing capacity for carbon monoxide (DL_{CO}). When pulmonary infiltrates are present on chest radiography, restrictive impairment with reduction in lung volumes, FVC and FEV_1, or a reduction in DL_{CO} is found in 40–70% of cases. Obstructive impairment is found in <30–50% of patients,

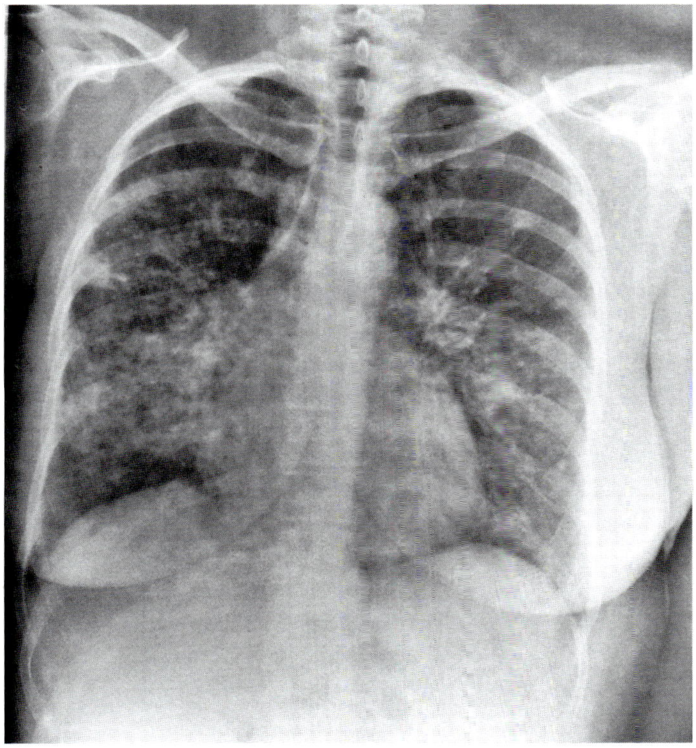

Figure 85.3 Chest radiograph demonstrating a stage II pattern with bilateral hilar adenopathy and reticulonodular infiltrates.

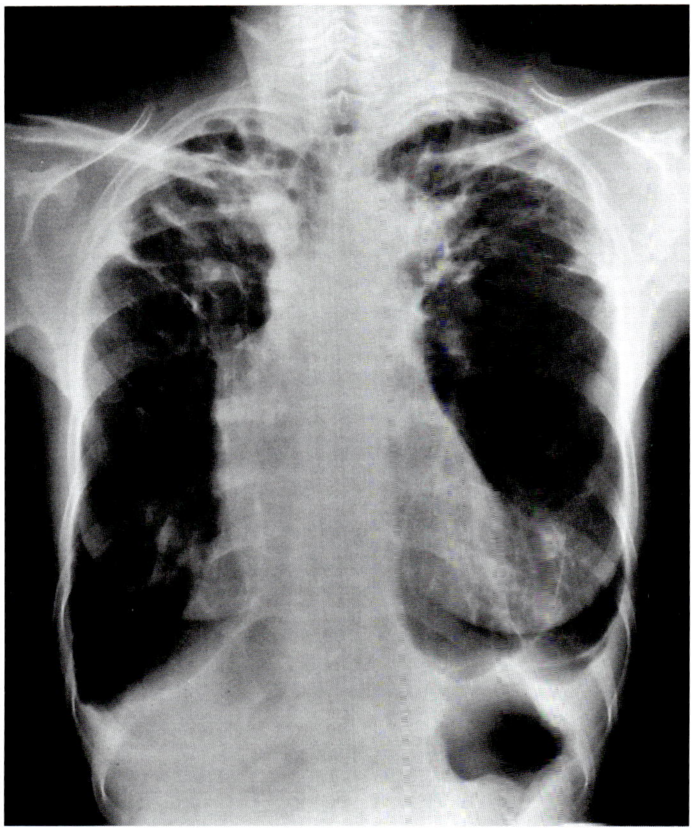

Figure 85.4 Fibrocystic (stage IV) pulmonary sarcoidosis with typical upward hilar retraction and multiple cystic and bullous changes.

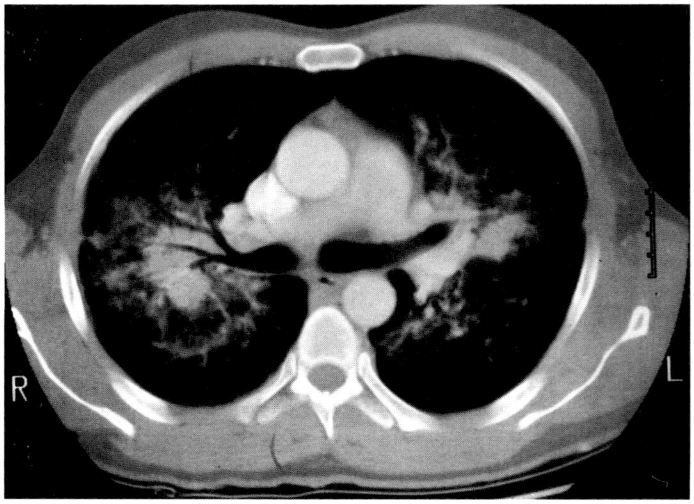

Figure 85.5 CT scan of the chest in a patient with biopsy-proven pulmonary sarcoidosis, demonstrating bilateral hilar, paratracheal and paraaortic lymphadenopathy with interstitial infiltrates in a dominantly central bronchovascular distribution.

most often in advanced fibrocystic sarcoidosis. Bronchial hyperreactivity is present in 10–30% of patients. Gas exchange is usually preserved until extensive fibrocystic changes are evident.

Extrapulmonary sarcoidosis

Although pulmonary symptoms are the most common presenting complaint, many patients have clinically important involvement of one or more organs systems, either with or without pulmonary sarcoidosis (Table 85.1).[3]

Sarcoidosis of the upper respiratory tract occurs in approximately 5–10% of patients, usually those with long-standing disease.[57] Involvement of the mucosa of the nasal septum, inferior turbinates and nasopharynx may lead to nasal congestion, dizziness, crusting, epistaxis, anosmia or rhinorrhea. Nasal septal perforation, a 'saddle nose' deformity or palatal perforation may occur, particularly in patients with previous submucous resections. Sarcoidosis may affect the maxillary, ethmoid and sphenoid sinuses, leading to obstruction and sinusitis. Direct invasion into contiguous bone may be seen on CT scan. Laryngeal sarcoidosis is an uncommon feature of sarcoidosis, occurring in <1–5% of patients, and rarely as the sole manifestation of disease. Patients usually present with hoarseness, dysphonia, dysphagia, dyspnea or, rarely, stridor and acute respiratory failure.

Ocular sarcoidosis

Unilateral or bilateral anterior uveitis is the most common presentation of ocular sarcoidosis and is often associated with bilateral hilar adenopathy. Chronic uveitis occurs in as many as 20% of patients with chronic sarcoidosis, more frequently in Black populations. Other manifestations include posterior uveitis, granulomatous conjunctivitis or severe chorioretinitis, or optic neuritis; these latter conditions may present acutely with blindness.

Cutaneous sarcoidosis

Erythema nodosum may be seen as a component of Löfgren's syndrome. Chronic skin sarcoidosis usually manifests as nontender and nonpruritic plaques and subcutaneous nodules around the hairline, eyelids, ears, nose, mouth, and the extensor surfaces of the arms and legs. Lupus pernio is a particularly disfiguring form of cutaneous sarcoidosis of the face, with violaceous plaques and nodules covering the nose, nasal alae, malar areas, and around the eyes.

Cardiac sarcoidosis

Cardiac sarcoidosis is clinically apparent in 5% or fewer patients with sarcoidosis in North America and Europe, but appears to be more common in Japan.[9,58] In one large study complete heart block was the most common manifestation; ventricular arrhythmias, bundle branch blocks, sudden death, cardiomyopathy, supraventricular arrhythmias and valvular dysfunction were less common.[59] Arrhythmias, heart block or congestive heart failure are responsible for most of the deaths related to cardiac sarcoidosis.

Hepatic sarcoidosis

Symptomatic hepatic sarcoidosis manifests with fever, tender hepatomegaly or pruritis. Characteristically, the serum alkaline phosphatase and γ-glutamyl transferase are elevated proportionately higher than the aspartate aminotransferase (AST) and alanine aminotransferase (ALT) and bilirubin, though all patterns can be seen. Hepatic sarcoidosis may mimic primary biliary cirrhosis, except that antimitochondrial antibodies are absent.

Joints and bones

Arthralgias are common in active multisystem sarcoidosis, although joint radiographs are usually negative. Acute, often incapacitating, migratory polyarthritis involving the ankles, feet, knees and wrists is seen in Löfgren's syndrome; usually the polyarthritis regresses within weeks to several months with or without therapy. Persistent joint disease is found in less than 5% of patients with chronic sarcoidosis. Pain, swelling and tenderness of the phalanges of the hands and feet are most common. Joint radiographs may demonstrate 'punched-out' lesions with cystic changes and marked loss of trabeculae but without evidence of erosive chrondritis. Cystic lesions of the long bones, pelvis, sternum, skull and vertebrae rarely occur.

Neurosarcoidosis

Neurosarcoidosis occurs in approximately 5% of patients with sarcoidosis. The most common manifestation is cranial neuropathy, with bilateral or unilateral seventh-nerve (Bell's) palsy or, less commonly, glossopharyngeal, auditory, oculomotor or trigeminal palsies.[60] The palsy may resolve spontaneously or with corticosteroids, but sometimes recurs years later. Optic neuritis can result in blurred vision, field defects and blindness. Manifestations of central nervous system (CNS) involvement include mass lesions, aseptic meningitis, obstructive hydrocephalus and hypothalamic/pituitary dysfunction. Seizures, headache, change in mental status, confusion and diabetes insipidus may be presenting symptoms. Spinal cord compression syndromes are rare, but paraparesis, hemiparesis and back and leg pain have been described. Peripheral neuropathies account for about 15% of cases of neurosarcoidosis, often presenting as mononeuritis multiplex or a primary sensory neuropathy.

Salivary, parotid and lacrimal gland sarcoidosis

Parotid or lacrimal gland enlargement or sicca syndrome can occasionally be the dominant clinical manifestations of sarcoidosis. Herefordt's syndrome, also known as uveoparotid fever, manifests as fever, parotid and lacrimal gland enlargement, uveitis and bilateral hilar adenopathy. This uncommon presentation of acute sarcoidosis can be associated with cranial neuropathies, usually facial palsy.

Hematologic sarcoidosis

Peripheral lymph node enlargement occurs in 20–30% of patients as an early manifestation of sarcoidosis, but then typically undergoes spontaneous remission. Persistent, bulky lymphadenopathy occurs less than 10% of the time. Splenomegaly, occasionally massive, occurs in less than 5% of cases and is often associated with hepatomegaly and, less frequently, hypercalcemia. Nonclonal hypergammaglobulinemia is present in 25% or more of patients.

Sarcoid myopathy

Although random muscle biopsies in autopsy series demonstrate muscle granulomas in a majority of patients with sarcoidosis, symptomatic myopathy with weakness and tenderness is uncommon. Rarely, sarcoidosis can present as a polymyositis with profound weakness and elevated serum creatine kinase and aldolase.

Hypercalcemia, hypercalciuria and renal disease

Hypercalcemia is present in 2–5% of patients; hypercalcuria is more common. Abnormal calcium regulation is thought to be due to an increased conversion of 1-OH vitamin D_3 to the active 1,25-(OH)2 vitamin D_3 by macrophages and epithelioid cells from granulomas. Chronic hypercalcemia or hypercalciuria most commonly manifests as kidney stones. Renal failure from chronic, clinically silent, nephrocalcinosis may occur. Granulomatous involvement of the kidneys is uncommon and usually not a cause of renal failure.

Diagnosis

A diagnosis of sarcoidosis is based on a compatible clinical picture, histologic evidence of noncaseating granulomas and the absence of other known causes of this pathologic response. Tuberculosis, fungal disease and lymphoma are usually the most important diseases to be excluded in patients with chest disease. Chronic beryllium disease and hypersensitivity pneumonitis must be excluded when there is a compatible history and clinical findings are confined to the lung. Collagen vascular disease or vasculitis, such as Wegener's granulomatosis, must be considered in the context of pulmonary disease and a multisystem disorder. In the absence of defined multisystem disease a diagnosis of sarcoidosis should be presumed, as local 'sarcoid' reactions may occur in response to infection, tumor or foreign material. Biopsy confirmation of sarcoidosis is usually not necessary in Löfgren's syndrome, except in regions where histoplasmosis is endemic, and fungal infection must be excluded prior to initiating corticosteroid therapy.

In general, biopsy of the easiest, most accessible abnormal tissue site is used to confirm the diagnosis. Biopsy of a skin nodule, superficial lymph node, lacrimal gland, nasal mucosae, conjunctivae or salivary gland (lip biopsy) can often establish a diagnosis. Biopsy of the liver or bone marrow is nonspecific and should be used to support a diagnosis of sarcoidosis only after malignancy, infectious granulomatous diseases or other organ-specific diagnoses have been excluded.

Biopsy by fiberoptic bronchoscopy is frequently used to diagnose pulmonary sarcoidosis because of its relative safety and high yield. The yield of transbronchial biopsy is operator dependent, but approaches 80–90% when pulmonary infiltrates are seen radiographically (Figs 85.3–85.5). The yield is less than 50% in patients with a stage 1 chest radiograph.[61] Endobronchial or transbronchial needle aspiration biopsies may increase the yield further. Mediastinoscopy or thoracoscopic or open lung biopsy should be considered in cases where lymphoma or other intrathoracic malignancy cannot be reasonably excluded.

An initial diagnostic evaluation of a patient with possible sarcoidosis should consist of tests to evaluate the presence and extent of pulmonary involvement and screen for extrathoracic disease.[2] Specialized testing is indicated when symptoms or signs suggest extrapulmonary involvement. In the presence of cardiac symptoms, a 2D echocardiogram and Holter monitor are usually indicated to evaluate wall motion abnormalities and potentially dangerous arrhythmias.[60] Radionuclide imaging with gated 201-thallium scanning may show segmental areas of decreased uptake that correspond to areas involved with granulomatous inflammation or fibrosis. Gallium or technetium pyrophosphate scans may also show abnormalities, but are nonspecific. A diagnosis of cardiac sarcoidosis is usually made clinically, with biopsy confirmation of a site other than the heart. Endomyocardial biopsy is positive in only 20–30% of cases of cardiac sarcoidosis, owing to the patchiness of the granulomatous inflammation; thus, a negative biopsy never excludes the diagnosis.

When CNS sarcoidosis is considered, MRI with gadolinium enhancement is now considered the optimal test to detect characteristic inflammatory lesions that have a propensity for periventricular and leptomeningeal areas.[60] The images are nonspecific and can be produced by infectious (tuberculosis, fungal disease) or malignant (lymphoma, carcinomatosis) disease. A normal scan does not exclude neurosarcoidosis, particularly for cranial neuropathies or in the presence of corticosteroid therapy. Cerebral spinal fluid characteristically demonstrates lymphocytic pleocytosis and/or elevated protein levels. A diagnosis of neurosarcoidosis is usually confirmed by biopsy of a non-CNS site, generally by bronchoscopic or lymph node biopsy. Rarely, brain biopsy is needed to exclude infectious or malignant disease. In suspected cases of peripheral neuropathy or myopathy, EMG or nerve conduction studies should be considered.

CLINICAL PEARLS

Tests recommended for an initial evaluation of a patient with sarcoidosis

- Chest radiograph
- Pulmonary function tests
  - Spirometry
  - Diffusing capacity
  - Lung volumes
  - Flow–volume loop (if suspected upper airway obstruction)
- Slit-lamp examination (to exclude subclinical uveitis)
- Liver and renal function tests
- Calcium level
- Complete blood count
- Electrocardiogram
- Purified protein derivative skin test

Other diagnostic studies

Several noninvasive tests have been proposed to assist the clinician in making a diagnosis of sarcoidosis.[2,62] For example, many studies have examined the usefulness of BAL results.[2] Although >90% of nonsmoking patients with pulmonary sarcoidosis have increased proportions of $CD4^+$ BAL T cells, typically with a CD4:CD8 ratio of 3–10:1 compared to 2:1 in healthy individuals, and a CD8 T-cell predominance in hypersensitivity pneumonitis, viral infections and many drug reactions, these findings are not sufficiently specific to establish a diagnosis of sarcoidosis. Levels of serum angiotensin-converting enzyme (SACE) have also been proposed as a diagnostic aid, as this enzyme is elevated in 40–90% of patients with clinically active disease.[63] However, elevated SACE levels are found both in other granulomatous diseases (e.g. chronic beryllium disease, fungal and mycobacterial infections) and in some nongranulomatous conditions, such as Gaucher's disease, hyperthyroidism, hepatic cirrhosis, diabetes mellitus and Hodgkin's disease. The lack of specificity of SACE elevations in sarcoidosis limits its usefulness for diagnosis.[62] Gallium-67 scans almost always demonstrate enhanced uptake in the lungs and mediastinal lymph node area in patients with active pulmonary sarcoidosis, but are nonspecific.

PREVENTION AND PATIENT MANAGEMENT

The clinical course of sarcoidosis is highly variable.[4,5] Overall, 50–65% of patients undergo spontaneous remission, usually (>85%) within the first 2 years. The prognosis is best for those with Löfgren's syndrome, >80% of whom have a spontaneous remission. Peripheral adenopathy, salivary and parotid gland enlargement and Bell's palsy generally subside spontaneously or with treatment, and do not recur. Elevated serum liver function tests also can revert to normal without treatment. The rate of spontaneous remission in pulmonary sarcoidosis differs according to the initial chest X-ray pattern. Approximately 50–80% of patients with a stage I chest radiograph have remission, whereas 30–60% with a stage II radiograph and 20–30% with a stage III undergo remission. Patients who present with a stage IV chest radiograph with fibrocystic changes rarely (<5%) undergo remission. Extrapulmonary disease that is symptomatic and severe on presentation tends to persist and require treatment. Patients with lupus pernio, bony involvement, nephrocalcinosis and hepatosplenomegaly rarely undergo spontaneous remission.

The intensity of surveillance of sarcoidosis depends on the severity of clinical presentation, but should include serial tests of organ-specific function. The first 2 years of follow-up are critical, given that this interval usually separates those with acute, remitting versus chronic disease. When sarcoidosis undergoes remission, the disease rarely recurs. Noninvasive tests such as BAL, SACE, gallium scanning and other biochemical measurements have not been shown to be useful in management decisions.[2,64]

TREATMENT

Corticosteroids remain the mainstay of therapy for serious or progressive pulmonary or extrapulmonary sarcoidosis (Table 85.2).[65] Corticosteroids acutely provide symptomatic relief and reverse organ dysfunction in >90% of patients with symptomatic disease. Although there is controversy regarding their overall effectiveness in altering the long-term course of the disease, there is widespread agreement that early treatment is indicated for serious pulmonary or extrapulmonary disease. When there is not serious or organ-threatening involvement, a period of observation is often indicated to evaluate whether the patient will undergo spontaneous remission.

The optimal doses and duration of corticosteroid treatment have not been established by rigorous clinical studies. Extensive clinical experience has shown that initial treatment with corticosteroids usually requires no more than 30–40 mg/day of prednisone for 2–4 weeks, followed by a slow tapering regimen over several months to a maintenance dose of 5–15 mg/day (Table 85.2).[65,66] Alternate-day therapy (e.g. 10–30 mg every other day) is suggested by some investigators, although such a regimen may not be effective in a subgroup of patients who then respond to daily dosing. Treatment should ordinarily be continued for a minimum of 8–12 months, as premature tapering is likely to result in relapse. Intermittent attempts to taper steroids are appropriate in the first several years of treatment, but patients with repetitive relapses usually require indefinite suppressive therapy. Inhaled corticosteroids may be helpful in reducing symptoms of endobronchial sarcoidosis, such as cough or airway irritability, but have not been proven useful as sole agents in pulmonary sarcoidosis, except possibly in mild disease.[67]

Low-dose corticosteroid therapy is usually well tolerated. Weight gain, hypertension and hyperglycemia may be difficult to manage in some patients, and glaucoma and osteoporosis are serious long-term complications of corticosteroid therapy. To avoid the potential for hypercalcemia and hypercalciuria, routine use of supplemental calcium and vitamin D is often avoided. The benefit of newer antiosteoporosis medications (bisphosphonates) seems likely, but clinical studies are lacking.

THERAPEUTIC PRINCIPLES

Indications for corticosteroid therapy in patients with sarcoidosis

- Pulmonary involvement
  - Moderate or severe, symptomatic pulmonary disease
  - Progressive, symptomatic pulmonary disease
  - Persistent pulmonary infiltrates or abnormal lung function for 1–2 years with mild symptoms to assess reversibility
  - Advanced fibrocystic disease
- Extrapulmonary involvement
  - Threatened organ failure: severe ocular, cardiac or CNS disease
  - Posterior uveitis or anterior uveitis not responding to local steroids
  - Persistent hypercalcemia
  - Persistent renal or hepatic dysfunction
  - Pituitary disease
  - Myopathy
  - Palpable splenomegaly or evidence of hypersplenism such as thrombocytopenia
  - Severe fatigue and weight loss
  - Painful lymphadenopathy
  - Disfiguring skin disease

Medications and doses used in the treatment of sarcoidosis		
Drug	**Typical dose**	**Major adverse effects**
Corticosteroids	Prednisone 30–40 mg/day for 2 wks Decrease by 5 mg/day every 2 wks until 10–15 mg/day; maintain for 8–12 months then taper 2.5 mg/day every 2–4 wks; Reinstitute for relapse	Weight gain Hypertension Hyperglycemia Osteoporosis Cataracts
Antimalarial drugs		
Hydroxychloroquine	200 mg daily to b.i.d.	Ocular toxicity (rare) Gastrointestinal upset
Chloroquine	250 mg daily (500 mg every 2 days) for 6 months, followed by 6-month drug holiday	Ocular toxicity (retinopathy)
Azathioprine	100–200 mg/day	Hematologic suppression Hepatic toxicity ?Oncogenic potential
Methotrexate	10–20 mg/wk	Hepatic toxicity Bone marrow suppression Pulmonary toxicity
Pentoxifylline	400 mg 3–4 times daily	Gastrointestinal upset Headache
Thalidomide	100–200 mg nightly	Terotogenicity Peripheral neuropathy Sedation

Table 85.2 Medications and doses used in the treatment of sarcoidosis.

Specific situations

Löfgren's syndrome

Nonsteroidal anti-inflammatory drugs are recommended for the relief of constitutional symptoms and joint pains. For disabling arthritis or severe constitutional symptoms, corticosteroids are almost immediately effective. Generally, the steroids can be tapered over a few weeks to months without recrudescence of symptoms.

Mucocutaneous sarcoidosis

The antimalarial drugs chloroquine and hydroxychloroquine have been used as first-line treatment for mucocutaneous disease, including lupus pernio, other disfiguring skin disease and nasal, sinus and laryngeal sarcoidosis. The beneficial effects may not be evident for 2–3 months, with an overall 40–50% response rate. Hydroxychloroquine is less effective than chloroquine, but because of its lower potential for ocular toxicity is usually tried first and may be used without interruption (Table 85.2).

Ocular sarcoidosis

Anterior uveitis can often be treated effectively with topical corticosteroids alone. Oral corticosteroids are usually necessary for posterior uveitis, chorioretinitis and optic neuritis. The latter two may present as ocular emergencies requiring high doses of intravenous corticosteroids initially.

Cardiac sarcoidosis

Treatment consists of antiarrhythmic therapy, diuretics and afterload-reducing agents for heart failure, in addition to anti-inflammatory drugs.[58] Corticosteroids are recommended in moderate doses based on observations that such treatment may reverse heart block, reduce arrhythmias and improve ejection fraction. An overall improvement in mortality has not been proved by prospective study. Initial therapy often begins with prednisone 40–60 mg/day, followed by a slow taper to a maintenance dose of 10–20 mg/day. Automatic implantable defibrillators or pacemakers are indicated in patients at risk for sudden death from serious arrhythmias or heart block.

Neurosarcoidosis

High doses of oral corticosteroids (60–80 mg/day) or high-dose pulse intravenous therapy are often employed for serious CNS involvement.[60] Tapering should be performed over several months after evidence of suppression of inflammation by objective criteria (e.g. serial MRI scans). With the exception of cranial neuropathies, neurosarcoidosis tends to be chronic and requires long-term therapy. Endocrine deficiency from hypopituitarism may not respond to steroid therapy.

Hepatic sarcoidosis

Persistently elevated liver function tests (e.g. alkaline phosphatase >2–3 times normal) may require treatment with low-dose corticosteroids in order to prevent progressive hepatic dysfunction and cirrhosis. Hyperglycemia is a frequent complication of corticosteroid therapy in hepatic sarcoidosis, and should be prospectively monitored.

Hypercalcemia

Persistent hypercalcemia is an indication for treatment because of the risk of nephrocalcinosis or, rarely, acute hypercalcemic crisis. Low-dose prednisone is almost always effective. Chloroquine, hydroxychloroquine (below) and ketoconazole can also be effective treatment for hypercalcemic sarcoidosis.

Bone and joint sarcoidosis

Corticosteroids usually result in a dramatic improvement in symptoms. New bone formation can occur over months, with a return to a normal radiographic bone appearance. Chloroquine and hydroxychloroquine can also be effective.

Hematologic sarcoidosis

Corticosteroids are usually effective in partially shrinking an enlarged spleen. Hypersplenism also frequently responds, at least in part, to low or moderate doses of corticosteroids.

Role of cytotoxic and other alternative therapies

Methotrexate has been used to treat severe skin disease, with a 30–50% success rate. More recently, methotrexate in low weekly doses (10–20 mg/day) has been proposed as an alternative therapy in corticosteroid-recalcitrant pulmonary, cardiac, ocular (panuveitis) and neurologic sarcoidosis.[68] Randomized clinical trials have not yet been reported, and the overall effectiveness of the drug in these situations remains unclear. Hepatic toxicity, opportunistic infections, bone marrow suppression and pulmonary toxicity are serious complications of this drug.

Azathioprine

Anecdotal experience and limited clinical studies suggest that azathioprine in a dose of 100–200 mg/day may be useful in corticosteroid-recalcitrant sarcoidosis.[69] Low doses of corticosteroids often are prescribed concomitantly. Beneficial effects usually are apparent by 2–3 months. Potential drug toxicities include bone marrow suppression, gastrointestinal symptoms, skin rashes, arthralgias, and possibly a slightly increased risk of malignancy. Nonetheless, because azathioprine is often tolerated well for prolonged periods it remains the first drug used by many clinicians for severe corticosteroid-resistant sarcoidosis.[70]

Other cytotoxic and immunosuppressive agents

Chlorambucil and cyclophosphamide have had anecdotal success in treating steroid-recalcitrant sarcoidosis, particularly refractory neurosarcoidosis, though their oncogenic potential should severely limit their use. Cyclosporine, a drug known to inhibit T-cell activation, appears to be ineffective, except possibly in a few cases of severe neurosarcoidosis.

Pentoxifylline

A recent clinical study found that pentoxifylline was beneficial when used alone or with corticosteroids in the initial treatment of sarcoidosis.[71] The author's anecdotal experience is that the drug is beneficial in a small minority of patients with mild pulmonary or hepatic disease, or as a steroid-sparing agent. Gastrointestinal side-effects often limit the dose that is tolerated, but given its relative safety a trial of the drug may be considered in patients who do not require urgent treatment.

Thalidomide

Anecdotal case reports suggest that thalidomide may be beneficial in pulmonary or cutaneous sarcoidosis.[72] Peripheral neurotoxicity and the well known terotogenicity of the drug mandate careful patients selection.

Role of transplantation in sarcoidosis

Lung, heart, kidney and liver transplantations have been performed successfully in small numbers of patients with sarcoidosis.[73] Recurrent granulomas are found in the transplanted organs of some patients.[74] However, the recurrence of granulomas is generally transient, self-limited and responsive to an increase in immunosuppression. The survival rate for lung transplantation for end-stage pulmonary sarcoidosis appears to be similar to that of other organ-specific diseases.

CONTROVERSIES

The long-term benefits of corticosteroid therapy in sarcoidosis are controversial.[75] Several prospective studies failed to find any long-term benefit as regards altered outcomes in pulmonary sarcoidosis, but the patients in these studies had a high likelihood of spontaneous remission.[76] Retrospective studies from centers treating patients at high risk for chronic disease provide data that corticosteroids delay the progression of chronic pulmonary sarcoidosis.[65] In support of this view, a recent prospective study of patients with stage II or III disease found that chronic maintenance corticosteroid therapy significantly improved long-term pulmonary function compared to a group that was treated intermittently for symptomatic disease.[77] Further studies are needed to corroborate these results, but most authorities favor the view that corticosteroid therapy improves outcome in patients with chronic pulmonary and serious extrapulmonary disease.

The overall effectiveness and benefit of methotrexate, azathioprine and other alternative agents in steroid-resistant sarcoidosis also continues to be debated. Controlled clinical trials have not been performed and there is disparity regarding the effectiveness of these agents in different centers. Multicenter clinical trials will be needed to evaluate their overall benefit and that of newer therapies rapidly emerging from the current biotechnology revolution.

REFERENCES

1. Mitchell DN, Scadding JG. Sarcoidosis. Am Rev Respir Dis 1974;110:774.
2. Costabel U, Hunninghake GW. ATS/ERS/WASOG statement on sarcoidosis. Sarcoidosis Statement Committee. American Thoracic Society. European Respiratory Society. World Association for Sarcoidosis and Other Granulomatous Disorders. Eur Respir J 1999;14:735.
3. Mayock RL, Bertrand P, Morrison CE. Manifestations of sarcoidosis. Am J Med 1963;35:67.
4. Siltzbach LE, James DG, Neville E. Course and prognosis of sarcoidosis around the world. Am J Med 1974;57:847.
5. Neville E, Walker AN, James DG. Prognostic factors predicting the outcome of sarcoidosis: an analysis of 818 patients. Q J Med 1983;208:525.
6. Hillerdal G, Nou E, Osterman K. Sarcoidosis: epidemiology and prognosis. A 15-year European study. Am Rev Respir Dis 1984;130:29.
7. Longcope WT, Freiman DG. A study of sarcoidosis based on a combined investigation of 160 cases including 30 autopsies from the Johns Hopkins Hospital and the Massachusetts General Hospital. Medicine 1952;31:1

8. Löfgren S. Erythema nodosum. Studies on etiology and pathogenesis in 185 adult cases. Acta Med Scand 1946;124:1.
9. Hosoda Y, Yamaguchi M, Hiraga Y. Global epidemiology of sarcoidosis. What story do prevalence and incidence tell us? In: Sharma OP (ed) Clinics in chest medicine, 18th edn. Philadelphia, WB Saunders, 1997, p 681.
10. Henke CE, Henke G, Elveback LR. The epidemiology of sarcoidosis in Rochester, Minnesota: a population-based study of incidence and survival. Am J Epidemiol 1986;123:840.
11. Bresnitz EA, Strom BL. Epidemiology of sarcoidosis. Epidemiol Rev 1983;5:124.
12. Gideon NM, Mannino DM. Sarcoidosis mortality in the United States, 1979–1981: an analysis of multiple-cause mortality data. Am J Med 1996;100:423.
13. Rybicki BA, Maliarik M, Major M, Popovich JJ, Iannuzzi MC. Genetics of sarcoidosis. In: Sharma OP (ed) Clinics in chest medicine, 2nd edn. Philadelphia, WB Saunders, 1997: p 707.
14. Rybicki BA, Harrington D, Major M, et al. Heterogeneity of familial risk in sarcoidosis. Genet Epidemiol 1996;13:23.
15. Muller-Quernheim J. Sarcoidosis: immunopathogenetic concepts and their clinical application. Eur Respir J 1998;12:716.
16. Berlin M, Fogdel-Hahn A, Olerup O, Eklund A, Grunewald J. HLA-DR predicts the prognosis in Scandinavian patients with pulmonary sarcoidosis. Am J Respir Crit Care Med 1997;156:1601.
17. Lympany PA, Petrek M, Southcott AM, Newman Taylor AJ, Welsh KI, du Bois RM. HLA-IDPLB polymorphisms: Glu 69 association with sarcoidosis. Eur J Immunogenet 1996;23:353.
18. Richeldi L, Sorrentino R, Saltini C. HLA-DPB1 glutamate 69: a genetic marker of beryllium disease. Science 1993;262:242.
19. Maliarik MJ, Chen KM, Major ML, et al. Analysis of HLA-DPB1 polymorphisms in African-Americans with sarcoidosis. Am J Respir Crit Care Med 1998;158:111.
20. Seitzer U, Swider C, Stuber F, et al. Tumour necrosis factor alpha promoter gene polymorphism in sarcoidosis. Cytokine 1997;9:787.
21. Newman LS, Rose CR, Maier LA. Sarcoidosis. N Engl J Med 1997;336:1224.
22. Mangiapan G, Hance AJ. Mycobacteria and sarcoidosis: an overview and summary of recent molecular biological data. Sarcoidosis 1995;12:20.
23. Ishige I, Usui Y, Takemura T, Yoshinobu E. Quantitative PCR of mycobacterial and propionibacterial DNA in lymph nodes of Japanese patients with sarcoidosis. Lancet 1999;354:120.
24. Burke W, Keogh A, Maloney P, Delprado W, Bryant D, Spratt P. Transmission of sarcoidosis via cardiac transplantation. Lancet 1990;336:1579.
25. Munro CS, Mitchell DN. The Kveim response: still useful, still a puzzle. Thorax 1987;42:321.
26. Wiesenhutter CW, Sharma OP. Is sarcoidosis an autoimmune disease? Report of four cases and review of the literature. Semin Arthritis Rheum 1979;9:124.
27. Moller DR. Etiology of sarcoidosis. In: Sharma OP (ed.) Clinics in chest medicine, 18th edn. Philadelphia, WB Saunders, 1997, p 1695.
28. Moller DR. Involvement of T cells and alterations in T cell receptors in sarcoidosis. Semin Resp Infect 1998;13:174.
29. Thomas PD, Hunninghake GW. Current concepts of pathogenesis of sarcoidosis. Am Rev Respir Dis 1987;135:747.
30. Hunninghake GW, Crystal RG. Pulmonary sarcoidosis: a disorder mediated by excess helper T-lymphocyte activity at sites of disease activity. N Engl J Med 1981;305:429.
31. DuBois RM, Kirby M, Balbi B, Saltini C, Crystal RG. T-lymphocytes that accumulate in the lung in sarcoidosis have evidence of recent stimulation of the T-cell receptor. Am Rev Respir Dis 1992;145:1205
32. Bergeron A, Bonay M, Kambouchner M et al. Cytokine patterns in tuberculous and sarcoid granulomas: correlations with histopathologic features of the granulomatous response. J Immunol 1997;159:3034.
33. Moller DR, Konishi K, Kirby M, Balbi B, Crystal RG. Bias toward use of a specific T cell receptor beta-chain variable region in a subgroup of individuals with sarcoidosis. J Clin Invest 1988;82:1183
34. Grunewald J, Janson CH, Eklund A et al. Restricted Va2.3 gene usage by CD4+ T lymphocytes in bronchoalveolar lavage fluid from sarcoidosis patients correlates with HLA-DR3. Eur J Immunol 1993;22:129.
35. Forrester JM, Wang Y, Ricalton N et al. TCR expression of activated T-cell clones in the lungs of patients with pulmonary sarcoidosis. J Immunol 1994;153:4291.
36. Forman JD, Klein JT, Silver RF, Liu MC, Greenlee BM, Moller DR. Selective activation and accumulation of oligoclonal V beta-specific T-cells in active pulmonary sarcoidosis. J Clin Invest 1994;94:1533.
37. Grunewald J, Hultman T, Bucht A, Eklund A, Wigzell H. Restricted usage of T cell receptor V alpha/J alpha gene segments with different nucleotide but identical amino acid sequences in HLA-DR3^{+} sarcoidosis patients. Molec Med 1995;1 297.
38. Balbi B, Moller DR, Kirby N, Crystal RG. Increased numbers of T lymphocytes with γδ-positive antigen receptors in a subgroup of individuals with pulmonary sarcoidosis. J Clin Invest 1990;85:13531.
39. Forrester JM, Newman LS, Wang Y, et al. Clonal expansion of lung V gamma 1+ T cells in pulmonary sarcoidosis. J Clin Invest 1993;91:292.
40. Wilsher ML, Hallowes M, Birchall NM. Gamma/delta T lymphocytes in the blood of patients with sarcoidosis. Thorax 1995;50:858.
41. Tazi A, Fajac I, Soler P, Valeyre D, Battesti JP, Hance AJ. Gamma/delta T-lymphocytes are not increased in number in granulomatous lesions of patients with tuberculosis or sarcoidosis. Am Rev Respir Dis 1991;144:1373.
42. Agostini C, Semenzato G, James DG. Immunologica , clinical and molecular aspects of sarcoidosis. Mol Aspects Med 1997;18:91.
43. Nicod LP, Isler P. Alveolar macrophages in sarcoidosis coexpress high levels of CD86 (B7.2), CD40, and CD30L. Am J Respir Cell Mol Biol 1997;17:91.
44. Lem VM, Lipscomb MF, Weissler JC, et al. Bronchoalveolar cells from sarcoid patients demonstrate enhanced antigen presentation. J Immunol 1985;135:1766.
45. Bachwich PR, Lynch JP, Larrick J, Spengler M, Kunkel SL. Tumor necrosis factor production by human sarcoid alveolar macrophages. Am J Pathol 1986;125:421.
46. Moller DR, Forman JD, Liu MC, et al. Enhanced expression of IL-12 associated with Th1 cytokine profiles in active pulmonary sarcoidosis. J Immunol 1996;145:4952.
47. Agostini C, Trentin L, Facco M, et al. Role of IL-15, IL-2, and their receptors in the development of T cell alveolitis in pulmonary sarcoidosis. J Immunol 1996;157:910.
48. Standiford TJ, Rolfe MW, Kunkel SL. Macrophage inflammatory protein-1a expression in interstitial lung disease. J Immunol 1988;131:191.
49. Moller DR. Cells and cytokines involved in the pathogenesis of sarcoidosis. Sarcoidosis Vasc Diffuse Lung Dis 1999;16:24.
50. Walker C, Bauer W, Braun RK, et al. Activated T cells and cytokines in bronchoalveolar lavages from patients with various lung diseases associated with eosinophilia. Am J Respir Crit Care Med 1994;150:1038
51. Rogge L, Papi A, Presky DH, et al. Antibodies to the IL-12 receptor beta 2 chain mark human Th1 but not Th2 cells in vitro and in vivo. J Immunol 1999;162:3926.
52. Pietropaoli A, Modrak J, Utell M. Interferon-alpha therapy associated with the development of sarcoidosis. Chest 1999;116:569.
53. Zissel G, Homolka J, Schlaak J, Schlaak M, Muller-Quernheim J. Anti-inflammatory cytokine release by alveolar macrophages in pulmonary sarcoidosis. Am J Respir Crit Care Med 1996;154:713.
54. Kunkel SL, Lukacs NW, Strieter RM, Chensue SW. Th1 and Th2 responses regulate experimental lung granuloma development. Sarcoidosis Vasc Diffuse Lung Dis 1996;13:120.
55. Limper AH, Colby TV, Sanders MS, Asakura S, Roche PC, DeRemee RA. Immunohistochemical localization of transforming growth factor-beta 1 in the nonnecrotizing granulomas of pulmonary sarcoidosis. Am J Respir Crit Care Med 1994;149:197.
56. Lynch JP, Kazerooni EA, Gay SE. Pulmonary sarcoidosis. In: Sharma OP (ed) Clinics in chest medicine, 18th edn. Philadelphia, WB Saunders, 1997, p 755.
57. Neville E, Mills RGS, Jash DK, MacKinnon DM, Carstairs LS, James GD. Sarcoidosis of the upper respiratory tract and its association with lupus pernio. Thorax 1976;31:660.

58. Sharma OP. Myocardial sarcoidosis. Chest 1993;103:253.
59. Robert WC, McAllister HA, Ferrans VJ. Sarcoidosis of the heart. A clinicopathologic study of 35 necropsy patients (group I) and review of 78 previously described necropsy patients (group II). Am J Med 1977;63:86.
60. Sharma OP. Cardiac and neurologic dysfunction in sarcoidosis. In: Sharma OP (ed) Clinics in chest medicine, 18th edn. Philadelphia, WB Saunders, 1997; p 813.
61. Gilman MJ, Wang KP. Transbronchial lung biopsy in sarcoidosis: an approach to determine the optimal number of biopsies. Am Rev Respir Dis 1980;122:721.
62. Costabel U, Teschler H. Biochemical changes in sarcoidosis. In: Sharma OP (ed) Clinics in chest medicine, 18th edn. Philadelphia, WB Saunders, 1997; p 827.
63. Lieberman J. Elevation of serum angiotensin-converting-enzyme (ACE) level in sarcoidosis. Am J Med 1975;59:365.
64. Turner-Warwick M, McAllister W, Lawrence R, Britten A, Haslam PL. Corticosteroid treatment in pulmonary sarcoidosis: do serial lavage lymphocyte counts, serum angiotensin converting enzyme measurements, and gallium-67 scans help management? Thorax 1986;41:903.
65. Johns CJ, Michele TM. The clinical management of sarcoidosis – a 50-year experience at the Johns Hopkins Hospital. Medicine 1999;78:65.
66. Winterbauer RH, Kirtland SH, Corley DE. Treatment with corticosteroids. In: Sharma OP (ed) Clinics in chest medicine, 18th edn. Philadelphia, WB Saunders, 1997; p 843.
67. Milman N. Oral and inhaled corticosteroids in the treatment of pulmonary sarcoidosis – a critical reappraisal. Sarcoidosis Vasc Diffuse Lung Dis 1998;15:150.
68. Lower EE, Baughman RP. Prolonged use of methotrexate for sarcoidosis. Arch Intern Med 1995;155:846.
69. Hof DG, Hof PC, Godfrey WA. Long-term use of azathioprine as a steroid-sparing treatment for chronic sarcoidosis. Am J Respir Crit Care Med 1996;153:A870.
70. Muller-Quernheim J, Kienast K, Held M, Pfeifer S, Costabel U. Treatment of chronic sarcoidosis with an azathioprine/prednisolone regimen. Eur Respir J 1999;14:1117.
71. Zabel P, Entzian P, Dalhoff K, Schlaak M. Pentoxifylline in treatment of sarcoidosis. Am J Respir Crit Care Med 1997;155:1665.
72. Carlesimo M, Giustini S, Rossi A. Treatment of cutaneous and pulmonary sarcoidosis with thalidomide. J Am Acad Dermatol 1995;32:866.
73. Barbers RG. Role of transplantation (lung, liver, and heart) in sarcoidosis. In: Sharma OP (ed) Clinics in chest medicine, 18th edn. Philadelphia, WB Saunders, 1997;865.
74. Martinez F, Orens JB, Deeb MO et al. Recurrence of sarcoidosis following allogeneic lung transplantation. Chest 1994;106:1597.
75. DuBois RM. Corticosteroids in sarcoidosis: friend or foe? Eur Respir J 1994;7:1203.
76. Hunninghake GW, Gilbert S, Pueringer R. Outcome of the treatment for sarcoidosis. Am J Respir Crit Care Med 1994;149:893.
77. Gibson GJ, Prescott RJ, Muers MF. British Thoracic Society Sarcoidosis Study: Effects of long-term corticosteroid treatment. Thorax 1996;51:238.

Chapter 86

Immunologic Ocular Disease

James T. Rosenbaum, Matthias D. Becker and Justine R. Smith

INTRODUCTION

The immune system can induce disease in virtually any portion of the eye. Examples include conjunctivitis, keratitis, keratoconjunctivitis, uveitis, scleritis, optic neuritis and orbital inflammation. The anatomy of the eye is depicted schematically in Figure 53.1. Before considering those disorders that are the most visually significant, it is critical to review some unique considerations related to ocular immunology.

OCULAR IMMUNE PRIVILEGE

Many of the mechanisms that drive inflammation within the eye are identical to those operating at other tissue sites. The major difference between the immunopathology of intraocular inflammation and that of systemic inflammatory disease relates to the fact that the eye, like the brain and the testis, is an immunologically privileged site. During uveitis, keratitis and scleritis, as well as following corneal transplantation, a variety of local immunosuppressive mechanisms act to limit the damage caused by infiltrating leukocytes and, consequently, to influence the patient's clinical course. One of the most important factors is the constitute expression of Fas ligand (FasL) within the eye. In addition, normal ocular tissues express an immunosuppressive cytokine profile. Other factors include the blood–aqueous and blood–retinal anatomical barriers, limited MHC expression, a paucity of lymphatic drainage channels and, in the case of the cornea, the complete absence of blood vessels. Anterior chamber-associated immune deviation (ACAID) is a research tool which has greatly facilitated the study of these mechanisms.

FAS LIGAND

Many cells, including neutrophils, monocytes, macrophages and lymphocytes, express Fas (CD95) on their surface. The interaction between Fas and its ligand, FasL (CD95L) triggers apoptosis of the Fas-bearing cell. FasL is constitutively expressed within the eye, being detected in normal cornea, anterior uvea and retina.[1] The importance of FasL to ocular immune privilege has been demonstrated primarily in experimental models of ocular inflammation. Corneal allografts from FasL-negative mice into recipients of normal phenotype are rejected in all cases, whereas around half of FasL-positive grafts survive.[2] When injected into the eyes of FasL-deficient mice, herpes simplex virus causes a severe invasive infection.[1] A similar procedure in normal phenotype control animals results in relatively minor inflammation. Levels of FasL in aqueous humor during human acute anterior uveitis are capable of inducing apoptosis in Fas-positive lymphoid cells.[3] In this self-limiting condition, as well as in relevant rodent models, apoptosis of infiltrating T cells is observed early in the course of the inflammation.[3,4]

CYTOKINE NETWORK

Tissues in both the anterior and the posterior segments of the human eye constitutively express the immunomodulatory cytokine transforming growth factor β (TGF-β).[5,6] The concentration of TGF-β in the aqueous humor is sufficient to inhibit T-cell activation and proliferation in a variety of assays.[7] As might be anticipated, significantly lower levels of activated cytokine are measured in the aqueous of patients with a variety of uveitis syndromes compared to levels present in normal eyes.[8] The pro-inflammatory cytokine interleukin (IL)-1 has been implicated in the pathogenesis of various ocular inflammatory diseases. There is expression of IL-1 receptor antagonist (IL-1Ra) in normal cornea[9] and retinal pigment epithelium,[10] implying that this tissue contains a control mechanism for responses mediated by IL-1. Interestingly, topical application of IL-1Ra has a significantly positive effect in promoting experimental corneal allograft survival.[11]

ANTERIOR CHAMBER-ASSOCIATED IMMUNE DEVIATION

Anterior chamber-associated immune deviation is 'a stereotypic, systemic immune response to antigens placed in the anterior chamber [of the eye] in which delayed hypersensitivity is avoided and suppressed'.[12] The molecular events responsible for this phenomenon, a manifestation of ocular immune privilege, can be summarized as follows:[13]

1. Entry of an antigen into the eye stimulates the production of tumor necrosis factor-α and, as a result, the up-regulation of cell adhesion molecules, secretion of IL-10 by the infiltrating T cells, and sensitization of these cells for FasL-mediated killing. TGF-β also induces ocular antigen-presenting cells to secrete IL-10 during antigen processing.[14]
2. Apoptotic T cells pass in the bloodstream to the spleen, where they are phagocytosed and, on presentation in the MHC class II pathway, induce the activation of Th2-type CD4-positive T cells.
3. The Th2-type cells control Th1 function by secreting various immunomodulatory cytokines.
4. T-cell receptor α-chain fragments from apoptosed cells are presented in the MHC class I pathway.
5. This event generates CD8-positive killer cells, which are capable of deleting the CD4-positive T cells that would

KEY CONCEPTS

- Immune-mediated diseases can affect virtually any portion of the eye. Uveitis, scleritis, keratoconjunctivitis sicca, conjunctivitis, optic neuritis, keratitis and orbital pseudotumor are examples of eye diseases that are frequently immune-mediated.
- The immune privilege of the eye does not prevent immune-mediated eye disease.
- Uveitis and scleritis are frequently associated with a systemic illness. These illnesses can usually be diagnosed by history without resorting to extensive laboratory testing.

otherwise mediate a delayed-type hypersensitivity response. CD8-positive T cells, which secrete immunomodulatory cytokines including IL-10 and TGF-α, are also generated.

UVEITIS

Uveitis as a diagnostic entity

The uveal tract is the middle layer of the eye, divided into the anterior uvea (iris, ciliary body) and the posterior uvea (choroid). The uvea is sandwiched between an outer layer (sclera) and an inner layer (retina). The anterior segment is separated from the posterior segment by the lens. Uveitis is an extremely variable spectrum of different diseases that includes a variety of infections and immune-mediated diseases (Table 86.1). It is the third leading cause of preventable blindness worldwide. Inflammatory disorders of the retina (retinitis) and sclera (scleritis) frequently involve the adjacent uveal tract. Many different immune mechanisms could result in uveitis, as evidenced in animal models. They include an immune response to a sequestered self-antigen, molecular mimicry, immune complex deposition, and the response to a toxin.

Identifying characteristic clinical features facilitates the differential diagnosis of uveitis. Uveitis can be classified by location: anterior (iritis, iridocyclitis), intermediate (pars planitis, vitritis) or posterior (retinitis, choroiditis, retinochoroiditis, chorioretinitis, retinal vasculitis). The incidence rate of anterior uveitis is approximately four times that of posterior uveitis. Some forms of uveitis involve all portions of the uveal tract (panuveitis). Uveitis can be classified by course (self-limited, chronic or recurrent); by onset (sudden, insidious); by symmetry (unilateral, bilateral); by associated complications such as glaucoma, cystoid macular edema (Fig. 86.1A), synechiae (for example adhesion of the iris to the lens) (Fig. 86.1B), retinal detachment or band keratopathy (the deposition of calcium in the epithelium of the cornea) (Fig. 86.1C); and by the appearance of inflammatory keratic precipitates on the endothelium of the cornea within the eye (granulomatous, nongranulomatous) (Fig. 86.1D). Granulomatous diseases with large cellular concretions on the cornea or nodules within the iris include tuberculosis, syphilis, sarcoidosis, Vogt–Koyanagi–Harada disease and sympathetic ophthalmia. The group of nongranulomatous diseases includes ankylosing spondylitis, reactive arthritis and juvenile rheumatoid arthritis (JRA). Table 86.2 shows how these parameters contribute to the differential diagnosis. In addition, ethnic and geographic considerations factor into the differential diagnosis. For example, sarcoidosis, Behçet's syndrome

Diagnostic categories of uveitis

Diagnostic group	Diagnosis
Infectious causes	
Viral	Herpes simplex Herpes zoster Cytomegalovirus HTLV-1 Mumps
Bacterial or spirochetal	Atypical mycobacterium Bacterial endocarditis Bartonella Brucellosis Leprosy Leptospirosis Lyme disease Propionibacterium Tuberculosis Leprosy Syphilis Whipple's disease
Parasitic (protozoan or helminthic)	Acanthameba Cysticercosis Onchocerciasis *Pneumocystis carinii* Toxoplasmosis Toxocariasis
Fungal	Histoplasmosis Coccidioidomycosis Candidiasis Aspergillosis Sporotrichosis Blastomycosis Cryptococcosis
Suspected immune-mediated	Ankylosing spondylitis Behçet's disease Crohn's disease Drug or hypersensitivity reaction (such as rifabutin or cidofovir) Familial granulomatous synovitis with uveitis Interstitial nephritis Juvenile rheumatoid arthritis Kawasaki disease Multiple sclerosis Psoriatic arthritis Reactive arthritis Relapsing polychondritis Rheumatic fever Sarcoidosis Scleritis Sjogren's syndrome Sweet's syndrome Systemic lupus erythematosus Ulcerative colitis Vasoulitis Vogi–Koyanagi–Harada syndrome
Syndromes confined primarily to the eye	Acute multifocal placoid pigmentary epitheliopathy Birdshot choroidopathy Fuchs' heterochromic cyclitis Glaucomatocyclitic crisis Lens-induced uveitis Multifocal choroiditis Multifocal evanescent white dot syndrome Pars planitis Punctate inner choroidopathy Serpiginous choroiditis Sympathetic ophthalmia Trauma

Table 86.1 Diagnostic categories of uveitis.

Diagnostic categories of uveitis	
Diagnostic group	**Diagnosis**
Masquerade syndromes	Ischemia Iris melanoma Juvenile xanthogranuloma Leukemia Lymphoma Melanoma Retinitis pigmentosa Retinoblastoma

Table 86.1 Diagnostic categories of uveitis. (*contd*)

Uveitis – characteristies

Location
- **Anterior**: ankylosing spondylitis, Reiter's syndrome, juvenile chronic arthritis
- **Intermediate**: pars planitis
- **Posterior**: Vogt–Koyanagi–Harada syndrome

Onset
- **Sudden**: ankylosing spondylitis, reactive arthritis
- **Insidious**: pars planitis, juvenile rheumatoid arthritis

Symmetry
- **Unilateral**: ankylosing spondylitis, toxoplasmosis
- **Bilateral**: pars planitis, lymphoma, juvenile chronic arthritis

Course
- **Self-limited**: toxoplasmosis
- **Recurrent**: Behçet's disease, ankylosing spondylitis
- **Chronic**: pars planitis

Table 86.2 Characteristic features of common forms of uveitis.

and Vogt–Koyanagi–Harada disease have very strong ethnic predispositions, whereas certain infections, such as cytomegalovirus in association with AIDS, leprosy, or onchocerciasis, vary in prevalence depending on geographic area. Together with a medical history, gender and age, these findings help to narrow the differential diagnosis of uveitis.

The following case studies illustrate how important a precise and critical history and examination is. A 22-year-old man with low back pain and a red painful eye due to episodic, unilateral sudden-onset anterior uveitis is highly likely to have a spondyloarthropathy. A 6-year-old girl with no ocular complaints but biomicroscopic findings of bilateral band keratopathy and leukocytes

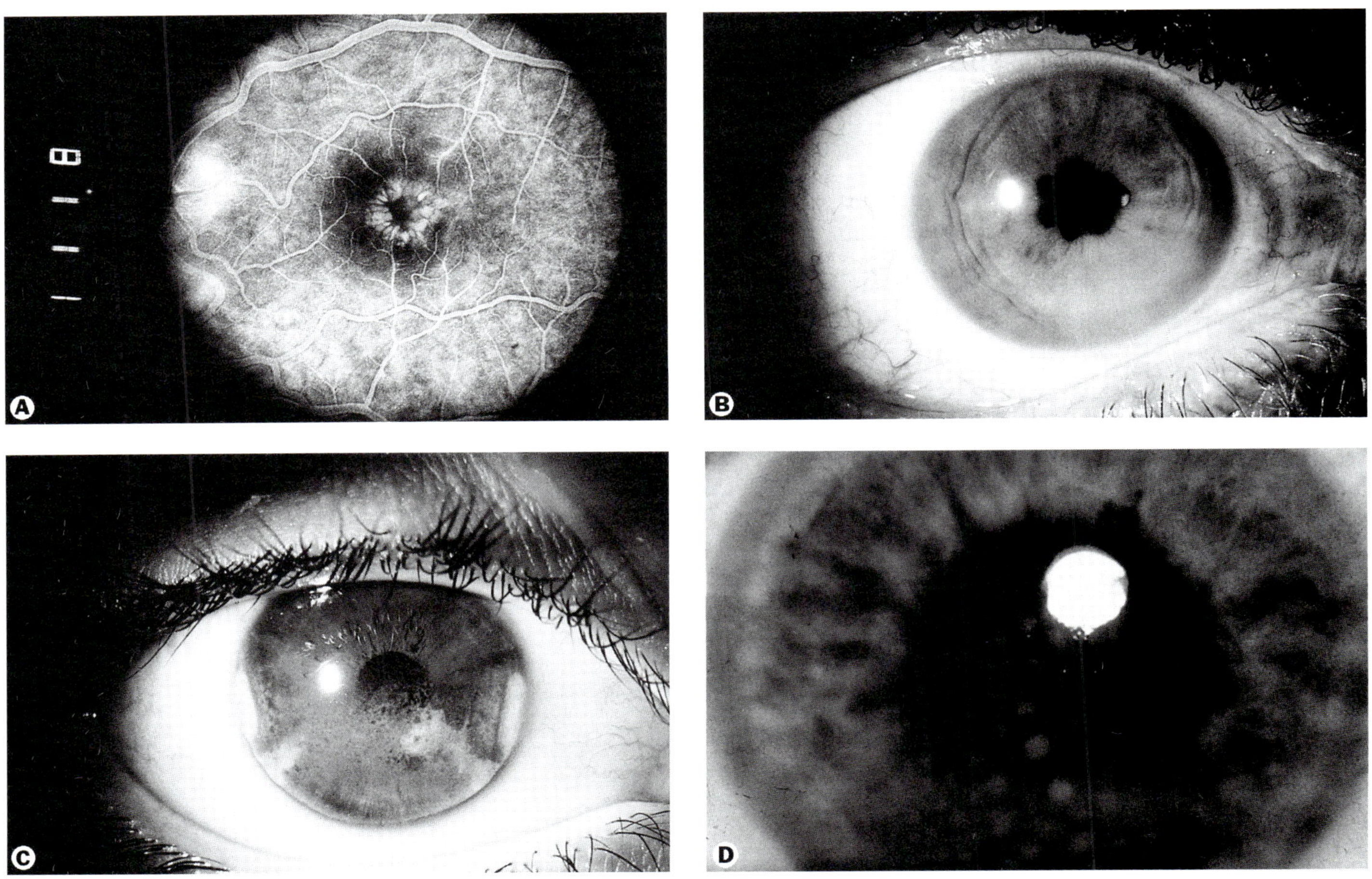

Figure 86.1 Physical findings in uveitis. (A) Fundus fluorescein angiogram showing cystoid macular edema. Fluorescein, which appears as a white stain, should be absent from the center of this photograph because the macular area is avascular. **(B)** Posterior synechiae. The cloverleaf appearance of the pupil is caused by the iris adhering to the lens. **(C)** Band keratopathy. Calcium deposition in the corneal endothelium complicates the iridocyclitis in a patient with juvenile rheumatoid arthritis. **(D)** Granulomatous keratic precipitates. Round white dots are scattered in a triangular shape. The dots represent concretions of leukocytes adherent to the corneal endothelium. (See also colour plate 86.1.)

in the anterior chamber, is likely to suffer from the pauciarticular subset of JRA.

The most obvious sign of uveal inflammation is the presence of biomicroscopically visible leukocytes, in either the anterior or the posterior chamber of the eye, or both. Most patients with anterior uveitis will experience pain, redness, photophobia, miosis and a variable degree of visual loss. In contrast, many forms of uveitis that affect the posterior segment will cause no redness, no pain and no change in pupil size (no macroscopically apparent signs of an inflamed eye). Disturbances in visual acuity may vary from normal vision to seeing floaters, to blurred vision to blindness.

Epidemiology

The incidence and prevalence of the different types of uveitis vary among different regions of the world, depending on numerous factors: level of socioeconomic development, HLA distribution, prevalence of different infectious diseases in each region, prevalence of various associated systemic diseases (Table 86.3), and also the methodology employed by each physician to evaluate and classify uveitis.[15] However, a considerable portion of all epidemiological studies is the contribution of unclassified or idiopathic uveitis.

Prevention and patient management

Uveitis can be the first sign of occult, potentially severe systemic disease (sarcoidosis, syphilis, tuberculosis, vasculitis). Despite the difficulty of successful systemic anti-inflammatory/immunosuppressive treatment, there are some diagnoses that can be treated to complete recovery (infectious uveitis, e.g. syphilis). Therefore, it is essential to identify as accurately as possible the cause of uveitis. A targeted approach is preferable, with limited work-ups guided by the type and severity of uveitis and the presence of systemic findings. The history assumes a greater importance than with any other ophthalmic entity. The minimal work-up for uveitis of unknown etiology requires an extensive and careful review of systems, a complete blood count with differential, syphilis serology and a chest X-ray.[16]

Most practitioners use a stepladder approach to uveitis therapy. The first step is treatment with corticosteroids for all patients with noninfectious uveitis. This can be topical, especially for anterior uveitis, local peribulbar injection, or systemic. Systemic immunosuppressive therapy should be used in cases of inadequate benefit from corticosteroids or unacceptable steroid side-effects. Immunosuppression is usually reserved for bilateral forms of uveitis with a severity sufficient to alter activities of daily living, and is frequently chosen for eye involvement with Behçet's disease. Immunosuppression is contraindicated by active infection in the eye or elsewhere.

Uveitis/disease associations

Diagnosis	Likelihood (%)
Ankylosing spondylitis	30
Sarcoidosis	25–50
Behçet's disease	80
Inflammatory bowel disease	1–9
Psoriatic arthritis	7
Juvenile rheumatoid arthritis	<2–53*
Multiple sclerosis	0–3

*The wide range reflects variable likelihood depending on the subset of JRA.

Table 86.3 Likelihood of developing uveitis in association with a specific disease.

CLINICAL PEARLS

Uveitis and systemic disease
- Uveitis can be the first sign of an occult and potentially severe systemic disease.
- It is essential to identify as accurately as possible the cause of uveitis.
- The minimal work-up for uveitis of unknown etiology requires a careful history with complete review of systems, complete blood count with differential, syphilis serology, and a chest X-ray.

THERAPEUTIC PRINCIPLES

Stepladder approach for uveitis therapy
- Local corticosteroids
  - Topical for anterior uveitis
  - Local peribulbar injection
- Systemic corticosteroids
- Additional systemic immunosuppressive therapy
  - Bilateral and severe uveitis with alteration of activities of daily living
  - Inadequate benefit or unacceptable side-effects from corticosteroids
  - Contraindicated by active infection in the eye or elsewhere

Overview of the most common uveitis diagnoses

Ankylosing spondylitis (AS)

This is the most common systemic diagnosis associated with uveitis in western nations (Chapter 66). A genetic predisposition with the inheritance of HLA-B27 is found in 88–96% of patients with AS. About 30% of AS patients develop anterior uveitis transiently during a lifetime; conversely, 30% of anterior uveitis patients have AS. Approximately 50% of patients with a sudden-onset anterior uveitis are HLA-B27 positive.[17] In some studies 80–90% of individuals with HLA-B27-associated iritis have a systemic disease, either ankylosing spondylitis or reactive arthritis.[18] Ankylosing spondylitis should be sought in any patient with sudden-onset primarily anterior unilateral uveitis associated with redness and pain. The iritis associated with HLA-B27 follows a very reproducible pattern.[18–20] The majority of patients are male. A bilateral sacroiliitis is the sine qua non for AS. Characteristically, the low back pain begins insidiously, is associated with morning stiffness and improves with exercise. Sacroiliac x-ray films show sclerosis and eventual narrowing of the joint

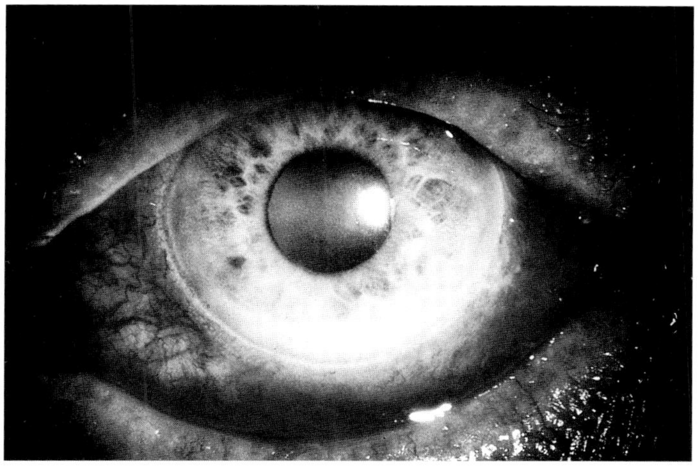

Figure 86.2 Hypopyon. Intense inflammation has resulted in a creamy exudate (pus), seen as whitening over the inferior portion of the anterior chamber. (See also colour plate 86.2.)

space. Cells can be seen in the anterior chamber on slit-lamp examination. Inflammation is sometimes so severe that inflammatory cells layer out in the anterior chamber and a hypopyon (Fig. 86.2) develops. The posterior segment of the eye is not commonly involved in this disease, except for the development of a vision-reducing cystoid macular edema (Fig. 86.1A), which is a more frequent complication than with other forms of anterior uveitis. The disease usually shows a good response to topical corticosteroids. In frequently recurrent cases therapy with sulfasalazine has shown to be effective in reducing the frequency and severity of the attacks.

Inflammatory bowel disease (IBD)

Ocular manifestations of IBD (Crohn's disease and ulcerative colitis; Chapter 87) include iritis, episcleritis and scleritis (1–9% of all cases).[21–23] Twenty per cent of patients with IBD may have sacroiliitis. 60% of these are HLA-B27 positive. The anterior uveitis in patients with IBD is often similar to that seen with the HLA-B27 spectrum of joint diseases (AS): sudden in onset, unilateral and self-limited. However, Crohn's disease is a granulomatous process; like sarcoidosis, it may result in intraocular inflammation that is insidious in onset, bilateral, posterior, chronic, or associated with a retinal vasculitis.[24]

Psoriasis

One per cent of the population has psoriasis; 7% of psoriasis patients have arthritis, and 7% of patients with psoriasis and arthritis have uveitis. The diagnosis is made clinically with the typical findings of cutaneous changes (erythematous, hyperkeratotic rash) and joint disease. Patients with sacroiliac disease and psoriatic arthritis are especially likely to develop uveitis.[25]

Sarcoidosis

Ocular disease is the initial manifestation of sarcoidosis in 20% of patients (Chapter 85). The systemic illness begins as ocular inflammation almost as often as it initially presents as pulmonary disease. Between 25% and 50% of patients with systemic sarcoidosis exhibit ocular inflammatory disease. In most case series sarcoidosis accounts for 3–10% of all patients with uveitis, and it therefore follows spondyloarthropathy as the second most common systemic illness associated with uveitis in North America and Europe. The diagnosis of sarcoidosis should always be considered in any patient presenting with a uveitis of unknown etiology. Sarcoidosis has a strong ethnic relationship: it occurs in the United States 10 times more frequently among African-Americans than among whites.[26] Because ocular sarcoidosis can affect almost every part of the eye symptoms vary widely, depending on the distribution of pathology. Most commonly patients will have a bilateral chronic granulomatous iridocyclitis.[27–29] The disease might disappear, so that two-thirds of patients are symptom free after 10 years. Typical findings include 'mutton-fat' keratic precipitates of the cornea (Fig. 86.1D), Koeppe and Busacca iris nodules, posterior synechiae (Fig. 86.1B) and white clumps of cells ('snowballs') in the inferior anterior vitreous. A chest X-ray (or CT scan[30]) should be included in every basic work-up. The diagnosis is most reliably established by a biopsy that demonstrates the noncaseating granuloma in the absence of an infection or beryllium exposure. Possible biopsy sites include the lymph nodes, lung, skin, oral mucosa and conjunctiva. Serological abnormalities are not sufficiently unique to establish a diagnosis. They include elevated serum angiotensin-converting enzyme and lysozyme levels. In general, the combination of uveitis and symmetrical hilar adenopathy, however, is sufficiently specific for sarcoidosis. It is therefore not necessary to obtain tissue confirmation when this presentation occurs. Topical, periocular and systemic corticosteroids are the mainstay of therapy.

Behçet syndrome

Behçet syndrome is a generalized occlusive vasculitis of unknown cause that accounts for about 2.5% of patients at a North American referral uveitis clinic.[31] It has a strong ethnic relationship, being most common in Japan (20% of uveitis patients) and prevalent in Middle Eastern countries along the silk road. The classic complex includes aphthous stomatitis, genital ulceration and iritis, sometimes with hypopyon (30% of patients), and skin lesions. Involvement of the posterior segment is more common than the anterior, and includes an occlusive retinal vasculitis (Fig. 86.3).[32] Extraocular manifestations most commonly include arthritis, erythema nodosum, diarrhea (mimicking inflammatory bowel disease) and sterile meningitis. There is a strong tendency for the symptoms to remit and exacerbate spontaneously. HLA-B5, or its subset Bw51, is more commonly found in Behçet patients.[33] Behçet syndrome may lead to blindness if ischemic optic neuropathy and retinopathy are not adequately treated. Patients are often inadequately managed by corticosteroids alone. A regimen with immunosuppressive drugs (cyclosporine A,[34] azathioprine[35] or chlorambucil[36]) has been proved to be useful.

Multiple sclerosis

Although retrobulbar optic neuritis is the ocular inflammation most clearly associated with multiple sclerosis, both intermediate uveitis (pars planitis) and a granulomatous anterior uveitis are well described in association with this demyelinating central nervous system disease.[37–39] The granulomatous inflammation is typically bilateral, and may indicate a worse prognosis for the neurologic disease. The HLA-DR2 antigen, strongly associated with MS, is associated with uveitis as well.[39]

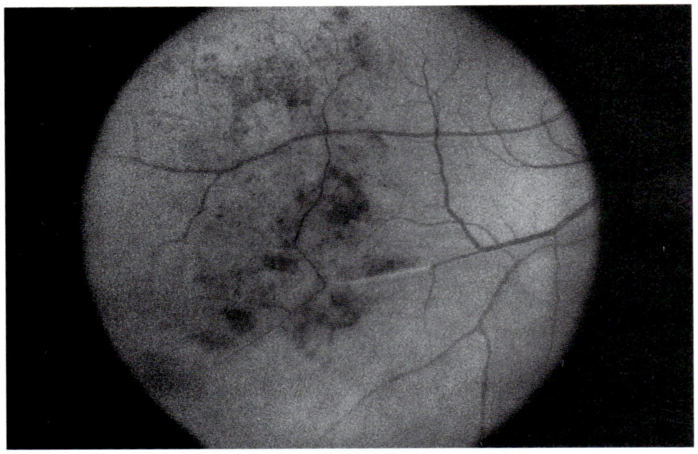

Figure 86.3 Fundus photograph showing retinal vasculitis. The scattered hemorrhages are secondary to the vasculitis. The patient has Behçet's syndrome. (See also colour plate 86.3.)

Juvenile rheumatoid arthritis

Patients with JRA need special consideration as the disease often does not present with a 'red eye'. It is often a smoldering, silent inflammation with a quiet, white eye. These young patients need to be screened on a routine basis every 3–4 months to avoid structural damage to the eye from even low-grade inflammation, with resulting blindness. In 20% of all JRA cases the joint involvement is pauciarticular (five or fewer joints affected). Uveitis occurs far more commonly in this pauciarticular subset. Girls are four times more often affected than are boys. Eighty per cent of uveitis cases are positive for antinuclear antibodies (ANA) and negative for rheumatoid factor. The onset of ocular disease is usually within 5 years of arthritis. Ophthalmologic evaluation may demonstrate bilateral fine keratic precipitates, band keratopathy (Fig. 86.1C), flare and cells in the anterior chamber, posterior synechiae, glaucoma and cataract formation. Topical and periocular corticosteroid treatment with a slow taper is the mainstay of therapy. Systemic therapy with methotrexate as a substitute for corticosteroids can be used in selected cases. Cataract surgery is a special challenge and may require intense perioperative immunosuppression.

SCLERITIS

Description/natural history

Scleritis is a relatively uncommon inflammation that affects the sclera, the white tunic that encases the posterior eye. It is usually presumed to represent a vasculitis of scleral vessels. Approximately 50% of patients with scleritis will have clinical evidence for a systemic vasculitis elsewhere in the body. The most common systemic disease is rheumatoid arthritis (RA), especially the subset of patients with rheumatoid nodules, high-titer rheumatoid factor, and sometimes pleuropericarditis, as well as small vessel vasculitis in the skin of the lower extremities.[40] Other commonly associated systemic diseases are listed in Table 86.4. The epidemiology of scleritis has not been adequately reported. However, rheumatoid arthritis accounts for about one-third of all cases. Because only 1% of patients with rheumatoid arthritis develop scleritis, and about 1% of the population has RA, one can estimate that the prevalence of scleritis is $0.01 \times 0.01 \times 3$, or 3 per 10 000.

Systemic immune-mediated diseases associated with scleritis
Rheumatoid arthritis
Wegener's granulomatosis
Inflammatory bowel disease
Polyarteritis nodosa
Temporal arteritis/giant cell arteritis
Systemic lupus erythematosus
Ankylosing spondylitis
Rheumatic fever
IgA nephropathy

Table 86.4 Systemic immune-mediated diseases associated with scleritis.

Scleritis is frequently divided into five subsets based on the clinical presentation: diffuse anterior (Fig. 86.4A); nodular anterior; necrotizing; scleromalacia perforans (Fig. 86.4B); and posterior. Scleromalacia perforans is also known as necrotizing without inflammation. The clinical presentation varies depending on the type, but usually scleritis is a very painful and persistent condition. Even with treatment, one large series reported a median duration of 7 years.[41]

Genetic/environmental factors

Genetic factors affecting scleritis have not been adequately studied. Genes that affect the associated systemic diseases, such as RA, Wegener's granulomatosis and polyarteritis, presumably also influence the susceptibility to scleritis. Environmental triggers for scleritis have not been defined, except that some cases of scleritis can follow infection with, for example, herpes zoster, syphilis or Lyme disease, as well as other bacterial and fungal infections.

Immunology/pathology

Biopsy of the sclera entails some risk. Accordingly, many of the published histological observations are based on end-stage or extremely severe disease. In one pathology study of 55 examples of necrotizing scleritis, the histology was divided into four types: zonal necrotizing granulomatous; nonzonal diffuse; necrotizing with microabscess; and sarcoidal granulomatous.[42] Eighty-five per cent of patients with zonal necrotizing granulomatous pathology had a systemic disease, usually rheumatoid arthritis. The pathology associated with RA was not distinct from other systemic diseases such as Wegener's granulomatosis. None of 19 patients with nonzonal diffuse scleral inflammation had a systemic disease. Just over half of the patients with microabscesses had an identifiable infection as the cause of scleritis. Only one patient had 'sarcoidal granulomatous inflammation', and that patient had sarcoidosis.

Prevention/management

Topical medications are only slightly beneficial for most patients with scleritis. Topical nonsteroidal anti-inflammatory drugs (NSAIDs) such as ketorolac have not been proved to be efficacious in a controlled study. A topical corticosteroid can sometimes help in symptomatic control[43] but also has risk, especially the promotion of cataract formation and elevation of intraocular pressure. The role for topical cyclosporine has not been adequately evaluated but the authors' clinical experience has not been favorable.

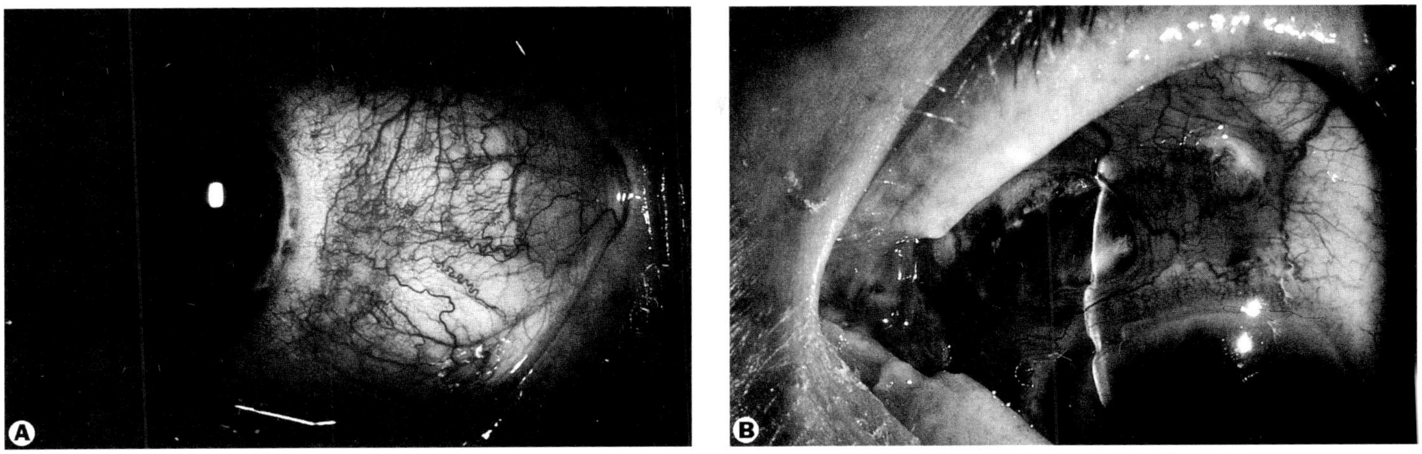

Figure 86.4 **Clinical presentation of scleritis. (A)** Diffuse anterior scleritis. The blue, thinned sclera is visible beneath the inflamed vessels. **(B)** Scleromalacia perforans. Blue sclera is visible secondary to inflammation resembling a rheumatoid nodule in the eye. (See also colour plate 86.4.)

Although most forms of scleritis represent a vasculitis, oral NSAIDs can be immensely beneficial. Whereas not all patients derive adequate control from an NSAID, a subset of patients will benefit sufficiently such that no other medication is required. Indomethacin is the NSAID most frequently reported to be effective,[44] but others have simply not been tested on a sufficient sample size.

Many patients with scleritis will not benefit adequately from an NSAID and will require immunosuppression. In general, for those with an associated systemic disease the control of that disease will lead to control of the scleritis. For those without a systemic illness, oral corticosteroid is an accepted initial approach to treatment. For example, therapy might begin with a dose of prednisone of 1 mg/kg body weight per day. The use of calcium, vitamin D, estrogen and other measures to preserve bone mineral density should be considered for any patient who will be receiving corticosteroid on a chronic basis. If prednisone is not adequate for disease control, or if the medication is toxic, poorly tolerated and cannot be safely tapered to a modest dosage, it is reasonable to add a steroid-sparing medication such as methotrexate, azathioprine, cyclosporin,[45,46] mycophenolate, or even an alkylating agent such as cyclophosphamide.

Periocular corticosteroids are very effective for uveitis but are relatively contraindicated for patients with necrotizing scleritis. The steroid probably promotes reduced wound healing and thus enhances the likelihood that the sclera might perforate as a result of the inflammation. Inflammation limited to the posterior sclera can probably be safely treated with a periocular steroid injection. Anterior scleritis that is nonnecrotizing also responds to the cautious use of periocular corticosteroid injections[47,48]

In choosing to treat with systemic corticosteroid or immunosuppressive drugs the clinician will of course weigh the risk/benefit ratio. The rationale for aggressive therapy is much stronger if the disease is bilateral and affecting activities of daily living, because of either pain or a reduction in visual acuity.

Evaluation/differential diagnosis

Patients with scleritis generally have characteristic findings, which allow an accurate diagnosis; scleritis can usually be readily distinguished from other causes of a red, painful eye. The most difficult distinction is between scleritis and episcleritis. The episclera overlies the sclera. In general patients with episcleritis do not experience pain, do not have an associated systemic disease, do not have complications such as iritis or glaucoma, and have an excellent prognosis, with complete resolution usually within weeks.

CLINICAL PEARLS

Contrasting features of scleritis and episcleritis

	Scleritis	*Episcleritis*
Pain	Prominent	Minimal
Duration	Years	Days to several months
Association with systemic disease	Frequent	Rare
Vessels blanch with topical vasoconstrictor	No	Yes
Associated ocular complications including visual loss	Sometimes present	Never
Vessel color	Deep pink to violaceous	Light pink

The scleritis associated with a systemic vasculitis is often more severe than that not associated with a systemic illness.[49] When associated with Wegener's granulomatosis it may be particularly destructive and refractory to therapy.[50] Scleritis in association with rheumatoid arthritis is often a poor prognostic sign for the joint disease. For example, the small subset of patients with scleritis in association with rheumatoid arthritis have a shortened life expectancy compared to other patients with RA who have no evidence for scleritis.[51]

Posterior scleritis can be extremely difficult to diagnose. If the anterior sclera is uninvolved there is no redness. Pain with posterior scleritis is much more variable. The examination may show elevation of the adjacent retina and choroid. The diagnosis can be confirmed with ultrasound or, less commonly, with a CT scan of the orbit, demonstrating thickening of the sclera. Posterior scleritis is treated similarly to anterior scleritis except that topical corticosteroids are not useful, and a periocular corticosteroid injection can be given safely.

Pitfalls/controversy

Some experts believe that scleritis is often a *forme fruste* of Wegener's granulomatosis. Scleritis clearly occurs in association with Wegener's, and patients with scleritis, a positive ANCA test but no other evidence for Wegener's granulomatosis have been well described.[52–54]

With the exception of the ANCA, laboratory studies are generally selected according to the history and general physical examination. For example, although rheumatoid arthritis is associated with scleritis, the patients almost always have long-standing severe RA. A rheumatoid factor would not be an appropriate test if no joint disease is present clinically. Similarly, systemic lupus erythematosus can be associated with scleritis, but one would not diagnose lupus on the basis of a positive ANA, scleritis, and the absence of other findings to suggest lupus. An erythrocyte sedimentation rate can sometimes be helpful in reassuring that no systemic process is present. The medication that is chosen and how that medication is monitored largely dictate other laboratory tests.

KERATITIS

The cornea is the anteriorly situated window to the eye. Normally it should be clear, but it can become opacified as a result of trauma, toxin, infection, dryness, calcium deposition or genetic disease such as corneal dystrophies. The three main presumably autoimmune diseases that affect the cornea are corneal melt, Mooren's ulcer and Cogan syndrome.

Corneal melt is also known as marginal keratolysis (Fig. 86.5). The majority of patients have an associated systemic form of vasculitis and usually scleritis. The medical therapy is basically the same as that described for scleritis, with emphasis on controlling the underlying systemic illness and the use of immunosuppression. Corneal melt often leads to perforation of the eye. This is usually treated surgically with tissue adhesives, conjunctival flaps or corneal transplantation. Corneal melt is fortunately very rare. It must also be distinguished from other causes of corneal thinning, such as Terrien's marginal degeneration or a senile marginal furrow, both of which are generally more benign and rarely lead to perforation.

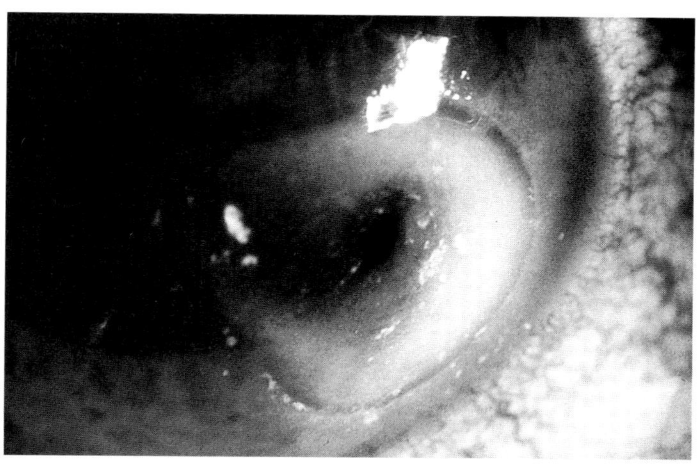

Figure 86.5 Corneal melt. A pie shaped wedge of the cornea is thinned. The eye is red secondary to an associated scleritis. (See also colour plate 86.5.)

Mooren's ulcer is clinically very similar to a melt except that there is no accompanying scleritis and no evidence for a systemic illness. The superior cornea is especially likely to be involved. Mooren's ulcer is too rare for therapeutic options to be studied with randomized clinical trials. It may respond to oral immunosuppression, which is warranted if the severity threatens visual acuity because of impending perforation of the eye. One small study suggested that Mooren's ulcer is frequently associated with evidence for previous infection with hepatitis C but this was not confirmed by subsequent investigators.[55] Some patients with Mooren's ulcer have an autoantibody to calgranulin C.[56] This antigen is expressed in the cornea, in neutrophils, and by filarial nematodes. The cornea is divided into three layers: the epithelium facing the atmosphere; the stroma; and the endothelium abutting on aqueous humor. Opacification of the stroma is known as interstitial keratitis. Congential syphilis and other infections such as herpes simplex are important causes of interstitial keratitis. Cogan's syndrome is characterized by an autoimmune disease of the eighth nerve and interstitial keratitis which presumably also has an autoimmune basis.[57] Some ophthalmologists also recognize autoimmune eighth-nerve disease associated with other forms of ocular inflammation such as uveitis as examples of Cogan's disease.[58–60] The pathogenesis of Cogan's syndrome is presumed to be a vasculitis, and many patients will have evidence for vasculitis elsewhere in the body. The treatment usually requires aggressive use of systemic immunosuppressive medications.

CORNEAL TRANSPLANTATION AND TRANSPLANT REJECTION

Corneal transplantation involves the replacement of a diseased cornea with one from a healthy cadaver. Since the 1970s, advances in microsurgical techniques and eye banking procedures have led to widespread acceptance of this procedure. Currently 40 000 corneal transplantations are performed annually in the United States alone. The usual indication for a corneal graft is poor vision, although the operation may also be undertaken to relieve ocular pain. Keratoconus, a condition in which myopic astigmatism develops as the cornea becomes progressively more conical in shape, corneal edema often following intraocular surgery, and a failed previous corneal graft are the must common medical conditions leading to corneal transplantation.[61]

Although the eye is an immune privileged site, and corneal transplants enjoy a 91% 1-year Kaplan–Meier survival, only 62% of grafts are functional at 10 years,[61] the commonest cause of failure being immunological rejection.[61] Corneal allograft rejection rarely occurs within 2 weeks, and may occur as late as 20 years following surgery. Animal studies using monoclonal antibodies directed against different T-cell subsets indicate that CD4 T cells play a critical role in the rejection response.[62] However, the exact mechanisms responsible for this process have yet to be elucidated.

Early recognition of a rejection episode is the most important factor in achieving survival of the corneal transplant. In its most florid form the anterior eye is obviously inflamed, with intense conjunctival injection, a cellular anterior chamber reaction and a Khodadoust line. The latter, which is visible with the slit-lamp biomicroscope, is a classic sign of corneal graft rejection. It appears as a linear formation of inflammatory precipitates stretching across the corneal endothelium and represents a wave of lymphocytes marching across the cornea and destroying the endothelium in their path.[63] As the endothelial pump function is lost, the cornea becomes waterlogged and opaque. At an early stage of rejection the patient may be asymptomatic, but later ocular redness, photophobia, halos and blurred vision are frequent complaints. An intensive and extended course of topical corticosteroids is the mainstay of treatment for rejection, and in severe cases intravenous and/or oral corticosteroids may also be required.[64] Patients considered to be at high risk for transplant rejection, such as those with corneal neovascularization or a history of other anterior segment inflammation, are often given perioperative systemic immunosuppression. The ideal prophylactic regimen has not been defined, although various combinations of prednisone, cyclosporin and azathioprine may be used. Despite the critical influence of donor–recipient histocompatibility matching for solid organ transplant survival, the probability of corneal graft survival is not significantly improved by a HLA matching.[65]

CANCER-ASSOCIATED RETINOPATHY

Cancer-associated retinopathy (CAR) is a rare paraneoplastic syndrome most commonly induced by small cell carcinoma of the lung. The disease has also been documented in association with various tumors of the female reproductive tract, carcinoma of the breast and neuroendocrine bronchial carcinoma. For 50% of patients CAR is the presenting feature of their malignancy.[66] Interestingly, there is a recent report of retinopathy mimicking CAR but occurring in an apparently healthy individual.[67] Melanoma-associated retinopathy is a related syndrome, occurring in patients with metastatic cutaneous melanoma.

Histopathological examinations of postmortem specimens taken from patients with CAR consistently demonstrate loss of inner and outer segments of the retinal photoreceptors.[68] This destruction was initially attributed to the release of a hormone-like substance from the malignant cells, but evidence has now accumulated in support of an autoimmune etiology. Affected individuals produce antibodies against one or more retinal photoreceptor antigens,[69] and when injected into laboratory animals these antibodies induce experimental CAR.[70] Although over 15 antigens have been described in relation to CAR, the commonest is the so-called CAR antigen.[69] This 23-kDa protein has been identified as recoverin, a photoreceptor protein which participates in visual adaptation. There is experimental work to support the hypothesis that a single mutational event simultaneously activates the recoverin gene and eliminates functional p53, a tumor-suppressor protein.[71] Consequently, a tumor develops which encodes for CAR antigen and stimulates the formation of antirecoverin antibody. Antirecoverin antibodies are capable of inducing photoreceptor apoptosis, leading to the characteristic loss of both rods and cones.[72]

Cancer-associated retinopathy generally occurs after the age of 60. Patients usually complain of decreased vision, although other symptoms may include transient visual obscurations, various positive visual phenomena, night blindness, scotomata, glare and photosensitivity. Although visual acuity may be dramatically reduced, other clinical signs are often subtle. Color vision may be impaired. The presence of an afferent pupillary defect requires asymmetry of the retinopathy. There may be mild iridocyclitis and/or vitritis, narrowing of retinal arterioles, mottling of retinal pigment epithelium and optic disc pallor. Visual field abnormalities occur, the most common being several midperipheral scotomata, which later join up as a ring scotoma or central defect.

Electroretinography shows either reduced or completely flattened amplitudes. The disease must be differentiated from optic neuritis which, unlike CAR, typically occurs in younger people, some of whom suffer from multiple sclerosis, and is painful. In contrast to CAR, optic neuritis is typically abrupt in onset. In patients with malignancy, direct tumor spread and the effects of drugs, including chemotherapy agents, must be excluded before CAR is diagnosed.

The natural history of CAR is one of progressive visual loss, although this occurs over a variable period. Treatment directed towards curing or palliating the malignancy does not appear to prevent this loss. A series of case reports have documented an improvement of vision in response to systemic corticosteroid therapy.[68] High doses (60–80 mg) of prednisone have been used, but the minimum dose for preservation of vision is uncertain. It is suggested that monitoring serum antibody levels can be used to guide the corticosteroid dose.[68] However, in some cases advanced photoreceptor damage may be irreversible despite corticosteroid therapy.

IMMUNOLOGIC ETIOLOGICAL FACTORS IN 'NONIMMUNOLOGIC' OCULAR DISEASE

The eye contains many unique proteins that are sequestered from the immune system in early development, and which, if released systemically during adulthood, could act as autoantigens. Autoantibodies directed against certain ocular proteins have been detected in the serum of patients with a variety of ocular diseases traditionally regarded as nonimmunologic. Examples of such conditions include cataract, glaucoma, age-related macular degeneration (ARMD), and retinal degenerative diseases such as retinitis pigmentosa (RP). The unanswered question is whether these antibodies contribute to the pathogenesis of the disease or merely coexist as an epiphenomenon.

Cataract is an opacification of the crystalline lens of the eye. It is the most frequent cause of blindness worldwide and most commonly occurs as an age-related phenomenon. The prevalence is approximately 70% in those over 75 years of age. Pathogenesis is poorly understood, and many varied mechanisms, including autoimmunity, have been hypothesized. Autoantibodies to sequestered lens proteins termed crystallins are present in some normal individuals, but occur significantly more frequently in patients with cataract.[73] Immune complexes have also been demonstrated in human cataractous lenses.[73] Immunization of rabbits with human lens protein can induce cataract formation, which is suppressed by systemic corticosteroid therapy.[73] Human sera containing autoantibodies against lens proteins are cytotoxic for lens epithelial cells in culture.[74] On the other hand, it has not been possible to demonstrate T-cell-mediated immune responses to lens proteins experimentally, suggesting that a process of active tolerance might prevent these autoantigens from inducing significant inflammation.[75]

In glaucoma a relative elevation of intraocular pressure is associated with optic nerve damage and visual field loss. More than

3 million people in the world are irreversibly blind because of this disease, the basic mechanisms of which continue to puzzle clinicians and scientists despite very extensive research. There is recent evidence that autoimmunity may play a role in glaucoma, at least for a subgroup of affected individuals with so-called normal-tension glaucoma, in which there is no apparent elevation in intraocular pressure above population normal levels. Increased titers of various autoantibodies, including antibodies directed against extractable nuclear antigens,[76] retinal heat-shock proteins[77] and the retinal photoreceptor protein rhodopsin,[78] have been measured in patients with normal-tension glaucoma. In addition, autoantibodies to optic nerve head glycosaminoglycans have been detected in the serum and optic nerve of patients with glaucoma, including the normal-pressure form.[79] It is postulated that these antiglycosaminoglycan antibodies may increase susceptibility of the optic nerve head to glaucomatous disease by altering physical characteristics of the tissue.

Age-related macular degeneration is the leading cause of irreversible visual loss in the elderly in western nations. A spectrum of pathologies may occur at the macula, ranging from relatively benign focal hypo- and hyperpigmentation of the retinal pigment epithelium to sinister subretinal neovascularizations, which may leak serous fluid and blood. The pathogenic stimulus for these changes is unknown. There is a single report documenting the presence of antibodies to an apparent retinal neuronal cytoskeletal protein in the serum of some patients with ARMD.[80] Interestingly, subretinal scar tissue removed from patients with advanced disease may contain immunoglobulins and complement components.[81] At the same time there are few inflammatory cells, including lymphocyte subsets, although local cell populations may express class II MHC antigens. Macular drusen, seen early in the course of ARMD, may also contain immunoglobulin.[82]

Retinitis pigmentosa is a hereditary pigmentary degeneration of the retina, although just under half of patients have no family history. Various antiretinal antibodies have been detected in approximately one-half of patients with this disease, including antibodies directed against the enzymes carbonic anhydrase II and enolase.[83] Interestingly, there is a significant association between the occurrence of cystoid edema at the macula, a dreaded vision-threatening complication of RP, and the presence of the circulating antiretinal antibodies. The complication has been reported in 90% of affected individuals with antibodies, compared with only 13% of those who do not make these antibodies.[84] A less convincing association is that between an accelerated rate of visual field loss and the presence of antiretinal antibodies.[83]

REFERENCES

1. Griffith TS, Brunner T, Fletcher SM, Green DR, Ferguson TA. Fas-ligand induced apoptosis as a mechanism of immune privilege. Science 1995;270:1189.
2. Stuart PM, Griffith TS, Usui N, Pepose J, Yu X, Ferguson TA. CD95 ligand (FasL)-induced apoptosis is necessary for corneal allograft survival. J Clin Invest 1997;99:396.
3. Dick AD, Siepmann K, Dees C, et al. Fas–Fas ligand-mediated apoptosis within aqueous during idiopathic acute anterior uveitis. Invest Ophthalmol Vis Sci 1999;40:2258.
4. Smith JR, Hart PH, Standfield SD, Coster DJ, Wing S, Williams KA. Apoptosis is a prominent feature of acute anterior uveitis in the Fischer 344 rat. Br J Ophthalmol 2000;84:205.
5. Pasquale LR, Dorman-Pease ME, Lutty GA, Quigley HA, Jampel HD. Immunolocalization of TGF-beta1, TGF-beta2, and TGF-beta3 in the anterior segment of the human eye. Invest Ophthalmol Vis Sci 1993;34:23.
6. Lutty GA, Merges C, Threlkeld AB, Crone S, McLeod DS. Heterogeneity in localization of isoforms of TGF-beta in human retina, vitreous, and choroid. Invest Ophthalmol Vis Sci 1993;34:477.
7. Cousins SW, McCabe MM, Danielpour D, Streilein JW. Identification of transforming growth factor-beta as an immunosuppressive factor in aqueous humor. Invest Ophthalmol Vis Sci 1991;32:2201.
8. de Boer JH, Limpens J, Orengo-Nania S, de Jong PT, La Heij E, Kijlstra A. Low mature TGF-beta 2 levels in aqueous humor during uveitis. Invest Ophthalmol Vis Sci 1994;35:3702.
9. Kennedy MC, Rosenbaum JT, Brown J, et al. Novel production of interleukin-1 receptor antagonist peptides in normal human cornea. J Clin Invest 1995;95:82.
10. Holtkamp GM, de Vos AF, Kijlstra A, Peek R. Expression of multiple forms of IL-1 receptor antagonist (IL-1ra) by human retinal pigment epithelial cells: identification of a new IL-1ra exon. Eur J Immunol 1999;29:215.
11. Dana MR, Yamada J, Streilein JW. Topical interleukin 1 receptor antagonist promotes corneal transplant survival. Transplantation 1997;63:1501.
12. Okamoto S, Streilein JW. Role of inflammatory cytokines in induction of anterior chamber-associated immune deviation. Ocul Immunol Inflamm 1998;6:1.
13. Ferguson TA. The molecular basis of anterior associated immune deviation (ACAID). Ocul Immunol Inflamm 1997;5:213.
14. D'Orazio TJ, Niederkorn JY. A novel role for TGF-beta and IL-10 in the induction of immune privilege. J Immunol 1998;160:2089.
15. Vadot E, Barth E, Billet P. Epidemiology of uveitis – preliminary results of a prospective study in Savoy. In: Saari KM (ed) Uveitis update. New York, Excerpta Medica, 1994, p 13
16. Rosenbaum JT. An algorithm for the systemic evaluation of patients with uveitis: guidelines for the consultant. Semin Arthritis Rheum 1990;19:248.
17. Brewerton DA, Caffrey M, Nicholls A, Walter D, James DCO. Acute anterior uveitis and HLA B27. Lancet 1973;2:994.
18. Rosenbaum JT. Characterization of uveitis associated with spondyloarthritis. J Rheum 1989;16:792.
19. Feltkamp TEW. HLA B27, acute anterior uveitis, and ankylosing spondylitis. Adv Inflam Res 1985;9:211.
20. Rosenbaum JT. Acute anterior uveitis and spondyloarthropathies. Rheum Dis Clin North Am 1992;18:143.
21. Knox DL, Schachat AP, Mustonen E. Primary, secondary, and coincidental ocular complications of Crohn's disease. Ophthalmology 1984;91:163.
22. Billson FA, Dombal FTD, Watkinson G, Goligher JC. Ocular complications of ulcerative colitis. Gut 1967;8:102.
23. Hopkins DJ, Horan E, Burton IL, et al. Ocular disorders in a series of 332 patients with Crohn's disease. Br J Ophthalmol 1974;58:732.
24. Lyons JL, Rosenbaum JT. Uveitis associated with inflammatory bowel disease compared with uveitis associated with spondyloarthropathy. Arch Ophthalmol 1997;115:61.
25. Paiva ES, Macaluso DC, Edwards A, Rosenbaum JT. Characterisation of uveitis in patients with psoriatic arthritis. Ann Rheum Dis 2000;59:67.
26. Rothova A, Alberts C, Glasius E, Kijlstra A, Buitenhuis HJ, Breebaart AC. Risk factors for ocular sarcoidosis. Doc Ophthalmol 1989;72:287.
27. Jabs DA, Johns C. Ocular involvement in chronic sarcoidosis. Am J Ophthalmol 1986;102:297.
28. Obenauf CD, Shaw HE, Sydnor CF, Klintworth GK. Sarcoidosis and its ophthalmic manifestations. Am J Ophthalmol 1978;86:648.
29. James DG. Ocular sarcoidosis. Ann NY Acad Sci 1986;465:551.

30. Kosmorsky GS, Meisler DM, Rice TW, Mezaine M, Lowder CY. Chest computed tomography and medianoscopy in the diagnosis of sarcoid-associated uveitis. Am J Ophthalmol 1998;126:132.
31. Rodriguez A, Calonge M, Pedroza-Seres M, et al. Referral patterns of uveitis in a tertiary eye care center. Arch Ophthalmol 1996; p 114.
32. Michelson JB, Chisari FV. Behçet's disease. Surv Ophthalmol 1982;26:190.
33. Ohno S, Ohguchi M, Hirose S, Matsuda H, Wakisaka A, Aizawa M. Close association of HLA-Bw51 with Behçet's disease. Arch Ophthalmol 1982;100:1455.
34. Nussenblatt RB, Palestine AG, Chan CC, et al. Effectiveness of cyclosporin therapy for Behçet's disease. Arthritis Rheum 1985;28:671.
35. Yazici H, Pazarli H, Barnes CG, et al. A controlled trial of azathioprine in Behçet's syndrome. N Engl J Med 1990;322:281.
36. Tricoulis D. Treatment of Behçet's disease with chlorambucil. Br J Ophthalmol 1976;60:55.
37. Meisler DM, Tomsak RL, Khoury S, Hanson MR, Schwab IR, Ransohoff RM. Anterior uveitis and multiple sclerosis. Cleveland Clin J Med 1989;56:535.
38. Lim JI, Tessler HH, Goodwin JA. Anterior granulomatous uveitis in patients with multiple sclerosis. Ophthalmology 1991;98:142.
39. Malinowski SM, Pulido JS, Goeken NE, Folk JC. The association of HLA-B8, B51, DR2 and multiple sclerosis in pars planitis. Ophthalmology 1993;100:1199.
40. Jayson MIV, Jones DEP. Scleritis and rheumatoid arthritis. Ann Rheum Dis 1971;30:343.
41. Watson PG, Hazleman BL. Clinical presentation of inflammatory episcleral and scleral disease. In: Watson PG, Hazleman BL (eds) The sclera and systemic disorders. London, WB Saunders, 1976; p 90.
42. Riono WP, Hidayat AA, Rao NA. Scleritis: a clinicopathologic study of 55 cases. Ophthalmology 1999;106:1328.
43. McMullen M, Kovarik G, Hodge WG. Use of topical steroid therapy in the management of nonnecrotizing anterior scleritis. Can J Ophthalmol 1999;34:217.
44. Rosenbaum JT, Robertson JE Jr. Recognition of posterior scleritis and its treatment with indomethacin. Retina 1993;13:17.
45. Hakin KN, Ham J, Lightman SL. Use of cyclosporin in the management of steroid dependent non-necrotising scleritis. Br J Ophthalmol 1991;75:340.
46. Wakefield D, McCluskey P. Cyclosporin therapy for severe scleritis. Br J Ophthalmol 1989;73:743.
47. Croasdale CR, Brightbill FS. Subconjunctival corticosteroid injections for nonnecrotizing anterior scleritis. Arch Ophthalmol 1999;117:966.
48. Hakin KN, Ham J, Lightman SL. Use of orbital floor steroids in the management of patients with uniocular non-necrotising scleritis. Br J Ophthalmol 1991;75:337.
49. Sainz de la Maza M, Foster CS, Jabbur NS. Scleritis associated with rheumatoid arthritis and other systemic immune-mediated diseases. Ophthalmology 1994;101:1281.
50. Sainz de la Maza M, Foster CS, Jabbur NS. Scleritis associated with systemic vasculitic diseases. Ophthalmology 1995;102:687.
51. Foster SC, Forstot SL, Wilson LA. Mortality rate in rheumatoid arthritis patients developing necrotizing scleritis or peripheral ulcerative keratitis. Ophthalmology 1984;91:1253.
52. Nolle B, Coners H, Duncker G. ANCA in ocular inflammatory disorders. Adv Exp Med Biol 1993;336:305.
53. Kalina PH, Garrity JA, Herman DC, DeRemee RA, Specks U. Role of testing for anticytoplasmic autoantibodies in the differential diagnosis of scleritis and orbital pseudotumor. Mayo Clin Proc 1990;65:1110.
54. Soukiasian SH, Foster S, Niles JL, Raizman MB. Diagnostic value of antineutrophil cytoplasmic antibodies in scleritis associated with Wegener's granulomatosis. Ophthalmology 1992;99:125.
55. Zegans ME, Srinivasan M, McHugh T, et al. Mooren ulcer in South India: serology and clinical risk factors. Am J Ophthalmol 1999;128:205.
56. Gottsch JD, Liu SH. Cloning and expression of human corneal calgranulin C (CO-Ag). Curr Eye Res 1998;17:870.
57. Cogan DG. Syndrome of nonsyphilitic interstitial keratitis and vestibuloauditory symptoms. Arch Ophthalmol 1945;33:144.
58. Allen NB, Cox CC, Cobo M, et al. Use of immunosuppressive agents in the treatment of severe ocular and vascular manifestations of Cogan's syndrome. Am J Med 1990;88:296
59. Haynes BF, Kaiser-Kupfer MI, Mason P, Fauci AS. Cogan syndrome: studies in thirteen patients, long-term follow-up, and a review of the literature. Medicine 1980;59:426.
60. Vollersten RS, McDonald TJ, Younge BR, Banks PM, Stanson AW, Ilstrup DM. Cogan's syndrome: 18 cases and a review of the literature. Mayo Clin Proc 1986;61:344.
61. Williams KA, Muehlberg SM, Lewis RF, Coster DJ. Long-term outcome in corneal allotransplantation. The Australian Corneal Graft Registry. Transplant Proc 1997;29:983.
62. Ayliffe W, Alam Y, Bell EB, McLeod D, Hutchinson IV. Prolongation of rat corneal graft survival by treatment with anti-CD4 monoclonal antibody. Br J Ophthalmol 1992;76:602
63. Khodadoust AA, Silverstein AM. Transplantation and rejection of individual cell layers of the cornea. Invest Ophthalmol 1969;8:180.
64. Larkin DF. Corneal allograft rejection. Br J Ophthalmol 1994;78:649.
65. (CCTS) Tccts. Effectiveness of histocompatibility matching in high-risk corneal transplantation. The Collaborative Corneal Transplantation Studies Research Group. Arch Ophthalmol 1992;110:1392.
66. Chung SM, Selhorst JB. Cancer-associated retinopathy. Ophthalmol Clin North Am 1992;5:587.
67. Whitcup SM, Vistica BP, Milam AH, Nussenblatt RB, Gery I. Recoverin-associated retinopathy: a clinically and immunologically distinctive disease. Am J Ophthalmol 1998;126:230.
68. Cohen RG, Rizzo J III, Lou P. New developments in cancer-associated retinopathy. Int Ophthalmol Clin 1997;37:233.
69. Thirkill CE, Keltner JL, Tyler NK, Roth AM. Antibody reactions with retina and cancer-associated antigens in 10 patients with cancer-associated retinopathy. Arch Ophthalmol 1993;111:931.
70. Thirkill CE, FitzGerald P, Sergott RC, Roth AM, Tyler NK, Keltner JL. Cancer-associated retinopathy (CAR syndrome) with antibodies reacting with retinal, optic-nerve, and cancer cells. N Engl J Med 1989;321:1589.
71. McGinnis JF, Austin B, Klisak I, et al. Chromosomal assignment of the human gene for the cancer-associated retinopathy protein (recoverin) to chromosome 17p13.1. J Neurosci Res 1995;40:165.
72. Adamus G, Machnicki M, Elerding H, Sugden B, Blocker YS, Fox DA. Antibodies to recoverin induce apoptosis of photoreceptor and bipolar cells in vivo. J Autoimmun 1998;11:523.
73. Angunawela I. The role of autoimmune phenomena in the pathogenesis of cataract. Immunology 1987;51:363.
74. Ibaraki N, Lin LR, Dang L, et al. Anti-beta-crystallin antibodies (mouse) or sera from humans with age-related cataract are cytotoxic for lens epithelial cells in culture. Exp Eye Res 1997;64:229.
75. Goldschmidt L, Goldbaum M, Walker SM, Weigle WO. The immune response to homologous lens crystallin. I. Antibody production after lens injury. J Immunol 1982;129:1652.
76. Wax MB, Barrett DA, Pestronk A. Increased incidence of paraproteinemia and autoantibodies in patients with normal-pressure glaucoma. Am J Ophthalmol 1994;117:561.
77. Tezel G, Seigel GM, Wax MB. Autoantibodies to small heat shock proteins in glaucoma. Invest Ophthalmol Vis Sci 1998;39:2277.
78. Romano C, Barrett DA, Li Z, Pestronk A, Wax MB. Anti-rhodopsin antibodies in sera from patients with normal-pressure glaucoma. Invest Ophthalmol Vis Sci 1995;36:1968.
79. Tezel G, Edward DP, Wax MB. Serum autoantibodies to optic nerve head glycosaminoglycans in patients with glaucoma. Arch Ophthalmol 1999;117:917.
80. Gurne DH, Tso MO, Edward DP, Ripps H. Antiretinal antibodies in serum of patients with age-related macular degeneration. Ophthalmology 1991;98:602.
81. Baudouin C, Peyman GA, Fredj-Reygrobellet D, et al. Immunohistological study of subretinal membranes in age-related macular degeneration. Jpn J Ophthalmol 1992;36:443.
82. Newsome DA, Hewitt AT, Huh W, Robey PG, Hassell JR. Detection of specific extracellular matrix molecules in drusen, Bruch's membrane, and ciliary body. Am J Ophthalmol 1987;104:373.

83. Heckenlively JR, Aptsiauri N, Nusinowitz S, Peng C, Hargrave PA. Investigations of antiretinal antibodies in pigmentary retinopathy and other retinal degenerations. Trans Am Ophthalmol Soc 1996;94:179.

84. Heckenlively JR, Jordan BL, Aptsiauri N. Association of antiretinal antibodies and cystoid macular edema in patients with retinitis pigmentosa. Am J Ophthalmol 1999;127:565.

Section 7 Organ-Specific Inflammatory Disease

Chapter 87

Immunologic Disease of the Gastrointestinal Tract

Markus F. Neurath, Susetta Finotto and Warren Strober

INTRODUCTION

Immunologic processes at the interface between the mucosal surface and the external environment represent the sum of a carefully balanced mechanism of immune response and non-response. An appropriate mucosal immune response is critical to the maintenance of host and the regulation of responses to ubiquitous antigens that could otherwise co-opt the mucosal and the systemic immune systems for unnecessary, or even harmful, immune responses. Conversely, dysfunction of the immune system frequently leads to disorders of the gastrointestinal system, including recurrent or chronic infections, malabsorption, and an increased risk of cancer.

GASTROINTESTINAL DISORDERS ASSOCIATED WITH IMMUNODEFICIENCY DISEASES

X-linked agammaglobulinemia

The prototype B-cell immunodeficiency is X-linked agammaglobulinemia (XLA, Chapter 34), a disease that results from dysfunction of the gene encoding Bruton's tyrosine kinase (BTK).[1] XLA is strictly a B-cell disorder, with absent or nearly absent B cells and normal T-cell numbers. Although acute gastrointestinal infections are common in XLA, patients are surprisingly free of chronic GI infections.[2] Thus, although patients are at greater risk for *Giardia*, *Campylobacter*, *Salmonella*, *Escherichia coli* or rotavirus infections, chronic GI infection is the exception rather than the rule. However, XLA patients are at risk for recurrent to chronic *subclinical* GI infections, which can have pathologic consequences. For example, XLA patients often suffer with lactase deficiency, which can reflect an altered bacterial flora in the upper GI tract.[3] XLA patients are also at greater risk of chronic infections with enteroviruses, which can lead to severe neurologic syndromes and scleroderma-like conditions.[4] Finally, an apparent increase in rapidly progressive colon cancer in XLA has recently been reported.[5]

Common variable immunodeficiency

With an estimated incidence of 1:30 000–1:60 000, common variable immunodeficiency (CVID) is the most frequent type of primary immune deficiency under the care of clinical immunologists (Chapter 34).[6] Most CVID patients of northern European descent exhibit a distinctive phenotype, characterized by a broad deficiency of immunoglobulin isotypes in spite of the presence of normal numbers of surface immunoglobulin bearing B-cell precursors in the peripheral blood. Some patients present during childhood, but most are diagnosed in the third decade of life.[7] Although CVID thus appears to be an acquired disorder, family studies have clearly documented that susceptibility for the disease can be inherited, and the manifestations of the disorder can change with time. In particular, CVID is associated with certain HLA haplotypes (HLA-B8 and -DR3) that are similar to those associated with gluten-sensitive enteropathy and other autoimmune states.[8]

Infections are more frequently seen in CVID than in XLA.[9] The major clinical manifestation of CVID is recurrent sinopulmonary infection, placing the patient at risk for pulmonary insufficiency and a respiratory death. However, 10–30% of patients have severe GI disease, which may take any of several forms.

CVID patients frequently have gastric atrophy and achlorhydria, which in some is associated with pernicious anemia.[9,10] The achlorhydria of CVID undoubtedly contributes to the observation that patients sometimes display a mild increase in upper intestinal bowel flora and the presence of anaerobes in the upper part of the GI tract. Because gastric atrophy is associated with an increased incidence of gastric cancer, subtle infection of the stomach may ultimately be responsible for the increased incidence of gastric cancer in patients with CVID.

CVID patients can develop a malabsorption syndrome associated with partial villous atrophy and a chronic mononuclear inflammatory infiltrate, which is similar to that seen in intestinal enteropathy caused by food hypersensitivity. This syndrome can occur with biliary abnormalities (gallstones), secondary bile salt malabsorption and intestinal nodular lymphoid hyperplasia (i.e. extensive intestinal lymphadenopathy characterized by nodules of surface membrane immunoglobulin M+[sIgM+] B cells) (Fig. 87.1). The origin of these nodules is unknown, but they may represent B-cell proliferation, which occurs because of the lack of feedback control that would accompany normal B-cell differentiation. Intestinal nodular lymphoid hyperplasia does not in itself lead to clinical problems, but it is possible that the lymphadenopathy may place the patient at greater risk for intestinal lymphoma.[11] Finally, in about 5–10% of patients with CVID the malabsorption syndrome can be quite severe, leading to a relentless diarrhea with impaired absorption of fat, D-xylose, minerals and vitamin-B_{12}, a severe protein-losing enteropathy, and a progressive weight loss that eventually dominates the clinical picture. The etiology of this syndrome is not well understood.[12]

Treatment of malabsorption and villous atrophy in patients with CVI is usually difficult. Immunoglobulin replacement therapy is ineffective in this condition, although it is quite effective in the prevention of respiratory infection. Patients respond to steroids, but this treatment is somewhat immunosuppressive and may increase the risk of opportunistic infections. At present severely affected patients are being treated with milder immunosuppressive therapy on an experimental basis. Symptomatic treatment

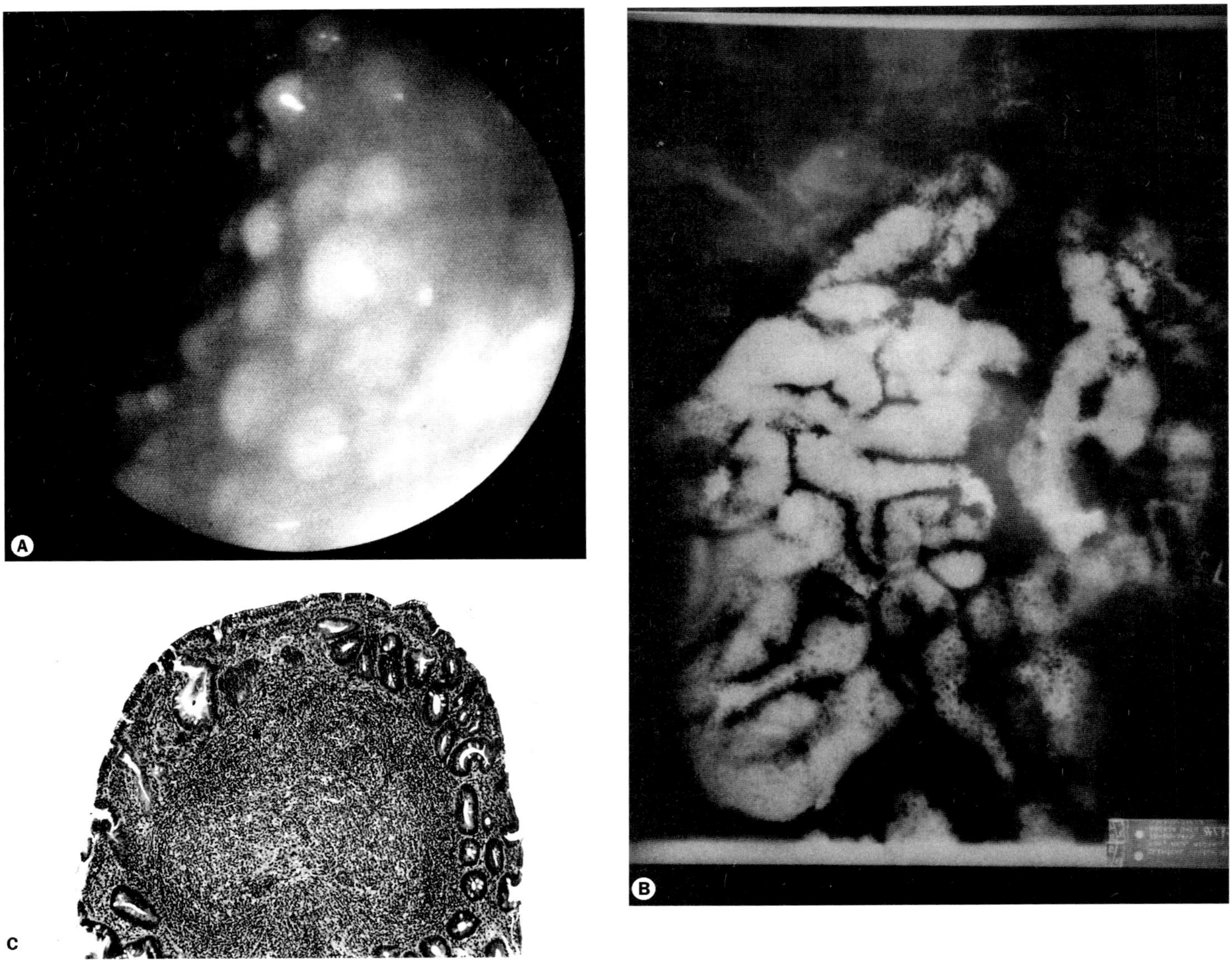

Figure 87.1 Intestinal nodular hyperplasia in CVID. (**A**), Endoscopic appearance of nodules. (**B**) Radiologic appearance of nodules. (**C**) Microscopic appearance of nodules. The nodules are composed of B cells, rather than plasma cells as in normal germinal centers.

modalities include an elemental diet, total parenteral nutrition, and vitamin supplementation.

CVID patients often suffer from recurrent infections of the GI tract. These may be with 'conventional' (nonopportunistic) pathogens, such as *Salmonella* and *Campylobacter*; opportunistic pathogens such as *Cryptosporidia* or cytomegalovirus; or unusual organisms such as the gramnegative bacterium dysgonic fermentor-3 (DF-3).[13] In the past, infections with conventional pathogens, particularly *Giardia*, were quite common in patients with CVID, but they appear to be less common with the advent of effective immunoglobulin replacement therapy. Nevertheless, such pathogens must be excluded in all patients with the previously described villous atrophy/malabsorption syndrome, because they may greatly aggravate symptoms.

Finally, CVID patients may develop colonic inflammation, which typically consists of low-grade 'microscopic' colitis but may occasionally manifest as overt ulcerative colitis or transmural granulomatous colitis, which is indistinguishable from inflammatory bowel disease (IBD).[14] The low-grade colitis is marked pathologically by infiltration of the lamina propria with lymphocytes and neutrophils, and by an increase in intraepithelial lymphocyte numbers. However, the classic features of IBD, such as granuloma formation or crypt abscesses, are typically absent. The cause of such colitis is unknown.

Selective IgA deficiency

Selective IgA deficiency is the most common primary immunodeficiency, and can represent a more benign form of the same disease process seen in CVID (Chapter 34).[15] When clinical GI problems occur, they are often similar to those seen in patients with CVID, i.e. villous atrophy/malabsorption syndrome, or infection by conventional pathogens. IgA deficiency is found with an increased frequency in gluten-sensitive enteropathy.[16] In addition, patients with IgA deficiency tend to absorb intestinal macromolecules and fail to clear the latter from the circulation once they are absorbed. These findings are attributable to the important role IgA plays in maintaining the intestinal barrier and in the clearance of antigens from the circulation (Chapter 4).

Chronic granulomatous disease

Chronic granulomatous disease (CCD) is characterized by a defect in the enzymatic pathway that generates superoxide anions and other oxygen species in neutrophils and other phagocytic cells, which limits the ability of these cells to kill ingested organisms (Chapter 37).[17] In response to infection, affected patients often generate granulomatous lesions in the soft tissues, bones, liver and lung. Somewhat surprisingly, the GI tract is generally free of infection, and chronic diarrhea and malabsorption are uncommon. However, a small proportion of patients have intestinal obstruction caused by the accumulation of macrophages containing lipid-rich cellular debris.[18] Patients with CGD may have typical granulomas in the rectum or other areas of the large bowel that resemble those seen in Crohn's disease; however, these probably represent an abnormal response to one or more infectious agents, and not idiopathic inflammatory disease.

Severe combined immunodeficiency (SCID)

Disorders affecting both limbs of the immune system arise from a number of genetically defined and undefined disorders (Chapter 35).[19] Patients with SCID are subject to severe and overwhelming infections with conventional and opportunistic pathogens and die quite early, unless they undergo transplantation with normal bone marrow. In the vast majority of patients these infections include those affecting the GI tract and those caused by a variety of opportunistic agents, such as *Candida*, *Cryptosporidia* and viral organisms. In addition, it should be noted that such patients have malabsorption syndrome and lactose deficiency, as noted in patients with CVID, suggesting that these manifestations are fundamentally related to a T-cell defect.

Despite the attention to HLA matching, SCID patients who have undergone bone marrow transplantation frequently experience a graft-versus-host (GVH)[20] reaction in the post-transplant period, which is accompanied by GI symptoms. Such GVH is marked during its acute phase by watery diarrhea, loss of fluids and electrolytes, and ulceration that can lead to blood loss. In the GI tract a GVH lesion is characterized by a mixed inflammatory infiltrate, epithelial cell necrosis and crypt abscesses. In its more chronic phase the lesion has features of villous atrophy, such as those associated with the villous enteropathies described below. The cause of these lesions is both B- and T-cell-mediated tissue damage aggravated by infectious agents.

HUMAN IMMUNODEFICIENCY VIRUS INFECTION

The mucosal surface of the GI tract plays a fundamental role in the pathogenesis of human immunodeficiency virus type 1 (HIV-1) infection. In the early phase of disease HIV-1 may gain initial access to lymphoid tissues through mucosal surfaces. Upon infection, the mucosa, as the largest lymphoid organ of the body, is a potential reservoir for HIV-1-infected mononuclear cells. Ultimately the mucosal immune system becomes sufficiently impaired by HIV infection to allow infection with conventional and opportunistic pathogens and neoplasms.[21] The importance of HIV infection has led to a growing interest in the development of an effective vaccine that induces protective antibodies or cytotoxic lymphocytes at mucosal surfaces.

Early phase of HIV infection

The GI tract serves as a potential portal of entry of HIV. In homosexual transmissions the virus may enter the host through the rectal mucosa during receptive anal intercourse. The upper gastrointestinal tract mucosa may also be involved in the acquisition of the virus during receptive orogenital contact.[22] However, oral transmission of HIV-1 in humans appears to be infrequent, perhaps owing to the presence of viral inhibitors (e.g. secretory leukocyte protease inhibitor) in saliva.[23]

HIV may enter the gut wall via breaks in the mucosal surface. M cells, which are scattered over the epithelial surfaces of lymphoid follicles in the rectal area and the tonsils, and intestinal epithelial cells represent potential alternative points of transport and entry into the underlying lamina propria.[24,25] If mucosal lymphoid follicles are the site of initial viral entry into the body they could be the site of primary infection of CD4 T cells and macrophages. The latter, however, exhibit a low prevalence of virus-expressing cells in the intestine, possibly because of their low expression of CCR5 (the principal coreceptor for gp120-mediated entry of macrophage-tropic virus strains).[26] CCR5 ligands are β-chemokines such as RANTES, MIP-1α, MIP-1β (Chapter 13). In contrast, the corresponding coreceptor for lymphocyte-tropic strains is CXCR4, and its ligand is stromal-derived factor 1. Finally, it should be noted that T cells developing in mucosal lymphoid follicles traffic widely to other mucosal areas and to the systemic lymphoid tissues as well. Therefore, a primary infection of the GI tract could be an efficient means of viral dissemination throughout the body.

Early HIV infection often manifests with an acute mononucleosis-like syndrome (days to weeks after inoculation) with viremia that includes various GI manifestations such as diarrhea, nausea and anorexia. Although the precise mechanism of this syndrome is unknown, it is likely to involve the release of various inflammatory cytokines such as interleukin-1 (IL-1) and tumor necrosis factor (TNF), which may mediate febrile responses and possibly diarrhea. The acute syndrome resolves after 1–3 weeks, with a decline in viremia.

Intermediate phase of HIV infection

The intermediate phase of HIV infection can last for many years. During this period, infection in the mucosal immune system is probably causing the depletion of local CD4 T cells and progressive damage that eventually results in severe GI infection.[27–30] A somewhat controversial manifestation of intermediate-stage HIV infection is the so-called HIV or AIDS enteropathy syndrome. Originally this was thought to occur in patients with AIDS associated with severe GI syndromes in which no pathogen could be identified as the causative agent. HIV infection itself was believed to be the underlying etiologic factor. Over the course of time, however, GI symptoms in such patients could be increasingly explained by infection with opportunistic pathogens such as various protozoa, adenoviruses and atypical mycobacteria. It is now recognized that subtle evidence of malabsorption (abnormal Schilling tests, partial villous atrophy, epithelial enzyme deficiencies) may occur relatively early in the course of disease, well before the appearance of very low CD4 T-cell counts in the periphery and the onset of opportunistic infections.[31,32] Thus it seems likely that AIDS enteropathy does exist, albeit in a less severe and earlier form than formerly believed.

Late stage of HIV infection

In the late stage of HIV infection there is widespread impairment of T-cell and B-cell function. Levels of CD4 T cells in the lamina propria are low and CD8 T-cell levels are increased or, at a very late stage, decreased as well. The patients are subject to myriad opportunistic and nonopportunistic infections that produce a variety of GI manifestations, ranging from esophageal ulcers caused by *Candida albicans* (which often heralds the onset of late-stage HIV infection), to large-bowel ulceration caused by cytomegalovirus infection, or to the severe protracted diarrhea caused by various protozoan infections (Table 94.1).[33] These infections lead to the progressive weight loss and wasting of HIV infection and to 'slim disease' in Africa. Unchecked, these GI manifestations are fatal.

Late HIV infection is a cause of GI neoplasms in about 12% of patients with AIDS. These include Kaposi sarcoma (about 60%) and non-Hodgkin lymphoma. Kaposi sarcoma-associated herpesvirus (KSHV) (also called human herpesvirus-8 – HHV8) appears to be the etiological agent in Kaposi sarcoma,[34,35] which typically manifests as a multifocal mucosal lesion with spindle cells. Tumor cell growth is probably augmented by cytokine and growth factor release, as HIV-1-infected mononuclear cells release a transactivator of transcription (Tat) protein and various cytokines such as TNF, which are known to stimulate the proliferation of Kaposi sarcoma-derived spindle cells. The spindle cells produce IL-1, FGF and IL-6, which stimulate their own growth and that of other cells, including the vascular and lymphatic cells that help form the lesions of Kaposi sarcoma.

Non-Hodgkin lymphoma is the second most common neoplasm of the GI tract in AIDS patients. It has recently been suggested that HHV8 may also play an etiologic role in AIDS-related lymphomas, possibly in association with Epstein–Barr virus (EBV) infections, which are commonly seen in AIDS patients. Because EBV infection is known to immortalize B cells in vitro, and as EBV-specific cytotoxic T-cell responses are suppressed in HIV-infected individuals, it has been proposed that the development of GI lymphoma in HIV-1-infected persons could represent the malignant transformation of EBV-infected mucosal B lymphocytes.[36]

Infectious agents in late HIV disease

	Type of agent	
	Nonopportunistic	**Opportunistic**
Bacterial	*Salmonella* species *Shigella flexneri* *Mycobacteria* Spirochetes	*Mycobacterium avium* *Mycobacterium intracellulare* *Campylobactor jejuni*
Fungal		*Candida albicans* *Histoplasma capsulatum*
Protozoal	*Giardia lamblia* *Entamoeba dispar*	*Cryptosporidia* *Microsporidia* *Isospora belli* *Cyclospora*
Viral	Rotavirus Norwalk agent	Cytomegalovirus Herpes simplex virus Adenovirus

Table 87.1 Infectious agents encountered in late HIV disease.

KEY CONCEPTS

Gastrointestinal manifestations of HIV infection

- Early phase:
  - The GI tract is a major portal of entry.
  - The mucosal system is a disseminator and reservoir of infected cells.
- Intermediate phase:
  - Progressive mucosal CD4 T-cell depletion precedes CD4 T-cell depletion in peripheral blood.
  - HIV enteropathy – partial villous atrophy syndrome associated with malabsorption.
- Late disease phase:
  - Multiple opportunistic and conventional infections.
  - GI neoplasia (Kaposi sarcoma and lymphoma).

GASTROINTESTINAL DISEASES CAUSING IMMUNODEFICIENCY

Certain GI diseases can lead to immunodeficiency. In general, immunodeficiency occurs when immune elements are lost into the gut lumen as part of protein-losing enteropathy (PLE). PLE is brought about by several different types of disease states, including inflammation of the mucosa, allergic reactions involving the GI tract, and lymphatic blockage abnormalities. In PLE associated with inflammation or allergic reactions, only proteins are lost into the gastrointestinal tract and the chief manifestation is hypoalbuminemia and hypogammaglobulinemia. Although the hypoalbuminemia can be sufficiently severe as to cause edema, the hypogammaglobulinemia rarely, if ever, is severe enough to lead to immunodeficiency. In contrast, in patients with PLE associated with lymphatic blockage there is loss of both serum proteins and lymphoid cells into the GI tract, which does result in immunodeficiency. Intestinal lymphangiectasia and Whipple's disease are protein-losing states characterized by loss of both protein and lymphocytes into the GI tract.

Intestinal lymphangiectasia (IL)

Intestinal lymphangiectasia (IL) is a disorder of the intestinal lymphatics associated with loss of protein-rich and lymphocyte-rich fluid into the GI tract and hence the production of a lymphocytopenic, protein-losing gastroenteropathy.[37] IL occurs either as a primary form caused by a congenital defect in lymphatic development, or as a secondary form caused by an acquired lesion that affects lymphatic function. Primary IL is part of a spectrum of idiopathic lymphatic abnormalities that range from generalized disorders affecting the central and peripheral lymphatics to those affecting central or peripheral lymphatics selectively. Secondary IL is due to an acquired abnormality affecting lymphatic flow. Cardiac conditions, such as pericarditis or right-sided cardiac lesions, that impair the emptying of major lymphatics into the major veins are one common cause of secondary IL. Secondary IL can also result from specific infection (such as Whipple's disease), nonspecific inflammation (such as Crohn's disease), neoplasms, or intestinal conditions associated with lipophage infiltration and obstruction to the drainage tract (such as hypolipoproteinemia) or fibrosis (sclerosing mesenteritis/ retroperitonitis, postradiation fibrosis). One interesting inflammatory process of this sort is associated with a lupus-like syndrome ('inflammatory' IL); in this case the obstruction may be due to a vasculitic process affecting the lymphatics.[38]

Primary IL usually has its onset in the second or third decade, and is marked by edema, various GI symptoms and fatigue. The edema may be due to parenchymal lymphatic abnormalities and/or to protein-losing enteropathy and hypoalbuminemia; when peripheral lymphatic abnormalities are present, a very characteristic asymmetric edema is found. Patients with long-standing chylous ascites develop peritoneal fibrosis. Stasis dermatitis with peripheral ulcer formation may occur in the extremities. GI symptoms may consist of diarrhea, steatorrhea or malabsorption, but these are relatively uncommon because of the presence of a normal epithelial cell lining. In addition, in some patients cutaneous or intradermal lymphangiomas and/or vascular and nerve tumors are observed.

Secondary IL differs clinically from primary IL. The edema of secondary IL is invariably symmetric, and patients may show signs indicative of the underlying cause of the disease, e.g. the jugular venous distention of constitutive pericarditis, the hyperpigmentation of Whipple's disease or the butterfly rash of lupus erythematosus.

The diagnosis of IL rests on the presence of severe hypoalbuminemia (<2.0–2.5 g/dl) and lymphopenia (<1000–1500 cells/mm^2), in concert with a jejunal biopsy demonstrating characteristic dilated lymphatics (Fig. 87.2); however, the absence of the latter finding does not exclude the diagnosis, because the lesion may be patchy. Patients invariably have a severe protein-losing enteropathy as measured by α_1-antitrypsin clearance. They can be losing 5–40% of the intravascular fluid volume each day (normal <2% per day),[39] making IL the most severe of the protein-losing enteropathies.

Treatment of primary IL is symptomatic and only marginally effective. Patients are placed on a very low-fat diet, which has the effect of reducing intestinal lymphatic blockage. In contrast, the treatment of secondary IL can be dramatically effective if the underlying abnormality can be found and corrected. For example,

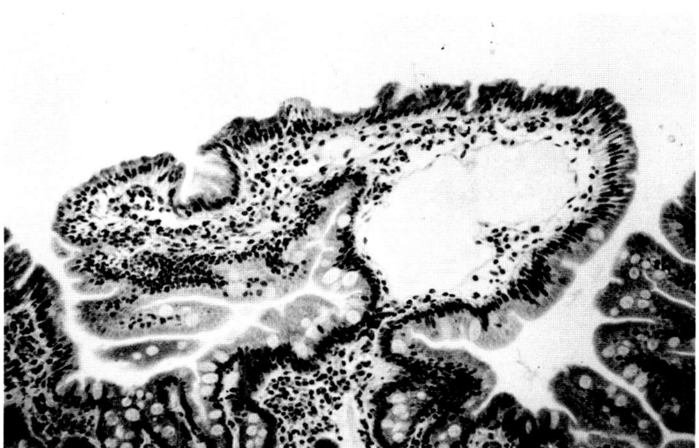

Figure 87.2 Intestinal lymphangiectasia. Jejunal biopsy showing dilated lymphatics at a villus tip.

pericardiectomy in patients with constrictive pericarditis can completely reverse secondary IL and its attendant protein-losing enteropathy.[40] Similarly, treatment of Whipple's disease with antibiotics and systemic lupus erythematosus (SLE)-like inflammatory disease with steroids can lead to dramatic resolution of secondary IL.

The loss of lymphocytes into the bowel lumen in IL can lead to a severe lymphocytopenia, with a massive depletion of T cells in the lymphoid tissues.[40,41] The lymphocyte loss is selective in that it affects T cells more than B cells, and CD4 T cells more than CD8 T cells.[42] This selectivity probably reflects the circulation pattern of the various cellular subsets, and thus the risk for loss into the bowel lumen as a result of lymphatic blockage. The residual cell population responds poorly in vitro even when stimulated at normal cell concentrations, indicating that the T-cell loss results in both a quantitative and a qualitative deficiency of responsive cells.[43] B-cell immunity in IL is far less affected than is T-cell immunity. IgG is the immunoglobulin most subject to the bulk loss process of IL (levels about 30% of normal), whereas IgA and IgM levels are about 50% of normal. These levels are typically sufficient to support substantive antibody responses.

Overall, IL is associated with a moderately severe T-cell immunodeficiency state. Although there is a measurable loss of immune elements, enough capacity to mount host defense responses is retained and most patients are not subject to infection with low-grade pathogens.

KEY CONCEPTS

Whipple's disease

- *Presentation*: hyperpigmentation of unknown cause, lymphadenopathy, hepatosplenomegaly, ascites, endocarditis, pleuropericarditis, pulmonary infiltrates, and central nervous system (CNS) manifestations such as ophthalmoplegia, uveitis, cerebellar symptoms and dementia.
- *Diagnosis*: intestinal biopsy followed by detection of *Trophyrema whippelii*, or PCR amplification of *T. whippelii* DNA from the tissue.
- *Treatment*: antibiotics (e.g. trimethoprim–sulfamethoxazole). Additive immunotherapy with IFN-γ or IL-12 in patients with refractory disease.
- *Potential complications of therapy*: failure to treat CNS, resulting in recurrent disease.

Whipple's disease

Whipple's disease is an infectious disease caused by a unique member of the actinobacteria family, *Trophyrema whippelii*.[44] The actinomycete *T. whippelii* appears in biopsies as a gram-positive and periodic acid–Schiff (PAS)-positive bacillary rod. The main focus of infection is the small intestine, where free bacteria and large numbers of 'foamy' macrophages filled with PAS-positive bodies consisting of intact bacteria and bacterial remnants can be found (Fig. 87.3). A curious feature of the histopathologic condition is that, other than the macrophage reaction, the bacteria evoke little inflammatory response and the intestinal damage is mainly due to the consequence of cellular infiltration. The disease is characterized by clubbed and distorted villi, lymphatic

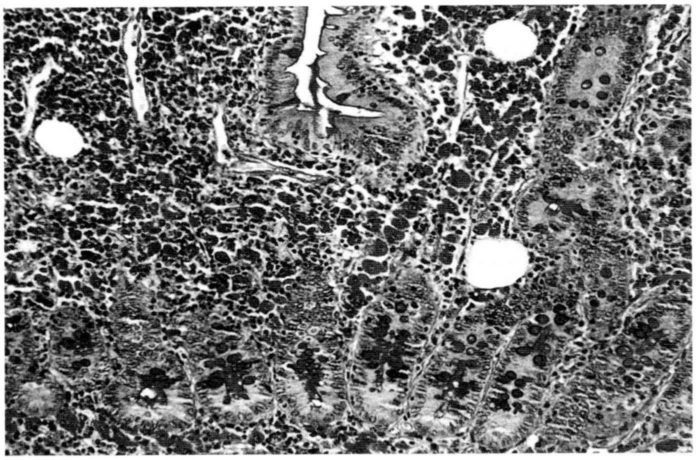

Figure 87.3 Whipple's disease (infection with *Trophyrema whippelii*). Jejunal biopsy showing macrophages filled with PAS-positive bacteria.

obstruction/dilatation, malabsorption and protein-losing enteropathy. As a result, patients with untreated disease have progressive weight loss that can be fatal. Although infection of the GI tract is the most prominent and well-known aspect of Whipple's disease, infections of the lymphatic system, heart, lung, kidney, serosal surfaces and central nervous system also occur. Joint involvement is common, but rarely if ever leads to deformity.

Whipple disease occurs predominantly in caucasian males (~80% of cases; 25% HLA-B27 positive) as a sporadic disease in their fourth or fifth decade of life. Diarrhea, progressive weight loss and other manifestations of malabsorption are the major presenting symptoms, although arthralgias occur. Patients typically have hyperpigmentation of unknown cause, lymphadenopathy (especially involving mesenteric nodes) and, less frequently, hepatosplenomegaly or even ascites. In addition, they may have endocarditis, pleuropericarditis, pulmonary infiltrates, and central nervous system (CNS) manifestations such as ophthalmoplegia, uveitis, cerebellar symptoms and dementia. The diagnosis is made by intestinal biopsy or polymerase chain reaction-based detection of *T. whippelii* from intestinal tissues. Whipple's disease responds to antibiotics (e.g. trimethoprim–sulfamethoxazole), but care must be taken to use an antibiotic that crosses the blood–brain barrier so as to eliminate CNS infection. Failure to do so may lead to recurrent disease.

Although the etiology of Whipple's disease is now established, its nontransmissibility suggests the presence of host immunologic abnormalities. Immunologic studies in Whipple's disease have so far been centered on the elucidation of general immune defects.[45] In these studies it has been shown that patients frequently have a number of T-cell abnormalities, including lymphocytopenia, reduced or absent delayed skin test responses, and decreased response to various T-cell mitogens. In addition, the lamina propria of patients contains decreased numbers of CD4 T cells and increased numbers of CD8 IEL. These T-cell abnormalities can persist into the post-treatment period and probably occur because Whipple's disease causes a secondary intestinal lymphangiectasia, resulting in a loss of T cells into the intestinal lumen and leading to an acquired lymphocyte loss immunodeficiency. B-cell function appears normal.

Impaired delayed-type hypersensitivity responses in Whipple's disease are accompanied by persistent immunologic alterations of peripheral blood mononuclear cells (PBMC), such as reduced surface expression of complement receptor type 3 α chain CD11b, a molecule mainly expressed on monocytes involved in phagocytosis and respiratory burst. Marth and co-workers[46] described reduced IL-12 production by PBMC in Whipple's disease. These data may indicate a primary monocyte defect that results in a secondary reduction of IFN-γ and IgG_2 serum levels, and thus provide a rationale for additive immunotherapy with IFN-γ or IL-12 in patients with chronic therapy-refractory Whipple's disease.

FOOD HYPERSENSITIVITIES (INTESTINAL ENTEROPATHY)

Reactions to food proteins may have several causes, the most easily understood being IgE-mediated allergic hypersensitivity (Chapter 52). This is generally an immediate-type hypersensitivity that gives rise to acute GI symptoms and to associated allergic symptoms, such as skin rash (urticaria, eczema), pharyngeal edema and bronchospasm. It is almost always associated with a positive skin test to the offending substance. The mechanism of disease is mast cell degranulation via IgE antibody cross-linking, with subsequent release of mediators that induce a typical type 1 immune response. Mediator release can result in changes in vascular permeability, and thus this form of sensitivity can be associated with massive protein-losing enteropathy and hypoalbuminemia.[47]

Other types of food hypersensitivities consist of nonallergic, nonimmunologic sensitivities to certain ingested chemicals that have pharmacologic effects (e.g. cheese, tyramine, caffeine) or cause mast cell mediator release directly. This category also includes toxic chemicals such as hexachlorobenzene, which produces acquired porphyria, and acetanilide in rapeseed oil, which causes respiratory failure. Finally, this category contains those substances that cause GI difficulties because of genetically determined enzyme deficiencies in the host, such as lactose in patients who are lactase-deficient and fava bean components that induce hemolytic anemia in patients who have glucose 6-phosphate dehydrogenase deficiency.

A third type of food hypersensitivity is non-IgE-mediated immunologic sensitivity.[48,49] This is mediated by T cells, and possibly B cells, producing non-IgE antibodies. The most prominent of these conditions is gluten-sensitive enteropathy (celiac disease), but other forms such as cow-milk 'allergy' also occur.

Gluten-sensitive enteropathy

Gluten-sensitive enteropathy (GSE), also known as celiac disease, celiac sprue or idiopathic sprue, is a small-intestinal disease characterized by villous atrophy and attendant malabsorption.[50] It results from a hypersensitivity to various cereal grain storage proteins, most commonly those found in wheat gluten or, more precisely, a substance derived from wheat gluten known as gliadin. Initially GSE was believed to be due to an intestinal enzyme deficiency, causing toxic accumulation of undegraded gluten peptides, but recent evidence now strongly favors the idea that it is an immunologic disorder.

Clinical aspects

GSE occurs either as a disease limited to the GI tract or as an abnormality that accompanies the skin disease dermatitis herpetiformis. In the former, more common form of GSE (ordinary GSE), the clinical course is dominated by GI symptoms and the consequences of malabsorption: fatty diarrhea, weight loss, various nutritional deficiencies, and growth failure in children. In the GSE associated with dermatitis herpetiformis (GSE-DH), a skin disease characterized by a vesicular pruritic lesion on the extensor and exposed surfaces of the body, is the main manifestation, and a GSE-type GI condition, although present in most if not all cases, is usually quite mild or unapparent.

The GI lesions of GSE consist of a villous atrophy marked by blunted, shortened, or even absent villi, and a surface epithelium made up of disarrayed, morphologically abnormal epithelial cells (Fig. 87.4). The villous atrophy is associated with elongated crypts in which immature epithelial cells are being generated at an increased rate; thus the disease process does not affect all epithelial cells, and the mucosa retains an intact, nonulcerated epithelial cell lining, albeit one that does not function normally.[51] The skin disease of GSE-DH consists of a subepidermal collection of acute inflammatory cells that causes local fluid accumulation and hence the typical vesicular lesion of GSE-DH.[52] Both lesional and nonlesional skin contains granular IgA and complement deposits in the basement membrane zone, which are believed to initiate an inflammatory process under certain circumstances. Although such IgA deposits are not present in the skin of patients with ordinary GSE and cannot be shown to contain gliadin, their relation to gluten ingestion indicates that they are composed of immunoglobulin that originated in the gastrointestinal tract.

Marsh has identified several histopathologic forms of GSE that define the progression of disease and its severity.[51] In the infiltrative stage the mucosal architecture is normal, but the villous epithelial cells are infiltrated with increased numbers of IEL. This minimal lesion is associated with normal intestinal function and is most often found in patients with GSE-DH or asymptomatic relatives of GSE patients with GSE. In the hyperplastic stage the villi remain normal in length, but the crypts are elongated and are also infiltrated with IEL. This lesion is presumably a 'compensated' form of GSE in which the epithelial proliferation in the crypts compensates for increased epithelial cell loss in the villi. In the destructive stage of disease one sees

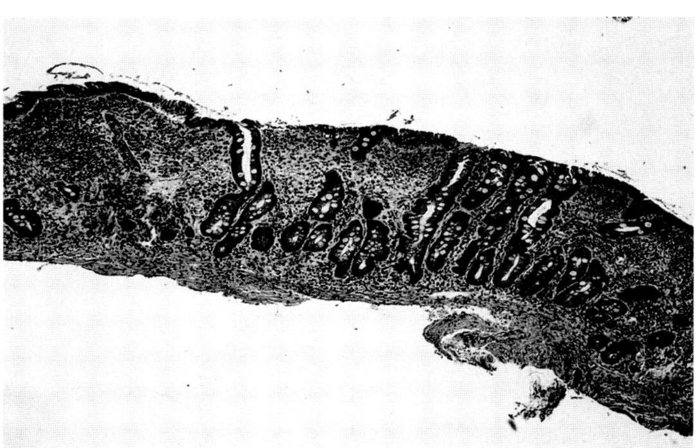

Figure 87.4 Gluten-sensitive enteropathy. Jejunal biopsy showing severe villous atrophy. The lamina propria is infiltrated with mononuclear cells but the epithelia cell layer is intact.

the typical villous atrophy of GSE. This uncompensated form of GSE leads to malabsorption and related gastrointestinal symptoms. Finally, in the hypoplastic/atrophic stage of disease there is severe villous atrophy without crypt cell hyperplasia. In this 'end stage' the patient is no longer completely responsive to gluten withdrawal because of a permanent disturbance in the generative function of the crypt epithelial cells. Occasionally this lesion is associated with ulcerations (known as ulcerative jejunitis) or with lymphoma. When this stage occurs without a previous history of gluten responsiveness, as it sometimes does, its relationship with GSE may be difficult to establish.

The gastrointestinal lesion in both ordinary GSE and GSE-DH responds rapidly to gluten exclusion, both clinically and histopathologically. The only exceptions to this rule are those patients with long-standing disease who have the hypoplastic/atrophic type lesion mentioned previously. In contrast, the skin disease of GSE-DH is quite slow to respond to a gluten-free diet and often requires months of strict gluten exclusion to achieve a complete resolution of symptoms. For this reason, patients with GSE-DH are more often treated with anti-inflammatory agents. GSE is generally a condition that requires constant (lifelong) treatment with a gluten-free diet. If untreated or partially treated, subclinical enteropathy and covert nutritional deficiency may result. In addition, GSE that is untreated or partially treated for a long time is quite clearly associated with an increased incidence of gastrointestinal lymphoma or carcinoma. Cases of transient GSE have been described, usually in children, in which the hypersensitivity to gluten appeared to resolve completely and did not return when gluten was reintroduced into the diet. In view of the threat of neoplasia, however, such transient cases must be carefully documented before a gluten-free diet can be safely abandoned.

GSE may manifest quite early in life, with the introduction of cereal grains into the diet. However, it can also have a delayed onset, occurring for the first time in adulthood or even in advanced age. The reason for the variable age of onset is unknown and is probably related to individual differences in genetic or environmental factors. There appears to be a recent tendency to more frequent oligo- or even monosymptomatic GSE cases, leading to the hypothesis that the condition is underdiagnosed. GSE must be differentiated from several other gastrointestinal conditions that also produce villous atrophy and malabsorption. These conditions include sensitivities to other food substances, other immunodeficiencies, and lymphoma. In addition, rare patients with 'idiopathic' villous atrophy are encountered whose disease is unrelated to gluten hypersensitivity or to hypersensitivity to other food substances.

Given the necessity for lifelong gluten exclusion in GSE, the diagnosis of the disease requires definitive evidence of gluten sensitivity. This may include biopsy procedures and serologic testing. Endoscopic biopsies are important to confirm the diagnosis and assess the severity of the disease. Tissue samples are taken from multiple sites to reduce false-negative results (because of the patchy nature of the lesions) and from the duodenum in the area beyond the ampulla of Vater to avoid false positives (because of the distortion of villous architecture as a result of the presence of Brunner's glands). If the biopsy results are positive, the patient is put on a strict gluten-free diet for several weeks and is then subjected to a repeat endoscopic biopsy to confirm that duodenal histology has improved. Alternatively, a second biopsy is not done and instead the patient is monitored with tests of intestinal absorption (fat excretion, D-xylose absorption) and by serologic tests to ensure that improvement has occurred.

This diagnostic regimen establishes the presence of GSE with a fair degree of certainty; however, it does not exclude the real possibility (applicable mainly to pediatric patients) that the intestinal changes have been caused by a transient infection that just happens to improve with the institution of a gluten-free diet. This possibility can be eliminated with a short gluten challenge followed by serologic studies to determine the presence of an abnormal immunologic response to gluten exposure. The serologic tests available are based on the association of GSE with antigliadin antibody, antiendomesial antibody and antireticular antibody.[53] IgA antigliadin antibodies are quite specific for GSE, particularly when present at high titer, and are detectable with an enzyme-linked immunosorbent assay (ELISA) technique.[54] IgG antigliadin antibodies also occur, but they are far less disease specific than are IgA antigliadin antibodies.

The most disease-specific of these antibodies is the antiendomesial antibody detected by immunofluorescence of muscle cell basement membranes in monkey esophagus or human umbilical cord (sensitivity >90%, specificity nearly 100%). Dieterich et al.[55] identified the autoantigen of these antibodies by showing that they are directed against a specific tissue transglutaminase. The identification of this antigen will soon allow serologic ELISA testing for transglutaminase antibodies on a routine basis. Based on the availability of serologic testing, the presumptive diagnosis of GSE can be made and further evaluated by endoscopic biopsy and response to gluten-free diet. Other uses of GSE-specific serologic testing are the detection of latent (subclinical) GSE in relatives of patients and other at-risk individuals; in the workup of patients with symptoms suggestive of malabsorption who are being considered for jejunal biopsy and finally, in monitoring established patients for adherence to a gluten-free diet.[56,57] Detection of subclinical disease is important, because the intestinal lesion in GSE predisposes to the occurrence of neoplasia.

The use of serologic techniques and other noninvasive diagnostic procedures has led to the identification of a group of patients who have subclinical GSE, as defined by the fact that their intestinal abnormality is not associated with overt malabsorption. This group may include as many as 50% of patients with gluten sensitivity, who must be considered at risk for conversion to active disease. It should be noted, however, that not all serologically positive patients have an abnormal intestinal mucosa. Thus in some patients with subclinical disease it may be difficult to identify gluten sensitivity unequivocally.

The gluten component responsible for GSE

Gliadin is not a single protein, but rather a heterogeneous group of proline- and glutamine-rich proteins in the alcohol–water-extractable portion of wheat gluten.[58] Major advances in our understanding of gliadin structure came with the identification of distinct classes of gliadin based on their primary structure (ω_5-, $\omega_{1,2}$-, γ- and α-gliadins). Although the toxicity of the α-gliadin fraction has been shown most clearly, it is likely that all gliadin fractions contain toxic components.[59] In recent years studies have narrowed the range of suspects to peptides containing the tetramer sequences QQQP or PSQQ, although the flanking regions of these sequences may also be important.[60,61] One may speculate that this finding is due to the fact that peptides active in GSE must fit into the groove of certain MHC class II antigen-presenting molecules, thereby favoring the generation of a specific polyclonal T-cell response to gliadin fractions.

Immunopathologic features of GSE

The inflammatory lesion in patients with GSE is restricted to the small-intestinal mucosa, because this is the site ordinarily in contact with gliadin that has not yet been broken down into constituent amino acids.[62] The earliest histologic changes take place in the lamina propria beneath the epithelial cell layer.[63] There is evidence of increased vascular permeability, including swelling of capillary endothelia, tissue edema and extravascular fibrinogen deposition, which is followed by an influx of polymorphonuclear leukocytes that cause a second round of vascular permeability changes. At 36–96 hours after gluten exposure, lymphocytes, plasma cells and complement appear in the lesion.[64] Of considerable interest is the fact that epithelial cell injury clearly does not occur as an early event, and thus does not initiate the pathologic process of GSE.

The mature lesion of GSE is characterized by infiltration of B cells and T cells. The B cells synthesize IgA, IgM and IgG, with IgM and IgG plasma cells somewhat disproportionately increased relative to IgA plasma cells. Approximately 5–10% of the B cells are producing antigliadin antibodies, especially of the IgG isotype.[65] The presence of both IgG and complement raises the possibility that IgG-complement-mediated epithelial damage plays a role in the disease.

The second cellular component in the mature GSE lesion is a T-cell infiltrate that is evident both in the lamina propria and in the intraepithelial layer. The lamina propria T cells are TCRαβ CD4 or CD8, and are enriched cells bearing markers for memory (CD45RO) and activation (IL-2R).[66] In contrast, intraepithelial T cells bear a marker associated with proliferation.[67] These data support the view that in GSE, gliadin activates lamina propria T cells and thereby induces lymphokine production, but not proliferation. Evidence that T cells infiltrating GSE lesions produce large amounts of Th1 cytokines such as IFN-γ supports this possibility.[68]

A major immunologic feature of GSE is a qualitative and quantitative change in IEL. Patients with GSE have an increase in the proportion of IEL T cells bearing the γδ T-cell receptor.[69] However, the contribution of these γδ T cells to the pathogenesis of GSE remains unclear. The number of γδ IEL is not related to gluten ingestion; occurs in patients before the onset of villous atrophy; and persists after successful treatment. The γδ IEL in GSE are polyclonal, with a normal V repertoire. Finally, increased numbers of γδ IEL occur in unaffected relatives of GSE patients, particularly those who have similar MHC class II types.[70] The increase in γδ IEL may thus reflect underlying expansion of γδ T cells in the intraepithelial compartment. Patients with GSE show increased number of TCRαβ IEL bearing markers of proliferation and memory.[71] The number of αβ IEL waxes with gluten ingestion and wanes with gluten restriction,[72] suggesting that in contrast to the γδ IELs, αβ IELs may play a role in disease pathogenesis.

Humoral immunity in patients with GSE

Serum and secretory IgA levels are increased and tend to fall when the patient is on a gluten-free diet. IgG levels are only minimally elevated, and IgM levels are decreased. IgA deficiency occurs far more often in patients with GSE than in normal individuals, and various members of several families have been reported with multiple forms of autoimmunity, GSE and IgA deficiency.[73] On this and other bases, it is likely that susceptibility to GSE and IgA deficiency is genetically related.

Virtually all patients with GSE have antigliadin antibodies in the circulation,[74] the level of which is broadly correlated with disease severity and falls when the patient is on a gluten-free diet. High titers of IgA antigliadin antibodies are quite specific for GSE and occur in the vast majority of patients,[75] supporting the view that the antigliadin response in GSE is a major manifestation of the disease and is indicative of a primary hyperresponsiveness to gliadin.

Cellular immunity in GSE

In vitro responses to mitogens and common environmental antigens are essentially normal in patients with GSE, indicating that no general defect in T-cell immunity is present. However, rather than proliferate, patient T cells respond to gliadin with the production of a lymphokine, leukocyte migration inhibition factor (LMIF), and an increase in the surface expression of IL-2 receptor (Fig. 87.5).[76]

Mechanism of tissue injury in patients with GSE

Organ cultures of intestinal tissue from patients with GSE who were in remission are not injured by the addition of gliadin, whereas tissue from patients with active disease is injured.[77] This suggests that gliadin is not directly toxic to GSE tissue: instead, its toxicity appears to depend on the presence of an activated endogenous effector mechanism, which is most likely immunologic. Although T cells are probably the key mechanism of villous atrophy in patients with GSE, humoral antibody reaction with complement may also contribute to GSE pathogenesis.[78]

Genetic factors in patients with GSE

GSE frequently occurs in association with other autoimmune diseases, such as type I diabetes mellitus. Moreover, within families close relatives may exhibit either GSE or autoimmune manifestations, or both. The observation that GSE is closely associated with certain HLA genes helps explain this familial pattern.[79] GSE is associated with the HLA-A1, -B8, -DR3, -DQ2 haplotype (Chapter 6), a haplotype that is also associated with susceptibility to diabetes mellitus, autoimmune thyroiditis, myasthenia gravis, IgA deficiency and CVID. GSE is also frequently found in patients who express both the HLA-DR5 and DR7 alleles. A common factor in these patients is the frequent inheritance (~95%) of a specific HLA-DQ allele, DQ2 (~95% of patients vs 12% of control groups). DQ2 is a heterodimer composed of a DQα chain determined by the DQA1*0501 allele and a DQβ chain determined by the DQB1*0201 allele.[80] It is the DQB1*0201 that specifies the DQ2 antigenic determinant. The DQA1*0501 and DQB1*0201 alleles can be on the same chromosome (in which case they are associated with DR3) or on opposite chromosomes (in which case they are associated with DR5 and DR7, respectively).[81] This finding explains the fact that GSE is associated with either the DR3 or the DR5/7 serologic specificities. Although the association of GSE with HLA-DQ2 (i.e. the *DQB1*0201* gene) is strong, it is not absolute, suggesting that alternative *DQ* genes can act as GSE-predisposing genes.

Pathogenesis of GSE

Based upon the above observations a possible scenario for the pathogenesis of this disease is suggested (Fig. 87.5). The first step involves the ingestion of gliadin protein, which is then taken up by dendritic cells that process the protein into peptides containing the Gln-Gln-Gln-Pro sequence. These dendritic cells present these peptides to Peyer's patch T cells in the context of the HLA-DQ heterodimer (encoded by *DQA1*0501/DQB1*0201*) and thereby induce gliadin-specific Th1 T cells. The activated T cells migrate to the lamina propria and are restimulated by gliadin peptides that have penetrated the epithelial cell barrier in the context of DQ2. In the final step, the Th1 T cells secrete cytokines such as IFN-γ and TNF, thereby inducing matrix metalloproteinases (e.g. MMP-1: collagenase; MMP-3: stromelysin), which cause villous atrophy and the other immunopathologic manifestations of GSE.

A key question that remains unanswered in this scenario concerns the phenomenon of oral antigen-induced unresponsiveness, or tolerance. The vast majority of protein antigens that

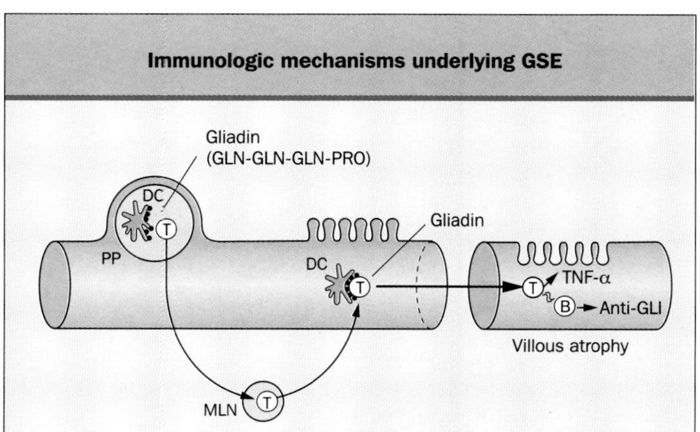

Figure 87.5 Immunologic mechanisms underlying GSE. Gliadin peptides (GLN-GLN-GLN-PRO) induce T-cell activation in Peyer's patches via specific HLA-DQ restriction molecules. T cells migrate to the lamina propria where, on restimulation, they secrete cytokines and cause villous atrophy.

KEY CONCEPTS

Gluten-sensitive enteropathy (GSE)/celiac disease

- *Definition*: intestinal enteropathy caused by immunologic hypersensitivity to the gliadin component of wheat and other cereal grains.
  - Occurs as GSE limited to GI manifestation.
  - Occurs as dermatitis herpetiformis (skin disease associated with mild GI disease).
- *Pathophysiology*: villous atrophy caused by T-cell-mediated immune damage to the small intestinal mucosa. Autoantigen in GSE: Tissue transglutaminase.
- *Diagnosis*: biopsy, response to gluten-free diet, high titers of IgA antigliadin and antitissue transglutaminase/antiendomyosin antibodies.
- *Clinical effects*: malabsorption, fatty diarrhea; tumors of the GI tract in long-term disease.
- *Immunologic basis*: immune response gene (HLA)-mediated hyperresponsiveness to gliadin.

encounter T cells in the mucosal immune system elicit a 'negative' immune response that leads to either the elaboration of suppressor T cells or T-cell anergy. Thus, the suggestion that gliadin elicits a positive immune response in patients with GSE would suggest that the central defect in GSE is the subversion of immune unresponsiveness to gliadin.

Other food-induced intestinal enteropathies

Additional food-induced enteropathies are best represented by cow-milk enteropathy, but in fact can be due to other food proteins (such as soy protein) as well.[82] Patients with cow-milk enteropathy have a villous atrophy and consequent malabsorption that resolves when they are placed on a milk-free diet. The offending substance appears to be β-lactalbumin, and patients do have cell-mediated immunity to this antigen. Cow-milk enteropathy differs from GSE in that it is almost invariably a disease of early childhood and disappears as the child matures, whereas GSE can become clinically manifest at any age and persists for life. Furthermore, cow-milk enteropathy appears to be associated with certain environmental factors, such as a preceding history of infectious gastroenteritis or various types of intestinal obstruction.

Antigen-nonspecific intestinal enteropathies

Another form of intestinal enteropathy is antigen-nonspecific intestinal enteropathy. This is characterized by severe villous atrophy and malabsorption that is apparently unrelated to any ingested substance and persists despite the institution of a strict elimination diet or even total parenteral nutrition.[83] In some cases antigen-nonspecific intestinal enteropathy occurs de novo without any apparent cause or antecedents, whereas in other cases it appears to be the result of a pre-existing gastrointestinal condition. Examples include ulcerative ileojejunitis[84] and certain forms of eosinophilic gastroenteropathy.[85] The latter condition is uniquely defined by eosinophilic infiltration of the lamina propria of the stomach antrum and upper small intestine. In some cases this is due to an IgE-mediated allergic reaction to a particular food substance that responds to elimination of that substance from the diet, whereas in other cases it appears to be a nonallergic reaction to many foods and is unresponsive to elimination diets. It is this second form of eosinophilic gastroenteropathy that is associated with villous atrophy and shades into antigen-nonspecific intestinal enteropathy. The pathogenesis of antigen-nonspecific intestinal enteropathy is unclear and its treatment rests mainly on the use of anti-inflammatory and immunosuppressive agents.

THE INFLAMMATORY BOWEL DISEASES

The inflammatory bowel diseases (IBD) are defined as inflammations of the GI tract *not* due to specific pathogens.[86] Although there is excellent evidence that these diseases are immunologically mediated, it remains unclear whether the primary cause is an immunologic defect. By virtue of their relatively common occurrence, their severity and chronicity, IBD are the most important of the immunologically mediated GI diseases.

IBD has two forms: ulcerative colitis (UC), which is an inflammation limited to the large bowel; and Crohn disease (CD), which is an inflammation that can occur anywhere along the alimentary canal but is most often localized in the terminal ileum and ascending colon. UC and CD appear to be the products of very different immunopathologic processes; however, their grouping under a single heading is justified because of their clinical overlap, the genetic factors they have in common, and their shared immunologic findings.

Ulcerative colitis originates as a distal (rectal) inflammation that gradually spreads up the colon in a contiguous fashion. In about half of the cases the disease remains distal (an ulcerative proctitis), but in up to one-fifth it will ultimately involve the entire large bowel (pancolitis). In the latter case the disease is far more severe and debilitating and carries an increased risk for colonic carcinoma. Colonic inflammation in UC is relatively superficial; however, ulcer formation leads gradually to the loss of mucosal absorptive function (Fig. 87.6A). Endoscopy reveals mucosal granularity and superficial ulcers covered with mucopurulent exudate. The clinical course is marked by abdominal pain, painful defecation, bloody diarrhea, weight loss and, in children, poor growth.

In contrast, CD is a transmural inflammation with hallmark granulomatous lesions (Fig. 87.6*B*). Unlike UC, the CD lesion is discontinuous and characteristically leads to obstructive symptoms, abscess formation, and fistulas leading from the bowel to other organs or to the body wall. Ulcers also occur in CD, but these tend to be linear and extend deep into the bowel wall. The clinical course of CD is marked by severe abdominal pain and symptoms referable to intestinal obstruction or abscess formation. Patients may have excessive diarrhea caused by motility disturbances, or malabsorption and constipation caused by obstruction. Severe bleeding occurs more frequently because of the involvement of deeper tissues. These differences notwithstanding, in up to one-tenth of cases UC and CD can be indistinguishable, particularly when CD is limited to the large bowel and the inflammation is not associated with granulomas (indeterminate colitis).

In the absence of a better understanding of the mechanisms that underlie these diseases, medical treatment of IBD is limited to control of the symptoms, especially the inflammatory process. For both diseases, treatment can be medical or surgical, a choice that is influenced by the stage and severity of the disease. At low levels of inflammation both diseases can be controlled with anti-inflammatory agents, such as sulfasalazine and related 5-aminosalicylic acid compounds. In patients with UC, anti-inflammatory agents can be administered per rectum by the use of enemas. At intermediate levels of inflammation corticosteroids can provide relief. Steroids may be given continuously at low doses or intermittently in large doses. Unfortunately, many patients become dependent on steroids to suppress ongoing inflammation (steroid dependent). At the highest level of inflammation and in situations where surgery is not required, patients can be aggressively treated with immunosuppressants. This strategy is particularly relevant to CD, because in this case surgical therapy is less definitive. Among the immunosuppressants that have been used with some success are 6-mercaptopurine in both CD and UC, and cyclosporin in acute UC. Anti-TNF antibodies have proved effect in the treatment of acute CD. CD in acute stages is also treatable with parenteral nutrition, although the disease tends to recur after parenteral nutrition is discontinued.

When IBD can no longer be controlled with medical therapy, surgery should be considered. In UC this usually involves total colectomy, because the disease at this stage affects the entire large bowel. Moreover, the patient is at an increased risk for the development of colonic adenocarcinoma. Colectomy for UC is

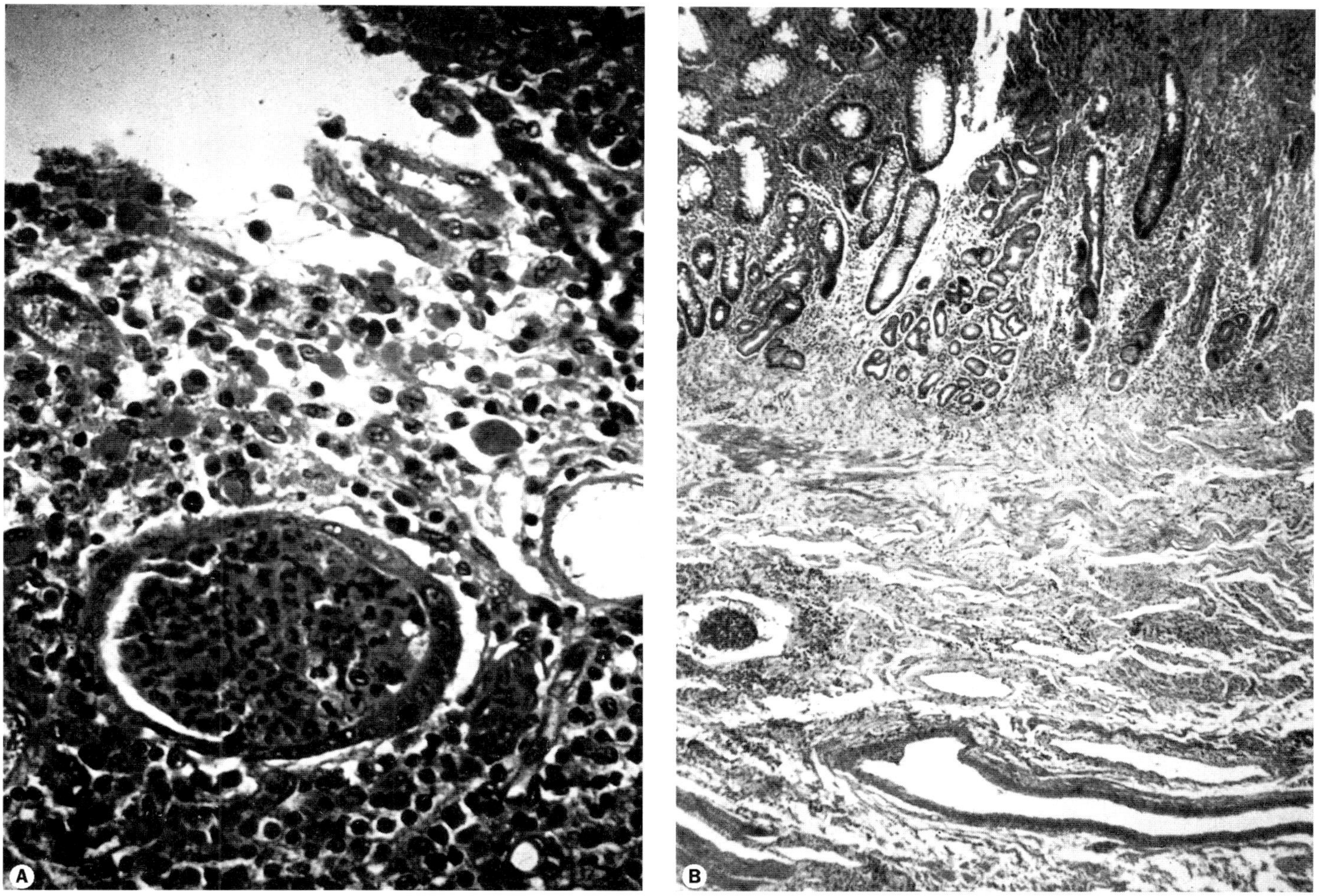

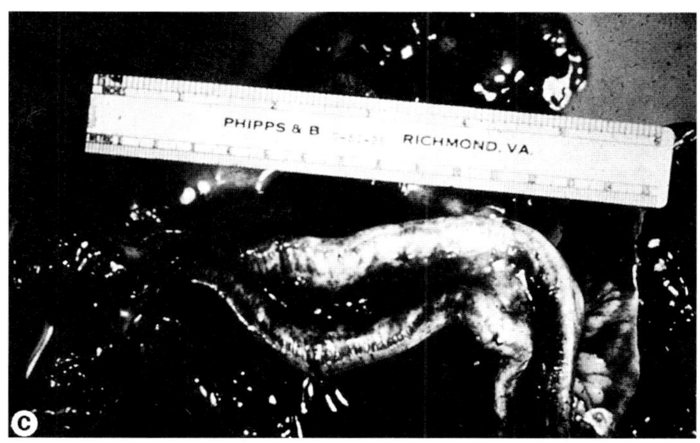

Figure 87.6 Pathologic conditions of UC and CD. (**A**) Pathologic condition in UC: ulcerated surface and underlying crypt abscess. (**B**) Pathologic condition in CD: granulomatous infiltrate associated with a linear ulcer. (**C**) Gross pathologic condition in CD: thickened intestinal wall leading to obstruction.

definitive, because the disease never involves the small intestine. Colectomy is accompanied by either an ileostomy or, more frequently, the formation of a small intestinal pouch (J pouch) that will serve as a neorectum. Unfortunately, patients may develop inflammation in the pouch (pouchitis) after surgery. In CD surgery consists of segmental resection, which is done when severe obstruction develops and is not reversed by the medical therapy. Abdominal abscesses or fistulas may also require surgical intervention. In general there is a reluctance to perform surgery in CD, because it is well established that the disease tends to recur very frequently in uninvolved residual bowel at the anastomosis. Thus, profligate surgery may lead to a short bowel syndrome.

Environmental factors in IBD

The inflammatory bowel diseases are 'diseases of civilization', occurring more commonly in industrialized urbanized societies than in rural or nomadic ones. This observation strongly implies that the diseases result from causative environmental factors, which remain poorly defined.[87] For example, UC incidence is inversely related and CD directly related to smoking incidence; however, the mechanism by which tobacco smoke influences IBD is unknown. Exacerbations of CD have also been related to analgesic intake.[88,89] A number of investigators have sought evidence of a pathogenic organism, but none has ever been found.

Genetic factors in IBD

Familial and ethnic studies indicate a high degree of heritability in IBD. The risk of disease is greater in monozygotic than dyzygotic twins, in children with two affected parents rather than those with one affected parent, and in first-degree relatives of patients.[90] Within ethnic groups there is a greater occurrence in Jews version non-Jews and also in first-degree relatives of Jewish probands as opposed to non-Jewish probands.[91] These studies indicate that genetic factors play a major role in IBD.

Additional support for the genetic basis of IBD comes from the statistically significant association of the disease with certain HLA class II specificities (e.g. HLA-DR2 with UC and DR1/DQ5 with CD).[92] Within families, the type of IBD that develops tends to be similar (UC vs CD, time of onset etc.). There is also an association of IBD with subclinical markers in both patients and relatives. These markers include abnormalities of intestinal permeability, certain types of intestinal mucins, and the occurrence of antineutrophil antibodies (ANCA). The latter occur in 70–80% of patients with UC (but only ~20–25% of patients with CD) and 16% of healthy relatives with UC. ANCA-positive UC is associated with HLA-DR2, whereas ANCA-negative UC is not.[93] The presence of subclinical markers of IBD in otherwise unaffected relatives suggests the presence of susceptibility genes of IBD, genes that set the stage for the development of disease but do not cause it directly. Gene mapping studies point to the existence of CD susceptibility genes on chromosomes 3, 7, 12 and 16.[94] The identification and characterization of these genes could provide important new insights in IBD pathogenesis in subgroups of patients.

Immunopathologic features of IBD

CD lesions begin as an accumulation of lymphocytes and plasma cells next to a mucosal crypt.[95] This is followed by an influx of macrophages that ultimately assume the appearance of epithelioid cells and are distributed as nascent granulomas. Cellular accumulations at the bottom of the crypt develop into abscesses, whereas accumulations at the top of the crypt ulcerate. Accumulations of these ulcers, which span several adjacent crypts, give rise to an 'aphthous ulcer', which is considered the earliest macroscopic evidence of CD. Thus CD begins as a de novo inflammatory process that ultimately results in epithelial cell damage, rather than as epithelial cell damage that leads to inflammation of deeper layers of tissue. This observation implies that an immunologic process directed at the epithelial cells is not a primary feature of the disease. A similar type of immunopathologic study has yet to be conducted for UC, where ulceration is a much more prominent part of the inflammatory process. It remains possible that UC, in contrast to CD, initiates an anti-epithelial cell immune reaction.

The mature lesions of IBD are characterized by a mixed cellular infiltrate in one of two patterns. In some cases the lesion consists of a loose follicular arrangement composed of B cells surrounded by T cells. In others, the lesion presents as a diffuse infiltration of cells, with B cells in the more superficial layers and T cells in the deeper layers. The B-cell component includes both non-Ig-producing B cells and Ig-producing plasma cells. The plasma cell fraction is not representative of a normal mucosal population, being enriched for IgM and IgG, rather than IgA.[86] Among the IgA-producing cells IgA_1 is favored, and among the IgG-producing cells IgG_1 is prominent in UC and IgG_2 in CD.[97] Finally, J-chain production is decreased, with a compensatory increase in monomeric IgA. This pattern is more typical of the systemic humoral response and may reflect an influx of systemic cells into the mucosal lesion. Alternatively, they may be due to inflammation-induced expansion of a separate fraction of mucosal B cells.

The expanded B-cell population in the lamina propria of IBD tissues is theoretically capable of producing antibodies with specificity for epithelial cell components, and thus of mediating tissue damage via complement-mediated or antibody-dependent cellular cytotoxicity mechanisms. Support for complement-mediated damage comes from observations that in UC, complement components indicative of activation (terminal C complex and C3c) are readily identified in IBD tissues, in blood vessel walls, along the luminal surface of epithelial cells, in crypt abscesses, and in the subepithelial layer of severely inflamed tissue.[98] Nevertheless, it is unclear whether antibody-mediated damage is a major immunologic effector mechanism in IBD.

T-cell populations within IBD lamina propria also differ from those in normal individuals. In UC there is a disproportionate increase in CD4 cells, and an increased fraction of the T cells express activation markers such as HLA-DR. T cells bearing antigens associated with memory cells (CD45RO) are increased, whereas T cells bearing antigens associated with naive cells (CD45RA) are decreased.[99] These observations support the view that the lamina propria T cells in IBD are antigen stimulated and play a role in the inflammatory process, whereas the IEL T-cell populations do not.[99]

Inflammatory cells other than lymphocytes also contribute to the IBD infiltrate. Neutrophils and eosinophils accumulate around the crypts to form abscesses, especially in UC. There is also enrichment for macrophages, especially in CD, and for mast cells. The macrophages frequently bear activation surface markers, and there is enrichment for mast cells in the fibrotic lesions. Mast cells appear to facilitate the influx of additional inflammatory cells into an already established lesion.

Autoimmune mechanisms in IBD

A number of studies have examined the hypothesis that IBD is an organ-specific autoimmune disease and that autoantibodies mediate its course.[100] For example, UC is an organ-specific disease (restricted to the colon): it is associated with other potentially autoimmune diseases such as sclerosing cholangitis, and autoantibodies specifically for very defined epithelial cell antigens are found in UC patients. Among these are antibodies against so-called epithelial cell-associated components (ECAC), and antibodies against members of the topomyosin family of proteins.[101,102] This latter autoantibody has been found in virtually all patients with UC, but not in patients with CD or in normal individuals.

Similarly, the majority of patients with UC and a significant number of those with CD express antineutrophil cytoplasmic antibodies (pANCA).[103] This antibody is rare in normal individuals but is found in approximately one-third of close relatives of

UC patients, and persists after colectomy. These latter findings suggest that pANCA may not be involved in disease pathogenesis. The antigen recognized by pANCA is myeloid specific and appears to be associated with neutrophil granules. pANCA differs from the antineutrophil cytoplasmic antibody cANCA found in Wegener's granulomatosis, which is directed against proteinase-3.[104] Although the titers of pANCA antibodies are higher in UC than in CD, they cannot be used to distinguish the two diseases in indeterminate cases.

The discovery of antibodies against pANCA led to a search for additional autoantibodies in UC and CD. A summary of many of these is given in Table 87.2. It should be noted, however, that these antibodies generally do not occur in all patients and frequently occur in patients with other diseases, including those with infections of the gastrointestinal tract. These observations suggest that the production of autoantibodies in IBD may represent the effect of the disease, rather than a cause, perhaps owing to the loss of the intestinal barrier and hence the exposure of the internal immune system to environmental antigens.

It has been suggested that autoantibodies in IBD play a role in the cell-mediated immune destruction of intestinal epithelial cells. For example, natural killer (NK) cells (or related non-specific cytotoxic cells) could be armed with antiepithelial cell antibodies and engage in epithelial cell lysis. Recent studies have cast doubt on this hypothesis as well. In fact, NK-cell activity is quite low in IBD patients.[105] Moreover, when stable epithelial cell populations are examined, both patient and control peripheral lymphocytes exhibit low (and equal) cytotoxicity for the epithelial cells.[106] In addition, the earliest pathologic lesions in CD do not involve epithelial cells. Finally, the antibodies that are presumably necessary for cytotoxicity are present in the secretions of unaffected relatives who do not have disease. Thus, it is likely that epithelial cell damage mediated by antiepithelial cell antibodies plays at best an adjunct role in tissue injury in patients with IBD, and that the tissue injury is more importantly related to the accumulation of inflammatory cells capable of causing injury on a purely nonspecific basis.

Autoantibodies in IBD

Antoantibody	Occurrence[a]	
	Type of IBD	Other diseases
Antierythrocyte	UC, CD (~25%)[b]	*C. jejuni* enterocolitis
Antimycobacterial stress protein (65 kDa)	CD	
Anticardiolipin	CD (~20%)	
Antigoblet cell (?anti-MUC-1)	UC, CD (~30%)	
Anticathepsin G (?ANCA)	UC	Sclerosing cholangitis Autoimmune hepatitis
Rheumatoid factor	CD	

[a] Reflects patient groups studied, rather than all possible patient groups.
[b] Approximate percentage of patients with antibody.

Table 87.2 Autoantibodies in IBD.

Regulatory lymphokine production in IBD

The question of whether IBD T cells display a cytokine production pattern indicative of Th1 (IL-2 and IFN-γ) or Th2 cells (IL-4, IL-5) has been addressed in a number of different ways. This question is important because these patterns of T-cell differentiation give rise to very different pathophysiologic outcomes (Chapter 16). The results have been contradictory. For example, CD and UC lamina propria T cells produce less than half the amount of IL-2 as do controls.[107] However, in the lesions both IL-2 mRNA levels and the number of IL-2-secreting T cells are increased in CD, but not in UC.[108,109] Similarly, some studies have shown decreased IFN-γ production by phytohemagglutinin (PHA)-stimulated CD lamina propria T cells, whereas other studies demonstrated increased secretion of IFN-γ in resting cells and no difference from controls in stimulated cells.[110,111]

The nature of the stimulus can influence the T-cell response. Compared with peripheral T cells, lamina propria T cells proliferate poorly in response to CD2/CD28 accessory pathway stimulation, whereas lymphokine production is increased. In IBD the proliferative response to CD2/CD28 stimulation by lamina propria T cells from UC and CD patients is relatively preserved.[112] However, UC lamina propria T cells produce normal amounts of IFN-γ less IL-4 and more IL-5 than controls; whereas stimulated CD lamina propria T cells produce less IL-2 and IL-4, but more IFN-γ, than controls. Although activation of the transcription factor STAT-4 has been implicated in the augmented IFN-γ production by CD T cells, a reduced expression of the Th2 T-cell-associated transcription factors NFATc1 and GATA-3 appears to be responsible for decreased production of IL-4 in CD.[113] Thus, CD T cells manifest an abnormal lymphokine profile, characterized by an increase in IFN-γ and a decrease in IL-2 production (Fig. 87.7), which may represent a unique immunoregulatory defect.

Inflammatory cytokine production in IBD

Studies of inflammatory cytokine production in the lamina propria of patients with IBD have been performed *pari passu* with the previously mentioned regulatory lymphokine studies. This type of cytokine production occurs primarily in macrophages and is a constant feature in all types of inflammatory states. It therefore comes as no surprise that the production of these lymphokines is increased in active IBD lesions and, indeed, usually mirrors disease activity. Thus in various studies, IL-1β production by lamina propria mononuclear cells was found to be elevated, and this elevation was abolished by macrophage depletion.[114] Similarly, IL-6 and TNF production by lamina propria cells is increased in IBD (both CD and UC), and IL-8 production is increased in UC.[115] TNF is an important proinflammatory cytokine that activates via TNF-R1/2 macrophages, T cells and stroma cells. In turn, stroma cells can produce matrix metalloproteinases (MMP-1: collagenase; MMP-3: stromelysin) and keratinocyte growth factor (KGF), which cause tissue destruction and epithelial hyperplasia, respectively. The key pathogenic role of TNF in CD is supported by the observation that treatment with a neutralizing TNF antibody induces clinical remission and closure of draining fistulas.[116,117] The increased production of proinflammatory cytokines by lamina propria macrophages in both CD and UC appears to be due, at least in part, to activation and nuclear translocation of the NF-κB transcription factor, which controls the promoter activity of the respective genes.[118]

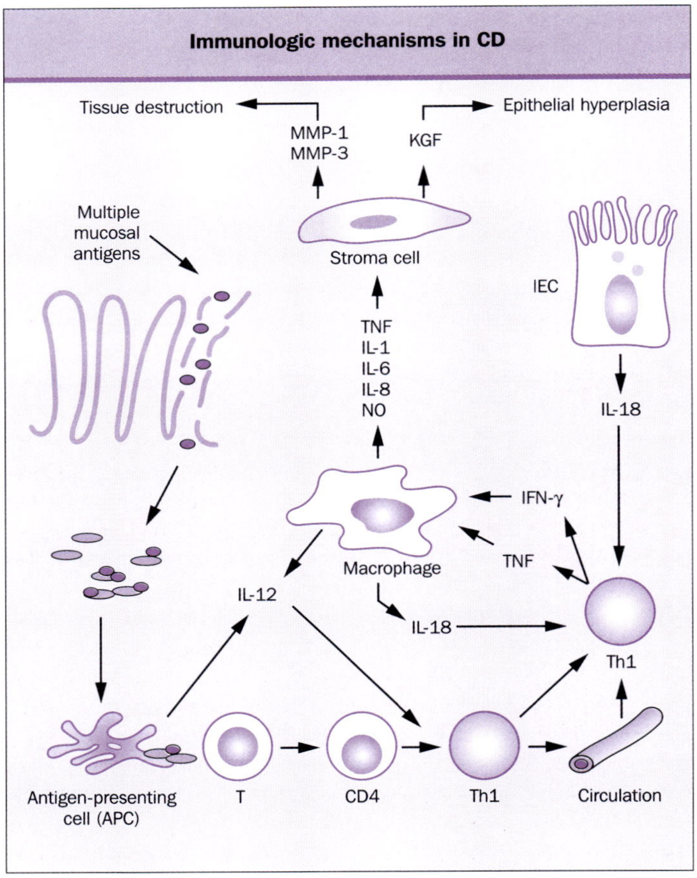

Figure 87.7 Immunologic mechanisms in CD. Mucosal antigens induce T cells in Peyer's patches that migrate to the lamina propria. In the lamina propria T cells produce proinflammatory cytokines such as IFN-γ.

A potentially important difference between CD and UC cytokine production by lamina propria macrophages relates to the production of IL-12, a proinflammatory cytokine that induces Th1 T-cell differentiation, and IFN-γ production of T cells. Increased IL-12 production has been shown in CD, but not UC. This provides an explanation for the Th1 cytokine profile in CD. Evidence for increased IL-12 signaling in CD is provided by activation of the IL-12-related signaling protein STAT-4 in CD lamina propria T cells. The relevance of these findings for intestinal inflammation in CD is underlined by the recent observations that chronic intestinal inflammation in various Th1 animal models is suppressed or even abrogated by antibodies to IL-12, and that transgenic mice overexpressing the STAT-4 protein develop chronic intestinal inflammation in response to bacterial antigens.[119,120] Finally, elevated production of the IFN-γ-inducing cytokine IL-18 has been observed in CD, but not in UC, further explaining why effector T cells in the former disease may produce large amounts of IFN-γ.[121]

The increased production of inflammatory cytokines in IBD lesions provides a possible mechanism for tissue injury. Following stimulation by T-cell lymphokines, the production of inflammatory cytokines by macrophages in IBD lesions leads to an influx of granulocytes and the release of additional inflammatory mediators. In turn, the granulocytes cause injury to normal cellular constituents. It appears possible that proinflammatory cytokines contribute to the recently observed resistance of IBD lamina propria T cells against apoptosis, a phenomenon that may contribute to the perpetuation of these diseases.

Pathogenesis of inflammatory bowel disease: an overview

IBD appears primarily to be an immunologic disease. The inflammation begins as a lymphocytic infiltration in the bowel wall (seen clearly in Crohn's disease, if not in ulcerative colitis) and unfolds as either a classic granulomatous immune reaction (Crohn's disease) or as a more diffuse and disorganized lymphocyte-dominated infiltrate that secondarily brings in granulocytic inflammatory cells (ulcerative colitis). The skeptic would object that although an immunologic reaction undoubtedly occurs in IBD and is the proximate cause of tissue injury, another, as yet unidentified 'first cause' must exist to initiate the immunologic reaction, such as an occult infection. However, very extensive efforts to identify an infectious agent in IBD have repeatedly failed, and it seems unlikely that an infection sufficiently potent and persistent to cause IBD would not leave serologic or other footprints. It remains possible, of course, that an infectious agent could trigger the development of disease in susceptible individuals and be long gone by the time the patient is examined for its presence. In fact, the finding that early/relatively mild CD patients display increased levels of CD8/CD57 T cells with heightened suppressor or cytotoxic function supports this hypothesis, as such cells are commonly seen in the setting of chronic infection. It should be emphasized, however, that such cells are not found in more advanced disease, nor in lesional tissues, and so it appears unlikely that infection is the continuing cause of the persistent inflammatory lesion.

Having posited an immunologic basis for IBD, one cannot immediately assume that IBD inflammation is solely due to an immunologic defect. Genetic and environmental cofactors may contribute to disease. One potential factor is a genetically determined abnormality in mucosal permeability arising from a biochemical defect in the array of mucins produced at the mucosal surface.[122] Such a defect could conceivably interact with an immunologic abnormality by increasing the exposure of immune elements to mucosal antigens.

A second major question relates to the nature of the immunologic defect leading to IBD. The mucosal system (Chapter 20) is characterized by a well developed immunoregulatory mechanism that down-regulates responses to ubiquitous food or bacterial antigens while retaining the ability to respond to pathogens. IBD may be due to a fundamental derangement in mucosal immunoregulation. For example, in IBD the mucosal immune system may respond to a host of usually ignored mucosal antigens, and thus engage in an immune response that cannot end because the inciting stimulus is always present. A number of observations support this view. First, there is evidence that IBD patients hyperrespond to mucosal antigens of any type.[123] Second, there are a number of animal models of mucosal inflammation where immunologic dysregulation leads to hyperresponsiveness to normal gut constituents and subsequent mucosal inflammation.[124,125]

Finally, the source of the many autoantibodies produced in IBD, particularly in UC, remains uncertain. This phenomenon may represent a fundamental inability to down-regulate mucosal responses – in this case B-cell responses – to exogenous or endogenous gut constituents.

CLINICAL PEARLS

Inflammatory bowel disease

- *Definition*: chonic inflammation of the GI tract not due to infection:
  - Ulcerative colitis (UC): relatively superficial ulcerative disease limited to the large bowel. UC affects the mucosa and submucosa.
  - Crohn disease (CD): transmural granulomatous disease occurring in the GI tract, most commonly in the terminal ileum and ascending colon.
- *Diagnosis*: endoscopy (UC), colon biopsy (UC & CD); currently no diagnostic serologic tests. Many UC patients have anticytoplasmic antibodies (pANCA).
- *Probable cause*: hyperresponsive (loss of oral tolerance) to multiple mucosal antigens.
- *Treatment*: anti-inflammatory agents, immunosuppressants (e.g. azathioprine, anti-TNF antibodies), surgery.

AUTOIMMUNITY AND THE GASTROINTESTINAL TRACT

Systemic autoimmune diseases often affect the GI tract. These may take the form of a small-vessel vasculitis such as that seen in Henoch–Schönlein purpura, in which IgA immune complexes are present in the circulation and are deposited in the skin, joints, kidneys and GI tract. GI symptoms include abdominal pain, gastrointestinal bleeding, and ulceration resulting from vasculitis initiated by immune complex deposition. A similar GI picture occurs in patients with systemic lupus erythematosus and periarteritis nodosa, although in these cases larger vessels may be involved, leading to ischemia, intestinal necrosis and perforation. Finally, in systemic sclerosis, with or without CREST syndrome (Chapter 64), a somewhat different GI presentation is seen, involving motor dysfunction of the esophagus and stomach, smooth muscle atrophy, and collagen deposition all along the gastrointestinal tract. This involvement leads to impaired intestinal motility and consequent stasis and dilatation of the intestine, which may be associated with bacterial overgrowth and malabsorption.

Pernicious anemia

Pernicious anemia (PA) is an autoimmune state that affects the GI tract in particular. The disease is characterized by a megaloblastic haematopoiesis, a neuropathy caused by cobalamin (vitamin B_{12}) deficiency, or both. In humans the sole source of cobalamin is the methylcobalamin that is found in the diet and is nonspecifically bound to proteins. After the ingestion and release of cobalamin by acid proteolysis in the stomach, cobalamin binds to R protein (haptocorrin) at high-affinity binding sites and, when in excess, to intrinsic factor (IF) at lower-affinity binding sites. Both proteins are produced by the parietal (oxyntic) cells of the gastric fundus. Both cobalamin–R and cobalamin–IF complexes pass through the duodenum, where pancreatic proteases degrade the cobalamin–R complexes. The cobalamin–IF complexes, in the form of oligomers and dimers, pass through the jejunum and eventually arrive in the distal ileum, where they bind to membrane-associated receptors on the microvilli of mucosal cells and are taken up. Cobalamin–IF complex receptors in humans comprise two subunits: a pair of lumen-facing hydrophilic subunits connected to a pair of membrane-anchored hydrophobic β subunits by disulfide bonds. The cobalamin is transferred to transcobalamin II (TC II) and is transcytosed to the basal portion of the cell, where it is delivered to the portal blood.

Patients with PA exhibit a megaloblastic anemia and its associated symptoms. In addition, because cobalamin is necessary for nerve cell function, severe cobalamin deficiency is associated with neuropathy. The disease generally presents later in life, with only about one-tenth of patients being younger than 40 years. Women are more frequently affected than men. Of interest is the fact that PA may be part of a syndrome of autoimmune abnormalities. In particular, it has been associated with primary myxedema and thyroid disease, particularly Hashimoto's disease, marked by the presence of antithyroid antibodies. It may also occur as a component of an autoimmune state known as Schmidt syndrome: PA, Hashimoto's thyroiditis, vitiligo, diabetes mellitus and hypoadrenalism. Finally, PA has been associated with an increased incidence of carcinoid tumors (4%) and gastric carcinoma (3%).

Whereas PA is always the result of cobalamin deficiency, the latter can have multiple causes. One set of causes relates to factors that decrease cobalamin availability independent of any affect on IF, whereas another set relates to problems with the availability of IF itself. In the former category are decreased intake of cobalamin resulting from a deficient diet (very rare), competition for uptake (fish tapeworm, bacterial overgrowth as in blindloop syndrome), or small-intestinal diverticulosis and selective cobalamin malabsorption. In the latter category are the many defects affecting IF availability: congenital IF defect, gastrectomy, terminal ileal disease or resection. IF production may be secondarily affected by atrophic gastritis caused by chronic *Helicobacter pylori* infection (see below) or unapparent infections associated with CVID. The most common cause of PA, however, is an autoimmune process that directly targets the cells producing IF, or IF itself.

The evidence supporting an autoimmune etiology in PA comes primarily from the observation that most patients with the disease have antibodies against either gastric parietal cells, IF or both. In addition, these patients frequently exhibit cell-mediated immunity to IF and other gastric constituents. It is believed that the antiparietal cell antibodies are cytotoxic and thus impair IF production by parietal cell depletion. Alternatively, anti-IF antibodies may act by blocking cobalamin binding to IF, or by blocking the uptake of cobalamin–IF complexes by ileal cells.

The autoimmune process just described produces a gastric atrophy characterized by a thinning of the stomach wall and the

THERAPEUTIC PRINCIPLES

Pernicious anemia

- *Diagnosis*: megaloblastic anemia associated with decreased cobalamin levels. Confirmatory studies include a Schilling test and gastric biopsies that verify the presence of atrophic gastritis.
- *Treatment*: parenteral vitamin B_{12}.
- *Potential complications of therapy*: uric acid levels may rise and cause renal toxicity; potassium levels may decline and lead to cardiac arrythmias and sudden death.

replacement of columnar secretory mucosa by mucosa containing an irregular array of mucus-producing cells, a process known as intestinal metaplasia. The mucosa also exhibits a lymphocytic infiltrate composed of both IgA- and IgG-producing plasma cells and T cells (type A gastritis). This pathologic process involves mainly the fundus of the stomach, spares the antrum, and results in a severe loss of secretory cells and a marked reduction in output of gastric juice. Gastric production by antral cells is relatively unaffected, and serum gastrin levels may be raised because of reduced feedback inhibition by acid.

Megaloblastic anemia associated with decreased cobalamin levels strongly supports the diagnosis of PA. Confirmatory tests include a Schilling test, which measures the ability to absorb labeled cobalamin and thus assesses IF dysfunction; and gastric biopsies to verify the presence of atrophic gastritis. It should be noted that the detection of achlorhydria by gastric analysis also helps to establish the presence of atrophic gastritis, but this finding is nonspecific because achlorhydria is not unusual in older individuals without PA. In addition, although the presence of antibodies against parietal cells and IF (found in 90% and 54% of patients, respectively) helps establish the diagnosis of PA, the absence of these antibodies does not exclude this diagnosis, for reasons already mentioned.

Before the advent of effective substitution therapy, PA was usually fatal. Life expectancy was less than 3 years from the time of diagnosis, and survival for longer than 5 years was unusual. It is now well established, however, that patients with PA strongly benefit from vitamin B_{12} supplementation. Although patients with PA will respond to oral treatment with animal IF, they usually become resistant and ultimately require parental vitamin B_{12}. Elevated uric acid levels (sometimes enough to cause kidney damage) and low potassium levels (very rarely causing cardiac arrythmias and sudden death) have been observed after vitamin B_{12} treatment. Therefore, patients with severe megaloblastic anemia require close observation of serum uric acid and potassium levels during therapy.

HELICOBACTER PYLORI

A little more than 15 years ago the world was reintroduced to *Helicobacter pylori* (previously called *Campylobacter pylori*), with the finding that a causal relationship might exist between *H. pylori* infection and inflammation of the upper gastrointestinal tract.[126,127] This relationship is now well documented: ingestion of live bacteria in both humans and animals leads to clinical and histological signs of gastritis (thus fulfilling Koch's postulate). The bacteria are invariably present when antral gastritis is present. Finally, successful treatment of the infection leads to resolution of the gastritis.

Infection with *H. pylori* is a worldwide problem, with infection rates in developed countries of 20% by the age of 30 years, increasing to 50% by the age of 60 years. In developing countries infection rates of more than 80% of the adult population are seen. The bacteria are capable of long-term persistence and may exist in the mucosa for the lifetime of the host. These facts taken together establish *H. pylori* infection as a major pathologic factor in gastrointestinal disease.

Helicobacter pylori infection and gastrointestinal disease

H. pylori infection should be considered a risk factor for the development of various upper gastrointestinal diseases, rather than as a factor invariably leading to disease. Thus, although many individuals in developed countries are infected with *H. pylori*, most do not have clinical symptoms and not all individuals who have chronic active gastritis because of infection go on to have gastric ulceration. In a similar vein, *H. pylori* infection is a risk factor for the occurrence of duodenal ulcers (prevalence of *H. pylori* in duodenal ulcers >90%), albeit an obligate factor in the absence of other risk factors such as nonsteroidal anti-inflammatory drug therapy or Zollinger–Ellison syndrome. Finally, *H. pylori* infection is a risk factor for the development of upper gastrointestinal tumors: individuals serologically positive for antibodies to *H. pylori* have an almost fourfold increased risk for distal gastric adenocarcinoma. In addition, infection with this organism predisposes to the occurrence of mucosa-associated lymphoid tumors (MALT lymphoma; see below). Based on these observations, the World Health Organization has recently classified *H. pylori* as a human carcinogen.

Helicobacter pylori-associated inflammation is influenced by a variety of factors, including host responsiveness, the phase of the disease and the virulence of the bacteria. The initial phase of the infection with the spiral shaped gram-negative bacteria is thought to involve ingestion, followed by penetration of the gastric mucus layer and attachment to the mucosal surface. It has been shown that such adherence to the cells is mediated by fucosylated blood-group antigens associated with blood-group O phenotype, thereby explaining the higher prevalence of stomach ulcers in individuals with this blood group. The ability of *H. pylori* to adhere is probably a critical virulence factor and is related to ulcerogenesis, because the *Helicobacter* species associated with ulceration are ones that have the ability to adhere. The attachment phase of the *H. pylori* infection is followed by an acute inflammatory process, whose perpetuation leads to infiltration of various inflammatory cells. In addition to mononuclear cells (monocytes/macrophages), B cells and T cells, the *H. pylori*-associated gastritis exhibits a variable component of neutrophil activity. These cell types produce a variety of potent mediators (including TNF, IFN-γ, platelet-activating factor, IL-6, IL-8, leukotrienes and oxygen radicals) that are responsible for the development of the chronic inflammatory reaction. Evidence to support this concept came from animal studies in C57BL/6 mice, in which infection with *H. felis* induced production of large amounts of Th1 cytokines by both splenic and gastric lymphocytes that correlated with gastric inflammation.[128] Furthermore, T lymphocytes from patients infected with *H. pylori* are known to recognize a spectrum of *Helicobacter* antigens (including urease, CagA, VacA, heat-shock proteins), and B lymphocytes produce antibodies to *Helicobacter* that may cross-react with antigens on gastric epithelial cells, and thus may contribute to *H. pylori*-induced tissue damage in the stomach.

H. pylori infection in the highly unfavorable environment of the gastric mucosa is made possible by its ability to produce a variety of enzyme and cytokines that facilitate the initiation and maintenance of infection. Perhaps most importantly, *H. pylori* organisms synthesize a urease whose activity is optimal at low pH and which acts on one or more substrates to produce substances that neutralize acid gastric juices and thus establish a neutral pH environment. The enzyme is loosely bound to the bacterial surface and seems to be essential for colonization, but not for survival after colonization has been established. Urease is one of the main bacterial antigens that induce antibody production;

such antibodies may be one of the ways that the body limits *H. pylori* infection. *H. pylori* also produces catalase, oxidase and phospholipase C, enzymes that also help the organism to survive in inflamed tissues. The former enzyme splits oxygen species produced by phagocytes that would otherwise kill the organism. The latter enzyme degrades the phospholipids embedded in mucus, and thereby decreases mucus hydrophobicity.

Clinical isolates of *H. pylori* can be classified into two groups, based on the ability of the organism to produce a cytotoxin that causes massive vacuolation of several mammalian cell lines. Thus it has been suggested that the vacuolated gastric epithelial cells observed in patients with chronic gastritis associated with *H. pylori* infection are due to the secretion of this cytotoxin. This view is supported by the fact that cytotoxin expression is very closely associated with a surface antigen with high molecular mass (denoted cytotoxin-associated gene – CagA), and that high titers of CagA protein are found in the serum of all patients with duodenal ulcers and in most of those with gastric carcinomas. In addition, administration of the purified cytotoxin to mice causes ulcerations and gastric lesions that resemble those seen in human disease.[129] These various findings suggest that *H. pylori* infection leads to ulcer formation by virtue of its ability to produce an epithelial cell cytotoxin, and thus that the disease-producing potential of *H. pylori* strains resides with the cytotoxin production. However, it should be noted that *H. pylori* strains are highly diverse at the genetic level, and that major phenotypic differences (in addition to cytotoxin and CagA production) comprise lipopolysaccharide (LPS) structure and antigenicity.

The *H. pylori* cytotoxin gene has been cloned. Its product is a 140 kDa precursor that is processed into a 94 kDa cytotoxin. The cell vacuoles produced by the toxin can be blocked by inhibitors of Na-K-adenosine triphosphate (ATP)ases, suggesting that its mechanism of action is the induction of aberrant ion transport. The cytotoxin contains an antigenic determinant (CagA) that evokes a strong immune response in the host, leading to the induction of anti-CagA antibodies.

The presence of *H. pylori* infection of the gastric mucosa can be established by urease testing, or by histologic examination of gastric biopsy material. Direct culturing of the organism has proved difficult and is not considered a standard diagnostic procedure. Serologic testing of antibodies to *Helicobacter* antigen is an excellent noninvasive method to detect *Helicobacter*; however, its use is limited because antibody levels may persist for many years after successful treatment of the infection.

The most important noninvasive test for *H. pylori* is the urea breath test, in which ^{13}C- or ^{14}C-labeled urea is given by oral administration and is hydrolyzed by the *Helicobacter* urease enzyme, resulting in the production of labeled carbon dioxide that diffuses into the blood and is excreted by the lungs. The amount of exhaled labeled carbon dioxide is then measured. Time–course studies allow evaluation regarding the successful eradication of *H. pylori* infections.

Treatment of *H. pylori* is challenging because the organism lives in a protected environment beneath the mucus layer. Nevertheless, a triple-drug therapy (inhibitors of the acid pump, such as omeprazole, metronidazole and clarithromycin or amoxicillin) leads to successful cure in 85–98% of cases. In this context, antibiotic therapy appears to be optimal when administered for 2 weeks and then followed by 4 weeks of antisecretory therapy. Side-effects are usually mild and rarely require the patient to discontinue the therapy. Treatment of the infection solely to prevent cancer is not currently recommended.

CLINICAL PEARLS

***Helicobacter* infections**

- Common, usually occult, infection of the stomach.
- Causes gastric atrophy, a risk factor for gastric and duodenal ulcer.
- Pathogenesis: organism produces urease, which leads to neutralization of stomach acid; it also produces a cytotoxin that destroys epithelial cells.
- Infection is limited by an immune response, but nevertheless persists indefinitely.
- Infection can lead to B-cell lymphomas of the mucosa-associated lymphoid tissue (MALT).
- *H. pylori* colonization also predisposes individuals to increased risk of developing gastric cancer.

MUCOSA-ASSOCIATED LYMPHOID TISSUE (MALT) LYMPHOMA

The term [('mucosa-associated lymphoid tissue' (MALT)] evolved from the finding that mucosal surfaces share organizational and functional similarities (Chapter 20). MALT can be separated into several components, among them the gut-associated lymphoid tissue (GALT = Peyer's patches, the appendix, mesenteric lymph nodes, IEL and lamina propria lymphocytes in the gut).

Distinctive lymphoid tumors arise from the MALT and occur as monofocal or multifocal tumors. Included in this group is the so-called Mediterranean lymphoma (MTL). MALT lymphomas have been shown to be clonal B-cell malignancies. MALT lymphomas frequently present as gastric ulcers with marginal indurations. In most cases, MALT lymphoma occurs after an indolent course and responds well to chemotherapy. However, malignant forms with metastases or progression to large-cell lymphoma have also been reported. The latter condition is frequently marked by the occurrence of nausea, vomiting, hematemesis, melena and weight loss.

In recent studies an association between *Helicobacter* infection, MALT and lymphoma has been established.[130,131] Eradication of the *Helicobacter* infection results in remission of some MALT lymphomas. One possible mechanism of MALT lymphoma development in the presence of *H. pylori* infection is that the chronic infection induces a neoplastic effect in B cells and the proliferation of B cells specific for an organism-related antigen. In this regard, chronic *H. pylori* infection by its very persistence takes the role of multiple organisms in the development of Mediterranean lymphoma. Once established, the monoclonal B cells are further induced by T cells that are also specific for *Helicobacter* antigens. Evidence for this view is the recent demonstration that, at least in the early stages of disease, the proliferation of gastric MALT lymphoma B cells is stimulated by IL-2 and other cytokines produced by *H. pylori*-specific T cells.

Diagnostic procedures comprise endoscopic examinations and biopsies. Histologic examination of the material thus obtained usually reveals infiltrates of lymphoid cells and plasma cells that can cause characteristic lymphoepithelial lesions. Some plasma

CLINICAL PEARLS

Heavy-chain disease (HCD) and immunoproliferative small-intestinal disease (IPSD)

- *Definition*: small-intestinal B-cell lymphomas producing primarily incomplete Cα heavy chains devoid of light chains and, rarely, monoclonal or polymeric IgA
- *Diagnosis*: serum immunoelectrophoresis, immunoselection or immunofixation
- *Probable cause*: abnormal monoclonal response to a mucosal infection, especially *Giardia lamblia*
- *Treatment*: antibiotic and antiparasitic therapy in early disease, chemotherapy in late disease

cells may contain so-called Dutcher bodies (intranuclear pseudo-inclusions). In addition to conventional histologic examination, immunohistochemistry (i.e. staining for Ig production) and molecular studies (Southern blots for Ig light chains) can be performed.

MALT lymphomas usually respond well to chemotherapy. Eradication of the associated *H. pylori* infection can cause remission of some early MALT lymphomas, suggesting that early tumors (at a stage preceding autonomous tumor growth) may be responsive to withdrawal of this stimulus. However, the re-remergence of *Helicobacter* and the recurrence of MALT lymphomas after initial eradication have been reported, suggesting that a careful follow-up of treated patients for residual lymphoma is critical after initial successful antibiotic therapy. The phenomenon of re-emerging bacteria in such cases seems to be almost always due to bacteriologic relapse of *Helicobacter*, rather than to reinfection by a different strain. Because chemotherapy, radiation or both, has been found to cause an increased incidence of perforation, therapy for gastric lymphoma associated with large ulcers often entails gastrectomy. In this context, preoperative antibiotic therapy may substantially reduce tumor bulk and reduce associated morbidity.

HEAVY-CHAIN DISEASE (HCD) AND IMMUNOPROLIFERATIVE SMALL-INTESTINAL DISEASE (IPSID)

The group of small-intestinal lymphomas comprising the immunoproliferative small intestinal diseases (IPSIDs) largely consists of B-cell lymphomas that commonly produce incomplete heavy chains devoid of light chains, and rarely secrete monoclonal or polymeric IgA.[132] The disease has also been referred to as α-heavy-chain disease (αHCD). The molecular basis for the occurrence of isolated heavy chains is the fact that the Cα gene contains deletions in the Cα1–Cα2 regions that would normally contain the binding site for L chains.

Patients with HCD are usually young (15–35 years) and in a low socioeconomic group. Most patients in western Europe show chronic diarrhea and evidence of malabsorption. Physical findings include abdominal masses, clubbing, enlarged peripheral nodes and ascites. Many patients also have fever, weight loss and abdominal pain.

HCD usually involves the whole length of the small intestine and, in more advanced cases, the mesenteric lymph nodes. The spread of HCD to other lymph nodes or organs is rare. On histologic examination HCD can be divided into three stages. In stage A the cellular infiltrate is mainly in the mucosa, the intestinal villi are shortened and wide, and plasma cells massively infiltrate the lamina propria. Stage C is characterized by an immunoblastic lymphoma with plasmacytoid features that forms either discrete ulcerated tumors or extensive infiltrates in long segments of the small intestine. Stage B is intermediate between A and C.

The identification of HCD proteins relies on serum immunoelectrophoresis, immunoselection or immunofixation. In addition, immunohistochemical studies of intestinal tissue can be performed and usually demonstrate the presence of intracytoplasmic heavy chains in the absence of light chains. *Giardia lamblia* is present in one-third of cases, and antiparasitic therapy may reduce the symptoms. Radiographs usually show enlarged duodenal and jejunal folds in a polypoid pattern, and rarely demonstrate stenoses, ulcerations or fistulas.

Patients with stage A lesions should be treated with oral antibiotics, including metronidazole, which also eradicates the frequent *Giardia lamblia* parasites. The duration of treatment before complete remission may vary between 5 and 36 months. However, chemotherapy should not be delayed too long in unresponsive patients. At stage B, chemotherapy should be performed in patients who show no improvement after 6 months of antibiotic and antiparasitic therapy. All patients in stage C with disseminated immunoblastic lesions of the small intestine require intensive chemotherapy. Because patients with HCD are usually young, those with disseminated stage C lesions who show a good response after chemotherapy can be considered for autologous bone marrow transplantation.

REFERENCES

1. Conley ME. X-linked immunodeficiencies. Curr Opin Genet Dev 1994;4:401.
2. Ament MB. Immunodeficiency syndromes and the gut. Scand J Gastroenterol 1985;114:127.
3. Dubois RS, Roy CC, Fulginiti VA, et al. Disaccharidase deficiency in children with immunologic defects. J Pediatr 1970;76:377.
4. Misbah A, Spickett GP, Clyba PC, et al. Chronic enterovirus meningoencephalitis in agammaglobulinemia; case report and literature review. J Clin Immunol 1992;12:266.
5. Van der Meer JW, Weening RS, Schellekens PT, van Munster IP, Nagengast FM. Colorectal cancer in patients with X-linked agammaglobulinemia. Lancet 1993;341:1439.
6. Sneller MC, Strober W, Eisenstein EM, et al. NIH Conference: New insights into common variable immunodeficiency. Ann Intern Med 1993;118:720.
7. Cunningham-Rundles C. Clinical and immunological analyses of 103 patients with common variable immunodeficiency. J Clin Immunol 1989;9:22.
8. Eisenstein EM, Jaffe JS, Strober W: Reduced interleukin-2 (IL-2) production in common variable immunodeficiency is due to primary abnormality of CD4+ T cells. J Clin Immunol 1993;13:247.
9. Twomey JJ, Jordan PH, Laughter AH, Meuwissen HJ, Good RA. The gastric disorder in immunoglobulin-deficient patients. Ann Intern Med 1970;72:499.

10. Borriello SP, Reed PJ, Dolby JM, et al. Microbial and metabolic profile of achlorhydric stomach: comparision of pernicious anemia and hypogammaglobulinemia. J Clin Pathol 1985;38:946.
11. Castellano G, Moreno D, Galves O, et al. Malignant lymphoma of jejunum with common variable hypogammaglobulinemia and diffuse nodular hyperplasia of the small intestine: a case study and literature review. J Clin Gastroenterol 1992;15:281.
12. Catassi C, Mirakian R, Natalini G, et al. Unresponsive enteropathy associated with circulating enterocyte autoantibodies in a boy with common variable hypogammaglobulinism and type I diabetes. J Pediatr Gastroenterol Nutr 1988;7:608.
13. Wagner DKK, Wright JJ, Onsher AF, et al. Dysgonic fermenter 3-associated gastrointestinal disease in a patient with common variable hypogammaglobulinemia. Am J Med 1988;84:315.
14. Teahon K, Webster AD, Price AB, et al. Studies on the enteropathy associated with primary hypogammaglobulinemia. Gut 1994;35:1244.
15. Johnson ML, Keeton LG, Zhu Z-B, et al. Age-related changes in serum immunoglobulins in patients with familial IgA deficiency and common variable immunodeficiency (CVID). Clin Exp Immunol 1997;108:477.
16. Tomkin GH, Mawhinnedy H, Nevin NC. Isolated absence of IgA with autosomal dominance inheritance. Lancet 1971;2:124.
17. Dinauer MC, Orkin SH. Chronic granulomatous disease. Annu Rev Med 1992;43:117.
18. Neuman SL, Lindahl JA. Chronic granulomatous disease: a model for gastrointestinal manifestations of immunodeficiency. J Clin Gastroenterol 1985;7:470.
19. Voss SD, Hong R, Sondel PM. Severe combined immunodeficiency, interleukin-2 (IL-2) and the IL-2 receptor: experiments of nature continue to point the way. Blood 1994;83:626.
20. Kersey J, Filipovich A, McGlave P, et al. Donor and host influence in bone marrow transplantation for immunodeficiency disease and leukemia. Semin Hematol 1993;30:105.
21. Smith PD, Quinn TC, Strober W, et al. Gastrointestinal infections of AIDS. Ann Intern Med 1992;116:63.
22. Schacker T, Collier AC, Hughes J. Clinical and epidemiologic features of primary HIV infection. Ann Intern Med 1996;125:257.
23. Wahl SM, McNeely TB, Janoff EN, Shugars D, Worley P, Tucker C, Orenstein JM. Secretory leukocyte protease inhibitor (SLPI) in mucosal fluids inhibits HIV-1. Oral Dis 1997; 3(Suppl):64.
24. Amerongen HM, Weltzin R, Farnet CM, et al. Transepithelial transport of HIV-1 by intestinal M cells: a mechanism for transmission of AIDS. AIDS 1991;4:760.
25. Smith PD, Quinn TC, Strober W, Janoff EN, Masur H. Gastrointestinal infections of AIDS. Ann Intern Med 1992;116:63.
26. Doranz BJ, Rucker J, Yi Y, et al. A dual-tropic primary HIV-1 isolate that uses fusin and the beta-chemokine receptors CKR-5, CKR-3 and CKR-2b as fusin cofactors. Cell 1996;85:1149.
27. Lim SG, Condez A, Lee CA, et al. Loss of mucosal CD4 lymphocytes is an early feature of HIV infection. Clin Exp Immunol 1993;92:448.
28. Kotler DP, Scholes JV, Tierney AR. Intestinal plasma cell alterations in acquired immuno-deficiency syndrome. Dig Dis Sci 1984;32:129.
29. Eriksson K, Kilander A, Hagberg L, Norkrans G, Homgren J, Czerkinsky C. Virus-specific antibody production and polyclonal B-cell activation in the intestinal mucosa of HIV-infected individuals. AIDS 1995;9:695.
30. Janoff EN, Jackson S, Wahl SM, et al. Intestinal mucosal immunoglobulin during human immunodeficiency virus type 1 infection. J Infect Dis 1994;170:2399.
31. Harriman GR, Smith PD, Horne MK, et al. Vitamin B12 malabsorption in patients with acquired immunodeficiency syndrome. Arch Intern Med 1989;149:2039.
32. Ullrich R, Zeitz M, Heise W, et al. Small intestinal structure and function in patients infected with immunodeficiency virus (HIV): evidence of HIV-induced enteropathy. Ann Intern Med 1989;3:15.
33. Budhraja M, Levendoglu H, Kocka F, et al. Duodenal mucosal T cell subpopulation and bacterial cultures in acquired immune deficiency syndrome. Am J Gastroenterol 1987;82:427.
34. Moore PS, Chang Y. Detection of herpes virus-like DNA sequences in Kaposi's sarcoma in patients with and those without HIV infection. N Engl J Med 1995;332:1181.
35. Gao SJ, Kinsley L, Hoover DR, et al. Seroconversion to antibodies against Kaposi's sarcoma-associated herpesvirus-related latent nuclear antigens before the development of Kaposi's sarcoma. N Engl J Med 1996;335:233.
36. Katz BZ, Raub-Traub N, Miller GGG. Latent and replicating forms of Epstein–Barr Virus DNA in lymphomas and lymphoproliferative diseases. J Infect Dis 1989;160:589.
37. Strober W. Protein-losing enteropathy. In: Bouchier IAD, Allan RN, Hodgson HJF, et al. (eds.) Gastroenterology, clinical science and practice, 2nd edn. Philadelphia, WB Saunders, 1993.
38. Fleisher TA, Strober W, Muchmore AV, et al. Corticosteroid-responsive intestinal lymphangiectasia, secondary to an inflammatory process. N Engl J Med 1979;300:605.
39. Waldmann TA, Wochner RD, Strober W. The role of the gastrointestinal tract in plasma protein metabolism studies with 51Cr-albumin. Am J Med 1969;46:275.
40. Nelson DL, Blaese RM, Strober W, et al. Constructive pericarditis, intestinal lymphangiectasia and reversible immunologic deficiency. J Pediatr 1975;86:548.
41. Strober W, Wochner RD, Carbone PP, et al. Intestinal lymphangiectasia: a protein-losing enteropathy with hypogammaglobulinemia, lymphocytopenia and impaired homograft rejection. J Clin Invest 1967;46:1643.
42. Sorensen RU, Halpin TC, Abramowsky CR, et al. Intestinal lymphangiectasia and thymic hypoplasia. Clin Exp Immunol 1985;59:217.
43. Weiden PL, Blaese RM, Strober W, et al. Impaired lymphocyte transformation in intestinal lymphangiectasia: evidence of at least two functionally and distinct lymphocyte populations in man. J Clin Invest 1972;51:1319.
44. Rilman DA, Schmidt TM, MacDermott RR, et al. Identification of the uncultured bacillus of Whipple's disease. N Engl J Med 1992;327:293.
45. Dobbins WO III: Whipple's disease. Springfield, IL, CC Thomas, 1987.
46. Marth T, Neurath MF, Cuccherini B, Strober W. Defects in monocyte interleukin-12 production and humoral immunity in Whipple's disease. Gastroenterology 1997;113:442.
47. Waldmann TA, Wochner RD, Laster L, et al. Allergic gastroenteropathy: a cause of excessive gastrointestinal protein loss. N Engl J Med 1967;276:762.
48. Mowat AM, Felstein MV, Borland A, et al. Experimental studies of immunologically mediated enteropathy: development of cell-mediated immunity and intestinal pathology during a graft-versus-host reaction in irradiated mice. Gut 1988;29:949.
49. Piguet PF. GVHR elicited by products of class I or class II loci of the MHC: analysis of the response of mouse T lymphocytes to products of class I and class II loci of the MHC in correlation with GVHR-induced mortality, medullary aplasia and enteropathy. J Immunol 1985;135:1637.
50. Strober W. Gluten-sensitive enteropathy: an abnormal immunologic response of the gastro-intestinal tract to a dietary protein. In: Kirsner JR, Shorter RG (eds) Gastrointestinal immunity for the clinician. New York, Grune & Stratton, 1985.
51. Marsh MN. Gluten, major histocompatibility complex, and the small intestine: a molecular and immunobiologic approach to the spectrum of gluten-sensitivity (celiac sprue). Gastroenterology 1992;102:330.
52. Cooke WT, Holmes GKT. Skin manifestations and dermatitis herpetiformis. In: Cooke WT, Holmes GKT (eds) Coeliac disease. London, Churchill Livingstone, 1970.
53. Mascart-Lemone F, van den Broeck J, Cadranel S, et al. Serological aspects of coeliac disease. Acta Gastroenterol Belg 1992;45:200.
54. Lindquist BL, Rogozinski T, Moi H, et al. Endomysial and gliadin IgA antibodies in children with coeliac disease. Scand J Gastroenterol 1994;29:452.
55. Dieterich W, Ehnis T, Bauer M, et al. Identification of tissue transglutaminase as the autoantigen in celiac disease. Nature Med 1997;3:797.
56. Catassi C, Kotsch IM, Fabiani E, et al. Coeliac disease in the year 2000: exploring the iceberg. Lancet 1994;343:200.
57. Volta U, Corozza GR, Grisoni M, et al. IgA antigliadin antibodies and persistence of jejunal lesions in adult coeliac disease. Digestion 1990;47:111.

58. Kasarda DD. Structure and properties of alpha-gliadins. Ann Technol Agric 1980;29:151.
59. Ciclitira PJ, Evans DJ, Fagg NLK, et al. Clinical testing of gliadin fractions of coeliac disease. J Clin Sci 1984;66:357.
60. de Ritis G, Auricchio S, Jones HW, et al. In vitro (organ culture) studies of the toxicity of specific-gliadin peptides in celiac disease. Gastroenterology 1988;94:41.
61. Sturgess R, Day P, Ellis HJ, et al. Wheat peptide challenge in coeliac disease. Lancet 1994;343:758.
62. Ensari A, Ager A, Marsh MN, et al. Time-course of adhesion molecule expression in rectal mucosa of gluten-sensitive subjects after gluten challenge. Clin Exp Immunol 1993;92:303.
63. Shiner M. Ultrastructural changes suggestive of immune reactions in the jejunal mucosa of coeliac children following gluten challenge. Gut 1973;14:1.
64. Halstensen TS, Hvatumn M, Scott H, et al. Association of subepithelial deposition of activated complement and immunoglobulin G and M response to gluten in celiac disease. Gastroenterology 1992;102:751.
65. Brandtzaeg P, Halstensen TS, Kett K, et al. Immunobiology and immunopathology of human gut mucosa: humoral immunity and intraepithelial lymphocytes. Gastroenterology 1989;97:1562.
66. Halstensen TS, Brandtzaeg P. Mucosal T cells subsets in coeliac disease: expression of T cell receptor and CD45 isoforms. Immunol Res 1991;10:493.
67. Halstensen TS, Brandtzaeg P. Activated T cells in the celiac lesion: non-proliferative activation (CD25) of CD4+ β cells in the lamina propria but proliferation (Ki-67) of β cells in the epithelium. Eur J Immunol 1993;23:505.
68. Breese EJ, Kumar P, Farthing MJ, MacDonald TT. Interleukin-2 and interferon-gamma producing cells in the lamina propria in celiac disease. Dig Dis Sci 1994;39:2243.
69. Spencer J, Isaacson PG, MacDonald TT, et al. T cells and the diagnosis of coeliac disease. Clin Exp Immunol 1991;85:109.
70. Holm K, Maki M, Savilachti E, et al. Intraepithelial T cell receptor lymphocytes and genetic susceptibility to coeliac disease. Lancet 1992;339:1500.
71. Halstensen TS, Scott H, Brandtzaeg P. Intraepithelial T cells of the Tcr $\gamma\delta^{+}$ $CD8^{-}$ and $V\delta 1/J\delta 1^{+}$ phenotypes are increased in coeliac disease. Scand J Immunol 1989;30:665.
72. Leigh RJ, Marsh MN, Crowe P, et al. Studies of intestinal lymphoid tissue. IX. Dose-dependent gluten-induced lymphoid infiltrates of coeliac jejunal epithelium. Scand J Gastroenterol 1985;20:715.
73. van Thiel DH, Smith WI, Rabin BS, et al. A syndrome of immunoglobulin A deficiency, diabetes mellitus, malabsorption and a common HLA haplotype: immunologic study of 43 family members. Ann Intern Med 1977;86:10.
74. Stern M, Fisher K, Gruttner K. Immunofluorescent serum gliadin antibodies in children with coeliac disease and various malabsorptive disorders. II. Eur J Pediatr 1979;130:165.
75. Unsworth DJ, Walker-Smith JA, Holbrow EJ. Gliadin and reticulin antibodies in childhood coeliac disease. Lancet 1983;1:874.
76. Crowe JP, Phelan JJ, Cleere WF, et al. The lymphocyte transformation test in coeliac disease: effect of gliadin and detoxified gliadin. Digestion 1980;20:95.
77. Falchuk ZM, Gebhard RL, Sessoms C, et al. An in vitro model of gluten-sensitive enteropathy: effect of gliadin on intestinal epithelial cells of patients with gluten-sensitive enteropathy in organ culture. J Clin Invest 1974;53:487.
78. Webster AD, Slavin G, Shiver M, et al. Coeliac disease with severe hypogammaglobulinemia. Gut 1981;22:153.
79. Strober W. Gluten-sensitive enteropathy. In: King RA, Rotter JI, Motulsky AG (eds) The genetic basis of common diseases. New York, Oxford University Press, 1992.
80. Tosi R, Vismara D, Tonigaki N, et al. Evidence that celiac disease is primarily associated with a DC locus allele specificity. Clin Immunol Immunopathol 1985;28:395.
81. Sollid LM, Markussen G, Ek J, et al. Evidence for a primary association of celiac disease to a particular HLA-DQ/β heterodimer. J Exp Med 1989;169:345.
82. Polanco I. Current status of digestive intolerance to foods. J Pediatr 1992;121:S108.
83. Ferguson A. Models of immunologically driven small intestinal damage. In: Marsh MM (ed) Immunopathology of the small intestine New York, John Wiley & Sons, 1987.
84. Baer AN, Bayless TM, Yardley JH. Intestinal ulceration and malabsorption syndrome. Gastroenterology 1980;79:754.
85. Talley NH, Shorter RG, Phillips SF, et al. Eosinophilic gastroenteritis: a clinicopathological study of patients with disease of the mucosa, muscle layer and subserosal tissues. Gut 1990;31:54.
86. Podolsky DK. Inflammatory bowel disease. N Engl J Med 1991;325:928.
87. Yardley JH, Lazenby AJ, Giardiallo FM, et al. Collagenous 'microscopic' lymphocytic and other gentler and more subtle forms of colitis. Hum Pathol 1990;21:1089.
88. Calkins BM. A meta-analysis of the roles of smoking in inflammatory bowel disease. Dig Dis Sci 1989;34:1841.
89. Rampton DS, McNeil NI, Garner M. Analgesic ingestion and other factors preceding relapse in ulcerative colitis. Gut 1982;24:187.
90. Bennett RA, Rubin PH, Prisent DH. Frequency of inflammatory bowel disease in offspring of couples both presenting with inflammatory bowel disease. Gastroenterology 1991;100:1638.
91. Yang H, McElree C, Roth M-P, et al. Familial empiric risks for inflammatory bowel disease: differences between Jews and non-Jews. Gut 1992;34:517.
92. Yang H, Shobat T, Rotter JI. The genetics of inflammatory bowel disease. In: MacDermott RP, Stenson WF (eds) Inflammatory bowel disease. New York, Elsevier, 1992.
93. Yang H, Rotter RI, Toyoda H, et al. Ulcerative colitis: a genetically heterogenous disorder defined by genetic (HLA dass II) and subclinical (antineutrophil cytoplasmic antibodies). J Clin Invest 1993;92:1080.
94. Hugot J, Laurent-Puig P, Gowe-Rousseau C, et al. Mapping of a susceptibility locus for Crohn's disease on chromosome 16. Nature 1996;379:821.
95. Schmitz-Moorman P, Becker H. Histologic studies on the formal pathogenesis of the epithelial cell granuloma in Crohn's disease. In: Pena AS, Weterman IT, Booth CC, Strober W (eds) Recent advances in Crohn's disease. The Hague, Martinus Nijhoff, 1991.
96. Brandtzaeg P, Halstensen TS, Kitt K, Rognum TO. Local immunopathology in inflammatory bowel disease. In: Järnerot G (ed) Inflammatory bowel disease. New York, Raven Press, 1987.
97. MacDermott RP, Nash GS, Bertovich MS, et al. Altered patterns of secretion of monomeric IgA and IgA subclass I by intestinal mononuclear cells in inflammatory bowel disease. Gastroenterology 1986;91:379.
98. Halstensen TS, Mollnes TE, Garred P, Fausa O, Brandtzaeg P. Epithelial deposition of immunoglobulin GI and activated complement (C3b and terminal complement complex) in ulcerative colitis. Gastroenterology 1989;98:1264.
99. Moore K, Walters MT, Jones DB, Harvey J, Cawley MI, Smith JL. An immunohistological study of CD4+ lymphocyte subsets with inflammatory lesions with special reference to rheumatoid arthritis and inflammatory bowel disease. Immunology 1988;65:457.
100. Perlmann P, Hammarstrom S, Lagercrantz R. Immunologic features of idiopathic ulcerative colitis and Crohn's disease. Rendic Gastroenterol 1973;5:17.
101. Roche JK, Fiocchi C, Youngman K. Sensitization to epithelial antigens in chronic mucosal inflammatory disease: characterization of human intestinal mucosa-derived mononuclear cells relative with purified epithelial cell-associated components in vitro. J Clin Invest 1985;75:522.
102. Das KM, Dasgupta A, Mandal A, Geng X. Autoimmunity to cytoskeletal protein tropomyosin: a clue to the pathogenetic mechanism for ulcerative colitis. J Immunol 1993;150:2487.
103. Snook JA, Chapman RW, Fleming K, Jewell DP. Anti-neutrophil nuclear antibody in ulcerative colitis, Crohn's disease and primary sclerosing cholangitis. Clin Exp Immunol 1989;76:30.
104. Hauschild S, Schmidt WH, Csemok E, Flesch BK, Rautmann A, Gross WL. ANCA in systemic vasculitides collagen vascular disease, rheumatic disorders and inflammatory bowel disease. Adv Exp Med Biol 1994;336:245.

105. MacDermott RP, Bragdon MJ, Kodner IJ, Bertovich MJ. Deficient cell-mediated cytotoxicity and hypo-responsiveness to interferon and mitogenic lectin activation by inflammatory bowel disease peripheral blood and intestinal mononuclear cells. Gastroenterology 1986;90:6.
106. Gibson PR, van de Pol E, Pullman W, Doe WF. Lysis of colonic epithelial cells by allogeneic mononuclear and lymphokine activated killer cells derived from peripheral blood and intestinal mucosa: evidence against a pathogenic role in inflammatory bowel disease. Gut 1988;29:1076.
107. Fiocchi C, Hilfiker ML, Youngman KR, Doerder NC, Finke JH. Mucosa mononuclear cell: decreased levels in inflammatory bowel disease. Gastroenterology 1984;86:734.
108. Mullin GE, Lazinby AJ, Harris ML, et al. Increased interleukin-2 messenger RNA in the intestinal mucosal lesion of Crohn's disease but not ulcerative colitis. Gastroenterology 1992;102:1620.
109. Breese E, Braegger CP, Corrigan CJ, et al. Interleukin-2- and interferon-gamma-secreting T cells in normal and diseased human intestinal mucosa. Immunology 1993;78:127.
110. Lieberman BY, Fiocchi C, Youngman KR, et al. Interferon-gamma production by human intestinal mucosal mononuclear cells decreased levels in inflammatory bowel disease. Dig Dis Sci 1988;33:1297.
111. Fais S, Capobianchi MR, Pallone F, et al. Spontaneous release of interferon-gamma by intestinal lamina propria lymphocytes in Crohn's disease: kinetic of in vitro response to infection inducers. Gut 1991;32:403.
112. Fuss I, Neurath MF, Boirivant M, Klein JS, et al. Disparate CD4+ lamina propria (LP) lymphocyte secretion profiles in inflammatory bowel disease. J Immunol 1996;157:1261.
113. Finotto S, Schürmann G, Mudter J, Galle PR, Neurath MF. Unpublished data.
114. Mahida YR, Wu K, Jewell DP. Enhanced production of interleukin 1-beta by mononuclear cells isolated from mucosa with active ulterative colitis or Crohn's disease. Gut 1989;30:835.
115. Mahida YR, Kurlac L, Gallagher A, Hawkey JC. High circulating concentrations of interleukin 6 in active Crohn's disease, but not ulcerative colitis. Gut 1991;32:1531.
116. Targan SR, Hanauer SB, Deventer SJV, et al. A short-term study of chimeric monoclonal antibody cA2 to tumor necrosis factor alpha for Crohn's disease. N Engl J Med 1997;337:1029.
117. Stack W, Mann S, Roy A, Heath P, et al. Randomised controlled trial of CDP571 antibody to tumour necrosis factor-alpha in Crohn's disease. Lancet 1997;349:521.
118. Neurath MF, Pettersson S, Meyer zum Büschenfelde KH, Strober W. Local administration of antisense phosphorothioate oligonucleotides to the p65 subunit of NF-kappaB abrogates established experimental colitis in mice. Nature Med 1996;2:998.
119. Neurath MF, Fuss I, Kelsall BL, Stuber E, Strober W. Antibodies to IL-12 abrogate established experimental colitis in mice. J Exp Med 1995;182:1280.
120. Wirtz S, Finotto S, Kanzler S, et al. Cutting edge: chronic intestinal inflammation in STAT-4 transgenic mice: characterization of disease and adoptive transfer by TNF-plus IFN-gamma-producing CD4+ T cells that respond to bacterial antigens. J Immunol 1999;162:1884.
121. Pizarro TT, Michie MH, Bentz M, et al. IL-18, a novel immunoregulatory cytokine, is up-regulated in Crohn's disease: expression and localization in intestinal mucosal cells. J Immunol 1999;162:6829.
122. Podolsky DK, Fourmier DA. Alterations in mucosal content of colonic glycoconjugates in inflammatory bowel disease defined by monoclonal antibodies. Gastroenterology 1988;95:379.
123. Pirzer V, Schönhaer A, Fleisher B, et al. Reactivity of infiltrating T lymphocytes with microbial antigens in Crohn's disease. Lancet 1991;338:1238.
124. Allison KC, Strober W, Harriman GR. Induction of IL-5 reteptors on normal B cells by cross-linking surface Ig with Ig-Dextran. J Immunol 1991;146:4197.
125. Elson CO, Sartor RB, Tennyson GS, Riddell RH. Experimental models of inflammatory bowel disease. Gastroenterology 1995;109:1344.
126. Peura DA, Graham DY. *Helicobacter pylori*: consensus reached: peptic ulcer is on the way to becoming an historic disease. Am J Gastroenterol 1994;89:1137.
127. Marshall BJ. Unidentified curved bacilli on gastric epithelium in active chronic gastritis. Lancet 1983;i:1273.
128. Mohammadi M, Nedrud J, Redline R, Lycke N, Czinn S. Murine CD4+ T cell responses to *Helicobacter* infection: TH1 cells enhance gastritis and TH2 cells reduce bacterial load. Gastroenterology 1997;113:1848.
129. Telford JL, Ghiara P, Dell'Orco M, et al. Gene structure of the *Helicobacter pylori* cytotoxin and evidence to its key role in gastric disease. J Exp Med 1994;179:1653.
130. Hussell T, Isaacson PG, Crabtree JE, Spencer J. The response of cells from low-grade B-cell gastric lymphoma of mucosa-associated lymphoid tissue to *Helicobacter pylori*. Lancet 1993;342:571.
131. Wotherspoon AC, Doglioni C, Diss TC, et al. Regression of primary low-grade B-cell gastric lymphoma of mucosa-associated lymphoid tissue type after eradication of *Helicobacter pylori*. Lancet 1993;342:575.
132. Rambaud JC, Brouet JC, Seligmann M. Alpha chain disease and related lymphoproliferative disorders. In: Ogra P, Mestecky J, Lamm ME, et al. (eds) Handbook of mucosal immunology. Academic Press, 1994.

Chapter 88

Inflammatory Hepatobiliary Cirrhosis

Patrick S.C. Leung, Petra Obermayer-Straub, Michael P. Manns, Aftab Ansari and M. Eric Gershwin

PRIMARY BILIARY CIRRHOSIS

Primary biliary cirrhosis (PBC) is a liver disease characterized by autoimmune-mediated destruction of intrahepatic bile ducts with progressive inflammatory scarring followed by liver failure and the presence of high titer of antimitochondrial autoantibodies (AMA).[1] The initial characterization of the reactive mitochondrial antigens was limited to a trypsin-sensitive moiety in the inner mitochondrial membrane designated as M2. In the mid 1980s, the autoantigens in human PBC were identified as members of the 2-oxoacid dehydrogenase complexes (2-OADC), of which pyruvate dehydrogenase-E2 (PDC-E2) is the most prominent antigenic component.[2] Other mitochondrial antigens of PBC include the E2 subunit of the branched chain 2-oxo-acid dehydrogenase complex (BCOADC-E2), the E2 subunit of oxoglutarate dehydrogenase complex (OGDC-E2), E3 binding protein (E3BP, previously known as protein X), and the E1α subunit of PDC (Table 88.1).

KEY CONCEPTS

Primary biliary cirrhosis (PBC)

- PBC is an autoimmune disease of the liver that primarily affects women and is associated with a high titer of antimitochondrial autoantibodies (AMA).
- The autoantigens recognized by AMA are part of the 2-oxoacid dehydrogenase pathway, including the E2 subunits of pyruvate dehydrogenase, branched chain 2-oxoacid dehydrogenase, 2-oxo-glutarate dehydrogenase, E3 binding protein, and the E1 alpha subunit of pyruvate dehydrogenase.
- PBC is marked by progressive inflammatory destruction and obliteration of intrahepatic bile ducts, followed by development of cirrhosis and liver failure.

Clinical features

PBC has a strong gender predominance, affecting women up to 10–20 times more frequently than men. PBC is virtually the only autoimmune disease that has never been reported in children, and its incidence gradually rises with age. (In 1997, an AMA-positive autoimmune hepatitis was reported in a 12-year-old girl, but the clinical symptoms did not indicate a true autoimmune hepatitis/PBC overlap syndrome.[3])

Predominant clinical features in patients with PBC include jaundice, pruritus, fatigue, persistent ill-defined abdominal discomfort, and hepatomegaly. The onset of clinical jaundice usually precedes other manifestations of hepatic decomposition and the degree of jaundice is correlated with the degree of liver failure.[4] Pruritus is the predominant symptom in up to 57% of PBC patients, however the intensity of pruritus is not correlated with other clinical features and is not a reflection of the severity of the lesion. It may even resolve during the later stage of the disease.[5] Approximately 10% of PBC patients have persistent fatigue, but

Characteristics of antimitochondrial autoantibodies and mitochondrial antigens in PBC

Antigen	MW (kDa)[a]	Frequency in PBC (%)[b]	Lipoyl domain	B-cell epitope	Major Ig isotype and IgG subclass	Inhibition of enzyme function by AMA	T-cell epitope
PDC-E1α	41	41–66	–	TPP binding and phosphorylation sites	NR	+	NR
PDC-E1β	36	2–7	–	NR	NR[c]	NR	NR
PDC-E2	74	95	+	Outer and inner lipoyl domains	IgG_3, IgM	+	Lipoyl domain
BCOADC-E2	52	53–55	+	Lipoyl domain	NR	+	NR
OGDC-E2	48	39–88	+	Lipoyl domain	IgG_2, IgM	+	NR
E3BP	55	95	+	Lipoyl domain	IgG	+	NR

[a]Determined by SDS-PAGE.
[b]Determined by immunoblotting or ELISA.
[c]NR – not reported.

Table 88.1 Characteristics of antimitochondrial autoantibodies and mitochondrial antigens in PBC.

this symptom also has no significant relation to disease severity. Serum bilirubin levels usually increase gradually over the course of the disease. Xanthomas are evident during the life-time course in up to one fourth of PBC patients, but represent the first symptom in less than 1%.[6] Interestingly, up to 60% of patients may not have any liver-related symptoms at the time of diagnosis.

Other symptoms and clinical features include gastrointestinal bleeding, portal hypertension, ascites, spider nevi, increased skin pigmentation, and encephalopathy. These symptoms, however, are generic to any chronic liver disease. Renal tubular acidosis, hepatomas, and breast carcinomas have been found in PBC patients, but the relationship between these disorders and PBC remains uncertain.

An elevated alkaline phosphatase and AMA are characteristic clinical laboratory features of PBC. Although the presence of AMA is a serological hallmark of PBC, 5–10% of PBC patients with definite clinical, histological and biochemical diagnostic criteria of PBC are AMA-negative by immunofluorescence.[7] However, other features, including liver histology and prevalence of other autoimmune disorders, were indistinguishable from AMA-positive PBC.[8]

Origin

Studies of the origin of PBC include the search for a potential microbial association with the disease, an extensive analysis of epidemiological data, and studies of the genetic and environmental backgrounds of PBC patients. Several lines of serological evidence support a role of infectious agents in the pathogenesis of PBC especially enteric bacteria and mycobacteria.[9] In addition, it has been reported that a protein located in the membrane of *Neisseria meningitidis* consists of 11 amino acid residues that are highly homologous with the lipoyl domain of the PDH-E2 component.[10]

Cross-reactivity between human PDC-E2 and *E. coli* PDC-E2 at the T-cell level has also been demonstrated. Amino acids E, D, and K, at positions 170, 172, and 173 respectively, of the human PDC-E2 are found to be the essential amino acid residues required for T-cell recognition and activation. This sequence EXDK is also found in *E. coli* PDC-E2. It was also reported that PDC-E2 163–176 specific T-cell clones cross-reacted with PDC-E2 peptide 36–49 and OGDC-E2 peptide 100–113, both of which include EXDK sequences. These findings suggest that molecular mimicry between human PDC-E2 and *E. coli* PDC-E2 is possible at the T-cell level.[11]

A number of independent studies have attempted to detect evidence of microbes in PBC, but in spite of extensive analyses of cross-reactive epitopes between PDC-E2 and a number of infectious agents, an association between microbes and PBC has yet to be proven. For example, Tanaka et al[12] used primers specific for *gro*EL for the detection of mycobacterial DNA, and primers for the 16s rRNA gene for the detection of helicobacterial DNA. Mycobacterial DNA was not found in any of PBC livers, and helicobacterial DNA was found only in 1 of 29 PBC livers, which turned out to be *H. pylori* by sequencing. Furthermore, PCR primers for another region of the 16s rRNA gene of *E. coli* (which is well conserved in all eubacteria), failed to define 'consensus' bacteria detected only in PBC livers. Mason et al[13] investigated seroreactivity of HIV-1 p24 gag and human intracisternal A-type particle (HIAP) proteins using sera from patients with PBC and other liver diseases, as well as SLE and healthy controls. Reactivity against these two proteins was found not to be PBC specific, making it unlikely that mitochondrial antigens, which are disease-specific autoantigens in PBC, share epitopes with the HIV-1 p24 and HIAP retroviral proteins.

PBC is present among various ethnic and racial populations, but the incidence and prevalence vary quite widely. It is found with the highest frequency among Northern European populations with a prevalence of over $100/10^6$ in Sweden, Norway, England, Wales and Scotland,[14–19] and a lower frequency in Japan[20] and other parts of Asia. Moreover, even among populations derived from Northern European stock, there is a striking difference in prevalence[21–24] (Table 88.2).

Incidence and prevalance of primary biliary cirrhosis

Geographical location	Number of patients	Incidence per million	Point prevalence per million
Victoria, Australia[21]	71	–	19
Ontario, Canada[24]	206	3	22
Sheffield, England[25]	34	5.8	54
Northeast England[16]	117	10	37–144
Northeast England[17]	347	11–18	129
Newcastle England[19]	99	14–32	240
Dundee, Scotland[18]	21	10.6	40.2
Swansea, Wales[17]	65	20	200
Malmo, Sweden[16]	33	4–24	92
Orebro, Sweden[15]	43	14	128
Umea, Sweden[16]	111	13	151
Estonia, Russia[22]	69	2	27

Table 88.2 Incidence and prevalance of primary biliary cirrhosis.

The possible genetic and environmental backgrounds of PBC patients in relation to AMA and other autoantibodies have been studied by a number of laboratories. There is an increase in the prevalence of various autoantibodies among otherwise normal relatives of PBC patients.[25] Moreover, there is evidence of familial clustering.[26] Indeed, the overall prevalence of PBC in first-degree relatives is between 4% and 6%, which is significantly higher than the general population prevalence.[19] An analysis of the inheritance patterns of HLA and the pro-inflammatory cytokine tumor necrosis factor-alpha (TNF-α), which are closely linked on chromosome 6 (Chapter 6), has failed to identify a definite genetic association to disease susceptibility in PBC. Studies attempting to link promoter polymorphisms of the natural resistance – associated macrophage protein 1 (NRAMP1) and search for fetal microchimerism, an alternative mechanism that could explain familial clustering, have also been unproductive.

Pathogenesis

Many immunologic abnormalities are found in PBC patients, suggesting that the disease is caused by abnormalities of immune regulation. The most striking abnormality is high-titer AMA. The targets of the AMA are proteins within the 2-oxoacid dehydrogenase pathway and include PDC-E1α, PDC-E1β, PDC-E2, E3BP (protein X), BCOADC-E2, and OGDC-E2. Accordingly, significant attention has been focused on the role of AMA in both B-cell and T-cell mediated immune reactivity.

The structures of PDC, E3BP, BCOADC, and OGDC are similar to one another. Each consists of multiple copies of three functionally equivalent subunits that have structural similarities but act on different substrates. More than 90% of the sera from patients with PBC react against PDC-E2[1] which has four structural and functional regions: two lipoyl domains near the N-terminal, a binding site for the other subunits E1 and E3, and, at the C terminus, a catalytic site which is interconnected by an alanine-proline rich region. *E. coli* PDC-E2 contains three lipoyl regions, and mammalian PDC has two such regions, outer and inner. E3BP, BCOADC-E2, and OGDC-E2 are similar to PDC-E2, but have only one lipoyl-binding binding region (Fig. 88.1).

Among these 2-OADC, the antigenic determinants of PDC-E2 are currently the best characterized. Immunoassays of multiple overlapping recombinant fusion proteins from human PDC-E2 cDNA indicate at least three autoepitopes on human PDC-E2: the cross-reactive outer and inner lipoyl domains, and a site surrounding the E1–E3 binding region. The dominant epitope is localized to the inner lipoyl region. Analysis of recombinant fusion proteins expressed from cDNA encoding the inner lipoyl domain has revealed that 75 amino acids (residues 146–221) of the protein are required for detectable autoantibody binding and 93 amino acids (residues 128–221) are necessary for strong binding,[27] strongly suggesting that a conformational autoepitope is involved.

Studies using genetically engineered variants of *E. coli* PDC-E2 have shown that the immunoreactivity of PBC sera depends on the presence of the lipoic acid moiety.[28] Sera from PBC patients appeared to recognize specifically an octadecapeptide of the inner lipoyl domain (amino acid residue 167–184) when it was covalently attached to lipoic acid.[29] The same peptide also absorbed reactivity from PBC sera, preventing the sera from reacting with rat kidney, stomach, and liver and human HEp-2 cells. However, while 95% of the PBC sera reacted with either recombinant or native PDC-E2, half of the tested sera reacted with the peptide 167–184. In contrast, removal of lipoic acid did not affect antibody recognition by PBC sera.[30] Thus, the role of lipoic acid as an epitope and in the pathogenesis of PBC remains to be defined.

The lipoyl-binding region of PDC, the major PBC autoepitope, is homologous with corresponding regions of the E2 subunits of OGDC-E2 and BCOADC-E2. Using purified antigens, antibodies to OGDC-E2 and BCOADC-E2 were detected in the sera of approximately 90% and 50% of PBC patients examined, respectively.[7] Epitope mapping studies showed that AMA recognize conformational epitopes within residues 1–227 of BCOADC-E2 and residues 67–147 of OGDC-E2 of their lipoyl domains.[31,32] Likewise, the E3BP epitope was mapped to the lipoyl domain (Table 88.1, Fig. 88.1).[33] Other components of the enzymes PDC-E1α (41 kDa) and PDC-E1β (36 kDa), which do not contain lipoic acid, are recognized by antibodies in sera of approximately 50% and approximately 5%, respectively, of patients.[34] Although no systematic studies have been reported with E1 subunits of OGDC and BCOADC, reactivity to E1 of OGDC has been described. Low-titer (dilutions of 1:100) antibodies to E3 (dihydrolipoamide dehydrogenase), a shared subunit of the three 2-OADC enzyme complexes, have also been reported. These antibodies are of the IgG class but may be 'natural', since they occur with nearly equal frequency in the sera of not only patients with PBC but also in sera from normal individuals. Recent reports have demonstrated the presence of AMA IgG and IgA as well as mitochondrial antigens in the bile as well as saliva of PBC patients but not in controls, providing evidence for a locally driven mucosal response.[35] It is possible that membrane expression of these mitochondrial autoantigens by salivary epithelial cells can lead to enhanced susceptibility to immune-mediated damage similar to that noted against biliary epithelial cells. Although the titer of AMA does not correlate with the stages or prognosis of the disease, the specific reactivity of AMA and their inhibition of enzyme function make AMA unlikely to be simply an epiphenomenon.

The mononuclear cell infiltrate surrounding the bile duct of PBC patients consists primarily of T cells that appear to be oligoclonal and appear to respond to both the lipoyl domain and the

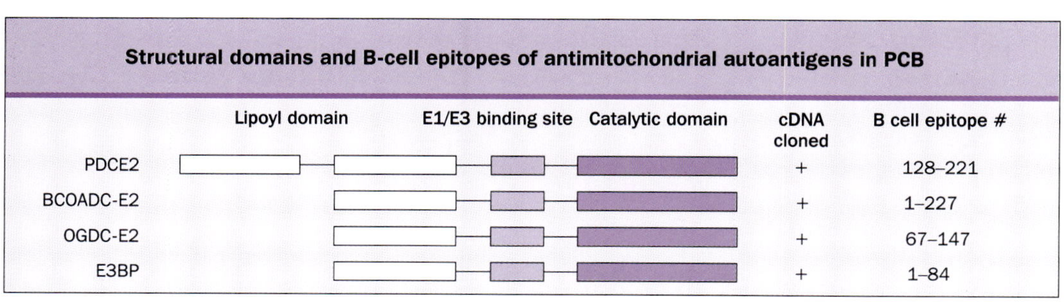

Figure 88.1 Schematic diagram of the structural domains and B-cell epitopes of antimitochondrial autoantigens in PBC. The amino acid residues of the B-cell epitope are shown on the right.

core/E1 domain of PDC-E2.[36] Analysis of T-cell clones from the blood has helped map these minimal autoepitopes. These epitopes include peptides 163–176 (GDLLAEIETDKATI), which corresponds to the inner lipoyl domain of human PDC-E2,[37] and peptide 36–49 (GDLIAEVETDKATD), which is derived from the outer lipoyl domain. Peripheral blood mononuclear cells (PBMC) from those patients showing no response to whole PDC-E2 also did not respond to either the lipoyl domain or the core/E1 domain.

Recent studies indicate that PDC-E2-specific T-cell lines are not eliminated from the PBMC by thymic selection, and suggest that tolerance against PDC-E2 is normally established in the periphery. PDC-E2 specific T-cell lines can be obtained from the blood of both normal individuals and PBC patients. The precursor frequency is only 2–4-fold higher in patients with PBC when compared with healthy controls.[11] In PBC patients, however, the frequency of T-cell precursor specific for peptide 163–176 of PDC-E2 was 100–150-fold higher in the hilar lymph nodes and liver than in the blood, pointing to failure of peripheral tolerance and proliferation of autoreactive T-cell populations. Moreover, T-cell lines that reacted with PDC-E2 peptide 163–176 also showed reactivity against PDC-E2 peptide 36–49 (GDLIAEVETDKATV) and the OGDC peptide 100–113 (DEVVCEIETDKTSV), suggesting the presence of cross-reactivity (plasticity of the TCR) among these three mitochondrial enzymes of the T-cell level. Since these three peptides share ExETDK amino acid sequences, this may be a common T-cell epitope motif that could serve as a focus for therapeutic intervention.

It has been hypothesized that T-cell recognition of peptide 163–176 can be affected by the tertiary structure of human PDC-E2. Data from X-ray crystallography and 2-D NMR of human as well as bacterial PDC-E2 showed that the peptide 163–176 of the lipoyl domain is located at a structurally exposed region of the molecule,[38] which may partly explain the particular immunogenicity of this sequence. Future identification of the tertiary structure of other mitochondrial autoantigens (e.g. BCOADC-E2 or OGDC-E2) will allow the prediction and determination of T-cell autoepitopes of these additional autoantigens and may yield further clues regarding their role in the pathogenesis of PBC.

Natural history

Although the natural history of PBC is extraordinarily variable, in many patients with symptomatic PBC the disorder is progressive and leads to end-stage cirrhosis of the liver. Classical PBC often presents with jaundice and syndromes such as pruritus, fatigue, portal hypertension, and abdominal pain. Histopathologically, duct damage and periportal fibrosis precede the development of end-stage cirrhosis.

Christensen et al[39] reported that symptomatic PBC is primarily a progressive order. A cohort of symptomatic PBC patients with a median disease duration of 2.1 years at the time of their entry into the study were followed for a median 18 months. After 4 years, the proportion of patients with cirrhosis rose from 27% to 82%. Over 5 years, the proportion of patients with pruritus rose from 75% to 95% and the proportion with jaundice rose from 9% to 82%. A later study by Metcalf et al[40] followed a cohort of 29 AMA-positive patients without symptoms or cholestasis for nearly 18 years. They found that in asymptomatic patients PBC was also a progressive disease. The median time from the first AMA-positive test to the development of cholestasis was 5.6 years, and at the end of the study cholestasis was evident in 24 of the 29 patients. Additional studies have confirmed the progressive nature of asymptomatic PBC, with up to half of initially asymptomatic patients becoming symptomatic over a 24-year period.[41] Once they develop symptoms, the survival rate of PBC patients who were originally identified with asymptomatic disease is indistinguishable from that of patients who were first identified with symptomatic PBC. Nonetheless, up to 33% of patients who are asymptomatic at time of diagnosis may remain asymptomatic during a median follow-up period of 12 years, and patients with asymptomatic disease maintain a higher survival rate as long as they remain asymptomatic.[41]

Where gender differences exist in the prevalence of many autoimmune diseases, patients who belong to the gender with lower prevalence exhibit more serious manifestations. However, in PBC no significant gender-related differences have been observed either in the clinical course or in the survival rate among symptomatic patients with stage III or stage IV disease.[6,39]

Sequestration of antigen is one mechanism by which peripheral tolerance can be maintained, and it would appear logical that mitochondrial antigens might not be easily seen by the immune system. However, several studies have suggested that in patients with PBC, these specific mitochondrial autoantigens may be present on the surface of hepatocytes or biliary epithelium. For example, one study showed that cultured biliary epithelial cells from PBC patients have luminal surface membrane-bound E2.[42] Similarly, another study showed that antibodies to PDC-E2 uniquely stain the luminal region of bile duct epithelial cells from patients with PBC but not in specimens from normal controls.[43] The sequences of a number of antibodies specific for PDC-E2 and OGDC-E2 have been reported.[7] Cloning and sequencing of the additional human AMA and analysis of their immunoglobulin gene usage are expected to be helpful in determining the role of AMA in the natural history of PBC.

Despite our increasing knowledge of the molecular immunology of PBC, the natural history of patients has undergone very little change and orthotopic liver transplant (OLT) continues to be the major form of treatment for end-stage cirrhosis. It remains unclear whether the autoimmune response continues after transplantation. Mattalia et al[44] have assayed a well-defined collection of 35 PBC sera collected serially before and after liver transplantation for quantitative and isotype-specific titers of antibodies against a set of recombinant mitochondrial autoantigens and gp210. Following OLT, the frequency of sera that responded to PDC-E2 alone increased from 7/35 to 12/35. Similarly, reactivity to BCOADC-E2 slightly increased from 2/35 to 4/35. However, there was an overall decrease in sera that responded to more than one antigen. Neither immunoglobulin isotype nor subclass of the autoimmune response changed following OLT. Findings with gp210 were similar. Overall, the titers of AMAs decline slightly during the first year post OLT (which could be a reflection of the effect of immunosuppressive drugs), but are equivalent to pre-OLT values by 6 months. Moreover, the antibody subclass/isotype remained unchanged. These data suggest that the removal of a diseased PBC liver has little, if any, impact on the serological characteristics of PBC.

Diagnosis

Patients with PBC present with a wide range of clinical patterns. The classical pattern includes jaundice and syndromes in which pruritus, fatigue, portal hypertension, and abdominal pain predominate. Indeed, up to 60% of PBC patients are without any liver-related symptoms at the time of their initial presentation. The diagnosis of PBC is a clinical one that is based upon the appearance of painless jaundice and the absence of mechanical biliary obstruction. The histologic features of portal inflammation and the presence of AMA confirm the diagnosis.[45] There is usually reactivity against two or more of the 2-OADC enzymes, but serologic cross-reactivity is found only between PDC-E2 and E3BP.

Measurement of serum alkaline phosphatase, serum bilirubin, serum ceruloplasmin, and serum lipid levels play an important role in the diagnosis of PBC. Generally, patients with PBC show a cholestatic pattern, with a significant elevation of serum alkaline phosphatase concentrations.[45] An increase in the serum bilirubin level is observed in patients with advanced disease and often correlates with poor prognosis.[46] In addition, a rise in serum ceruloplasmin levels is common among patients with PBC. Finally, patients with early PBC demonstrate a mild elevation of low-density and very low density lipoproteins lipoproteins, and a marked elevation of high-density lipoproteins. In contrast, patients with advanced disease have marked elevations in low-density lipoproteins and decreased high-density lipoproteins.[47]

Genetically engineered recombinant molecules (pML-MIT3) containing epitopes derived from PDC-E2, BCOADC-E2, and OGDC-E2 sequence have been used for the refinement of measurements of AMA by ELISA and provide a highly sensitive diagnosis of PBC (Fig. 88.2).[48] Using these techniques, it has been possible to detect AMA by testing saliva. The specificity of the salivary IgA in the vast majority of patients tested was found to reside against PDC-E2.[35] The use of genetically engineered autoantigenic epitopes, combined with the ability to utilize excretory fluid such as saliva, clearly provides a much less invasive and sensitive method for the detection of AMA, which may potentially replace conventional indirect immunofluorescence based assays for the detection of AMA in the future.

Treatment

Corticosteroids and immunosuppressive drugs that were widely used in the past for the treatment of PBC failed to show a significant benefit to the natural history of the disease while enhancing the potential for other pathologies, e.g. osteoporosis with corticosteroid therapy. Penicillamine was another treatment failure. This drug not only produced an increased incidence of significant toxicity, it had no significant influence on the progression of the disease, including survival.[49] Although several studies have suggested a beneficial effect of colchicine in improving some aspects of liver function, the overall results are not dramatic and the effect on survival have not been thoroughly assessed.[50] Studies of methotrexate and cyclosporine have also been disappointing.[45]

Treatment with ursodeoxycholic acid (UCDA) has recently received a great deal of attention. UCDA increases the transport of exogenous bile acids across the liver cell and the canalicular membrane, thereby reducing the concentrations of retained membrane-damaging bile acids.[51] Data from three different randomized controlled trials showed that 13–15 mg/kg/day of UCDA can significantly delay the time to liver transplantation in patients with PBC.[52]

At present, liver transplantation remains the most successful form of therapy for PBC. Unfortunately, liver transplantation is reserved for patients with end-stage organ disease and is difficult and expensive. However, AMA titers return to pretransplantation levels by 6 months after transplantation. Future therapy of PBC will largely depend on the identification of the underlying etiology of the disease. As long as the etiology is unknown, empirical therapies with the use of newly identified immunosuppressive drugs, antibiotics, and anticholestatic agents (with fewer side-effects) need to be identified and evaluated. If PBC is caused by infectious agents, antimicrobial therapy will be needed. On the

THERAPEUTIC PRINCIPLES

Primary biliary cirrhosis
- Therapy begins with immunosuppressive agents.
- Anticholestatic agents can be useful, e.g. ursodeoxycholic acid (UCDA)
- Liver transplantation is a viable option with patients demonstrating dramatic clinical improvement. Unfortunately, recent data show that AMA can recur after transplantation.

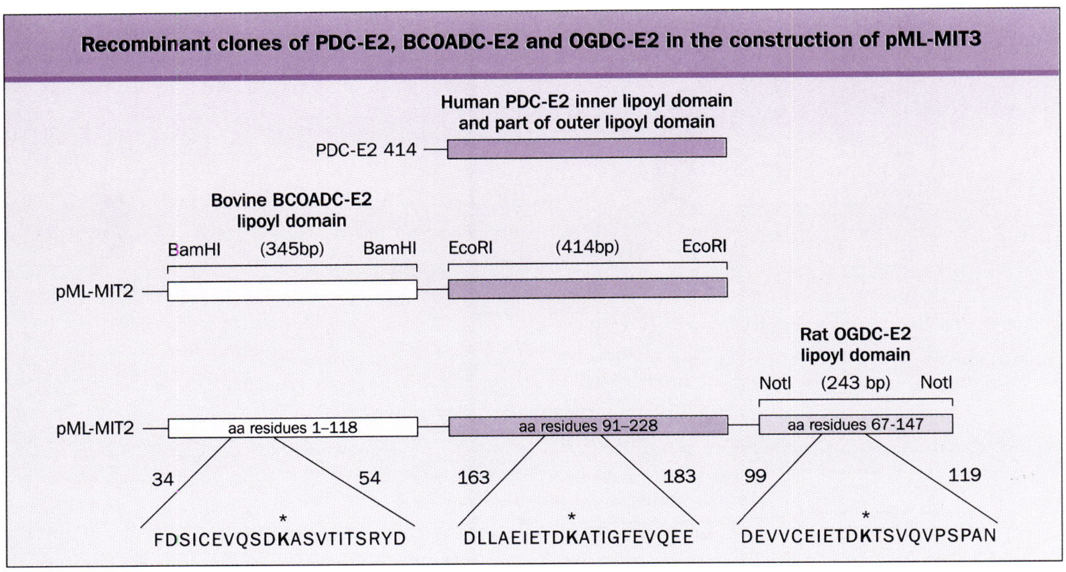

Figure 88.2 Diagrammatic representation of recombinant clones of PDC-E2, BCOADC-E2 and OGDC-E2 in the construction of pML-MIT3. Note that PDC-414 contains the human PDC-E2 inner lipoyl domain and part of the outer lipoyl domain, pML-MIT2 contains the bovine BCOADC-E2 lipoyl domain and PDC-414 and pML-MIT3 contains the lipoyl domains of PDC-E2, BCOADC-E2 and OGDC-E2. The number of base pairs and amino acid residues of each of the lipoyl domain are shown. *Indicates the lysine residue to which the lipoic acid is bound.

other hand, if PBC is an autoimmune disorder, future directions aimed at gene therapy and tolerance will be sought.

AUTOIMMUNE HEPATITIS

Clinical features and diagnosis of autoimmune hepatitis

Autoimmune hepatitis (AIH) is defined as a chronic disease that results from an immune-mediated destruction of hepatic tissues. In the absence of known viruses as etiologic agents, a loss of tolerance against autologous liver tissue is regarded as the main pathogenetic mechanism. AIH is characterized by female preponderance, hypergammaglobulinemia, extrahepatic autoimmune syndromes, an increased prevalence of HLA-DR3 and/or HLA-DR4, a good response to immunosuppressive treatment, and the presence of characteristic autoantibodies. Features typical for AIH and criteria for exclusion of other causes of hepatitis have been summarized in a scoring system, which is accepted as a valid tool for the diagnosis of hepatitis (Table 88.3).[53]

AIH may be subdivided into two subtypes. Autoimmune hepatitis type 1 (AIH-1) is characterized by antinuclear autoantibodies (ANA), smooth muscle autoantibodies (SMA), and/or autoantibodies against soluble liver antigen (SLA/LP). Autoimmune hepatitis type 2 (AIH-2) is characterized by liver and kidney microsomal (LKM1) antibodies and/or anti-liver

CLINICAL PEARLS

Primary biliary cirrhosis and autoimmune hepatitis

- PBC and AIH both present with jaundice, pruritis, lethargy and fatigue, malaise and nausea, persistent ill-defined abdominal discomfort, and a skin rash or an increase in skin pigmentation.
- PBC is more likely to present with portal hypertension, an increase in serum bilirubin, elevated alkaline phosphatase, and elevated cholesterol.
- AIH is more likely to present with pale stools, dark urine, loss of appetite and loss of weight, arthralgia, pyrexia, an increase in serum transaminases (ALP/AST<1.5), and hypergammaglobulinemia.

KEY CONCEPTS

Autoimmune hepatitis (AIH)

- AIH is an autoimmune disease of the liver that primarily affects women and in 80% of cases is associated with autoantibodies to either (type 1) ANA, SMA, and/or SLA/LP or (type 2) LKM-1, LKM-3, and LC1.
- The disease is marked by progressive inflammatory destruction of hepatocytes, followed by the development of cirrhosis and liver failure.
- There is generally a good response to immunosuppressive therapy.
- There is an association between AIH and the HLA (MHC) class II alleles DR3 and/or DR4.
- First-degree relatives of AIH patients are more likely to demonstrate other autoimmune diseases.

Scoring system for diagnosis of autoimmune hepatitis: minimum required parameters

Parameter	Score
Gender	
Female	+2
Male	0
Serum biochemistry	
Ratio of elevation of serum alkaline phosphatase vs aminotransferase	
<1.5	+2
1.5–3.0	0
>3.0	–2
Total serum globulin, γ-globulin or IgG (times upper normal limit)	
>2.0	+3
1.5–2.0	+2
1.0–1.5	+1
<1.0	0
Autoantibodies (titers by immunofluorescence on rodent tissues)	
Adults	
ANA, SMA or LKM-1	
>1:80	+3
1:80	+2
1:40	+1
<1:40	0
Antimitochondrial antibody	
Positive	–4
Viral markers	
Positive	–3
Negative	+3
Drug history	
Positive	–4
Negative	+1
Alcohol intake (average consumption)	
<25 g/day	+2
>60 g/day	–2
Other autoimmune diseases	+2
Liver histology	
Interface hepatitis	+3
Predominantly lympohocytic infiltrate	+1
Rosetting liver cells	+1
None of the above	–5
Biliary changes	–3
Other changes	–3
Optional additional parameters	
Seropositivity for other *defined* autoantibodies	+2
HLA-DR3 or DR4	+1
Response to therapy	
Complete	+2
Relapse	+3

Interpretation of aggregate scores:

- Pretreatment: >15: definite AIH and 10–15 probable AIH
- Post-treatment: >17 definite AIH, 12–17 probable AIH

ANA – antinuclear antibody; SMA – smooth muscle antibodies; LKM-1 – type 1 liver/kidney microsomal antibody.

Table 88.3 Scoring system for diagnosis of autoimmune hepatitis: minimum required parameters. Modified from Alvarez F, Berg PA, Bianchi FB, et al. International Autoimmune Hepatitis Group Report: review of criteria for diagnosis of autoimmune hepatitis. *J Hepatology* 1999;31:929.

cytosolic autoantibodies (anti-LC1). Patients with AIH-2 are typically younger at the time of disease onset, exhibit higher inflammatory activity, suffer more frequent relapses under immunosuppressive treatment, and are more likely to progress to cirrhosis.[54,55] Preliminary data on HLA associations indicate that there may also be genetic differences.

Autoantibodies in autoimmune hepatitis

Antinuclear and anti-smooth muscle antibodies (ANA and SMA)

Antinuclear (ANA) and/or smooth muscle antibodies (SMA) autoantibodies are common in AIH-1, but rare in AIH-2. By indirect immunofluorescence, ANA may show various staining patterns of the nuclei. These variations in staining pattern likely reflect the heterogeneity of the ANA targets, which include a wide spectrum of different nuclear proteins and nucleic acids. SMA are mostly directed against actin filaments and associated proteins. Autoantibody patterns and titers are subject to fluctuations over the course of the disease, and loss of autoantibodies may be associated with improved laboratory parameters. However, disappearance of autoantibodies is not a prognostic marker for a positive outcome of the immunosuppressive treatment. Neither autoantibody titers at presentation nor autoantibody behavior during therapy are accurate markers for severity or prognosis of disease.[58]

Autoantibodies directed against soluble liver protein (SLA) and liver pancreas antigen (LP)

Antibodies against soluble liver antigen (SLA) recognize one or two bands of about 50 kDa and closely associate with autoimmune hepatitis. Approximately 30% of AIH-1 patients are SLA positive and some overlap is seen with SMA and ANA, but not with LKM-1 autoantibodies. An autoantibody with properties similar to SLA, which recognizes an antigen of 50 kDa in homogenates of liver and pancreas, was described in literature as liver pancreas autoantibody (anti-LP).[57] Recent cloning experiments demonstrated that SLA and anti-LP autoantibodies recognize an identical autoantigen, which may be a UGA-suppressor tRNA-associated protein. The two different bands recognized represent splice variants of the anti-SLA/LP antigen. Amino acids 371–409 appear critical for immune recognition.

Antineutrophil cytoplasmic antibodies (ANCA)

Antineutrophil cytoplasmic antibodies (ANCA) recognize cytoplasmic components of neutrophilic granulocytes. P-ANCAs, characterized by a perinuclear staining pattern, are detected with a high prevalence in patients with autoimmune liver diseases. Significant titers of p-ANCA are recognized in 65–96% of AIH-1 sera, while p-ANCA are not detected by sera from patients with AIH-2. In general, titers of p-ANCA are significantly higher in AIH-1 than in other liver diseases.[58] No correlation of p-ANCA with asparare aminotransferase (AST), IgG levels or presence and absence with concurrent autoimmune disorders has been detected. Several antigens have been described as molecular targets of p-ANCA, e.g. cathepsin G, high mobility group (HMG) nonhistone chromosomal proteins, HMG1 and HMG2 and lactoferrin.

Anti-asialoglycoprotein receptor autoantibodies

The asialoglycoprotein receptor (ASGP-R) is a glycoprotein that is located in the plasma membrane of hepatocytes and mediates the internalization of asialoglycoproteins. Autoantibodies directed against ASGP-R are frequently detected in sera from patients with chronic liver diseases.[59] About three fourths of patients with AIH exhibit anti-ASGP-R autoantibodies, versus about one fifth of patients with PBC and one tenth of patients with viral hepatitis or other liver diseases. Titers of anti-ASGP-R autoantibodies are typically significantly higher in AIH than in PBC or chronic virus hepatitis. In autoimmune hepatitis, titers of anti-ASGP-R autoantibodies appear to correlate with disease activity.

Liver-kidney microsomal autoantibodies type I (LKM-I)

LKM-1 autoantibodies are the serological markers of AIH-2.[54] LKM-1 autoantibodies are characterized by an even cytoplasmic staining of the entire liver lobule and the exclusive staining of the proximal renal tubules.

Cytochrome P450 2D6 (CYP2D6), a protein of 50 kDa, is detected in almost all sera from patients with AIH-2. LKM-1 autoantibodies inhibit the enzymatic activity of their major target protein, CYP2D6, in vitro.[60] CYP2D6 is a drug-metabolizing enzyme active in phase 1 of detoxification. The enzyme is polymorphic in the Caucasian population. Ten per cent of Caucasians are void of enzymatic activity, which results in a slow metabolizer phenotype for all drugs metabolized by CYP2D6, e.g. debrisoquine or sparteine. Using sparteine as a test substrate, the measurement of CYP2D6 activity can be determined in vivo. Interestingly, all patients with LKM-1 antibodies tested so far have been of the extensive metabolizer phenotype, which expresses functionally intact CYP2D6 protein.[61] Therefore, an adequate expression of CYP2D6 seems to be necessary for the development of LKM-1 autoantibodies.

Sera from patients with AIH recognize at least four different linear epitopes for LKM-1 autoantibodies: amino acids 257–260, 321–351, 373–389 and 419–429.[62] The major linear CYP2D6 epitope is comprised of amino acids 257–269 and is recognized in almost three fourths of patients with AIH-2. This major linear epitope of LKM-1 autoantibodies shows a six amino acid sequence identity with an immediate early protein (IEP 175) of herpes simplex virus. A pair of identical twins has been reported with a discordant manifestation of LKM-1-positive AIH-2, i.e. only one sister was affected by the disease. Interestingly, the healthy twin was negative for herpes simplex virus (HSV) infection, while the child affected by AIH-2 had antibodies directed against HSV. Anti-CYP2D6 specific antibodies isolated from the girl with AIH-2 were used to immunoprecipitate proteins from HSV-infected cells, demonstrating cross-reactivity with HSV-derived IEP175.[63] This case raises the possibility that viral infections by HSV and related viruses may trigger autoimmune hepatitis by the mechanism of molecular mimicry.

LKM-3 autoantibodies

LKM-3 autoantibodies, either alone or in combination with LKM-1 autoantibodies, are detected in 10% of patients with AIH-2. LKM-3 autoantibodies are directed against family 1 UDP-glucuronosyltransferases (UGT1A).[64] Epitope mapping of UDP-glucuronosyltransferases in autoimmune hepatitis revealed a large minimal epitope from amino acids 264–373. The epitope is destroyed upon removal of any further sequence, suggesting that the autoantibodies may recognize a conformation-dependent domain that requires stabilizing sequence to refold after denaturation.

It is interesting to note that two AIH-2 autoantigens, UGTs and CYP2D6, are both active in phases 1 and 2 of drug metabolism and that both may work on the same substrates. One can speculate that CYP2D6 may metabolically activate a substrate that covalently modifies CYP2D6 itself and also binds to the active center of family 1 UGTs. Metabolic modification by CYPs has been shown to be the critical event leading to drug-induced hepatitis and may also contribute to the induction of AIH-2.

Antibodies to liver cytosolic protein type I (LC I)

Autoantibodies directed against liver-cytosolic protein (anti-LC1) are characterized by cytoplasmic staining in indirect immunofluorescence of periportal, but not perivenal compartments. This suggests that the target is not evenly distributed in the liver. Under denaturing conditions, western blot analysis with human LC1 autoantibodies detects a 58–62 kDa protein from liver. By gel filtration, the target protein appears at 240–290 kDa, indicating that the native protein is a tetramer. The molecular target of anti-LC1 autoantibodies has been identified as the foramiminotransferase cyclodeaminase.[65]

Anti-LC1 autoantibodies are closely associated with AIH-2. Between one fifth and one half of patients with anti-LKM autoantibodies produce anti-LC1 autoantibodies as a second disease marker. However, anti-LC1 autoantibodies may also be the only disease marker in patients with AIH-2. Compared to LKM-1 autoantibodies, titers of LC-1 autoantibodies seem to correlate better with disease activity. When titers of anti-LC1 were compared at onset of AIH and after remission under immunosuppressive therapy, anti-LC1 titers had considerably decreased during immunosuppressive therapy.[66]

Cellular immune reactions

LKM-1 autoantibodies are widely used as diagnostic markers for AIH-2.[54] However, their contribution to the pathogenesis of AIH remains unclear. It is possible that these autoantibodies play a pathogenetic role by binding to CYP2D6, which appears to be transported to the cell surface in this disease. Alternatively, liver cell injury may be induced by liver-infiltrating T lymphocytes. T-cell responses to CYP2D6 have been described,[67] and CYP2D6 has been shown to induce proliferation in peripheral blood lymphocytes from some patients with LKM-1 autoantibodies while a proliferative response was not detectable in LKM-1-negative patients with chronic liver diseases and in healthy controls. A peptide consisting of amino acids 262–285 of CYP2D6 can induce a proliferative response in all AIH-2 patients tested; however, a similar response can be found in about half of patients with AIH-1 and one eighth of patients with chronic HCV infection. Still, after the start of immunosuppressive treatment, T-cell responses to this epitope decreased. Thus it is possible that this epitope plays a role in the immune response in AIH. Intriguingly, T-cell lines generated from responsive T cells of these patients showed characteristics compatible with a Th1-phenotype.[68]

Genetic predisposition for autoimmune hepatitis

HLA associations in caucasian patients

Among patients of European descent, the HLA-A1; B8; DR3 haplotype (Chapter 6) was identified as a particular susceptibility marker for AIH-1. All DR3-linked alleles appear to predispose patients to AIH, but homozygosity for DRB3*0101 increases the relative risk from 4.2 to 14.7 and is associated with a reduction of 10-year survival.[69] When all DR3-positive patients were eliminated, a secondary association of DR4 (especially DRB1*0401) with AIH-1 was also detected.[69] HLA-DR alleles did not only confer increased risk for AIH-1, but were also associated with different clinical profiles. Patients with the HLA-A1; B8; DR3 haplotype tend to be younger at the onset of disease, exhibit more frequent relapses under immunosuppressive treatment, and are more likely to require liver transplantation. HLA-DR4-positive patients show a higher prevalence for concurrent autoimmune diseases. Autoimmune diseases associated with the highest prevalences were autoimmune thyroiditis, Graves disease, ulcerative colitis, and pernicious anemia.[70]

HLA associations in the Japanese and Argentinian populations

In Japanese patients, where the HLA-A1; B8; DR3 haplotype is uncommon, susceptibility is similarly associated with DR4. Japanese patients are characterized by a strong female preponderance (female:male ratio 8:1) and a late age of onset of hepatitis (32–72 years).[71] In addition to DR4, significant associations of AIH with HLA-Bw54, DR53 and DQ4 have been reported.

Among Argentinians of European descent, linkage of AIH-1 to HLA alleles appears to differ from that observed in North America. Although a week association of AIH-1 with DR4 was detected, the major association was with HLA-A11. Extrahepatic autoimmunity was significantly increased in HLA-A11-positive patients. When HLA-A11 and HLA-DR4 occurred together, a synergistic effect was noted, yielding a relative risk of 357. This synergistic effect was not noted for HLA-A11 and HLA-DR3. Among children with AIH-1, an association with HLA-DR6 was found.[72]

Polymorphisms in human complement C4 genes in Caucasians

AIH-1 is frequently associated with persistently low serum complement levels. C4 phenotyping revealed association of null allotypes at the *C4A* or the *C4B* loci with AIH-1 and that serum C4 levels are indeed lower in patients with *C4A* deletions. *C4A* deletions are associated with increased mortality and a tendency to relapse while on treatment. Homozygosity for *C4A* deletion allele correlated with a stronger increase in the relative risk for hepatitis (RR = 18.1) than did a single deletion (RR = 3.3).[73] The *C4A* deletion allele is in strong linkage disequilibrium with the HLA-A1, B8; DR3 haplotype, however, making it difficult to assess which gene or genes are responsible for the increased susceptibility for disease.

Treatment and prognosis

Treatment with prednisone or prednisolone alone or in combination with azathioprine

Without treatment, the prognosis of patients with autoimmune hepatitis is poor. About one half of untreated patients with biochemical or histological indicators of severe autoimmune hepatitis are dead after 5 years, and about 9 in 10 are dead after 10 years.[74]

Currently, the most effective therapy for autoimmune hepatitis is immunosuppression.[75] Prednisone or prednisolone in combination with azathioprine or a higher dose of prednisone or prednisolone alone are the treatments of choice (Table 88.4). Responders to this therapy experience 5- and 10-year life expectancies of 94% and 90%, respectively.[76] Unfortunately, a complete remission, which can be defined as a complete disappearance of biochemical, serological, and histological disease, is ultimately achievable by only one third of patients. Moreover,

Table 88.4 Treatment of autoimmune hepatitis.

Treatment of autoimmune hepatitis		
Therapeutic stages	**Single drug regimen**	**Combination regimen**
Induction therapy		
Week 1	40–60 mg prednisone/day[a]	40–60 mg prednisone/day + 1–2 mg azathioprine/kg body weight
Week 2	40 mg prednisone/day	15 mg prednisone/day + 1–2 mg azathioprine/kg body weight
Week 3	30 mg prednisone/day	15 mg prednisone/day + 1–2 mg azathioprine/kg body weight
Week 4	Taper down 5 mg every week, until maintenance therapy	
Maintenance therapy	5–15 mg/day are common dosages	10 mg prednisone/day + 1–2 mg azathioprine/kg body weight *alternative option*: 2 mg/kg azathioprine as monotherapy
Upon relapse	Like induction therapy	Like induction therapy

[a]Prednisolone may be taken instead of prednisone.

THERAPEUTIC PRINCIPLES

Autoimmune hepatitis

- Standard treatment begins with corticosteroids ± azathioprine for immunosuppression. The prognosis is favorable in responders (77%). The prognosis is poor among partial responders (14%) and nonresponders (9%).
- Several alternative immunosuppressive treatments (e.g. cyclosporine, tacrolimus (FK-506), budesonide, 6-mercaptopurine, cyclophosphamide, mycophenolate mofetil) are under investigation for poor and partial responders.
- Liver transplantation is the therapeutic option after progression of AIH to end-stage cirrhosis. The prognosis for liver transplantation in AIH is good.

about three fourths of patients with histological remission and a complete response to therapy relapse if their drugs are withdrawn. Thus, for most patients a remission is not a cure.

Thirteen per cent of patients experience an incomplete response after a 3-year treatment period and 9% of patients experience treatment failure. After failure to achieve remission in 4 years, these patients should be considered for liver transplantation.

Monotherapy and combination therapy are associated with side-effects that lead to a discontinuation of treatment in about 13% of patients. Common side-effects of prednisone treatment are usually mild. They include cosmetic changes such as facial rounding, acne, hirsutism, dorsal hump formation, and obesity and are reversible with reduction of drug dosage or drug withdrawal. Severe adverse side-effects that necessitate withdrawal of treatment include osteoporosis, diabetes, cataracts, and psychosis. These side-effects are mostly due to prednisone. However, azathioprine has its own spectrum of side-effects, including nausea, emesis, rash, hepatotoxicity, and bone marrow suppression. Complications develop in less than 10% of patients receiving azathioprine at a dosage of 50 mg/day and they improve with dosage reduction or drug withdrawal.[76]

Response to other drugs

If standard treatment with prednisone or prednisolone alone or in combination with azathioprine fails to induce remission, other immunosuppressive compounds such as cyclosporine, tacrolimus (FK506), budesonide, cyclophosphamide or mycophenolic acid represent experimental therapeutic options that are most appropriately administered within controlled treatment trials.

Liver transplantation

Liver transplantation represents the ultimate therapeutic option for end-stage cirrhosis caused by autoimmune hepatitis, which may develop despite complete biochemical remission under long-term immunosuppressive treatment. Autoimmune hepatitis is among the best indications for liver transplantation and accounts for 4% of liver transplants in Europe. Five-year survival rates of more than 90% have been reported.[77]

Hepatitis in the autoimmune polyglandular syndrome type I (APS I)

Clinical features of APS I

The autoimmune polyglandular syndrome type 1 (APS1) is a rare autosomal recessive disorder caused by mutations in the *AIRE* (autoimmune regulator) gene.[78] The AIRE protein contains two PHD ring finger motifs, as well as several other domains that are common among genes that regulate transcription.

Patients with APS1 present with a variable combination of mucocutaneous candidiasis, autoimmune tissue destruction, and ectodermal dystrophy.[79] Typically, onset of APS1 occurs in childhood and multiple autoimmune diseases evolve in a single patient (Table 88.5).

AIRE is expressed in rare cells of lymphoid tissues, e.g. thymus medulla, lymph nodes, spleen, and the fetal liver.[80] All AIRE-positive cells strongly express HLA-DR. Thymic medullary epithelial cells are believed to be involved in clonal deletion of a subset of high-affinity T cells and in the induction of anergy in low-affinity subsets. These results and the disease spectrum seen in APS1 indicate that *AIRE* may be involved in the establishment and maintenance of tolerance.

The first APS1-associated hepatic autoantigen identified was CYP1A2.[81] By indirect immunofluorescence, anti-CYP1A2 stain perivenous rat hepatocytes, and, by western blot, these autoantibodies recognize a band of 54 kDa that is contained within human hepatic microsomes. Approximately 7% of APS1 Finnish patients studied expressed CYP1A2 autoantibodies, and all of these patients were affected by hepatitis (Obermayer-Straub, unpublished results). Anti-CYP1A2 antibodies were not detected in the sera of German patients with idiopathic AIH-2, and anti-

Disease components	Prevalence (%)		
	Neufeld[84] 1981	Ahonen[79] 1990	Betterle[85] 1998
Endocrine components			
Hypoparathyroidism	76	79	93
Adrenal failure	100	72	73
IDDM	4	12	2
Parietal cell atrophy	13	13	15
Autoimmune thyroid disease	11	2	10
Gonadal failure	17	50	43
Nonendocrine components			
Mucocutaneous candidiasis	73	100	83
Alopecia	32	29	37
Vitiligo	8	13	15
Keratoconjunctivitis	–	35	12
Chronic hepatitis	13	12	20
Intestinal malabsorption	22	18	15
Enamel hypoplasia	–	77	–
Nail dystrophy	–	52	–

Table 88.5 Disease components in the autoimmune polyglandular syndrome type 1 (APS 1). Modified from Betterle C, Greggic NA, Volpato M. Autoimmune polyglandular syndrome type 1. *J Clin Endocrinol Metab* 1998;83:1049.

CYP2D6 autoantibodies were not detected among Finnish patients with APS1. These findings indicate that idiopathic AIH-2 and APS1 are characterized by different autoantibodies, and that AIH-2 and hepatitis in APS1 may be distinguished on the basis of differences in autoantibody patterns (Obermayer-Straub, unpublished results).

Aromatic-L-aminoacid decarboxylase (AADC), a pyridoxal phosphate-dependent enzyme, was the second hepatic autoantigen identified in APS1.[82] AADC is expressed in the hepatic cytosol. In contrast to anti-CYP1A2 autoantibodies, which are relatively rare, fully half of Finnish patients with APS1 expressed AADC autoantibodies. The prevalence of AADC autoantibodies was significantly increased in APS1 patients with vitiligo and hepatitis, where 88% and 92% of patients were found to express AADC autoantibodies.

DRUG-INDUCED HEPATITIS

Detoxification reactions usually require two steps (Fig. 88.3). In phase 1 of detoxification, hydrophobic drugs are hydroxylated by cytochrome P450 enzymes. In phase 2, hydroxylated products are conjugated with hydrophilic compounds, e.g. glucuronic acid. Most of these conjugates are hydrophilic and may be excreted via bile or kidney. Usually detoxification reactions are beneficial and lead to the detoxification of a wide variety of diet-borne components and environmental chemicals. Sometimes, however, a reactive metabolite may be generated as a consequence of a 'detoxification' reaction (Fig. 88.3). This reactive metabolite may bind directly to the active center the enzyme that generated the metabolite. If the metabolite is more stable, it may leave the active center and bind to other hepatic proteins (adduct formation). With repeated exposure to such metabolites, the immune system may be activated against modified CYPs and other liver proteins. Antibodies directed against proteins modified by the drug are then produced. Since the majority of proteins active in detoxification are expressed by hepatocytes, adduct formation frequently is seen in hepatocytes, which become targets of immune-mediated cytotoxic processes, resulting in severe hepatitis.[83] Well-documented examples of hepatitis induced by drugs are dihydralazine hepatitis with autoantibodies directed against CYP1A2, tienilic acid-induced hepatitis with antibodies directed against CYP2C9, and halothane hepatitis with antibodies directed against CYP2E1 and several other liver proteins (rev. 83). While adduct formation occurs in many patients, drug-induced immune-mediated hepatitis is a rare event. It is likely that certain genetic polymorphisms (genetic predisposition) may render the

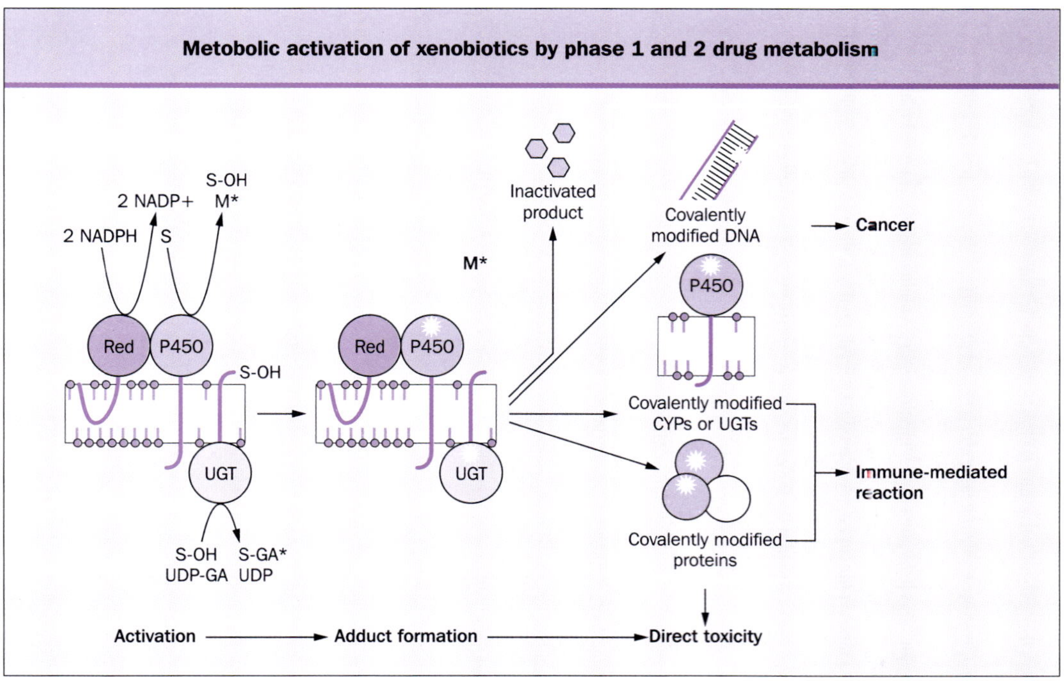

Figure 88.3 Metabolic activation of xenobiotics by enzymes of phase 1 and phase 2 drug metabolism. (Modified from Manns & Obermayer-Straub. Cytochromes P450 and UDP-glucuronosyltransferases: model autoantigens to study drug-induced, virus-induced and autoimmune liver disease. *Hepatology* 1997;26:1054.

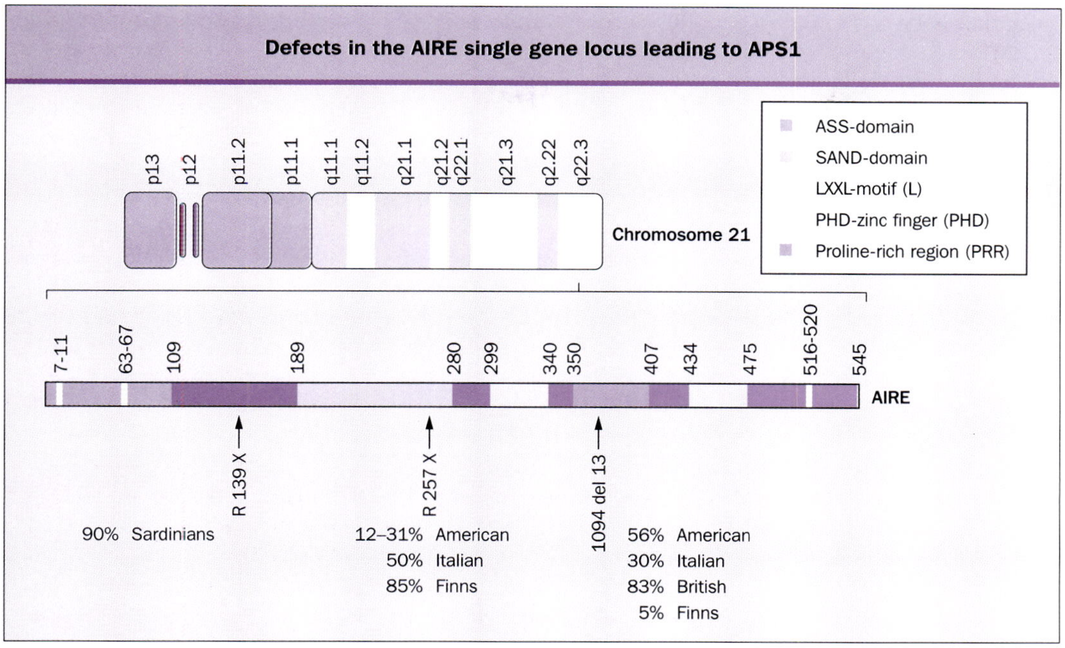

Figure 88.4 The autoimmune polyglandular syndrome type 1 (APS1) is caused by defects in the *AIRE* single gene locus. (Modified from Manns & Obermayer-Straub. Immunological mechanisms in liver injury. In: Kaplowitz N, DeLeve L (eds) *Drug induced liver disease*. New York, Marcel Dekker, 2000.

individual more susceptible to develop immune-mediated drug-induced hepatitis.

SUMMARY

Autoimmune hepatitis is a rare autoimmune disease that reflects a loss of tolerance to normal hepatic proteins. About one third of patients and one third of their first-degree relatives also are affected with a second organ-specific autoimmune disease, pointing to the existence of a common genetic predisposition to autoimmunity. Part of this predisposition can be attributed to known risk factors, such as HLA-DR3 and HLA-DR4, C4A-Q0 alleles and female gender. However, other as yet unknown genetic factors are also likely to play a role in the induction of AIH. It is possible that these genes may also be involved in the induction and maintenance of tolerance in general.

APS1 can be viewed as a model for the investigation of autoimmune hepatitis and other organ-specific autoimmune diseases. In this disease, homozygosity for a defect in a single gene (*AIRE*) leads to a broad spectrum of organ-specific autoimmune diseases, among them a form of autoimmune hepatitis. APS1 hepatitis shares a number of the features of AIH-2. For example, it affects patients in the pediatric age range and it is characterized by the presence of antibodies directed against CYPs. In Finland, 90% of APS1 cases are caused by a common *AIRE* mutation (Fig. 88.4). However, in spite of a very homogeneous genetic background concerning the primary gene defect, a wide spectrum of disease manifestations is seen. This spectrum includes patients with transient increases in transaminase values, patients with chronic corticoid-treated hepatitis, and patients who ultimately die from fulminant hepatitis. Diversity of manifestation of APS1 demonstrates the importance of other genes and the environment in the outcome of this monogenic autoimmune syndrome. APS1 is not unique. Even in identical twins, the concordance rate for idiopathic autoimmune diseases is typically 30–40%.

The differences in the clinical manifestations of these disorders have raised the possibility that environmental triggers are involved in precipitating these autoimmune diseases. Potential triggers include infections with hepatotropic viruses and exposure to nutritional compounds or drugs (Fig. 88.5).

A number of autoimmune hepatitis case studies have demonstrated induction of hepatitis after infection with a wide range of hepatotropic viruses. Infection with one specific hepatotropic virus has yet to be consistently correlated with autoimmune hepatitis, suggesting that hepatitis results from mechanisms that are common to most virus infections, rather than a unique response to a specific virus.

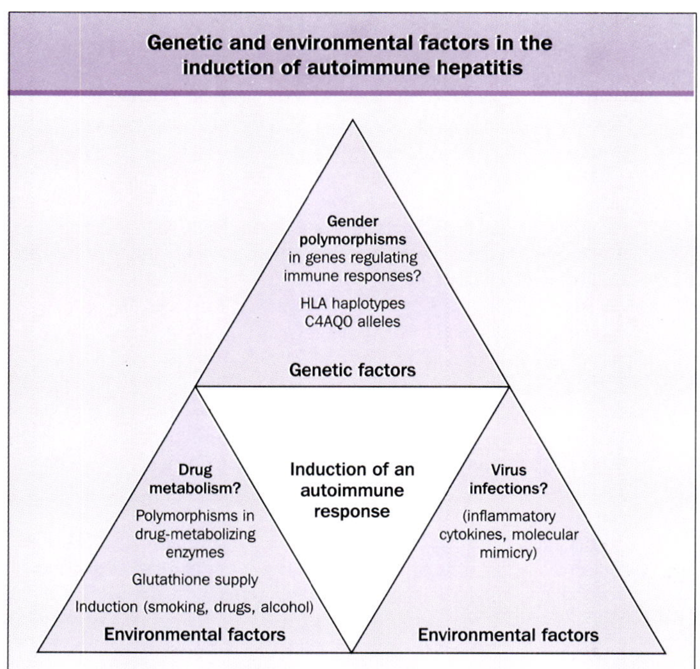

Figure 88.5 Genetic and environmental factors are involved in the induction of autoimmune hepatitis.

Factors common to viral infections that have been proposed to influence the development of hepatitis include production of inflammatory cytokines and molecular mimicry. Inflammatory cytokines are often produced as a first line of defense against virus infections, yet their presence can have unintended side-effects. For example, treatment with interferon-α has been shown to induce thyroid autoimmunity or to exacerbate hepatitis in patients with chronic hepatitis C. Viruses occasionally use molecular mimicry to hide surface proteins and viral enzymes from the immune system. For functional reasons molecular mimicry by viral components cannot be complete. Therefore viruses often express epitopes that are similar but not identical to host epitopes. It is thus possible that during an infection the immune system may accidentally break tolerance against 'virus-like' self-epitopes and induce an autoimmune reaction against noninfected, normal hepatocytes.

An alternative potential mechanism for the induction of hepatitis is chemical modification of hepatic proteins during drug therapy or by nutritional components, i.e. environmental exposures. For example, in drug-induced hepatitis, autoimmune reactions evolve by adduct formation with reactive metabolites of 'detoxification reactions'. Interestingly, cytochrome P450 enzymes, which mediate the generation of reactive metabolites, are the preferred targets of these autoimmune reactions. Similarly, in AIH-2, autoantibodies directed against drug-metabolizing enzymes of phase 1 (CYP2D6) and phase 2 (UGT1A) are formed. This raises the question whether the presence of these autoantibodies is an accidental finding or whether LKM autoantibodies provide us with an important hint on potential triggers of AIH-2. Answers to these questions may yield new insights into both the pathogenesis and therapy of autoimmune hepatitis and cirrhosis.

ACKNOWLEDGMENTS

This work was supported by NIH grant DK 39588, AI31585 and a grant of the Deutsche Forschungsgemeinschaft SFB 244, project C11.

REFERENCES

1. Gershwin ME, Mackay IR. Primary biliary cirrhosis: paradigm or paradox for autoimmunity. Gastroenterology 1991;100:822.
2. Mackay IR, Gershwin ME. Molecular basis of mitochondrial autoreactivity in primary biliary cirrhosis. Immunol Today 1989;10:315.
3. Gregorio GV, Portmann B, Mowat AP, Vergani D, Mieli-Vergani G. A 12-year-old girl with antimitochondrial antibody positive autoimmune hepatitis. J Hepatol 1997;27:751.
4. Heathcote J. The clinical expression of primary biliary cirrhosis. Semin Liver Dis 1996;17:23.
5. Nyberg A, Loof L. Primary biliary cirrhosis: clinical features and outcome, with special reference to asymptomatic disease. Scand J Gastroenterol 1989;24:57.
6. Lucey MR, Neuberger JM, Williams R. Primary biliary cirrhosis in men. Gut 1986;27:1373.
7. Leung PSC, Coppel RL, Ansari A, Munoz S, Gershwin ME. Antimitochondrial antibodies in primary biliary cirrhosis. Semin Liver Dis 1997;17:61.
8. Invernizzi P, Crosignani A, Battezzati PM, et al. Comparison of the clinical features and clinical course of antimitochondrial antibody-positive and -negative primary biliary cirrhosis. Hepatology 1997;25:1090.
9. Vilagut L, Pare A, Vinas O, Vila J, Jimenez de Anta T, Rodes J. Antibodies to mycobacterial 65-kD heat shock protein cross-react with the main mitochondrial antigens in patients with primary biliary cirrhosis. Eur J Clin Invest 1997;27:667.
10. De la Sierra IL, Pernot L, Prange T, Saludjian P, Schitz M, Fourme R, Padrong G. Molecular structure of the lipoamide dehydrogenase domain of a surface antigen from *Neisseria meningitidis*. J Mol Biol 1997;269:129.
11. Shimoda S, Van de Water J, Ansari A, et al. Identification and precursor frequency analysis of a common T cell epitope motif in mitochondrial autoantigens in primary biliary cirrhosis. J Clin Invest 1998;102:1831.
12. Tanaka A, Prindiville TP, Gish R, et al. Are infectious agents involved in primary biliary cirrhosis? A PCR approach. J Hepatol 1999;31:664.
13. Mason AL, Xu L, Guo L, et al. Detection of retroviral antibodies in primary biliary cirrhosis and other idiopathic biliary disorders. Lancet 1998;351:1620.
14. Hamlyn AN, Macklon AF, James O. Primary biliary cirrhosis: geographical clustering and symptomatic onset seasonality. Gut 1983;24:940.
15. Myszor M, James OF. The epidemiology of primary biliary cirrhosis in north-east England: an increasingly common disease? Quart J Med 1990;75:377.
16. Danielsson A, Boqvist L, Uddenfeldt P. Epidemiology of primary biliary cirrhosis in a defined rural population in the northern part of Sweden. Hepatology 1990;11:458.
17. Kinghan JGC, Parker DR. The association between primary biliary cirrhosis and coeliac disease, a study of relative prevalences. Gut 1998;42:120.
18. Hislop WS, Main G, Robertson AJ. Primary biliary cirrhosis: experience in a non-referral centre. Lancet 1981;2(8238):144.
19. Metcalf JV, Bhopal RS, Gray J, James OJ. Incidence and prevalence of primary biliary cirrhosis in the city of Newcastle upon Tyne, England. Int J Epidemiol 1997;26:830.
20. Yasutoshi M. Annual of hepatitis research committee of Japan. 1989;8.
21. Watson R, Angun PW, Dewan M, Goss B, Sewell RB, Smallwood RA. Low prevalence of primary biliary cirrhosis in Victoria, Australia. Gut 1995;36:927.
22. Remmel T, Remmel H, Uibo R, Salupere V. Primary biliary cirrhosis in Estonia with special reference to incidence, prevalence, abnormal features and outcome. Scand J Gastroenterol 1995;30:367.
23. Triger DR. Primary biliary cirrhosis: an epidemiological study. Br Med J 1980;281:772.
24. Witt-Sullivan H, Heathcote J, Cauch K, et al. The demography of primary biliary cirrhosis in Ontario, Canada. Hepatology 1990;12:98.
25. Galbraith RM, Smith M, Mackenzie RM, Tee DE, Doniach D, Williams R. High prevalence of seroimmunologic abnormalities in relatives of patients with active chronic hepatitis or primary biliary cirrhosis. N Engl J Med 1974;290:63.
26. Jaup BH, Zettergren LS. Familial occurrence of primary biliary cirrhosis associated with hypergammaglobulinemia in descendants: a family study. Gastroenterology 1980;78:549.
27. Surh CD, Coppel R, Gershwin ME. Structural requirement for autoreactivity on human pyruvate dehydrogenase-E2, the major autoantigen of primary biliary cirrhosis. Implication for a conformational autoepitope. J Immunol 1990;144:3367.
28. Fussey SP, Ali ST, Guest JR, James OF, Bassendine MF, Yeaman SJ. Reactivity of primary biliary cirrhosis sera with *Escherichia coli* dihydrolipoamide acetyltransferase (E2p): characterization of the main immunogenic region. Proc Natl Acad Sci U S A 1990;87:3987.
29. Tuaillon N, Andre C, Briand JP, Penner E, Muller S. A lipoyl synthetic octadecapeptide of dihydrolipoamide acetyltransferase specifically recognized by anti-M2 autoantibodies in primary biliary cirrhosis. J Immunol 1992;148:445.
30. Leung PS, Iwayama T, Coppel RL, Gershwin ME. Site-directed mutagenesis of lysine within the immunodominant autoepitope of PDC-E2. Hepatology 1990;12:1321.

31. Leung PSC, Chuang DT, Wynn RM, et al. Autoantibodies to BCOADC-E2 in patients with primary biliary cirrhosis recognize a conformational epitope. Hepatology 1995;22:505.
32. Moteki S, Leung PSC, Dickson ER, et al. Epitope mapping and reactivity of autoantibodies to the E2 component of 2-oxoglutarate dehydrogenase complex (OGDC-E2) in primary biliary cirrhosis using recombinant OGDC-E2. Hepatology 1996;23:436.
33. Dubel L, Tanaka A, Leung PS, et al. Autoepitope mapping and reactivity of autoantibodies to the dihydrolipoamide dehydrogenase-binding protein (E3BP) and the glycine cleavage proteins in primary biliary cirrhosis. Hepatology 1999;29:1013.
34. Fussey SP, Bassendine MF, Fittes D, Turner IB, James OF, Yeaman SJ. The E1 alpha and beta subunits of the pyruvate dehydrogenase complex are M2'd' and M2'e' autoantigens in primary biliary cirrhosis. Clin Sci 1989;77:365.
35. Reynosa-Paz S, Leung PSC, Van de Water J, et al. Evidence for a local driven mucosal response and the presence of mitochondrial antigens in saliva in primary biliary cirrhosis. Hepatology 2000;31:24.
36. Jones DEJ, Palmer JM, James OFW, Yeaman SJ, Bassendine MF, Diamond AG. T-Cell responses to the components of pyruvate dehydrogenase complex in primary biliary cirrhosis. Hepatology 1995;21:995.
37. Moebius U, Manns M, Hess G, Kober G, Meyer zum Buschenfelde KH, Meuer SC. T cell receptor gene rearrangements of T lymphocytes infiltrating the liver in chronic active hepatitis B and primary biliary cirrhosis (PBC): oligoclonality of PBC-derived T cell clones. Eur J Immunol 1990;20:889.
38. Howard MJ, Fuller C, Broadhurst RW, et al. Three-dimensional structure of the major autoantigen in primary biliary cirrhosis. Gastroenterology 1998;115:139.
39. Christensen E, Crowe J, Doniach D, et al. Clinical pattern and course of disease in primary biliary cirrhosis based on an analysis of 236 patients. Gastroenterology 1980;78:236.
40. Metcalf JV, Mitchison HC, Palmer JM, Jones DE, Bassendine MF, James OF. Natural history of early primary biliary cirrhosis. Lancet 1996;348 1399.
41. Mahl TC, Shockcor W, Boyer JL. Primary biliary cirrhosis: survival of a large cohort of symptomatic and asymptomatic patients followed for 24 years. J Hepatol 1994;20:707.
42. Joplin R, Lindsay JG, Johnson GD, Strain A, Neuberger J. Membrane dihydrolipoamide acetyltransferase (E2) on human biliary epithelial cells in primary biliary cirrhosis. Lancet 1992;339:93.
43. Cha S, Leung PS, Coppel RL, Van de Water J, Ansari AA, Gershwin ME. Heterogeneity of combinatorial human autoantibodies against PDC-E2 and biliary epithelial cells in patients with primary biliary cirrhosis. Hepatology 1994;20:574.
44. Mattalia A, Luttig B, Rosia F, et al. Persistence of autoantibodies against recombinant mitochondrial and nuclear pore proteins after orthotopic liver transplantation for primary biliary cirrhosis. Autoimmunity 1997;10:491.
45. Kaplan MM. Primary biliary cirrhosis. N Engl J Med 1987;316:521.
46. Shapiro JM, Smith H, Schaffner F. Serum bilirubin: a prognostic factor in primary biliary cirrhosis. Gut 1979;20:137.
47. Jahn CE, Schaefer EJ, Taam LA, et al. Lipoprotein abnormalities in primary biliary cirrhosis. Association with hepatic lipase inhibition as well as altered cholesterol esterification Gastroenterology 1985;89:1266.
48. Moteki S, Leung PSC, Coppel RL, Dickson ER, Kaplan MM, Munoz S, Gershwin ME. Use of Designer triple expression hybrid clone for three different lipoyl domains for the detection of anti-mitochondrial antibodies Hepatology 1996;24:97.
49. Bodenheimer H Jr, Schaffner F, Sternlieb I, Klion FM, Vernace S, Pezzullo J. A prospective clinical trial of D-penicillamine in the treatment of primary biliary cirrhosis. Hepatology 1985;5:1139.
50. Kaplan MM, Alling DW, Zimmerman HJ, et al. A prospective trial of colchicine for primary biliary cirrhosis. N Engl J Med 1986;315:1448.
51. Setchell KDR, Rodrigues CMP, Cleric C, Solinas A, Morelli A, Gartung C, Boyer J. Bile acid concentrations in human and rat liver tissue and hepatocyte nuclei. Gastroenterology 1997;112:226.
52. Poupon RE, Lindor KD, Cauch-Dudek K, Dickson ER, Poupon R, Heathcore EJ. Combined analysis of randomised controlled trails of ursodeoxycholic acid in primary biliary cirrhosis. Gastroenterology 1997;113:884.
53. Alvarez F, Berg PA, Bianchi FB, et al. International Autoimmune Hepatitis Group Report: review of criteria for diagnosis of autoimmune hepatitis. J Hepatology 1999;31:929.
54. Homberg JC, Abuaf N, Bernard O, et al. Chronic active hepatitis associated with anti liver/kidney microsome type 1: a second type of 'autoimmune' hepatitis. Hepatology 1987;7:1333.
55. Gregorio GV, Portman B, Reid F, et al. Autoimmune hepatitis in childhood: a 20-year experience. Hepatology 1997;25:541.
56. Czaja AJ. Behavior and significance of autoantibodies in type 1 autoimmune hepatitis. J Hepatol 1999;30:394.
57. Stechemesser E, Klein R, Berg PA. Characterization and clinical relevance of liver-pancreas antibodies in autoimmune hepatitis. Hepatology 1993;18:1.
58. Targan SR, Landers C, Vidrich A, Czaja AJ. High titer antineutrophil cytoplasmic antibodies in type-1 autoimmune hepatitis. Gastroenterology 1995;108:1159.
59. Treichel U, McFarlane BM, Seki T, et al. Demographics of anti-asialoglycoprotein receptor autoantibodies in autoimmune hepatitis. Hepatology 1994;107:799.
60. Zanger UM, Hauri HP, Loeper J, Homberg JC, Meyer UA. Antibodies against human cytochrome P-450db 1 in autoimmune hepatitis type 2. Proc Natl Acad Sci USA 1988;85:8256.
61. Manns M, Zanger U, Gerker G, Sullivan KF, Meyer zum Büschenfelde K, Eichelbaum M. Patients with type II autoimmune hepatitis express functionally intact cytochrome P450 db1 that is inhibited by LKM1 autoantibodies in vitro but not in vivo. Hepatology 1990;12:127.
62. Yamamoto AM, Cresteil D, Boniface O, Clerc FF, Alvarez F. Identification and analysis of cytochrome P450IID6 antigenic sites recognized by anti-liver-kidney microsome type-1 antibodies (LKM1). Eur J Immunol 1993;23:1105.
63. Manns MP, Griffin KJ, Sullivan KF, Johnson EF. LKM-1 autoantibodies recognize a short linear sequence in P450llD6, a cytochrome P-450 monooxygenase. J Clin Invest 1991;88:1370.
64. Strassburg C, Obermayer-Straub P, Alex B, Durazzo M, Rizzetto M, Tukey RH, Manns MP. Autoantibodies against glucuronosyltransferases differ between viral hepatitis and autoimmune hepatitis. Gastroenterology 1996;11:1582.
65. Lapierre P, Hajoui O, Homberg J-C, Alvarez F. Fomiminotransferase cyclodeaminase is an organ specific autoantigen recognized by sera of patients with autoimmune hepatitis. Gastroenterology 1999;116:643.
66. Muratori L, Cataleta M, Muratori P, Lenz M, Bianchi FB. Liver/kidney microsomal antibody type 1 and liver cytosol antibody type 1 concentrations in type 2 autoimmune hepatitis. Gut 1998;42:721.
67. Löhr H, Manns M, Kyriatsoulis A, Lohse AW, Trautwein C, Meyer-zum-Büschenfelde KH, Fleischer B. Clonal analysis of liver infiltrating cells in patients with chronic active hepatitis (Al-CAH). Clin Exp Immunol 1991;84:297.
68. Löhr HF, Schlaak JF, Lohse AW, Böcher WO, Arenz M, Gerken G, Meyer zum Büschenfelde K-H. Autoreactive CD4+ LKM-specific and anticlonotypic T-cell responses in LKM-1 antibody-positive autoimmune hepatitis. Hepatology 1996;24:1416.
69. Donaldson P, Doherty D, Underhill J, Williams R. The molecular genetics of autoimmune liver disease. Hepatology 1994;20:225.
70. Czaja AJ, Carpenter HA, Santrach PJ, Moore SB. Significance of HLA DR4 in type 1 autoimmune hepatitis. Gastroenterology 1993;105:1502.
71. Seki T, Ota M, Furuta S, Fukushima H, Kondo T, Hino K, Mizuki N. HLA Class II molecules and autoimmune hepatitis susceptibility in Japanese patients. Gastroenterology 1992;103:1041.
72. Marcos Y, Fainboim HA, Capucchio M, et al. Two locus involvement in the association of human leukocyte antigen with the extrahepatic manifestations of autoimmune chronic active hepatitis. Hepatology 1994;19:1371.
73. Scully LJ, Toze C, Sengar DPS, Goldstein R. Early-onset autoimmune hepatitis is associated with a C4A gene deletion. Gastroenterology 1993;104:1478.
74. Soloway RD, Summerskill WHJ, Baggenstoss AH, Geall MG, Gitnick GL, Elveback ER, Schoenfield LJ. Clinical, biochemical and histologic

remission of severe chronic active liver disease: A controlled study of treatments and early prognosis. Gastroenterology 1972;63:820.
75. Summerskill WHJ, Korman MG, Ammon HV, Baggenstoss AH. Prednisone for chronic active liver disease: dose titration, standard dose and combination with azathioprine compound. Gut 1975;16:876.
76. Czaja AJ. Drug therapy in the management of type 1 autoimmune hepatitis. Drugs 1999;57:49.
77. Sanchez-Urdazpal L, Czaja AJ, Van Holk B. Prognostic features and role of liver transplantation in severe corticoid-treated autoimmune chronic active hepatitis. Hepatology 1991;15:215.
78. Nagamine K, Peterson P, Scott HS, et al. Positional cloning of the APECED gene. Nat Genet 1997;17:393.
79. Ahonen P, Myllärniemi S, Sipilä I, Perheentupa J. Clinical variation of autoimmune polyendocrinopathy-candidiasis-ectodermal dystrophy (APECED) in a series of 68 patients. N Engl J Med 1990;322:1829.
80. Heino M, Peterson P, Kudoh J, et al. Autoimmune regulator is expressed in the cells regulating immune tolerance in thymus medulla. Biochem Biophys Res Commun 1999;257:821.
81. Clemente MG, Obermayer-Straub P, Meloni A, et al. Cytochrome P450 1A2 is a hepatic autoantigen in autoimmune polyglandular syndrome type 1. J Clin Endocrinol Metabol 1997;82:1353.
82. Rorsman F, Husebye ES, Winquist O, Björk F, Karlsson FA, Kämpe O. Aromatic-L-aminoacid decarboxylase, a pyridoxal phosphate-dependent enzyme, is a beta-cell autoantigen. Proc Natl Acad Sci USA 1995;92:8626.
83. Beaune PH, Pessayre D, Dansette P, Mansuy D, Manns MP. Autoantibodies against cytochromes P450: Role in human diseases. Adv Pharmacol 1994;30:199.
84. Neufeld M, Maclaren NK, Blizzard RM. Two types of autoimmune Addison's disease associated with different polyglandular autoimmune (PGA) syndromes. Medicine 1981;60:355.
85. Betterle C, Greggic NA, Volpato M. Autoimmune polyglandular syndrome type 1. J Clin Endocrinol Metab 1998;83:1049.
86. Manns MP, Obermayer-Straub P. Cytochromes P450 and UDP-glucuronosyltransferases: model autoantigens to study drug-induced, virus-induced and autoimmune liver disease. Hepathology 1997;26:1054.
87. Manns MP, Obermayer-Straub P. Immunological mechanisms in liver injury. In: Kaplowitz N, DeLeve L (eds) Drug induced liver disease. New York, Marcel Dekker, 2000.

Chapter 89 Concepts and Challenges in Solid Organ Transplantation

Barry D. Kahan

Although transplantation as a cure for disease is richly described in mythic literature, its clinical practice spans only four decades. The legendary exchange of hearts by the Chinese practitioner Pien Ch'iao restored the proper balance of Yin and Yang elements in each recipient; the xenotransplantation of the elephant's head on to the boy corrected the mistaken decapitation by the Hindu god Shiva; and the limb transplant from the cadaveric Ethiopian gladiator to their devout sacristan by the Saints Cosmas and Damien replaced a gangrenous appendage.[1] The powerful symbolism of the chimeric patient in whom diseased organs are replaced by normal ones represents not only the pantheistic ideal of renewal and 'rebirth' of the recipient, but also the immortality of at least remnants of a frequently unexpectedly and catastrophically terminated donor life.

The barrier to transplant success remained a mystery until this century, when the local resistance 'athrepsia' theory of Ehrlich, which had been reinforced by Loeb's concept of incompatible protein templates, was superseded by the observations of Jensen, Schoene, Holman and, most elegantly, Medawar, that rejection was due to acquired immunity:[1] foreign grafts confer a state of donor-specific systemic resistance transferable by lymphocytes and abrogated by neonatal exposure. Our present failures to ensure graft success and to achieve full host rehabilitation are due both to gaps in our knowledge of the immunological events, and to a lack of understanding of the pathophysiology of transplanted organs.

ALLOGRAFT REJECTION

Immune mechanisms

Antigenic signals

The transplant presents a mosaic of antigens foreign to the host. Incompatibility for major blood group ABH antigens triggers rapid rejection, due in most cases to the onslaught of natural antibodies. However, if it survives the first month the ABH-incompatible allograft can enjoy survival similar to an ABH-compatible transplant. The incompatibility is not absolute: blood group O recipients display far less violent reactions toward grafts from donors of the ABO-A2 than from the -A1 erythrocyte subgroup.

A second system determining transplant outcome is encoded by the 'classic loci' within the major histocompatibility complex (MHC), which encode surface glycoprotein products (Chapter 6). The human Class I MHC genes HLA-A and -B heavy chains complexed with β_2-microglobulin are assembled with endogenously generated peptide fragments into heterotrimers. Expression on donor-type antigen-presenting cells (APCs) in the graft interstitium–dendritic cells – powerfully triggers CD8 T cells. In contrast, each Class II MHC gene (HLA-DP, -DQ, -DR) encodes two polypeptide chains which, upon cytoplasmic assembly, bind exogenous, endocytosed and endosomally processed antigenic peptides for indirect presentation primarily to CD4 T cells (Chapters 6, 7). Determination of the patient's phenotype for the three MHC loci of greatest import to transplant outcomes – HLA-A, -B and -DR – has evolved from the use of serologic microcytotoxicity reactions to DNA amplification reactions using selective primers. A six-antigen ('full') match assures most living related transplant recipients of a postoperative course free of serious rejection episodes, provided that the patient has not been presensitized. Evidence of presensitization would be provided by the presence of cytotoxic antibodies, toward donor-type non-MHC antigens encoded by endothelial, tissue or Lewis erythrocyte markers. The undeniable benefit of HLA identity for living related donor transplants may be explained by the fact that not only the HLA-A, -B and -DR, but also other, as yet incompletely defined, classic and nonclassic MHC genes encoded on the short arm of human chromosome 6 are shared between donor and recipient. However, even these patients require immunosuppression to counter the modest immunogenicity of non-MHC – so-called 'minor' – histocompatibility loci that, in aggregate, can trigger prompt allograft rejection. Only a graft from an identical twin donor fails to evoke alloimmunity, and thus does not require immunosuppression (unless the recipient's original disease was autoimmune in nature).

In contrast, the impact of HLA matching on the survival of cadaveric donor grafts is controversial. Although it is generally believed that there is a hierarchical relation between the number of HLA matches and the rate of graft survival, data from the large US Renal Data System document little difference between the outcomes of one- versus six-antigen mismatched kidney grafts. The difference in outcomes between six-antigen matched and living versus cadaveric donor transplants probably reflects the impact of antigens not currently detected by available HLA reagents. The variable impact of HLA mismatch may be obfuscated by three additional factors: chemical microheterogeneity of individual determinants causing seemingly identical HLA disparities to evoke a spectrum of responses; distinctive host immune repertoires; and interindividual differences in pharmacodynamic responses to immunosuppressive agents. Indeed, the current approach utilizing multiple types of agents has substantially reduced the impact of matching on kidney (but possibly not on heart) transplant survival.[2]

The graft's antigenic mosaic includes a variety of tissue factors. In the past decade, renal-specific antigens have been identified on the surface of proximal tubular cells and on vascular endothelium (with possible specialization on arterial versus capillary versus venous cells). It seems unlikely that these antigens elicit primary

KEY CONCEPTS

Variables determining transplant outcome
- Donor–host antigenic disparity
- Strength of host antidonor response
- Immunosuppressive regimen
- The condition of the allograft

immune reactions in immunosuppressed hosts, but the emergence of a rejection episode may trigger augmented release and enhanced immunogenicity of tissue antigens or passenger microbes, producing 'epitope spreading'. Although these immune responses are more likely to affect long-term graft survival/function, they may lead to presensitization that is undetectable using lymphocyte targets in cross-match procedures (see below). In summary, despite the availability of the organ donor, it has neither been possible to identify the precise antigenic stimulus that incites rejection, nor to predict the type and/or severity of the host immune response.

Evolution of host responses to the allograft

Four factors interact to determine transplant outcome: the antigenic disparity between host and donor; the host's donor-specific immune response; the immunosuppressive regimen; and the condition of the allograft. Just as the graft presents an antigenic mosaic, the host mounts a pleomorphic response directed by a variety of T- and B-cell clones that recruit an array of nonspecific inflammatory mediators. The multiple alternative pathways not infrequently circumvent the inhibitory effects of immunosuppressive agents. As T cells are the pivotal elements in the induction of both cellular and humoral responses, the major focus of transplantation biology is to identify the switch that determines whether T cells pursue an alloaggressive pathway or the clinically desirable peripheral tolerance cascades – programmed cell death (apoptosis), inactivation (anergy), differentiation into negative regulatory elements (suppression), or balanced chimerism. The chemical nature and presentation form of the foreign antigen, the host's T-cell repertoire, the presence of costimulatory cytokine or surface membrane signals, and the array of therapeutic immunosuppressive agents presumably influence the selection of the response mechanism – alloimmunity versus allotolerance.

Ischemia–reperfusion injuries

The ischemic injuries consequent upon organ retrieval cause ion and water fluxes, cellular and interstitial edema, the generation of reactive oxygen species in concentrations greater than the capacity of inherent salvage mechanisms, and the activation of apoptotic cascades. These processes are compounded by the reperfusion syndrome owing to the effects of the release of multiple chemokines and cytokines, triggered by the brain-death process in the donor prior to organ retrieval, and by the adverse effects on the poorly oxygenated, substrate-deprived graft during cold storage. These pathologic pathways produce vascular effects, not only constriction, but also up-regulated expression of ligand pairs on lymphocytes and on endothelial cells that promote leukocyte rolling, tethering and emigration, namely L-, P- and E-selectins, intercellular adhesion molecule-1 (ICAM-1), and α/β integrins, as well as chemokine homing receptors, respectively (Fig. 89.1). Host lymphocyte contact with donor endothelial and interstitial dendritic cells produces an initial and powerful immune stimulus. The cytokines, particularly tumor necrosis factor-α (TNF-α) and interferon-γ (IFN-γ), increase the expression of MHC antigens, augmenting graft immunogenicity; produce endothelial cell dysfunction, causing cytosolic swelling, proliferative and/or cytotoxic effects; and augment the nonspecific inflammatory response of monocytes and granulocytes. All of these antigen-dependent immune and antigen-independent inflammatory processes contribute to the condition of the transplant, and may conspire to delay recovery and impair long-term graft function.

KEY CONCEPTS

Peripheral mechanisms of tolerance
- Apoptosis
- Anergy
- Negative regulation
- Balanced chimerism

Because of the increasing demand by transplant candidates and the diminishing supply of cadaveric donors, an increasing proportion of organs are derived under 'marginal' circumstances – advanced age, concomitant hypertensive and cardiovascular disease, reduced graft functional reserve, and/or adverse procurement conditions. Thus, antigen-*independent* inflammatory reactions play an increasing role among the causes of short- and long-term graft failure.

T-helper cell responses

Foreign alloantigens are presented by both the direct and the indirect pathways to host T cells.[3] Most organs are endowed with efficient interstitial donor-type dendritic APCs capable of providing costimulatory signals. In contrast, the liver bears 'nonprofessional' APCs that cannot deliver critical signals, owing either to their failure to produce costimulatory cytokines such as

The adhesion–migration paradigm: events and interdictions

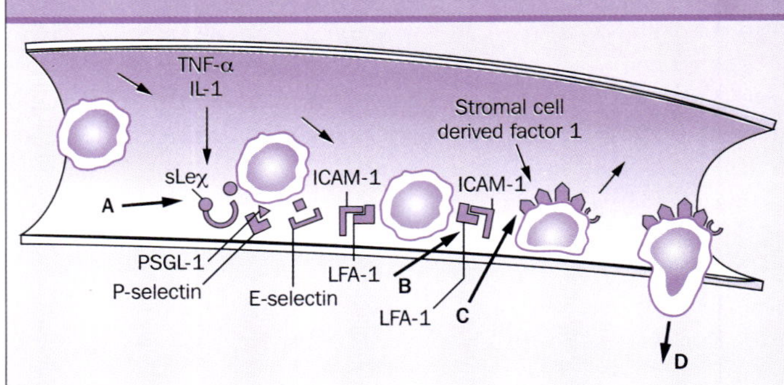

Figure 89.1 The adhesion–migration paradigm: events and interdictions. Events **A:** Lymphocytes entering the graft roll based on selectin interactions (sLe^x, PSGL-1, P-, E- and L-selectins) up-regulated by TNF-α and/or IL-1. Events **B:** Up-regulation of ICAM-1 leads to adhesion to lymphocyte LFA-1. Events **C:** In the presence of chemokines there is selective up-regulation of chemokine receptors, which promote adhesion. Event **D:** Diapedesis into tissues.

interleukins (IL)-12, IL-1 and IL-6, or to the absence of the B7 and/or CD40 ligands, which bind the CD28 and CD154 coreceptors, respectively (Chapter 12). In addition, the weak primary linkage of host TCRs to donor antigen on APCs requires amplification by coreceptor pairs, including CD8/MHC Class I molecules or CD4/MHC Class II molecules, lymphocyte function antigen (LFA)-1/ICAM-1, and CD2 (LFA-2)/LFA-3 (CD58), respectively.

The alternative, indirect route of alloantigen presentation demands that host APCs endocytose and endosomally process released donor antigen into peptides, which are assembled with Class II MHC molecules. In contrast to the direct route, which triggers a high frequency of allospecific T cells, the indirect route, akin to stimulation by nominal antigens, elicits only a low frequency of cells. The type and intensity of the host response to foreign alloantigens depend on (1) utilization of the direct and/or the indirect modes of antigen presentation; (2) the potential capacities and activation status of the APCs; and (3) the nature and strength of the cytokine signals.

TCRs are primarily α/β heterodimers that are present on the majority of mature peripheral blood T cells, with γ/δ heterodimers on a smaller number of lymphocytes, many of which do not appear to be classic T cells (Chapter 5). The nature of peptide binding may determine whether the T-cell engagement is stimulatory or inhibitory. The cell surface events involved in signal transduction and T-cell activation are discussed in Chapter 12.

A major function of primed helper T cells is the synthesis of lymphokines – IL-2 and -15, which predominantly expand T cells; IFN-γ, macrophages; IL-4, -5 and -7, B and, to a lesser extent, T cells; as well as IL-10, which may inhibit APCs and CD4 T cells. There is considerable controversy as to whether the progression toward alloaggression versus acceptance depends upon the lymphokine profile, namely, a preponderance of IL-2/IFN-γ–synthesizing T-helper 1 (Th1) versus IL-4/IL-10 Th2 elements that are Fc receptor (FcR) positive, negative regulatory cells.[4] However, some recent findings call into question whether this balance generally explains the mechanisms of graft acceptance. Clearly, the predominant response of naive hosts to an allograft includes the synthesis of IL-2, TNF-α and IFN-γ, which recruit not only immunocompetent donor-specific elements, but also nonspecific inflammatory cells, which form the majority of cells infiltrating an allograft (Fig. 89.2).

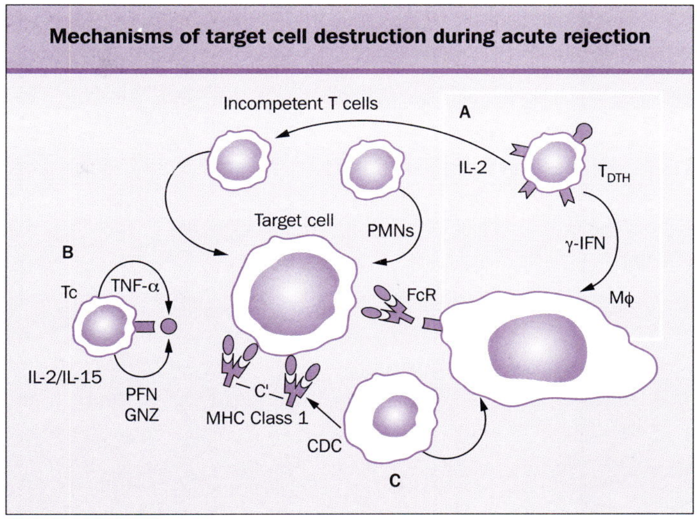

Figure 89.2 Mechanisms of target cell destruction during acute rejection. A: Cytokines produced by delayed-type hypersensitivity T cells (T_{DTH}) recruit granulocytes (PMN) and macrophages (MΦ) to attack graft. **B:** Specific T cells directly kill targets via TNF-α, granzyme (GNZ) and perforin (PFN). **C:** Humoral response includes Abs that directly fix C′ (CDC) or attach to MΦ to attack graft cells (antibody-dependent cell-mediated cytotoxicity).

Cytotoxic lymphocytes (CTL)

CD8 T cells, which recognize antigenic peptides displayed on MHC Class I molecules, mature into a major cytotoxic effector population. Foreign Class I epitopes, presented as intact surface molecules on donor dendritic cells, directly activate CTL. Following antigen recognition in conjunction with a costimulatory second and an IL-2 third signal, CD8 cells proliferate and mature into specific alloreactive clones capable of releasing the humoral mediators granzyme (serine esterase), perforin and cytokines, including TNF-α. Alternatively, CTL activation may be interdicted by 'exhaustive' differentiation following 'superantigen' stimulation, by apoptosis upon contact with cognate peptide, or by the negative regulatory behaviors of 'backward' killing of Th cells, fratricide of other CTLs, and bystander killing of inflammatory elements.

CTL activity in naive hosts is readily demonstrable after in vivo (or even in vitro) priming. Lymphocytes obtained by fine needle aspirates of allografts proliferate in vitro, generating CTL clones that display broad usage of the TCR repertoire, thus confirming the overlapping and redundant nature not only of stimulatory cytokines, but also of alloreactive host elements. Although estimation of the frequency of CTL precursors/mature elements in naive hosts does not forecast the severity of subsequent rejection events, one stigma of an immune response is an increased CTL frequency. Despite the critical role of donor-reactive CD8 CTLs, it has been impossible to diagnose the presence or to prognosticate the outcome of rejection episodes based upon the number of peripheral blood, or even graft-infiltrating, CD8 T cells.

B lymphocytes

Class I antigen-bearing donor cells may serve as APCs to trigger antibody synthesis. Host antidonor presensitization, as a result of prior blood transfusions, pregnancy or exposure to cross-reactive infectious agents, may presage a poor prognosis. Although donor-directed IgM antibodies produce target cell lysis in vitro, they rarely cause graft loss. In contrast, the presence in recipient serum of complement-fixing host antidonor IgG antibodies, particularly directed toward Class I antigens – a 'positive cross-match' – represents an absolute contraindication to renal transplantation, owing to its proclivity to produce hyperacute rejection. However, liver and heart grafts may be less vulnerable to this outcome.

Clinical rejection responses

The four major forms of allograft rejection are discerned based upon time of onset, pathophysiology and vulnerability to therapeutic reversal[5] (Table 89.1). Renal allograft rejection is described herein as the paradigm, as similar types of immune responses may occur in all organ transplants. *Hyperacute rejection* occurs within the first 48 hours posttransplant. The binding of cytotoxic antibodies to vascular endothelial cells produces thrombosis following local complement activation and aggregation of

Rejection characteristics of renal allografts							
Type	**Timing**	**Symptoms**	**Time frame of onset**	**Vector**	**Histopathology**	**Treatment**	**Success rate of treatment (%)**
Hyperacute	<24 h	Fever, anuria	Hours	Ab + complement	Polymorph deposition and thrombosis	None	0
Accelerated	3–5 days	Fever, graft swelling, oliguria, tenderness	1 day	Non-complement fixing Ab	Vascular disruption with hemorrhage	Antilymphocyte reagents	60
Acute	6–90 days	Decreased urine output, salt retention, graft swelling/tenderness, infrequently fever	Days to weeks	T cells	'Tubulitis'	Steroids	80
						Antilymphocyte reagents	90
				Ab	Endovasculitis	Antilymphocyte reagents	60
Chronic	>60 days	Peripheral edema, hypertension, proteinuria, occasional hematuria	Months to years	Ab	Vascular onion-skinning	None	0

Table 89.1 Rejection characteristics of renal allografts.

FcR-positive leukocytes (PMN) and platelets onto the antibody-coated endothelial cells. These events are frequently heralded by fever, as well as by severe allograft dysfunction and markedly reduced graft perfusion. Because this response is not amenable to treatment, the condition demands emergency transplant removal. Histopathologic examination showing polymorphonuclear leukocyte infiltration, particularly in the glomeruli of renal allografts, confirms an immunologic vector, as opposed to a 'bland' thrombosis resulting from a technical misadventure during the vascular anastomoses.

Accelerated rejection occurs between 3 and 5 days postoperatively and results from the deposition of noncomplement-fixing antibodies that act via FcR-positive K cells and monocytes to produce vascular disruption and interstitial hemorrhage. These events tend to evolve rapidly (within a day), resulting in a clinical picture of fever, graft swelling and tenderness, as well as rapidly progressive dysfunction. Because of the involvement of a cellular vector and the rapid pace of events, antilymphocyte antibodies represent the best therapeutic option. In cases where a positive *post*-transplant cross-match is observed, plasmapheresis offers a useful adjunct. Frequently, the condition is only partially reversed and recurs as progressively more severe bouts, until transplant removal becomes the most appropriate option. Hyperacute and accelerated rejections are anamnestic responses, wherein the antibody vector was either in the circulation at the time of, or its production is immediately triggered after, transplantation. In contrast, acute and chronic rejections result from primary immune responses.

Acute rejection generally occurs between 6 and 90 days post-transplant, but may begin later in the transplant course, particularly when triggered by patient or physician noncompliance with the immunosuppressive regimen. Mild and moderate acute rejection episodes produce clinical syndromes of progressive graft dysfunction, swelling and tenderness, infrequently accompanied by fever. The characteristic histopathologic appearance includes a cellular infiltrate containing CD8 cytolytic T cells, and a polymorphic inflammatory response elicited by lymphokine release by

KEY CONCEPTS

Rejection vector/treatment/prognosis (% 5-year graft survival)

Anamnestic responses
- Hyperacute/none/irreversible (0%)
- Accelerated/intense antilymphocyte antibody ± plasmapheresis/poor (40%)

Primary immune responses
- Acute cellular/steroids ± antilymphocyte antibody/fair (60%)
- Chronic/none/irreversible (50%)

CD4 T cells. Although perivenous lymphocyte collections characteristic of delayed-type hypersensitivity reactions are frequently present, the typical histopathologic lesion results from direct lymphocyte contact with parenchymal elements, often accompanied by interstitial edema. For example, in the kidney, lymphocyte penetration of peritubular basement membranes produces 'tubulitis', a lesion that is almost always reversed by the administration of large doses of steroids. Severe bouts of acute rejection frequently include a humoral antibody component that produces endovasculitis, with the deposition of lymphoid cells on swollen, ischemic endothelial cells. Although the administration of antilymphocyte antibodies may reverse humoral as well as steroid-refractory cell-mediated lesions, some cases show only transient benefit, followed by recurrent acute episodes and evolution to chronic rejection.

Chronic rejection usually appears at least 60 days post-transplant. This insidious condition, which is generally believed to be antibody mediated, includes histopathologic features of smooth muscle cell invasion and proliferation in the intima, disruption of the internal elastic lamina, and vascular immuno-obliteration. Interstitial cicatricial changes are also observed, either associated with or independent of the vascular events. Although the molecular mechanisms by which antibodies trigger these changes are uncertain, cytokines, eicosanoids and growth factors have been documented to participate in the process. In renal transplantation the clinical picture includes vasculopathic hypertension and glomerulopathy with accelerating proteinuria, followed by microscopic and then gross hematuria. Liver allografts undergo the 'vanishing bile duct' syndrome; heart transplants, a pernicious form of coronary artery disease; and lung transplants, bronchiolitis obliterans. The chronic rejection lesion shows a treatment-resistant, indolent but progressive course of stepwise deterioration of allograft function over a period of months to years.

IMMUNOSUPPRESSION

Immunosuppressive strategies have evolved slowly during the past century, from the cytotoxic agents benzene and toluene to the antiproliferative modalities of radiation or antimetabolites, to the present era of disrupting the production, reception and transduction of cytokine signals. However, despite this progress, the pharmacologic and antibody reagents currently available are merely nonspecific bludgeons that can engender serious disease. First, most agents display at least some degree of inhibition of nonspecific host resistance by macrophages, monocytes and polymorphonuclear leukocytes. Second, excessive immunodepression of T and B cells can result in the emergence of occult viral infections in, or neoplastic diseases of, lymphoid cells. Third, adverse effects on nonimmune organs not infrequently result from the high drug doses that must be administered to achieve adequate immunosuppression. The antiproliferative and steroid combination used in the original pharmacologic strategies exemplifies the first problem; the monoclonal antibody (mAb) OKT3, the second problem; and cyclosporine (CsA), tacrolimus (TRL), and sirolimus (SRL), the third problem. Indeed, in some cases the 'diseases' produced by immunosuppression are of greater consequence than that of allograft rejection. Avoidance of adverse outcomes is currently difficult owing to the *lack* of assays to quantify the effects of individual immunosuppressive agents; intermediate immunologic endpoints for early rejection diagnosis prior to tissue damage, and for monitoring reversal to avoid excessive treatment; and quantitative, scientifically based algorithms to tailor the induction, maintenance and antirejection therapies to individual patient needs. Thus, current clinical practice utilizes an array of nonspecific therapies of low immunosuppressive or low therapeutic index, rather than strategies that induce donor-specific unresponsiveness.

Agents interfering with allorecognition

Interruption of ischemia/adhesion/migration

Although no agents are currently available to interdict the initial events in the injury response – leukocyte adhesion and emigration into the graft interstitium – this area represents a major focus for new therapeutic strategies. In experimental animal models some agents seem to dampen these injuries: endothelin-A receptor antagonists,[6] molecular antagonists or mAbs blocking selectins[5,7,8] or LFA-1;[9,10] or ICAM-1.[11] However, clinical trials using murine mAb directed against ICAM-1 or against LFA-1 failed to show beneficial effects in human renal transplantation. One exciting new agent is the synthetic sphingosine analog FTY720,[12] which seems to up-regulate the expression of chemokine receptor (CCR)7,[13] thereby producing sequestration of lymphocytes in secondary lymphoid structures – peripheral and mesenteric lymph nodes, as well as Peyer's patches. Many of these agents are likely to be delivered initially ex vivo to saturate the graft, and then administered continuously in the recipient (Fig. 89.3A).

Depletion of graft antigen

A variety of strategies have sought to eliminate 'passenger' dendritic APC elements within the graft and thereby subvert direct allorecognition (Fig. 89.3B). Only modest depletion has been observed after donor pretreatment with a methylprednisolone/cyclophosphamide cocktail administered in vivo,[14] or after exposure of the isolated graft to irradiation or to pan-leukocyte cell anti-CD45 mAbs.[15] In contrast, reducing the T-cell component of bone marrow or small bowel transplants by purging these grafts with large doses of selective lectins, polyclonal sera or mAbs has been shown to improve outcomes, as the donor lymphoid contingent mediates alloaggressive graft-versus-host reactions that are particularly resistant to existent immunosuppressants.

Inhibition of APC function (Fig. 89.3C)

At the present time steroids are used to dampen APC functions (Fig. 89.3C). The complexes of steroids with their cytoplasmic

Potential sites of action of immunosuppressive interventions

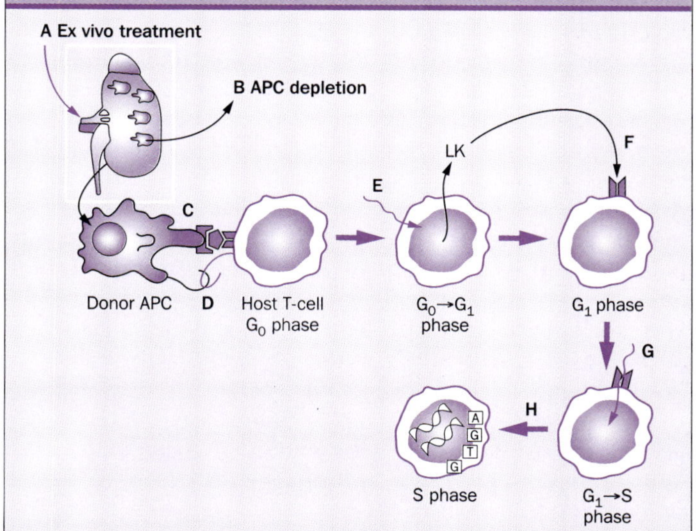

Figure 89.3 Potential sites of action of immunosuppressive interventions. A: Ex vivo treatment to mitigate ischemia–reperfusion injuries. **B:** APC depletion to reduce immunogenicity. **C:** Dampening of donor APC activity. **D:** Disruption of coreceptor interactions. **E:** Inhibition of antigen-driven activation events generating cytokine proteins up-regulating DNA transcription. **F:** Blockade of cytokine reception. **G:** Dampening of cytokine receptor signal transduction. **H:** Antimetabolite action to block nucleoside synthesis necessary for DNA synthesis.

THERAPEUTIC PRINCIPLES

Limitations of immunosuppressive therapy
- Paresis of nonspecific host resistance
- Excessive T-cell depression
- Collateral toxicities

and nuclear receptors interact with glucocorticoid reactive elements (GRE) within the DNA sequences of a variety of gene promoters, such as the enhancer region of IL-1. However, similar GRE sequences enhance (or repress) the functions of many genes, resulting in what has long been regarded as the Achilles' heel of clinical immunosuppression: the pernicious side-effect profile associated with steroid therapy.

The experimental drug 15-deoxyspergualin (15-DSG; molecular weight 500 Da) binds to intracellular heat shock proteins (HSP) 40 and 90, which are involved in cytoplasmic shuttling and MHC-loading of peptides. 15-DSG inhibits APC processing and presentation, thereby dampening antigen-specific, but not mitogenically driven, T-cell proliferation. Neither IL-1 or IL-6 synthesis, nor the expression of B7 or CD28 costimulatory signals, is reduced by 15-DSG.[16] However, the compound blocks the secretion of hydrolytic enzymes, the generation of oxygen radicals, the expression of MHC Class II surface antigens and the production of cytokines. Preliminary trials of 15-DSG at doses of 40–220 mg/m^2 revealed modest clinical activity, primarily for the reversal[17] rather than the prophylaxis of acute rejection episodes. However, because of the toxicities of leukopenia, thrombocytopenia, nausea, vomiting, anorexia, facial numbness and headache, only short courses of therapy are recommended.

Blockade of surface T-cell receptor/coreceptor molecules (Fig. 89.3D)

A variety of rodent antihuman mAbs have been exploited to bind surface epitopes, either for cell depletion from the peripheral blood or for 'covering' to prevent interaction(s) critical for T-cell activation. The only Food and Drug Administration (FDA)-approved agent, OKT3 (Ortho, Raritan, NJ), is an IgG_{2a} mouse mAb directed against the ε chain of the pentapeptide CD3 complex. In large doses it purges T cells from the circulation. In the more reasonable 'approved' 5 mg doses, OKT3 modulates cell function by interrupting the transduction of the TCR signal. Approved for the reversal of acute cellular rejection episodes,[18] the agent is also claimed to delay their onset and possibly decrease their incidence. OKT3 displays toxic effects owing to its propensity to initially activate T cells releasing TNF-α and IL-2 cytokines.[19] The clinical syndrome includes fever, chills, myalgias, dyspnea, aseptic meningitis etc. Furthermore, OKT3 treatment may be limited by host production of human antimouse antibodies (HAMA) that bind to circulating reagent molecules, neutralizing their activity. This obstacle is being addressed by engineering antibodies to contain a majority of human amino acid sequences, particularly in the Fc region, with xenogeneic murine sequences, either as $F(ab)_{2'}$ (chimeric) or as only the complementarity-determining regions (humanized). Alternatively, less toxic mouse isotypes or IgA variants that cannot bind human FcR are being proposed as reagents that do not cause the activation processes seen with OKT3.

A broad array of mAbs reactive with other epitopes are under clinical investigation. The first group is directed toward monomorphic common determinants on human α/β TCR: the T10B9 IgM reagent displays equivalent potency in rejection reversal, but less toxicity than OKT3.[20] The IgG_{2b} BMA 031 reagent (Behringwerke, Marburg, Germany) delays the onset and reduces the 30-day incidence of, but does not reverse ongoing, rejection episodes.[21] In contrast to these broad reagents directed against all TCRs, specific anti-TCR idiotype reagents have been demonstrated to avert transplant rejection or to reverse autoimmune disease in experimental animal models.[22] Unfortunately, the pleomorphic array of TCR idiotypes exploited by various patients in alloimmune rejection responses probably precludes this approach.

A second group of reagents are directed against APC: T-cell coreceptors that strengthen the antigen–TCR signal. Although anti-CD4 mAbs produce a durable distortion of alloimmunity with consequent transplantation tolerance in rodents,[23] preliminary trials of an anti-CD4A mAb (Ortho) failed to demonstrate a benefit in clinical trials. However, dose and schedule considerations warrant further investigation. Because anti-CD8 mAbs produce only modest effects in animal models, they have not been tested in humans. The report of transplantation tolerance induction in mice using a cocktail of two mAbs directed toward the third pair of costimulatory markers – ICAM-1/LFA-1 – led to disappointing results in clinical trials using these mAbs individually. Whereas studies in experimental animal models suggested the utility of mAbs directed against CD2, a pan-T-cell marker present both in the resting and the activated states, or against CD7, an activation marker on lymphocytes, these reagents seem to display little clinical promise for effective rejection prophylaxis.

Recent attention has focused on reagents that disrupt costimulatory interactions. The administration to mice of an IgG conjugate of a CD28 homolog, cytotoxic T-lymphocyte antigen-4 Ig (CTLA-4Ig; Schering, NJ), disrupts interactions between the APC B7-1/-2 and the T-cell CD28 markers. It only modestly prolonged allograft survival, but did induce tolerance to xenogeneic human pancreatic islets. Furthermore, only at high (40 mg/kg) doses did the agent ameliorate psoriasis in a clinical trial. Unfortunately, interruption of the interaction of CD40 with CD154 using anti-CD154 mAbs (Biogen; Boston, MA), which appeared to be even more effective than CTLA-4 Ig in experimental animal models, produced an array of thrombotic events, leading to its withdrawal from clinical trials. The alternative approach using mixtures of anti-B7-1/-2 mAbs is currently in clinical trials.

Agents that interfere with cytoplasmic activation from G_0 to G_1: inhibition of regulatory proteins for gene transcription

Despite the numerous and multifaceted independent pathways that mediate the initial activation of resting T cells (G_0 phase), only one therapeutic strategy is currently available, namely, to inhibit the Ca^{2+}-dependent cascade which generates the regulatory proteins that control DNA transcription of a range of m-RNAs encoding proinflammatory cytokines, including IL-2, IL-3, IL-4, and IFN-γ. Cyclosporine (CsA; Sandimmune or Neoral formulation, Novartis, Basel, Switzerland), a fungally derived cyclic endecapeptide of molecular weight 1202 Da, and tacrolimus (TRL; FK506; Prograf, Fujisawa, Japan), an actinomycete macrocyclic lactone of molecular weight 750 Da, act via a similar mechanism. Because of their hydrophobic nature, the drugs readily penetrate plasma membranes and bind to the cytoplasmic *cis-trans* prolyl isomerases, cyclophilins and FK-binding proteins, respectively.[24] These complexes inhibit the enzymatic actions of calcineurin to dephosphorylate and transport the nuclear factor of activated T cells (NF-AT) to the nucleus, thereby disrupting the generation of an initial regulatory protein that promotes the transcription of cytokine genes (Fig. 89.3E).

The introduction of CsA improved 1-year cadaveric renal graft survival from 51% to 88%, and reduced the rate of acute rejection episodes from 85% to 50%.[25] The pharmacokinetic limitations of the original, oil-based CsA formulation, including poor oral bioavailability and great inter- and intrapatient variability, have been addressed by the introduction of a microemulsion formulation.[26] In vitro experiments and in vivo animal transplant models suggest that TRL displays a 25- to 50-fold greater immunosuppressive effect than CsA; however, this benefit has been difficult to document in humans owing to the equally narrow therapeutic window of the two agents. TRL and Sandimmune CsA-based immunosuppressive therapy, in conjunction with azathioprine (Aza) and prednisone (Pred), produced equal graft survival rates in renal[27] or liver recipients,[28,29] although the incidence of acute rejection episodes was significantly reduced, namely, 30.7% versus 46.6% (P=0.001) in the US and 25.9% versus 45.7% (P=0.001) in the European multicenter trials, respectively. Size-limited and therefore anecdotal experiences in pancreas,[30] heart,[31] and lung[32] transplantation suggest similar results.

However, both CsA[25] and TRL display pleiotropic toxicities, possibly related to the wide tissue distribution both of calcineurins and of drug-binding isomerase proteins. Both drugs produce similar degrees of nephrotoxicity. On the one hand, TRL causes a more severe neurotoxicity, and on the other hand CsA causes hypertrichosis and gingival hyperplasia. One alternative strategy has been advocated to reduce the toxicities: a peptide analog of NF-AT (nuclear factor of activated T cells) that competes with calcineurin action only for this and not for other substrates. However, this approach is unlikely to overcome all of the toxicities associated with CsA and TRL, as NF-AT is expressed in many tissues, including cardiac muscle. Thus, neither NF-AT nor calcineurin is an ideal therapeutic target. It may be anticipated that ongoing biochemical dissection of lymphocyte activation pathways will provide insight into the future design of more selective agents acting in the G_0–G_1 transition.

Agents interfering with cytokine reception

Because IL-2 is a prominent (albeit neither necessary nor sufficient) vector of rejection responses, anti-IL-2 receptor (R) mAbs have been developed to block activation driven by this cytokine. In contrast to the high degree of xenosensitization caused by, and the low efficacy of, the original polyclonal antibodies, humanized[33] or chimeric[34] reagents directed towards epitopes on the activation-induced IL-2R α chain display greater tolerability and better rejection prophylaxis (Fig. 89.3F). Two multicenter trials (US and worldwide) using the same protocol documented that the administration of two 20 mg doses of the mouse–human chimeric mAb basiliximab (Simulect, Novartis, East Hanover, NJ) in combination with CsA and steroids decreased both the incidence (33% basiliximab group versus 48% placebo group; P=0.012) and the severity of acute rejection episodes, as well as improved renal function over 12 months.[34] In contrast, the addition of five biweekly 1 mg/kg doses of the humanized anti-IL-2R mAb daclizumab (Zenapax, Hoffman-LaRoche, Nutley, NJ) to a regimen of CsA, Aza and steroids significantly reduced the incidence of biopsy-proven acute rejection within the first 6 months to 28%, compared to 43% for the placebo-treated group in the US trial (with Aza–Pred) and to 47% in the European cohort (without Aza; P=0.03).[33] However, at 12 months patients treated with CsA–Aza–Pred failed to display a benefit of adjunctive daclizumab treatment on either rejection episodes or renal function (Daclizumab Product Insert). The immunosuppressive activity of both reagents is limited by two shortcomings. First, the antibodies do not compete effectively with the IL-2 ligand for binding to the IL-2R. Thus, they must be used in circumstances when the IL-2 production is low and cannot reverse acute rejection episodes. Second, the specificity of the antibodies for CD25 (IL-2Rα), despite ensuring their reactivity with only activated T cells, does not prevent immune activation generated via other cytokines, such as IL-7 and IL-15, which do not share the α chain and which can be independently recruited to mediate allorejection in IL-2 knockout animals.

> **THERAPEUTIC PRINCIPLES**
>
> **The cytokine paradigm of modern immunosuppressive therapy**
> - Calcineurin antagonists
>   - Cyclosporine
>   - Tacrolimus
> - Anti-IL-2 monoclonal antibodies
>   - Basiliximab (chimeric)
>   - Daclizumab (humanized)
> - Cytokine signal transduction inhibitors
>   - Sirolimus
>   - SDZ-RAD

Agents disrupting cytokine-stimulated G_1 activation

Two agents act on the calcium-independent cytokine transduction events during the G_1 phase. Sirolimus (SRL; rapamycin; Rapamune; Wyeth-Ayerst, Princeton, NJ; molecular weight 950 Da),[35] a macrocyclic lactone produced by an actinomycete, forms complexes with the immunophilin FKBP12, thereby inhibiting a multifunctional kinase–mammalian target of rapamycin (mTOR). This inhibition disables the transduction of cytokine signals in the G_1 phase (Fig. 89.3g), both at the relatively early stage of activation of $p70^{S6}$ kinase kinase, and later at the generation of the elongation factor for ribosomal protein synthesis, and at steps necessary for cyclin activation. SRL thus inhibits the transduction of a variety of cytokine signals in addition to those of the IL-2 family, namely, the hematologic–vascular stem cell growth factor, vascular endothelial growth factor, and fibroblast-derived growth factor. Whereas the inhibition of the latter group of mediators may explain the myelosuppressive effects of SRL, particularly in the early post-transplant period, blockade of vascular cytokines may produce beneficial effects that blunt arteriopathic chronic rejection processes.

We believe that SRL acts in synergistic fashion with CsA, due to its effects on both G_1 progression and, as recently discovered, the costimulatory signal 2 cascade, namely, blockade of the kinase necessary for generation of c-Rel transcription factors. Thus, we formulated the matrix of CsA, anti-IL-2R mAbs and SRL as the three components of the cytokine paradigm (Fig. 89.4).

Recently completed clinical trials have documented the immunosuppressive activity of SRL.[36] The pivotal phase III US and global trials showed that the rates of efficacy failure (a composite of the occurrences of acute rejection episodes, graft loss and/or death) were significantly reduced (P<0.0001) in patients treated with either SRL 2 mg/day (n=511) or SRL 5 mg/day (n=493), versus either placebo (n=130) or azathioprine (Aza;

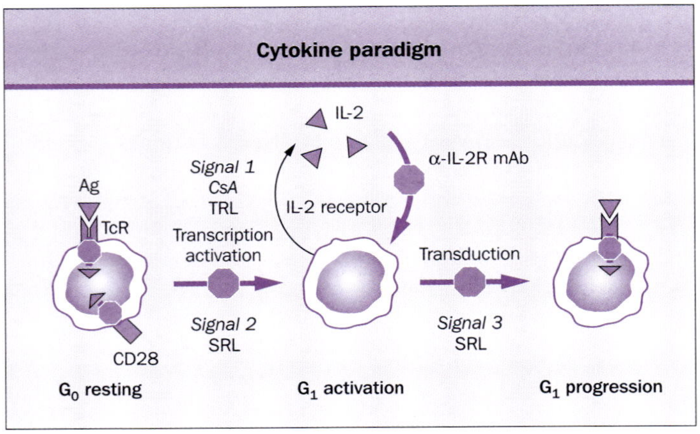

Figure 89.4 Cytokine paradigm. Complementary sites of action of immunosuppressive drugs during lymphocyte activation. Cyclosporine (CsA) and tacrolimus (TRL) inhibit transcription of T-cell growth-promoting genes (e.g. IL-2). Anti-IL-2 mAbs block binding of IL-2 to its receptor. SRL blocks growth factor-initiated signal transduction.

n=161). Furthermore, fewer patients treated with SRL displayed acute rejection episodes that were graded as moderate or severe by the Banff system, or required antibody therapy for rejection reversal. Because of the 90–96% overall patient and graft survival rates, it was not possible to discern a difference in these outcomes between the groups. As is the case for other immunosuppressive agents, higher (5 mg/day) doses of SRL were necessary to show a therapeutic effect in African-American patients.[37]

SDZ RAD (Certican, Novartis, Basel, Switzerland), a 25-hydroxy-ethyl derivative of SRL, is slightly more hydrophilic than the parent compound and displays a more rapid clearance rate. Like SRL, the analog drug is rapidly absorbed, reaching a maximum concentration (C_{max}) within 2 hours but, in contrast, SDZ RAD displays a half-life of 16–19 hours, which is significantly shorter than that of SRL (30 hours) and thus necessitates twice-daily dosing. SDZ RAD concentrations reach steady state by 4 days, in contrast to 7 days for SRL. The pharmacokinetic parameters of both drugs show dose proportionality, with a good correlation between trough and area under the curve (AUC) concentrations.[38] Future studies must gauge whether the SDZ RAD analog confers any benefits beyond those achieved with SRL. In a phase I study in stable renal transplant patients[38] SDZ RAD displayed a similar spectrum of side-effects to that observed with SRL, and in a preliminary phase II dose-finding trial the 2 mg/day SDZ RAD cohort showed a similar incidence of acute rejection episodes to that of the SRL 2 mg/day group.

Recently, attention has focused on disrupting membrane-proximal signal transduction events that are relatively specific for the IL-2 family of lymphokine receptors – IL-2, -4, -7, -9, -13 and -15. A nonspecific inhibitor of Lck and Fyn tyrosine kinases of the Src family, the isoxazol derivative leflunomide (Hoechst, Basel, Switzerland), has been shown to prolong rodent as well as canine renal allograft survival times.[39] However, its toxic effects in animal models necessitate caution in de novo administration to human transplant recipients, a trial that is currently under way. An alternative target is Jak3, a kinase responsible for transducing signals from the γ chain of the IL-2R family to STAT transcription factors.

Another target is the protein translation process. The selective class of agents – DNA oligonucleotides (oligos) – bind homologous regions of mRNA, thereby disrupting ribosomal synthesis of a specific protein. Oligos that selectively disrupt TNF-α-driven up-regulation of ICAM-1 synthesis have been shown to inhibit in vitro proliferation, block expression of this tethering molecule upon perfusion ex vivo, and prolong the survival of vascularized heterotopic cardiac or renal allografts in vivo. Although the stability of oligos has been enhanced by substitution of sulfuryl for phosphoryl groups, the clinical application of these agents has been limited by their high negative charge, leading to poor cytoplasmic penetration, an obstacle that is being addressed by methoxyethoxy substitutions on the terminal nucleotides.

De novo nucleoside synthesis inhibitors

The slightly reduced activity of purine salvage enzymes in lymphocytes compared to other rapidly dividing cell types suggests that these immune elements are more dependent on de novo nucleoside synthesis of DNA and RNA building blocks (Fig. 89.3H). However, the inhibition of de novo nucleoside synthesis produces a low immunosuppressive index because this effect also inhibits a variety of cell types. Azathioprine (Aza; Burroughs-Wellcome, Research Triangle, NC), mizorbine (MZB; Bredinin, Toyo Jozo, Tokyo, Japan) and mycophenolic acid (MPA) all inhibit the generation of guanosine monophosphate (GMP), thus mimicking the Lesch–Nyhan syndrome. Aza, a competitive inhibitor of a variety of synthetic pathways, including inosine monophosphate dehydrogenase (IMPDH), the target of MPA and MZB, was developed following the pioneering animal work of Schwartz and Dameshek[40] using 6-mercaptopurine, as well as the clinical trials of its imidazole analog by Calne et al.[41] After 20 years of clinical use Aza was displaced by CsA as the cornerstone of pharmacologic therapy; however, some physicians combine Aza with CsA in order to enhance the immunosuppressive effect. Although MZB is widely used in Japan, the morpholinylethyl analog of MPA, mycophenolate mofetil (MMF; Roche, Basel, Switzerland) is used throughout the rest of the world, where it is approved for the prophylaxis of acute rejection episodes in combination with CsA. Although non-nephrotoxic, MMF is associated with diarrhea and gastrointestinal complaints, neutropenia, and an increased incidence of cytomegalovirus (CMV) infections.

Randomized, double-blind, multicenter clinical trials conducted in the US, Canada, Europe and Australia showed that the addition to CsA and Pred of either 2 or 3 g daily doses of MMF, compared to Aza or placebo, significantly reduced the incidence and severity of acute renal allograft rejection episodes during the first 6 months.[42] However, the addition of MMF had less effect on African-American than on Caucasian recipients.[43] Furthermore, non-blinded studies have reported that MMF provides better prophylaxis of acute rejection episodes than does Aza in the settings of liver, simultaneous pancreas–kidney,[44] heart[45] and lung[46] transplantations. However, MMF treatment failed to improve patient or graft survivals at 1 or 3 years following cadaveric kidney transplantation, suggesting that the drug did not impede the occurrence or the progression of chronic rejection, a clinical observation that does *not* support the preliminary findings claiming benefits in animal models.[47] The frequent gastrointestinal intolerance encountered with the use of MMF may be overcome with a new enteric-coated formulation of mycophenolic acid (MPA; ERL080A, Novartis, Basel, Switzerland) that does not produce diarrhea. A 720 mg dose of ERL080A resulted in an MPA exposure bioequivalent to that of 1000 mg of MMF. ERL080A is currently being assessed for clinical efficacy in phase III trials.

A second type of nucleoside synthesis inhibitor is one that blocks dihydro-orotate dehydrogenase, the third enzyme in the pyrimidine de novo synthesis pathway. Because of the critical role of UDP sugars in the synthesis of glycoproteins, these agents may possess additional immunosuppressive properties beyond antiproliferative effects. The original drug of this type was brequinar (BQR; DuPont-Merck, Wilmington, DE);[48] recently, it has been claimed that leflunomide also displays this activity.[49] The occurrence of the principal toxicity of BQR, thrombocytopenia, correlates with high plasma concentrations, but proved to be so dose-limiting as to vitiate any benefit when added to a CsA/steroid-based immunosuppressive regimen. Owing to their lack of lymphocyte specificity and to their failure to display synergistic interactions that would permit dose reduction of calcineurin antagonists, the nucleoside synthesis inhibitors are unlikely to become permanent members of a T-cell-selective immunosuppressive armamentarium.

Induction immunosuppression strategies for renal transplantation

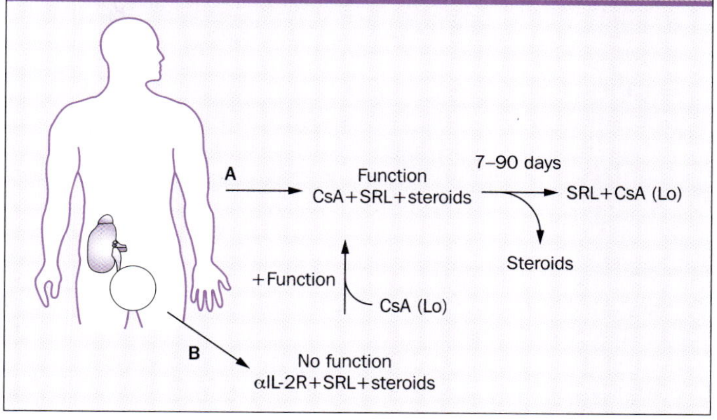

Figure 89.5 Induction immunosuppression strategies for renal transplantation. A: Regimen for immediate function includes CsA in low doses, SRL and steroids, with steroid withdrawal. **B**: Regimen for delayed graft function: αIL-2R mAbs + SRL + steroids, with delayed introduction of low-dose CsA.

The clinical immunosuppressive matrix

Unfortunately, the current therapeutic matrix is based upon empirical rather than scientific foundations. Indeed, despite the widely disparate intrinsic immunogenicity of various organs, the various degrees of donor versus host incompatibility, and the well recognized interindividual variations in host immunoresponsiveness, transplant centers tend to use relatively uniform schedules for initial induction and early maintenance immunosuppressive regimens.

Induction immunosuppression

The first 2 post-transplant weeks pose the greatest therapeutic challenge, owing to the requirement to establish adequate immunosuppression promptly and thus avert an acute allograft rejection episode. Although CsA may exert maximal benefit when delivered at the time of antigen presentation, the proclivity of the drug to produce renal and/or hepatic dysfunction suggests the need for delayed administration, particularly in cases of poor graft function. The brief window provided by antilymphocyte antibodies, either monoclonal (anti-IL-2R or OKT3) or polyclonal, has now been widened by simultaneous treatment with SRL or MMF, both of which are non-nephrotoxic.

We prefer to use anti-IL-2Rα mAbs for induction therapy, as they do not carry the potentially severe penalties of OKT3 or polyclonal Abs, namely, excessive global immunodepression, enhancing the proclivity to viral infection and/or post-transplant lymphoproliferative disease (PTLD). Whereas induction immunosuppression with daclizumab and MMF was attended by an almost 50% incidence of acute rejection episodes,[50] the combination of basiliximab with SRL has permitted extended periods (mean 33 days) of freedom from concomitant CsA treatment, a particularly useful period for grafts displaying poor initial function (Fig. 89.5). Only 18% of patients experienced acute rejection episodes, which occurred almost exclusively in retransplant or African-American patients.[51] In the future the induction period will be the stage for selective immunoregulation. Indeed, a recent preliminary report observed that one injection of anti-CD154 mAb provided a 'window of opportunity' for donor–host interactions, facilitating the induction of 'almost tolerance', namely, a state of graft acceptance despite only low doses of immunosuppressive agents.[52]

Acute rejection prophylaxis

The early immunosuppressive regimen from 2 to 12 weeks seeks to avert allograft rejection episodes, as their mere occurrence, particularly if not totally reversed, presages a greatly increased rate of eventual graft loss. During the past decade, when CsA and TRL were the therapeutic linchpins, successful rejection prophylaxis reflected, at least in part, the clinician's expertise to deliver

CLINICAL PEARLS

Antilymphocyte antibodies
- Avoid cytokine release syndrome with pretreatment with anti-inflammatory agents, and by initial administration of small divided doses
- Reduce viral complications with prophylactic ganciclovir treatment
- Biopsy transplant prior to and at the end of treatment

CLINICAL PEARLS

Cyclosporine
- Mechanism of action to inhibit proinflammatory cytokine m-RNA synthesis
- Assure adequate levels of drug: use 2-hour or absorptive phase (0–4)/full area under the curve concentrations
- Avoid use in damaged kidney/liver; prefer induction therapy
- Synergistic immunosuppressive effect with sirolimus

CLINICAL PEARLS

Sirolimus

- Mechanism of action to block transduction of virtually every cytokine signal
- Non-nephrotoxic: use for induction therapy
- Hyperlipidemia, particularly in diabetics, a major side-effect
- Pharmacokinetic interaction with CsA (cytochrome P450 3A4; p-glycoprotein)

adequate doses of the calcineurin inhibitors tailored to achieve target drug concentrations. For example, the initial 8–10 mg/kg CsA oral dose divided as a twice daily (b.i.d.) regimen, was adjusted thereafter based upon measured trough levels. Although a variety of measurement methods/matrices are available, most workers strive for whole-blood CsA concentration targets of 175–350 ng/ml, measured with specific mAbs either in an automated fluorescence device (TDx, Abbott, IL) or in radioimmunoassays with ^{3}H or ^{131}I tracers. The major challenge posed by this dose-finding strategy is the 54-fold interindividual variation in CsA (and probably TRL) pharmacokinetic parameters and the limited correlation between CsA trough levels and the AUC, a measure of drug exposure during the dosing interval.[53] As pharmacokinetic studies are beyond the expertise of most centers, an abbreviated strategy utilizing a single 2-hour concentration (target ≥ 800 ng/ml) has been advocated as a method to assure adequate exposure during the critical drug absorption phase.

Some clinicians seek to compensate for the pharmacokinetic variability by adding 1 g b.i.d. doses of MMF (1.5 g b.i.d. in African-Americans) to augment the immunosuppressive effect of full doses of the calcineurin antagonist. However, this strategy may result in overimmunosuppression. Because SRL acts in synergistic fashion with CsA, combination therapy permits substantial reductions in exposure to each drug, namely, dose ratios of 10–5 mg q.d. with 50–150 mg b.i.d., respectively. When TRL is used as base therapy, initial oral doses of 10 mg b.i.d. are followed by adjustments targeting a trough concentration of 10 ng/ml. The addition of SRL to the TRL regimen permits the use of 10–2 mg q.d. with 1–4 mg b.i.d., respectively. Anecdotal experience, primarily in liver transplant patients, suggests that SRL monotherapy[54] or in combination with TRL may provide good initial rejection prophylaxis.

The strategy of combining steroids with a calcineurin inhibitor is based upon both clinical and experimental data.[55] Steroids inhibit the generation of the IL-1 cytokine, and of inhibitor κ-kinase (IκK)-α, which would be otherwise activated by costimulation, thereby generating NF-κB, a critical transcription factor. Almost all steroid regimens include a massive (250–1000 mg) intraoperative dose of methylprednisolone to dampen graft tissue injury, drive lymphocytes out of the circulation and away from the allograft, and reduce T-cell activation. During the immediate postoperative phase steroid doses are rapidly tapered from 200 mg to 20–30 mg/day, followed by a more gradual taper to 15 mg between 30 and 90 days, 10 mg by 180 days, and 5 mg by 1 year.

Immunosuppression to reverse acute rejection episodes

The principles of treatment of rejection episodes are relatively uniform across organs and among transplant centers. Whereas some physicians empirically initiate treatment with increased doses of steroids, most centers demand histopathologic confirmation of an immune injury, owing to the significant penalties of excessive treatment of an adequately immunosuppressed patient. Steroid regimens combine large i.v. doses of methylprednisolone with an oral Pred taper. The delivery of i.v. steroids achieves high plasma concentrations and rapid reversal of symptoms, particularly fever, graft swelling and tenderness. The risks of steroid therapy include exacerbating or inducing diabetes mellitus, producing gastrointestinal irritation/perforation, and triggering psychoses. Administration of more than 7 g of methylprednisolone within the first 30 days post-transplant constitutes a risk factor for survival, owing to the pronounced depression of nonspecific host resistance. Recycling of oral steroids tends to follow a twofold slower version of the taper used during the first post-transplant week. It is important to reduce the level of steroids to the pre-therapy dose within 1 month, as long-term administration of high doses predisposes to gastrointestinal bleeding, myopathy, osteoporosis, bacterial/fungal infections and hypertension. The advantages of steroid treatment are the low medication costs and the 90% efficacy of rejection reversal.

Acute rejection episodes may also be treated with OKT3. However, the administration of doses over 75 mg has been associated with the development of PTLD among cardiac transplant recipients.[56] Furthermore, as discussed above, the production of neutralizing HAMA occurs in nearly 50% of patients following the initial course of OKT3 and may render a patient resistant to a second course of OKT3 treatment. Thus, before initiating repeat treatment with OKT3, it is useful to rule out the presence of HAMA. The laboratory at The University of Texas at Houston currently uses OKT3 covalently bound to tosylated dynabeads (M-280) to test for the presence of HAMA. The binding of patient serum to the coated beads is evaluated by flow cytometry after incubation with a fluorescein-conjugated goat anti-human antibody (Jackson ImmunoResearch Laboratories, West Grove, PA).

Refractory rejection therapy

There are considerable differences in the timing at which various transplant centers deem a rejection episode to be actually or potentially steroid resistant. For example, acute rejection episodes that display evidence of vascular injury on histopathologic examination are unlikely to respond to steroids. Some workers define a rejection episode as 'refractory' if it does not reverse after steroid treatment, and suggest a benefit of TRL or MMF in this setting.[57] A few centers believe that the benefits of steroids, even in the setting of mild rejection episodes, are modest, and favor initial treatment with antilymphocyte preparations. After 2–5 days of steroid treatment most centers assess treatment success based upon the remission of symptoms and the onset of improved graft function. In the clinical setting this assessment may be difficult to make. On the one hand, blood chemistry values reflect tissue damage endpoints, which only slowly reverse even after control of the immune process; on the other hand, delay in the delivery of adequate immunosuppression may condemn the graft to failure or severe permanent impairment.

If the response to steroids is deemed inadequate, the physician proceeds to administer an antilymphocyte preparation; most workers use OKT3 rather than polyclonal sera. To minimize OKT3 toxicity, a modest and graded cytokine release is required.

Our regimen employs a split-dose approach, delivering 1, 2 and 2 mg i.v. every 8 hours for the first day, followed by 2.5 mg every 12 hours on the second day, and 5 mg per day thereafter. Each dose is administered with an anti-inflammatory pretreatment cocktail of 100 mg hydrocortisone, 50 mg benadryl and 120 mg acetaminophen. Enumeration of the $CD3^+$ T cells in the peripheral circulation provides an intermediate endpoint for the efficacy of OKT3 therapy: values of $<10\%$ are deemed to represent a good therapeutic effect. In addition to the acute complications of cytokine release, excessive OKT3 therapy predisposes to CMV infections and PTLD despite routine antiviral prophylaxis. Unfortunately, there are no secure algorithms to guide the duration of OKT3 treatment, as the therapeutic effect is delayed by 7–10 days and the long-term toxic effects by 14–30 days. On balance, OKT3 therapy has an established role in reversing 80% of steroid-resistant acute rejection episodes.[18]

Deterioration in transplant function during OKT3 therapy may be due to the emergence of host HAMA that neutralize the therapeutic agent. However, in most instances OKT3 failures reflect pharmacodynamic resistance caused by the emergence of immune mechanisms not susceptible to the modulation of T-cell function. In these cases some physicians advocate a switch to treatment with polyclonal xenogeneic antibodies in an attempt to obtain lymphocyte depletion; however, because of the limited possibility of success, and the morbidity associated with an additional course of treatment, this strategy is rarely justified. ‘Refractory’ rejection episodes that fail to respond to a 14- (or preferably 21)-day course of an antilymphocyte antibody place the patient at high risk for graft loss. Thus, a rigorous definition of a refractory rejection episode is one that is both steroid- and antilymphocyte antibody-resistant, as documented by the presence of a positive transplant biopsy at the end of these treatments.[58] In this setting the addition of SRL to a CsA–Pred or a TRL–Pred regimen has been shown to ameliorate renal function.

Long-term maintenance immunosuppression

Although calcineurin inhibitors without or with concomitant MMF administration have reduced the incidence and severity of acute rejection episodes, they have not improved the 5% annual rate of graft attrition previously observed under Aza–Pred therapy.[59] Although it is possible that this failure reflects chronically inadequate or variable CsA exposure owing to reductions in the calcineurin antagonist doses in response to impaired renal function, it is more likely that the host B-cell responses that mediate chronic rejection are less sensitive to these agents than are T-cell responses.

Owing to a lack of knowledge concerning the pathophysiologic mechanisms of chronic rejection, long-term immunosuppressive regimens, including CsA, TRL, steroids, MMF, Aza and SRL, show greater intercenter variations than do the short-term strategies. In the chronic rejection setting long-term SRL administration may confer novel advantages based upon the capacity of this agent to block the effects of hematologic–vascular cytokines that stimulate endothelial and smooth muscle cell proliferation, resulting in immuno-obliterative lesions. Although there are no data at present to support this hypothesis, four observations suggest that SRL may prevent the occurrence or slow the progression of chronic rejection.[60] First, SRL inhibits growth factor-driven proliferation of endothelial and smooth muscle cells in vitro,[61–63] presumably by blocking the action of cytokines critical to producing the immuno-obliterative vascular and bronchial lesions – the histologic hallmarks of chronic rejection. Second, SRL exerts a beneficial effect on the smooth muscle and endothelial cell responses to vascular injury provoked in vivo by balloon catheter injury or observed in aortic allografts.[64] Third, SRL mitigates chronic rejection in rat renal allografts.[41,65–67] Fourth, used in combination with CsA in humans, SRL reduces the incidence of acute rejection episodes, which are widely believed to forecast an increased risk of chronic rejection.[68,69] Further, the administration of SRL permits either minimization or the elimination of CsA, thereby promoting renal recovery during the early postoperative period and possibly mitigating chronic CsA-induced renal dysfunction, which may exacerbate other processes that contribute to graft attrition.

There is a general impression that drug doses can be reduced over time owing to ‘adaptation’ of the graft to the host; this phenomenon has been attributed to repopulation of the donor vasculature with host elements. However, transplantation of long-term accepted grafts back into syngeneic donor-strain animal hosts fails to elicit rejection responses, a finding that suggests that the host rather than the donor ‘adapts’ to this artificial situation. Although the usual strategy is to attempt steroid withdrawal upon patient request, good HLA matching or evidence of drug-induced morbidities, the clinician’s decision must be based upon a perception of the safety of steroid withdrawal. A delay in withdrawal may compromise some of the potential benefits to be gained from a steroid-free regimen, specifically the prevention of cataract formation, amelioration of diabetes mellitis[70] and mitigation of bone destruction. However, virtually every patient who discontinues all immunosuppressive medications rejects the graft; there is at present no clinically applicable strategy for tolerance induction.

TRANSPLANT TOLERANCE

Immunounresponsiveness

The ultimate goal of transplantation research is to achieve selective tolerance toward donor, but not third-party, foreign allografts. Tolerance is distinguished from immunounresponsiveness, a state that demands at least some concomitant immunosuppression. Although the treatment of experimental animals with relatively abbreviated courses of immunosuppressants produces a proclivity toward tolerance induction, such an evolution occurs only rarely in humans. Evidence of host antidonor hyporesponsiveness in mixed lymphocyte cultures, cell-mediated cytotoxic effector and precursor assays,[71] and suppressor ‘three-cell’ reactions, has provided indices to withdraw steroids from or otherwise modulate CsA- or TRL-based regimens. Recently, the presence of donor-type putatively dendritic elements in numerous tissues of organ transplant recipients has been attributed to the presence of an unresponsive state,[72] indicating a ‘truce’ between host-versus-graft and graft-versus-host reactions. These findings led to the postulate that the facile acceptance of liver grafts reflects their rich passenger cell component. This hypothesis has not yet been supported by clinical trials: infusion of supplemental donor bone marrow elements concomitant with transplantation of passenger cell-poor cardiac or renal allografts, or even rich orthotopic liver transplants, has neither improved graft survival nor rendered patients tolerant of their grafts.[73] Indeed, the significance of chimerism as a marker for unresponsiveness is controversial: some patients displaying donor cell chimerism have been reported to undergo rejection episodes. Calne and colleagues[52] offer a more conservative proposal: after T-cell depletion with an anti-CD154 mAb, a 1-day interval is allowed to elapse before initiating treatment with low-dose CsA in the absence of steroids. These workers suggest that the modest (18%) incidence of rejection reflects 'prope' (almost) tolerance.

Immunologic tolerance

The concept of immunologic tolerance evolved from observations that hosts exposed to foreign cells during the fetal/neonatal stages of life subsequently accepted donor-type tissue transplants.[1] In 1914, Murphy reported that duck or pigeon embryos permit the unrestricted growth of Rous chicken sarcoma cells, unless the embryo had been previously inoculated with adult chicken lymphoid cells. Owen in 1945 demonstrated that nonidentical freemartin calf twins show erythrocyte chimerism, which he attributed to the exchange of placental blood. Tissue transplant tolerance was demonstrated in fetal or newborn mice by Billingham, in chicken egg embryos by Hasek, and in the first 2 weeks of life of rats by Woodruff.

These phenomena have been explained as an alteration of the 'central' thymic process, which naturally eliminates putatively self-reactive T-cell clones present in the thymus[74] (Chapter 10). A similar cellular 'macro' chimerism has been produced in adult animals following 'debulking' of the immune system by total-body or total-lymphoid[75] irradiation to recreate the 'pristine' fetal state and allow 'space' for reconstitution with donor or F_1 bone marrow cells. Adult allogeneic T cells are 'purged' from the donor bone marrow inoculum with anti-T-cell sera, with anti-CTLA-4Ig receptor conjugates[76] or with anti-CD40 ligand (-CD154) mAbs[77] to prevent graft-versus-host disease. Hosts displaying this 'macrochimeric' type of tolerance show either an absent or an altered T-cell repertoire, presumably owing to the effects of the newly seeded donor-type dendritic cells in the host thymus. Clinical induction of macrochimerism is limited by the hazards and logistical demands of pretransplant radiotherapy, as well as by the mature state of the primate thymus, such that donor-specific tolerance is not readily produced by intrathymic injection of donor materials combined with peripheral lymphoid depletion using polyclonal antisera.[78]

A critical question for the clinical enterprise is whether tolerance can be produced peripherally without the bludgeon of 'debulking' and/or the reversion to the pristine fetal state. The 'horror autotoxicus' concept of Ehrlich postulated that tolerance is a natural immune process that lymphocytes undergo after leaving the thymus. This 'peripheral' form of tolerance occurs despite the persistence of alloantigen-reactive host T cells,[79,80] an observation elegantly confirmed in transgenic mouse models. The expression of foreign MHC Class II (I-E) molecules restricted to the acinar pancreas and kidney,[81] or to pancreatic islet β cells, failed to elicit rejection responses, although adoptive transfer of naive T lymphocytes killed the transgenic cells.[82]

Several mechanisms may explain post-thymic 'peripheral' unresponsiveness: 'veto' cell generation, T-cell anergy, ignorance, deletion, blocking antibodies, and/or regulatory cell activity. Anergy represents an unresponsive state of antigen-reactive lymphocytes. Bretscher and Cohn[83] proposed that this unresponsiveness is due to the absence of an appropriate second humoral activation signal. Th cells recognize alloantigen, but neither proliferate nor secrete IL-2,[84] the addition of which reverses the anergy.[85] Although in animal models anergy emerges after the abrogation of helper–inducer function using nonspecific bludgeons, such as massive doses of a single or multiple mAb(s) in combination with CsA or, alternatively, high CsA doses alone, this progression has not been documented in humans. On the one hand, anergy may result from ineffective stimulation by modified antigen – for example following treatment with immunogens modified by cross-linking fixation[86] or by planer membrane array.[87] On the other hand, anergy can be produced by direct contact of immature T or B cells with antigen in the absence of costimulatory signals, such as due to treatment with anti-B7 or anti-CD154 mAbs or CTLA-4 Ig. The critical role of Th cell-generated cytokine signals was documented by the failure of B cells expressing the transgene-encoded membrane immunoglobulin to secrete antibody upon confrontation with the corresponding chicken lysozyme epitope. Anergic cells appear to have a proclivity to apoptosis, particularly when the induction strategy – for example anti-B7 mAbs – is combined with a proapoptotic drug such as SRL (but not CsA or TRL).[88]

The 'infectious' tolerance mechanism suggests that lymphoid 'regulatory' cells adoptively transfer unresponsiveness. Waldmann[23] observed that treatment with large amounts of anti-CD4 mAb elicited a novel negative regulatory response, which he proposed is integral to the differentiation repertoire of all cells.

Regulatory cell activity has been implicated in seven other tolerance models. Animals rendered neonatally tolerant to Class II MHC antigens show a higher frequency of tolerogen-reactive lymphocytes than normal mice in vitro, yet in vivo their cells transfer unresponsiveness but neither cytotoxicity[89] nor delayed-type hypersensitivity to naive mice. Total lymphoid irradiation (TLI) treatment induces both donor-specific and nonspecific negative regulatory elements.[90] 'Debulking' strategies of tolerance induction using cyclophosphamide produce initial deletion, followed by regulatory mechanisms.[91] Regulatory cells mediate the unresponsiveness produced by antilymphocyte serum combined with bone marrow,[92] as well as by high-dose CsA treatment,[93] particularly in combination with extracted antigen.[94] Finally, regulatory T cells – possibly of the $CD4^+$ phenotype[95] – mediate classic humoral unresponsiveness associated with 'enhancing' antibody.[96]

These regulatory anti-idiotypic α/β TCR^+ $CD3^+$ $CD8^+$ cells seem to proliferate upon confrontation with specific alloantigen,[97,98] as demonstrated by Batchelor et al.[99] In order to understand the mechanism of induction of regulatory cells investigators have used 'processed' donor antigens that display putatively tolerogenic epitopes; mAbs that alter coreceptor activities; selective activation of IL-4- and IL-10-producing Th2 cells, rather than the IL-2- and IFN-γ-producing Th1 cells;[100] or anti-idiotype reagents that eliminate cells bearing donor-specific TCRs.

Clinical trials to induce tolerance demand that the manipulation be performed within the context of appropriate baseline immunosuppression so as not to jeopardize patient outcome if the strategy is unsuccessful. This requirement presents two potential obstacles: first, the possible inhibitory effect of the immunosuppressant to prevent lymphocyte differentiation along a tolerogenic pathway; and second, the extreme caution that must be exercised in the withdrawal of baseline immunosuppression, particularly in view of the lack of assays to document the tolerant state. Thus, the present success of the transplant enterprise creates seemingly daunting obstacles to the exploration of specific immunologic tolerance.

THE FUTURE

Because our knowledge of the immunologic processes that trigger allograft rejection is limited, the clinical success of the transplant enterprise seems outrageous. This success has, however, been achieved at the price of appreciable patient morbidity, usually owing to excessive immunosuppression, which is frequently administered in the overzealous treatment of nonexistent or mild/moderate alloimmune reactions. The tenuous balance between dampened host resistance and the threat of viral/fungal pathogens, as well as the pleiotropic array of drug toxicities, almost inevitably leads clinicians to reduce the degree of immunosuppression, a measure that is often followed by the emergence of chronic rejection. Thus, the recent spectacular improvements in cadaveric donor transplant outcomes have been short term rather than long term: only a minority of patients retain their grafts for 10 years. A more secure strategy seems to be forthcoming with the use of synergistic drug combinations, such as CsA/SRL.

Although animal models proffer excellent tools to test scientific hypotheses, they have yielded few basic insights into human transplant immunology, owing to distinctive alloresponses. Incisive dissection of alloimmunity in humans demands the development of quantitative indices of graft function, diagnostic tools to detect alloresponses, and reliable surrogates of the pharmacodynamic effects of as well as pharmacokinetic interactions between immunosuppressive agents. These indices could be used to shape an era of hypothesis-testing clinical research that moves the present 'art' of transplant care to firm scientific foundations, and brings us to the eventual goal to immunodeviate alloaggressive host responses toward allotolerance. Thus, transplantation offers a fertile field for basic and applied investigation by clinical immunologists.

REFERENCES

1. Kahan BD. Transplantation timeline. Transplantation 1991;51:1.
2. Kerman RH, Van Buren CT, Lewis RM, Frazier OH, Cooley D, Kahan BD. The impact of HLA A, B, and DR blood transfusions and immune responder status on cardiac allograft recipients treated with cyclosporine. Transplantation 1988;45:333.
3. Auchincloss H Jr, Lee R, Shea S, Markowitz JS, Grusby MJ, Glimcher LH. The role of 'indirect' recognition in initiating rejection of skin grafts from major histocompatibility complex Class II-deficient mice. Proc Natl Acad Sci USA 1993;90:3373.
4. Fiorentino DF, Bond MW, Mosmann TR. Two types of mouse T helper cell. IV. Th2 clones secrete a factor that inhibits cytokine production by Th1 clones. J Exp Med 1989;170:2081.
5. Schmid C, Heemann U, Tilney NL. Factors contributing to the development of chronic rejection in heterotopic rat heart transplantation. Transplantation 1997;64:222.
6. Braun C, Conzelmann T, Vetter S, Schaub M, Back WE. Prevention of chronic renal allograft rejection in rats with an oral endothelin A receptor antagonist. Transplantation 1999;68:739.
7. Snapp KR, Ding H, Atkins K, Warnke R, Luscinskas FW, Kansas GS. A novel P-selectin glycoprotein ligand-1 monoclonal antibody recognizes an epitope within the tyrosine sulfate motif of human PSGL-1 and blocks recognition of both P- and L-selectin. Blood 1998;91:154.
8. Takada M, Nadeau KC, Hancock WW, et al. Effects of explosive brain death on cytokine activation of peripheral organs in the rat. Transplantation 1998;65:1533.
9. Yamazaki S, Isobe M, Suzuki J-I, et al. Role of selectin-dependent adhesion in cardiac allograft rejection. J Heart Lung Transplant 1998;17:1007.
10. Harlan JM, Winn RK, Doerschuk CM, et al. In vivo models of leukocyte adherence to endothelium. In: Harlan JM, Liu D (eds) Adhesion: its role in inflammatory disease. New York, WH Freeman & Co, 1992, p 117.
11. Stepkowski SM, Wang ME, Condon TP, et al. Protection against allograft rejection with ICAM-1 antisense oligodeoxynucleotides. Transplantation 1998;66:699.
12. Suzuki S, Enosawa S, Kakefuda T, et al. A novel immunosuppressant, FTY720, with a unique mechanism of action, induces long-term graft acceptance in rat and dog allotransplantation. Transplantation 1996;61:200.
13. Chiba K, Yanagawa Y, Masubuchi Y, et al. FTY720, a novel immunosuppressant, induces sequestration of circulating mature lymphocytes by acceleration of lymphocyte homing in rats. I. FTY720 selectively decreases the number of circulating mature lymphocytes by acceleration of lymphocyte homing. J Immunol 1998;160:5037.
14. Guttmann RD, Lindquist RR. Renal transplantation in the inbred rat. XI. Reduction of allograft immunogenicity by cytotoxic drug pretreatment of donors. Transplantation 1969;8:490.
15. Brewer Y, Palmer A, Taube D, et al. Effect of graft perfusion with two CD45 monoclonal antibodies on incidence of kidney allograft rejection. Lancet 1989;2:935.
16. Nadler SG, Tepper MA, Schacter B, Mazzucco CE. Interaction of the immunosuppressant deoxyspergualin with a member of the Hsp 70 family of heat shock proteins. Science 1992;258:484.
17. Amemiya H, Dohi K, Otsuba O, et al. Markedly enhanced therapeutic effect of deoxyspergualin on acute rejection when combined with methylprednisolone in kidney recipients. Transplant Proc 1991;23:1087.
18. Ortho Multicenter Transplant Study Group. A randomized clinical trial of OKT3 monoclonal antibody for acute rejection of cadaveric renal transplants. N Engl J Med 1985;313:337.
19. Abramowicz D, Schandene L, Goldman M, et al. Release of tumor necrosis factor, interleukin-2, and gamma-interferon in serum after injection of OKT3 monoclonal antibody in kidney transplant recipients. Transplantation 1989;47:606.
20. Waid TH, Lucas BA, Thompson JS, et al. Treatment of acute cellular rejection with T10B9.1A-31 or OKT3 in renal allograft recipients. Transplantation 1992;53:80.
21. Knight RJ, Kurrle R, McClain J, et al. Clinical evaluation of induction immunosuppression with a murine IgG2b monoclonal antibody (BMA 031) directed toward the human α/β-T cell receptor. Transplantation 1994;57:158.
22. Lanzavecchia A. Identifying strategies for immune intervention. Science 1993;260:937.
23. Qin S, Cobbold SP, Pope H, et al. 'Infectious' transplantation tolerance. Science 1993;259:974.
24. Fischer G, Wittmann-Liebold B, Lang K, et al. Cyclophilin and peptidyl-prolyl *cis-trans* isomerase are probably identical proteins. Nature 1989;337:476.
25. Kahan BD. Cyclosporine. N Engl J Med 1989;321:1725.
26. Keown P, Niese D. Cyclosporine microemulsion increases drug exposure and reduces acute rejection without incremental toxicity in de novo renal transplantation. International Sandimmune Neoral Study Group. Kidney Int 1998;54:938.
27. Pirsch JD, Miller J, Deierhoi MH, Vincenti F, Filo RS. A comparison of tacrolimus and cyclosporine for immunosuppression after cadaveric renal transplantation. Transplantation 1997;63:977.
28. European FK506 Multicentre Liver Study Group. Randomized trial: comparing tacrolimus (FK506) and cyclosporine in prevention of liver allograft rejection. Lancet 1994;344:423.

29. US Multicenter FK506 Liver Study Group. A comparison of tacrolimus (FK506) and cyclosporine for immunosuppression in liver transplantation. N Engl J Med 1994;331:1110.
30. Gruessner RWG, Burke GW, Stratta R, et al. A multicenter analysis of the first experience with FK506 for induction and rescue therapy after pancreas transplantation. Transplantation 1996;61:261.
31. Reichart B, Meiser B, Vigano M, et al. European Multicenter Tacrolimus (FK506) heart pilot study: one-year results European Tacrolimus Multicenter Heart Study Group. J Heart Lung Transplant 1998;17:775.
32. Keenan RJ, Konishi H, Kawai A, et al. Clinical trial of tacrolimus versus cyclosporine in lung transplantation. Ann Thorac Surg 1995;60:580.
33. Vincenti F, Kirkman R, Light S, et al. Interleukin-2-receptor blockade with daclizumab to prevent acute rejection in renal transplantation. Daclizumab Triple Therapy Study Group. N Engl J Med 1998;338:161.
34. Kahan BD, Rajagopalan PR, Hall M. Reduction of the occurrence of acute cellular rejection among renal allograft recipients treated with basiliximab, a chimeric anti-interleukin-2-receptor monoclonal antibody. United States Simulect Renal Study Group. Transplantation 1999;67:276.
35. Kahan BD, Chang JY, Seghal SN. Preclinical evaluation of a new potent immunosuppressive agent, rapamycin. Transplantation 1991;52:185.
36. Kahan BD, Gibbons S, Tejpal N, Stepkowski SM, Chou T-C. Synergistic interactions of cyclosporine and rapamycin to inhibit immune performances of normal human peripheral blood lymphocytes in vitro. Transplantation 1991;51:232.
37. Kahan BD, for the USA Rapamune Study Group. Sirolimus (Rapamune, rapamycin) is more effective than azathioprine to reduce the incidence of acute renal allograft rejection episodes when used in combination with cyclosporine and prednisone: a phase III US multicenter trial. Lancet 2000;356:194.
38. Kahan BD, Wong RL, Carter C, Katz SH, Von Fellenberg J, Van Buren CT. A phase I study of a four-week course of SDZ-RAD (RAD) in quiescent cyclosporine-prednisone-treated renal transplant recipients. Transplantation 1999;68:1100.
39. Chong AS, Finnegan A, Jiang X. Leflunomide, a novel immunosuppressive agent. The mechanism of inhibition of T cell proliferation. Transplantation 1993;55:1361.
40. Schwartz RS, Dameshek W. Drug-induced immunological tolerance. Nature 1959;183:1682.
41. Calne RY, Collier DS, Lim S, et al. Rapamycin for immunosuppression in organ allografting. Lancet 1989;2:227.
42. Mathew T, for the Tricontinental Mycophenolate Mofetil Renal Transplantation Study Group. A blinded, long term, randomized multicenter study of mycophenolate mofetil in cadaveric renal transplantation. Transplantation 1998;65:1450.
43. Schweitzer EJ, Yoon S, Fink J, et al. Mycophenolate mofetil reduces the risk of acute rejection less in African-American than in Caucasian kidney recipients. Transplantation 1998;65:242.
44. Odorico JS, Pirsch JD, Knechtle SJ, D'Alessandro AM, Sollinger HW. A study comparing mycophenolate mofetil to azathioprine in simultaneous pancreas-kidney transplantation. Transplantation 1998;66:1751.
45. Kobashigawa J, Miller L, Renlund D, et al. A randomized active-controlled trial of mycophenolate mofetil in heart transplant recipients. Mycophenolate mofetil investigators. Transplantation 1998;66:507.
46. Ross DJ, Waters PF, Levine M, Kramer M, Ruzevich S, Kass RM. Mycophenolate mofetil versus azathioprine immunosuppressive regimens after lung transplantation: preliminary experience. J Heart Lung Transplant 1998;17:768.
47. Azuma H, Binder J, Heemann V, Schmid C, Tullius SG, Tilney NL. Effects of RS61443 on functional and morphological changes in chronically rejecting rat kidney allografts. Transplantation 1995;59:460.
48. Cramer DV, Chapman FA, Jaffee BD, et al. The effect of a new immunosuppressive drug, brequinar sodium, on heart, liver, and kidney allograft rejection in the rat. Transplantation 1992;53:303.
49. Davis JP, Cain GA, Pitts WJ, Magolda RL, Copeland RA. The immunosuppressive metabolite of leflunomide is a potent inhibitor of human dihydroorotate dehydrogenase. Biochemistry 1996;35:1270.
50. Vincenti F, Grinyó J, Ramos E, et al. Can antibody prophylaxis allow sparing of other immunosuppressives? Transplant Proc 1999;31(1–2):1246.
51. Hong JC, Kahan BD. Use of anti-CD25 monoclonal antibody in combination with rapamycin to eliminate cyclosporine treatment during the induction phase of immunosuppression. Transplantation 1999;68:701.
52. Calne R, Moffatt SD, Friend PJ, et al. Campath IH allows low-dose cyclosporine monotherapy in 31 cadaveric renal allograft recipients. Transplantation 1999;68:1613.
53. Kahan BD, Grevel J. Overview: optimization of cyclosporine therapy in renal transplantation by a pharmacokinetic strategy. Transplantation 1988;46:631.
54. Watson CJ, Friend PJ, Jamieson NV, et al. Sirolimus: a potent new immunosuppressant for liver transplantation. Transplantation 1999;67:505.
55. Vathsala A, Chou T-C, Kahan BD. Analysis of the interactions of immunosuppressive drugs with cyclosporine in inhibiting DNA proliferation. Transplantation 1990;49:463.
56. Swinnen LJ, Costanzo-Nordin MR, Fisher SG, et al. Increased incidence of lymphoproliferative disorder after immunosuppression with the monoclonal antibody OKT3 in cardiac transplant recipients. N Engl J Med 1990;323:1723.
57. Sollinger HW, Belzer FO, Deierhoi MH, et al. RS-61443 (mycophenolate mofetil). A multicenter study for refractory kidney transplant rejection. Ann Surg 1992;216:513.
58. Slaton JW, Kahan BD. Case report: Sirolimus rescue therapy for refractory renal allograft rejection [Brief Communication]. Transplantation 1996;61:977.
59. Knight RJ, Kerman RH, Welsh M, et al. Chronic rejection in primary renal allograft recipients under cyclosporine-prednisone immuno-suppressive therapy. Transplantation 1991;51:355.
60. Kahan BD. The role of rapamycin in chronic rejection prophylaxis: a theoretical consideration. Graft 1998;1(2 Suppl.II):93.
61. Graves LM, Bornfeldt KE, Argast GM, et al. cAMP- and rapamycin-sensitive regulation of the association of eukaryotic initiation factor 4E and the translational regulator PHAS-I in aortic smooth muscle cells. Proc Natl Acad Sci USA 1995;92:7222.
62. Scott PH, Belham CM, Al-Hafidh J, et al. A regulatory role for cAMP in phosphatidylinositol 3-kinase/p70 ribosomal S6 kinase-mediated DNA synthesis in platelet-derived-growth-factor stimulated bovine airway smooth-muscle cells. Biochem J 1996;318(Pt 3):965.
63. Mohacsi PJ, Tuller D, Hullinger B, Wijngaard PL. Different inhibitory effects of immunosuppressive drugs on human and rat aortic smooth muscle and endothelial cell proliferation stimulated by platelet-derived growth factor or endothelial cell growth factor. J Heart Lung Transplant 1997;16:484.
64. Geerling RA, de Bruin RWF, Scheringa M, et al. Suppression of acute rejection prevents graft arteriosclerosis after allogenic aorta transplantation in the rat. Transplantation 1994;58:1258.
65. Meiser BM, Billingham ME, Morris RE. Effects of cyclosporin, FK506, and rapamycin on graft-vessel disease. Lancet 1991;338:1297.
66. Schmid RA, Yamashita M, Boasquevisque CH, et al. Carbohydrate selection inhibitor CY-1503 reduces neutrophil migration and reperfusion injury in canine pulmonary allografts. J Heart Lung Transplant 1997;16:105.
67. Gallo R, Padurean A, Jayaraman T, et al. Inhibition of intimal thickening after balloon angioplasty in porcine coronary arteries by targeting regulators of the cell cycle. Circulation 1999;99:2164.
68. Almond PS, Matas A, Gillingham K, Dunn DL, Payne WD, et al. Risk factors for chronic rejection in renal allograft recipients. Transplantation 1993;55:752.
69. Kahan BD, Welsh M, Schoenberg L, et al. Variable oral absorption of cylosporine: a biopharmaceutical risk factor for chronic renal allograft rejection. Transplantation 1996;62:599.
70. Hricik DE, Bartucci MR, Moir EJ, Mayes JT, Schulak JA. Effects of steroid withdrawal on posttransplant diabetes mellitus in cyclosporine-treated renal transplant recipients. Transplantation 1991;51:374.
71. Herzog WR, Zanker B, Irschick E, et al. Selective reduction of donor-specific cytotoxic T-lymphocyte precursors in patients with a well-functioning kidney allograft. Transplantation 1987;43:384.
72. Starzl TE, Demetris AJ, Murase N, Ilstad S, Ricordi C, Trucco M. Cell migration, chimerism, and graft acceptance. Lancet 1992;339:1579.

73. Rolles K, Burroughs AK, Davidson BR, Karatapanis S, Prentice HG, Hamon MD. Donor-specific bone marrow infusion after orthotopic liver transplantation. Lancet 1994;343:263.
74. Kappler JW, Roehm N, Marrack P. T cell tolerance by clonal elimination in the thymus. Cell 1987;49:273.
75. Slavin S, Strober S, Fuks Z, et al. Induction of specific tissue transplantation tolerance using fractionated total lymphoid irradiation in adult mice: long-term survival of allogeneic bone marrow and skin grafts. J Exp Med 1977;146:34.
76. Blazar BR, Taylor PA, Panoskaltsis-Mortari A, Sharpe AH, Vallera DA. Opposing roles of CD28:B7 and CTLA-4:B7 pathways in regulating in vivo alloresponses in murine recipients of MHC disparate T cells. J Immunol 1999;162:6368.
77. Buhlmann JE, Gonzalez M, Ginther B, et al. Cutting edge: sustained expansion of CD8+ T cells requires CD154 expression by Th cells in acute graft versus host disease. J Immunol 1999;162:4373.
78. Odorico JS, Barker CF, Posselt AM, Naji A. Induction of donor-specific tolerance to rat cardiac allografts by intrathymic inoculation of bone marrow. Surgery 1992;112:370.
79. Schwartz RH. Acquisition of immunologic self-tolerance. Cell 1989;57:1073.
80. Nossal GJ. Immunologic tolerance: collaboration between antigen and lymphokine. Science 1989;245:147.
81. Lo D, Burkly LC, Flavell RA, et al. Tolerance in transgenic mice expressing Class II major histocompatibility complex on pancreatic acinar cells. J Exp Med 1989;170:87.
82. Jones-Youngblood SL, Wieties K, Forman J, Hammer RE. Effect of the expression of a hepatocyte-specific MHC molecule in transgenic mice on T cell tolerance. J Immunol 1990;144:1187.
83. Bretscher P, Cohn M. A theory of self-nonself discrimination. Science 1970;169:1042.
84. Mueller DL, Jenkins MK, Schwartz RH. Clonal expansion is functional clonal inactivation: a costimulatory signalling pathway determines the antigen receptor occupancy. Annu Rev Immunol 1989;7:445.
85. Stockinger B. Cytotoxic T-cell precursors revealed in neonatally tolerant mice. Proc Natl Acad Sci USA 1984;81:220.
86. Jenkins MK, Schwartz RH. Antigen presentation by chemically modified splenocytes induces antigen-specific T cell unresponsiveness in vitro and in vivo. J Exp Med 1987;165:302.
87. Quill H, Schwartz RH. Stimulation of normal inducer T cell clones with antigen presented by purified Ia molecules in planar lipid membranes: specific induction of a long-lived state of proliferative nonresponsiveness. J Immunol 1987;138:3704.
88. Li Y, Li XC, Zheng XX, Wells AD, Turka LA, Strom TB. Blocking both signal 1 and signal 2 of T-cell activation prevents apoptosis of alloreactive T cells and induction of peripheral allograft tolerance. Nature Med 1999;5:1298.
89. Streilein JW, Mohler KM. Suppression in Class II MHC tolerance is mediated by Ia-specific lymphocytes that fail to mature into allodestructive effectors. Transplant Proc 1989;21:236.
90. Strober S. Natural suppressor cells, neonatal tolerance, and total lymphoid irradiation: exploring obscure relationships. Annu Rev Immunol 1984;2:219.
91. Mayumi H, Good RA. Long-lasting skin allograft tolerance in adult mice induced across fully allogeneic (multimajor H-2 plus multiminor histocompatibility) antigen barriers by a tolerance inducing method using cyclophosphamide. J Exp Med 1989;169:213.
92. Wood ML, Monaco AP. Suppressor cells in specific unresponsiveness to skin allografts in ALS-treated, marrow-injected mice. Transplantation 1980;29:196.
93. Hall BM, Pearce NW, Gurley KE, Dorsch SE. Specific unresponsiveness in rats with prolonged cardiac allograft survival after treatment with cyclosporine: III. Further characterization of the CD4+ suppressor cell and its mechanisms of action. J Exp Med 1990;171:141.
94. Yoshimura N, Kahan BD. Nature of the suppressor cells mediating prolonged graft survival after administration of extracted histocompatibility antigen and cyclosporine. Transplantation 1985;39:162.
95. Pearce NW, Spinelli A, Gurley KE, Dorsch SE, Hall BM. Mechanisms maintaining antibody-induced enhancement of allografts: II. Mediation of specific suppression by short-lived CD4+ T cells. J Immunol 1989;143:499.
96. Batchelor JR, Welsh KI. Mechanisms of enhancement of kidney allograft survival: a form of operational tolerance. Br Med Bull 1976;32:113.
97. Mohagheghpour N, Damle NK, Takada S, Engleman EG. Generation of antigen receptor-specific suppressor T cell clones in man. J Exp Med 1986;164:950.
98. Lamb J, Feldmann M. A human suppressor T cell clone which recognizes an autologous helper T cell clone. Nature 1982;300:45.
99. Batchelor JR, Phillips BE, Grennan D. Suppressor cells and their role in the survival of immunologically enhanced rat kidney allografts. Transplantation 1984;37:43.
100. Takeuchi T, Lowry RP, Konilerzny B. Heart allografts in murine systems. The differential activation of Th2-like effector cells in peripheral tolerance. Transplantation 1992;53:1281.

Section 8 Solid Organ Transplantation

Chapter 90

Renal Transplantation

Mohamed H. Sayegh and Charles B. Carpenter

Compared to long-term dialysis maintenance a successful kidney transplant improves the quality of life and reduces the mortality risk for most patients with end-stage renal disease. There are three donor sources: cadavers, living related and living unrelated. Graft survival depends on different risk factors in the short (1 year) and long terms (5–10 years). The use of powerful nonspecific immunosuppressive therapies can prevent acute rejection and provide 85–90% short-term survival for HLA nonidentical grafts from both living and cadaveric donors. There is, however, a loss of grafts over the long term which is much less responsive to current drug therapy. The challenge is to develop novel strategies that induce tolerance to the donor, thus leading to prevention of acute and chronic rejection with no or only minimal, immunosuppression.

PATIENT AND DONOR SELECTION

Recipient selection

There are a few generally accepted contraindications to transplantation: malignancy with short life expectancy; poorly controlled psychosis; proven habitual medical noncompliance; active substance abuse; and HIV infection. Conditions that require careful evaluation and prior therapy, if possible, include cardiovascular disease, active infections, metabolic bone disease, active hepatitis and elderly patients. Although age over 60 years is not considered a contraindication, graft survival is shortened because of the naturally lower life expectancy. Patients with diabetes have a particularly high risk of coronary artery disease. Patients with hepatitis B antigenemia or hepatitis C antibodies are at risk for progressive liver disease after transplantation, presumably because of the aggravating effects of immunosuppression.

Donor evaluation

The criteria for brain-death in cadaveric donors have become standardized under the system of organ procurement agencies supervised by the national transplantation network of the USA, administered by the United Network of Organ Sharing (UNOS). Individual physician judgment is operative in matters of age, history of hypertension, length of time after death and anatomic features, and testing to exclude the risk of transmission of HIV and hepatitis viruses has become standard. Living related donors have an extensive work-up to establish the presence of two normal kidneys and ureters, and to rule out both operative risks to the donor and infectious diseases that could threaten the recipient. The scarcity of cadaveric donors in relation to demand has prompted the use of living unrelated donors in selected circumstances. These donors receive the same medical evaluation, with consideration also to medicolegal issues. Many centers currently limit such donations to spouses and very close friends. Follow-up for up to 20 years after living donation in several donor cohorts has shown no signs of renal insufficiency or hypertension in the group as a whole. Should such a donor acquire a renal disease, its progression might be hastened.

DIAGNOSIS AND THERAPY OF RENAL ALLOGRAFT DYSFUNCTION

The most common complication of renal transplantation is allograft dysfunction, which in some cases leads to graft loss. The causes of renal allograft dysfunction vary with the time after transplantation. Hence, the differential diagnosis is best approached by considering the time periods separately.

Immediate post-transplant period

Delayed graft function (DGF) is defined as anuria or the requirement for dialysis immediately after transplantation. Less than 5% of kidneys with DGF never function (primary nonfunction).[1] Postischemic acute tubular necrosis (ATN) is the most common cause of DGF. The incidence of this complication increases with a cold ischemia time exceeding 24 h, with induction therapy including calcineurin inhibitors (cyclosporine or tacrolimus), and with prior sensitization in retransplanted patients, indicating that some cases of DGF may be mediated by immunologic injury. Other identified risk factors include older donors (above age 50), low mean arterial blood pressure in the recipient (<100 mmHg) and a gender mismatch (female kidney to male recipient).[2]

Hyperacute rejection[3] is a rare and generally preventable cause of primary nonfunction. It is caused by unrecognized ABO incompatibility or antibodies to HLA class I (positive cross-match), both of which are contraindications to kidney transplantation. The diagnosis of hyperacute rejection is usually made by the surgeon in the operating room, as the pink kidney becomes mottled and cyanotic. There is little or no urine output, and no renal blood flow on renal scan or duplex Doppler. Renal biopsy shows intrarenal coagulopathy with thrombi occluding the small arteries and glomeruli, and neutrophils are prominent. The differential diagnosis includes pulsatile perfusion-induced endothelial injury, cryoglobulinemia, disseminated intravascular coagulation, fat emboli and anti-GBM (glomerular-basement) disease. There is no effective therapy for this disorder, although plasmapheresis has been tried in uncontrolled reports.

Accelerated rejection occurs 2–5 days after transplantation in patients with or without DGF. It is caused by prior sensitization to donor antigens, but may not be avoided by the most sensitive cross-matching techniques, and is mediated by a rapid antibody response or sensitized T cells. Retransplanted recipients

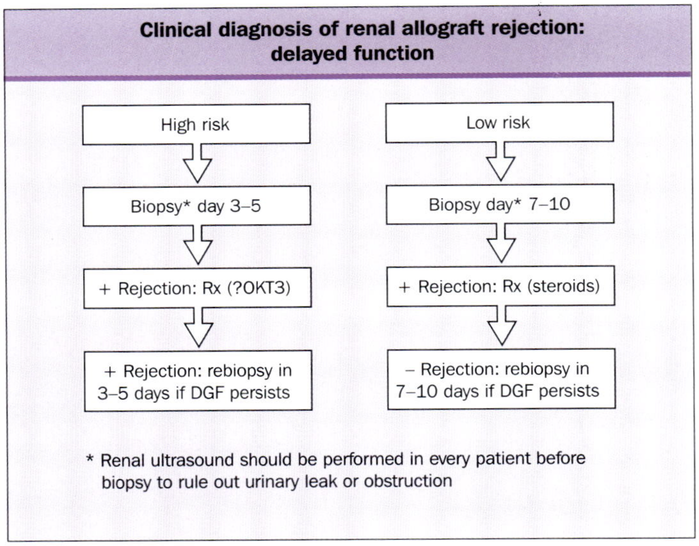

Figure 90.1 Clinical diagnosis of renal allograft rejection: delayed function. Patients at high risk for rejection (sensitized to HLA, previous transplant rejection) should have an earlier biopsy than low risk patients. The presence of acute rejection is treated with high dose corticosteroids or OKT3. If there is no rejection, rebiopsy is indicated if delayed graft function persists. Rejection may start at any time, even in the presence of acute tubular necrosis or cyclosporine toxicity.

are at greater risk. The diagnosis of allograft rejection in patients with DGF can be made only by renal biopsy. High-risk factors for rejection include sensitization and retransplantation (especially in those who lost the previous graft within the first 3 months). The presence of DGF increases the likelihood of acute rejection and resulting poorer graft function at 1 year, but does not lower the 1-year graft survival rate.[2] Figure 90.1 summarizes a practical approach to the diagnosis of allograft dysfunction in patients with DGF.

Early post-transplant period (1–12 weeks)

The most common cause of renal allograft dysfunction in patients with initial function is acute rejection. This is defined as an acute deterioration in allograft function associated with specific pathologic changes in the graft. The incidence of acute rejection and its timing vary with the induction therapy protocol used for immunosuppression, but it can occur in as many as 50–60% of recipients. Early acute rejection episodes can have a major effect on allograft survival, which is decreased at 1 year by 18 and 27% in living- and cadaver-graft recipients, respectively. Some of these kidneys will not regain function even with maximal antirejection therapy.[4] Acute rejection episodes also have a negative impact on long-term graft survival, being the major predictor of the occurrence of chronic rejection, which is responsible for most grafts lost after the first year post transplant.[5]

Clinically, patients typically have decreased urine output and increased blood pressure, associated with a serum creatinine which is either rising or failing to decline towards normal. Fever, graft pain and/or tenderness and graft swelling are uncommon. The differential diagnosis includes ongoing ischemic ATN, drug nephrotoxicity, urinary tract obstruction, and rarely, recurrent disease and infections such as urinary tract infections or cytomegalovirus (CMV). Urinary tract obstruction can usually be ruled out by renal ultrasonography, which should be performed in every transplant recipient with a rising serum creatinine; false negative results are seen rarely when local scarring limits the degree of ureteral and pelvic dilatation.

The most difficult issue related to the diagnosis of acute rejection is the clinical distinction from calcineurin inhibitor-mediated nephrotoxicity and, in patients with delayed allograft function, from ischemic ATN. Calcineurin inhibitors induce renal vasoconstriction and can worsen ischemic injury to the grafts. Figure 90.2 summarizes a practical approach to the diagnosis of allograft dysfunction in patients with initial allograft function. The pathologic changes that occur with acute cellular rejection (Fig. 90.3) include interstitial infiltration with mononuclear cells and occasionally eosinophils, and disruption of the tubular basement membranes (tubulitis) by the infiltrating cells. The presence of patchy mononuclear cell infiltrates without tubulitis is not uncommon in normal functioning renal allografts, and is not sufficient to make the diagnosis of acute rejection. Acute vascular

KEY CONCEPTS

Differential diagnosis of delayed allograft function

- Postischemic acute tubular necrosis (ATN)
- Cyclosporine or tacrolimus nephrotoxicity
- Hyperacute rejection, antibody mediated
- Accelerated or acute rejection superimposed on ischemic ATN
- Urinary tract obstruction due to ureteral necrosis with a urinary leak or hematoma
- Vascular catastrophe or thrombosis of the renal artery or vein

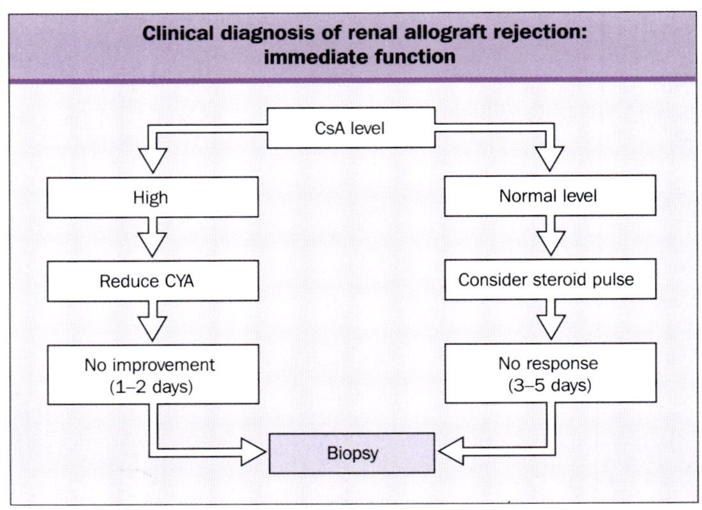

Figure 90.2 Clinical diagnosis of renal allograft rejection: immediate function. These patients initially have a diuresis and a falling serum creatinine, and then a plateau or a rising creatinine level. Although there may be decreased urine volume or increased blood pressure, the creatinine pattern may be the only indication of rejection. Cyclosporine (CsA) levels, if elevated, may be responsible, and a short trial of dose reduction may be useful. Otherwise, biopsy and rejection treatment is indicated. If the clinical picture is clearcut, biopsy may be deferred and done only for assessment of a poor response.

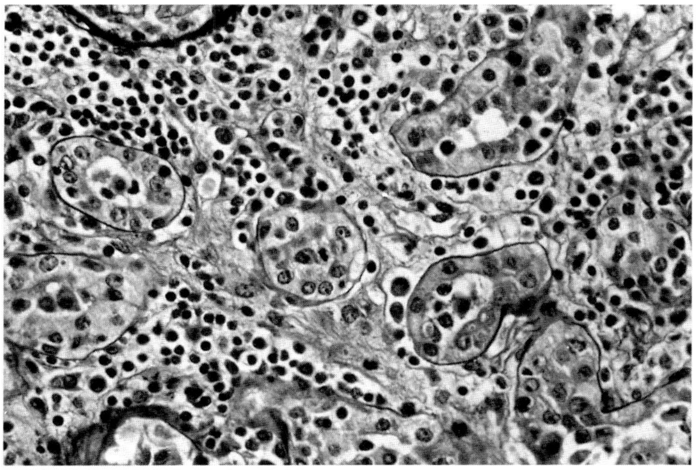

Figure 90.3 Acute rejection, tubulointerstitial. The interstitium is diffusely expanded by an inflammatory infiltrate composed predominantly of mononuclear cells (lymphocytes, monocytes). Most of the tubule profiles also contain inflammatory cells located between epithelial cells or within the lumen (tubulitis). PAS strain, 500×. (Courtesy of Helmut G. Rennke.)

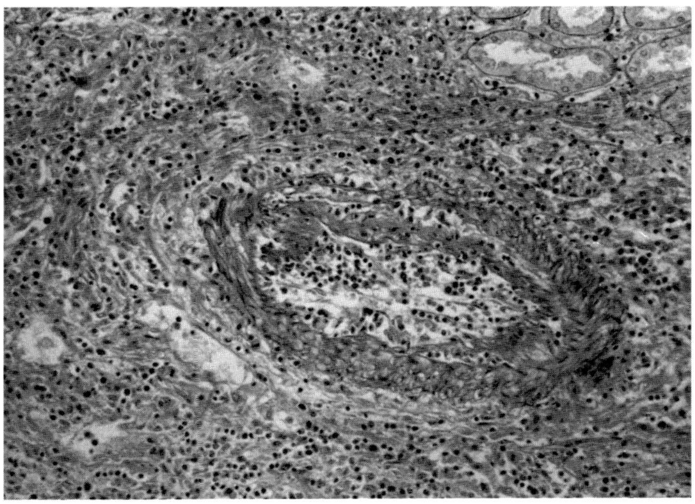

Figure 90.4 Acute rejection, vascular. The interlobular artery depicted here shows prominent infiltration of mononuclear cells within the expanded intima. Isolated inflammatory cells can also be identified in the media. The peri-arterial tissue is edematous and also contains inflammatory infiltrates. PAS strain, 200×. (Courtesy of Helmut G. Rennke.)

rejection (Fig. 90.4), on the other hand, is characterized pathologically by capillary endothelial swelling, arteriolar fibrinoid necrosis, fibrin thrombi in glomerular capillaries, and frank cortical necrosis in severe cases. Interstitial mononuclear cell infiltration may be present in this setting, suggesting mixed cellular and vascular rejection. These pathological changes have also been seen in accelerated rejection occurring earlier than 1 week post transplantation.[3] Complications of percutaneous renal allograft biopsy include macroscopic hematuria (6.6%), transient anuria due to obstructing blood clots (1.2%) and perirenal hematoma (0.7%).[6]

Late post-transplant period

Tapering or stopping immunosuppressive therapy for noncompliance or economic reasons can lead to late acute rejection and graft loss. The differential diagnosis of late acute dysfunction includes prerenal azotemia due to volume depletion, calcineurin inhibitor nephrotoxicity, urinary tract obstruction, and recurrence or de novo renal disease.[1,7] Slowly progressive chronic renal allograft dysfunction is commonly called chronic rejection, but may have elements of chronic calcineurin inhibitor nephrotoxicity, hypertensive nephrosclerosis from poorly controlled hypertension, urinary tract obstruction, and recurrent or de novo renal disease.[7] It is often difficult to determine whether the dysfunction is caused by these disorders or by concurrent chronic rejection. There is currently no therapy for late chronic dysfunction other than adequate blood pressure control and reducing the calcineurin inhibitor dose if there is clear evidence of drug toxicity on renal biopsy. Chronic rejection, defined pathologically as transplant nephropathy or transplant glomerulopathy, is manifested by gradual deterioration of graft function, with slowly rising plasma creatinine concentration, increasing proteinuria and worsening hypertension. The pathologic changes involve all parts of the renal parenchyma, including the blood vessels, glomeruli, interstitium and tubules. The vessel walls are thickened by the subintimal accumulation of loose or organized connective tissue, variable mononuclear cellular infiltration, and disruption and duplication of the internal elastic lamina. The glomerular capillary walls are thickened, with an occasional double-contour appearance (Fig. 90.5). The glomeruli may be enlarged and show a lobular pattern; segmental or, in severe cases, global sclerosis may also be seen. The interstitium shows variable degrees of patchy fibrosis and focal cellular infiltrates with lymphocytes and plasma cells, associated with a variable degree of tubular atrophy and tubular cell dropout (Fig. 90.6). Nonimmunologic mechanisms that can exacerbate the immunologic injury in chronic rejection include hypertension, hyperlipidemia, glomerular hyperfiltration (as the graft contains only about half the number of nephrons in two normal native kidneys), abnormal prostaglandin metabolism, and superimposed recurrent or de novo renal parenchymal disease. Immunosuppressive therapy is generally ineffective, except for patients in whom the precipitating cause is inadequate immunosuppression owing to noncompliance or aggressive drug tapering. Nonimmunologic interventions should be focused primarily on aggressive control of the blood pressure, and possibly of hyperlipidemia. It remains to be determined whether angiotensin-converting enzyme inhibitors provide any special benefit (because of preferential lowering of the intraglomerular pressure) over other antihypertensive drugs. A short-term (3 months) study showed that lisinopril reduced protein excretion in transplant recipients with hypertension and proteinuria without adversely affecting renal hemodynamics or

KEY CONCEPTS

Acute rejection
- Creatinine increasing or failing to decrease
- Decreased urine output, increased blood pressure
- Pathology: cellular and/or vascular rejection pattern
- Therapy: increased immunosuppression
- Differential: acute tubular necrosis (ATN), CsA or tacrolimus toxicity, urinary tract obstruction, infection, dehydration
- Outcome: usually reversed; some loss of renal function

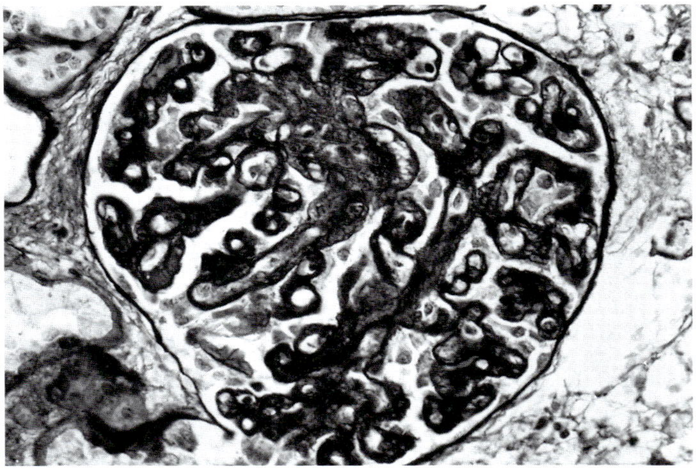

Figure 90.5 Transplant glomerulopathy. This pattern of injury is most likely the result of endothelial injury followed by repair. This results in a double contoured basement membrane which can resemble a membranoproliferative pattern of injury. The mesangium is expanded and may show variable degrees of hypercellularity. This pattern of capillary wall injury is often associated with damage of larger vessels (chronic vascular rejection). PAS stain, 500×. (Courtesy of Helmut G. Rennke.)

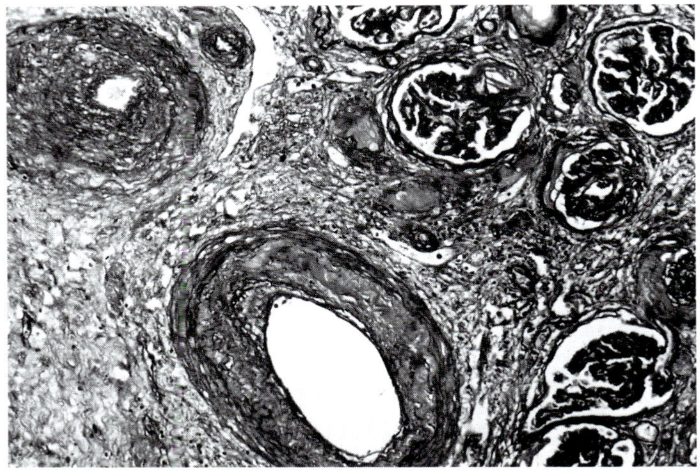

Figure 90.6 Chronic rejection. The arteries reveal prominent narrowing of the lumen by dense connective tissue, most likely the result of organized inflammatory infiltrates from previous episodes of active rejection. There is also extensive tubular atrophy, as evidenced by the crowding of the glomeruli. The glomerular profiles are small and reveal partially collapsed capillaries with wrinkled basement membranes, a sign of glomerular hypoperfusion. PAS stain, 200×. (Courtesy of Helmut G. Rennke.)

KEY CONCEPTS

Chronic rejection
- Slow, progressive renal allograft dysfunction
- Differential: prerenal azotemia, CsA or tacrolimus toxicity, hypertensive nephrosclerosis, urinary tract obstruction, recurrent or de novo renal disease
- Pathology: vasculopathy and fibrosis
- Therapy: immunosuppression generally ineffective, results with sirolimus not yet evaluated, strict management of hypertension

causing significant hyperkalemia.[8] The long-term impact of such therapy on the progression of allograft dysfunction is unknown.

IMMUNOSUPPRESSION IN RENAL TRANSPLANTATION

Induction and maintenance

The optimal induction and maintenance immunosuppressive therapy in renal transplantation is not established. In general, induction strategies used by transplant centers fall into one of two categories. The first relies upon high doses of conventional immunosuppressive agents, and the second uses antibodies directed against lymphocytes, especially T cells, combined with lower doses of conventional agents. A number of trials have been and are being conducted to look at the effects of the different prophylactic antibody induction therapies. These include perioperative administration of antilymphocyte globulin or the monoclonal antibody OKT3. Humanized anti-IL-2 receptor antibodies, daclizumab or basiliximab, or other antibody-like agents, such as CTLA4Ig, that impair T-cell costimulatory signals, will improve the prospects for preventing all acute and chronic rejection and lead to a more tolerant state.

A fundamental feature of all clinically useful drugs for the prevention of rejection and long-term maintenance is their ability to suppress primary, but not memory, responses. The three immunosuppressive agents used in most centers for nearly two decades were corticosteroids (primarily oral prednisone), azathioprine (Imuran) and cyclosporine (CsA). In the past few years several new agents have been introduced (Table 90.1). Myophenolate mofetil has essentially replaced azathioprine, having a similar but more effective mode of action, with much less bone marrow suppression. Tacrolimus, a second calcineurin inhibitor with an action and side-effect profile similar to cyclosporine, is being increasingly used for rescue from cyclosporine failures and as primary therapy. Sirolimus, more recently licensed, has a unique mode of action in preventing the cell-cycle progression in activated T cells.

Corticosteroids

These are the most commonly used component of various combinations with other drugs to prevent acute rejection. There is no consensus on the optimal dose or maintenance schedule of steroids following renal transplantation. Patients are usually discharged on oral prednisone in a dose of 0.5 mg/kg/day. This is tapered slowly, beginning 1 month after successful transplantation to a maintenance dose of 10 mg/day by 6 months. In an attempt to minimize toxicity and to decrease the overall immunosuppression, slow tapering and ultimate withdrawal of steroids has been attempted. Cessation of steroid therapy is often associated with a fall in blood pressure and, in diabetic patients, better glycemic control; total cholesterol levels also fall, but there is an equivalent reduction in HDL-cholesterol and therefore an uncertain effect on cardiovascular risk.[9]

Immunosuppressive drugs				
Agent	**Pharmacology**	**Mechanism of action**		**Side-effects**
		Molecular target	**Molecular effect**	
Corticosteroids	Increased bioavailability with hypoalbuminemia and liver disease	Bind cytosolic receptors & heat-shock proteins	Blocks transcription of cytokine genes e.g. IL-1, 2, 3, 6, TNF-α and IFN-γ	Hypertension Glucose intolerance Dyslipidemia Osteoporosis
Cyclosporine (CsA)	Lipid soluble polypeptide oral absorption poor Microemulsion – more predictable bioavailability	Binds cyclophilin Inhibits calcineurin Blocks cytokine production	Inhibits IL-2 production Stimulates TGF-β production	Nephrotoxicity Hypertension Dyslipidemia Glucose intolerance
Tacrolimus (FK506)	Lipid-soluble macrolide Good absorption	Binds FKBP-12 Inhibits calcineurin Blocks cytokine production	Inhibits IL-2 production	Similar to CsA but less hirsutism/gum enlargement Up to 15% incidence of IDDM
Azathioprine	Analog of 6-mercaptopurine Hepatic metabolism to active product	Inhibits purine synthesis	Blocks DNA and RNA synthesis	Marrow suppression
Mycophenolate mofetil	Good bioavailability Hepatic metabolism to form active product	Inhibits inosine monophosphate dehydrogenase	Blocks de novo pathway of purine synthesis (selective for lymphocytes) Blocks glycosylation	Diarrhea/GI upset Leukopenia less than with azathioprine
Sirolimus (rapamycin)	Lipid-soluble macrolide Poor oral bioavailability	Binds FKBP12 Blocks p70 S6 kinase	Blocks IL-2-induced cell-cycle progression	Hyperlipidemia Thrombocytopenia, mild

Table 90.1 Induction and maintenance immunosuppressive drugs.

Azathioprine

The usual maintenance dose of azathioprine is 1.5 mg/kg/day. Leukopenia is the most serious side-effect. The immunosuppressive effect of azathioprine is not related to the reduction in white blood cell count, and the drug should be temporarily withheld if the white cell count falls below 4000/mm^3. Recovery usually occurs within 2–3 days. The drug can then be restarted at a lower dose and increased gradually to the usual maintenance dose while monitoring the white cell count. Severe leukopenia can occur if allopurinol is given with azathioprine. As a result, these two medications should not be used together or, if necessary, the azathioprine dose should be reduced and the white blood cell count closely monitored.

Mycophenolate mofetil

This inhibitor of nucleic acid metabolism is given orally, 1500–3000 mg/day in divided doses. It has dose-related gastrointestinal side-effects (usually a mild diarrhea) and may need to be reduced if leukopenia develops. It is much less likely than azathioprine to impair bone marrow function, and can be used with allopurinol. Overall, the substitution of mycophenolate for azathioprine has reduced acute rejection episodes by 50%.[10]

Cyclosporine (CsA)

This fungal peptide, after binding to an intracellular molecule called cyclophilin, inhibits the calcineurin pathway initiated by contact of T-cell receptors with antigen, with the result that the cell's ability to synthesize cytokines such as IL-2 is impaired (Chapter 111). The optimal maintenance dose of cyclosporine is unknown, as no controlled trials have been performed;[11] however, periodic trough blood levels are useful in the extremes of >300 ng/ml and <150 ng/ml, and also in relation to significant changes in the patient's baseline levels, especially in interpreting a decline in renal function. The two limiting factors associated with chronic cyclosporine administration are cost and nephrotoxicity. The starting dose is 8–10 mg/kg/day. This is usually tapered gradually over the first 6 months to a maintenance dose of 3–5 mg/kg/day. The withdrawal of cyclosporine is associated with an increased incidence of late acute rejection and a possible decrease in long-term allograft survival. Black patients appear to be at particular risk after discontinuing cyclosporine.[12] Another important consideration in patients maintained on cyclosporine is that several drugs interfere with its metabolism and may therefore cause either overdosing, with deterioration of renal function, or underdosing with an increased incidence of rejection.[13–15] Common drugs that will elevate blood levels include diltiazem, verapamil, erythromycin, ketoconazole and fluconazole; nafcillin, rifampin, phenytoin, carbmazepine and St John's Wort accelerate catabolism. In general, dosage adjustments are not recommended unless the patient has a rising plasma creatinine concentration and CsA levels that are persistently elevated (>300 ng/ml in whole blood) or reduced (<150 ng/ml in whole blood).

Cyclosporine causes vasoconstriction of the afferent and efferent glomerular arterioles and reductions in renal blood flow and glomerular filtration rate (GFR).[11] The exact mechanism of vasoconstriction is unclear, but increased cell calcium, reduced production of vasodilator prostaglandins, and endothelial injury leading to the release of vasconstricting hormones (such as endothelin or thromboxane) may all contribute. Increased sympathetic tone may also be present,[16] although renal vasoconstriction occurs even in denervated kidneys. Clinically, patients have elevated plasma creatinine concentration and hypertension. In addition, cyclosporine-induced renal vasoconstriction can cause delayed recovery from early ATN and, in severe cases, primary nonfunction. These complications are most likely to occur with prolonged ischemic time and high cyclosporine doses (14–17 mg/kg/day). Acute cyclosporine nephrotoxicity is usually reversible on reduction of the dose or after cessation of therapy. There are no specific pathologic changes of acute cyclosporine nephrotoxicity, although the absence of cellular or vascular rejection on biopsy strongly suggests cyclosporine nephrotoxicity. Rarely, vascular lesions of thrombotic angiopathy can be seen (Fig. 90.7). This lesion is idiosyncratic and is presumably initiated by injury to the vascular endothelial cells. It may be reversible if cyclosporine is discontinued promptly, but frequently results in graft loss or only partial recovery. Chronic CsA excess may lead to an obliterative arteriolopathy (suggesting primary endothelial damage) (Fig. 90.8), ischemic collapse or scarring of glomeruli, vacuolization of tubules, and focal areas of interstitial fibrosis, referred to as 'striped'. Whether there is a 'safe' dose that is effective immunologically but does not cause progressive renal dysfunction is difficult to answer because of the lack of well controlled prospective trials. Retrospective longitudinal studies of cadaveric transplant recipients suggest that most patients maintained on 3–5 mg/kg day of cyclosporine after the first year have stable plasma creatinine levels and glomerular filtration rates for up to 5–9 years.[17] In addition to potential glomerular and vascular injury, a number of other renal effects may be induced by cyclosporine, including hypertension and tubular dysfunction manifested by hyperkalemia, hyperuricemia and gout, metabolic acidosis and hypomagnesemia.

Tacrolimus

This is a fungal macrolide which, after combining with FK-binding protein, also inhibits the calcineurin pathway of T-cell cell activation and has the same immunosuppressive effects and major side-effects as CsA.[18] It is demonstrably more effective than CsA in some patients and differs in not causing abnormal hair growth and gum hyperplasia, although in high doses it is more likely to induce diabetes than is CsA. Its dosing is in the 0.1 mg/kg/day range, with whole blood levels maintained between 8 and 16 ng/ml.

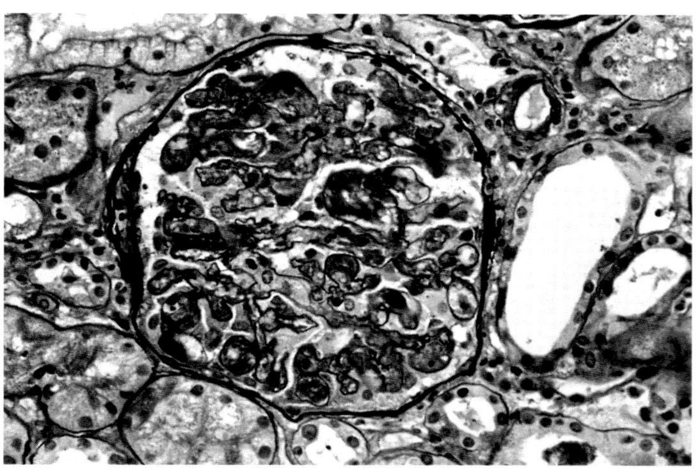

Figure 90.7 Acute cyclosporine toxicity. This glomerulus shows numerous intravascular thrombi that have resulted as an expression of capillary injury secondary to cyclosporine toxicity. The absence of inflammation in the tubulointerstitial and vascular compartments and the presence of other degenerative changes in the tubules (vaucuolization, giant mitochondria, and micro-calcifications) help to distinguish this form of injury from active rejection. PAS stain, 500×. (Courtesy of Helmut G. Rennke.)

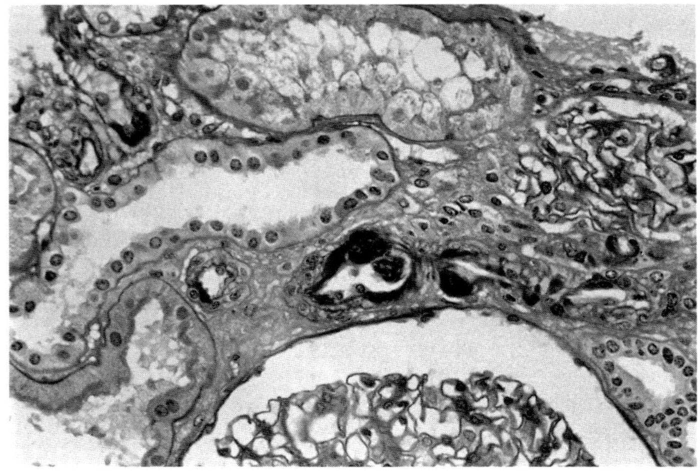

Figure 90.8 Chronic cyclosporine toxicity. The vascular changes depicted here have been ascribed to cyclosporine treatment. There is prominent accumulation of PAS positive material in the vessel wall, often replacing necrotic smooth muscle cells of the media. PAS stain, 500×. (Courtesy of Helmut G. Rennke.)

When administered perioperatively, calcineurin inhibitors can be associated with an increased incidence and duration of delayed allograft function (DGF). Therefore, a number of centers administer prophylactic antilymphocyte globulin (ALG) or monoclonal OKT3, while withholding cyclosporine, until the graft begins to function.[19] Although the incidence of delayed function is lower and acute rejection episodes are delayed with this regimen, overall graft survival and function are no different. In a recently completed multicenter study prophylactic OKT3 appears to be most effective in high-risk cadaveric transplant recipients, defined as those who are sensitized or who have two HLA-DR mismatches or a prolonged cold ischemic time.[20]

Sirolimus

This drug, most recently approved for clinical use, is another fungal macrolide that initially binds to the FK-binding protein but then inhibits a pathway called TOR, resulting in a block in the ability to respond to cytokines, such as IL-2. It has a fundamentally different mode of action from the preceding drugs. Given in daily oral doses of 3–5 mg its efficacy is comparable to that of CsA, and some synergy when these drugs are combined has been shown.[21] Its main side-effect is elevation of blood lipids.

Over time, a reduction in the dose of immunosuppressive drugs is often well tolerated in stable rejection-free patients, but the patient must be carefully monitored and complete withdrawal of all maintenance therapy is never recommended, as it may lead to late acute or accelerated chronic rejection. However, it is likely that combinations of new and old drugs will be more effective, thereby allowing the avoidance of long-term toxicities of calcineurin inhibitors and corticosteroids.

Treatment of acute rejection

Except for low-grade rejection activity, which can best be managed by changing azathioprine to mycophenolate mofetil, or cyclosporine to tacrolimus, for example, active cellular rejection requires major intervention. The three major modalities that have been used are pulse corticosteroids, polyclonal antibodies to lymphocytes (ALG) or thymocytes (ATG), and monoclonal OKT3.[22]

Pulse corticosteroids

The first-line therapy for acute rejection in most centers is pulse methylprednisolone, 500–1000 mg/day given intravenously for 3–5 days. After completing the steroid pulse, oral steroids are restarted using the previous maintenance dose. The cyclosporine dose should be increased if the serum levels are subtherapeutic. The expected reversal rate for the first episode of acute cellular rejection is 60–70% with this regimen. The urine output increases and the serum creatinine starts decreasing within 5 days after the start of therapy. The mechanism of action of steroids in reversing acute rejection is incompletely understood. Steroids probably act in part by suppressing the production of IL-1 and IL-6 by macrophages. This in turn leads to diminished production of IL-2 by activated T cells, thereby lessening the entire cellular immune response. The major complication of pulse steroids is increased susceptibility to infection, especially oral candidiasis. Other potential problems include acute hyperglycemia, hypertension, peptic ulcer disease and psychiatric disturbances, including euphoria and depression. Prophylactic antacids, as well as local mouth antifungal therapy, are generally recommended. Steroid resistance is defined as a lack of improvement in urine output or plasma creatinine concentration within 5 days. In this setting, second-line therapy consists of the administration of antilymphocyte antibodies, either as polyclonal antilymphocyte globulin (ALG) or monoclonal OKT3.

Antilymphocyte globulins

ALG or ATG is prepared by immunizing horses or rabbits with human lymphoid cells derived from cultured B-cell lines or thymus cells, respectively. These polyclonal antibody products, administered intravenously for 7–10 days, have been used both for prophylaxis against and for the primary treatment of acute rejection.[23] The reversal rate varies from 75 to 100% in different series, with the serum creatinine returning to baseline several days after initiating therapy. During the period in which antibodies are given, calcineurin inhibitors are usually discontinued and the dose of azathioprine/mycophenolate is reduced, to decrease the overall immunosuppression and therefore the risk of infection. Complications of such antibody therapy include fever and chills during the initial infusion. Anaphylactic reactions, including respiratory distress and hypotension, are exceedingly rare. A pruritic skin rash (20%) and presumed antiplatelet antibody-induced thrombocytopenia of varying severity (50%) can occur later in the course. Both CMV and herpes infections may also be seen, but with current prophylactic antiviral therapy are now rarely life-threatening. In contrast to murine monoclonal antibodies (such as OKT3), polyclonal antibodies do not generally induce a host antibody response to the horse or rabbit serum. As a result, there is a greater opportunity for successful readministration. In some cases these products have been used to reverse rebound rejection following OKT3 administration in patients with high titers of antimouse antibodies, which can limit retreatment with OKT3.

OKT3

OKT3 is the first mouse monoclonal antibody licensed for antirejection therapy.[24] Its mechanism of action is related to the inhibition of cell-mediated immunity via modulation/clearing of CD3+ T cells. OKT3 has been used both as the primary treatment of acute rejection and as rescue therapy for resistant rejection. The usual dose is 5 mg intravenously daily for 10–14 days. Cyclosporine is usually discontinued during this period and then restarted 3 days before the end of the course. The expected reversal rate with OKT3 is between 70 and 90% for steroid- and/or ALG-resistant rejection. The plasma creatinine concentration typically increases for the first 2–3 days of OKT3 therapy and then declines. However, rebound rejection occurs in approximately 30% of cases; roughly 75% of these episodes can be reversed by pulse steroids. OKT3 is also used as primary induction therapy in the minority of patients who have predominantly vascular rejection,[25] a process that is generally more resistant to steroids and ALG. The reversal rate of cellular acute episodes is 80–90%; however, ultimate allograft function is worse than in patients with milder steroid sensitive rejections. OKT3 is associated with a common first-dose reaction, which may include fever (70–100%), rigors (30%), nausea, vomiting and diarrhea (15–20%), hypotension, and chest pain, dyspnea or wheezing (10–20%). Most of these symptoms are thought to be mediated by T-cell release of cytokines, such as tumor necrosis factor, IL-2, and interferon-γ. Dyspnea, on the other hand, may be related to neutrophil sequestration in the pulmonary circulation. Two other serious complications can occur. First, fatal pulmonary edema has rarely developed in patients whose weight at the start of therapy was more than 3% above their dry weight. Fluid removal with diuretics or ultrafiltration is therefore recommended in fluid-overloaded patients prior to OKT3. Second, aseptic meningitis has been reported in 3–5% of patients. OKT3 can predispose the patients to potentially life-threatening infections, especially those due to CMV. The incidence of infection increases from 16% after one exposure to 62% after two exposures, to almost 100% after three exposures. Patients receiving multiple courses may also develop Epstein–Barr virus-related lymphoproliferative disorders.[26] Approximately 15–20% of renal transplant patients have recurrent episodes of acute rejection. The success rate of retreatment with OKT3 in this setting is related to its ability to modulate/clear CD3+ T cells.[27] This is determined by two factors: circulating antimouse antibody titers and the timing of the rejection episode. Low antibody titers (<1:100) do not affect the response to retreatment if the rejection episode occurs within 90 days after transplantation. On the other hand, titers above 1:100, or recurrent rejection beyond 90 days, are associated with a reversal rate of less than 25%.

KEY CONCEPTS

Immunosuppression

- Induction and maintenance: corticosteroids, CsA or tacrolimus, mycophenolate mofetil or azathioprine, sirolimus, monoclonal antibodies to IL-2 receptor (various combinations)
- Acute rejection:
  - first-line, pulse corticosteroids
  - second-line, polyclonal antilymphocyte or antithymocyte globulin, monoclonal OKT3

INFECTIONS IN RENAL TRANSPLANTATION

Infections are the leading cause of morbidity and mortality in the early post-transplant period, as more than 80% of recipients suffer at least one episode of infection in the first year. The level of overall immunosuppression used for induction therapy, maintenance therapy and the treatment of acute rejection episodes is the major risk factor. The occurrence of certain types of infections, as well as the organisms involved, tends to follow a general temporal pattern in the post-transplant period. In the first month are the usual postoperative surgical infections, bacterial or fungal organisms causing wound infection, bacterial pneumonia, and bacterial or fungal infections related to urinary catheters or central venous lines. In the period from 1 to 6 months after transplantation, infections with immunomodulating viruses, particularly CMV, are most important. In addition to the clinical syndromes induced by these viruses, their immunomodulating properties predispose to opportunistic infections with such organisms as *Pneumocystis carinii*, *Listeria monocytogenes* and *Aspergillus fumigatus*. Most patients in the late post-transplant period who have stable allograft function and are maintained on minimal immunosuppressive therapy have a low infection risk, similar to that seen in the general population (influenza, pneumococcal pneumonia, benign urinary tract infections etc.). A small number of patients (5–15%) having a history of multiple acute rejection episodes necessitating high levels of immunosuppression are at risk for serious opportunistic infections, with significant morbidity and mortality.

Overall, the most common serious infections are hepatitis, urinary tract infections and CMV.

Hepatitis

Liver disease is an important cause of morbidity and mortality in renal transplant recipients, with abnormalities in liver function occurring in up to 24% of patients in the early post-transplant period,[28,29] and death due to liver failure occurring in 8–28% of long-term survivors.[30] Many factors have been implicated in the etiology of post-transplantation liver disease, including drug toxicity and viral infection. Early focus was on the hepatitis B virus, because of the available assays for antibodies and antigens relevant to this virus, but when exposure to hepatitis C could be documented by an assay to detect antibody against a recombinant viral antigen [c100] from the hepatitis C virus,[31] it was possible to trace the transmission of HCV, and its role in acute and chronic liver disease and hepatocellular carcinoma is now better understood.[32,33] Transmission by transfusion of blood products has been unequivocally demonstrated, and preliminary data suggest that sexual, vertical and intrafamilial spread also occurs.

Transplant recipients are potentially at risk of developing HCV owing to *reactivation* of pretransplantation HCV infection or to infection *acquired* from blood products received at the time of transplantation or from HCV-infected organ donors. Stored sera from 716 consecutive cadaver organ donors from 1986 to 1990 were screened for anti-HCV using the ELISA-1: 13 anti-HCV-positive donors were identified,[32,33] and these provided organs for 29 recipients. Fourteen (48%) of these recipients developed non-A, non-B hepatitis after transplantation; 12 had chronic liver disease and one had subfulminant hepatic failure. Post-transplantation sera tested positive for HCV RNA in all of the recipients from HCV RNA-positive donors, suggesting that almost all patients are at risk in this setting. In view of the high risk of both infection and progressive liver disease, most organ banks have adopted a policy restricting the use of HCV-positive donors to life-saving transplants (heart, liver or lung). A similar policy has been recommended by the United States Public Health Service Inter-agency Guidelines.[34]

The natural history of HCV infection and the host response to the virus in transplant recipients[32] are different from those observed in healthy individuals with post-transfusion hepatitis.[35] A large proportion of nontransplanted patients with HCV infection have no evidence of liver disease, whereas approximately 50% of patients with post-transfusion non-A, non-B hepatitis progress to chronic liver disease; in contrast, a majority of patients with post-transplantation liver disease progress to chronic hepatitis or develop subfulminant liver failure, and none clear the virus from the serum. Immunosuppression impairs the anti-HCV response in transplant recipients with HCV, as only 62% of recipients originally HCV RNA-negative show evidence of seroconversion, despite the almost uniform presence of HCV RNA.[32,33] Interferon (IFN)-α has been used with considerable success in nontransplant patients with chronic active hepatitis due to HCV,[36] apparently including those with mixed cryoglobulinemia or HCV-induced glomerular disease. Unfortunately, therapy with IFN-α carries the risk of inducing or facilitating rejection in the allograft, and the efficacy of IFN-α in treating HCV infection in the immunosuppressed transplant recipient is unproven.

Urinary tract infections

Urinary tract infections (UTIs) are the most common bacterial infections occurring in the renal transplant recipient, affecting approximately 30–40% of patients.[37] The major risk factors include indwelling bladder catheters, which are routinely used for at least 2–3 days after transplantation; handling and trauma to the kidney and ureter during surgery; anatomic abnormalities of the native or transplanted kidneys (such as vesicoureteral reflux; stones, or stents placed for the relief of urinary tract obstruction); neurogenic bladder, especially in diabetic patients; and possibly rejection injury and the effects of immunosuppression. Hospital-acquired infections are more serious, with bacteremia occurring in approximately 12% and graft infection in 90% of recipients. UTIs developing more than 3–6 months after transplantation are usually more benign and are clinically indistinguishable from UTIs in the general population. In the absence of pyelonephritis or bacteremia they can be treated with a conventional 10–14-day course of oral antibiotics. The typical microorganisms causing post-transplant UTI are the enteric gram-negative bacilli and enterococci. In addition, *Corynebacterium urealyticum* (group D2) has been recognized as a potential new pathogen that may be responsible for up to 10% of cases, versus less than 2% of UTIs in the general population.[38] This observation is clinically important because C. *urealyticum* is difficult to isolate and is not sensitive to conventional oral antibiotics. The treatment of choice is with vancomycin. Routine administration of trimethoprim–sulfamethoxazole is common practice for prophylaxis against *Pneumocystis carinii*, and it has also been shown to reduce the incidence of UTI and resultant bacteremia in renal transplant recipients.[39] The dose should be adjusted according to renal function.

Cytomegalovirus

Cytomegalovirus (CMV) is the most important infection in renal transplant recipients.[40] Onset of the febrile illness is usually delayed until 3–4 weeks after transplantation. It is characteristically a disease of the second and third months, but may occur at any time thereafter. Previous exposure to the virus, as indicated by the presence of detectable IgG anti-CMV antibodies in the plasma, increases with age in the general population and is present in more than one-third of donors and recipients prior to transplantation. It is therefore common for the donor and/or the recipient to be CMV positive at the time of transplantation. The virus can be transmitted from the donor either by blood transfusion or by the transplanted kidney; the concurrent administration of immunosuppressive drugs to prevent rejection further increases the risk of infection. Thus, both the recipient and the donor are routinely tested for anti-CMV antibodies prior to transplantation. There is an important distinction between CMV infection and CMV disease. Infection is considered to be present if one or more of the following are noted: seroconversion, with the appearance of anti-CMV IgM antibodies; a fourfold increase in pre-existing anti-CMV IgG titers; and/or isolation of the virus. CMV disease, in contrast, requires clinical signs of infection, such as fever, leukopenia or organ involvement, including hepatitis, pneumonitis, pancreatitis, colitis, meningoencephalitis and, rarely, myocarditis. Active CMV infection itself has an immunosuppressive effect and can set the stage for clinically important infections, such as other viruses, bacteria and *Pneumocystis carinii*.[40] CMV disease risk has been established in renal transplant recipients to be particularly high when CMV antibody-positive kidney donors are used for CMV antibody-negative recipients. Because in the absence of prophylactic therapy the mortality rate is 15%, it has been recommended that these patients receive prophylactic therapy with CMV hyperimmune globulin;[41] however, prophylaxis with ganciclovir has been used more generally. Reactivation of latent virus occurs in approximately 50% of cases, especially when OKT3 or ALG is included in the antirejection protocol.[42]

MALIGNANCIES

Lymphoproliferative disorders

Lymphoproliferative disorders are among the most serious and potentially fatal complications of chronic immunosuppression in renal transplant recipients, second only to nonmelanoma skin cancer and in situ cervical cancer, and accounting for 21% of all malignancies versus 5% of malignancies in the general population.[43] Non-Hodgkin's lymphoma (NHL) accounts for 65% of lymphomas in the general population, compared to 93% in transplant recipients. These tumors are mostly large-cell lymphomas, the great majority of which are of the B-cell type. Extranodal involvement is common, occurring in approximately 70% of cases. Twenty to 25% have central nervous system disease, which is rare in the general population, and a similar proportion have infiltrative lesions in the allograft itself. The pathogenesis of post-transplant NHL appears to be related to B-cell proliferation induced by Epstein–Barr virus (EBV) infection in the setting of chronic immunosuppression.[44] Furthermore, the degree of overall immunosuppression appears to be a major determinant of the development of a lymphoproliferative disorder.[45] In particular, transplant patients who are at increased risk for the development of NHL or other lymphoproliferative disorders are those treated with cyclosporine or polyclonal (antilymphocyte serum) or monoclonal (OKT3) antilymphocyte antibodies.[46,47] The progression appears to be one of EBV-driven proliferation leading to fully malignant monoclonal expansion.

Other cancers

The most common malignancy in renal transplant patients is skin cancer, which has been increasing in incidence over the years. Careful monitoring of skin lesions for removal is essential, and patients should be instructed to avoid direct exposure to sunlight or to use heavy sunscreens when exposed. In females cervical cancer is also more frequent, and requires Pap smear monitoring. Another malignancy related to states of immunosuppression, Kaposi's sarcoma, is uncommon in organ transplant recipients.

SPECIAL ISSUES IN KIDNEY TRANSPLANTATION

Dialysis versus transplantation

Direct comparison between morbidity and mortality figures for patients who remain on chronic dialysis and those who receive transplants is difficult because there is some selection bias towards younger and healthier patients as transplant candidates. A recent study of a large end-stage renal disease cohort of over 220 000 patients on long-term dialysis showed that of the more than 46 000 who were placed on the waiting list for transplantation between 1991 and 1996, half received cadaveric transplants before the end of 1997.[48] Although the early mortality rates up to 3 months were higher in the transplanted patients, the overall projected life expectancy was 10 years in the nontransplanted group and 20 years in those who were transplanted. This study, made possible by the merging of the end-stage renal disease and transplant databases, confirmed previous estimates from cross-sectional data on different sets of patients.[49,50] A small cohort of 226 transplanted patients followed for 3 years revealed an improved level of general health with successful transplantation: 64% with functioning transplants were capable of working part or full time, whereas only 32% of the patients with failed transplants were so classified. If the failures were retransplanted successfully, however, this figure rose to 73%.[50]

HLA matching

Antigens of the major histocompatibility complex system, called HLA in humans, provide the major barrier to acceptance of renal transplants. Proof of this was first obtained with living related donor transplants, wherein graft survival was found to be superior in sibling pairs inheriting the same HLA antigens, compared to randomly matched cadaveric donors treated with the same immunosuppressive drugs. There was an intermediate level of graft survival in haploidentical parent–child or sibling–sibling transplants, in which one but not both of the haplotypes matched (Table 90.2). Although there have been numerous reports on the benefits of HLA antigen matching in cadaveric transplantation over the years, there have also been some negative studies. These discordant results have been due in part to the fact that most single-center studies have not included sufficient numbers of well-matched cases to establish the role of such matching. Furthermore, widespread competence in both class I and class II typing, particularly the latter, has been achieved only in the past

HLA mismatching and graft survival			
Types of donor	**Mismatches***	**Half-life (yrs)**	**10-yr graft survival (%)**
Living			
Related (HLA identical)	0	24.0	74
Related (1-HLA haplotype)	3	12.0	54
Unrelated (spouse)	4	12.0	54
Cadaver			
1992 (6-antigen match)	0	20.3	65
1996 (0 antigen mismatch)	0	14.0	57
any mismatch	1–6	9.0	40
	1–2	10.4	45
	3–4	8.4	38
	5–6	7.7	34

*Total number of antigens considered = 6 (2 HLA-A, 2 HLA-B, and 2 HLA-DR).

Table 90.2 HLA mismatching effects on renal graft survival.*

decade. The most valuable databases now in existence are those with pooled information from a large number of collaborating centers. Although such pooled data may suffer from variations in protocols and undocumented selection factors, the power becomes compelling when several thousands of patients are included. Two international registries[50–52] have collected data for several years on tens of thousands of cases, and provide insights into risk factors related to donor source, blood transfusion, immunosuppressive modality, and HLA matching and sensitization. Most transplants that will be lost from acute rejection will be so within the first year; later graft loss is primarily due to chronic progressive dysfunction, generally lumped together as 'chronic rejection', but not responsive to current immunosuppressive regimens. Log-linear plots of graft survival after the first year show a straight-line decline, making it possible to calculate a transplant half-life and to project probable future survival. For grafts that have survived 1 year, long-term survival is best in HLA-identical kidneys and worst in cadaver kidneys (Table 90.2). Mismatches for HLA antigens of the A, B, DR loci are commonly scored equally, but do not in fact have equal weight. The major impact comes from the DR antigens, with smaller additional effect from the A and B antigens.[51,53] Therefore, priority for HLA-DR matching (avoidance of mismatches) is used in many European centers. In contrast, avoidance of all HLA-A, -B and -DR mismatches ('6-antigen match') is the only mandatory sharing rule for cadaveric kidney grafts in the USA. Such grafts have a 14–20-year half-life,[50,54] a result superior to that with one-haplotype-matched living related and unrelated donors (Table 90.2). If zero mismatched recipients are defined by DNA typing techniques, the results are at the 20-year half-life level. Long-term graft survival may also be related to the presence or absence of early rejection episodes. As an example, an 18-center study evaluated the relationship between rejection episodes in first cadaveric grafts within the first 60 days after transplantation, 1-year graft survival, and HLA-B and HLA-DR mismatches.[4] A strong matching effect was found in 689 patients who experienced early rejection, with a spread in 1-year survival rates from 78 to 59% for 0–4 mismatches, respectively; the spread was less – from 96 to 85% – in 1576 patients without an early rejection episode. This finding suggests that early rejection

KEY CONCEPTS

HLA matching in renal transplantation
- HLA-identical grafts from siblings have greatest survival (74% survival at 10 yrs)
- HLA-zero mismatched cadaveric donors (57% at 10 yrs, and 65% if identical by DNA typing)
- HLA-half identical living donors, and living unrelated donors (54% at 10 yrs)
- HLA-mismatched cadaveric donors (40% at 10 yrs)

increases the risk of future graft failure, which is less likely to occur with a reduction in the HLA barrier. Despite the importance of HLA matching, some seemingly well-matched kidneys are still rejected, particularly in patients sensitized by previous transplants or transfusions, and in some cases non-HLA antigens expressed on endothelial cells are targets for rejection. An important limitation of HLA matching is the difficulty in finding well-matched kidneys (15% of the national pool) and the logistic constraints of shipping very large numbers of kidneys between centers for improvements of only 2–5% in graft survival when HLA antigens are only partially matched.

Presensitization

Antibodies against HLA class I (A, B, C) or class II (DR, DQ) are found in subjects who have been immunized to these glycoproteins. They develop as a result of pregnancy, blood transfusion, or a prior HLA-mismatched allograft. The risk of generalized sensitization is higher in multiparous women who are subsequently transfused, and in dialysis patients with a history of a failed renal allograft.[55] Testing is performed periodically on serum samples reacted against lymphocytes from individual reference panel members. Such panel-reactive antibodies (PRA) are expressed as a percentage of cells positive. Highly sensitized patients (PRA >50%) have a lesser chance of being transplanted because of their high likelihood of a positive pretransplant cross-match. Such patients now wait 2–5 years or more for a cross-match-compatible donor. Highly sensitized patients also have somewhat lower 1- and 2-year allograft survival, despite the presence of a negative pretransplant cross-match. More sensitive techniques involving fluorescence with flow cytometry[56] may be useful, especially in previously transplanted patients. Anticlass II antibodies are also not typically predictive of early graft failure. Rare exceptions can occur when, for some reason, the donor organ endothelium is up-regulated for expression of HLA class II antigens.[57] Finally, the excess failure rate of 5–10% may not be from antibodies, but from the associated T-lymphocyte sensitivity, which is difficult to test for in the pretransplant hours.

Blood transfusion and sensitization

Approximately 30% of transfused individuals develop anti-HLA antibodies, with a higher rate in previously pregnant women and a lower rate in males.[58] Responders and nonresponders to blood transfusions declare themselves fairly early after the initiation of a series of blood transfusions, with very few nonresponders converting after the first 6 months on dialysis. It is possible that a major effect of blood transfusions is to reveal strong immune response preferences, at least in terms of antibody formation in responders. In this view, blood transfusions provide a process of negative selection, with the result that transplants destined to early failure are avoided. Close attention to rejection events provides evidence that transfusions are beneficial in patients destined to have rejection activity, and nontransfused patients have more early rejection episodes.[59] Unfortunately, there are at present no reliable predictive tests to show who needs to have transfusions prior to transplantation. When the HLA type of both blood donor and recipient is known, it has been shown that a one-HLA-DR antigen match results in a lower PRA after a single transfusion than with a complete HLA-mismatched transfusion. Furthermore, both kidney and heart transplant recipients had reduced rejection frequency and superior graft survival when they were transfused prior to transplantation with 1–3 units from donors who matched for one DR antigen with the recipient. As an example, the 5-year kidney survival was 81% with the one-DR match, versus 57% with zero DR match and 45% with no transfusions. In this study, having a one-DR match between the recipient and the *blood* donor was more important than a one-DR match between the recipient and the *graft* donor.[60,61] Careful periodic antibody screening of sera from patients waiting for transplantation, in order to define the specificities of anti-HLA antibodies in sensitized cases, is a useful way to select donors who bear antigens to which a patient has never made antibodies.[62]

Immunological monitoring

The most useful laboratory tests are antibody screens and crossmatches performed prior to the transplant to avoid disastrous hyperacute rejections. A large number of immunological phenomena have been described which correlate with acute rejection in the immediate post-transplant period; however, close monitoring of renal function and graft histology are most reliable clinically. States of T-cell activation (e.g. IL-2 receptors) may be discerned in stable patients, and are not always indicative of rejection.

Infections, both clinical and subclinical, may also cause activation changes in T cells. The long-term stable patient with a selectively depressed mixed leukocyte response or reduction in precursor frequencies of donor-directed CD4 or CD8 T-cell activity may be a candidate for reduction of immunosuppressive drug therapy; however, such observations have been made in only a small number of patients. Assessment of graft biopsies for RNA transcripts reflecting activation states of cytokine and other genes may have application to the earlier detection of rejection activity,[63,64] and demonstration of the presence of peripheral blood T cells primed to polymorphic peptide fragments of donor HLA antigens in patients with chronic vasculopathy[65] may also lead to clinically useful applications. It is likely that future therapies involving attempts to produce donor-specific unresponsiveness in the absence of generalized immunosuppression will depend upon immunological monitoring to assess the results of the tolerance strategies.[66]

Overall status of renal transplantation

Many factors affect the prognosis for successful transplantation. The existence of kidney transplant databases containing tens of thousands of cases is a relatively unique resource in clinical medicine. Multivariant analyses of databases have been mentioned above. Figure 90.9 is a summary of all first cadaveric kidney grafts in the USA for over two decades, showing 1-year graft survival and the subsequent half-life of survival for cohorts of patients transplanted in each year. These data are inclusive and not adjusted for known risk factors.[67] For cadaveric transplantation there has been a year-by-year increase in 1-year graft survival from 45% in the mid-1970s to 90% at present. The known contributing early risk factors include having antibodies to HLA, antigen mismatches for HLA-DR and -B, donors aged over 50, donor death with increased intracranial pressure, and long cold storage times before transplantation. When these and other known factors are normalized, there still remains an unaccounted-for annual increase in the 1-year success rate,[68] most probably the result of a number of clinical selection and management factors. These certainly include better prophylaxis of infections and treatment of hypertension and other comorbid conditions. There is an indication that the half-life – in the 7–9-year range for many years (Fig. 90.9) – has started to improve to a level of 10–12 years.[68] Although mortality rates have also been falling, when deaths with functioning grafts are not counted there remains an overall positive trend in both short- and long-term survival. The data shown are not significantly affected by the introduction of the newer immunosuppressive agents described above, and so further beneficial effects, especially in the promotion of long-term tolerance, may soon be realized.

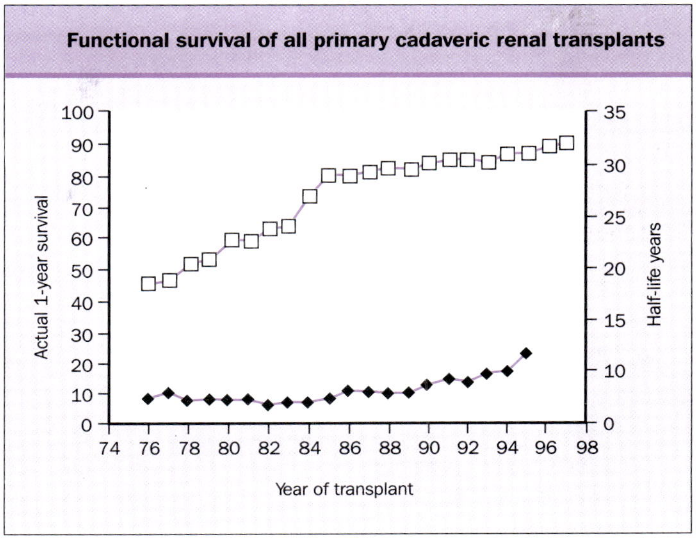

Figure 90.9 Functional survival of all primary cadaveric renal transplants. These are data from the United States, 1976–1997. The registry was founded at UCLA and has evolved into the national repository for data submission on all cases, under the Organ Procurement and Transplantation Network program of the Department of Health and Human Services/United Network for Organ Sharing. There are now more than 10 000 new cases added annually. The upper curve shows the actual 1-year graft survival rate (%), and the lower curve the projected long-term half-life, for each annual cohort. The period from 1983–1985 marked the introduction of cyclosporine with an improvement in 1-year survival that was not matched by the rates of long-term survival, although the latter is now improving. (From Carpenter CB, Milford EL, Sayegh MH. *Harrison's principles of internal medicine*, 15th edn 2001, in press, with permission.)

REFERENCES

1. McKay DB, Milford EL, Tolkoff-Rubin NE. Clinical aspects of renal transplantation. In: Brenner BM (ed) Brenner and Rector's The Kidney, 6th edn. Philadelphia, WB Saunders, 2000, p. 2542.
2. Boom H, Mallat MJK, deFijter JW, Zwinderman AH, Paul LC. Delayed graft function influences renal function, but not survival. Kidney Int 2000;58:859.
3. Braun WE. The immunobiology of different types of renal allograft rejection. In: Milford EL (ed) Renal transplantation: contemporary issues in nephrology. New York, Churchill Livingstone, 1989;19:45.
4. Cecka JM, Terasaki PI. Early rejection episodes. In: Terasaki PI (ed) Clinical transplants. Los Angeles, UCLA Tissue Typing Laboratory, 1989, p 425.
5. Basadonna GP, Matas AJ, Gillingham KJ, et al. Early versus late acute renal allograft rejection: impact on chronic rejection. Transplantation 1993;55:993.
6. Huraib S, Goldberg H, Katz A, et al. Percutaneous needle biopsy of the transplanted kidney: technique and complications. Am J Kidney Dis 1989;14:13.
7. Ramos EL. Recurrent disease in the renal allograft. J Am Soc Nephrol 1991;2:109.
8. Traindl O, Falger S, Reading S, et al. The effects of lisinopril on renal function in proteinuric renal transplant recipients. Transplantation 1993;55:1309.
9. Hricik DE, Whalen J, Lautman J, et al. Withdrawal of steroids after renal transplantation – predictors of outcome. Transplantation 1992;53:41.
10. Renal Transplant Mycophenolate Mofetil Study Group. Mycophenolate mofetil in cadaveric renal transplantation. Am J Kidney Dis 1999;34:296.
11. Kahan BD. Cyclosporine. N Engl J Med 1989;321:1725.
12. Sanders CE, Curtis JJ, Julian BA, et al. Tapering or discontinuing cyclosporine for financial reasons – a single-center experience. Am J Kidney Dis 1993;21:9.
13. Lake KD. Management of drug interactions with cyclosporine. Pharmacotherapy 1991;11:110S.
14. First MR, Schroeder TJ, Michael A, et al. Cyclosporine–ketoconazole interaction. Long-term follow-up and preliminary results of a randomized trial. Transplantation 1993;55:1000.
15. Chrysostomou A, Walker, RG, Russ GR, et al. Diltiazem in renal allograft recipients receiving cyclosporine. Transplantation 1993;55:300.1.
16. Scherrer U, Vissing SF, Morgan BJ, et al. Cyclosporine-induced sympathetic activation and hypertension after heart transplantation. N Engl J Med 1990;323:693.
17. Lewis L, Podbielski J, Sprayberry S, et al Stability of renal allograft glomerular filtration associated with long-term use of cyclosporine A. Transplantation 1993;55:1014.
18. Pirsch JD, Miller J, Deierhoi MH, Vincenti S, Filo RS. A comparison of tacrolimus (FK506) and cyclosporine for immunosuppression after cadaveric renal transplantation. Transplantation 1997;63:977.
19. Steinmuller DR, Hayes JM, Novick AC, et al. Comparison of OKT3 with ALG for prophylaxis for patients with acute renal failure after renal transplantation. Transplantation 1991;52:67.
20. Norman DJ, Kahana L, Stuart FP Jr, et al. A randomized clinical trial of induction therapy with OKT3 in kidney transplantation. Transplantation 1993;55:44.
21. Kahan BD, Julian BA, Pescovitz MD, Vanrenterghem Y, Neylan J for the Rapamune Study Group. Sirolimus reduces the incidence of acute rejection episodes despite lower cyclosporine doses in caucasian recipients of mismatched primary renal allografts: a phase II trial. Transplantation 1999;67:1526.
22. Delmonico FL, Tolkoff-Rubin N. Treatment of acute rejection. In: Milford EL (ed) Renal transplantation: contemporary issues in nephrology. New York, Churchill Livingstone, 1989,19:129.
23. Streem SB, Novick AC, Braun WE, et al. Low dose maintenance prednisone and antilymphocyte globulin for the treatment of acute rejection. Transplantation 1983;35:420.
24. Goldstein G. An overview of orthoclone OKT3. Transplant Proc 1986;18:927.
25. Schroeder TJ, Weiss MA, Smith RD, et al. The efficacy of OKT3 in vascular rejection. Transplantation 1991;51:312.
26. Swinnen JJ, Costanza-Nordin MR, Fisher SG, et al. Increased incidence of lymphoproliferative disorders after immunosuppression with the monoclonal antibody OKT3 in cardiac transplant recipients. N Engl J Med 1990;323:1723.
27. Norman DJ, Shield CF, Henell KR, et al. Effectiveness of a second course of OKT3 monoclonal anti-T cell antibody for treatment of renal allograft rejection. Transplantation 1988; 46:523.
28. LaQuaglia MP, Tolkoff-Rubin NE, Dienstag JL, et al. Impact of hepatitis on renal transplantation. Transplantation 1981;32: 504.
29. Boyce NW, Holdsworth SR, Hooke D, et al. Non-hepatitis B-related liver disease in a renal transplant population. Am J Kidney Dis 1988;11:307.
30. Braun WE. Long-term complications of renal transplantation. Kidney Int 1990;37:1363.
31. Kuo G, Choo QL, Alter HJ, et al. An assay for circulating antibodies to a major etiologic virus of human non-A non-B hepatitis. Science 1989;244:362.
32. Pereira BJG, Milford EL, Kirkman RL, Levey AS. Transmission of hepatitis C virus by organ transplantation. N Engl J Med 1991;325:454.
33. Pereira BJG, Milford EL, Kirkman RL, et al. Prevalence of HCV RNA in hepatitis C antibody positive cadaver organ donors and their recipients. N Engl J Med 1992;327:910.
34. Public Health Service inter-agency guidelines for screening donors of blood, plasma, organs, tissues and semen for evidence of hepatitis B and hepatitis C. MMWR 1991;40:1.
35. Koretz RL, Stone O, Mousa M, Gitnick GL. Non-A, non-B post-transfusion hepatitis – a decade later. Gastroenterology 1985;88:1251.
36. Black M. Alpha-interferon treatment of chronic hepatitis C: need for accurate diagnosis in selecting patients. Ann Intern Med 1992;116:86.
37. Rubin RH. Infectious disease complications of renal transplantation. Kidney Int 1993;44:221.
38. Aguado JM, Salto E, Morales JM, et al. *Corynebacterium urealyticum*: a new and threatening pathogen for the renal transplant patient. Transplant Proc 1993;25:1493.
39. Fox BC, Sollinger HW, Belzer FO, Maki DG. A prospective, randomized, double-blind study of trimethoprim–sulfamethoxazole for prophylaxis of infection in renal transplantation: clinical efficacy, absorption of trimethoprim–sulfamethoxazole, effects on microflora, and the cost benefit of prophylaxis. Am J Med 1990; 89:255.
40. Farrugia E, Schwab TR. Management and prevention of cytomegalovirus infection after renal transplantation. Mayo Clin Proc 1992;67:879.
41. Snydman DR, Rubin RH, Werner BG. New developments in cytomegalovirus prevention and treatment. Am J Kidney Dis 1993; 21:217.
42. Hibberd PL, Tolkoff-Rubin NE, Cosimi AB, et al. Symptomatic cytomegalovirus disease in the cytomegalovirus antibody seropositive renal transplant recipient treated with OKT3. Transplantation 1992;53:68.
43. Penn I. Cancers complicating organ transplantation. N Engl J Med 1990;323:1767.
44. Patton DF, Wilkowski CW, Hanson CA, Shapiro R. Epstein–Barr virus determines clonality in post-transplant lymphoproliferative disorders. Transplantation 1990;49:1080.
45. Penn I (ed) Immunosuppression and lymphoproliferative disorders. PRO/COM, University of Cincinnati Medical Center, 1992.
46. Swinnen LJ, Costanza-Nordin MR, Fisher SG, et al. Increased incidence of lymphoproliferative disorders after immunosuppression with the monoclonal antibody OKT3 in cardiac transplant recipients. N Engl J Med 1990;323:1723.
47 Cockfield SM, Preiksaitis JK, Jewell LD, Parfrey NA. Post-transplant lymphoproliferative disorder in renal allograft recipients. Clinical experience and risk factor analysis in a single center. Transplantation 1993;56:88.
48 Wolfe RA, Ashby VB, Milford EL, et al. Comparison of mortality in all patients on dialysis. Patients on dialysis awaiting transplantation, and

recipients of a first cadaveric transplant. New Engl J Med 1999; 341:1725.
49 USRDS 1992 Annual Data Report. Ch. VII. Mortality rate comparisons of never, previously and currently transplanted ESRD patients.
50. Cecka JM. The UNOS Scientific Renal Transplant Registry. In: Cecka JM, Tersaki PI (eds) Clinical transplant 1998. Los Angeles, UCLA Tissue Typing Laboratory, p 1.
51. Opelz G, Wujciak T, Dohler B, Scherer S, Mytilineos J. HLA compatibility and organ transplant survival. Rev Immunogenet 1999;1:334–342
52. Opelz G, Mytilineos J, Wujciak T, Schwarz V, Back D. Current ststus of HLA matching in renal transplantation. The Collaborative Transplant Study. Clin Invest 1992;70:767.
53. Leivestad T, Reisaeter AV, Brekke IB, Vartdal F, Thorsby E. The role of HLA matching in renal transplantation: experience from one center. Rev Immunogenet 1999;1:343.
54. Takemoto S, Terasaki, PI, Cecka JM, et al. Survival of nationally shared HLA-matched kidney transplants from cadaveric donors. N Engl J Med 1992;327:834.
55. Braun WE. Laboratory and clinical management of the highly sensitized organ transplant recipient. Hum Immunol 1989;26:245.
56. Ogura K, Terasaki C, Johnson R, et al. The significance of positive flow cytometry crossmatch test in primary kidney transplantation. Transplantation 1993;56:294.
57. Halloran PF, Wadgymar A, Autenreid P. The regulation of MHC products. Prog Allergy 1986;38:258.
58. Opelz G, Graver B, Mickey MR, Terasaki PI. Lymphocytotoxic antibody responses to transfusions in potential kidney transplant recipients. Transplantation 1981;32:177.
59. Iwaki Y, Cecka M, Terasaki PI. The transfusion effect in cadaver kidney transplants. Transplantation 1990;49:56.
60. Lagaaij EL, Hennemann PH, Ruigrok M, et al. Effect of one HLA-DR antigen matched and completely HLA-DR mismatched blood transfusions on survival of heart and kidney allografts. N Engl J Med 1989;321:701.
61. Van Twuyver E, Mooijaart RJ, Ten Berge IJ, et al. Pretransplantation blood transfusion revisited. N Engl J Med 1991; 325:1210
62. Claas FHJ, DeMeester J, Witvliet MD, Smits JMA, Persijn GG, Doxiadis IIN. Acceptable HLA mismatches for highly immunized patients. Rev Immunogenet 1999;1:351.
63. Suthanthiran M. Molecular analysis of human renal allografts: differential intragraft gene expression during rejection. Kidney Int 1997; Suppl. 58:S–15.
64. Strehlau J, Pavlakis M, Lipman M, et al. Quantitative detection of immune activation transcripts as a diagnostic tool in kidney transplantation. Proc Natl Acad Sci USA 1997;94:695–700
65. Vella JP, Ferreira M, Murphy B, et al. Indirect allorecognition of MHC allopeptides in human renal transplant recipients with chronic graft dysfunction. Transplantation 1997;64:795.
66. Denton MD, Magee CC, Sayegh MH. Immunosuppressive strategies in transplantation. Lancet 1999;353:1083.
67. Cho YW, Cecka JM. Center effect in the UNOS Renal Transplant Registry. In: Terasaki PI, Cecka JM (eds) Clinical transplants 1992. UCLA 1993, p 333.
68. Hariharan S, Johnson CP, Brenahan BA, Taranto SE, McIntosh MJ, Stablein D. Improved graft survival after renal transplantation in the United States, 1988 to 1996. N Engl J Med 2000;342:605.

Section 8 Solid Organ Transplantation

Chapter 91 Thoracic Organ Transplantation: Heart, Heart–Lung, and Lung Transplantation – a Decade of Change

James B. Young

Solid organ transplantation is well accepted as one treatment option for highly select patients with end-stage diseases having high morbidity and poor survival. It is important to gain insight into heart, heart–lung, and lung transplantation so that these operations can be placed into their proper therapeutic perspective. The goals of this chapter are to define outcomes after thoracic organ transplantation; to describe patients most likely to benefit; to overview current clinical practice; and to discuss the limitations of these procedures. Although the results of thoracic organ transplantation are variable (particularly with heart–lung transplantation), outcomes compare quite favorably with other solid organ transplant procedures and are clearly superior to the natural history of patients with advanced disease otherwise meeting transplant criteria but not undergoing these procedures. A great deal of data has been gathered by the United Network of Organ Sharing (UNOS) and the United States Department of Health and Human Services with respect to clinical solid organ transplantation in general.[1,2] The registries of UNOS, as well as those of the International Society of Heart and Lung Transplantation (ISHLT) and the Cardiac Transplant Research Database (CTRD) Group, are a rich resource that allows the characterization of clinical thoracic organ transplantation practice, particularly over the last decade.[1–4]

THORACIC ORGAN TRANSPLANTATION CHARACTERISTICS

Table 91.1 details the number of heart, heart–lung and lung transplants performed in the United States from 1989 to 1998. This is the most recent UNOS data set and demonstrates several interesting trends. Overall, the number of heart transplants performed has increased from 1705 in 1989 to 2345 in 1998. However, the number of heart transplants actually decreased in 1996 and 1997, and increased by only 2% between 1997 and 1998 (from 2294 to 2345), which was still less than the number performed in 1995 and 1996. It is apparent that the number of heart transplant procedures has, at best, plateaued, and this probably reflects characteristics of the donor organ pool. Heart–lung transplant procedures were never common, with 67 performed in 1989 and even fewer recently. Indeed, in 1998 only 47 heart–lung transplant procedures were carried out. With few data available it is difficult to draw many definitive conclusions from the heart–lung transplant experience. It is likely that the number of transplants of this sort performed has changed because of the ability to perform single lung transplantation successfully in patients who previously would have undergone combined heart–lung transplantation. The annual number of lung recipients has fluctuated over the last several years, but has risen dramatically over time with 93 lung transplants performed in 1989 and 862 procedures in 1998. Overall, 3254 total thoracic organ transplants were performed in 1998, and this represents 16% of all solid organ transplants done that year in the United States, with little change in this proportion occurring in the last decade.

> **CLINICAL PEARLS**
>
> **Trends in thoracic organ transplantation**
> - Over the last decade thoracic organ transplants have accounted for 14–18% of all solid organs transplanted annually.
> - There has been a plateau in the number of hearts transplanted annually, at about 2300 procedures.
> - Combined heart–lung transplant procedures were never common, but recently even fewer are have been performed (47 in 1998).
> - Single and double lung transplant procedures appear to have peaked at around 800 per year, with living related donor transplants increasing in number but still only representing a few dozen procedures.

Table 91.2 details the number of patients on The Organ Procurement and Transplantation (OPTN) waiting list for heart, heart–lung and lung transplants in the United States: overall, on December 31, 1998 there were 7613 registrants waiting for thoracic organ transplantation. There has been a dramatic increase in numbers on the list over the decade analyzed, with heart registrants rising from 1320 to 4185. Interestingly, although annualized mortality for patients awaiting heart transplantation is about 20%, the death rate per 1000 patient-years at risk has dramatically declined for thoracic organ transplant registrants. For example, the death rate fell from 462 in 1989 to 192 in 1998 for patients awaiting heart allocation. The fall in death rate per 1000 patient-years at risk is difficult to explain, but is probably multifactorial. First, many programs are extraordinarily aggressive during the waiting period and when egregious hemodynamic compromise presents, ventricular assist device insertion is the norm. This intervention can successfully bridge patients to transplantation about 60% of the time, and these patients would surely have died had they not been transplanted or so supported. Also over the decade, new medications and more sophisticated therapeutic approaches to heart failure have evolved. In addition, it is likely that less ill patients have been registered more recently as perceptions of long waiting periods emerge. This is an important issue because the therapeutic benefit of cardiac transplantation has never been evaluated with a randomized clinical trial. None the less, we believe that benefit appears in decompensated, unstable patients

Number of thoracic organ transplants										
	1989	1990	1991	1992	1993	1994	1995	1996	1997	1998
Heart	1705	2107	2126	2171	2297	2340	2361	2393	2294	2345
Heart–lung	67	52	51	48	60	71	69	39	61	47
Lung (LRD)	93 (0)	203 (1)	405 (4)	535 (0)	667 (7)	723 (15)	872 (23)	810 (20)	929 (18)	862 (24)
Total thoracic	1865	2362	2582	2754	3024	3134	3402	3192	3284	3254
Total solid	13082	14931	15687	16048	17530	18172	19214	19465	19988	20989
% Thoracic	14	16	17	17	17	17	18	16	16	16

LRD, Living related donor; Thor, Thoracic organ; Total solid, Total number of solid organ transplants performed.

Table 91.1 Number of thoracic organ transplants.

Organ Procurement and Trandplantation Network (OPTN) waiting list at year end 1989–1998			
Year	Heart	Heart–lung	Lung
1989	1320 (462)	240 (468)	94 (421)
1990	1788 (403)	225 (334)	308 (241)
1991	2267 (406)	154 (277)	670 (297)
1992	2690 (322)	180 (195)	942 (287)
1993	2839 (278)	202 (242)	1240 (242)
1994	2933 (256)	205 (264)	1625 (213)
1995	3468 (244)	208 (151)	1932 (204)
1996	3700 (210)	237 (246)	2318 (194)
1997	3899 (207)	236 (207)	2672 (174)
1998	4185 (192)	257 (105)	3171 (173)

Figures in parentheses are deaths/1000 patient-years at risk.

Table 91.2 Organ Procurement and Transplantation Network (OPTN) waiting list at year end 1989–1998.

with profound hemodynamic compromise that can be stabilized enough to allow them to proceed to transplantation. The benefits of cardiac transplantation in less ill, stable outpatients with heart failure are yet to be established. The reasons for the decline in death rates while waiting lung and heart–lung transplantation are probably similar, but more difficult to characterize precisely. Despite this observation, the number of patients dying while awaiting thoracic organ transplantation is large and tragic.

Donor characteristics for heart and lung transplant recipients are summarized in Table 91.3. The number of hearts recovered from cadaveric donors was slightly greater in 1998, after decreases for each of the previous 3 years. The 2450 hearts recovered in 1998 are, however, still fewer than the number recovered in 1994, 1995 and 1996. Furthermore, only 1385 lungs were recovered in 1998, down from 1554 in 1997 and 1695 in 1994. As can be seen from Table 91.3, driving the number of heart and lung donors has been a change in donor characteristics that is most noted for the use of older donors for both heart and lung transplantation. Over the decade, heart donors over the age of 50 increased from 3% to almost 10% of donors used. Also interesting is the fact that the percentage of male donors fell from 72% to 65% for hearts, and the percentage of white donors fell from 82% to 77%. It does not appear that a great deal of difference exists with respect to the cause of brain death when 1998 donors are compared to 1989 donors. Moreover, when transplant recipients of donor hearts less than or more than 63 years of age were compared, 2-year mortality rates were not different, although recipients of younger hearts did have a lower incidence of focal coronary stenosis and less frequent cytomegalovirus infection.[5]

Recipient characteristics of thoracic organ transplant recipients are detailed in Table 91.4. There has been a decrease in the percentage of males undergoing heart transplantation over the last decade (80% in 1989 to 74% in 1998). This is an interesting observation, as the incidence of advanced heart failure is seemingly equal in male and female populations. The reasons for fewer transplants being performed in women are unclear, but may represent impaired access to transplant centers. In contrast, both heart–lung and lung transplants are performed relatively more frequently in women, as reflected by the fact that in 1998 only 51% of lung and 52% of heart–lung recipients were male. Also interesting is the fact that the percentage of white heart recipients fell from 85% to 79% between 1989 and 1998. Minorities may be better represented more recently in the rank of thoracic organ recipients. Repeat transplantation procedures have not increased dramatically for heart or heart–lung recipients, but rose from 2% in 1989 to 11% in 1998 for lung transplantation. Great concern has been raised about the retransplantation issue. As will be seen, the half-life of a heart transplant, for example, is between 8 and 10 years. If transplantation is performed at a young age, patients are likely to present with increasing frequency for consideration of repeat transplantation at the 10–15-year follow-up mark. Adding these patients to the list of individuals awaiting transplantation for the first time will increase the registration list burden. Another dramatic change over the last decade with respect to recipient characteristics is the number of heart patients on life support at the time of transplantation. This has risen from 15% in 1989 to 59% in 1998. A highly significant increase in lung transplant recipients on life support has also occurred, from 2% in 1989 to 35% in 1998. This trend probably reflects the fact that, although the registrant list is dramatically increasing, death

Table 91.3 Donor characteristics.

Donor characteristics	1989		1991		1993		1995		1998	
	Ht	L	Ht	L	Ht	L	Ht	L	Ht	L
% Male	72	69	68	67	69	67	67	64	65	60
% White	82	80	80	80	76	76	76	76	77	76
Brain death										
% Trauma	12	9	12	9	13	15	*7	7	*10	10
% GSW	22	32	23	33	22	26	21	24	17	21
% MVA	34	27	31	25	29	24	34	30	35	30
% Anoxia/Asphyxia	2	1	3	1	3	2	8	5	10	7
% CVA	30	26	29	27	29	29	29	30	31	34
% Cardiac	1	1	1	0	1	2	1	2	2	2
% Age <1	2	1	4	1	3	1	3	2	3	2
% Age <17	22	28	25	30	27	26	26	28	24	25
% Age 18–50	72	73	70	67	64	66	66	68	67	68
% Age 50–64	3	1	5	4	8	8	8	10	9	8
% Age >64	0	0	0	0	0	1	1	0	0	1

Ht, heart; L, lung; GSW, Gunshot wound; MVA, motor vehicle accident; CVA, cerebrovascular accident; cardiac, cardiac arrest.

Table 91.4 Recipient characteristics.

Recipient characteristics	1989			1992			1995			1998		
	Ht	HL	L	Ht	HL	L	Ht	HL	L	Ht	HL	L
% Male	80	51	46	79	46	35	77	48	32	74	52	51
% White	85	92	94	81	93	87	80	88	81	79	91	85
% BT O	38	41	36	37	40	48	38	48	38	39	44	26
% ReTx	3	5	2	3	2	3	3	2	3	4	3	11
% Life support	15	2	2	35	3	8	57	7	16	59	6	35
% Age <1	4	1	2	5	3	0	4	1	3	3	8	11
% Age <17	9	3	11	12	5	24	11	8	17	11	7	19
% Age 18–50	40	63	83	33	49	64	30	45	72	28	40	66
% Age 50–64	48	34	6	51	45	13	53	45	10	52	50	15
% Age>64	2	0	0	5	2	0	6	3	0	9	4	0

Ht, heart; HL, heart–lung; L, lung; BT O, blood type O; ReTx, = repeat transplant.

rates are decreasing and patients ultimately undergoing heart and lung transplantation are clearly more ill than a decade ago. Another important observation is the fact that older heart transplant patients are being seen. Indeed, only 2% of heart recipients in 1989 were over the age of 64, whereas almost 10% in 1998 were older than this. Interestingly, very few older patients are considered to be lung transplant candidates, with only 15% being over the age of 50 in the 1998 experience, and no patients over the age of 64 undergoing lung transplantation in the last decade.

The primary indications for thoracic organ transplantation are summarized in Tables 91.5, 91.6 and 91.7. As might be expected, the majority of heart transplants are done for either end-stage heart failure due to coronary heart disease (45% in 1998) or for dilated cardiomyopathy (42%) (Table 91.5). In 1998, 41% of heart–lung transplants (Table 91.6) were done for congenital heart disease, with pulmonary hypertension accounting for 17% of the cohort. This is up from 31% in 1989, whereas combined heart–lung transplants for primary pulmonary hypertension,

Table 91.5 Heart transplantation – primary diagnosis (percentage of patients).

Heart transplantation – primary diagnosis	1989	1990	1991	1992	1993	1994	1995	1996	1997	1998
CAD	47	49	41	41	43	43	46	45	45	45
DCM	38	37	42	44	42	45	42	42	41	42
Congenital	6	7	9	8	8	7	7	7	8	7
Valvular	4	4	3	3	3	3	2	3	2	2
Retransplant	2	3	3	3	3	2	3	3	3	4

CAD, coronary artery disease; DCM, dilated cardiomyopathy.

Table 91.6 Heart–lung transplantation – primary diagnosis (percentage of patients).

Heart–lung transplantation – primary diagnosis	1989	1990	1991	1992	1993	1994	1995	1996	1997	1998
Congenital	30	25	49	46	38	49	54	54	45	41
PPH	31	29	28	25	27	25	17	10	20	17
Cystic F	16	17	8	4	2	7	3	5	2	0
α_1-anti-T	12	10	4	2	2	0	0	0	0	0
COPD	0	4	2	4	5	1	0	5	0	5
Retransplant	2	4	2	0	3	0	3	5	0	5

PPH, primary pulmonary hypertension; Cystic F, cystic fibrosis; α_1-anti-T, α_1-antitryspin; COPD, chronic obstructive pulmonary disease.

Table 91.7 Lung transplantation – primary diagnosis.

Lung transplantation – primary diagnosis	1989	1990	1991	1992	1993	1994	1995	1996	1997	1998
Congenital	7	5	5	3	6	3	2	2	1	2
PPH	10	17	13	11	8	9	6	5	5	5
Cystic F	7	7	14	13	15	15	18	17	19	18
α_1-anti-T	19	20	14	15	11	9	9	8	10	8
COPD	20	20	27	33	41	39	32	36	36	39
IPF	23	12	12	12	11	11	13	16	14	15
Retransplant	5	4	4	3	2	3	2	3	4	3

PPH, primary pulmonary hypertension; Cystic F, cystic fibrosis; α_1-anti-T, α_1-antitrypsin; COPD, chronic obstructive pulmonary disease; IPF, idiopathic pulmonary fibrosis.

cystic fibrosis and α_1-antitrypsin disease all decreased dramatically over time. This decline is because single and double lung transplants have proved quite satisfactory for treating these maladies. In 1998, 39% of lung transplants (Table 91.7) were performed for chronic obstructive pulmonary disease, 18% for cystic fibrosis and 15% for idiopathic pulmonary fibrosis. A major difference between heart and lung recipients is the percentage not hospitalized prior to transplantation. In sharp contrast to heart recipients, the percentage of lung recipients not hospitalized just prior to transplantation increased from 79% in 1989 to 87% in 1998.

Tables 91.8 and 91.9 summarize thoracic organ transplant patient survival rates at 1 month, and at 1, 3 and 5 years. There was little difference between graft and patient survival rates at all points for all solid organs because of rare opportunities to retransplant when thoracic organ grafts fail. One-year heart transplant survival (Table 91.8) overall is 86%, and 5-year actuarial survival is 70%. ISHLT data registry analysis suggests that the half-life survival for a heart transplant patient is now 9.7 years. Long-term survival rates are highest for recipients in the 35–49-years age range, although older recipients clearly do well when

Survival – Heart transplant	1 Month	1 Year	3 Years	5 Years
Overall	93	86	77	70
Race				
White	94	87	78	71
Black	91	79	68	58
Hispanic	90	84	76	70
Gender				
Female	93	85	75	67
Male	93	86	77	70
Prior Tx	93	86	57	47
Tx Type				
Not hospitalized	93	87	79	71
On life support	93	85	75	68
Diagnosis				
CAD	93	85	77	69
DCM	95	88	78	71
VHD	90	86	76	71
Cong	86	79	68	65
Heterotopic	80	75	57	53

CAD, coronary artery disease; DCM, dilated cardiomyopathy; VHD, valvular heart disease; Cong, congenital heart disease.

Table 91.8 Survival – Heart transplant.

Survival – lung transplant	1 Month	1 Year	3 Years	4 Years
Overall	89	75	58	44
Race				
White	90	76	59	45
Black	81	66	51	41
Hispanic	93	79	47	34
Gender				
Female	90	76	60	47
Male	89	74	56	41
Prior Tx	84	62	35	32
Status				
Not hospitalized	90	77	60	45
On life support	75	62	47	ND
Tx Type				
Single	90	74	57	41
Double	88	77	60	51
Diagnosis				
Cong	69	53	44	39
PPH	80	65	55	44
Cystic-F	93	81	58	49
α_1-anti-T	93	75	58	47
COPD	92	81	62	43
IPF	85	67	52	35

See previous tables for abbreviations.

Table 91.9 Survival – Lung transplant.

they are carefully selected. However, Black heart recipients had lower survival rates than other races. For example, the 1-year survival rate for Black receipients was 79%, and at 5 years only 50%, compared to White recipients having survival of 87% at 1 year and 71% at 5 years. Patients who had a previous transplant had the lowest survival rates at 3- and 5-years time points (47% at 5 years). Among recipients on life support just prior to transplant, survival did not seem significantly compromised. There was little difference in survival rates by UNOS waiting list acuity status at the time of transplant. Long-term patient survival was highest for recipients whose donors were between the ages of 11 and 34 years of age. Patients with a primary diagnosis of congenital heart disease had the lowest survival rates at all time points.

For the 1996–1997 heart–lung transplant cohort, the 1-year, survival rate was 63% overall. Recipients between the ages of 11 and 17 years had the best 3-year survival rates (69%) of all age groups. Females had higher survival rates at all time points.

The 1-year lung transplant survival rate for the 1996–1997 follow-up cohort (Table 91.9) was 75%. Female recipients had higher short- and long-term survival rates than did males. Survival rates were lowest at all time points for recipients who had had a previous transplant. Lung recipients with a primary diagnosis of congenital heart disease had low survival rates at all time points, and idiopathic pulmonary fibrosis patients had low long-term survival rates. Single and double lung survival was similar to 3 years, but double lung survival rates were better at 5 years (51% versus 41%). The long-term survival rates after lung and heart–lung transplantation are substantially worse than for heart transplantation alone. The lung is apparently a more challenging organ to transplant because it is so susceptible to ischemic and reperfusion injury, with peculiar alacrity to have both acute and chronic rejection (bronchiolitis obliterans).[6] These harvesting and immunosuppression management challenges are reflected in outcomes.

It is important to note that long-term patient survival rates appear to increase as center volume increases. For example, at 3 years post heart–lung transplant graft survival ranged from a low of 39% for centers performing fewer than three transplants per year, to 61% for those performing 19 or more transplants per year. A less obvious, but still statistically significant, impact is noted in heart and lung transplant centers performing few (generally less than a dozen) cases annually.

A subcomponent of the UNOS transplant registry is the ISHLT registry. Table 91.10 summarizes portions of a multiple variable logistic regression analysis performed on that database in order to identify donor and recipient characteristics that had an impact on patient survival following heart, heart–lung and lung transplantation in the United States between 1 October 1987 and 30 September 1998. This analysis is consistent with other individual center and registry reports and demonstrates that patients receiving a second or subsequent heart transplant had a much higher likelihood of dying than did those receiving their first heart. Factors related to higher odds of mortality at the 1-year point included a patient being in an intensive care unit prior to transplantation; a patient intubated and on a mechanical ventilator; a patient having received a ventricular assist device; or a patient on an intra-aortic balloon counterpulsation pump. Interestingly, none of these factors had a significant impact on conditional 5-year survival when that analysis was performed, suggesting that even though a patient's medical condition prior

Risk factor	Heart 1 Year RR	Heart–lung 1 Year RR	Lung 1 Year RR
On ventilator	1.96*	5.38	1.78
In ICU	1.11		2.46
Prior Tx	2.57	3.65	1.81
Congenital Dx	1.49		2.32
Tx center volume	1.30		0.82
Donor gender Fem	1.12		0.83
Black vs. Non-black	1.37	3.40	1.32
Donor age (yrs)			
0	0.98		1.70
15	0.94		1.12
30	1.03		1.00
45	1.31		1.21
60	1.91		1.97
Recipient age (yrs)			
0	1.34	0.43	0.35
15	1.00	0.65	0.49
30	0.90	0.96	0.70
45	0.99	1.43	1.00
60	1.32	2.12	1.42
Ischemic time			
0	0.74		0.72
3	1.02		0.90
6	1.41		1.11
9	1.94		1.39
12	2.67		1.73

Multivariable prediction of mortality – thoracic transplant

RR, Risk ratio (all $P < 0.05$ at least).

Table 91.10 Multivariable prediction of mortality: Thoracic transplant.

to transplantation reduced the probability of short-term survival, when they survived the first year later survival was not adversely effected. The only factors, other than repeat transplantation, that had an effect on both short- and long-term survival were the year of transplantation (earlier transplant experience not producing as high survival likelihood), donor age, recipient race and donor race. The largest effect of donor age on survival was seen, naturally, at older ages. In the immediate post-transplant period there appears to be a very slight increase in the odds of mortality for infant donors compared to adolescent and young adults, but this effect dissipates with time. Recipient age and ischemia time had an impact on mortality at 1 year, with an increased risk at both the youngest and oldest ages. As might be anticipated, ischemia time had a linear relationship with mortality. Other factors affecting mortality include diagnosis, transplant center volume, donor gender, recipient gender, level of histocompatibility mismatch, and cause of donor death.

The factors having the largest impact on mortality after lung transplantation relate to either the patient's medical condition (that is, in the intensive care unit prior to transplantation or requiring mechanical ventilation) or diagnosis. At 1 year, patients with an anatomic congenital diagnosis (such as Eisenmenger's syndrome due to congenital heart disease) or primary pulmonary hypertension had a greatly increased mortality compared with other diagnoses, but particularly when compared to emphysema and α_1-antitrypsin deficiency. Patients with chronic obstructive pulmonary disease had decreased odds of mortality compared to those with idiopathic pulmonary fibrosis. As with hearts, higher transplant center volume was related to lower odds of mortality at the 1-year point. An increasing level of histocompatibility mismatch modestly increased the odds of mortality at 1, 3 and 5 years after transplantation. However, other covariates, such as repeat transplantation, transplantation for congenital heart disease, advanced recipient age, and an early era of transplantation, were stronger predictors of mortality. In addition, there was no significant association between ALA mismatching and the development of obliterative bronchiolitis.[7]

Owing to small numbers, multivariant analyses of factors relating to death after heart–lung transplantation were more difficult to interpret. As with the other thoracic transplant procedures, mechanical ventilation and having a previous transplant seemed to have the largest impact on mortality. Other significant factors included recipient race and age, with older recipients having increased odds of mortality.

With the success of solid organ transplantation generally, and an interrelationship between thoracic organ failure and end-stage liver and kidney disease, an occasional foray has been made into combinations of intra- and extrathoracic solid organ transplants. Table 91.11 summarizes such procedures. Combined heart–lung transplantation accounts for most combination procedures over the past decade (565 total). Over the last decade, combined heart and kidney transplant has been performed 164 times, heart–liver 15 times, heart–kidney–pancreas six times, heart–pancreas and lung–kidney four times each, heart–liver–lung twice, and heart–liver–kidney only once. These are transplant procedures generally done at one operation or sequentially within a few days, often using organs from the same donor. None the less, this total represents only 761 patients undergoing solid organ

Multiorgan transplants 1989–1998

Combinations	Total
Heart–lung	565
Heart–kidney	164
Heart–liver	15
Heart–kidney–pancreas	6
Heart–pancreas	4
Lung–kidney	4
Heart–liver–lung	2
Heart–liver–kidney	1
Total	761*

* Representing 0.4% of 174 916 solid organ transplants during observation period.

Table 91.11 Multiorgan transplants – thoracic combination (1989–1998).

transplants between 1989 and 1998, which is 0.4% of the 174 916 solid organ transplants performed during the observation period. Because of the few numbers, anecdotes can be the only description of outcomes. It appears that lower long-term survival is seen after multiorgan transplantation. Because of this, and the negative impact multiple organs going into one patient has on overall organ allocation dynamics, it is unlikely that multiorgan transplants will be embraced with any significant frequency in the future. This concept, however, needs to be addressed more formally because of the association of renal and hepatic failure to the immunosuppressive drugs used during the management of heart and lung transplant recipients. In the future, many patients are likely to present with end-stage renal and hepatic disease after having had a cardiac allograft in place for a decade or two.

WAITING LIST CHARACTERISTICS AND MEDIAN WAIT TIMES

The heart transplant waiting list more than tripled between 1989 and 1998 (Table 91.2), with the number increasing 21% between 1995 and 1998. Pediatric registrants accounted for 3% of the heart transplant wait list in 1989, and for 6% in 1998. Registrants 65 years and older also increased, from 2% in 1989 to 7% in 1998. Black registrants increased from 9% of all registrants in 1989 to 14% in 1998. Although females were only a small number of total heart registrants, the percentage grew from 15% in 1989 to 22% in 1998. At the end of 1999 only 4% of registrants had been on the waiting list for 2 years or more, but at the end of 1998 this group accounted for 36% of the list. On 31 December 1998 temporarily inactive registrants (UNOS Status VII) accounted for 39% of the heart transplant waiting list, and presumably represented those who had either become 'too well' to undergo transplantation at that time or had developed contraindications to transplantation.

The lung transplant waiting list grew more than 30-fold from 1989 to 1998, and increased 19% between 1997 and 1998. The percentage of older registrants has increased over time, with those aged 50–64 increasing from 27% in 1989 to 42% in 1998. Black registrants grew from 3% in 1989 to 9% in 1998, whereas Hispanic registrants decreased from 6% to 2% over the same period. Female registrants increased from 55% in 1989 to 59% in 1998. The length of time spent waiting for a lung transplant has increased dramatically. In 1989, 14% of registrants waited 1 year or longer for a lung transplant, and by 1998 the rate had grown to 51%. Temporarily inactive on the waiting list for lung transplantation were 27% of the patients in 1998.

The heart–lung waiting list has remained small, with nearly the same number of registrants at the end of 1998 (257) as in 1989 (240). This number has probably not increased because single and double lung transplants have replaced heart–lung transplants as effective treatment options for certain pulmonary conditions. The percentage of registrants who had waited 3 years or more for a heart–lung transplant increased from 4% in 1989 to 31% in 1998. Temporarily inactive on the heart–lung transplant list was 29% in 1998.

As alluded to, the death rate for the heart waiting list (Table 91.2) has decreased dramatically over time, from 462 per 1000 patient-years at risk in 1989 to 192 in 1998. Asian registrants, interestingly, had higher death rates than did those of other races. In 1998, the death rate for Asians was 279, compared to 204 for Black and 189 for White registrants. Registrants in the most mechanically urgent status (UNOS Status I) had much higher death rates than others: 671 in 1998, compared to 163 for UNOS Status II patients. Over the last several years, death rates of White lung transplant recipients have been lower than those for all other races: 161 for White registrants in 1998 compared to 254 for Blacks and 247 for Hispanics. Males generally had higher death rates than females. In 1998 the death rate among heart–lung recipients was 180, the second lowest yearly death rate in the last 10 years.

IMMUNOSUPPRESSION STRATEGIES

In a recent analysis of a retrospective multicenter heart transplant database created from experience in 10 centers with over 250 transplant patients followed for the last year (ending January 2000), an insight into current immunosuppressive strategies can be gained. Overall, patient survival 1 year was 89%, with major causes of death being infection (20%), graft failure (12%), cerebrovascular accident (8%), multiorgan system failure (8%) and allograft arteriopathy (4%). The mean time post transplant per patient death in this cohort was 131 days, with a median of 69 days. 'Induction' therapy was utilized in only 16% of patients initially started on cyclosporine and in 17% of those initially started on tacrolimus. OKT3 was used in 24 of 27 patients receiving an induction agent. Three patients received Zenapax. Virtually all patients receiving induction therapy had low urine output and renal insufficiency as the reason for treatment with monoclonal antibodies. This represents a substantial shift in philosophy away from the use of induction cytolytic therapy, which permeated post heart transplant immunosuppressive protocols in the mid-1980s. At the 1-year point maintenance immunosuppression generally included azathioprine or mycophenolate mofetil and cyclosporine or tacrolimus in addition to prednisone.[8–10] Several institutions aggressively attempted to wean patients off prednisone, such that only about half of the cohort were taking maintenance prednisone therapy at that time. Approximately

KEY CONCEPTS

Characteristics of thoracic organ allograft recipients

- In order to maintain adequate thoracic organ transplants (particularly heart transplants) the age of donors has increased, as have the number of comorbid conditions once thought to compromise post-transplant outcomes.
- Despite the increasing number of registrants on the thoracic organ transplants waiting list, annualized mortality per 1000 patient-years at risk has actually decreased.
- Thoracic organ transplant probably only benefits in substantive fashion those patients with the most critical illnesses and at high risk of dying within 6 months of listing if transplant or life-support system utilization does not occur.
- Long-term outcomes are best for heart recipients (86% 1-year and 70% 5-year survival), whereas heart–lung 1-year survival was only 63% (too few patients to calculate 5-year rates) and lung 1- and 5-year survival was 75% and 44%, respectively.

two-thirds were on a cyclosporine-based protocol. There is some suggestion that when tacrolimus was used fewer patients required antihypertensive therapy, fewer had rejection episodes requiring therapies in ad hoc fashion, and more patients could be weaned from prednisone. When biopsy-proven rejection was manifest the vast majority of patients received intravenous pulsed prednisone therapy. Oral pulses of prednisone were used for less severe rejection levels, and cytolytic therapy to treat rejection was invariably used only when multiple episodes of repeated rejection occurred or hemodynamic compromise in association with significant rejection was noted. Steroid-resistant rejection episodes have been successfully treated with tacrolimus.[9] Contemporary lung transplant immunosuppression strategies appear to parallel those of heart transplantation.

DEVELOPMENTS IN THORACIC ORGAN TRANSPLANTATION

Mechanical cardiac assist devices

As the donor availability situation worsens, with more patients being registered for heart transplantation yet relatively fewer procedures being performed, a great deal of attention is being paid to the successful development of mechanical cardiac assist devices to be used as 'bridges' to heart transplantation, or even as permanent alternatives.[11,12] Most systems are either pneumatically activated and driven or use an electrical power source. The Abiomed ventricular assist device (VAD) was the first US FDA-approved ventricular assist device (1992) and was generally employed as a bridge to recovery in patients with postcardiotomy cardiogenic shock. It is an extracorporeal pulsatile device that fills by gravity and is suitable for only short durations of support (days to weeks). The device has been used as a bridge either to transplant or to a more permanent mechanical bridging system. The Thoratec extracorporeal ventricular assist device was approved in 1995 for use in hospitalized patients as a bridge to transplant when the risk of death was extraordinarily high. The HeartMate pneumatic ventricular assist device was the first intracorporeal system approved by the FDA (1994) for use in hospitals as a bridge to transplant. This and the Novacor portable ventricular assist device (also electric) were both approved as bridges to transplant and can be used outside the hospital. Both of these devices have been employed rarely for permanent implantation (that is, without the intent to transplant). Total artificial heart systems have been long in development and slow to be used with any frequency. The CardioWest total artificial heart is a biventricular pneumatic system that has been used as a bridge to transplant and is the only total artificial heart currently under clinical evaluation, although several newer artificial heart systems are getting close to clinical trials. The CardioWest device is the direct descendant of the Jarvik-7 total artificial heart (which was subsequently known as the Symbion total artificial heart). Smaller, possibly less expensive and less complicated continuous-flow impeller-driven ventricular assist devices are entering trials as bridge-to-transplant systems, including the NASA-Baylor MicroMed pump and the latest Jarvik device.

THERAPEUTIC PRINCIPLES

Management of patients with thoracic organ allografts

- In order to optimize thoracic organ allograft function, ischemia–reperfusion injury and chronic rejection (allograft arteriopathy and bronchiolitis obliterans) must be attenuated.
- Aggressive 'triple-drug' maintenance immunosuppression is generally pursued in thoracic organ transplants, and usually includes tacrolimus or cyclosporine, imuran or mycophenolate mofetil, and prednisone.
- Lymphocytotoxic maneuvers with monoclonal or polyclonal antibodies early post transplant to induce tolerance have largely been abandoned recently.
- Mechanical ventricular assist devices are more likely to become alternatives to heart transplant than are xenographic allografts.

Xenotransplantation

At present one cannot be optimistic that xenotransplantation will be a suitable alternative to thoracic organ transplantation. Despite the development of genetically engineered pigs, experiments in primates indicate that adequate performance can only last a few hours for thoracic organs. Of particular concern is the potential risk of infectious disease transmission, especially of retroviruses, from these animals.[5]

Cardiac transplantation research direction

A bellwether of important areas for progress are the major areas of research funded by the US National Heart, Lung, and Blood Institute (NHLBI). Federal support for cardiac transplantation is focusing on the development of coronary allograft vasculopathy or accelerated graft arteriosclerosis (also referred to as chronic rejection), tolerance induction and organ preservation. Chronic rejection is probably the result of multiple perturbations, including the activities of lymphocyte subpopulations, inflammatory cytokines and alloantibodies,[13–16] The harmful effects of organ preservation (ischemia and reperfusion injury), and the role of cytomegalovirus infection, as well as traditional atherosclerotic cardiovascular risk factors such as dyslipidemia, hypertension and diabetes. Chronic allograft vasculopathy is the single greatest cause of graft loss long term after heart transplantation.[16,17] Interestingly, transplant coronary artery disease is not only seen in adult patients, but is also common in infants and children after heart transplantation.[18] A better understanding of its pathophysiology might allow strategies to be developed that would attenuate graft loss from this problem. A greater understanding of allograft arteriopathy would probably also give insight into native-vessel atherosclerotic cardiovascular disease.[19] Several clinical trials designed to induce tolerance of the cardiac allograft are ongoing. Of particular interest is a technique being pursued in animal models for tolerance induction using bone marrow transplantation in conjunction with heart transplantation.[20] If tolerance can be achieved by concomitant bone marrow transplantation, theoretically the cost and morbidity associated with immunosuppression could be attenuated. Tolerance induction via gene therapy is also being explored in animal models,[21] and potentially offers a new approach to long-term cardiac allograft acceptance.

Lung transplantation

NHLBI support for lung transplantation focuses on the preservation of donor lungs, cellular and molecular mechanisms involved in chronic rejection (bronchiolitis obliterans), and strategies for optimal immunosuppression post transplant. Obviously, support of studies on xenotransplantation has implications for lung transplantation as well, as do studies focusing on pulmonary vascular regulation, lung growth, and the development of living related lobar lung transplant procedures. Techniques utilizing gene therapy are being developed to prevent ischemia–reperfusion injury in transplanted rat and dog lungs. Inducible nitric oxide synthase and prostaglandin G/H synthase enzyme levels being increased through the use of gene therapy is being pursued in an attempt to reduce leukocyte adherence and reperfusion injury.[22] Additional studies include those addressing the role of cyclic adenosine monophosphate (cAMP) and the nitric oxide/cyclic guanosine monophosphate (cGMP) pathways in an attempt to understand the pulmonary vascular response, with a focus on the response of the endothelium to ischemia and reperfusion.[23] The role of allogeneic lung macrophages and dendritic cells in mediating allograft rejection is being studied in lung transplant patients,[24] as well as in animal models. The role of cytomegalovirus infection and T-lymphocyte response in the development of bronchiolitis obliterans or chronic lung rejection is being explored.[25,26] A trial of aerosolized cyclosporine versus placebo aerosol as an adjuvant to oral immunosuppression with tacrolimus, prednisone and azathioprine is under way, as is another clinical trial comparing tacrolimus and mycophenolate mofetil with standard therapy consisting of cyclosporine, prednisone and azathioprine. It is specifically hoped that newer and more aggressive immunotherapeutic strategies will reduce the mortality of lung transplantation, and particularly the problem of developing bronchiolitis obliterans.

SUMMARY

Thoracic organ transplantation has provided remarkable options for end-stage lung and heart disease patients at the brink of death. Major limitations to these procedures focus on the development of allograft arteriopathy for heart transplant recipients and bronchiolitis obliterans for lung transplant recipients. These forms of chronic rejection contribute to substantial morbidity and account for the majority of graft loss after thoracic organ transplantation. A new understanding of their pathophysiology, coupled to a better ability to induce tolerance, will undoubtedly improve post-thoracic organ transplant morbidity and mortality. Also critical will be the development of better patient selection criteria, which will help focus organ distribution (as they are rare) to the most ill patients likely to benefit most.

REFERENCES

1. United States Department of Health and Human Services. Report to Congress on the Scientific and Clinical Status of Organ Transplantation, September 1999.
2. United States Scientific Registry of Transplant Recipients and Organ Procurement and Transplantation Network 1999 Annual Report, Transplant Data 1989–1998. United States Department of Health and Human Services, 1999.
3. Keck BM, Bennett LE, Rosendale J, et al. Worldwide Thoracic Organ Transplantation: a Report from the UNOS/ISHLT International Registry for Thoracic Organ Transplantation. In: Cecka P, Terasaki P (eds) Clinical transplants 1999. UCLA Immunogenics Center, Los Angeles, 2000.
4. Working Group of Transplant Cardiologists. Cardiac Transplant Research Database (CTRD): 1999 annual report. University of Alabama, Birmingham, November 1999.
5. Potapov EV, Loebe M, Hubler M, et al. Medium-term results of heart transplantation using donors over 63 years of age. Transplantation 1999;68:1834.
6. Boehler A, Estenne M. Obliterative bronchiolitis after lung transplantation. Curr Opin Pulm Med 2000;6:133.
7. Quantz MA, Bennett LE, Meyer DM, et al. Does human leukocyte antigen matching influence the outcome of lung transplantation? An analysis of 3,549 lung transplantations. J Heart Lung Transplant 2000;19:473.
8. Yamani MH, Starling RC, Goormastic M, et al. The impact of routine mycophenolate mofetil drug monitoring on the treatment of cardiac allograft rejection. Transplantation 2000;69(11):2326.
9. Yamani MH, Starling RC, Pelegrin D, et al. Efficacy of tacrolimus in patients with steroid-resistant cardiac allograft cellular rejection. J Heart Lung Transplant 2000;19(4):337.
10. Mathieu P, Carrier M, White M, et al. Effect of mycophenolate mofetil in heart transplantation. Can J Surg 2000;43:202.
11. Scherr K, Jensen L, Koshal A. Mechanical circulatory support as a bridge to cardiac transplantation: toward the 21st century. Am J Crit Care 1999;8:324.
12. Bank AJ, Mir SH, Nguyen DQ, et al. Effects of left ventricular assist devices on outcomes in patients undergoing heart transplantation. Ann Thorac Surg 2000;69:1369.
13. Cooper DKC, Lanza RP. Xeno: the promise of transplanting animal organs into humans. Oxford University Press, Oxford, 2000.
14. Braun MY, Desalle F, Le Monie A, et al. IL-5 and eosinophils mediate the rejection of fully histoincompatible vascularized cardiac allografts: regulatory role of alloreactive CD8(+) T lymphocytes and IFN-gamma. Eur J Immunol 2000;30:1290.
15. Derhaag JG, Duijvestijn AM, Damoiseaux JG, et al. Effects of antibody reactivity to major histocompatibility complex (MHC) and non-MHC alloantigens on graft endothelial cells in heart allograft rejection. Transplantation 2000;69:1899.
16. Weis M, von Scheidt W. Coronary artery disease in the transplanted heart. Annu Rev Med 2000;51:81.
17. Julius BK, Attenhofer Jost CH, Sutsch G, et al. Incidence, progression and functional significance of cardiac allograft vasculopathy after heart transplantation. Transplantation 2000;69:847.
18. Dent CL, Canter CE, Hirsch R, Balzer DT. Transplant coronary artery disease in pediatric heart transplant recipients. J Heart Lung Transplant 2000;19:240.
19. Young JB. Perspective on cardiac allograft vasculopathy. Current Atherosclerosis Reports 2000;2:259.
20. Gammie JS, Pham SM. Simultaneous donor bone marrow and cardiac transplantation: can tolerance be induced with the development of chimerism? Curr Opin Cardiol 1999;14:126.
21. Guillot C, Mathieu P, Coathalem H, et al. Tolerance to cardiac allografts via local and systemic mechanisms after adenovirus-mediated CTLA4Ig expression. J Immunol 2000;164:5258.
22. Suda T, Mora BN, D'Ovidio F, et al. In vivo adenovirus-mediated endothelial nitric oxide synthase gene transfer ameliorates lung allograft ischemia–reperfusion injury. J Thorac Cardiovasc Surg 2000;119:297.
23. Pinsky DJ. The vascular biology of heart and lung preservation for transplantation. Thromb Haemost 1995;74:58.
24. Leonard CT, Soccal PM, Singer L, et al. Dendritic cells and macrophages in lung allografts: a role in chronic rejection? Am J Resp Crit Care Med 2000;161:1349.
25. Husain AN, Siddiqui MT, Holmes EW. Analysis of risk factors for the development of bronchiolitis obliterans syndrome. Am J Resp Crit Care Med 1999;159:829.
26. Milne DS, Moy JV, Corris PA, et al. Intragraft proliferating T lymphocytes are associated with moderate acute pulmonary rejection. Transplantation 2000;69:1981.

Section 8 Solid Organ Transplantation

Chapter 92 Transplantation of the Liver and Pancreas

John Renz and Chris E. Freise

Extrarenal abdominal organs that have been successfully transplanted include the liver, pancreas and small bowel. This chapter focuses on liver and pancreas transplantation, two procedures that are widely utilized today and which have enjoyed improved success over the last decade.

LIVER TRANSPLANTATION

Since Starzl's successful orthotopic liver transplant (LTX) in a human in 1963,[1] liver transplantation has evolved from being an experimental procedure to optimal therapy for the treatment of patients with end-stage liver disease. Advances in surgical technique, immunosuppression and medical management have contributed to improved long-term survival and universal acceptance of the procedure.[2] As long-term survival following LTX has increased, indications for the procedure have expanded to include metabolic, viral, malignant and acquired liver failure.

Indications and patient selection

Liver transplantation is inherently limited by organ-donor supply. As demand for the procedure has increased, the number of patients awaiting transplantation has exceeded the supply of cardaveric organs available, resulting in increasing numbers of patients dying while waiting (Fig. 92.1).

Currently an estimated 20 000 patients per year are candidates for approximately 4000 cadaveric organs[3] in the United States. Small increases in organ availability have been realized secondary to the use of older donors,[4] marginal donors,[5] living donors[6] and the use of split liver transplantation,[7,8] but the above techniques combined represent a relatively small percentage of the total number of liver transplants performed annually. Besides increasing organ availability, future progress in transplantation will depend on advances in our understanding of the human immune system and the development of techniques to regulate a patient's response to transplanted tissue or to 'mask' transplanted tissues from a patient's immune surveillance.

The indications for liver transplantation have expanded over the last decade (Table 92.1). Typically, potential recipients need to undergo extensive work-up to evaluate other comorbidities. Once placed on the waiting list, patients may progress with their liver disease and develop complications that could then eliminate them as a candidate for transplant. As waiting times have grown more patients receive transplants while critically ill in intensive care units. Although excellent results are still possible, more resources are necessary to support a critically ill patient through the recovery period from transplantation.

Summary of US data for liver transplant procedures performed for years 1988–1998

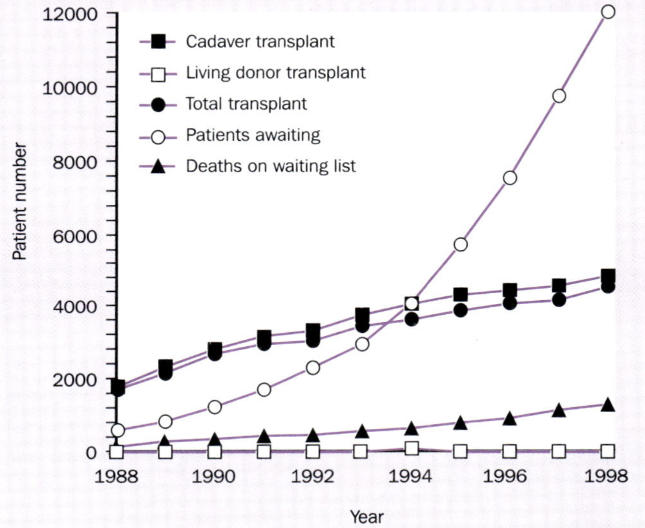

	1988	1989	1990	1991	1992	1993	1994	1995	1996	1997	1998
Cadaver donor	1833	2372	2868	3165	3334	3764	4094	4325	4459	4584	4816
Living donor	0	2	14	22	33	36	60	47	54	73	70
Total transplant	1713	2201	2690	2953	3064	3440	3652	3925	4066	4172	4487
No. waiting	616	827	1237	1676	2323	2997	4059	5691	7467	9637	12056
No. deaths	196	282	317	435	495	560	655	797	956	1130	1319

Figure 92.1 Summary of US data for liver transplant procedures performed for years 1988–1998. Actual cadaveric liver donors, living-donor liver transplants, total liver transplant procedures performed, patients awaiting liver transplantation, and deaths while awaiting liver transplantation are illustrated. The demand for liver transplantation has dramatically exceeded current and projected supply, resulting in increased waiting times, increased morbidity while waiting, and increased deaths from end-stage liver failure, while awaiting transplantation. In addition, transplantation of patients who are critically ill from chronic liver failure as a result of a long waiting period is associated with a poorer outcome. (United Network for Organ Sharing. www.UNOS.org, 2000.)

Anatomy and immunology of the liver

The liver occupies the right upper quadrant of the abdomen and in a normal-sized adult weighs 1500 g (2% of body weight). Its functions include nutrient metabolism, hormone and protein synthesis, drug detoxification and the elimination of metabolic

Indications for liver transplantation
Fulminant liver disease
Viral hepatitis (A,B)
Drug induced
Toxin induced
Metabolic
Wilson's disease
Organic aciduria
Chronic liver disease
Cholestatic disease
Primary biliary cirrhosis
Primary sclerosing cholangitis
Secondary biliary cirrhosis
Biliary atresia
Hepatocellular disease
Autoimmune disease
Alcoholic liver disease
Drug induced
Viral hepatitis (B, C, others)
Vascular disease
Budd–Chiari disease
Veno-occlusive disease
Malignancy
Metabolic disorders

Table 92.1 Indications for liver transplantation.

THERAPEUTIC PRINCIPLES

Parameters indicating need for liver transplantation

- Clinical signs:
  - Recurrent variceal bleeding
  - Encephalopathy
  - Spontaneous bacterial peritonitis
  - Deteriorating nutritional status
  - Ascites
  - Hepatorenal syndrome
- Laboratory signs:
  - Prothrombin time elevation
  - Albumin decline
  - Bilirubin elevation

waste products. Vascular anatomy includes the dual blood supply of the portal vein and hepatic artery, as well as the draining hepatic veins. The biliary system originates as bile canaliculi in the portal triads, which eventually coalesce into the right and left bile duct.

Two cellular components of the liver are generally recognized: hepatic parenchymal and nonparenchymal cells. Parenchymal cells are hepatocytes that endogenously express MHC Class I molecules. Transplanted allogeneic hepatocytes do not elicit a strong immune response and are not involved in antibody-mediated graft rejection. Furthermore, hepatocytes are not early targets of acute rejection, but only become involved in the very late stages of cell-mediated graft rejection.

In contrast, the nonparenchymal cell fraction, composed of bile duct epithelium, dendritic cells, Kupffer cells, Ito cells, interstitium and vascular endothelium, are immunogenetically active. These cells express both MHC Class I and Class II molecules and are also active in antigen presentation; The MHC Class II$^+$ cells are integral to the initiation of the rejection response. The nonparenchymal cell fraction is the immediate target of antibody-mediated rejection and the earliest site of cell-mediated organ rejection.[9]

Surgical technique

Surgical advances within the past decade have resulted in several options for transplantation of the adult patient with end-stage liver disease. These include: cadaveric (brain-dead organ donor) whole-organ, cadaveric split liver, living donor, and auxiliary liver transplantation. Split-liver, living-donor and auxiliary liver transplantations are innovative techniques that have been developed as a response to increasing organ demand. A principal challenge in the use of these techniques is the creation of a graft that optimizes the transplanted liver volume without prohibitively increasing the technical difficulty or significantly increasing graft complications.

Adult cadaveric liver transplantation is the original technique described by Starzl and remains the most common liver transplant procedure performed today. It comprises the removal of the recipient's entire liver and replacement with a whole organ obtained from a cadaveric donor. The liver is routinely placed in the anatomic position of the native liver (orthotopic), but in unusual clinical situations may be placed in a nonanatomic position (heterotopic).

For split-liver transplantation a whole cadaveric donor liver is split into two approximately equal halves, each of which is transplanted into a separate recipient, either two adults or an adult and a child (Fig. 92.2). Thus, one adult cadaver can

Utilization of a whole liver for two recipients

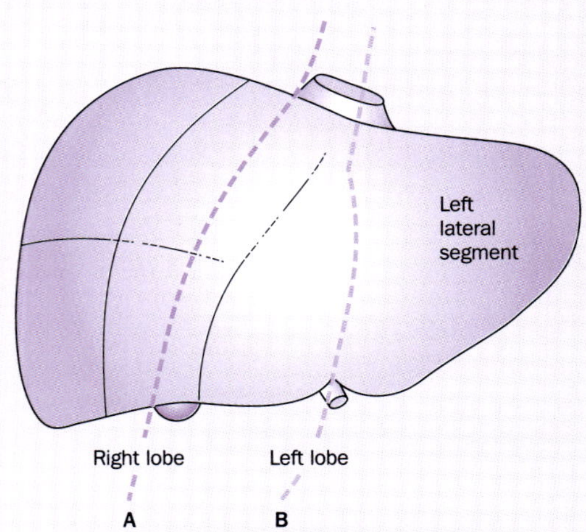

Figure 92.2 Utilization of a whole liver for two recipients. With increasing organ shortages, novel techniques to utilize a single organ for two patients have been developed. A whole liver may be split along line A to allow for transplant of a right lobe and a left lobe into two adult recipients. Alternatively, a liver can be separated along line B, allowing for a left lateral segment to be transplanted into a child and the remaining liver into an adult. These concepts have been applied to the use of live donors, as well as with the removal of a left lateral segment, left lobe or right lobe.

potentially donate to two recipients. This technique is possible because of the unique ability of the liver to regenerate after transplantation. Following transplantation, each liver half will grow and remodel to form a complete liver. Split-liver transplantation has been performed for over 10 years, with excellent results.[2,7] At present split-liver transplantation is reserved for optimum cadaveric grafts to maximize their regenerative potential.

Living-donor liver transplantation in adults is a new technique that evolved from the successes of living-donor liver transplantation in children and split-liver transplantation.[6,7] Living-donor liver transplantation in children (Fig. 92.3) has been performed for over 10 years with excellent results, and frequently accounts for as many as half of all liver transplant procedures performed upon children at larger pediatric transplant centers.[2] The surgical technique of adult living-donor liver transplantation is identical to the split-liver procedure, except that it is performed in a live donor, typically with removal of the anatomic right lobe of the liver.

The principal advantage of living-donor liver transplantation is the ability to optimize the timing of transplantation and thereby avoid long waiting periods and the progression of disease. As in split-liver transplantation, both donor and recipient will grow and remodel their liver in the post-transplant period. At present living-donor liver transplantation is only performed in selected transplant centers within the United States; the results have been comparable to those of other techniques.

Auxiliary liver transplantation is a specialized technique whereby a small piece of liver is removed from the recipient and replaced with a small piece from a cadaver liver or a living donor to 'temporarily' assist the recipient's native liver. This technique is indicated in situations where short-term augmentation of liver function is necessary, such as fulminant liver failure in a patient recovering from exposure to drugs or toxins. In these situations the donated piece of liver provides enough function for the recipient's native liver to recover. After recovery, the donated piece of liver can be removed, allowing the recipient to discontinue immunosuppression and live with only their native liver.

Complications following liver transplantation can be classified as technical, medical, and problems directly related to immunosuppression. Complications of immunosuppression include not only early infectious problems, but also the long-term risks of metabolic problems and malignancy (Table 92.2).

Complications following liver transplantation

- Immediate postoperative complications
  - Medical problems
    - Renal failure
    - Cardiac failure
    - Pulmonary failure
    - Overwhelming sepsis
    - Intracerebral bleed
  - Surgical problems
    - Primary non-function of graft
    - Hepatic artery thrombosis
    - Wound infections/breakdown
    - Intra-abdominal abscess
    - Biliary complications
    - Venous stenosis
    - Bleeding
  - Immunosuppression related
    - Neurologic changes
    - Renal failure
    - Infections
    - Diabetes
- Long-term complications
  - Medical problems
    - Hypertension
    - Bone disease
    - Cardiac disease
    - Recurrence of original disease
  - Surgical problems
    - Biliary complications
    - Hepatic artery thrombosis
    - Hernias/wound problems
  - Immunosuppression related
    - Infections
    - Malignancy
    - Renal insufficiency
    - Metabolic complications

Table 92.2 Complications following liver transplantation.

Completed living related transplant in a pediatric recipient

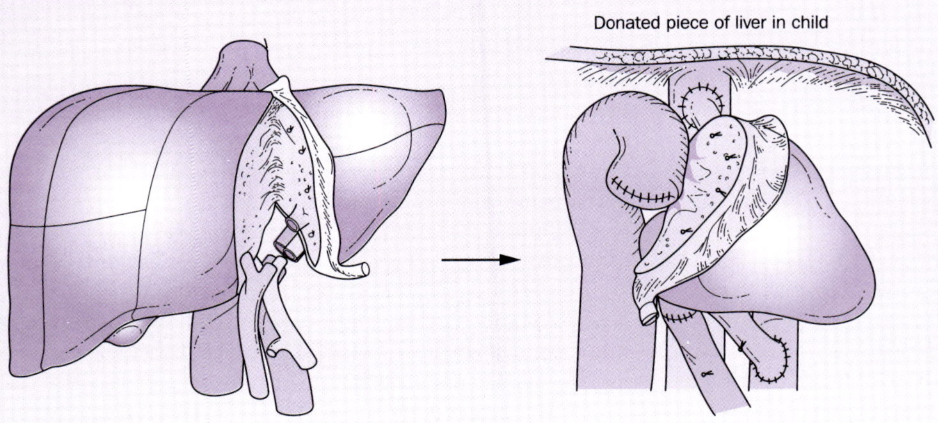

Figure 92.3 Completed living related transplant in a pediatric recipient. Removal of a left lateral segment from an adult and transplant into a pediatric recipient, illustrating the use of a loop of bowel for the bile duct drainage. The use of this technique has dramatically reduced waiting times for pediatric recipients and allowed for improved results.

Immunology of rejection

Understanding of the mechanisms of human liver allograft rejection derives from the interpretation of in vivo animal studies; the evaluation of in vitro human mixed lymphocyte/hepatocyte coculture systems; in vitro assay of 'local environment' lymphocytes from end-stage rejection explants; assay of serum, bile and biopsy material; and the extrapolation of mechanisms underlying the rejection of other human organs (kidney, heart, bone marrow).

Rejection of human liver allografts is dependent on recognition of donor antigen by the recipient's immune system. Donor alloantigen is recognized by recipient T-helper cells which initiate a cytokine cascade resulting in the clonal expansion of allospecific, cytotoxic T lymphocytes (CTL) and the recruitment of inflammatory cells consisting of macrophages, granulocytes, natural killer, CD4, CD8 and other lymphocyte subsets.[10–12] Histologically, acute rejection is first diagnosed as a mixed inflammatory infiltrate within the portal triads, with a loss of biliary epithelium and vascular endotheliitis. As rejection proceeds there is parenchymal destruction with secondary fibrosis, which is primarily a consequence of the activities of proinflammatory cytokines.[10,13–15] Cytokines mediate allograft rejection in experimental models through a variety of mechanisms, including enhanced MHC antigen expression on allograft tissue; activation, differentiation and clonal expansion of allospecific CTL; enhanced expression of cell surface adhesion molecules on allograft tissue; direct damage upon the graft; and nonspecific recruitment and priming of inflammatory cells to the allograft.[10–12] However, the relative importance of each of the above mechanisms in human liver allograft rejection has not been defined.

Phenotypic analysis of intragraft lymphocyte traffic suggests characteristic patterns of CD4 and CD8 T-cell infiltration in acute and chronic rejection. In addition, lymphocyte traffic patterns of $CD8^+CD45RO^+$ (memory) versus $CD8^+$ $CD45RA^+$ (naive) T cells may predict the severity of the rejection episode and the response to immunosuppressive therapy.[12]

Post-LTX rejection is confirmed histologically by percutaneous liver biopsy, either when clinically indicated, as in the setting of elevated liver function studies, or by biopsy at protocol time intervals. A National Institutes of Health Consensus Conference has established uniform pathologic grading criteria to diagnose rejection and guide immunosuppressive therapy.[16] The pathologic diagnosis of acute cellular rejection requires observation of at least two of the three following criteria: mixed portal inflammatory infiltrate, bile duct damage, or venous endotheliitis. Mixed portal inflammatory infiltrates consist predominantly of lymphocytes but may also contain neutrophils, eosinophils or plasma cells. Duct damage is identified by loss of epithelial nuclei, irregular nuclei, or inflammatory cells in the bile duct wall, and endotheliitis is manifested by mononuclear cells within the venous wall or near the endothelial surface which appear to lift the surface endothelium from the vessel wall.

Post-transplant immunosuppression

Lifelong immunosuppression is currently a prerequisite for successful liver transplantation. Although advances in the potency and safety of immunosuppressive medications have led to significant increases in short- and long-term patient and graft survival, immunosuppressive therapy remains a significant cause of morbidity and mortality among patients undergoing LTX.[17] The challenge is to achieve a therapeutic immunosuppressive drug level that inhibits acute cellular rejection but does not result in the sequelae of overimmunosuppression, including sepsis, cancer, drug toxicities and graft-versus-host disease.

Modern immunosuppression can be functionally categorized into induction therapies, maintenance immunosuppression, and medications for the treatment of rejection (Chapter 89). Difficulty in achieving therapeutic immunosuppressive drug levels in the immediate post-transplant period may necessitate the use of induction therapy to prevent acute cellular rejection. The aim of induction therapy is the immediate inhibition of T-cell responses. This is commonly achieved through the administration of anti-T-cell antibody preparations, high-dose glucocorticoids or a combination. Although it is effective in the prevention of acute cellular rejection, the profound immunosuppression associated with induction therapy predisposes to significant short- and long-term morbidity. Moreover, recent formulations of maintenance immunosuppressants now result in rapid therapeutic drug levels with oral administration. Thus, induction therapy is now reserved for unusual clinical circumstances.[17,18]

Maintenance immunosuppression can be subcategorized as calcineurin inhibitors (cyclosporine, tacrolimus), antimetabolites (azathioprine, mycophenolate mofetil), and low-dose glucocorticoids. Most liver transplant centers in the Unites States currently employ a maintenance immunosuppressive regimen of at least a calcineurin inhibitor plus either low-dose corticosteroids or an antimetabolite.

The treatment of acute cellular rejection is guided by biopsy criteria[16] and the interval since the last treatment. Initial episodes are frequently treated with a steroid bolus, followed by a rapid taper or conversion to a tacrolimus-based immunosuppressive regimen. Second episodes or steroid-resistant acute cellular rejection are commonly treated with antilymphocyte therapy, in addition to conversion to tacrolimus-based immunosuppression. Antilymphocyte therapy for the treatment of acute cellular rejection may employ polyclonal antilymphocyte preparations. However, the most common antilymphocyte preparation for the treatment of acute rejection is OKT3, a purified murine monoclonal antibody preparation that inhibits T-lymphocyte function by binding to the CD3 T-cell surface receptor. Because OKT3 is a murine-derived antibody patients do develop neutralizing antibodies with repeated exposure, which limits the applicability of the drug. Recently, a human-hybrid antibody mating the murine CD3-binding hypervariable region with a human immunoglobulin heavy and light chain has been developed to reduce the antigenic profile of OKT3 while retaining its functional properties.

In the scenario of chronic rejection or retransplantation of recipients who have lost a previous allograft from rejection, tacrolimus-based immunosuppression is the preferred regimen.

Specific disease states and liver transplantation

Autoimmune diseases of the liver and biliary system

Autoimmune diseases of the liver or biliary system are a significant cause of end-stage liver disease and account for approximately 20% of all liver transplants performed annually in the United States. Autoimmune diseases that lead to liver failure requiring LTX include primary biliary cirrhosis, primary sclerosing cholangitis and autoimmune hepatitis.

Primary biliary cirrhosis (PBC) is a chronic progressive cholestatic liver disease most commonly diagnosed in middle-aged women.

Histologically, it is characterized by the progressive destruction of small and middle-sized bile ducts, with the eventual development of a portal-type cirrhosis.[19] A variety of immunologic anomalies have been described for PBC, with antimitochondrial antibody occurring in 95% of patients, which is pathognomonic for PBC.[20] The most common early presenting symptoms are fatigue and pruritus. Later, manifestations of chronic liver disease with hepatocellular dysfunction and/or portal hypertension can occur.[21] PBC is staged histologically and follows a natural history that can be based upon clinical models using biochemical and pathological parameters to predict disease progression.[20–22]

There has been considerable debate regarding the clinical significance of recurrent PBC in the transplanted liver. Whereas Neuberger's group has reported clinically significant disease recurrence over time using protocol biopsies,[23,24] the Pittsburgh group has not observed PBC recurrence in patients not subjected to protocol biopsies,[25] and Gouw et al did not observe recurrence in patients over an 11-year period.[26] Furthermore, Neuberger's group reported recurrence more frequently in patients treated with tacrolimus-based immunosuppression.[24,27] The diagnosis of recurrent PBC included clinical symptoms of fatigue and pruritus, biochemical evidence of transaminitis, increased alkaline phosphatase, and histologic evidence of direct injury to bile ducts. At the University of California, San Francisco, recurrent PBC was diagnosed in 14% of recipients receiving liver transplantation for PBC, with a small fraction of patients requiring retransplantation for recurrent PBC.[28]

Primary sclerosing cholangitis is a chronic cholestatic process characterized by intra- and extrahepatic periductular fibrosis.[29–32] Although PSC accompanies inflammatory bowel disease infrequently (~15%), the conjunction is seen 80% of the time. The disease typically occurs in males in association with ulcerative colitis or Crohn's disease. The natural history of the disease is progressive biliary obstruction, recurrent infection, and hepatic fibrosis with the development of portal hypertension. In Scandinavian longitudinal studies the natural history of the disease process from diagnosis to death from progressive liver insufficiency ranged from 10 to 15 years, with the majority of patients clustered around 12 years.[33] The increase in diagnosis of this disease in the last decade has been attributed to increased clinical awareness and increased use of endoscopic retrograde pancreatography.[34,35] The average age at diagnosis is 40 years.[30,31] PSC must be differentiated from cholangiocarcinoma, which is an infrequent but important complication. In a large series of patients undergoing liver transplantation for PSC, 7% demonstrated unsuspected cholangiocarcinoma.[36,37] The diagnosis of a concomitant cholangiocarcinoma is essential prior to liver transplantation, as LTX in the setting of cholangiocarcinoma is associated with a poor prognosis.[37]

The diagnosis of PSC is made by histologic and radiographic findings. Typical histology is that of a portal-based hepatitis, periductular inflammation, and fibrosis with eventual bile duct obliteration and portal-based cirrhosis.[30–32] The radiographic findings of extra- and intrahepatic duct stricture and dilatation form the basis for diagnosis and may be difficult to differentiate from cholangiocarcinoma, depending on the extent and location of disease. The clinical manifestations of PSC relate to obstruction and infection of the biliary tree, portal hypertension and hepatocellular dysfunction. Signs and symptoms of biliary obstruction and infection are the most common sequelae of PSC: though rarely life-threatening, these complications are a significant source of morbidity. Hepatocellular decompensation is a late finding in PSC relative to other disease processes that directly affect hepatocyte function; morbidity relating to recurrent infection becomes relatively more important in determining the timing for liver transplantation.

Complications relating to portal hypertension may be seen prior to cirrhosis as the liver becomes inflamed from cholangitis. Indeed, recurrent cholangitis may become the principal indication for LTX.[38,39] The diagnosis of recurrent PSC posttransplantation may be made by radiographic or histologic means. In a large group of LTX recipients studied at the University of Pittsburgh, PSC with the development of biliary stricture post transplantation occurred in approximately 14% of cases.[40]

Autoimmune chronic active hepatitis (AICH) is a progressive inflammatory liver disease of unknown etiology which accounts for approximately 5% of all liver transplants performed annually in the United States.[41] The most common clinical presentation is a middle-aged woman with an insidious history of fatigue, malaise, myalgia and anorexia;[42] however, Davis et al reported that approximately 25% of patients present with symptoms of acute viral hepatitis, including hepatomegaly, cholestasis and a mild transaminitis.[43] Initial treatment involves steroids or combination steroid/azathioprine therapy; however, long-term follow-up data involving 111 AICH patients from the Mayo Clinic show that as many as 20% of AICH patients exhibit disease progression despite medical therapy.[44] Although several reports have demonstrated an increased incidence of medical therapy failure among AICH patients with HLA-A1 and -B8 phenotypes,[44,45] to date no clinical, biochemical or histologic features have been conclusively demonstrated to predict disease progression or prognosticate the efficacy of medical therapy for individual patients.[41] Untreated, disease progression is the rule, with hepatitis, intrahepatic fibrosis and the ultimate development of cirrhosis. Indications for liver transplantation in the patient with AICH stem from the development of decompensated cirrhosis or complications thereof, and include hepatic encephalopathy, variceal hemorrhage or intractable ascites.

Biochemically, AICH is characterized by a polyclonal hyperglobulinemia, circulating autoantibodies, including antinuclear, antidouble-strand deoxyribonucleic acid, and antismooth muscle or antimicrosomal antibodies.[41,46] Following LTX, autoantibody titers frequently persist but do not portend disease recurrence.[47] Histologically, the mononuclear cellular infiltrate observed in AICH consists predominantly of lymphocytes, plasma cells and macrophages, with rare isolated eosinophils.[41] The inflammatory cells violate the limiting hepatocyte plate, which is the interface between parenchymal cells and portal tracts, and extend into hepatic parenchyma causing inflammation and hepatocyte necrosis, termed piecemeal necrosis. As the inflammatory infiltrate further disrupts the lobular hepatic architecture, hepatocyte necrosis becomes contiguous between central veins or portal tracts, producing bridging necrosis which ultimately triggers a reactive, intrahepatic fibrotic response and the development of cirrhosis. The histology of autoimmune hepatitis, allograft rejection and viral hepatitis has multiple overlapping features which complicate the pathologic diagnosis of recurrent autoimmune hepatitis. Neuberger et al were the first to report post-transplant recurrence of AICH in a 26-year-old woman who developed clinical, serologic and histologic features of AICH 18 months after liver transplantation.[48]

AICH recurrence followed a reduction in immunosuppression, with symptoms resolving after a subsequent increase in steroid administration. Results from other large centers have varied, from several groups reporting no recurrence of histologic, serologic or clinical disease, to the University of Pittsburgh reporting histologic evidence of disease recurrence in up to 26% of patients with a median of 18 months post LTX.[47] Van Thiel et al further demonstrated that AICH recurrence was significantly increased in HLA-DR-3-positive recipients of HLA-DR-3-negative grafts, but was unaffected by the associated HLA-B8 phenotype.[47]

Viral hepatitis

Hepatitis C-induced cirrhosis is currently the most common indication for liver transplantation in the United States. Unfortunately, all patients who undergo transplant have evidence of ongoing viral infection within the transplanted liver on biopsy. The majority of these patients, however, will do well, with no clinical evidence of advancing liver disease. The use of combination therapy with interferon-α and ribavirin may help to minimize the number of patients who develop recurrent liver failure following transplantation although interferon therapy does have the theoretical risk of flaring a rejection episode.[49,50] Early survival of both patient and graft appears to be equivalent to results in patients transplanted for other reasons. Important in management is tapering immunosuppression to minimal doses to avoid aggressive recurrence of the virus.

Hepatitis B-related cirrhosis is also a common reason for liver transplantation. Unlike hepatitis C, there are excellent agents available to control the virus posttransplant. These include passive immunization with hepatitis B hyperimmune globulin, as well as the use of the antiviral agent lamivudine.[51]

Because of the high incidence of hepatocellular carcinoma in patients with chronic viral hepatitis and cirrhosis (approximately 4% per year with hepatitis C; somewhat higher for hepatitis B), these patients should have serial ultrasound examinations and α-fetoprotein measurements. The discovery of a small tumor (<5 cm) does not eliminate the patient as a candidate for transplantations. Consequently, early detection is critical and, if a tumor is discovered, this may mandate earlier transplantation.

> **CLINICAL PEARLS**
>
> **Liver transplantation for viral hepatitis-induced cirrhosis**
> - Hepatitis C
>   - Most common indication for liver transplantation in the US.
>   - Continuing viral infection is consistently observed within the transplanted liver.
>   - Combination therapy with ribavirin and interferon-α significantly reduces the risk of recurrent liver failure in transplant recipients.
>   - Patients in Japan and the western hemisphere are at increased risk for hepatocellular carcinoma.
> - Hepatitis B
>   - Combination therapy with lamivudine and hepatitis B hyperimmune globulin is generally successful in controlling viral infection post transplant and reducing the risk of recurrent liver failure.
>   - Chronic hepatitis B infection is a major risk factor associated with hepatocellular carcinoma worldwide.

Future directions: chimerism and tolerance

The highest aspiration in the field of transplantation is the development of immunologic education and tolerance. Advances in immune education/tolerance would not only reduce the need for immunosuppressive medications, but also enable the practical use of xenografts. The 'immunologic privilege' endowed by the body upon the liver has been widely recognized since the beginning of human and animal transplantation experiments. Indeed, multiorgan transplants such as combined liver/kidney or liver/small bowel demonstrate an 'immunoprotective' function of the liver, with a lower incidence of observed rejection than with isolated kidney or small bowel organ transplants. Furthermore, tolerance has been observed in select human liver allograft recipients who demonstrate a stable population of donor-derived cells functioning outside the transplanted allograft. Studies aimed at characterizing the chimeric cell indicate a subpopulation of bone marrow-derived liver nonparenchymal cells that are capable of translocation to the thymus. Therefore, the liver-derived dendritic cell has been proposed as a putative target for the mediation of tolerance.[52] Currently, liver dendritic cell isolation protocols which will facilitate targeted cell transplantation experiments are being developed to examine the role of dendritic cells in T-lymphocyte education and the development of tolerance. A better understanding of these tolerizing mechanisms in liver transplantation will probably benefit all types of transplant.

PANCREAS TRANSPLANTATION

Diabetes mellitus is prevalent in about 5% of the general population. The complications of diabetes, including retinopathy, microvascular disease and renal disease, are a significant cause of morbidity and mortality; diabetes and its complications are the eighth leading cause of death in the United States. It is the leading cause of renal failure and blindness in adults, as well as the most frequent underlying disease leading to amputations.

Approximately 30% of patients with diabetes require daily insulin injections. The administration of insulin in this fashion prevents the serious metabolic derangements that can occur with hyperglycemia, and tight control of serum glucose can slow or prevent the secondary complications of diabetes. However, no exogenous insulin administration can compare to the physiologic delivery of insulin that occurs with an intact pancreas. For this reason, transplantation of whole-organ pancreas grafts was first attempted in humans in 1966. The development of the surgical techniques for successful transplantation, the use of newer immunosuppression agents and an understanding of the pitfalls and complications following pancreas transplantation have allowed the graft and patient survival to reach levels that are far superior to early results. This justifies offering the procedure to carefully selected patients, with the possibility that earlier intervention in the course of the disease will result in better prevention of secondary complications. Worldwide experience with pancreas transplantation has continued to increase over the last 20 years as these concepts have become more widely accepted (Fig. 92.4).

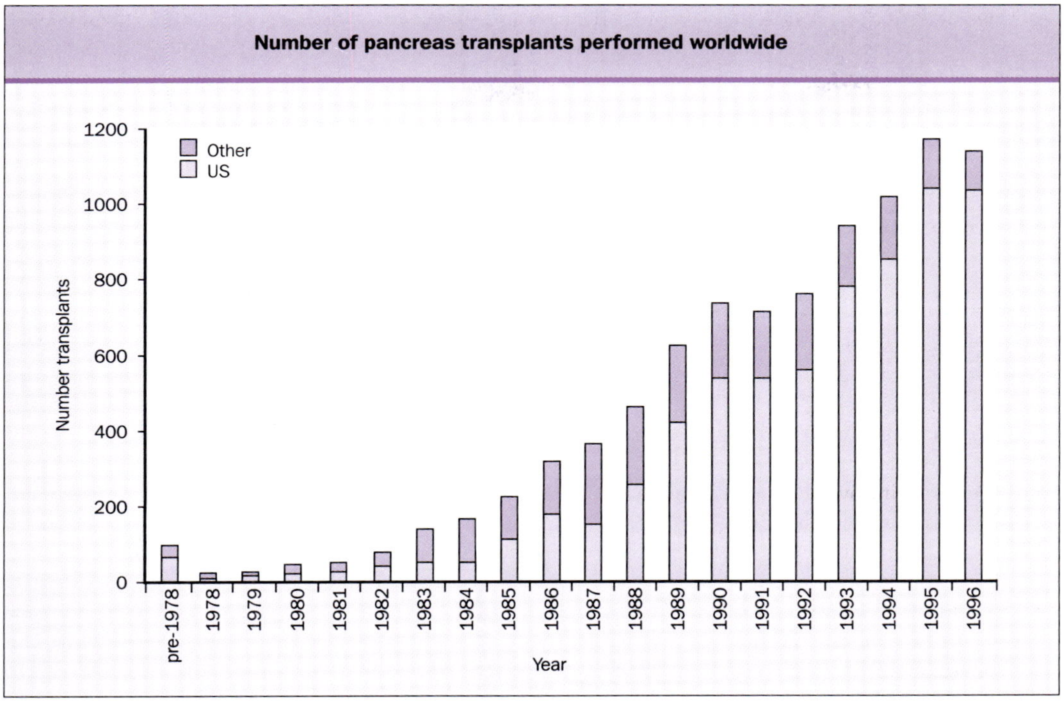

Figure 92.4 Number of pancreas transplants performed worldwide. There has been a steady increase in the total number of pancreas transplants performed worldwide, with the majority in the United States. Of this total more than 90% continue to be simultaneous pancreas–kidney transplants, a procedure which still has the best long-term results. (Data from International Pancreas Transplant Registry.)

Indications and patient selection

Simultaneous pancreas–kidney transplantation is typically offered to patients with insulin-dependent diabetes mellitus who by definition have developed at least diabetic nephropathy and renal insufficiency at the time of transplant. Many of these potential recipients have other manifestations of diabetes, including retinopathy, neuropathy and gastropathy. Patients who may benefit from the simultaneous pancreas–kidney (SPK) procedure must be carefully selected so as to best utilize scarce organs.

Isolated pancreas transplantation may be done following a successful live or cadaver donor kidney transplant (pancreas after kidney; PAK), or may be undertaken before renal failure has developed (pancreas transplant alone; PTA). These two types of isolated pancreas transplant have recently seen improved results, approaching the graft survival rates of SPK, and for that reason are being performed with increasing frequency.

KEY CONCEPTS

Risk/benefit of simultaneous kidney pancreas (SPK) versus kidney alone

- Risks SPK
  - More complex procedure, higher complication rate
  - Longer hospitalization, greater readmission rate
  - More immunosuppression required
  - Postoperative monitoring more involved
- Benefits SPK
  - Stabilization retinopathy/neuropathy in many patients
  - Prevents recurrence of diabetic nephropathy in transplanted kidney
  - Kidney long-term survival similar to kidney-only transplant
  - Improved quality of life

The selection process involves the identification of a potential recipient by the nephrologist or endocrinologist, and then referral for evaluation by the transplant surgeon. Absolute contraindications to SPK include active infection, a recent or current history of malignancy, and HIV positivity. Morbid obesity, advanced cardiovascular or peripheral vascular disease, advanced age and a history of poor compliance or substance abuse are relative contraindications. Although some centers have reported favorable results in patients with coronary artery disease who have undergone revascularization,[53] we typically recommend kidney transplantation alone in this patient group. For patients receiving an isolated pancreas transplant, a suitable amount of renal function must be demonstrated. In the case of PTA or PAK, a creatinine clearance greater than 70 ml/min is desirable, as these patients will receive a calcineurin inhibitor which may worsen renal function.

The surgical procedure

The first clinically successful combined kidney – pancreas transplants were performed at the University of Minnesota in 1966 by Lillihei and Kelly.[54] This initial report demonstrated the feasibility of pancreas transplantation, although length of survival was limited to less than 3 months. However, there were fewer than 100 pancreas transplants performed in the next decade, and further advancement in the field was only possible after the introduction of improved surgical techniques, newer immunosuppressive agents and a better understanding of the rejection of pancreas allografts.

Early technical issues that needed to be resolved included the management of exocrine drainage of the pancreas allograft, location of the venous drainage of the allograft, the prevention of graft thrombosis, and timing of the pancreas transplant relative to the renal transplant. The management of exocrine drainage was initially accomplished by anastomosing the donor duodenum to a loop of recipient bowel. A high incidence of anastomotic breakdown, with abscess formation and subsequent graft loss, was seen early in this experience. Other techniques included occlusion of the pancreatic duct with injected neoprene, often leading to early graft fibrosis. The technique of bladder drainage, whereby the donor's duodenum at the level of the ampulla of Vater is directly anastomosed to the recipient's bladder,[55] was the most widely accepted technique until recently. This allows exocrine secretions to be expelled with the urine and monitoring of urinary amylase, which is helpful to detect rejection early in its course. This technique is accompanied by its own set of problems, including fluid and electrolyte losses, especially bicarbonate; urinary tract complications; and the potential for the development of leaks if the bladder becomes overdistended. These problems have led to a recent return to the technique of enteric drainage at most centers, with more favorable results than in the early experience.[56]

The pancreas allograft is now commonly placed in the right iliac fossa, with anastomosis of the donor portal vein to the recipient external iliac vein for venous outflow. Arterial inflow is established from the recipient external iliac artery to the superior mesenteric and splenic arteries of the donor pancreas via an extension graft of donor iliac artery. This results in insulin delivery to the systemic circulation. Careful studies of postprandial glucose metabolism indicate that carbohydrate metabolism is relatively unaffected, but that a state of hyperinsulinemia is created. This appears to be secondary to decreased insulin clearance, as C-peptide levels are not increased.[57] A few groups have questioned this route of delivery of insulin and have devised a procedure to allow for anastomosis of the donor portal vein to the recipient portal circulation via the superior mesenteric vein.[58] The long-term benefit of this more physiologic positioning of the graft remains to be seen.[59]

The pancreas graft is a low-flow organ compared to a kidney or liver allograft. Therefore, thrombosis of either the arterial supply or the splenic/portal vein occurred at a significant rate in most centers' early experience.[60] Initial attempts at decreasing graft thrombosis rates focused on anticoagulation in the early postoperative period. Many programs continue to use aspirin and dipyridamole immediately postoperatively. Better attention to the vascular anastomoses, with proper orientation of the arterial bifurcation graft and shortening of the portal vein to eliminate kinking, improved preservation solution, better organ recovery techniques, and proper selection of donors and recipients, has resulted in a graft thrombosis rate of less than 5% in most current series. With isolated pancreas transplants in the nonuremic patient, the thrombosis risk is even greater, and protocols using heparin or dextran in the early recovery period are common.

The timing of the pancreas transplant in relation to the renal transplant has also been evolving. Thrombosis rates are clearly lower when a simultaneous kidney–pancreas transplant is done. In addition, there are immunologic advantages to the simultaneous transplant procedure. As concurrent rejection of the kidney and pancreas is frequently seen in recipients of SPK transplants, and as rejection of the pancreas can be difficult to diagnose, parameters of kidney rejection are usually used to trigger the initiation of rejection therapy. Therefore, the presence of a simultaneously transplanted kidney may result in more prompt treatment of rejection. The recipient of an SPK transplant is also exposed to only one set of HLA antigens, which may have implications regarding sensitization should retransplantation be necessary. In the last 15 years the majority of pancreas transplants have been simultaneous pancreas–kidney transplants. However, waiting times for organs have been increasing and the scenario of living related kidney transplant followed by pancreas transplant from a cadaver donor has become more popular. Ultimately, transplantation of an isolated pancreas before the secondary complications of diabetes have begun would be ideal.[61]

In general, potential pancreas cadaver donors tend to be younger, have no underlying history of cardiovascular disease or diabetes, and have no hemodynamic instability during the pre-recovery phase. They are typically less than 50 years old, with no absolute cutoff at the lower age limit, although donors weighing less than 45 kg tend to have smaller-caliber arteries, which may increase the rate of technical complications. A careful medical and social history is obtained, as for any potential donor, but the ideal donor has no underlying medical conditions that might contribute to pancreatitis, acute tubular necrosis or infection in the immediate post-transplant period. Because of the increased need for immunosuppression in pancreas recipients, attention to these donor factors is critical.

The preoperative preparation of the recipient consists of several phases. Final cross-matching with current and several historical recipient serum specimens is completed, using conventional T-cell cross-matching in unsensitized patients. Potential sensitized recipients also undergo cross-matching using flow cytometric techniques.[62] The recipient undergoes standard laboratory screening, EKG and chest X-ray. Preoperative antibiotics are given and continue postoperatively to prevent clinical infection from organisms that frequently reside in the donor duodenum.

The perioperative immunosuppression consists of an antimetabolite, methylprednisolone, and a calcineurin inhibitor, most commonly tacrolimus. The calcineurin inhibitor is usually held in the setting of an SPK until the new kidney is clearly functioning. Many programs continue to use induction therapy, with either a monoclonal or a polyclonal anti-T-cell antibody. This is typically continued until adequate levels of the calcineurin inhibitor are reached.

The pancreas graft is implanted first. After the vascular anastomoses are completed, blood sugars are carefully monitored on an hourly basis as serum glucose levels typically drop 50 mg/dl each hour, and dextrose infusion may be necessary. The duodenal segment is then anastomosed to the dome of the bladder or the distal small bowel, allowing exocrine secretions to drain with the urine or into the gut. The kidney is then implanted on the left side using standard techniques with an extravesicular bladder anastomosis (Fig. 92.5). Because SPK donors are carefully selected, the rate of delayed graft function of the kidney is less than 5% and the majority of patients leave the operating room producing urine.

For isolated pancreas transplants the graft is ideally placed on the right side, where the vascular arrangement of the recipient is more favorable. The pancreas is typically bladder drained, and a final opening to the peritoneum is created to help prevent the accumulation of peripancreatic fluid collections in an extraperitoneal space.

Postoperatively, patients are monitored in the intensive care unit for 24 hours. A nasogastric tube is left in place until there is evidence of bowel function, and a diet is typically started by postoperative day 5. Dipyridamole and aspirin are administered for 2–3 weeks to reduce the risk of graft thrombosis. Serum glucose is carefully monitored four times a day after a diet is started. We have not found the need for perioperative insulin administration in the majority of patients, as has been described at some other

Completed simultaneous pancreas–kidney transplant

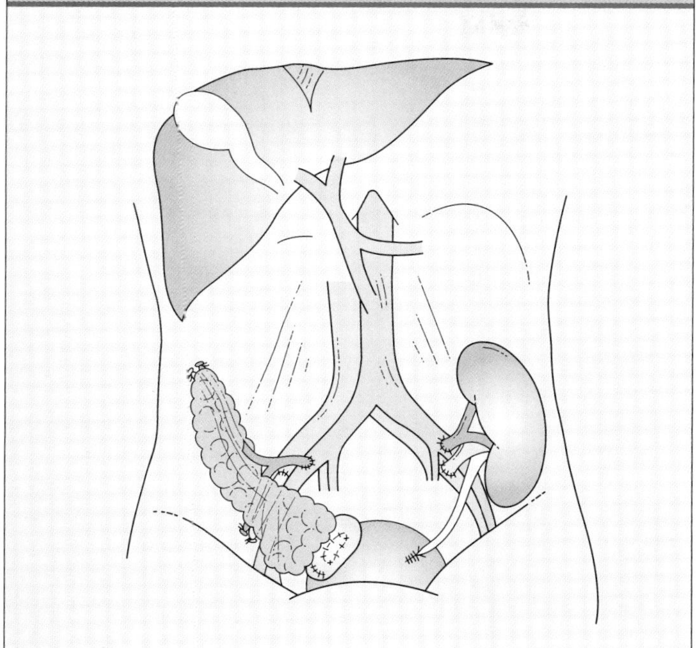

Figure 92.5 Completed simultaneous pancreas–kidney transplant. This diagram illustrates bladder drainage of the exocrine secretion of the pancreas via a duodenocystostomy. Direct drainage of the pancreas into the bowel has again become popular, thereby avoiding the metabolic and infectious complications associated with bladder drainage.

centers.[63] When the patient is tolerating a liquid diet, oral immunosuppressive agents are introduced and other intravenous medications are converted to the oral route. Prophylactic antibacterial antibiotics are continued for 5 days postoperatively, unless a specific organism is cultured from the donor duodenal segment or from a drain culture, in which case appropriate antibiotics are continued for 2 weeks. Drains are typically removed when the drain amylase values have dropped to low levels. Lastly, serum and urine amylase values are monitored daily to detect any evidence of graft pancreatitis, rejection, or other technical problems.

Laboratory indicators of renal and pancreatic function, including urinary amylase for bladder-drained grafts, are followed two to three times a week initially. Prednisone is gradually tapered over the first 6–12 months to 10 mg a day as the patient tolerates. Some recent reports have suggested that complete steroid withdrawal may be possible in selected patients.

The diagnosis of pancreas rejection can be difficult, especially in the enteric-drained situation. Evidence for rejection may be as subtle as fever or pain over the allograft. If the pancreas is bladder drained, a drop in urine amylase to <50% of baseline suggests rejection. Hyperglycemia is usually a late sign of rejection, and may also indicate thrombosis. In an enteric-drained pancreas serum amylase elevation may be the only laboratory sign of rejection. The use of percutaneous ultrasound-guided biopsies of the pancreas graft has become more common, and is helpful in grading the degree of rejection and dictating therapy.[64] Simultaneous kidney and pancreas rejection is not always apparent on clinical grounds, but when biopsies have been done of the kidney in the face of pancreas rejection there is a high rate of concurrent histologically identified rejection. In general, with newer immunosuppressive protocols, mostly based on tacrolimus, rejection rates have fallen to less than 30% in the first year, and rejection has become more steroid responsive.

Complications following pancreas transplantation include bleeding, thrombosis, anastomotic leaks and wound infections. Other complications are primarily related to the immunosuppression and include infections and malignancies. Despite these potential problems, 1-year graft survival of SPK approaches 90%, and that for for isolated pancreas transplants 75%.

Effect of SPK on secondary complications of diabetes

The greatest potential benefit of pancreas transplantation is the prevention of secondary complications of diabetes. By definition, most patients who undergo simultaneous pancreas–kidney transplantation have already progressed to end-stage renal disease as a result of diabetic nephropathy. These patients often display features of neuropathy, retinopathy, gastropathy and diabetic microangiopathy, with myriad vascular diseases. The effect of optimal glucose control following pancreas transplantation has been evaluated for its ability to either halt progression or reverse some of these complications.

The recurrence of diabetic nephropathy in transplanted kidneys of patients who do not receive a pancreas transplant has been documented in many series. An increase in the mesangial matrix density is seen in diabetic recipients of isolated kidney transplants, and this lesion is prevented when a pancreas is transplanted simultaneously.[65] Initial reports indicated that a successful solitary pancreas transplant was unable to reverse the established lesions of diabetic nephropathy in native kidneys However, histologic improvement in the lesions of diabetic nephropathy has been documented after more than 5 years of normoglycemia with a successful isolated pancreas transplant.[66] Additionally, long-term kidney survival in simultaneous pancreas–kidney transplant recipients tends to be better than in diabetic patients receiving kidneys alone. This may be explained by the fact that the quality of the donor kidneys and the underlying health of the recipient of a simultaneous kidney–pancreas transplant are often better. This improved long-term graft survival is in spite of a higher acute rejection rate and the requirement for increased doses of immunosuppression.[67]

Retinopathy is often far advanced by the time patients undergo pancreas transplantation. In one series comparing the degree of retinopathy in patients with successful pancreas transplants versus failed grafts, there was no difference in visual symptoms over the first 3 years. After that time, in patients with successful grafts the retinopathy had stabilized, whereas patients with failed grafts had further deterioration in their vision.[68] It appears that by the time nephropathy has developed retinopathy is also far advanced, such that stabilization of retinal lesions is the best outcome that can be anticipated.[69]

The effect of successful pancreas transplantation on the polyneuropathy of diabetes has been evaluated.[70,71] Symptomatic improvement and measurable increases in nerve conduction velocities and sensory action potentials are seen following successful pancreas transplantation. Symptoms of gastroparesis are also often improved. It must be remembered, however, that improvement of uremia alone can have an impact on both gastropathy and neuropathy. The degree of autonomic dysfunction has a negative impact on long-term survival. In patients with autonomic dysfunction quantified by cardiorespiratory reflexes, survival is improved in those with functioning pancreas grafts verses failed grafts or no transplant.[72]

Potential recipients of pancreas–kidney transplants are carefully screened for evidence of cardiovascular disease. It has clearly been shown that there is a high morbidity and mortality rate in patients with underlying cardiac disease who receive a pancreas transplant.[73] A successful pancreas–kidney transplant may be able to affect the progression of cardiovascular lesions in patients who undergo the procedure and who do not have far advanced baseline disease. Serum sialic acid, a risk factor for cardiac disease, has been shown to fall more in patients receiving a successful kidney pancreas transplant than in those receiving a kidney transplant alone.[74] Carotid lesions were compared in patients following SPK versus isolated kidney transplant. There was a progression of lesions in both groups, but it was less pronounced in the kidney–pancreas recipients.[75] In general it is difficult to compare these two groups, as many potential kidney–pancreas recipients with advanced cardiac or vascular disease are typically advised to undergo a kidney transplant alone. In addition, differences in disease progression may be diluted by the adverse effects of increased steroids and hyperinsulinemia in the kidney–pancreas group.

Pancreas–kidney transplantation alters lipid profiles, with an increase in HDL cholesterol and a decrease in plasma concentrations of cholesterol and triglycerides.[76] The use of immunosuppressive agents such as cyclosporine and tacrolimus has been associated with worsening lipid profiles in recipients of kidney or liver transplants. It is interesting, however, that lipid profiles are markedly improved in SPK patients receiving tacrolimus.[77]

Quality of life measurements also indicate an advantage to patients receiving a successful pancreas–kidney transplant. In a self-reporting questionnaire, patients with a successful transplant reported a more positive health perception, less pain and a greater ability to function socially.[78] In addition there is a strong willingness of patients with failed grafts to repeat the procedure.

Recurrence of diabetes in recipients

Because autoimmunity is believed to play a role in the development of diabetes, pancreas transplantation represents an interesting set of circumstances to observe for the recurrence of diabetes in the transplanted graft. Of course, patients typically receive high doses of immunosuppression, which would probably prevent recurrent damage to the grafted pancreas if autoimmunity were important. Interestingly, three pancreas transplant recipients receiving their grafts from identical twins in a procedure performed at the University of Minnesota were not given immunosuppression postoperatively. Diabetes recurred within 6–12 weeks and biopsy confirmed isletitis with β-cell destruction. One of the patients was immediately treated with immunosuppression, and evidence of graft function continued for 10 years.

Recurrence has not been seen in cadaveric grafts, probably because of the increased immunosuppression in this setting. This phenomenon suggests the possibility that immunosuppression administered early enough to patients with preclinical diabetes mellitus may prevent β-cell destruction.[79]

ISLET TRANSPLANTATION

The results of transplantation of a whole or partial pancreas graft continue to improve, but it is appreciated by all transplant physicians that only the pancreatic islets are necessary to achieve a reversal of diabetes. Therefore, the ultimate goal is to develop a protocol that allows for islet transplantation only. An obvious benefit would be to avoid the invasive surgical procedure required for a solid organ transplant, as a cellular transplant utilizing islets injected into the portal vein would require minimally invasive techniques. Not only would this allow the more debilitated patient to undergo a procedure to reverse diabetes, but it may be more suitable for newly diagnosed patients as an effective therapy to prevent the secondary complications of diabetes. Unfortunately, despite many different attempts and protocols, until recently reliable results have been lacking.

The techniques for isolating islets from pancreatic tissue were developed over 30 years ago, using collagenase digestion and purification with gradient separation.[80] Islets recovered in this manner can be infused via the portal vein and embolize to the liver, where they are able to remain viable. The procedure has been applied to patients with severe pancreatitis using their own resected pancreatic tissue, which is processed for islets and then autotransplanted.[81] Normoglycemia can be demonstrated if a critical mass of islets is infused, and in many cases is long-lasting. These clinical successes have allowed for the determination of optimal conditions for the recovery of islets, the perfection of injection techniques, and the characterization of secretory function after intrahepatic implantation. Unfortunately, the immunologic barriers have proved more difficult in the application of this technology to transplantation between unrelated individuals.

Early encouraging results in the allotransplant setting were demonstrated when islets were injected into the portal vein at the time of transplantation of a whole liver graft in patients with diabetes and liver failure.[82] However, complete insulin independence was not accomplished in all patients at the time of the islet infusion, and long-term survival was difficult to achieve. The concept that the transplanted liver may provide some immune privilege was intriguing, although clearly not relevant to most patients with type 1 diabetes.

A major breakthrough in the field was reported by a group from Edmonton utilizing a new immunosuppressive protocol consisting of sirolimus, tacrolimus and daclizumab (a monoclonal humanized antibody to the human IL-2 receptor). This protocol deliberately avoided glucocorticoids, given their diabetogenic potential secondary to β-cell damage and increased insulin resistance.[83] Of seven patients undergoing the procedure, all had normal glycosylated hemoglobin values after transplantation, as well as detectable C-peptide values at 3 and 6 months post transplant. There were no rejection episodes documented, and infectious complications were not seen in the early follow-up. This report has sparked a renewed interest in clinical islet programs, and further trials are under way in several US centers.

Although the use of islets may prove to be a less invasive procedure to cure diabetes, the problems of tissue availability remain. Many investigators have looked at alternative sources of islet tissue, including fetal tissue[84] and xenogeneic sources. Encapsulation of porcine islets has shown some promise in animal models, although indefinite survival has not been achieved.[85] The possibility of manufacturing a β cell has been the focus of several laboratories using genetic engineering techniques.[86] Regardless of approach, it seems likely that a source of tissue beyond the standard cadaver donor will need to be secured before islet transplantation can be expected to have a significant impact on the conventional management of diabetes.

One of the most interesting facets of islet transplantation and cellular transplantation in general is the possibility of modifying the tissue prior to transplant. The potential to decrease the immunogenicity of islets has been an area of active research with very exciting results in animal models, including some regimens that may allow for the development of tolerance. Infection of rat islets with an adenovirus expressing CTLA4-Ig (a potent inhibitor of the costimulation pathway) allows for prolonged survival of the islets when transplanted across a xenogeneic barrier into mice.[87] Alternatively, cotransplantation of islets with dendritic cells modified to express CTLA4-Ig has resulted in prolonged survival in a murine model.[88] As these innovative strategies are refined, the immunologic risk of islet transplantation will probably decrease, making the procedure even more acceptable. Finally, a further benefit of this research may be a better understanding of the mechanisms leading to diabetes in the first place, as the alloimmune response leading to the destruction of transplanted islets must be separated from the autoimmune response responsible for the initial disease.

REFERENCES

1. Starzl TE, Groth CG, Brettschneider L et al. Extended survival in 3 cases of orthotopic homotransplantation of the human liver. Surgery 1968;63:549.
2. Heffron TG. Living related liver transplantation. Semin Liver Dis 1995;15:165.
3. Belle SH, Beringer KC, Detre KM. An update on liver transplantation in the United States: recipient characteristics and outcome. In: Terasaki PI, Cecka JM (eds) Clinical transplants 1995. Los Angeles, UCLA Tissue Typing Laboratory, 1996.
4. Teperman L, Podesta L, Mieles L, Starzl TE. The successful use of older donors for liver transplantation. JAMA 1989;262:2837.
5. Loinaz C, Gonzales EM. Marginal donors in liver transplantation. Hepatogastroenterology 2000;47:256.
6. Broelsch CE, Whitington PF, Emond JC, et al. Liver transplantation in children from living related donors. Ann Surg 1991;214:428.
7. Broelsch CE, Emond JC, Whitington PF, Thistlethwaite JR, et al .Application of reduced-size liver transplants as split grafts, auxiliary orthotopic grafts, and living related segmental transplants. Ann Surg 1990;212:368.
8. Goss JA, Yersiz H, Shackleton CR, et al. In situ splitting of the cadaveric liver for transplantation. Transplantation 1997;64:871.
9. Clemmings SM, Hoffman RA, Cahill DR, Simmons RL, Ascher NL. Compartmentalization of lymphocyte traffic after allograft challenge. Transplant Proc 1987;19:391.
10. Bumgardner GL, Orosz CG. Transplantation and cytokines. Semin Lives Dis 1999;19:189.
11. Hart J, Lewin KJ. Liver allograft pathology. Pathology (Phila) 1994;3:207.
12. Ibrahim S, Dawson DV, Killenberg PG, Sanfilippo F. The pattern and phenotype of T-cell infiltration associated with human liver allograft rejection. Hum Pathol 1993;24:1365.
13. Imagawa DK, Millis JM, Seu P, et al. The role of tumor necrosis factor in allograft rejection I. Transplantation 1990;50:219.
14. Martinez OM, Krams SM, Sterneck M, et al. Intragraft cytokine profile during human liver allograft rejection. Transplantation 1992;53:449.
15. Baan CC, Weimer W. Intragraft cytokine gene expression: implications for clinical transplantation. Transplant Int 1998;11:1691.
16. Demetris JA, Seaberg EC, Batts KP, et al. Reliability and predictive value of the National Institute of Diabetes and Digestive and Kidney Diseases liver transplantation database nomenclature and grading system for cellular rejection of liver allografts. Hepatology 1995;21:408.
17. Klintmalm GB. Induction and maintenance of immunosuppression. In: Busuttil RW, Klintmalm GB (eds) Transplantation of the liver. Philadelphia, WB Saunders, 1996, p. 741.
18. Ascher NL. Immunosuppressive therapy in liver transplantation: principles and practice. Prog Liver Dis 1995;13:381.
19. Mitchison HC, Lucey MR, Kelly PJ, Neuberger JM, Williams R, James OF. Symptom development and prognosis in primary biliary cirrhosis: a study in two centers. Gastroenterology 1990;99:778.
20. Gershwin ME, Ansari AA, Mackey IR, et al. Primary biliary cirrhosis: an orchestrated immune response against epithelial cells. Immunol Rev 2000;174:210.
21. Roll J, Boyer JL, Barry D, Klatskin G. The prognostic importance of clinical and histological features in asymptomatic and symptomatic biliary cirrhosis. N Engl J Med 1983;308:1.
22. Prince MI, Jones DE. Primary biliary cirrhosis: new perspectives in diagnosis and treatment. Postgrad Med J 2000;76:199.
23. Polson RJ, Portmann F, Neuberger J, Calne RY, Williams R. Evidence for disease recurrence after liver transplantation for primary biliary cirrhosis. Gastroenterology 1989;97:715.
24. Neuberger J. Transplantation for primary biliary cirrhosis. Semin Liver Dis 1997;17:137.
25. Demetris AJ, Markus BH, Esquivel C, et al. Pathologic analysis of liver transplantation for primary biliary cirrhosis. Hepatology 1988;4:939.
26. Gouw ASH, Haagsma EB, Manns M, Klompmaker IJ, Sloof MJH, Gerber MA. Is there recurrence of primary biliary cirrhosis after liver transplantation? A clinicopathologic study in long-term survivors. J Hepatol 1994;20:500.
27. Dmitrewski J, Hubscher SG, Mayer D, Neuberger JM. Recurrence of primary biliary cirrhosis in the liver allograft: the effect of immunosuppression. J Hepatol 1996;24:253.
28. Ascher NL, Renz JF. Liver transplantation for non-viral, non-malignant diseases: the problem of recurrence. World J Surg (in press).
29. Crippin JS, Lindor KD. Primary sclerosing cholangitis: etiology and immunology. Eur J Gastroenterol Hepatol 1992;4:261.
30. Farrant JM, Hayllar KM, Wilkinson M, et al. Natural history and prognostic variables in primary sclerosing cholangitis. Gastroenterology 1991;100:1710.
31. Harrisen PM. Diagnosis of primary sclerosing cholongitis. J Hepatobiliary Pancreat Surg 1999;6:356.
32. Angulo P, Larson DR, Therneau TM, et al. Time course of histological progression in primary sclerosing cholangitis. Am J Gastroenterol 1999;94:3310.
33. Aadland E, Schrumpf E, Fausa O, et al. Primary sclerosing cholangitis: a long-term follow-up study. Scand J Gastroenterol 1987;22:655.
34. Gaing AA, Geders JM, Cohen SA, Siegal JH. Endoscopic management of primary sclerosing cholangitis: review, and report of an open series. Am J Gastroenterol 1993;88:2000.
35. Lee JG, Schutz SM, England RE, Leung JW, Cotton PB. Endoscopic therapy of sclerosing cholangitis. Hepatology 1995;21:661.
36. Knechtle SJ, D'Alessandro AM, Harms BA, Pirch JD, Belzer FO, Kalayoglu M. Relationship between sclerosing cholangitis, inflammatory bowel disease, and cancer in patients undergoing liver transplantation. Surgery 1995; 118:615.
37. Abu-Elmegd KM, Selby R, Iwatsuki S, et al. Cholangiocarcinoma and sclerosing cholangitis: clinical characteristics and effect on survival after liver transplantation. Transplant Proc 1993;25:1124.
38. Lee YM, Kaplan MM. Primary sclerosing cholangitis. N Engl J Med 1995; 332:924.
39. Narumi S, Roberts JP, Emond JC, Lake J, Ascher NL. Liver transplantation for sclerosing cholangitis. Hepatology 1995;22:451.
40. Lerut J, Demetris AJ, Stieber AC, et al. Intrahepatic bile duct strictures after human orthotopic liver transplantation: recurrence of primary

sclerosing cholangitis or unusual presentation of allograft rejection? Transplant Int 1988;1:127.
41. Yarze JC, Martin P. Liver transplantation for idiopathic autoimmune chronic active hepatitis. In: Busuttil RW, Klintmalm, GB (eds) Transplantation of the liver. Philadelphia, WB Saunders, 1996, p 113.
42. Keating JJ, O'Brien CJ, Stellon AJ, et al. Influence of etiology, clinical and histologic features on survival in chronic active hepatitis: an analysis of 204 patients. Q J Med 1987;237:59.
43. Davis G, Czaja AJ, Baggenstoss AH, Taswell HF. Prognostic and therapeutic implications of extreme serum aminotransferase elevation in chronic active hepatitis. Mayo Clin Proc 1982;57:303.
44. Sanchez-Urdazpal L, Czaja AJ, Rakela J, Ludwig J. Prognostic features and role of liver transplantation in severe corticosteroid-treated autoimmune chronic active hepatitis. Hepatology 1992;15:215.
45. Donaldson PT, Doherty DG, Hayllor KM, McFarlane IG, Johnson PJ, Williams R. Susceptibility to autoimmune chronic active hepatitis: Human leukocyte antigens DR4 and A1-B8-DR3 are independent risk factors. Hepatology 1991;13:701.
46. Obermayer-Straub P, Strassburg CP, Manns MP. Autoimmune hepatitis. J Nepatol 2000;32 (Suppl 1):181.
47. Wright HL, Bou-Abboud CF, Hassanein T, et al. Disease recurrence and rejection following liver transplantation for autoimmune chronic active liver disease. Transplantation 1992; 53:136.
48. Neuberger J, Portmann B, Calne R, Williams R. Recurrence of autoimmune chronic active hepatitis following orthotopic liver grafting. Transplantation 1984; 37:363.
49. Daevis GL. Current therapy for chronic hepatitis C. Gastroenterology 2000;118 (Suppl 2):S104.
50. Terrault NA. Hepatitis C virus and liver transplantation. Semin Gastrointest Dis 2000;11:96.
51. Yoshida EM, Erb SR, Partovi N, et al. Liver transplantation for chronic hepatitis B infection with the use of combination lamivudine and low-dose hepatitis B immune globulin. Liver Transplant Surg 1999;5:520.
52. Thomson AW, Drakes ML, Zahorchak, et al. Hepatic desdritic cells: immunobiology and role in liver transplantation. J Leukoc Biol 1999;66:322.
53. Schweitzer EJ, Anderson L, Kuo P, et al. Safe pancreas transplantation in patients with coronary artery disease. Transplantation 1997;63:1294.
54. Lillehei RC, Idezuki Y, Feemster JA, et al. Transplantation of stomach, intestine and pancreas; experimental and clinical observations. Surgery 1967;62:721.
55. Sollinger HW, Ploeg RJ, Eckhoff DE, et al. Two hundred consecutive simultaneous pancreas–kidney transplants with bladder drainage. Surgery 1993;114:736.
56. Corry RJ, Egidi MF, Shapiro R, et al. Pancreas transplantation with enteric drainage under tacrolimus induction therapy. Transplant Proc 1997;29:642.
57. Matte J, Fery F, Lankoande C, Schinohoritis P, De Pauw L. Insulin secretion and glucose tolerance evolution in kidney-pancreas graft. Transplant Proc 1995; 27:3073.
58. Gaber AO, Shokouh-Amiri MH, Grewel HP, Britt LG. A technique for portal pancreas transplantation with enteric drainage. Surg Gynecol Obstet 1993;177:417.
59. Newell KA, Woodle ES, Millis JM, et al. Pancreas transplantation with portal venous drainage and enteric exocrine drainage offers early advantages without compromising safety or allograft function. Transplant Proc 1995;27:3002.
60. Troppmann C, Gruessner AC, Benedetti E, et al. Vascular graft thrombosis after pancreatic transplantation: univariate and multivariate operative and nonoperative risk factor analysis. J Am Coll Surg 1996;182:285.
61. Bartlett ST, Schweitzer EJ, Johnson LB, et al. Equivalent success of simultaneous pancreas kidney and solitary pancreas transplantation. Ann Surg 1996;224:440.
62. Pelletier RP, Orosz CG, Adams PW, et al. Clinical and economic impact of flow cytometry crossmatching in primary cadaveric kidney and simultaneous pancreas–kidney transplant recipients. Transplantation 1997;63:1639.
63. Troppmann C, Gruessner AC, Papalois BE, et al. Delayed endocrine pancreas graft function after simultaneous pancreas–kidney transplantation. Transplantation 1996;61:1323.
64. Drachenberg CB, Papadimitriou JC, Klassen DK, et al. Evaluation of pancreas transplant needle biopsy. Transplantation 1997;63:1579.
65. Wilczek HE, Jaremko G, Groth CG. Evolution of diabetic nephropathy in kidney grafts. Transplantation 1995;59:51.
66. Fioretto P, Steffes M, Sutherland DER, Goetz F, Mauer M. Reversal of lesions of diabetic nephropathy after pancreas transplantation. New Engl J Med 1998;339:69.
67. El-Gebely S, Hathaway DK, Elmer DS, Gaber LW, Acchiardo S, Gaber AO. An analysis of renal function in pancreas–kidney and diabetic kidney-alone recipients at two years following transplantation. Transplantation 1995;59:1410.
68. Ramsey RC, Goetz FC, Sutherland DER, et al. Progression of diabetic retinopathy after pancreas transplantation for insulin-dependant diabetes mellitus. N Engl J Med 1988;318:208.
69. Sutherland DER. Effect of pancreas transplants on secondary complications of diabetes: review of observations at a single institution. Transplant Proc 1992; 24:859.
70. Laftavi MRA, Chapuis F, Vial C, et al. Diabetic polyneuropathy outcome after successful pancreas transplantation; 1 to 9 year follow up. Transplant Proc 1995;27:1406.
71. Trojaborg W, Smith T, Jakobsen J, Rasmussen K. Effect of pancreas and kidney transplantation on the neuropathic profile in insulin-dependent diabetics with end-stage nephropathy. Acta Neurol Scand 1994;90:5.
72. Navarro X, Kennedy WR, Loewenson RB, Sutherland DER. Influence of pancreas transplantation on cardiorespiratory reflexes, nerve conduction, and mortality in diabetes mellitus. Diabetes 1990;39:802.
73. Manske CL, Wang Y, Thomas W. Mortality of cadaveric kidney transplantation verus combined kidney–pancreas transplantation in diabetic patients. Lancet 1995; 346:1658.
74. Auersvald LA, Perez RV, Lorber MI, et al. Serum sialic acid, a risk factor for cardiovascular disease, improves following pancreas transplantation. Transplant Proc 1995;27:3037.
75. La Rocca E, Minicucci F, Secchi A, et al. Evolution of carotid vascular lesions in kidney–pancreas and kidney-alone transplanted insulin-dependent diabetes patients. Transplant Proc 1995;27:3072.
76. Foger B, Konigsrainer A, Palos G, et al. Effects of pancreas transplantation on distribution and composition of plasma lipoproteins. Metabolism 1996;45:856.
77. Burke GW, Alejandro R, Roth D, et al. Use of FK506 in simultaneous pancreas/kidney transplantation: lack of impairment of glycemic or lipid metabolism. Transplant Proc 1995;27:3119.
78. Gross CR, Zehrer CL. Health-related quality of life outcomes of pancreas transplant recipients. Clin Transplant 1992;6:165.
79. Sutherland DE, Gruessner R, Gores P. Pancreas and islet transplantation: an update. Transplant Rev 1994;8:85.
80. Lacy PE, Kostianovsky M. Method for the isolation of intact islets of Langerhans from the rat pancreas. Diabetes 1967;16:35.
81. Wahoff DC, Papalois PE, Najarian JS. Autologous islet transplantation to prevent diabetes after pancreatic resection. Ann Surg 1995;222:562.
82. Angelico MC, Alejandro R, Tzakis AG, et al. Transplantation of islets of Langerhans in patients with diabetes mellitus undergoing orthotopic liver transplantation – the Miami experience. J Mol Med 1999;77:144.
83. Shapiro AM, Lakey J, Ryan E, et al. Islet transplantation in seven patients with type 1 diabetes mellitus using a glucocorticoid-free immunosuppressive regimen. New Engl J Med 2000;343:230.
84. Mandel TE. Fetal islet xenotransplantation in rodents and primates. J Mol Med 1999;77:155.
85. De Vos P, Van Straaten J, Schilfgaarde R, et al. Why do microencapsulated islet grafts fail in the absence of fibrotic overgrowth? Diabetes 1999;48:1381.
86. Bailey CJ, Davies EL, Docherty K. Prospects for insulin delivery by ex-vivo somatic cell gene therapy. J Mol Med 1999;77:244.

87. Feng S, Quickel RR, Weir GC, et al. Prolonged xenograft survival of islets infected with small doses of adenovirus expressing CTLA4-Ig. Transplantation 1999;67:1607.

88. O'Rourke RW, Kang SM, Stock PG, et al. A dendritic cell line genetically modified to express CTLA4-Ig as a means to prolong islet allograft survival. Transplantation 2000;69:1440.

Section 9 Immunology of Neoplasia

Chapter 93 A Molecular Genetic Analysis of Lymphoid Neoplasia

Shai Izraeli and Ilan Kirsch

INTRODUCTION

Cancer is a genetic disease that results from subversion or dysregulation of the normal genes that govern cell growth and development. This process is what makes cancer so difficult both conceptually and therapeutically. Much of what a cancer cell does was also done before its malignant transformation. With transformation comes a loss of control of its growth and developmental pathway(s), rather than a fundamental change in course.

This is not to say that a cancer cell is no different from the 'normal' cells from which it arises. In every tumor cell that has been studied in sufficient depth, molecular genetic analyses have demonstrated that DNA is altered compared to its nonmalignant 'normal' counterpart. The mechanistic consequence of many of the point mutations, deletions, transpositions, amplifications, insertions and translocations that can comprise these DNA alteration(s) (Fig. 93.1) represents the gene disruption/dysregulation that contributes to malignant transformation.

KEY CONCEPTS

Genetic instability

- Cancer is a disease of genetic instability.
- The mechanism that generates functional immune responsiveness is at least partly responsible for the generation of malevolent translocation frankly associated with the development of lymphoid malignancy.

GENETIC INSTABILITY

The fact that cancer is not a rare event underscores the point that DNA is not a static and immutable structure. It is the inherent instability of DNA that accounts for evolutionary development and this same inherent instability that is the basis of cancer. The instability of DNA has two components, one of which is inherited and represents the physiologic 'program' with which an organism is born. This is a function of the specific nucleotide sequence, the structure and level of various histones and other chromatin-covering proteins, repair enzymes, recombinases, nuclear matrix components etc. The other aspect of genetic instability is acquired, a function of stabilizing or destabilizing influences from the environment, diet, medication and other factors. These influences act in combination with the underlying 'baseline' level of genetic instability to make DNA alteration more or less likely at any given time. Corresponding to this level of DNA instability, there is an accompanying level of risk for the development of a particular malignancy.

GENETIC INSTABILITY IN LYMPHOCYTES

It is not just in evolution and cancer that the force of genetic instability dominates. Normal development requires that DNA be able to reconfigure itself. The classic example of this is the rearrangement of DNA in vertebrate organisms that is required

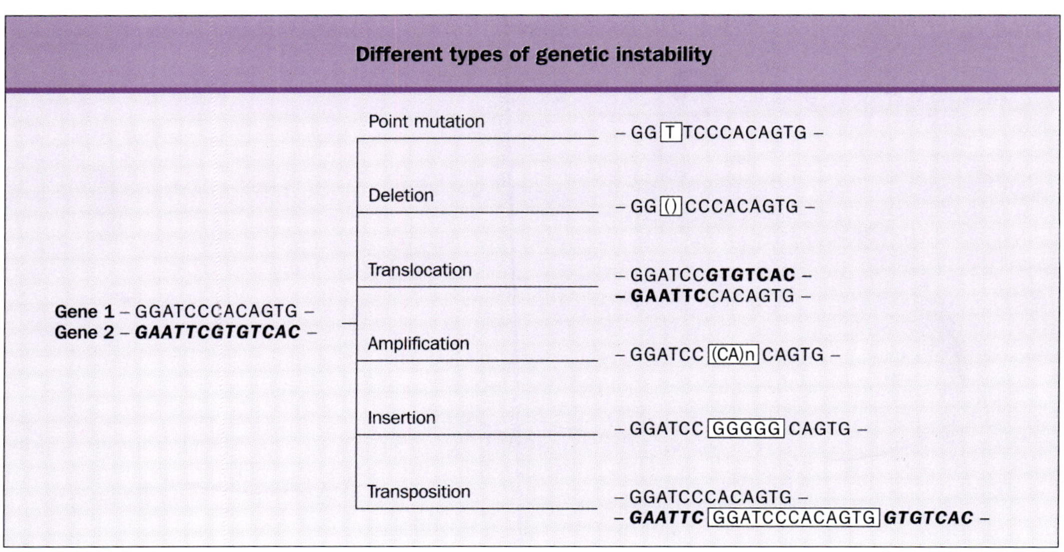

Figure 93.1 Examples of different types of genetic instability. Two hypothetical segments of DNA corresponding to two genetic loci are shown (one in plain text, one bold and italicized). Alterations in the primary sequence caused by point mutation, deletion, translocation, amplification, insertion and transposition are demonstrated. Although the example of amplification shown consists of amplification of a dinucleotide repeat, much larger segments of the genome can also be part of an amplified unit (amplicon).

for the generation of the immune response. The role of lymphocytes in the generation of the immune response depends on the elaboration of a group of particularly 'destabilizing' enzymes, and probably also requires the organization of chromatin (at least in certain regions) into a state that makes it particularly amenable to DNA breakage and rejoining events. This 'lymphocyte-specific' genetic instability becomes an important factor in considering the process of malignant transformation of these cells.

IMMUNE RECEPTOR REARRANGEMENT

As is discussed in detail in Chapters 4 and 5, the DNA that eventually codes for a functional immune receptor (immunoglobulin (Ig) or T-cell antigen receptor (TCR)) initially exists in germline DNA as a series of discrete noncontiguous segments (Fig. 93.2). Within a prototypical immune receptor locus there are multiple variable (V) segments separated by one to hundreds of kilobases

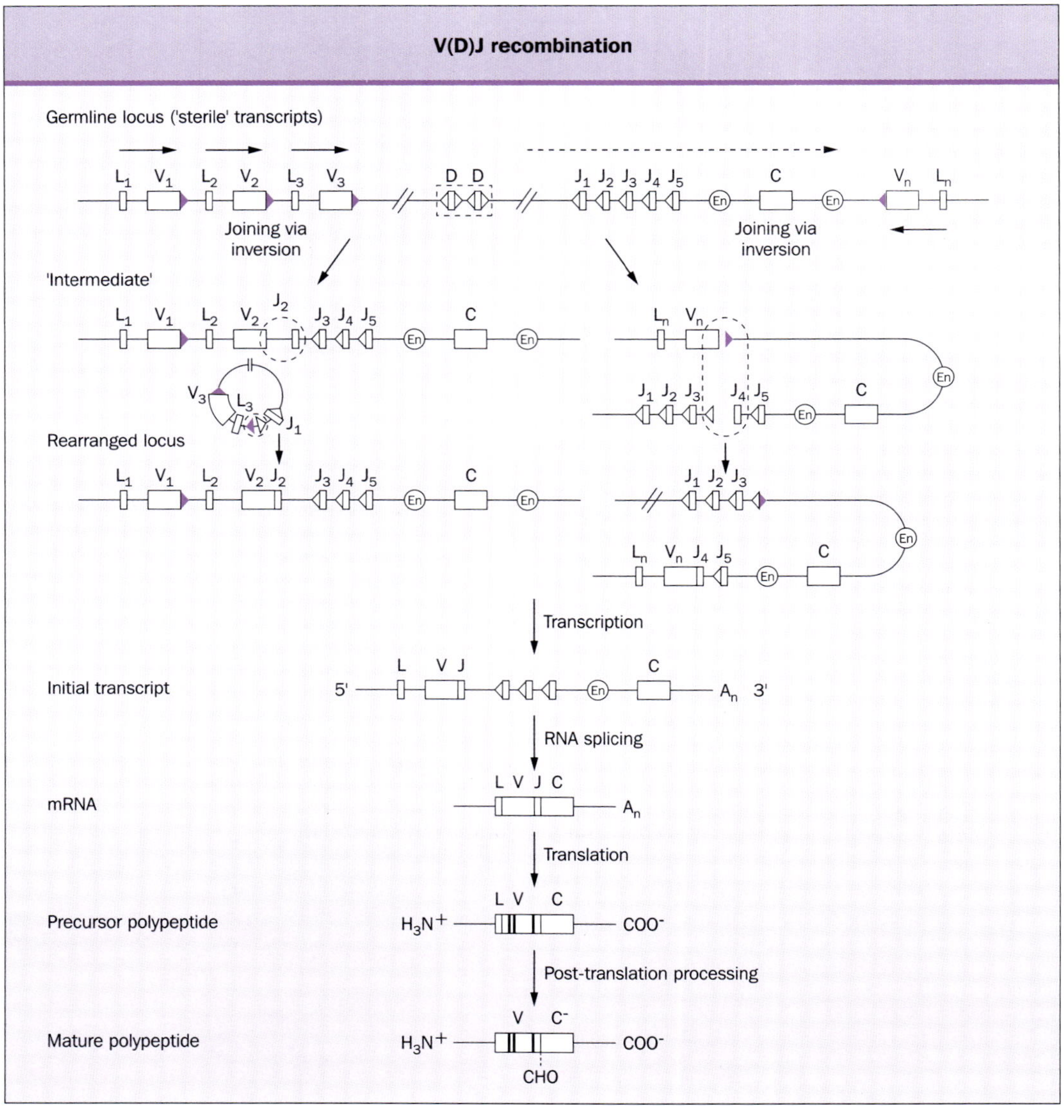

Figure 93.2 V(D)J recombination. The structural reconfigurations of immune receptor loci that are a prerequisite to the formation of a functional polypeptide and therefore to the generation of immune diversity. The gene that eventually constitutes the immune receptor exists initially in germline DNA as a set of discrete, noncontiguous segments. There are multiple variable (V) segments with their upstream leader (L) exons that mediate transport of the polypeptide into or through a membrane. For certain of the immune receptor loci (IgH, TCRβ, TCRδ) there are diversity (D) segments. All the loci joining (J) segments are found upstream from constant (C) segments. Before gene rearrangement, 'sterile' transcription (solid and dashed arrows over the first line of the diagram) of the loci about to be rearranged occurs, probably indicative of a change in the status and 'accessibility' of the chromatin at these sites (see text). Structural and irreversible rearrangement of the DNA occurs either by deletion of the DNA between the rearranging segments or by inversion. The reaction is essentially site specific, mediated by a recombinase enzyme complex that recognizes heterologous signal sequences (solid and open triangles) that flank the rearranging segments. Following recombination, a now contiguous V(D)J region is formed and still can begin from the promoter located 5′ to the rearranged V segment, with transcriptional activity 'enhanced' by enhancer elements (En) that are found around the DNA flanking the C segment. A precursor RNA is transcribed up to the point where the addition of a run of adenosine residues (A_n) is sited. RNA intervening between coding segments is spliced out, yielding the mature messenger RNA (mRNA). The mRNA is translated into protein and transported to its position in the membrane. The mature polypeptide is finished after additional processing, which includes cleavage of the leader peptide and possible glycosylation (CHO) of certain sites within the peptide. (From Kirsch IR. In: Pizzo P, Poplack D (eds) *Principles and practice of pediatric oncology*, 2nd edn. Philadelphia, J. B. Lippincott, 1993; with permission.)

(kb) of intervening DNA from multiple joining (J) segments. These, in turn, are located a few thousand nucleotides upstream of one or a small number of constant (C) segments.[1] For the Ig heavy-chain (H) locus and the TCR β and δ loci there are also diversity (D) segments interposed between the V and J segments. As a prerequisite to the formation of a functional immunoglobulin or T-cell antigen receptor, one of the V segments undergoes a site-specific rearrangement with a J (or previously site-specifically rearranged DJ) segment to form a now contiguous VJ (VDJ) region, still upstream from the C segment. The segments appear to be targeted for rearrangement because they are flanked by particular signal sequences, consisting of a nucleotide heptamer with consensus CACAGTG separated by 12 or 23 nucleotides from a nonamer with consensus ACAAAAACC. In most cases the rearrangement is accompanied by deletion of the intervening DNA between the rearranging segments. The DNA in the rearranged cell is therefore fundamentally different from that in the germline cell, and this process is irreversible.

This rearrangement reaction is catalyzed by a complex of enzymes (recombinase complex) that includes the products of the *RAG1* and *RAG2* genes, DNA bending high-mobility group proteins HMG1 and HMG2, DNA breakage and repair genes (e.g. DNA-dependent protein kinase gene, which is mutated in the SCID mouse), the Ku proteins and, in some cases, terminal deoxynucleotidyl transferase, TdT.[1,2] This complex of enzymes targets the specific signal sequences that flank the rearranging segments. The presence of the recombinase complex in a cell is not, by itself, sufficient for V(D)J rearrangement. The segments to be rearranged must be accessible to the complex. Within nonlymphoid cells it appears that, in general, the immune receptor loci are not accessible. The accessibility of these segments within lymphocytes is observed as a change in chromatin status heralded by an increased DNase sensitivity, an alteration in the pattern of methylation and the production of 'sterile' transcripts (transcripts that do not appear to encode a protein) from the locus about to be rearranged.[3,4] These transcripts are not believed to be necessary for the recombination event itself. Instead, their presence suggests that accessibility to an RNA polymerase is accompanied by accessibility to the recombinase complex.

B-LYMPHOCYTE-SPECIFIC GENOMIC INSTABILITY

Receptor editing, switch recombination and somatic hypermutation are three additional DNA-altering events restricted to B cells[5] (Chapter 4). Receptor editing involves the replacement of one V(D)J region by a secondary V(D)J rearrangement. The IgH locus is subject to 'switch' recombination, in which the immunoglobulin isotype changes from μ to γ, ε or α. In the germinal centers of the lymphoid organs the rearranged V genes commonly undergo extensive somatic mutations. Most of these occur in B cells that have 'switched' from a primary IgM response to a secondary IgG or IgA response.

OTHER V(D)J RECOMBINASE-MEDIATED GENOMIC REARRANGEMENTS

Interlocus rearrangements

Classically, the V(D)J recombination process has been viewed as occurring within a given immune receptor locus. However, the process can also occur between two distinct immune receptor loci, leading to the formation of a 'hybrid' immune receptor with a V segment from one locus and (D)J and C segments from another (Fig. 93.3). The formation of such hybrids is not a freak event but a routine occurrence. All normal humans that have been studied carry such hybrid genes in a small fraction of their peripheral blood lymphocyte population.[6]

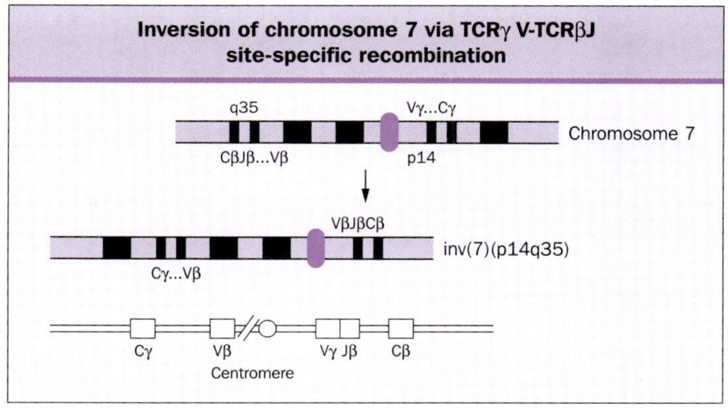

Figure 93.3 A model for the mechanism of inversion of chromosome 7 via TCRγ V-TCRβJ site-specific recombination. Idiograms of normal and inverted chromosomes 7 are depicted. Orientations and locations of the TCRγ and TCRβ chain loci in both germline and inverted states are illustrated. A schematic representation of the interlocus rearrangement and hybrid gene formation is shown below. (From Stern MH, et al. *Blood* 1989;74:2076, with permission.)

These hybrid genes have a number of implications. First, from a strictly mechanistic point of view, they demonstrate that the V(D)J recombinase complex does not require linear contiguous DNA to mediate recombination. Second, the formation of hybrid genes raises certain issues from the standpoint of development and immunology. Based on the study of intralocus rearrangement, the finding of hybrid genes strongly suggests that two disparate immune receptors must have been simultaneously accessible both temporally and topologically. In addition, the occurrence of such hybrids is of interest in terms of clonal selection of immune receptor-bearing lymphocytes (Chapters 8 and 9). In the peripheral blood 30–50% of these hybrid immune receptor genes are in-frame at the level of genomic DNA, and over 90% are in-frame at the detectable mRNA level. This is similar to the situation for normal intralocus rearrangements, and suggests that hybrid genes are capable of being functional and positively selected. One might speculate that combinations of Vs and Js that were routinely beneficial to an organism would lead to their being brought together within the same locus, and thus be favored for recombinatorial joining. The actual role that interlocus hybrids play in the normal immune response remains to be determined.

Hybrid immune receptors as markers of genetic instability and possible cancer risk

The hybrid genes that we carry are a polyclonal population. Multiple independent interlocus rearrangements have occurred in each individual. The sum total of all these clones defines the frequency of these genes in the peripheral blood. For example, for a hybrid involving the recombination of a V segment from the TCRγ locus with a J segment from the TCRβ locus, the frequency in normal individuals is in the range of 0.001–0.0001% of circulating T cells.

In the autosomal recessive disease ataxia telangiectasia (AT) there is an approximately 100-fold increase in the frequency of interlocus hybrid genes found in the peripheral blood lymphocyte population.[6] AT is a complex disease with the homozygotes demonstrating oculocutaneous telangiectasia, progressive cerebellar degeneration, premature aging, radiosensitivity, immunodeficiency, and a predisposition to the development of cancer, particularly lymphoid malignancies (Chapter 35). The risk to an AT patient of developing lymphoma is approximately 100 times that of the unaffected population. The V(D)J recombination machinery and process appears normal in an AT patient. At the nucleotide sequence level, the hybrid genes formed in an AT patient are indistinguishable from the hybrids found in an unaffected individual. The increased frequency of these hybrids and the increased risk of lymphomas in AT may reflect an increased accessibility of these loci to the recombinase complex. This implies a difference in chromatin structure or organization between AT patients and unaffected individuals. Such a qualitative difference in chromatin has also been suggested based on an increased frequency in the conversion of double-strand DNA breaks into chromosome breaks following irradiation of AT patient-derived cell lines.[7]

An increase in the frequency of hybrid gene formation can be acquired as well as inherited. In a pilot study, agriculture workers exposed to pesticides, fumigants and herbicides were shown, as a group, to have an increased incidence of hybrid genes in their peripheral blood lymphocytes compared to a control population. Interestingly, these workers were representative of a population that also demonstrated an increased risk for the development of lymphoid malignancy. Similar findings were reported in people and mice exposed to DNA-destabilizing agents.[8]

Hybrid gene formation may not just be a fortuitous marker for the risk of developing lymphoid malignancy. The mechanism that mediates the formation of hybrid genes, V(D)J recombination, is, at least in part, the same that mediates the formation of many of the malevolent translocations frankly associated with the development of lymphoid malignancy. Indeed, the occurrence of lymphomas in the ATM knockout mouse, the mouse model for AT, is completely dependent on the activity of the V(D)J recombinase. Mice that lack both the ATM and the *Rag-1* genes do not develop thymic lymphomas.[9]

At any time we have a finite risk of developing lymphoid malignancy and a certain level of genetic instability as measured by, among other things, a particular frequency of hybrid gene formation. The level of these hybrids at any moment seems to be a function of the inherited propensity for the interlocus recombination event to occur. This propensity is a summation of chromatin accessibility, topographic (the relative positions of genes in the nucleus), and topologic (the configuration of one locus vis-à-vis another) organization of DNA in the interphase nucleus, and exposure to stabilizing or destabilizing agents that can alter these reaction prerequisites. Thus, the frequency of hybrid gene formation may be a marker for the risk of developing lymphoid malignancy. An increased level of hybrid genes does not mean that a person has leukemia or lymphoma or will develop one of these diseases: it only means that the conditions are more favorable than usual for the generation of the kind of chromosomal rearrangements that appear to facilitate cellular transformation.

CHROMOSOMAL ABERRATIONS ASSOCIATED WITH LYMPHOID MALIGNANCY

Table 93.1 lists chromosomal aberrations that have been specifically associated with the development of lymphoid malignancy. Only those that have been cloned and analyzed at the level of the DNA are included, whereas purely descriptive cytogenetic data are not included. The list is extensive but it is not all inclusive, and other chapters in this section focus on some of the disease-specific aberrations that are listed. Throughout the remainder of this chapter various entries are taken from this list to provide examples of the particular phenomenon or mechanism being described.

V(D)J RECOMBINASE-MEDIATED REARRANGEMENTS

Immunoglobulins and T-cell receptors as oncogenes

Immunoglobulins and T-cell receptors are cell-surface receptors that transduce ligand-dependent (antigenic) stimuli at the cell surface into differentiative and proliferative activity of these cells. Were it not for the varied nature of the ligands (antigens) that they bind and the consequences of that binding, these molecules would simply be a variation on the theme of growth-factor–growth-factor receptor. One basic paradigm of cancer biology is that cellular transformation can be promoted because of aberrant expression or binding of a growth factor, as well as aberrant or structurally altered expression of a growth-factor receptor. It is plausible that under certain circumstances the presence of a particular idiotype, together with specific antigenic stimulation, may lead to unremitting stimulus for cellular proliferation.

Mutations in the Ig or TCR effector domains that interact with the intracellular transduction machinery are also potential targets for transforming alterations. When hybrid genes are considered, the concept of immune receptors as oncogenes can also be raised. These hybrids were initially appreciated because of their rare presence on the surfaces of frank leukemias. Having a V segment of one locus associated with a J segment of a different locus does not look the same as the more common intralocus rearrangements. Here again, because of either its specificity or its peculiar conformation, a hybrid gene may provide an aberrant signal for cellular proliferation.

There is some evidence implicating immune receptors as occasionally part of the transformation process. Antigen stimulation is required for the growth of gastric MALT lymphoma, which is almost always associated with *Helicobacter pylori* infection and may disappear after treatment of the infection.[10] A rather restricted pattern of Ig receptor expression on the surface of B-type chronic lymphocytic leukemia (B-CLL) cells is consistent with a potential role of antigenic stimulation in the development of B-CLL.[11] There are also examples of certain lymphoid malignancies – follicular lymphoma being the most notable – where the presence of a functional immunoglobulin on the surface of the lymphoma cells appears to be a requirement for continued expansion of the malignant clone.[12] This is consistent with the role of the Ig receptor in maintaining the survival of normal mature B cells.[13]

Rearrangements between immune receptors and oncogenes

The field of molecular cytogenetics began with the cloning and characterization of a particular group of chromosomal break-

Chromosomal translocations in lymphoid malignancies

Category	Phenotype	Characteristic translocation	Translocated genes	Comments
Acute lymphoblastic leukemia (ALL)	Pre-B	t(1;19)(q23;p13)	*E2A–PBX1 fusion*	Intermediate prognosis
	Early pre-B	t(17;19)(q22;p13)	*E2A–HLF fusion*	Poor prognosis
	Early pre-B	t(12;21)(p13;q22)	*TEL–AML1 fusion*	Good prognosis
	Early pre-B	t(9;22)(q34;q11)	*BCR–ABL fusion*	Poor prognosis
	Early pre-B	t(4;11)(q21;q23)	*MLL–AF4 fusion*	Infants; poor prognosis
	Early pre-B	t(11;19)(q23;p13)	*MLL–ENL fusion*	MLL involved in multiple other translocations
	Early pre-B	t(5;14) (q31;q32)	*IL3–IGH*	Hypereosonophilia
	B	t(8;14)(q24;q32.3)	*MYC–IGH*	
	T	t(1;7)(p34;q35)	*LCK–TCRβ*	
	T	t(1;14)(p33;q11.2)	*SCL (TAL1)–TCRα/δ*	
	T	del 1(p33)	*SIL–SCL*	
	T	t(7;9)(q35;q34.2)	*TCRβ–TAL2*	
	T	t(7;10)(q35;q24)	*TCRβ–HOX11*	
	T	t(10;14)(q23;q11)	*HOX11–TCRα/δ*	
	T	t(7;19)(q35;p13)	*TCRβ–LYL-L*	
	T	t(7;9)(q35;q34)	*TCRβ–TAN1*	
	T	t(8;14)(q24;q11)	*MYC–TCRα/δ*	
	T	t(11;14)(q13;q11)	*LMO2–TCRα/δ*	
	T	t(11;14)(p15;q11)	*LMO1–TCRα/δ*	
Lymphoma/CLL	LCL, CD30+	t(2;5)(p23;q35)	*NPM–ALK fusion*	ALK involved in multiple translocations
	Burkitt lymphoma	t(8;14)(q24;q32.3)	*MYC–IGH*	
	HIV associated	t(2;8)(p12;q24)	*IGκ–MYC*	
		t(8;22)(q24;q11)	*C-MYC–IGλ*	
	DLCL	t(3;14)(q27;q32.3)	*BCL6–IGH*	BCL6 also involved in other translocations
	High and low grade B-NHL	t(10;14)(q24;q32)	*LYT10–IGH*	
	MCL; MM; CLL	t(11;14)(q13;q32.3)	*CCND1–IGH*	CCND1 = Cyclin D1
	FL	t(14;18)(q32.3;q21)	*IGH–BCL2*	
	CLL	t(14;19)(q32;q11.3)	*IGH–BCL3*	
	MM	t(4;14)(p16.3;q32.3)	*FGER3&MMSET–IGH*	Activating mutation in FGFR3
	MM	t(14;16)(q32.3;q23)	*IGH–C-MAF*	
	MM; LPL	t(9;14)(p13;q32)	*PAX5–IGH*	
	MALT	t(1;14)(p22;q32)	*BCL10–IGH*	
	T-PLL	inv(14)(q11.2;q32.1)	*TCRα/δ–TCL1*	
	T-PLL	t(X;14)(q28;q11.2)	*MTCP1*	
	T-cell lymphoproliferation	inv(14)(q11.2;q32.1)	*TCRα/δ–TCL1*	Ataxia–telangectasia
	T cell lymphoproliferation	t(X;14);(q28;q11.2)	*TCRα/δ–MTCP*	Ataxia–telangectasia
	T-CLL	t(14;14)(q11.2;q32.1)	*TCRα/δ–TCL1*	

CLL, chronic lymphocytic leukemia; B-CLL, B-cell CLL; PLL, prolymphocytic leukemia; MM, multiple myeloma; LPL, lymphoplasmacytic lymphoma; DLCL, diffuse large cell lymphoma; LCL, large cell lymphoma; MCL, mantle cell lymphoma; FL, follicular lymphoma.

Table 93.1 Chromosomal translocations associated with lymphoid malignancies.

points. These defined the translocations associated with the development of human Burkitt lymphoma and BALB/c murine plasmacytoma. This represented the first cloning of a translocation associated with the development of a malignancy. Flanking the translocation on one side was the immunoglobulin heavy-chain locus and on the other was the c-*MYC* oncogene. One group identified the translocation by studying the c-*MYC* gene, discovering an unexpected structural rearrangement of the gene in murine plasmacytomas.[14] Several other groups, building on their knowledge of the organization and structure of the immunoglobulin loci, probed the IgH locus. They arrived at the translocation by cloning and characterizing all the immunoglobulin rearrangements found in tumors or cell lines carrying this particular cytogenetically detectable translocation.[15,16] The precedent of using probes from the Ig and TCR loci for the cloning and characterization of chromosomal aberrations in lymphocytes was thus established. It has been a highly useful and productive strategy, resulting in the elucidation of dozens of karyotypic as well as cytogenetically undetectable aberrations, the discovery of numerous growth-affecting genes, and insight into the fundamental mechanism of DNA breakage and rejoining.

> **KEY CONCEPTS**
>
> **Immune receptors (Ig and TCR) as oncogenes**
> - Stimulation of normal or abnormal growth factor receptors can serve as a trigger for cellular transformation.
> - Immune receptors are often juxtaposed to proto-oncogenes by translocations associated with the development of lymphoid malignancies.

It is notable that immunoglobulins and T-cell receptors, the fundamental products of differentiated lymphocytes, are frequently involved in the chromosomal aberrations that contribute to malignant transformation of these cells. The reason for this involvement has to do with both the expressive quality and the quantity of these genes in lymphocytes. In addition, powerful enzyme systems, including the V(D)J and 'switch' recombinase complexes, are found in these cells, which actively engage in DNA breakage and rejoining events within these loci. This clearly seems to put these loci at greater risk for aberrant ligation than other parts of the genome. There is no clear evidence that all rearrangements involving an immune receptor locus are mediated by one or the other of these recombination systems, but the majority are. The product of a translocation such as the t(1;14) involving the *SCL* gene and the TCRδ locus, or the t(14;18) involving the *BCL2* gene and the IgH locus, suggests site specificity at a D or J signal sequence, exonucleolytic 'nibbling' of coding sequence, and nontemplated N-region addition of nucleotides. These three findings are all hallmarks of the V(D)J recombinase complex (including TdT).[1] Any other explanation for this breakage event requires a far more complicated model.

Can the V(D)J recombinase target DNA conformations other than recognition signal sequences (RSS)? In certain circumstances accounting for the breakage of an oncogene-carrying chromosome presents a problem because of the absence of appropriate signal sequences at the sites of chromosome breakage. Occasionally, DNA in the translocation breakpoints is notable for containing alternating stretches of purine and pyrimidine nucleotides compatible with the model for formation of Z (left-handed helical turn) DNA.[17] Perhaps this conformational change is recombinogenic. This implies that either there is more recognition ambiguity, allowing the action of V(D)J recombinase, or that a different set or subset of recombinase enzymes is involved in this DNA breakage. Insight into this problem has now been derived from analysis of recombinase-mediated transposition, demonstrating that the intermediates created by the activity of the RAG proteins are capable of insertion into non-RSS-containing DNA. These data suggest that the recombinase complex alone and its DNA byproducts can explain the occurrence of the potentially oncogenic DNA rearrangements. The genomic structure and activity of the *RAG* genes are consistent with their origin as a transposable element which became fortuitously incorporated into an early vertebrate genome and evolved as the recombination machinery generating immune diversity and, occasionally, oncogenic chromosomal translocations.[18,19]

It is still possible that the occurrence of chromosomal aberrations is a random event. In this model DNA breaks would occur anywhere in the genome and selection would be based on the fortuitous juxtaposition of particular DNA sequences conferring a growth advantage on the cell. Although formally a possibility, certain observations seem to make this less likely as a dominant mechanism. There are stringent requirements for chromosomal accessibility, allowing for routine immune receptor rearrangements. Chromosomal aberration in lymphocytes appears to be a variation on this theme. Furthermore, the translocations are often reciprocal: that is, a t(1;14) generates a derivative chromosome 1 and a complementary derivative chromosome 14. The fact that so many of the chromosomal aberrations are reciprocal makes a random and chaotic model problematic. If a chromosome breaks and its ends are 'floating free', a random model would suggest that one end could religate to the end of a subsequently disrupted chromosome, whereas the other end might be lost or united with a completely different, fortuitously disrupted part of the genome. The reciprocity actually observed implies that the breakage and rejoining events occur specifically at a point in time and space. This seems to favor the concept of certain parts of the genome being more predisposed to undergo chromosomal aberration in specific cell lineages at certain times during lineage development or differentiation.

Taken together, the overall structure and specificity of these various translocations, their association with distinctive malignant phenotypes representing particular stages of lymphocyte development, and their overall structural consistency suggest that these events are not random. These findings imply that in a given cell type certain parts of the genome, because of structure, function and differential accessibility, are more likely to undergo chromosomal translocation than other parts. This conclusion is reinforced and strengthened by an understanding of the constraints and prerequisites for normal immune receptor rearrangement previously discussed. Perhaps the V(D)J (and switch) recombinase complexes are sequestered in a particular part of the lymphocyte nucleus, and DNA of a particular transcriptional state and chromatin structure is more likely to participate in this recombinational event (Fig. 93.4).

V(D)J recombinase-mediated rearrangements that do not involve immune receptors

Although many of the chromosomal translocations in lymphocytes involve an immune receptor locus and a nonimmune receptor locus, several chromosomal aberrations associated with lymphoid malignancy, where neither locus is an immune receptor, appear to involve V(D)J recombinase mediation (Fig. 93.5). The *SIL–SCL* rearrangement is formed by an interstitial deletion of chromosome 1 and represents a clear example of V(D)J recombinase-mediated rearrangement between two nonimmune receptor loci. *SIL–SCL* juxtaposition is the most frequent genetic alteration associated with the development of T-cell ALL.[20] The *SCL* gene, which appears not to be significantly expressed in T cells, is placed under the control of the *SIL* promoter, which is active in proliferating T cells.[21–23] The rearrangement results in an approximately 90 kb deletion of DNA intervening between these two loci on chromosome 1. There are two major sites of DNA breakage within the *SCL* gene with regard to this deletion, both of which are sites of classic heptamer and nonamer sequences separated by appropriate spacing. On the *SIL* side a sequence quite consistent with the consensus heptamer is found at the site of DNA breakage. Again, in these rearrangements exonucleolytic removal of nucleotides and nontemplated nucleotide addition are both found. Thus the sequences, site specificity and structure of the junction between these two nonimmune receptor loci bear unequivocal hallmarks of the action of the V(D)J recombinase complex. Another example of V(D)J-mediated chromosomal rearrangements is a deletion of a multiple tumor-suppressor gene locus in T-cell leukemia.[24]

GENOMIC REARRANGEMENTS IN THE GERMINAL CENTERS

Somatic hypermutation

The presence of somatic hypermutation in a rearranged IgH or IgL V region provides a genotypic marker for passing through a germinal center. The majority of B-cell lymphomas carry hypermutated rearranged immunoglobulin genes that are generated during or after passage in the germinal centers. It has been suggested that the frequent deletions, insertions and duplications that occur during somatic hypermutation cause breaks that could

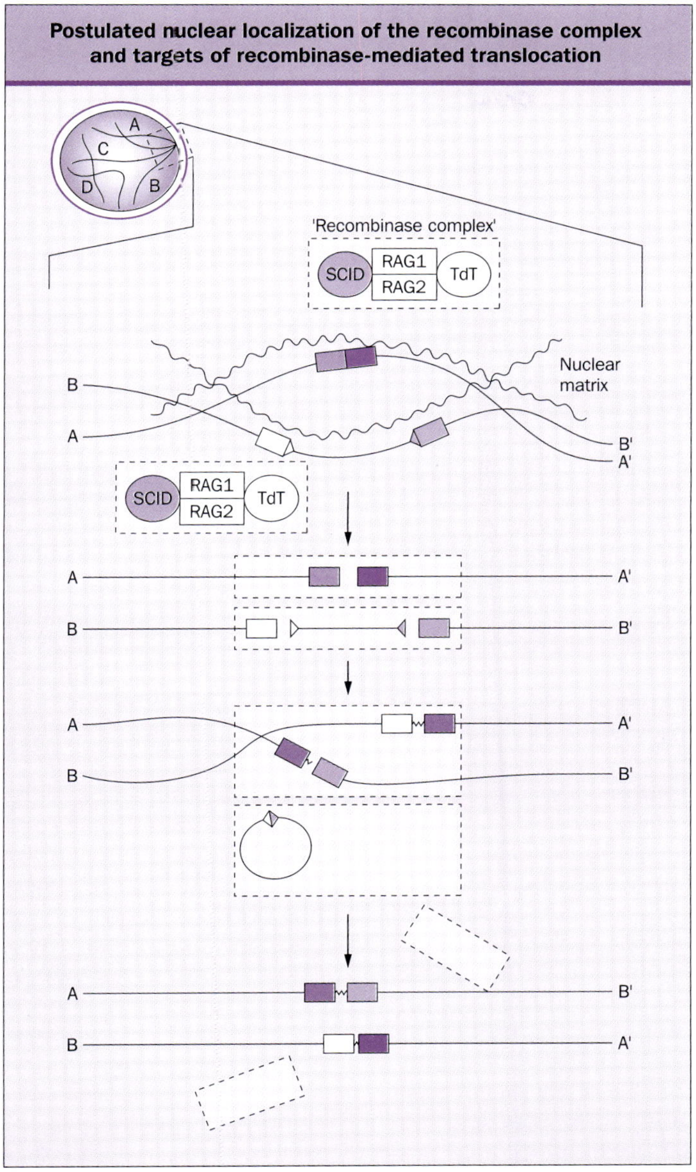

Figure 93.4 Postulated nuclear localization of the recombinase complex and targets of recombinase-mediated translocation. The circle at the top of the figure represents a cell (for example, a lymphocyte) in which a part of chromosome A and a part of chromosome B are sequestered in a portion of the nucleus, perhaps attached to the nuclear matrix (wavy line) because of their particular structure, function, chromatin status or accessibility, or by chance. The recombinase complexes are operative in this part of the nucleus and act on the two chromosomes to cause breakage and rejoining events. The complex (dashed line box) consists of targeting, nucleolytic and repair enzymes, including *RAG1*, *RAG2*, the *SCID* gene product and TdT. The hatched and open boxes delineate 'coding' segments, the triangle, 'signal' sequences. The structure shown on chromosome B in the upper part of the figure is consistent with an immune receptor locus. Part of the recombination reaction proceeds normally; the ends of the intervening sequence carrying the signal segments are joined together in an extrachromosomal circle. However, the topography and topology of chromosomes A and B cause an interchromosomal rather than an intralocus rearrangement, which results in a chromosomal translocation. (From Kirsch IR. In: Pizzo P, Poplack D (eds) *Principles and practice of pediatric oncology*, 2nd edn. Philadelphia, J. B. Lippincott, 1993; with permission.)

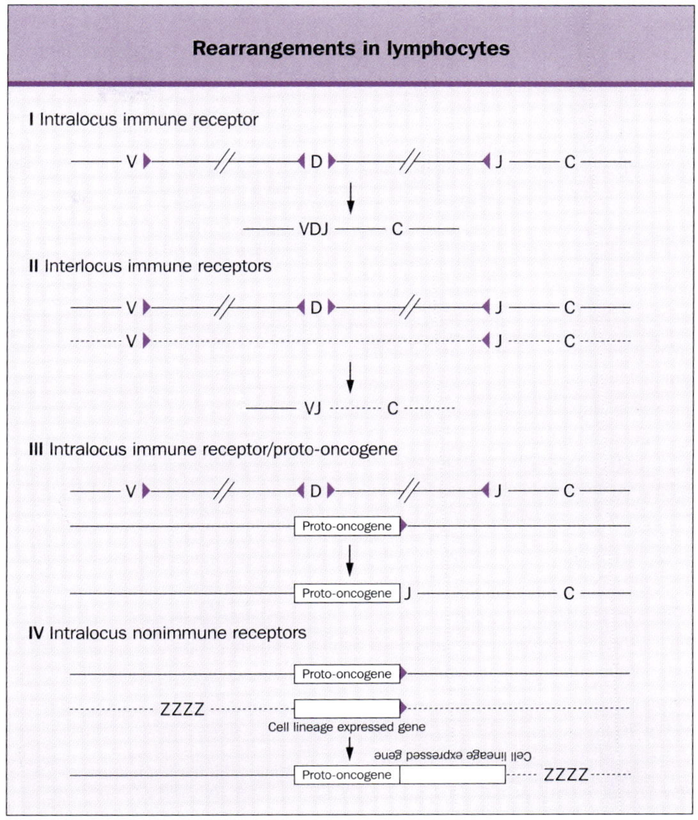

Figure 93.5 Rearrangements in lymphocytes. Four types of genomic rearrangements that have been characterized in lymphocytes. I, Intralocus rearrangements that generate immune receptor diversity. II, Rearrangements mediated by the same process as I (above) but occurring between two immune receptor loci rather than within one or another of the loci. III, Rearrangements between an immune receptor locus and a protooncogene (e.g. IgH–*BCL2* rearrangements in B-cell follicular lymphoma). IV, Rearrangements between two loci, neither of which is an immune receptor. This kind of rearrangement can still involve the lymphocyte-specific recombinase enzymes if appropriate signal sequences are present flanking the loci and if the loci are accessible (e.g. *SIL–SCL(TAL1)* rearrangements in T-ALL).

result in chromosomal translocations. The machinery of somatic hypermutation can be also responsible for somatic mutations of *BCL6*, c-*MYC* and *FGFR3*, genes translocated into the IgH locus in diffuse large cell lymphoma, Burkitt's lymphoma or myeloma, respectively.[5]

Translocations that utilize the immunoglobulin 'switch' mechanism

As previously noted, there is an additional inherent mechanism of destabilization in lymphocytes that mediates the switch of immunoglobulin isotype from IgM to IgG, IgE or IgA. This also involves DNA breakage and rejoining, in this case being targeted to regions of repeating pentamers of DNA (switch regions) which are found in the intervening DNA between the J and C segments of the μ gene and 5′ from the other heavy-chain C segments, γ, ε and α. Certain characteristic translocations do routinely occur within the heavy-chain switch regions.[25,26] The most notable of these is the t(8;14)(q24;q32.3) associated with the development of sporadic (as opposed to the disease endemic to central Africa)

Burkitt lymphoma and B-cell leukemia. By contrast, translocation breakpoints associated with endemic Burkitt lymphoma are usually near JH or JL regions and thus are probably mediated by the V(D)J recombinase. As switch recombination usually seems to follow the formation of an immunoglobulin gene, it has been suggested that the transformed cell in sporadic Burkitt lymphoma is at a later stage of development than that in the endemic form. However, both sporadic and endemic Burkitt's lymphoma cells have IgH and IgL with extensive somatic hypermutations, indicating that they are germinal center or postgerminal center B-cell tumors. It now seems likely that the translocations in endemic Burkitt lymphoma are caused either by somatic hypermutation or by errors in process of V(D)J-mediated receptor editing that can occur in the germinal centers.[5]

OTHER MECHANISMS OF CHROMOSOMAL TRANSLOCATIONS

Chromosomal aberrations are not restricted to cells carrying the V(D)J or 'switch' recombinase systems. Therefore, there must be other mechanisms capable of mediating reciprocal or unidirectional chromosomal breakage and rejoining. These mechanisms may be particularly relevant to the formation of translocations that result in the fusion between two nonimmune genes. The t(9;22)(q34;q11) is associated with blast crisis in patients with CML or de novo development of ALL. It is a reciprocal translocation from which the derivative chromosome 22 is the so-called 'Philadelphia' chromosome, identification of which is one of the founding observations in the field of cancer cytogenetics.[27,28] The translocation event juxtaposes the *ABL* gene on chromosome 9 with the *BCR* gene on chromosome 22.[29] There are no obvious signal or switch sequences that suggest recombinase targeting. Proximate to some of the breakpoints within the *BCR* gene are *'alu'* repetitive sequences.[30] These are found dispersed throughout the genome and a number of these segments are transcribed by RNA polymerase III. Thus, for certain of these repeat elements, their presence may confer accessibility upon the local chromatin. The topographical distance between the *BCR* and the *ABL* genes in the interphase nucleus is cell type-specific and appears differentially minimized in hematopoietic precursor cells.[31] Cell type-specific nuclear topography may therefore be another unifying mechanistic theme required for the formation of reciprocal chromosomal translocations.

An intriguing link between site-specific DNA breakage during the early stages of apoptosis and the generation of oncogenic chromosomal translocations has recently been suggested by a study of the *MLL* and *AML1* genes. The *MLL* gene (also known as *ALL1* or *HRX*) at chromosome 11q23, and the *AML1* (also called *CBFA2*) at chromosome 21q22 are frequently involved in chromosomal translocations with multiple independent partners in both lymphoid and myeloid leukemias.[32] Chromosomal rearrangements of either gene are found in therapy-related acute myeloid leukemia (t-AML) following treatment of the primary malignancy with chemotherapy that often includes topoisomerase II (topo II) inhibitors such as etoposide or adriamycin. Accordingly, it has been shown that topo II inhibitors can cause site-specific double-strand DNA breaks within the areas of the translocation's associated breakpoints.[33] Stanulla et al[34] demonstrated that the same breaks could be induced in intact living cells by exposing them to a variety of apoptosis-inducing agents. These breaks within the *MLL* and the *AML1* genes are associated with the cleavage of large (50–100 kb) DNA loops at their anchorage sites to the nuclear matrix during the initial stages of apoptosis. This cleavage, mediated by topo II, is reversible at its earliest stages before the activation of other DNA nucleases and the occurrence of extensive apoptotic DNA degradation.[35]

The hypothesis that some oncogenic chromosomal translocations are generated by the repair of site-specific DNA breaks during aborted apoptosis is particularly attractive for lymphoid malignancies. These malignancies arise on the background of normal extensive developmental apoptosis of lymphoid precursors. In this model a lymphoid precursor cell rarely may be rescued from apoptotis by the generation of a survival-promoting chromosomal rearrangement. Consistent with this model is the reported analysis of single Reed–Sternberg cells, the malignant cell of Hodgkin's lymphoma, that revealed crippling mutations in their Ig genes and suggested that these cells were rescued from apoptosis.[5] Also consistent with translocations resulting from DNA breakage followed by DNA repair is the finding of extensive DNA repair at the junctions of the t(4;11), fusing the *MLL* with the *AF4* genes in infant ALL, and the t(12;21), fusing the *TEL* with the *AML1* genes in childhood common ALL.[36,37]

FUNCTIONAL CONSEQUENCES OF GENETIC INSTABILITY IN LYMPHOCYTES

In most cases cancer is caused not by a foreign entity taking control of the cell, but by mutation of the cell's own growth-regulating machinery. An emerging paradigm suggests that many 'solid' epithelial tumors arise after a series of mutational events that sufficiently disrupt the normal checks and balances on cellular growth, resulting in malignant transformation.[38] These events have been charted and elucidated for a variety of tumors, and involve combinations in the activation of dominant growth-promoting genes or death-preventing genes, and deletion or dysfunction of growth-arresting genes. At times it appears that the number of mutational events found in a colon or lung carcinoma are so many as to defy current concepts of mutational frequencies in eukaryotic cells. Part of the solution to this paradox is suggested by the finding that mutation of certain genes (e.g. p53) seems to result in loss of a checkpoint control at the cell cycle transition from G1 to S and from G2 to M phases.[39] These checkpoints appear to be used by the cell to repair DNA damage or alteration and restore genomic integrity. With their loss the ability to accumulate additional mutations may increase substantially.[40] Thus, in many solid tumors there appears to be a step specifically required to destabilize the genome, after which follows a series of additional mutational events that, in combination, contribute to cellular transformation. The question of whether there is a programmed sequence of mutational events that must, more or less, be followed to transform a cell is still under investigation.[41] Whether there is a fundamental difference between leukemias, lymphomas and other solid tumors with regard to this destabilization step deserves further discussion.

Although there are examples of hematopoietic malignancies, such as multiple myeloma and HIV-related lymphoma, in which multiple mutational events have occurred, it is striking that for a number of hematopoietic malignancies (particularly certain lymphoid malignancies), a vast accumulation of mutations has not been observed at the time of first presentation. These observ-

KEY CONCEPTS

Genetic instability
- Many lymphoid malignancies are caused in part by a dysregulation of one or more transcription factors.
- Genes that function at any point in a growth-regulatory cascade can also be involved.

ations are not consistent with a multistep model of carcinogenesis. In many cases of lymphoid malignancy there is often one predominant genetic alteration, frequently consisting of a specific chromosomal aberration, that can be a diagnostic marker for that type of malignancy. There are examples of similar diagnostic chromosomal changes that allow the identification of certain pediatric sarcomas and occasional adult cancers, but the general picture in carcinomas is not as simple as that of the hematopoietic malignancies.[42] Perhaps the inherent targeted mechanisms of genetic instability in lymphocytes makes the de novo generation of early destabilizing mutations unnecessary in the progression to malignancy. This would somewhat limit the average number of alterations that are required to initiate transformation in lymphocytes, compared to other types of cancer.

This apparent simplicity is somewhat deceptive. For most, if not all, of the lymphoid neoplasms the primary chromosomal aberration is necessary but not sufficient for the development of frank malignancy. This conclusion is based on several observations. First, with sensitive methodologies it is possible to detect in normal people many of the chromosomal translocations typically associated with hematopoietic malignancies (e.g. t(14;18), t(4;11), t(9;22), t(2;5)).[43–46] Second, in experimental mouse models there is usually a significant time lag between the introduction of the translocation and the development of lymphoma, suggesting the need for additional transforming steps.[47,48] Third, and most striking, is the observation that at least some of the translocations associated with childhood lymphoblastic leukemia originate in utero. Clonospecific translocations have been detected simultaneously in blood collected routinely at birth, and in diagnostic blood samples from six of nine children who presented with TEL/AML1-positive leukemia at the age of 2–5 years.[49] A description of identical twins who developed the same t(12;21)-positive leukemias at different ages (as far as 5 and 14 years) suggests that the leukemic clone originated in one twin and passed to the other in utero.[50] Similar findings have been reported for the t(4;11), a translocation characteristic of infant leukemia.[51] Finally, identical clonal immune receptor gene rearrangements have been found in paired neonatal and subsequent diagnostic blood samples from children with cytogenetically negative ALL, suggesting that a prenatal origin of childhood leukemia is a documentable phenomenon (R. Panzer-Gruemayer, personal communication).

It is likely that additional mutational events occur in the interval between the formation of a translocation in utero and the development of frank leukemia years later. Two pathways regulating cell cycle progression that are frequently – perhaps universally – disrupted in carcinomas appear also to be targeted in lymphoid malignancies. The retinoblastoma pathway controls the progression from the G1 to the S phase of the cell cycle. Cyclin D1, a positive regulator of this pathway, is dysregulated through its involvement in several translocations (see Table 93.1), whereas in other instances $p16^{ink4}$ and $p15^{ink4}$, inhibitors of this pathway, are frequently inactivated.[52] As mentioned earlier, the deletion of these tumor-suppressing genes in T-ALL is probably mediated by the V(D)J recombinase. The same genomic locus is also home to $p19^{ARF}$, whose role is to stabilize p53 by inhibiting MDM2, a protein that targets p53 for degradation. When $p19^{ARF}$ is deleted, wild-type p53 is destabilized. Thus, despite the low frequency of *p53* mutations at diagnosis, its pathway is functionally inactivated in many cases of T-ALL.[53] Inactivation of $p19^{ARF}$ has also been identified as an important secondary event in the generation of lymphomas in c-*myc* transgenic mice.[54] It appears, therefore, that despite diverse mechanisms of genomic instability and strikingly different magnitudes of genomic disruption, basic cellular growth controlling pathways are targeted in both lymphoid and epithelial malignancies.

ANALYSIS OF GENES CLONED FROM TRANSLOCATION BREAKPOINTS

The apparent simplicity suggested by distinct chromosomal aberrations that correlate with specific subtypes of lymphoid malignancies has provided an obvious target for studying genes critical to lymphoid growth and development. Strategically, numerous investigators have viewed the cloning and characterization of the genes flanking various leukemia-associated or lymphoma-associated chromosomal aberrations as a way to examine malignant transformation as well as normal lymphoid proliferation and development. Table 93.2 offers a partial list of the genes that have been found flanking the chromosomal breakpoints of specific leukemia or lymphoma subtypes. This represents a slightly different way of looking at the data presented in Table 93.1.

Many of the genes discovered at the junctions of chromosomal aberrations associated with the development of lymphoid malignancy are transcription factors (e.g. *SCL*, *E2A*) or nuclear proteins that interact with transcription factors (e.g. LMO1, LMO2). These transcription complexes bind to DNA at the promoter sites of genes and recruit chromatin-remodeling proteins that regulate transcription by controlling accessibility to the RNA polymerase. Activating complexes 'open' the local chromatin through chemical modifications such as histone acetylation, whereas repressing proteins 'close' the local chromatin by reversing these chemical modifications. The net result of this interplay can be the inhibition or activation of entire programs and cascades of gene expression governing cellular developmental programs, proliferation and differentiation.[55] The other genes listed in Table 93.2 cover almost all other facets of a growth-regulatory cascade, including growth factors, growth-factor receptors, signal-transducing factors and apoptosis-preventing proteins.

With the advancement in genetic knockout techniques in mice it has become clear that many of the genes cloned from cancer-associated chromosomal translocations play fundamental roles in development. Some are important for the development of the same lineage in which their disruption occurs. For example, the proteins encoded by the *E2A* gene, E12 and E47, are required for early development of B cells.[56] Translocations involving the *E2A* gene are associated with early B-cell leukemias.[57] Similarly, *BCL6* is required for the development of germinal centers and is translocated in lymphomas originated in the germinal centers.[58] Other

Functional characterization of transforming genes at functional breakpoints

Gene family		Gene	Developmental role	Characteristic translocation	Malignancy
Transcription factors	Homeodomain	*PBX1*	ND	t(1;19)(q23;p13)	Pre-B ALL
		PAX5	B-cell development	t(9;14)(p13;q32)	MM, LPL
		HOX11	Spleen formation	t(10;14)(q24;q11); others	T-ALL
	Trithorax	*MLL*	Embryonic patterning; hematopoiesis	11q23 translocations	ALL and AML
	Helix–loop–helix	*LYL1*	ND		
		MYC	Embryonic, generalized	8q24 translocations	Burkitt and T-ALL
		SCL(TAL1)	Hematopoiesis, angiogenesis	t(1;14)(p33;q11.2) del(1p33)	T-ALL
		TAL2	ND	t(7;9)(q35;q34.2)	T-ALL
		E2A	Lymphopoiesis	19p13 translocations	Pre B ALL
	NFκB/Rel	*BCL3*	T and B cell functions; secondary lymphoid organs	t(14;19)(q32;q11.3)	CLL
		NFkB2/lyt10κ	ND	t(10;14)(q24;q32)	B and T-NHL
	LIM	*LMO1*	Hematopoiesis	t(11;14)(p15;q11)	T-ALL
		LMO2	Hematopoiesis	t(11;14)(q13;q11)	T-ALL
	Zinc finger	*BCL6*	Germinal centers	t(3;14)(q27;q32.3)	DLCL
	Ets	*TEL*	Angiogenesis	t(12;21)(p13;q22)	Early pre-B ALL
	Runt homology	*AML1*	Hematopoiesis	t(12;21)(p13;q22)	Early pre-B ALL
	Leucine zipper	*HLF*	ND	t(17;19)(q22;p13)	Early pre-B ALL
Tyrosine kinases		*ABL*	B-cell development and more	t(9;22)(q34;q11)	CML/ALL
		LCK	T-cell development	t(1;7)(q34;q35)	T-ALL
Serine kinases		*BCR*	Neutrophil function	t(9;22)(q34;q11)	CML; ALL
Cell cycle regulatory (cyclins)		*Cyclin D1*	General growth; breast; retina	t(11;14)(q13;q32.3) t(11;22)(q13;q11)	MM; CLL
Growth factor receptors		*TAN1 (Notch)*	Lymphopoiesis; fate determination of multiple tissues	t(7;9)(q35;q34)	T-ALL
		FGFR-3	Osteogenesis	t(4;14)(q16.3;q32.3)	MM
Growth factors		*IL-3*	Hematopoiesis	t(5;14) (q31;q32)	ALL with eosinophilia
Apoptosis regulatory (*BCL2* family)		*BCL-2*	Antiapoptosis; general growth. T-cell survival, renal development	t(14;18)(q32.3;q21) and others	FL; MM; CLL
		BCL10	ND	t(1;14)(p22;q32)	MALT
Other phosphoproteins		*SIL*	Embryonic midline and left/right asymmetry	del(1p33)	T-ALL
		NPM	ND	t(2;5)(p23;q35)	LCL

ALL, acute lymphoblastic leukemia; CLL, chronic lymphocytic leukemia; MM, multiple myeloma; LPL, lymphoplasmacytic lymphoma; DLCL, diffuse large cell lymphoma; FL, follicular lymphoma; LCL, large cell lymphoma; NHL, non-Hodgkin's lymphoma; MALT, mucosa-associated lymphoid tumor; ND, not defined.

Table 93.2 Functional characterization of transforming genes at translocation breakpoints.

genes are required for the development of hematopoietic lineages, but are not expressed in lymphoid progenitors. *SCL*, for example, is a transcription factor critical for the earliest stage of hematopoietic and blood vessel development.[23] Similarly, *LMO1*, *LMO2*, *AML1* and the *TEL* genes have various developmental roles in hematopoietic development.[32] Other genes are involved in the determination of nonhematopoietic tissues.[32,59] *MLL* and *PBX1* are unique in their role of regulating *HOX* genes, genes that encode homeotic proteins critical for spatial patterning during embryonic development.[60] Their orthologs in Drosophila, *trithorax* and *extradenticle*, respectively, are critical for the determination of segmental and anterior posterior identities. Mice lacking one allele of the *mll* genes are small, anemic and thrombocytopenic, and demonstrate segmental abnormalities with disordered identity of their vertebrae. Mice lacking both copies of the *mll* gene die in utero, lacking expression of the *hox* genes.[61] The translocation-induced misexpression of these developmentally important genes leads to the hypothesis that their role in tumorigenesis is through subversion of the normal developmental program of the cells in which the translocations reside.

Mechanisms of gene disruption via chromosomal aberrations

Chromosomal translocations disrupt genes either by altering the expression of a normal gene or by altering gene structure (Fig. 93.6). The expression level is altered by chromosomal aberrations through the insertion of regulatory sequences upstream or downstream from the transcription unit. Alternatively, one transcription unit is fused with another, creating a gene encoding a novel chimeric protein. Misexpression of a normal or chimeric protein alters the dynamic equilibrium of protein–protein interaction in the cell, leading to the emergence of the malignant cell phenotype: differentiation arrest coupled with enhanced cellular proliferation and survival.

The functional consequences of chromosomal translocations have been studied in some detail for transcription factors.

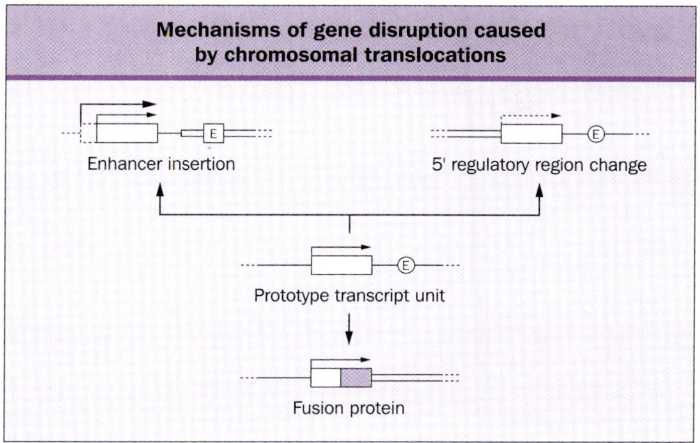

Figure 93.6 Mechanisms of gene disruption caused by chromosomal translocations. A prototype transcript unit is disrupted in its 3′ region (upper left) by a translocation that removes one and substitutes a different enhancer sequence. This enhancer causes transcription to start upstream of its usual position and also increases the quantity of transcript emanating from the locus. A different kind of translocation (upper right) removes the normal 5′ regulatory region and substitutes a different region that changes the transcriptional regulation of the locus. Yet another way in which chromosomal translocation can alter a gene is by structurally changing it so as to create a novel protein composed of segments from the two loci formerly separate, but now contiguous.

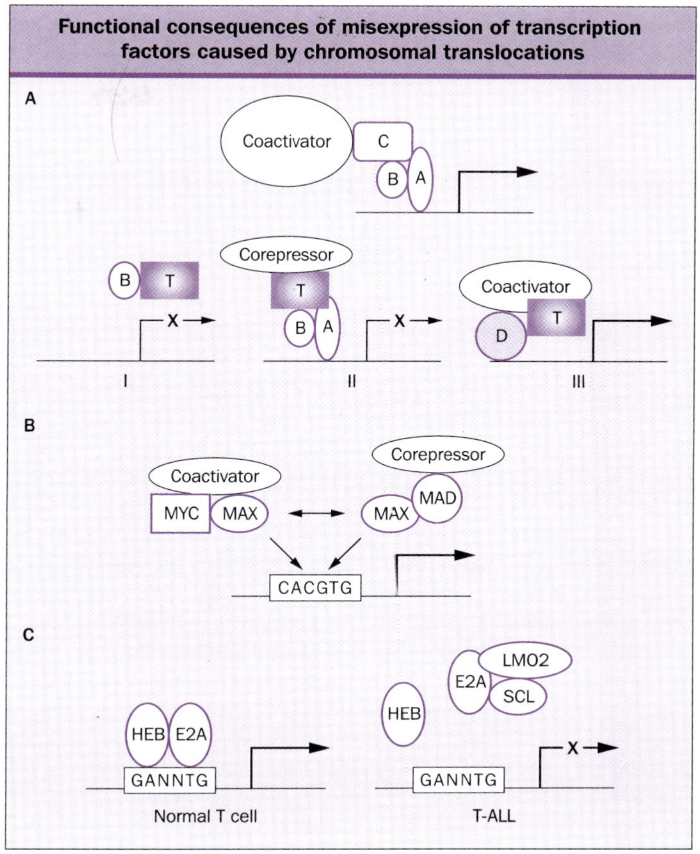

Figure 93.7 Functional consequences of misexpression of transcription factors caused by chromosomal translocations. (**A**) Transcriptional complex of proteins binds to promoter sequences and regulates gene expression through recruitment of a coactivator or corepressor chromatin-remodeling protein complex. When a transcription factor 'T' is misexpressed, the transcriptional complex may be disrupted by (I) sequestration of one or more of its components, or (II) recruitment of a chromatin-remodeling complex of an opposite activity (e.g. AML1 fusion proteins cause exchange of a corepressor with a coactivator). Alternatively (III) a new aberrant transcription complex is formed, regulating a different set of genes. (**B**) A simplified scheme of MYC transcriptional network. MAX can dimerize either with MYC to form transcriptional activating complexes or with MAD to inhibit transcription. Constitutive expression of MYC secondary to its placement under the control of an immune receptor locus would have substantial effects on this dynamic equilibrium. (**C**) Proposed mechanism of leukemogenesis by dysregulation of SCL (TAL1) and LMO2, in T-cell ALL. E2A proteins direct T-cell development by regulating transcription through binding to E-BOX promoter sequences as heterodimers with the bHLH1 protein HEB. Abnormally expressed SCL and/or LMO bind and sequester E2A, thereby disrupting the normal T-lymphocyte developmental program.

Misexpressed or chimeric transcription factors can disrupt the transcription complex in several ways (Fig. 93.7).[48,55,60] The complex can be disrupted entirely, or may recruit chromatin-remodeling proteins with the opposite regulatory effects, e.g. from activation to repression, or vice versa. The net result is the reversal of the normal expression pattern of regulated downstream genes. A variation on this theme occurs when the misexpression of a particular factor leads to sequestration of one or more of the normally interactive components of a lineage-specific transcription complex. Alternatively, a new transcription complex can be formed, regulating a different set of genes that normally are not regulated in that particular cell, thereby altering the normal cellular growth and developmental program.

Identifying the downstream genes and cellular pathways targeted by the oncogenic events remains a significant challenge. Even for a protein such as MYC, which has been studied intensively for the last two decades, very few downstream genes have been identified with certainty. Microarray technology enabling the simultaneous analysis of the levels and patterns of expression of thousands of genes may dramatically expedite the delineation of these pathways.[62]

A few well-studied examples of gene disruption by chromosomal translocations in lymphoid malignancies include the following.

Promoter truncation and/or enhancer introduction

Translocations involving the *c-MYC* proto-oncogene (Fig. 93.8)

These translocations provide dramatic examples of how chromosomal aberrations can lead to dysregulated expression.[63] c-*MYC* is characteristically juxtaposed with an immunoglobulin locus in L3-ALL, Burkitt lymphoma, and a subgroup of other nonHodgkin lymphomas. It is also juxtaposed with the TCRα locus in a subgroup of T-ALL. In each of these cases it appears that the c-*MYC* gene is placed within the range of influence of a region resulting in enhanced transcription of the locus. The break within the immune receptor occurs in the neighborhood of J or switch sequences, but not always with a precision that can be explained simply by invoking the known recombinases. Perhaps the lability of these loci makes them also more susceptible to other types of DNA breakage and rejoining processes. In some cases the normal promoter sequences of c-*MYC* are left intact; in other cases they are mutated or removed to the other derivative chromosome.

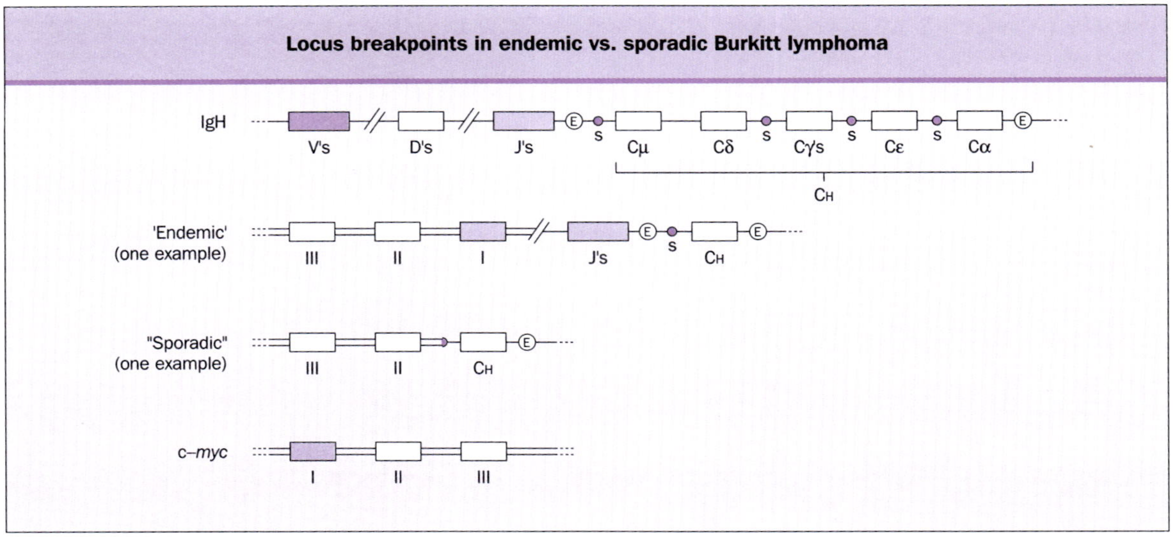

Figure 93.8 Locus breakpoints in endemic vs. sporadic Burkitt lymphoma. A schematic of the IgH locus is shown in the top line (Vs, Ds, Js and Cs; E, enhancers; s, 'switch' regions) and of the c-*myc* proto-oncogene (coding segments shown in clear boxes, noncoding first exon in hatched box) in the bottom line. In endemic Burkitt lymphoma the c-*MYC* gene is often disrupted far 5′ of its first exon and joined head to head with the IgH locus disrupted within or upstream of the J segments. In sporadic Burkitt lymphoma the c-*MYC* gene is often disrupted within its first noncoding exon or between exons I and II, and joined to the IgH locus within the Ig 'switch' region (half of a switch region is shown juxtaposed to the truncated c-*MYC*).

The net effect appears to be that c-*MYC* is regulated like an immune receptor and not like a powerful growth-promoting gene that must be precisely tuned. The *MYC* gene on the untranslocated allele is usually quiescent, whereas the translocated allele is expressed.[64] Presumably a program for continued cell growth is therefore kept active, providing a powerful contribution to malignant transformation.

In cases in which all three exons of the c-*MYC* gene remain together during the translocation associated with B-cell malignancy, additional structural changes in the c-*MYC* gene have been noted. An approximately 400 bp region that stretches from within the first exon into the first intron appears to be targeted for mutation accompanying or shortly following the translocation event. Within this region are sites that are normally involved in blocking the elongation of the *MYC* transcript, one mechanism of control of c-*MYC* during normal growth and development.[65] This same mutational 'hotspot' also contains a potential binding site of a c-*MYC* regulatory protein, MIF.[66] Mutations of this region could therefore be at least partly responsible for c-*MYC* dysregulation.[67] In addition, somatic mutation of the second exon of the translocated c-*MYC* gene within regions that encode the transactivation domain of the protein have been reported.[68] The mechanism by which these regions of the c-*MYC* gene become targets for somatic hypermutation has not been determined. It is tempting to speculate that placing the c-*MYC* gene in the context of the IgH locus leads to these mutational events. In that light, it is relevant that in a small number of sequence analyses of c-*MYC* genes translocated in T-cell malignancies, these mutational events were not noted (R. Dalla-Favera, personal communication). T-cell antigen receptors are not subject to somatic hypermutation.[58]

The direct connection has not yet been made between c-*MYC* dysregulation by chromosomal translocation and transformation of the cell in which the translocation occurs. However, a great deal of circumstantial information is accumulating regarding the role of c-*MYC* in lymphoid transformation. Strong evidence comes from a recent study of transgenic mice conditionally expressing c-*myc* in hematopoietic cells. Sustained expression of c-*myc* caused clonal T-cell lymphomas.[69] These lymphomas regressed when the expression of c-*myc* was turned off. Because the lymphomas were clonal, despite the overexpression of c-*myc* in every lymphoid cell, it is clear that secondary oncogenic events must have occurred. This is consistent with the model of multistep tumorigenesis. It is striking, however, that the lymphomas remained dependent on c-*myc* expression, suggesting that c-*myc* may be a good target for therapy of malignancies in which it is overexpressed.

MYC is one of those transcription factors with both DNA binding and protein–protein interactive capabilities, diverse function and complicated regulation.[70] The c-*MYC* gene encodes a protein with both a basic DNA-binding domain (b) and two distinct motifs mediating protein dimerization, a helix–loop–helix (HLH) and a leucine zipper (LZ). The presence of these two dimerization motifs suggests a complex panoply of interactions of this gene product with numerous other transcription factors within the cell. MYC dimerizes with MAX and binds to specific DNA sequences in promoters of downstream genes (Fig. 93.7B). MYC:MAX dimers activate transcription through the recruitment of a large chromatin-remodeling complex with histone acetyltransferase activity. MAX, in turn, can inhibit transcription through dimerization with two additional partners, MAD or MXI-1. Depending on the dynamic equilibrium among all these proteins, transcriptional activation or inhibition results. Clearly, the constitutive expression of c-MYC secondary to its placement under the control of an immune receptor locus would have substantial effects on this dynamic equilibrium.

Which genes under the control of c-MYC might contribute to malignant transformation? Many have been proposed as candidate targets for c-MYC.[70] These genes link c-MYC to cell cycle and apoptosis, to DNA and cellular metabolism, and to intercellular communication. Their validity as true targets is disputed and their importance in malignant transformation is unclear. Interestingly, c-MYC was found to induce anerobic metabolism through the induction of lactic dehydrogenase (LDH-A), a key enzyme in anerobic glycolysis. This associates c-MYC with the Warburg effect.[71] Warburg described the ability of cancer cells to survive in anerobic conditions, an essential property for survival in the hypoxic environment within tumor masses. Interestingly, the serum level of LDH is a strong indicator of tumor burden in several malignancies, including B-cell lymphomas.[72]

Dysregulation of SCL (TAL1), LMO1 and LMO2 in T-cell malignancies[48,73]

This intriguing example is chosen because it represents a potentially general mechanism for the development of precursor T-cell leukemia and lymphoma through dominant negative suppression of a normal development pathway (Fig. 93.7C). *SCL* encodes a transcription factor containing a carboxy-terminal bHLH DNA-binding and protein interaction domain and an amino-terminal transactivation domain. Like other type 2 bHLH transcription factors it binds to bHLH1 proteins, such as E2A or HEB, to regulate the expression of genes. Although normally not expressed in T lymphocytes, SCL is detected in over 60% of childhood T-cell ALL. Aberrant expression in T-cell leukemia is caused either by translocations of the *SCL* coding sequences into the proximity of TCR enhancers or, more commonly, by promoter substitution caused by the chromosomal rearrangement with the *SIL* gene described earlier. In many cases the mechanism leading to SCL overexpression has not been characterized.

LMO and LMO2 (Lim Only) are small nuclear adaptor proteins that do not bind DNA. Their pattern of expression in normal hematopoietic and in leukemic cells and their developmental role are similar to those of SCL. As suggested by the similar expression pattern, a pentameric activation complex containing SCL, LMO2, LDB1, GATA1 and E2A can be detected in hematopoietic precursors in vivo. Like SCL, LMO1 and LMO2 are not expressed normally in the thymus, but they are expressed in the majority of human T-cell precursor leukemia/lymphomas. Their aberrant expression is caused by translocations into the TCR region or by other uncharacterized mechanisms. Interestingly, LMO2 and SCL are also aberrantly expressed in the majority of T-cell lymphoblastic lymphomas in mice defective in the mismatch repair gene *msh2*. Their expression in other murine models of T-cell lymphomas has not been analyzed. The wide expression of SCL and LMO2 in human and mouse precursor T-cell lymphoma suggests a similar and critical role in lymphomagenesis.

> **KEY CONCEPTS**
>
> **Mechanisms of gene disruption**
> - Mechanisms of altering function of proto-oncogenes in lymphoid malignancies include:
>   - The assumption of transcriptional control by an enhancer element introduced by chromosomal translocation
>   - The redirection of transcription by the alteration of the usual 5′ regulatory and promoter sequences
> - The formation of a fusion between two genes that formerly had distinct and separate functions.

Mice transgenic for *scl*, *lmo1* or *lmo2* develop T-cell lymphoma after a very long latency. However, when crossed with either *lmo1* or *lmo2*, transgenic mice with thymic expression of *scl* develop T-cell lymphomas at young age, with a high degree of penetrance. Remarkably, identical lymphomas develop at the same rate when the *scl* transgene lacks the transactivating domain. This suggests a dominant negative mechanism of lymphomagenesis. Indeed, biochemical analysis of mouse and human thymic lymphoma cells revealed that the SCL and LMO1 (or LMO2) proteins sequester E2A and inhibit normal E2A activity. In T-cell development E2A dimerizes with another bHLH1 transcription factor, HEB, to regulate genes critical for T-cell development.[56] Mice lacking E2A develop T-cell lymphomas that are similar to those observed in the *scl/lmo1* transgenic mice. Restoration of E2A in cell lines derived from patients with T-ALL, or in mice lacking the *e2a* gene, result in growth suppression and apoptosis of the lymphoma cells.[74,75] These combined observations strongly suggest that *SCL, LMO1* and *LMO2* induce T-cell lymphomas by disrupting the normal developmental program mediated by *E2A*. Because several other genes dysregulated by chromosomal translocations in T-ALL either bind E2A (e.g. *TAL2, LYL1*) or inactivate it (*TAN1*, the human ortholog of *Notch*), abrogation of the contribution of *E2A* to a developmental pathway may be a unifying mechanism of T-cell lymphomagenesis.[76] It is perplexing, however, that genomic disruption of the *E2A* or the *HEB* genes has not been described in T-cell malignancies.

Dysregulation of BCL2

Study of *BCL2* has revealed or supported novel and fundamental principles of growth and development. *BCL2* is a prime example of this. This gene is dysregulated by its translocation to the IgH locus coincident with the t(14;18) translocation associated with the development of follicular lymphoma.[77] The *BCL2* gene product appears to abrogate the apoptotic pathway that normally occurs in B lymphocytes that are not positively selected.[78] As in the case of the transcription factors mentioned above, the action of BCL2 appears to be mediated through its interaction with a variety of dimerizing partners.[79] Depending on the relative levels of the various proteins, apoptosis is favored or suppressed. Thus constitutive expression of the BCL2 protein may be a mechanism by which the program is directed toward the maintenance of cells that normally are destined to die.

THE FORMATION OF FUSION PROTEINS

In B-cell precursor leukemias the *E2A* gene is involved in at least two chromosomal translocations.[57] In the t(1;19)(q23;p13), associated with 25% of cases with pre-B ALL, several fusion proteins are formed in which the E2A transactivation domain is fused with the homeodomain of PBX1. In the extremely rare t(17;19)(q22;p13), reported in seven patients with pro-B ALL, the bHLH of the *E2A* gene is again removed and the transactivation domain is fused with the DNA-binding and dimerization domain of HLF. Thus in both translocations the fusion proteins carry a strong activating domain from *E2A* and a DNA-binding and protein interaction domains from a different gene. The mixing together of different DNA-binding, protein dimerization capabilities and transactivation domains could result in abnormal activation or repression of a variety of growth and proliferative pathways. Both chimeric proteins have transforming ability in vitro and induce lymphomas in transgenic mice. As commonly happens in mouse models, however, the lymphomas are of T and not B lineage. Surprisingly, the DNA binding of PBX1 is dispensible, and the only parts required for transformation are the protein-interacting domain of PBX1 and the transactivation domain of E2A.[80] E2A/PBX1 activity is mediated by the interaction of PBX1 with HOX proteins. Thus it is likely that the oncogenic activity of E2A–PBX1 is caused by the inappropriate activation of genes normally regulated by PBX1–HOX complexes. The Drosophila ortholog of *PBX1*, *extradenticle*, induces the wnt signaling pathway. Similarly, WNT-16, a new member of the WNT family of secreted growth factors, was recently identified as a downstream target of E2A–PBX1 in pre-B leukemia cells. As WNT receptors are expressed on pre-B cells it appears that the t(1;19) leads to the development of leukemia through the induction of a WNT-16 mediated autocrine growth.[81]

The t(12;21), creating the *TEL–AML1* (also named *ETV6–CBFA2*) fusion gene, is the most common chromosomal translocation in childhood B-cell precursor leukemia and is associated with an especially favorable outcome.[82,83] This translocation is unique because it involves two genes that are common targets of chromosomal rearrangement in human leukemias. AML1 is a transcription factor that forms a tight complex with CBFβ and activates the expression of many hematopoietic specific genes. This complex is frequently interrupted by translocations in myeloid leukemias. The *TEL* gene is characterized by a C-terminal ETS DNA-binding domain and an N-terminal HLH protein-interacting domain, and is involved in close to 20 different translocations in human hematopoietic malignancies. The t(12;21) translocation fuses the HLH domain of TEL to almost all of AML1. The normal *TEL* gene on the other chromosome is usually lost, suggesting that loss of normal TEL activity is important for leukemogenesis. The chimeric protein dominantly inhibits the AML1–CBFβ complex, possibly by recruiting a repressor chromatin-remodeling complex (Fig 93.7A).

In the *BCR–ABL* fusion the contribution of the *ABL* gene is relatively constant, whereas the contribution of the *BCR* gene is somewhat variable. This variability results in the production of two varieties of fusion proteins, p210 (containing more *BCR* exons), seen in CML and ALL, and P190 (containing fewer *BCR* exons), noted in juvenile and adult Philadelphia chromosome-positive ALL.[84] *ABL* is a well established proto-oncogene that encodes a nuclear tyrosine kinase. The BCR–ABL fusion protein localizes to the cytosol and has a constitutive increased activity. Transgenic mice carrying expressed *bcr–abl* fusion genes and mice transplanted with bone marrow infected by *bcr–abl* succumb to hematopoietic malignancies.[85,86] However, the fusion gene does not appear to be highly oncogenic in nonhematopoietic tissues. Transformation by *BCR–ABL* appears to involve the activation of multiple genes, including *JUN*, *STAT5*, c-*MYC* and Cyclin D1.[82]

GENE REARRANGEMENTS AS TUMOR-SPECIFIC MARKERS

As is clear from the preceding discussion, the DNA in a malignant lymphocyte is not the same as that in other tissues or in nontransformed lymphocytes. Irreversible reconfigurations of the DNA have occurred, reconfigurations that are unique to the transformed cell. One class of these rearrangements is the specific immunoglobulin and T-cell receptor locus rearrangements that the cell has elaborated in the process of generating a functional antigen-binding moiety. The other is the rearrangements of growth-affecting genes whose disruption has contributed to the process of malignant transformation. Recognition of these molecular fingerprints is finding increased use in the diagnosis, classification and staging of an individual patient's malignancy. Furthermore, the high sensitivity and specificity of the molecular genetic tests now being used are promoting the application of tumor-specific gene rearrangements as a means of following a given patient's response to therapy, residual tumor burden during or after therapy, and early diagnosis of relapse. For example, until the advent of these sophisticated tests a patient with leukemia was said to be 'in remission' when less than 5% leukemic blasts could be identified morphologically on a stained preparation of their bone marrow. Current polymerase chain reaction (PCR)-based techniques are capable of detecting one leukemic cell in a background of 100 000 to 1 000 000 normal cells, and allow quantitative estimation of the level of residual disease.

The realization that certain chromosomal rearrangements in ALL are strong prognostic factors has led to the development of treatment protocols tailored for specific molecular subtypes.[87] For example, ALL with *TEL-AML1* rearrangements are treated less intensively than leukemias carrying the *E2A–PBX1*, *BCR–ABL* or *MLL–AF4* translocations, which are associated with a worse prognosis. Molecular techniques are applied for diagnosis because several translocations, especially the t(1;19) and the t(12;21), are frequently missed by conventional cytogenetics[82,88] (Chapter 125). Sensitive multiplex RT-PCR techniques are used to detect most of the common, prognostically significant fusion genes[89,90]. Southern analysis of genomic DNA is also useful in detecting gene rearrangements and is used, for example, for the detection of *MLL* rearrangements, and of translocations into the switch locus in multiple myeloma.[26,91] Molecular cytogenetics, such as spectral karyotyping (chromosome painting) and fluorescent in situ hybridization (FISH), are very useful for diagnosing and stratifying lymphoid malignancies on the basis of novel genomic juxtapositions brought about by chromosomal translocations, delections, insertions or amplifications.[92,93] These techniques do not require prior knowledge of the precise primary DNA sequences involved in the reconfigurations. They are also useful in identifying cryptic translocations, not appreciated in routine karyotypic examination (Fig. 93.9).

CLINICAL RELEVANCE

Molecular and cytogenetic characterization of lymphoid malignancies

- The lymphocyte-specific chromosomal rearrangements provide molecular fingerprints useful in the diagnosis, classification and staging of an individual patient's malignancy.
- Certain chromosomal rearrangements in ALL are strong independent prognostic factors. New treatment protocols are tailored for specific molecular subtypes.
- Modern molecular and cytogenetic techniques are available for the detection of chromosomal translocation at diagnosis and for quantification of residual disease during and after therapy.

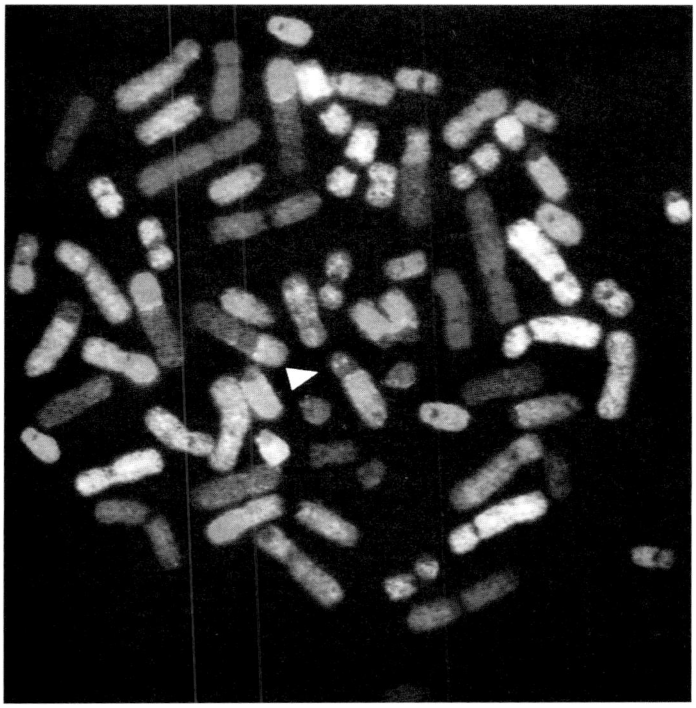

Figure 93.9 Molecular cytogenetics. Example of spectral karyotyping (SKY) combined with fluorescence in-situ hybridization (FISH) with IgH probe, of a metaphase cell from a myeloma cell line. Each chromosome is stained with distinct color after hybridization with 24 combinatorially labeled chromosome painting probes. Chromosome painting probes were prepared in a two-step degenerate oligonucleotide-primed (DOP) PCR of a human chromosome library using combinations of different fluorochromes for labeling. Spectral image acquisition and analysis were performed on a Leica DMRXA microscope equipped with the SD200 SpectraCube system and related software (Applied Spectral Imaging). The arrow points to a complex t(8;14) translocation in which a piece of chromosome 8 (blue) is inserted between two pieces of chromosome 14. The fluorescent dots represent the IgH locus. Several other translocations are easily detected by the presence of chromosomes painted by more than one color. (Courtesy of Dr Giovanni Tonon.) (See also color plate 93.9.)

For detection of residual disease, either the tumor-specific translocation or the clonotypic immune receptor gene rearrangement is used.[94,95] When an immunoglobulin or T-cell receptor locus rearrangement is being used as the tumor-specific marker, primers are chosen that flank the hypervariable segment of the V region. An oligonucleotide that encompasses that particular cell's hypervariable segment is then defined as the tumor-specific marker. The advantage of using these 'normal' gene rearrangements as tumor-specific markers is that over 99% of all lymphoid malignancies carry a rearrangement of one or more of the immune receptor loci. Some malignancies, for example B-cell precursor (pre-B) ALL of childhood, often have rearrangements of multiple loci from both the T-cell and the Ig loci.[96] Other lymphoid malignancies, for example the B-cell follicular lymphoma, show a pattern of rearrangements more restricted to the Ig locus and consistent with a classic view of B-cell lineage determination. Acute leukemias of infancy (children less than 1 year of age) can present a problem with regard to use of this V segment tumor-specific marker because many of these leukemias (up to 50%) lack Ig or TCR locus rearrangement,[97] suggesting transformation of a very early lymphoid progenitor and, by definition, not providing an Ig or TCR blast-specific target. However, the overall number of lymphoid leukemias where the Ig and TCR loci are found to be retained in the germline configuration is very small.

There are problems with the use of the 'normal' Ig and TCR rearrangements carried in leukemic blasts as tumor-specific markers. First, the detection method must be individualized for each patient, which can be time-consuming and expensive. Second, the targeted hypervariable region can, under certain circumstances, continue to undergo somatic mutation. This would result in poor recognition by the specific probe and allow leukemic cells to go unmeasured or undetected.

When identification of the rearrangement is focused on the chromosomal aberration that contributes to cellular transformation, it is easier to relate this directly as a tumor-specific marker. The advantage of studying these events is that they are leukemia or lymphoma type specific but not patient specific. Once such a chromosomal aberration is known, it may be amenable to PCR analysis using the same (or a small set of) primers in the analyses of all patients with that particular type of malignancy. The problem is that despite the ever-increasing number of chromosomal aberrations that are correlated with lymphoid malignancy, and whose breakpoints and involved loci have now been cloned and characterized (see Table 93.1), there are still a large number of malignancies that have not been sufficiently defined or characterized to allow for PCR primer design and analysis.

Recent large studies using (semi) quantitative PCR techniques have established that residual disease can be reliably followed, and the level of residual leukemic cells and the rate of the change in their level is correlated with disease-free survival.[98,99] Large prospective studies that are under way will determine whether therapeutic decisions based on a slow reduction in residual leukemia during therapy or a gradual increase in residual disease during remission will change the final outcome.

Interestingly, minimal residual disease is sometimes identified in patients who have been in remission for such a long time that they are considered cured. Although these may be quiescent leukemic stem cells which may one day give rise to frank leukemia, there are other interpretations related to the nature of PCR-based techniques. The mere presence of amplifiable DNA in a patient does not necessarily mean that DNA is present in a blast capable of continued proliferation. It is certainly possible that amplifiable DNA could be extracted from cells that are no longer able to undergo cellular division and remain viable. Thus, in such cases a patient could be determined to have a residual tumor burden when, actually, the viable tumor burden may be much lower or nonexistent. Another intriguing possibility is that such cells may not be the fully transformed cells but the precursors of the first leukemic cell carrying the clonospecific immune gene rearrangement or the fusion oncogenic gene.[100] The detection of such cells in normal healthy people leads to the questions discussed earlier regarding the origin of human lymphoid neoplasia.

CONCLUSION

The primary differentiated and expressed products of lymphocytes are immunoglobulins and T-cell antigen receptors. When considering the molecular genetics of lymphoid malignancies, it is often observed that the transformation event includes the juxtaposition of one of these immune receptors with a growth-affecting gene. This may lead to the constitutive expression of a growth-stimulatory protein. In certain cases there may also be a requirement for the elaboration of a functional immune receptor whose antigen reactivity may provide an additional essential proliferative stimulus. The mechanisms by which these transformation events occur are diverse, but often reflect the genome-destabilizing and gene-rearranging enzymes present during normal lymphocyte development. Whether this inherent genetic instability of lymphocytes distinguishes the etiology of lymphoid malignancies from that of solid tumors, or instead focuses attention on universal prerequisites of transformation, is an issue that continues to provoke thought and experimentation. The DNA in a transformed lymphocyte is not the same as that of its normal counterpart. The recognition of this fact provides a ready tool for leukemia and lymphoma diagnosis, staging, classification, minimal residual disease determination and gene discovery.

REFERENCES

1. Kirsch IR, Kuehl WM. Gene rearrangements in lymphoid cells. In: Stamatoyannopoulos G, et al. (eds) The molecular basis of blood diseases. Philadelphial, W.B. Saunders, 2001, p. 389.
2. Oettinger MA, Schatz DG, Gorka C, Baltimore D. RAG-1 and RAG-2, adjacent genes that synergistically activate V(D)J recombination. Science 1990;248:1517.
3. Blackwell TK, Moore MW, Yancopoulos GD, et al. Recombination between immunoglobulin variable region segments is enhanced by transcription. Nature 1986;324:585.
4. Cherry SR, Baltimore D. Chromatin remodeling directly activates V(D)J recombination. Proc Natl Acad Sci USA 1999;96:10788.
5. Kuppers R, Klein U, Hansmann ML, Rajewsky K. Review Articles: Mechanisms of disease: cellular origin of human B-cell lymphomas. N Engl J Med 1999;341:1520.
6. Lipkowitz S, Stern MH, Kirsch IR. Hybrid T cell receptor genes formed by interlocus recombination in normal and ataxia–telangiectasia lymphocytes. J Exp Med 1990;172:409.
7. Pandita TK, Hittelman WN. Initial chromosome damage but not DNA damage is greater in ataxia telangiectasia cells. Radiat Res 1992;130:94.
8. Kirsch IR, Lista F. Lymphocyte-specific genomic instability and risk of lymphoid malignancy. Semin Immunol 1997;9:207.
9. Liao MJ, Van Dyke T. Critical role for Atm in suppressing V(D)J recombination-driven thymic lymphoma. Genes Dev 1999;13:1246.
10. Wotherspoon AC, Doglioni C, Diss TC, et al. Regression of primary low-grade B-cell gastric lymphoma of mucosa-associated lymphoid tissue type after eradication of *Helicobacter pylori*. Lancet 1993;342:575.
11. Fais F, Ghiotto F, Hashimoto S, et al. Chronic lymphocytic leukemia B cells express restricted sets of mutated and unmutated antigen receptors. J Clin Invest 1998;102:1515.
12. Bahler DW, Levy R. Clonal evolution of a follicular lymphoma: evidence for antigen selection. Proc Natl Acad Sci USA 1992;89:6770.
13. Lam KP, Kuhn R, Rajewsky K. In vivo ablation of surface immunoglobulin on mature B cells by inducible gene targeting results in rapid cell death. Cell 1997;90:1073.
14. Shen-Ong GLC, Keath EJ, Piccoli SP, Cole MD. Novel c-*myc* oncogene RNA from abortive immunoglobulin gene recombination in mouse plasmacytomas. Cell 1982;31:443.
15. Dalla-Favera R, Bregni M, Erikson J, Patterson D, Gallo RC, Croce CM. Human c-*myc* oncogene is located on the region of chromosome 8 that is translocated in Burkitt lymphoma cells. Proc Natl Acad Sci USA 1982;79:7824.
16. Taub R, Kirsch I, Morton C. et al. Translocation of the c-*myc* gene into the immunoglobulin heavy chain locus in human Burkitt lymphoma and murine plastacytoma cells. Proc Natl Acad Sci USA 1982;79:7837.
17. Boehm T, Mengle-Gaw L, Kees UR, et al. Alternating purine–pyrimidine tracts may promote chromosomal translocations seen in a variety of human lymphoid tumors. EMBO J 1989;8:2621.
18. Hiom K, Melek M, Gellert M. DNA transposition by the RAG1 and RAG2 proteins: a possible source of oncogenic translocations. Cell 1998;94:415.
19. Gabrea A, Bergsagel PL, Chesi M, Shou Y, Kuehl WM. Insertion of excised IgH switch sequences causes overexpression of cyclin D1 in a myeloma tumor cell. Molec Cell 1999;3:119.
20. Aplan PD, Lombardi DP, Reaman GH, Sather HN, Hammond GD, Kirsch IR. Involvement of the putative hematopoietic transcription factor SCL in T-cell acute lymphoblastic leukemia. Blood 1992;79:1327.
21. Aplan PD, Lombardi DP, Ginsberg AM, Cossman J, Bertness VL, Kirsch IR. Disruption of the human SCL locus by 'illegitimate' V(D)J recombinase activity. Science 1990;250:1426.
22. Izraeli S, Colaizzo-Anas T, Bertness VL, Mani K, Aplan PD, Kirsch IR. Expression of the SIL gene is correlated with growth induction and cellular proliferation. Cell Growth & Differentiation 1997;8:1171.
23. Begley CG, Green AR. The SCL gene: from case report to critical hematopoietic regulator. Blood 1999;93:2760.
24. Cayuela JM, Gardie B, Sigaux F. Disruption of the multiple tumor suppressor gene MTS1/p16(INK4a)/CDKN2 by illegitimate V(D)J recombinase activity in T-cell acute lymphoblastic leukemias. Blood 1997;90:3720.
25. Neri A, Barriga F, Knowles DM, Magrath IT, Dalla-Favera R. Different regions of the immunoglobulin heavy-chain locus are involved in chromosomal translocations in distinct pathogenetic forms of Burkitt lymphoma. Proc Natl Acad Sci USA 1988;85:2748.
26. Bergsagel PL, Chesi M, Nardini E, Brents LA, Kirby SL, Kuehl WM. Promiscuous translocations into immunoglobulin heavy chain switch regions in multiple myeloma. Proc Natl Acad Sci USA 1996;93:13931.
27. Nowell PC, Hungerford D. A minute chromosome in human chronic granulocytic leukemia. Science 1960;132:1497.
28. Rowley JD. Letter: A new consistent chromosomal abnormality in chronic myelogenous leukaemia identified by quinacrine fluorescence and Giemsa staining. Nature 1973;243:290.
29. de Klein A, van Kessel AG, Grosveld G, et al. A cellular oncogene is translocated to the Philadelphia chromosome in chronic myelocytic leukaemia. Nature 1982;300:765.
30. Denny CT, Shah NP, Ogden S, et al. Localization of preferential sites of rearrangement within the BCR gene in Philadelphia chromosome-positive acute lymphoblastic leukemia. Proc Natl Acad Sci USA 1989;86:4254.
31. Neves H, Ramos C, da Silva MG, Parreira A, Parreira L. The nuclear topography of ABL, BCR, PML, and RARalpha genes: evidence for gene proximity in specific phases of the cell cycle and stages of hematopoietic differentiation. Blood 1999;93:1197.
32. Rowley JD. The critical role of chromosome translocations in human leukemias. Annu Rev Genet 1998;32:495.
33. Broeker PL, Super HG, Thirman MJ, et al. Distribution of 11q23 breakpoints within the MLL breakpoint cluster region in de novo acute leukemia and in treatment-related acute myeloid leukemia: correlation with scaffold attachment regions and topoisomerase II consensus binding sites. Blood 1996;87:1912.
34. Stanulla M, Wang J, Chervinsky DS, Thandla S, Aplan PD. DNA cleavage within the MLL breakpoint cluster region is a specific event which occurs as part of higher-order chromatin fragmentation during the initial stages of apoptosis. Mol Cell Biol 1997;17:4070.
35. Li TK, Chen AY, Yu C, Mao Y, Wang H, Liu LF. Activation of topoisomerase II-mediated excision of chromosomal DNA loops during oxidative stress. Genes Dev 1999;13:1553.

36. Wiemels JL, Greaves M. Structure and possible mechanisms of TEL-AML1 gene fusions in childhood acute lymphoblastic leukemia. Cancer Res 1999;59:4075.
37. Gillert E, Leis T, Repp R, et al. A DNA damage repair mechanism is involved in the origin of chromosomal translocations t(4;11) in primary leukemic cells. Oncogene 1999;18:4663.
38. Fearon ER, Vogelstein B. A genetic model for colorectal tumorigenesis. Cell 1990;61:759.
39. Kuerbitz SJ, Plunkett BS, Walsh WV, Kastan MB. Wild-type p53 is a cell cycle checkpoint determinant following irradiation. Proc Natl Acad Sci USA 1992;89:7491.
40. Hartwell L. Defects in a cell cycle checkpoint may be responsible for the genomic instability of cancer cells. Cell 1992;71:543.
41. Hahn WC, Counter CM, Lundberg AS, Beijersbergen RL, Brooks MW, Weinberg RA. Creation of human tumour cells with defined genetic elements. Nature 1999;400:464.
42. Sandberg A. The chromosomes in human cancer and leukemia. Amsterdam, Elsevier Science, 1990.
43. Limpens J, de Jong D, van Krieken JH, et al. Bcl-2/JH rearrangements in benign lymphoid tissues with follicular hyperplasia. Oncogene 1991;6:2271.
44. Bose S, Deininger M, Gora-Tybor J, Goldman JM, Melo JV. The presence of typical and atypical BCR–ABL fusion genes in leukocytes of normal individuals: biologic significance and implications for the assessment of minimal residual disease. Blood 1998;92:3362.
45. Kim-Rouille MH, MacGregor A, Wiedemann LM, Greaves MF, Navarrete C. MLL–AF4 gene fusions in normal newborns. Blood 1999;93:1107.
46. Pulford K, Lamant L, Morris SW, et al. Detection of anaplastic lymphoma kinase (ALK) and nucleolar protein nucleophosmin (NPM)-ALK proteins in normal and neoplastic cells with the monoclonal antibody ALK1. Blood 1997;89:1394.
47. Dedera DA, Waller EK, LeBrun DP, et al. Chimeric homeobox gene E2A–PBX1 induces proliferation, apoptosis, and malignant lymphomas in transgenic mice. Cell 1993;74:833.
48. Rabbitts TH. LMO T-cell translocation oncogenes typify genes activated by chromosomal translocations that alter transcription and developmental processes. Genes Dev 1998;12:2651.
49. Wiemels JL, Cazzaniga G, Daniotti M, et al. Prenatal origin of acute lymphoblastic leukaemia in children. Lancet 1999;354:1499.
50. Wiemels JL, Ford AM, Van Wering ER, Postma A, Greaves M. Protracted and variable latency of acute lymphoblastic leukemia after TEL-AML1 gene fusion in utero. Blood 1999;94:1057.
51. Gale KB, Ford AM, Repp R, et al. Backtracking leukemia to birth: identification of clonotypic gene fusion sequences in neonatal blood spots. Proc Natl Acad Sci USA 1997;94:13950.
52. Drexler HG. Review of alterations of the cyclin-dependent kinase inhibitor INK4 family genes p15, p16, p18 and p19 in human leukemia-lymphoma cells. Leukemia 1998;12:845.
53. Gardie B, Cayuela JM, Martini S, Sigaux F. Genomic alterations of the p19ARF encoding exons in T-cell acute lymphoblastic leukemia. Blood 1998;91:1016.
54. Eischen CM, Weber JD, Roussel MF, Sherr CJ, Cleveland JL. Disruption of the ARF-Mdm2-p53 tumor suppressor pathway in myc-induced lymphomagenesis. Genes Dev 1999;13:2658.
55. Redner RL, Wang J, Liu JM. Chromatin remodeling and leukemia: new therapeutic paradigms. Blood 1999;94:417.
56. Bain G, Murre C. The role of E-proteins in B- and T-lymphocyte development. Semin Immunol 1998;10:143.
57. Hunger SP. Chromosomal translocations involving the E2A gene in acute lymphoblastic leukemia: clinical features and molecular pathogenesis. Blood 1996;87:1211.
58. Dalla-Favera R, Migliazza A, Chang CC, et al. Molecular pathogenesis of B cell malignancy: the role of BCL-6. Curr Topics Microbiol Immunol 1999;246:257; discussion 263.
59. Izraeli S, Lowe LA, Bertness VL, et al. The SIL gene is required for mouse embryonic axial development and left–right specification. Nature 1999;399:691.
60. Look AT. Oncogenic transcription factors in the human acute leukemias. Science 1997;278:1059.
61. Yu BD, Hanson RD, Hess JL, Horning SE, Korsmeyer SJ. MLL, a mammalian trithorax-group gene, functions as a transcriptional maintenance factor in morphogenesis. Proc Natl Acad Sci USA 1998;95:10632.
62. Alizadeh A, Eisen M, Botstein D, Brown PO, Staudt LM. Probing lymphocyte biology by genomic-scale gene expression analysis. J Clin Immunol 1998;18:373.
63. Dalla-Favera R. Chromosomal translocations involving the c-myc oncogene in lymphoid neoplasia. In: Kirsch IR (ed.) The causes and consequences of chromosomal aberrations. New York, CRC Press, 1993, p 313.
64. Grignani F, Lombardi L, Inghirami G, Sternas L, Cechova K, Dalla-Favera R. Negative autoregulation of c-*myc* gene expression is inactivated in transformed cells. EMBO J 1990;9:3913.
65. Bentley DL, Groudine M. A block to elongation is largely responsible for decreased transcription of c-myc in differentiated HL60 cells. Nature 1986;321:702.
66. Zajac-Kaye M, Gelmann EP, Levens D. A point mutation in the c-*myc* locus of a Burkitt lymphoma abolishes binding of a nuclear protein. Science 1988;240:1776.
67. Cesarman E, Dalla-Favera R, Bentley D, Groudine M. Mutations in the first exon are associated with altered transcription of c-*myc* in Burkitt lymphoma. Science 1987;238:1272.
68. Bhatia K, Huppi K, Spangler G, Siwarski D, Iyer R, Magrath I. Point mutations in the c-*Myc* transactivation domain are common in Burkitt's lymphoma and mouse plasmacytomas. Nature Genet 1993;5:56.
69. Felsher DW, Bishop JM. Reversible tumorigenesis by MYC in hematopoietic lineages. Molec Cell 1999;4:199.
70. Dang CV. c-*Myc* target genes involved in cell growth, apoptosis, and metabolism. Mol Cell Biol 1999;19:1.
71. Warburg O. On the origin of cancer cells. Science 1956;123:309.
72. Reiter A, Schrappe M, Tiemann WD, et al. Improved treatment results in childhood B-cell neoplasms with tailored intensification of therapy: a report of the Berlin–Frankfurt–Munster Group trial (NHL-BFM-90). Blood 1999;94:3294.
73. Chervinsky DS, Zhao XF, Lam DH, Ellsworth M, Gross KW, Aplan PD. Disordered T-cell development and T-cell malignancies in SCL LMO1 double-transgenic mice: parallels with E2A-deficient mice. Mol Cell Biol 1999;19:5025.
74. Engel I, Murre C. Ectopic expression of E47 or E12 promotes the death of E2A-deficient lymphomas. Proc Natl Acad Sci USA 1999;96:996.
75. Park ST, Nolan GP, Sun XH. Growth inhibition and apoptosis due to restoration of E2A activity in T cell acute lymphoblastic leukemia cells. J Exp Med 1999;189:501.
76. Ordentlich P, Lin A, Shen CP, et al. Notch inhibition of E47 supports the existence of a novel signaling pathway. Mol Cell Biol 1998;18:2230.
77. Tsujimoto Y, Finger LR, Yunis J, Nowell PC, Croce CM. Cloning of the chromosome breakpoint of neoplastic B cells with the t(14;18) chromosome translocation. Science 1984;226:1097.
78. McDonnell TJ, Deane N, Platt FM, et al. bcl-2-immunoglobulin transgenic mice demonstrate extended B cell survival and follicular lymphoproliferation. Cell 1989;57:79.
79. Adams JM, Cory S. The Bcl-2 protein family: arbiters of cell survival. Science 1998;281:1322.
80. Chang CP, de Vivo I, Cleary ML. The Hox cooperativity motif of the chimeric oncoprotein E2a-Pbx1 is necessary and sufficient for oncogenesis. Mol Cell Biol 1997;17:81.
81. McWhirter JR, Neuteboom ST, Wancewicz EV, Monia BP, Downing JR, Murre C. Oncogenic homeodomain transcription factor E2A-Pbx1 activates a novel WNT gene in pre-B acute lymphoblastoid leukemia. Proc Natl Acad Sci USA 1999;96:11464.
82. Rubnitz JE, Look AT. Molecular basis of leukemogenesis. Curr Opin Hematol 1998;5:264.
83. Rubnitz JE, Behm FG, Wichlan D, et al. Low frequency of TEL-AML1 in relapsed acute lymphoblastic leukemia supports a favorable prognosis for this genetic subgroup. Leukemia 1999;13:19.
84. Clark SS, McLaughlin J, Crist WM, Champlin R, Witte ON. Unique forms of the abl tyrosine kinase distinguish Ph1-positive CML from Ph1-positive ALL. Science 1987;235:85.

85. Elefanty AG, Hariharan IK, Cory S. bcr-abl, the hallmark of chronic myeloid leukaemia in man, induces multiple haemopoietic neoplasms in mice. EMBO J 1990;9:1069.
86. Pear WS, Miller JP, Xu L, et al. Efficient and rapid induction of a chronic myelogenous leukemia-like myeloproliferative disease in mice receiving P210 bcr/abl-transduced bone marrow. Blood 1998;92:3780.
87. Pui CH, Evans WE. Acute lymphoblastic leukemia. N Engl J Med 1998;339:605.
88. Izraeli S, Janssen JW, Haas OA, et al. Detection and clinical relevance of genetic abnormalities in pediatric acute lymphoblastic leukemia: a comparison between cytogenetic and polymerase chain reaction analyses. Leukemia 1993;7:671.
89. Izraeli S, Lion T. Multiprimer-PCR for screening of genetic abnormalities in acute lymphoblastic leukaemia. Br J Haematol 1991;79:645.
90. Pallisgaard N, Hokland P, Riishoj DC, Pedersen B, Jorgensen P. Multiplex reverse transcription polymerase chain reaction for simultaneous screening of 29 translocations and chromosomal aberrations in acute leukemia. Blood 1998;92:574.
91. Thirman MJ, Gill HJ, Burnett RC, et al. Rearrangement of the MLL gene in acute lymphoblastic and acute myeloid leukemias with 11q23 chromosomal translocations. N Engl J Med 1993;329:909.
92. Hilgenfeld E, Padilla-Nash H, Schrock E, Ried T. Analysis of B-cell neoplasias by spectral karyotyping (SKY). Curr Topics Microbiol Immunol 1999;246:169.
93. Tonon G, Roschke A, Stover K, Shou Y, Kuehl W, Kirsch I. Spectral karyotyping combined with locus-specific FISH simultaneously defines genes and chrmosomes involved in chromosomal translocations. Genes Chromosomes and Cancer 2000;27:418.
94. Pongers-Willemse MJ, Seriu T, Stolz F, et al. Primers and protocols for standardized detection of minimal residual disease in acute lymphoblastic leukemia using immunoglobulin and T cell receptor gene rearrangements and TAL1 deletions as PCR targets: report of the BIOMED-1 Concerted Action: investigation of minimal residual disease in acute leukemia. Leukemia 1999;13:110.
95. Pallisgaard N, Clausen N, Schröder H, Hokland P. Rapid and sensitive minimal residual disease detection in acute leukemia by quantitative real-time RT-PCR exemplified by t(12;21) TEL-AML1 fusion transcript. Genes Chromosomes Cancer 1999;26:355.
96. Felix CA, Poplack DG, Reaman GH, et al. Characterization of immunoglobulin and T-cell receptor gene patterns in B-cell precursor acute lymphoblastic leukemia of childhood. J Clin Oncol 1990;8:431.
97. Felix CA, Reaman GH, Korsmeyer SJ, et al. Immunoglobulin and T cell receptor gene configuration in acute lymphoblastic leukemia of infancy. Blood 1987;70:536.
98. Roberts WM, Estrov Z, Ouspenskaia MV, Johnston DA, McClain KL, Zipf TF. Measurement of residual leukemia during remission in childhood acute lymphoblastic leukemia. N Engl J Med 1997;336:317.
99. van Dongen JJ, Seriu T, Panzer-Grumayer ER, et al. Prognostic value of minimal residual disease in acute lymphoblastic leukaemia in childhood. Lancet 1998;352:1731.
100. Greaves M. Silence of the leukemic clone. N Engl J Med 1997;336:367.

Chapter 94 Virus-induced T-cell Malignancies and Associated Diseases

Takashi Uchiyama

HTLV-I-ASSOCIATED T-CELL MALIGNANCIES

Adult T-cell leukemia (ATL) is a distinct T-cell leukemia/lymphoma that develops in adults after a long latent period in a small proportion of people infected with the human T-cell leukemia virus type I (HTLV-I). Clinical features consist of lymph node enlargement, hepatomegaly, splenomegaly, skin lesions, and the appearance of morphologically characteristic leukemia cells. The most common complications are hypercalcemia and various infections and the prognosis is very poor. Studies on the cell surface properties of T and B cells in human lymphoid neoplasms led to the first description of ATL.[1] A few years later, a novel human retrovirus termed human T-cell leukemia virus type I was discovered. This was followed by epidemiological and molecular studies that demonstrated a causative role for HTLV-I in the development of ATL and established ATL as a new disease entity.[2–6]

The mean age of the onset of ATL is 58 years, with a male to female ratio of 1:2.[7] The age at diagnosis ranges from 25 to 94 years. It is estimated that about 700 new cases of ATL are diagnosed every year in Japan,[7] where the occurrence of ATL is the highest in the world.

Subtypes

ATL is classified into at least four clinical subtypes: acute, lymphoma, chronic and smoldering. Classification is based on the number of abnormal T cells in the peripheral blood, together with serum lactic acid dehydrogenase (LDH) level, serum calcium level, tumor lesions in various organs, and clinical course.[8,9]

Clinical manifestations of acute-type ATL include acute presentation of symptoms and signs, including general malaise, fever, cough, dyspnea, abdominal fullness, thirst, drowsiness, lymph node enlargement, hepatosplenomegaly and jaundice.[1,8,9] Abnormal laboratory findings include marked leukocytosis, hypercalcemia, high serum LDH levels, increased amounts of the soluble form of interleukin-2 receptor (IL-2R) α chain and the appearance of characteristic leukemic cells with deeply convoluted or lobulated nuclei.[1,7–9]

The predominant feature of lymphoma-type ATL is histologically proven lymphadenopathy without leukemic manifestations (peripheral blood lymphocyte count less than 4×10^9/l, and 1% or less abnormal T lymphocytes). The involvement of skin, lung, lymph node, liver, spleen, central nervous system, bone or gastrointestinal tract may be seen.

Chronic-type ATL is characterized by mild symptoms and signs and a longer clinical course. Peripheral blood lymphocyte count is more than 4×10^9/l, with more than 5% abnormal T lymphocytes. Serum LDH level can be up to twice the normal limit. Patients may have lymphadenopathy, hepatomegaly, splenomegaly, and skin and pulmonary lesions. However, neither hypercalcemia nor involvement of the central nervous system or gastrointestinal tract is observed.

Patients with smoldering type ATL have a few leukemic cells in their peripheral blood. They frequently present with skin lesions such as papules, nodules and erythema, but lymph node enlargement and splenomegaly are minimal and serum LDH level is either slightly elevated (up to 1.5 times the normal upper limit) or normal. They do not have tumor lesions in the lymph nodes, liver, spleen, central nervous system, bone or gastrointestinal tract.

The distribution of each type of case is approximately 55% acute type, 20% lymphoma type, 20% chronic type and 5% smoldering type.

> **KEY CONCEPTS**
>
> **Clinical characteristics of ATL**
> - T-cell leukemia of adults
> - HTLV-I is a causative agent
> - Four clinical subtypes (acute, chronic, smoldering and lymphoma type)
> - Major clinical manifestations: lymph node enlargement, hepatosplenomegaly, skin lesions, leukemic cells with deeply indented nuclei, hypercalcemia, infectious complications, poor prognosis

Clinical features

Symptoms and signs

Symptoms at the onset of the disease can include general malaise, fever, cough, dyspnea, abdominal fullness, abdominal pain, jaundice, superficial lymph node swelling, skin manifestations, thirst and drowsiness. Malaise, thirst, drowsiness and constipation are usually due to the hypercalcemia. Physical findings frequently detectable at the time of diagnosis include lymphadenopathy, hepatomegaly, splenomegaly, various skin lesions, jaundice and ascites. Skin lesions include papules, nodules, nodes, tumors, erythema and erythroderma, but none of these findings is pathognomonic for ATL.

Pulmonary changes often detectable by radiological examinations of the chest include neoplastic cell infiltration into pulmonary tissue, or pulmonary infections by bacteria, fungi and/or viruses. The most commonly observed pulmonary infections are pneumonias due to *Pneumocystis carinii*, *Aspergillus* sp. or cytomegalovirus.

Hepatomegaly with abnormal findings, including hyperbilirubinemia and elevated levels of serum GPT/ALT and GOT/AST, are usually due to the infiltration of leukemic cells into the liver. Leukemic cell infiltration and/or tumor formation in the gastrointestinal tract can sometimes be found. Leptomeningeal involvement is observed in about 10% of patients, but CNS involvement is uncommon.

Laboratory findings

Peripheral blood lymphocyte count is high, particularly in acute-type ATL. A marked leukocytosis of more than 30×10^9/l is observed in about 40% of acute-type and 20% of chronic-type cases. Peripheral blood smears usually show the characteristic leukemic cells, with large, deeply indented or lobulated nuclei with clear nucleolei and basophilic cytoplasm (Fig. 94.1). The typical leukemic cells sometimes bear a flower-like configuration. The mechanism responsible for the development of these morphologically peculiar cells remains unknown. Another characteristic finding in peripheral blood smears is the pleomorphism of leukemic cells, with variable sizes and morphologies observed in the same blood smear. The relative proportion of the morphologically characteristic ATL cell is usually highest in acute-type ATL and lower in other types. Patients with smoldering or lymphoma-type ATL do not have leukocytosis. Neutrophilia (30% of all cases) or eosinophilia are common. Anemia and thrombocytopenia are uncommon, although severe anemia and thrombocytopenia are seen in rare cases.

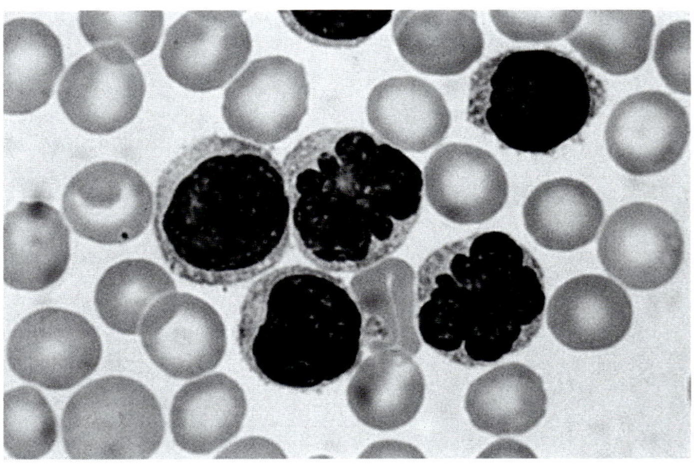

Figure 94.1 Peripheral blood leukemic cells from a patient with acute-type ATL. Note the cells with deeply indented nuclei. (See also color plate 94.1.)

CLINICAL PEARLS

Diagnosis of ATL
- Symptoms and signs
- Appearance of morphologically characteristic lymphocytes ('flower cells')
- Serum antibodies to HTLV-I
- Demonstration of monoclonal integration of HTLV-I provirus into tumor cells
- Markedly high levels of serum soluble IL-2 receptor α chain

The leukemic cells from ATL patients are $CD3^+CD4^+CD8^-$ in the majority (80–90%) and either $CD3^+CD4^+CD8^+$, $CD3^+CD4^-CD8^+$ or $CD3^+CD4^-CD8^-$ in the remaining 10–20%.[10,11] It was reported that the latter unusual cell surface phenotype was associated with poor prognostic signs, including marked organomegaly and a bulky tumor mass.[11] The expression of so-called T-cell activation antigens, including IL-2R α chain (CD25), Ki67, transferrin receptor (CD71) and HLA-DR is common in leukemic cells. The T-cell receptor expressed on leukemic cells is usually a heterodimer of α and β chains. Restricted expression of TCR β-chain variable genes has not been observed, suggesting that leukemic cells are not derived from particular antigen-specific T-cell clones. Leukemic cells from the patients with ATL constitutively express IL-2R-α chain on their surface, which is easily detectable by flow cytometry. This observation contrasts with the inducible expression seen in normal T lymphocytes.[12–14]

Cytogenetic study of ATL cells reveals various chromosomal abnormalities, although ATL-specific abnormalities have not been described. The frequently detectable chromosomal abnormalities are trisomy of chromosomes 3 (21% of all cases examined), 7 (10%) and 21 (9%), monosomy of the X chromosome (38%), loss of the Y chromosome (17%), translocation involving 14q32 (28%) or 14q11 (14%), and deletion of 6q (23%).[15] Chromosomal abnormalities are more common in acute or lymphoma-type ATL than the chronic or smoldering type.

Bone marrow aspiration reveals an increase in the proportion of lymphoid cells, including the characteristic leukemic cells. However, this is not marked in a small proportion of acute-type and a majority of chronic and lymphoma-type ATL.

Serum LDH levels are usually moderately to markedly elevated in both acute and lymphoma-type ATL. Serum levels of the soluble IL-2 receptor α chain are markedly elevated (usually more than 10–100 times higher than normal) except in smoldering-type ATL, and serve as very useful indicators of the patient's neoplastic cell mass.[16] Serum levels of total bilirubin, transaminases (GOT/AST, GPT/ALT) and alkaline phosphatase are elevated when leukemic cells infiltrate the liver. Liver dysfunction with hypoalbuminemia (<40 g/l) is detectable in approximately 60% and 74% of acute-type ATL, respectively. Renal dysfunction, as evidenced by elevated levels of blood urea nitrogen and serum creatinine, is observed in about 30% of acute-type, 15% of lymphoma-type and 10% of chronic-type cases. Hypercalcemia (corrected serum level > 2.74 mmol/l) is detectable in 50% of acute-type and 15% of lymphoma-type ATL.[7–9]

Histological examination of the affected skin usually shows infiltration of leukemic cells into the dermis and subcutaneous tissue (Fig. 94.2). The leukemic cell infiltration into epidermal tissue typically observed in Sézary syndrome is also occasionally detected. Histopathological examination of the biopsy specimens of enlarged lymph nodes shows the destruction of normal structure, as evidenced by burned-out lymphatic follicles, uncertain peripheral sinus and a predominant distribution of atypical lymphoid cells. There is a diffuse proliferation of atypical lymphoid cells, which vary in size and shape and have irregular or convoluted nuclear contours, stippled chromatin patterns and amphophilic cytoplasm. Giant cells with cerebriform or Reed–Sternberg-type nuclei and mitoses are occasionally observed.

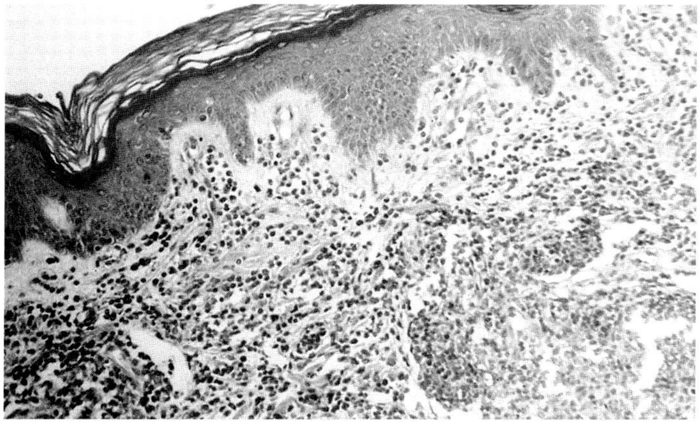

Figure 94.2 Skin lesions in ATL. Leukemic cells infiltrate predominantly into the dermis and subcutaneous tissue. (See also color plate 94.2.)

Complications and prognosis

Infections with bacteria, fungi, protozoa and viruses are common in ATL. Approximately half of patients with ATL die of severe infections, with pneumonia the most frequent (80%) cause of death, followed by sepsis. Bacterial, fungal (*Aspergillus*, *Candida*), viral (including interstitial pneumonitis) and protozoal (*Pneumocystitis carinii*) pneumonias represent 50%, 10%, 40% and 5% respectively of these infections.[8] Strongyloidiasis is often observed in HTLV-I infected carriers and ATL patients in Okinawa.[9] It is considered that frequent infectious complications are due to the immunodeficient state of ATL patients.

Hypercalcemia, one of the most serious acute serious complications, is observed in 40–50% of all patients throughout the entire clinical course. Hypercalcemia is due to the excessive production of parathyroid hormone-related protein (PTHrP), the transcription of which is enhanced by the HTLV-I regulatory protein, Tax.[17] Because PTHrP mobilizes calcium ion from bones, marked osteolytic lesions may be demonstrated by roentgenological examination in some cases (Fig. 94.3). Histopathological examination of the affected bone shows the proliferation of osteoclasts and the resultant bone resorption. Other cytokines, such as interleukin-1α (IL-1α), IL-1β, tumor necrosis factor-β (TNF-β) and tumor growth factor-β (TGF-β), abnormally produced in HTLV-I-infected cell line cells and/or fresh leukemic cells, may also have a role in inducing hypercalcemia.

The prognosis of the disease is generally very poor. The median survival time calculated from the analysis of 818 ATL cases was 9.0 months.[18] Survival rates at 2 and 4 years were 26.8% and 10.3%, respectively. Acute and lymphoma-type ATL had the worst prognosis, while the prognosis of chronic and smoldering types was less grave. The median survival time was 6.2 months for the acute type, 10.2 months for the lymphoma type, 24.3 months for the chronic type, and has not yet been established for the smoldering type. Two- and 4-year survival rates were 16.7% and 5.0% for the acute type, 21.3% and 5.7% for the lymphoma type, 52.4% and 26.9% for the chronic type, and 77.7% and 62.8% for the smoldering type, respectively. Adverse prognostic factors in ATL include age (>40 years), poor performance status, total tumor lesions, hypercalcemia and elevated serum LDH level.[18,19]

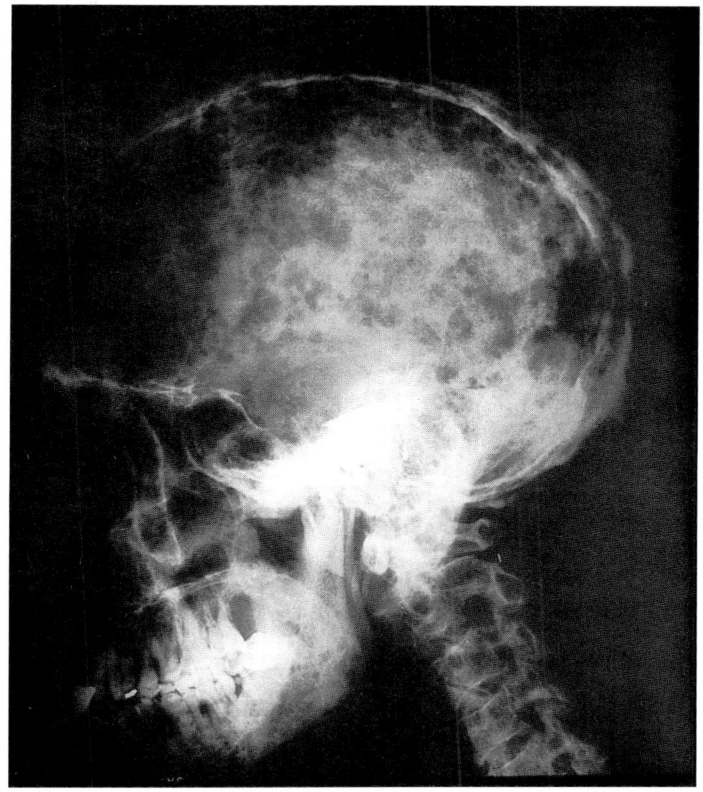

Figure 94.3 Marked osteolytic lesions in a patient with lymphoma-type ATL who had a severe hypercalcemia.

Genetic and environmental factors

It is now established that HTLV-I is an etiologic agent of ATL. HTLV-I was first identified in a T-cell line (Hut 102) established from a patient originally diagnosed as having an aggressive form of cutaneous T-cell lymphoma (CTCL).[2] Early studies subsequently failed to find the association between HTLV-I infection and CTCL. In 1981, it was demonstrated that the MT-1 cell line derived from an ATL patient harbored the virus and expressed an antigen that reacted with the sera from ATL patients.[3] The viruses isolated from Hut102 and MT-1 were subsequently shown to be the same, clarifying its role as the etiologic agent of ATL.[2,6]

The entire genetic structure of HTLV-I is similar to that of other animal retroviruses, except for a novel portion initially referred to as the X region (pX)[20] (Fig. 94.4). The HTLV-I provirus genome is 9032 bp long and contains *gag*, *pol* and *env* genes that encode the viral matrix (p19), capsid (p24) and nucleocapsid proteins (p15), enzymes including reverse transcriptase, integrase and protease, and envelope proteins consisting of a surface glycoprotein (gp46) and a transmembrane protein (p21). In addition to the viral structural genes, the HTLV-I genome contains unique genes principally encoded by sequences at the 3′ end of the genome that are called pX.[20] The proteins encoded by these genes are not viral structural but regulatory proteins, and are identified as Tax, Rex and $p21^{rexIII}$. Other proteins, including p12, $p13^{II}$ and $p30^{II}$, are also encoded within the X region located between the end of the envelope gene and the beginning of *Tax/Rex*.[21] Tax and Rex proteins regulate viral expression both positively and negatively, a finding that helps explain the transient expression of HTLV-I.

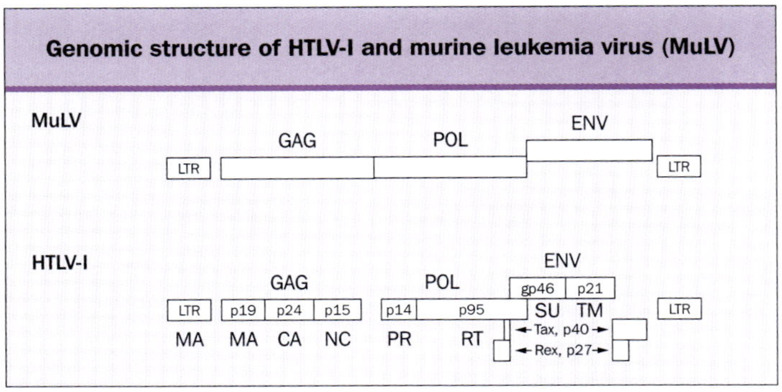

Figure 94.4 Genomic structure of HTLV-I and murine leukemia virus (MuLV), which is an animal retrovirus producing leukemia in a mouse.

KEY CONCEPTS

Tax of HTLV-I

- 40 kDa nuclear phosphoprotein
- Oncogenic protein of HTLV-I
- Tax transactivates various cellular genes, including IL-2 and IL-2 receptor α chain
- One of the major epitopes of anti-HTLV-I CTL
- Tax may play an important role in early stage of the development of ATL

Tax is a 40 kDa nuclear phosphoprotein that transactivates the transcription of HTLV-I and a variety of cellular genes, including those for IL-2, IL-2R α chain, c-*fos* and PTHrP.[22–25] The direct repeats of the 21 bp enhancer in the long terminal repeat (LTR) are needed for Tax to exert its transactivation activity. However, Tax protein does not bind directly to the enhancer elements but exerts its effect through interaction with transcription factors that bind the sites contained in the three repeats of the enhancer elements in the LTR. Tax can bind to the members of CREB (c-AMP-responsive element binding) ATF (activating transcription factor) family which form homo- or heterodimers and bind to CRE (c-AMP-responsive element) or the 21 bp enhancer. Tax interacts with the basic region leucine zipper (bZIP) DNA-binding domain of cellular transcription factors that bind to the CRE target sites to promote peptide dimerization. No specific sequence of the leucine zipper is required for a Tax response. In contrast, the basic region is essential for the Tax-mediated increase in DNA binding. Tax alters the relative affinity of a bZIP for different DNA-binding sites.[26,27]

It has been demonstrated that many heterogeneous promoters other than the HTLV-I LTR are transactivated by Tax (Fig. 94.5). The promoters of the genes for cellular IL-2, IL-2R α chain, TGF-β, granulocyte–macrophage colony-stimulating factor (GM-CSF), c-*myc*, vimentin, TNF-β and gp34 (OX40 ligand) all contain NF κB binding sites and are transactivated through the interaction of NF-κB/Rel proteins with Tax protein. Similarly, Tax forms a complex with $p67^{SRF}$ and binds indirectly to CArG box enhancer for the genes of c-*fos*, c-*egr* (*egr-1,2*) and *fra*-1, enhancing the transcription of these genes. The transcriptions of the genes for IL-1, IL-6, nerve growth factor (NGF), major histocompatibility complex Class I (MHC-I), PTHrP and OX40 are also activated by Tax protein, although the mechanism is not clear. In addition to its transactivation of HTLV-I LTR, it has recently been shown that Tax can activate cellular CREs through the transcriptional coactivator CREB-binding protein (CBP).

Furthermore, Tax binds to cytoplasmic inhibitor NF-κB proteins or NF-κB precursor proteins and promotes nuclear translocation of NF-κB and precursor proteins, providing another mechanism of transactivation. In a similar way, it has been reported that Tax prevents the formation of $p16^{INK4A}$/cyclin-dependent kinase 4 (CDK4) complex by interacting with cyclin-dependent kinase inhibitor $p16^{INK4A}$, possibly through the ankyrin motifs, resulting in CDK4 activation (Fig. 94.5). Furthermore, the gene expression of DNA polymerase-β, a DNA repair enzyme, was reported to be suppressed by Tax.

Dysregulated expression of a variety of cellular genes in HTLV-I-infected cells may play a key role in the development of HTLV-I-associated diseases and may be responsible for some of their characteristic clinical features. Enhanced expression of the

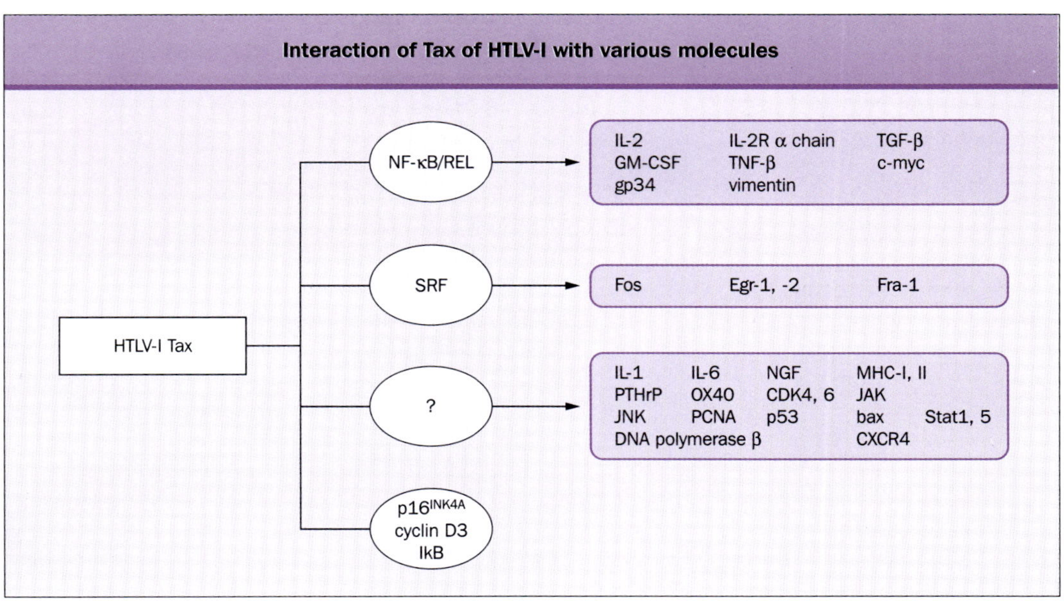

Figure 94.5 Interaction of Tax of HTLV-I with various molecules. Tax of HTLV-I transactivates various cellular genes through the interaction with NF-κB/Rel, SRF, or unknown factors. In addition, Tax directly interacts with $p16^{INK4A}$, cyclin D3 and IκB.

genes for cell growth-, cell cycle- or cell death-associated molecules, such as IL-2, IL-2R α chain, p16^{INK4A} and DNA polymerase β may be crucially involved in the transformation of T cells expressing *TAX* gene products.

It has been shown that transfection with the *TAX* gene resulted in the immortalization of normal human peripheral blood T cells activated by phytohemagglutinin (PHA) in the presence of IL-2 in vitro.[28] In addition, rodent fibroblasts transformed by the *TAX* gene were reported to lose anchorage-dependent proliferation and to be able to grow and form a tumor in nude mice. The oncogenic potential of *TAX* has also been demonstrated in *TAX* transgenic mice that revealed different phenotypes, including mesenchymal tumors, brain tumors, lymphoid tumors and large granular lymphocyte leukemia.[29,30] Thus, the *TAX* gene is clearly oncogenic both in vitro and in vivo, although it remains unclear whether Tax expression alone is sufficient for the development of ATL or responsible for the leukemic cell growth of ATL cells.

HTLV-I infects various types of cells, including T cells, B cells, macrophages, cells of neural origin and immature cells from bone marrow. Direct cell-to-cell contact is required for efficient infection, but the cellular receptor for HTLV-I has not been identified.

HTLV-I is transmitted through three major routes: mother to child via milk; transfusion; and sexual intercourse (male to female). It is thought that transmission requires the presence of virally infected cells. There remains a controversy as to whether the virus is transmitted across the placenta and from female to male, although data indicating such possibilities have been reported. Areas where HTLV-I is endemic are Japan (Kyushu, Okinawa, Shikoku, Ainu Aborigines), the South Pacific (Papua New Guinea, Solomon Islands and Australian Aborigines), South America (Brazil, Andes Mountain Highland Indians), the Caribbean and West Africa. In Japan, approximately 1.2 million people are infected and the estimated lifetime risk of ATL is about 5% in individuals infected before the age of 20.[7] Thus, most virally infected individuals do not develop leukemia or lymphoma, and in view of the long latent period, HTLV-I infection alone does not appear to be sufficient for the development of overt ATL. Indeed, it was reported that the stochastic analysis of the age-specific occurrence of ATL using 357 cases suggested the presence of an age-dependent accumulation of leukemogenic events estimated to number five for HTLV-I-infected T cells to develop ATL.[31] The average age of onset of ATL is 60 years in Japan, but only 40 years in Jamaica, suggesting that genetic or environmental factors as well as HTLV-I infection may play a role in the development of ATL.

HTLV-I is also associated with a neurological disease called HTLV-I-associated myelopathy (HAM)/tropical spastic paraparesis (TSP), which is characterized by spasticity of the lower extremities, urinary bladder disturbances, lower extremity muscle weakness, and sensory disturbances with poorly defined thoracic sensory levels.[32,33] Because ATL and HAM/TSP rarely coincide, host factors may be involved in the different expression of disease. It has been reported that certain HLA haplotypes are closely associated with either ATL or HAM/TSP.[34]

Immunology/pathogenesis

HTLV-I-infected healthy carriers, as well as ATL patients usually produce antibodies to various viral structural proteins, including gag proteins (p15, p24, p19) and their precursor (p55), envelope glycoprotein (gp46), the transmembrane protein (p21) and their precursors (gp61/69). In addition to these structural proteins, antibodies are also produced against the *TAX* gene product (p40). The amino terminal of HTLV-I gp46 contains type-specific linear neutralizing determinants. The time course of seroconversion was studied in HTLV-I-contaminated blood recipients.[35] Early after transfusion, antibodies to gag proteins and then to envelope transmembrane protein were detected, and anti-gp46 and anti-gp61 antibodies developed later. Anti-Tax antibodies appeared several months after viral infection. It does not appear that seroconversion with the development of antibodies to both gag and envelope proteins leads to elimination of HTLV-I. There is no clinical syndrome associated with acute seroconversion to HTLV-I. Antibody titers examined in serial samples over a 10-year period among asymptomatic carriers were persistent and stable.[4] The levels were highest in patients with HAM/TSP, somewhat lower in ATL, and generally lowest in asymptomatic carriers. There is a strong correlation between antibody titer and serum HTLV-I proviral level. In addition, a direct correlation between antibody titer and the presence of anti-Tax antibody was reported.[36]

Cellular immunity to HTLV-I has also been described. Cytotoxic T lymphocytes (CTL) against HTLV-I have been demonstrated in patients with ATL, HAM/TSP and HTLV-I uveitis, and in HTLV-I-infected asymptomatic carriers.[37–39] The reported epitopes recognized by these CTL have been localized to Tax protein and gp46 envelope protein. Recent studies revealed the high frequency of circulating CD8 CTL reactive with Tax11-19 peptide in HAM/TSP patients. It has been considered that HTLV-I remains latent for long periods in infected individuals, partly because of the sophisticated regulation of virus expression by Tax and Rex regulatory proteins, resulting in the emergence of escape virus mutants. However, according to recent reports, HTLV-I is persistently replicating at a high level in vivo, despite the relative constancy of its genome sequence. In addition, there is a persistently activated CTL response to the Tax protein that is maintained by active replication of the virus in the majority of HTLV-I-infected individuals.[40]

In the Miyazaki prefecture cohort study, delayed-type hypersensitivity to purified protein derivative (PPD) was diminished in HTLV-I carriers.[41] Other reports also described diminished humoral and cellular immune responses in ATL patients, in contrast to high responses in HAM/TSP patients. The mechanism of immunosuppression in asymptomatic HTLV-I carriers and ATL patients remains unclear, although various cytokines produced by HTLV-I-infected T cells, including IL-1, IL-6, TNF-β and TGF-β, may play a partial role in the development of immunosuppression.

Shortly after the first description of ATL, the intermediate state or a preleukemic state was proposed as a clinical condition characterized by the appearance of abnormal lymphocytes in the peripheral blood similar to the typical ATL leukemic cells. Some of the carriers with such clinical features eventually developed ATL, indicating the monoclonal proliferation of HTLV-I-infected T cells in an intermediate state or preleukemic state. Subsequent studies examining monoclonal proliferation using the random HTLV-I provirus integration site or the diversity of T-cell repertoire with reverse polymerase chain reaction (PCR) have demonstrated the clonal expansion of CD4$^+$ T cells and polyclonal expansion of $CD8^+$ T cells in asymptomatic HTLV-I carriers and patients with HAM/TSP.[42,43]

Although the precise mechanism(s) that induces ATL following HTLV-I infection is unknown, the expression of Tax protein is felt to play a major role. This appears to result from the transactivation of various cellular genes causing dysregulation of cell proliferation or cell death, at least in the early stage of the development of ATL. It was initially reported that IL-2R α chain was constitutively expressed by leukemic cells from ATL patients and HTLV-I-infected cell line cells,[12,14] and it was also demonstrated that Tax protein transactivated the transcription of the genes for IL-2 and IL-2R.[23,24] Furthermore, suggestive evidence was reported that leukemic cells from some ATL patients proliferate in vitro by an IL-2 autocrine mechanism, although freshly isolated leukemic cells from a majority of patients did not proliferate in response to exogenous IL-2, and IL-2 production was hardly detectable. Recently it has been shown that the intracellular IL-2 signal transducing molecules, including JAK1, JAK3, STAT3 and STAT5, are constitutively activated in some HTLV-I-infected cell lines. The transition from IL-2-dependent to IL-2-independent cell growth in vitro correlated with the acquisition of a constitutively activated JAK-STAT pathway in HTLV-I-infected cord blood lymphocytes.[44] Based on these observations, it is considered that the constitutive expression of IL-2 and its receptor, or dysregulated intracellular IL-2 signaling which is caused by HTLV-I infection, may play a crucial role at least in the early stage of ATL development.

The Miyazaki cohort study determining risk factors for ATL among HTLV-I carriers revealed the greatest risk for ATL development in carriers was a high anti-HTLV-I antibody titer and a lower anti-Tax reactivity.[45] This supports the hypothesis that persistent expression of the TAX gene product is not required for the maintenance of the malignant phenotype. The high frequency of defective HTLV-I provirus, incapable of producing Tax protein in acute or lymphoma-type ATL, may also indicate that Tax protein is not needed for the neoplastic proliferation of leukemic cells in advanced and aggressive ATL.[46]

Prevention and patient management

As previously noted, HTLV-I is transmitted via three major routes: maternal milk, transfusion, and sexual intercourse. In most developed countries, donor blood is now screened for anti-HTLV-I antibody. Intervention studies recommending HTLV-I-infected mothers refrain from breast feeding have markedly reduced this mode of transmission although approximately 3% of Japanese children who were not breast-fed have been found to be HTLV-I infected. Owing to these programs directed at preventing new viral infection, the number of the HTLV-I-infected carriers has been gradually decreasing in Japan. There are currently no effective means to prevent the occurrence of ATL in HTLV-I-infected individuals. Factors associated with the risk of developing ATL have been identified and include high anti-HTLV-I antibody levels, low anti-Tax antibody titer, a high viral load and monoclonal proliferation of T cells.[32,42,43]

Treatment

Combination chemotherapy using different regimens in the treatment of non-Hodgkin lymphoma has been tried in acute or lymphoma-type ATL.[47] The tumor is usually responsive, but the remission induced by such combination chemotherapy is very short compared to other malignant lymphomas. Typically relapses are observed within 4–10 months.

THERAPEUTIC PRINCIPLES

- Combination chemotherapy such as CHOP, VEPA, MACOP-B and LSG4 may provide a transient remission, but early relapse is common.
- Hematopoietic stem cell transplantation and immunotherapy is a potentially effective treatment in younger patients.
- Treatment for hypercalcemia (hydration, furosemide, corticosteroids, bisphosphonates and calcitonin) and management of infections are important.

The first-generation combination chemotherapy consisted of VEPA (vincristine, cyclophosphamide, prednisolone, adriamycin), VEPA-M (VEPA + methotrexate), standard or biweekly CHOP (cyclophosphamide, adriamycin, vincristine, prednisolone) and others. The second- or third-generation combination chemotherapy consisted of LSG4 (alternating therapy using three different regimens, VEPA-B (vincristine, cyclophosphamide, adriamycin, prednisolone, bleomycin) + M-FEPA (an intermediate dose of methotrexate, vindesine, cyclophosphamide, prednisolone, adriamycin) + VEPP-B (vincristine, cyclophosphamide, procarbazine, prednisolone, bleomycin)); MACOP-B (methotrexate, adriamycin, cyclophosphamide, vincristine, prednisolone, bleomycin) and others. The complete remission rates for first-generation and second or third-generation combination chemotherapies are 21% and 41%, respectively, indicating some improvement in the induction of remission using the combination of intensified doses of these drugs.[47] Nevertheless, the disease-free and overall survival times have not been improved with new-generation combination chemotherapy (mean disease-free survival time 5.0 versus 6.0 months, and mean survival time 7.5 versus 8.0 months, respectively.)

Deoxycoformycin (DCF), an adenosine deaminase inhibitor, was found to be effective in about a half of cases of Sézary syndrome and T-prolymphocytic leukemia. DCF was tested in ATL and showed a response rate of about 30%. It was reported that the combination of interferon-α and zidovudine elicited responses in a substantial fraction of patients with ATL.[48] Other treatment trials, including bone marrow transplantation, low-dose total body irradiation, leukapheresis, and administration of interferon-β, γ and IL-2, were unsuccessful. However, recent clinical trials treating a small number of younger ATL patients with bone marrow transplantation were encouraging, suggesting the potential efficacy of cell therapy combined with immunotherapy, similar to some EB virus-associated lymphoproliferative diseases.

Trials of IL-2 receptor-targeted therapy have been performed in ATL patients in the United States. The administration of mouse monoclonal antibody, anti-Tac, which reacts with human IL-2 receptor α chain, resulted in clinical improvement in seven of 19 patients examined.[49] Humanized anti-Tac antibody conjugated with ^{90}Y has also been effective in 10 of 15 patients with ATL. Anti-Tac antibody conjugated with ricin A chain, *Pseudomonas* exotoxin, or ^{212}Bi and the fusion protein composed of IL-2 and diphtheria toxin or *Pseudomonas* exotoxin, has been studied in vitro and selectively killed HTLV-I infected T-cell line cells expressing large numbers of IL-2 receptor α chains.

Smoldering-type ATL should not be treated intensively and it is controversial whether chronic-type ATL should be treated or not. However, the rapid elevation of serum LDH or soluble IL-2 receptor α chain, the rapid increase in the number of circulating abnormal lymphocytes and the rapid enlargement of lymph nodes indicate the need to initiate treatment.

Bacterial, viral and fungal infections that are common in ATL must be treated accordingly.

Hypercalcemia is often encountered as the disease accelerates, and can be fatal. This complication requires immediate treatment, including hydration and furosemide to relieve acute symptoms. Second-generation bisphosphonates are the preferred agents to control severe hypercalcemia in ATL. Bisphosphonates are analogs of pyrophosphate and have a high affinity for bone, especially in areas of increased turnover, acting to inhibit osteoclast activity. Calcitonin, which has a rapid onset of action, is also useful as an adjuvant in severe hypercalcemia. It is important to reduce the tumor mass using combination chemotherapy to control severe hypercalcemia at the same time as initiating anti-hypercalcemia treatment.

Patient evaluation and differential diagnosis

It is not difficult to establish the diagnosis in cases of typical acute or lymphoma-type ATL. The combination of clinical symptoms and signs, including lymph node enlargement, hepatomegaly, splenomegaly and skin lesions, together with the finding of morphologically characteristic tumor cells expressing IL-2R α chain (CD25), elevated serum levels of LDH, calcium and soluble IL-2R α chain and the presence of serum antibody to HTLV-I are helpful in establishing the diagnosis. This can be confirmed by the demonstration of monoclonal proliferation of HTLV-I-infected T cells. Studies of T-cell receptor β-chain gene rearrangement and/or HTLV-I provirus integration by Southern blot analysis of tumor cell DNA are necessary, because these differ in each HTLV-I-infected T-cell clone. Adverse prognostic factors (age more than 40, poor performance status, total tumor burden, hypercalcemia and elevated serum LDH level) as well as the clinical type (acute, chronic, lymphoma or smoldering) must be established in order to determine the prognosis.

Acute lymphoblastic leukemia with T-cell properties, malignant T-cell lymphoma, chronic lymphocytic leukemia of T-cell origin and cutaneous T-cell lymphoma are sometimes difficult to differentiate from ATL solely by symptoms, signs and ordinary laboratory findings. The detection of monoclonal HTLV-I provirus integration in leukemic cells is crucial to make a differential diagnosis in such cases. Very rare patients have been reported with the typical clinical manifestations of ATL and leukemic cells with characteristic morphology and immunophenotype, but lacking serum antibodies to HTLV-I.[50] Southern blot analysis of leukemic cell DNA using probes covering the whole region of HTLV-I failed to demonstrate the provirus integration into leukemic cells. This suggests the possibility that a factor other than HTLV-I infection can also result in the development of disease that is clinically indistinguishable from typical ATL.

Cutaneous T-cell lymphoma (CTCL), including mycosis fungoides and Sézary syndrome, is a malignancy of CD4 T cells and has clinical and histopathological features similar to those of ATL. As mentioned above, one of the findings helpful for differentiating these two diseases is the presence of HTLV-I infection in ATL but not in CTCL. However, several groups in countries where HTLV-I is not endemic have recently reported that HTLV-I provirus integration into neoplastic cells is detectable in a minority of CTCL patients, although the provirus is mostly deleted or defective and the patients are routinely seronegative.[51,52] In addition, the provirus may contain deletions and may be defective in rare cases of ATL which are seronegative. Therefore, it has now become important to establish criteria that clearly differentiate such cases of CTCL from ATL, and elucidate the role of HTLV-I infection in the pathogenesis of CTCL.

HTLV-II-ASSOCIATED T-CELL MALIGNANCIES

HTLV-II was first isolated from a phenotypic T-cell line derived from a patient with an unusual variant of hairy cell leukemia (HCL).[53,54] HCL is characterized by the presence of typical 'hairy' cells in the peripheral blood and bone marrow, pancytopenia and splenomegaly. The typical leukemic cells are mononuclear, with relatively abundant blue-gray cytoplasm and a variable number of elongated (hairy) projections. The immunophenotype of HCL cells is that of a B cell in most cases. Studies subsequent to the discovery of HTLV-II failed to demonstrate the association of the virus with HCL. The second HCL patient from whom HTLV-II was isolated had a biphenotypic malignancy with a monoclonal B-cell population that had morphological features of HCL and an atypical clonal CD8 T-cell population containing integrated HTLV-II.[55] HTLV-II may be associated with such a rare T-cell variant of HCL. The genomic structure of HTLV-II is closely homologous to that of HTLV-I, and their biological and antigenic similarity has also been demonstrated. Recent epidemiological studies have shown higher rates of HTLV-II infection in intravenous drug users and native Americans residing in North, Central and South America. In addition, HTLV-II infection has been suggested to be associated with other diseases including HAM/TSP, glomerular nephritis in children, large granular lymphocyte leukemia, eczema and asthma. However, in contrast to HTLV-I, there is very limited evidence showing an etiological role for HTLV-II in any human disease except for unusual cases of HCL. Further studies will be needed to reveal any additional relationship between HTLV-II and human disease.

OTHER HTLV-I-ASSOCIATED DISEASES (Table 94.1)

HTLV-I-associated myelopathy (HAM)/tropical spastic paraparesis (TSP)

The onset of HAM/TSP is insidious, with clinical features that include muscle weakness or stiffness of one or both legs, hyperreflexia, clonus, extensor plantar responses, back pain, sensory disturbances, urinary incontinence and impotence. Laboratory examination reveals antibodies to HTLV-I in the serum and cerebrospinal fluid.[32,33] Magnetic resonance imaging (MRI) demonstrates lesions in both the white matter and the paraventricular regions of the brain, as well as the spinal cord. Histopathological findings of the spinal cord include mononuclear cell infiltration, marked myelin and axonal destruction and astrocytic gliosis. The average age at diagnosis is 40 years and the lifetime risk in HTLV-I carriers is estimated to be less than 2%, which is lower than that

HTLV-I-associated diseases
Adult T-cell leukemia/lymphoma (ATL) acute type, lymphoma type, chronic type, smoldering type
HTLV-I-associated myelopathy (HAM)/Tropical spastic paraparesis (TSP)
HTLV-I-uveitis (HU)
HTLV-I-associated infective dermatitis
HTLV-I-associated arthropathy?
HTLV-I-associated Sjögren syndrome?
HTLV-I-associated polymyositis?
HTLV-I-associated lymphadenitis?

Table 94.1 HTLV-I-associated diseases.

of ATL. In contrast to ATL, HAM/TSP affects females disproportionately more. The mechanism(s) underlying the development of HAM/TSP remains unclear, although at least two hypotheses explaining the role of HTLV-I have been proposed. One is that persistent central nervous system infection with HTLV-I results in chronic activation and destruction of tissue by a cellular immune attack by HTLV-I-specific CTLs. A second hypothesis is that HTLV-I infection promotes the activation of autoreactive T cells, which migrate to the CNS, recognize target antigens in the CNS and secrete various cytokines, inducing inflammation and tissue damage.

Systemic or intrathecal administration of corticosteroids provides a transient beneficial effect in some patients, especially during the early stage of disease. HAM/TSP is a progressively disabling disorder and the complications during the clinical course, including infection, may lead to death.

HTLV-I uveitis (HAU)

A specific form of uveitis has been proposed to be associated with HTLV-I infection.[56] Its clinical features include blurred vision or myodesopsia with acute or subacute onset, relatively preserved visual acuity in most cases, iritis, vitreous opacities, retinal vasculitis, and retinal exudates and hemorrhages. The mean age of the patients is 44 years in men and 49 in women. HTLV-I proviral DNA has been demonstrated in about 60% of T-cell clones established from the intraocular fluid of patients with HTLV-I uveitis. PCR analysis showed infiltration of HTLV-I-infected T cells in the affected eye and a higher HTLV-I provirus load in the peripheral blood. In addition, the data suggested a correlation between a previous history of Graves' disease and HTLV-I uveitis. HTLV-I uveitis usually responds well to ocular or oral administration of corticosteroids, although recurrence is observed in approximately half of the cases.

HTLV-I-associated infective dermatitis

Infective dermatitis with unique clinical manifestations was first described in Jamaican children in 1966 and was later found to be associated with HTLV-I.[57] The clinical features of the disease include a severe exudative dermatitis of the scalp, external ear and retroauricular areas, eyelid margins, paranasal skin, neck, axillae and groin, as well as a generalized fine papular rash. Chronic watery nasal discharges without other signs of rhinitis are also common. *Staphylococcus aureus* and β-hemolytic streptococci are usually cultured from the anterior nares and skin. The administration of antibiotics produces a prompt response, but relapse occurs on their withdrawal. The pathogenesis of the disease is unknown, although lymphocyte infiltration into the skin lesions suggests a strong anti-HTLV-I immune response. The average age of the onset was 2 years, with 60% of the patients reported to be female. Familial clustering was also observed.

HTLV-I-associated arthropathy (HAAP)

HTLV-I-associated arthropathy (HAAP) was proposed as a new disease entity defined as an arthropathy developing in HTLV-I-infected individuals.[58] It was reported that HTLV-I antibodies were detectable in the synovial fluid of the affected joints, and HTLV-I proviral DNA was also demonstrable by PCR both in synovial tissue and in synovial fluid lymphocytes.

In addition, it was reported that mice transgenic for HTLV-I demonstrated swelling of the ankles with redness and/or swelling of the adjacent footpad, caused by chronic inflammatory lesions closely resembling the changes observed in human rheumatoid arthritis.[59] However, subsequent studies by others reported that most patients with rheumatoid arthritis are seronegative for HTLV-I and -II. Taken together, HTLV-I may be involved in rare cases of chronic arthritis in humans.

REFERENCES

1. Uchiyama T, Yodoi J, Sagawa K, Takatsuki K, Uchino H. Adult T-cell leukemia: clinical and hematologic features of 16 cases. Blood 1977;50:481.
2. Poiesz BJ, Ruscetti FW, Gazdar AF, Bunn PA, Minna JD, Gallo RC. Detection and isolation of type C retrovirus particles from fresh and cultured lymphocytes of a patient with cutaneous T-cell lymphoma. Proc Natl Acad Sci USA 1980;77:7415.
3. Hinuma Y, Nagata K, Hanaoka M, et al. Adult T-cell leukemia: antigen in an ATL cell line and detection of antibodies to the antigen in human sera. Proc Natl Acad Sci USA 1981;78:6476.
4. Blattner WA, Kalyanaraman VS, Robert GM, et al. The human type-C retrovirus, HTLV, in blacks from the Caribbean region, and relationship to adult T-cell leukemia/lymphoma. Int J Cancer 1982;30:257.
5. Hinuma Y, Komoda H, Chosa T, et al. Antibodies to adult T-cell leukemia-virus-associated antigen (ATLA) in sera from patients with ATL and controls in Japan: a nation-wide sero-epidemiologic study. Int J Cancer 1982;29:631.
6. Yoshida M, Seiki M, Yamaguchi K, Takatsuki K. Monoclonal integration of human T-cell leukemia provirus in all primary tumors of adult T-cell leukemia suggests causative role of human T-cell leukemia virus in the disease. Proc Natl Acad Sci USA 1984;81:2534.
7. Tajima K. The fourth nation-wide study of adult T-cell leukemia/lymphoma (ATL) in Japan: estimates of risk of ATL and its geographical and clinical features. The T- and B-cell Malignancy Study Group. Int J Cancer 1990;45:237.
8. Shimoyama M. Diagnostic criteria and classification of clinical subtypes of adult T-cell leukaemia–lymphoma. A report from the Lymphoma Study Group (1984–87). Br J Haematol 1991;79:428.
9. Takatsuki K, Matsuoka M, Yamaguchi K. ATL and HTLV-I related diseases. In: Takatsuki K (ed.) Adult T cell leukemia and related diseases. Oxford, Oxford University Press, 1994, 1.

10. Hattori T, Uchiyama T, Toibana T, Takatsuki K, Uchino H. Surface phenotype of Japanese adult T-cell leukemia cells characterized by monoclonal antibodies. Blood 1981;58:645.
11. Kamihira S, Sohda H, Atogami S, et al. Phenotypic diversity and prognosis of adult T-cell leukemia. Leuk Res 1992;16:435.
12. Uchiyama T, Hori T, Tsudo M, et al. Interleukin-2 receptor (Tac antigen) expressed on adult T cell leukemia cells. J Clin Invest 1985;76:446.
13. Uchiyama T. Human T cell leukemia virus type I (HTLV-I) and human diseases. Annu Rev Immunol 1997;15:15.
14. Waldmann TA. The IL-2/IL-2 receptor system: a target for rational immune intervention. Immunol Today 1993;14:264.
15. Kamada S, Sakurai M, Miyamoto K, et al. Chromosome abnormalities in adult T-cell leukemial lymphoma: a karyotype review. Cancer Res 1992;52:1481.
16. Marcon L, Rubin LA, Kurman CC, et al. Elevated serum levels of soluble Tac peptide in adult T-cell leukemia: correlation with clinical status during chemotherapy. Ann Intern Med 1988;109:274.
17. Watanabe T, Yamaguchi K, Takatsuki K, Osame M, Yoshida M. Constitutive expression of parathyroid hormone-related protein gene in human T cell leukemia virus type 1 (HTLV-1) carriers and adult T cell leukemia patients that can be trans-activated by HTLV-1 tax gene. J Exp Med 1990;172:759.
18. Shimoyama M, Ota K, Kikuchi M, et al. Major prognostic factors of adult patients with advanced T-cell lymphomal leukemia. J Clin Oncol 1988;6:1088.
19. Lymphoma Study Group (1984–1987). Major prognostic factors of patients with adult T-cell leukemia-lymphoma: a cooperative study. Leukemia Res 1991;15:81.
20. Seiki M, Hattori S, Hirayama Y, Yoshida M. Human adult T-cell leukemia virus: complete nucleotide sequence of the provirus genome integrated in leukemia cell DNA. Proc Natl Acad Sci USA 1983;80:3618.
21. Koralnik IJ, Fullen J, Franchini G. The p12^{I}, p13^{II} and p30^{II} proteins encoded by human T-cell leukemia/lymphotropic virus type I open reading frames I and II are localized in three different cellular compartments. J Virol 1993;67:2360.
22. Sodroski JG, Rosen CA, Haseltine WA. Trans-acting transcriptional activation of the long terminal repeat of human T lymphotropic viruses in infected cells. Science 1984;225:381.
23. Leung K, Nabel GJ. HTLV-1 transactivator induces interleukin-2 receptor expression through an NF-kappa B-like factor. Nature 1988;333:776.
24. Ballard DW, Bohnlein E, Lowenthal JW, Wano Y, Franza BR, Greene WC. HTLV-I Tax induces cellular proteins that activate the kappa B element in the IL-2 receptor alpha gene. Science 1988;241:1652.
25. Fujii M, Sassone CP, Verma IM. c-fos promoter trans-activation by the tax 1 protein of human T-cell leukemia virus type I. Proc Natl Acad Sci USA 1988;85:8526.
26. Perini G, Wagner S, Green MR. Recognition of bZIP proteins by the human T-cell leukaemia virus transactivator Tax. Nature 1995;376:602.
27. Baranger AM, Palmer CR, Hamm MK, et al. Mechanism of DNA-binding enhancement by the human T-cell leukaemia virus transactivator Tax. Nature 1995;376:606.
28. Akagi T, Shimotohno K. Proliferative response of Tax 1-transduced primary human T cells to anti-CD3 antibody stimulation by an interleukin-2-independent pathway. J Virol 1993;67:1211.
29. Nerenberg M, Hinrichs SH, Reynolds RK, Khoury G, Jay G. The *tat* gene of human T-lymphotropic virus type 1 induces mesenchymal tumors in transgenic mice. Science 1987;237:1324.
30. Grossman WJ, Kimata JT, Wong FH, Zutter M, Ley TJ, Ratner L. Development of leukemia in mice transgenic for the tax gene of human T-cell leukemia virus type I. Proc Natl Acad Sci USA 1995;92:1057.
31. Okamoto T, Ohno Y, Tsugane S, et al. Multi-step carcinogenesis model for adult T-cell leukemia. Jpn J Cancer Res 1989;80:191.
32. Gessain A, Barin F, Vernant JC, et al. Antibodies to human T-lymphotropic virus type-I in patients with tropical spastic paraparesis. Lancet 1985;2:407.
33. Osame M, Usuku K, Izumo S, et al. HTLV-I associated myelopathy, a new clinical entity. Lancet 1986;1:1031.
34. Sonoda S, Fujiyoshi T, Yashiki S. Immunogenetics of HTLV-I/II and associated diseases. J AIDS Hum Retrovirol 1996;13 Supl:S119.
35. Manns A, Murphy EL, Wilks R, et al. Detection of early human T-cell lymphotropic virus type I antibody patterns during seroconversion among transfusion recipients. Blood 1991;77:896.
36. Shioiri S, Tachibana N, Okayama A, et al. Analysis of anti-tax antibody of HTLV-I carriers in an endemic area in Japan. Int J Cancer 1993;53:1.
37. Kannagi M, Harada S, Maruyama I, et al. Predominant recognition of human T cell leukemia virus type I (HTLV-I) pX gene products by human CD8^{+} cytotoxic T cells directed against HTLV-I-infected cells. Int Immunol 1991;3:761.
38. Jacobson S, Shida H, McFarlin DE, Fauci AS, Koenig S. Circulating CD8^{+} cytotoxic T lymphocytes specific for HTLV-I pX in patients with HTLV-I associated neurological disease. Nature 1990;348:245.
39. Parker CE, Nightingale S, Taylor GP, Weber J, Bangham CR. Circulating anti-Tax cytotoxic T lymphocytes from human T-cell leukemia virus type I-infected people, with and without tropical spastic paraparesis, recognize multiple epitopes simultaneously. J Virol 1994;68:2860.
40. Wondarz D, Nowak MA, Bangham CR. The dynamics of HTLV-I and the CTL response. Immunol Today 1999;20:220.
41. Tachibana N, Okayama A, Ishizaki J, et al. Suppression of tuberculin skin reaction in healthy HTLV-I carriers from Japan. Int J Cancer 1988;42:829.
42. Etoh K, Tamiya S, Yamaguchi K, et al. Persistent clonal proliferation of human T-lymphotropic virus type I-infected cells in vivo. Cancer Res 1997;57:4862.
43. Eiraku N, Hingorani R, Ijicji S, et al. Clonal expansion within CD4^{+} and CD8^{+} T cell subsets in human T lymphotropic virus type I-infected individuals. J Immunol 1998;161:6674.
44. Xu X, Kang SH, Heidenreich O, Okerholm M, O'Shea JJ, Nerenberg MI. Constitutive activation of different Jak tyrosine kinases in human T cell leukemia virus type 1 (HTLV-1) tax protein or virus-transformed cells. J Clin Invest 1995;96:1548.
45. Hisada M, Okayama A, Shioiri S, Spiegelman DL, Stuber S, Muller NE. Risk factors for adult T-cell leukemia among carriers of human T-lymphotropic virus type I. Blood 1998;92:3557.
46. Tamiya S, Matsuoka M, Etoh K, et al. Two types of defective human T-lymphotropic virus type I provirus in adult T-cell leukemia. Blood 1996;88:3065.
47. Shimoyama M. Chemotherapy of ATL. In: Takatsuki K (ed) Adult T cell leukemia. Oxford, Oxford University Press, 1994;221.
48. Gill PS, Harrington W, Kaplan M, et al. Treatment of adult T-cell leukemia-lymphoma with a combination of interferon alfa and zidovudine. N Engl J Med 1995;332:1744.
49. Waldmann TA, Goldman CK, Bongiovanni KF, et al. Therapy of patients with human T-cell lymphotrophic virus I-induced adult T-cell leukemia with anti-Tac, a monoclonal antibody to the receptor for interleukin-2. Blood 1988;72:1805.
50. Shimoyama M, Kagami Y, Shimotohno K, et al. Adult T-cell leukemia/lymphoma not associated with human T-cell leukemia virus type I. Proc Natl Acad Sci USA 1986;83:4524.
51. Hall WW, Liu CR, Schneewind O, et al. Deleted HTLV-I provirus in blood and cutaneous lesions of patients with mycosis fungoides. Science 1991;253:317.
52. Zucker-Franklin D, Coutavas EE, Rush MG, Zouzias DC. Detection of human T-lymphotropic virus-like particles in cultures of peripheral blood lymphocytes from patients with mycosis fungoides. Proc Natl Acad Sci USA 1991;88:7630.
53. Kalyanaraman VS, Sarngadharan MG, Robert-Guroff M, et al. A new subtype of human T-cell leukemia virus (HTLV-II) associated with a T-cell variant of hairy cell leukemia. Science 1982;218:571.
54. Saxon A, Stevens RH, Golde DW. T-lymphocyte variant of hairy cell leukemia. Ann Intern Med 1978;88:323.
55. Rosenblatt JD, Golde DW, Wacksman W, et al. A second HTLV-II isolate associated with atypical hairy-cell leukemia. N Engl J Med 1986;315:372.
56. Mochizuki M, Watanabe T, Yamaguchi K, et al. HTLV-I uveitis: a distinct clinical entity caused by HTLV-I. Jpn J Cancer Res 1992;83:236.
57. LaGrenade L, Hanchard B, Fletcher V, Cranston B, Blattner W. Infective dermatitis of Jamaican children: a marker for HTLV-I infection. Lancet 1990;1:1345.

58. Nishioka K, Maruyama I, Sato K, Kitajima I, Nakajima Y, Osame M. Chronic inflammatory arthropathy associated with HTLV-I. Lancet 1989;1:441.

59. Iwakura Y, Tosu M, Yoshida E, et al. Induction of inflammatory arthropathy resembling rheumatoid arthritis in mice transgenic for HTLV-I. Science 1991;253:1026.

Section 9 Immunology of Neoplasia

Chapter 95 Mechanisms of Lymphoid Malignant Transformation by Herpes Group of Viruses

Kishor Bhatia and Gianluca Gaidano

Herpesviruses are large DNA viruses that infect a wide spectrum of hosts, including – though not restricted to – primates and humans. A few of the 100 members of these viruses are also implicated in causing or promoting malignancy in their natural hosts. These include the Luke virus, associated with carcinomas in the frog, the Marek's disease virus associated with lymphomas in chickens, Epstein–Barr virus (EBV) associated with Burkitt's lymphoma and nasopharyngeal carcinoma in humans, and human herpesvirus type-8 (HHV-8), associated with primary effusion lymphoma and Kaposi sarcoma.

Based on studies of infection prevalence, human herpesviruses have been very successful, as more than 90% of the human population is infected by members of this group. The success of herpesviruses derives from their unique ability to establish a non-symptomatic association with their human host. Following primary infection, these viruses persist in the infected individual for life, and also sustain their tenacious association with the human species through a process of strategic and controlled replication and shedding of progeny viruses. The ability of these viruses to coexist with the human population is a result of intricate interactions between the genetic programs that control expression of viral proteins and the host immune system. When the host immune system fails, however, these complex DNA viruses do carry the potential to cause disease.

Eight herpes viruses are known to infect humans and share common structural features (Fig. 95.1), including an inner core of double-stranded DNA, a protein capsid, a tegument and a lipid envelope embedded with glycoproteins derived from the host cells. They are transmitted from host to host by direct intimate contact and are shed into the saliva of infected individuals, thus allowing their subsistence in the human population. Based upon their biologic properties and tissue tropism, human herpesviruses are grouped into three subfamilies, i.e. the alphaherpesvirinae, the betaherpesvirinae and the gammaherpesviriniae. The α-herpes viruses include the herpes simplex viruses types 1 and 2 and the varicella zoster virus. The subfamily of β-herpes viruses include cytomegalovirus (CMV), human herpesvirus 6 (HHV-6) and human herpesvirus 7 (HHV-7). The human γ herpesviruses include Epstein–Barr virus (EBV) and human herpesvirus 8 (HHV-8). The α herpesviruses are neurotropic, whereas CMV infects lymphocytes, monocytes and neutrophils. The remainder of the β- and γ-herpesviruses (HHV-6, HHV-7, HHV-8 and EBV) are lymphotropic.

A schematic representation of a herpes viron structure

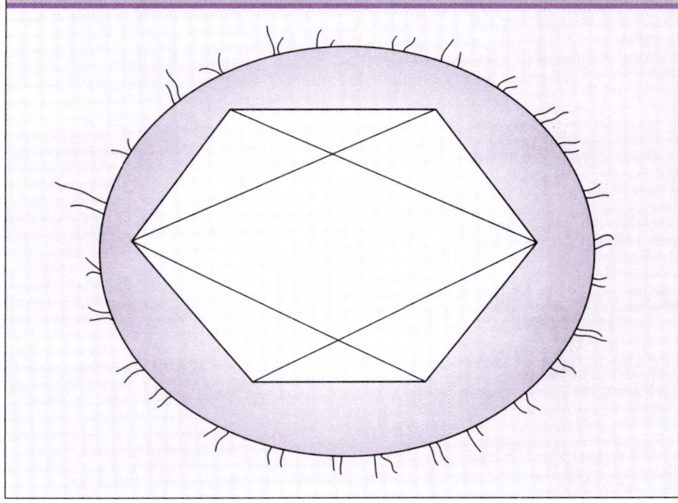

Figure 95.1 A schematic representation of a herpes viron structure. The size of the particle is 180–200 nm. The outer lipid envelope with its associated glycoproteins contains an inner protein tegument. A toroidal core that contains the genomic DNA wrapped about a protein is encased in an icosahedral nucleoprotein consisting of 162 hexagonal capsomeres.

KEY CONCEPTS

Human herpesviruses

- Consist of three subfamilies: alpha-, beta- and gamma-herpesviruses.
- Alphaherpesviruses are neurotropic.
- Beta- and gammaherpesviruses are lymphotropic (CMV also infects monocytes and neutrophils).
- Alphaherpesvirus: herpes simplex 1 & 2, varicella zoster.
- Betaherpesvirus: CMV, HHV-6, HHV-7.
- Gammaherpesvirus: EBV, HHV-8.

Human herpesviruses are associated with lymphoproliferative disorders (Table 95.1). Several studies have attempted to link herpesviruses to human malignancies, although studies based solely on seroepidemiologic evidence and/or detection of viral DNA in the tumor cells cannot be considered conclusive. Examples of such proposed associations include HSV-2 and cervical carcinoma, CMV and cancers of the prostate, colon and cervix, as well as HHV-6 and some types of lymphoid malignancy. Conversely, the association of EBV with Burkitt's lymphoma and nasopharyngeal carcinoma, and that of HHV-8 with Kaposi sarcoma and primary effusion lymphoma, are firmly established.

Human lymphotropic herpesviruses and associated conditions

Virus/subfamily	Target lymphoid cells	Lymphoproliferation
Epstein–Barr virus (HHV4; Herpesvirus γ_1)	B lymphocytes, T lymphocytes	Burkitt's lymphoma T-cell/NK cell lymphomas Hodgkin's disease X-linked lymphoproliferation Infectious mononucleosis Post-transplant lymphoproliferative disorder AIDS-associated NHL
HHV8-Kaposi sarcoma virus (Herpesvirus γ_2)	B-lymphocytes, macrophages, variety of leukocytes	Primary effusion lymphomas Multicentric Castleman's disease
HHV-6 (Herpesvirus β)	CD4 lymphocytes	?
HHV-7 (Herpesvirus β)	CD4 lymphocytes	?

Table 95.1 Human lymphotropic herpesviruses and associated lymphoproliferative conditions.

This chapter reviews the biologic and transforming properties of the lymphotropic herpesviruses and emphasizes the molecular mechanisms the viruses utilize to persist in their target tumor cells.

EPSTEIN–BARR VIRUS

The discovery of EBV was a result of seminal observations made by Burkitt during his investigations of jaw tumors in Africa. In reviewing the incidence of this malignancy from old hospital records, he noted that the distribution of this tumor was dependent upon geographic factors of altitude and temperature, reflecting the possibility that insect vectors played a role in transmitting a viral agent responsible for Burkitt's lymphoma.[1] In 1964, Epstein, Achong and Barr described herpesvirus particles in cells cultured from these tumors. Subsequent seroepidemiologic and electron microscopy studies provided evidence that the virus associated with Burkitt's lymphoma was a novel and unique human herpesvirus. The indirect immunofluorescent assay developed by Henle et al demonstrated that antibodies to EBV were prevalent in the sera of normal adults, suggesting that a large proportion of healthy individuals are infected with EBV. Of note was the observation that sera from African children with Burkitt's lymphoma (but not of children with other malignancies) were uniformly seropositive for EBV. In addition, Henle et al also demonstrated that EBV from Burkitt's lymphoma cells could be transmitted to normal peripheral blood lymphocytes, causing immortalization of previously quiescent B cells.[2]

EBV structure, genome and gene products

EBV is a typical herpesvirion and consists of a protein core that is wrapped with DNA and protected by an icosahedral capsid with 162 capsomeres. This nucleocapsid is surrounded by a protein tegument. The outer envelope, derived from the host cell membranes, bears numerous glycoprotein spikes. Taxonomists have suggested a designation of HHV-4 for EBV.[3]

The EBV genome is a linear double-stranded DNA molecule of about 172 kb in length and encodes more than 85 genes (Fig. 95.2). The genome contains five domains of unique sequences, separated by four domains of repeated internal sequences and bordered at the extreme ends by terminal repeats.

A linear representation of a herpesvirus genome

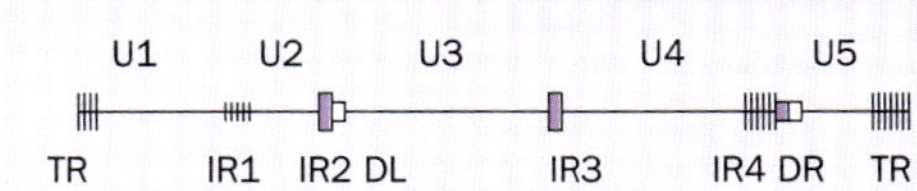

Figure 95.2 A linear representation of a herpes virus genome. The 172 kb long EBV genome, like the genome of other herpes viruses contains unique regions (U1–5) bounded by inverted repeats (IR1–4). The termini of the genome contains multiple repeat elements (TR).

The latter are the site at which the linear genome circularizes during the establishment of a latent infection in a host cell and persists as an episome. Because the exact size of the recombination between the terminal repeat at the two extreme ends is random, the fused terminal region for each circularized event, and hence for each infecting particle, is unique. During the process of latent infection the genome persists via DNA synthesis, mediated by the host cell DNA polymerase, thus allowing the progeny of the infected cell to maintain the same number of terminal repeats as the parental cell. Because of this property, the recombined fused termini have been used as an accurate marker for monoclonality of EBV infection. Under rare circumstances it may be possible for the EBV genome to integrate into the host cell chromosomes. The few examples of EBV-infected cells carrying only the integrated EBV genome did not show a preference for or restriction of the integration site. Because integration of the EBV genome may not be conducive to a productive lytic infection, integration is not a regular event in the biology of EBV infection.

The full complement of 85–90 viral genes is expressed during replicative infection. The expression of gene products is strictly regulated in latent infection. The nuclear antigen EBNA-1 is essential for the persistence of the viral genome and is thus the only protein universally expressed in all EBV-containing cells. Based upon the type of latency, as many as 10 additional EBV genes may be expressed. These include the five other nuclear antigens, EBNA 2–6, two small nonpolyadenylated RNAs termed EBER 1 and 2, and the three latent membrane proteins (LMP)

1, 2A and 2B. This full spectrum of latent gene expression is observed in vivo only in immunosuppressed individuals. When EBV infects B cells in vitro an identical pattern of gene expression is seen, and this also results in the immortalization of B cells. These latently expressed genes are designated transformation-associated proteins. The differences in the expression of latency genes in vivo and in vitro demonstrate the interplay between the host immune system and the ability of the virus to evade immunosurveillance.

In immunocompetent hosts the pattern of expression is lesion dependent (Table 95.2). Expression is restricted to either EBNA-1, and EBERs, defined as latency I and exemplified by EBV in Burkitt's lymphomas,[4] or to EBNA-1, EBERs and LMPs, defined as latency II, and observed in nasopharyngeal carcinomas[5] and Hodgkin's disease. A latency III pattern, characterized by broad expression of EBNAs and LMPs is observed in patients with post-transplant lymphoproliferation and infectious mononucleosis. Although latency I is the expression pattern observed with EBV-positive Burkitt's lymphomas, most (though not all) Burkitt's lymphomas shift to a latency III phenotype when explanted into tissue culture. This observation highlights the pressure encountered by infected cells to down-regulate EBV gene products that may provide epitope targets for cytotoxic T lymphocytes (CTL). This notion is further reinforced by the example of primary EBV infection. In this setting there is a transitory phase of type III latency, which is the pattern of gene expression also observed in acute infectious mononucleosis.[7] The mounting of an effective immune response by the host cell immune system conceivably forces the infected cells to shift to a pattern of gene expression that allows escape from CTL.

A restricted pattern of gene expression different from the previous ones has been reported in leiomyosarcomas, which are tumors of smooth muscle cells.[8] In these tumors the latent virus expresses EBNA-2 in addition to the genes expressed in type I latency. Interestingly, these tumors have been described in an immunocompromised setting. Thus, it is likely that the pattern of gene expression is influenced not only by the host immune system but also by the cell type infected. In general, type II latency is the prevalent pattern in non-B-cell malignancies.

Although latency is strictly regulated, it is apparent that latent infection alone does not suffice to maintain EBV in the human population. The latent virus retains the capacity for viral replication both in tumors and in lymphoblastoid cell lines.[9] The shift to lytic infection is principally controlled by the expression of Zta, a transactivator that is both necessary and sufficient for this switch.[10] In productive infection the viral genome is amplified via the origin of lytic replication (OriLyt), whereas the maintenance and replication of the episomal form of viral DNA during latent infection utilizes OriP sequences. The full complement of viral genes expressed during the replicative phase has been categorized as immediate early genes, which include genes that are expressed independently of de novo protein synthesis. The three major proteins expressed as immediate early products are all transactivators and include the open reading frames (ORF) BZLF1, BRLF1 and B1LF4. Exogenous expression of BZLF1, also known as Zebra or Zta, is sufficient to induce the lytic cycle, and therefore it is probably the main initiator of the lytic cascade.

The early genes expressed in lytic infection are those involved in DNA metabolism and in initiating cell lysis.[11] As the virus uses its own DNA synthesizing machinery, the complement of these genes includes a DNA-binding protein, ribonucleotide reductases, the viral DNA polymerase, primase, helicase, uracil DNA glycosylase, alkaline exonuclease and a transactivating protein encoded by the ORF BMRF1. The expression of these early lytic genes is resistant to inhibitors of viral DNA synthesis. Therefore, it is likely that at this stage the actual lysis of the host cell occurs irrespective of virion production. The final set of genes expressed during the lytic cycle are termed late genes, and their synthesis can be blocked by the inhibition of viral DNA synthesis. The majority of the late gene products are the virion structural proteins, that also include proteins such as BHRF1, which may maintain host cell survival.

EBV infection

Although EBV primarily infects humans, lymphocytes from several primates can be efficiently transformed in vitro. Experimental infection of New World monkeys with EBV has resulted in either the induction of lymphomas or the induction of a mononucleosis-like syndrome.[12] EBV has clearly been associated with malignancies of both B and T lymphocytes, as well as epithelial cell cancers. Under normal circumstances, however, EBV is thought to be a B-cell tropic virus.

EBV proteins expressed in lymphoproliferative lesions

Disease	EBV proteins expressed	Pattern of latency
Endemic Burkitt's lymphomas	EBNA-1	I
Sporadic Burkitt's lymphoma	EBNA-1	I
AIDS-associated Burkitt's lymphomas	EBNA-1	I
AIDS-associated CNS lymphomas	EBNA-1, LMP-1, LMP-2	II
Hodgkin's disease	EBNA-1, LMP-1, LMP-2	II
T-cell lymphomas	EBNA-1, LMP-1, LMP-2	II
Post-transplant lymphoproliferation	EBNAs-1, -2, -3A(3), -3B(4), EBNA-3C(6), -LP(5), LMP-1, LMP-2	III
Infectious mononucleosis	EBNAs-1, -2, -3A(3), -3B(4), EBNA-3C(6), -LP(5), LMP-1, LMP-2	III

Table 95.2 EBV proteins expressed in various lymphoproliferative lesions.

In vitro EBV infection models

Although in vitro infection with EBV has been successfully reported in several cell types, the virus has an apparent predilection for infecting lymphoid B cells. This tropism may be due, at least in part, to quantitative differences in the receptor for the virus on these cells. The B-cell lymphotropism of EBV is mediated through the interactions between the CR2 receptor CD21 and the glycoprotein gp350 on the viral envelope.[13] In addition to infecting of mature B cells, EBV also infects B-lymphocyte precursors, including those highly immature precursors that have not yet rearranged their immunoglobulin loci.[14]

Several groups have also been successful in infecting T cells and immature thymocytes with EBV.[15] The infection of T cells with EBV is consistent with the frequent detection of this virus in T-cell lymphomas. The EBV latency programs are not significantly different in mature versus progenitor B cells, whereas latent infection of immature thymocytes is less tightly regulated than infection of mature T cells. In addition, a significant fraction of infected immature thymocytes enter the lytic phase.

Among nonlymphoid cells, epithelial cells can be infected by EBV.[16] Exogenous expression of the B-cell EBV receptor CR2 may be required for the infection of keratinocytes. Other cell types that have been shown to be permissive for EBV infection under defined conditions include colon carcinoma, hepatoma, monocytes and an endothelial cell line.[17] It is unclear whether the CR2 receptor alone confers EBV tropism and the distribution of this receptor is not restricted to B cells.[18] CD21 has also been detected on follicular dendritic cells,[19] although these cells are not known to be associated with the virus in vivo, and attempts to infect dendritic cells in vitro have had limited success.

In vivo EBV infection

Paralleling the ease of infectability seen in vitro, B cells are also particularly receptive to infection in vivo. Proliferation of EBV-infected B cells has been observed in the germinal center,[20] suggesting that the presence of EBV does not impair the ability of these cells to respond to antigenic stimuli. EBV-carrying B cells are readily identified in patients with both acute and chronic forms of infectious mononucleosis.[21] These B cells can be detected both in peripheral blood and in lymphoid tissues, particularly in paracortical areas. The detection of EBV in B cells is consistent with the well documented association of the virus with B-cell lymphomas. Plasmacytic differentiation is observed in a small fraction of EBV-containing B cells.

Although EBV is also associated with various T-cell lymphomas, the detection of nonneoplastic T cells infected with EBV has been controversial.[22] Some reports indicate that T cells are infected following primary EBV infection. Several reports also indicate that patients with chronic EBV infection carry EBV in their T and NK cells, in addition to B cells. In one study the predominant population of EBV-infected cells was represented by NK cells.[23]

Although the presence of EBV in nasopharyngeal carcinoma is a clear indication that EBV can infect epithelial cells in vivo, there is significant controversy as to whether EBV infects epithelial cells in the normal course of its lifecycle.[24] An earlier model for EBV persistence and spread in the human population was based on studies reporting that EBV DNA could be detected in oropharyngeal epithelial cells, and that EBV replication also occurred at this site.[25] As primary infection occurs via the transmission of viral particles in saliva, the hypothesis that emerged was that oropharyngeal epithelial cells represent the primary target for EBV infection, as well as the site for its persistence and replication.[26] Recent reports, however, have failed to demonstrate the presence of the virus in tonsillar epithelium either from patients with infectious mononucleosis or from healthy individuals.[27,28] Therefore, the issue of EBV infection of epithelial cells in vivo during the normal virus lifecycle is still a matter of debate, and might be clarified by studies comparing multiple approaches of EBV detection.[29]

Total elimination of the EBV reservoir from seropositive individuals following severe eradication of their lymphoid cells during bone marrow transplants make it less likely that epithelial cells serve a central role in the maintenance and spread of viral infection.[30] Therefore, the present working hypothesis centers around B cells as the reservoir for EBV persistence. It is probable that, at the time of primary infection, EBV infects mucosa-associated B cells in the oropharynx. Because an effective immune response has not yet developed at this stage, the virus initiates a transcription program resulting in the expression of a complete complement of latent genes. It is likely that in the absence of any challenge from T cells this results in a rapid proliferation of EBV-infected B cells. B-cell proliferation is, however, self-limiting and is effectively curtailed by a concurrent development of an effective T-cell response. Viral persistence in the face of a strong T-cell response necessitates the switch in the latency program to allow down-regulation of genes that serve as immunogenic epitopes. Thus, the virus modulates transcription from the expression of full complement of latent genes to the expression of EBNA-1 and LMP-2A mRNAs only.

EBV immortalization-related genes and their function

EBV is very efficient at immortalizing B cells and this function must therefore be critical to the EBV–host interaction, as well as to the overall EBV lifecycle. In contrast to the latency associated with EBV-infected B cells in vivo, EBV infection in vitro is dependent upon the expression of all latent gene products. Also, whereas the infected B cell in vivo is quiescent, the in vitro immortalized B cell has a lymphoblastoid phenotype. EBV-infected lymphoblastoid B cells are said to be transformed and express CD19, CD20, CD23, CD30, CD39, CD54, CD58, CD70 and CD80. Cell growth is sustained and enhanced by an autocrine mechanism that is dependent upon one or more cytokines, including IL-5, IL-6 and IL-10. The sustained growth of EBV-infected B cells is similar to the long-term maintenance of B-cell lines resulting from concerted interactions of CD40-ligand and IL-4.[31]

It is probable that only some genes expressed in latency III infection are directly involved in immortalization (Table 95.3). Experiments using mini-EBV genomes, antisense directed strategies and recombinational knockouts of viral genes have implicated six genes as essential for EBV immortalization. These include EBNA-1, -2, -3A and -3C, as well as LP and LMP-1.[32]

LMP-1 is one of the EBV proteins with proven oncogenic potential, inducing the transformation of rodent fibroblasts. The expression of LMP-1 in transgenic mice results in hyperplasia when the transgene is targeted to the skin,[33] and in lymphomas when the transgene is targeted to B cells.[34] LMP-1 is a 386 amino acid transmembrane protein belonging to the family of the tumor necrosis factor receptor proteins. Proteins that interact with the

Table 95.3 EBV genes with a potential to immortalize, influence cell proliferation and survival.

EBV genes that influence cell survival					
Gene	**Locus**	**Function**	**Transformation**	**Interaction with cellular genes**	**Evidence of oncogenic activity**
EBNA-1	BKRF-1	Maintenance of EBV episome	Yes	Partners with p32, EBP2	Lymphomagenic in mice
EBNA-2	BYRF-1	Transactivator	Yes	Interacts with the Cp-binding factor	–
EBNA-3A	BERF-1	Transactivating	Yes	Interacts with the Cp-binding factor	–
EBNA-3B(4)	BERF2	Transactivating	No	Interacts with the Cp-binding factor	–
EBNA-3C(6)	BERF3/4	Transactivating	Yes	Interacts with the Cp-binding factor	Cooperates in in vitro transformation assay
EBNA-LP(5)	BWRF1	Transactivating	Partially	Stimulates EBNA-2 transactivation	–
LMP-1	BNLF-1	Transforming	Yes	Up-regulates cellular gene expression	Hyperplasia and lymphomas in transgenic mice
V-IL10	BCRF-1	Cytokine	No	–	–
V-bcl-2	BHRF-1	Anti-apoptotic	No	Inhibits cellular death pathways	–

rather large cytoplasmic domain of LMP-1 include TRAF-1, TRAF-3 and TRADD.[35] These interactions lead to the activation of the NFκB-mediated signaling pathways. Forced expression of LMP-1 into B cells upregulates the expression of several markers associated with the transformation phenotype caused by EBV infection. These include CD23, CD30, CD70 and several adhesion molecules, including LFA-1, LFA-3 and ICAM-1.[36] The expression of these molecules on the cell surface is responsible for the characteristic clumping seen in B-cells infected with EBV. LMP-1 probably mimics those B cell activation processes that are physiologically triggered by T-cell signals aimed at sustaining B-cell growth. In addition, LMP-1 also up-regulates host survival genes, including *bcl-2* and *A20*.[37] It has been suggested that this antiapoptotic function of LMP-1 contributes to some extent to the lymphomagenic potential of EBV.

Several variants of EBV with deletions in LMP-1 have been described: the most common carries a 30 bp deletion proximal to one of the functional domains in the cytoplasmic region of LMP-1. Although experimental evidence suggests that EBV variants with deleted LMP-1 may be more oncogenic and less immunogenic,[38] studies have failed to find tumor-specific associations of this variant.[39]

EBNA-1 is the only known viral protein that is consistently expressed in all forms of EBV-associated infections. EBNA-1 is a 641 amino acid protein with unique N and C termini separated by a 239 amino acid polymer of alanine and glycine residues. The amino terminus contains 89 residues and is rich in basic amino acids. The carboxy terminus of EBNA-1 consists of a basic domain and a long hydrophobic domain. This domain encompasses residues 459–607 and functions as the DNA-binding and dimerization domain. EBNA-1 also carries RNA-binding properties, probably mediated via several RGG repeats within the protein-unique domains. The main function of EBNA-1 is to maintain the viral episome via interaction with the origin of replication of the EBV genome. The cognate sequence to which EBNA-1 binds is a partial palindrome. Within the origin of replication these sequences can be found both as tandem repeats and as dyad symmetry sites. In addition, EBNA-1 is a transactivating protein and its binding to the tandem repeat component enhances transcription from neighboring promoters. Binding sites for EBNA-1 are also present adjacent to promoters regulating lytic genes, and EBNA-1 is the only EBNA gene expressed in the lytic cycle, suggesting that EBNA-1 is involved in the regulation of the lytic cycle.

The crystal structure of the DNA-binding and dimerization domain of EBNA-1 has revealed a remarkable similarity to the structure of the papillomavirus E2 protein.[40] Recent studies have also identified host cell proteins that interact with EBNA-1, including p32, a protein that may be involved in transcriptional regulation, and EBNA-2, a 35 kDa protein that appears to be necessary for stable segregation of episomes following replication.[41,42]

Because EBNA-1 is the only viral protein expressed in several EBV-associated malignancies, it is a likely candidate to play a role in the development or maintenance of the tumor phenotype. Variants of EBNA-1 have been reported to segregate with disease,[43] although other reports have suggested that the distribution of the variants is geographically influenced.[44] At least one study has reported the development of B-cell lymphomas in mice expressing EBNA-1 as a transgene in the B-cell compartment.[45] The transactivating properties of EBNA-1 may cause inappropriate regulation of some host genes, thereby influencing the oncogenic process. In this regard, EBNA-1 has been suggested to up-regulate recombinase-activating genes.[46] As the products of recombinase-activating genes are involved in the recombination of immunoglobulin genes, a role for EBNA-1 in influencing illegitimate recombination can be hypothesized. Indeed, EBV infection of pro-B cell lines has been associated with the presence of translocations involving chromosome 14.[47]

EBNA-2 is a transactivating protein that is essential for immortalization. It is characterized by genetic heterogeneity and has been used to classify EBV in subtypes 1 and 2. The EBNA-2 protein of EBV subtype 1 is 484 amino acids long, whereas EBNA-2 of EBV subtype 2 is 41 amino acids shorter. Both versions carry two internal repeats, a stretch of poly-proline that can be up to 40 amino acids in length, and an arginine–glycine repeat in the carboxy terminus. Insights into the essential role for EBNA-2 were originally obtained from the isolation of virions of a Burkitt's lymphoma cell line which did not possess transforming potential. The strain of EBV (P3-HR1) associated with this cell line carried a deletion affecting the entire stretch of EBNA-2 coding sequences. Complementation with the missing sequences allowed for the restoration of the transforming abilities.[48]

The transactivating ability of EBNA-2 provides the basis for much of the phenotypic change associated with transformation. EBNA-2 transactivates both cellular genes, e.g. the C-*FGE* proto-oncogene[49], and viral genes, e.g. LMP-1 and LMP-2.[50] It is responsible for the up-regulation of B-cell markers, including CD21 and CD23.[51] Although most unique domains of EBNA-2 have overlapping roles in transformation and transactivation, the deletion of the domain carrying the Arg–Gly reiterations results in an increase in the protein-transactivating properties while at the same time decreasing its transformation efficiency.

The interaction of EBNA-2 with its cognate sequences is indirect and the transactivating potential of EBNA-2 is mediated by its interaction with various cellular proteins. Critical among these are CBF-1, an adapter of transcriptional regulatory proteins, and PU-1, which is frequently involved in the transcription of lymphoid-specific genes. Recent data suggest that EBNA-2 and other viral proteins (viral-interferon regulatory factor) may use the coadapters to up-regulate *c-myc*.[52]

EBNA-3A and EBNA-3C are similar in sequence and structure and also share homology with a third EBV protein, EBNA-3B. These three proteins are located in a tandem rearrangement within a 10 kb stretch of the EBV genome. EBNA-3A, -3B and -3C also vary in sequence between EBV subtypes 1 and 2. Because the EBNA-3 proteins provide the most effective target epitopes for CTL recognition in the context of specific HLA subtypes, it has been suggested that the geographical distribution of EBV subtypes and the sequence divergence of EBNA-3 are modulated in response to immune surveillance.[53] In spite of the structural and sequence similarities, EBNA-3A and -3C are not redundant in mediating B-lymphocyte immortalization, suggesting that they act by triggering independent molecular events. All EBNA-3 proteins can interfere with the transactivating properties of EBNA-2, via interaction with CBF-1. EBNA-3B and EBNA-3C may also have transcriptional promoting properties. EBNA-3B facilitates the up-regulation of CD40 and vimentin, and EBNA-3C can up-regulate CD21 and LMP-1 expression.[54] Thus it is likely that all the three EBNA-3 proteins are intricate components of a transcriptional regulatory mechanism.

EBNA-LP is variable in size between different viral isolates. This variation derives from the fact that the open reading frame (ORF) of EBNA-LP is encoded within the internal repeat regions of the EBV genome. The transcript consists of exons from the W1 and W2 repeats spliced to unique Y1 and Y2 exons at the 3′ end. However, the splicing events that regulate EBNA-LP expression are poorly understood and can result in several spliced variants. Cotransfection of EBNA-LP with EBNA-2 suggest that the two proteins may cooperate in inducing cells to cycle by inducing cyclin D2. It is possible that the mechanisms of this cooperativity are transcriptional.[55]

EBV interactions with host cell genes in promoting transformation

Unlike other viruses that interact directly with the host cell cycle regulatory mechanisms, no single dominant strategy for directly influencing cell growth is apparent in EBV biology. It is likely that the EBV transformation mechanisms are directly linked to the ability of the virus to establish a long-term association with the human host.

There are several mechanisms that EBV uses to evade immune surveillance. One such mechanism involves the down-regulation of viral genes that can potentially elicit CTL responses. For those viral genes that cannot be down-regulated the virus interferes with antigen processing, as exemplified by the effects of the Ala–Gly polymeric region of EBNA-1.[56] Finally, EBV can also interfere with other immune recognition pathways by down-regulating MHC Class I-associated proteins and transporter-associated proteins in the host cell, thus affording these cells some protection against CTLs.[57]

EBV has pirated mammalian genes that provide additional strategies to modulate the survival of the infected cell, namely the BCRF-1 and BHRF-1 ORFs. The EBV gene product BCRF-1 shares high homology with the human cytokine IL-10. Viral IL-10 functions in much the same fashion as human IL-10, and can promote the outgrowth of EBV-transformed B cells by interfering with the synthesis of interferon-γ, IL-1 and IL-12.[58] BHRF-1 is a viral homolog of the antiapoptotic protein bcl-2, and may thus function to extend cell survival. As most data on the expression of these products implicate a role in the productive phase of the lytic cycle, it is unclear whether these gene products have any role in the maintenance of the transformed phenotype.

Cellular genes involved in the host–virus loop include the cellular *BCL-2*, which is up-regulated by the viral LMP-1, and *c-MYC*, which may be regulated via EBNA-1. It is possible that the contribution of the virus to the immortalization of infected cells is dependent on separate mechanisms that operate in the context of the specific microenvironment of the host cell. EBV may be capable of setting up an interactive loop between the immune mechanisms that operate to destroy the infected cell, while at the same time extending the survival of the infected cell

KEY CONCEPTS

Viral strategies of immune evasion

- Modulate expression of viral genes – limiting expression to nonimmunogenic proteins.
- Inhibit T-cell proliferation via expression of viral homologs of cellular cytokines.
- Down-regulate expression of transporter-associated proteins and MHC Class I associate proteins.
- Impair antigen processing.
- HLA-dependent polymorphic variation of antigenic epitopes.

by interfering with death pathways and promoting pathways that induce cell proliferation.[59]

HUMAN HERPESVIRUS TYPE 8

Prior to the emergence of HIV, the mesenchymal tumor Kaposi sarcoma was prevalent only in specific geographic populations. Kaposi sarcoma occurs in an endemic form which is common in Africa,[60] and in a classic form which occurs in individuals from the Mediterranean region and generally spares the viscera.[61] Kaposi sarcoma is an AIDS-defining cancer which, in the pre-HAART era, occurred in more than one-fifth of AIDS patients[62] (Chapter 38). Similar to the endemic form, AIDS-associated Kaposi sarcoma is disseminated and aggressive. Among HIV-infected individuals the risk of Kaposi sarcoma is highest in homosexuals and lower in children, hemophiliacs, i.v. drug users and heterosexual AIDS patients, suggesting that a sexually transmitted agent may be involved. Several reports identified various viruses in Kaposi sarcoma samples, including CMV and HPV. However, it was the amplification of novel DNA sequences from Kaposi sarcoma biopsies by Chang et al[63] that paved the way for the isolation and characterization of a novel herpesvirus termed Kaposi sarcoma-associated herpesvirus (KSHV). The sequences of the DNA isolated from the Kaposi sarcoma biopsies suggested significant homology to sequences from the DNA of other gammaherpes viruses, specifically EBV and herpesvirus samiri.[64] Further analyses demonstrated that Kaposi sarcoma biopsies are infected with a novel γ_2 herpesvirus. KSHV thus became the first known human herpesvirus of this group. The DNA sequences from this virus can be identified in all forms of Kaposi sarcoma, supporting the hypothesis that KSHV, now renamed HHV-8, is involved in the pathogenesis of Kaposi sarcoma.

HHV-8 structure and genome

Electron microscopic studies have revealed that HHV-8 has the typical structure of herpesviruses. The virion, which is about 100–150 nm in size, consists of a central core surrounded by a capsid and an envelope. The layout of the genome is similar to the group β herpesviruses, including herpesvirus samiri, herpesvirus ateles and the murine herpesvirus-4, and consists of terminal repeats that enclose a unique region. Unlike the EBV genome, the genomic DNA bounded by the terminal repeats is not interspersed with internal repeat regions. This long unique region is about 140 kb and the flanking repeat termini may add another 25 kb, giving an overall size of about 165 kb.[65]

The terminal repeat (TR) region appears to be a characteristic feature of herpesviruses and is involved in the packaging of the viral DNA. The HHV-8 genome has about 30 repeating units, each approximately 800 bp in length and these provide a good target for detection of the virus by hybridization methodologies. The HHV-8 genome, like the EBV genome, is maintained as an extrachromosomal episome in infected cells. The replication of the genome during the productive phase is thought to be mediated via the rolling circle mechanism, with individual genomes cleaved at the TR region. The individual genomes are packaged as linear molecules, which circularize at the TR regions following infection of the host cell. Because the integrity of the TR region is maintained in episomal replicative cycles, clonality in the context of HHV-8 can be assessed using restriction-based analysis of the TR region.

> **KEY CONCEPTS**
>
> **Human herpesvirus-8 (HHV-8)**
> - Detected in Kaposi sarcoma and primary effusion lymphoma.
> - Genome carries genes with homology to human growth control genes, including IL-6, MIP-I, MIP-II, cyclin D and bcl-2.
> - Serologic data demonstrates the highest prevalence is in Africa (50–70%) and lower in the US and northern Europe (1–20%).

HHV-8 gene products

Sequence analysis of the long unique region of the HHV-8 genome suggests that the virus encodes at least 81 potential ORFs.[66] Studies of the characterization and function of these genes are just emerging, and it is likely that additional proteins, resulting from alternative processing and splicing of viral transcripts, will add to this repertoire. The nomenclature of the gene products is based upon numbering of the ORFs from left to right, with a prefix of K for ORFs that are unique to HHV-8.

Several of the encoded genes have homology to corresponding genes in the herpesvirus samiri genome. Several genes encode structural proteins. Others encode enzymes involved in DNA metabolism and replication. The functions of several of these genes suggest that they would be expressed during the viral lytic cycle. Interspersed among these conserved ORFs, the HHV-8 genome harbors additional subsets of genes which are either unique to HHV-8 or homologous to genes from other rhadinoviruses. It is probable that these account for the oncogenic potential of the virus (Table 95.4). Several of these genes demonstrate significant homology to human growth control genes, and may have thus been incorporated in the viral genome as an adaptive strategy of molecular piracy during viral evolution. Many of these proteins are also expressed during viral latency. These include the homolog of the growth factor IL-6,[67] the homolog of the cell cycle regulator cyclin D,[68] the homolog of the antiapoptotic protein bcl-2,[69] and the homologs of two chemokines, the macrophage inflammatory proteins I and II.[70] The functions of some ORFs remain to be elucidated. These include K1, which appears to be a type I transmembrane receptor, and the latency-associated nuclear antigen (LANA) encoded by ORF 73.

Patterns of viral gene expression in host cells supporting HHV-8 infection

The genome of HHV-8 has been detected in a wide variety of cell types, including endothelial cells in Kaposi sarcoma,[71] B cells from primary effusion lymphomas,[72] dendritic cells, macrophages[71] and prostatic epithelial cells.[73] HHV-8 has been implicated in the pathogenesis of Kaposi sarcoma, primary effusion lymphoma and multicentric Castleman's disease.[74]

Although HHV-8 can be clearly detected in biopsy samples of Kaposi sarcoma, explanted cultures of the tumor fail to maintain viral persistence. Consequently, most of the information regarding the expression of the viral genes in endothelial cells comes from study of Kaposi sarcoma biopsies. The persistence of viral infection in Kaposi endothelial or spindle cells is correlated with the expression of ORF 72 (homolog of mammalian cyclin D),

HHV-8 genes that influence cell survival			
Open reading frame	**Cellular homolog**	**Functional feature**	**Expression in lymphomas**
ORF K1	–	Transmembrane protein	?
ORF K2	IL-6	Cytokine	yes
ORF 4	MIP-II	Chemokine	yes
ORF 6	MIP-I	Chemokine	yes
ORF K9	IRF	Modulates transcription	yes
ORF K13	FLIP	Blocks Fas-mediated signals	yes
ORF 16	bcl-2	Antiapoptic	yes
ORF 72	Cyclin D	Induces cell cycle	yes
ORF 73	–	Transcriptional protein	yes
ORF 74	IL8 Receptor	Signal transduction	yes

Table 95.4 HHV-8 genes with a potential to influence cellular proliferation and survival.

ORF 73 (LANA) and ORF 74 (homolog of chemokine receptor). Expression of K12, a gene unique to HHV-8 encoding a 60 amino acid protein of unknown function, has also been detected. In addition, a subpopulation of spindle cells that show evidence of lytic infection also express an untranslated RNA T1.1.

The availability of cultured cell lines from biopsies of primary effusion lymphomas has provided a significant resource for the study of the expression of viral genes in B cells. In addition to the genes expressed in Kaposi sarcomas, primary effusion lymphomas also express ORF 16 (bcl-2 homolog), ORF K2 (homolog of IL-6), the homologs of the chemokines MIPI and II (K-4 and K-6), and the ORF K9 (homolog of the interferon regulatory factor).

Reservoirs of HHV-8 infection

The persistence of the virus in nonneoplastic cells in high-risk individuals and its prevalence in the overall human population are not fully elucidated. Serological studies indicate that viral infection is most prevalent (50–70% seropositivity) in African countries, and more common in Mediterranean countries than in the United States. The prevalence of infection in the US and northern Europe ranges from 1 to 20%.[75] Immunosuppression is clearly one risk factor contributing to viral spread in geographic areas of low prevalence. However, the low frequency of Kaposi sarcoma in HIV-infected hemophiliacs suggests that other cofactors, principally sexual practices, may significantly contribute to the prevalence of viral infection.

Early studies indicated that the virus can be detected in peripheral blood mononuclear cells of individuals from geographical regions associated with Kaposi sarcoma: 40–50% of HIV-positive individuals, as well as a similar percentage of all Kaposi sarcoma patients, demonstrate the presence of virus in their peripheral blood cells. Because viral transmission has also been associated with sexual practices, several studies have attempted to detect HHV-8 in semen.[76] Some studies indicate that semen samples from as many as one-third of HIV-infected men, with or without Kaposi sarcoma, test positive for HHV-8. Varying rates of viral detection have also been reported in semen from HIV-negative semen donors. Consistent with the presence of the virus in semen, other reports have demonstrated the presence of the virus in prostatic epithelium,[73] suggesting that the prostate may be a major site of viral persistence and infection.

Lymphoproliferations associated with HHV-8 infections

The ability of HHV-8 to transform lymphoid cells is exemplified by its association with a novel type of B-cell lymphoma termed primary effusion lymphoma.[77] This neoplastic condition is mainly found in the context of AIDS, and presents as a primary malignant lymphomatous effusion in pleural, pericardial or peritoneal body cavities, without significant tumor mass or lymphadenopathy. The morphological features of the neoplastic B cells bridge those of immunoblastic large cell and anaplastic large cell lymphomas. Although the cells have a null phenotype, B-cell lineage is clearly indicated by rearrangements of the B-cell immunoglobulin loci and by the monoclonality of expressed κ or λ light chains. Specific nonrandom chromosomal aberrations that may implicate c-*myc*, *bcl-6* or *bcl-2* have not been associated with these lymphomas. In addition, no mutations in other loci, including *p53* and *K-ras*, have been reported in the neoplastic B cells.

Coinfection with EBV is a common feature of primary effusion lymphoma. It is possible that EBV and HHV-8 contribute to set up a synergistic paracrine mechanism for continued proliferation of the B cell. Consistent with this hypothesis is the finding that the levels of both IL-6 (a viral homolog of this protein is encoded in HHV-8) and IL-10 (a viral homolog of this protein is encoded in EBV) are elevated in primary effusion lymphomas.[78] However, the fact that a fraction of primary effusion lymphomas are devoid of EBV infection suggests that EBV is dispensable for the pathogenesis of the disease.

Potential genetic pathways corruptible by HHV-8-mediated transformation

Several genes encoded by HHV-8 have sequence similarities to known human genes regulating cell growth and survival. It is conceivable that the expression of these genes contributes to the transformation of lymphoid cells infected with HHV-8. The viral ORF 4 and ORF 6 encode proteins with sequence similarity to the chemokines MIP I and II. Both these viral genes are expressed in latently infected primary effusion lymphomas. In addition, the virus encodes ORF K2, a gene with about 25% identity to the human IL-6 gene. The viral IL-6 functions in a highly similar fashion to human IL-6 and is capable of supporting the growth of cell lines dependent upon human IL-6. Similar to the human IL-6, HHV-8 viral IL-6 is also capable of activating the JAK/STAT pathway.[79] The protein encoded by ORF K9 is homologous to a family of cellular cytokines, the interferon regulatory factors (IRF). Although viral IRF is expressed in primary effusion lymphomas its role in lymphomagenesis is not yet known.

Two viral proteins are directly involved in antiapoptotic functions. The ORF 16 of HHV-8 encodes a homolog of the cellular *BCL-2* gene and can interfere functionally with bax-mediated apoptosis. Similar to the *BCL-2* homolog encoded by EBV, i.e. BHRF1, the expression of ORF 16 is up-regulated during lytic infection. ORF K13 encodes a protein with a death effector domain that may act as a dominant negative inhibitor of cell death in a manner similar to cellular Flip (c-Flip). Other rhadinoviruses also carry homologs of c-Flip. At present there are insufficient data to demonstrate whether the HHV-8 v-Flip is expressed in latently infected B cells.[80]

The HHV-8 ORF 72 is a homolog of a cellular gene (cyclin D) that has been implicated in the pathogenesis of human malignancies. ORF 72 is expressed in latently infected cell lines and tumor biopsies of primary effusion lymphomas. The ORF 72 of HHV-8 has about 30% amino acid identity with the human cellular cyclin D2. It has conserved the region of the protein responsible for interactions with the cyclin-dependent kinases, and has been shown to interact with both cyclin-dependent kinase 6 and 4. Exogenous expression of the HHV-8 v-cyclin in SAOS cells can override cell cycle arrest induced by forced expression of the Rb protein. The v-cyclin and cyclin-dependent kinase complexes have in fact been shown to properly phosphorylate Rb. Thus it is likely that the expression of ORF 72 plays a significant role in the malignant transformation of B cells by HHV-8.

The ORF 74 of HHV-8 is a homolog of a G-protein-coupled receptor with sequence homology to the IL-8 chemokine receptor. Transient expression of ORF 74 suggests that this protein is constitutively active.[81] In experimental models in vitro, the expression of ORF 74 induced cell growth of rat kidney fibroblasts. However, like other growth-promoting genes pirated by HHV-8, a direct role for this protein in malignant transformation in vivo is unclear, principally because the temporal expression of this protein correlates with induction of the lytic cycle rather than latency.

CLINICAL PEARLS

EBV and HHV-8

- These members of the herpesvirus family are linked to human tumors.
- Infection establishes a state of latency.
- These viruses have pirated genes from the host that encode proteins important in cell growth and survival.
- The tumors associated with these viruses most commonly emerge in the setting of altered host immunity.

HUMAN HERPESVIRUS TYPES 6 AND 7

Both HHV-6 and HHV-7 were discovered in the late 1980s and early 1990s.[82,83] Although they belong to the β family of herpes viruses, HHV-6 and HHV-7 display the lymphotropism typical of gammaherpesviruses, with an affinity for CD4 lymphocytes. They have a similar genomic architecture, with a large sequence repeated at both the termini. Infection is thought to take place early in life, as HHV-7 is quite prevalent in the human population, with a reported seropositivity of over 80% in adults. There is, however, little information on the pathways these viruses utilize in establishing persistent reservoirs.

CONCLUSIONS

Lymphotropic human herpesviruses have provided significant insights into the potential molecular pathways that the viruses may use in lymphomagenesis. As the herpesviruses do not target tumor suppressor pathways directly, alternative or indirect mechanisms of inducing cellular proliferation must be considered. The two possible scenarios that can be hypothesized include a role in expanding the population of preneoplastic target cells, or direct participation in both induction and maintainance of the lymphoma phenotype.

Conceivably, the ability of these viruses to cause malignant transformation is tied to their adaptive strategies to hitch a long-term ride with the lymphocytes. Both the EBV and HHV-8 genomes carry several examples of genes pirated from the host cellular gene repertoire. Viral homologs of cellular genes are often implicated in the control of cell growth and survival. Thus, a putative scenario is that the viruses use the expression of these genes to induce inappropriate proliferation or survival at times when the homologous host genes are either shut off or under controlled regulation. One problem with this hypothesis is that several of these genes are temporally linked to the productive phase of the lytic cycle, which is not conducive to lymphomagenesis. It seems sensible to suggest that the contribution of the virus to inducing and/or maintaining a transformed phenotype must be mediated by viral genes expressed in the lymphomas. If this is the case, then only a handful of genes could be the culprits. Indeed, many genes expressed in latent viral infection also deregulate cellular proliferation by altering the expression of host cellular genes. As several of these genes are also 'flags' for CTL-mediated destruction, the virus has to down-regulate their expression in order to maintain itself. How does the virus then sustain the lymphoma phenotype? Further examination of EBV and HHV-8 biology, as well as the identification of interactive loops between infected cells and the surrounding microenvironment, will continue to provide clues to this intricate process of viral lymphomagenesis.

REFERENCES

1. Burkitt D. Determining the climatic limitations of a children's cancer common in Africa. Br Med J 1962;ii:1019.
2. Henle W, Diehl V, Kohn G, zur hausen H, Henle G. Herpes-type virus and chromosome marker in normal leukocytes after growth with irradiated Burkitt's cells. Science 1967;157:1064.
3. Roizman B, Herpesviridae. In: Fields BN, Knipe DM, Howley PM (eds) Fields virology, 3rd edn. Philadelphia, Lippincott-Raven, 1996, p 2221.
4. Rowe M, Rowe DT, Gregory CD, et al. Differences in B cell growth phenotype reflect novel patterns of Epstein–Barr virus latent gene expression in Burkitt's lymphoma cells. EMBO J 1987;9:2743.
5. Brooks L, Yao QY, Rickinson AB, Young LS. Epstein–Barr virus latent gene transcription in nasopharyngeal carcinoma cells: coexpression of EBNA1, LMP1, and LMP2 transcripts. J Virol 1992;66:2689.
6. Deacon EM, Pallesen G, Niedobitek G, et al. Epstein–Barr virus and Hodgkin's disease: transcriptional analysis of virus latency in the malignant cells. J Exp Med 1993;177:339.
7. Tierney RJ, Steven N, Young LS, Rickinson AB. Epstein–Barr virus latency in blood mononuclear cells: analysis of viral gene transcription during primary infection and in the carrier state. J Virol 1994;68:7374.
8. Lee ES, Locker J, Nalesnik M, et al. The association of Epstein–Barr virus with smooth-muscle tumors occurring after organ transplantation. N Engl J Med 1995;332:19.
9. Gutierrez MI, Bhatia K, Magrath I. Replicative viral DNA in Epstein–Barr virus associated Burkitt's lymphoma biopsies. Leuk Res 1993;17:285.
10. Gutierrez MI, Judde JG, Magrath IT, Bhatia KG. Switching viral latency to viral lysis: a novel therapeutic approach for Epstein–Barr virus-associated neoplasia. Cancer Res 1996;56:969.
11. Baer R, Bankier AT, Biggin MD, et al. DNA sequence and expression of the B95-8 Epstein–Barr virus genome. Nature 1984;310:207.
12. Emini EA, Luka J, Armstrong ME, Banker FS, Provost PJ, Pearson GR Establishment and characterization of a chronic infectious mononucleosis like syndrome in common marmosets. J Med Virol 1986;18:369.
13. Lowell CA, Klickstein LB, Carter RH, Mitchell JA, Fearon DT, Ahearn JM. Mapping of the Epstein–Barr virus and C3dg binding sites to a common domain on complement receptor type 2. J Exp Med 1989;170:1931.
14. Katamine S, Otsu M, Tada K, et al. Epstein–Barr virus transforms precursor B cells even before immunoglobulin gene rearrangements. Nature 1984;309:369.
15. Kelleher CA, Dreyfus DH, Jones JF, Gelfand EW. EBV infection of T cells: potential role in malignant transformation. Semin Cancer Biol 1996;7:197.
16. Shapiro IM, Volsky DJ. Infection of normal human epithelial cells by Epstein–Barr virus. Science 1983;219:1225.
17. Jones K, Rivera C, Sgadari C, et al. Infection of human endothelial cells with Epstein–Barr virus. J Exp Med 1995;182:1213.
18. Birkenbach M, Tong X, Bradbury LE, Tedder TF, Kieff E. Characterization of an Epstein–Barr virus receptor on human epithelial cells. J Exp Med 1992;176:1405.
19. Schriever F, Freeman G, Nadler L. Follicular dendritic cells contain a unique gene repertoire demonstrated by single-cell polymerase chain reaction. Blood 1991;77:787.
20. Anagnostopoulos I, Hummel M, Kreschel C, Stein H. Morphology, immunophenotype, and distribution of latently and/or productively Epstein–Barr virus-infected cells in acute infectious mononucleosis: implications for the interindividual infection route of Epstein–Barr virus. Blood 1995;85:744.
21. Niedobitek G, Agathanggelou A, Herbst H, Whitehead L, Wright DH, Young LS. Epstein–Barr virus (EBV) infection in infectious mononucleosis: virus latency, replication and phenotype of EBV-infected cells. J Pathol 1997;182:151.
22. Kanegane H, Bhatia K, Gutierrez M, et al. A syndrome of peripheral blood T-cell infection with Epstein–Barr virus (EBV) followed by EBV-positive T-cell lymphoma. Blood 1998;91:2085.
23. Kanegane H, Wado T, Nunogami K, Seki H, Taniguchi N, Tosato G. Chronic persistent Epstein–Barr virus infection of natural killer cells and B cells associated with granular lymphocytes expansion. Br J Haematol 1996;95:116.
24. Magrath I, Bhatia K. Breast cancer: a new Epstein–Barr virus-associated disease? J Natl Cancer Inst 1999;91:1349.
25. Niedobitek G, Young LS, Lau R, et al. Epstein–Barr virus infection in oral hairy leukoplakia: virus replication in the absence of a detectable latent phase. J Gen Virol 1991;72: 3035.
26. Allday MJ, Crawford DH. Role of epithelium in EBV persistence and pathogenesis of B-cell tumours. Lancet 1988;1:855.
27. Karajannis MA, Hummel M, Anagnostopoulos I, Stein H. Strict lymphotropism of Epstein–Barr virus during acute infectious mononucleosis in non immunocompromised individuals. Blood 1997;89:2856.
28. Tao Q, Srivastava G, Chan AC, Chung LP, Loke SL, Ho FC. Evidence for lytic infection by Epstein–Barr virus in mucosal lymphocytes instead of nasopharyngeal epithelial cells in normal individuals. J Med Virol 1995;45:71.
29. Wen S, Shimizu N, Yoshiyama H, Mizugaki Y, Shinozaki F, Takada K. Association of Epstein–Barr virus (EBV) with Sjogren's syndrome: differential EBV expression between epithelial cells and lymphocytes in salivary glands. Am J Pathol 1996;149:1511.
30. Gratama JW, Oosterveer MA, Zwaan FE, Lepoutre J, Klein G, Ernberg I. Eradication of Epstein–Barr virus by allogeneic bone marrow transplantation: implications for sites of viral latency. Proc Natl Acad Sci USA 1988;85:8693.
31. Banchereau J, de Paoli P, Valle A, Garcia E, Rousset F. Long-term human B cell lines dependent on interleukin-4 and antibody to CD40. Science 1991;251:70.
32. Kempkes B, Pich D, Zeidler R, Hammerschmidt W. Immortalization of human primary B lymphocytes in vitro with DNA. Proc Natl Acad Sci USA 1995;92: 5875.
33. Wilson JB, Weinberg W, Johnson R, Yuspa S, Levine AJ. Expression of the BNLF-1 oncogene of Epstein–Barr virus in the skin of transgenic mice induces hyperplasia and aberrant expression of keratin 6. Cell 1990;61:1315.
34. Kulwichit W, Edwards RH, Davenport EM, Baskar JF, Godfrey V, Raab-Traub N. Expression of the Epstein–Barr virus latent membrane protein 1 induces B cell lymphoma in transgenic mice. Proc Natl Acad Sci USA 1998;95:11963.
35. Izumi KM, McFarland EC, Ting AT, Riley EA, Seed B, Kieff ED. The Epstein–Barr virus oncoprotein latent membrane protein 1 engages the tumor necrosis factor receptor-associated proteins TRADD and receptor-interacting protein (RIP) but does not induce apoptosis or require RIP for NF-kappaB activation. Mol Cell Biol 1999;19:5759.
36. Wang D, Liebowitz D, Wang F, et al. Epstein–Barr virus latent infection membrane protein alters the human B-lymphocyte phenotype: deletion of the amino terminus abolishes activity. J Virol 1988;62:4173.
37. Handerson S, Rowe M, Gregory C, et al. Induction of bcl-2 expression by Epstein–Barr virus latent membrane protein 1 protects infected B cells from programmed cell death. Cell 1991;65:1107.
38. Kingma DW, Weiss WB, Jaffe ES, Kumar S, Frekko K, Raffeld M. Epstein–Barr virus latent membrane protein-1 oncogene deletions: correlations with malignancy in Epstein–Barr virus-associated lymphoproliferative disorders and malignant lymphomas. Blood 1996;88:242.
39. Barozzi P, Luppi M, Cagossi K, et al. The oncogenic 30 and 69 bp deletion variants of the EBV LMP-1 gene are common in HIV-negative lymphoproliferations, both malignant and benign. Ann Oncol 1999;10:467.
40. Bochkarev A, Barwell JA, Pfuetzner RA, Bochkareva E, Frappier L, Edwards AM. Crystal structure of the DNA-binding domain of the Epstein–Barr virus origin-binding protein, EBNA1, bound to DNA. Cell 1996;84:791.
41. Wang Y, Finan JE, Middeldorp JM, Hayward SD. P32/TAP, a cellular protein that interacts with EBNA-1 of Epstein–Barr virus. Virology 1997;236:18.
42. Shire K, Ceccarelli DF, Avolio-Hunter TM, Frappier L. EBP2, a human protein that interacts with sequences of the Epstein–Barr virus nuclear antigen 1 important for plasmid maintenance. J Virol 1999;73:2587.

43. Bhatia K, Raj A, Guitierrez MI, et al. Variation in the sequence of Epstein–Barr virus nuclear antigen 1 in normal peripheral blood lymphocytes and in Burkitt's lymphomas. Oncogene 1996; 13:177.
44. Habeshaw G, Yao QY, Bell AI, Morton D, Rickinson AB. Epstein–Barr virus nuclear antigen 1 sequences in endemic and sporadic Burkitt's lymphoma reflect virus strains prevalent in different geographic areas. J Virol 1999;73:965.
45. Wilson JB, Bell JL, Levine AJ. Expression of Epstein–Barr virus nuclear antigen-1 induces B cell neoplasia in transgenic mice. EMBO J 1996;15:3117.
46. Srinivas SK, Sixbey JW. Epstein–Barr virus induction of recombinase-activating genes RAG1 and RAG2. J Virol 1995;69:8155.
47. Kuhn-Hallek I, Sage DR, Stein L, Groelle H, Fingeroth JD. Expression of recombination activating genes (RAG-1 and RAG-2) in Epstein–Barr virus-bearing B cells. Blood 1995;85:1289.
48. Pfitzner AJ, Tsai EC, Strominger JL, Speck SH. Isolation and characterization of cDNA clones corresponding to transcripts from the BamHI H and F regions of the Epstein–Barr virus genome. J Virol 1987;61:2902.
49. Knutson JC. The level of c-fgr RNA is increased by EBNA-2, an Epstein–Barr virus gene required for B-cell immortalization. J Virol 1990;64:2530.
50. Zimber-Strobl U, Suentzenich KO, Laux G, et al. Epstein–Barr virus nuclear antigen 2 activates transcription of the terminal protein gene J Virol 1991;65:415.
51. Cordier M, Calender A, Billaud M, et al. Stable transfection of Epstein–Barr virus (EBV) nuclear antigen 2 in lymphoma cells containing the EBV P3HR1 genome induces expression of B-cell activation molecules CD21 and CD23. J Virol 1990;64:1002.
52. Uchida J, Yasui T, Takaoka-Shichijo Y, et al. Mimicry of CD40 signals by Epstein–Barr virus LMP1 in B lymphocyte responses. Science 1999;286:300.
53. de Campos-Lima PO, Gavioli R, Zhang Q-J, et al. HLA-A11 epitope loss isolates of Epstein–Barr virus from a highly A11+ population. Science 1993;260:98.
54. Robertson ES. The Epstein–Barr virus EBNA 3 protein family as regulators of transcription. Epstein–Barr Virus Report 1997;4:143.
55. Sinclair AJ, Palmero I, Peters G, Farrell PJ. EBNA-2 and EBNA-LP cooperate to cause G0 to G1 transition during immortalization of resting human B lymphocytes by Epstein–Barr virus. EMBO J 1994;13:3321.
56. Levitskaya J, Coram M, Levitsky V, et al. Inhibition of antigen processing by the internal repeat region of the Epstein–Barr virus nuclear antigen-1. Nature 1995;375:685.
57. Khanna R, Burrows SR, Moss DJ. Immune regulation in Epstein–Barr virus-associated diseases. Microbiol Rev 1995;59:387.
58. Stuart AD, Stewart JP, Arrand JR, Mackett M. The Epstein–Barr virus encoded cytokine viral interleukin-10 enhances transformation of human B lymphocytes. Oncogene 1995;11:1711.
59. Klein G. EBV-B cell interactions: immortalization, rescue from apoptosis, tumorigenicity (a short review). Acta Microbiol Immunol Hung 1996;43:97.
60. Cook-Mozaffari P, Newton R, Beral V, Burkitt DP. The geographical distribution of Kaposi's sarcoma and of lymphomas in Africa before the AIDS epidemic. Br J Cancer 1998;78:1521.
61. Franceschi S, Geddes M. Epidemiology of classic Kaposi's sarcoma, with special reference to Mediterranean population. Tumori 1995;81:308.
62. Rabkin CS. Association of non-acquired immunodeficiency syndrome-defining cancers with human immunodeficiency virus infection. J Natl Cancer Inst Monogr 1998;23:23.
63. Chang Y, Cesarman E, Pessin MS, et al. Identification of herpesvirus-like DNA sequences in AIDS-associated Kaposi's sarcoma. Science 1994;266:1865.
64. Russo JJ, Bohenzky RA, Chien MC, et al. Nucleotide sequence of the Kaposi sarcoma-associated herpesvirus (HHV8). Proc Natl Acad Sci USA 1996;93:14862.
65. Nicholas J, Zong JC, Alcendor DJ, et al. Novel organizational features, captured cellular genes, and strain variability within the genome of KSHV/HHV8. J Natl Cancer Inst Monogr 1998;23:79.
66. Sarid R, Flore O, Bohenzky RA, Chang Y, Moore PS. Transcription mapping of the Kaposi's sarcoma-associated herpesvirus (human herpesvirus 8) genome in a body cavity-based lymphoma cell line (BC-1). J Virol 1998;72:1005.
67. Burger R, Neipel F, Fleckenstein B, et al. Human herpesvirus type 8 interleukin-6 homologue is functionally active on human myeloma cells. Blood 1998;91:1858.
68. Li M, Lee H, Yoon DW, et al. Kaposi's sarcoma-associated herpesvirus encodes a functional cyclin. J Virol 1997; 71:1984.
69. Cheng EH, Nicholas J, Bellows DS, et al. A Bcl-2 homolog encoded by Kaposi sarcoma-associated virus, human herpesvirus 8, inhibits apoptosis but does not heterodimerize with Bax or Bak. Proc Natl Acad Sci USA 1997;94:690.
70. Nicholas J, Ruvolo VR, Burns WH, et al. Kaposi's sarcoma-associated human herpesvirus-8 encodes homologues of macrophage inflammatory protein-1 and interleukin-6. Nature Med 1997;3:287.
71. Ascherl G, Hohenadl C, Monini P, et al. Expression of human herpesvirus-8 (HHV-8) encoded pathogenic genes in Kaposi's sarcoma (KS) primary lesions. Adv Enzyme Regul 1999;39:331.
72. Said W, Chien K, Takeuchi S, et al. Kaposi's sarcoma-associated herpesvirus (KSHV or HHV8) in primary effusion lymphoma: ultrastructural demonstration of herpesvirus in lymphoma cells. Blood 1996;87:4937.
73. Diamond C, Brodie SJ, Krieger JN, et al. Human herpesvirus 8 in the prostate glands of men with Kaposi s sarcoma. J Virol 1998;72:6223.
74. Gaidano G, Castanos-Velez E, Biberfeld P. Lymphoid disorders associated with HHV-8/KSHV infection: facts and contentions. Med Oncol 1999;16:8.
75. Chatlynne LG, Ablashi DV. Seroepidemiology of Kaposi's sarcoma-associated herpesvirus (KSHV). Semin Cancer Biol 1999;9:175.
76. LaDuca JR, Love JL, Abbott LZ, Dube S, Freidman-Kien AE, Poiesz BJ. Detection of human herpesvirus 8 DNA sequences in tissues and bodily fluids. J Infect Dis 1998;178:1610.
77. Nador RG, Cesarman E, Chadburn A, et al. Primary effusion lymphoma: a distinct clinicopathologic entity associated with the Kaposi's sarcoma-associated herpes virus. Blood 1996;88:645.
78. Drexler HG, Meyer C, Gaidano G, Carbone A. Constitutive cytokine production by primary effusion (body cavity-based) lymphoma-derived cell lines. Leukemia 1999;13:634.
79. Molden J, Chang Y, You Y, Moore PS, Goldsmith MA. A Kaposi's sarcoma-associated herpesvirus-encoded cytokine homolog (vIL-6) activates signaling through the shared gp130 receptor subunit. J Biol Chem 1997;272:19625.
80. Djerbi M, Screpanti V, Catrina AI, Bogen B, Biberfeld P, Grandien A. The inhibitor of death receptor signaling, FLICE-inhibitory protein defines a new class of tumor progression factors. J Exp Med 1999;190:1025.
81. Arvanitakis L, Geras-Raaka E, Varma A Gershengorn MC, Cesarman E. Human herpesvirus KSHV encodes a constitutively active G-protein coupled receptor linked to cell proliferation. Nature 1997;385:347.
82. Kimberlin DW. Human herpesviruses 6 and 7: identification of newly recognized viral pathogens and their association with human disease. Pediatr Infect Dis J 1998;17:59.
83. Levy JA. Three new human herpesviruses (HHV6, 7, and 8). Lancet 1997;349:558.

Section 9 Immunology of Neoplasia

Chapter 96

Lymphomas, Including Hodgkin's Disease

Stefania Pittaluga and Elaine S. Jaffe

The classification of the malignant lymphomas has undergone significant reappraisal over the past 40 years. These changes have resulted from insights gained through the application of immunological and molecular techniques, as well as better understanding of the clinical aspects of lymphoma through advances in diagnosis, staging and treatment.

Early classifications were based on architectural and cytological characteristics of the neoplastic elements; however, with increasing knowledge of the complexity of the immune system a more functional approach was sought.[1] This attempt was only partially successful, owing to the limited array of tools available to the pathologist in the 1970s and 1980s. The integration of immunological functions with morphological descriptions is best exemplified by the Kiel classification and its updated versions. The identification of morphologically distinct cell types within normal lymphoid tissue provided a conceptual framework into which malignant lymphomas could be placed and matched with their normal counterparts. However, the proposed differentiation scheme was not always supported by experimental evidence and, despite extensive study, the definition of lymphoid compartments in humans and the movement of cells between these compartments still contains many uncertainties. Ideally, lymphomas, like most other tumors, should be classified according to their presumed normal counterpart, as far as possible. This approach should provide the best information about disease biology, natural history and response to treatment. However, there are difficulties in defining the full extent of the neoplastic clone in individual cases of lymphoma, and some well defined lymphoma types lack obvious normal counterparts. Consequently, although differentiation schemes provide useful conceptual frameworks for understanding lymphomas (Fig. 96.1), and suggest important new lines of research, current understanding of both the immune system and the lymphomas appears inadequate to support a biologically 'correct' lymphoma classification. Thus, a classification of human lymphomas based strictly on a theoretical relationship of tumors to normal stages of differentiation is both unrealistic and unnecessary. Such an approach also overlooks the relationship of molecular pathogenesis to disease definition.

> **KEY CONCEPTS**
>
> **Somatic mutation in relation to normal B-cell development**
> - Premutational stage: circulating naive B cells (IgM/D^+) prior to antigen exposure
> - Stage of somatic mutation, antigen selection and isotype switch: at the germinal center
> - Postmutational stage: selected B cells move to the periphery (postgerminal center), to the recirculating pool, or undergo terminal differentiation

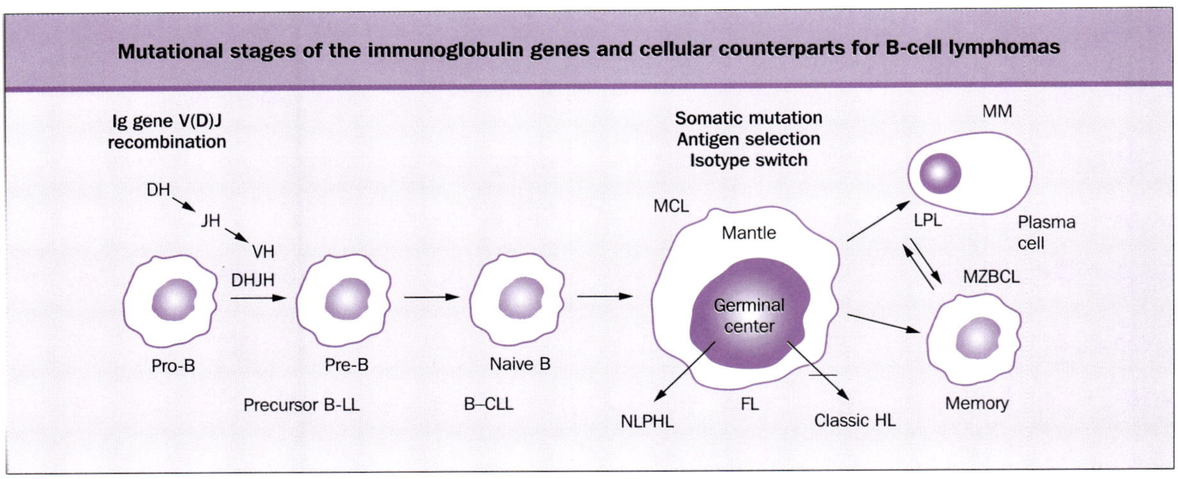

Figure 96.1 Normal B-cell differentiation, mutational stages of the immunoglobulin genes and cellular counterparts for B-cell lymphomas. Simplified version of B-cell development indicates points at which VDJ recombination and somatic muations occur. B-cell lymphomas are related to different stages of B-cell differentiation and function. Precursor B-LL, precursor B-lymphoblastic leukemia/lymphoma; CLL, chronic lymphocytic leukemia; MCL, mantle cell lymphoma; FL, follicular lymphoma; MM, multiple myeloma; LPL, lymphoplasmacytic lymphoma; MZBCL, marginal-zone lymphoma; Classic HL, classic Hodgkin lymphoma; NLPHL, nodular lymphocyte-predominant Hodgkin lymphoma.

The International Lymphoma Study Group in 1994 concluded that the most practical approach to lymphoma categorization was to define the diseases that could be recognized with the currently available morphologic, immunologic and genetic techniques.[2] The resulting Revised European American Lymphoma (REAL) classification departed from previous traditional schemes and represented a new paradigm for the classification of lymphomas. Each variant could be distinguished by a combination of morphologic, immunophenotypic and genotypic analyses, and each was associated with a characteristic clinical behavior, pattern of spread and response to therapy. In addition it stressed the distinction between histologic grade and clinical aggressiveness, and emphasized that histologic grade should be applied within individual diseases and not across the entire spectrum of lymphoid neoplasms. It further noted that the site of involvement (e.g. nodal vs. extranodal) was often an indicator of important biologic distinctions. It stressed that many disease entities are associated with distinctive clinical presentations and natural histories, even though treatment options may still be limited.

To test the validity of this approach, an international study sought to determine the applicability and reproducibility of the REAL classification among a group of independent expert pathologists.[3] Other goals included defining the role of immunophenotyping and clinical data in the classification and determining the usefulness of clinical groupings for clinical trials and practice. This study concluded that indeed the REAL classification enhanced diagnostic accuracy and reduced subjectivity. Immunophenotyping improved reproducibility and was essential in some specific entities, such as most peripheral T-cell lymphomas.[4] This study also stressed the importance of clinical factors, such as the International Prognostic Index (IPI) for predicting prognosis and providing a guide to clinical management.[5] Applying the IPI, a wide range of survival was observed across most disease entities. This observation suggests that it can be misleading to stratify different diseases into risk groups based only on histologic criteria. Moreover, when diseases were grouped according to post-treatment survival (as previously done in the Working Formulation, WF), it was noted that not only were the entities included in each group heterogeneous, but they required markedly different treatment modalities. It became evident that there was a need to approach each disease individually, considering the diagnosis, the patient's risk factors and the known idiosyncrasies of each disease with regard to treatment.

Utilizing the principles of the REAL classification, a new World Health Organization (WHO) classification for hematological malignancies was developed (Table 96.1). There are strong similarities between the WHO and the REAL classification schemes. However, since the publication of the REAL, new data have been generated for some categories. These studies allowed the resolution of entities that were previously listed as provisional; some were retained, whereas others were eliminated from the classification scheme.

This chapter focuses on the classification of neoplasms derived from mature B cells, T cells and NK cells, with emphasis on malignant lymphomas.

WHO classification for lymphoid neoplasia

B-cell neoplasms
- *Precursor B-cell lymphoblastic leukemia/lymphoma*
- Mature B-cell neoplasms
  - *B-cell chronic lymphocytic leukemia/small lymphocytic lymphoma*
  - B-cell prolymphocytic leukemia
  - Lymphoplasmacytic lymphoma
  - *Mantle cell lymphoma*
  - *Follicular lymphoma*
  - *Marginal-zone B-cell lymphoma of mucosa-associated lymphoid tissue (MALT) type*
  - Nodal marginal zone B-cell lymphoma with or without monocytoid B cells
  - Splenic marginal zone B-cell lymphoma
  - Hairy cell leukemia
  - *Diffuse large B-cell lymphoma*
    - Subtypes: mediastinal (thymic), intravascular, primary effusion lymphoma
  - Burkitt's lymphoma
  - Plasmacytoma
  - *Plasma cell myeloma*

T-cell neoplasms
- *Precursor T-cell lymphoblastic leukemia/lymphoma*
- Mature T-cell and NK cell neoplasms
  - T-cell prolymphocytic leukemia
  - T-cell large granular lymphocytic leukemia
  - NK-cell leukemia
  - Extranodal NK/T-cell lymphoma, nasal type
  - *Mycosis fungoides*
  - Sézary syndrome
  - *Angioimmunoblastic T-cell lymphoma*
  - *Peripheral T-cell lymphoma (unspecified)*
  - Adult T-cell leukemia/lymphoma
  - *Systemic anaplastic large cell lymphoma (T- and null cell types)*
  - Primary cutaneous anaplastic large cell lymphoma
  - Subcutaneous panniculitis-like T-cell lymphoma
  - Enteropathy-type intestinal T-cell lymphoma
  - Hepatosplenic T-cell lymphoma

Hodgkin's lymphoma (Hodgkin's disease)
- Nodular lymphocyte-predominant Hodgkin's lymphoma
- Classic Hodgkin's lymphoma
  - *Hodgkin's lymphoma nodular sclerosis (grades I and II)*
  - Classic Hodgkin's lymphoma, lymphocytes-rich
  - *Hodgkin's lymphoma, mixed cellularity*
  - Hodgkin's lymphoma, lymphocytic depletion

Most common entities are in italics.
Morphologic and clinical variants are not listed.
In this chapter we will discuss disease entities that do not appear in other chapters.

Table 96.1 Proposed World Health Organization classification for neoplastic diseases of the lymphoid tissue.

KEY CONCEPTS

Lymphoma
- Classification consists of a list of individual disease entities defined by morphologic, immunophenotypic, genetic and clinical features
- Neoplastic cells related to the postulated normal counterpart, when possible
- Histologic grade should be applied within individual diseases
- Clinical factors for individual patients as measured by the International Prognostic Index (IPI) are useful in predicting clinical outcome

MATURE B-CELL NEOPLASMS

Lymphoplasmacytic lymphoma (LPL)

The definition of LPL is still controversial as specific genetic and immunophenotypic markers have not yet been identified. The previously used terms (lymphoplasmacytoid lymphoma, plasmacytoid lymphocytic lymphoma, or immunocytoma) do not appear to define a single entity, as used in the literature. Many B-cell neoplasms occasionally show maturation to plasmacytoid or plasma cells containing cytoplasmic immunoglobulin (cIg), including B-cell chronic lymphocytic leukemia (B-CLL), and mantle cell, follicle center and marginal-zone cell lymphomas. We suggest that these cases be classified according to their major features, and not as lymphoplasmacytic lymphomas. There does appear to be a distinct disorder of small lymphoid cells that show maturation to plasma cells without features of other lymphoma types, which corresponds to most cases of Waldenström's macroglobulinemia (WM). The term LPL should be restricted to these cases.

This is a disease of adult life (median age 61) that usually presents with generalized lymphadenopathy, vague constitutional symptoms, anemia and splenomegaly. Autoimmune hemolytic anemia is a common complication. Peripheral blood involvement with an absolute lymphocytosis is less common in LPL than in B cell chronic lymphocytic leukemia/small lymphocytic lymphoma. IgM monoclonal gammopathy may be associated with increased serum viscosity, leading to neurologic and vascular complications.[6,7] However, this phenomenon can also be observed in other lymphomas. The course is chronic and indolent, and the disease is not generally curable with the available treatments; median survival is 78 months. Similar to other indolent lymphomas, the survival curve does not show any plateau. The treatment options, which depend on the clinical presentation, include plasmapheresis, the use of alkylating agents and more aggressive chemotherapy.[8]

The tumor consists of a diffuse proliferation of small lymphocytes, plasmacytoid lymphocytes (cells with abundant basophilic cytoplasm but lymphocyte-like nuclei) and plasma cells, with or without Dutcher bodies. The growth pattern is often interfollicular, with sparing of the sinuses.

The cells have surface and cytoplasmic Ig, usually of IgM type, usually lack IgD, and express B-cell-associated antigens (CD19, 20, 22, 79a). They are negative for CD5, CD10 and CD43; CD25 or CD11c may be faintly positive in some cases.[6,7] A lack of CD5 and the presence of strong cytoplasmic Ig are useful in distinction from B-CLL.

A recurrent chromosomal abnormality t(9;14)(p13;q32) has been detected in approximately 50% of LPL, most commonly in patients with WM.[9] The *PAX5* gene is involved in this translocation and encodes for a B-cell-specific transcription factor involved in the control of B-cell differentiation and proliferation.[10] The postulated normal counterpart is thought to be a postfollicular medullary cord B cell,[7,11] based in part on the presence of somatic mutations in the Ig heavy and light-chain variable region genes.[12]

Mantle cell lymphoma (MCL)

MCL is a distinct clinicopathologic entity that has been more precisely defined in recent years through the integration of immunophenotypic, molecular genetic and clinicopathologic studies.[13] This tumor was recognized in the Kiel classification as centrocytic lymphoma and in the modified Rappaport scheme as lymphocytic lymphoma of intermediate differentiation. It tended to surround residual naked germinal centers, and a derivation from the follicular lymphoid cuff was postulated.[14] Tumors with a very conspicuous mantle zone pattern of growth were also termed 'mantle zone lymphoma'.

MCL occurs in adults (median age 62), with a high male-to-female ratio. Most patients present with advanced stage at diagnosis.[15–18] Common sites of involvement include the lymph nodes, spleen, bone marrow, and lymphoid tissue of Waldeyer's ring. Gastrointestinal tract involvement is common and is associated with the picture of lymphomatous polyposis.[19] This tumor appears to be incurable with the available treatments. In data collated from several retrospective studies the prognosis is poor, with a median survival ranging from 20 months to 52 months. The relapse rate is high, with a median disease-free survival between 10.2 and 25.5 months.[15–18] The use of interferon (IFN) as maintenance or consolidation therapy may be of value.[16] Purine analogs have produced a low response rate compared to other indolent lymphomas. A subset of patients may benefit from a more aggressive regimen using high-dose chemotherapy with autologous stem cell transplantation. However, because of the frequent bone marrow involvement, purging of the neoplastic cells is difficult to achieve.[20]

The hallmark of MCL is a very monotonous cytologic composition. In the typical case the cells are slightly larger than a normal lymphocyte, with finely clumped chromatin, scant cytoplasm and inconspicuous nucleoli. The nuclear contour is usually irregular or cleaved. Cytological (blastoid or blastic) and architectural variants (mantle zone, nodular and diffuse) have been described and associated with a more aggressive clinical course (blastoid variant) or with a longer median survival (mantle zone pattern).[21] However, because of the overall poor prognosis and the lack of statistical significance of these architectural/cytological changes, the WHO classification considers mantle cell lymphoma and its variants to be one group.[15,17,21,22]

Immunophenotypic and genotypic studies have been helpful in precisely defining MCL. The immunophenotype is distinctive (IgM/IgD$^+$; CD5$^+$, CD10$^-$ and CD23$^-$). In addition, the chromosomal translocation t(11;14) involving *CYCLIN D1* located at the *BCL-1/PRAD1* locus is associated with MCL, but is absent in most other low- and high-grade B-cell malignancies.[23] By Northern analysis virtually 100% of cases of MCL have shown overexpression of cyclin D1, which has not been identified to the same degree in other B-cell malignancies.[24] Additional alterations involving other cell cycle regulatory molecules, such as RB, p53 and CDK inhibitors (p16 and p27), have been described in the more aggressive forms of MCL.[22,25–27]

The postulated normal counterpart is the CD5$^+$ 'virgin' B cell, sIgM$^+$ and sIgD$^+$ that can be found in the peripheral blood and in the mantle of reactive germinal centers. Mutational analysis of the rearranged immunoglobulin variable region genes shows few or no somatic mutations.[28]

Follicular lymphoma (FL)

FL is the most common subtype of non-Hodgkin's lymphoma in the United States and accounts for approximately 45% of all newly diagnosed cases. It has a peak incidence in the fifth and sixth decades, and is rare under the age of 20. Men and women are equally affected. FL is less common in Black and Asian populations. Most patients have stage 3 or 4 disease at diagnosis, with generalized lymphadenopathy[39] and staging evaluation usually detects bone marrow involvement.[29] Approximately 10% of patients have circulating malignant cells.[30] However, careful immunophenotypic or molecular analyses may disclose peripheral blood involvement in a higher proportion of patients.

CLINICAL PEARLS

Indolent lymphomas
- Natural history: survival measured in years
- Least sensitive to therapy
- Good response to low-dose oral alkylating agents, radiotherapy and steroids
- Partial remissions are frequently seen; fewer complete remissions, but almost no curability
- New therapeutic approaches: immunotherapy (monoclonal antibodies with or without chemotherapy, labeled with radioisotopes, vaccination strategies)
- High-dose chemotherapy and autologous stem cell transplantation in selected patients is a potentially curative modality

FL is indolent, but currently incurable with available therapeutic modalities. The natural history of the disease, with frequent relapses and relatively long survival[31] has led to different therapeutic approaches (watchful waiting vs chemotherapy).[32] More recently, new therapeutic avenues have been explored as, following relapses, patients become resistant to chemotherapy. A more aggressive approach with intent to eradicate the disease at the first or second relapse has been tested in clinical trials.[33,34]

The natural history of the disease is associated with histologic progression in both pattern and cell type (Fig. 96.2). A heterogeneous cytologic composition is one of the hallmarks of FL. Usually, all of the follicle center cells are represented, but in varying proportions.

This variation in cytologic composition is the basis for the subclassification of follicular lymphoma. It should be stressed that the variation in cytologic grade is a continuum, and therefore precise morphologic criteria for subclassification are difficult to establish. Most studies have shown that the subclassification of follicular lymphoma is difficult to reproduce among groups of pathologists. According to the WHO clinical advisory committee, follicular lymphomas should be graded and for most clinical purposes the distinction into two grades is sufficient (grade 1, predominantly small cleaved cell together with grade 2, mixed small cleaved and large cell; as distinct from grade 3, predominantly large cell). However, the distinction into three grades continues, with a recommendation for the use of the 'Berard' counting method.[35]

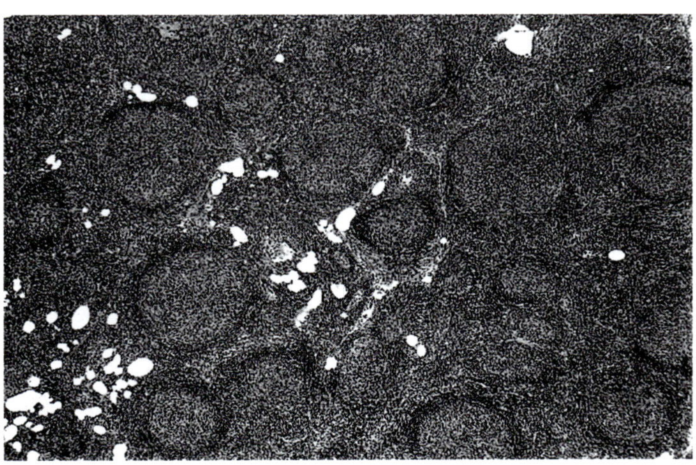

Figure 96.2 Follicular lymphoma. The neoplastic follicles are similar in size and are partially surrounded by lymphoid cuffs. They lack the starry sky histiocytes seen in reactive germinal centers.

The vast majority of FL (approximately 85%) are associated with a t(14;18) involving rearrangement of the *BCL2* gene.[36] This translocation appears to result in constitutive expression of BCL-2 protein, which is capable of inhibiting apoptosis in lymphoid cells.[37] The cells of FL accumulate and are at risk for secondary mutations, which may be associated with histologic progression. It is interesting that the small subset of grade 3 follicular lymphomas (large cell) are less commonly associated with the *BCL2* translocation.[38] Thus, some forms of FL may have a different pathogenesis. It is thought that the *BCL2* translocation occurs at a very early stage of B cell development, during immunoglobulin gene rearrangement. This fact may contribute to the difficulty of eradicating the neoplastic clone with chemotherapy.

Most FL present in lymph nodes. A subset of cases with the morphologic features of FL present in skin.[39] Clinically, these tumors are usually localized and infrequently associated with lymph node involvement. They have an excellent prognosis; complete remissions may be obtained with either surgical excision or local radiation therapy.[40] Interestingly, these cutaneous FL frequently lack the *BCL2* translocation associated with nodal FL. Biologically, the cutaneous FL may be part of the mucosa-associated lymphoid tissue (MALT) lymphoma spectrum[41] (see below).

The cells have a mature B-cell phenotype with expression of the B cell antigens CD19, CD20 and CD22. Surface Ig is positive, most commonly with IgM expression, but IgG or IgA can be seen in many cases. CD10 is positive but CD5 is negative.

FL represents the neoplastic counterpart of the reactive germinal center cells[41] and was one of the first lymphomas demonstrating an immunophenotypic derivation from a normal lymphoid equivalent.[42] Consistent with their normal counterparts, intraclonal heterogeneity with high numbers of somatic mutations and ongoing mutations of the Ig genes was detected in these cells.[43]

Marginal-zone B-cell lymphoma of mucosa-associated lymphoid tissue (MALT) type

Most lymphomas of marginal-zone derivation present in extranodal sites and have histopathologic and clinical features that are part of the spectrum of MALT lymphomas.[44] MALT lymphomas are characterized by a heterogeneous cellular composition that includes marginal-zone or centrocyte-like cells, monocytoid B cells, small lymphocytes and plasma cells. In most cases large transformed cells are uncommon, but reactive germinal centers are nearly always present. Therefore, it is not surprising that, based on the heterogeneous cellular composition and the presence of reactive follicles, most MALT lymphomas were in the past diagnosed as pseudolymphomas or atypical hyperplasias. However, recent studies have shown the majority to be composed of monoclonal B cells. The follicles usually contain reactive germinal centers, but the germinal centers may become colonized by neoplastic cells. When follicular colonization occurs the process can simulate follicular lymphoma.[45] The plasma cells are usually found in the subepithelial zones and are monoclonal in up to 50% of cases.

MALT lymphomas have been described in nearly every anatomic site, but are most frequent in the stomach, lung, thyroid, salivary gland and lacrimal gland.[11,46] Other less common sites of involvement include the orbit, breast, conjunctiva, bladder, kidney and thymus. Most patients present with localized disease, although regional lymph node involvement is common in gastric and salivary gland MALT lymphoma. The involved lymph nodes in those cases resemble monocytoid B cell lymphoma, and it is thought that monocytoid B cell lymphoma is the nodal equivalent of a MALT lymphoma.[47,48] Widespread nodal involvement is infrequent, as is bone marrow involvement. The clinical course is usually quite indolent and many patients are asymptomatic. MALT lymphomas tend to relapse in other MALT-associated sites.[11]

MALT lymphomas of the salivary gland and thyroid are usually associated with a history of autoimmune diseases. *Helicobacter* gastritis is common in most patients with gastric MALT lymphomas, and it has been suggested that antigen stimulation is critical to both the development of a MALT lymphoma and the maintenance of the neoplastic state.[49] Indeed, in some cases antibiotic therapy and the eradication of *Helicobacter pylori* has led to the spontaneous remission of gastric MALT lymphoma.[50] Antibiotic treatment is currently advocated as first-line therapy. However, the therapy of MALT lymphomas remains controversial. Isolated lesions readily amenable to surgical excision should be removed. Systemic chemotherapy may be warranted for more widespread disease, and local radiation therapy may play a role in the control of localized tumor masses, especially for gastric and orbital MALT lymphomas.

Immunophenotyping is helpful in the differential diagnosis of MALT lymphomas from cytologically similar lymphomas such as B-CLL/SLL and MCL. MALT lymphomas are positive for B-cell-associated antigens CD19, CD20 and CD22 but, in contrast to most systemic small lymphocytic malignancies, are negative for CD5.

MALT lymphomas also have a commonly recurring cytogenetic abnormality, t(11;18), which is observed in 50% of extranodal cases.[51–53] The genes involved in the translocation have been identified as *c-IAP2*, a gene encoding for an inhibitor of apoptosis, and a novel gene on 18q21 named *MLT* (of unknown function).[53] It has been speculated that the fusion protein may lead to increased inhibition of apoptosis, conferring a survival advantage to the neoplastic cells.[52]

The translocation t(11;18)(q21;q21) is associated exclusively with low-grade extranodal MALT and is not detected in cases with simultaneous low and high-grade tumors, or in 'primary' extranodal large cell lymphomas, raising the question of whether these primary extranodal lymphomas are in fact related to low-grade MALT.[53] In the WHO Clinical Advisory Committee the term extranodal marginal-zone lymphoma of MALT type applies only to low-grade MALT, and it was recommended that the term high-grade MALT not be used for extranodal large cell lymphomas in a 'MALT' site. The putative cell of origin of marginal-zone lymphomas is a memory B cell (postgerminal center).[54,55]

Nodal marginal-zone lymphoma (MZL) with or without monocytoid B cells

Monocytoid B cell lymphoma is seen most often in association with an extranodal MALT lymphoma.[56] However, the existence of the primary extranodal disease may not be immediately apparent. Relapses in nodal sites can occur many years after the primary diagnosis. Patients who present with nodal disease, often with bone marrow involvement and no evidence of extranodal disease, tend to have a more aggressive clinical course than those with extranodal MALT.[3,15,57]

The neoplastic proliferation is composed mostly of monocytoid B cells with interspersed large blast-like cells. There is an expansion of the marginal-zone area, often with preservation of the nodal architecture. The mantle zone can be intact, attenuated or effaced.

Immunophenotype is similar to that of other marginal-zone B-cell lymphomas, $CD20^+$, $CD5^-$, $CD10^-$, with variable IgD expression (weak to negative). Some nodal MZL have a morphology and immunophenotype similar to those of splenic marginal zone (see below) and in these cases the tumour cells are IgD positive.[58] A morphologically similar but different phenomenon is monocytoid B cell differentiation in a primary nodal lymphoma. Cells resembling monocytoid B lymphocytes have been described in many low-grade lymphomas, most commonly FL.[59] The monocytoid B-cell component appears to occupy the marginal zone. Nevertheless, the immunophenotype and genotype of the neoplastic cells are those of FL. Monocytoid differentiation is an interesting morphologic variant but does not yet have proven clinical or biological significance. However, one study suggested that cases with MZL differentiation have a more aggressive clinical course.[60]

Splenic marginal-zone lymphoma

Splenic marginal-zone lymphomas (SMZL) present in adults and are slightly more common in women than in men. The clinical presentation is splenomegaly, usually without peripheral lymphadenopathy. The majority of patients have bone marrow involvement, but there is usually only a modest lymphocytosis, with elevations in the lymphocyte count usually less than in B-CLL. Some evidence of plasmacytoid differentiation may be seen and patients may have a small M protein. The abundant pale cytoplasm evident in tissue sections may also be seen in peripheral blood smears. The cytologic features may be mistaken for those of hairy cell leukemia. The disorder described as splenic lymphoma with villous lymphocytes (SLVL) appears equivalent to splenic marginal-zone lymphoma.[61] The course is reported to be indolent, and splenectomy may be followed by a prolonged remission.

Immunophenotypic studies are useful in distinguishing SMZL from B-CLL/SLL involving the spleen. Whereas typical B-CLL/SLL cells are $CD5^+$, SMZL cells are $CD5^-$. Careful attention to the cytologic features in these cases indicates that the cells have somewhat more abundant cytoplasm than those of typical B-CLL/SLL and resemble the lymphocytes of the normal splenic marginal zone. The nuclei are usually predominantly round but may be slightly irregular and have a moderate amount of pale cytoplasm. Histologically, the spleen shows expansion of the white pulp, but usually some infiltration of the red pulp is present as well.[62] In early cases preferential involvement of the marginal zone may be seen, with residual mantle cells present.[63] A characteristic biphasic pattern in the neoplastic white pulp has been described[61] in which a central zone of small lymphocytes is surrounded by a peripheral zone of larger cells that resemble marginal zone cells. In this instance the residual polytypic mantle is no longer present. The phenotype of these cells resembles that of the other marginal zone B-cell lymphomas; however, sIgD expression is more frequently positive.[62] Studies of the Ig variable genes have also revealed the presence of mutations suggesting a postfollicular origin.[64]

Diffuse large B-cell lymphoma (DLBCL)

DLBCL is one of the more common subtypes of non-Hodgkin lymphoma, representing up to 40% of cases. It has an aggressive natural history but responds well to chemotherapy. The complete remission rate with modern regimens is 75–80%, with long-term disease-free survival approaching 50% or more in most series.[65] This lymphoma may present in lymph nodes or in extranodal sites, including bone, skin, thyroid, gastrointestinal tract and lung.

Because of the variation in the response to chemotherapy and the frequency of DLBCL, there has been great interest in identifying morphologic or immunophenotypic features that might be prognostically important. In most studies there is some suggestion that tumors composed of large cleaved or large noncleaved follicular center cells have a slightly better prognosis than those composed predominantly of immunoblasts.[29] However, the differences have been neither statistically significant nor consistently reproducible. Some data suggest that a high growth fraction is an adverse prognostic marker,[66] but other studies have reached an opposite conclusion, suggesting that lymphomas with a high growth fraction may be more sensitive to chemotherapy.[67] It is likely that in the future the use of immunophenotypic and/or genotypic markers will yield useful information in the subclassification of large B-cell lymphoma.[68–70] The prognostic significance of BCL-2 protein expression and *BCL2* rearrangement in DLBCL is controversial. However, in several studies the expression of BCL-2 (irrespective of the presence of t(14;18)) has been associated with a reduced disease-free survival.[71,72] This result may be related to the antiapoptotic effect of BCL-2, abrogating apoptosis induced by chemotherapy. The presence of *BCL6* rearrangement was originally described mainly in cases of DLBCL with extranodal involvement, and it was associated with a better prognosis.[73] However, these data were not confirmed by other studies. At present, although morphologic features are useful in identifying the spectrum of appearances that are encountered diagnostically, they do not appear to be important prognostically.

DLBCL are composed of large, transformed lymphoid cells with nuclei at least twice the size of a small lymphocyte (Fig. 96.3). The nuclei generally have vesicular chromatin, prominent nucleoli, basophilic cytoplasm and a moderate to high proliferation fraction. Marked variation in the nuclear contour can be seen. In the majority of cases the cells are round to oval. However, in some cases they are polylobated or cleaved. The expression of B-cell-associated antigens, especially CD20, is a consistent feature.

Most aggressive lymphomas show a spectrum in cytologic appearance, and in any given field the predominant cell could be large cell or large cell immunoblastic. The designation of immunoblastic lymphoma of B-cell type is reserved for cases in which more than 90% of the cells have an immunoblastic appearance. If only 10% of the cells resemble centroblasts the case is classified as a centroblastic lymphoma. Using these criteria only 4% of all non-Hodgkin lymphomas are classified as B immunoblastic; cases with an immunoblastic appearance have a worse prognosis.[74]

DLBCL may be associated with sclerosis, particularly in extranodal sites.[29] Sclerosis is more common in tumors with large cleaved cell morphology, and is also seen in mediastinal or thymic large B cell lymphoma[75] (see below).

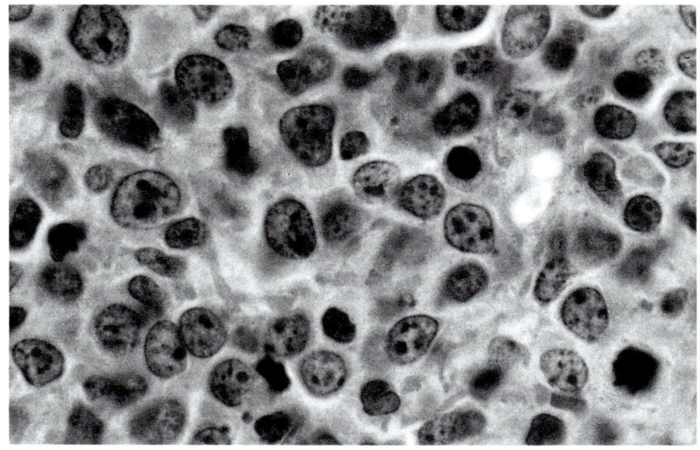

Figure 96.3 Diffuse large B-cell lymphoma. The neoplastic cells have large round to oval nuclei with vesicular chromatin. Usually multiple eosinophilic nucleoli are present

> **CLINICAL PEARLS**
>
> **Aggressive lymphomas**
> - Natural history: survival measured in months
> - Successful therapy can be achieved with combination chemotherapy
> - Relapses from chemotherapy-induced remission may be cured with high-dose chemotherapy with hematopoietic support
> - The International Prognostic Index and the age-adjusted international index (age, tumor stage, serum lactate dehydrogenase concentration, performance status and number of extranodal disease sites) identified four risk groups with significantly different responses to therapy and survival. It is significantly more accurate than the Ann Arbor classification in predicting long-term survival.

Some large B-cell lymphomas are rich in either small T lymphocytes or histiocytes or both. Histologically, they can resemble peripheral T-cell lymphomas or Hodgkin's disease.[76,77] They are clinically aggressive, with a prognosis comparable to that of DLBCL.[78] The admixture of small lymphocytes and histiocytes is a variable phenomenon, and the inflammatory background can be absent on second biopsies. These tumors have been referred to in the literature as 'pseudoperipheral T-cell lymphomas'[76] or T-cell-rich B-cell lymphoma.[79] T-cell-rich B-cell lymphoma, as currently defined, does not appear to be a distinct clinical pathologic entity but rather a variant that can be seen in association with several different subtypes of DLBCL.[80] Histiocyte-rich large B-cell lymphoma has a more aggressive clinical behavior, tends to occur in younger patients compared to other DLBCL, and often presents with advanced stage and bone marrow involvement.[77]

Distinct subtypes of DLBCL include primary mediastinal (thymic) large B-cell lymphoma (PMBCL), intravascular large B-cell lymphoma and primary effusion lymphoma (HHV-8 associated).

PMBCL has emerged in recent years as a distinct clinicopathologic entity.[75] Cytologically it resembles many other large B-cell lymphomas and is composed of large transformed cells that can resemble large noncleaved cells, large cleaved cells, multilobated cells and even immunoblasts. A constant feature is relatively abundant pale cytoplasm, often with distinct cytoplasmic membranes. Many cases have fine compartmentalizing sclerosis, which can even lead to misdiagnosis as an epithelial tumor, such as thymoma. The tumor appears to be derived from medullary B cells within the thymus gland. These cells express CD20 and CD79a, but not surface Ig.[81,82] Recently, the expression of the *MAL* gene has been detected in PMBCL and not in other DLBCL.[83] This observation further supports the distinctive nature of this lymphoma. PMBCL usually lack rearrangement for *BCL2* and *BCL6*; however, *c-MYC* abnormalities and *c-REL* amplification have been described.[84,85]

Clinically, mediastinal large B-cell lymphoma is much more common in females than males. It is common in adolescents and young adults, with a median age at presentation in the fourth decade. The clinical presentation is that of a rapidly growing anterior mediastinal mass with frequent superior vena cava syndrome and/or airway obstruction. Nodal involvement is uncommon at presentation and also at relapse. Frequent extranodal sites of involvement, particularly at relapse, include the liver, kidneys, adrenal glands, ovaries, gastrointestinal tract and central nervous system. Earlier studies suggested that the tumor was associated with an unusually aggressive clinical course, with poor responses to conventional chemotherapy. More recent studies have reported cure rates similar to those seen for other large B-cell lymphomas with the use of combined chemotherapy and irradiation.[86]

Burkitt's lymphoma (BL)

Burkitt's lymphoma is most common in children and accounts for up to one-third of all pediatric lymphomas in the United States.[87] It is the most rapidly growing of all lymphomas, with 100% of the cells in cell cycle at any time. It usually presents in extranodal sites. In nonendemic regions, such as the United States, common sites of presentation are the ileocecal region, ovaries, kidneys or breasts. Jaw presentations, as well as the involvement of other facial bones, are common in African or endemic cases and are occasionally seen in nonendemic regions. Some cases present as acute leukemia with diffuse bone marrow infiltration and circulating Burkitt tumor cells (L3-ALL). Even in patients with typical extranodal disease bone marrow involvement is a poor prognostic sign.

Burkitt's lymphoma is one of the more common tumors associated with the human immunodeficiency virus (HIV).[88] It can present at any time during the clinical course. In some patients with HIV infection Burkitt's lymphoma is the initial AIDS-defining illness.

The pathogenesis of Burkitt's lymphoma is undoubtedly related to the translocations involving the *c-MYC* oncogene, which are seen in virtually 100% of cases.[89] Most of the translocations involve the Ig heavy-chain gene on chromosome 14. Less commonly the light-chain genes on chromosomes 2 and 22 are involved. African Burkitt's lymphoma occurs in regions endemic for malaria, and it has been postulated that immunosuppression associated with malarial infection puts patients at increased risk.[36] In this regard, the pathogenesis appears similar to that seen with HIV infection.

> **CLINICAL PEARLS**
>
> **Highly aggressive lymphomas**
> - More common in children
> - Natural history similar to acute leukemia
> - Successful treatment includes high-dose chemotherapy (induction, consolidation and maintenance phases) with CNS prophylaxis

Epstein–Barr virus (EBV) is closely linked to Burkitt's lymphoma in endemic regions but is less frequently seen (15–20%) in Europe and North America.[87] In other regions, characterized by low socioeconomic status and EBV infection at an early age Burkitt's lymphoma is often EBV positive, in the range of 50–70%. These data support the concept the EBV is a cofactor for the development of Burkitt's lymphoma. Differences in the proportion of cases associated with the two EBV strains (types 1 and 2) have also been shown in sporadic and endemic EBV-positive Burkitt's lymphomas.[90]

Cytologically, Burkitt's lymphoma is monomorphic with cells of medium size, round nuclei, moderately clumped chromatin and multiple (2–5) basophilic nucleoli. The cytoplasm is deeply basophilic and moderately abundant. These cells contain cytoplasmic lipid vacuoles, which are probably a manifestation of the high rates of proliferation and spontaneous cell death. The starry sky pattern characteristic of Burkitt's lymphoma is a manifestation of the numerous benign macrophages that have ingested karyorrhectic or apoptotic tumor cells.

Burkitt's lyphoma has a mature B-cell phenotype. The cells express CD19, CD20, CD22, CD79a and monoclonal surface Ig, nearly always IgM. CD10 is positive in nearly all cases, and CD5 and CD23 are consistently negative.

In the WHO classification Burkitt-like lymphomas (BLL) have been more narrowly defined and are included in the Burkitt lymphoma group as a variant. BLL should have a growth fraction of essentially 100% and show cytologic similarities to classic BL, but a greater variation in nuclear size and shape.

A number of clinical studies have suggested that both BL and BLL have an aggressive clinical course.[66,91] Therefore, it was felt that the separation of such tumors from diffuse large B-cell lymphoma was warranted on clinical grounds. Nevertheless, with current chemotherapeutic regimens a complete continuous remission can be obtained in many cases.[91]

T-CELL AND PUTATIVE NK-CELL NEOPLASMS

Overview of the classification of T-cell neoplasms

Whereas the definition of precursor T cell or lymphoblastic neoplasms is straightforward, the classification of peripheral T-cell lymphomas has been controversial. These are uncommon, representing less than 15% of all non-Hodgkin lymphomas. Most previously published classification schemes for the malignant lymphomas in the United States or Europe have been based on the far more common B-cell malignancies.

The revised Kiel classification does include T-cell lymphomas.[92] However, the REAL classification differs from the approach utilized in the Kiel scheme in several respects. For one, it recognizes adult T-cell leukemia/lymphoma (ATLL) as a distinct clinicopathologic entity.[93] The Kiel classification describes T-cell lymphomas in morphologic terms and independently notes the status as HTLV-1 positive or negative.

The REAL classification also recognizes the distinctive nature of many extranodal T-cell lymphomas. These include the nasal and nasal-type angiocentric lymphomas, enteropathy-associated T-cell lymphoma, and subcutaneous panniculitic T-cell lymphoma. Clinical features play an important role in the definition of many T-cell lymphoma entities, as it is felt that cytologic features alone are not sufficient to delineate many of these diseases.

Finally, T-zone lymphoma and lymphoepithelioid cell lymphoma were not felt to be distinct clinicopathologic entities, although they do represent morphologic variations that can be seen in peripheral T-cell lymphoma. In addition, previous studies have suggested that they are difficult to distinguish reliably from other nodal T-cell lymphomas.[94] Cytogenetic studies also have suggested an overlap between these categories of nodal T cell lymphoma in the Kiel classification.[95] Therefore, they were left within the category of peripheral T-cell lymphomas, unspecified. Moreover, although the Kiel classification considered these variants histologically 'low grade', clinically they have an aggressive course.

The WHO classification retains most of the categories described in the REAL classification, but also incorporates new data that have been accumulated since its publication.

Extranodal NK/T-cell lymphoma, nasal-type previously angiocentric lymphoma

Extranodal NK/T-cell lymphoma, nasal type, is a distinct clinicopathologic entity highly associated with EBV.[96] It affects adults (median age 50) and the most common clinical presentation is a destructive nasal or midline facial lesion. Palatal destruction, orbital swelling and edema can be prominent.[97] NK/T-cell lymphomas have been reported in other extranodal sites, including the skin, soft tissue, testis, upper respiratory tract and gastrointestinal tract. A leukemic form of the disease also has been reported, with similar morphologic, immunophenotypic and genotypic features.[98] The clinical course is usually highly aggressive, with a slightly improved median survival in patients with localized disease. However, with current chemotherapy the outcome remains poor. Radiation therapy may be effective in localized disease.

Extranodal NK/T cell lymphoma, nasal type, is characterized by a broad cytologic spectrum. The atypical cells can be small or medium in size. Large atypical and hyperchromatic cells can be admixed, or may predominate. If the small cells are in the majority the disease can be difficult to distinguish from an inflammatory or infectious process. In early stages there can also be a prominent admixture of inflammatory cells, causing further difficulty in diagnosis.

Although the cells express some T-cell-associated antigens, most commonly CD2, other T-cell markers, such as surface CD3, are usually absent.[99] Cytoplasmic CD3 can be found in paraffin-embedded sections, but cytoplasmic CD3 can be found in NK cells and is not specific for a T-cell lineage tumor. In addition, molecular studies have not shown a clonal T-cell gene rearrangement, despite clonality being shown by other methods.[99–101] In favor of an NK cell origin, the cells are nearly always $CD56^+$, although CD16 and CD57 are usually negative. EBV is invariably positive by EBER in situ hybridization.

Extranodal NK/T-cell lymphoma, nasal type, is much more common in Asians than in those of European background. Clusters of the disease also have been reported in Central and South America in individuals of Native American heritage, suggesting that ethnic background may play a role in the pathogenesis of these lymphomas.

A hemophagocytic syndrome is a common clinical complication, and adversely affects survival in extranodal NK/T-cell lymphoma, nasal type.[102] It is likely that EBV plays a role in the pathogenesis of the hemophagocytic syndrome.

Angioimmunoblastic T-cell lymphoma (AILT)

AILT was initially proposed as an abnormal immune reaction or form of atypical lymphoid hyperplasia with a high risk of progression to malignant lymphoma.[103] Because the majority of cases show clonal rearrangements of T-cell receptor genes, it is now regarded as a variant of T-cell lymphoma. The median survival is usually less than 5 years, so that the designation as lymphoma is also warranted on clinical grounds.[104]

The nodal architecture is generally effaced, but peripheral sinuses are often open and even dilated. The abnormal infiltrate usually extends beyond the capsule into the surrounding tissue. Hyperplastic germinal centers are absent. However, there can be regressed follicles containing a proliferation of dendritic cells and blood vessels. These regressed follicles are referred to as 'burned out'. At low power there is usually a striking proliferation of post capillary venules with prominent arborization. The cellularity of the lymph node usually appears reduced or depleted at low power. Clusters of lymphoid cells with clear cytoplasm may be seen and their nuclei exhibit moderately condensed chromatin with a slightly irregular nuclear contour. These are admixed with a polymorphous cellular background containing small normal-appearing lymphocytes, basophilic immunoblasts, plasma cells and histiocytes, with or without eosinophils. The abnormal cells are usually $CD4^+$ T cells. In paraffin-embedded sections a helpful diagnostic feature is the presence of numerous $CD21^+$ dendritic reticulum cells, which are especially prominent around post-capillary venules Polyclonal plasma cells may be numerous.

AILT presents in adults; most patients have generalized lymphadenopathy with prominent systemic symptoms, including fever, weight loss and skin rash. There is usually a polyclonal hypergammaglobulinemia. Patients may respond initially to steroids or mild cytotoxic chemotherapy, but progression usually occurs. More aggressive combination chemotherapeutic regimens have led to a higher remission rate but patients are prone to secondary infectious complications.[105] Progression to a more monomorphic T-cell immunoblastic lymphoma occurs in some cases, and the proportion of large immunoblastic cells appears to correlate with the clinical course. Rarely, B-cell immunoblastic lymphomas positive for EBV occur in patients with AILT; These latter malignancies appear secondary to the underlying immunodeficiency.

Peripheral T-cell lymphomas, unspecified (PTCL)

PTCL is a diagnosis of exclusion and is admittedly a heterogeneous category with most cases being nodal in origin. PTCL are characterized by a heterogeneous cellular composition. There is usually a mixture of small and large atypical lymphoid cells. An inflammatory background is common, consisting of eosinophils, plasma cells and histiocytes. If the epithelioid histiocytes are numerous and clustered, the neoplasm fulfills the criteria for lymphoepithelioid cell lymphoma or Lennert's lymphoma.[106] In the REAL classification lymphoepithelioid cell lymphoma was considered a morphologic variant of PTCL and not a distinctive clinicopathologic entity. It has not been associated with any specific immunophenotypic, cytogenetic or molecular features that would permit distinction from other PTCL.[95]

PTCL may show preferential involvement of the paracortical region of lymph nodes. In some cases this architectural pattern is striking, with sparing of follicles. Such cases have been referred to as T-zone lymphoma.[92] However, on cytologic grounds they resemble other peripheral T cell lymphomas of medium or mixed cytologic types. The neoplastic cells usually have a moderate amount of pale cytoplasm.

Clinically, PTCL most often present in adults. Most patients exhibit generalized lymphadenopathy, hepatosplenomegaly and frequent bone marrow involvement. Constitutional symptoms, including fever and night sweats, are common, as is pruritus. The clinical course is aggressive, although complete remissions may be obtained with combination chemotherapy.[107] However, the relapse rate is higher in PTCL than in B-cell lymphomas of comparable histologic grade.[107]

PTCL, as defined in the WHO classification, remains heterogeneous. It is likely that individual clinicopathologic entities will be delineated in the future from this broad group of malignancies. Thus far, immunophenotypic criteria have not been helpful in delineating subytpes. Most cases have a mature T-cell phenotype and express one of the major subset antigens, with CD4 expression seen more frequently than CD8. These are not clonal markers, and antigen expression can change over time. Loss of one of the pan-T-cell antigens (CD3, CD5, CD2, or CD7) is seen in 75% of cases, with CD7 most frequently being absent.

Systemic, anaplastic large cell lymphoma (ALCL) (T- and null cell types)

ALCL is characterized by pleomorphic or monomorphic cells that have a propensity to invade lymphoid sinuses.[108] Because of the sinusoidal location of the tumor cells and their lobulated nuclear appearance, this disease was previously interpreted as a variant of malignant histiocytosis. Misdiagnosis as metastatic carcinoma or melanoma was also common.

A consistent feature is the expression of the CD30 antigen, which is a hallmark of this disease. It has been referred to as Ki-1$^+$ lymphoma.[109] However, CD30 expression is not specific for ALCL and may also be seen in other forms of malignant lymphoma, including Hodgkin's disease.[110] Systemic ALCL is associated with a characteristic chromosomal translocation, t(2;5)(p23;q35), involving *ALK/NPM* genes, respectively.[111] Polyclonal and monoclonal antibodies to the cytoplasmic portion of ALK protein have been made, and they stain tumor cells carrying the translocation.[112]

The cells of classic ALCL have large, often lobulated nuclei with nucleoli that are usually not prominent and are frequently basophilic. In some cases the nuclei may be round. The cytoplasm is usually abundant, amphophilic, with distinct cytoplasmic borders. A prominent Golgi region is generally visible. Immunohistochemistry is very valuable in the correct diagnosis of ALCL. The prominent Golgi region usually shows intense staining for CD30 and epithelial membrane antigen (EMA). In the majority of cases the neoplastic cells show nuclear and cytoplasmic staining with ALK-1 antibody. In about 15–20% of cases the presence of only cytoplasmic staining with ALK-1 suggests that a variant translocation has occurred.[113]

The cells exhibit an aberrant phenotype with loss of many of the T-cell-associated antigens. Both CD3 and CD45RO, the most widely used pan-T-cell markers, are negative in more than 50% of cases. CD2 and CD4 are positive in the majority of cases, whereas CD8 is usually negative. ALCL cells, despite the CD4$^+$/CD8$^-$ phenotype, do express the cytotoxic associated antigens TIA-1, granzyme B and perforin.[114] Molecular studies in most cases demonstrate T-cell receptor rearrangement, confirming a T-cell origin.

ALCL is most common in children and young adults. However, in elderly patients the t(2;5)/ALK-1 expression is lacking, suggesting that these cases may be part of a different clinicopathologic entity. A marked male predominance, usually presenting with nodal disease, has been noted. However, a high incidence of extranodal site involvement also has been reported (involving skin, bone and soft tissue). About 75% of cases present with advanced stage and systemic symptoms.[115] Although these lymphomas have an aggressive natural clinical history they respond well to chemotherapy; overall survival and disease-free survival are significantly better in ALK-1$^+$ than in ALK-1$^-$cases.[115] Recent studies suggest that the IPI is prognostically useful, in contrast to early reports.[115]

Primary cutaneous anaplastic large cell lymphoma

A primary cutaneous form of ALCL is closely related to lymphomatoid papulosis and differs clinically, immunophenotypically and at the molecular level from the systemic form.[116,117] Indeed, lymphomatoid papulosis and cutaneous ALCL appear to represent a histologic and clinical continuum of 'CD30$^+$ cutaneous lymphoproliferative diseases'. Small lesions are likely to regress, whereas patients with large tumor masses may develop disseminated disease with lymph node involvement. However, primary cutaneous ALCL is a more indolent disease than other T-cell lymphomas of the skin. Most patients with primary cutaneous ALCL have multiple skin lesions. Because the skin nodules may show spontaneous regression, a period of observation is usually warranted before the institution of any chemotherapy.[118] Cutaneous ALCL is CD30$^+$, but usually ALK-1 and EMA negative, and also lacks the t(2;5) translocation.[116,117]

Subcutaneous panniculitis-like T-cell lymphoma

Subcutaneous panniculitis-like T-cell lymphoma is sufficiently distinct to warrant separation from other forms of peripheral T-cell lymphoma.[119] The disease usually presents with subcutaneous nodules, primarily affecting the extremities and ranging in size from 0.5 cm to several centimeters in diameter. Larger nodules may become necrotic. In its early stages the infiltrate may appear deceptively benign, and lesions are often misdiagnosed as panniculitis.[119] However, histologic progression usually occurs and subsequent biopsies show more pronounced cytologic atypia, permitting the diagnosis of malignant lymphoma.

The cytologic composition of subcutaneous panniculitis-like T-cell lymphoma varies. The lesions may contain a predominance of small to medium-sized lymphoid cells with clear cytoplasm, or larger cells with hyperchromatic nuclei. Admixed reactive histiocytes are frequently present, particularly in areas of fat infiltration and destruction. The histiocytes are frequently vacuolated, owing to ingested lipid material. Vascular invasion is seen in some cases, and necrosis and karyorrhexis are common.

The neoplastic cells are $CD8^+$ cytotoxic T cells that are also positive for the cytotoxic proteins perforin, granzyme B and TIA-1.[120] These proteins may be responsible for the cellular destruction seen in these tumors.

A hemophagocytic syndrome is a frequent complication of subcutaneous panniculitis-like T-cell lymphoma.[119] Patients present with fever, pancytopenia and hepatosplenomegaly. It is most readily diagnosed in bone marrow aspirate smears, where histiocytes containing erythrocytes, platelets and other blood elements may be observed. The hemophagocytic syndrome usually heralds a fulminant downhill clinical course. However, if therapy for the underlying lymphoma is instituted and is successful, the hemophagocytic syndrome may remit. A hemophagocytic syndrome is the cause of death in the majority of patients with subcutaneous panniculitis-like T-cell lymphoma. Dissemination to lymph nodes and other organs is uncommon and usually occurs late in the clinical course. The cause of the hemophagocytic syndrome appears to be related to cytokine production by the malignant cells. Interferon-γ, granulocyte–monocyte colony-stimulating factor and MIP-1α have been identified.[121]

It is likely that subcutaneous panniculitis-like T-cell lymphoma is the process previously described as histiocytic cytophagic panniculitis. It had been thought that histiocytic cytophagic panniculitis was a malignant histiocytic proliferation. Although histiocytes may be numerous in these lesions, the malignant cells have a mature T-cell phenotype. Evidence for an association with EBV has been lacking.

Enteropathy-type T-cell lymphoma (ETL)

ETL was originally termed malignant histiocytosis of the intestine.[122] However, the demonstration of clonal T-cell gene rearrangement indicated that it was a T-cell lymphoma. The small bowel usually shows ulceration, frequently with perforation. A mass may or may not be present. The infiltrate shows a varying cytologic composition with an admixture of small, medium and larger atypical lymphoid cells. Anaplastic cells strongly positive for CD30 can be present. The adjacent small bowel can show villous atrophy associated with celiac disease.[123] The neoplastic cells are $CD3^+$, $CD7^+$ T cells that also express the homing receptor CD103 (HML-1).[124] The cells express cytotoxic molecules, a feature shared by nearly all extranodal T-cell lymphomas.

This disease occurs in adults, the majority of whom have either overt or clinically silent gluten-sensitive enteropathy. Patients usually present with abdominal symptoms such as pain, small bowel perforation and associated peritonitis. The clinical course is aggressive.

Hepatosplenic T-cell lymphoma (HSTCL)

The majority of peripheral T lymphocytes belong to the αβ TCR subset, whereas only a minority express the γδ TcR. Similarly, most peripheral T-cell lymphomas are of αβ T-cell derivation. However, there is a unique subtype of peripheral T-cell lymphoma that is derived in most cases from γδ T cells.

HSTCL presents with marked hepatosplenomegaly.[125] The homing pattern manifested by the malignant cells is similar to that of normal γδ T cells, which also populate the sinusoidal areas of the spleen.

HSTCL shows a marked male predominance and most patients are young adults.[126] The clinical presentation is that of marked hepatosplenomegaly in the absence of lymphadenopathy. Abnormal cells are usually present in the bone marrow but may be difficult to identify. They selectively infiltrate the bone marrow sinusoids and can be most easily recognized with immunohistochemical stains.

The cells of HSTCL are usually moderate in size, with a rim of pale cytoplasm. The nuclear chromatin is loosely condensed, with small inconspicuous nucleoli, and usually some irregularity of the nuclear contour can be seen. The liver and spleen show marked sinusoidal infiltration, with sparing of both portal triads and white pulp, respectively. The neoplastic cells have a phenotype that resembles that of normal γδ T cells, usually expressing neither CD4 nor CD8. CD56 is often positive.[125,126] In situ hybridization for EBV is negative.[126] Isochromosome 7 is a consistent cytogenetic abnormality.[127] Rare cases with similar morphological and biological festurers are derived from αβ T cells.

Clinically, HSTCL is aggressive.[126] Although patients may respond initially to chemotherapy, relapse occurs in the vast majority of cases and the median survival is less than 3 years. Other γδ TCL exist, usually presenting in extranodal sites such as the skin and intestine but they are unrelated to HSTCL.

> **CLINICAL PEARLS**
>
> **Hodgkin lymphoma**
> - B-cell lineage established in nearly all cases.
> - Reed-Sternberg cell, the hallmark of the disease, represents a 'crippled' germinal center B cell.
> - Nodular lymphocyte-predominant Hodgkin lymphoma considered a related but distinct entity.
> - Eighty percent of patients are curable with current therapy.
> - Stage of disease guides the choice of therapy; even patients with advanced-stage disease may be cured.
> - Late complications from treatment include acute leukemia (alkylating agents with extended field radiation therapy), second solid tumors (radiation therapy) and premature atherosclerotic coronary artery disease (radiation therapy).
> - Cause of death in the first 5–10 years is mainly Hodgkin lymphoma; after 10 years, mainly secondary malignant tumors.

HODGKIN LYMPHOMA (HODGKIN'S DISEASE)

Hodgkin's disease (HD) and non-Hodgkin lymphoma have long been regarded as distinct disease entities based on their differences in pathology, phenotype, clinical features and response to therapy. In recent years evidence has been accumulating that the malignant cell of HD is in nearly all cases an altered B cell.[128,129] Therefore, it is not surprising that both biological and clinical overlaps should occur between these two lymphoma groups. Although we have become aware of this closer relationship from the histogenetic point of view (hence the name Hodgkin lymphoma, HL), these disorders are still treated with different modalities. The diagnosis of classic HL depends on the identification of classic Reed-Sternberg (RS) cells with an appropriate growth pattern (often interfollicular) in an inflammatory background composed of small T lymphocytes, plasma cells, histiocytes and granulocytes (often eosinophils).

All cases of classic HL share certain immunophenotypic and genotypic features. The phenotype is $CD30^+$, $CD15^{+/-}$, $CD45^-$

and EMA⁻ Expression of B-cell-associated antigens is seen in up to 75% of cases. However, when present, CD20 staining is weaker than the normal B cells and variable in intensity among individual tumor cells. CD79a is usually negative. Ig and TCR genes are usually germline, but rearrangements of Ig genes are reported in some cases, usually with faint bands.[130,131] More recently, using microdissection and single-cell PCR amplification for Ig, several groups have shown clonal rerrangement of the Ig gene accompanied by frequent somatic mutations.[128,129] Epstein–Barr virus is associated with classic HL in about 15–70% of cases, depending on the subtype.

Sufficient evidence has emerged in recent years to warrant the recognition of nodular lymphocyte-predominant Hodgkin's disease as a distinct entity.[132] Although it resembles other types of HL in having a minority of putative neoplastic cells on a background of benign inflammatory cells, it differs morphologically, immunophenotypically and clinically from classic HD.[133–135] The older term paragranuloma has been used by some as synonym for this distinctive tumor.

The category of diffuse lymphocyte predominance in the Rye classification probably includes cases more closely related to classic HL (see lymphocyte-rich classic HL, below).

The proposed WHO classification retains the basic division of Hodgkin's disease into classic Hodgkin's disease and nodular lymphocyte-predominant Hodgkin's disease, which was already proposed by the REAL classification. The renamed Hodgkin lymphoma (HL) reflects the acknowledgment that this disease is indeed a lymphoma and not an atypical reactive process.

Nodular lymphocyte-predominant Hodgkin lymphoma (NLPHL)

NLPHL usually has a nodular growth pattern, with or without diffuse areas; it is rarely purely diffuse. Nodularity may be more easily recognized using immunohistologic stains with anti-B-cell or anti-FDC antibodies. Progressively transformed germinal centers are often seen in partially involved lymph nodes or other lymph node sites. The atypical cells have vesicular, polylobated nuclei and small nucleoli; these have been called L&H cells (lymphocytic and/or histiocytic), or 'popcorn' cells. Although these cells may be very numerous, usually no diagnostic Reed-Sternberg cells are found. The background is predominantly lymphocytes with or without epithelioid histiocyte clusters. Plasma cells are infrequent, and eosinophils and neutrophils are rarely seen.[136] Occasionally sclerosis may cause lesions to resemble nodular sclerosis.

The atypical cells are CD45⁺-expressing B-cell-associated antigens (CD19, 20, 22, 79a), CDw75⁺, EMA⁺/⁻ CD15⁻, CD30⁻/⁺ and usually SIg⁻ by routine techniques, although one study reported light-chain restriction.[137] J chain has been demonstrated in many cases.[138] Small lymphocytes in the nodules are predominantly B cells with a mantle-zone phenotype. However, numerous T cells are present, with CD57⁺ T cells surrounding the L&H cells. The proportion of T cells tends to increase over time in sequential biopsies. A prominent meshwork of FDC is present within the nodules.[133,135,137] Ig and TCR genes are germline by Southern blot analysis. However, by single-cell polymerase chain reaction (PCR) amplification for Ig it has been shown that the L & H cells are either polyclonal and/or clonal.[139,140] Large cells are EBV⁻ in most cases.[141]

NLPHL occurs at all ages, in adults more commonly than in children and in males more than in females. It usually involves peripheral lymph nodes, with sparing of the mediastinum. It is usually localized at diagnosis, but rarely may be disseminated. Survival is long, with or without treatment, for localized cases. Late relapses have been reported to be more common than in other types of HL;[142] it may be associated with or progress to large B-cell lymphoma.[143,144] Prospective clinical studies using different forms of treatment should be attempted to determine the optimal approach to this disorder.

Classic Hodgkin lymphoma, nodular sclerosis (NSHL)

This variant is most common in adolescents and young adults, but can occur at any age; female cases equal or exceed those in males. The mediastinum is commonly involved; stage and bulk of disease have prognostic importance. NSHL is often curable. However, in longterm survivors the risk of secondary malignancies is increased, especially in those receiving both radiation and chemotherapy.

The tumor has at least a partially nodular pattern, with fibrous bands separating the nodules in most cases. Diffuse areas may be present, as is necrosis. The characteristic cell is the lacunar-type RS cell, which may be very numerous. Diagnostic RS cells are usually also present. The background contains lymphocytes, histiocytes, plasma cells, eosinophils and neutrophils. Subclassification according to the number of atypical cells may be clinically relevant; several grading schemes exist (NSI/II,[145] syncytial variant,[146] lymphocyte depleted, cellular phase). However, clinical trials have shown conflicting results. For routine clinical purposes grading will not be required according to the WHO clinical advisory report. However, grading may be useful for clinical trials. The grading scheme of the BNLI (NSI/II) is recommended.[147] The immunophenotype and genotype are characteristic of classic HD.

Classic Hodgkin lymphoma, mixed cellularity (HLMC)

Patients are usually adults; males outnumber females and the stage may be more advanced than in NS or LP types, involving lymph nodes, spleen, liver or marrow. The course is moderately aggressive but is often curable.

The infiltrate is diffuse, without band-forming sclerosis, although fine interstitial fibrosis may be present (Fig. 96.4). RS cells are of the classic type, although some lacunar cells may be seen. The inflammatory background is similar to that of other subtypes

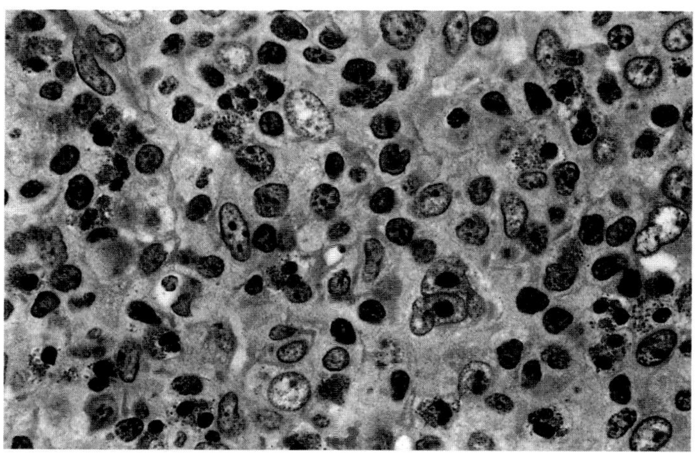

Figure 96.4 Classic Hodgkin lymphoma, mixed cellularity subtype. A classic Reed-Sternberg cell is shown in an inflammatory background with eosinophils, plasma cells and histiocytes.

of classic HL and the immunophenotype and genotype are also similar. The diagnosis is made on routine sections, and immunophenotyping studies are at best an adjunct to the diagnosis.

Classic Hodgkin lymphoma, lymphocyte depletion (HLLD)

This is the least common variant of HL and is most common in older people, in HIV$^+$ individuals[148] and in nonindustrialized countries. It frequently presents with abdominal lymphadenopathy, spleen, liver and bone marrow involvement, without peripheral adenopathy. The stage is usually advanced at diagnosis; however, response to treatment is reported not to differ from other subtypes.[149]

The infiltrate is diffuse and often appears hypocellular, owing to the presence of diffuse fibrosis and necrosis. Relative to the number of normal lymphocytes there are large numbers of RS cells and occasional bizarre 'sarcomatous' variants, with a paucity of other inflammatory cells. Confluent sheets of RS cells and variants may occur and rarely predominate ('reticular' variant, or 'Hodgkin's sarcoma').

The immunophenotype is characteristic of classic HL. Since the histologic differential diagnosis often includes B- or T-large cell lymphoma or ALCL, immunohistochemistry should be performed in most cases. EBV is positive in the majority of cases.

Classic Hodgkin lymphoma, lymphocyte rich (HLLR)

This type of classic HL may be nodular or diffuse and contains relatively infrequent RS cells, which are of the classic type, rather than the variants seen in NLPHL. Some lacunar cells may be present, in a background of lymphocytes, with infrequent eosinophils or plasma cells. In the past many cases of HLLR were misdiagnosed as nodular or diffuse lymphocyte-predominant HL. In contrast to NLPHL, the RS cells have the morphology and immunophenotype of classic RS cells. The immunophenotype and genetic features are similar to those of the other variants of classic HL. Patients usually present with localized disease.[144] This variant of HL was a provisional form of HD in the REAL classification and has been retained in the WHO classification. The nodular form has been recognized more recently.[150]

REFERENCES

1. Lukes R, Collins R. Immunologic characterization of human malignant lymphomas. Cancer 1974;34:1488.
2. Harris NL, Jaffe ES, Stein H, et al. A revised European-American classification of lymphoid neoplasms: a proposal from the International Lymphoma Study Group. Blood 1994;84:1361.
3. The Non-Hodgkin's Lymphoma Classification Project. A clinical evaluation of the International Lymphoma Study Group classification of non-Hodgkin's lymphoma. Blood 1997;89:3909.
4. Gisselbrecht C, Gaulard P, Lepage E, et al. Prognostic significance of T-cell phenotype in aggressive non-Hodgkin's lymphomas. Groupe d'Etudes des Lymphomes de l'Adulte (GELA). Blood 1998;92:76.
5. Shipp MA. Prognostic factors in aggressive non-Hodgkin's lymphoma: who has 'high risk' disease? Blood 1994;83:1165.
6. Lennert K, Tamm I, Wacker H-H. Histopathology and immunocytochemistry of lymph node biopsies in chronic lymphocytic leukemia and immunocytoma. Leuk Lymphoma 1991;7 (Suppl):157.
7. Zukerberg L, Medeiros L, Ferry J, Harris N. Diffuse low-grade B-cell lymphomas: four clinically distinct subtypes defined by a combination of morphologic and immunophenotypic features. Am J Clin Pathol 1993;100:373.
8. Desikan R, Dhodapkar M, Siegel D, et al. High-dose therapy with autologous haemopoietic stem cell support for Waldenstrom's macroglobulinemia. Br J Haematol 1999;105:993.
9. Offit K, Parsa NZ, Filippa D, Jhanwar SC, Chaganti RS. t(9;14)(p13;q32) denotes a subset of low-grade non-Hodgkin's lymphoma with plasmacytoid differentiation. Blood 1992;80:2594.
10. Iida S, Rao P, Nallasivam P, et al. The t(9;14)(p13;q32) chromosomal translocation associated with lymphoplasmacytoid lymphoma involves the PAX-5 gene. Blood 1996;88:4110.
11. Sundeen J, Longo D, Jaffe E. CD5 expression in B-cell small lymphocytic malignancies: correlations with clinical presentation and sites of disease. Am J Surg Pathol 1992;16:130.
12. Aoki H, Takishita M, Kosaka M, Saito S. Frequent somatic mutations in D and/or JH segments of Ig gene in Waldenstrom's macroglobulinemia and chronic lymphocytic leukemia (CLL) with Richter's syndrome but not in common CLL. Blood 1995;85:1913.
13. Banks P, Chan J, Cleary M, et al. Mantle cell lymphoma: a proposal for unification of morphologic, immunologic, and molecular data. Am J Surg Pathol 1992;16:637.
14. Jaffe ES, Bookman MA, Longo DL. Lymphocytic lymphoma of intermediate differentiation – mantle zone lymphoma. Hum Pathol 1987;18:877.
15. Fisher RI, Dahlberg S, Nathwani BN, Banks PM, Miller TP, Grogan TM. A clinical analysis of two indolent lymphoma entities: mantle cell lymphoma and marginal zone lymphoma (including the mucosa-associated lymphoid tissue and monocytoid B-cell subcategories): a Southwest Oncology Group study. Blood 1995;85:1075.
16. Teodorovic I, Pittaluga S, Kluin-Nelemans J, et al. Efficacy of four different regimens in 64 mantle-cell lymphoma cases: clinicopathologic comparison with 498 other non-Hodgkin's lymphoma subtypes. J Clin Oncol 1995;13:2819.
17. Argatoff LH, Connors JM, Klasa RJ, Horsman DE, Gascoyne RD. Mantle cell lymphoma: a clinicopathologic study of 80 cases. Blood 1997;89:2067.
18. Velders G, Kluin-Nelemans J, De Boer C, et al. Mantle-cell lymphoma: a population-based clinical study. J Clin Oncol 1996;14:1269.
19. O'Briain D, Kennedy M, Daly P, et al. Multiple lymphomatous polyposis of the gastrointestinal tract: a clinicopathologically distinctive form of non-Hodgkin's lymphoma of centrocytic type. Am J Surg Pathol 1989;13:691.
20. Freedman A, Neuberg D, Gribben J, et al. High-dose chemoradiotherapy and anti-B-cell monoclonal antibody-purged autologous bone marrow transplantation in mantle-cell lymphoma: no evidence for long-term remission. J Clin Oncol. 1998;16:13.
21. Lardelli P, Bookman MA, Sundeen J, Longo DL, Jaffe ES. Lymphocytic lymphoma of intermediate differentiation. Morphologic and immunophenotypic spectrum and clinical correlations. Am J Surg Pathol 1990;14:752.
22. Greiner T, Moynihan M, Chan W, et al. p53 mutations in mantle cell lymphoma are associated with variant cytology and predict a poor prognosis. Blood 1996;87:4302.
23. Raffeld M, Sander CA, Yano T, Jaffe ES. Mantle cell lymphoma: an update. Leuk Lymphoma 1992;8:161.
24. Bosch F, Jares P, Campo E, et al. PRAD-1/cyclin D1 gene overexpression in chronic lymphoproliferative disorders: a highly specific marker of mantle cell lymphoma. Blood. 1994;84:2726.
25. Jares P, Campo E, Pinyol M, et al. Expression of retinoblastoma gene product (pRb) in mantle cell lymphomas. Correlation with cyclin D1 (PRAD1/CCND1) mRNA levels and proliferative activity. Am J Pathol 1996;148:1591.
26. Quintanilla-Martinez L, Thieblemont C, Fend F, et al. Mantle cell lymphomas lack expression of p27Kip1, a cyclin-dependent kinase inhibitor. Am J Pathol 1998;153:175.

27. Pinyol M, Hernandez L, Cazorla M, et al. Deletions and loss of expression of p16INK4a and p21Waf1 genes are associated with aggressive variants of mantle cell lymphomas. Blood 1997;89:272.
28. Hummel M, Tamaru J, Kalvelage B, Stein H. Mantle cell (previously centrocytic) lymphomas express VH genes with no or very little somatic mutations like the physiologic cells of the follicle mantle. Blood 1994;84:403.
29. Non-Hodgkin's Lymphoma Pathologic Classification Project. National Cancer Institute sponsored study of classifications of non-Hodgkin's lymphomas: summary and description of a Working Formulation for clinical usage. Cancer 1982;49:2112.
30. Come ES, Jaffe ES, Andersen JC, et al. Non-Hodgkin's lymphomas in leukemic phase: Clinicopathologic correlations. Am J Med 1980;69:667.
31. Horning S, Rosenberg S. The natural history of initially untreated low-grade non-Hodgkin's lymphomas. N Engl J Med 1984;311:1471.
32. Young R, Longo D, Glatstein E, Ihde D, Jaffe E, DeVita VJ. The treatment of indolent lymphomas: watchful waiting v aggressive combined modality treatment. Semin Hematol 1988;25:11.
33. Rohatiner A, Johnson P, Price C, et al. Myeloablative therapy with autologous bone marrow transplantation as consolidation therapy for recurrent follicular lymphoma. J Clin Oncol 1994;12:1177.
34. Liu S, Eary J, Petersdorf S, et al. Follow-up of relapsed B-cell lymphoma patients treated with iodine-131-labeled anti-CD20 antibody and autologous stem-cell rescue. J Clin Oncol 1998;16:3270.
35. Mann R, Berard C. Criteria for the cytologic subclassification of follicular lymphomas: a proposed alternative method. Hematol Oncol 1982;1:187.
36. Croce C, Nowell P. Molecular basis of human B cell neoplasia. Blood 1985;65:1.
37. Hockenbery D, Zutter M, Hickey W, Nahm M, Korsmeyer S. BCL2 protein is topographically restricted in tissues characterized by apoptotic cell death. Proc Natl Acad Sci USA. 1991;88:6961.
38. Gaulard P, d'Agay M, Peuchmaur M, et al. Expression of the bcl-2 gene product in follicular lymphoma. Am J Pathol 1992;140:1089.
39. Garcia CF, Weiss LM, Warnke RA, Wood GS. Cutaneous follicular lymphoma. Am J Surg Pathol 1986;10:454.
40. Santucci M, Pimpinelli N, Arganini L. Primary cutaneous B-cell lymphoma: a unique type of low-grade lymphoma. Clinicopathologic and immunologic study of 83 cases. Cancer 1991;67:2311.
41. Jaffe ES, Raffeld M, Medeiros LJ. Histopathologic subtypes of indolent lymphomas: caricatures of the mature B-cell system. Semin Oncol 1993;20:3.
42. Jaffe ES, Shevach EM, Frank M, Berard CW, Green I. Nodular lymphoma: evidence for origin from follicular B lymphocytes. N Engl J Med 1974;290:813.
43. Kuppers R, Zhao M, Hansmann ML, Rajewsky K. Tracing B cell development in human germinal centres by molecular analysis of single cells picked from histological sections. *EMBO* J 1993;12:4955.
44. Isaacson P, Wright D. Malignant lymphoma of mucosa associated lymphoid tissue. A distinctive B cell lymphoma. Cancer 1983;52:1410.
45. Isaacson P, Wotherspoon A, Diss T, Pan L. Follicular colonization in B cell lymphoma of mucosa associated lymphoid tissue. Am J Surg Pathol 1991;15:819.
46. Pelstring R, Essell J, Kurtin P, Banks P. Diversity of organ site involvement among malignant lymphomas of mucosa-associated tissues. Am J Clin Pathol 1991;96:738.
47. Cogliatti S, Lennert K, Hansmann M, Zwingers T. Monocytoid B cell lymphoma: clinical and prognostic features of 21 patients. J Clin Pathol 1990;43:619.
48. Ortiz-Hidalgo C, Wright DH. The morphological spectrum of monocytoid B-cell lymphoma, and its relationship to lymphomas of mucosa-associate lymphoid tissue. Histopathology 1992;21:555.
49. Hussell T, Isaacson P, Crabtree J, Spencer J. The response of cells from low-grade B-cell gastric lymphomas of mucosa-associated lymphoid tissue to *Helicobacter pylori*. Lancet 1993;342:571.
50. Wotherspoon A, Doglioni C, Diss T, et al. Regression of primary low-grade B-cell gastric lymphoma of mucosa-associated lymphoid tissue type after eradication of *Helicobacter pylori*. Lancet. 1993;342:575.
51. Auer IA, Gascoyne RD, Connors JM, et al. t(11;18)(q21;q21) is the most common translocation in MALT lymphomas. Ann Oncol 1997;8:979.
52. Dierlamm J, Baens M, Wlodarska I, et al. The apoptosis inhibitor gene API2 and a novel 18q gene, MLT, are recurrently rearranged in the t(11;18)(q21;q21)p6ssociated with mucosa-associated lymphoid tissue lymphomas. Blood 1999;93:3601.
53. Rosenwald A, Ott G, Stilgenbauer S, et al. Exclusive detection of the t(11;18)(q21;q21) in extranodal marginal zone B cell lymphomas (MZBL) of MALT type in contrast to other MZBL and extranodal large B cell lymphomas. Am J Pathol 1999;155:1817.
54. Quin Y, Greiner A, Trunk M, Schmausser B, Ott MM, Muller-Hermelink HK. Somatic hypermutation in low-grade mucosa-associated lymphoid tissue-type B-cell lymphoma. Blood 1995;86:3528.
55. Tierens A, Delabie J, Pittaluga S, Driessen A, De Wolf-Peeters C. Mutation analysis of the rearranged immunoglobulin heavy chain genes of marginal zone cell lymphomas indicates an origin from different marginal zone B cell subsets. Blood 1998;91:2381.
56. Sheibani K, Burke J, Swartz W, Nademanee A, Winberg C. Monocytoid B cell lymphoma. Clinicopathologic study of 21 cases of a unique type of low grade lymphoma. Cancer 1988;62:1531.
57. Nathwani BN, Anderson JR, Armitage JO, et al. Marginal zone B-cell lymphoma: a clinical comparison of nodal and mucosa-associated lymphoid tissue types. Non-Hodgkin's Lymphoma Classification Project. J Clin Oncol 1999;17:2486.
58. Campo E, Miquel R, Krenacs L, Sorbara L, Raffeld M, Jaffe ES. Primary nodal marginal zone lymphomas of splenic and MALT type. Am J Surg Pathol 1999;23:59.
59. Ngan B-Y, Warnke R, Wilson M, Takagi K, Cleary M, Dorfman R. Monocytoid B-cell lymphoma: a study of 36 cases. Hum Pathol 1991;22:409.
60. Nathwani BN, Anderson JR, Armitage JO, et al. Clinical significance of follicular lymphoma with monocytoid B cells. Non-Hodgkin's Lymphoma Classification Project. Hum Pathol. 1999;30:263.
61. Isaacson PG, Matutes E, Burke M, Catovsky D. The histopathology of splenic lymphoma with villous lymphocytes. Blood 1994;84:3828.
62. Mollejo M, Menarguez J, Lloret E, et al. Splenic marginal zone lymphoma: a distinctive type of low-grade B-cell lymphoma. A clinicopathological study of 13 cases. Am J Surg Pathol 1995;19:1146.
63. Schmid C, Kirkham N, Diss T, Isaacson P. Splenic marginal zone cell lymphoma. Am J Surg Pathol 1992;16:455.
64. Zhu D, Oscier DG, Stevenson FK. Splenic lymphoma with villous lymphocytes involves B cells with extensively mutated Ig heavy chain variable region genes. Blood 1995;85:1603.
65. Longo DL, Duffey PL, DeVita VJ, et al. Treatment of advanced-stage Hodgkin's disease: alternating noncrossresistant MOPP/CABS is not superior to MOPP. J Clin Oncol 1991;9:1409.
66. Miller TP, Grogan TM, Dahlberg S, et al. Prognostic significance of the Ki-67 associated proliferative antigen in aggressive non-Hodgkin's lymphomas: a prospective Southwest Oncology Group trial. Blood 1994;83:1460.
67. Wilson WH, Teruya-Feldstein J, Fest T, et al. Relationship of p53, bcl-2, and tumor proliferation to clinical drug resistance in non-Hodgkin's lymphomas. Blood 1997;89:601.
68. Hall PA, Richards MA, Gregory WM, d'Ardenne AJ, Lister TA, Stansfeld AG. The prognostic value of Ki67 immunostaining in non-Hodgkin's lymphoma. J Pathol 1988;154:223.
69. Gerdes J, Stein H, Pileri S, et al. Prognostic relevance of tumour-cell growth fraction in malignant non-Hodgkin's lymphomas [letter] (published erratum appears in Lancet 1987; 2(8561):756). Lancet 1987;2:448.
70. Piris MA, Pezzella F, Martinez MJ, et al. p53 and bcl-2 expression in high-grade B-cell lymphomas: correlation with survival time [published erratum appears in Br J Cancer 1994; 69(5):978). Br J Cancer 1994;69:337.
71. Gascoyne RD, Adomat SA, Krajewski S, et al. Prognostic significance of Bcl-2 protein expression and Bcl-2 gene rearrangement in diffuse aggressive non-Hodgkin's lymphoma. Blood 1997;90:244.
72. Kramer M, Hermans J, Wijburg E, et al. Clinical relevance of BCL2, BCL6, and MYC rearrangements in diffuse large B-cell lymphoma. Blood 1998;92:3152.

73. Offit K, Lo CF, Louie DC, et al. Rearrangement of the bcl-6 gene as a prognostic marker in diffuse large-cell lymphoma. N Engl J Med 1994;331:74.
74. Engelhard M, Brittinger G, Huhn D, et al. Subclassification of diffuse large B-cell lymphomas according to the Kiel classification: distinction of centroblastic and immunoblastic lymphomas is a significant prognostic risk factor. Blood 1997;89:2291.
75. Lamarre L, Jacobson J, Aisenberg A, Harris N. Primary large cell lymphoma of the mediastinum. Am J Surg Pathol 1989;13:730.
76. Jaffe E. Post-thymic lymphoid neoplasia. In: Jaffe E (ed) Surgical pathology of the lymph nodes and related organs. Philadelphia, WB Saunders, 1985, p 218.
77. Delabie J, Vandenberghe E, Kennes C, et al. Histiocyte-rich B-cell lymphoma. A distinct clinicopathologic entity possibly related to lymphocyte predominant Hodgkin's disease, paragranuloma subtype. Am J Surg Pathol 1992;16:37.
78. Macon W, Williams M, Greer J, Stein R, Collins R, Cousar J. T-cell-rich B-cell lymphomas. A clinicopathologic study of 19 cases. Am J Surg Pathol 1992;16:351.
79. Ramsay A, Smith W, Isaacson P. T-cell-rich B-cell lymphoma. Am J Surg Pathol 1988;12:433.
80. Krishnan J, Wallberg K, Frizzera G. T-cell rich large B-cell lymphoma: a study of 30 cases supporting its histologic heterogeneity and lack of clinical distinctiveness. Am J Surg Pathol 1994;18:455.
81. Hofmann WJ, Momburg F, Moller P. Thymic medullary cells expressing B-lymphocyte antigens. Hum Pathol 1988;19:1280.
82. Kanavaros P, Gaulard P, Charlotte F, et al. Discordant expression of immunoglobulin and its associated molecule mb-1/CD79a is frequently found in mediastinal large B-cell lymphomas. Am J Pathol 1995;146:735.
83. Copie-Bergman C, Gaulard P, Maouche-Chretien L, et al. The MAL gene is expressed in primary mediastinal large B-cell lymphoma. Blood 1999;94:3567.
84. Scarpa A, Borgato L, Chilosi M, et al. Evidence of c-myc gene abnormalities in mediastinal large B-cell lymphoma of young adult age. Blood 1991;78:780.
85. Joos S, Otano-Joos MI, Ziegler S, et al. Primary mediastinal (thymic) B-cell lymphoma is characterized by gains of chromosomal material including 9p and amplification of the REL gene. Blood 1996;87:1571.
86. Zinzani PL, Martelli M, Magagnoli M, et al. Treatment and clinical management of primary mediastinal large B-cell lymphoma with sclerosis: MACOP-B regimen and mediastinal radiotherapy monitored by 67gallium scan in 50 patients. Blood 1999;94:3289.
87. Magrath I, Shiramizu B. Biology and treatment of small non-cleaved cell lymphoma. Oncology 1989;3:41.
88. Ballerini P, Gaidano G, Gong JZ, et al. Multiple genetic lesions in acquired immunodeficiency syndrome-related non-Hodgkin's lymphoma. Blood 1993;81:166.
89. Pelicci P, Knowles D, Magrath I, Dalla-Favera R. Chromosomal breakpoints and structural alterations of the c-myc locus differ in endemic and sporadic forms of Burkitt lymphoma. Proc Natl Acad Sci USA 1986;83:2984.
90. Goldschmidts WL, Bhatia K, Johnson JF, et al. Epstein–Barr virus genotypes in AIDS-associated lymphomas are similar to those in endemic Burkitt's lymphomas. Leukemia 1992;6:875.
91. Longo DL, Duffey PL, Jaffe ES, et al. Diffuse small noncleaved-cell, non-Burkitt's lymphoma in adults: a high-grade lymphoma responsive to ProMACE-based combination chemotherapy. J Clin Oncol 1994;12:2153.
92. Suchi T, Lennert K, Tu L-Y. Histopathology and immunohistochemistry of peripheral T-cell lymphomas: a proposal for their classification. J Clin Pathol 1987;40:995.
93. Levine PH, Cleghorn F, Manns A, et al. Adult T-cell leukemia/lymphoma: a working point-score classification for epidemiological studies. Int J Cancer 1994;59:491.
94. Hastrup N, Hamilton-Dutoit S, Ralfkiaer E, Pallesen G. Peripheral T-cell lymphomas: an evaluation of reproducibility of the updated Kiel classification. Histopathology 1991;18:99.
95. Schlegelberger B, Himmler A, Godde E, Grote W, Feller AC, Lennert K. Cytogenetic findings in peripheral T-cell lymphomas as a basis for distinguishing low-grade and high-grade lymphomas. Blood 1994;83:505.
96. Ho F, Choy D, Loke S, et al. Polymorphic reticulosis and conventional lymphomas of the nose and upper aerodigestive tract – a clinicopathologic study of 70 cases, and immunophenotypic studies of 16 cases. Hum Pathol 1990;21:1041.
97. Ferry JA, Sklar J, Zukerberg LR, Harris NL. Nasal lymphoma: a clinicopathologic study with immunophenotypic and genotypic analysis. Am J Surg Pathol 1991;15:268.
98. Imamura N, Kusunoki Y, Kawa-Ha K, et al. Aggressive natural killer cell leukaemia/lymphoma: report of four cases and review of the literature. Possible existence of a new clinical entity originating from the third lineage of lymphoid cells [see comments]. Br J Haematol 1990;75:49.
99. Jaffe ES, Chan JKC, Su IJ, et al. Report of the workshop on nasal and related extranodal angiocentric T/NK cell lymphomas: definitions, differential diagnosis, and epidemiology. Am J Surg Pathol 1996;20:103.
100. Medeiros LJ, Peiper SC, Elwood L, Yano T, Raffeld M, Jaffe ES. Angiocentric immunoproliferative lesions: a molecular analysis of eight cases. Hum Pathol 1991;22:1150.
101. Ho F, Srivastava G, Loke S, et al. Presence of Epstein–Barr virus DNA in nasal lymphomas of B and T cell type. Hematol Oncol 1990;8:271.
102. Jaffe ES, Costa J, Fauci AS, Cossman J, Tsokos M. Malignant lymphoma and erythrophagocytosis simulating malignant histiocytosis. Am J Med 1983;75:741.
103. Frizzera G, Moran E, Rappaport H. Angio-immunoblastic lymphadenopathy with dysproteinemia. Lancet 1974;i:1070.
104. Feller A, Griesser H, Schilling C, et al. Clonal gene rearrangement patterns correlate with immunophenotype and clinical parameters in patients with angioimmunoblastic lymphadenopathy. Am J Pathol 1988;133:549.
105. Siegert W, Agthe A, Griesser H, et al. Treatment of angioimmunoblastic lymphadenopathy (AILD)-type T-cell lymphoma using prednisone with or without the COPBLAM/IMVP-16 regimen. A multicenter study. Kiel Lymphoma Study Group. Ann Intern Med 1992;117:364.
106. Patsouris E, Noel H, Lennert K. Histological and immunohistological findings in lymphoepithelioid cell lymphoma (Lennert's lymphoma). Am J Surg Pathol 1988;12:341.
107. Coiffier B, Brousse N, Peuchmaur M, et al. Peripheral T-cell lymphomas have a worse prognosis than B-cell lymphomas: a prospective study of 361 immunophenotyped patients treated with the LNH-84 regimen. Ann Oncol 1990;1:45.
108. Stein H, Lennert K, Feller A, Mason D. Immunological analysis of tissue sections in diagnosis of lymphoma. In: Hoffbrand A (ed) Recent advances in haematology. New York, Churchill Livingstone, 1985; p 127.
109. Agnarsson B, Kadin M. Ki-1 positive large cell lymphoma: a morphologic and immunologic study of 19 cases. Am J Surg Pathol 1988;12:264.
110. Piris M, Brown D, Gatter K, Mason D. CD30 Expression in non-Hodgkin's lymphoma. Histopathology 1990;17:211.
111. Morris SW, Kirstein MN, Valentine MB, et al. Fusion of a kinase gene, ALK, to a nucleolar protein gene, NPM, in non-Hodgkin's lymphoma [published erratum appears in Science 1995; 267(5196):316]. Science 1994;263:1281.
112. Pulford K, Lamant L, Morris SW, et al. Detection of anaplastic lymphoma kinase (ALK) and nucleolar protein nucleophosmin (NPM) ALK proteins in normal and neoplastic cells with the monoclonal antibody ALK1. Blood 1997;89:1394.
113. Falini B, Pulford K, Pucciarini A, et al. Lymphomas expressing ALK fusion protein(s) other than NPM-ALK. Blood 1999;94:3509.
114. Krenacs L, Wellmann A, Sorbara L, et al. Cytotoxic cell antigen expression in anaplastic large cell lymphomas of T- and null-cell type and Hodgkin's disease: evidence for distinct cellular origin. Blood 1997;89:980.
115. Falini B, Pileri S, Zinzani PL, et al. ALK+ lymphoma: clinicopathological findings and outcome. Blood 1999;93:2697.
116. DeCoteau JF, Butmarc JR, Kinney MC, Kadin ME. The t(2;5) chromosomal translocation is not a common feature of primary cutaneous CD30+ lymphoproliferative disorders: comparison with anaplastic large-cell lymphoma of nodal origin. Blood 1996;87:3437.

117. Wellmann A, Otsuki T, Vogelbruch M, Clark HM, Jaffe ES, Raffeld M. Analysis of the t(2;5) (p23;q35) translocation by reverse transcription-polymerase chain reaction in CD 30+ anaplastic large-cell lymphomas, in other non-Hodgkin's of T-cell phenotype, and in Hodgkin's disease. Blood 1995;86:2321.
118. Paulli M, Berti E, Rosso R, et al. CD30/Ki-1-positive lymphoproliferative disorders of the skin – clinicopathologic correlation and statistical analysis of 86 cases: a multicentric study from the European Organization for Research and Treatment of Cancer Cutaneous Lymphoma Project Group. J Clin Oncol 1995;13:1343.
119. Gonzalez CL, Medeiros LJ, Braziel RM, Jaffe ES. T-cell lymphoma involving subcutaneous tissue: a clinicopathologic entity commonly associated with hemophagocytic syndrome. Am J Surg Pathol 1991;15:17.
120. Kumar S, Krenacs L, Elenitoba-Johnson K, et al. Subcutaneous panniculitic T-cell lymphoma is a tumor of cytotoxic T-lymphocytes. Hum Pathol 1998;29:397.
121. Teruya-Feldstein J, Setsuda J, Yao X, et al. MIP-1 alpha expression in tissues from patients with hemophagocytic syndrome. Lab Invest 1999;79:1583.
122. Isaacson P, Spencer J, Connolly C, et al. Malignant histiocytosis of the intestine: a T-cell lymphoma. Lancet 1985;ii:688.
123. Chott A, Dragosics B, Radaszkiewicz T. Peripheral T-cell lymphomas of the intestine. Am J Pathol 1992;141:1361.
124. Spencer J, Cerf-Bensussan N, Jarry A, et al. Enteropathy-associated T-cell lymphoma is recognized by a monoclonal antibody (HML-1) that defines a membrane molecule on human mucosal lymphocytes. Am J Pathol 1988;132:1.
125. Farcet J, Gaulard P, Marolleau J, et al. Hepatosplenic T-cell lymphoma: sinusal/sinusoidal localization of malignant cells expressing the T-cell receptor gd. Blood 1990;75:2213.
126. Cooke CB, Krenacs M, Stetler-Stevenson M, et al. Hepatosplenic gamma/delta T-cell lymphoma: a distinct clinicopathologic entity of cytotoxic gamma/delta T-cell origin. Blood 1996;88:4265.
127. Wang CC, Tien HF, Lin MT, et al. Consistent presence of isochromosome 7q in hepatosplenic T gamma/delta lymphoma: a new cytogenetic-clinicopathologic entity. Genes Chromosom Cancer 1995;12:161.
128. Kuppers R, Rajewsky K, Zhao M, et al. Hodgkin's disease: Hodgkin and Reed Sternberg cells picked from histological sections show clonal immunoglobulin gene rearrangements and appear to be derived from B cells at various stages of development. Proc Natl Acad Sci USA 1994;91:1092.
129. Kanzler H, Kuppers R, Hansmann ML, Rajewsky K. Hodgkin and Reed-Sternberg cells in Hodgkin's disease represent the outgrowth of a dominant tumor clone derived from (crippled) germinal center B cells. J Exp Med 1996;184:1495.
130. Knowles D, Neri A, Pelicci P, et al. Immunoglobulin and T-cell receptor beta-chain gene rearrangement analysis of Hodgkin's disease: implications for lineage determination and differential diagnosis. Proc Natl Acad Sci USA 1986;83:7942.
131. Sundeen J, Lipford E, Uppenkamp J, et al. Rearranged antigen receptor genes in Hodgkin's disease. Blood 1987;70:96.
132. Mason D, Banks P, Chan J, et al. Nodular lymphocyte predominance Hodgkin's disease: a distinct clinico-pathological entity. Am J Surg Pathol 1994;18:528.
133. Pinkus G, Said J. Hodgkin's disease, lymphocyte predominance type, nodular – further evidence for a B cell derivation: L&H variants of Reed-Sternberg cells express L26, a pan B cell marker. Am J Pathol 1988;133:211.
134. Schmid C, Pan L, Diss T, Isaacson P. Expression of B-cell antigens by Hodgkin's and Reed-Sternberg cells. Am J Pathol 1991;139:701.
135. Pinkus G, Said J. Hodgkin's disease, lymphocyte predominance type, nodular – a distinct entity? Unique staining profile of L&H variants of Reed-Sternberg cells defined by monoclonal antibodies to leukocyte common antigen, granulocyte specific antigen, and B-cell specific antigen. Am J Pathol 1985;116:1.
136. Burns B, Colby T, Dorfman R. Differential diagnostic features of nodular L&H Hodgkin's disease, including progressive transformation of germinal centers. Am J Surg Pathol 1984;8:253.
137. Schmid C, Sargent C, Isaacson P. L and H cells of nodular lymphocyte predominant Hodgkin's disease show immunoglobulin light-chain restriction. Am J Pathol 1991;139:1281.
138. Stein H, Hansmann M, Lennert K, Brandtzaeg P, Gatter K, Mason D. Reed-Sternberg and Hodgkin cells in lymphocyte-predominant Hodgkin's disease of nodular subtype contain J chain. Am J Clin Pathol 1986;86:292.
139. Delabie J, Tierens A, Wu G, Weisenburger DD, Chan WC. Lymphocyte predominance Hodgkin's disease: lineage and clonality determination using a single-cell assay. Blood 1994;84:3291.
140. Marafioti T, Hummel M, Anagnostopoulos I, et al. Origin of nodular lymphocyte-predominant Hodgkin's disease from a clonal expansion of highly mutated germinal-center B cells. N Engl J Med 1997;337:453.
141. Weiss L, Chen Y, Liu X, Shibata D. Epstein–Barr virus and Hodgkin's disease: a correlative in situ hybridization and polymerase chain reaction study. Am J Pathol 1991;139:1259.
142. Regula D, Hoppe R, Weiss L. Nodular and diffuse types of lymphocyte predominance Hodgkin's disease. N Engl J Med 1988;318:214.
143. Bennett M, MacLennan K, Hudson G, Hudson B. Non-Hodgkin's lymphoma arising in patients treated for Hodgkin's disease in the BNLI: a 20-year experience. Ann Oncol 1991;2 (Suppl 2):83.
144. Diehl V, Sextro M, Franklin J, et al. Clinical presentation, course, and prognostic factors in lymphocyte-predominant Hodgkin's disease and lymphocyte-rich classical Hodgkin's disease: report from the European Task Force on Lymphoma Project on Lymphocyte-Predominant Hodgkin's Disease [see comments]. J Clin Oncol 1999;17:776.
145. Ferry JA, Linggood RM, Convery KM, Efird JT, Eliseo R, Harris NL. Hodgkin disease, nodular sclerosis type. Implications of histologic subclassification. Cancer 1993;71:457.
146. Strickler J, Michie S, Warnke R, Dorfman R. The 'syncytial variant' of nodular sclerosing Hodgkin's disease. Am J Surg Pathol 1986;10:470.
147. Harris NL, Jaffe ES, Diebold J, et al. World health organization classification of neoplastic diseases of the hematopoietic and lymphoid tissues: report of the clinical advisory committee meeting – Airlie House, Virginia, November 1997. J Clin Oncol 1999;17:3835.
148. Pelstring R, Zellmer R, Sulak L, Banks P, Clare N. Hodgkin's disease in association with human immunodeficiency virus infection. Cancer 1991;67:1865.
149. Kant JA, Hubbard SM, Longo DL, Simon RM, DeVita VT, Jaffe ES. The pathologic and clinical heterogeneity of lymphocyte-depleted Hodgkin's disease. J Clin Oncol 1986;4:284.
150. Ashton-Key M, Thorpe PA, Allen JP, Isaacson PG. Follicular Hodgkin's disease. Am J Surg Pathol 1995;19:1294.

Section 9 Immunology of Neoplasia

Chapter 97

Monoclonal Gammopathies

Robert A. Kyle and Angela Dispenzieri

The monoclonal gammopathies (paraproteinemias, dysproteinemias) are a group of disorders characterized by the proliferation of a single clone of plasma cells that produce an immunologically homogeneous (monoclonal) protein (M-protein, paraprotein). Each M-protein consists of two heavy polypeptide chains of the same class, designated as γ in IgG, α in IgA, μ in IgM, δ in IgD and ε in IgE, and two associated light chains of the same type (κ or λ).

The monoclonal gammopathies include monoclonal gammopathy of undetermined significance (MGUS), multiple myeloma (MM), smoldering multiple myeloma (SMM), plasma cell leukemia, nonsecretory myeloma, solitary plasmacytoma (bone or extramedullary), osteosclerotic myeloma (POEMS syndrome), Waldenström's macroglobulinemia (WM), heavy-chain diseases (HCD), and primary systemic amyloidosis (AL).

The distribution of serum M-proteins in 1050 new cases at the Mayo Clinic during 1998 is shown in Figure 97.1 and the diseases associated with them in Figure 97.2.

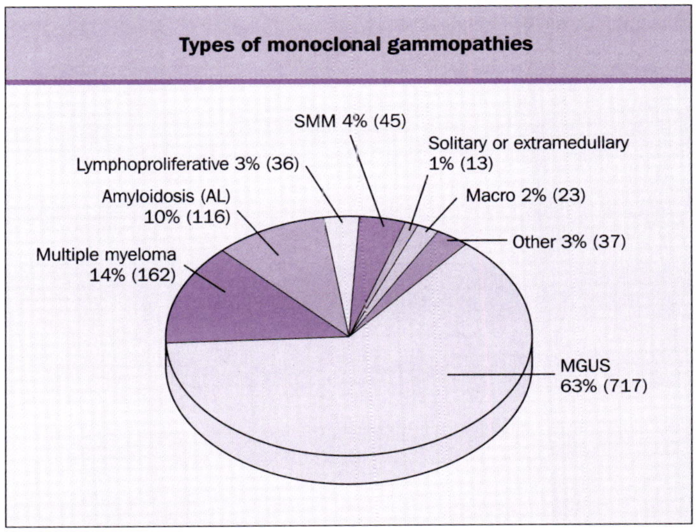

Figure 97.2 Types of monoclonal gammopathies. Data are from 1149 Mayo Clinic cases in 1998. Macro, macroglobulinemia; MGUS, monoclonal gammopathy of undetermined significance; SMM, smoldering multiple myeloma. (From Kyle RA, Rajkumar SV. Monoclonal gammopathies of undetermined significance. *Hematol Oncol Clin North Am* 1999;13:1181 with permission.)

RECOGNITION OF M-PROTEINS IN SERUM AND URINE

High-resolution agarose gel electrophoresis is preferred for the detection of an M-protein. Immunofixation should be used to confirm the presence of an M-protein and to identify the heavy-chain type and the light-chain class.[1] Serum protein electrophoresis should be performed whenever MM, WM or AL is suspected and, if clinical suspicion is high, immunofixation studies should be done despite a normal serum electrophoretic pattern. These studies are also indicated in the presence of unexplained back pain, weakness or fatigue, recurrent infections, anemia, hypercalcemia, renal insufficiency, osteoporosis or lytic lesions. It should also be performed in all patients with a sensorimotor peripheral neuropathy, nephrotic syndrome, orthostatic hypotension, refractory congestive heart failure, carpal tunnel syndrome or malabsorption of unknown cause, because the presence of an M-protein in one of these syndromes strongly suggests AL.

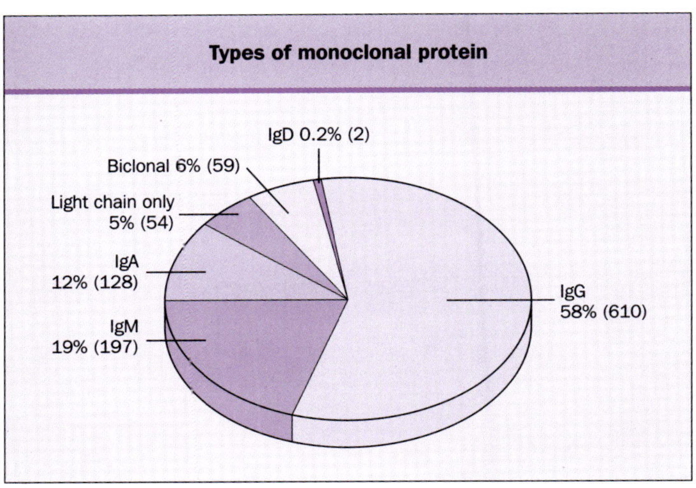

Figure 97.1 Types of monoclonal proteins. Data are from 1050 Mayo Clinic cases in 1998.

An M-protein appears as a narrow peak or spike in the densitometer tracing or as a discrete band on agarose gel (Fig. 97.3).[2] In contrast, an excess of polyclonal immunoglobulins (having one or more heavy-chain types and both κ and λ light chains) produces a broad-based peak or band. It is important to differentiate an M-protein from a polyclonal increase because the former is associated with a neoplastic process or a potentially malignant condition, whereas a polyclonal increase in immunoglobulins is associated with a reactive or inflammatory process. An M-protein may exist even when the total protein level, β and γ globulin concentrations and quantitative immunoglobulin values are all within the normal limits. A monoclonal light chain in the serum (Bence Jones proteinemia) is rarely recognized with agarose gel

KEY CONCEPTS

Classification of monoclonal gammopathies
- Monoclonal gammopathy of undetermined significance (MGUS) (benign monoclonal gammopathy)
- Multiple myeloma (MM)
- Multiple myeloma variants: smoldering multiple myeloma (SMM), plasma cell leukemia, nonsecretory myeloma, osteosclerotic myeloma (POEMS syndrome)
- Plasmacytoma: solitary plasmacytoma of bone, extramedullary plasmacytoma
- Waldenström's macroglobulinemia
- Heavy-chain diseases (α, γ and μ)
- Primary amyloidosis (AL) (Chapter 71)

From Kyle RA. Classification and diagnosis of monoclonal gammopathies. In: Rose NR, Friedman H, Fahey JL (eds). *Manual of clinical laboratory immunology*, 3rd edn. Washington DC, American Society for Microbiology, 1986, 152–167, with permission.

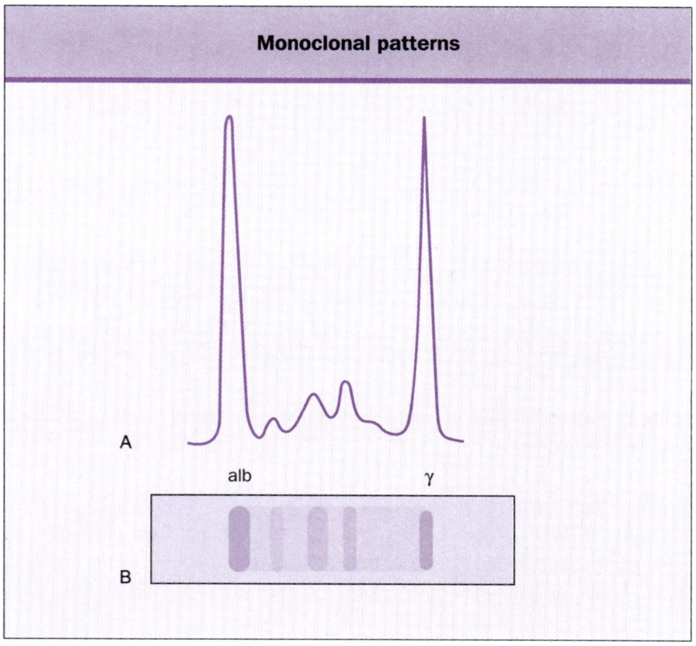

Figure 97.3 Monoclonal patterns. (A) Monoclonal pattern of serum protein as traced by densitometer after electrophoresis on agarose gel; tall, narrow-based peak of γ mobility. **(B)** Monoclonal pattern from electrophoresis of serum on agarose gel (anode on left); dense, localized band representing monoclonal protein of γ mobility. (From Kyle RA, Katzmann JA. Immunochemical characterization of immunoglobulins. In: Rose NR, de Macario EC, Folds JD, Lane HC, Nakamura RM (eds.) *Manual of clinical laboratory immunology*, 5th edn. Washington DC, ASM Press, 1997, p. 156, with permission.)

electrophoresis. Immunofixation is recommended for identification of an M-protein. The κ:λ ratio obtained from nephelometry will detect a large M-protein, but small M-proteins will have a normal ratio and will not be recognized.

Rate nephelometry is the preferred method for quantitation of immunoglobulins because it is not affected by molecular size. The nephelometry value for IgM, and occasionally IgG or IgA, is higher than that obtained with the densitometer tracing of serum protein electrophoresis.[3] However, we have also found that the densitometer tracing underestimates the amount of IgG when the M spike is >3–4 g/dl. One must use either electrophoresis or nephelometric quantitation of immunoglobulins throughout the course of a patient's illness, instead of alternating the techniques, because of the differences in results.

Immunofixation is the preferred technique for identifying a monoclonal light chain. A 24-hour urine specimen should be collected and the amount of M protein calculated on the basis of the densitometer tracing and the 24-hour urine protein content. The amount of M-protein is a direct reflection of the size of the tumor mass. The heat test for Bence Jones (monoclonal light chain) proteinuria is unsatisfactory.

MONOCLONAL GAMMOPATHY OF UNDETERMINED SIGNIFICANCE

The term 'monoclonal gammopathy of undetermined significance' (MGUS; benign monoclonal gammopathy) indicates the presence of an M-protein in persons without evidence of MM, WM, AL or related disorders.[4] MGUS is characterized by an M-protein concentration < 3 g/dl; fewer than 10% plasma cells in the bone marrow; no or only small amounts of M-protein in the urine; absence of lytic bone lesions, anemia, hypercalcemia and renal insufficiency; and, most importantly, the stability of the M-protein and the failure of other abnormalities to develop. Although this disorder has been considered benign, it is known that symptomatic MM or related disorders can develop in many patients, and for this reason the term MGUS is more appropriate.[5]

MGUS occurs in 3% of patients over 70 years old and 1% of persons older than 50.[6–8] The incidence increases with advancing age and is higher in African-Americans than in Caucasians.[9]

Because of its frequency, it is of great importance to know whether the M-protein will remain stable or will progress. At the Mayo Clinic, 241 patients with an apparently benign monoclonal gammopathy have been followed for 25–39 years. The median age at diagnosis was 64 years. The initial M-protein level (median 1.7 g/dl) consisted of IgG (74%), IgA (10%) and IgM (16%). The bone marrow contained 1–10% plasma cells (median 3%). After follow-up of 25–39 years, the 241 patients were classified into four groups (Table 97.1). The hemoglobin level, amount of M-protein and number of plasma cells in the bone marrow at the

Course of MGUS in 241 cases

Group	Description	Follow-up (25–39 yrs)	
		n	%
1	No substantial increase in M-protein (benign)	26	11
2	Increase in M-protein ≥ 3 g/dl	25	10
3	Died of unrelated causes	127	53
4	Development of myeloma, macroglobulinemia, amyloidosis, etc.	63	26
Total		241	100

Table 97.1 Course of 241 patients with monoclonal gammopathy of undetermined significance. (Modified from Kyle RA. 'Benign' monoclonal gammopathy. A misnomer? *JAMA* 1984;251:1849–54, with permission.)

time of diagnosis of MGUS did not differ substantially between the stable group and those who developed serious disease.

Only 11% of the patients are still alive with a stable M-protein, thus fulfilling the criteria of benign monoclonal gammopathy. Ten per cent of the patients had an increase in M-protein to 3 g/dl or more, but did not require chemotherapy. The median interval from the recognition of the M-protein to the level of 3 g/dl or more was 0–21 years (median 9 years). More than half of the patients died of an unrelated cause, with cardiac and cerebrovascular diseases the most common causes of death. MM, AL, macroglobulinemia, or a malignant lymphoproliferative process developed in 26% of the 241 patients during follow-up. The actuarial risk of malignant transformation was 16% at 10 years, 33% at 20 years, and 40% at 25 years (Fig. 97.4). The interval from recognition of M-protein to the diagnosis of serious disease ranged from 2 to 29 years (median 10 years). In seven patients MM was diagnosed more than 20 years after detection of the M-protein. The mode of development of MM was variable, in that some patients remained stable for many years and MM developed gradually or suddenly, whereas in others there was a steady increase in the M-protein level until they became symptomatic. The median duration of survival after the diagnosis of MM was 34 months, which is not different from those who develop myeloma de novo.

WM developed in seven patients at a median interval of 8.5 years after recognition of the M-protein (Table 97.2) whereas AL occurred in eight patients 6–19 years (median 9 years) after recognition of the M-protein. A malignant lymphoproliferative process (chronic lymphocytic leukemia or lymphoma) developed in five patients 9–22 years (median 10.5 years) after detection of the M-protein (Fig. 97.5). The rate of development of serious disease did not differ according to the presence of an IgG, IgA or IgM monoclonal gammopathy.[5] Similar findings have been reported in other series: the actuarial risk was 8.5% at 5 years and 19.2% at 10 years in one series of 128 patients with MGUS.[10] In a report of 335 patients with MGUS, the frequency of progression after a median follow-up of 70 months was 6.8%.[11]

Myeloma or other diseases in MGUS

	n	%	Interval to diagnosis (yrs)* Median	Range
Multiple myeloma	43	68	10.0	2–29
Macroglobulinemia	7	11	8.5	4–20
Amyloidosis	8	13	9.0	6–19
Lymphoproliferative	5	8	10.5	6–22
Total	63	100		

*Actuarial rate: 10 years, 16%; 20 years, 33%; 25 years, 40%.

Table 97.2 Development of myeloma or related disease in 63 patients with monoclonal gammopathy of undetermined significance. Modified from Kyle RA. Monoclonal gammopathy of undetermined significance. *Bailliére's Clin Hematol* 1995;8:761, with permission.)

Incidence of monoclonal gammopathies

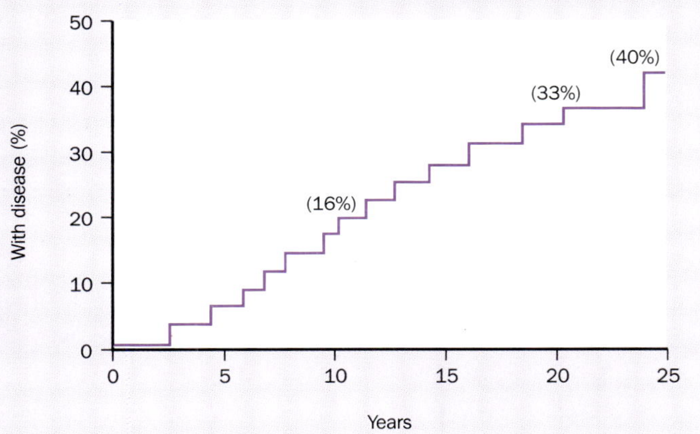

Figure 97.4 Incidence of monoclonal gammopathies. Rates are for multiple myeloma, macroglobulinemia, amyloidosis or lymphoproliferative disease after recognition of monoclonal protein. (From Kyle RA. Monoclonal gammopathy of undetermined significance. *Baillière's Clin Hematol* 1995;8:761, with permission.)

Follow-up results of monoclonal gammopathies

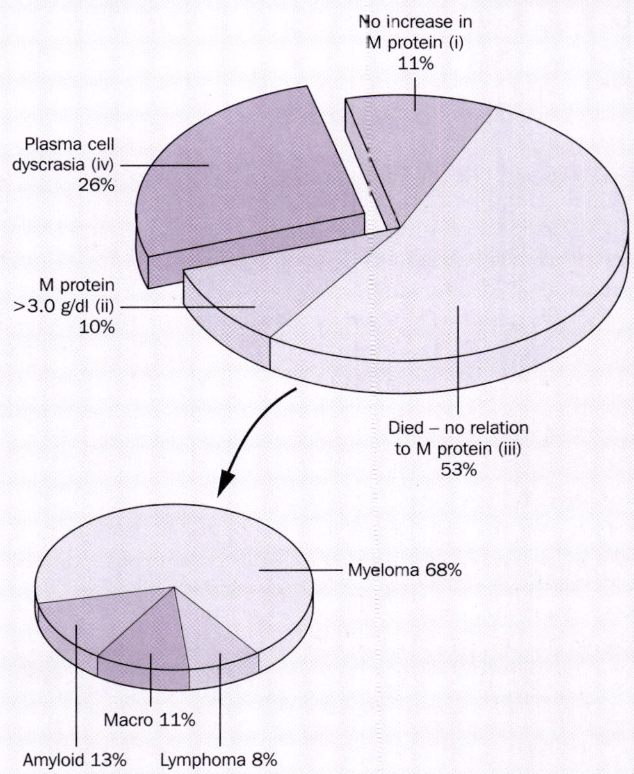

Figure 97.5 Follow-up results of monoclonal gammopathies. Results of long-term follow-up of monoclonal gammopathy of undetermined significance. Macro, macroglobulinemia. (Modified from Kyle RA. Monoclonal gammopathy of undetermined significance. *Baillière's Clin Hematol* 1995;8:761, with permission.)

Although MGUS frequently exists without any other abnormalities, certain diseases are associated with it, as would be expected in an older population. There may be an apparent association because of differences in the referral practices or in other selected patient groups. Appropriate control populations are essential for determining whether the association is merely a coincidence. For example, the association of monoclonal gammopathy and hyperparathyroidism has been reported.[12] In an effort to clarify this relationship, we reviewed our cases of surgically proven parathyroid adenoma in which serum protein electrophoresis had been performed within 6 months preceding parathyroidectomy. Among 911 patients older than 50 years who met these criteria, nine (1%) had MGUS.[13] This prevalence is similar to that expected in a normal population and indicates that the association of MGUS and hyperparathyroidism is probably the result of chance.

M-proteins have been noted in lymphoproliferative disorders, leukemia, other hematologic diseases, connective tissue disorders, and neurologic conditions such as peripheral neuropathy. Dermatologic diseases, including lichen myxedematosus, pyoderma gangrenosum, necrobiotic xanthogranuloma and plane xanthomatosis, have been associated with an M-protein.[14] M-proteins also have been found after renal, bone marrow or liver transplantation as a result of immunosuppressive therapy.

An M-protein may exhibit an unusual specificity to various antigens, including dextran, antistreptolysin O, riboflavin, von Willebrand factor, thyroglobulin, insulin, double-stranded DNA, apolipoprotein, thyroxin, human immunodeficiency virus (HIV), actin and antibiotics. Transient M-proteins have been recognized after infections. Binding of calcium, copper or phosphate by the M-protein may produce spurious laboratory values. M-proteins with antibody activity in plasma cell dyscrasias have been reviewed.[15]

Biclonal gammopathies

Biclonal gammopathies occur in approximately 4% of patients with monoclonal gammopathies and have similar clinical features. Two-thirds of cases of biclonal gammopathy are of undetermined significance.[16] The remainder have MM, AL, macroglobulinemia or other lymphoproliferative disorders. In some patients the M-proteins arise from two separate plasma cell clones, whereas in others they behave in a concordant fashion, consistent with incomplete class switching of a single plasma cell clone.[17] More than 25 cases of triclonal gammopathy have been reported.[18]

Idiopathic Bence Jones proteinuria

In most patients the presence of Bence Jones proteinuria indicates MM, AL, WM or other lymphoproliferative disorders. However, it may follow a benign course for many years. Patients with 'idiopathic' Bence Jones proteinuria must be observed indefinitely, because MM or AL will eventually develop in most of those with more than 1 g of Bence Jones protein in the urine per 24 hours.[19]

> **CLINICAL PEARLS**
>
> **Monoclonal gammopathies**
> - Monoclonal gammopathy of undetermined significance (MGUS) (benign monoclonal gammopathy) occurs in almost two-thirds of all patients with a monoclonal gammopathy.
> - MGUS occurs in 3% of patients older than 70 years.
> - Multiple myeloma, primary amyloidosis, macroglobulinemia or related disorders develop in 25% of patients with MGUS during long-term follow-up.

MULTIPLE MYELOMA

MM (myelomatosis, Kahler's disease) is characterized by the neoplastic proliferation of a single clone of plasma cells producing an M-protein. This proliferation often results in skeletal destruction, with osteolytic lesions or pathologic fractures producing pain, hypercalcemia and anemia. An excess of M-protein can contribute to renal failure, the hyperviscosity syndrome or recurrent bacterial infections.

Epidemiology

The annual incidence of MM is 4 per 100 000.[20] The apparent increased incidence during the past few decades is probably related more to the increased availability and use of medical facilities in the elderly and to improved diagnostic techniques, rather than an actual increased incidence. MM represents 1% of all malignant disease and slightly more than 10% of hematologic malignancies. Its incidence in African-Americans is twice that in Caucasians, and it is slightly more frequent in men than in women. MM occurs in all races and all geographic regions, but rates are lower in Asian populations. Only 18% of patients are younger than 50 years, and 3% are younger than 40. The median age is 65 years.

Etiology

The cause of MM is unknown. Radiation may play a role in some patients, with an increased risk of MM being reported in atomic bomb survivors exposed to more than 5 Gy.[21] An increased risk has been reported in farmers, especially those who use herbicides and insecticides, and in people exposed to other organic solvents.[22] MM has been reported in familial clusters of two or more first-degree relatives[23] and in identical twins. Some have postulated that repeated chronic antigenic stimulation may contribute to the development of MM. However, a case–control study provided no support for this hypothesis.[24] Human herpesvirus 8 has been reported in dendritic cells and has been suggested to play a role in the pathogenesis of MM.[25]

Biologic aspects

Plasma cells contain cytoplasmic Ig (cIg$^+$) and express surface CD38 and PCA-1. A small subset of myeloma cells expresses CD10, and 15–20% express CD20. CD56 (N-CAM) is expressed on the majority of malignant plasma cells, but CD34 is not. The

> **CLINICAL PEARLS**
>
> **Multiple myeloma**
> - Interleukin-6 (IL-6) is a major growth factor in multiple myeloma.
> - Ninety-eight per cent of patients have a monoclonal protein in the serum or urine at the time of diagnosis.
> - The most important prognostic factors are plasma cell labeling index, β_2-microglobulin level and cytogenetic changes.

clonogenic cell in MM has not been demonstrated with certainty.[26] There is evidence that plasma cell precursors of myeloma cells circulate in the peripheral blood.[27] The current hypothesis is that, by means of adhesion molecules, circulating clonogenic myeloma cells, home to the bone marrow, where they find an appropriate microenvironment in which to differentiate and further expand.[28]

In patients with MM, CD4 T cells often are reduced in both percentage and absolute numbers. They are particularly reduced with chemotherapy.[29] Interleukin-6 (IL-6) is a potent plasma cell growth factor in MM. IL-6 levels correlate with disease activity and tumor cell mass, and increased IL-6 serum levels occur in almost all patients in an aggressive terminal phase of MM resistant to chemotherapy and in those with plasma cell leukemia. This observation supports the concept that IL-6 is an important factor in the progression of MM.[30] The overproduction of IL-1β, which has bone-resorbing activity, is important in the pathogenesis of myeloma bone disease.[31] Approximately 15% of patients with MM have a point mutation of *p53*, a tumor suppressor gene.

Cytogenetic studies in MM are difficult because of the low proliferative activity of plasma cells. Conventional cytogenetic studies show abnormal karyotypes in only 30–40% of patients. Partial or complete deletion of chromosome 13 or 11q represents an adverse prognostic factor.[32] Newer techniques using interphase fluorescence in situ hybridization (FISH) (Chapter 125) have detected a higher frequency of abnormalities. In 59 patients studied before therapy, the presence of a *p53* gene deletion, identified by FISH, was associated with stage III disease and a significantly shorter survival time than in patients without a deletion.[33] The most common chromosome translocation in MM involves 14q32, the site of IgH (heavy-chain) locus.[34]

Clinical manifestations

Bone pain, usually in the back or chest, is present at the time of diagnosis in two-thirds of patients and is usually aggravated by movement.[35] The patient's height may be reduced by several inches because of vertebral collapse. Weakness and fatigue are common and usually associated with anemia. Fever is rarely caused by myeloma and, when present, is usually from an infectious process. The major symptoms may result from an acute infection, renal failure, hypercalcemia or AL. Pallor is the most frequent physical finding. In about 15% of patients the liver is palpable, but the spleen is rarely enlarged. Extramedullary plasmacytomas, when present, are usually observed late in the course of the disease and appear as large, purplish, subcutaneous masses.

Renal involvement

The serum creatinine level is 2 mg/dl or more in one-fifth of patients at diagnosis. Two major causes of renal failure are 'myeloma kidney' and hypercalcemia. Myeloma kidney is characterized by the presence of large, dense, waxy, laminated casts in the distal and collecting tubules. They are composed mainly of precipitated monoclonal light chain (Bence Jones protein) and a small amount of albumin, Tamm–Horsfall protein, fibrinogen and polyclonal light chains. The casts are surrounded by giant cells that originate from macrophages. Dilatation and atrophy of the tubules develop, and the entire nephron becomes distorted and nonfunctional. Extensive cast formation correlates directly with the severity of renal insufficiency. The mechanism of nephrotoxicity from Bence Jones proteinuria is unclear. The isoelectric point, the type of light chain and the specific amino acid sequence play no recognized role in nephrotoxicity. Hypercalcemia, which is present in 15% of patients initially, is a major and treatable cause of renal insufficiency. Dehydration, infections or nonsteroidal anti-inflammatory agents may all contribute to renal failure. The infusion of contrast material rarely produces acute renal failure if dehydration is avoided.[36] Amyloidosis occurs in 10–15% of patients with myeloma and produces renal insufficiency and nephrotic syndrome. Deposition of monoclonal light chains, especially κ chains, in the renal glomeruli (light-chain deposition disease) may be responsible for nephrotic syndrome or renal failure.[37]

Skeletal involvement

Three-quarters of patients have lytic lesions, osteoporosis or fractures shown on conventional radiographs at diagnosis. The vertebrae, skull, thoracic cage, pelvis and proximal humeri and femora are the most frequent sites of involvement. ^{99m}Tc bone scanning is inferior to conventional radiography and is not advised. MRI of the thoracolumbar spine may be of value in distinguishing between MGUS and overt MM. In one series thoracolumbar MRI was normal in patients with MGUS and abnormal in more than 80% of those with overt MM.[38] MRI or CT is most helpful in the detection of extramedullary plasmacytomas in patients with severe back pain but no abnormalities on routine radiographs.[39]

Neurologic involvement

Radiculopathy from nerve compression by an extradural plasmacytoma or by the collapsed bone itself is the most frequent neurologic complication. Compression of the spinal cord occurs in 5–10% of patients and must be recognized and treated without delay. Peripheral neuropathy is rare in MM and, when present, is usually due to amyloidosis. Leptomeningeal myelomatosis is uncommon, but is being recognized more frequently.[40] Intracranial plasmacytomas are rare.

Other systemic involvement

The incidence of infections is increased in MM. The most common are gram-negative organisms and *Streptococcus pneumoniae*. Impairment of antibody response, reduction of normal immunoglobulins, neutropenia and treatment with glucocorticoids all contribute to infection. Hepatomegaly from plasma cell infiltration is rare. Plasmacytomas of the ribs are often present. Diffuse pulmonary involvement and pleural effusion from plasma cell infiltration are rare and usually occur late in the course of the disease.

Laboratory findings

Approximately two-thirds of patients have a normocytic, normochromic anemia at diagnosis. Hypercalcemia occurs in 15%, and 20% have an increase of the serum creatinine to 2.0 mg/dl or more. The serum protein electrophoretic pattern shows a spike or localized band in 80% of patients at diagnosis. Hypogammaglobulinemia is found in about 10%, and the remainder have a normal electrophoretic pattern. An M-protein is found in the serum in 90% of patients, of which about half have an IgG M-protein, approximately a fifth have IgA, and almost 20% have a free monoclonal light chain (Bence Jones proteinemia). Immunofixation of the urine reveals an M-protein in 75% of patients. An M-protein is found in the serum or urine in 98% of patients with MM at the time of diagnosis and the relative frequency of κ:λ is 2:1.

Plasma cells usually constitute more than 10% of all nucleated cells in the bone marrow, but the number may range from less than 5% to almost 100%. Bone marrow involvement may be more focal than diffuse, and repeat bone marrow examinations may be necessary. The presence of a monoclonal immunoglobulin in the cytoplasm of plasma cells is helpful in differentiating a monoclonal plasma cell proliferation from reactive plasmacytosis.

Differential diagnosis

The diagnosis of MM depends on the presence of an increased number of plasma cells in the bone marrow (usually >10%), an M-protein in the serum (usually >3 g/dl), a monoclonal light chain in the urine, or osteolytic lesions. Clinical features of MM must also be present. Metastatic carcinoma, connective tissue disorders or lymphoma must be considered in the differential diagnosis.

Patients with MM must be differentiated from those with MGUS, SMM and AL. Patients with MGUS have an M-protein <3 g/dl, a bone marrow containing fewer than 10% plasma cells, and no anemia, lytic lesions, hypercalcemia, renal insufficiency or Bence Jones proteinuria. SMM is characterized by a serum M-protein value >3 g/dl or more than 10% plasma cells in the bone marrow, but no skeletal bone lesions, anemia or renal insufficiency. Patients with SMM or MGUS should not be treated until symptoms of MM develop or laboratory abnormalities progress.

The differential diagnosis of MGUS from MM or WM may be difficult. The concentration of the serum M-protein, the amount of urine M-protein, the number of bone marrow plasma cells, the hemoglobin, calcium and creatinine levels, and the presence of lytic lesions are all helpful in differentiating MGUS and SMM from MM. The level of uninvolved serum immunoglobulins is not helpful because in one-third of patients with MGUS the uninvolved immunoglobulins are reduced. The plasma cell labeling index, which measures the synthesis of DNA, is helpful in differentiating MGUS or SMM from MM.[41] An increased value suggests that the patient has, or will soon have, symptomatic MM, as this finding is rare in patients with MGUS or SMM. However, the labeling index is normal in about 40% of patients with MM requiring therapy. Monoclonal plasma cells can be detected in the peripheral blood of 80% of patients with active MM. In contrast, patients with MGUS or SMM have few or no circulating plasma cells. In one series of 57 patients with SMM, 16 showed signs of progression within 12 months.[42] Almost two-thirds of these had increased plasma cells of the same isotype in the peripheral blood, compared to only 10% of those who remained stable. Other laboratory determinations, such as β_2-microglobulin or reduced numbers of CD4 T lymphocytes, are unreliable for differentiating MM from SMM or MGUS.

Differentiation of AL from MM is arbitrary because both diseases are plasma-cell-proliferative disorders with different manifestations. In AL, the proportion of bone marrow plasma cells is usually less than 20%, there are no osteolytic lesions, and the amount of Bence Jones proteinuria is modest. However, AL and MM also have overlapping features in the spectrum of plasma-cell-proliferative disorders. Systemic amyloidosis will develop during the course of disease in approximately 10% of patients with MM, but MM rarely develops in patients with AL. In a series of 1596 patients with AL seen at the Mayo Clinic, only 6 (0.4%) developed overt MM during follow-up.[43]

No single test reliably differentiates a patient with MGUS from one in whom MM or other malignant disease will subsequently develop. The most reliable means of differentiation is serial measurement of the M-protein value in thê serum and urine and periodic evaluation of the pertinent clinical and laboratory features.

Prognostic factors

The median duration of survival in MM is approximately 3 years, but there is a great deal of variability between patients. Approximately 25% survive 5 years or more, but less than 5% live longer than 10 years.

The Durie–Salmon clinical staging system is based on a combination of factors that correlate with the myeloma cell mass.[44] However, the unreliability of this system and its many shortcomings have led to the search for other prognostic factors.

The bone marrow plasma cell labeling index (PCLI) and β_2-microglobulin levels are the most important prognostic factors in previously untreated patients.[45] Patients with a low PCLI and low β_2-microglobulin have a median duration of survival of almost 6 years when treated with conventional chemotherapy. The presence of plasmablastic morphologic features is an important adverse diagnostic finding in patients with MM.[46] Increased soluble IL-6 receptor, lactate dehydrogenase or C-reactive protein levels, older age, increased numbers of circulating plasma cells in the peripheral blood, reduced numbers of CD4 T cells, increased thymidine kinase levels and increased levels of IL-6 are all associated with a poorer prognosis. Cytogenetic abnormalities are important prognostic factors. The deletion of chromosome 13 or 11q and the presence of translocations are both predictors of poor outcome.[32]

Treatment

Most patients with MM have symptomatic disease at diagnosis and require chemotherapy. However, not all patients who fulfill the minimal criteria for the diagnosis of MM should be treated, and patients with SMM or MGUS should be observed until progression occurs. An increasing level of the M-protein in the serum or urine, the development of anemia, hypercalcemia, or renal insufficiency, and the occurrence of lytic bone lesions or extramedullary plasmacytomas are all indications for therapy. If there is doubt about whether to begin therapy, the most reasonable approach is to re-evaluate the patient in 2 months and to delay treatment until progressive disease is evident. There is no evidence that early treatment of MM is advantageous.[47]

If the patient is younger than 70 the physician should discuss the possibility of autologous peripheral blood stem-cell transplantation. Peripheral stem cells should be collected before the patient is exposed to alkylating agents. Most investigators prefer vincristine, doxorubicin (Adriamycin) and dexamethasone (VAD) as the initial therapy because these drugs do not damage hematopoietic stem cells. Generally, patients over 70 should be treated with melphalan and prednisone, or a combination of chemotherapeutic agents.

Radiotherapy

Palliative radiation in a dosage of 20–30 Gy should be limited to patients with disabling pain who have a well defined focal process that has not responded to chemotherapy. Analgesics in combination with chemotherapy usually can control the bone pain. This approach is preferred to local radiation, because pain frequently occurs in another site and local radiation does not benefit the patient with systemic disease.

Chemotherapy

Chemotherapy is the preferred initial treatment for overt symptomatic MM in patients over 70 or in younger patients in whom transplantation is not feasible. Melphalan and prednisone, given orally, produce an objective response in only 50–60% of patients. Melphalan must be given when the patient is fasting because food interferes with absorption. Leukocyte and platelet counts should be determined at 3-week intervals after beginning therapy, because the melphalan dosage must be altered until midcycle neutropenia or thrombocytopenia occurs. The melphalan and prednisone treatment should be repeated every 6 weeks. At least three courses of melphalan and prednisone should be given before therapy is discontinued, unless the patient has evidence of progressive disease, because an objective response may not be achieved for 6–12 months. The natural course of MM is one of progression, and if the patient's pain is alleviated and there is no evidence of progressive disease, the therapy may prove to be beneficial despite failure to reach an objective response.

Because of the obvious shortcomings of melphalan and prednisone, various combinations of therapeutic agents have been used. Vincristine, carmustine (BCNU), melphalan, cyclophosphamide and prednisone (VBMCP)[48] is a useful combination. Doxorubicin (Adriamycin), BCNU, cyclophosphamide and melphalan (ABCM)[49] have been reported to be superior to melphalan. In an overview of individual data of 4930 persons from 20 randomized trials comparing melphalan and prednisone with various combinations of therapeutic agents, response rates were significantly higher with combination chemotherapy (60%) than with melphalan and prednisone (53%) ($P < 0.00001$). However, there was no significant difference in response duration or overall survival. Furthermore, there was no evidence that any group of patients benefited from receiving combination chemotherapy. In fact, there was nothing to indicate that high-risk patients benefited from combination therapy.[50]

Chemotherapy should be continued for at least 1 year or until the patient is in a plateau state with stable serum and urine M-protein levels and no progression of disease. Continued chemotherapy may lead to the development of myelodysplastic syndrome or acute leukemia.[51] Patients should be followed closely during the plateau state, and the same chemotherapy should be reinstituted if relapse occurs after 6 months.

The role of α_2-interferon (IFN-α_2) in the treatment of MM is controversial. After induction chemotherapy, IFN-α_2 produced a superior response duration.[52] This finding has been confirmed by some studies but not others. A large meta-analysis is being performed on the individual patient data in all prospective IFN-α_2 trials by the Myeloma Trial Collaborative Group. If IFN-α_2 is used, the dose must be altered so undesirable side effects do not interfere with the patient's quality of life.

Autologous transplantation

Autologous peripheral blood stem-cell transplantation has virtually replaced autologous bone marrow transplantation because engraftment is more rapid and there is less contamination of myeloma cells. Autologous peripheral stem-cell transplantation is applicable for more than half of patients with MM. The two major shortcomings are that myeloma is not eradicated even with large doses of chemotherapy and total body radiation, and that autologous peripheral blood stem cells are contaminated by myeloma cells or their precursors. The mortality rate with autologous transplantation is currently 1–2% if patients are appropriately selected. The role of intensive therapy was recently reviewed.[53–55]

Standard treatment consists of VAD for 3–4 months to reduce the number of tumor cells in the bone marrow and peripheral blood. The peripheral stem cells are then collected after high-dose cyclophosphamide and granulocyte colony-stimulating factor. The patient is given high-dose chemotherapy or total body radiation, followed by infusion of the peripheral blood stem cells. The other choice is to treat the patient with alkylating agents after stem cell collection until a plateau is reached; at the time of relapse the patient is given high-dose melphalan with or without total body radiation and the previously collected peripheral blood stem cells are infused. A French study showed no difference in survival whether the patient had an early or a delayed stem-cell transplant.[56]

A randomized trial performed by the French Myeloma Group compared high-dose chemotherapy and autologous bone marrow transplantation with conventional chemotherapy. A higher rate of 5-year event-free survival (28% vs. 10%) and overall survival (52% vs. 12%) occurred in the transplant group.[57] However, in another study the median survival of 77 patients with MM who were potential candidates for transplantation (age < 66 years, stage II or III disease, good performance status and disease responsive to initial chemotherapy) but who were given conventional chemotherapy had similar overall survival.[58]

The largest single-institution experience with autologous transplantation in myeloma included 496 patients enrolled in a tandem transplant program.[59] In a recent report of 231 patients receiving tandem transplants, the overall median survival was 68 months.[60] In a randomized trial of 400 patients in France there was no difference in event-free or overall survival between double and single autologous stem-cell transplantation when evaluated at 2 years.[61]

The preparatory regimen for the autologous stem-cell transplantation must be improved because it is probably the source of relapse in most patients. In addition, removal of myeloma cells and their precursors from the peripheral blood is desirable. $CD34^+$ selection reduces the number of tumor cells but appears to have no effect on the duration of response or survival. The use of dendritic cell vaccines may be of benefit in delaying or reducing relapse after autologous transplantation.

Allogeneic bone marrow transplantation

Allogeneic bone marrow transplantation is advantageous because the graft contains no tumor cells and there may be a graft-versus-tumor effect. However, there is a mortality rate of at least 25%. Furthermore, 90–95% of patients with MM are ineligible because of their age, lack of an HLA-matched sibling donor, or inadequate renal, pulmonary or cardiac function. In a series of 266 patients from the European Bone Marrow Transplantation Registry, 51% achieved a complete response but the overall treatment mortality was approximately 40%. Furthermore, patients continued to have relapse throughout observation. The use of donor lymphocyte infusions after allogeneic transplantation produces an objective response in more than half of patients.[62]

The mortality rate for allogeneic transplantation must be reduced before it can assume a major role in therapy. The use of T-cell-depleted allogeneic stem cells and nonmyeloablative regimens with fludarabine and melphalan may result in a lower mortality. At present, allogeneic transplantation is associated with an excess of mortality and cannot be recommended as a routine procedure.

Refractory multiple myeloma

Cure rarely occurs, so that almost all patients who respond to chemotherapy will eventually have a relapse if they do not die from another disease. Furthermore, at least one-third of patients treated initially do not obtain an objective response. The highest response rates reported for patients with MM resistant to alkylating agents have been with VAD, approximately 80% of the activity of which is from dexamethasone.[63] The major shortcomings of VAD are that vincristine and doxorubicin must be given by central venous catheter, there is significant steroid toxicity, and the median duration of response is less than 1 year. Other alternatives include methylprednisolone: we find this has fewer side effects than does dexamethasone. VBAP (vincristine, BCNU, doxorubicin [Adriamycin] and prednisone) given every 3–4 weeks produces some benefit in more than a third of patients. Cyclophosphamide plus prednisone followed by granulocyte–macrophage colony-stimulating factor may be useful for refractory myeloma. Results with IFN-α_2 or topotecan are disappointing. Thalidomide has produced impressive responses in about a third of refractory patients, with recent data suggesting at least the possibility of long-term remissions with treatment.[64]

The multidrug-resistant phenotype of myeloma cells is characterized by the expression of glycoprotein P-170. These cells are low in intracellular drug concentrations. Attempts to prevent or overcome multidrug resistance in myeloma with a calcium channel blocker such as verapamil have been disappointing. The efficacy of the combination of VAD with the cyclosporine analog PSC-833, which blocks the activity of the glycoprotein pump, in refractory myeloma is being investigated.

Treatment of complications

Hypercalcemia

Hypercalcemia is present in 15% of patients at diagnosis. It should be suspected in the presence of anorexia, nausea, vomiting, polyuria, polydipsia, constipation, confusion or stupor. Hypercalcemia also contributes to the development of renal insufficiency. Hydration and prednisone, 25 mg four times a day, provide effective therapy in most cases. If not, a bisphosphonate such as pamidronate or etidronate should be given. Patients with MM should be encouraged to be as active as possible because prolonged bed rest contributes to osteopenia and hypercalcemia.

Skeletal lesions

Complications related to lytic skeletal lesions are common in MM. Patients should be encouraged to be as active as possible but to avoid trauma. Fixation of fractures or impending fractures of long bones with an intramedullary rod and methyl methacrylate has produced good results.

Bisphosphonates are beneficial for skeletal disease. In a prospective placebo-controlled study, pamidronate showed a significant reduction in skeletal events (pathologic fractures, need for radiation or surgery to treat or prevent pathologic fractures, or spinal cord compression associated with compression fractures). There was also a significant reduction in bone pain, a lower requirement for analgesic drugs, and an improved quality of life in the pamidronate group.[65]

THERAPEUTIC PRINCIPLES

Treatment of multiple myeloma

- If patient is ≤ 70 years of age the physician should discuss the possibility of an autologous peripheral blood stem-cell transplantation.
- Oral melphalan and prednisone are indicated for patients >70 years of age.
- Combinations of alkylating agents produce a higher response rate but no significant difference in survival compared to melphalan and prednisone.
- Autologous peripheral blood stem-cell transplantation is not curative. Eradication of multiple myeloma in the patient and removal of myeloma cells and their precursors from the bone marrow or peripheral blood are major challenges.
- Allogeneic bone marrow transplantation has a significant early mortality and is not recommended unless T-cell depletion or nonmyeloablative approaches are used to reduce mortality.

Renal insufficiency

A reduction in renal function is present in one-fifth of patients initially, and may develop insidiously or acutely. Maintenance of a high (3 l/day) urine output is important for preventing renal failure in patients with Bence Jones proteinuria. Allopurinol is helpful for the prevention and treatment of hyperuricemia. Hemodialysis is necessary for patients with symptomatic azotemia. Plasmapheresis may be useful in acute renal failure, but patients with irreversible renal changes are unlikely to benefit.[66]

Other complications

Anemia occurs in almost all patients during the course of MM. Symptomatic anemia during the plateau phase is benefited in at least half of patients by the administration of erythropoietin.[67,68] There are no side-effects and the major disadvantage is its cost. Red cell transfusions may also be needed for anemia.

Prompt and appropriate therapy for bacterial infection is essential. Prophylactic daily penicillin (oral) often benefits patients with recurrent pneumococcal pneumonia infections. Pneumococcal and influenza vaccines should be given to all patients despite their suboptimal antibody response. Intravenous immunoglobulin may be helpful for patients with recurrent infections but is very expensive. The daily use of trimethoprim–sulfamethoxazole during the first 2 months of chemotherapy may be helpful.[69]

Spinal cord compression should be suspected in patients with severe back pain, weakness or paresthesias of the lower extremities, or bowel dysfunction. MRI or CT must be performed immediately. Radiation therapy and dexamethasone are usually helpful and surgical compression is rarely necessary.

Variants of multiple myeloma

Smoldering multiple myeloma (SMM)

SMM is characterized by the presence of an M-protein value > 3 g/dl or more than 10% plasma cells in the bone marrow, but no evidence of anemia, hypercalcemia, skeletal lesions or renal insufficiency.[70] Biologically, patients with SMM have a benign monoclonal gammopathy, but they must be followed because symptomatic MM frequently develops. Treatment should not be given unless progression occurs.

Plasma cell leukemia

Plasma cell leukemia is defined as the presence of more than 20% plasma cells in the peripheral blood and an absolute plasma cell count >2 × 10^9/l. When it presents de novo (60% of cases) it is classified as primary, and when it presents as a leukemic transformation of a previously recognized MM it is secondary (40%).[71] Patients with primary plasma cell leukemia are younger and have a greater incidence of hepatosplenomegaly and lymphadenopathy, fewer bone lesions, a smaller serum M-component and a longer survival than patients with secondary plasma cell leukemia. Cytogenetic abnormalities are more common than in patients with MM.[72] Autologous stem-cell transplantation after response to high-dose chemotherapy has been beneficial for some patients. Those with secondary plasma cell leukemia rarely respond to chemotherapy because they have already received treatment for MM and are refractory.

Nonsecretory myeloma

Patients with nonsecretory myeloma have no M-component in either the serum or the urine and account for only 2% of patients with MM. The diagnosis is established by identification of an M-protein in the plasma cells by immunofluorescence or immunoperoxidase. The behavior of nonsecretory myeloma is similar to that of MM, except there is less renal involvement.[73]

Solitary plasmacytoma of bone

The diagnosis of solitary plasmacytoma of bone is based on the presence of a skeletal plasma cell tumor without evidence of MM. The hemoglobin, calcium and creatinine values are normal, there are no other bone lesions, and the bone marrow contains no increase in monoclonal plasma cells. Small amounts of M-protein may be present in the serum or urine, but they usually disappear after tumoricidal radiation (40–50 Gy). MRI is useful because of the high incidence of MM if additional lesions are seen, in contrast to patients with no additional lesions on MRI.[74] Overt MM develops in approximately 55% of patients during long-term follow-up. New bone lesions or local recurrences develop in about 10%.[75] There is no convincing evidence that chemotherapy affects the incidence of conversion to MM. Progression, when it occurs, usually is evident within 3–4 years.[76]

Extramedullary plasmacytoma

The diagnosis is based on the finding of a plasma cell tumor in an extramedullary location and the absence of MM on bone marrow examination, radiography, and appropriate studies of serum and urine. Approximately 80% of cases involve the upper respiratory tract, producing epistaxis, nasal discharge or nasal obstruction.[77] Central nervous system involvement may produce localized symptoms. Primary plasmacytoma of the lung often presents as a pulmonary nodule or hilar mass. There is a predominance of IgA M-proteins.

Treatment consists of tumoricidal radiation. Adjuvant chemotherapy does not appear to lower the relapse rate or increase disease-free survival. Local recurrence is approximately 5% or less if tumoricidal radiation is given. A review of 400 publications between 1905 and 1997 found 800 cases. Patients who had combined surgery and radiation had better results than those who had only surgery or only radiation. There was local recurrence in 22% of patients, whereas MM developed in 15%.[77]

OSTEOSCLEROTIC MYELOMA (POEMS SYNDROME)

The major clinical findings in POEMS syndrome are characterized by *p*olyneuropathy, *o*rganomegaly, *e*ndocrinopathy, *M*-protein and *s*kin changes.[78,79] The major clinical findings are chronic inflammatory demyelinating polyneuropathy with predominantly motor disability and sclerotic skeletal lesions. Papilledema may occur. Hepatosplenomegaly and lymphadenopathy may be present. Skin hyperpigmentation and hypertrichosis may be prominent. Gynecomastia, testicular atrophy, and clubbing of the fingers and toes may occur. Pulmonary hypertension has been recognized in several instances. Ascites, pleural effusion and peripheral edema may be present. The hemoglobin level is usually normal or increased, and thrombocytosis is common. Hypercalcemia and renal insufficiency rarely occur, and the bone marrow usually contains less than 5% plasma cells. Most patients have a λ protein, and IgA is common. The diagnosis is confirmed by the presence of monoclonal plasma cells in an osteosclerotic lesion. Radiation to the localized osteosclerotic lesion usually produces improvement of the neuropathy, but if the lesions are widespread, chemotherapy or autologous stem cell transplantation is necessary.

WALDENSTRÖM'S MACROGLOBULINEMIA (WM)

WM is a consequence of a malignant proliferation of plasma cells and B-cell lymphocytes producing a monoclonal IgM protein. In a study from the United States, the incidence of WM was 0.3/100 000 in white men and 0.17/100 000 in white women, and approximately 1400 new cases occur each year.[80] The median age at diagnosis is 63 years; less than 1% of our patients are younger than 40 years, and approximately 60% are males.[81]

Clinical manifestations

The onset is usually insidious and characterized by weakness and fatigue. There may be oozing from the oronasal area or blurring of vision. Weight loss, fever and night sweats, resembling lymphoma, may occur. Peripheral neuropathy, pulmonary infiltration with cough and dyspnea, or skin lesions may be evident. Dyspnea and congestive heart failure may be an initial finding. In contrast to MM, renal failure, osteolytic lesions and amyloidosis are rare.

Pallor is a frequent finding on physical examination. Hepatomegaly, splenomegaly and lymphadenopathy occur in about a third of cases. Hyperviscosity is often present in WM and can produce oronasal bleeding, blurred vision, headache, vertigo, dizziness, sudden deafness, diplopia or ataxia.[82] Confusion, dementia and disturbances of consciousness may occur. Clinical manifestations are rarely due to hyperviscosity if the serum viscosity is less than 4 centipoises (normal ≤ 1.8). The correlation between the serum viscosity and clinical manifestations is not precise. Clinical symptoms and retinal lesions, including hemorrhages, exudates and venous congestion, are more important in making a therapeutic decision.

Laboratory findings

A normocytic, normochromic anemia occurs in almost all cases during the course of the disease. The hemoglobin and hematocrit values are often spuriously reduced because of the increased plasma volume. Serum protein electrophoresis reveals a sharp narrow spike or dense localized band consisting of monoclonal IgM. Quantitative IgM levels obtained by nephelometry may be 2–3 g/dl more than that found in the serum protein electrophoretic spike. Therefore, the serum protein abnormality must be measured by the same technique during follow-up. Seventy-five per cent of the IgM proteins are the κ light-chain type. Approximately 10% precipitate in the cold (cryoglobulin). In 80% of cases the urine contains a small monoclonal light chain. A bone marrow aspirate is often hypocellular, but the biopsy specimen is hypercellular and extensively infiltrated by lymphocytes, plasma cells, lymphoplasmacytoid cells and mast cells. In contrast to MM, lytic lesions and fractures are found in fewer than 5% of patients.

Differential diagnosis

Diagnosis depends on the presence of typical symptoms, physical findings, IgM protein in the serum, and a lymphoplasma cell proliferation in the bone marrow. It must be differentiated from MGUS of the IgM type, smoldering WM, lymphoma, other lymphoproliferative diseases, MM and chronic lymphocytic leukemia.

Treatment

Therapy should be withheld until the patient has constitutional symptoms such as weakness, fatigue, night sweats, weight loss, features of hyperviscosity, anemia, significant hepatosplenomegaly or lymphadenopathy. Plasmapheresis should be performed based on the patient's symptoms and physical findings, rather than on the magnitude of the viscosity measurement (Chapter 118). Plasmapheresis will alleviate symptoms quickly, but has no effect on the disease process. Therapeutic options include the nucleoside analogs fludarabine and cladribine (2-chlorodeoxyadenosine, 2-CdA), alkylating agents such has chlorambucil or cyclophosphamide, and corticosteroids.

Chlorambucil has been used in WM for more than 35 years. Patients should be treated until the disease has reached a plateau state, which occurs in about 70% of cases.[83] Cyclophosphamide or combinations of alkylating agents such as the M-2 protocol (vincristine, BCNU, melphalan, cyclophosphamide and prednisone; VBMCP) have also been beneficial.

2-CdA has been reported to produce an objective response in 85% of previously untreated WM patients,[84] but it is unsatisfactory for previously treated patients. The combination of 2-CdA, cyclophosphamide and prednisone may be beneficial.[85]

Fludarabine has been reported to produce a high incidence of response, but a recent study revealed partial responses in only 34% of 117 patients.[86] Rituximab (Rituxan), an anti-CD20 monoclonal antibody, produces a 50% reduction in measurable disease in refractory WM.[87]

Transfusion of packed red cells should be given for symptomatic anemia and erythropoietin may be of help. The median duration of survival for patients with WM is approximately 5 years.

HEAVY-CHAIN DISEASES

The heavy-chain diseases (HCD) are lymphoplasma-cell proliferative disorders characterized by the production of an M-protein consisting of an incomplete heavy chain devoid of light chains. There are three major types, α, γ and μ.

α Heavy-chain disease

α Heavy-chain disease (α-HCD) is the most common type and is characterized by the presence of a monoclonal α chain with extensive internal deletions encompassing the V_H region and the entire first constant domain.[88] It usually occurs in the second or third decade of life, and about 60% of patients are male. Most have been from the Mediterranean region and Middle East. Gastrointestinal tract involvement is most common and is manifested by malabsorption with weight loss, diarrhea and steatorrhea. It is similar to 'immunoproliferative small intestinal disease' (IPSID), but patients with IPSID do not synthesize α heavy chains. Poor hygiene and low socioeconomic status are important risk factors. Rarely, the respiratory tract is involved.

The serum protein electrophoretic pattern typically shows a broad band in the α_2 or β regions in half of patients and is normal in the remainder. There is no visible spike. The diagnosis depends on the recognition of a monoclonal α heavy chain in the serum, the jejunal fluid or the lymphocytes and plasma cells. The amount of α chain in the urine is small and Bence Jones proteinuria is absent. The bone marrow is normal. The course of α-HCD is variable but generally progressive. Surprisingly, antibiotics may produce remission. In patients who do not respond to antibiotics and in those with extensive intestinal or mesenteric involvement, chemotherapy with cyclophosphamide, doxorubicin (Adriamycin), vincristine and prednisone should be given.[89]

γ Heavy-chain disease

In γ heavy-chain disease (γ-HCD) the γ chain is incomplete, with large deletions of amino acids, including the C_H1 domain and a portion of the V_H1 of the constant region. The median age at diagnosis is approximately 60 years, but several patients younger than 20 years have been recognized. The clinical picture of γ-HCD has been described as a lymphoma-like illness but its features are variable, ranging from an aggressive lymphoproliferative process to an asymptomatic state.[90] The most frequent presenting symptoms are weakness, fatigue and fever, but edema of the uvula and palate from Waldeyer's ring involvement, skin infiltration, and enlargement of the parotid gland or thyroid have been reported. It usually presents as a lymphoproliferative disorder, with hepatosplenomegaly and lymphadenopathy in about 60% of patients. Autoimmune disorders such as rheumatoid arthritis, Sjögren's syndrome, systemic lupus erythematosus, Hashimoto's thyroiditis and myasthenia gravis have been noted.

Normocytic, normochromic anemia is found in 80% of cases. In several instances Coombs-positive autoimmune hemolytic anemia has been recognized. Lymphocytosis and thrombocytopenia have been observed. All patients have a monoclonal γ heavy chain in the serum, but the serum protein electrophoretic pattern often shows a broad-based γ band or hypogammaglobulinemia rather than the expected localized band. The amount of γ heavy-chain protein in the urine ranges from nondetectable to 20 g/24 h; more than half of patients excrete less than 1 g of protein. Bence Jones proteinuria is not found. The bone marrow and lymph nodes contain an increased number of plasma cells, lymphocytes and lymphoplasmacytoid cells. The diagnosis depends on the demonstration of a monoclonal γ heavy chain in the serum or urine.

The prognosis of γ-HCD is variable because the clinical course may range from an asymptomatic state to a rapidly progressive disease. The median duration of survival in 49 patients for whom such data were available was 12 months (range 1–264 months).[16]

Therapy with cyclophosphamide, vincristine and prednisone is a reasonable choice, but if there is no response doxorubicin should be added.

μ Heavy-chain disease

μ Heavy-chain disease (μ-HCD) is characterized by a monoclonal μ heavy chain in which the V_H domain is absent. Other deletions also may occur. Most patients have a chronic lymphoproliferative process resembling chronic lymphocytic leukemia or lymphoma. A monoclonal peak is found in the serum of 40% of patients. Two-thirds have Bence Jones proteinuria. Increases in lymphocytes, plasma cells and lymphoplasmacytoid cells in the bone marrow are common. Vacuolization of the plasma cells is an important clue for the diagnosis of μ-HCD, which depends on the demonstration of a μ heavy chain in the serum. The course of the disease is variable; the duration of survival ranges from less than 1 month to 11 years (median 24 months).[91] Treatment with corticosteroids and alkylating agents has shown benefit.

ACKNOWLEDGMENT

Supported in part by Grant CA 62242 from the National Cancer Institute.

REFERENCES

1. Kyle RA. Sequence of testing for monoclonal gammopathies. Arch Pathol Lab Med 1999;123:114.
2. Kyle RA, Katzmann JA. Immunochemical characterization of immunoglobulins. In: Rose NR, de Macario EC, Folds JD, Lane HC, Nakamura RM (eds) Manual of clinical laboratory immunology, 5th edn. Washington DC, ASM Press, 1997, p. 156.
3. Riches PG, Sheldon J, Smith AM, Hobbs JR. Overestimation of monoclonal immunoglobulin by immunochemical methods. Ann Clin Biochem 1991;28:253.
4. Kyle RA. Monoclonal gammopathy of undetermined significance. Natural history in 241 cases. Am J Med 1978;64:814.
5. Kyle RA. 'Benign' monoclonal gammopathy – after 20 to 35 years of follow-up. Mayo Clin Proc 1993;68:26.
6. Axelsson U, Bachmann R, Hällén J. Frequency of pathological proteins (M-components) in 6,995 sera from an adult population. Acta Med Scand 1966;179:235.
7. Kyle RA, Finkelstein S, Elveback LR, Kurland LT. Incidence of monoclonal proteins in a Minnesota community with a cluster of multiple myeloma. Blood 1972;40:719.
8. Saleun JP, Vicariot M, Deroff P, Morin JF. Monoclonal gammopathies in the adult population of Finistère, France. J Clin Pathol 1982;35:63.
9. Cohen HJ, Crawford J, Rao MK, Pieper CF, Currie MS. Racial differences in the prevalence of monoclonal gammopathy in a community-based sample of the elderly. Am J Med 1998;104:439.
10. Bladé J, Lopez-Guillermo A, Rozman C, et al. Malignant transformation and life expectancy in monoclonal gammopathy of undetermined significance. Br J Haematol 1992;81:391.
11. Baldini L, Guffanti A, Cesana BM, et al. Role of different hematologic variables in defining the risk of malignant transformation in monoclonal gammopathy. Blood 1996;87:912.
12. Schnur MJ, Appel GB, Bilezikian JP. Primary hyperparathyroidism and benign monoclonal gammopathy. Arch Intern Med. 1977;137:1201.
13. Mundis RJ, Kyle RA. Primary hyperparathyroidism and monoclonal gammopathy of undetermined significance. Am J Clin Pathol 1982;77:619.
14. Bladé J, Kyle RA. Monoclonal gammopathies of undetermined significance. In: Malpas JS, Bergsagel DE, Kyle RA, Anderson KC (eds) Myeloma: biology and management, 2nd edn. New York, Oxford University Press, 1998, p.135.
15. Merlini G, Farhangi M, Osserman EF. Monoclonal immunoglobulins with antibody activity in myeloma, macroglobulinemia and related plasma cell dyscrasias. Semin Oncol 1986;13:350.
16. Kyle RA, Robinson RA, Katzmann JA. The clinical aspects of biclonal gammopathies. Review of 57 cases. Am J Med 1981;71:999.
17. Riddell S, Traczyk Z, Paraskevas F, Israels LG. The double gammopathies. Clinical and immunological studies. Medicine (Baltimore) 1986;65:135.
18. Grosbois B, Jégo P, de Rosa H, et al. Triclonal gammopathy and malignant immunoproliferative syndrome [in French]. Rev Méd Interne 1997;18:470.
19. Kyle RA, Greipp PR. 'Idiopathic' Bence Jones proteinuria: long-term follow-up in seven patients. N Engl J Med 1982;306:564.
20. Kyle RA, Beard CM, O'Fallon WM, Kurland LT. Incidence of multiple myeloma in Olmsted County, Minnesota: 1978 through 1990, with a review of the trend since 1945. J Clin Oncol 1994;12:1577.
21. Ichimaru M, Ishimaru T, Mikami M, Matsunaga M. Multiple myeloma among atomic bomb survivors in Hiroshima and Nagasaki, 1950–76: relationship to radiation dose absorbed by marrow. J Natl Cancer Inst 1982;69:323.
22. Riedel DA, Pottern LM. The epidemiology of multiple myeloma. Hematol Oncol Clin North Am 1992;6:225.
23. Grosbois B, Jégo P, Attal M, et al. Familial multiple myeloma: report of fifteen families. Br J Haematol 1999;105:768.
24. Doody MM, Linet MS, Glass AG, et al. Leukemia, lymphoma, and multiple myeloma following selected medical conditions. Cancer Causes Control 1992;3:449.
25. Rettig MB, Ma HJ, Vescio RA, et al. Kaposi's sarcoma-associated herpesvirus infection of bone marrow dendritic cells from multiple myeloma patients. Science 1997;276:1851.
26. Epstein J. Myeloma phenotype: clues to disease origin and manifestation. Hematol Oncol Clin North Am 1992;6:249.
27. Billadeau D, Van Ness B, Kimlinger T, et al. Clonal circulating cells are common in plasma cell proliferative disorders: a comparison of monoclonal gammopathy of undetermined significance, smoldering multiple myeloma, and active myeloma. Blood 1996;88:289.
28. Hallek M, Bergsagel PL, Anderson KC. Multiple myeloma: increasing evidence for a multistep transformation process. Blood 1998;91:3.
29. Kay NE, Leong T, Bone N, et al. T-helper phenotypes in the blood of myeloma patients on ECOG phase III trials E9486/E3A93. Br J Haematol 1998;100:459.
30. Zhang XG, Klein B, Bataille R. Interleukin-6 is a potent myeloma-cell growth factor in patients with aggressive multiple myeloma. Blood 1989;74:11.
31. Lacy MQ, Donovan KA, Heimbach JK, Ahmann GJ, Lust JA. Comparison of interleukin-1 beta expression by in situ hybridization in monoclonal gammopathy of undetermined significance and multiple myeloma. Blood 1999;93:300.
32. Tricot G, Sawyer JR, Jagannath S, et al. Unique role of cytogenetics in the prognosis of patients with myeloma receiving high-dose therapy and autotransplants. J Clin Oncol 1997;15:2659.
33. Drach J, Ackermann J, Fritz E, et al. Presence of a p53 gene deletion in patients with multiple myeloma predicts for short survival after conventional-dose chemotherapy. Blood 1998;92:802.
34. Chesi M, Nardini E, Brents LA, et al. Frequent translocation t(4;14)(p16.3;q32.3) in multiple myeloma is associated with increased expression and activating mutations of fibroblast growth factor receptor 3. Nature Genet 1997;16:260.
35. Kyle RA. Multiple myeloma: review of 869 cases. Mayo Clin Proc 1975;50:29.

36. McCarthy CS, Becker JA. Multiple myeloma and contrast media. Radiology 1992;183:519.
37. Heilman RL, Velosa JA, Holley KE, Offord KP, Kyle RA. Longterm follow-up and response to chemotherapy in patients with light-chain deposition disease. Am J Kidney Dis 1992;20:34.
38. Bellaïche L, Laredo J-D, Lioté F, et al. Magnetic resonance appearance of monoclonal gammopathies of unknown significance and multiple myeloma. The GRI Study Group. Spine 1997;22:2551.
39. Libshitz HI, Malthouse SR, Cunningham D, MacVicar AD, Husband JE. Multiple myeloma: appearance at MR imaging. Radiology 1992;182:833.
40. Leifer D, Grabowski T, Simonian N, Demirjian ZN. Leptomeningeal myelomatosis presenting with mental status changes and other neurologic findings. Cancer 1992;70:1899.
41. Greipp PR, Witzig TE, Gonchoroff NJ, et al. Immunofluorescence labeling indices in myeloma and related monoclonal gammopathies. Mayo Clin Proc 1987;62:969.
42. Witzig TE, Gertz MA, Lust JA, Kyle RA, O'Fallon WM, Greipp PR. Peripheral blood monoclonal plasma cells as a predictor of survival in patients with multiple myeloma. Blood 1996;88:1780.
43. Rajkumar SV, Gertz MA, Kyle RA. Primary systemic amyloidosis with delayed progression to multiple myeloma. Cancer 1998;82:1501.
44. Durie BG, Salmon SE. A clinical staging system for multiple myeloma. Correlation of measured myeloma cell mass with presenting clinical features, response to treatment, and survival. Cancer 1975;36:842.
45. Greipp PR, Lust JA, O'Fallon WM, Katzmann JA, Witzig TE, Kyle RA. Plasma cell labeling index and beta 2-microglobulin predict survival independent of thymidine kinase and C-reactive protein in multiple myeloma. Blood 1993;81:3382.
46. Greipp PR, Leong T, Bennett JM, et al. Plasmablastic morphology – an independent prognostic factor with clinical and laboratory correlates: Eastern Cooperative Oncology Group (ECOG) myeloma trial E9486 report by the ECOG Myeloma Laboratory Group. Blood 1998;91:2501.
47. Hjorth M, Hellquist L, Holmberg E, Magnusson B, Rodjer S, Westin J. Initial versus deferred melphalan–prednisone therapy for asymptomatic multiple myeloma stage I – a randomized study. Myeloma Group of Western Sweden. Eur J Haematol 1993;50:95.
48. Oken MM, Harrington DP, Abramson N, Kyle RA, Knospe W, Glick JH. Comparison of melphalan and prednisone with vincristine, carmustine, melphalan, cyclophosphamide, and prednisone in the treatment of multiple myeloma: results of Eastern Cooperative Oncology Group Study E2479. Cancer 1997;79:1561.
49. MacLennan IC, Chapman C, Dunn J, Kelly K. Combined chemotherapy with ABCM versus melphalan for treatment of myelomatosis. The Medical Research Council Working Party for Leukaemia in Adults. Lancet 1992;339:200.
50. Myeloma Trialists' Collaborative Group. Combination chemotherapy versus melphalan plus prednisone as treatment for multiple myeloma: an overview of 6,633 patients from 27 randomized trials. J Clin Oncol 1998;16:3832.
51. Kyle RA, Gertz MA. Second malignancies after chemotherapy. In: Perry MC (ed) The chemotherapy source book. Baltimore, Williams & Wilkins, 1992, p. 689.
52. Mandelli F, Avvisati G, Amadori S, et al. Maintenance treatment with recombinant interferon alfa-2b in patients with multiple myeloma responding to conventional induction chemotherapy. N Engl J Med 1990;322:1430.
53. Kyle RA. High-dose therapy in multiple myeloma and primary amyloidosis: an overview. Semin Oncol 1999;26:74.
54. Gahrton G, Björkstrand B. High-dose treatment of multiple myeloma. Crit Rev Oncol Hematol 1999;30:173.
55. Lokhorst HM, Sonneveld P, Verdonck LF. Intensive treatment for multiple myeloma: where do we stand? Br J Haematol 1999;106:18.
56. Fermand JP, Ravaud P, Chevret S, et al. High-dose therapy and autologous peripheral blood stem cell transplantation in multiple myeloma: upfront or rescue treatment? Results of a multicenter sequential randomized clinical trial. Blood 1998;92:3131.
57. Attal M, Harousseau JL, Stoppa AM, et al. A prospective, randomized trial of autologous bone marrow transplantation and chemotherapy in multiple myeloma. Intergroupe Français du Myelome. N Engl J Med 1996;335:91.
58. Bladé J, San Miguel JF, Fontanillas M, et al. Survival of multiple myeloma patients who are potential candidates for early high-dose therapy intensification/autotransplantation and who were conventionally treated. J Clin Oncol 1996;14:2167.
59. Vesole DH, Tricot G, Jagannath S, et al. Autotransplants in multiple myeloma: what have we learned? Blood 1996;88:838.
60. Barlogie B, Jagannath S, Desikan KR, et al. Total therapy with tandem transplants for newly diagnosed multiple myeloma. Blood 1999;93:55.
61. Attal M, Payen C, Facon T, et al. Single versus double transplant in myeloma: a randomized trial of the 'Inter Groupe Français du Myélome' (IFM) (abstract). Blood 1997;90 Suppl 1:418a.
62. Lokhorst HM, Schattenberg A, Cornelissen JJ, Thomas LL, Verdonck LF. Donor leukocyte infusions are effective in relapsed multiple myeloma after allogeneic bone marrow transplantation. Blood 1997;90:4206.
63. Alexanian R, Dimopoulos MA, Delasalle K, Barlogie B. Primary dexamethasone treatment of multiple myeloma. Blood 1992;80:887.
64. Singhal S, Mehta J, Desikan R, et al. Antitumor activity of thalidomide in refractory multiple myeloma. N Engl J Med 1999;341:1565.
65. Berenson JR, Lichtenstein A, Porter L, et al. Long-term pamidronate treatment of advanced multiple myeloma patients reduces skeletal events. Myeloma Aredia Study Group. J Clin Oncol 1998;16:593.
66. Johnson WJ, Kyle RA, Pineda AA, O'Brien PC, Holley KE. Treatment of renal failure associated with multiple myeloma. Plasmapheresis, hemodialysis, and chemotherapy. Arch Intern Med 1990;150:863.
67. Garton JP, Gertz MA, Witzig TE, et al. Epoetin alfa for the treatment of the anemia of multiple myeloma. A prospective, randomized, placebo-controlled, double-blind trial. Arch Intern Med 1995;155:2069.
68. Osterbörg A, Boogaerts MA, Cimino R, et al. Recombinant human erythropoietin in transfusion-dependent anemic patients with multiple myeloma and non-Hodgkin's lymphoma – a randomized multicenter study. The European Study Group of Erythropoietin (Epoetin Beta) Treatment in Multiple Myeloma and Non-Hodgkin's Lymphoma. Blood 1996;87:2675.
69. Oken MM, Pomeroy C, Weisdorf D, Bennett JM. Prophylactic antibiotics for the prevention of early infection in multiple myeloma. Am J Med 1996;100:624.
70. Kyle RA, Greipp PR. Smoldering multiple myeloma. N Engl J Med 1980;302:1347.
71. Noel P, Kyle RA. Plasma cell leukemia: an evaluation of response to therapy. Am J Med 1987;83:1062.
72. Garcia-Sanz R, Orfão A, Gonzalez M, et al. Primary plasma cell leukemia: clinical, immunophenotypic, DNA ploidy, and cytogenetic characteristics. Blood 1999;93:1032.
73. Cavo M, Galieni P, Gobbi M, et al. Nonsecretory multiple myeloma. Presenting findings, clinical course and prognosis. Acta Haematol 1985;74:27.
74. Liebross RH, Ha CS, Cox JD, Weber D, Delasalle K, Alexanian R. Solitary bone plasmacytoma: outcome and prognostic factors following radiotherapy. Int J Radiat Oncol Biol Phys 1998;41:1063.
75. Frassica DA, Frassica FJ, Schray MF, Sim FH, Kyle RA. Solitary plasmacytoma of bone: Mayo Clinic experience. Int J Radiat Oncol Biol Phys 1989;16:43.
76. Dimopoulos MA, Goldstein J, Fuller L, Delasalle K, Alexanian R. Curability of solitary bone plasmacytoma. J Clin Oncol 1992;10:587.
77. Alexiou C, Kau RJ, Dietzfelbinger H, et al. Extramedullary plasmacytoma: tumor occurrence and therapeutic concepts. Cancer 1999;85:2305.
78. Bardwick PA, Zvaifler NJ, Gill GN, Newman D, Greenway GD, Resnick DL. Plasma cell dyscrasia with polyneuropathy, organomegaly, endocrinopathy, M protein, and skin changes: the POEMS syndrome. Report on two cases and a review of the literature. Medicine (Baltimore) 1980;59:311.
79. Waldenström JG. POEMS: a multifactorial syndrome [editorial]. Haematologica 1992;77:197.
80. Groves FD, Travis LB, Devesa SS, Ries LA, Fraumeni JF Jr. Waldenström's macroglobulinemia: incidence patterns in the United States, 1988–1994. Cancer 1998;82:1078.

81. Kyle RA, Garton JP. The spectrum of IgM monoclonal gammopathy in 430 cases. Mayo Clin Proc 1987;62:719.
82. Gertz MA, Kyle RA. Hyperviscosity syndrome. J Intensive Care Med 1995;10:128.
83. Kyle RA, Greipp PR, Gertz MA, et al. Waldenström's macroglobulinemia: a prospective study comparing daily with intermittent oral chlorambucil. Br J Haematol 2000;108:737.
84. Dimopoulos MA, Alexanian R. Waldenström's macroglobulinemia. Blood 1994;83:1452.
85. Laurencet FM, Zulian GB, Guetty-Alberto M, Iten PA, Betticher DC, Alberto P. Cladribine with cyclophosphamide and prednisone in the management of low-grade lymphoproliferative malignancies. Br J Cancer 1999;79:1215.
86. Dhodapkar M, Jacobson J, Gertz M, et al. Phase II intergroup trial of fludarabine (FAMP) in Waldenström's macroglobulinemia (WM): results of Southwest Oncology Group trial (SWOG 9003) in 220 patients (abstract). Blood 1997;90 Suppl 1:577a.
87. Byrd JC, White CA, Link B, et al. Rituximab therapy in previously treated Waldenström's macroglobulinemia: preliminary evidence of activity. Blood 1998;92 Suppl 1:106a.
88. Rambaud JC, Halphen M, Galian A, Tsapis A. Immunoproliferative small intestinal disease (IPSID): relationships with α-chain disease and 'Mediterranean' lymphomas. Springer Semin Immunopathol 1990;12:239.
89. Ben-Ayed F, Halphen M, Najjar T, et al. Treatment of alpha chain disease. Results of a prospective study in 21 Tunisian patients by the Tunisian–French Intestinal Lymphoma Study Group. Cancer 1989;63:1251.
90. Wahner-Roedler DL, Kyle RA. Heavy-chain diseases. In: Malpas JA, Bergsagel DE, Kyle RA, Anderson KC (eds) Myeloma: biology and management, 2nd edn. New York, Oxford University Press, 1998, p 604.
91. Wahner-Roedler DL, Kyle RA. Mu-heavy chain disease: presentation as a benign monoclonal gammopathy. Am J Hematol 1992;40:56.

Chapter 98

Acute Lymphoblastic Leukemia

Dario Campana and Ching-Hon Pui

Acute lymphoblastic leukemia (ALL) is a malignant proliferation and accumulation of immature lymphoid cells. The leukemic cell population is clonal, as evidenced by cytogenetics, glucose-6-phosphate dehydrogenase enzyme studies, analysis of antigen–receptor gene rearrangements and of X-linked restriction fragment-length polymorphisms.[1]

Although leukemic cells generally do not proliferate as actively as their normal hematopoietic counterparts,[2] they accumulate inexorably and compete successfully with normal cells. Their inability to differentiate and their increased resistance to apoptosis may explain this phenomenon. At diagnosis, leukemic cells have usually already replaced normal bone marrow cells and disseminated to various extramedullary sites.[1,3] Therefore, the presenting features of ALL typically reflect the degree of bone marrow replacement and the extent of extramedullary spread.

EPIDEMIOLOGY AND ETIOLOGY

ALL is the most common malignancy in patients under 15 years of age. In developed countries, incidence peaks in children aged 2–5 years, remains low during later childhood, adolescence and young adulthood, and then rises again during and after the sixth decade. Males are generally affected more often than females in all age groups. The incidence is higher in Whites than in Blacks in most age groups, and especially among children 2–5 years of age. ALL rates are higher in northern and western Europe, North America and Oceania, and lower in Asia and Africa.[4]

A small number (5%) of cases are associated with inherited genetic syndromes.[1] Children with Down syndrome have a 10–30-fold increased risk of leukemia; ALL predominates among those older than 3 years of age. Patients who have autosomal recessive genetic diseases associated with increased predisposition to chromosomal breakage, such as ataxia–telangiectasia and Bloom syndrome, are also at increased risk of ALL, as are patients with other congenital immunodeficiencies, such as X-linked agammaglobulinemia, immunoglobulin A deficiency, and common variable immunodeficiency.[1]

Fraternal twins and siblings of affected children are at a 2–4-fold greater risk of developing leukemia during the first decade of life than are unrelated children.[1] When leukemia occurs in one identical twin, the other twin generally has a 20% chance of developing the disease. However, if leukemia develops before the index twin is 1 year of age, it almost invariably develops in the other twin, typically within a few months. Molecular studies have demonstrated that intrauterine metastasis from one twin to the other via their shared placental circulation is responsible for the concordant leukemia.[5]

Although environmental agents such as ionizing radiation and chemical mutagens have been implicated in the induction of ALL, almost all cases lack discernible etiologic factors.[4] Associations of childhood ALL with maternal exposure to various potential mutagens, neonatal administration of vitamin K, and vicinity to electromagnetic fields have not been proven.[4] As the risk of B-lineage ALL is increased by higher socioeconomic status and isolation, Greaves[6] hypothesized that many childhood cases are the consequence of an abnormally late immunologic response to common infections, enhancing the likelihood of leukemogenic genetic mutations.

PATHOGENESIS

The lymphoblasts in virtually all cases of ALL have acquired genetic changes believed to be central to the development of leukemia.[7] These include changes in both the number (ploidy) and the structure of chromosomes; structural changes consist of translocations, inversions, deletions, point mutations and amplifications. The dysregulation of transcription factors that regulate hematopoietic cell homeostasis provides a plausible mechanism for the generation of leukemia (Table 98.1). Notably, many of these are involved in the regulation of the major clusters of homeobox-containing *HOX* genes, whose expression is tightly regulated during hematopoietic cell differentiation.[7] In addition, chimeric protein products of gene fusions can directly interfere with normal apoptotic pathways, as has been demonstrated in the case of the E2A-HLF protein.[8] Cell survival requirements can also be altered by the dysregulated activity of tyrosine kinases, as in the case of the *BCR–ABL* gene fusion.[9] Finally, there may be alterations affecting the expression and function of molecules that regulate apoptosis, such as increased BCL2 expression or mutations in the *BAX* gene in leukemic lymphoblasts.[10,11]

KEY CONCEPTS

Pathogenesis of ALL

- ALL arises from a clonal expansion of B- or T-lymphoid progenitors.
- Most cells have nonrandom genetic changes, including numerical and structural chromosomal abnormalities; these are believed to be central to leukemogenesis.
- Genetic changes affect factors that regulate hematopoietic cell homeostasis.
- ALL can have a long period of latency; in some cases, the associated genetic abnormalities are acquired before birth.

Proteins involved in ALL development

Dysregulated proteins	Function	Translocation	Involved genes	ALL phenotype	Frequency (%)	
					Children	Adults
TEL and AML1	Transcription factors	t(12;21)(p13;q22)	*TEL/AML1*	Early pre-B	20–25	<1
E2A and PBX1	Transcription factors	t(1;19)(q23;p13.3)	*E2A/PBX1*	Pre-B	5–6	3
E2A and HLF	Transcription factors	t(17;19)(q22;p13.3)	*E2A/ HLF*	Early pre-B	<1	<1
HOX11	Transcription factors	t(10;14)(q24;q11.2) t(7;10)(q35;q24)	*HOX11/TCRD* *TCRB/HOX11*	T-cell T-cell	<1 <1	3–7 <1
LMO1 and LMO2	Transcription factors	t(11;14)(p15;q11.2) t(11;14)(p13;q11.2) t(7;11)(q35;p13)	*LMO1/TCRD* *LMO2/TCRD* *TCRB/LMO2*	T-cell T-cell T-cell	<1 <1 <1	<1 5–7 <1
SCL	Transcription factor	t(1;7)(p32;q35) t(1;14)(p32;q11.2)	*SCL/TCRB* *SCL/TCRD*	T-cell T-cell	<1 0.5	<1 ~20
MLL	Regulation of transcription and kinase activity	t(4;11)(q21;q23) t(11;19)(q23;p13.3)	*MLL/AF4* *MLL/ENL*	Early pre-B Early pre-B	2 1	3–5 <1
MYC	Transcription factor	t(8;14)(q24.1;q32) t(2;8)(p12;q24.1) t(8;22)(q24.1;q11) t(8;14)(q24.1;q11.2)	*MYC/IGH* *IGK/MYC* *MYC/IGL* *MYC/TCRA*	B-cell B-cell B-cell T-cell	2–3 <1 <1 <1	3–4 <1 <1 <1
ABL	Tyrosine kinase	t(9;22)(q34;q11.2)	*BCR/ABL*	Early pre-B	3–4	20–30
IL-3	Cytokine	t(5;14)(q31;q32)	*IL3/IGH*	Early pre-B	<1	<1
TAN1	Notch receptor	t(7;9)(q34;q34)	*TCRB/TAN1*	T-cell	<1	<1

Table 98.1 Proteins dysregulated by chromosomal translocations and involved in the development of ALL.

The time lapse between genetic lesion and overt leukemia is unknown, but a prolonged latency is likely. Indeed, genetic abnormalities seen in children diagnosed with ALL at ages 2–5 years were found to be present in their blood cells at birth,[12] suggesting that childhood ALL may initiate in utero.

CLINICAL FEATURES

Physical examination may reveal pallor, petechiae, ecchymoses, and bone tenderness caused by leukemic infiltration or hemorrhage. Anemia may cause fatigue and lethargy, dyspnea, angina and dizziness. If thrombocytopenia is severe there may be life-threatening bleeding (e.g. intracranial hematoma). Neutropenia may lead to severe infection. Approximately half the patients present with fever, which may be induced by pyrogenic cytokines (e.g. interleukin (IL)-1, IL-6 and tumor necrosis factor (TNF)) released from the leukemic cells, or by infection.

The liver, spleen and lymph nodes are common sites of extramedullary involvement. An anterior mediastinal (thymic) mass is typical of T-cell ALL. Painless enlargement of the scrotum can be a sign of testicular leukemia or hydrocele resulting from lymphatic obstruction. Arthralgia and bone pain may be especially severe in young children. Very rarely, ALL produces no signs or symptoms and is detected during routine examination.

LABORATORY FEATURES

Anemia, neutropenia and thrombocytopenia are common findings, and their severity reflects the degree of bone marrow replacement by leukemic lymphoblasts. The presenting leukocyte counts range from 0.1 to 1500×10^9/l (median $10–12 \times 10^9$/l); hyperleukocytosis ($>100 \times 10^9$/l) occurs in up to 16% of patients (Fig. 98.1). Profound neutropenia ($<0.5 \times 10^9$/l) is found in 20–40% of patients. Most patients have circulating leukemic blast cells. Elevated serum lactate dehydogenase activity, and uric acid and phosphorous concentrations are common in patients with a large leukemic cell burden.

Leukemic blast cells can be identified at diagnosis in the cerebrospinal fluid (CSF) of as many as one-third of childhood ALL patients, most of whom have no neurologic symptoms.[1] Traditionally, central nervous system (CNS) leukemia is defined by the presence of at least 5 leukocytes per microliter of CSF and the detection of leukemic blast cells, or by the presence of cranial nerve palsy.

DIAGNOSIS AND CELL CLASSIFICATION

Morphologic and cytochemical analysis

Morphologic analysis of leukemic lymphoblasts in Romanowsky (Wright–Giemsa or May–Grünwald–Giemsa)-stained bone marrow smears distinguishes three subtypes of ALL (L1, L2 and L3) according to the French–American–British (FAB) classification (Fig. 98.2).[13] Cells with L3 morphology (typical of B-cell ALL; see below) are large and homogeneous, have regularly shaped nuclei with prominent nucleoli, and have basophilic cytoplasm with prominent vacuoles. L1 blast cells are distinguished from the L2 variety by their smaller size, more regular nuclear shape, higher nucleocytoplasmic ratio, and fewer and less distinct

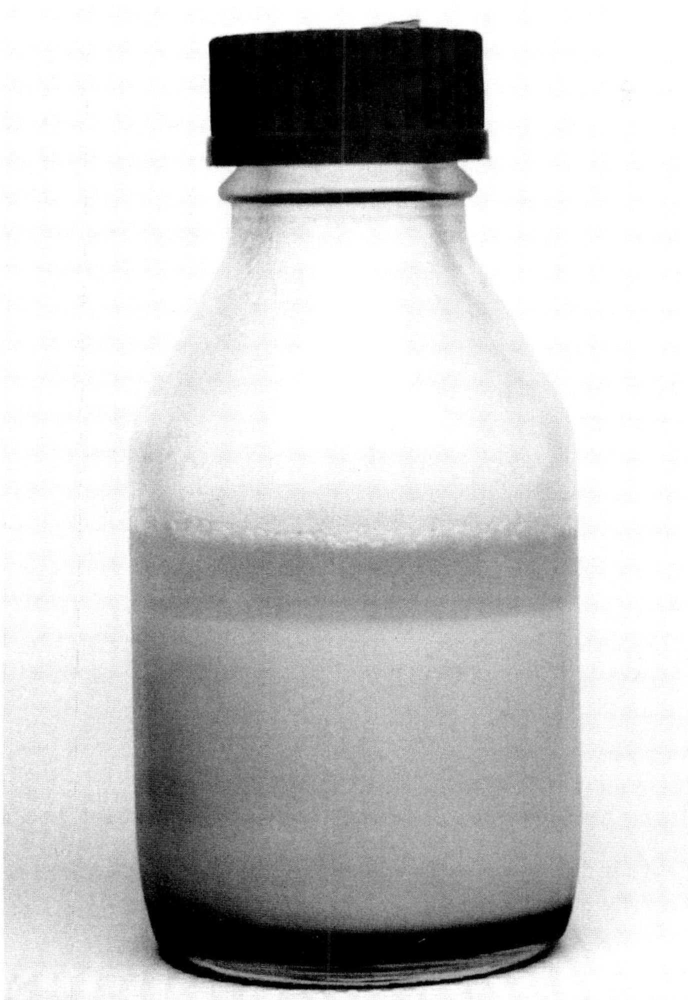

Figure 98.1 Leukapheresis product from a patient with ALL at diagnosis. The upper layer is plasma; red blood cells constitute the bottom layer; the large middle layer is constituted by leukemia cells, illustrating well the term 'leukemia' (white blood). (See also color plate 98.1.)

CLINICAL PEARLS

Diagnosis and risk classification

- Common physical signs of ALL include pallor, petechiae and ecchymoses; anemia, neutropenia, and thrombocytopenia are common laboratory findings.
- Romanowsky-stained bone marrow smears typically reveal replacement of normal hematopoietic cells by leukemic lymphoblasts.
- Cytochemical stains and immunophenotyping are used to establish the diagnosis.
- The most useful risk factors are age and leukocyte count at diagnosis, specific genetic abnormalities and early response to treatment; the most reliable methods to assess treatment response are flow cytometric identification of aberrant immunophenotypes and PCR detection of antigen receptor genes.

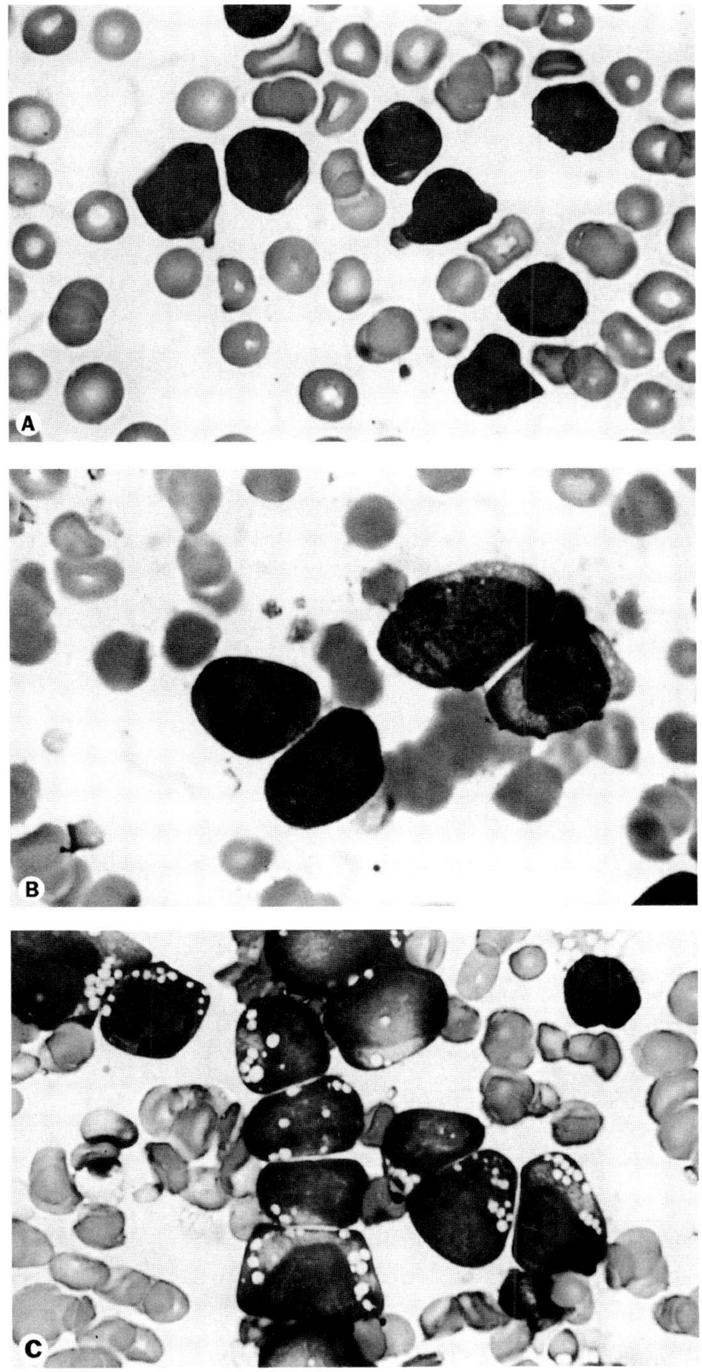

Figure 98.2 ALL cell morphology. (**A**) small regular blast cells (FAB L1). (**B**) Large blast cells with moderate amounts of cytoplasm admixed with smaller blast cells (FAB L2). (**C**) Blast cells in a case of B-cell ALL with basophilic cytoplasm, prominent nucleoli and cytoplasmic vacuoli (FAB L3). (See also color plate 98.2.)

nucleoli. The distinction between these two subtypes lacks clinical or biologic correlates.

Analysis of a Romanowsky-stained smear cannot accurately distinguish between ALL and acute myeloid leukemia. Cytochemical stains help this distinction. Myeloperoxidase, Sudan black and nonspecific esterases, including α-naphthyl butyrate and α-naphthyl acetate esterase, react with myeloid blast cells, whereas periodic acid–Schiff reagent reacts positively in over 70% of ALL cases.

Immunologic classification

The subtypes of ALL are usually identified by their immunophenotype (Table 98.2).

Early pre-B ALL and pre-pre-B ALL

Leukemic blast cells of early pre-B ALL resemble normal B-lymphoid cell precursors. The leukemic cells of early pre-B ALL express CD19, CD22 and CD79a.[14] CD10 and terminal deoxynucleotidyl transferase (TdT) are detectable in 90% of cases, and CD34 in more than 75% of cases.[14]

Leukemias that involve rearrangements of the *MLL* gene are sometimes called pre-pre-B or pro-B ALL because of their expression of CD19 and CD34 without CD10.[14] These cases also typically express CD15 and CD65, and surface chondroitin protoglycan sulfate.[14]

Pre-B ALL

In pre-B ALL cases lymphoblasts accumulate cytoplasmic immunoglobulin μ heavy chains but have no detectable surface immunoglobulins.[14] This subtype also expresses CD19, CD22 and CD79a. Rearrangement of immunoglobulin light-chain genes is evident in some of these leukemias, but κ and λ proteins are not detectable. More than 95% of these leukemias express CD10 and TdT, but only two-thirds express CD34.

Transitional (or late) pre-B ALL

Leukemic cells that express both cytoplasmic and surface immunoglobulin μ heavy chains without κ or λ light chains have been designated transitional pre-B ALL.[14] The surface μ chains on these leukemic cells are linked to pseudo-light chains (Chapter 4) as well as to CD79a and CD79b. As in pre-B ALL, the blast cells express CD19, CD10, usually TdT, and sometimes CD34.

B-cell ALL

In cases of B-cell ALL cells express surface immunoglobulin μ heavy chains plus either κ or λ light chains.[14] In most cases cells have L3 morphology and express CD19, CD22, CD20, and frequently CD10 and CD23; CD34 is absent. Often these cases represent the leukemic phase of Burkitt lymphoma arising in the abdomen or the head and neck.

In a less common subtype of B-cell ALL, blast cells have L1 or L2 morphology, may express TdT and CD34, and express CD20 only weakly.[14] Extramedullary masses are not seen at presentation, and rearrangements of the c-*MYC* (typical of the more common B-cell ALL variety) gene are absent.

T-cell ALL

T-cell ALL cells have surface CD7 and cytoplasmic CD3 (cCD3) antigens;[4] more than 90% of T lymphoblasts express CD2, CD5 and TdT.[15]

Three stages of immunophenotypic differentiation can be determined: early ($CD7^+$, $cCD3^+$, surface $CD3^-$, $CD4^-$ and $CD8^-$), intermediate ($cCD3^+$, surface $CD3^-$, $CD4^+$, $CD8^+$ and $CD1^+$) and late (surface $CD3^+$, $CD1^-$, and either $CD4^+$ or $CD8^+$). However, in as many as 25% of T-lineage ALL cases, immunophenotype does not conform to any of these maturation stages. The prognostic significance of surface CD2, CD3, CD5 or CD10 expression is controversial.[15] T-lineage ALL cases that are $CD2^-$ are sometimes called 'pre-T ALL'. This subset is more common in adults than in children, and is associated with an unfavorable outcome.[3]

T-cell receptor (TCR) proteins are heterogeneously expressed in T-lineage ALL.[16] In approximately two-thirds of cases membrane CD3 and TCR proteins are absent. In half of these cases, however, TCR proteins (TCRβ, TCRα, or both) are present in the cytoplasm. When membrane CD3 and TCR chains are expressed, the αβ form of the TCR predominates; a minority of cases express TCRγδ proteins.

ALL with myeloid-associated antigen expression

The expression of myeloid-associated antigens, such as CD13, CD15, CD33 or CD65, in leukemic lymphoblasts confounded leukemia classification in early studies. However, the diagnosis of B-lineage ALL should be made when leukemic cells express cytoplasmic immunoglobulin, CD79a, or CD19 plus CD22, regard-

Table 98.2 Immunophenotypes of ALL subtypes.

Immunophenotypes of ALL subtypes

	Leukocyte antigen expression (% of cases positive)										Frequency (%)	
Subtype	CD19	cCD22	CD79a	CD10	CD7	CD2	cCD3	cIg μ	sIg μ	sIg κ or γ	Children	Adults
Pre-pre-B	100	>95[a]	>95	0	0	0	0	0	0	0	5	10
Early pre-B	100	>95[a]	>95	95	5	<5	0	0	0	0	60–65	50–55
Pre-B	100	100[a]	100	>95	0	0	0	100	0	0	20–25	10
Transitional pre-B	100	100[a]	100	50	0	0	0	100	100	0	1–3	?
B	100	100[a]	100	50	0	0	0	>95	>95	>95	2–3	4
Pre-T	<5	0	0–20	45	100	0	100	0	0	0	1	5
T	<5	0	0–20	45	100	95	100[a]	0	0	0	10–15	15–20

c, cytoplasmic; cIg μ, cytoplasmic immunoglobulin μ chain; sIg μ, surface immunoglobulin μ chain; sIg κ or λ, surface immunoglobulin κ or λ chains.
[a]Detectable on the cell surface membrane in some cases.

less of myeloid-associated antigen expression. Likewise, the diagnosis of T-lineage ALL should be made when leukemic cells express CD7 plus either surface or cytoplasmic CD3.

Myeloid-associated antigen expression in ALL has no independent prognostic significance, but it is associated with molecular genetic abnormalities.[17] For example, atypical expression of the myeloid-associated antigen CD15 is characteristic of B-lineage ALL with the t(4;11) translocation, whereas expression of the myeloid-associated antigens CD13 and CD33 is more frequent in cases with the *TEL–AML1* gene fusion.[14]

Cytogenetic and molecular classification

Hyperdiploid ALL

In approximately half of ALL cases leukemic blast cells have a modal chromosomal number greater than 46. In approximately 50% of hyperdiploid cases the leukemic cells have additional structural chromosomal abnormalities, including duplication of 1q and isochromosome of 17q; however, no consistent structural abnormality has been identified.

Hyperdiploid cases with a modal chromosome number of 51–65 represent a distinct biologic subset with an excellent prognosis.[1] Leukemic lymphoblasts with this karyotype have a marked propensity to undergo apoptosis,[18] and they accumulate greater quantities of methotrexate and its active polyglutamate metabolites.[19] These features explain the relatively small presenting tumor burden and the good prognosis of this subtype of ALL.

ALL with E2A-PBX1 *and* E2A-HLF *rearrangements*

The translocation t(1;19)(q23;p13) is found in 20–25% of pre-B ALL cases. The affected genes are those encoding the E2A transcription factor on chromosome 19 and the PBX1 homeodomain-containing transcription factor on chromosome 1.[20] The resulting E2A–PBX1 fusion protein contains the transcriptional activation domains of E2A linked to the DNA-binding domain of PBX1. Thus, the protein should inappropriately activate the transcription of genes normally regulated by PBX1. Ectopic expression of the E2A–PBX1 chimeric protein in mice leads to the development of lymphomas and myeloid leukemias.[21,22]

A second *E2A* fusion gene is created by the t(17;19), in which *E2A* is fused to the gene that encodes hepatic leukemia factor (*HLF*).[23] HLF is a member of the bZip family of transcription factors. The E2A–HLF fusion protein contains the transcriptional activation domains of E2A linked to the DNA-binding and protein–protein interaction motifs of HLF. Therefore, this chimeric protein should activate the transcription of genes normally regulated by HLF. In addition, E2A–HLF itself appears to inhibit apoptosis.[23]

ALL with TEL-AML1 *rearrangements*

The t(12;21) translocation forms a chimeric gene consisting of the 5′ portion of the *TEL* gene (also known as *ETV6*) and the nearly complete *AML1* gene (also known as *CBFA2*).[24] This translocation can rarely be identified by conventional cytogenetic banding techniques, but can frequently be detected by fluorescence in situ hybridization (FISH) (Chapter 125). The *TEL–AML1* gene fusion is the most common genetic abnormality in pediatric ALL (approximately 20% of cases), but is extremely rare in adult ALL. In children, it defines a subgroup with an excellent prognosis.[24]

The *TEL* gene belongs to the *Ets* family of transcription factors. TEL functions as a sequence-specific DNA-binding transcription regulator. It is normally widely expressed and appears to have an essential role in yolk sac angiogenesis, neuronal development and the establishment of bone marrow hematopoiesis.[24] *AML1* encodes a transcription factor that binds DNA as a heterodimer with core-binding factor B, and is essential for the development of definitive hematopoiesis.[24] In addition, the TEL–AML1 protein represses AML1-mediated transcriptional activation through a dominant negative mechanism.[24] The non-translocated *TEL* allele is frequently deleted in cases with the t(12;21); this deletion may be important for leukemogenesis.[24]

ALL with MLL *gene rearrangements*

Structural alterations involving band 11q23 of chromosome 11 are the most frequent cytogenetic abnormality in infant ALL.[25] In most cases the target is a gene designated *MLL*, for mixed-lineage leukemia (also known as *HRX*, *ALL1* and *HTRX1*).[25] The most common 11q23 abnormality in ALL is the t(4;11), which produces a chimeric protein that contains the N-terminal portion of MLL linked in-frame to the C-terminal portion of AF-4.

MLL normally maintains expression of specific *HOX* genes by binding to DNA and recruiting a histone acetylase that keeps chromatin in an open conformation, accessible to transcriptional activators.[25] In addition to interacting with DNA, MLL also interacts directly with the antiphosphatase Sbf1,[26] which positively regulates kinase signaling pathways. The leukemia-associated alterations in MLL directly disrupt both of these crucial activities.

ALL with BCR-ABL *rearrangements*

The t(9;22)(q34;q11) encodes a chimeric gene consisting of the 5′ portion of *BCR* fused to the 3′ portion of *ABL*.[9] Whereas in chronic myelogenous leukemia breaks occur most often within the major breakpoint cluster region and encode a 210-kDa BCR–ABL chimeric tyrosine kinase, breaks in ALL tend to occur in the minor breakpoint cluster regions, forming a 190-kDa BCR–ABL. In each fusion protein, N-terminal sequences of ABL are replaced by BCR sequences. This alteration results in a constitutively active ABL tyrosine kinase that induces aberrant signaling and activates multiple cellular pathways. Expression of either chimeric protein results in malignant hematopoietic cell transformation and leukemia in murine experimental systems.[27]

ALL with c-MYC *rearrangements*

The majority of B-cell ALL cases have the t(8;14) translocation or, less frequently, t(2;8) and t(8;22). These translocations juxtapose the c-*MYC* proto-oncogene on chromosome 8 with the *IgH*, *Igκ* and *Igλ* loci on chromosomes 14, 2 and 22, respectively. These rearrangements dysregulate the expression of c-MYC (a transcription factor), resulting in altered cell proliferation and survival.[28] Dysregulated c-MYC expression in mice, in the presence of other genetic alterations, results in the generation of B-lineage leukemia/lymphoma.[29]

Genetic abnormalities in T-cell ALL

Genes that are dysregulated in T-cell ALL include *SCL* (*TAL1*), *LMO1* (*TTG1*), *LMO2* (*TTG2*), and *HOX11*. As a result of the t(1;14), *SCL* (a gene involved in early hematopoiesis) is inserted into the *TCRδ* locus on chromosome 14; an internal deletion in the 5′ untranslated region of *SCL* is found in an additional 25% of T-lineage ALL cases.[30] This deletion juxtaposes a locus called *SIL* with the *SCL* coding region, resulting in the expression of a fused *SIL–SCL* transcript that encodes a normal SCL protein.

The t(11;14)(p15;q11) inserts *LMO1* into the *TCRα/δ* locus, whereas the t(11;14)(p13;q11) rearranges *LMO2* into this locus. The LMO1 and LMO2 proteins, which are then inappropriately expressed, contain two zinc-binding domains and participate in multiprotein DNA-binding complexes. LMO2, like SCL, plays an essential role in the development of primitive and definitive hematopoiesis.[31]

An additional alteration found in T-cell ALL cases is the deletion of the *INK4a* and *INK4b* genes, which encode the $p16^{INK4a}$ and $p15^{INK4b}$ inhibitors of the Cdk4 cyclin D-dependent kinase, from chromosome 9p21.[32] This locus, which is deleted in more than 50% of T-lineage cases, also encodes another cell-cycle regulatory protein, $p19^{ARF}$, which arrests cell-cycle progression through p53.[33]

DIFFERENTIAL DIAGNOSIS

The acute onset of petechiae, ecchymoses and bleeding may suggest idiopathic thrombocytopenic purpura (often associated with a recent viral infection, large platelets in blood smears and no evidence of anemia). Both ALL and aplastic anemia may present with pancytopenia and complications associated with bone marrow failure, but in aplastic anemia hepatosplenomegaly and lymphadenopathy are rare and the skeletal changes associated with leukemia are absent.

Infectious mononucleosis and other viral infections can be confused with leukemia. Detection of atypical lymphocytes or elevated viral titers aid in the diagnosis. Patients with pertussis or parapertussis may have marked lymphocytosis, but the affected cells are mature lymphocytes rather than lymphoblasts. Bone pain, arthralgia and occasionally arthritis may mimic juvenile rheumatoid arthritis, rheumatic fever, other collagen diseases or osteomyelitis.

Childhood ALL should also be distinguished from pediatric small round-cell tumors that involve the bone marrow, including neuroblastoma, rhabdomyosarcoma and retinoblastoma. Generally, in patients with solid tumors a primary lesion can be found by routine diagnostic studies, and any disseminated tumor cells tend to form clumps.

OUTLINE OF THERAPY

B-cell ALL

The most effective treatment regimens for B-cell ALL are based on high-dose cyclophosphamide, methotrexate and intrathecal therapy given over a relatively short time (3–6 months). The addition of high-dose cytarabine, etoposide or ifosfamide may further improve cure rates. Currently, 70–80% of children with B-cell ALL[34,35] and 50% of adults may be cured with this treatment approach.[36]

B-cell precursor and T-cell ALL

Treatment for B-cell precursor or T-cell ALL consists of three standard phases: remission induction, intensification (consolidation) and prolonged continuation therapy. CNS-directed therapy is begun early and is given for lengths of time that reflect the patient's risk of relapse and the intensity of the primary systemic regimen.

THERAPEUTIC PRINCIPLES

- Risk-directed therapy is necessary to avoid overtreatment or undertreatment. Childhood ALL usually comprises low-, standard- and high-risk groups, whereas adults have either standard- or high-risk leukemia.
- B-cell ALL is treated with intensive combination chemotherapy given over a relatively short time. Treatment of B-precursor or T-cell ALL consists of three standard phases: remission induction, intensification (consolidation), and prolonged continuation therapy.
- Allogeneic stem-cell transplantation is indicated for patients with early bone marrow relapse, induction failure or clinicobiologic features indicating a very high risk of relapse.
- The emergence of agents that differ radically from conventional treatment may require new approaches to clinical testing.

Typical remission induction regimens include a glucocorticoid (prednisone, prednisolone or dexamethasone), vincristine, and either L-asparaginase (for children) or an anthracycline (for adults).[1,3,37] The rate of complete remission now ranges from 97% to 99% in children and from 75% to 90% in adults.

Intensification therapy either uses high doses of multiple agents not used during the induction phase or repeats the induction regimen.[1] Regimens used for children include high-dose methotrexate with or without 6-mercaptopurine; high-dose L-asparaginase given for an extended period; an epipodophyllotoxin plus cytarabine; or a combination of dexamethasone, vincristine, L-asparaginase, doxorubicin and thioguanine, with or without cyclophosphamide. Intensification treatment has improved the outcomes of children with ALL.[1] Its value is less certain for adults, although several studies have suggested that it is beneficial.[3,37,38]

In childhood ALL continuation therapy generally lasts 2–2.5 years for girls and 3 years for boys. In adult trials continuation therapy is given for 2–3 years. The usual continuation regimen for children with ALL is a combination of methotrexate administered weekly and mercaptopurine administered daily, with intermittent pulses of vincristine and dexamethasone.[1] Another integral component of many protocols is reinduction therapy. This treatment employs drugs similar to those used during the initial phase of induction therapy and has improved the outcomes of both children and adults with ALL.[1,37]

Cranial irradiation (24 Gy) plus intrathecal methotrexate, introduced after the induction of complete remission, became the cornerstone of ALL therapy in the 1970s.[39] More recently, because of concerns about neurotoxicity and the occurrence of brain tumors, intensive intrathecal and systemic chemotherapy are used instead for most patients. For the approximately 10% of patients at a high risk of CNS relapse, cranial irradiation is still used by many investigators, albeit at a reduced dosage (12–18 Gy).

Allogeneic stem-cell transplantation

Allogeneic stem-cell transplantation is usually reserved for patients with relapsed or refractory leukemia. Because of their dismal prognosis, patients with the t(9;22) or induction failure also commonly receive allogeneic stem-cell transplantation during the first remission (Chapter 102).[40] With improvements in the prevention of transplant-related toxicities, suitable marrow donors are not only HLA-identical siblings or one-antigen mismatched family members, but also matched unrelated donors and, in some situations, two- and three-antigen mismatched family members. Umbilical cord blood and peripheral blood stem cells have also been used successfully.

COURSE AND PROGNOSIS

Relapse

Relapse is defined as the reappearance of leukemic cells at any site in the body after remission has occurred. Most relapses occur during treatment or within the first 2 years after its completion, although they have been observed 10 years or more after diagnosis.[1] The bone marrow is the most common site of relapse in ALL. The frequency of relapse in extramedullary sites, such as the CNS and testes, has decreased to 5% or less. Leukemic relapse occasionally occurs at other sites, including the eye, ear, ovary, uterus, bone, muscle, tonsil, kidney, mediastinum, pleura and paranasal sinuses.

Bone marrow relapse, with or without extramedullary involvement, predicts a poor outcome for most patients.[41] Factors indicating an especially poor prognosis include relapse on therapy, intensive primary therapy, T-cell immunophenotype, translocation t(9;22), and the presence of circulating blast cells or a high leukocyte count at relapse. Although chemotherapy may secure prolonged second remissions in many patients who relapse late (i.e. >6 months after completion of therapy), allogeneic hematopoietic stem-cell transplantation is the treatment of choice for those who experience hematologic relapse during therapy or shortly thereafter.[40]

Although extramedullary relapse frequently presents as an 'isolated' finding, most occurrences are associated with minimal residual disease in the bone marrow.[42] Hence these patients require intensive systemic treatment to prevent subsequent hematologic relapse.

Treatment sequelae

Improvements in supportive care have reduced the rate of early death to less than 2% in the 1990s.[43] However, the death rate among elderly patients during remission induction therapy can be as high as 30% because of hematologic, hepatic and cardiac toxicity.[3,37]

Induction therapy with prednisone, vincristine and L-asparaginase may cause hyperglycemia and thrombosis. The intensified use of methotrexate and glucocorticoids has caused an increased frequency of neurotoxicity and, in older children and adults, aseptic necrosis of bone. Treatment with anthracyclines at high cumulative doses can produce severe cardiomyopathy, especially in young children. Cranial irradiation causes neuropsychologic deficits and endocrine abnormalities, leading to obesity, short stature, precocious puberty and osteoporosis.

The development of therapy-related acute myeloid leukemia has been linked to the use of topoisomerase II inhibitors (teniposide and etoposide), and the risk is apparently dependent on the treatment schedule and the concomitant use of other agents (e.g. L-asparaginase, alkylating agents, and perhaps antimetabolites).[44] Children who received cranial irradiation at 6 years of age or younger are most susceptible to the development of brain tumors. This risk is increased by the intensive use of antimetabolite drugs before and during cranial irradiation.[45]

PROGNOSTIC FACTORS

Modern therapy for childhood ALL is based on assessment of the relapse hazard. Standard- and high-risk cases are treated with intensive therapy, and less toxic treatments are reserved for low-risk cases. In contrast, virtually all adult patients are candidates for intensive therapy.

Presenting age between 1 and 9 years and a leukocyte count less than 50×10^9/l are widely considered the minimal criteria for low-risk ALL.[1] In adults the outcome of therapy worsens with increasing age and leukocyte count; patients older than 60 and/or leukocyte count $>100 \times 10^9$/l have a particularly poor treatment response.[3,36] Boys fare worse than girls, a disparity partially explained by the higher frequency of T-cell ALL in boys;[1] sex has less influence in adult ALL. The historically poor prognosis for Black children with ALL has been eliminated by more effective treatment.[46]

Certain genetic subtypes of ALL are strongly correlated with age and prognosis. For example, infants with *MLL* gene rearrangements, especially the *MLL–AF4* fusion, have a very low survival rate. In adolescent and adult age groups the frequency of *MLL* rearrangements and the t(9;22) is relatively high, which partly accounts for the overall low long-term survival.[43] In contrast, two favorable genetic abnormalities – hyperdiploidy (> 50 chromosomes) and the *TEL–AML1* fusion – occur mainly in children 1–9 years of age.[43] However, genetic abnormalities are not precise in predicting outcome. For example, as many as 15% of children with hyperdiploid or *TEL–AML1*-positive ALL eventually relapse.[43] Moreover, there are subgroups of patients with *MLL* rearrangements and a favorable age, or with the t(9;22) fusion and either low initial leukocyte counts or a good response to early treatment who fare well on contemporary protocols.[43]

To further refine risk assessment oncologists have used early response to treatment as a factor predictive of outcome. A rapid clearance of leukemic cells from the blood or bone marrow confers a favorable prognosis.[47] More recently, the level of minimal residual disease after the induction of clinical remission has emerged as a powerful tool for gauging treatment response and predicting outcome (see below).

MINIMAL RESIDUAL DISEASE

ALL is considered to be in remission when a patient's bone marrow sample contains less than 5% leukemic cells (the sensitivity limit of morphologic examination). However, patients may have as many as 10^{10} undetectable neoplastic cells when in remission by this criterion.[48] Several methods based on leukemic cell genetic or phenotypic characteristics have been developed to detect minimal (i.e. submicroscopic) residual disease (MRD).[49]

MRD measurements by detection of karyotypic abnormalities

Conventional cytogenetic banding techniques lack sufficient sensitivity for MRD detection. Even FISH has a sensitivity of only 1–5% because of inherent technical artifacts, variations in probe features and variable hybridization efficiency.[49]

The breakpoint fusion regions of chromosomal aberrations can serve as tumor-specific targets for MRD detection by polymerase chain reaction (PCR). PCR amplification of breakpoint fusion sequences at the DNA level can be used only for chromosomal aberrations in which the breakpoints in different cases cluster in a relatively small area (e.g. less than 2 kb), such as deletions in the *SIL/SCL* region in T-cell ALL. For most translocations the breakpoints in different cases cover larger regions. However, the genes involved may be transcribed into fusion-gene mRNA molecules that are similar despite different breakpoints at the DNA level. These transcripts can be used as targets for PCR analysis after reverse transcription (RT) to cDNA. Examples include *BCR–ABL* transcripts in cases with the t(9;22), *E2A–PBX1* mRNA in cases with the t(1;19), and *MLL–AF4* transcripts in cases with the t(4;11).[49]

RT-PCR can consistently detect one leukemic cell among 10^4 or more normal cells. Quantification of PCR products has been significantly improved by the development of 'real-time' PCR technology. The stability of the breakpoint–fusion regions of chromosomal aberrations during the disease course makes them useful tumor-specific PCR targets for MRD detection. However, only approximately 40% of ALL cases have specific chromosomal aberrations with well defined breakpoint–fusion regions.

MRD measurement by detection of junctional regions of Ig and TCR genes

The junctional regions of rearranged *Ig* and *TCR* genes are unique 'fingerprint-like' sequences for each lymphoid clone. They can therefore be used as tumor-specific targets for PCR analysis.

For PCR studies, *Ig* or *TCR* gene rearrangements must be identified in each patient's malignant cells at diagnosis. The sequence information allows the design of junctional region-specific oligonucleotides. These can be used as probes that specifically hybridize to the PCR products derived from the malignant cells, or as primers in the PCR procedure to specifically amplify the rearrangements of the malignant clone (Fig. 98.3).[49]

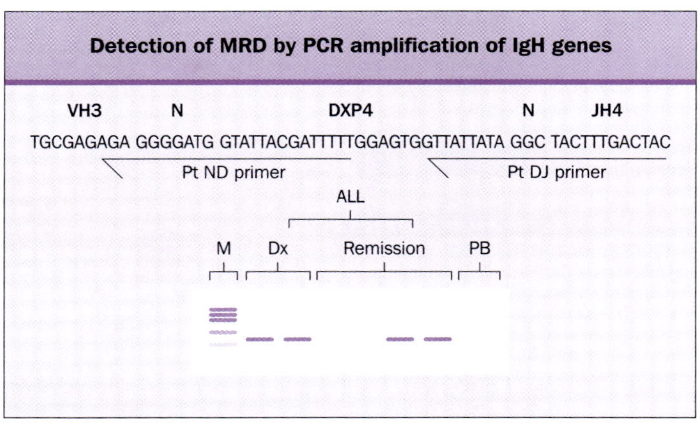

Figure 98.3 Detection of MRD by PCR amplification of immunoglobulin μ heavy-chain genes. The sequence of the patient-specific primer combination used in the PCR reaction is indicated at the top.[52] The bottom panel illustrates the results of the PCR reaction in two aliquots of the bone marrow sample obtained at diagnosis (Dx), and in five aliquots of a sample obtained from the same patient during clinical remission, showing residual leukemia. Two aliquots of a normal peripheral blood sample (PB) used as a control are also shown. M, molecular weight markers.

In most cases PCR amplification of antigen–receptor genes can achieve a sensitivity of at least $1/10^4$. Approximately 90% of B-lineage ALL cases have rearranged *IgH* genes.[50] Almost all T-cell ALL cases have rearranged *TCRβ*, *TCRγ* or *TCRδ* genes; *TCR* rearrangements are also found in many cases of B-lineage ALL.[50]

MRD measurements by flow cytometry

Current strategies for flow cytometric detection of MRD rely on combinations of leukocyte markers that do not normally occur in cells of the peripheral blood and bone marrow. Such leukemia-associated phenotypes can be identified by two-, three- or four-color staining techniques (Fig. 98.4).[51] Flow cytometric analysis of these immunophenotypes allows the detection of one leukemic cell among 10^4 or more normal cells.

A recent review provides a detailed list of the markers used for MRD detection in our laboratory.[51] Briefly, for T-cell ALL, antibodies to TdT are combined with antibodies to T-cell markers such as CD3 or CD5. Quantitative differences between leukemic and normal cells in the expression of CD19, CD10 and CD34 or TdT can be used to distinguish leukemic cells from normal lymphoid cells in approximately 30–50% of B-lineage ALL cases. Other useful markers whose expression may differ quantitatively in leukemic and normal immature B cells are CD38, CD45 and CD22.[51] Qualitative differences between normal and leukemic cells can be detected by using antibodies to myeloid- and NK-associated molecules, or to molecules expressed by mature but not by immature normal B cells. anti-CD66c and monoclonal antibody 7.1 are also informative. If all of these marker combinations are used, MRD can be monitored with a sensitivity of 1 in 10^4 cells in approximately 80% of B-lineage ALL cases.[51] Comparative gene expression studies using DNA microarrays may identify new markers of leukemia, thereby increasing the number of patients for whom MRD studies can be performed.

Neither immunologic nor molecular techniques can at present be applied to all patients, but either can be used for approximately 85–90% of ALL cases. We have found that immunologic and molecular techniques are equally reliable for detecting clinically significant residual leukemia,[52] and that the two methods used in tandem allow universal monitoring of minimal residual ALL.

Clinical studies of MRD

Although MRD monitoring of *BCR–ABL* fusion transcripts predicted treatment outcome in patients with t(9;22) who underwent allogeneic or autologous bone marrow transplantation,[53] detection of *E2A–PBX1* fusion transcripts at the end of consolidation treatment failed to correlate with clinical outcome in a study of childhood t(1;19) cases.[54]

In two recent prospective multicenter studies using PCR amplification of *Ig* and *TCR* genes to monitor MRD in children with ALL,[55,56] the presence or absence and the level of MRD were significantly correlated with the risk of early relapse at each of the time points studied. In both studies a high level ($\geq 10^{-2}$) of leukemic cells was associated with a higher rate of relapse.

The potential clinical value of MRD studies with flow cytometry was demonstrated by a prospective study of MRD in 158 children with ALL treated at our institution.[57] The flow cytometric finding of MRD at any point during clinical remission was highly associated with subsequent clinical relapse (Fig. 98.5).

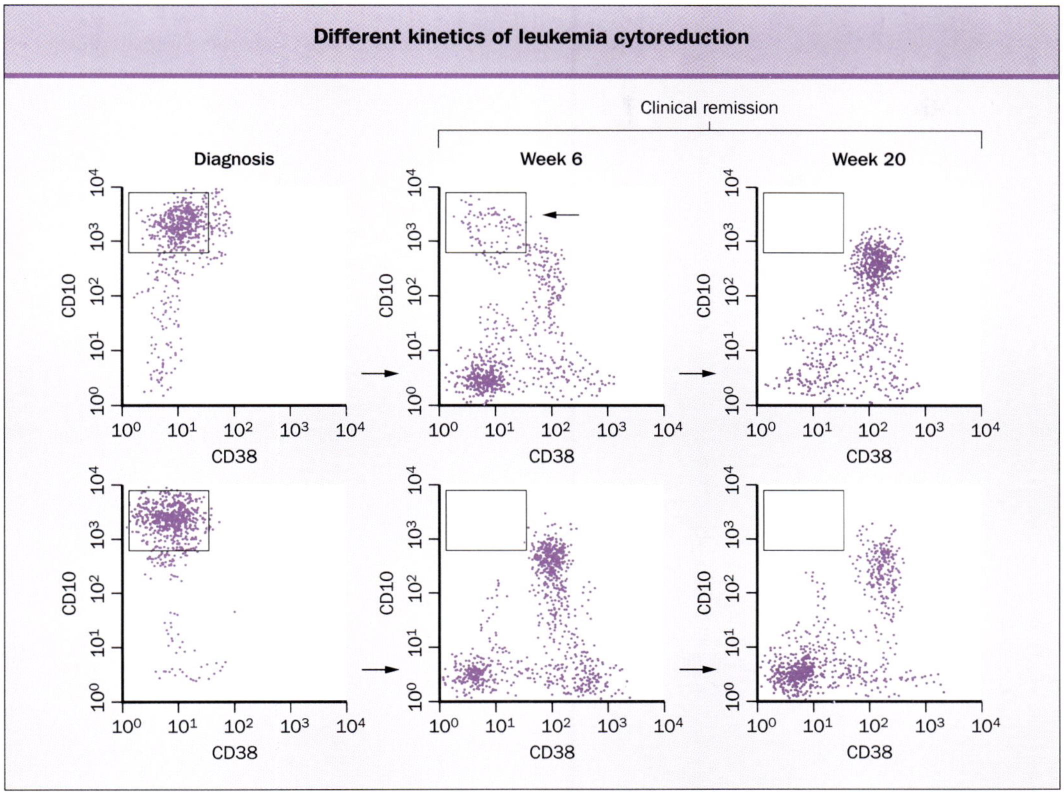

Figure 98.4 Different kinetics of leukemia cytoreduction revealed by MRD studies with flow cytometry.[51] Left panels illustrate the leukemia-specific immunophenotype ($CD10^+$,$CD38^-$) determined at diagnosis in two children with ALL. This phenotype is not found in normal bone marrow. Bone marrow samples were collected during clinical remission from both patients. In one patient (top panels) 0.04% of mononuclear cells expressed the leukemia-specific phenotype at week 6; MRD became undectable by week 20. In the other patient (bottom panels) a profound remission (MRD <0.01%) was already achieved by week 6 and maintained at week 20.

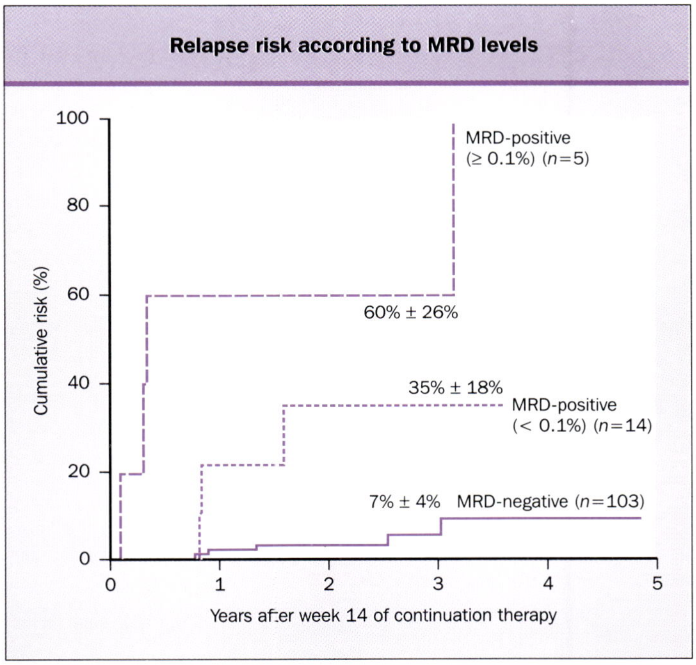

Figure 98.5 Cumulative incidence of relapse in children with ALL according to MRD levels at week 14 of continuation chemotherapy. (From Coustan-Smith E, Behm FG, Sanchez J, et al. Immunological detection of minimal residual disease in children with acute lymphoblastic leukaemia. Lancet 1998;351:550.)

These results strongly suggest that MRD studies should be incorporated into treatment protocols. Single measurements at informative time points during therapy (e.g. at the end of remission induction, after consolidation therapy, and at the end of therapy) may be sufficient for most patients. However, patients who have had positive MRD findings may benefit from more frequent MRD tests during clinical remission.

CURRENT CONTROVERSIES AND FUTURE PERSPECTIVE

The current cure rates in patients with ALL (nearly 80% in children and 40% in adults) attest to the steady progress that has been made in treating this disease (Fig. 98.6). A further increase in cure rates will require efforts to maximize the efficacy and minimize the toxicity of current therapy. However, the methods of achieving optimal treatment are the subject of intense debate. For example, there is considerable disagreement about the optimal risk criteria and the terminology for defining prognostic subgroups. In the future, it may be possible to identify more accurate and universally acceptable variables for risk classification, perhaps through the use of large-scale gene expression analysis.[58] Although MRD monitoring now allows the objective and sensitive assessment of treatment response, it is not yet clear how the results of MRD assays should be used to guide treatment. Should they overrule the predictions of traditional presenting features? Should the intensity or duration of treatment be reduced for patients with consistently negative MRD results?

Although allogeneic transplantation benefits some high-risk cases the value of autologous transplantation is unclear, but its utility could conceivably be improved by the development of effective techniques for purging the graft of leukemic cells, coupled with sensitive methods for the detection of MRD.

The development of new treatments for ALL, beginning with preclinical evaluations, has been at the core of progress in

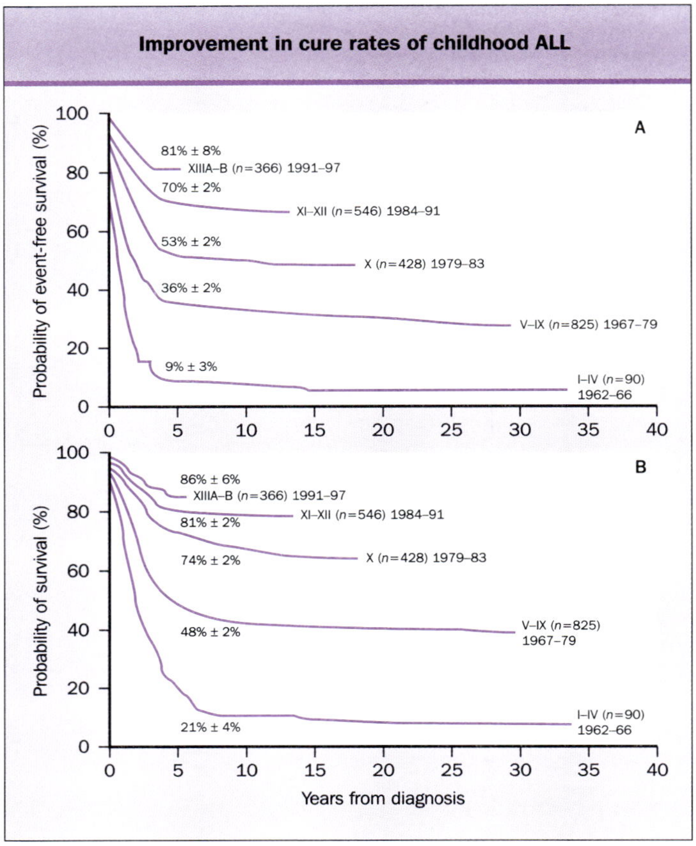

Figure 98.6 Improvement in cure rates of childhood ALL. Probability of event-free survival **(A)** and of survival **(B)** for children with ALL treated at St. Jude Children's Research Hospital in consecutive Total Therapy treatment protocols. (From Pui CH, Evans WE.[43] Drug therapy: acute lymphoblastic leukemia. *N Engl J Med* 1998;339:605 with permission.)

leukemia research. Recently developed compounds with potential clinical value include GW506U78 (a prodrug of arabinosylguanine) for the treatment of T-lineage ALL,[59] and STI571 (formerly CGP 57148, an inhibitor of the Abl tyrosine kinase) for the treatment of ALL with the t(9;22).[60] Other potentially useful therapeutic approaches that are being investigated include biologic response modifiers, monoclonal antibodies, adoptive T cells, compounds interfering with oncogenic molecular aberrations, and inhibitors of angiogenic growth factors. Testing of these approaches may mean modifying the way in which anticancer treatments have traditionally been tested. It may soon be necessary to extend efficacy studies of these agents to patients who have not yet been heavily treated, and perhaps to use MRD measurements to assess tumor response.

REFERENCES

1. Pui CH, Crist WM. Acute lymphoblastic leukemia. In: Pui CH (ed) Childhood leukemias. Cambridge, Cambridge University Press, 1999, p. 288.
2. Campana D, Janossy G. Proliferation of normal and malignant human immature lymphoid cells. Blood 1988;71:1201.
3. Cortes JE, Kantarjian HM. Acute lymphoblastic leukemia. A comprehensive review with emphasis on biology and therapy. Cancer 1995;76:2393.
4. Bhatia S, Ross JA, Greaves MF, Robison LL. Epidemiology and etiology. In: Pui CH (ed). Childhood leukemias. Cambridge, Cambridge University Press, 1999, p. 38.
5. Ford AM, Ridge SA, Cabrera ME, et al. In utero rearrangements in the trithorax-related oncogene in infant leukaemias. Nature 1993;363:358.
6. Greaves MF. Aetiology of acute leukaemia. Lancet 1997;349:344.
7. Look AT. Oncogenic transcription factors in the human acute leukemias. Science 1997;278:1059.
8. Inukai T, Inoue A, Kurosawa H, et al. SLUG, a ces-1-related zinc finger transcription factor gene with antiapoptotic activity, is a downstream target of the E2A-HLF oncoprotein. Mol Cell 1999;4:343.
9. Gotoh A, Broxmeyer HE. The function of BCR/ABL and related proto-oncogenes. Curr Opin Hematol 1997;4:3.
10. Coustan-Smith E, Kitanaka A, Pui CH, et al. Clinical relevance of BCL-2 overexpression in childhood acute lymphoblastic leukemia. Blood 1996;87:1140.
11. Meijerink JP, Mensink EJ, Wang K, et al. Hematopoietic malignancies demonstrate loss-of-function mutations of BAX. Blood 1998;91:2991.
12. Wiemels JL, Cazzaniga G, Daniotti M, et al. Prenatal origin of acute lymphoblastic leukaemia in children. Lancet 1999;354:1499.
13. Bennett JM, Catovsky D, Daniel MT, et al. Proposals for the classification of the acute leukaemias. French–American–British (FAB) cooperative group. Br J Haematol 1976;33:451.
14. Campana D, Behm FG. Immunophenotyping. In: Whittaker JA, Holmes JA (eds). Leukaemia and related disorders. Oxford, Blackwell Science, 1998, p. 71.
15. Pui CH, Behm FG, Singh B, et al. Heterogeneity of presenting features and their relation to treatment outcome in 120 children with T-cell acute lymphoblastic leukemia. Blood 1990;75:174.
16. Campana D, van Dongen JJ, Mehta A, et al. Stages of T-cell receptor protein expression in T-cell acute lymphoblastic leukemia. Blood 1991;77:1546.
17. Pui CH, Rubnitz JE, Hancock ML, et al. Reappraisal of the clinical and biologic significance of myeloid-associated antigen expression in childhood acute lymphoblastic leukemia. J Clin Oncol 1998;16:3768.

18. Ito C, Kumagai M, Manabe A, et al. Hyperdiploid acute lymphoblastic leukemia with 51 to 65 chromosomes: a distinct biological entity with a marked propensity to undergo apoptosis. Blood 1999;93:315.
19. Synold TW, Relling MV, Boyett JM, et al. Blast cell methotrexate–polyglutamate accumulation in vivo differs by lineage, ploidy, and methotrexate dose in acute lymphoblastic leukemia. J Clin Invest 1994;94:1996.
20. Hunger SP. Chromosomal translocations involving the *E2A* gene in acute lymphoblastic leukemia: clinical features and molecular pathogenesis. Blood 1996;87:1211.
21. Dedera DA, Waller EK, LeBrun DP, et al. Chimeric homeobox gene E2A-PBX1 induces proliferation, apoptosis, and malignant lymphomas in transgenic mice. Cell 1993;74:833.
22. Kamps MP, Baltimore D. E2A-Pbxl, the t(1;19) translocation protein of human pre-B-cell acute lymphocytic leukemia, causes acute myeloid leukemia in mice. Mol Cell Biol 1993;13:351.
23. Inaba T, Inukai T, Yoshihara T, et al. Reversal of apoptosis by the leukaemia-associated E2A-HLF chimaeric transcription factor. Nature 1996;382:541.
24. Rubnitz JE, Pui CH, Downing JR. The role of TEL fusion genes in pediatric leukemias. Leukemia 1999;13:6.
25. Rowley JD. The critical role of chromosome translocations in human leukemias. Annu Rev Genet 1998;32:495.
26. De Vivo I, Cui X, Domen J, Cleary ML. Growth stimulation of primary B cell precursors by the anti-phosphatase of Sbf1. Proc Natl Acad Sci USA 1998;95:9471.
27. Daley GQ, Van Etten RA, Baltimore D. Induction of chronic myelogenous leukemia in mice by the P210bcr/abl gene of the Philadelphia chromosome. Science 1990;247:824.
28. Nowell P, Finan J, Dalla-Favera R, et al. Association of amplified oncogene c-myc with an abnormally banded chromosome 8 in a human leukaemia cell line. Nature 1983;306:494.
29. Adams JM, Harris AW, Pinkert CA, et al. The c-myc oncogene driven by immunoglobulin enhancers induces lymphoid malignancy in transgenic mice. Nature 1985;318:533.
30. Brown L, Cheng JT, Chen Q, et al. Site-specific recombination of the tal-1 gene is a common occurrence in human T cell leukemia. EMBO J 1990;9:3343.
31. Rabbitts TH. LMO T-cell translocation oncogenes typify genes activated by chromosomal translocations that alter transcription and developmental processes. Genes Dev 1998;12:2651.
32. Drexler HG. Review of alterations of the cyclin-dependent kinase inhibitor INK4 family genes p15, p16, p18 and p19 in human leukemia–lymphoma cells. Leukemia 1998;12:845.
33. Kamijo T, Zindy F, Roussel MF, et al. Tumor suppression at the mouse INK4a locus mediated by the alternative reading frame product p19ARF. Cell 1997;91:649.
34. Patte C. Non-Hodgkin's lymphoma. Eur J Cancer 1998;34:359.
35. Reiter A, Schrappe M, Tiemann M, et al. Improved treatment results in childhood B-cell neoplasms with tailored intensification of therapy: a report of the Berlin–Frankfurt–Munster group trial NHL-BFM 90. Blood 1999;94:3294.
36. Hoelzer D, Ludwig WD, Thiel E, et al. Improved outcome in adult B-cell acute lymphoblastic leukemia. Blood 1996;87:495.
37. Laport GF, Larson RA. Treatment of adult acute lymphoblastic leukemia. Semin Oncol 1997;24:70.
38. Ludwig WD, Rieder H, Bartram CR, et al. Immunophenotypic and genotypic features, clinical characteristics, and treatment outcome of adult pro-B acute lymphoblastic leukemia: results of the German multicenter trials GMALL 03/87 and 04/89. Blood 1998;92:1898.
39. Pinkel D, Woo S. Prevention and treatment of meningeal leukemia in children. Blood 1994;84:355.
40. Appelbaum FR. Allogeneic hematopoietic stem cell transplantation for acute leukemia. Semin Oncol 1997;24:114.
41. Gaynon PS, Qu RP, Chappell RJ, et al. Survival after relapse in childhood acute lymphoblastic leukemia: impact of site and time to first relapse – the Children's Cancer Group Experience. Cancer 1998;82:1387.
42. Neale GA, Pui CH, Mahmoud HH, et al. Molecular evidence for minimal residual bone marrow disease in children with 'isolated' extramedullary relapse of T-cell acute lymphoblastic leukemia. Leukemia 1994;8:768.
43. Pui CH, Evans WE. Drug therapy: acute lymphoblastic leukemia. N Engl J Med 1998;339:605.
44. Pui CH, Relling MV. Topoisomerase II inhibitor-related acute myeloid leukemia. Br J Haematol 2000 (in press).
45. Relling MV, Rubnitz JE, Rivera GK, et al. High incidence of secondary brain tumours after radiotherapy and antimetabolites. Lancet 1999;354:34.
46. Pui CH, Boyett JM, Hancock ML, Pratt CB, Meyer WH, Crist WM. Outcome of treatment for childhood cancer in black as compared with white children. The St Jude Children's Research Hospital experience, 1962 through 1992. JAMA 1995;273:633.
47. Gajjar A, Ribeiro R, Hancock ML, et al. Persistence of circulating blasts after 1 week of multiagent chemotherapy confers a poor prognosis in childhood acute lymphoblastic leukemia. Blood 1995;86:1292.
48. Campana D, Pui CH. Detection of minimal residual disease in acute leukemia: methodologic advances and clinical significance. Blood 1995;85:1416.
49. Campana D, van Dongen JJ, Pui CH. Minimal residual disease. In: Pui CH (ed) Childhood leukemias. Cambridge, Cambridge University Press, 1999, p.413.
50. van Dongen JJ, Langerak AW. Immunoglobulin and T-cell receptor gene rearrangements. In: Pui CH (ed) Childhood leukemias. Cambridge, Cambridge University Press, 1999, p.145.
51. Campana D, Coustan-Smith E. Detection of minimal residual disease in acute leukemia by flow cytometry. Cytometry 1999;38:139.
52. Neale GA, Coustan-Smith E, Pan Q, et al. Tandem application of flow cytometry and polymerase chain reaction for comprehensive detection of minimal residual disease in childhood acute lymphoblastic leukemia. Leukemia 1999;13:1221.
53. Radich J, Gehly G, Lee A, et al. Detection of bcr-abl transcripts in Philadelphia chromosome-positive acute lymphoblastic leukemia after marrow transplantation. Blood 1997;89:2602.
54. Hunger SP, Fall MZ, Camitta BM, et al. E2A-PBX1 chimeric transcript status at end of consolidation is not predictive of treatment outcome in childhood acute lymphoblastic leukemias with a t(1;19)(q23;p13): a Pediatric Oncology Group study. Blood 1998;91:1021.
55. Cave H, van der Werff ten Bosch, Suciu S, et al. Clinical significance of minimal residual disease in childhood acute lymphoblastic leukemia. European Organization for Research and Treatment of Cancer – Childhood Leukemia Cooperative Group. N Engl J Med 1998;339:591.
56. van Dongen JJ, Seriu T, Panzer-Grumayer ER, et al. Prognostic value of minimal residual disease in acute lymphoblastic leukaemia in childhood. Lancet 1998;352:1731.
57. Coustan-Smith E, Behm FG, Sanchez J, et al. Immunological detection of minimal residual disease in children with acute lymphoblastic leukaemia. Lancet 1998;351:550.
58. Golub TR, Slonim DK, Tamayo P, et al. Molecular classification of cancer: class discovery and class prediction by gene expression monitoring. Science 1999;286:531.
59. Gandhi V, Plunkett W, Rodriguez COJ, et al. Compound GW506U78 in refractory hematologic malignancies: relationship between cellular pharmacokinetics and clinical response. J Clin Oncol 1998;16:3607.
60. Druker BJ, Tamura S, Buchdunger E, et al. Effects of a selective inhibitor of the Abl tyrosine kinase on the growth of Bcr-Abl positive cells. Nature Med 1996;2:561.

Section 9 Immunology of Neoplasia

Chapter 99 Chronic Lymphocytic Leukemia

Geraldine P. Schechter

For reasons still not well understood B-lymphocyte malignancies predominate over T-cell leukemias and lymphomas in most of the world. The most common leukemia in the western hemisphere and Europe is B-cell chronic lymphocytic leukemia (B-CLL), an indolent malignancy of small to medium-sized morphologically mature lymphocytes. It was first recognized by Virchow in 1847, and the initial description based on histochemical stains was made by Turk in 1903. In 1924 Minot and Isaacs[1] reported the first clinical series of CLL, describing its natural history and responsiveness to therapeutic radiation. In the 1960s Dameshek[2] in the United States and Galton[3] in Great Britain separately presented the concept of CLL as an immunoproliferative disorder developing from a gradual accumulation of immunologically incompetent lymphocytes, predominantly in G_0/G_1 of the cell cycle, infiltrating blood, bone marrow, spleen and lymph nodes. During the following decades the leukemia was shown to be a clonal B-cell malignancy in over 90% of patients with this presentation, first on the basis of the restricted light-chain type of the surface membrane immunoglobulin (sIg),[4] and subsequently by the demonstration of restricted G6PD isoenzymes[5] and clonal immunoglobulin gene rearrangements[6] and karyotypic abnormalities.[7] The ability to identify T cells by the E-rosette receptor (CD2) revealed that a small percentage of chronic lymphocytic leukemias are T-cell tumors.[8] With the advent of monoclonal antibodies, these leukemias of differentiated B and T cells could be further subclassified on the basis of their membrane antigens as well as their morphologic and clinical presentations[9] (Table 99.1). B-CLL, the most prevalent of these leukemias, is the main focus of this chapter.

Differentiated lymphocytic leukemias
B-cell type (>90%)
B-cell chronic lymphocytic leukemia (>90%)
small cell type (80%)
pleomorphic variants (20%)
Hairy cell leukemia
B-prolymphocytic leukemia
Lymphoma with a leukemic phase
Lymphoplasmacytic (Waldenström's macroglobulinemia)
Mantle-zone lymphoma
Splenic lymphoma with villous lymphocytes (marginal zone lymphoma)
Follicular lymphoma
T-cell or large granular lymphocyte type (<10%)
Cutaneous T-cell lymphoma
Sézary syndrome/mycosis fungoides
(Small cell variant, mixed cell variant)
Adult T-cell leukemia–lymphoma (HTLV-I associated)
T-helper cell leukemia
T-cell prolymphocytic leukemia
T-cell large granular lymphocyte leukemia
Natural killer (NK) large granular lymphocyte leukemia

Adapted from Newman RA, Peterson B, Davey FR, et al: *Blood* 1993;82:1239. Loughran TP Jr. *Blood* 1993;82:1. Bennett JM, Catovsky D, Daniel M-T, et al. *J Clin Pathol* 1989;42:567. Catovsky D. In: Cheson B (ed) *Chronic lymphocytic leukemia: scientific advances and clinical development*, New York, Marcel Dekker, 1993. Dick FR. In: Jaffe E, (ed) *Surgical pathology of the lymph nodes and related organs*, Philadelphia, Saunders, 1985. Schechter GP, Sausville E, Fischmann AB, et al. *Blood* 1987;69:841.

Table 99.1 The differentiated lymphocytic leukemias.

EPIDEMIOLOGY

B-CLL is the most common leukemia in adults, except for those of Asian origin. The annual age-adjusted incidence rate is 2.9 per 100 000 in the United States and is almost as high in African-Americans as in Caucasians.[10] The incidence is low in Japanese and does not increase substantially after emigration to the United States. CLL is highly unusual under the age of 40, and vanishingly rare under the age of 30. The median age at diagnosis is in the mid-60s to early 70s, and the age-adjusted incidence climbs to 20 per 100 000 over the age of 65 years, reaching a high of 50 per 100 000 after age 85. It is found more commonly in men than women, with a ratio of about 2:1.[10]

PATHOGENESIS AND CELLULAR CHARACTERISTICS

The etiology of B-CLL is not known, however there appears to be a weak genetic predisposition. Familial chronic lymphocytic leukemia has been sporadically reported, and relatives of patients with CLL appear to have an increased propensity to develop CLL itself or other lymphoproliferative or autoimmune disorders.[11] In the familial cases the tumor frequently occurs at an earlier age in subsequent generations.[12] CLL has also been described in a pair of monozygotic twin sisters, but the leukemias differed in their immunoglobulin gene rearrangements, suggesting different transforming somatic events.[13]

In contrast to other leukemias, exposure to ionizing radiation has not been implicated in the etiology of B-CLL. An excess incidence in rural areas has raised the possibility of a role for pesticides and other chemicals which has not been further defined. The human T-cell lymphotropic virus type I (HTLV-I) is an important factor in the pathogenesis of the adult T-cell leukemia–lymphoma endemic to Japan and the Carribbean (Chapter 94). There is no definitive evidence for a viral etiology for other B- or T-cell differentiated leukemias.

The chromosomal abnormalities observed in B-CLL have indicated considerable heterogeneity in this disorder. Clonal abnormalities have been found in more than 80% of leukemias with fluorescence in situ hybridization.[14] More than 50% of cytogenetic abnormalities involve deletions or translocations of 13q14. Trisomy 12 and aberrations of 11q22.3–23.1 (site of the ataxia–telangiectasia mutated *ATM* locus) occur with a frequency of less than 20%. Other structural aberrations occurring with decreasing frequency involve 6q, 17p13 (site of the *p53* gene) and, more rarely, 14q32 (site of the IgH locus) and 11q13 (site of the *BCL1* or *PRAD1* oncogene) (reviewed in Ref. 14). The *BCL1* oncogene, a member of the cyclin gene family involved in the control of the cell cycle, is more frequently associated with mantle zone (centrocytic) lymphomas,[15] but overexpression of the gene has been noted in 11q13 bearing B-CLL.[16] Whether the latter cases represent B-CLL or mantle zone lymphoma with peripheral blood involvement remains controversial. Trisomy 12 appears to be a result of clonal evolution rather than an initiating oncogenetic stimulus, as the karyotypic abnormality is only found in a subset of the clonal B cells.

At the molecular level the identity of the genes involved at the 13q14 deletion and trisomy 12 remains undefined. Although monoallelic deletion of the retinoblastoma tumor suppressor gene *RB1* occurs frequently in leukemias with the 13q deletion,[17] normal levels of the RB1 protein have been detected. This finding suggests that the loss of a second more distal locus, rather than *RB1*, may be playing the pathogenetic role.[18] The *ATM* gene, which is located at 11q22–23, has been shown to be mutated in some B-CLL patients[19] and the discovery of mutations in the germline as well as the tumor has raised speculation that carriers of the ataxia–telangiectasia mutation may be at increased risk of developing CLL.[19]

Interestingly, the cytogenetic abnormalities have defined two different origins of B-CLL and have been correlated with prognosis. 13q14 tumors have increased somatic mutations in the variable regions of their IgH genes (V_H), indicating that the cell of origin is most likely a memory B cell that had previously been exposed to antigen.[20] Intraclonal diversity, such as is seen in follicular lymphoma cells, however, is not present. In contrast, trisomy 12 tumors have little evidence of somatic mutation and appear to represent a naive B cell.[20] Patients with 13q14 tumors are less likely to require treatment, and their survival is similar to that of age-matched controls. Trisomy 12 patients are more likely to show atypical morphology, to require treatment for progressive disease, and to have a shorter survival. Patients with 11q22–23 and 17p abnormalities are also associated with advanced disease and poor prognosis (reviewed in Ref. 14).

Immunophenotypic markers in B-CLL

The surface membrane antigens commonly found on B-CLL cells are illustrated in Figure 99.1. Typically, the leukemic cells express pan-B antigens and monoclonal sIg but exhibit considerable heterogeneity in the expression of antigens normally found on differentiated B cells[21] (Table 99.2). The monoclonal sIg is most often IgM, usually accompanied by IgD. It is characteristically of very low density and, when reacted with fluorescein isothiocyanate (FITC)-labeled anti-Ig antisera, exhibits dim, rapidly fading fluorescence, in contrast to the bright sIg on most normal B cells.[4] Normal B cells which have been anergized by exposure to self-antigen may exhibit similar low levels of sIg. It

Frequency of membrane antigens in B-CLL

Type of antigen	Expression	% CLL patients
Pan B		
Ia	+++	100
CD19 (B4)	+++	100
CD20 (B1)	++ to +++	100
CD24 (BA-1)	+++	100
CD40	++	100
CD45RA (Leukocyte common antigen)	+	100
Mature B		
IgM/IgD	+ (dim)	80
CD21 (C3dR, EBVR)	++	90
CD1c	—	20–40
CD35 (C3bR)	+	<20
FMC7	—	<20
Activation antigens		
CD5	+ to ++	90
CD23 (FcR-IgE)	++	60
CD25 (IL2-R)	—	50
CD48 (Blast-1)	++	50
Adhesion, myeloid & other		
CD44 (homing receptor, adhesion molecule-1)	+++	76–98
CD62L (L-selectin, homing receptor mediates binding to HEV)	+	28–55
CD11c/CD18	++	35
CD14 (My4)	—	35
CD22 (BL-CAM)	—	20
CD54 (ICAM-1)	—	<20
cCLLa (common CLL antigen)	+++	100

Adapted from Freedman AS, Boyd AW, Bieber FR, et al. *Blood* 1987;70:418. Freedman AS, Nadler LM. In: Cheson B (ed) *Chronic lymphocytic leukemia: scientific advances and clinical developments*. New York, Marcel Dekker, 1993; Newman RA, Peterson B, Davey FR, et al. *Blood* 1993;82:1239. Agee JF, Garver FA, Faguet GB. *Blood* 1986;68:62. Faguet GB, Agee JF, Marti GE. *Leukem Lymphoma* 1992;6:335. Sembries S, Pahl H, Stilgenbauer S, et al: *Blood* 1999;93:624.
+, weak; ++, moderate; +++, strong; —, degree of expression not given; EBVR, Epstein–Barr virus receptor; HEV, high endothelial venule; BL-CAM, B lymphocyte-cell adhesion molecule; ICAM, intercellular adhesion molecule.

Table 99.2 Membrane antigens in B-cell chronic lymphocytic leukemia.

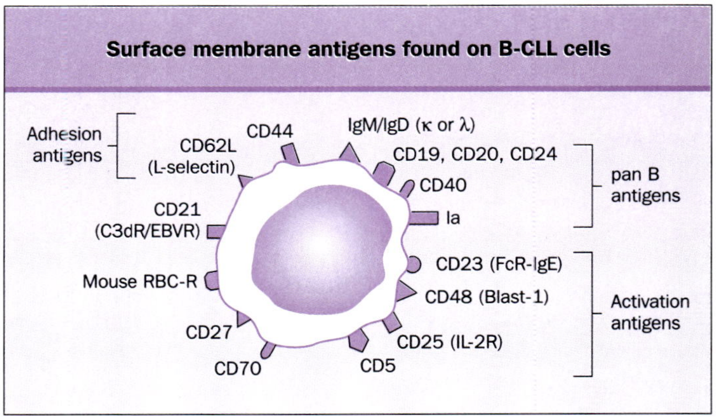

Figure 99.1 Surface membrane antigens found commonly on B-CLL cells. Characteristic B-cell antigens not commonly found on B-CLL cells include CD11a/CD18 (LFA-1), CD35 (C3bR), and CD54 (ICAM-1), CD 79b (of the B cell receptor), CD 80 and CD86. Adapted from Freedman AS, et al. In: Cheson B (ed), *Chronic lymphocytic leukemia: scientific advances and clinical developments*, New York, Marcel Dekker, 1993).

has been suggested that B-CLL may represent a tumor of anergic B cells.[22]

Occasional monoclonal sIgG-bearing leukemias occur, but more often the sIgG reflects either Fc receptor binding of circulating immunoglobulin, or rheumatoid factor activity of the monoclonal sIgM. The ratio of leukemias exhibiting κ light-chain sIg to those with λ sIg is approximately equal, although some series show a κ predominance.[4,23] In up to 20% of B-CLL patients sIg cannot be detected, although the presence of other differentiation antigens indicates the B-cell origin of the leukemia.[21]

Early investigators assumed that CLL was derived from an unstimulated peripheral blood B cell; however, subsequent demonstrations of the coexpression of CD5 with sIg or other B-cell membrane antigens in 95% of CLL patients pointed to another B-cell subset as the normal counterpart.[21] CD5 is a 67 kDa protein originally thought to be a unique T-cell antigen until its discovery on CLL cells.[24] It is now understood to be an identifying characteristic of a subset of normal B lymphocytes. The CD5$^+$ B cell develops early in ontogeny and is prevalent in fetal spleen and other embryonal lymphoid tissues.[25] In normal adult tissues it occurs in very small percentages, e.g. in the mantle zones of secondary germinal follicles in lymph node, spleen and tonsil. CD5$^+$ B cells are known to produce polyreactive, low-affinity autoantibodies. Increased percentage of CD5$^+$ B cells have been noted in patients recovering from allogeneic transplantation and in those with autoimmune diseases.[21]

Other B-cell differentiation antigens frequently coexpressed on CLL cells include the pan-B antigens CD19, CD20, CD24, CD40 and HLA Class II; antigens found on resting mature B cells including CD21 (containing the C3d receptor and the Epstein–Barr virus receptor); and two adhesion molecules involved in lymphocyte homing, CD44 and CD62L (L-selectin) (Fig. 99.1, Table 99.2). One group has described an antigen specific for B-CLL and two other clonal B-cell disorders, hairy cell leukemia and B-prolymphocytic leukemia: the chronic lymphocytic leukemia antigen (cCLLa), which is not found on normal B or T lymphocytes.[26]

Antigens found on normal B cells but missing from the B-CLL cell membrane include CD79b (part of the B-cell receptor, a multimeric complex containing sIg), which is important for antigen presentation, and CD80 and CD86, which are costimulatory molecules for T-cell activation. Their absence is considered a major factor in the immunodeficiency characteristic of B-CLL (reviewed in Ref. 22). B-CLL cells also lack Fas/APO (CD95), a molecule important for signaling the induction of apoptosis. The absence of the cell–cell adhesion molecules ICAM-1 (CD54) and LFA-1 (CD11a/CD18) normally found on mature B cells may play a role in the propensity of CLL cells to circulate in high levels in the blood. On the other hand, CD11b/CD18, CD11c/CD18 and CD14 (My4), which are more typically found on myeloid cells and monocytes and not on normal B cells, have frequently been described on CLL cells.[21]

Normal CD5$^+$ B cells exhibit a high proliferative rate, with up to 10% synthesizing DNA, indicating a state of activation. CD5 is a ligand for another B-cell antigen, CD72, and may thereby mediate B-cell interaction and activation. Another T-cell antigen, CD27, a member of the nerve growth factor family, and its ligand CD70, are also coexpressed on B-CLL cells, which can influence interactions with T cells.[27] B-CLL cells also frequently exhibit other 'activation' antigens such as interleukin-2 receptor (IL-2R) α chain (CD25), CD23 (the Fc receptor for IgE) and CD48 (Blast-1) antigens (Fig. 99.1, Table 99.2). The loss of CD79b on the B-CLL membrane is due to truncation of the molecule, a form that is also found in activated normal B cells.[28] However, despite the presence of these activation proteins the percentage of CLL cells undergoing DNA synthesis and mitosis is extremely low. Generally 1% or less of the cells are in cycle, accounting for the indolent natural history of the majority of patients with this leukemia.

Ig gene rearrangements and cross-reacting idiotypes in B-CLL

The sIg found on CLL cells differs significantly in a number of ways from that of most normal B cells. CLL sIg frequently demonstrates rheumatoid factor reactivity, the ability to bind the Fc portion of IgG molecules.[25] Other autoreactivities of CLL sIgM include the ability to bind single- and double-stranded DNA, histones, cardiolipin and other cytoskeletal proteins. These autoantibody features are similar to those of the immunoglobulins produced by normal CD5$^+$ B cells and generally do not have clinical importance.[25] However, rarely the autoantibodies on the red cells of CLL patients with autoimmune hemolytic anemia have been shown to have the same restricted light-chain type as the sIg of the leukemic cells.[29] A rare patient whose leukemic cells' sIg exhibited anti-cardiolipin activity was reported to manifest the anticardiolipin syndrome with vasculitis and thrombosis.[30]

An important discovery relating to the CLL sIg is the high frequency of shared or 'cross-reacting' idiotypes in up to 25% of patients. The reasons for this lack of diversity have been shown to be both restrictions in the use of the variable (V) genes and a lack of somatic mutation in a large subset of B-CLL patients.[20,25]

The immunoglobulin gene rearrangements found in CLL patients therefore differ in substantial ways from those found in most normal B cells, where the process generates a high degree of antibody diversity (Chapter 4). In the CLL cell and the normal B cell there is initially rearrangement of a heavy-chain gene (V_H) with the DJ_H complex to form a V_HDJ_H exon, which will encode for the variable region of the heavy chain of the IgM.[6] Most normal B cells appear to have a random choice of any of six subgroups containing 100–200 V_H genes. CLL tumors differ in having an increased percentage of rearrangements involving V_H4, V_H5 and the single-copy V_H6 gene and a lower percentage of V_H3, the largest subgroup, than would be expected if these rearrangements were occurring randomly. Furthermore, when the rearrangement involves V_H1, a specific gene called *51p1* is most likely to be used in the rearrangement.[25] Similarly, there appears

KEY CONCEPTS

B-CLL sIg characteristics

- Low density (IgM +/– IgD)
- Restricted light-chain type
- Frequent autoimmune features:
  - Rheumatoid factor activity
  - Anti-DNA, anti-cardiolipin reactivity
- Preferential use of certain V_H and V_L genes
- Variable absence of somatic mutation of V_H and V_L genes
- Increased frequency of cross-reacting idiotypes

to be preferential use of certain κ light-chain genes (but not V_κ gene families) in the rearrangements.

The lack of somatic mutation in the CLL V genes found following recombination, particularly in trisomy 12 tumors, is strikingly different from normal B cells and the follicular non-Hodgkin lymphomas, where somatic hypermutation of the V genes is the rule.[25] The normal $CD5^+$ B cell has a similar restricted immunoglobulin diversity. It has been speculated that the restricted idiotopes or complementarity-determining regions found in the sIg of the normal $CD5^+$ B cell may define certain antibodies that are prone to antigen-triggered expansions which increase the susceptibility for malignant transformation.[25]

The autocrine and paracrine growth factors and cytokines that may play a role in promoting and maintaining the expansion of the leukemic cells has been extensively investigated (reviewed in Refs 22,31). Tumor necrosis factor-α (TNF-α), IL-1α, IL-1β, IL-6, IL-7, IL-8, IL-10, granulocyte–macrophage colony-stimulating factor, transforming growth factor-β (TGF-β) and interferon-γ (INF-γ) have been shown to be produced by B-CLL cells. Plasma levels of some of these cytokines, such as TGF-β, INF-γ and IL-8, as well as the soluble forms of CD23 and CD27 (sCD23, sCD27), are elevated in CLL patients but their role as autocrine negative or positive modulators remains undefined. TNF-α has been shown to stimulate in vitro proliferation of CLL cells as well as hairy cell leukemia cells,[32] and may play a role in inhibiting the growth of normal hematopoietic stem cells.[33] IL-2 and IL-4 are not produced by CLL cells but may play important roles in paracrine growth loops affecting proliferation of the leukemic cells.[31]

A more important role for IL-4 may be its capacity to block apoptosis (programmed cell death) in CLL cells and increase cellular levels of BCL-2.[34] Resistance to apoptosis in vivo is thought to be an important factor promoting the survival of CLL cells and their gradual accumulation. The members of the *BCL2* gene family that block apoptosis, *BCL2*, *BCLxL* and *MCL1*, are overexpressed in B-CLL. Although the proapoptotic *BAX* is also increased, the ratio of *BCL2* to *BAX* is in favor of repression of apoptosis.[35] There is also in vitro evidence of a protective effect of adhesion to bone marrow stroma via β_1 and β_2 integrins for promoting the survival of CLL cells.[36] Figure 99.2 illustrates a hypothetical schema of control of proliferation and apoptosis of B-CLL by these cytokines, as well as the interferons, chemotherapeutic agents and other factors.[22,31] The role that the BCL-2 protein family and these autocrine and paracrine growth loops play in the progression of B-CLL and its response to therapy remains to be elucidated.

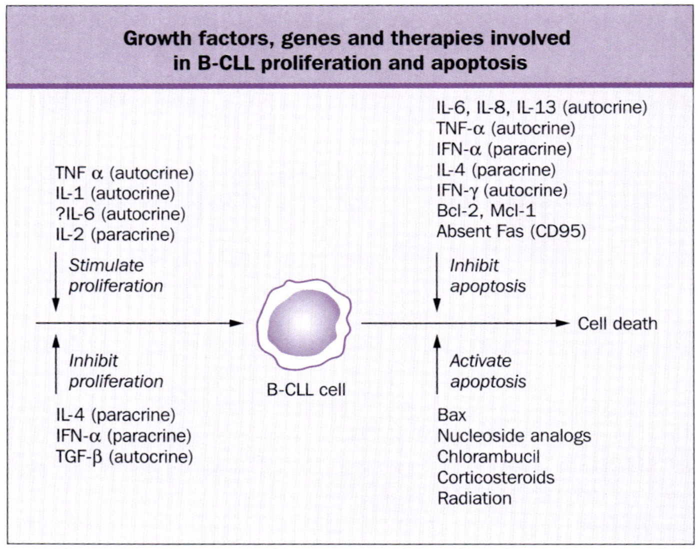

Figure 99.2 Hypothetical schema of growth factors, genes and therapies involved in cell proliferation and apoptosis in B-CLL BCL2 and *BAX* are members of the *BCL2* family. IFN, interferon: TNF, tumor necrosis factor. Modified from Hoffbrand et al. *Semin Hematol* 1993; 30:306.

KEY CONCEPTS

B-cell CLL: cellular characteristics
- Clonal $CD5^+$ B cell
- Low-density sIgM and sIgD
- SIg exhibits rheumatoid factor and autoimmune reactivity
- Restricted V_H and V_L gene usage
- Subsets with somatic mutations ('memory' B cells) or absent somatic mutations ('naive' B cells)
- Cross-reacting idiotypes frequent
- Heterogenous adhesion, activation and other mature B membrane antigens
- Low mitotic rate despite presence of activation membrane antigens
- Heterogeneous chromosomal abnormalities

CLINICAL FEATURES OF B-CLL

Differential diagnosis

A large immunophenotyping study of patients with minor elevations of absolute lymphocyte counts (ranging between 4500 and 10 000/mm³) found that about 20% were clonal B-cell expansions usually consistent with B-CLL. The remainder were mainly due to reactive T-cell lymphocytosis.[37] Patients with a relative lymphocytosis or an absolute lymphocytosis consisting of more than 10 000/mm³ morphologically mature lymphocytes will have B-CLL more than 90% of the time.[37] The diagnosis of B-CLL can be readily confirmed by the presence of low-density monoclonal sIg or CD5 positivity in the absence of other T-cell markers (Table 99.3). In B-CLL the bone marrow is invariably infiltrated with more than 30% lymphocytes.

The uncommon B- and T-cell malignancies make up less than 10% of 'chronic' lymphocytic leukemias (more appropriately termed leukemias of differentiated lymphocytes). The cellular and clinical features that distinguish these uncommon tumors of differentiated B and T cells from classic B-CLL are found in Tables 99.3 and 99.4. The B-cell leukemias that are occasionally confused with CLL include hairy cell leukemia and prolymphocytic leukemia, although the morphologic characteristics are generally sufficient to distinguish between them (Fig. 99.3). Lymphomas presenting with circulating tumor cells can also mimic CLL, particularly small-cell lymphomas of varying types, including mantle-cell (centrocytic), lymphoplasmacytic and follicular lymphomas. These B-cell malignancies usually have high density, bright sIgM and often lack CD5; however, in a small percentage of cases the surface markers may be similar to B-

Table 99.3 Leukemias of differentiated lymphocytes.

Leukemias of differentiated lymphocytes	Markers	Morphology	Other Features
B Cell			
CLL	Ig genes rearranged SIg dim CD5⁺, CD23⁺	Small to medium mature lymphocytes <10% prolymphocytes (large cells with fine nuclear chromatin and nucleoli	Indolent course Adenopathy and splenomegaly common
CLL/prolymphocytoid transformation	Same	>10% prolymphocytes	Accelerating course
Prolymphocytic leukemia	SIg bright $CD5^{-/+}$ $FMC7^{+}$	>55% prolymphocytes	Isolated splenomegaly common Rapid progression
Hairy cell leukemia	SIg bright $CD5^{-}$, $IL2R^{+}$ $TRAP^{+}$, $CD103^{+}$	'Hairy' membrane; nuclear/cytoplasmic ratio decreased	Splenomegaly common; Adenopathy unusual Increased serum soluble IL-2R
Mantle-zone lymphoma	SIg bright $CD5^{+}$, $CD23^{-}$ BCL-1 rearranged	Atypical lymphocytes, nuclear folding, cleaves	Nodes and spleen more prominent than blood involvement
Splenic lymphoma with villous lymphocytes (marginal zone lymphoma)	$CD5^{-}$, $CD23^{-}$	Villi less conspicuous than in hairy cells Often polar	Splenomegaly Adenopathy unusual
Lymphoma, follicular	SIg bright $CD5^{-}$, $CD10^{+}$ BCL-2 rearranged	Atypical lymphocytes	Same as mantle zone Paratrabecular bone marrow infiltration
T Cell			
T-cell leukemia/T-cell PLL	TCR gene rearranged $CD2^{+}$, $CD3^{+}$, $CD4^{+/-}$ $CD7^{+}$, $CD8^{-/+}$	Variable	Indolent to aggressive
Cutaneous T-cell lymphoma (Sezary syndrome Mycosis fungoides)	$CD2^{+}$, $CD3^{+}$, $CD4^{+}$, $CD7^{-/+}$, $CD8^{-}$	Marked nuclear convolutions hyperchromatic, pleomorphic large or small cell variants	Leukemia common in erythrodermic CTCL (Sézary syndrome)
Adult T-cell leukemia/ lymphoma (HTLV-I)	$CD2^{+}$, $CD3^{+}$, $CD4^{+}$ $IL2R^{+}$, $CD7^{-}$, $CD8^{-}$	Multilobed, pleomorphic	Hypercalcemia Skin infiltration Often aggressive Increased serum soluble IL-2R
T-cell LGL leukemia	$CD2^{+}$, $CD3^{+}$, $CD8^{+}$ $CD16(FcR\text{-}IgG)^{+}$ $CD57\ (HNK1)^{+}$ $TCR\alpha/\beta^{+/-}$	Large granular lymphocytes	Indolent Neutropenia Rheumatoid arthritis Red cell aplasia
NK-LGL			
	$TCR\ \alpha/\beta^{-}$ $CD2^{+}$, $CD3^{-}$, $CD8^{-}$ $CD56(NCAM)^{+}$ $CD57^{+/-}$, $CD16^{+}$	Large granular lymphocytes	Aggressive; thrombocytopenia; hepatomegaly

TRAP, tartrate-resistant acid phosphatase; LGL, large granular lymphocyte; NCAM, neural cell adhesion molecule; PLL, prolymphocytic leukemia.

CLL cases.[38] Prominent lymphadenopathy and splenomegaly in the face of a minor lymphocytosis, often with atypical morphology, points to a diagnosis of lymphoma rather than CLL. Lymph node and bone marrow biopsies frequently distinguish these lymphoma cases from CLL. The typical lymph node biopsy in uncomplicated CLL shows a diffuse infiltration with small, well differentiated lymphocytes, with occasional proliferation centers (pseudofollicular growth centers) and isolated prolymphocytes.[39]

T-cell leukemias and lymphomas form the other group of relatively uncommon malignancies that must be distinguished from B-CLL. The Sézary syndrome, the leukemic form of mycosis fungoides or cutaneous T-cell lymphoma (CTCL), is distinguished by prominent erythrodermal skin involvement and highly convoluted nuclear morphology.[40] A small percentage of patients with tumor or the plaque form of CTCL (classic mycosis fungoides) may have blood involvement as well.[40] Adult T-cell lymphoma–leukemia, the helper T-cell lymphoma associated with the HTLV-I virus endemic to southern Japan and the Carribbean, is generally easily distinguished by the prominent multilobated nuclei of the tumor cells and frequent clinical findings of hypercalcemia and skin involvement[41] (Chapter 94). Other T-helper chronic lymphocytic leukemias require immunophenotyping or gene rearrangement studies to distinguish them from B-CLL.[42] The large granular lymphocyte and natural killer

Leukemias of differentiated lymphocytes	
B-cell leukemias	**T-cell or LGL leukemias**
SIg positive Dim (CLL) Bright (hairy cell leukemia, PLL, lymphomas)	SIg negative
Ig genes rearranged	TCR β chain gene rearranged (T-cell leukemias)
Variable B antigens positive CD23 (CLL)	B antigens negative
CD5 positive (weak to moderate) (CLL, mantle-zone lymphoma, some PLLs)	CD5 positive (weak to strong) (T-cell leukemias)
Other T-cell antigens negative	T- or NK-cell antigens positive CD2 (T, NK leukemias) CD3 (T leukemias) CD4 (helper T-cell leukemias: CTCL, Sézary syndrome, HTLV-I ATLL) CD7 (T leukemias, T-PLL) CD8 (cytotoxic–suppressor/LGL leukemias) CD56 (NK-LGL leukemia) CD57 (T-LGL or NK-LGL leukemia)
IL-2 receptor positive Weak to moderate positivity: (CLL, hairy cell leukemia)	IL-2 receptor positive Strongly positive, (HTLV-I ATLL)

CLL, chronic lymphocytic leukemia; PLL, prolymphocytic leukemia; CTCL, cutaneous T-cell lymphoma; NK, natural killer; LGL, large granular lymphocyte; HTLV-I, human T-cell lymphoma virus; ATLL, adult T-cell leukemia–lymphoma.

Table 99.4 Cellular and molecular characteristics of leukemias of differentiated lymphocytes.

cell leukemias can usually be distinguished by the presence of cytoplasmic granules as well as the T cell and NK antigens.[43] T-cell leukemias usually demonstrate rearrangement of the gene for the β chain of the T-cell receptor (TCR) and germline unrearranged IgH genes.[42] However, a small number of B-CLL patients will show both IgH and TCR-β gene rearrangements.[42]

Clinical manifestations and prognostic features of B-CLL

There is a spectrum of clinical presentations of B-CLL that is nicely delineated in the staging system proposed by Rai in 1975 (Table 99.5).[44] All patients have infiltration of the peripheral blood and bone marrow with B lymphocytes of mature morphology. About 40% are asymptomatic at diagnosis, having been discovered accidentally after a routine blood count. Over half of the patients with findings restricted to blood and bone marrow lymphocytosis only (Rai stage 0) will remain asymptomatic and never require treatment for their leukemia. The median survival of stage 0 patients is more than 10 years.[44] Some patients will have stable blood counts for up to 20 years and their condition has been likened to the plasma-cell dyscrasia of benign mono-

CLINICAL PEARLS

Clinical history of B-CLL

- Indolent to slowly progressive in the majority of patients
- Progression associated with increasing leukemia, anemia, thrombocytopenia, hepatosplenomegaly, and immune deficits
- Clonal evolution with prolymphocytic transformation or aggressive large cell lymphoma (Richter's syndrome) in a minority of patients

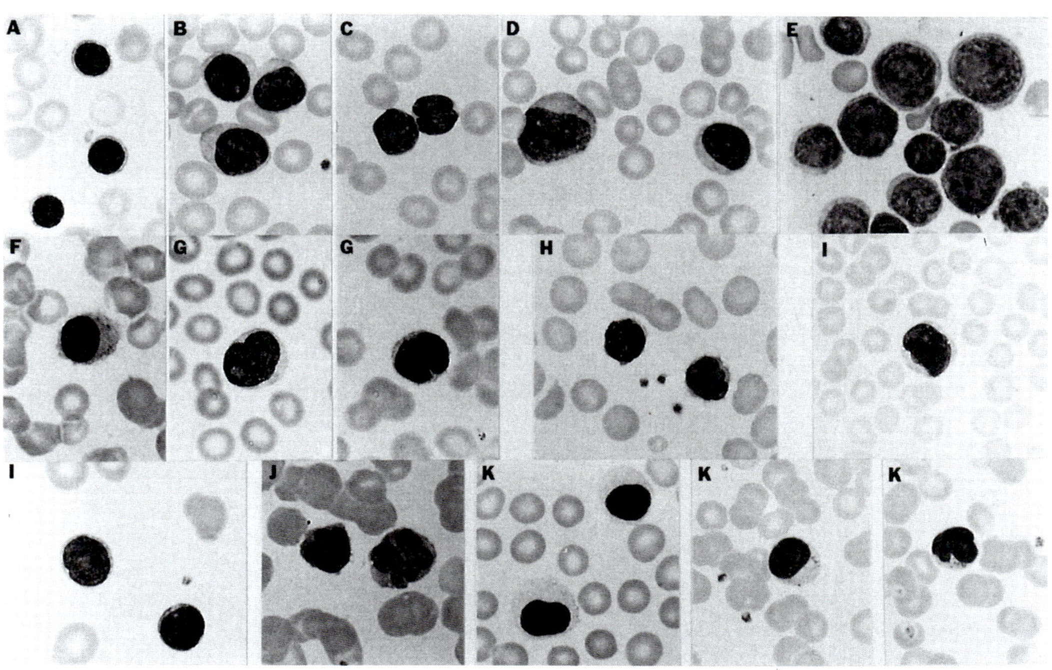

Figure 99.3 Light microscopic morphology of B-cell chronic lymphocytic leukemia and other differentiated lymphocytic leukemias. (A) B-CLL, small lymphocytes. **(B)** B-CLL with medium lymphocytes. **(C)** B-CLL, atypical variant with cleaved cells; **(D)** B-CLL with prolymphocytoid transformation, **(E)** Prolymphocytic leukemia. **(F)** Hairy cell leukemia: **(G)** Mantle-zone lymphoma. **(H)** Sézary leukemia (cutaneous T cell lymphoma), small cell variant. **(I)** Sézary leukemia, mixed cell variant. **(J)** HTLV-1-associated adult T-cell leukemia. **(K)** T-cell large granular lymphocyte leukemia. Wright–Giemsa ×1000.

Prognosis	Clinical Status[a]	Never treated (%)	Median survival (yrs)
Low risk			
Stage 0	Blood and marrow lymphocytosis	59	>10
Intermediate risk			
Stage I	Lymph node enlargement	21	>8
Stage II	Spleen or liver enlargement	23	>6
High risk			
Stage III	Anemia (Hb <11.0 g/dl)	5	<2
Stage IV	Thrombocytopenia (<100 000/mm³)	0	<2

Rai staging system for B-CLL

[a] Only blood and bone marrow lymphocytosis is required for stage I–IV, in addition to the clinical finding specified. For example, stage II patients may or may not have node involvement.

Table 99.5 Rai clinical staging system for B-CLL. Modified from Rai KR, Sawitsky A, Cronkite EP, et al: *Blood* 1975;46:219.

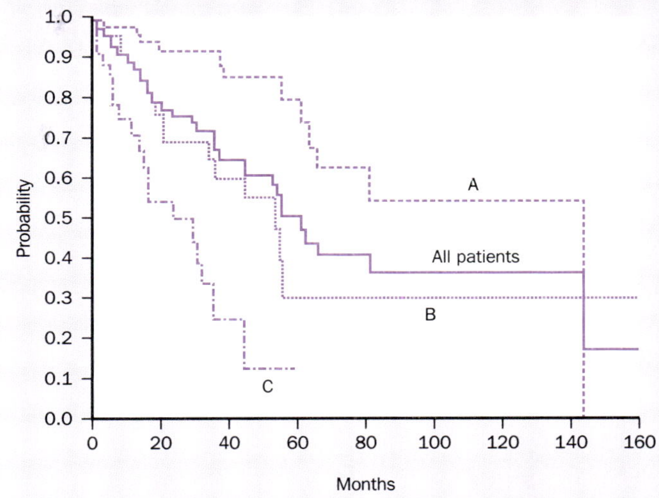

Figure 99.4 Actuarial survival of 150 consecutively staged B-CLL patients according to the Binet International Clinical Staging System. Stage A, fewer than three areas of involvement; stage B, three or more areas of involvement; stage C, hemoglobin less than 10 g/dl or platelets <100 000/mm.[3] Areas of involvement include enlargement of cervical, axillary or inguinal nodes, or hematomegaly or splenomegaly. (From Rozman et al. *Blood* 1982;59:1001.)

clonal gammopathy. Women with stage 0 disease and patients with white blood cell counts <30 000/mm³ at diagnosis are most likely to have the nonprogressive 'benign monoclonal B-cell lymphocytosis'.[23]

In the majority of patients the tumor burden will gradually increase, and palpable lymphadenopathy (Rai stage I) and/or splenomegaly with or without hepatomegaly (Rai stage II) will develop. The median survival of this group of intermediate-risk patients (Rai stages I and II) approaches 6–8 years.

Lymphadenopathy is usually generalized, nontender, and may be massive. The spleen may be just palpable or massively enlarged. As the lymphocytic infiltration of nodes and spleen increases so does the peripheral lymphocytosis and the percentage of patients who become symptomatic and require treatment. Increasing bone marrow infiltration by leukemic cells results in the anemia (hemoglobin <11 g/dl) and thrombocytopenia (platelet counts <100 000/mm³) that respectively characterize the high-risk groups Rai stages III and IV. Blood counts are frequently further compromised by red cell and platelet sequestration due to splenomegaly. In the initial report Rai stage III and IV patients had very short median survivals of less than 2 years.[44] More recent studies report survivals of approximately 4 years, possibly relating to improved supportive care.[23]

Binet et al. in France developed a second staging system, the International Clinical Staging System for CLL, which condensed the Rai stages and has received wide acceptance.[45] This system depends on the number of areas of involvement (cervical, axillary, inguinal adenopathy, hepatomegaly or splenomegaly). Stage A patients have fewer than three and stage B patients have three or more areas of involvement. Anemia (hemoglobin <10 g/dl) or thrombocytopenia (platelets <100 000/mm³) advances patients to stage C. The actuarial survival curves of a large series of patients consecutively staged in this manner are shown in Figure 99.4.[46] The survival of the majority of stage A patients is similar to that of an age- and sex-matched nonleukemic French population.[47]

Weakness, easy fatiguability, night sweats, weight loss, fever, discomfort from growing adenopathy and abdominal organomegaly, and bleeding secondary to thrombocytopenia are among the symptoms that may lead the patient to seek medical attention initially, or may develop years after the diagnosis was first made as the tumor burden gradually increases. Frequent bacterial and viral infections can result from progressive hypogammaglobulinemia and cellular immune deficits that progress as the tumor burden increases. A small percentage of patients may also develop autoimmune hemolytic anemia or immune thrombocytopenia at any Rai stage. Rarely autoimmune neutropenia or pure red cell aplasia may occur. The immunologic complications of CLL are discussed later in this chapter.

Laboratory features in B-CLL

The peripheral blood B-cell concentration at diagnosis is generally more than 10 000/mm³, with a median under 50 000/mm³. The white blood cell count may exceed 100 000/mm³. Counts above 200 000/mm³ are unusual, and hyperviscosity due to hyperleukocytosis is rare but amenable to prompt treatment by leukapheresis. The peripheral blood lymphocyte doubling time is an important prognostic feature. Patients whose doubling times are shorter than a year are more likely to become symptomatic, to advance in clinical stage and to require treatment.[48]

The majority of the leukemic cells are small to medium in size and exhibit the clumped heterochromatin typical of normal lymphocytes. A small percentage of the lymphoid cells may be large and have features typical of prolymphocytes, exhibiting finely divided nuclear chromatin and prominent nucleoli (Fig. 99.3). A classification of CLL based on the frequency of prolymphocytes,

> **CLINICAL PEARLS**
>
> **Hematologic manifestations of B-CLL**
> - Monoclonal blood lymphocytosis (> 4000/mm^3)
> - Morphology: normal small to medium lymphocytes
> - Tissue infiltration
>   - Bone marrow lymphocytosis (>30% of total cells)
>   - Interstitial, nodular or diffuse pattern
>   - Lymph nodes, spleen, liver
>   - Other sites of symtomatic involvement uncommon

> **CLINICAL PEARLS**
>
> **Immunologic manifestations of B-CLL**
> - Hypogammaglobulinemia
> - Impaired cellular immunity
> - Increased risk of bacterial and viral infections
> - Exuberant anglioedematous reactions
> - Increased risk for autoimmune disorders:
>   - Autoimmune hemolytic anemia
>   - Autoimmune thrombocytopenia
>   - Pure red-cell aplasia

large lymphocytes and cleaved lymphocytes has been proposed.[38] In more than 80% of patients more than 90% of the leukemic cells will be small and there will be less than 10% prolymphocytes or large lymphocytes. Occasional patients will have a variant morphology, for example exhibiting high percentages of small cleaved lymphocytes, prolymphocytes or large lymphocytes. These patients may represent the trisomy 12 subset of B-CLL or, alternatively, other B-cell lymphoproliferative disorders such as mantle-cell lymphoma.

The distribution of the lymphocytic infiltration in the bone marrow has been shown to correlate with survival, perhaps because it reflects tumor burden.[49] Preservation of the normal architecture with interstitial infiltrates or small nodules of leukemic cells is associated with longer survival than is diffuse involvement with loss of the normal bone marrow fat spaces.

Immunologic abnormalities in B-CLL

CLL is unique among the B-cell malignancies in having profound immune deficits. A broad spectrum of B- and T-cell immune deficits are associated with a significantly increased propensity to bacterial and viral infections and autoimmune disorders, particularly in patients with advanced-stage diseases. Hypogammaglobulinemia is the most common deficit, with more than 50% of patients developing low levels of polyclonal immunoglobulins.[50] Low levels of IgM and IgA precede the decline in IgG, and all IgG subclasses are decreased. Immunoglobulin concentrations fall progressively with advanced disease, putting the patient at high risk for infections caused by encapsulated organisms. Small monoclonal IgM paraproteins with the same light chain found on the membrane Ig are found in a small percentage of patients on routine protein electrophoresis. When agarose gel electrophoresis and immunofixation are used a paraprotein can be detected in serum or urine in more than 50% of patients, indicating that the clonal B cell has some ability to differentiate to a secretory B cell. Frequently the monoclonal IgM is of low molecular weight in the form of monomeric or oligomeric molecules.[51] In a small percentage of CLL patients the paraprotein is an IgG with the same light-chain type as the sIg, suggesting the capability of an isotype switch by the leukemic cells.[29] However, nonclonal B cells are also dysfunctional or inhibited, as even patients with early disease have deficient primary antibody responses to both T-cell-dependent and T-cell-independent antigens.[52] Secondary antibody responses are typically progressively impaired with advancing disease.

T-cell responses are also significantly impaired. The ability to develop delayed hypersensitivity to new antigens is significantly diminished, although T-cell responses to recall antigens may remain intact. The cellular immune deficits most probably account for the increased susceptibility of CLL patients to herpesvirus infections, both simplex and zoster, and their significantly increased risk for disseminated varicella and severe reactions to live virus vaccines such as vaccinia.[52] Disturbing but less threatening are the exuberant angioedematous reactions to insect bites that occur in some CLL patients, which are probably related to abnormal regulation of cellular immune responses.

The mechanisms underlying the hypogammaglobulinemia and the impairment of delayed hypersensitivity remain poorly understood, although multiple cellular abnormalities have been detected.[53] Even though the percentage of T cells is low in CLL owing to dilution by the expansion of clonal B cells, the absolute numbers are actually elevated. Absolute concentrations of both $CD4^+$ and $CD8^+$ cells are normal or elevated, but the ratio of $CD4^+$ to $CD8^+$ cells is reversed.[54] Elevated percentages of $CD4^+$, $CD8^+$ and $CD16^+$ cells bearing HLA-DR and exhibiting low levels of CD4 and CD8 antigen on the T cells have been reported.[55] These findings have been interpreted as indicating a state of activation or reactivity against the leukemia.[55] There are T-cell functional abnormalities as well: mitogen and antigen responses of isolated T cells, separated from leukemic cells, are

> **KEY CONCEPTS**
>
> **Cellular immune alterations in B-CLL**
> - Impaired in vitro and in vivo synthesis of normal immunoglobulins
> - Impaired in vitro proliferative responses to T- and B-cell mitogens and antigens and the mixed leukocyte reaction
> - Dilution of T cells, normal B cells, NK cells and other cytotoxic and accessory cells by the monoclonal B-cell leukemia
> - Increased absolute concentrations of T-helper ($CD4^+$) and T-cytotoxic ($CD8^+$) cells
> - Acquired deficiency of CD40 ligand (CD154) on T-helper cells
> - Increased concentrations of 'activated' T-helper and cytotoxic subsets (HLA-DR^+ cells)
> - Reversed CD4:CD8 ratio
> - In vitro impaired T-helper, NK, ADCC and LAK activity
> - Impaired generation and availability of IL-2
> - Increased serum levels of TNF-α, IL-1, IL-6, interferon-γ
> - Increased serum levels of soluble IL-2 and TNF-α receptors.

ADCC, antibody-dependent cytotoxicity; LAK, lymphokine-activated killer; TNF, tumor necrosis factor.

diminished.[56] IL-2 generation is abnormal or possibly limited in its availability, owing to binding to the IL-2 receptors present on the large pool of malignant cells.[53] Natural killer cells are increased in some patients, and have been shown to suppress B-cell immunoglobulin synthesis in vitro in some patients with hypogammaglobulinemia.[57]

An acquired deficiency of the CD40 ligand (CD154) in helper T cells of patients with B-CLL has been demonstrated. This deficiency appears to be due to down-regulation of CD40L by the mass of CD40$^+$ B cells.[58] It has been suggested that T-cell deficiency of CD40L, coupled with the defective B-cell receptor complex (BCR) on B-CLL cells and their loss of the costimulatory molecules CD80 and CD86, is the major cause of the failure of effective antibody production in these patients[22] (Fig. 99.5). The relative importance of the various immune alterations in the pathogenesis of the profound dysfunction of the normal, nonclonal B cells remains to be elucidated.

The treatment of hypogammaglobulinemia in CLL with immunoglobulin infusions has been disappointing. A controlled study of 400 mg/kg intravenous immunoglobulin vs. placebo showed a diminution in mild to moderate infections but no difference in serious bacterial infections, viral or fungal infections, or survival.[59] Subsequent analysis of the data found that routine immunoglobulin infusions were enormously costly, calculated at $6 million per year of life gained.[60] In a randomized double-blind study patients were shown to be equally protected by high- and low-dose intravenous immunoglobulin (500 mg/kg vs. 250 mg/kg every 4 weeks).[61] However, even at the lower dose the cost-effectiveness of prophylactic immunoglobulin in CLL is questionable. Its use is probably justified only for patients with repeated bacterial infections who have advanced disease.[9,60]

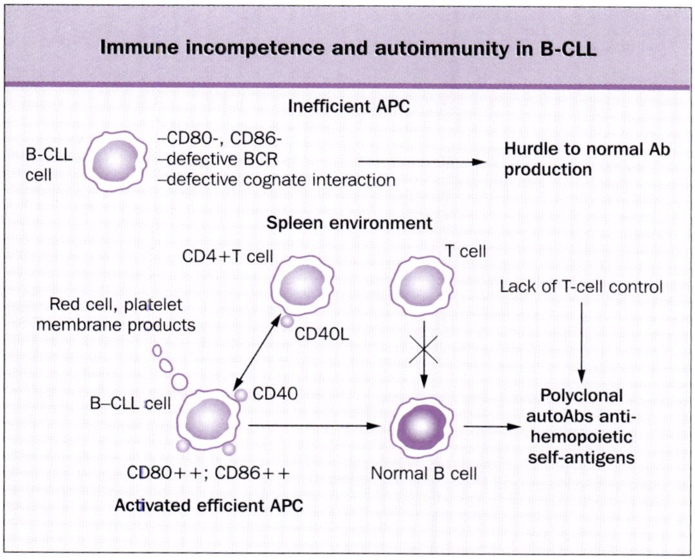

Figure 99.5 Hypothetical schema of the events involved in immune incompetence and autoimmunity in B-CLL. B-CLL cells have a defective B-cell receptor complex (BCR) and suboptimal expression of the costimulatory molecules CD80 and CD86, and therefore are inefficient antigen-presenting cells (APC). However, in the spleen B-CLL cells can be stimulated by nearby CD4$^+$ T cells through CD40–CD40 ligand (CD40L, CD154) interaction and become efficient APC for normal B cells. The lack of effective T-cell control can result in autoantibodies to the abundant red cell and platelet membrane products in the spleen.

Autoimmune disorders

B-CLL presents the paradox of a high frequency of autoimmune disorders in the face of profound hypogammaglobulinemia. Curiously, the most frequent and clinically important autoantibodies are directed against hematologic cells, resulting in autoimmune hemolytic anemia and immune thrombocytopenia.[62] Autoimmune hemolytic anemia (AIHA) occurs in approximately 10–20% of CLL patients at some point during the course of their disease. It may occur at any stage, but tends to increase in frequency with advanced stages. Treatment with the nucleoside fludarabine, which can markedly suppress CD4$^+$ T-cell concentrations, has been associated with an increased risk for AIHA. This problem has been noted primarily in patients who have been given the drug as salvage treatment after previous therapy.

Most studies of CLL patients with AIHA have found IgG or 'warm-reacting' antibodies on the red blood cells. The antibodies are almost always polyclonal in origin, and presumed to be the result of abnormal immunoregulation of nonclonal B cells.[62] It has been speculated[22] that the red cell and platelet membranes sequestered in the splenic environment, and other unknown factors, may permit the B-CLL cell to become a more efficient antigen-presenting cell for the normal splenic B cells and CD4$^+$ T cells. The lack of T-cell regulation (particularly after treatment with the immunosuppressive fludarabine) results in a failure to suppress antibody against the self-antigens (Fig. 99.5). There also appears to be a bias in favor of particular V_H genes (particularly overrepresentation of the *51p1* gene) in patients with AIHA, suggesting a role for certain B-CLL tumors in stimulating the induction of the polyclonal autoantibodies.[63]

The clinical course of AIHA in CLL may be quite variable. Occasional patients can exhibit markedly positive direct antiglobulin tests without hemolysis. Some patients may have a single episode of hemolysis that quickly responds to prednisone, whereas others have recurrent bouts which are responsive to prednisone and cytotoxic treatment.[64] More refractory patients may require additional measures, including high-dose immunoglobulin infusions, splenectomy, or immunosuppressive drugs such as azathioprine, cyclosporine or vinca alkaloids. Occasional patients continue to be refractory despite these measures, and have a shortened survival.[64] Fludarabine-associated hemolytic anemia has been reported to be particularly difficult to treat and associated with fatalities.

Immune thrombocytopenic purpura (ITP) occurs less frequently than does AIHA. Approximately 2% of CLL patients will develop the clinical picture of ITP, with moderate to marked thrombocytopenia associated with increased megakaryocytes in the marrow, and the absence of significant splenomegaly.[62] Patients with clinical ITP regularly demonstrate platelet-associated IgG. However, up to 45% of CLL patients have been reported to exhibit platelet-associated IgG not clearly associated with shortened platelet survival.[65] It is not uncommon for patients with ITP to exhibit red cell autoantibodies as well, often with evidence of hemolysis (Evan's syndrome). Treatment is similar to that for AIHA. Most patients respond to steroids and alkylating agents with or without splenectomy. Refractory patients may respond to trials of vincristine infusions, danazol or cyclosporine.[66]

Pure red cell aplasia is a rare cause of anemia in CLL. It is also believed to occur on an autoimmune basis.[62] Tγ cells expressing

FcR-IgG have been reported to suppress erythroid colony growth, suggesting abnormal immunoregulation as an etiology.[67] Other studies have implicated toxicity associated with alkylating agents. Dramatic remissions after the administration of cyclosporine have been reported in patients refractory to standard immunosuppressive therapy.[68] Chronic parvovirus infection should be considered as well in the differential diagnosis of pure red cell aplasia, as the hypogammaglobulinemic CLL patient is unlikely to have a normal response to this infection.

CLONAL EVOLUTION IN B-CLL: PROLYMPHOCYTOID TRANSFORMATION AND RICHTER SYNDROME

In a small number of patients, rapid progression in symptoms and increasing tumor burden have been associated with the gradual or abrupt appearance of increasing numbers of circulating prolymphocytes (termed prolymphocytic transformation).[69] The prolymphocyte is larger than the typical B-CLL cell and contains less dense nuclear chromatin and prominent nucleoli (Fig. 99.3). It commonly exhibits the same surface membrane characteristics as the original tumor, and probably results from clonal evolution.[69] A second type of clonal evolution, Richter syndrome, features a change in lymph node pathology to that of aggressive large cell lymphoma, accompanied by systemic symptoms, progressive lymphadenopathy and extranodal involvement without any change in peripheral blood lymphocyte morphology.[70] Over the years there has been controversy about whether Richter syndrome represents clonal evolution or a second malignancy resulting from impaired immunosurveillance.[70] Frequently the new tumors are CD5 negative, and occasionally the light-chain subtype differs from that of the original leukemia. Nevertheless, the results of a number of studies comparing nucleotide analysis of the complementarity-defining region 3 (CDR3) of the hypervariable region of the primary CLL and the large cell lymphoma are consistent with clonal evolution.[71] In one case somatic changes in the CDR3 of the Richter tumor suggested that abrupt changes indicating genetic instability may have accounted for transformation.

GENERAL APPROACHES TO ANTILEUKEMIC THERAPY

Chronic lymphocytic leukemia remains an incurable tumor, although the leukemia is responsive to a number of chemotherapeutic agents as well as to radiation. For more than 35 years alkylating agents – usually chlorambucil – have been the standard of therapy; however, these agents result in complete remission in less than 10% of patients. A large randomized study of early treatment with chlorambucil vs postponement of therapy until progression in stage A (fewer than three areas of lymph node involvement) patients showed that early treatment resulted in an inferior outcome, mainly because of excess mortality associated with an increased incidence of second epithelial malignancies.[47] Chlorambucil appeared to increase the underlying propensity of CLL patients to develop epithelial malignancies, which has been attributed to an impairment of immune surveillance.[47] Chemotherapy is generally not indicated for patients who are asymptomatic and have low tumor burdens until they show signs of tumor progression. A second study from the same group of combined prednisone and chlorambucil vs no treatment showed no difference in survival in stage A patients.[72]

Randomized studies in patients with more advanced disease have shown little advantage to the addition of prednisone and vincristine to the alkylating agent cyclophosphamide (CVP or COP), compared to chlorambucil with or without prednisone.[73] A small randomized study showed an improved response rate and survival with the addition of the anthracycline doxorubicin to COP (low-dose CHOP) over COP in stage C patients.[74]

Splenectomy has been useful in selected patients with splenic pain due to marked splenomegaly or cytopenia due to hypersplenism.[75] As these patients rarely respond adequately to pneumococcal vaccines, daily antibiotic therapy is recommended to prevent overwhelming postsplenectomy pneumococcal sepsis. Some investigators recommend splenic irradiation for symptomatic splenomegaly; however, there is a significant risk of worsening cytopenias, particularly thrombocytopenia. Radiotherapy is also occasionally useful for the treatment of bulky refractory lymph node masses.

The introduction of the nucleoside analogs fludarabine, 2-chlorodeoxyadenosine and the adenosine deaminase inhibitor 2-deoxycoformycin (pentastatin) led to a revival of interest in the treatment of CLL.[76–78] These agents have a profound lymphopenic effect in many patients and may induce the tumor lysis syndrome, which can occasionally be fatal.[79] The cytotoxicity of the agents is mediated through induction of apoptosis in the leukemic cells by mechanisms which are not well understood (Fig. 99.2). Remarkable clinical responses to fludarabine have included complete clinical responses with normalization of blood and bone marrow findings in over 10% of relapsed or refractory patients and 30% of previously untreated patients, as well as partial responses of over 40% in both groups.[77] Large randomized studies carried out in North America and Europe have shown that fludarabine treatment showed a superior complete and overall response rate but no difference in survival compared to chlorambucil or to CHOP.[80,81] In small studies similar high remission rates have been achieved with 2-chlorodeoxyadenosine, which may also be effective in fludarabine-resistant patients.[78] Although clinical complete remissions occur with the nucleoside analogs, evidence of immunophenotypic and molecular studies show persistence of $CD5^+$ B cells and immunoglobulin rearrangements consistent with the presence of residual tumor in such patients.[82]

Unfortunately, the profound lymphopenia induced by the nucleoside analogs includes normal lymphocytes as well. Patients who have been treated with fludarabine may have persistently low CD4 counts – $<200/mm^3$ – for 1–2 years. Nor are there significant improvements in the serum immunoglobulin levels. An increase in bacterial and opportunistic infections has been reported, particularly in patients treated in relapse or treated with both prednisone and fludarabine.[83]

Experimental innovative therapies for B-CLL include monoclonal antibodies targeted to B-cell antigens such as CD20 (rituximab)[84] or lymphocyte antigens such as CD52 (Campath-1H).[9] Bone marrow transplantation has also been performed in unusual young patients with chronic lymphocytic leukemia,[85] and non-myeloablative approaches are being explored in older patients.[86]

A valuable supportive therapy has been the use of erythropoietin to improve the anemia in these patients. The role of other cytokines and growth factors, both in supportive care and as immunostimulants, remains for future studies.

LEUKEMIAS OF DIFFERENTIATED T CELLS OR NK CELLS

As noted above, 'chronic' T-cell leukemias, i.e. leukemias of differentiated post-thymic T cells, are infrequently encountered. Most helper T-cell leukemias are related to cutaneous T-cell lymphoma or HTLV-I-associated leukemia–lymphoma, or are leukemias of prolymphocytes. T-cell leukemias that are clinically and morphologically indistinguishable from B-CLL are extremely rare.[38,87] Indeed, most of the early reports of T-cell CLL were actually of patients with T-cell prolymphocytic leukemia (T-PLL) or T-cell large granular lymphocytic (T-LGL) leukemia.[8,43,88] Most T-PLL derive from helper T cells, and the LGL leukemias from cytotoxic–suppressor cells or NK cells (Table 99.3).

T-helper leukemias

Consistent with their post-thymic state, helper T-cell leukemias do not exhibit the nuclear enzyme terminal deoxynucleotidyl transferase or CD1a membrane antigen. Generally the helper T-PLL exhibit the immunophenotype $CD2^+$ $CD3^+$ $CD4^+$ $CD5^+$ $CD7^+$ $CD8^-$. Occasional T-PLL exhibit both CD4 and CD8 positivity, similar to the normal mature thymocyte.[88] The leukemic cells associated with cutaneous T-cell lymphoma and the HTLV-I associated ATLL differ from T-PLL in that they frequently lack CD7.[88,89] Occasionally there appears to be aberrant loss of T-cell-defining antigens in these helper T-cell malignancies, for example CD2, CD3 and CD4.[40,88]

Patients with T-cell prolymphocytic leukemia frequently have inversion or translocations of chromosome 14, with breakpoints at q11 and q32.[88] The breakpoint at band 14q11 is of note in that the genes for the TCR α- and δ-chains have been mapped at this site. Little is known about chromosome abnormalities of the very rare helper T-CLL.

The clinical course of the T-helper leukemias is variable. T-PLL and HTLV-I ATLL are usually rapidly progressive and, when responsive to chemotherapy, remissions are of short duration.[88] Patients with Sézary syndrome generally have a more indolent course, the median survivals of patients with the mixed cell variant and small cell variant being approximately 2 and 5 years from recognition of blood involvement.[40] Cytologic transformation from the small to medium convoluted lymphocytes usually found in cutaneous T-cell lymphoma to large nonconvoluted immature lymphoid cells is associated with rapid progression and a very short median survival of 2 months.[90]

Leukemias of LGL cells

Most leukemias of differentiated lymphocytes bearing T-cell antigens derive from granular lymphocytes.[43] These leukemic cells generally contain prominent cytoplasmic azurophilic granules and exhibit a high nuclear/cytoplasmic ratio similar in morphology to normal granular lymphocytes (Fig. 99.3). Most of these leukemias derive from the normal cytotoxic–suppressor T cell and generally bear similar membrane antigens, $CD2^+$ $CD3^+$, $CD4^-$, $CD8^+$ $CD57\ (NCAM)^+$ (Table 99.3). A smaller group with similar morphologies appear to derive from natural killer (NK) cells and exhibit an NK phenotype, $CD2^+$, $CD3^-$, $CD4^-$, $CD8^-$, $CD56^+$. Both leukemias often show positivity for CD16(IgG-FcR), and NK-LGL leukemias may be $CD57^+$.[43] Both leukemias also express the p75 subunit of the IL-2 receptor and lack expression of the high-affinity p55 IL-2R.[43] It has been suggested that the two LGL leukemias may be best distinguished by the presence or absence of CD3 and TCRα/β positivity; however, occasional T-LGL leukemias are TCRα/β negative and express TCRγ/δ.[43]

> **CLINICAL PEARLS**
>
> **T-LGL leukemia: clinical manifestations**
> - Indolent lymphoproliferative disorder
> - Modest lymphocytosis with prominent cytoplasmic granulation
> - Cytotoxic suppressor immunophenotype
> - Neutropenia and recurrent infections
> - Mild to moderate splenomegaly
> - Immunologic abnormalities

Clinically, T-LGL leukemia is usually an indolent process characterized by onset in middle age. The lymphocytosis is usually modest and rarely rises above 20 000/mm^3. Mild to moderate splenomegaly may be found, but adenopathy and hepatomegaly are infrequent. The most typical presentation is related to neutropenia, which is occasionally severe. Anemia and thrombocytopenia may also occur. The hematologic abnormalities may be related to autoimmune processes; antineutrophil and antiplatelet antibodies have been frequently demonstrated, and occasionally Coombs-positive hemolytic anemia or pure red-cell aplasia occurs. Positive tests for rheumatoid factor, antinuclear antibodies and polyclonal hyperglobulinemia are common, and hypogammaglobulinemia is occasionally found.[43] A rheumatoid arthritis-like picture may be a prominent finding and mimic the features of Felty syndrome, with neutropenia, splenomegaly and rheumatoid arthritis. Demonstrating that the LGL cells are clonal by gene rearrangement studies of TCRβ or TCRγ chain or by cytogenetic studies may be helpful in distinguishing Felty syndrome from the leukemia. Treatment with prednisone, cyclophosphamide, methotrexate or cyclosporine has been useful in improving neutropenia and anemia.

T-LGL must be distinguished from benign proliferations of large granular lymphocytes. Reactive proliferation of LGL is not uncommon after viral infections, and may be seen following infectious mononucleosis, HIV infection, bone marrow transplantation and other disorders. Although usually transient, these benign proliferations may be prolonged and mimic clonal T-LGL.

Since the initial report of Tγ leukemia the functional attributes of the LGL cells have been implicated in the neutropenia and anemia frequently found in this disorder. The leukemic cells frequently display antibody-mediated cytotoxicity,[43] and may produce γ-interferon. Numerous defects of cellular immunity have also been demonstrated, including impaired NK activity, diminished responses to T-cell mitogens and impaired formation of high-affinity IL-2 receptors.[43]

NK leukemias tend to be more aggressive, with higher levels of leukemic cells, prominent hepatosplenomegaly and evidence of systemic illness. The presence of CD56, a neural cell adhesion molecule, has been implicated in the prevalence of central nervous system involvement in aggressive NK leukemia and peripheral T-cell lymphoma.[91] Immune abnormalities and severe neutropenia are less likely in NK–LGL leukemia than in T-LGL leukemia. Patients with NK leukemia frequently require urgent treatment with chemotherapy, but have poor or only transient responses and ultimately succumb to disseminated disease or multiorgan failure.[43]

REFERENCES

1. Minot GR, Isaacs R. Lymphatic leukemia; age incidence, duration and benefit derived from irradiation. Boston Med Surg J 1924;191:1.
2. Dameshek W. Chronic lymphocytic leukemia – an accumulative disease of immunologically incompetent lymphocytes. Blood 1967;29:566.
3. Galton DAG. The pathogenesis of chronic lymphocytic leukemia. Can Med Assoc J 1966;94:1005.
4. Preud'homme JL, Seligmann M. Surface bound immunoglobulin as a cell marker in human lymphoproliferative diseases. Blood 1972;40:777.
5. Fialkow PJ, Najfeld V, Reddy A, et al. Chronic lymphocytic leukemia: clonal origin in a committed B-lymphocyte progenitor. Lancet 1978;2:444.
6. Korsmeyer SJ. Hierarchy of immunoglobulin gene rearrangements in B cell leukemias. In: Waldmann TA (ed) Molecular genetic analyses of human lymphoid neoplasms: immunoglobulin gene and the c-myc oncogene. Ann Intern Med 1985;102:497.
7. Gahrton G, Robert K-H, Friberg K, et al. Non-random chromosomal aberrations in chronic lymphocytic leukemia revealed by polyclonal B-cell mitogen stimulation. Blood 1980;56:640.
8. Brouet JC, Flandrin G, Sasportes M, et al. Chronic lymphocytic leukaemia of T-cell origin. Immunological and clinical evaluation in eleven patients. Lancet 1975;ii:890.
9. Rai KR, Patel DV. Chronic lymphocytic leukemia. In: Hoffman R, Benz EJ Jr, Shattil SJ et al. (eds) Hematology, basic principles and practice. New York, Churchill Livingstone, 2000, p 1350.
10. Miller BA, Ries LAG, Hankey BF, et al (eds) Cancer Statistics Review: 1973–1989, National Cancer Institute. NIH Pub. No. 92–2789, 1992.
11. Conley CL, Misiti J, Laster AJ. Genetic factors predisposing to chronic lymphocytic leukemia and to autoimmune disease. Medicine 1980;59:323.
12. Payelle-Brogard, Magnac C, Mauro FR, et al. Analysis of the B-cell receptor B29 (CD79b) gene in familial chronic lymphocytic leukemia. Blood 1999;94:3516.
13. Brok-Simoni F, Rechavi G, Katzir N, Ben-Bassat I. Chronic lymphocytic leukemia in twin sisters: monozygous but not identical. Lancet 1987;i:329.
14. Dohner H, Stilgenbauer S, Dohner K, et al. Chromosome aberrations in B-cell chronic lymphocytic leukemia: reassessment based on molecular cytogenetic analysis. J Molec Med 1999;77:266.
15. Williams ME, Meeker TC, Swerdlow SH. Rearrangement of the chromosome 11 bcl-1 locus in centrocytic lymphoma: analysis with multiple breakpoint probes. Blood 1991;78:493.
16. Rimokh R, Berger F, Delsol G, et al. Rearrangement and overexpression of the BCL-1/Prad-1 gene in intermediate lymphocytic lymphomas and in t(11q13)-bearing leukemias. Blood 1993; 81:3063.
17. Stilgenbauer S, Dohner H, Bulgay-Morschel M, et al. High frequency of monoallelic retinoblastoma gene deletion in B-cell chronic lymphoid leukemia shown by interphase cytogenetics. Blood 1993;81:2118.
18. Corcoran MM, Rasool O, Liu Y, et al. Detailed molecular delineation of 13q14.3 loss in B cell chronic lymphocytic leukemia. Blood 1998;91:1382.
19. Bullrich F, Rasio D, Kitada S, et al. *ATM* mutations in B-cell chronic lymphocytic leukemia. Cancer Res 1999;59:24.
20. Oscier DG, Thompsett A, Zhu D, Stevenson FK. Differential rates of somatic hypermutation in V_H genes among subsets of chronic lymphocytic leukemia defined by chromosomal abnormalities. Blood 1997;89:4153.
21. Freedman AS, Boyd AW, Bieber FR, et al. Normal cellular counterparts of B cell chronic lymphocytic leukemia. Blood 1987;70:418.
22. Caligaris-Cappio F, Hamblin TJ. B-cell chronic lymphocytic leukemia: a bird of a different feather. J Clin Oncol 1999;17:399.
23. Catovsky D, Fooks J, Richards S, et al. Prognostic factors in chronic lymphocytic leukemia: the importance of age, sex and response to treatment in survival. Br J Haematol 1989;72:141.
24. Royston I, Majda JA, Baird SM, et al. Human T cell antigens defined by monoclonal antibodies: The 65000 dalton antigen of T cells (T65) is also found on chronic lymphocytic leukemia cells bearing surface immunoglobulin. J Immunol 1980;125:275.
25. Kipps TJ, Carson DA. Autoantibodies in chronic lymphocytic leukemia and related systemic autoimmune diseases. Blood 1993;81:2475.
26. Faguet GB, Agee JF, Marti GE. CD5 and cCLLa expression in chronic lymphocytic leukemia (CLL): demonstration of their relative prevalence and that of other common B-CLL markers. Leukem Lymphoma 1992;6:335.
27. Ranheim EA, Cantwell M, Kipps TJ. Expression of CD27 and its ligand, CD70, on chronic lymphocytic leukemia cells. Blood 1995; 85:3556.
28. Alfarano A, Indraccolo S, Circosta P, et al. An alternatively spliced form of CD79b gene may account for altered B-cell receptor expression in B-chronic lymphocytic leukemia. Blood 1999;93:2237.
29. Shtoeger ZM, Shtoeger D, Shtairid M, et al. Mechanism of autoimmune hemolytic anemia in chronic lymphocytic leukemia. Am J Hematol 1993;43:259.
30. Meriette X, Levy Y, Dubreuil ML, et al. Characterization of a human monoclonal autoantibody directed to cardiolipin/beta 2 glycoprotein I produced by chronic lymphocytic leukaemia B cells. Clin Exp Immunol 1993;94:385.
31. Hoffbrand AV, Panayiotidis P, Reittie J, Ganeshaguru K. Autocrine and paracrine growth loops in chronic lymphocytic leukemia. Semin Hematol 1993;30:306.
32. Foa R, Massaia M, Cardona S, et al. Production of tumor necrosis factor-α by B-cell chronic lymphocytic leukemia cells: a possible regulatory role of TNF in the progression of the disease. Blood 1990;76:393.
33. Lindemann A, Ludwig WD, Oster W, et al. High level secretion of tumor necrosis factor-alpha contributes to the hematopoietic failure in hairy cell leukemia. Blood 1988;73:880.
34. Danescu M, Rubop-Tryillo M, Biron G, et al. Interleukin-4 protects chronic lymphocytic leukemia B-cells from death by apoptosis and upregulates Bcl-2 expression. J Exp Med 1992;176:1319.
35. Kitada S, Andersen J, Akar S, et al. Expression of apoptosis-regulating proteins in chronic lymphocytic leukemia: correlations with in vitro and in vivo chemoresponses. Blood 1998;91:3379.
36. Lagneaux L, Delforge A, Bron D, De Bruyn C, Strychmans P. Chronic lymphocytic leukemic B cells but not normal B cells are rescued from apoptosis by contact with normal bone marrow stromal cells. Blood 1998;91:2387.
37. Hunt KM, Steed A, Morgan MAM, et al. Chronic B-cell malignancies in patients with lymphocytosis. Leuk Lymphoma 1990;2:257.
38. Bennett JM, Catovsky D, Daniel M-T, et al. Proposals for the classification of chronic (mature) B and T lymphoid leukaemias. J Clin Pathol 1989;42:567.
39. Harris NL, Jaffe ES, Stein H, et al. Perspective: a revised European–American classification of lymphoid neoplasm: a proposal from the International Lymphoma Study Group. Blood 1994;84:1361.
40. Schechter GP, Sausville E, Fischmann AB, et al. Evaluation of circulating malignant cells provides prognostic information in cutaneous T cell lymphoma. Blood 1987;69:841.
41. Bunn PA, Jr, Schechter GP, Jaffe E, et al. Clinical course of retrovirus-associated adult T-cell lymphoma in the United States. N Engl J Med 1983;309:257.
42. Waldmann TA, Davis MM, Bongiovanni KF, Korsmeyer SJ. Rearrangements of genes for the antigen receptor on T cells as markers of lineage and clonality in human lymphoid neoplasms. N Engl J Med 1985;313:776.
43. Loughran TP Jr. Clonal diseases of large granular lymphocytes. Blood 1993;82:1.
44. Rai KR, Sawitsky A, Cronkite EP, et al. Clinical staging of chronic lymphocytic leukemia. Blood 1975;46:219.
45. Binet J-L, Catovsky D, Chandra P, et al. Chronic lymphocytic leukemia: proposals for a revised prognostic staging system. Br J Haematol 1981;48:365.
46. Rozman C, Montserrat E, Feliu E, et al. Prognosis of chronic lymphocytic leukemia: a multivariate survival analysis of 150 cases. Blood 1982;59:1001.

47. French Cooperative Group on Chronic Lymphocytic Leukemia. Effects of chlorambucil and therapeutic decision in initial forms of chronic lymphocytic leukemia (stage A): results of a randomized clinical trial on 612 patients. Blood 1990;75:1414.
48. Montserrat E, Sanchez-Bisono J, Vinolas N, Rozman C. Lymphocyte doubling time in chronic lymphocytic leukaemia: analysis of its prognostic significance. Br J Haematol 1986;62:567.
49. Rozman C, Montserrat E, Rodriguez-Fernandez JM, et al. Bone marrow histologic pattern – the best single prognostic parameter in chronic lymphocytic leukemia: a multivariate survival analysis of 329 cases. Blood 1984;64:642.
50. Rozman C, Montserrat E, Vinolas N. Serum immunoglobulin and B-chronic lymphocytic leukemia. Natural history and prognostic significance. Cancer 1988;61:279.
51. Xu HJ, Roberts-Thomson FJ. Low molecular weight IgM in the sera of patients with chronic lymphocytic leukemia. Pathology 1993;25:52.
52. Chapel HM, Bunch C. Mechanisms of infection in chronic lymphocytic leukemia. Semin Hematol 1987;24:291.
53. Foa R. Pathogenesis of the immunodeficiency in B-cell chronic lymphocytic leukemia. In: Cheson B (ed) Chronic lymphocytic leukemia: scientific advances and clinical development. New York, Marcel Dekker, 1993, p 147.
54. Kay NE, Johnson JD, Stanek R, Douglas SD. T-cell subpopulations in chronic lymphocytic leukemia: abnormalities in distribution and in in vitro receptor maturation. Blood 1979;54:540.
55. Totterman TH, Carlsson M, Simonsson B, et al. T-cell activation and subset patterns are altered in B-CLL and correlate with the stage of the disease. Blood 1989;74:786.
56. Foa R, Lauria F. Reduced T lymphocyte colonies in B chronic lymphocytic leukemia. III Evidence of a proliferative abnormality of the T helper cell population. Clin Exp Immunol 1982;50:336.
57. Kay NE, Perri RT. Evidence that large granular lymphocytes from B-CLL patients with hypogammaglobulinemia down-regulate B-cell immunoglobulin synthesis. Blood 1989;73:1016.
58. Cantwell M, Hua T, Pappas J, Kipps TJ. Acquired CD40-ligand deficiency in chronic lymphocytic leukemia. Nature Med 1997;3:984.
59. Cooperative Group for the Study of Immunoglobulin in Chronic Lymphocytic Leukemia. Intravenous immunoglobulin for the prevention of infection in chronic lymphocytic leukemia. N Engl J Med 1988;319:902.
60. Weeks JC, Tierney MR, Weinstein MC. Cost effectiveness of prophylactic intravenous immune globulin in chronic lymphocytic leukemia. N Engl J Med 1991;325:123.
61. Gamm H, Huber C, Chapel H, et al. Intravenous immune globulin in chronic lymphocytic leukemia. Clin Exp Immunol 1994;97:17–20.
62. Hamblin TJ, Oscier DJ, Young BJ. Autoimmunity in chronic lymphocytic leukemia. J Clin Pathol 1986;39:713.
63. Efremov DG, Ivanovski M, Siljanovski N, et al. Restricted immunoglobulin Vh region repertoire in chronic lymphocytic leukemia patients with autoimmune hemolytic anemia. Blood 1996;87:3869.
64. Majumdar G, Brown S, Slater NG, Singh AK. Clinical spectrum of autoimmune haemolytic anaemia in patients with chronic lymphocytic leukemia. Leuk Lymphoma 1993;9:149.
65. De Rossi G, Granati L, Girelli G, et al. Incidence and prognostic significance of autoantibodies against erythrocytes and platelets in chronic lymphocytic leukemia (CLL). Nouv Rev Fr Hematol 1988;30:403.
66. Diehl LF, Ketchum LH. Autoimmune disease in chronic lymphocytic leukemia: autoimmune hemolytic anemia, pure red cell aplasia and autoimmune thrombocytopenia. Semin Oncol 1998;25:80.
67. Mangan KF, Chikkappa G, Farley PC. T gamma (Tγ) cells suppress growth of erythroid colony-forming units *in vitro* in the pure red cell aplasia of B-cell chronic lymphocytic leukemia. J Clin Invest 1982;70:1148.
68. Chikkappa G, Pasquale D, Mangan K, et al. Successful treatment of pure red cell aplasia in a patient with chronic lymphocytic leukemia with cyclosporine A. Blood 1986;68(suppl 1):1069.
69. Enno A, Catovsky D, O'Brien M, et al. 'Prolymphocytoid' transformation of chronic lymphocytic leukemia. Br J Haematol 1979;9:41.
70. Robertson LE, Pugh W, O'Brien S, et al. Richter's syndrome: a report on 39 patients. J Clin Oncol 1993;11:1985.
71. Cherepakhin V, Baird SM, Meisenholder GW, Kipps TJ. Common clonal origin of chronic lymphocytic leukemia and high-grade lymphoma of Richter's syndrome. Blood 1993;82:3141.
72. Dighiero G, Maloum K, Desablens B et al. Chlorambucil in indolent chronic lymphocytic leukemia. NEJM 1998;338:1506.
73. French Cooperative Group on Chronic Lymphocytic Leukemia. A randomized clinical trial of chlorambucil versus COP in stage B chronic lymphocytic leukemia. Blood 1990;75:1422.
74. French Cooperative Group on Chronic Lymphocytic Leukemia. Effectiveness of 'CHOP' regimen in advanced untreated chronic lymphocytic leukaemia. Lancet 1986;i:1346.
75. Coad JE, Matutes E, Catovsky D. Splenectomy in lymphoproliferative disorders. A report of 70 cases and review of the literature. Leukem Lymphoma 1993;10:245.
76. Grever MR, Leiby JM, Kraut EH, et al. Low-dose deoxycoformycin in lymphoid malignancy. J Clin Oncol 1985;3:1196.
77. Keating MJ, O'Brien S, Lerner S, et al. Long term follow-up of patients with chronic lymphocytic leukemia (CLL) receiving fludarabine regimens as initial therapy. Blood 1998;92:1165.
78. Juliusson G, Liliemark J. High complete remission rate from 2-chloro-2'-deoxyadenosine in previously treated patients with B-cell chronic lymphocytic leukema: response predicted by rapid decrease of blood lymphocyte count. J Clin Oncol 1993;11:679.
79. Dann EJ, Gillis S, Polliack A, et al. Brief report: tumor lysis syndrome following treatment with 2-chlorodeoxyadenosine for refractory chronic lymphocytic leukemia. N Engl J Med 1993;329:1547.
80. Rai KR, Peterson B, Elias L, et al. A randomized comparison of fludarabine and chlorambucil for patients with previously untreated chronic lymphocytic leukemia: a CALGB, SWOG, CTG/NCI-C and ECOG Intergroup study. Blood 1996;88(Suppl 1):141a.
81. Leporrier M, Chevret S, Cazin B, et al. Randomized clinical trial comparing two anthracyclin-containing regimens (CHOP and CAP) and fludarabine (FDR) in advanced chronic lymphocytic leukemia (CLL). Blood 1999;94(Suppl 1):603a.
82. Magnac C, Sutton L, Cazin B, et al. Detection of minimal residual disease in B chronic lymphocytic leukemia (CLL). Hematol Cell Ther 1999;41:13.
83. Anaissie EJ, Kontoyiannis DP, O'Brien S, et al. Infections in patients with chronic lymphocytic leukemia treated with fludarabine. Ann Intern Med 1998;129:559.
84. Byrd JC, Waselenko JK, Meatis TJ, et al. Rituximab therapy in hematologic malignancy patients with circulating blood tumor cells: association with increased infusion-related side effects and rapid blood tumor clearance. J Clin Oncol 1999;17:791.
85. Khouri IF, Przepiorka D, Van Besien K, et al. Allogeneic blood or marrow transplantation for chronic lymphocytic leukemia: timing of transplantation and potential effect of fludarabine on graft-vs-host disease. Br J Haematol 1997;97:466.
86. Waselenko JK, Flynn JM, Byrd JC. Stem cell transplantation in chronic lymphocytic leukemia: the time for designing randomized studies has arrived. Semin Oncol 1999;26:48.
87. Neame PB, Soamboonsrup P, Giesbrecht J. T-cell form of chronic lymphocytic leukemia. Leukemia 1993;7:916.
88. Matutes E, Brito-Babapulle B, Swansbury J, et al. Clinical and laboratory features of 78 cases of T-prolymphocytic leukemia. Blood 1991;78:3269.
89. Haynes BA, Metzgar RS, Minna JD, Bunn PA. Phenotypic characterization of cutaneous T-cell lymphoma. N Engl J Med 1981;304:1319.
90. Dmitrovsky E, Matthews MJ, Bunn PA, et al. Cytologic transformation in cutaneous T cell lymphoma: a clinicopatholic entity associated with poor prognosis. J Clin Oncol 1987;5:208.
91. Kern WF, Spier CM, Hanneman EH, et al. Neural cell adhesion molecule-positive peripheral T-cell lymphoma: a rare variant with a propensity for unusual sites of involvement. Blood 1992;79:2432.

Section 9 Immunology of Neoplasia

Chapter 100 Tumor Immunology

James C. Yang

In the last decade there have been unparalleled advances in our understanding of the nature of the immune responses of cancer patients to their malignancies. New technology has led to the identification of T- and B-cell responses to autologous tumors and the delineation of the precise antigens and epitopes that are being recognized. In parallel with this scientific effort, clinical trials begun in the 1980s demonstrated that therapies with purely immunological bases could, in some cases, mediate the total and durable regression of metastatic cancer. An improved understanding of the molecular nature of the immune response has also allowed the creation of new immune reagents and vaccine strategies which arose from the genetic manipulation of components of the immune system and its mediators. This chapter reviews the current status of our understanding of the immune response and immunotherapy as it pertains to patients with cancer.

HISTORY

There has been a long-standing interest in using inflammatory responses, antibodies and immune cells to mediate the rejection of cancer in patients. In the 1800s William Coley at the New York Hospital began injecting the tumors of patients with a preparation of *Streptococcus pyogenes* and *Serratia marcescens* known as Coley's toxins. He reported that some tumors regressed after a brisk inflammatory and febrile reaction. It was nearly a century later that Carswell and Old[1] reported the identification of a protein produced by T cells in response to lipopolysaccharide (LPS) from bacterial cell walls that could mediate the regression of tumors in mice. They called this cytokine tumor necrosis factor (TNF).[1] In the early 1900s, leading immunologists first formulated the concept that immune cells might be used in the therapy of cancer. These approaches were hampered by the inability to demonstrate convincingly that cancer patients mounted classic cellular or humoral responses to their growing cancers. Despite the demonstration that transplanted murine tumors could show specific protection in immunization experiments, there were reports as recently as 1979 that such responses against spontaneously arising human tumors did not occur.[2] Beginning in the 1970s, our understanding of the humoral and cellular immune responses changed dramatically with the cloning of cytokines such as TNF, interleukin-2 (IL-2) and interferon (IFN)-α and -γ; the elucidation of the nature of the T- and B-cell receptors and the mechanisms that generate their diversity and repertoire; and the clarification of antigen processing and presentation in the context of MHC molecules. Each of these advances in immunology spawned dramatic new approaches in treating patients with cancer. That process continues today.

CYTOKINE THERAPIES FOR CANCER

Interferon was the first cytokine to see widespread use in the treatment of cancer. It was originally available as a purified product of stimulated peripheral blood mononuclear cells (lymphoblastoid interferon) and produced largely by methods developed by Cantell at the State Serum Institute in Helsinki. Initial clinical trials involved patients with advanced cancers of many different histologies.[3,4] Although largely disappointing, this effort did demonstrate that some patients with, for example, renal cell carcinoma, could show regression of their tumors. Larger studies eventually established that the overall response rate for patients with metastatic renal cancer was approximately 10–15%, and consisted largely of partial responses of short duration (Table 100.1).[4–8] With the myriad actions attributed to IFN, including direct antimitotic activity, it was difficult to classify these responses as clearly resulting from immunotherapy. A more definitive answer was obtained when IL-2 was employed in clinical trials beginning in 1983.[9] Again, most tumor types did not show a significant response but some patients with advanced renal cell cancer and melanoma had partial or complete regression of their tumors (Fig. 100.1). Although many of these initial patients also received in vitro-generated lymphokine-activated

Responses to interferon therapy

Reference	IFN	*n*	Partial responses (%)	Complete responses (%)
deKernion[4]	IFN-α IM	48	13	2
Quesada[5]	IFN-α IM	50	20	6
Umeda[6]	IFN-α IM	153	13	2
	Lymphoblastoid IM	73	22	1
Muss[7]	IFN-α2b SC	58	7	2
	IFN-α2b IV	54	4	2
Minasian[8]	IFN-α2a IM	42	17	0
	IFN-α2a SC	117	6	2
Totals		595	12.4	2.0

IFN given 2–7 times per week at widely varying doses.

Table 100.1 Response rates of patients with metastatic renal cell cancer treated with interferon

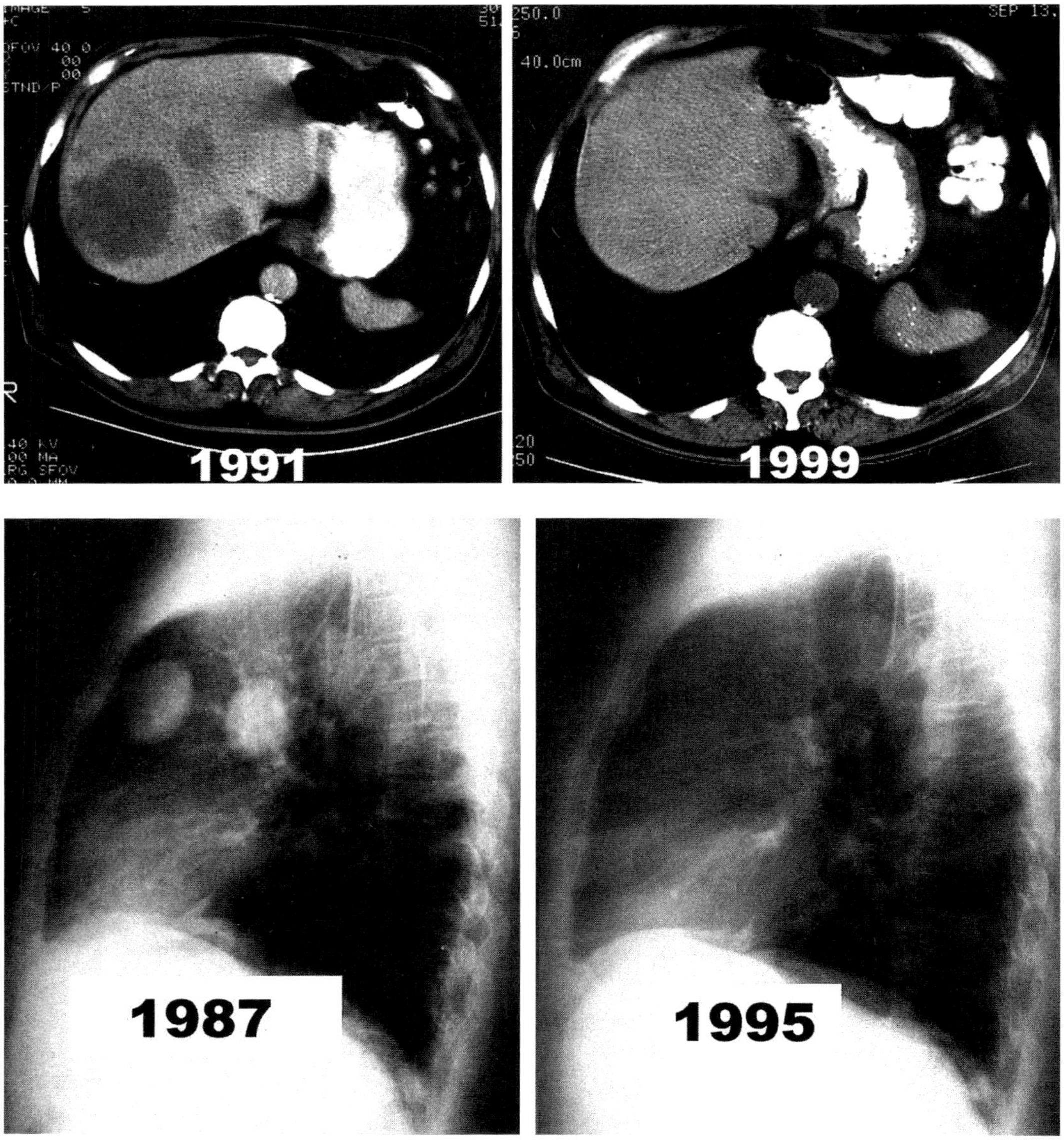

Figure 100.1 Patients with metastatic melanoma and renal cancer who receive high-dose intravenous IL-2 can achieve clinically significant tumor regressions. A patient with extensive liver metastases from renal cancer (top) had complete regression of tumor at all known sites and remains disease free over 9 years later. A patient with metastatic renal cancer to the lungs had a similar complete response, now sustained over 13 years.

killer (LAK) cells[10,11] (based on preclinical data), it was later demonstrated that these responses were largely due to the IL-2 administered.[12] In view of the fact that IL-2 has never been shown to have direct antitumor activity, and because it was ineffective in immunosuppressed animals, this clinical experience demonstrated conclusively that a purely immune-based therapy could mediate clinically significant tumor regressions in certain patients. A remarkable feature of some of these responses was their durability. Overall, approximately 15–20% of patients with melanoma or renal cancer responded to a regimen containing high doses of IL-2 (600 000–720 000 IU/kg every 8 h by IV bolus administered to the maximum number of doses tolerated) (Table 100.2).[13–22] Approximately 7–9% of patients went on to have a complete response, with all evidence of disease disappearing. Only 19% of these patients ever relapsed, with a median follow-up of over 7 years (maximum > 13 years) (Fig. 100.2).[13] These data proved for the first time that immune therapy was capable of mediating the complete regression of metastatic cancer in patients, and that some of these regressions appear to be potentially curative.

Although much effort has been expended, there is still no significant understanding of the factors involved in mediating these responses, nor any practical parameters helpful in predicting which patients will respond to IL-2. Histology of regressing lesions often showed intense lymphocytic infiltrates within both tumors and normal tissues, but a variety of other infiltrating cells such as eosinophils and macrophages was also seen in some cases. There is also diverse multisystem toxicity seen with high-dose IL-2 therapy. With continued intravenous administration a systemic vascular leak syndrome with multiorgan system dysfunction is induced which can be fatal in 0.4–2.5% of treatment courses. These toxicities and their management have been extensively reviewed.[23,24] Experience, screening for occult coronary artery disease and the appropriate application of prophylactic antibiotics can reduce this treatment-related mortality to the point where some investigators have treated over 800 consecutive patients without a death.[25] Nevertheless, this toxicity has resulted in a major effort to develop effective regimens using lower doses of IL-2. Non-randomized data have suggested that low-dose IL-2 regimens for metastatic melanoma do not attain significant

Responses to IL-2 therapy				
Reference	**IL-2 regimen**	***n***	**Response rate (%)**	**CR (%)**
Renal cancer				
Rosenberg[13]	High-dose IV bolus	227	19	9
Cytokine Working Group[14,15]	High-dose IV bolus	71	17	7
Gold[16]	High-dose continuous IV	47	13	6
Escudier[17]	Moderate-dose continuous IV	104	19	4
Yang[18]	Low-dose IV bolus	112	10	4
Lissoni[19]	Low-dose daily SC	91	23	2
Buter[20]	Low-dose daily SC	47	19	4
Yang[18]	Low-dose daily SC	53	11	6
Total		752	17.0	6.4
Melanoma				
Rosenberg[13]	High-dose IV bolus	182	15	7
Parkinson[21]	High-dose IV bolus	46	22	4
Sparano[22]	High-dose IV bolus	44	5	0
Total		272	14.3	5.1

Table 100.2 Response of patients with metastatic cancer to interleukin-2 therapy.

Survival in patients achieving complete responses with IL–2

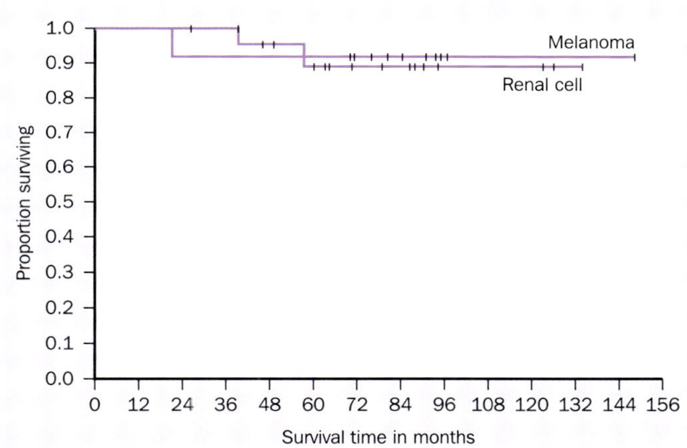

Figure 100.2 If patients achieve a complete regression of tumor with high-dose IL-2 therapy it is likely to be durable. Overall survival is shown for patients with metastatic melanoma and renal cell cancer who had complete responses to IL-2 at 720 000 IU/kg by IV bolus every 8 hours.[13]

response rates. On the other hand, response rates for metastatic renal cancer treated with these low-dose regimens have been reported which are comparable to high-dose therapy.[26,27] Patient selection in such nonrandomized trials may affect outcome and a randomized trial is under way to determine the optimally effective regimen for the healthy patient with measurable metastatic renal cancer who has no other significant limiting medical problems. The reported interim results suggest that high-dose bolus IL-2 (19% partial and complete responses) may be superior to a low-dose regimen (1/10th the dose, given by the same route and schedule) which showed much less toxicity but a 10% response rate; however, the difference is of borderline significance.[18] In addition, the durability of complete responses may also differ, although more complete data and follow-up will be necessary to determine this.

Clinical trials with IL-1, IL-4, IL-6 and IL-12, as well as IFN-β and IFN-γ, show only sporadic or no responses.[28,29] A variety of combination regimens have been tested and, despite initial reports of improved response rates (especially with IL-2 and IFN-α for renal cancer),[30,31] wider experience has produced response rates that overlap with those of IL-2 alone.[14,32] One widely used outpatient regimen reported by Atzpodien and co-workers combined subcutaneous IL-2 and IFN-α with 5-FU (5-fluorouracil) chemotherapy and was reported to have a major response rate of 39% consisting of 14% complete and 25% partial responses.[33] A subsequent trial by the Eastern Cooperative Oncology Group using the regimen described by Atzpodien resulted in only a 16% response rate, with 4% complete responses.[34] In addition, a different regimen using these same three agents administered to 111 patients by Ravaud et al resulted in only two major responses.[35] Thus there is currently no convincing evidence that combination therapy is superior to IL-2 therapy alone. This is most apparent when the end-point of durable complete responses is evaluated.[34] In view of the relatively low overall response rate to IL-2 (and current immunotherapy in general), this end-point constitutes the strongest argument in favor of the clinical value of this cytokine, and should be considered in evaluating competing regimens.

TUMOR ANTIGENS RECOGNIZED BY T CELLS

Despite the compelling proof of principle provided by IL-2, that patients with advanced metastatic melanoma and renal cancer could completely and durably respond to immunological therapies, little understanding of the precise nature of the immune responses to these cancers was available until 1991, when an antigen from a melanoma that was recognized by T cells was first identified, including precise delineation of its epitope.[36] Using peripheral blood from a patient with melanoma who had been vaccinated repeatedly with her own irradiated, mutagenized autologous tumor line, a CD8 T cell was cloned from a mixed tumor cell–lymphocyte culture. This clone was then used to screen a DNA library from this tumor that was expressed by a transfection target displaying the appropriate MHC restriction element for recognition (an immunoselected, antigen-loss variant of the autologous tumor was used). Transfectants were found that caused TNF release by the tumor-specific CTL. This screening identified a gene, *MAGE1*, which proved to be one of a larger family of similar genes. *MAGE1* was expressed in tumor tissue and testis, but not by other normal tissues. The 9-amino acid epitope from *MAGE1* that triggered the tumor-specific T-cell clone when bound to HLA-A1 was also identified (Fig. 100.3).[37]

KEY CONCEPTS

Tumor antigenic epitopes may be coded for:

- In open reading frames that are out of the native open reading frame
- By DNA sequences that extend into introns
- By transcription of antisense DNA

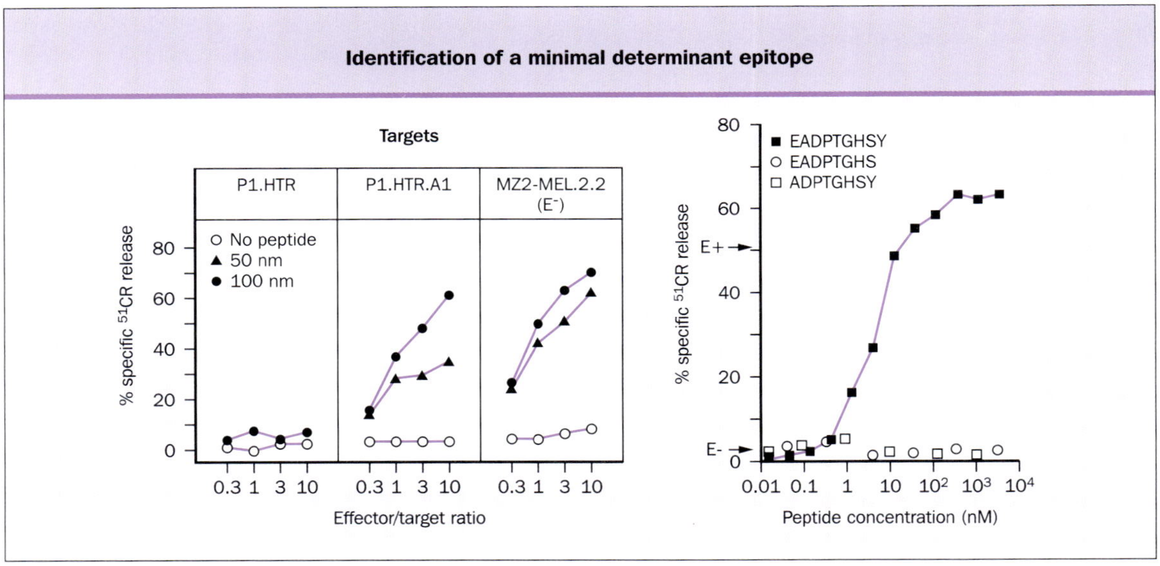

Figure 100.3 Identification of the minimal determinant epitope from the first cloned human tumor antigen recognized by T cells. A CTL clone from a patient repeatedly vaccinated with her own tumor was used to identify MZ2-E (encoded by the *MAGE1* gene) as the antigen being recognized in the context of HLA-A1. This figure demonstrates that the peptide EADPTGHSY, encoded by codons 161–169 of the open reading frame of MAGE-1, is the peptide that binds to HLA-A1 and is recognized by the patient's CTL. P1.HTR is a murine tumor cell line, P1.HTR-A1 is that line transfected with human HLA-A1 and MZ2-MEL.2.2 E- is an antigen-loss variant of the patient's autologous tumor line. When a target cell expressing HLA-A1 is exposed to low concentrations of EADPTGHSY it confers susceptibility to lysis by the autologous CTL clone. The right panel demonstrates that this is indeed the minimal determinant.

This groundbreaking work quickly led to the cloning of other antigens.[38,39] A simplified technique is most often used that involves screening a cDNA library from the recognized tumor and transfecting the cDNA into a target cell line (such as the COS monkey kidney cell line) that was previously stably transfected with the proper HLA restriction element (Fig. 100.4). At present, more than three dozen antigens expressed by melanoma as well as other tumors have been elucidated (Table 100.3).[39–51] Some of these have demonstrated unexpected and interesting immunological properties. Several have epitopes contained in polypeptides that are transcribed and translated out of their native open reading frame. For example, the HLA-A31-restricted determinant of tyrosinase-related protein-1 (TRP-1) consists of the peptide MSLQRQFLR, which arises from the third open reading frame of the *TRP1* gene, instead of the reading frame that yields the TRP-1 protein.[52] This phenomenon was also observed for two epitopes from *NY-ESO1*,[53] for intestinal carboxyl esterase[54] as well as for other antigens. Prior to these findings it was not clear that eukaryotic organisms transcribed and translated proteins from alternative reading frames, but the sensitivity of immunological detection has clearly established this fact. Other antigens appear to generate their minimal determinants from genomic coding sequences that extend into introns. This aberrant peptide translation has been demonstrated for *TRP2*[55] and *GP100*,[56] as well as other antigens; it implies that transcription and RNA splicing are quite inconsistent in tumors. A similar surprising development was described for the renal cancer antigen, RU1, which appears to encode its T-cell epitope by transcription from its antisense DNA strand.[49] This paradigm-disrupting array of findings illustrates that there is no shortage of means by which a tumor cell can generate immunogenic epitopes, and begs the question of why these tumors ever grew in immunocompetent

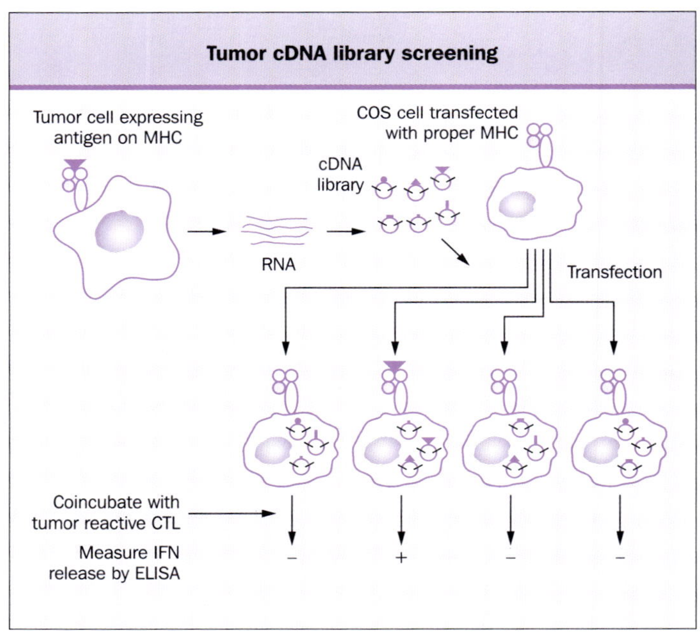

Figure 100.4 Method for screening a tumor cDNA library for antigens recognized in the context of Class I MHC molecules. A cytotoxic T-lymphocyte line with MHC-restricted recognition of the tumor is used to screen a cDNA expression library from the tumor. The cDNA is transfected in small pools into a recipient cell that expresses the appropriate MHC molecule (here a COS cell line stably transfected with the appropriate human MHC molecule is shown), which is not recognized by the tumor-reactive CTLs. The CTL line is added to these transfectants and the supernatant tested for IFN-γ release by ELISA. On identifying cDNA pools that induce recognition of the recipient target cell, these pools are subcloned to identify the cDNA encoding the tumor antigen that is being recognized.

Table 100.3 Human tumor antigens recognized by T cells.

Human tumor antigens recognized by T cells

	Tumors expressing antigen	HLA restriction	Peptide epitope
Tissue differentiation antigens			
MART-1/MelanA	Melanoma	A2	AAGIGILTV
		B45	AEEAAGIGILT
GP100	Melanoma	A2	KTWGQYWQV
		A2	AMLGTHTMEV
		A2	MLGTHTMEV
		A2	ITDQVPFSV
		A2	YLEPGPVTA
		A2	LLDGTATLRL
		A2	VLYRYGSFSV
		A2	RLMKQDFSV
		A2	SLADTNSLAV
		A2	RLPRIFCSC
		A3	SLIYRRRLMK
		A3	ALLAVGATK
		A3	LIYRRRLMK
		A24	VYFFLPDHL
		DR4[40]	QLYPEWTEAQRL
Tyrosinase	Melanoma	A1	KCDICTDEY
		A1	SSDYVIPIGTY
		A2	MLLAVLYCL
		A2	YM*D*GTMSQV
		A24	AFLPWHRLF
		B44	SEIWRDIDF
		DR4	QNILLSNAPLGPQFP
		DR4	SYLQDSDPDSFQD
TRP-1	Melanoma	A31	MSLQRQFLR
TRP-2	Melanoma	A2	SVYDFFVWL
		A31, A33	LLPGGRPYR
		A68, A33	EVISCKLIKR
MSH-1[41]	Melanoma	A2	TILLGIFFL
		A2	FLALIICNA
		A2	AIIDPLIYA
Tumor–testis antigens			
MAGE-1	Melanoma, lung, bladder and others	A1	EADPTGHSY
		A3	SLFRAVITK
		A28	EVYDGREHSA
		B53	DPARYEFLW
		Cw2	SAFPTTINE
		Cw3, Cw16	SAYGEPRKL
MAGE-2	Melanoma, lung, bladder	A24[42]	EYLQLVFGI
MAGE-3	Melanoma, lung, bladder, head and neck	A1	EVDPIGHLY
		A2	FLWGPRALV
		A24	IMPKAGLLI
		A24	TFPDLESEF
		B44	MEVDPIGHLY
		DR11[43]	TSYVKVLHHMVKISG
		DR13[44]	AELVHFLLLKYRAR
		DR13	LLKYRAREPVTKAE
MAGE-12	Melanoma	Cw7[45]	VRIGHLYIL
RAGE-1	Renal, sarcoma, bladder, melanoma, mesothelioma	B7	SPSSNRIRNT
GAGE-1 and -2	Melanoma, sarcoma, lung bladder, seminoma head and neck	Cw6	YRPRPRRY
BAGE	Melanoma, bladder, breast, squamous, lung	Cw16	AARAVFLAL
NY-ESO-1	Melanoma, breast, prostate, bladder	A2	SLLMWITQC
		A2	QLSLLMWIT
		A31	ASGPGGGAPR
		A31	AAQERRVPR (ORF2)
		DRB4*01[46]	VLLKEFTVSGNILTIRLT
		DRB4*01	AADHRQLQLSISSCLQQL
Mutated or unique tumor antigens			
β-Catenin	Melanoma, gastric	A24	SYLDSGIH*F*
CDC-27	Melanoma	DR4	FSWAMDLDPKGA
Triosephospate Isomerase	Melanoma	DR1[47]	IG*I*LNAAKVPADT

Table 100.3 Human tumor antigens recognized by T cells. (*contd*)

Human tumor antigens recognized by T cells

	Tumors expressing antigen	HLA restriction	Peptide epitope
Intestinal carboxyl esterase	Kidney	B7	SPRWWPTCL
CDK4	Melanoma	A2	ACDPHSGHFV
LDLR-FUT fusion[48]	Melanoma	DR1	*PVTWRRAPAPGA*
MUM-1	Melanoma	B44	EEKLIVVLF
Caspase-8	Head and neck	B35	FPSD*SWCYF*
KIAA0205	Bladder	B44	AEPINIQTW
Other antigens			
Telomerase	Multiple tumors	A2	ILAKFLHWL
SART-1	Squamous carcinoma (lung and esophagus)	A26	KGSGKMKTE
PRAME	Melanoma, lung, sarcoma, kidney, leukemia	A24	LYVDSLFFL
p15	Melanoma	A24	AYGLDFYIL
N-acetylglucosaminyl-transferase V (GnT-V)	Melanoma	A2	VLPDVFIRC
RU2	Kidney, multiple others	B7[49]	LPRWPPPQL
MN/carbonic anhydrase IX	Kidney	A2	HLSTAFARV

Single-letter abbreviations for the amino acid residues are as follows: A, Ala; C, Cys; D, Asp; E, Glu; F, Phe; G, Gly; H, His; I, Ile; K, Lys; L, Leu; M, Met; N, Asn; P, Pro; Q, Gln; R, Arg; S, Ser; T, Thr; V, Val; W, Trp; and Y, Tyr. Underlined amino acid residues are either mutated or aberrantly translated. Antigens without citations are reviewed in refs[39,51].

hosts. This latter question has several potential answers. Tumors have ways to temper the immunological responses to their antigens. An unusual modulation of a tumor-specific T cell was demonstrated when a CD8 T-cell clone that recognized the HLA-A24-restricted determinant of PRAME was shown to express a functional killer inhibitory receptor (KIR; originally described to participate in the regulation of NK and activated NK cell lysis) that inhibited lysis of the tumor target when HLA-Cw7 was expressed by the tumor and engaged by this KIR.[57] Other tumors seem to escape recognition by losing antigen expression, losing expression of their HLA molecules, or losing their ability to process antigens. They may also fail to costimulate T cells properly and produce immunosuppressive hormones or surface molecules.[58]

The defined tumor antigens appear to be grouped into several general categories. Some are tumor-specific mutations that generate unique epitopes, and consequently are likely to be of little general use as immunotherapy targets. This does not belie their potential as significant and possibly dominant mediators of clinical regression in those patients. Other antigens appear to be nonmutated 'self' proteins expressed, for example, by all tissues of melanocytic origin, and designated as tissue differentiation antigens. In this group, proteins probably involved in the generation of melanin pigment, such as tyrosinase, GP100, MART-1, TRP-1 and TRP-2, are prominent. A third group includes proteins expressed by tumor and testis or ovary, but not other normal tissues – the so-called tumor–testis antigens. These antigens are nonmutated and are hypothesized to have roles in embryogenesis, but not in normal adult tissues. MAGE-1 was the first such antigen described, but other MAGE family members, NY-ESO-1 and other antigens also belong to this category. The fourth category includes proteins overexpressed by tumor cells (compared to the vast majority of normal tissues), but occasionally expressed to a lesser extent on selected normal tissues. Many of these proteins are putatively involved in generating or maintaining the malignant phenotype. This newer class of antigens includes the catalytic subunit of telomerase, fibroblast growth factor-5 and possibly HER-2/*neu*.

The work in MHC Class I-restricted tumor antigens has been paralleled by advances in the identification of antigens recognized by CD4 cells and restricted by MHC Class II. Again, these antigens seem to be classified in the same overall groups as Class I antigens. The identification of Class II-restricted antigens has been more complicated because many tumor cells do not express MHC Class II. One approach has used tumor lysates fed to specialized antigen-presenting cells, such as matched or autologous EBV-B cells and biochemical fractionation and purification of these lysates,[47,59] but this only works for some proteins and not others. A recent innovation has been to use expression cloning very similar to that used for Class I antigens, but first cloning the cDNA library into a vector then incorporates the targeting sequence from the first 80 amino acids of the invariant chain (Ii). When a cell expressing the appropriate Class II molecule (and certain other components of the Class II processing pathway) is transfected with this Ii-fusion construct, the tumor antigens are targeted into the appropriate endosomal compartment for successful presentation by the Class II molecule.[60]

For both Class I and Class II-restricted antigens there is much current controversy over which types of antigens are clinically most relevant and mediate tumor regression. Support for the tissue differentiation antigens is found in the striking association of vitiligo with a clinical response to IL-2 in patients with melanoma (but not

KEY CONCEPTS

Tumor antigens include:

- Tumor-specific mutations that generate unique epitopes
- Nonmutated 'self' antigens that are differentiation antigens (e.g. GP100, MART-1 TRP-1)
- Nonmutated 'self' antigens that are found only in testis and tumor (e.g. MAGE-1, NY-ESO-1)
- Antigens overexpressed by tumor cells compared to normal tissue (e.g. telomerase)

Vitiligo and melanoma regression

	Total number of patients	Patients with vitiligo (%)	P_2 value
Patients with renal cancer	104	0 (0)	0.0001
Patients with melanoma	74	11 (15)	
Patients responding to IL-2 therapy	43	11 (26)	0.0002
Patients not responding to IL-2 therapy	27	0 (0)	
Not evaluable	4		

Table 100.4 The association of vitiligo with IL-2-induced regression of melanoma. Rosenberg SA, White DE.[61] Vitiligo in patients with melanoma: normal tissue antigens can be targets for cancer immunotherapy. J Immunother Emphasis Tumor Immunol 1996;19:81.

patients with renal cancer responding to IL-2) (Table 100.4).[61] Counterarguments point out that 'self' tolerance paradigms imply that responses against mutated tumor proteins would be less susceptible to the deletion of high-affinity T cells during thymic maturation, and thus might be superior antigens. The present challenge is not only to resolve this issue, but to discover the means to exploit the entire list of antigens in order to increase the frequency of clinical responses to immunotherapy.

For nonmelanoma tumors the discovery of tumor-associated T-cell antigens has been much more difficult. Some antigens expressed by renal cancer, head and neck cancer and bladder cancer have been identified, but many of these have been limited in utility by low frequency of expression on these cancers. RAGE-1 was identified from a cDNA library using standard expression screening with a T-cell clone generated by in-vitro mixed tumor cell–lymphocyte culture and limiting dilution cloning.[62] Unfortunately, it may only be expressed on 2% of renal cancers. Caspase-8 was identified in a similar fashion screening a cDNA library from a head and neck cancer.[63] SART-1 and PRAME (both on tumors of multiple histological types) were also identified with this method.[57,64] Much of the difficulty has been in generating tumor-reactive T cells against nonmelanoma cancers. The search for melanoma antigens has occasionally identified a protein expressed not only by melanoma cells but by other tumors as well. In this fortuitous but tangential manner MAGE-3 was recognized as a T-cell antigen expressed and recognized on a variety of tumors, including lung cancer, bladder cancer and hepatoma. Another approach to finding antigens expressed by tumors has been to select proteins known to be overexpressed by these tumors and then attempt to generate T cells in vitro, using candidate peptide epitopes from these proteins that are predicted by MHC-binding algorithms. This approach has been tried for Her-2-*neu*, prostate-specific antigen (PSA), carcinoembryonic antigen (CEA), p53, the melanocyte-stimulating hormone receptor (MC1R) and the catalytic subunit of telomerase. Peptide reactivity was often achieved in vitro, but not all peptide-reactive T cells generated in vitro could recognize tumor cells, implying that the candidate peptides selected were not being naturally processed and presented on tumor cells in adequate amounts. One successful example of the application of this technique has been in the identification of an HLA-A2-restricted epitope in the catalytic subunit of telomerase that was expressed on tumors of many different histologies and recognized by T cells directed at this epitope.[65] This approach was also successful with the melanoma candidate antigen MC1R.[41] Nevertheless, the majority of efforts studying candidate proteins from nonmelanoma tumors have not convincingly identified epitopes that could consistently mediate MHC-restricted immune recognition of native antigen-expressing tumors.

Some tumors, by virtue of their progenitor cell, can express unique proteins. One such tumor is B-cell lymphoma. These cells typically express a unique immunoglobulin receptor that can be targeted by cellular and humoral anti-idiotypic responses. Humoral responses have dominated immunotherapeutic approaches to this antigen (see Humoral responses to cancer). Recently, investigators have demonstrated that CD4 and CD8 T-cell responses to idiotype vaccines may to be important in generating complete clinical responses, and they are currently devising strategies that include vaccination using these determinants.[66]

A special note should be made on the potential use of viral antigens as therapeutic targets in the few human tumors with viral etiologies. Cervical cancer is one of the most common cancers in areas of the world where Papanicolaou screening is not generally utilized. A compelling body of evidence has been accumulated indicating that the majority of cervical cancer is caused by infection and transformation of cervical epithelium by human papillomavirus (HPV), particularly serotypes 16 and 18. Not only is there a strong epidemiological association between viral infection and disease, but viral DNA can be found in nearly all cervical cancers, and the E6 and E7 genes from HPV are potent transforming agents for epithelial cells. In view of this, many investigators have hypothesized that these viral proteins would be attractive targets for immunotherapy for cervical cancer. Not only are they tumor specific, but as foreign viral products they might be particularly immunogenic. Specific epitopes from the E6 and E7 proteins have been identified as potential targets, as have T cells that recognize tumors based on these viral epitopes.[67] Much of the clinical effort is directed at vaccine trials attempting to prevent the spread of these oncogenic viruses, a goal that is likely to be more easily attained than the therapy of advanced cervical cancer. The major remaining obstacles to clinical trials are to define the immune responses that best prevent viral infection and spread, and to determine the optimal methods of vaccinating a patient against a particular epitope or antigen. Another tumor that is extremely common worldwide (especially in Asia) is hepatoma. Two agents implicated in the genesis of a large proportion of hepatomas are the hepatitis B and C viruses. Although a vaccine against hepatitis B is widely available and would have a major impact on the incidence of hepatoma if widely used, this vaccine is directed at generating a neutralizing humoral response to a viral surface component and is not intended as a therapy for patients with hepatoma. Although prevention of viral infection through vaccination is likely to have the greatest impact on these tumors in the long term, other approaches involve the generation of cytolytic T cells for the purposes of treating patients who already have hepatoma or cervical cancer. An example of the success of such an approach in another virus-associated malignancy that involves Epstein–Barr virus (EBV). This is clearly a virus with oncogenic potential, as seen in African Burkitt's lymphoma and nasopharyngeal carcinoma in Asia. These tumors are characterized by the expression of EBV proteins in tumor cells, and epidemiological evidence again strongly supports a causative role for EBV. In the United States and Europe, patients receiving allogeneic bone marrow and organ transplantation with the attendant immunosuppression have a significant risk for post-transplant lymphoproliferative disease (LPD) and lymphoma that appears to be EBV associated. This risk appears to increase with the use of anti-T-cell agents. In the setting of bone marrow transplantation, the malignancies appear to be donor derived. In this situation, investigators have hypothesized that the restoration of anti-EBV T-cell reactivity through donor lymphocyte infusions might have therapeutic activity against these malignancies. This was subsequently confirmed in several clinical trials in a prophylactic setting. Rooney and co-workers reported that donor lymphocyte infusions in 42 patients at high risk for LPD resulted in none developing this complication, compared to 8 of 53 patients (15%) who did not receive donor lymphocyte transfusions.[68] This approach has also been utilized in the setting of established post-transplant lymphoma. In these cases not only are complete clinical responses seen, but when the donor lymphocytes are genetically marked prior to infusion, homing of donor lymphocytes to tumor sites and the recovery of gene-marked CTL with anti-EBV activity have been demonstrated.[69] This concept is being expanded to the treatment of EBV-positive Hodgkin's disease, using autologous T cells with specific antiviral reactivity.

Several other viral agents are under study as contributing agents to human cancer. The finding that exogenous and endogenous retroviral sequences can serve as tumor-associated antigens in murine cancers[70,71] has led to the consideration of a role for these viral agents in human cancer. Acute human T-cell lymphomas can be caused by HTLV-1 suggesting that therapy of this malignancy could include antiviral-based immunotherapy. However, the immunosuppression associated with this malignancy (as well as HIV infection and its associated malignancies) presents a formidable obstacle to effective immunotherapy directed at retroviral antigens. There is also recent evidence that mesothelioma frequently contains integrated SV40 genomic sequences, and even speculation that this DNA virus may be etiologically implicated in this and other malignancies.[72,73] Further work is needed to determine whether viral epitopes are expressed by these tumors which then might be targeted by immunotherapies.

CLINICAL TRIALS WITH TUMOR-REACTIVE IMMUNE CELLS

The recent ability to identify and expand immune cells with antitumor reactivity has had ramifications not only for antigen discovery, but also for adoptive cellular therapy. It is currently possible to produce both T cells with specific MHC-restricted reactivity and also nonspecific cells with innate tumor reactivity from most patients with melanoma. The latter population of nonspecific cells can in fact be generated in normal volunteers, as well as all patients with all types of malignancy. Initially, lymphokine-activated killer (LAK) cells were described as a cytolytic lymphoid cell generated by the incubation of peripheral blood mononuclear cells in high levels of IL-2.[74] These cells appeared to be phenotypically related to natural killer cells, but could kill fresh and cultured murine and human tumors (but not fresh normal tissues) in an indiscriminatory and MHC-non restricted fashion. It is now known that such cells recognize target cells via a receptor, and that this killing is inhibited by families of killer inhibitory receptors expressed on their surfaces which ligate a variety of MHC molecules. Murine studies suggested that the addition of LAK cell transfer to IL-2 therapy significantly augmented the therapeutic benefit, and so clinical trials administering IL-2 and up to 2×10^{11} LAK cells were performed in patients with advanced melanoma and renal cell cancer. Although complete and partial tumor regressions were seen, subsequent randomized studies attributed these responses to IL-2 and no evidence for a benefit of LAK cells in patients has been demonstrated.[12,75]

Another source of tumor-reactive immune cells in patients with cancer has been the tumors themselves. When tumors are excised, enzymatically dispersed and cultured in IL-2, tumor-infiltrating lymphocytes (TIL) will expand from these cultures and, in many cases, proliferate extensively. In patients with melanoma these TIL cultures frequently demonstrate specific CTL with MHC-restricted tumor recognition,[76] which (as noted above) have been used to clone the melanoma-associated antigens responsible for this recognition. These TIL have also been expanded to large numbers and administered by adoptive cellular transfer along with systemic IL-2 (Fig. 100.5). In one large experience, 29 of 86 patients (34%) showed a complete or partial response to this therapy.[77] Not only was this response rate higher than the historical response rate for IL-2 alone, but was the same (32%) in patients who had previously failed to respond to IL-2 alone. In addition, these expanded T cells could be labeled with ^{111}In and documented to localize to tumor deposits. It appeared

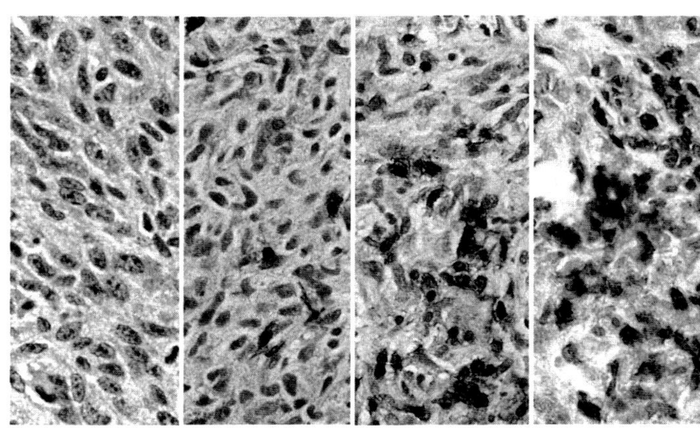

Figure 100.5 Histologic appearance of metastatic melanoma in a patient treated with high-dose IL-2 and a transfusion of cultured, autologous tumor-infiltrating lymphocytes recognizing her tumor. Pretreatment biopsy (left) shows viable melanoma with no infiltrating cells. Successive biopsies of other lesions from the same patient on days 3, 5 and 19 after the beginning of therapy are shown. Sections are immunostained for leukocyte common antigen to identify infiltrating leukocytes. This histological appearance of dense lymphocytic infiltrates is not significantly different from that seen in some patients after IL-2 therapy only. (See also color plate 100.5.)

THERAPEUTIC PRINCIPLES

Tumor-reactive immune cells

- Lymphokine-activated killer cells: no evidence of benefit in patient studies
- Polyclonal or oligoclonal tumor specific T cells may provide clinical benefit; studies are currently under way

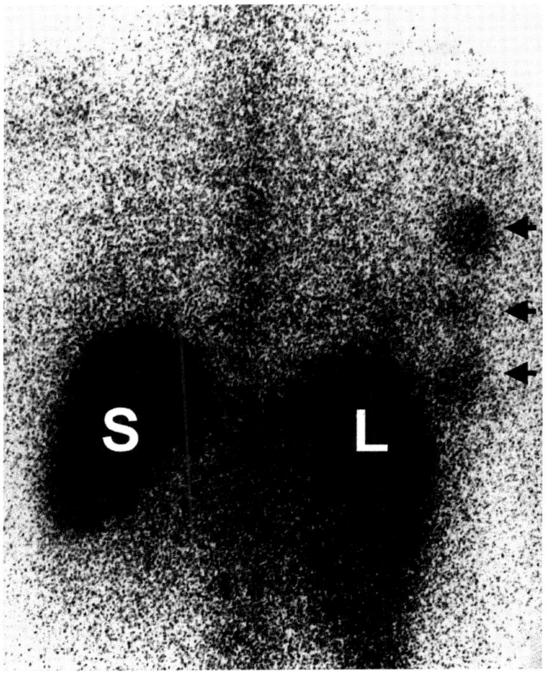

Figure 100.6 Localization of ^{111}In-labeled tumor infiltrating lymphocytes (TIL; expanded and activated in vitro with IL-2) to sites of metastatic melanoma in a patient undergoing therapy with adoptively transferred cells and IL-2. This gamma-camera image of the torso shows several foci of ^{111}In accumulation in tumors of the chest wall and axilla (arrows), 2 days after TIL infusion. (L, liver; S, spleen)

that such localization was associated with a higher probability of a major clinical response[78] (Fig. 100.6). These studies suggested that the use of polyclonal or oligoclonal tumor-specific T-cell populations might be more clinically effective than the use of nonspecifically lytic cells such as LAK. Techniques using anti-CD3 and large numbers of irradiated feeder peripheral blood lymphocytes and EBV-B cells to expand the normal antigen-specific T cells represent a major advance in our ability to generate adequate numbers of clonally reactive T cells for therapy.[79] This concept is currently being pursued with the use of monoclonal expanded T cells that have documented tumor reactivity combined with systemic IL-2 administration.[80]

HUMORAL RESPONSES TO CANCER

A large number of antibodies capable of binding human cancers with some degree of specificity have been identified. In early work many of these were generated in mice by vaccination with human tumors, followed by screening to eliminate reactivity based simply on species differences. Many of these antibodies were tested in clinical trials, infused alone or with cytokine adjuncts. These efforts were thwarted by the development of human antimurine antibody (HAMA) responses that neutralized these antibodies or truncated their survival in vivo. Initial reports of some striking responses against hematopoetic malignancies, especially B-cell lymphoma and occasional carcinomas, generated considerable interest in this approach.[81,82] Subsequent clinical trials have shown that responses are either rare or of short duration. These antibodies have also been widely used to deliver radiation therapy by conjugating them to radioisotopes. Trials utilizing the L6 antibody binding to multiple adenocarcinomas, the 17–1A antibody binding to a variety of gastrointestinal tumors and the B72.3 antibody recognizing a glycoprotein on several cancers, have shown only modest activity.[83–85]

Other vaccine approaches have targeted a humoral response to tumor-associated antigens in an effort to diversify the antibody response and to generate endogenous responses that would not be subject to the limitations of administering murine-derived immunoglobulins. This effort has been intensively pursued for certain melanoma antigens, particularly the ganglioside GM2. Vaccination with this agent seemed to induce brisk antibody responses in some patients, and in several publications these responses appeared to be associated with favorable survival. Only a randomized trial could discern whether these antibody titers were producing a survival benefit, or if better immune responses in general were simply being demonstrated by the healthier patients with less debility and better intrinsic survival. In a recently reported randomized trial, where patients with AJC stage III melanoma were randomized to receive either GM2 with low-dose cyclophosphamide and BCG or cyclophosphamide and BCG without GM2, disease-free and overall survival end-points favored patients vaccinated with GM2, but these differences were not statistically significant.[86]

Recently there has been a resurgence of interest in antibody therapy for cancer that is based on several developments. First, the technology to 'humanize' antibodies of murine origin to avoid the generation of HAMA has advanced significantly. The meticulous genetic assembly of human immunoglobulin framework regions combined with the complementary-determining regions from murine antibodies with specificity for human cancers has resulted in the creation of immunoglobulins with desired specificities, subtypes and affinities for clinical use.[87] In some cases the avoidance of a HAMA response has been documented in patients receiving these modified immunoglobulins repeatedly. Second, an antibody specific for a protein, HER-2/*neu*, expressed on many breast cancers as well as other tumors, has been demonstrated in randomized clinical trials to have efficacy both alone and in conjunction with cytotoxic chemotherapy in patients with advanced breast cancer.[88] Although the precise mechanisms of action of this antibody is unknown, it is likely that it intervenes in the signal transduction processes of susceptible cancer cells. Thus it functions less as an immunotherapeutic agent and more like a drug that happens to be an antibody. In the treatment of B-cell lymphoma, antibodies have had an increasing role. A chimeric monoclonal antibody against

THERAPEUTIC PRINCIPLES

Antitumor antibodies
- Humanized antitumor monoclonal antibody
  - Anti Her-2/*neu* approved for breast cancer
  - Anti-CD20 approved in B-cell lymphoma
  - Anti-CD25 approved in cutaneous T-cell lymphoma
- SEREX (serological identification of antigens by recombinant expression cloning) used to identify tumor antigens and patients with antitumor immune response
- Vaccine therapy: clinical trials under way; to date limited evidence for efficacy

CD20, a lymphocyte surface marker expressed on many B-cell lymphomas, has been demonstrated to have clinical efficacy against this class of hematopoietic tumors[89] and is approved for use by the US Food and Drug Administration. Ongoing studies are targeting other B-cell lymphoma surface antigens and coupling these antibodies to toxins or radioisotopes to increase efficacy.[90]

The third and potentially most significant development in the study of the humoral response to cancer is the development of the SEREX (*ser*ological identification of antigens by recombinant *ex*pression cloning) methodology for identifying tumor antigens that provoke humoral responses in cancer patients.[91] This technique uses diluted sera from patients with a variety of cancers to screen tumor cDNA libraries expressed in *Escherichia coli* as a means to identify antigens that have generated high-titer IgG responses. Initially used to identify the NY-ESO-1 antigen in serum from a patient with squamous cell carcinoma of the esophagus,[92] it has since been used to discover (and rediscover) a multitude of antigens from tumors of many histologies, including colon cancer, lung cancer, renal cancer and melanoma. In general, many of these screenings have identified new proteins of unknown function. Extensive work will be required to determine their antigen expression patterns and functions. Screening for high-titer IgG responses should identify patients who have CD4 T-cell responses to the tumor antigen as this is required for Ig class switching. There also appear to be collateral benefits from the SEREX technique. In some instances, T-cells with reactivity to the antigens defined by SEREX have been identified and HLA Class II restricted epitopes delineated.[46] In addition, these IgG responses may be indicative of a broader T-cell response, as some of these patients have also demonstrated Class I-restricted CD8 T-cell responses to these same tumor proteins.[53]

CLINICAL VACCINE EFFORTS

In spite of an imperfect understanding of the means of vaccinating patients against tumor antigens, and an even poorer understanding of the precise reactivity that must be generated to cause tumor regression, there have been several attempts at vaccinating patients with advanced disseminated cancer. Early efforts utilized whole tumor and tumor lysates of autologous or allogeneic origin. These efforts concentrated on melanoma and, in some cases, colon cancer, and although rare responses were described, little evidence of consistent efficacy was forthcoming. It was equally difficult to demonstrate that measurable or interpretable immune responses were occurring; without clinical responses there was little with which to correlate immunological evaluations. Several randomized trials involving patients in high-risk situations but without detectable disease (adjuvant therapy) also failed to demonstrate any survival value to whole-cell vaccines against colorectal cancer and melanoma. Long-term follow-up of patients with AJCC stage III melanoma who had been randomized to observation versus immunization with an allogeneic melanoma oncolysate showed no significant differences in overall or disease-free survival.[93] Immunization of patients with resected Duke's stage C colon cancer with tumor and BCG initially indicated a benefit in a small randomized pilot trial, but a larger confirmatory trial did not substantiate this finding.[94,95]

The advent of defined tumor antigens has greatly augmented the ability to perform immunological assessments in patients, but a shortage of clinical responses to vaccination has hindered the ability to interpret these in vitro assessments. Preclinical experiments suggested that a multitude of methods could be used to vaccinate against tumor-associated antigens. Evidence of immunization using in vivo murine models and in vitro human cells was demonstrated for minimal determinant peptides, recombinant viruses expressing a tumor antigen, naked DNA plasmids, and dendritic cells pulsed with whole tumor cells, proteins, peptides, DNA and even RNA. In patients, the use of minimal determinant peptides has proved an effective method of vaccination for some antigens and is also the least encumbered by necessary regulatory precautions. It has been discovered that modification and optimization of MHC-binding 'anchor' residues in these peptides can result in 'anchor-fixed' peptides, which are more immunogenic in vitro and in vivo and yet still generate T cells that cross-react with and recognize the native, unmodified peptides. For instance, the HLA-A2-restricted peptide at amino acid residues 209–217 in the melanoma protein gp100 has the sequence ITDQVPFSV, and many patients with melanoma can generate tumor-infiltrating lymphocytes that recognize this minimal determinant epitope. The classic HLA-A2-binding motif would suggest that at position 2 (aa 210), the optimal residue should be either methionine or leucine instead of threonine. If methionine is substituted for threonine at position 2, the resulting peptide, 209–217 (210M), is more immunogenic than the native peptide both in vitro and in vivo.[96] Ten of 11 melanoma patients vaccinated twice with this peptide in incomplete Freund's adjuvant developed CTL precursors with specificity for the native 209–217 peptide, and these CTL were also able to specifically recognize HLA-A2 tumors expressing gp100 as measured by several different assays (Table 100.5a). Only two of eight patients given the native peptide in an identical vaccination generated such CTL precursors (Table 100.5b). A preliminary clinical trial utilizing this peptide combined with high-dose IL-2 therapy reported a 42% response rate in patients with advanced melanoma (Fig. 100.7), compared to extensive nonrandomized historical cohorts where the response rates to either IL-2 alone or IL-2 with other vaccinations ranged from 15 to 17%.[97] This result is being retested in a larger, randomized trial. Other trials have administered the HLA-A1-restricted MAGE-3 peptide EVDPIGHLY monthly without adjuvant to patients with advanced melanoma. Seven of 39 patients were reported to have some evidence of tumor regression, with two durable complete responses.[98]

Sporadic reports have appeared on the use of dendritic cells pulsed with either minimal determinant peptides or tumor cell lysates that were then injected by a number of routes, including a study with intranodal injection. This latter study reported a 31% major response rate (5 of 16 patients) with vaccine alone in patients with metastatic melanoma, but this result has not yet been confirmed by others.[99] A trial using dendritic cells pulsed with the MAGE-3 A1-restricted peptide (along with a bystander recall antigen) also reported some evidence of clinical tumor regression.[100]

Extensive preclinical animal data have been generated in which the genetic introduction of an immunostimulatory cytokine or cell surface molecule into a tumor cell augmented the response to the tumor upon immunization.[101,102] This has been demonstrated for an extensive list of lymphokines, including IL-2, IL-4, IL-5, IL-6, IL-7 and IL-10, as well as for other molecules such

Peripheral blood lymphocyte reactivity in a patient immunized with the modified HLA-A2-restricted peptide 209-2M from GP100

	In-vitro stimulating peptide	IFN-γ release (pg/ml) in response to stimulator cells							
		T2	*T2+280*	*T2+flu*	*T2+209*	*501 Mel* (A2+)	*Sk23 mel* (A2+)	*624.28 mel* (A2−)	*888 mel* (A2−)
Preimmunization PBL	209 mod	135	102	230	146	195	180	89	115
	209	118	90	238	84	148	231	162	261
	flu	178	123	**35 570**	124	290	284	172	282
Postimmunization PBL	209 mod	86	74	61	**24 150**	**72 780**	**43 250**	124	33
	209	86	62	165	**9890**	**25 710**	**19 480**	104	98
	flu	121	118	**36 460**	132	313	448	85	362

Peripheral blood lymphocytes are incubated with the in vitro stimulating peptide for 10–12 days and then assayed for IFN-γ release in response to the stimulator cells indicated in a 24-hour assay. Bold values indicate IFN-γ release >2x control values. 209 mod is an anchor-modified peptide from gp 100, 209 is the native peptide and flu is a positive control using an influenza matrix peptide. T2 is an HLA-A2 expressing line that is pulsed with test peptides, and the various mel lines are cultured melanoma cell lines with their expression of HLA-A2 indicated.

Table 100.5a Peripheral blood lymphocyte reactivity in a patient immunized with the modified HLA-A2-restricted peptide 209-2M from GP100. Adapted from Rosenberg SA, Yang JC, Schwartzentruber DJ, et al. Immunologic and therapeutic evaluation of a synthetic peptide vaccine for the treatment of patients with metastatic melanoma [see comments]. *Nature Med* 1998;4:321.

Comparison of immunizations with the native 209–217 peptide from GP100 and the 210M-modified peptide in patients with melanoma

	Number of patients	Patients developing reactivity to the native 209–217 peptide	
Patients receiving native 209–217 in IFA	8	2 (25%)	
			P=0.006
Patients receiving 210M-modified 209–217 in IFA	11	10 (91%)	

Table 100.5b Comparison of immunizations with the native 209–217 peptide from GP100 and the 210M-modified peptide in patients with melanoma Adapted from Rosenberg SA, Yang JC, Schwartzentruber DJ, et al. Immunologic and therapeutic evaluation of a synthetic peptide vaccine for the treatment of patients with metastatic melanoma [see comments]. *Nature Med* 1998;4:321.

as GM-CSF, RANTES and others. Another twist on this approach has been to express T-cell costimulatory molecules such as CD80 and CD86 on tumors in order to provide the necessary 'second signal' for effective activation of T cells. Among these many attempts to combine gene therapy with immunotherapy, the most consistent data have been obtained with GM-CSF used in this manner. Three clinical trials have been published with this labor-intensive, individualized approach to developing vaccines. Patients must have tumor excised, established in culture, and then transduced with a high-efficiency retrovirus encoding hGM-CSF. In addition, preclinical models suggest that the production of GM-CSF must be quite substantial (of the order of 300 ng/10^6 tumor cells/24 h), and not all of these requirements can be accomplished in many patients. Nevertheless, a trial of autologous tumor vaccination with GM-CSF-transduced renal cell cancer in patients with metastatic disease has been reported based on 16 patients who were vaccinated and then immunologically and clinically assessed. One partial response was seen in a patient who generated a substantial DTH and CD4 response to autologous tumor.[103] In another trial of similar design in patients with metastatic melanoma, intense lymphocytic infiltrates were seen in all patients from whom biopsies could be obtained, although pre- and post-treatment biopsies could not be obtained from the same lesions. Despite these interesting biological findings, no clinical responses were seen in 21 evaluable patients.[104] Another trial in prostate cancer showed improvements demonstrable by PSA levels, but no major clinical responses.[105] This area of experimentation continues to be actively pursued in order to identify therapies that will result in clinically significant regressions.

GRAFT VERSUS TUMOR REACTIVITY AS CANCER IMMUNOTHERAPY

In patients undergoing bone marrow allotransplantation to deliver high doses of cytotoxic chemotherapy and to ablate hematopoietic malignancies infiltrating marrow, graft-versus-host disease (GVHD) is a major complication that results in morbidity and mortality for the recipient. It was noted paradoxically that the presence of this complication was associated with a better overall prognosis with respect to the hematopoietic malignancy. This observation led to the hypothesis that there was a graft-versus-tumor reaction that could assist in the obliteration of the hematopoietic malignancy. Extensive studies have confirmed this in lymphocytic lymphoma, chronic myelogenous leukemia, and other cancers. Limited clinical trials have attempted to augment this reactivity through modifications of immunosuppressive regimens, as well as the use of immunostimulants such as IL-2.[106] This concept has been extended by Childs et al to the treatment of solid tumors, most notably renal cell cancer.[107] In a pilot experience in which patients with metastatic renal cancer underwent a nonmyeloablative preparative chemotherapy regimen with cyclophosphamide and fludarabine, and allotransplantation from an HLA-matched sibling, several significant clinical responses were seen. These patients received chemotherapy and transplantation with G-CSF-mobilized peripheral blood stem cells followed by the requisite immunosuppression to allow engraftment and suppress acute GVHD. During this time most patients showed progressive growth of their renal cancers. Approximately 100 days later, after full engraftment, their immunosuppression was tapered (and in

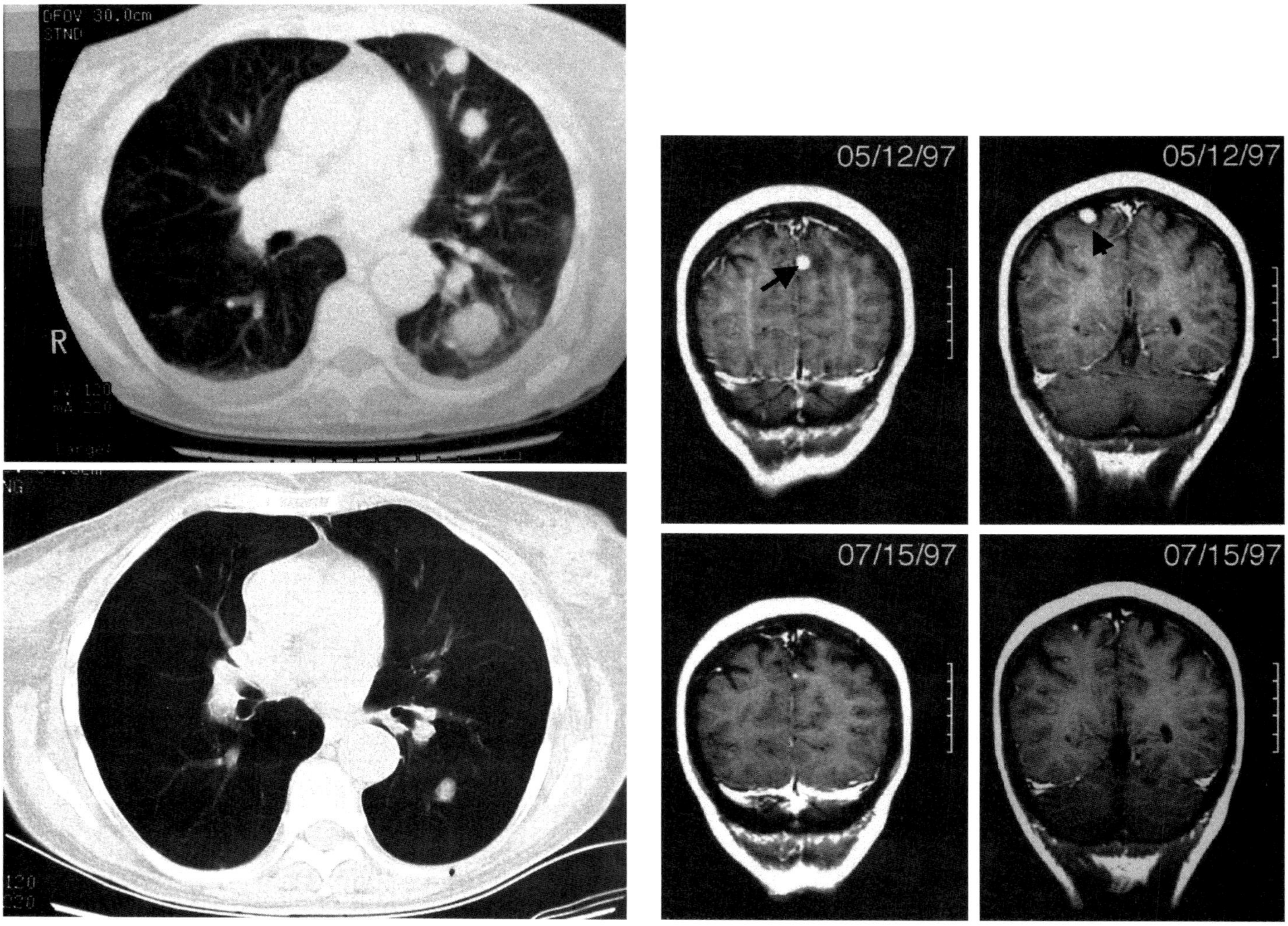

Figure 100.7 Rapid regression of metastatic lesions in patients vaccinated with anchor-modified antigenic peptides from the melanoma antigens MART-1 and GP100, followed by high-dose IL-2. (A) Extensive pulmonary metastases which regressed within 3 weeks. **(B)** An unusual regression of multiple brain metastases (arrows) in a patient who also had a response in extracranial sites. Randomized trials will be needed to determine the contribution of vaccination to regressions such as these.

some cases IFN or donor lymphocyte transfusions were given) until low-grade GVHD was evident. Among a total of 19 patients with renal cancer treated, 10 showed evidence of tumor regression and 3 attained a complete response.[107] In the face of an anticipated treatment-related mortality of over 10%, further experience in patients with renal cancer as well as other tumors is needed to fully evaluate this development.

OTHER APPROACHES TO IMMUNOTHERAPY

Several other experimental immunological approaches to cancer therapy are currently in use which are not readily classified. There have been many efforts to use gene therapy in the treatment of cancer. The current vectors for introducing genes into human cells in vivo are extremely inefficient, to the point that in vivo modification of tumor cells to treat cancers is not practical. Even under controlled in vitro conditions, current technology usually permits the introduction and expression of genes into human cells in, at best, a minority of the cells treated, necessitating selection or purification to enrich for successfully modified cells. With these limitations, molecular targets that can exert their action with only small numbers of molecules expressed by small percentages of cells represent the most attractive approaches to gene therapy. The receptors of the immune system, with their potent ability to transduce signals, and the ability of these activated cells to proliferate extensively and survive long term as memory cells, may be the best current route for exploiting gene therapy in cancer treatment. Two approaches for implementing this concept involve the introduction of native T-cell receptors with known tumor recognition into lymphocytes, and the fabrication of chimeric receptors that hybridize the antigen-binding domains of a tumor-reactive immunoglobulin with the intracytoplasmic signal transduction moieties of the T-cell–receptor complex. In the first approach, a T-cell with proven ability to recognize tumor is required, and its receptor α and β chains are sequenced and cloned into expression vectors. Preliminary in vitro work has demonstrated that when these constructs are introduced into activated T cells, the cells can be redirected to recognize the antigens specific for the introduced TCR. This technique may permit the introduction of large numbers of tumor antigen-specific T-cell precursors into patients. Other workers are investigating the introduction of these receptors into bone marrow stem cells to provide large numbers of in vivo-generated tumor-reactive T cells that can be readily renewed.[108] Further developments will require advances in the efficiency of introducing and expressing genes in lymphocytes, and a better understanding of the maturation and activation of such cells in humans. For most nonmelanoma tumors the major hurdle remains the identification of tumor-reactive T cells, so an alternative approach has been used which exploits the existence of monoclonal antibodies that bind to these tumors. First, single peptide chains that can bind antigen are fashioned by linking the variable portions of the immunoglobulin heavy and light chains with a peptide linker. Then the DNA encoding this peptide is ligated to the intracytoplasmic portion of the ζ-chain of the CD3 complex (or, in some cases, the Fc-receptor-γ), which normally transduces the signal after TCR ligation. This chimeric receptor DNA is then introduced into a suitable T cell and, when it is expressed and encounters its nominal antigen, it stimulates the T cell via an MHC-independent interaction. Despite the seeming unlikelihood of such a molecule functioning, it has been shown to stimulate both lysis and cytokine release by T cells, mediated by antigen binding to the antibody portion of the chimeric receptor. This approach is now entering clinical trials, beginning with a chimeric receptor utilizing the MOV-1 monoclonal antibody which binds the folate-binding protein expressed by most ovarian cancers.[109]

REFERENCES

1. Carswell EA, Old LJ, Kassel RL, Green S, Fiore N, Williamson B. An endotoxin-induced serum factor that causes necrosis of tumors. Proc Natl Acad Sci USA 1975;72:3666.
2. Hewitt HB. A critical examination of the foundations of immunotherapy for cancer. Clin Radiol 1979;30:361.
3. Quesada JR, Swanson DA, Trindade A, Gutterman JU. Renal cell carcinoma: antitumor effects of leukocyte interferon. Cancer Res 1983;43:940.
4. deKernion JB, Sarna G, Figlin R, Lindner A, Smith RB. The treatment of renal cell carcinoma with human leukocyte alpha-interferon. J Urol 1983;130:1063.
5. Quesada JR, Swanson DA, Gutterman JU. Phase II study of interferon alpha in metastatic renal-cell carcinoma: a progress report. J Clin Oncol 1985;3:1086.
6. Umeda T, Niijima T. Phase II study of alpha interferon on renal cell carcinoma. Summary of three collaborative trials. Cancer 1986;58:1231.
7. Muss HB, Costanzi JJ, Leavitt R, et al. Recombinant alfa interferon in renal cell carcinoma: a randomized trial of two routes of administration. J Clin Oncol 1987,5:286.
8. Minasian LM, Motzer RJ, Gluck L, Mazumdar M, Vlamis V, Krown SE. Interferon alfa-2a in advanced renal cell carcinoma: treatment results and survival in 159 patients with long-term follow-up. J Clin Oncol 1993;11:1368.
9. Lotze MT, Frana LW, Sharrow SO, Robb RJ, Rosenberg SA. In vivo administration of purified human interleukin 2. I. Half-life and immunologic effects of the Jurkat cell line-derived interleukin 2. J Immunol 1985;134:157.
10. Rosenberg SA, Lotze MT, Muul LM, et al. Observations on the systemic administration of autologous lymphokine-activated killer cells and recombinant interleukin-2 to patients with metastatic cancer. N Engl J Med 1985;313:1485.
11. Rosenberg SA, Lotze MT, Muul LM, et al. A progress report on the treatment of 157 patients with advanced cancer using lymphokine-activated killer cells and interleukin-2 or high-dose interleukin-2 alone. N Engl J Med 1987;316:889.
12. Rosenberg SA, Lotze MT, Yang JC, et al. Prospective randomized trial of high-dose interleukin-2 alone or in conjunction with lymphokine-activated killer cells for the treatment of patients with advanced cancer [published erratum appears in J Natl Cancer Inst 1993 Jul 7;85(13):1091]. J Natl Cancer Inst 1993;85:622.
13. Rosenberg SA, Yang JC, White DE, Steinberg SM. Durability of complete responses in patients with metastatic cancer treated with high-dose interleukin-2. Ann Surg 1998;228:319.
14. Atkins MB, Sparano J, Fisher RI, et al. Randomized phase II trial of high-dose interleukin-2 either alone or in combination with interferon alfa-2b in advanced renal cell carcinoma. J Clin Oncol 1993;11:661.
15. Fisher RI, Rosenberg SA, Sznol M, Parkinson DR, Fyfe G. High-dose aldesleukin in renal cell carcinoma: long-term survival update. Cancer J Sci Am 1997;3:S70.
16. Gold PJ, Thompson JA, Markowitz DR, Neumann S, Fefer A. Metastatic renal cell carcinoma: long-term survival after therapy with high-dose continuous-infusion interleukin-2. Cancer J Sci Am 1997;3:S85.
17. Escudier B, Ravaud A, Fabbro M, et al. High-dose interleukin-2 two days a week for metastatic renal cell carcinoma: an FNCLCC multicenter study. J Immunother 1994;16:306.
18. Yang JC, Rosenberg SA. An ongoing prospective randomized comparison of interleukin-2 regimens for the treatment of metastatic renal cell cancer. Cancer J Sci Am 1997;3:S79.
19. Lissoni P, Barni S, Tancini G, et al. Clinical response and survival in metastatic renal carcinoma during subcutaneous administration of interleukin-2 alone. Arch Ital Urol Androl 1997;69:41.
20. Buter J, Sleijfer DT, Winette TA, et al. A progress report on the out-patient treatment of patients with advanced renal cell carcinoma using subcutaneous recombinant interleukin-2. Semin Oncol 1993;20:16.
21. Parkinson DR, Abrams JS, Wiernik PH, et al. Interleukin-2 therapy in patients with metastatic malignant melanoma: a phase II study. J Clin Oncol 1990;8:1650.
22. Sparano JA, Fisher RI, Sunderland M, et al. Randomized phase III trial of treatment with high-dose interleukin-2 either alone or in combination with interferon alfa-2a in patients with advanced melanoma. J Clin Oncol 1993;11:1969.
23. Margolin KA, Rayner AA, Hawkins MJ, et al. Interleukin-2 and lymphokine-activated killer cell therapy of solid tumors: analysis of toxicity and management guidelines. J Clin Oncol 1989;7:486.
24. Schwartzentruber D. IL-2: Principles of administration and management of side effects. In: DeVita V, Hellman S, Rosenberg S (eds) Biologic therapy of cancer. Philadelphia, JB Lippincott, 1997, p 235.
25. Kammula US, White DE, Rosenberg SA. Trends in the safety of high dose bolus interleukin-2 administration in patients with metastatic cancer. Cancer 1998;83:797.
26. Sleijfer DT, Janssen RA, Buter J, et al. Phase II study of subcutaneous interleukin-2 in unselected patients with advanced renal cell cancer on an outpatient basis. J Clin Oncol 1992;10:1119.
27. Tourani JM, Lucas V, Mayeur D, et al. Subcutaneous recombinant interleukin-2 (rIL-2) in out-patients with metastatic renal cell carcinoma. Results of a multicenter SCAPP1 trial. Ann Oncol 1996;7:525.
28. Gleave ME, Elhilali M, Fradet Y, et al. Interferon gamma-1b compared to placebo in metastatic renal-cell carcinoma. N Engl J Med 1998;338:1265.
29. Sosman JA, Fisher SG, Kefer C, Fisher RI, Ellis TM. A phase I trial of continuous infusion interleukin-4 (IL-4) alone and following interleukin-2 (IL-2) in cancer patients. Ann Oncol 1994;5:452.
30. Rosenberg SA, Lotze MT, Yang JC, et al. Combination therapy with interleukin-2 and alpha-interferon for the treatment of patients with advanced cancer. J Clin Oncol 1989;7:1863.

31. Kruit WHJ, Lamers CHJ, Gratama JW, et al. High-dose regimen of interleukin-2 and interferon alpha in combination with lymphokine-activated killer cells in patients with metastatic renal cell cancer. J Immunother 1997;20:312.
32. Marincola FM, White DE, Wise AP, Rosenberg SA. Combination therapy with interferon alfa-2a and interleukin-2 for the treatment of metastatic cancer. J Clin Oncol 1995;13:1110.
33. Hanninen EL, Kirchner H, Atzpodien J. Interleukin-2 based home therapy of metastatic renal cell carcinoma: risks and benefits in 215 consecutive single institution patients. J Urol 1996;155:19.
34. Dutcher JP, Atkins M, Fisher R, et al. Interleukin-2-based therapy for metastatic renal cell cancer: the Cytokine Working Group experience, 1989–1997. Cancer J Sci Am 1997;3(Suppl 1)S73–8:S73.
35. Ravaud A, Audhuy B, Gomez F. Subcutaneous interleukin-2, interferon alfa-2a, and continuous infusion of fluorouracil in metastatic renal cell carcinoma: a multicenter phase II trial. Groupe Francais d'Immunotherapie. J Clin Oncol 1998;16:2728.
36. van der Bruggen P, Traversari C, Chomez P, et al. A gene encoding an antigen recognized by cytolytic T lymphocytes on a human melanoma. Science 1991;254:1643.
37. Traversari C, van der Bruggen P, Luescher IF, et al. A nonapeptide encoded by human gene MAGE-1 is recognized on HLA-A1 by cytolytic T lymphocytes directed against tumor antigen MZ2-E. J Exp Med 1992;176:1453.
38. Boon T, Coulie PG, Van den Eynde B. Tumor antigens recognized by T cells. Immunol Today 1997;18:267.
39. Robbins P, Wang R, Rosenberg S. Tumor antigens recognized by cytotoxic lymphocytes. In: Sitkovsky M, Henkart P (eds) Cytotoxic cells: basic mechanisms and medical applications. Philadelphia, Lippincott Williams and Wilkins, 2000, p 363.
40. Touloukian CE, Leitner WW, Topalian SL, Identification of a MHC Class II-restricted human gp100 epitope using DR4-IE transgenic mice. J Immunol 2000;164:3535.
41. Salazar-Onfray F, Nakazawa T, Chhajlani V, et al. Synthetic peptides derived from the melanocyte-stimulating hormone receptor MC1R can stimulate HLA-A2-restricted cytotoxic T lymphocytes that recognize naturally processed peptides on human melanoma cells. Cancer Res 1997;57:4348.
42. Tahara K, Takesako K, Sette A, Celis E, Kitano S, Akiyoshi T. Identification of a MAGE-2-encoded human leukocyte antigen-A24-binding synthetic peptide that induces specific antitumor cytotoxic T lymphocytes. Clin Cancer Res 1999;5:2236.
43. Manici S, Sturniolo T, Imro MA. Melanoma cells present a MAGE-3 epitope to CD4(+) cytotoxic T cells in association with histocompatibility leukocyte antigen DR11 [see comments]. J Exp Med 1999;189:871.
44. Chaux P, Vantomme V, Stroobant V, et al. Identification of MAGE-3 epitopes presented by HLA-DR molecules to CD4(+) T lymphocytes [see comments]. J Exp Med 1999;189:767.
45. Panelli MC, Bettinotti MP, Lally K. A tumor-infiltrating lymphocyte from a melanoma metastasis with decreased expression of melanoma differentiation antigens recognizes MAGE-12. J Immunol 2000;164:4382.
46. Jager E, Jager D, Karbach J, et al. Identification of NY-ESO-1 epitopes presented by human histocompatibility antigen (HLA)-DRB4*0101–0103 and recognized by CD4(+) T lymphocytes of patients with NY-ESO-1-expressing melanoma. J Exp Med 2000;1900;625.
47. Pieper R, Christian RE, Gonzales MI, et al. Biochemical identification of a mutated human melanoma antigen recognized by CD4(+) T cells [see comments]. J Exp Med 1999;189:757.
48. Wang RF, Wang X, Rosenberg SA. Identification of a novel major histocompatibility complex Class II-restricted tumor antigen resulting from a chromosomal rearrangement recognized by CD4(+) T cells. J Exp Med 1999;189:1659.
49. Van Den Eynde BJ, Gaugler B, Probst-Kepper M, et al. A new antigen recognized by cytolytic T lymphocytes on a human kidney tumor results from reverse strand transcription [see comments]. J Exp Med 1999;190:1793.
50. Kawakami Y, Robbins PF, Wang X, et al. Identification of new melanoma epitopes on melanosomal proteins recognized by tumor infiltrating T lymphocytes restricted by HLA-A1, -A2, and -A3 alleles. J Immunol 1998;161:6985.
51. Castelli C, Rivoltini L, Andreola G, Carrabba M, Renkvist N, Parmiani G. T-cell recognition of melanoma-associated antigens. J Cell Physiol 2000;182(3):323.
52. Wang RF, Parkhurst MR, Kawakami Y, Robbins PF, Rosenberg SA. Utilization of an alternative open reading frame of a normal gene in generating a novel human cancer antigen. J Exp Med 1996;183:1131.
53. Wang RF, Johnston SL, Zeng G, Topalian SL, Schwartzentruber DJ, Rosenberg SA. A breast and melanoma-shared tumor antigen: T cell responses to antigenic peptides translated from different open reading frames. J Immunol 1998;161:3598.
54. Ronsin C, Chung-Scott V, Poullion I, Aknouche N, Gaudin C, Triebel F. A non-AUG-defined alternative open reading frame of the intestinal carboxyl esterase mRNA generates an epitope recognized by renal cell carcinoma-reactive tumor-infiltrating lymphocytes in situ. J Immunol 1999;163:483.
55. Lupetti R, Pisarra P, Verrecchia A. Translation of a retained intron in tyrosinase-related protein (TRP) 2 mRNA generates a new cytotoxic T lymphocyte (CTL)-defined and shared human melanoma antigen not expressed in normal cells of the melanocytic lineage. J Exp Med 1998;188:1005.
56. Robbins PF, El-Gamil M, Li YF, Fitzgerald EB, Kawakami Y, Rosenberg SA. The intronic region of an incompletely spliced gp100 gene transcript encodes an epitope recognized by melanoma-reactive tumor-infiltrating lymphocytes. J Immunol 1997;159:303.
57. Ikeda H, Lethe B, Lehmann F, et al. Characterization of an antigen that is recognized on a melanoma showing partial HLA loss by CTL expressing an NK inhibitory receptor. Immunity 1997;6:199.
58. Marincola FM. The multiple ways to tumor tolerance [comment]. J Immunother 1997;20:178.
59. Topalian SL, Rivoltini L, Mancini M, Ng J, Hartzman RJ, Rosenberg SA. Melanoma-specific CD4+ T lymphocytes recognize human melanoma antigens processed and presented by Epstein–Barr virus-transformed B cells. Int J Cancer 1994;58:69.
60. Wang RF, Wang X, Atwood AC, Topalian SL, Rosenberg SA. Cloning genes encoding MHC Class II-restricted antigens: mutated CDC27 as a tumor antigen. Science 1999;284:1351.
61. Rosenberg SA, White DE. Vitiligo in patients with melanoma: normal tissue antigens can be targets for cancer immunotherapy. J Immunother Emphasis Tumor Immunol 1996;19:81.
62. Gaugler B, Brouwenstijn N, Vantomme V. A new gene coding for an antigen recognized by autologous cytolytic T lymphocytes on a human renal carcinoma. Immunogenetics 1996;44:323.
63. Mandruzzato S, Brasseur F, Andry G, Boon T, van der Bruggen P. A CASP-8 mutation recognized by cytolytic T lymphocytes on a human head and neck carcinoma. J Exp Med 1997;186:785.
64. Shichijo S, Nakao M, Imai Y. A gene encoding antigenic peptides of human squamous cell carcinoma recognized by cytotoxic T lymphocytes. J Exp Med 1998;187:277.
65. Vonderheide RH, Hahn WC, Schultze JL, Nadler LM. The telomerase catalytic subunit is a widely expressed tumor-associated antigen recognized by cytotoxic T lymphocytes. Immunity 1999;10:673.
66. Bendandi M, Gocke CD, Kobrin CB. Complete molecular remissions induced by patient-specific vaccination plus granulocyte–monocyte colony-stimulating factor against lymphoma [see comments]. Nature Med 1999;5:1171.
67. Ressing ME, Sette A, Brandt RM, et al. Human CTL epitopes encoded by human papillomavirus type 16 E6 and E7 identified through in vivo and in vitro immunogenicity studies of HLA-A*0201-binding peptides. J Immunol 1995;154:5934.
68. Rooney CM, Roskrow MA, Smith CA, Brenner MK, Heslop HE. Immunotherapy for Epstein–Barr virus-associated cancers. J Natl Cancer Inst Monogr 1998;89.
69. Rooney CM, Smith CA, Ng CY, et al. Infusion of cytotoxic T cells for the prevention and treatment of Epstein–Barr virus-induced lymphoma in allogeneic transplant recipients. Blood 1998;92:1549.

70. Sijts AJ, Ossendorp F, Mengede EA, van den Elsen PJ, Melief CJ. Immunodominant mink cell focus-inducing murine leukemia virus (MuLV)-encoded CTL epitope, identified by its MHC Class I-binding motif, explains MuLV-type specificity of MCF-directed cytotoxic T lymphocytes. J Immunol 1994;152:106.
71. Yang JC, Perry-Lalley D. The envelope protein of an endogenous murine retrovirus is a tumor-associated T-cell antigen for multiple murine tumors. J Immunother 2000;23:177.
72. Carbone M, Pass HI, Rizzo P, et al. Simian virus 40-like DNA sequences in human pleural mesothelioma. Oncogene 1994;9:1781.
73. Rizzo P, Carbone M, Fisher SG, et al. Simian virus 40 is present in most United States human mesotheliomas, but it is rarely present in non-Hodgkin's lymphoma. Chest 1999;116:470S.
74. Grimm EA, Mazumder A, Zhang HZ, et al. Lymphokine-activated killer cell phenomenon: lysis of natural killer-resistant fresh solid tumor cells by interleukin-2 activated autologous human peripheral blood lymphocytes. J Exp Med 1982;155:1832.
75. Law TM, Motzer R, Mazumdar M, et al. Phase III randomized trial of interleukin-2 with or without lymphokine activated killer cells in the treatment of patients with advanced renal cell carcinoma. Cancer 1995;76:824.
76. Topalian SL, Rosenberg SA. Tumor-infiltrating lymphocytes: evidence for specific immune reactions against growing cancers in mice and humans. Important Adv Oncol 1990;19.
77. Rosenberg SA, Yannelli JR, Yang JC, et al. Treatment of patients with metastatic melanoma with autologous tumor-infiltrating lymphocytes and interleukin-2. J Natl Cancer Inst 1994;86:1159.
78. Pockaj B, Sherry R, Wei J, et al. Localization of ^{111}Indium-labeled tumor infiltrating lymphocytes to tumor in patients receiving adoptive immunotherapy. Cancer 1994;73:1731.
79. Riddell SR, Watanabe KS, Goodrich JM, Li CR, Agha ME, Greenberg PD. Restoration of viral immunity in immunodeficient humans by the adoptive transfer of T cell clones [see comments]. Science 1992;257:238.
80. Yee C, Gilbert MJ, Riddell SR, et al. Isolation of tyrosinase-specific CD8+ and CD4+ T cell clones from the peripheral blood of melanoma patients following in vitro stimulation with recombinant vaccinia virus. J Immunol 1996;157:4079.
81. Miller RA, Maloney DG, Warnke R, Levy R. Treatment of B-cell lymphoma with monoclonal anti-idiotype antibody. N Engl J Med 1982;306:517.
82. Ragnhammar P, Fagerberg J, Frodin JE, et al. Effect of monoclonal antibody 17-1A and GM-CSF in patients with advanced colorectal carcinoma – long-lasting, complete remissions can be induced. Int J Cancer 1993;53:751.
83. DeNardo SJ, O'Grady LF, Richman CM, DeNardo GL. Overview of radioimmunotherapy in advanced breast cancer using I-131 chimeric L6. Adv Exp Med Biol 1994;353:203.
84. Meredith RF, Khazaeli MB, Plott WE, et al. Phase I trial of iodine-131-chimeric B72.3 (human IgG4) in metastatic colorectal cancer [see comments]. J Nucl Med 1992;33:23.
85. Meredith RF, Khazaeli MB, Plott WE, et al. Initial clinical evaluation of iodine-125-labeled chimeric 17-1A for metastatic colon cancer. J Nucl Med 1995;36:2229.
86. Livingston PO, Wong GY, Adluri S, et al. Improved survival in stage III melanoma patients with GM2 antibodies: a randomized trial of adjuvant vaccination with GM2 ganglioside. J Clin Oncol 1994;12:1036.
87. Presta LG, Chen H, O'Connor SJ, et al. Humanization of an anti-vascular endothelial growth factor monoclonal antibody for the therapy of solid tumors and other disorders. Cancer Res 1997;57:4593.
88. Norton L, Slamon D, Leyland-Jones B, et al. Overall survival (OS) advantage to simultaneous chemotherapy (CRx) plus the humanized anti-HER2 monoclonal antibody herceptin (H) in HER2-overexpressing (HER2+) metastatic breast cancer. Proc Am Soc Clin Oncol 1999;18:127a.[Abstract].
89. McLaughlin P, Grillo-Lopez AJ, Link BK, et al. Rituximab chimeric anti-CD20 monoclonal antibody therapy for relapsed indolent lymphoma: half of patients respond to a four-dose treatment program. J Clin Oncol 1998;16:2825.
90. Thrush GR, Lark LR, Clinchy BC, Vitetta ES. Immunotoxins: an update. Annu Rev Immunol 1996;14:49.
91. Sahin U, Tureci O, Schmitt H, et al. Human neoplasms elicit multiple specific immune responses in the autologous host. Proc Natl Acad Sci USA 1995;92:11810.
92. Chen YT, Scanlan MJ, Sahin U, et al. A testicular antigen aberrantly expressed in human cancers detected by autologous antibody screening. Proc Natl Acad Sci USA 1997;94:1914.
93. Wallack MK, Sivanandham M, Balch CM, et al. Surgical adjuvant active specific immunotherapy for patients with stage III melanoma: the final analysis of data from a phase III, randomized, double-blind, multicenter vaccinia melanoma oncolysate trial. J Am Coll Surg 1998;187:69.
94. Harris JE, Ryan L, Hoover HCJ, et al. Adjuvant active specific immunotherapy for stage II and III colon cancer with an autologous tumor cell vaccine: Eastern Cooperative Oncology Group Study E5283. J Clin Oncol 2000;18:148.
95. Hoover HCJ, Brandhorst JS, Peters LC, et al. Adjuvant active specific immunotherapy for human colorectal cancer: 6.5-year median follow-up of a phase III prospectively randomized trial [see comments]. J Clin Oncol 1993;11:390.
96. Parkhurst MR, Salgaller ML, Southwood S, et al. Improved induction of melanoma-reactive CTL with peptides from the melanoma antigen gp100 modified at HLA-A*0201-binding residues. J Immunol 1996;157:2539.
97. Rosenberg SA, Yang JC, Schwartzentruber DJ, et al. Immunologic and therapeutic evaluation of a synthetic peptide vaccine for the treatment of patients with metastatic melanoma [see comments]. Nature Med 1998;4:321.
98. Marchand M, van Baren N, Weynants P, et al. Tumor regressions observed in patients with metastatic melanoma treated with an antigenic peptide encoded by gene MAGE-3 and presented by HLA-A1. Int J Cancer 1999;80:219.
99. Nestle FO, Alijagic S, Gilliet M, et al. Vaccination of melanoma patients with peptide- or tumor lysate-pulsed dendritic cells [see comments]. Nature Med 1998;4:328.
100. Thurner B, Haendle I, Roder C. Vaccination with mage-3A1 peptide-pulsed mature, monocyte-derived dendritic cells expands specific cytotoxic T cells and induces regression of some metastases in advanced stage IV melanoma. J Exp Med 1999;190:1669.
101. Jaffee EM, Pardoll DM. Considerations for the clinical development of cytokine gene-transduced tumor cell vaccines. Methods 1997;12:143.
102. Baskar S. Gene-modified tumor cells as cellular vaccine. Cancer Immunol Immunother 1996;43:165.
103. Simons JW, Jaffee EM, Weber CE, et al. Bioactivity of autologous irradiated renal cell carcinoma vaccines generated by ex vivo granulocyte–macrophage colony-stimulating factor gene transfer. Cancer Res 1997;57:1537.
104. Soiffer R, Lynch T, Mihm M, et al. Vaccination with irradiated autologous melanoma cells engineered to secrete human granulocyte–macrophage colony-stimulating factor generates potent antitumor immunity in patients with metastatic melanoma. Proc Natl Acad Sci USA 1998;95:13141.
105. Simons JW, Mikhak B, Chang JF, et al. Induction of immunity to prostate cancer antigens: results of a clinical trial of vaccination with irradiated autologous prostate tumor cells engineered to secrete granulocyte–macrophage colony-stimulating factor using ex vivo gene transfer. Cancer Res 1999;59:5160.
106. Fefer A, Robinson N, Benyunes MC, et al. Interleukin-2 therapy after bone marrow or stem cell transplantation for hematologic malignancies [see comments] Cancer J Sci Am 1997; (Suppl 1): S48.
107. Childs R, Chernoff A, Contentin N, et al. Regression of metastatic renal-cell carcinoma after nonmyeloablative allogeneic peripheral-blood stem-cell transplantation. N Engl J Med 2000;343:750.
108. Clay TM, Custer MC, Spiess PJ, Nishimura MI. Potential use of T cell receptor genes to modify hematopoietic stem cells for the gene therapy of cancer. Pathol Oncol Res 1999;5:3.
109. Hwu P, Yang JC, Cowherd R, et al. In vivo antitumor activity of T cells redirected with chimeric antibody/T-cell receptor genes. Cancer Res 1995;55:3369.

Chapter 101

Bone Marrow Reconstitution in Primary Immunodeficiency

Rebecca H. Buckley

Shortly after discovery of the major human leukocyte antigen (HLA) chromosomal region in 1968,[1] immune function was conferred in two patients with invariably fatal genetically-determined immunodeficiency diseases by transplanting into them HLA-identical allogeneic bone marrow cells.[2,3] One patient had X-linked recessive severe combined immunodeficiency (SCID),[3] and the other had Wiskott–Aldrich syndrome.[2] The correction of those two very different defects, as well as the subsequent correction of many other types of primary immunodeficiency by bone marrow transplantation, has taught us that the defects in most such conditions are intrinsic to cells of one or more hematopoietic lineages and that they are not due to failure of the microenvironment to support the growth and development of those cells. The initial attempts also taught us that no chemotherapy or other pre-transplant conditioning was needed for SCID recipients to accept such transplants, as they are unable to reject grafts. Indeed, this is the basis for their extreme susceptibility to graft-versus-host disease (GVHD). However, the two early successes in immune reconstitution were followed over the next decade and a half by many disappointments due to the rare availability of HLA-matched sibling donors for patients with lethal primary T-cell defects. In the first report of the outcomes of bone marrow transplants for SCID in 1977, only 14 of 69 SCID patients given marrow or fetal tissue transplants worldwide were surviving with functional grafts.[4] The low availability of HLA-matched sibling donors for patients with lethal T-cell defects led to many different approaches being tried to avoid lethal GVHD when mismatched donors were used. From 1968 to 1980, all were unsuccessful except for fetal tissue transplants, which gave only marginal and/or unsustained immunologic improvement.[4] However, the fact that totally HLA-disparate fetal liver cells could partially correct the immune defect in a few such patients without causing GVHD gave hope that HLA-disparate marrow stem cells could effect immune reconstitution if cells with graft-versus-host (GVH) potential could be removed.

In the late 1970s, studies in rats[5] and mice[6] showed that removal of all (or nearly all) post-thymic T cells from *major histocompatibility complex (MHC) nonidentical* related donor marrow or spleen cell suspensions enabled successful rescue of lethally irradiated animals without causing fatal GVHD. This was accomplished in rats by treating donor marrow or spleen cells with anti-T-cell antisera[5] and in mice by agglutinating the unwanted cells with plant lectins.[6] The remaining immature marrow or splenic non-T cells restored lymphohematopoietic function in the ablated MHC-disparate animals. Similar T-cell depletion techniques now allow such haploidentical (half-matched) transplants in humans (see below).

CLINICAL PEARLS

Special transplantation circumstances for SCID patients

- SCID infants have no T-cell function, thus they cannot reject marrow grafts or T cells in blood products. They are, therefore, at very great risk for fatal graft-versus-host disease (GVHD) from anything infused into them that contains mature T cells.
- They cannot reject grafts, and so there is no need to give them any pre-transplant chemotherapeutic or antilymphocyte conditioning prior to giving them marrow or blood stem cell grafts. If they are allowed to keep their own neutrophils, platelets, and red blood cells, they will not have post-transplantation transfusion requirements, and they will not be as susceptible to fungal or bacterial infections because they have neutrophils.
- The kinetics of stem cell education by the SCID thymus are identical whether or not they are given pre-transplant chemotherapy. In addition, the use of pre-transplant chemotherapy does not ensure that B-cell function will develop. Therefore, there is no rationale for using pre-transplant chemotherapy or antithymocyte globulin prior to transplanting SCID infants with allogeneic marrow or blood stem cells.
- Since SCID infants do not need pre-transplant conditioning, this helps reduce the likelihood of GVHD if they are given unfractionated HLA-identical or T cell-depleted HLA-haploidentical related marrow or blood stem cell grafts. Thus, GVHD prophylaxis with cyclosporine and/or methotrexate can be omitted, so that immune function can develop without being impeded by these immunosuppressive drugs. This will also reduce the likelihood of their developing opportunistic infections.

PROBLEMS UNIQUE TO ALLOGENEIC MARROW TRANSPLANTATION

In addition to the usual problem of potential rejection of the graft by immune cells of the recipient, allogeneic marrow transplantation is complicated by specific problems not usually encountered in solid organ transplantation.

Susceptibility of reconstituting cells to immunosuppressive agents

Immunosuppressive agents commonly used to ensure the acceptance of solid organ grafts or the prevention of graft-versus-host disease have deleterious effects on the very cells one is trying to engraft in patients with genetically determined immunodeficiency. Therefore, immunosuppressive and myeloablative agents used to prevent graft rejection must be given *prior* to infusion of the marrow to avoid injury to the donor cells. Except in infants with SCID or complete DiGeorge syndrome who have absent T-cell function and are therefore unable to reject allografts, all other immunodeficient recipients need to be preconditioned with chemotherapeutic agents to prevent graft rejection. In those transplant recipients with some potential to reject grafts, factors influencing the likelihood of engraftment of donor marrow cells are: (1) the degree of immunocompetence of the recipient, (2) the degree of MHC disparity between donor and recipient, (3) the degree of presensitization of the recipient to the histocompatibility antigens of the donor, (4) the number of marrow cells administered, (5) the type of conditioning regimen given to the recipient, and (6) whether or not T-cell depletion techniques are used. Conditioning agents used most widely have included procarbazine, cyclophosphamide, busulfan, melphalan, and antithymocyte globulin (ATG). A combination of 2 or 4 mg/kg of busulfan daily for 4 days, followed by 50 mg/kg of cyclophosphamide daily for 4 days has been commonly employed.[7] In patients with primary immunodeficiency who do require conditioning, preparation of the recipient need only be directed at immunosuppression and myeloablation. Thus, total body irradiation (TBI), required to eradicate malignant cells, is not usually necessary. The toxicity of high-dose conditioning regimens, however, has resulted in considerable recent interest in using a minimally myelosuppressive conditioning regimen based on low-dose total body irradiation or fludarabine alone or in combination with other drugs, followed by a short course of immunosuppression and post-grafting cyclosporine and methotrexate or mycophenolate mofetil.[8–10]

KEY CONCEPTS

Rejection of marrow graft by host versus rejection of host by T-cell graft

- If host T-cell function is present to any degree in the immunodeficient transplanted host, the allogeneic marrow graft will probably be destroyed, no matter the apparent degree of HLA compatibility, and engraftment will fail unless pre-transplant chemotherapy is given.
- If host T-cell function is absent in the immunodeficient transplanted host (either because of the underlying defect or because of pre-transplant chemotherapy), the T cells in the graft may attack the host tissues, principally the skin, liver, and intestine (graft-versus-host reaction), depending upon the degree of HLA compatibility.
- Preconditioning the immunodeficient host who has any degree of T-cell function is done with agents designed to eliminate that function.
- GVHD risk factors include: HLA-mismatched donor, opposite sex of donor, older age of the recipient, pre-transplant conditioning, and previous viral infections.
- Prevention of GVHD is the best approach, since imperfect regimens make treatment of established acute or chronic GVHD difficult, and the immunodeficiency secondary to GVHD and the drugs used to treat it make the immunodeficient host even more susceptible to opportunistic infections for which there is no effective treatment.

Graft-versus-host disease

The most important problem unique to bone marrow transplantation is that donor T cells in the transplanted marrow can also 'reject' the recipient, causing GVHD. Earlier efforts to get around the lack of a match by fractionating HLA-nonidentical bone marrow on albumin density gradients or by using transplants of fetal liver and/or thymus were thwarted either by the recipient developing lethal GVHD from residual donor T cells in the HLA-nonidentical marrow fractions or by failure of immune reconstitution from fetal tissue transplants. These initial attempts thus taught us that, unlike the situation in solid organ transplantation, HLA identity (at least for Class II) between donor and recipient was required for successful unfractionated bone marrow transplantation. These unique problems entailed that bone marrow transplantation until the last two decades required strict HLA-D locus compatibility. Nevertheless, even in HLA-identical marrow transplantation, GVHD occurs and it is severe or fatal in a significant proportion of recipients who require pre-transplant conditioning with chemotherapeutic agents.

IMPORTANCE OF THE MAJOR HISTOCOMPATIBILITY COMPLEX IN BONE MARROW TRANSPLANTATION

It has long been known that Class II HLA antigens are important determinants in bone marrow transplantation, since successful transplantation of unfractionated marrow has been accomplished despite HLA Class I incompatibility (due to recombination)[3] but not when there is Class II incompatibility.[4] This is due to the fact that recipient Class II HLA antigens stimulate genetically different donor T cells to proliferate and become cytotoxic, causing GVHD. The reverse problem is also possible for the same reason in those recipients who have residual immunocompetence, i.e. host T cells recognize donor marrow HLA Class II antigens and effect marrow rejection. In addition, it is known that effective immune responses require the sharing of genetically identical Class II HLA antigens by interacting T, B, and antigen-presenting

KEY CONCEPTS

Importance of major histocompatibility complex (MHC) in bone marrow transplantation

- Immunologic attack of living tissue is governed by disparity of MHC antigens, especially Class II antigens, and is mediated by post-thymic T cells.
- Defects in SCID cause intrinsic abnormalities of T cells (and in some cases, B and NK cells), and reconstitution depends upon supplying an HLA-matched or half-matched (haploidentical) normal T cell and/or bone marrow stem cell capable of differentiating into a T cell, B cell or NK cell.
- Early attempts at bone marrow transplantation for SCID were hampered by lack of HLA-matched sibling donors.
- The latter problem was circumvented by removal of most post-thymic T cells from the donor marrow.

cells (APCs). The latter requirement is of particular importance for those nonablated immunodeficiency patients who become 'split' chimeras following bone marrow transplantation, i.e. they have genetically donor T cells but the B and APCs are of host origin. However, this sharing is still possible if only one of the two HLA haplotypes is identical between donor and recipient.[11]

GRAFT-VERSUS-HOST REACTIONS (GVHR)

Graft-versus-host reactions (GVHRs) are the major barrier to widespread successful application of bone marrow transplantation for the correction of many different diseases.[12–14]

Clinical features

Acute GVHRs begin 6 or more days post transplantation (or post transfusion in the case of nonirradiated blood products) with high unrelenting fever, a morbilliform maculopapular erythematous rash, and severe diarrhea.[13] The rash becomes progressively confluent and may involve the entire body surface; it is both pruritic and painful and eventually leads to marked exfoliation. Eosinophilia and lymphocytosis develop, followed shortly by hepatosplenomegaly, abnormal liver function tests, and elevation in blood conjugated bilirubin levels. The diarrhea is watery and voluminous and may become bloody as the disease progresses. Nausea, vomiting, and severe cramping abdominal pain occur as a consequence of the gastrointestinal involvement, which is also accompanied by a protein-losing enteropathy. The latter contributes to the marked generalized edema ('third spacing') seen in more severe acute GVHD. The most severe forms of acute GVHD are also characterized by bone marrow aplasia, marked susceptibility to infection, and death in a high proportion of cases.

Staging

Staging of GVHD is based on the severity and number of organ systems involved.[13] The four categories generally defined are:

Grade 1: 1+ to 2+ skin rash without gut involvement and with no more than 1+ liver involvement.

Grade 2: 1+ to 3+ skin rash with either 1+ to 2+ gastrointestinal involvement or 1+ to 2+ liver involvement or both.

Grade 3: 2+ to 4+ skin rash with 2+ to 4+ gastrointestinal involvement with or without 2+ to 4+ liver involvement. Decrease in performance status and fever also characterize grades 2 and 3, with increasing severity per stage.

Grade 4: the pattern and severity of GVHD is similar to that in grade 3 with extreme constitutional symptoms.

Chronic GVHD

If the patient does not succumb, and the acute GVHD persists, it is termed chronic after 100 days. Chronic GVHD may evolve from an acute GVHR or may develop in the absence of or after resolution of acute GVHD. It occurs in 45–70% of conditioned patients receiving HLA-matched bone marrow transplants.[15] Skin lesions of chronic GVHD resemble scleroderma, with hyperkeratosis, reticular hyperpigmentation, atrophy with ulceration, and fibrosis and limitation of joint movement. Other manifestations include the sicca syndrome and disordered immunoregulation – as evidenced by autoantibody and immune complex formation and poly and monoclonal hyperimmunoglobulinemia, idiopathic interstitial pneumonitis, and frequent infections.[16]

Etiology

The principal cause of GVHRs is that the recipient with absent T-cell function (or one made equally T-cell deficient by irradiation or chemotherapy) cannot reject bone marrow, matched or mismatched.[12] By contrast, engrafted genetically different immunocompetent donor T cells recognize foreign HLA antigens on the recipient's cells and respond to them.[12–14,16] In the case of unfractionated marrow transplants from HLA-D mismatched donors, this reaction of the donor T lymphocytes against the recipient is almost invariably fatal. Risk factors for GVHD include use of an HLA-mismatched donor, use of a matched unrelated donor, increasing age of the recipient, gender mismatch, and prior herpesvirus infections.[12]

Pathogenesis

In the case of HLA-identical marrow transplants, GVHRs are likely due to responses by donor T cells[17,18] to recipient minor locus histocompatibility or Y chromosome-associated transplantation antigens, since a significantly higher incidence of GVHD occurs in male patients given MHC-matched female marrows than in patients receiving MHC and sex-matched marrows.[4,12,16]

Natural history

GVHRs are usually mild and self-limited in SCID hosts not given pretransplant immunosuppression who receive unfractionated HLA-identical marrow. However, in 60% of recipients given pretransplant irradiation or immunosuppressive drugs, GVHD is moderate to severe and fatal in 15–20% despite HLA identity.[13,14] The severity of GVHD increases with the recipient's age, the use of HLA-matched unrelated donors, and, if a related donor is not HLA-identical, with the degree of genetic disparity.

Diagnosis

Although the diagnosis is strongly suspected when the above constellation of clinical manifestations is fully developed, histologic diagnosis is often necessary at earlier stages to exclude other causes of rash (such as drug rashes), hepatitis (such as infections with herpesviruses), or diarrhea (such as that due to infectious agents). Skin biopsies in acute GVHD reveal basal vacuolar degeneration or necrosis, spongiosis, single cell dyskeratosis, eosinophilic necrosis of epidermal cells, and a dermal perivascular round cell infiltration.[14] Similar necrotic changes occur in the liver and intestinal tract and eventually in most other tissues. However, in the early stages of GVHD the histology can resemble that of drug reactions or some forms of hepatitis, in which case the only definitive means of establishing a diagnosis is by identifying donor-derived cells in the blood or target organ. This has been facilitated greatly by the use of the polymerase chain reaction (PCR) to amplify DNA polymorphisms associated with variations in the length of dinucleotide or trinucleotide microsatellite repeats[19] (Chapter 125).

Treatment

Many regimens have been employed to mitigate GVHRs in both MHC-incompatible and compatible bone marrow transplants. In MHC-compatible bone marrow transplants into SCID or complete DiGeorge syndrome infants, it is usually unnecessary to give immunosuppressive agents to prevent or mitigate GVHD, although occasionally steroids are used to treat more severe forms of the condition. However, for unfractionated HLA-identical marrow transplants into all patients for whom pre-transplant chemotherapy is given to prevent rejection, it is necessary to use GVHD prophylaxis. Such patients are usually given cyclosporine daily for 6 months or methotrexate (15 mg/m^2 on the first day post-transplantation and 10 mg/m^2 on the third, sixth, and eleventh days and weekly thereafter until day 100) or both (in which case a shorter course of methotrexate is used.[20]

The best approach to GVHD is prevention. The above immunosuppressive agents have not prevented GVHRs entirely; moreover, as already mentioned, they can adversely affect the very cells one is trying to engraft. By far the best preventive approach is the removal of post-thymic T cells from the donor marrow (see below). Once severe GVHD has become established, it is extremely difficult to treat. Antithymocyte serum, steroids, cyclosporine and murine monoclonal antibodies to human T-cell surface antigens have ameliorated many, but the course has been inexorably fatal in others similarly treated.[14] Anticytokine and anti-cytokine receptor antibodies are being evaluated for their potential efficacy in mitigating GVHD.[14] Determination of the frequency of recipient-specific T-cell precursors in donor blood by limiting dilution analysis and identification of IL-2-producing cells after in vitro stimulation with recipient mononuclear leukocytes has been found to correlate with the severity of subsequent GVHD in HLA-identical sibling bone marrow transplants.[17,18] This approach could be used prospectively to intensify GVHD prophylaxis when the only available HLA-identical sibling donor has a high frequency of such recipient-specific T-cell precursors.[17,18]

INFECTIONS

Patients with primary immunodeficiency diseases affecting T cells are highly susceptible to opportunistic viral, fungal, and facultative intracellular microorganisms, and frequently develop an untreatable infection before their defect is diagnosed and prior to transplantation.[16] In addition, the immunodeficiency that occurs in the post-transplantation period for patients who have had conditioning regimens and who are receiving GVHD prophylactic drugs adds to the high incidence of infections in those patients during the first 100 days post transplantation, regardless of whether GVHD is present.[16] Another contributing factor is the profound granulocytopenia that occurs in conditioned patients for 11–18 days post transplantation. However, the use of granulocyte colony-stimulating factor (G-CSF) has reduced the severity of this problem. The advent of GVHD prolongs the impaired immunity and further heightens the susceptibility to infection. Protective isolation is necessary and some transplant groups utilize gut sterilization and laminar flow isolation units. The agents most problematic include *Candida albicans*, *Asperqillus* species, *Pneumocystis carinii*, cytomegalovirus (CMV), herpes simplex, varicella zoster virus, Epstein–Barr virus (EBV), parainfluenza, enteroviruses, and adenoviruses.[16] Bacterial infections with high-grade pathogens also occur but, if identified in time, can usually be treated effectively with antibiotics. Intravenous and oral gammaglobulin therapies have also helped to reduce the frequency and severity of infections with common bacterial and viral agents. Trimethoprim–sulfamethoxazole has vastly reduced the mortality from *Pneumocystis carinii* pneumonia and is an effective prophylactic agent for this infection. Ribavirin is somewhat effective against parainfluenza infections. Acyclovir is highly effective in treating varicella zoster and herpes simplex infections and may have some prophylactic effect for EBV infections, and ganciclovir and Cytogam are helpful in controlling CMV infections. Nevertheless, little other than the development of normal host T-cell function will attenuate ongoing infections with CMV, EBV, enteroviruses, and adenoviruses. Infections frequently lead to death before successful engraftment can occur; this is particularly true if severe GVHD occurs.

SOURCES OF STEM CELLS FOR BONE MARROW TRANSPLANTATION

The various potential sources of stem cells are listed in Table 101.1. It is known that all types of SCID and many other forms of primary immunodeficiency can be mitigated by bone marrow transplantation, but bone marrow is not the only source of stem cells that have the potential to do this.[21,22]

HLA-IDENTICAL BONE MARROW TRANSPLANTATION

Objective

The objective of marrow transplantation for primary immunodeficiency diseases is to restore immunocompetence by providing normal replicating immunocompetent cells. Normal bone marrow contains self-replicating cells that can give rise to erythrocytes, granulocytes, cells of the monocyte-macrophage lineage, megakaryocytes, and immunocompetent T and B cells.[23]

Indications

For over a decade, efforts have been underway worldwide to achieve correction of these defects by gene therapy, and spectacular success was achieved recently in infants with X-linked SCID.[24] However, at the time of writing, the only adequate therapy currently available for most patients with severe primary immunodeficiency affecting T cells is immunologic reconstitution by transplantation of immunocompetent tissue. Initially, fetal liver and thymus appeared ideal for this because they have very low GVH potential and are rich in precursors of immune cells; however, their success in conferring immune function on such

Sources of stem cells for treatment of primary immunodeficiency
HLA-identical sibling marrow
Haploidentical parental marrow • T-cell-depleted by soy lectin/SRBC • T-cell-depleted by monoclonal antibodies
Matched unrelated adult marrow • Unfractionated • T-cell-depleted
Unfractionated related or unrelated cord blood

Table 101.1 Sources of stem cells for treatment of primary immunodeficiency.

patients was, at best, only 10–15%. Moreover, the immune function that developed was incomplete and unsustained. Thus, except for infants with complete DiGeorge syndrome who have no HLA-identical donors and who therefore need a thymic transplant, the tissue used most successfully has been bone marrow. As noted above, it was first learned in 1968 that primary immunodeficiency can be treated effectively by HLA-matched bone marrow transplantation. Patients with many different types of immune defects have subsequently been given such transplants, with varying degrees of success. These defects include SCID, Wiskott–Aldrich syndrome, combined immunodeficiency (CID), Omenn syndrome, leukocyte adhesion deficiency (LAD), MHC antigen deficiency, Chediak–Higashi syndrome, chronic granulomatous disease, DiGeorge syndrome, purine nucleoside phosphorylase (PNP) deficiency, cartilage–hair hypoplasia, hyper-IgM syndrome, IL-2 deficiency, and X-linked lymphoproliferative disease.

Marrow transplant procedure

Unfractionated bone marrow transplantation is the simplest of all transplantation procedures, offering little risk to the donor as it involves removal of a tissue that is readily regenerated. The bone marrow cells are usually obtained by aspiration with a 14 or 16 guage needle from multiple sites along both iliac crests while the donor is under general anesthesia.[25] An alternative site in adults is the sternum, or (in children) the upper third of the tibia. The aspirate is placed in heparinized tissue culture medium, passed through metal screens with diminishing apertures to remove bone spicules, and the nucleated marrow cells are enumerated. The marrow cell suspension is then given intravenously in a manner similar to a blood transfusion.

Problems after transplant

Multiple problems occur during the post-transplant period, particularly in patients given pre-transplant conditioning, thus marrow transplantation should be carried out only by experienced teams. The dominant problems are infection and GVHD, as noted above. In addition, multiple red cell and platelet transfusions are usually necessary for chemoablated patients during the 7–20 days before erythroid and myeloid engraftment occurs. All transfusions that contain immunocompetent cells should be irradiated with 1500–3000 rads to prevent GVHRs and, if the recipient is CMV seronegative, they should be from CMV-seronegative donors. Family members can be used as blood donors during this period; they are preferred, so as to minimize the risk of hepatitis and human immunodeficiency virus (HIV) infections. The availability of G-CSF has shortened the time to development of neutrophils post transplantation.

Identification of engraftment

Four types of markers are used to identify donor cells in marrow recipients; chromosomal differences,[26,27] erythrocyte and leukocyte antigens, serum allotypes, and DNA sequence polymorphisms. If donor and recipient are of the opposite sex, karyotypic markers can be detected as early as 2 weeks after grafting. Serum immunoglobulin allotypic markers are particularly useful in documenting chimerism of B cells. The advantage of DNA sequence polymorphisms is that they do not require cell division, so that the origin of even nondividing cells such as monocytes or natural killer cells can be determined.[28]

Expected outcome

If a patient with a severe T-cell deficiency or other type of invariably fatal primary immunodeficiency is fortunate enough to have an HLA-identical sibling, unfractionated bone marrow cells can be given. Such marrow cell suspensions contain, in addition to stem cells, mature T and B cells. In most cases, both T-cell and B-cell immunity have been fully constituted by such matched transplants, with evidence of function detected as early as 2 weeks following transplantation when no pre-transplant conditioning and no post-transplant GVHR prophylaxis are required. Adoptive transfer of mature T cells is the explanation for the very rapid onset of immune function after matched unfractionated bone marrow transplantation. Unfractionated marrow cells will also become engrafted in HLA-disparate recipients who lack cellular immunity, but fatal GVHD can be anticipated.

HLA-HAPLOIDENTICAL BONE MARROW TRANSPLANTATION

Until 1980, only HLA-identical unfractionated bone marrow could be used for bone marrow transplantation because of the lethal GVHD that ensued if mismatched donors were used.[4] One of the most important advances over the past two decades has been the development of methods to transplant half-matched (haploidentical) parental stem cells.[22,29,30]

Rationale

Following the leads from his own work in mice[6] and from Muller-Ruchholtz et al's work in rats,[5] Reisner[29] demonstrated in the early 1980s that removal of most mature T cells from half-matched parental marrow allowed successful immune reconstitution of human infants with SCID by the remaining cells without subsequent GVHD. Since that time, this principle has been successfully applied many times to the treatment of SCID.[22,30–34] Moreover, the resulting chimeras have proven extremely useful in the study of human T- and B-cell ontogeny,[30,33–36] tolerance induction,[37] and mechanisms of MHC restriction for antigen presentation.[11]

Methods of T-cell depletion

Soybean lectin, sheep erythrocyte agglutination

This method for T-cell depletion involves agglutination of most mature marrow cells with soybean lectin, followed by sedimentation of clumped cells and subsequent removal of T cells from the unagglutinated marrow by sheep erythrocyte rosetting and density-gradient centrifugation.[29,38] For an adequate yield of stem cells, it is necessary to collect approximately one liter of bone marrow from the donor. This is usually not a problem, since a parent is usually used as the donor, and the donations are made under general anesthesia. Paradoxically, while soy lectin is very effective in removing most mature marrow cells, it does not bind to human T cells. Thus, after soy lectin agglutination, there are still numerous T cells in the nonagglutinated fraction.[38] To remove the T cells, two steps of sheep erythrocyte rosette depletion are required. The final cell preparation contains few if any lymphocytes, is nonresponsive to phytohemagglutin (PHA) and in mixed leukocyte culture (MLC) consists of immature myeloid cells, CD34+ stem cells, and dendritic cells, and represents less than 5–10% of the initial number of nucleated marrow cells.[38] Indeed, there is abundant evidence that such preparations contain stem cells, because they have immunologically reconstituted numerous SCID infants.

Monoclonal antibody and complement lysis

Another method of depleting post-thymic T cells from donor marrow is incubation with monoclonal antibodies to human T cells plus a source of complement.[39] Antibodies employed for this purpose have included T12, Leu 1, CT-2, and Campath-1.[40] T-cell depletion is not as effective with monoclonal antibody treatment as with the soy lectin, sheep erythocyte rosette-depletion method, possibly due to modulation of T-cell antigens from the surface of the T cells without destroying them. As a consequence, somewhat more frequent and severe GVHD has been observed, but fatal reactions have still been rare. Recently, better T-cell depletion has been achieved by using a solid-phase anti-CD34 monoclonal antibody for positive selection of stem cells, followed by purging with a monoclonal antibody to CD2.[41]

Sheep erythrocyte agglutination

A third approach has been to use sheep erythrocyte rosette-depletion alone to remove T cells from the donor marrow. Because different centers have used different numbers of rosette-depletions and different methods of modifying the sheep red cells (i.e. no modification, neuraminidase or amino-ethylisothiouronium treatment), there have been varying degrees of effectiveness of this approach to remove post-thymic T cells. In one center, only a single rosetting step is done, with the intent to leave a few post-thymic T cells.[42] GVH reactions are then modulated by giving the recipient cyclosporin A continuously for various time periods following the transplant. While somewhat more frequent and severe GVHRs have been seen in the recipients of only sheep erythrocyte T cell-depleted marrow, lethal GVHD has been unusual.

Indications

The indications for T cell-depleted haploidentical bone marrow cell transplantation in primary immunodeficiency are, with some exceptions, the same as those listed above for unfractionated HLA-identical marrow transplantation. One such exception is the complete DiGeorge syndrome, where T cell-depleted marrow cells are ineffective, since there is no thymus to educate the donor stem cells. The successful outcome after unfractionated HLA-identical marrow transplants into complete DiGeorge patients is due to the adoptive transfer of mature T and B cells that were 'educated' in the donor's thymus. T cell-depleted marrow transplants may also not be advisable in certain primary immunodeficiency diseases in which the patients can be sustained for many years by antibiotic and intravenous immunoglobulin therapy. The reason for this is that the ablation required for successful engraftment leaves them at risk for fatal opportunistic infection during the prolonged time it takes for T cell-depleted marrow to mature in the recipient's thymus, and there may also be resistance to engraftment.

Post-transplant problems and identification of engraftment

The problems are essentially the same as after HLA-identical unfractionated marrow transplantation, except that the period of vulnerability to infection is longer in recipients of T cell-depleted marrow due to the long period of time required for donor stem cells to develop into mature T cells in the recipient's thymus. In addition, the occurrence of fatal B-cell lymphoproliferative disease has been a problem with this type of transplantation, whereas it does not occur in recipients of unfractionated HLA-identical marrow.[43] Most of these proliferations have been EBV positive,[44] and most have occurred in recipients of monoclonal antibody T cell-depleted marrow. Again, the time required for stem cells to develop into normal T cells is felt to be related to the propensity to develop such tumors.

Expected outcome

The time to development of immune function following haploidentical stem cell grafts is quite different from that after unfractionated HLA-identical marrow. In contrast to the rapid development of immune function after the latter type of grafts, lymphocytes with mature T-cell phenotypes and functions fail to rise significantly until 3–4 months after transplantation of T cell-depleted marrow (Fig. 101.1 a–c).[22,30,32,34,35] This is true even if pre-transplant conditioning is given or if T cell-depleted HLA-

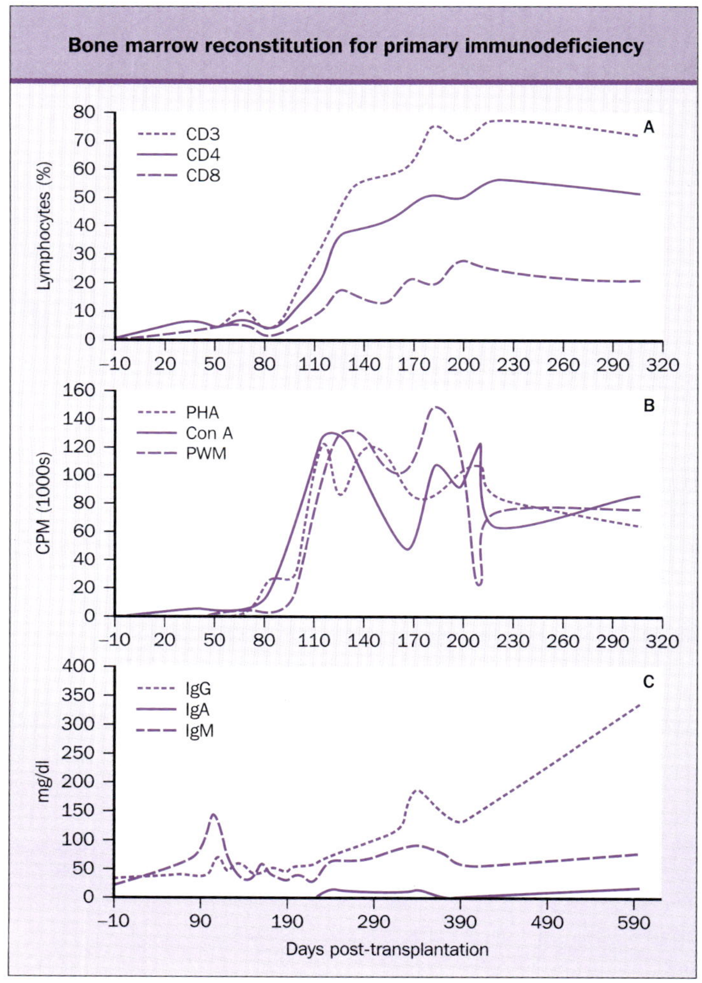

Figure 101.1 Bone marrow reconstitution for primary immunodeficiency. Results of sequential immunologic studies in a male infant with JAK3-deficient SCID before and after transplantation of T cell-depleted haploidentical maternal marrow stem cells, displaying: (**A**) T-cell phenotypes and (**B**) T-cell responses to mitogens, and (**C**) serum immunoglobulin concentrations. T-cell phenotypes and function appeared simultaneously, but not until more than 90 days post transplantation. All dividing T cells in (**B**) were of female karyotype. Serum immunoglobulin concentrations did not rise significantly until nearly 2 years post transplantation. The B cells were shown to be 100% male (i.e. of host origin).

identical sibling marrow is used (author, unpublished). Thus, whether the donor is HLA-identical or haploidentical, it still takes between 90 and 120 days for stem cells in T cell-depleted marrow to mature into functioning T cells in SCID infants. The time taken is not unlike that in intrauterine life, where PHA-responsive cells do not appear until around 12 weeks of gestation. The first to develop is T-cell function, and this function appears simultaneously with the development of phenotypically normal T cells. Karyotypic studies reveal that such T cells are always 100% of donor origin.[22,30] Thus, the vestigeal, architecturally abnormal epithelial thymi of all forms of SCID treated has the ability to cause normal stem cells to become phenotypically and functionally normal T cells.[36] B-cell function develops much more slowly, averaging 2–2.5 years for normalization in some; others fail to develop B-cell function altogether, despite normal T-cell function.[22,31-35,45] Genetic analyses of the cells from such chimeric patients have revealed all T cells to be genetically donor, whereas the B and antigen-presenting cells remain those of the recipient in a large majority of cases.[22,31] These observations indicate that the thymic microenvironment of most infants with SCID is capable of differentiating half-matched normal stem cells to become mature and functioning T lymphocytes that can cooperate effectively with host B cells for antibody production.[22,30,36] Thus, the SCID-causing genetic defects thus far identified appear not to affect the thymus except to the extent that it is small and morphologically abnormal, probably due to lack of interaction with normal stem cells. Patients with types of severe T-cell deficiency other than SCID who are not given pre-transplant conditioning fail to achieve engraftment because of sufficient recipient T-cell function to effect rejection.

MATCHED UNRELATED BONE MARROW OR CORD BLOOD TRANSPLANTATION

Rationale

The initial rationale for using HLA-identical unrelated donors for patients with primary immunodeficiency diseases was that fewer than 25% have HLA-identical siblings. Since matched related marrow was curative, the use of unrelated matched marrow could extend the possibility of this therapy to more patients. The first matched unrelated donor (MUD) transplant for primary immunodeficiency was done in a SCID infant in 1977;[46] although the transplant was eventually successful after booster transplantation, the recipient went on to develop severe, debilitating chronic GVHD. After the above-noted problems of longer time to development of immune function, resistance to engraftment, and the development of B-cell lymphoproliferative disease after T cell-depleted haploidentical marrow were appreciated, however, interest in MUD transplantation was renewed.[47-50] The principal reason was that it offered the possibility of giving unfractionated marrow, which would circumvent these three problems. However, the problem encountered in the first such patient, i.e. severe GVHD, continues to be the major limitation to the widespread application of this approach.

Recently, an alternative source of hematopoietic stem cells for transplantation has been proposed, i.e. unfractionated cord blood, which is a rich source of stem cells.[51] Part of the rationale for using cord blood is that the incidence of GVHD also appeared to be lower. Several successes with cord blood transplantation from HLA-identical siblings have been reported, notably in patients with genetic disorders – including immunodeficiencies[51-53] though graft failure rate could be increased.[51] In addition, in those who require pre-transplant chemoablation, there is a much longer period of thrombocytopenia (>100 days) than after HLA-identical unfractionated marrow transplants. More recently, matched unrelated cord blood has also been used successfully for certain immune disorders, particularly combined immunodeficiency (CID). The problem with both matched unrelated adult bone marrow donors and unrelated cord blood donors is that, because humans are an outbred population, the matching can never be perfect. Minor locus histocompatibility antigen differences are also much more likely to be present than in the related setting, resulting in a high probability of GVHD. GVHD prophylaxis is routinely given after transplants from either type of unrelated donor and this is continued for many months (9 months for cord blood transplants). If an infant with SCID is already infected, these drugs make them even more at risk for demise from these agents. In addition, most of the current protocols for cord blood transplantation call for pre-transplant conditioning regardless of the underlying diagnosis of the patient. The conditioning and GVHD prophylaxis both contribute to a long period of immune impairment post transplantation, seemingly defeating the purpose of such transplantations for immunodeficient hosts.

Indications

The indications for MUD adult marrow or cord blood transplantation in primary immunodeficiency are the same as for HLA-identical and haploidentical marrow transplantation, i.e. a lethal defect that cannot be effectively treated with replacement therapy and antibiotics. However, there is the additional requirement that there be a lack of an HLA-identical related donor. After that, a decision has to be made whether to give T cell-depleted haploidentical parental marrow, which is usually readily available within a short period of time, or to use a MUD adult donor, which is not always possible and, when available, takes on average 5 months to identify. Identification of suitable cord blood for transplantation takes somewhat less time. In the case of SCID, it is dangerous to wait at all, and, considering the high efficacy of T cell-depleted haploidentical parental marrow, MUD adult marrow or cord blood transplantation would be indicated only if a related haploidentical donor were not available. However, for those defects characterized by sufficient T-cell function to reject a graft (i.e. which would require pre-transplant conditioning) and by the presence of ongoing opportunistic infection, there is a theoretical advantage to the use of unfractionated MUD marrow or cord blood because of the ability to give mature T cells (even though immunosuppressed) that might help to resist infection. Examples of the latter conditions include Wiskott–Aldrich syndrome, combined immunodeficiency, Omenn syndrome, Chediak–Higashi syndrome, and chronic granulomatous disease.

Problems after transplant

The problems are similar to those encountered following HLA-identical and haploidentical marrow transplantation when pre-transplant chemotherapy is given, i.e. infection, GVHD, and the requirement for supportive transfusions of platelets and red cells. The principal problem with both MUD adult marrow and cord blood transplantation is the increased incidence and severity of GVHD when compared with that after unfractionated

HLA-identical sibling marrow transplants.[49] An analysis of 462 transplantations from MUD donors from the National Marrow Donor Program revealed that the probability of grade II, III, or IV acute GVHD was 64% and of chronic GVHD at one year, 55%. For patients with congenital immunodeficiency, the probability of survival was 52%. The most likely explanation for the high incidence and severity of GVHD is that there are other histocompatibility characteristics for which matching does not test when two unrelated individuals are typed in the standard manner. This GVHD occurs despite the use of at least 6 months of cyclosporin for MUD adult marrow transplants and steroids and 9 months of cyclosporin for MUD cord blood transplants.

Expected outcome

The outcome of MUD unfractionated marrow or cord blood transplantation would be expected to be the same as for unfractionated HLA-identical marrow transplants, i.e. the development of T- and B-cell immune functions from the adoptively transferred donor T and B cells. However, there is growing concern over the safety of leaving T cells in such marrow or cord blood preparations because of the above-noted problems with severe GVHD, and many centers are now T cell-depleting MUD marrows or cord blood before their administration. When that is done, the same problems noted with related T cell-depleted marrow grafts again emerge. The only advantage MUD marrow or cord blood transplantation has over the latter is the potential for adoptive transfer of donor immunity.

EFFECTIVENESS OF BONE MARROW TRANSPLANTATION FOR THE TREATMENT OF IMMUNODEFICIENCY DISEASES

Although precise figures are not available, more than 1055 patients worldwide with many different forms of genetically determined immunodeficiency have been given bone marrow transplants over the past 33 years in attempts to correct their underlying immune defects. From 1968 to 1977 only 14 (or 29%) of 48 infants with severe combined immunodeficiency (SCID) worldwide were long-term survivors of successful HLA Class II compatible bone marrow transplants.[4] Earlier diagnosis before untreatable opportunistic infections develop and the availability of better antimicrobials to treat infections may both have enabled the results of bone marrow transplantation to improve considerably over the last 15 years.[22,30,33,54–56] A worldwide survey conducted by the author from 1994 to 1997 with subsequent additions of published cases from the literature revealed that 239 of 302 or 79% of patients with primary immunodeficiency transplanted with HLA-identical marrow over a period of 29 years were surviving (Table 101.2).

Most encouraging, however, were the results of T cell-depleted haploidentical (half-matched) marrow transplants in patients with primary immunodeficiency. From the same survey, it was ascertained that 646 such transplants had been performed and, of these, 363 (or 56%) were surviving. The significance is even more impressive when it is realized that most of the 646 recipients would have died had not T-cell depletion techniques been developed.

Severe combined immunodeficiency (SCID)

Bone marrow transplantation has been more widely applied and more successful in infants with SCID than in any other primary immunodeficiency (Table 101.2). In the same survey and literature review, only 125 SCID patients were reported as having received HLA-identical marrow, and 105 or 84% were surviving. By contrast, 455 SCID infants had received haploidentical marrow, and 283 or 62% survived; however, the haploidentical transplants were not T cell-depleted until after 1980. Nevertheless, this is a major accomplishment, since SCID is invariably fatal without marrow transplantation or, in the case of ADA-deficient SCID, enzyme-replacement therapy. The latter is helpful for only a small percentage of SCID patients, since ADA deficiency accounts for only approximately 15% of SCID.[22,56,57] Only 17 SCID patients were reported as having received MUD transplants, and 12 or 71% were surviving. Six SCID patients were reported as having received related or unrelated cord blood transplants and 5 were surviving. The percentages of SCID patients who received either HLA-identical or haploidentical marrow and who were found to be surviving in the author's survey were roughly similar to those in reviews of the European experience with unfractionated HLA-identical and T cell-depleted haploidentical (or non-T depleted) bone marrow transplants in SCID.[58,59] The SCID survival rates in Europe ranged from 76% in the HLA-identical to 35–60% in the half-matched

CLINICAL PEARLS

Outcome of bone marrow transplantation in immunodeficiency

- Approximately 79% of HLA-identical, unfractionated bone marrow-transplanted immunodeficient patients survive; there is evidence for both donor post-thymic mature T-cell engraftment and donor stem cell-derived, thymus-selected T-cell engraftment.
- Approximately 56% of HLA-haploidentical bone marrow-transplanted immunodeficient patients survive; immune reconstitution in this type of transplant depends upon thymus-selected (both positive and negative) donor stem cell-derived T cells.
- The difference in time to development of T-cell function (14 days for unfractionated HLA-identical marrow or blood vs 90–120 days for T cell-depleted HLA-identical or haploidentical bone marrow transplants) is due to the fact that early immunity in recipients of unfractionated HLA-identical marrow is conferred by adoptive transfer of mature donor T and B cells. The time required for stem cells to be processed by the immunodeficient patient's thymus is a minimum of 90–120 days.
- Even the vestigeal thymus of SCID infants is able to process donor stem cells to become mature and functioning T cells.
- The use of HLA-matched unrelated (MUD) bone marrow or cord blood donors at this time offers no clear advantage over the use of HLA-haploidentical related donors; major problems of either type of MUD transplant are: long delay in identifying a donor, the need for heavy and prolonged GVHD prophylaxis with cyclosporine, methotrexate and/or steroids, a substantial rate of serious GVHD despite the use of the latter, and resultant prolongation of the immunodeficiency causing further susceptibility to opportunistic infections.

Bone marrow transplants in immunodeficiency diseases since 1968[a]					
Type of immune defect	Total number of patients[b]	Patients with HLA-identical donor	Patients with haplo-identical donor	Patients with unrelated donor	Patients with cord blood donor
SCID	616 (405)	125 (105)	455 (283)	17 (12)	6 (5)
Wiskott–Aldrich syndrome	153 (99)	65 (58)	58 (20)	29 (20)	4 (3)
CID	64 (32)	17 (13)	37 (14)	2 (0)	7 (5)
Omenn syndrome	42 (20)	12 (9)	24 (8)	6 (3)	0
LAD	32 (24)	8 (6)	20 (14)	2 (2)	3 (2)
MHC antigen deficiency	25 (14)	8 (4)	20 (7)	2 (2)	1 (1)
Chediak–Higashi syndrome	22 (17)	12 (10)	5 (1)	5 (5)	0
CGD	17 (22)	14 (10)	0	3 (2)	0
Hyper-IgM syndrome	12 (8)	6 (5)	3 (1)	3 (2)	0
Reticular dysgenesis	11 (9)	1 (1)	9 (7)	0	1 (0)
DiGeorge syndrome	11 (2)	3 (2)	3 (0)	0	0
PNP deficiency	8 (3)	5 (2)	2 (1)	1 (0)	1 (0)
Cartilage–hair hypoplasia	7 (4)	3 (3)	3 (1)	1 (0)	0
Immunodeficiency with albinism	7 (3)	7 (3)	0	0	0
X-linked lymphoproliferative syndrome	7 (4)	5 (3)	0	1 (0)	1 (1)
Other	21 (11)	11 (5)	7 (6)	2 (0)	0
All defects	*1055 (667)*	*302 (239)*	*646 (363)*	*74 (48)*	*24 (17)*

[a]Some of the information in this table was provided by the following physicians, listed alphabetically: the author; Douglas Barrett MD (Gainesville); Mary Ellen Conley MD (Memphis); Morton J. Cowan MD (San Francisco); A. Fasth MD (Goteborg); A. Filopovich MD (Minneapolis); Alain Fischer MD (Paris); William Friedrich MD (Ulm); Richard Hong MD (Wisconsin); Nina Kapoor MD (Oklahoma and Columbus); Hans Ochs MD (Seattle); F. Porta MD (Brescia, Italy); Reinhard Seger MD (Zurich); William Shearer MD (Houston); Trudy Small MD (Sloan-Kettering); Richard Stiehm MD (UCLA); Kenneth Weinberg MD (Los Angeles); Howard Weinstein MD (Boston Children's); John Zieglar MD (Australia). The remainder of the data were obtained from the published literature.
[b]Total numbers of patients transplanted; numbers of patients surviving are in brackets.

Table 101.2 Bone marrow transplants in immunodeficiency diseases worldwide since 1968[a].

transplants. A further retrospective analysis of the influence of the SCID phenotype on the outcome of haploidentical marrow transplants by the European Group for Bone Marrow Transplantation and the European Society for Immunodeficiency found the disease-free survival to be significantly better for patients with B^+ SCID (60%) than for those with B^- SCID (35%) (P=0.002).[45]

Over the past 18 years, the author and her associates have transplanted 107 infants with SCID, and 85 of these (79.4%) are currently surviving from one month to 18 years post transplantation (Fig. 101.2). No pre-transplant conditioning was given except to 2 infants who received cord blood transplants. Only 12 had HLA-identical donors; all of them survive with functioning grafts. Ninety-five SCID patients received half-matched related donor stem cells prepared by the soy lectin, sheep erythrocyte rosetting T-cell depletion technique,[29] and 73, or 77%, of these patients survive. Survival rates were similar whether the patients were ADA normal (79%) or ADA deficient (82%), and there was no significant difference in disease-free survival for B^+ versus B^- SCID. More importantly, Figures 101.3 and 101.4 demonstrate the clear ability of such transplants to provide normal numbers of T cells and to normalize T-cell function in all molecular types of SCID. Despite the fact that all SCID patients have a vestigeal thymus, we have recently demonstrated that the T cells that emerge post transplantation in these chimeras are thymically derived.[36] They are $CD45RA^+$ and they contain T-cell receptor extrachromosomal DNA circles (TRECs) formed during intrathymic T-cell development. Prior to transplantation, neither the few host T cells that are present nor any transplacentally transferred maternal T cells contain TRECs (Table 101.3) and they are $CD45RO^+$. However, after transplantation there is the gradual emergence of both $CD45RA^+$ and TREC-containing T cells, coinciding with the development of T-cell function (Fig. 101.5). Most impressive is the fact that 25/26 (96%) infants transplanted in the first 3.5 months of life survive. Thus, there appears to be no advantage in performing such transplants in utero as opposed to performing them soon after birth.[60,61] In utero transplants also carry the risks associated with injecting the fetus and the inability to detect GVHD during gestation.

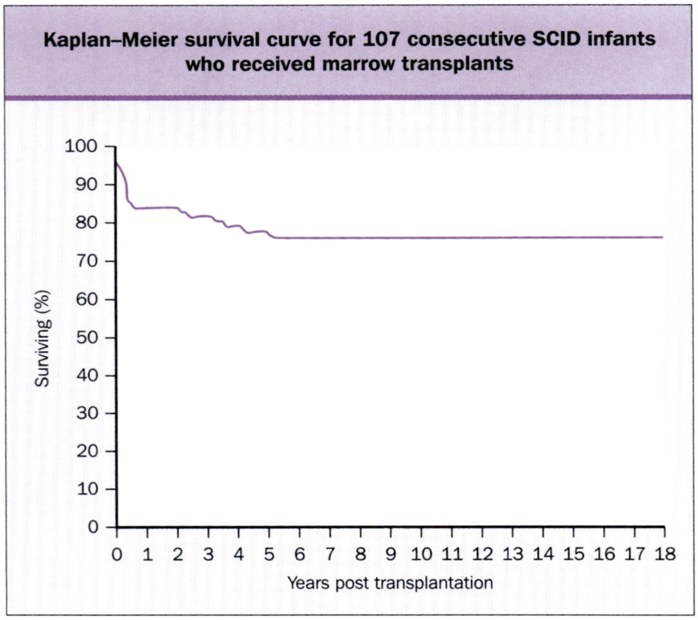

Figure 101.2 Kaplan–Meier survival curve for 107 consecutive SCID infants who received marrow transplants at the author's institution from HLA-identical (12) or haploidentical (95) donors without pre-transplant chemoablation and without post-transplant GVHD prophylaxis. Eighty-five (79.4%) survive for periods of 1 month to 18 years post transplantation. The 22 deaths occurred from opportunistic viral infections, most within the first 6 months after transplant.

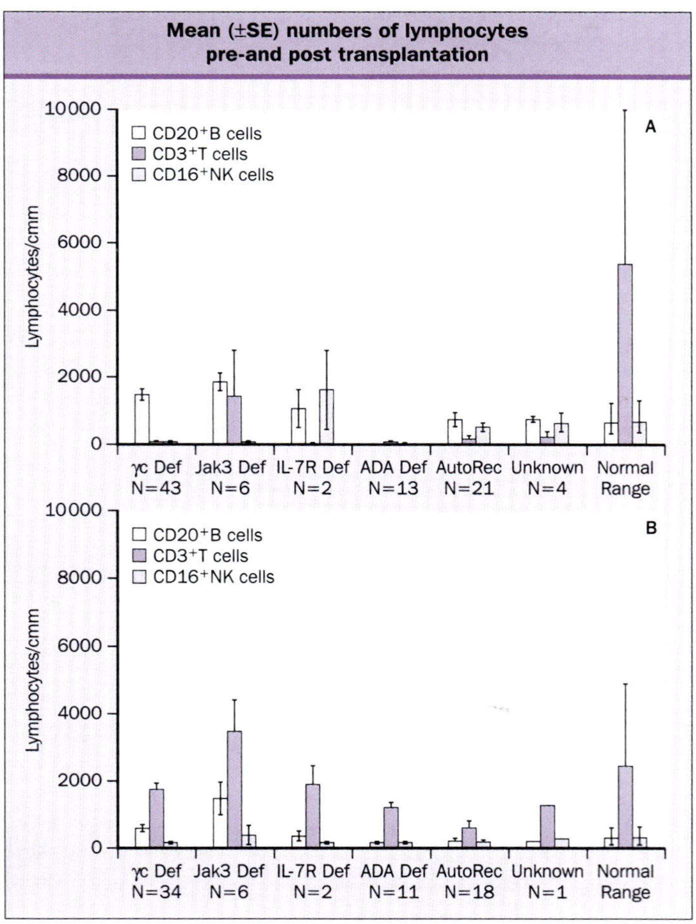

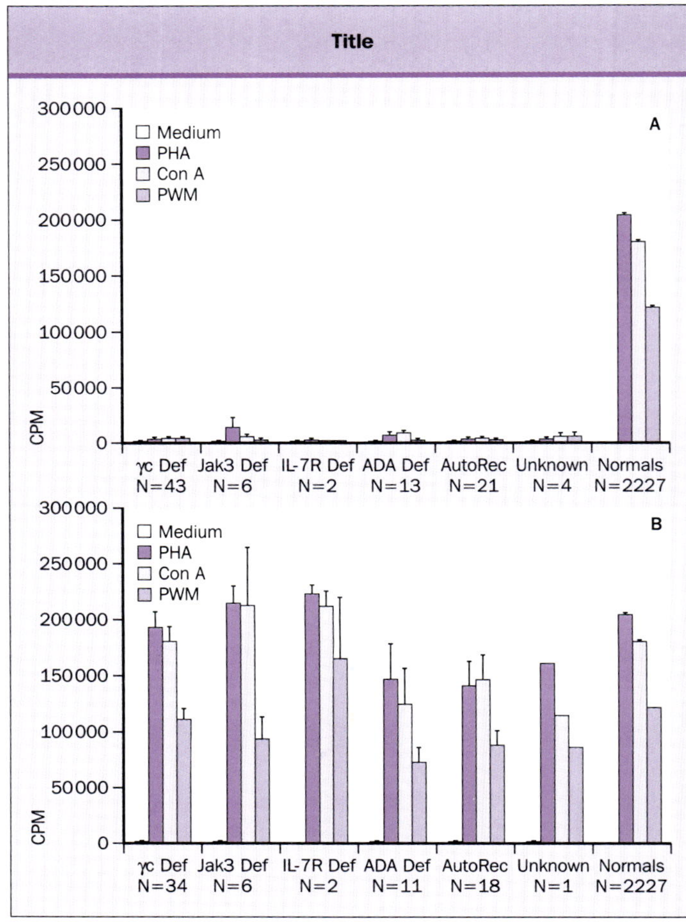

Figure 101.4 Tritium-labeled thymidine incorporated by proliferating lymphocytes in response to phytohemagglutinin, concanavalin A, and pokeweed mitogen before transplantation (**A**) and at the most recent evaluation after transplantation (**B**), according to the type of severe combined immunodeficiency. (From Buckley RH, Schiff SE, Schiff RI, et al. Hematopoietic stem cell transplantation for the treatment of severe combined immunodeficiency. *N Engl J Med* 1999;340:508 with permission.)

Figure 101.3 Mean (±SE) numbers of $CD20^+$ B cells, $CD3^+$ T cells, and $CD16^+$ natural killer cells before transplantation (**A**) and at the most recent evaluation after transplantation (**B**), according to the type of severe combined immunodeficiency. (From Buckley RH, Schiff SE, Schiff RI, et al. Hematopoietic stem cell transplantation for the treatment of severe combined immunodeficiency. *N Engl J Med* 1999;340:508 with permission.)

T-cell counts and thymic function before transplantation in infants with severe combined immunodeficiency (SCID)

Patients	SCID type	SjTRECs[a]	CD3$^+$ count[b]
1	Autosomal recessive	<100	100
2	JAK3$^{-/-}$	<100	8268[c]
3	X-linked	<100	17
4	X-linked	<100	21
5	X-linked	226	651[c]
6	X-linked	100	365[c]
7	X-linked	<100	15
8	X-linked	<100	42
9	X-linked	<100	570[c]
10	X-linked	<100	904[c]
11	X-linked	<100	23

[a] sjTRECs/mg PBMC DNA.
[b] CD3 count (CD3$^+$ lymphocytes/ml blood).
[c] Documented transplacental transfer of maternal T cells into the fetal circulation.

Table 101.3 T-cell counts and thymic function before transplantation in infants with severe combined immunodeficiency (SCID).

Kinetics of T-cell proliferation and thymic output after transplantation in infants with severe combined immunodeficiency

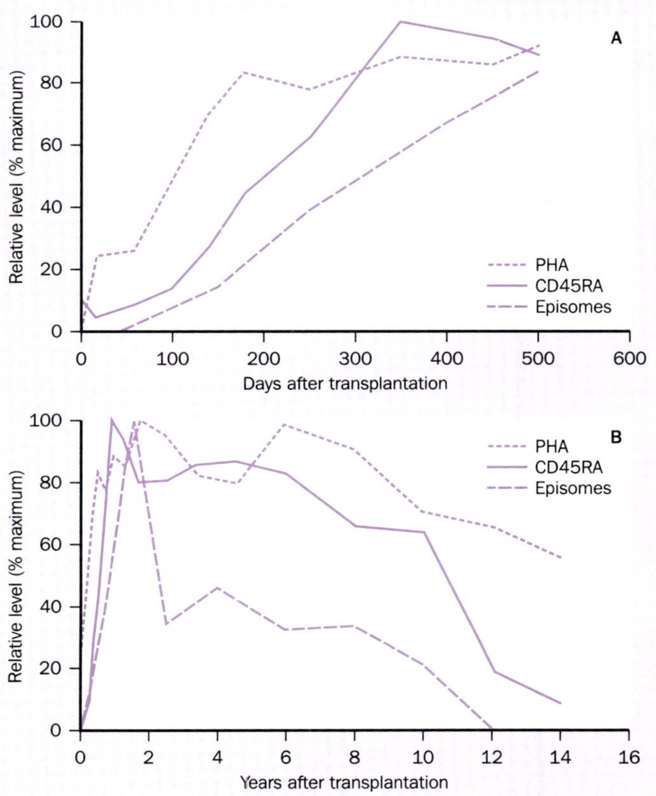

THERAPEUTIC PRINCIPLES

Recommendations for immune reconstitution in primary immunodeficiency

- For those immunodeficient patients for whom marrow or blood stem cell reconstitution has been shown to be effective, the earlier in life that a related stem cell transplant can be performed, the more likely it is that the outcome will be successful; for non-SCID defects, this is prior to the age of 5 years.
- SCID is a pediatric emergency. The potential exists for all forms of SCID to be diagnosed at the time of birth. However, the best screening tests for this syndrome, a white blood cell count and a manual differential to determine the absolute lymphocyte count, are not routinely done on cord blood. If the condition could be diagnosed at birth in all SCID infants, related donor transplants could be performed in all of them in the neonatal period, with a >95% probability of success – whether the related stem cell donor is HLA-identical or HLA-haploidentical.
- It is very likely that immune reconstitution will be accomplished by gene therapy in the future. At the time of this writing, gene therapy has been successful only in X-linked SCID in France. All efforts at gene therapy for ADA-deficient SCID have failed. Early diagnosis before the patient becomes infected with opportunistic infections for which there is no effective treatment will be of paramount importance. The latter is true regardless of whether the eventual treatment of choice for (some or all) patients with primary immunodeficiency is gene therapy or whether it is the currently available treatment of choice, i.e. related allogeneic stem cell transplantation.
- In gene therapy, autologous normal-gene-transduced stem cells will have to undergo thymus processing to become positively and negatively selected before they emerge as mature circulating T cells. Therefore, the kinetics of development of T-cell function will be similar to those of T cell-depleted allogeneic stem cell grafts. Gene therapy will also be constrained by the potential of the infant's thymus to generate T cells from stem cells and by the longevity of that potential.

Figure 101.5 Kinetics of T-cell proliferation and thymic output after successful bone marrow transplantation in infants with severe combined immunodeficiency. Shown are the levels of T-cell proliferation in response to phytohemagglutin (PHA), peripheral blood CD45RA counts, and T-cell antigen-receptor episomes (TRECs) as a percentage of the mean maximal level achieved during any period. The mean lengths of time needed to reach levels that were 50% of the maximum were 100 days for responsiveness to phytohemagglutinin, 200 days for CD45RA$^+$ cells, and 300 days for TRECs. (From Patel DD, Gooding ME, Parrott RE, Curtis KM, Haynes BF, Buckley RH. Thymic function after hematopoietic stem-cell transplantation for the treatment of severe combined immunodeficiency. *N Engl J Med* 2000;342:1325 with permission.)

Wiskott–Aldrich syndrome

The second largest group of immunodeficiency patients given bone marrow transplants since 1968 are those with the Wiskott–Aldrich syndrome (Table 101.2).[2,42,54,62–67] During this period, 153 patients were transplanted, and 99 or 65% were reported as surviving. However, in contrast to SCID patients, the survival rates for HLA-identical sibling marrow transplants in Wiskott–Aldrich patients (58 of 65 or 89%) and MUD marrow transplants (20 of 29 or 69%) were far superior to that for T cell-depleted haploidentical marrow transplants (20 of 58 or 34%). The facts that all such patients require myeloablation and cytoreduction to prevent graft rejection, that they have been multiply transfused with allogeneic platelets before transplantation resulting in resistance to engraftment, that they may have developed chronic herpesvirus infections prior to transplantation, and that they are prone to develop malignancy are all likely contributing factors to their failure to survive the 3–4 months required for stem cells to mature to functioning T cells from a T cell-depleted marrow graft. Many of the deaths were from EBV-associated B-lymphocyte lymphoproliferative disorders.[54]

Combined immunodeficiency (CID)

Patients with combined immunodeficiencies characterized by less severe T-cell defects than in SCID constituted the third largest group of patients given bone marrow transplants since 1968 (Table 101.2).[55] Thirty-two of 64 patients (50%) so treated were reported as surviving. HLA-identical marrow transplants were clearly more successful (13 of 17 or 76%) than T cell-depleted haploidentical (14 of 37 or 38%) or MUD adult marrow (0 of 2) transplants, but 5 of 7 recipients of cord blood transplants were surviving.[68]

Omenn syndrome

Forty-two patients with Omenn syndrome were reported in the literature[54,69,70] or to the author as having received marrow transplants since 1968, and 20 or 48% were alive at the time (Table 101.2). As with the other non-SCID defects, however, the greatest success was with HLA-identical sibling transplants, 9 of 12 (75%) of whom were surviving, whereas only 8 of 24 (33%) haploidentical marrow and 3 of 6 (50%) MUD marrow recipients were alive.

Leukocyte adhesion deficiency (LAD)

Twenty-four of 32 (75%) patients with leukocyte adhesion protein deficiency were alive after bone marrow transplantation at the time of the survey and review.[54,71,72] All types of marrow transplantation were successful in this condition: 6 of 8 (75%) HLA-identical sibling transplants, 14 of 20 (70%) T cell-depleted haploidentical marrow transplants, 2 of 2 (100%) MUD adult marrow transplants, and 2 of 3 cord blood transplants (Table 101.2).

MHC antigen deficiency syndromes

Fourteen of 25 (56%) patients with the bare lymphocyte syndrome were reported alive after having been given marrow transplants (Table 101.2).[54,73,74] These included 4 of 8 (50%) who received HLA-identical sibling marrow, but only 7 of 20 (35%) who received T cell-depleted haploidentical marrow, 2 of 2 (100%) who received MUD marrow, and 1 of 1 (100%) who received a related cord blood transplant.[54,73,75]

Chediak–Higashi syndrome

Seventeen of 22 (77%) patients with Chediak–Higashi syndrome who received bone marrow transplants were reported to be alive (Table 101.2).[42,54,76] These included 10 of 12 (83%) who received HLA-identical sibling marrow, 1 of 5 (20%) who received haploidentical marrow, and 5 of 5 (100%) who received MUD marrow.

Chronic granulomatous disease (CGD)

Twelve of 17 (71%) patients with CGD who had received bone marrow transplants were reported as surviving, and a majority of these were chimeric (Table 101.2).[77–81] The overall survival figures include 10 of 14 (71%) HLA-identical sibling marrow recipients and 2 of 3 recipients (67%) of MUD marrow.[82] Very recently, success has been reported in treating a patient with CGD with the 'mini-transplant' approach.[8]

DiGeorge syndrome

Eleven patients with the complete DiGeorge syndrome were reported to the author as undergoing marrow transplantation, while 4 more underwent fetal thymus or cultured mature thymic tissue transplantation (Table 101.2).[83,84] The only survivors were 2 of the 3 who received unfractionated HLA-identical sibling marrow, and 2 of 2 who were recipients of explants of cultured thymic epithelium. Twenty-six more were identified from the literature by Goldsobel et al[83] in 1987 as having undergone fetal thymus or cultured thymic epithelial transplantation, and at the time of their review only 8 were alive and well.

Other primary immunodeficiencies

Other disorders treated successfully by bone marrow transplantation include hyper-IgM (8 of 12 surviving),[85–88] reticular dysgenesis (9 of 11 surviving),[68,89] purine nucleoside phosphorylase (PNP) deficiency (3 of 8 surviving),[90,91] cartilage–hair hypoplasia (4 of 7 surviving), X-linked lymphoproliferative syndrome (4 of 7 surviving),[92–94] pigmentary dilution (Griscelli) syndrome (3 of 7 surviving),[95] IL-2 deficiency (2 of 2 surviving),[55] common variable immunodeficiency (CVID) (none of 4 surviving), chronic mucocutaneous candidiasis (none of 1 surviving), and ataxia telangiectasia (none of 4 surviving) (Table 101.2).

We have also transplanted 51 patients with non-SCID immunodeficiency at our institution, with the following survival rates: 11 of 26 with CID (42%), 5 of 7 with LAD (71%), 2 of 2 with Chediak–Higashi syndrome (100%), 2 of 2 with CGD (100%), 1 of 1 with ZAP-70 deficiency (100%), 2 of 5 with Omenn syndrome (40%), 1 of 3 with PNP deficiency (33%), 1 of 2 with Wiskott–Aldrich syndrome (50%), 1 of 1 with X-linked hyper-IgM (100%), and 1 each with Griscelli syndrome and IFNγR2 deficiency, neither of whom survive.

CAUSES OF DEATH

When we have lost infants with SCID, they have died from viral infections.[22] CMV and EBV infections are the major causes of death, but we have also had deaths from adenovirus, enteroviruses, respiratory syncytial virus, parainfluenza 3, and herpes simplex. Usually these viruses are already present in the infants when they present for therapy. The 90–120-day period required for stem cells to develop into T cells renders it very difficult to control these viral infections with the exception of those for which antibiotics are available, such as herpes simplex or varicella.

Ribavirin has also been helpful in the treatment of parainfluenza 3 and respiratory syncytial virus infections. Most of the non-SCID immunodeficient patients were given pre-transplant chemoablation and many were given GVHD prophylaxis. The 25 who died did so from gram-negative or fungal sepsis or GVHD, in contrast to the deaths predominantly from viral infections in our 22 SCID patients.

REMAINING PROBLEMS

A number of problems remain in T cell-depleted bone marrow transplantation. Clearly it is not nearly as effective when the recipient must be ablated by chemotherapy or irradiation, because of the 90–120-day period required for stem cells to mature into T cells. Even without chemotherapy, if SCID infants present with EBV or CMV infections, there is a very high probability that they will not survive until T cells emerge.

Another problem is that of resistance to engraftment, which we have seen in 8 SCID infants. Three of these were ADA-deficient patients who rejected their transplants. After booster transplants from the same or other parental donors also failed, they were begun on injections of polyethylene glycol-modified bovine ADA (PEG-ADA) and all are surviving. Of the 5 non-ADA-deficient patients who resisted engraftment, one was a female infant who first received a stem cell transplant from her father. At 180 days post transplantation she still had no evidence of T-cell phenotypes or function. We then gave T cell-depleted marrow from the mother, again without conditioning. Soon after we gave the mother's stem cells, we saw an increase in T-cell function. To determine whose cells the T cells were, we did karyotyping on the dividing cells and found that a majority of the cells were from the original donor, the father. Thus, even though we could not detect any function during the first 6 months after the first transplant, the cells that eventually developed function were from the first donor. Further sequential karyotyping demonstrated that this patient has double parental chimerism. A second SCID patient who demonstrated prolonged resistance to engraftment was a male infant who had received a transplant from his mother. By 6 months post transplantation, no T-cell phenotypes or function had developed, so we gave him a stem cell transplant from his father without pre-transplant conditioning. Shortly after that, there was a dramatic improvement in his T-cell function. In contrast to the first patient, a majority of the T cells were from the second donor, but some cells from the first donor were also found. Thus, both are double parental chimeras. Surprisingly, the B-cell function in these two patients is the best that we have seen in any of our reconstituted SCIDs. They both have normal serum immunoglobulin concentrations and normal antibody titers. Of the remaining 3 infants, all have had booster transplants from both parents, and only one has experienced improved T-cell function. One of the other two is a patient with X-linked SCID with an unusual mutation who failed to develop normal T-cell function despite two transplants from each parent. He is surviving at age 8 years, and gene therapy is being planned for him. The final patient was an autosomal recessive SCID of unknown molecular type who presented with disseminated varicella and who died at age 3.5 years with no T-cell function.

Resistance to engraftment has also been particularly difficult to overcome in patients with some pre-existing T-cell function given haploidentical stem cell transplants, even though they have received lethal conditioning regimens. Although the reasons for resistance to engraftment are not clear, some success in circumventing it has been reported by Fischer et al.[96,97] Following their observations that conditioned LAD patients readily accepted half-matched stem cell transplants, those authors employed in vivo pre-treatment of the recipient with a monoclonal antibody to the alpha chain of LFA-1 and achieved rapid engraftment of haploidentical marrow in 7 of 7 conditioned patients who had had some pre-treatment T-cell function.[96,97] Since LFA-1 is an adhesion protein important in immune cell interaction, they speculated that the antibody interfered with host recognition of the graft. Campath-1 has been used to treat the recipient in vivo to deplete residual lymphocytes (in addition to being used in vitro to deplete T cells from the donor marrow) with a resultant reduction in resistance to engraftment in patients with malignant diseases.[40]

Another problem is that some patients do not develop B-cell function post transplantation.[22,98,99] The B cells in most cases remain those of the host. Of the 12 SCID infants to whom we gave HLA-identical marrow, we have found some donor B cells in 5 and, among the half-matched SCID recipients, we have found some donor B cells in 21 of the 73 survivors. In many cases, those with donor B cells were infants who had received transplacental transfer of mature maternal T and B cells while they were in utero. Despite the fact that most have only host B cells, the half-matched T and B cells of many of the chimeras can cooperate for effective humoral and cellular immune responses. The latter also indicates that many patients with SCID have intrinsically normal B cells. In the case of the X-linked SCID patients, who paradoxically have the highest number of B cells pre-transplantation, the poor B-cell function post transplantation may be because the underlying molecular defect (i.e. mutations in the gamma chain of the IL-2 receptor) also affects other cytokine receptors that share that chain (IL-4, IL-7, IL-9, and IL-15 receptors) (Chapter 35). Because of this problem, some centers routinely condition SCID patients prior to half-matched marrow transplants with the hope of enhancing donor B-cell engraftment. However, when this is done, the probability of infection-related deaths increases, the agents used may have long-term undesirable effects on other body tissues, and the long-term survival rate is not improved.[42,59] Most centers, therefore, opt not to give pre-transplant conditioning and administer gamma-globulin to those recipients who remain B cell-deficient following haploidentical stem cell transplants despite normal T-cell function.

One question that arises is whether one stem cell transplant will be adequate to last these children for the rest of their lives. We plan to continue to monitor T-cell function throughout these patient's lives. Despite the fact that our recent studies of thymic function appear to demonstrate that thymic output may diminish sooner than in normal individuals (Fig. 101.5),[36] so far we see no evidence of waning T-cell function in these patients, the oldest of whom is now more than 18 years post transplantation.[22]

FETAL TISSUE AND THYMIC EPITHELIAL TRANSPLANTS

While transplantation of fetal liver and/or thymus has been attempted many times over the past three decades for the correction of SCID, DiGeorge syndrome, or other severe T-cell deficiency, it has rarely been permanently successful except possibly in patients with DiGeorge syndrome. Some or all of the improved immune function observed in patients with DiGeorge syndrome following fetal thymus transplantation could have been due to growth of autologous thymic tissue, since a majority of DiGeorge patients have tiny nests of autologous thymic tissue and some parathyroid glands in the mediastinum (i.e. they have 'partial' DiGeorge syndrome). Chimerism had rarely been proved in DiGeorge patients transplanted with fetal thymus. Recently, however, several patients with the complete DiGeorge syndrome have sustained immune reconstitution following partially matched transplants of unrelated donor cultured thymic epithelium, and thymopoiesis was demonstrated in the grafts.[84] In addition, the T cells that developed contained TRECs, indicating that they were recent thymic emigrants. As noted above, the complete DiGeorge syndrome has also been mitigated by unfractionated HLA-identical bone marrow transplantation.[83]

REFERENCES

1. Amos DB, Bach FH. Phenotypic expressions of the major histocompatibility locus in man (HL-A): leukocyte antigens and mixed leukocyte culture reactivity. J Exp Med 1968;128:623.
2. Bach FH, Albertini RJ, Joo P, Anderson JL, Bortin MD. Bone marrow transplantation in a patient with the Wiskott–Aldrich syndrome. Lancet 1968;2:1364.
3. Gatti RA, Meuwissen HJ, Allen HD, Hong R, Good RA. Immunological reconstitution of sex-linked lymphopenic immunological deficiency. Lancet 1968;2:1366.
4. Bortin MM, Rimm AA. Severe combined immunodeficiency disease. Characterization of the disease and results of transplantation. JAMA 1977;238:591.
5. Muller-Ruchholtz W, Wottge HU, Muller-Hermelink HK. Bone marrow transplantation in rats across strong histocompatibility barriers by selective elimination of lymphoid cells in donor marrow. Transplant Proc 1976;8:537.
6. Reisner Y, Itzicovitch L, Meshorer A, Sharon N. Hematopoietic stem cell transplantation using mouse bone marrow and spleen cells fractionated by lectins. Proc Natl Acad Sci USA 1978;75:2933.
7. Blazar DR, Ramsay NKC, Kersey JH, Krivit W, Arthur DC, Filipovich AH. Pretransplant conditioning with busulfan (Myleran) and cyclophosphamide for non malignant diseases. Assessment of engraftment following histocompatible allogeneic bone marrow transplantation. Transplantation 1985;39:597.
8. Nagler A, Ackerstein A, Kapelushnik J, Or R, Naparstek E, Slavin S. Donor lymphocyte infusion post-non-myeloablative allogeneic peripheral blood stem cell transplantation for chronic granulomatous disease. Bone Marrow Transplant 1999;24:339.
9. Carella AM, Giralt S, Slavin S. Low intensity regimens with allogeneic hematopoietic stem cell transplantation as treatment of hematologic neoplasia. Haematologica 2000;85:304.
10. Carella AM, Champlin R, Slavin S, McSweeney P, Storb R. Mini-allografts: ongoing trials in humans. Bone Marrow Transplant 2000;25:345.
11. Roberts JL, Volkman DJ, Buckley RH. Modified MHC restriction of donor-origin T cells in humans with severe combined immunodeficiency transplanted with haploidentical bone marrow stem cells. J Immunol 1989;143:1575.
12. Ferrara JL, Deeg HJ. Graft-versus-host disease. N Engl J Med 1991;324:667.
13. Glucksberg H, Storb R, Fefer A, et al. Clinical manifestations of graft-versus-host disease in human recipients of marrow from HLA-matched sibling donors. Transplantation 1974;18:295.
14. Deeg HJ, Henslee-Downey PJ. Management of acute graft-versus-host disease. Bone Marrow Transplant 1990;6:1.
15. Weisdorf D, Haake R, Blazar B, et al. Treatment of moderate/severe acute graft-versus-host disease after allogeneic bone marrow transplantation: an analysis of clinical risk features and outcome. Blood 1990;75:1024.
16. Skinner J, Finlay JL, Sondel PM, Trigg ME. Infectious complications in pediatric patients undergoing transplantation with T lymphocyte-depleted bone marrow. Pediatr Infect Dis 1986;5:319.
17. Theobald M, Nierle T, Bunjes D, Arnold R, Heimpel H. Host-specific interleukin-2-secreting donor T-cell precursors as predictors of acute graft-versus-host disease in bone marrow transplantation between HLA-identical siblings. N Engl J Med 1992;327:1613.
18. Schwarer AP, Jiang YZ, Brookes PA, et al. Frequency of anti-recipient alloreactive helper T-cell precursors in donor blood and graft-versus-host disease after HLA-identical sibling bone marrow transplantation. Lancet 1993;341:203.
19. Wang L, Juji T, Tokunaga K, et al. Polymorphic microsatellite markers for the diagnosis of graft-versus-host disease. N Engl J Med 1994;330:398.
20. Storb R, Deeg HJ, Whitehead J, et al. Methotrexate and cyclosporine compared with cyclosporine alone for prophylaxis of acute graft versus host disease after marrow transplantation for leukemia. N Engl J Med 1986;314:729.
21. Buckley RH, Fischer A. Bone marrow transplantation for primary immunodeficiency diseases. In: Ochs HD, Smith CIE, Puck JM (eds) Primary immunodeficiency diseases: A molecular and genetic approach. New York, Oxford University Press, 1999; p 459.
22. Buckley RH, Schiff SE, Schiff RI, et al. Hematopoietic stem cell transplantation for the treatment of severe combined immunodeficiency. N Engl J Med 1999;340:508.
23. Wu AM, Till JE, Siminovitch L, McCulloch EA. Cytological evidence for a relationship between normal hematopoietic colony-forming cells and cells of the lymphoid system. J Exp Med 1968;127:455.
24. Cavazzana-Calvo M, Hacein-Bey S, deSaint Basile G, et al. Gene therapy of human severe combined immunodeficiency (SCID)-X1 disease. Science 2000;288:669.
25. Thomas ED, Storb R, Clift RA, et al. Bone marrow transplantation. N Engl J Med 1975;292:823.
26. Vossen JM, van Leeuwen JE, van Tol MJ, et al. Chimerism and immune reconstitution following allogeneic bone marrow transplantation for severe combined immunodeficiency disease. Immunodeficiency 1993;4:311.
27. Van Den Berg H, Vossen JM, van den Bergh RL, Bayer J, van Tol MJD. Detection of Y chromosome by *in situ* hybridization in combination with membrane antigens by two-color immunofluorescence. Lab Invest 1994;64:623.
28. Blazar BR, Filipovich AH. Identification of transfused blood cells in children with SCID by analysis of multiple cell lineages using restriction fragment length polymorphisms. Bone Marrow Transplant 1990;5:327.
29. Reisner Y, Kapoor N, Kirkpatrick D, et al. Transplantation for severe combined immunodeficiency with HLA-A, B, D, DR incompatible parental marrow cells fractionated by soybean agglutinin and sheep red blood cells. Blood 1983;61:341.
30. Buckley RH, Schiff SE, Sampson HA, et al. Development of immunity in human severe primary T cell deficiency following haploidentical bone marrow stem cell transplantation. J Immunol 1986;136:2398.
31. O'Reilly RJ, Keever CA, Small TN, Brochstein J. The use of HLA-non-identical T cell depleted marrow transplants for correction of severe combined immunodeficiency disease. Immunodef Rev 1989;1:273.
32. Dror Y, Gallagher R, Wara DW, et al. Immune reconstitution in severe combined immunodeficiency disease after lectin-treated, T cell depleted haplocompatible bone marrow transplantation. Blood 1993;81:2021.
33. Giri N, Vowels M, Ziegler JB, Ford D, Lam-Po-Tang R. HLA non-identical T cell depleted bone marrow transplantation for primary immunodeficiency diseases. Aust N Z J Med 1994;24:26.
34. Wijnaendts L, LeDeist F, Griscelli C, Fischer A. Development of immunologic functions after bone marrow transplantation in

33 patients with severe combined immunodeficiency. Blood 1989;74:2212.
35. Moen RC, Horowitz SD, Sondel PM, et al. Immunologic reconstitution after haploidentical bone marrow transplantation for immune deficiency disorders: treatment of bone marrow cells with monoclonal antibody CT-2 and complement. Blood 1987;70:664.
36. Patel DD, Gooding ME, Parrott RE, Curtis KM, Haynes BF, Buckley RH. Thymic function after hematopoietic stem-cell transplantation for the treatment of severe combined immunodeficiency. N Engl J Med 2000;342:1325.
37. Schiff SE, Buckley RH. Modified responses to recipient and donor B cells by genetically donor T cells from human haploidentical bone marrow chimeras. J Immunol 1987;138:2088.
38. Schiff SE, Kurtzberg J, Buckley RH. Studies of human bone marrow treated with soybean lectin and sheep erythrocytes: stepwise analysis of cell morphology, phenotype and function. Clin Exp Immunol 1987;68:685.
39. Reinherz EL, Geha R, Rappeport JM, et al. Reconstitution after transplantation with T-lymphocyte-depleted HLA haplotype-mismatched bone marrow for severe combined immunodeficiency. Proc Natl Acad Sci USA 1982;79:6047.
40. Hale G, Waldmann H. Control of graft-versus-host disease and graft rejection by T cell depletion of donor and recipient with Campath-1 antibodies. Results of matched sibling transplants for malignant diseases. Bone Marrow Transplant 1994;13:597.
41. Martin-Hernandez MP, Arrieta R, Martinez A, Garcia P, Jimenez-Yuste V, Hernandez-Navarro F. Haploidentical peripheral blood cell transplantation with a combination of CD34 selection and T cell depletion as graft-versus-host disease prophylaxis in a patient with severe combined immunodeficiency. Bone Marrow Transplantation 1997;20:797.
42. Fischer A, Durandy A, De Villartay JP, et al. HLA-haploidentical bone marrow transplantation for severe combined immunodeficiency using E rosette fractionation and cyclosporine. Blood 1986;67:444.
43. Bhatia S, Ramsay NK, Steinbuch M, et al. Malignant neoplasms following bone marrow transplantation. Blood 1996;87:3633.
44. Shearer WT, Ritz J, Finegold MJ, et al. Epstein-Barr virus-associated B-cell proliferations of diverse clonal origins after bone marrow transplantation in a 12-year-old patient with severe combined immunodeficiency. N Engl J Med 1985;312:1151.
45. Bertrand Y, Landais P, Friedrich W, et al. Influence of severe combined immunodeficiency phenotype on the outcome of HLA non-identical T cell-depleted bone marrow transplantation. J Pediatr 1999;134:740.
46. O'Reilly RJ, Dupont B, Pahwa S, et al. Reconstitution in severe combined immunodeficiency by transplantation of marrow from an unrelated donor. N Engl J Med 1977;297:1311.
47. Filipovich AH, Shapiro RS, Ramsay NK, et al. Unrelated donor bone marrow transplantation for correction of lethal congenital immunodeficiencies. Blood 1992;80:270.
48. Ash RC, Casper JT, Chitambar CR, et al. Successful allogeneic transplantation of T cell depleted bone marrow from closely HLA-matched unrelated donors. N Engl J Med 1990;322:485.
49. Kernan NA, Bartsch G, Ash RC, et al. Analysis of 462 transplantations from unrelated donors facilitated by the National Marrow Donor Program. N Engl J Med 1993;328:593.
50. Dini G, Lanino E, Lamparelli T, et al. Unrelated donor marrow transplantation: initial experience of the Italian bone marrow transplant group (GITMO). Bone Marrow Transplant 1996;17:55.
51. Wagner JE, Kernan NA, Steinbuch M, Broxmeyer HE, Gluckman E. Allogeneic sibling umbilical-cord-blood transplantation in children with malignant and non-malignant disease. Lancet 1995;346:214.
52. Vowels MR, Tang RL, Berdoukas V, et al. Brief report: Correction of X-linked lymphoproliferative disease by transplantation of cord blood stem cells. N Engl J Med 1993;329:1623.
53. Stary J, Bartunkova J, Kobylka P, et al. Successful HLA-identical sibling cord blood transplantation in a 6 year old boy with leukocyte adhesion deficiency syndrome. Bone Marrow Transplant 1996;18:249.
54. Fischer A, Landais P, Friedrich W, et al. Bone marrow transplantation (BMT) in Europe for primary immunodeficiencies other than severe combined immunodeficiency: a report from the European Group for BMT and the European Group for Immunodeficiency. Blood 1994;83:1149.
55. Berthet F, Le Deist F, Duliege AM, Griscelli C, Fischer A. Clinical consequences and treatment of primary immunodeficiency syndromes characterized by functional T and B lymphocyte anomalies (combined immune deficiency). Pediatr 1994;93:265.
56. Stephan JL, Vlekova V, Le Deist F, et al. Severe combined immunodeficiency: a retrospective single-center study of clinical presentation and outcome in 117 cases. J Pediatr 1993;123:564.
57. Buckley RH, Schiff RI, Schiff SE, et al. Human severe combined immunodeficiency (SCID): Genetic, phenotypic and functional diversity in 108 infants. J Pediatr 1997;130:378.
58. Fischer A, Landais P, Friedrich W, et al. European experience of bone marrow transplantation for severe combined immunodeficiency. Lancet 1990;336:850.
59. Haddad E, Landais P, Friedrich W, et al. Long-term immune reconstitution and outcome after HLA-nonidentical T-cell-depleted bone marrow transplantation for severe combined immunodeficiency: a European retrospective study of 116 patients. Blood 1998;91:3646.
60. Wengler GS, Lanfranchi A, Frusca T, et al. In-utero transplantation of parental CD34 haematopoietic progenitor cells in a patient with X-linked severe combined immunodeficiency (SCIDX1). Lancet 1996;348:1484.
61. Flake AW, Roncarolo MG, Puck JM, et al. Treatment of X-linked severe combined immunodeficiency by in utero transplantation of paternal bone marrow. N Engl J Med 1996;335:1806.
62. Brochstein JA, Gillio AP, Ruggiero M, et al. Marrow transplantation from human leukocyte antigen-identical or haploidentical donors for correction of Wiskott–Aldrich syndrome. J Pediatr 1991;119:907.
63. Rumelhart SL, Trigg ME, Horowitz SD, Hong R. Monoclonal antibody T cell depleted HLA-haploidentical bone marrow transplantation for Wiskott–Aldrich syndrome. Blood 1990;75:1031.
64. Parkman R, Rappeport J, Geha R, et al. Complete correction of the Wiskott–Aldrich syndrome by allogenic bone-marrow transplantation. N Engl J Med 1978;298:921.
65. Mullen CA, Anderson KD, Blaese RM. Splenectomy and/or bone marrow transplantation in the management of the Wiskott–Aldrich syndrome: long-term follow-up of 62 cases. Blood 1993;82:2961.
66. Lenarsky C, Weinberg K, Kohn DB, Parkman R. Unrelated donor bone marrow transplantation for Wiskott–Aldrich syndrome. Bone Marrow Transplant 1993;12:145.
67. Ozsahin H, Le Deist F, Benkerrou M, et al. Bone marrow transplantation in 26 patients with Wiskott–Aldrich syndrome from a single center. J Pediatr 1996;129:238.
68. Knutsen AP, Wall DA. Kinetics of T-cell development of umbilical cord blood transplantation in severe T-cell immunodeficiency disorders. J Allergy Clin Immunol 1999;103(5 Pt 1):823.
69. Gomez L, Le Deist F, Blanche S, Cavazzana-Calvo M, Griscelli C, Fischer A. Treatment of Omenn syndrome by bone marrow transplantation. J Pediatr 1995;127:76.
70. Loechelt BJ, Shapiro RS, Jyonouchi H, Filipovich AH. Mismatched bone marrow transplantation for Omenn syndrome: a variant of severe combined immunodeficiency. Bone Marrow Transplant 1995;16:381.
71. LeDeist F, Blanche S, Keable H. Successful HLA non-identical bone marrow transplantation in three patients with leukocyte adhesion deficiency. Blood 1989;74:512.
72. Thomas C, LeDeist F, Cavazzana-Calvo M, et al. Results of allogeneic bone marrow transplantation in patients with leukocyte adhesion deficiency. Blood 1995;86:1629.
73. Casper JT, Ash RA, Kirchner P, Hunter JB, Havens PL, Chusid MJ. Successful treatment with an unrelated donor bone marrow transplant in an HLA-deficient patient with severe combined immune deficiency ('bare lymphocyte syndrome'). J Pediatr 1990;116:262.
74. Klein C, Cavazzana-Calvo M, Le Deist F, et al. Bone marrow transplantation in major histocompatibility complex Class II deficiency: a single center study of 19 patients. Blood 1995;85:580.
75. Bonduel M, Pozo A, Zelazko M, et al. Successful related umbilical cord blood transplantation for graft failure following T cell-depleted non-identical bone marrow transplantation in a child with major

histocompatibility complex Class II deficiency. Bone Marrow Transplant 1999;24:437.
76. Haddad E, Le Deist F, Blanche S, et al. Treatment of Chediak–Higashi syndrome by allogenic bone marrow transplantation: report of 10 cases. Blood 1995;85:3328.
77. Hobbs JR, Monteil M, McCluskey DR, Jurges E, El Tumi M. Chronic granulomatous disease 100% corrected by displacement bone marrow transplantation from a volunteer unrelated donor. Eur J Pediatr 1992;151:806.
78. Kamani N, August CS, Campbell DE, Hassan NF, Douglas SD. Marrow transplantation in chronic granulomatous disease: an update, with 6-year follow up. J Pediatr 1988;113:697.
79. di Bartolomeo P, Girolamo G, Angrilli P, et al. Reconstitution of normal neutrophil function in chronic granulomatous disease by bone marrow transplantation. Bone Marrow Transplant 1989;4:695.
80. Rappeport JM, Newburger PE, Goldblum RM, Goldman AS, Nathan DG, Parkman R. Allogeneic transplantation for chronic granulomatous disease. J Pediatr 1982;101:952.
81. Ozsahin H, von Planta M, Muller I, et al. Successful treatment of invasive aspergillosis in chronic granulomatous disease by bone marrow transplantation, granulocyte colony-stimulating factor-mobilized granulocytes, and liposomal amphotericin-B. Blood 1998;92:2719.
82. Seger RA, Ezekowitz RAB. Treatment of chronic granulomatous disease. Immunodeficiency 1994;5:113.
83. Goldsobel AB, Haas A, Stiehm ER. Bone marrow transplantation in DiGeorge syndrome. J Pediatr 1987;111:40.
84. Markert ML, Boeck A, Hale LP, et al. Thymus transplantation in complete DiGeorge syndrome. N Engl J Med 1999;341:1180.
85. Fasth A. Bone marrow transplantation for hyper-IgM syndrome. Immunodeficiency 1993;4:323.
86. Thomas C, de Saint Basile G, Le Deist F, et al. Brief report: correction of X-linked hyper-IgM syndrome by allogeneic bone marrow transplantation. N Engl J Med 1995;333:426.
87. Duplantier JE, Nelson RP Jr, Ochs HD, et al. Successful bone marrow transplantation (BMT) for X-linked hyper IgM (XHIM) syndrome. J Allergy Clin Immunol 1997;99S:102.
88. Scholl PR, O'Gorman MR, Pachman LM, Haut P, Kletzel M. Correction of neutropenia and hypogammaglobulinemia in X-linked hyper-IgM syndrome by allogeneic bone marrow transplantation. Bone Marrow Transplant 1998;22:1215.
89. De Santes KB, Lai SS, Cowan MJ. Haploidentical bone marrow transplants for two patients with reticular dysgenesis. Bone Marrow Transplant 1996;17:1171.
90. Broome CB, Graham ML, Saulsbury FT, Hershfield MS, Buckley RH. Correction of purine nucleoside phosphorylase deficiency by transplantation of allogeneic bone marrow from a sibling. J Pediatr 1996;128:373.
91. Carpenter PA, Ziegler JB, Vowels MR. Late diagnosis and correction of purine nucleoside phosphorylase deficiency with allogeneic bone marrow transplantation. Bone Marrow Transplant 1996;17:121.
92. Williams LL Rooney CM, Conley ME, Brenner MK, Krance RA, Heslop HE. Correction of Duncan's syndrome by allogeneic bone marrow transplantation. Lancet 1993;342:587.
93. Gross TG, Filipovich AH, Conley ME, et al. Cure of X-linked lymphoproliferative disease (XLP) with allogeneic hematopoietic stem cell transplantation (HSCT): report from the XLP registry. Bone Marrow Transplant 1996;17:741.
94. Pracher E, Panzer-Grumayer ER, Zoubek A, Peters C, Gadner H. Successful bone marrow transplantation in a boy with X-linked lymphoproliferative syndrome and acute severe infectious mononucleosis. Bone Marrow Transplant 1994;13:655.
95. Schneider LC, Berman RS, Shea CR, Perez-Atayde AR, Weinstein H, Geha RS. Bone marrow transplantation (BMT) for the syndrome of pigmentary dilution and lymphohistiocytosis (Griscelli's syndrome). J Clin Immunol 1990;10:146.
96. Fischer A, Friedrich W, Fasth A, et al. Reduction of graft failure by a monoclonal antibody (anti-LFA-1 CD11a) after HLA nonidentical bone marrow transplantation in children with immunodeficiencies, osteopetrosis and Fanconi's anemia: a European Group for Immunodeficiency/European Group for Bone Marrow Transplantation report. Blood 1991;77:249.
97. Jabado N, Le Deist F, Cant A, et al. Bone marrow transplantation from genetically HLA-nonidentical donors in children with fatal inherited disorders excluding severe combined immunodeficiencies: use of two monoclonal antibodies to prevent graft rejection. Pediatr 1996;98:420.
98. van Leeuwen JE, van Tol MJ, Joosten AM, et al. Relationship between patterns of engraftment in peripheral blood and immune reconstitution after allogeneic bone marrow transplantation for (severe) combined immunodeficiency. Blood 1994;84:3936.
99. Haddad E, Deist FL, Aucouturier P, et al. Long-term chimerism and B-cell function after bone marrow transplantation in patients with severe combined immunodeficiency with B cells: A single-center study of 22 patients. Blood 1999;94:2923.

Chapter 102 Hematopoietic Stem Cell Transplantation for Malignant Disease

Peter McSweeney and Rainer Storb

Over the last three decades hematopoietic stem cell transplantation (HSCT) has been transformed from an experimental therapy to a curative standard therapy for a number of diseases. HSCT has been used to treat hematopoietic malignancies, marrow failure syndromes, and genetic disorders of the immune and hematopoietic systems. Eighty per cent of allogeneic transplants[1] and nearly all autologous transplants have been undertaken for treatment of malignancy. Nowhere in clinical transplantation are the effects of donor–host immune incompatibility more routinely encountered than in allogeneic HSCT. Graft-versus-host disease (GVHD), graft rejection, and infection due to immune dysfunction remain major causes of treatment failure. Yet, as part of the GVH process, donor lymphocytes exert a cytotoxic effect on host immune cells and residual cancer cells not destroyed by conditioning therapy, thereby contributing to success of the procedure. Exploiting this 'allogeneic' effect is now a major goal of HSCT.

Initially HSCT was considered experimental and used as last, desperate procedure. Early results highlighted potential benefits and limitations of HSCT and set the stage for subsequent developments.[2] Conditioning regimens using cyclophosphamide (Cy) and total body irradiation (TBI) permanently eradicated leukemia in 30% of chemotherapy-resistant patients but overall long-term survival was only 10% due to a high incidence of transplant complications. Results improved when marrow grafting was used at earlier disease stages due to reduced transplant morbidity and lower relapse rates. HSCT has now progressed to a therapeutically effective modality for selected patients with malignant disease. The last two decades have seen a steadily increasing use of HSCT and broadening in the spectrum of its application (Table 102.1), reflecting increased acceptance of the procedure and relative lack of progress in conventional therapies for many hematological malignancies and solid tumors. Improved outcomes from HSCT documented during this period[3] have reflected progress primarily in management of transplant complications with less progress in eradicating malignancy. Advances in disease eradication are beginning to emerge due to research into tumor targeting with specific cytotoxic reagents and manipulations of host and/or donor immunity.

Malignancies treated by HSCT	
Hematological	**Solid tumors**
Acute lymphoblastic leukemia	Ewing sarcoma
Acute myelogenous leukemia	Neuroblastoma
Chronic myelogenous leukemia	Germ cell tumors
Chronic lymphocytic leukemia	Ovarian cancer
Hodgkin's disease	Breast cancer
Myelodysplastic syndromes	
Myeloproliferative syndromes	
Multiple myeloma	
NonHodgkin lymphoma	

Table 102.1 Malignancies treated by HSCT.

This chapter reviews the application of HSCT in the treatment of malignant disorders, contrasts autologous and allogeneic transplantation, highlights the principal problems that must still be overcome, and discusses some potential future solutions to these problems. Major recent developments include the increased use of peripheral blood stem cell (PBSC) allografting and the emergence of transplants that use nonmyeloablative, reduced-intensity conditioning regimens. The increased use of blood-derived hematopoietic stem cells renders the term 'bone marrow transplant' unsuitable to describe the varied sources of cells transplanted – HSCT is more appropriate.

GENERAL PRINCIPLES

Myelosuppression is frequently dose-limiting for conventional-dose cancer chemotherapy. HSCT allows treatment with significantly higher doses of cytotoxic therapy. By exploiting dose–response relationships that exist for radiation and chemotherapy, elimination of tumor cells resistant to conventional-dose chemotherapy is possible. Hematopoietic and immune elements, destroyed by the conditioning regimen, are reconstituted from the graft. HSCT allows systemic chemoradiotherapy doses to be increased approximately 10-fold, with further dose escalation limited by nonhematopoietic toxicities. This is in contrast to HSCT for some nonmalignant disorders, where the conditioning therapy is given primarily to ensure donor marrow engraftment and thus less intensive conditioning therapy may suffice. Unfortunately, currently tolerable conditioning regimens frequently fail to eradicate malignant disease permanently, particularly when malignancy is advanced.

The HSC graft usually comes from a healthy human leukocyte antigen (HLA)-matched sibling or unrelated donor (allogeneic transplant) or is taken from the patient (autologous transplant). After allogeneic transplants, immune-mediated graft-versus-tumor (GVT) reactions appear important in preventing relapses in a significant proportion of cases. After autologous HSCT, where the patient's HSC are stored before conditioning therapy, higher relapse rates occur due to a lack of GVT effects and possible graft contamination by tumor cells. Autologous transplants are safer because complications of donor–host immunological incompatibility are not encountered. Theoretically, autologous transplants should be ineffective in marrow-based malignancy because of contamination of the graft with malignant cells, and should be more useful in tumors that do not involve marrow. Nevertheless, autologous transplants have been successfully employed to treat acute leukemias even without attempts to remove leukemic cells from the graft, thus suggesting that autologous immune reactions may sometimes function to prevent relapse.

The sources of HSC

Genetically identical (syngeneic) donors are ideal from an immunological standpoint. However, such donors are rarely available and most related donors are HLA-A, -B, -DR, and -D identical siblings. Amongst siblings there is a 25% chance that a given sibling pair will be genotypically HLA identical (Chapter 6). In practice, approximately 20–30% of patients have an HLA-matched sibling donor. Alternative donors include partially HLA-matched related donors (found in approximately 10% of the cases) and phenotypically HLA-matched unrelated donors. Transplants of cryopreserved umbilical cord blood obtained from siblings or unrelated donors have also been investigated and are increasingly used, particularly in children. Autologous HSC grafts may be used when donors are not available or as the first choice of stem cells in some situations. Increasingly, autografts are being used to treat hematological malignancies and solid tumors. They have an established role in treating lymphomas and multiple myeloma.

HSC Collection, processing, and storage (rev. 4)

For bone marrow transplants, 10–20 ml/kg of a blood/marrow mixture is 'harvested' under general anesthesia by multiple aspirations from the iliac crests. This usually results in a total of $1–8 \times 10^8$ nucleated marrow cells per kilogram of patient weight. The marrow is heparinized and screened through wire mesh to remove bone and tissue particles. For PBSC transplants, cells are collected by leukapheresis. HSC are 'mobilized' into blood by treating the donor with growth factors such as granulocyte colony-stimulating factor (G-CSF) and granulocyte/macrophage colony-stimulating factor (GM-CSF). For autologous grafts, leukapheresis at the time of neutrophil recovery after 'mobilization' chemotherapy can enhance progenitor cell yields. The enumeration of $CD34^+$ cells by flow cytometry is an accepted measure of graft quality with $>2.0 \times 10^6$ $CD34^+$ cells/kg considered adequate for autografting and slightly higher values considered desirable for allografting. After infusion, HSC circulate in the blood, 'home' to the marrow microenvironment, and repopulate the marrow spaces. There is no significant or permanent loss of progenitor cells from the donor. While serious complications are rare, donors may experience temporary local pain and post-operative anemia after marrow harvesting, or hypocalcemia, bone pain, myalgias and thrombocytopenia during PBSC collections.

Autologous transplantation usually requires cryopreservation of HSC which involves freezing cells with a cryoprotective agent and storage in liquid nitrogen. The repopulating pluripotent HSC can survive such storage for years. Before cryopreservation, cells may be treated with monoclonal antibodies or certain chemicals to attempt to remove tumor cells. After completion of conditioning therapy, cells are rapidly thawed and infused intravenously.

Over the last decade, PBSC use has largely replaced use of bone marrow for autologous transplants. PBSC allow much faster recovery of neutrophils and platelets[5] thus reducing infections, transfusions, and hospitalization time. Rapid engraftment benefits have also been demonstrated for recipients of PBSC allografts.[6] Initial reports suggest that PBSC use improves allografting outcomes for patients with advanced malignancies. However, the approximately 10-fold higher T-cell doses infused with PBSC grafts predicted an increased risk of chronic GVHD which is now confirmed by initial results.[7] The overall benefits from using PBSC for allografting remain to be defined through longer follow-up.

A newer approach to HSC graft modification involves enrichment for $CD34^+$ progenitor cells. CD34 is a surface antigen expressed on hematopoietic progenitor cells (approximately 1% of marrow cells). Large-scale immunopurification techniques allow isolation of CD34-enriched cell populations for transplantation.[8] Currently this technology is mainly used for tumor-purging of HSC before autografting and to remove T cells from allografts to prevent GVHD. CD34 selection will be increasingly used as a first step in sophisticated graft engineering strategies which seek to modify outcomes through manipulating components of the grafts.

Another investigational approach has involved transplants of marrow maintained in long-term culture which favors survival of normal stem cells over leukemic cells, thereby permitting 'purging' of malignant cells.[9] Others have performed short-term progenitor cell 'expansion' in cytokine 'cocktails' to reduce the duration of neutropenia after HSCT.

Conditioning regimens used before transplantation

The conditioning programs are critical for the success of marrow grafting. Ideally they would: (1) fully suppress host immunity and facilitate engraftment in all cases, (2) eliminate all malignant cells, and (3) be well tolerated with no significant toxicity. Unfortunately, currently used regimens fall well short of these ideals. Most regimens include two or more agents, and many incorporate TBI. The most frequently used cytotoxic drugs include Cy, busulfan, bischloroethylnitrosourea (BCNU), cytosine arabinoside, etoposide, melphalan, carboplatin, and thiotepa. The pharmacology of these agents given in combination at high doses is not yet fully understood. Variations in metabolism or drug–drug interactions may partially account for differences in toxicity seen amongst patients. A commonly used regimen consists of Cy (60 mg/kg on each of 2 days) followed by TBI.[2] Radiation dose rates range from 2.5 to 85 cGy per minute delivered by either opposing ^{60}Cobalt sources or, more commonly, linear accelerators. Fractionation of TBI which reduces long-term toxicity, does not increase leukemic cell kill. Doses per fraction range from 1.25 to 3.3 Gy, fractionation intervals from 3 to 24 hours, and total doses from 5.0 to 15.75 Gy. Advantages of TBI include immunosuppressive properties that facilitate engraftment and an antitumor effect that can penetrate sanctuary sites for tumor (central nervous system and testicles) which are less accessible to chemotherapy. Other regimens include substitution of other chemotherapy for Cy in TBI-based regimens or use of multidrug regimens without irradiation, such as a combination of busulfan and Cy (Bu/Cy).[10,11] Many newer high-dose regimens with or without irradiation have been described. (Table 102.2), but there is little evidence for improved efficacy of these regimens.

Use of recombinant molecules in HSCT

Improved outcomes from HSCT could derive from effective manipulations of the hematopoietic and immune systems. The

Examples of conditioning regimens used for HSCT
Cy 120 mg/kg, TBI 1000 cGy[a], TBI 1200–1575 cGy[b] (Cy/TBI)
TBI 1320 cGy[b], etoposide 60 mg/kg
Melphalan 110 mg/m², TBI 950–1050 cGy[a]
Cytosine arabinoside 24 g/m², TBI 1125 cGy[b]
Busulfan 16 mg/kg, Cy 120 or 200 mg/kg (Bu/Cy)
Cy 6000 mg/m², etoposide 750 mg/m², BCNU 300 mg/m² (CBV)
BCNU 300 mg/m², etoposide 400 mg/m², melphalan 140 mg/m², cytosine arabinoside 800 mg/m² (BEAM)
Cy 5625 mg/m², cisplatin 165 mg/m², BCNU 600 mg/m² (STAMP I)

Cy = cyclophosphamide; TBI = total body irradiation; BCNU = bischloroethylnitrosurea.
[a]Single-dose TBI.
[b]Fractionated TBI.

Table 102.2 Examples of conditioning regimens used for HSCT.

recent cloning of genes for many cytokines, cell surface receptors, and their ligands promises much in this regard. Much work to date has focused on cytokine molecules. Although a great deal is known about their individual and combined actions in cell culture systems, much still remains to be learned about their clinical utility. Potential useful effects include stimulation of proliferation, differentiation, and function of hematopoietic and immune elements. To date, cytokines have been given primarily to hasten hematopoietic engraftment after transplant. GM-CSF[12] or G-CSF accelerate granulocyte recovery, reduce infections, and shorten hospitalizations and may favorably affect the usually poor outcome of patients with graft failure.[13] G-CSF and GM-CSF are well-tolerated agents, and concerns that GVHD and relapse rates would increase have not been demonstrated with these two factors. Factors evaluated for enhancing platelet recovery – including interleukin-3 (IL-3), IL-6, stem-cell factor, IL-11, and thrombopoietin – have had relatively weak effects after HSCT. Immunomodulating agents such as IL-2 and alpha-interferon have been given after transplant to try to prevent relapse. Flt-3 ligand is an interesting new molecule under investigation for various activities including stimulation of dendritic cell populations.

CLINICAL RESULTS OF MARROW GRAFTING

This section on specific diseases deals mainly with results of allogeneic transplants from HLA-matched sibling donors and with autologous transplants. A comparison of outcomes after conventional chemotherapy and allogeneic HSCT for hematological malignancies is shown in Table 102.3.

Acute myeloid leukemia (AML)

Initially allogeneic HSCT was used as a last resort for patients with refractory leukemia. Figure 102.1 shows long-term survival of the first 110 patients with refractory acute leukemia transplanted in Seattle[14] with follow-ups now at 28 years. Of 54

Comparison of allogeneic HSCT and conventional chemotherapy in treatment of hematological malignancies[a]

	HSCT		Chemotherapy[b]
	Disease-free survival (%)	Relapse (%)	Disease-free survival (%)
AML			
CR1[c]	50	22	20–30
First relapse/CR2	25–34	45	<10
Refractory	15	80	Incurable
ALL			
CR1[c]	54	35	40 (adults)
CR2	35	45	<5
Refractory	15	80	Incurable
CML			
Chronic phase	58	17	Incurable
Accelerated phase	30	45	Incurable
Blast crisis	15	70	Incurable
Myelodysplasia			
No excess blasts	54	<10	Incurable
With excess blasts	31	49	Incurable
Lymphoma (HD, aggressive NHL)			
CR2[c]	40	20	<10
Refractory[c]	15	70–80	Incurable

[a]Data mainly from references cited in this review. These do not necessarily reflect all reported outcomes.
[b]Patients failing conventional chemotherapy almost always die of leukemia.
[c]Similar disease-free survivals have been shown with autologous BMT, but relapse rates are higher.
AML = acute myeloid leukemia; ALL = acute lymphoblastic leukemia; CML = chronic myeloid leukemia; HD = Hodgkin's disease; NHL = nonHodgkin lymphoma; CR = complete remission.

Table 102.3 Comparison of allogeneic HSCT and conventional chemotherapy in treatment of hematological malignancies.[a]

Long-term survival after allogenic HSCT for refractory acute leukemia

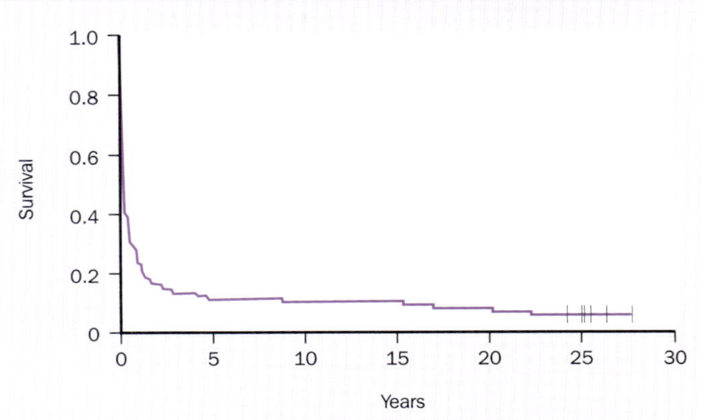

Figure 102.1 Kaplan–Meier estimates of disease-free survival showing long-term follow-up of 110 patients after allografting for refractory acute leukemia (54 AML patients and 56 ALL patients). Patients were given Cy and 10 Gy single-dose TBI followed by HLA-identical sibling marrow transplant. Seattle data[21] updated as of 2000. Late deaths were due to toxicities, not relapse.

patients with AML transplanted in Seattle before 1975, 4 were surviving 26–28 years later. The actuarial relapse rate was 65%. Survival improved in 132 subsequent patients[15] with a 34% 3-year survival for those grafted in untreated first relapse or second remission (Fig. 102.2) but only 24% for those grafted in resistant first relapse. In patients who never achieved a first remission, 21% long-term survivals and a relapse rate of 60% were reported.[16] In 1976 the Seattle Group began transplants for AML in first remission. Better results were expected because of a lower leukemia burden, less resistant disease, and patients in better condition to tolerate transplant. Results confirmed this with 12

Survival after allogeneic BMT for AML

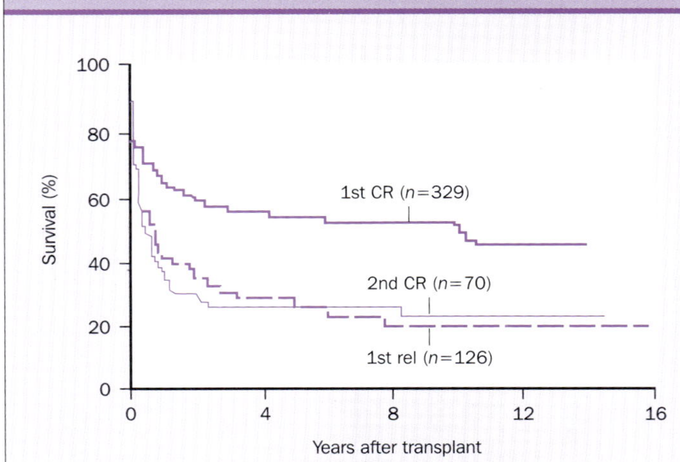

Figure 102.2 Survival after allogeneic BMT for AML. Outcome is dependent on disease stage at transplant with no difference between patients transplanted in first relapse or in second remission. Seattle data[22,32] as of 1993.

of the first 22 patients surviving 18–20 years after grafting. By 1986, 231 patients had been transplanted in Seattle with a 49% 3-year survival and a 25% relapse rate. Subsequent data from 329 patients have shown similar results (Fig. 102.2), as have reports from other transplant centers.[17–19]

An alternative to allografting is autologous HSCT. Autografting reports have shown 50% survivals at 2 years for AML in first remission, and 30% for AML in second remission,[20,21] results similar to those of allografting. However, many autografting recipients were treated late after their remissions were achieved, possibly selecting for patients with less aggressive disease and those already curved by chemotherapy. Regardless, these results are encouraging and suggest that in many cases the infused marrow lacks sufficient clonogenic leukemic cells to cause relapse. The value of marrow 'purging' to remove residual leukemia cells remains uncertain. Delayed engraftment, common after autografting for AML, is exacerbated after marrow manipulations to remove leukemia cells. The use of PBSC autografts may alleviate engraftment issues, but does not appear to improve overall outcomes.

The optimal timing of HSCT for AML remains controversial. Prospective studies comparing allografting and conventional chemotherapy for AML in first remission have shown advantages of transplantation.[22–24] However, transplant mortality may reach 25%, and 25–30% of patients may have been already cured by chemotherapy.[22–25] The two best approaches appear to be HSCT in first remission or in early first relapse. The latter allows for possible curve by chemotherapy and spares the patient risks associated with reinduction chemotherapy. Tumor cytogenetics and leukemia immunophenotypes are increasingly used to define prognosis and refine the timing of HSCT.

Acute lymphoblastic leukemia (ALL)

As for AML, allografting was first employed in ALL patients with advanced disease.[14] Of 56 patients transplanted in Seattle, 3 were alive between 25 and 28 years later (Fig. 102.1). The actuarial relapse rate was 75%. Data from the International Bone Marrow Transplant Registry (IBMTR) have showed relapse-free survivals of approximately 18% for patients treated in relapse.[1] Allografting in patients who failed to achieve a first remission led to a 23% survival and 59% relapse rate.[16] Results were better when marrow grafts were carried out in remission.[1, 18, 19, 26, 27] Overall, about 30% of patients transplanted in second remission were long-term survivors with a 50–60% relapse probability and with older age being an adverse prognostic feature.[27] Survival for patients transplanted in first remission has varied from 25% to 60%, with relapses at 20–40%. This variation might reflect differences in patients selected for transplant. After autografting, long-term survival has been reported to be 10–20% in second remission patients and 50% in first remission patients.[28] Often the marrow has been treated with monoclonal antibodies directed against lymphoid surface antigens to remove residual leukemia cells.

In children with ALL, the excellent results of conventional chemotherapy mean that HSCT is reserved for relapsed patients or first remission patients with adverse risk factors for chemotherapy failure. HSCT was superior to chemotherapy in children who relapsed[29] except for those who relapsed long after stopping chemotherapy.[30] In adults, conventional therapy leads to cure rates of 30–40%, significantly less than in children.[31, 32]

Again, HSCT is reserved for relapsed disease or first remission patients with adverse risk factors for relapse.

Chronic myelocytic leukemia (CML)

CML is a stem cell disorder, thus most interest has focused on allogeneic transplantation with little evidence to date that autologous transplants are curative. Results of allografting for CML in blast crisis were similar to those with advanced acute leukemia: long-term survival was approximately 15% and relapse rates were 50–75%.[33–35] Transplantation in the accelerated phase resulted in disease-free survivals of 15–30% with relapse rates of 40–50%. Subsequent studies showed that CML is significantly more sensitive to transplant conditioning regimens while in chronic phase. In 1976 the Seattle team began transplants in patients with syngeneic donors, and 12 of 19 patients were alive without evidence of CML 1–11.5 (median 8) years later. These results encouraged allogeneic transplantation from HLA-identical siblings.[33,34] Initial results showed 7–12-year disease-free survivals of 50% with actuarial probabilities of relapse of up to 30%.[36] With improved supportive care and better prevention of GVHD,[37] these figures have improved[38] (Fig. 102.3). A comparison between conditioning with BU/Cy and Cy/TBI showed no significant differences in event-free survivals.[39]

Although HSCT is the only curative treatment for CML, some patients treated with alpha-interferon may have a prolonged chronic phase and achieve sustained cytogenetic remissions. STI-571, a new drug that specifically targets the tyrosine kinase activity of the *bcr-abl* rearrangement, appears more effective than currently used conventional treatments. Patients may remain well with minimal treatment for long periods, thus the timing of HSCT remains a difficult question. Patients under 50 years of age with HLA-matched sibling donors should have transplant undertaken during the chronic phase. Results are best when transplants are performed within one year of diagnosis when greater than 80% of patients survive 6 years, 60–70% become relapse-free survivors, and transplant mortality is no more than 10%.[38]

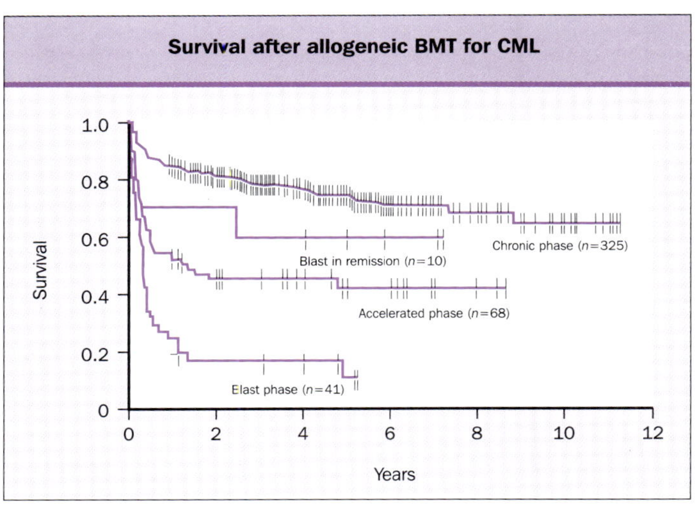

Figure 102.3 Survival after allogeneic BMT for CML according to disease stage at transplant. Patients were transplanted after 1985 with currently used regimens. (Reproduced with permission from Clift RA and Storb R. Marrow transplantation for CML: The Seattle experience. *Bone Marrow Transplant* 1996;17:S1.)

Chronic lymphocytic leukemia (CLL)

CLL is considered a disease of the elderly and is incurable with conventional therapy. Younger patients are encountered for whom the only potential cure is HSCT. CLL is usually an indolent form of leukemia, and there is therefore a reluctance to use aggressive strategies early in the disease. Although relatively few transplants have been done for CLL, reports show that sustained remissions can be achieved after allogeneic or autologous HSCT. Results are best in patients with less advanced disease.[40] Autologous transplants appear feasible and effective in patients who achieve disease remissions that minimize tumor involvement of bone marrow.

Lymphoma

Conventional chemotherapy cures a significant proportion of patients with Hodgkin's disease and aggressive nonHodgkin's lymphoma (NHL), and HSCT is usually reserved for relapsed patients. After relapse, most patients cannot be cured by conventional chemotherapy and HSCT is the most effective treatment. Between 1970 and 1985, Seattle transplanted 100 patients with recurrent lymphoma: 5-year disease-free survival was 22% with a 60% risk of relapse.[41] Patients in first relapse or second remission had a 2-year disease-free survival of 42% and a relapse rate of 41%, significantly better than for refractory lymphoma. Subsequent reports from other centers have shown similar outcomes for NHL. A prospective randomized study has shown that autologous transplants are superior to conventional therapy for treatment of relapsed NHL (Fig. 102.4).[42] Patients who are at high risk of relapse may benefit from transplant in first remission. Lower relapse rates are found in allograft recipients than in autograft recipients, suggesting a graft-versus-lymphoma effect.[43] However, allografting toxicities have offset gains from reduced relapse risk. In Hodgkin's disease, similar results to those with NHL have been reported, with survivals of 40–50% for good risk patients.[44]

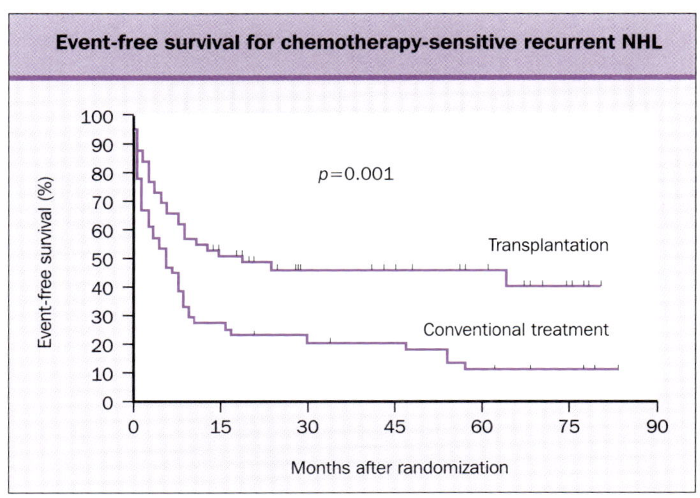

Figure 102.4 Event-free survival for chemotherapy-sensitive recurrent NHL randomized to treatment with high-dose chemotherapy with BCNU, cyclophosphamide, and etoposide (CBV) followed by autologous transplant or to sequential conventional chemotherapy. (Reproduced with permission from Philip T, Guglielmi C, Hagenbeek A, et al. Autologous bone marrow transplantation as compared with salvage chemotherapy in relapses of chemotherapy-sensitive non-Hodgkin's lymphoma. *N Engl J Med* 1995;333:1540.

Low-grade NHL have a long natural history, but are incurable with conventional treatment. In younger patients with progressive disease there is a rationale for HSCT. Most reported studies have involved autografting. It remains unclear whether this approach is curative or provides better survival than conventional therapy. Long-term disease-free survivals of up to approximately 60% have been reported, with patients in remission at time of transplant doing best.[45] A correlation between relapse risk and the presence of residual tumor in the graft has been reported,[46] suggesting the importance of successful marrow purging in this disease and perhaps for autografting as a whole. While allogeneic transplants have been used sparingly, low relapse rates have suggested that low-grade NHL are quite sensitive to GVT effects.

Myelodysplastic syndromes

Myelodysplastic syndromes are a heterogeneous group of clonal marrow failure syndromes found mostly in the elderly and with a predisposition to evolve to refractory AML. Conventional treatment is essentially supportive while allografting is curative in approximately 40% of patients transplanted, most of whom are less than 60 years of age. Best results were in patients with less than 5% marrow blasts, for whom a 54% disease-free survival was found, whereas with higher blast counts disease-free survival was 31% with a 49% relapse rate after transplant.[47]

Multiple myeloma

Myeloma is generally considered to be a chemosensitive tumor but median survival is only approximately 3 years with conventional therapy. A French randomized study established that high-dose chemotherapy followed by autologous transplant was superior to conventional chemotherapy in terms of overall and disease-free survivals.[48] Despite this benefit, high relapse rates were seen after autografting, which is rarely curative. Allografting may produce sustained remissions as survival curves show a plateau after transplant and patients are more likely to become negative by polymerase chain reaction (PCR) for tumor after allografting than after autografting.[49] Unfortunately, allografting for myeloma has been severely limited by a high early mortality risk (rev. 50).

Other hematological malignancies

Marrow grafting has been successful in treating a number of rare diseases including myeloproliferative syndromes, hairy cell leukemia, and hemophagocytic lymphohistiocytosis. Of these, there has been increasing interest recently in the use of HSCT for the treatment of primary myelofibrosis, where cures appear possible.

Solid tumors

High-dose therapy followed by autografting has been tested in chemosensitive solid tumors including neuroblastoma, breast, ovarian, testicular, and brain tumors and small cell lung cancer, usually after failure of other therapy. Results for metastatic disease were poor, with the exception of metastatic neuroblastoma and breast cancer, where some cures were achieved. Large randomized trials have tested high-dose chemotherapy versus conventional therapy as adjuvant therapy for high-risk stages II and III breast cancer after encouraging results in phase II studies.[51] Phase III studies have not yet matured sufficiently to provide a definitive answer.

HSCT from alternative donors

Data from experimental animals and human transplantation have shown best results with marrow from genotypically HLA-identical siblings and that HLA-nonidentity adversely affects engraftment, graft rejection, GVHD, and immune reconstitution. However, because only 20–30% of patients have an HLA-identical sibling, the application of allografting is limited unless other donors can be used.

HLA-nonidentical family members

HLA-nonidentical family donors usually share one HLA haplotype with the patient and are phenotypically matched at 0, 1, 2, or 3 HLA loci on the second haplotype. Transplant-related complications increase commensurate to the degree of HLA-disparity.[52,53] In earlier studies using unmodified bone marrow, the risk of graft rejection was as high as 20% for two-antigen-mismatched transplants. In patients with sustained engraftment, the rate of onset, severity, and overall incidence of acute GVHD were all increased. Recently, modifications of conditioning regimens to include greater immunosuppression combined with the use of CD34-selected PBSC grafts have improved engraftment rates with an acceptable incidence of GVHD in younger patients with HLA-haploidentical family donors. Recipients of phenotypically HLA-identical or one HLA-locus mismatched marrow grafts have similar survival to patients given genotypically HLA-identical grafts despite higher risk of graft failure and of GVHD.[53] This appears to be due to lower relapse rates associated with enhanced GVT effects from the HLA-nonidentical transplants.

Unrelated donors

Canine transplant studies suggested that marrow grafts from phenotypically DLA-identical unrelated donors, while better than those from DLA-haploidentical littermates, do worse than those from genotypically DLA-identical littermates. The clinical experience in humans concurs with those observations.[54] Molecular studies at HLA loci have shown sequence polymorphisms within serologically defined antigens, indicating that the likelihood of finding molecularly HLA-matched unrelated donors is much lower than finding serologically matched donors. Computerization has allowed development of an international database of donors' HLA types, thus facilitating an increasing use of unrelated donors.[1] More than 5 million donors are registered worldwide. Donors are readily found for patients with typical Caucasian HLA haplotypes but less readily for patients with other racial and ethnic backgrounds. Although a significant proportion of unrelated donor marrow recipients achieve prolonged disease-free survival, transplant-related mortality is higher than with matched sibling donors due to an increased incidence and severity of both acute and chronic GVHD.[54] Better matching of donors together with better supportive care improves outcomes through reductions in GVHD and graft rejection (Fig. 102.5).[55] For example, overall 5-year survival for patients with CML was 57%.[56] Amongst patients under age 50 years who were transplanted within 1 year of diagnosis and received prophylactic ganciclovir and fluconazole, 5-year survival was 74%.[56] Apart from increased GVHD risks, major drawbacks of unrelated donor transplants include the lack of suitable donors and the increased time taken to find the donors.

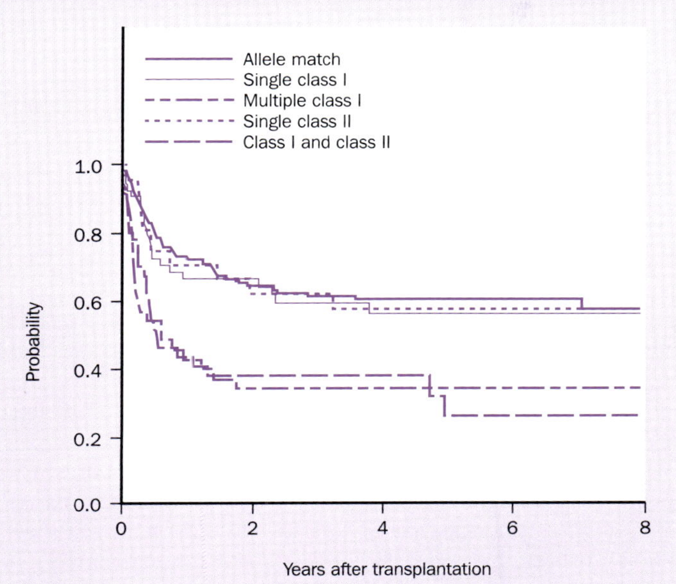

Figure 102.5 Effect of HLA matching on survival after unrelated donor HSCT for CML. Retrospective molecular matching was performed at HLA-A, B, C, DRB1 and DQB1 to resolve HLA differences not detected with serologic typing. Single Class I or Class II differences did not worsen outcomes as compared to fully matched transplants. Greater than one locus mismatched was associated with significantly poorer outcome. (Reproduced with permission from Petersdorf EW, Gooley TA, Anasetti C, et al. Optimizing outcome after unrelated marrow transplantation by comprehensive matching of HLA Class I and II alleles in the donor and recipient. *Blood* 1998;92:3515.)

An alternative for some patients is transplantation of umbilical cord blood. Large banks of HLA-typed cord blood units have recently been established. While used mainly in children,[57] transplants into adults are possible despite small cell numbers infused as compared to marrow and PBSC transplants. Potential advantages of cord blood include less GVHD risk, a relative freedom from transmitted viral pathogens, and rapid availability. Disadvantages include slow engraftment and a significant nonengraftment rate.

KEY CONCEPTS

Clinical results of marrow grafting for malignancy

- Outcomes depend primarily on age, disease, and disease stage.
- Immune-mediated graft-versus-leukemia effect appears important in reducing relapse rates, particularly in advanced leukemia.
- Allografting results in fewer relapses but greater peritransplant mortality than autografting.
- Overall outcomes after allografting and autografting are similar for patients with lymphoma and with acute leukemia in first remission.
- Allografting is the only way to cure CML, myelodysplasia, and multiple myeloma.

CLINICAL PEARLS

Planning transplant

- Patients with advanced malignancy have a high risk of transplant complications and relapse, and thus do poorly.
- Transplant options, including determining possible donors, should be evaluated early in the disease course of patients who are potential future transplant candidates.
- Unrelated donor transplants take months to set up if a donor has not been identified – frequently too long for patients with relapsed leukemia.
- Storage of bone marrow or PBSC while the patient is in remission may facilitate later autologous transplant for relapsed disease.

CURRENT PROBLEMS AND FUTURE APPROACHES

Successful marrow transplantation for malignant diseases requires the following: (1) permanent control of the malignancy, (2) immunological graft–host tolerance with restoration of normal immune responses, (3) stable normal hematopoiesis, (4) recovery of normal performance status with freedom from limiting organ toxicities. Achieving the above ideals requires avoiding toxicities from conditioning regimens, avoiding immunological sequelae from graft rejection and GVHD, and preventing tumor recurrence.

Transplant complications are influenced by age, underlying disease, and pre-existing medical problems. The principal complications of HSCT for leukemia are listed in Table 102.4 and are broadly categorized as follows: (1) toxicity from conditioning regimen, (2) infections due to granulocytopenia and immune depression, (3) immunological problems. The following section deals with recovery from transplant, associated complications, and relapse of malignancy after transplant. Outlined are current therapeutic approaches and some potential future solutions to these problems.

Major complications of allogeneic HSCT – incidence and mortality

Complication	Incidence (%)	Mortality (%)
Graft failure	<5[a]	>80
CMV pneumonia	<5	50
Interstitial pneumonia	3	30–85
Veno-occlusive disease	20	30–47
Acute GVHD	30–50[a]	15[a,b]
Chronic GVHD	17–50[a]	25[a]
Bacterial fungal infection	>50	5[a,b]

[a]Increases with HLA-mismatched/unrelated donors.
[b]Overall mortality.

Table 102.4 Major complications of allogeneic HSCT – incidence and mortality.

Recovery of hematopoiesis and immunity

Recovery to normal granulocyte and platelet levels usually occurs by day 40–50, and to normal hematocrit values by day 60–90. Recovery of monocytes and return of bronchoalveolar and hepatic macrophages are equally prompt. However, prolonged functional impairments may occur including deficient granulocyte chemotaxis, reduced clonogenic precursor numbers in the marrow, and impaired immunity (rev. 58). Hematopoietic elements are usually entirely of donor origin, whereas stromal elements of the marrow microenvironment are of host origin.[59] Some patients show a persistent mixture of donor and host cells known as mixed chimerism. Observations extending for over 25 years have shown stable hematopoiesis. Clonal hematopoiesis, suggesting reconstitution from a small number of pluripotent marrow stem cells, has been reported in animal experiments and in several patients.[60] However, a prospective study of 20 allograft recipients using X-linked clonal analysis techniques showed polyclonal reconstitution in all cases[61] and a recent analysis of patients more than 20 years after allografting also showed polyclonal hematopoiesis. Clonal hematopoiesis may occur more frequently after autografting because prior chemotherapy and/or ex-vivo marrow manipulations may damage or deplete stem cells.

Three components that contribute to the patient's immunologic status after transplantation may provide some protection against infections. First, vestiges of the host's immune system may persist as suggested by detection of host-type isohemagglutinin titers for as long as 12 months in ABO-incompatible graft recipients. Second, donor immune cells may convey 'instant' immune function as shown by transfer of immunity to keyhole-limpet hemocyanin, tetanus toxoid, measles, and diphtheria. Additionally, donor allergy may be transferred with the graft.[62] Finally, lymphocytes maturing from infused stem cells establish a new immune system. For adults in whom thymic function is minimal, most post-transplant T-cell immunity is from memory T-cells transferred with the graft with little production of naive T cells. Regardless of the type of transplant and underlying disease, profound deficits of most immune functions are present during the first 4–5 months. Exceptions include rapidly restored activity of monocyte-macrophages and of cytotoxic effector cells mediating natural killing, antibody-dependent and lectin-dependent killing, all of which are normal after 30 days. In the immediate post-transplant months, peripheral blood B-cell numbers are depressed. CD4-positive T-cell numbers and T-helper functions are also reduced. Concomitant with this is an increase in $CD8^+$ T-cell numbers and T-suppressor activity, and an inversion of the normal peripheral blood CD4:CD8 ratio. Beyond the first 4–5 months, recipients of autologous and syngeneic grafts, and those with allogeneic grafts and no GVHD, show gradual immunologic recovery. GVHD and its treatment can severely retard immune recovery. Some apparently healthy long-term survivors fail to produce appropriate humoral responses to neo- and recall-antigens, and 30–40% of these show persistent in vitro B-cell defects and decreased T-cell helper functions. In survivors with chronic GVHD, antibody responses and immunoglobulin class-switching after antigenic challenge are often defective; in vitro studies show B-cell dysfunction, lack of T-cell help, and, in many cases, T-cell suppression. Despite depressed B-cell immunity, normal or even elevated serum immunoglobulin levels may be found and immunoglobulin subclass deficiencies may be clinically important.

Unsuccessful attempts to hasten immune recovery have included grafts of thymic tissue and thymic epithelial monolayers, and injection of thymosin fraction V and thymopoietin. Recently, cloned CMV-specific donor T-cells restored immunity to CMV in the early post-transplant period,[63] suggesting that infusion of cloned donor T and B cells active against specific pathogens may be a future approach to reducing transplant-related infectious complications. Alternative or supplementary approaches would be to use recombinant cytokines and other immune response modifiers to correct immunological deficits.

Toxicities related to conditioning programs

Conditioning programs have been intensified to a point where serious nonhematopoietic toxicity occurs frequently (Table 102.5). Some effects occur early, are temporary, and do not have late sequelae. Others may persist long after treatment and contribute to late treatment failure (rev. 64). Painful mucositis of varying degrees of severity is common but usually subsides soon after day 14.[65] Similarly, diarrhea is frequent but reversible. The most frequent life-threatening toxicities are pancytopenia, interstitial pneumonitis, and veno-occlusive disease (VOD). Organ damage may contribute to GVHD and opportunistic infections. VOD of the liver is frequently encountered, particularly in patients with pre-existing liver disease.[65] It is caused by the conditioning programs but can be exacerbated by postgrafting immunosuppression with cyclosporine and methotrexate. Damage to endothelium of small liver venules appears to initiate local thrombosis leading to venous obstruction and hepatic dysfunction. Significant VOD may be seen in 15–28% of patients, with a case fatality rate as high as 30%. Attempts to prevent and treat VOD have mainly involved prophylaxis or treatment with anticoagulants. The incidence of idiopathic interstitial pneumonia was 8–10% after conditioning with single-dose TBI, but only 3% with the use of fractionated TBI.[66] Leukoencephalopathy can develop in children with ALL who have had previous cranial irradiation. Endocrine dysfunction

Toxicities associated with conditioning regimens
Early
Pancytopenia
Mucositis
Nausea/vomiting
Diarrhea
Acute myocarditis
Veno-occlusive disease of the liver
Interstitial pneumonia
Leukoencephalopathy
Hemorrhagic cystitis
Acute renal failure
Erythroderma
Alopecia
Late
Infertility
Neuroendocrine dysfunction
Delayed growth and development
Secondary malignancies
Cataracts
Leukoencephalopathy
Renal failure
Osteoporosis
Psychosocial maladjustment

Table 102.5 Toxicities associated with conditioning regimens.

is common including infertility and impaired growth and sexual development in children. Menopause almost invariably permanently occurred in females, and males are almost always infertile, after high-dose conditioning therapy for malignancy. Cataracts occurred in 80% of patients given single-dose TBI but only 18% of those given fractionated TBI. Late solid tumors occur in 6–7% of long-term survivors of HSCT which is approximately 3 times higher than for age-matched controls.[67] Myelodysplastic syndromes are an important severe late side-effect of autologous HSCT, occurring in up to 15% of patients.[68]

Opportunistic infections

Bacterial and fungal infections

Despite improved intensive supportive care including prophylaxis and treatment with potent broad-spectrum antibiotics and antifungal agents, bacterial and fungal infections remain an important cause of mortality, particularly after allografting.[69] Infections occur more frequently after transplants for HLA-nonidentical donors due to a higher incidence of GVHD and the frequent use of high-dose steroids. Furthermore, certain antibiotics and antifungal agents can exacerbate the organ toxicity of the conditioning programs and affect metabolism of immunosuppressive agents such as CSP and FK-506. The use of growth factor-mobilized PBSC grafts has shortened the period of pancytopenia, and after allografting appears to improve outcomes of patients with advanced malignancy, possibly through better control of infections. The use of fluconazole prophylaxis has reduced mortality from fungal infections and is now routine after allografting. Newer lipid preparations of amphotericin have less nephrotoxicity and are an improvement over conventional amphotericin B for treating fungal infections.

Viral and protozoan infections

The most important life-threatening infections during the immediate post-transplant months were of viral origin.[66,69] By far the most important virus is cytomegalovirus (CMV) which manifests itself primarily as pneumonia or gastrointestinal infection. CMV infections occurred in about 75% of CMV-seropositive patients within 3 months of transplant, mostly due to a reactivation of latent virus in host or transfused donor hematopoietic cells. Previously, CMV pneumonia occurred in about 15% of patients transplanted for malignancy and had a case mortality rate of about 85%. CMV infection can be prevented in CMV-seronegative patients who have CMV-seronegative donors by the exclusive use of CMV-seronegative blood products, or by use of leukocyte-depleted blood products. In other patients, ganciclovir is used as prophylaxis against CMV or started in response to detection of CMV reactivation by sensitive tests such as the antigenemia assay[70] or PCR, which effectively prevents most cases of overt clinical disease. Active CMV infections remain difficult to treat and only 50% of patients with CMV pneumonia respond to ganciclovir and immunoglobulin, the best available treatment.[71] Reactivation of herpes simplex virus immediately after grafting was common but is readily prevented with acyclovir. Varicella zoster infections, seen in approximately 40% of all patients, are treatable with acyclovir, and prevention studies with low-dose acyclovir are under way. *Pneumocystis carinii* infection, which formerly caused about 10% of interstitial pneumonias, can be prevented with prophylactic trimethoprim–sulfamethoxazole or pentamidine.

Immunological problems

Graft failure

After allografting, graft failure due to immunologic rejection is rare in recipients of unmodified HLA-identical sibling marrow or PBSC (<1% incidence). However, poor graft function is not uncommon and may be due to drug toxicity, e.g methotrexate, trimethoprim–sulfamethoxazole, interferon, ganciclovir, etc., or related to certain infections, e.g. CMV. When incriminating drugs are discontinued and/or recovery from viral infection occurs, graft function usually recovers. Persistent poor graft function is associated with poor outcome, and growth factors may improve outcomes.[13]

Graft failure from immunologic rejection occurs primarily after transplants from HLA-nonidentical donors[52] and/or when T-cell depleted marrow HSC grafts are used.[72] While graft rejection frequently leads to a fatal pancytopenia, some patients have autologous hematopoietic recovery and others may be salvaged with an emergency second transplant.

Understanding the mechanisms of graft failure is important in designing ways to overcome the problem. Canine studies implicated radioresistant non T cells in destruction of DLA-nonidentical marrow grafts, while T cells appeared to mediate rejection of DLA-identical grafts. While donor T cells appear important in facilitating allogeneic engraftment, it is unclear whether the same cells cause GVHD. Clinically, more intensive conditioning programs, including the addition of total lymphoid irradiation, reduce the incidence of graft rejection, but increased regimen-related toxicities may negate this advantage. Augmenting conditioning regimens with antibodies such as antithymocyte globulin (ATG) and anti-CD44, directed at immune cells, is being investigated. In canine studies neither G-CSF nor c-kit ligand given alone or in combination was able to prevent graft rejection.

After autologous transplants, particularly those for AML, problems with hematopoietic recovery are common and prolonged thrombocytopenia results in hemorrhagic fatality more frequently than after allogeneic transplants. Factors that may contribute to this problem include previous intensive chemotherapy, ex-vivo purging with cytotoxic agents and a clonal (possibly premalignant) marrow. The use of PBSC may reduce the risk of poor engraftment.

Acute GVHD (rev. 73–75)

Pathophysiology

Acute GVHD appears to be mediated by donor T cells reacting against non-MHC histocompatibility antigens presented by host antigen-presenting cells or alternatively directed against both non-MHC and MHC antigens when HLA incompatibility exists. While cytotoxic lymphocytes are the major effector mechanism in GVHD, cytokine elaboration also appears to play an important role in pathogenesis. Studies to date point to a complex series of cellular interactions generating a cascade of cytokine release. Cytokines may mediate tissue damage, drive effector cells of GVHD, and modulate the state of immunosuppression accompanying GVHD.[75] Different factors may operate at different times in the genesis of GVHD. For example, T cells requiring IL-2 appear to be active early in GVHD and may release cytokines that drive effector cells such as monocytes, macrophages, and natural killer cells. This may lead to further elaboration of cytokines such as tumor necrosis factor alpha (TNF-α), IL-1, IL-3, GM-CSF, and interferon gamma (IFN-γ) which sustain inflammation and cause tissue damage. Immunodeficiency may be mediated by factors such as transforming growth factor beta, prostaglandin E_2, and IFN-β which promote T-suppressor activity. Based on the proposed pathogenesis of GVHD, some investigators have tried to treat GVHD with specific antagonists to the implicated cytokines.

Clinical features

The clinical and histological criteria for acute GVHD have been described in detailed reviews.[73,74] There is a considerable range of severity, and a commonly used modification of the original Seattle clinical grading system is summarized in Table 102.6. Target organs are skin, gastrointestinal tract, and liver, and diagnosis usually depends on excluding concurrent toxicities from drugs, conditioning regimen and infection, often through biopsies of involved tissues. The principal risk factors for developing GVHD are listed in Table 102.7. Between 20% and 50% of patients given unmodified marrow grafts from HLA-identical siblings develop significant acute GVHD as a life-threatening complication. In 231 patients with AML transplanted in first remission in Seattle, clinically significant GVHD was associated with a 2.5 times higher risk of fatality.[15] Death is often due to infections, for which GVHD predisposes by creating portals of entry through lesions in skin and intestinal tract and through requirements for intensified immune suppression to treat GVHD. Prevention of infection by decontamination and laminar airflow room isolation can decrease the incidence and delay the onset of acute GVHD and increase survival.[73] Decontamination may prevent a process in which infections cause lymphocytes to secrete lymphokines, which in turn may increase the expression of Class II histocompatibility antigens on certain target cells, e.g. gut epithelium, thereby making them targets for GVHD. However, the practical difficulties and cost of decontaminating patients have limited enthusiasm for continued attempts to sterilize patients and their transplant rooms.

Major risk factors for developing GVHD

Acute	Chronic
HLA disparity	HLA disparity
Unrelated donor	Unrelated donor
Advanced malignancy	Preceding acute GVHD
Parous female donor	Increasing patient age
Increasing patient/donor age	CMV infection
Irradiation dose	

Table 102.7 Major risk factors for developing GVHD.

Clinical assessment of acute GVHD

1. Organ staging

Organ	Stage	Abnormality
Skin	1	Rash <25% BSA
	2	Rash 25–50% BSA
	3	Rash >50% BSA or generalized erythroderma
	4	Generalized erythroderma with bullae, desquamation
Liver	1	Total bilirubin 2–3 mg/dl
	2	Total bilirubin 3–6 mg/dl
	3	Total bilirubin 6–15 mg/dl
	4	Total bilirubin >15 mg/dl
Gut[a]	1	Diarrhea 500–1000 ml/24 hours
	2	Diarrhea 1000–1500 ml/24 hours
	3	Diarrhea >1500 ml/24 hours
	4	Diarrhea >1500 ml/24 hours plus severe abdominal pain, or ileus

2. Overall grade

Grade	Organ stage[b]					Performance status
	Skin		Gut		Liver	
I	1–2		0		0	Normal
II	1–3		1	and/or	1	Normal/reduced
III[c]	2–4		2–4	and/or	2–4	Moderately reduced
IV[d]	2–4	and/or	2–4	and/or	2–4	Severely reduced

BSA = body surface area.
[a]Upper gastrointestinal GVHD diagnosed if positive biopsy and nausea, anorexia or vomiting.
[b]Clinical stage.
[c]One organ system ≥ stage 3.
[d]Two or more systems ≥ stage 3.

Table 102.6 Clinical assessment of acute GVHD. (Modified from Glucksberg H, et al. *Transplantation* 1974; 18:295.)

Prevention of acute GVHD

Prevention of GVHD usually involves the temporary use of postgrafting immunosuppressive drugs. Most commonly used are cyclosporine, methotrexate, and corticosteroids, either alone or in combination (see Table 102.8 below). In contrast to patients with solid organ transplants, marrow graft recipients usually do not require indefinite immunosuppressive treatment. Immunosuppressive agents can often be discontinued 3–6 months after grafting when a stable state of graft–host tolerance has been reached. It is not entirely clear what maintains transplantation tolerance although specific suppressor cells of donor origin may be involved.[76] Omission of GVHD prophylaxis results in an unacceptably high incidence of acute GVHD and poor outcomes.[77] Prospective randomized trials showed methotrexate and cyclosporine to be equally effective in preventing GVHD; a combination of these two drugs was superior to either drug alone and is a commonly used prophylactic regimen.[78] For patients at low risk of relapse, outcomes were better with improved GVHD control[79] but, for aggressive malignancy, benefits of well-controlled GVHD are balanced in the long-term by increased relapse rates as illustrated in Figure 102.6.[37] While acute GVHD is lessened, the incidence of chronic GVHD does not appear to be reduced (Fig. 102.6). FK506 functions similarly to cyclosporine as a T-cell activation blocker, and randomized trials suggested similar or enhanced efficacy to CSP for GVHD prevention. Mycophenolate mofetil, an antimetabolite, has enhanced efficacy and possibly less toxicity than methotrexate and is currently being tested in combination with cyclosporine. Newer approaches being tested involving costimulation blockade by using CTLA4-IG and/or anti-CD40 ligand are theoretically very attractive because specific donor–host tolerance might be induced without broadly suppressing donor immunity.

Effect of GVHD prophylaxis after allogeneic BMT with HLA-identical sibling donors

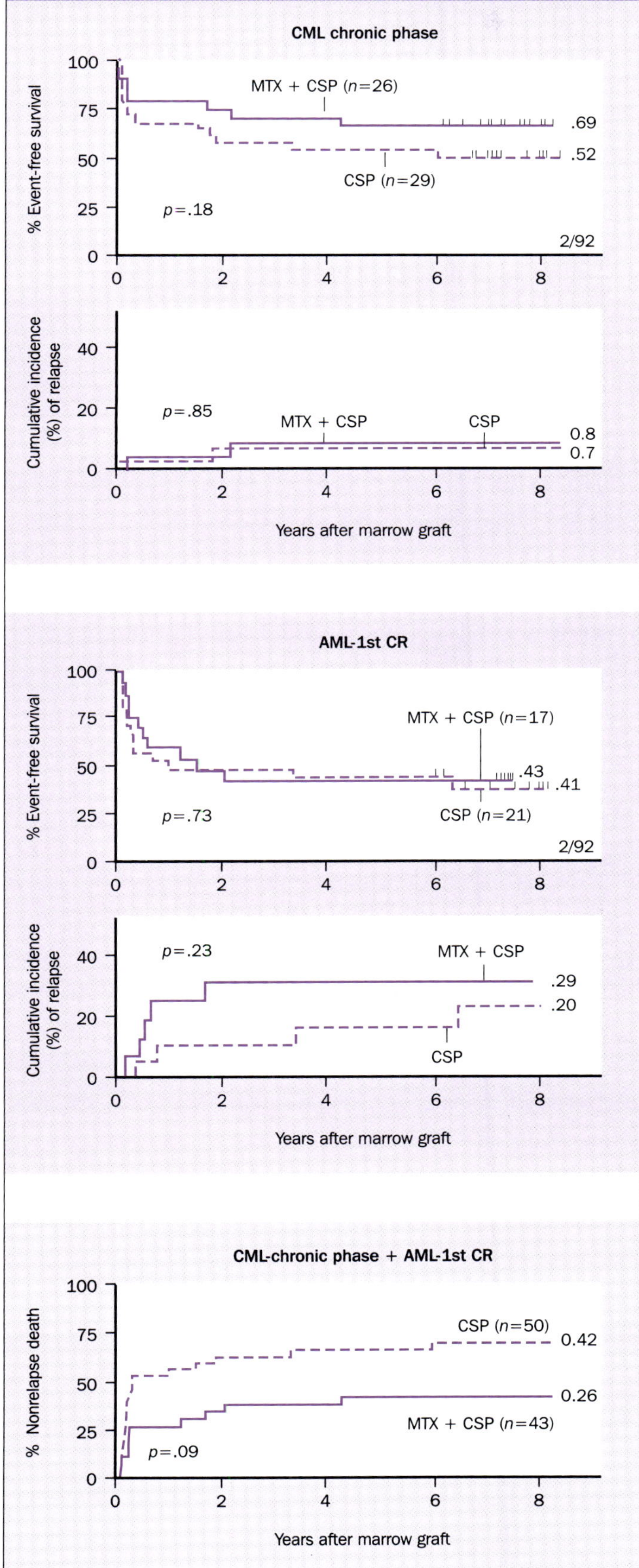

Figure 102.6 Effect of GVHD prophylaxis on outcomes after allogeneic BMT with HLA-identical sibling donors. Top panels show Kaplan–Meier event-free survival curves among patients with CML and AML. The center panels show cumulative incidence curves for relapse, and the bottom panel cumulative incidence curves for transplant-related mortality. (Reproduced with permission from Storb R, Pepe M, Deeg HJ, et al. Long-term follow-up of a controlled trial comparing a combination of methotrexate plus cyclosporine with cyclosporine alone for prophylaxis of graft-versus-host disease in patients administered HLA-identical marrow grafts for leukemia [Letter]. *Blood* 1992;80:560.)

Another strategy for GVHD prevention involves removal of T cells from the HSC graft, studies of which have delineated the role of T cells in allogeneic HSCT. Removal from the graft of virtually all differentiated T cells should result in return of the cellular immune system to an early prenatal state. Assuming normal thymic function, newly produced immune cells would accept the host antigenic environment as 'self' and become tolerant. T-cells depletion has worked well in preventing GVHD but has been associated with increased incidence of graft rejection, recurrent malignancy, and infections.[72] For patients given HLA-identical marrow, nearly all studies have demonstrated a significant reduction in acute GVHD if at least a 1.5 log T cell depletion is achieved, regardless of the technique used. Significant GVHD was seen in 11% of HLA-identical marrow graft recipients and only 28% of HLA-nonidentical recipients. However, the incidence of graft rejection in HLA-identical recipients increased from less than 1% to 10–20% and in HLA-nonidentical recipients from 5% to 35%. An increased risk of leukemic relapse following T-cell depletion appears due to a lack of GVT effects. A recent approach to overcoming rejection with haploidentical grafts involves transplanting high doses of CD34-selected (T-cell depleted) PBSC. This has been successfully employed in young patients with hematologic maligancies.[80]

Because graft rejection and leukemic relapse are often fatal complications, improved survival in patients given T-cell depleted HSCT from HLA-matched sibling donors has not been realized. Improved results with T-cell depletion are likely to come from two main approaches. One is through improved pretransplant conditioning programs leading to significantly better eradication of host malignant and immune cells. The second approach relies on the hypothesis that T cells causing GVHD are distinct from those that mediate engraftment and GVL effects. This might allow selective removal and/or addition of T-cell subpopulations to the graft that would facilitate engraftment and GVL activity, yet preserve the advantages of T-cell depletion in preventing GVHD. Initial attempts to study this have included clinical trials using selective depletion of specific T-cell populations from the HSC grafts.

Treatment of established acute GVHD

Based in part on animal studies, treatment of acute GVHD has been tried in humans with prednisone, antithymocyte globulin (ATG), cyclosporine, and monoclonal antibodies directed against T cells. Agents that block cytokine mediators of GVHD such as IL-2, TNF-α, and IL-1 have also been tested. Additionally, some agents may target specific organs affected by GVHD. PUVA has been used for skin GVHD, oral beclomethasone for gastrointestinal disease, and ursodeoxycholic acid for liver disease. The development of grade 2 or greater GVHD (Table 102.6) is

Agents used alone or in combination for prophylaxis and treatment of GVHD
Prophylaxis
Methotrexate
Cyclosporine
FK506
Mycophenolate mofetil
Prednisone
T-cell depletion
Selective T-cell depletion (CD8 or CD6)
Antithymocyte globulin
Monoclonal antibodies
Treatment
Prednisone
Cyclosporine
FK-506
Mycophenolate mofetil
Antithymocyte globulin
Cyclophosphamide
Azathioprine
Monoclonal antibodies, e.g. anti-CD3, anti-IL-2 receptor
Thalidomide
Psoralen ultraviolet A-range therapy
Topical corticosteroids (skin, gastrointestinal tract)
Investigational
Rapamycin
Anti-TNF antibody
Soluble IL-1 receptor antagonist
Deoxyspergualin
T-cell co-stimulation blockers, e.g. CTLA4-Ig, anti-CD40 ligand
Other monoclonal antibodies

Table 102.8 Agents used alone or in combination for prophylaxis and treatment of GVHD.

usually an indication for treatment. First-line systemic treatment of acute GVHD should be with methylprednisolone at a dose of 1–2 mg/kg, which appears more effective than other strategies.[81] Cyclosporine dose can usually be optimized by monitoring blood levels and renal function. Failure of GVHD to respond to first-line therapy indicates a need for additional therapy with ATG, higher steroid doses, or the newer agents in Table 102.8. In general, failure to respond to initial therapy has adverse prognostic implications and is associated with poor outcome.[81]

Chronic GVHD (rev. 73,74,82)

Pathophysiology

The major histological findings in tissues affected by chronic GVHD are epithelial injury, mononuclear cell infiltrates, and fibrosis. Clinically it resembles autoimmune systemic collagen vascular diseases such as scleroderma, Sjögren syndrome, and primary biliary cirrhosis. Manifestations include skin lesions, keratoconjunctivitis, buccal mucositis, esophageal and vaginal strictures, intestinal involvement, chronic liver disease, generalized wasting, sinus disease, and pulmonary insufficiency. T cells present in the donor marrow appear to be responsible for initiating this disease. A profound immunodeficiency accompanies chronic GVHD, and infection is the most common cause of death. Thymus, lymph nodes, and spleen show atrophy and hypocellularity. Circulating CD4 T cells are reduced as is IL-2 production by T cells. Increased numbers of circulating CD8 cells are present and T-suppressor activity is increased. Antibody responses are abnormal as a result of defective T-cell helper function, B-cell defects, or both.

Clinical features

Chronic GVHD occurs after 30–50% of HLA-matched sibling transplants with a higher incidence after mismatched-related or unrelated donor transplants. Manifestations vary from mild to severe, and while median onset is 4 months post transplant, it may occur as early as 70 days and as late as 15 months after transplantation. Acute GVHD predicts a high incidence of chronic GVHD, as does increasing patient age. In a retrospective analysis of data from the IBMTR, the 3-year probability of developing chronic GVHD was 28%, 49%, 59%, 80% and 85% for patients experiencing acute GVHD of grade 0, 1, 2, 3 and 4, respectively.[83] Thrombocytopenia (platelets less than 100 000/μl) is an adverse risk factor for treatment failure.[84] The mode of onset has prognostic value: patients who have de novo disease (no previous acute GVHD) do better than those with quiescent disease (previous acute GVHD having resolved). Patients with progressive disease, where acute GVHD merges into chronic GVHD, have the worst prognosis.[84] Untreated, chronic GVHD has a poor prognosis, and most patients die or become disabled. The most effective treatment is prednisone given alone or combined with cyclosporine.[84] A number of the agents listed in Table 102.8 have been used with variable success. For severe GVHD, prolonged therapy with combinations of drugs may be required. With current therapy, approximately half of the patients with extensive chronic GVHD are living with Karnofsky performance scores of 100%, and an additional 25% with scores of between 80% and 90%. In about half of the patients, therapy can be discontinued after 9–12 months. Despite improvements in treatment, the management of chronic GVHD remains unsatisfactory and 25% of affected patients die with infections, mainly from encapsulated gram-positive bacteria.

Relationship between GVHD and tumor recurrence: graft-versus-tumor effect

Many cures after allogeneic transplants appear to be due to graft-versus-leukemia (GVL) effects, immune reactions directed at normal and possibly leukemia-specific antigens expressed by the patient's leukemic cells. Initial support for this hypothesis came from animal studies, retrospective analyses of relapse rates in

CLINICAL PEARLS

Evaluation and treatment of GVHD

- Obtain histologic confirmation of GVHD whenever possible.
- Exclude and treat coexisting infections, especially CMV.
- Conditioning and drug toxicities are frequently difficult to separate clinically from GVHD, especially early after transplant.
- Prednisone is most effective primary therapy but avoid prolonged high-dose steroid therapy due to infectious and other complications.
- Consider organ-specific therapies e.g. topical steroids, PUVA, to spare use of systemic therapy.
- Consider newer agents such as monoclonal antibodies against T-cells, MMF, and rapamycin to spare toxicities from steroids or CSP.
- Fungal infections occur frequently after prolonged therapy for GVHD.

Graft-versus-leukemia effect

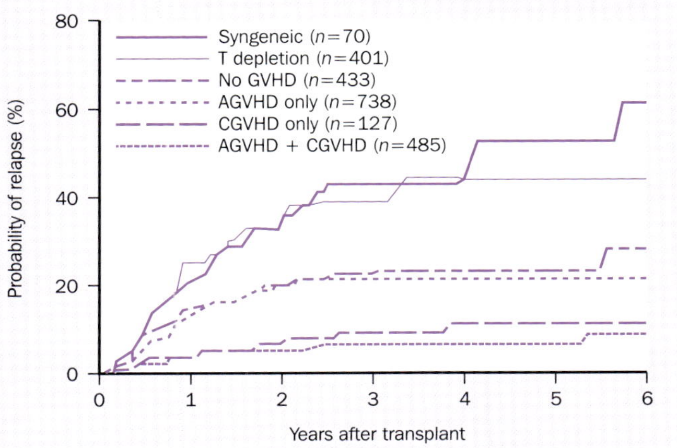

Figure 102.7 Graft-versus-leukemia effect Actuarial probability of relapse after HLA-identical sibling donor allogeneic BMT for good risk leukemia (ALL, AML in 1st remission, CML in chronic phase). Effect of (1) graft status (syngeneic, T-cell-depleted) and (2) development of acute and chronic GVHD. (Adapted with permission from Horowitz MM, Gale RP, Sondel PM, et al. Graft-versus-leukemia reactions after bone marrow transplantation. *Blood* 1990;75:555.)

patients with and without GVHD, and occasional clinical observations of active GVHD resulting in leukemia regression. Similar observations to suggest graft-versus-tumor (GVT) effects were also made in lymphoma and myeloma patients. In leukemia patients who survived at least 150 days after grafting, the likelihood of sustained remission was significantly higher in allogeneic recipients with acute or chronic GVHD than in those without GVHD or than in syngeneic recipients.[85] The impact on relapse of GVHD and the immunologic status of the graft is further illustrated in data from the IBMTR as shown in Figure 102.7.[86]

These data suggested that certain donor T cells can eliminate host leukemic cells. Direct evidence for this has come from studies that used donor leukocyte infusions (DLI) to treat malignancy that relapsed after allografting.[87] New strategies of nonmyeloblative stem cell transplantation attempt to exploit GVT effect as the primary antitumor modality (see later section). Murine studies suggested that GVT effects may be distinguished from GVHD in that some donor cells react specifically with surface antigens expressed on leukemic cells while others react more broadly with minor histocompatibility antigens expressed on host tissue.[88] Clinical GVT effects in the absence of clinical GVHD have been observed in some human patients but reliable methods for inducing such effects have not been developed. As suggested by some studies in murine models, it might be possible to expand in vitro donor T cells or specific T cells clones sensitized to tumor antigens, infuse these into the patients, and use IL-2 to potentiate cytotoxic antitumor function.

Nonmyeloablative stem cell transplants

The term 'nonmyeloablative' implies that conditioning therapy will not cause irreversible marrow suppression if the regimen is given without HSCT. Recent years have seen a remarkable change in allografting practice and theory with the testing of reduced-intensity nonmyeloablative regimens aimed not so much at disease eradication but at establishing engraftment of donor cells. Permanent eradication of malignancy is ultimately achieved by GVT reactions. Some investigators have used relatively intensive conventional chemotherapy while others have used attenuated conventional transplant regimens.[88–91] Fludarabine was used in many of these regimens because of its potent immunosuppressive properties at relatively non-toxic doses. The reduced toxicity of these approaches allows transplants in patients previously excluded due to older age or medical contraindications. To date, CML, CLL, and low-grade NHL have appeared very sensitive to GVT effects induced by these transplants.

Important principles leading to a well-tolerated clinical protocol were developed in preclinical canine studies.[90] In transplants from DLA-identical matched sibling donors, post grafting immunosuppression with a combination of cyclosporine and mycophenolate mofetil allowed stable engraftment as mixed chimerism after only 200 cGy of TBI, 720 cGy less than the TBI dose required without postgrafting immunosuppression (Fig. 102.8). Further, the dogs became stable mixed chimeras with minimal or no GVHD. Translation of this protocol to the clinic demonstrated successful engraftment in most patients with only mild myelosuppression, and powerful GVT reactions developed in some patients leading to complete molecular remissions.[91]

Recurrence of malignancy

Recurrent malignancy after HSCT is a frequent cause of treatment failure, occurring in 20–80% of cases depending on the disease and disease-stage of transplant. Almost always this means reappearance of the original tumor clone. Rarely, leukemia recurrences have involved donor-type cells, a poorly understood phenomenon. A small number of patients develop B-cell immunoblastic lymphomas in donor cells, usually after T-depleted transplants or treatment with monoclonal antibodies for steroid-resistant GVHD.[64,93] These are usually Epstein–Barr virus (EBV) driven B-cell lymphomas similar to those in AIDS and solid organ transplant recipients. Their occurrence suggests a more profound, more severe disturbance of T-cell function than usual in these patients.

While recurrent malignancy is usually detected by routine laboratory evaluation or imaging techniques, newer more sensitive methods of detection include multiparameter flow cytometry and PCR, which has a sensitivity far exceeding other techniques. Under optimal conditions PCR can detect one tumor cell in 10^5 or 10^6 normal cells. Tumor-specific markers include chimeric DNA or RNA sequences derived from chromosomal translocations or rearranged antigen receptor genes (which generate clone-specific unique sequences). PCR can detect recurrence of malignancy well before overt relapse[94,95] raising the prospect of testing post-transplant interventions before this occurs.

Recurrent malignancy usually has a poor prognosis with short survival. Second transplants have resulted in a high rate of severe regimen-induced toxicities. Nonetheless, some children and adults with CML have benefited from second transplants, possibly due to induction of effective GVT reactions.

Evidence of GVT effects, together with high mortality from second transplants, encouraged the testing of donor lymphocyte infusion (DLI) to treat relapses. At relapse, T cells are usually still of donor origin which allows additional donor cells to be given

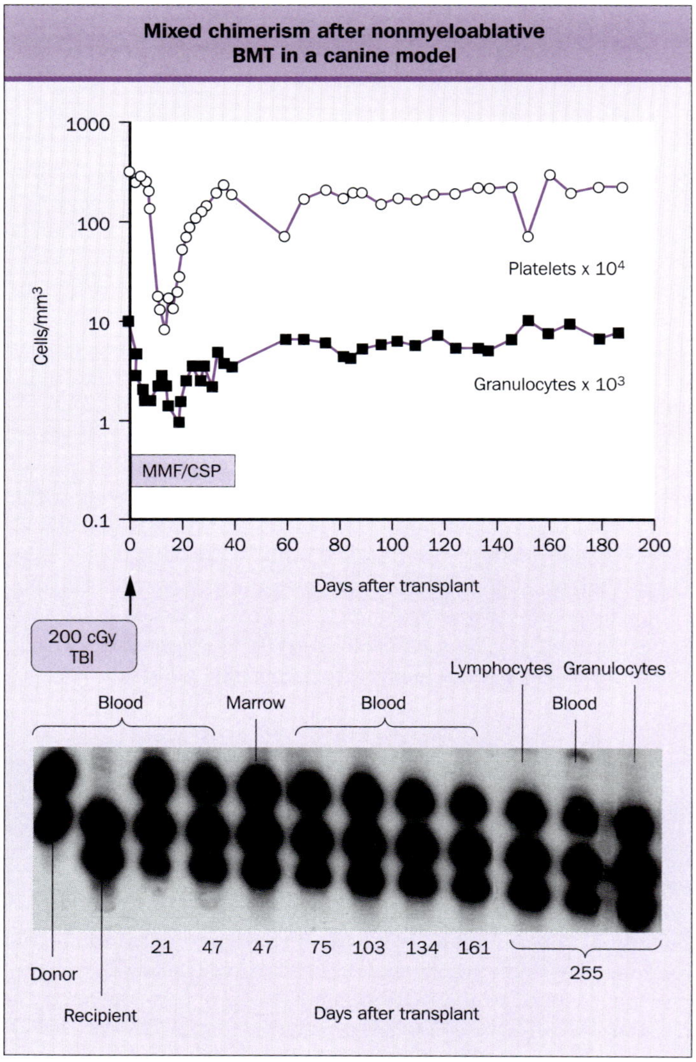

Figure 102.8 Sustained stable mixed chimerism after nonmyeloablative bone marrow transplant in a canine model. The dog received a marrow graft from a dog leukocyte antigen-matched littermate after conditioning with 200 cGy TBI and postgrafting immunosuppression with mycophenolate mofetil to day 27 and cyclosporine to day 35. The upper panel shows granulocyte and platelet counts and the lower panel chimerism testing using PCR-based detection of polymorphic dinucleotide repeats. (Reproduced with permission from Storb R, Yu C, Wagner JL, et al. Stable mixed hematopoietic chimerism in DLA-identical littermate dogs given sublethal total body irradiation before and pharmacological immunosuppression after marrow transplantation. *Blood* 1997;89:3048.)

without rejection. DLI have met with varied success. EBV-induced lymphoproliferative disorders and CML are usually effectively treated with DLI. Other diseases are less responsive although some patients with a variety of hematologic malignancies achieve sustained remissions.[87] Factors influencing responses to DLI are not yet well characterized but likely include remission status at DLI, rate of tumor growth, the expression of tumor-specific antigens, the nature of minor histocompatibilty differences between donor and recipients, and efficiency of antigen presentation by tumor cells.

Given the difficulty in effectively treating relapses, emphasis must remain on improving eradication of disease. Although many new combinations of chemotherapy and TBI have been tested, none has clearly proved superior to earlier conditioning regimens. Thus, with currently available agents the limits of nonhematopoietic toxicity may have been reached and no major breakthroughs should be expected. In order to augment antitumor responses and in the hope of avoiding additional toxicities to vital organs, some investigators have added monoclonal antibodies directed at hematopoietic cells, either alone or conjugated to radioisotopes, to the conditioning regimens.[96,97] Despite some initial promising results the feasibility of broadly applying this approach remains to be demonstrated. A similar approach involves the use of bone-seeking isotopes which localize to the bone and cause 'bystander' damage to hematopoietic and tumor cells.[98] Finally, to augment pretransplant therapy investigators have begun to test whether postgrafting immunity against tumors can be stimulated. This has involved treatment with agents such as interleukin-2 and interferon, and in some cases vaccinations against tumor antigens.

KEY CONCEPTS

Graft-versus-host disease

- Appears to be driven by alloreactive cytotoxic lymphocytes and, possibly, a complex cytokine network.
- Incidence and severity increase with unrelated donors and donor–recipient HLA incompatibility.
- Mortality from acute and chronic GVHD is largely due to associated infectious complications.
- Presence of GVHD is associated with lower relapse rates.
- T-cell depletion effectively prevents GVHD but is associated with increases in graft rejection and relapse.
- Most centers rely on pharmacologic GVHD prevention.
- Immunosuppression can generally be discontinued after 6–12 months without subsequent development of GVHD.

CONCLUSIONS AND OUTLOOK

While initially offered to younger patients with refractory acute leukemia, advances and refinements of HSCT have since broadened its acceptance as a treatment for patients with a variety of hematological malignancies. Despite impressive advances, treatment failure remains frequent – due mainly to recurrent malig-

THERAPEUTIC PRINCIPLES

Allografting for malignancy

- Conventional transplants rely on high-dose regimens to eradicate malignancy and prevent graft rejection.
- Graft-versus-tumor effects contribute to disease control.
- GVHD prevention is necessary and uses immunosuppressive agents and/or T-cell depletion of the graft.
- GVHD development confers increased risk of transplant mortality but less risk of relapse.
- HLA-identical siblings are the most frequently used donors.
- HLA-mismatched or HLA-matched unrelated donors are increasingly used for patients lacking related donors.
- Exploiting potent graft-versus-tumor effects is the concept underlying 'nonmyeloablative' transplants.

nant disease, acute and chronic GVHD, infections due to prolonged immunodeficiency, and late complications of conditioning programs. Critical to progress is the development of more effective and less toxic conditioning programs. This would allow broader use of T-cell depletion to prevent GVHD, thus extending transplantation from more HLA-nonidentical and unrelated donors, and would facilitate better outcomes in autologous HSCT. Another direction for improving outcomes is suggested by initial promising results of nonmyeloablative transplant studies in older patients. These results should stimulate vigorous investigation of strategies for exploiting donor immune reactions against a broad range of tumors. By exploiting GVT effects rather than high-dose therapies, allografting may be offered to many previously excluded patients and be a less toxic future option for many allografting candidates.

Progress will also depend heavily on continued preclinical and clinical research together with advances in biotechnology and drug development. The biosciences have continued to supply an exciting array of recombinant molecules with marrow-stimulating and immunomodulatory properties. Research with available agents and newly developed recombinant and pharmaceutical products should facilitate further advances in clinical HSCT.

REFERENCES

1. Bortin MM, Horowitz MM, Rimm AA. Progress report from the International Bone Marrow Transplant Registry. Bone Marrow Transplant 1992;10:113.
2. Thomas ED, Storb R, Clift RA, et al. Bone-marrow transplantation. N Engl J Med 1975; 292:895.
3. Frassoni F, Labopin M, Gluckman E, et al. Results of allogeneic bone marrow transplantation for acute leukemia have improved in Europe with time – a report of the acute leukemia working party of the European group for blood and marrow transplantation (EBMT). Bone Marrow Transplant 1996;17:13.
4. Thomas ED, Storb R. Technique for human marrow grafting. Blood 1970;36:507.
5. Langenmayer I, Weaver C, Buckner CD, et al. Engraftment of patients with lymphoid malignancies transplanted with autologous bone marrow, peripheral blood stem cells or both. Bone Marrow Transplant 1995;15:241.
6. Bensinger WI, Clift R, Martin P, et al. Allogeneic peripheral blood stem cell transplantation in patients with advanced hematologic malignancies: a retrospective comparison with marrow transplantation. Blood 1996;88:2794.
7. Storek J, Gooley T, Siadak M, et al. Allogeneic peripheral blood stem cell transplantation may be associated with a high risk of chronic graft-versus-host disease. Blood 1997;90:4705.
8. Berenson RJ, Bensinger WI, Hill RS, et al. Engraftment after infusion of CD34+ marrow cells in patients with breast cancer or neuroblastoma. Blood 1991;77:1717.
9. Barnett MJ, Eaves CJ, Phillips GL, et al. Successful autografting in chronic myeloid leukemia after maintenance of marrow in culture. Bone Marrow Transplant 1989; 4:345.
10. Santos GW, Tutschka PJ, Brookmeyer R, et al. Marrow transplantation for acute nonlymphocytic leukemia after treatment with busulfan and cyclophosphamide. N Engl J Med 1983;309:1347.
11. Tutschka PJ, Copelan EA, Klein JP. Bone marrow transplantation for leukemia following a new busulphan and cyclophosphamide regimen. Blood 1987;70:1382.
12. Nemunaitis J, Rabinowe SN, Singer JW, et al. Recombinant granulocyte-macrophage colony stimulating factor after autologous bone marrow transplant for lymphoid cancer. N Engl J Med 1991;324:1773.
13. Nemunaitis J, Singer JW, Buckner CD, et al. Use of recombinant human granulocyte-macrophage colony stimulating factor in graft failure after bone marrow transplantation. Blood 1990;76:245.
14. Thomas ED, Buckner CD, Banaji M, et al. One hundred patients with acute leukemia treated by chemotherapy, total body irradiation, and allogeneic marrow transplantation. Blood 1977;49:511.
15. Clift RA, Buckner CD, Thomas ED, et al. The treatment of acute non-lymphoblastic leukemia by allogeneic marrow transplantation. Bone Marrow Transplant 1987;2:243.
16. Biggs JC, Horowitz MM, Gale RP, et al. Bone marrow transplants may cure patients with acute leukemia never achieving remission with chemotherapy. Blood 1992;80:1090.
17. Clift RC, Buckner CD, Appelbaum FR, et al. Allogeneic marrow transplantation in patients with acute myeloid leukemia in first remission: a randomised trial of two irradiation regimens. Blood 1990;76:1867.
18. Champlin R, for the Advisory Committee of the International Bone Marrow Transplant Registry. Bone marrow transplantation for acute leukemia: A preliminary report from the International Bone Marrow Transplant Registry. Transplant Proc 1987;19:2626.
19. Gratwohl A, Hermans J, Lyklema A, Zwaan FE. Bone marrow transplantation for leukaemia in Europe: Report from the Leukaemia Working Party 1987. Bone Marrow Transplant 1987;2(Suppl 1):15.
20. Linch DC, Burnett AK. Clinical studies of ABMT in acute myeloid leukemia. Clin Hematol 1986;15:167.
21. Yeager AM, Kaizer H, Santos GW, et al. Autologous bone marrow transplantation in patients with acute nonlymphocytic leukemia, using ex vivo marrow treatment with 4-hydroperoxycyclophosphamide. N Engl J Med 1986;315:141.
22. Appelbaum FR, Dahlberg S, Thomas ED, et al. Bone marrow transplantation or chemotherapy after remission induction for adults with acute nonlymphoblastic leukemia: A prospective comparison. Ann Intern Med 1984;101:581.
23. Champlin RE, Ho WG, Gale RP, et al. Treatment of acute myelogenous leukemia: A prospective controlled trial of bone marrow transplantation versus consolidation chemotherapy. Ann Intern Med 1985;102:285.
24. Powles RL, Clink HM, Bandini G, et al. The place of bone-marrow transplantation in acute myelogenous leukaemia. Lancet 1980;i:1047.
25. Tallman MS, Appelbaum FR, Amos D, et al. Evaluation of intensive post-remission chemotherapy for adults with acute nonlymphocytic leukemia using high-dose cytosine arabinoside with L-asparaginase and amsacrine with etoposide. J Clin Oncol 1987; 5:918.
26. Thomas ED, Sanders JE, Flournoy N, et al. Marrow transplantation for patients with acute lymphoblastic leukemia: A long-term follow-up. Blood 1983;62:1139.
27. Barrett AJ, Horowitz MM, Gale RP, et al. Marrow transplantation for acute lymphoblastic leukemia: Factors affecting relapse and survival. Blood 1989;74:862.
28. Gorin NC, Aegerter P. Autologous bone marrow transplantation for acute leukaemia in remission: 4th EBMTG survey. Bone Marrow Transplant 1987;2(Suppl 1):320.
29. Johnson FL, Thomas ED, Clark BS, et al. A comparison of marrow transplantation with chemotherapy for children with acute lymphoblastic leukemia in second or subsequent remission. N Engl J Med 1981;305:846.
30. Rivera GK, Buchanan G, Boyett JM, et al. Intensive retreatment of childhood acute lymphoblastic leukemia in first bone marrow relapse. N Engl J Med 1986;315:273.
31. Hoelzer D, Thiel E, Loffler H, et al. Intensified therapy in acute lymphoblastic and acute undifferentiated leukemia in adults. Blood 1984;64:38.
32. Schauer P, Arlin ZA, Mertelsmann R, et al. Treatment of acute lymphoblastic leukemia in adults: Results of the L-10 and L-10M protocols. J Clin Oncol 1983;1:462.
33. Thomas ED, Clift RA, Fefer A, et al. Marrow transplantation for the treatment of chronic myelogenous leukemia. Ann Intern Med 1986;104:155.

34. Goldman JM, Apperley JF, Jones L, et al. Bone marrow transplantation for patients with chronic myeloid leukemia. N Engl J Med 1986;314:202.
35. Thomas ED, Clift RA. Indications for marrow transplantation in chronic myelogenous leukemia. Blood 1989;73:861.
36. Clift RA, Buckner CD, Appelbaum FA, et al. Allogeneic marrow transplantation in patients with chronic myeloid leukemia in the chronic phase. A randomized trial of two irradiation regimens. Blood 1991;77:1660.
37. Storb R, Pepe M, Deeg HJ, et al. Long-term follow-up of a controlled trial comparing a combination of methotrexate plus cyclosporine with cyclosporine alone for prophylaxis of graft-versus-host disease in patients administered HLA-identical marrow grafts for leukemia [Letter]. Blood 1992;80:560.
38. Clift RA, Storb R. Marrow transplantation for CML: The Seattle experience. Bone Marrow Transplant 1996;17:S1.
39. Clift RA, Buckner CD, Thomas ED, et al. Marrow transplantation for chronic myeloid leukemia: a randomized study comparing cyclophosphamide and total body irradiation with busulfan and cyclophosphamide. Blood 1994;84:2036.
40. Michallet M, Archimbaud E, Bandini G, et al. HLA-identical sibling bone marrow transplantation in younger patients with chronic lymphocytic leukemia. European Group for Blood and Marrow Transplantation and the International Bone Marrow Transplant Registry. Ann Intern Med 1996;124:311.
41. Appelbaum FR, Sullivan KM, Buckner CD, et al. Treatment of malignant lymphoma in one hundred patients with chemotherapy, total body irradiation and marrow transplantation. J Clin Oncol 1987;5:1340.
42. Philip T, Guglielmi C, Hagenbeek A, et al. Autologous bone marrow transplantation as compared with salvage chemotherapy in relapses of chemotherapy-sensitive non-Hodgkin's lymphoma. N Engl J Med 1995;333:1540.
43. Jones RJ, Ambinder FR, Piantadosa, et al. Evidence of a graft-versus-lymphoma effect associated with allogeneic bone marrow transplantation. Blood 1991;77:649.
44. Chopra R, McMillan AK, Linch DC, et al. The place of high-dose BEAM therapy and autologous bone marrow transplantation in poor-risk Hodgkin's disease. A single-center eight-year study of 155 patients. Blood 1993;81:1137.
45. Horning SJ. High-dose therapy and transplantation for low-grade lymphoma [Review]. Hematol Oncol Clin North Am 1997;11:919.
46. Freedman AS, Neuberg D, Mauch P, et al. Long-term follow-up of autologous bone marrow transplantation in patients with relapsed follicular lymphoma. Blood 1999; 94:3325.
47. Anderson JE, Appelbaum FR, Storb R. An update on allogeneic marrow transplantation for myelodysplastic syndrome. Leuk Lymphoma 1995;17:95.
48. Attal M, Harousseau JL, Stoppa AM, et al. A prospective, randomized trial of autologous bone marrow transplantation and chemotherapy in multiple myeloma. Intergroupe Francais du Myelome. N Engl J Med 1996;335:91.
49. Corradini P, Voena C, Tarella C, et al. Molecular and clinical remissions in multiple myeloma: role of autologous and allogeneic transplantation of hematopoietic cells. J Clin Oncol 1999;17:208.
50. Bensinger WI, Gahrton G. Allogeneic hematopoietic cell transplantation for multiple myeloma. In: Thomas ED, Blume KG, Forman SJ (eds) Hematopoietic cell transplantation. London, Blackwell Science, 1999;887.
51. Peters WP, Ross M, Vredenburgh JJ, et al. High-dose chemotherapy and autologous bone marrow support as consolidation after standard-dose adjuvant therapy for high-risk primary breast cancer. J Clin Oncol 1993;11:1132.
52. Beatty PG, Clift RA, Mickelson EM, et al. Marrow transplantation from related donors other than HLA-identical siblings. N Engl J Med 1985;313:765.
53. Anasetti C, Beatty PG, Storb R, et al. Effect of HLA incompatibility on graft-versus-host disease, relapse, and survival after marrow transplantation for patients with leukemia or lymphoma. Hum Immunol 1990;29:79.
54. Beatty PG, Hansen JA, Longton GM, et al. Marrow transplantation from HLA-matched unrelated donors for treatment of hematologic malignancies. Transplantation 1991; 51:443.
55. Petersdorf EW, Gooley TA, Anasetti C, et al. Optimizing outcome after unrelated marrow transplantation by comprehensive matching of HLA Class I and II alleles in the donor and recipient. Blood 1998;92:3515.
56. Hansen JA, Gooley TA, Martin PJ, et al. Bone marrow transplants from unrelated donors for patients with chronic myeloid leukemia. N Engl J Med 1998;338:962.
57. Gluckman E, Rocha V, Boyer-Chammard A, et al. Outcome of cord-blood transplantation from related and unrelated donors. Eurocord Transplant Group and the European Blood and Marrow Transplantation Group. N Engl J Med 1997;337:373.
58. Atkinson K. Reconstruction of the haemopoeitic and immune systems after marrow transplantation – review. Bone Marrow Transplant 1990;5:209.
59. Simmons PJ, Przepiorka D, Thomas ED, Torok-Storb B. Host origin of marrow stromal cells following allogeneic bone marrow transplantation. Nature 1987;328:429.
60. Turhan AG, Humphries RK, Phillips GL, et al. Clonal hematopoesis demonstrated by X-linked DNA polymorphisms after allogeneic bone marrow transplantation. N Engl J Med 1989;320:1655.
61. Nash R, Storb R, Neiman P. Polyclonal reconstitution of human marrow after allogeneic bone marrow transplantation. Blood 1988;72:2031.
62. Agosti JM, Sprenger JD, Lum LG, et al. Transfer of allergen-specific IgE-mediated hypersensitivity with allogeneic bone marrow transplantation. N Engl J Med 1988; 319:1623.
63. Riddell SR, Watanabe KS, Goodrich JM, et al. Restoration of viral immunity in immunodeficient humans by the adoptive transfer of T cell clones. Science 1992; 257:238.
64. Deeg HJ, Storb R, Thomas ED. Bone marrow transplantation: A review of delayed complications. Br J Haematol 1984;57:185.
65. McDonald GB, Shulman HM, Sullivan KM, et al. Intestinal and hepatic complications of human bone marrow transplantation. Gastroenterology 1986;90:770.
66. Meyers JD, Flournoy N, Thomas ED. Nonbacterial pneumonia after allogeneic marrow transplantation: A review of ten years' experience. Rev Infect Dis 1982;4:1119.
67. Curtis RE, Rowlings PA, Deeg HJ, et al. Solid cancers after bone marrow transplantation. N Engl J Med 1997;336:897.
68. Traweek ST, Slovak ML, Nademanee AP, Brynes RK, Niland JC, Forman SJ. Myelodysplasia and acute myeloid leukemia occurring after autologous bone marrow transplantation for lymphoma. Leuk Lymphoma 1996;20:365.
69. Bowden RA, Meyers JD. Infectious complications following marrow transplantation. Plasma Ther Transfus Technol 1985;6:285.
70. Boeckh M, Gooley TA, Myerson D, Cunningham T, Schoch G, Bowden RA. Cytomegalovirus pp65 antigenemia-guided early treatment with ganciclovir versus ganciclovir at engraftment after allogeneic marrow transplantation: a randomized double-blind study. Blood 1996;88:4063.
71. Reed EC, Bowden RA, Dandliker PS, et al. Treatment of cytomegalovirus pneumonia with ganciclovir and intravenous cytomegalovirus immunoglobulin in patients with bone marrow transplants. Ann Intern Med 1988;109:783.
72. Marmont AM, Horowitz MM, Gale RP, et al. T-cell depletion of HLA-identical transplants in leukemia. Blood 1991;78:2120.
73. Storb R, Thomas ED. Graft-versus-host disease in dog and man: The Seattle experience. In: Moller G (ed.) Immunological reviews, no. 88. Copenhagen, Munksgaard, 1985,p215.
74. Sale GE, Shulman HM (eds). The pathology of bone marrow transplantation. New York, Masson, 1984.
75. Jadus MR, Wepsic HT. The role of cytokines in graft-versus-host reactions and disease. Bone Marrow Transplant 1992;10:1.
76. Tsoi M-S, Storb R, Dobbs S, Thomas ED. Specific suppressor cells in graft-host tolerance of HLA-identical marrow transplantation. Nature 1981;292:355.
77. Sullivan KM, Deeg JH, Sanders J, et al. Hyperacute GVHD in patients not given immunosuppression after allogeneic marrow transplantation. Blood 1986;67:1172.

78. Storb R, Deeg HJ, Whitehead J, et al. Marrow transplantation for leukemia and aplastic anemia: Two controlled trials of a combination of methotrexate and cyclosporine versus cyclosporine alone or methotrexate alone for prophylaxis of acute graft-versus-host disease. Transplant Proc 1987;19:2608.
79. Storb R, Anasetti C, Appelbaum F, et al. Marrow transplantation for severe aplastic anemia and thalassemia major. Semin Hematol 1991;28:235.
80. Aversa F, Tabilic A, Velardi A, et al. Treatment of high-risk acute leukemia with T-cell-depleted stem cells from related donors with one fully mismatched HLA haplotype. N Engl J Med 1998;339:1186.
81. Martin PJ, Schoch G, Fisher L, et al. A retrospective analysis of therapy for acute graft-versus-host disease: Initial treatment. Blood 1990;76:1464.
82. Atkinson K. Chronic graft-versus-host disease – review. Bone Marrow Transplant 1990;5:69.
83. Atkinson K, Horowitz MM, Gale RP, et al. Risk factors for chronic graft-versus-host disease after HLA-identical sibling bone marrow transplantation. Blood 1990;75:2459.
84. Sullivan KM, Agura E, Anasetti C, et al. Chronic graft-versus-host disease and other late complications of bone marrow transplantation. Semin Hematol 1991;28:250.
85. Weiden PL, Sullivan KM, Flournoy N, et al. Antileukemic effect of chronic graft-versus-host disease: Contribution to improved survival after allogeneic marrow transplantation. N Engl J Med 1981;304:1529.
86. Horowitz MM, Gale RP, Sondel PM, et al. Graft-versus-leukemia reactions after bone marrow transplantation. Blood 1990;75:555.
87. Kolb HJ, Schattenberg A, Goldman JM, et al. Graft-versus-leukemia effect of donor lymphocyte transfusions in marrow grafted patients. European Group for Blood and Marrow Transplantation Working Party Chronic Leukemia. Blood 1995;86:2041.
88. Truitt RL, LeFever AV, Shih CC-Y. Graft-versus-leukemia reactions: Experimental models and clinical trials. In: Gale RP, Champlin R (eds) Progress in bone marrow transplantation. New York, AR Liss, 1987, p 219.
89. Giralt S, Estey E, Albitar M, et al. Engraftment of allogeneic hematopoietic progenitor cells with purine analog-containing chemotherapy: harnessing graft-versus-leukemia without myeloablative therapy. Blood 1997;89:4531.
90. Slavin S, Nagler A, Naparstek E, et al. Nonmyeloablative stem cell transplantation and cell therapy as an alternative to conventional bone marrow transplantation with lethal cytoreduction for the treatment of malignant and nonmalignant hematologic diseases. Blood 1998;91:756.
91. McSweeney P, Niederwieser D, Shizuru J, et al. Outpatient allografting with minimally myelosuppressive, immunosuppressive conditioning of low-dose TBI and postgrafting cyclosporine (CSP) and mycophenolate mofetil (MMF). [Abstract] Blood 1999;94:393a.
92. Storb R, Yu C, Wagner JL, et al. Stable mixed hematopoietic chimerism in DLA-identical littermate dogs given sublethal total body irradiation before and pharmacological immunosuppression after marrow transplantation. Blood 1997;89:3048.
93. Martin PJ, Hansen JA, Storb R, et al. Human marrow transplantation: An immunological perspective. In: Dixon FJ (ed.) Advances in immunology, vol. 40. Orlando, Academic Press, 1987,p379.
94. Radich JP, Gehly G, Gooley T, et al. Polymerase chain reaction detection of the BCR-ABL fusion transcript after allogeneic marrow transplantation for chronic myeloid leukemia: results and implications in 346 patients. Blood 1995;85:2632.
95. Radich J, Ladne P, Gooley T. Polymerase chain reaction-based detection of minimal residual disease in acute lymphoblastic leukemia predicts relapse after allogeneic BMT. Biol Blood Marrow Transplant 1995;1:24.
96. Press OW, Eary JF, Appelbaum FR, et al. Phase II trial of 131I-B1 (anti-CD20) antibody therapy with autologous stem cell transplantation for relapsed B cell lymphomas. Lancet 1995;346:336.
97. Matthews DC, Appelbaum FR, Eary JF, et al. Phase I study of (131)I-anti-CD45 antibody plus cyclophosphamide and total body irradiation for advanced acute leukemia and myelodysplastic syndrome. Blood 1999;94:1237.
98. Appelbaum FR, Brown PA, Sandmaier BM, et al. Specific marrow ablation before marrow transplantation using an aminophosphonic acid conjugate Ho-166-EDTMP. Blood 1992;80:1608.

Chapter 103 Immunoglobulin Treatment in Immunodeficiency Diseases

Charlotte Cunningham-Rundles

Antibody deficiency states can be successfully treated with immunoglobulin replacement. The available immunoglobulin concentrates contain mostly IgG with low but varying amounts of IgA and IgM; these concentrates provide antibodies commonly found in pooled human donor blood. In the years prior to immunoglobulin prophylaxis, patients with severe antibody deficits died of sepsis or other overwhelming infections. The introduction of intramuscular immunoglobulin permitted these patients to live longer and to suffer fewer infections, but the therapeutic dose of immunoglobulin was limited by the amount of the immunoglobulin solutions that could be given by an intramuscular injection. This problem was resolved by the introduction of immunoglobulin concentrates that could be administered intravenously (as reviewed in references 1–3). In the past two decades, the nearly universal use of intravenous immunoglobulins has demonstrated the efficacy of these preparations, although this therapy is particularly effective in patients who have not sustained chronic tissue damage and for whom there are no additional immunologic defects. New methods of manufacture and further considerations of biologic safety are still under investigation.

HISTORICAL CONSIDERATIONS

Von Behring and Kitasato determined that specific plasma substances are important in host defense in 1890, demonstrating that the plasma of animals immunized against tetanus and diphtheria contained substances that could neutralize these bacterial toxins.[4] The term 'antibody' first appeared in 1891 in the reports of Ehrlich, in connection with studies of plant toxins,[5] but was later used by other authors as a general term for soluble biologic factors. Later it was shown that placental extracts and plasma itself could be treated in such a way as to concentrate these active elements.[6,7] Cohn, whose work was carried out under contract with the US Navy to supply large quantities of stable albumin and IgG for wartime use, introduced the method of cold ethanol fractionation[6] to produce 'immune globulin (human)', as these substances were first termed.[8] 'Immunoglobulin globulin (human)' was first used in the prevention or amelioration of measles in 1935, and the alcohol-fractionated material was first used for prophylaxis against measles and hepatitis A in 1945.[8] In this method, antibodies are concentrated to between 15 and 25 times the usual serum concentration, supplying effective doses in relatively small volumes. The Cohn method, which effectively produces an IgG concentrate of relative purity, is expensive, in that a large amount of ethanol is necessary; additionally the yield of IgG is relatively small. Efforts to improve the yield have been developed, the Kistler–Nitschmann cold ethanol fractionation method being the best known.[7]

In 1952, immunoglobulin concentrates were first used in the treatment of human immunodeficiency disease, although the report of the first case did not equate 'antibody' with gammaglobulin. This report noted that 'to speak of gammaglobulin and antibody interchangeably is probably incorrect'.[9] The first immunodeficient patient treated with 'immunoglobulin (human)' was 8 years old. He received 3.2 g of gammaglobulin given subcutaneously at intervals of 1 month, since this dose increased the amount of the gammaglobulin fraction visible on serum electrophoresis. It was assumed that antipneumococcal antibody was contained in the gammaglobulin fraction, since the hypogammaglobulinemic child who was treated no longer had periodic pneumococcal sepsis. Immune antibodies to diphtheria and typhoid were believed to be present in the concentrates since immunity to these organisms was demonstrated in the serum of this patient only after treatment.[9]

The interval between doses of intramuscular immunoglobulin, first chosen on the basis of the gamma globulin peak on electrophoresis, was later confirmed in other studies by investigation in subjects with immunodeficiency. The half-life of immunoglobulin was found to range between 30 and 70 days.[8,10,11] The dose of intramuscular immunoglobulin given to the first patient was the same as that subsequently recommended for other immunodeficient patients – 100 mg/kg per month (or 25 mg/kg per week). This amount of the intramuscular preparation was found to increase the serum IgG level from near zero levels to 100–150 mg per 100 ml, a level found to be the minimum necessary to prevent serious infections.[12] Intramuscular immunoglobulin reduced both morbidity and mortality in hypogammaglobulinemic patients. In order to determine whether the dose was optimal, the Medical Research Council in Great Britain performed a trial in which patients treated with the usual dose of 25 mg/kg per week were compared with patients receiving 50 mg/kg per week. The results showed that patients receiving the higher dose developed significantly fewer infections.[13] However, the latter dose was impractical to administer since it required too large an injection (for example, 20 ml of a 15% solution would have to be administered every week to a 60 kg patient.) Thus, the eventually recommended dose for hypogammaglobulinemic patients was based more upon expediency than upon the available clinical data.

Plasma infusion has also been used in antibody replacement in the primary immunodeficiency diseases.[13] Although more nearly normal levels of serum immunoglobulins can be achieved by plasma infusions (including IgG and IgA), this method is cumbersome and requires donors of known medical history who must be screened for transmissible infectious diseases. Another drawback to plasma infusion is that the donated immunoglobulin confers the antigenic experience of only a single donor, and a broad range of antibodies in high titer is not likely to be present.

Development of intravenous immunoglobulins

Intravenous infusion of gammaglobulin concentrates was first attempted in the 1950s and 1960s; these infusions resulted in severe reactions in a number of instances. Various methods to modify the immunoglobulin solutions were devised to produce products suitable for intravenous use. Schultze and coworkers treated gammaglobulin with pepsin so that 80% of the resulting preparation was altered to $F(ab)'_2$ fragments;[14] Sgouris treated gammaglobulin with plasmin, resulting in less drastic reduction in the size of the molecule.[15] An additional early method was stabilization of immunoglobulin by exposure to acid at pH 4.0 with traces of pepsin, resulting in a widely used method, a version of which is still in use today.[16] Other methods included reduction, sulfonation, or reduction followed by alkylation, addition of stabilizers (maltose, sucrose, albumin), filtration, and precipitation of aggregates by polyethylene glycol.[17] Since enzyme-treated or reduced and alkylated immunoglobulin has reduced effector functions, in particular opsonic capacity[18] and complement fixation,[19,20] these treatments have not been favored.[21] There has also been a consensus that such concentrates should contain IgG subclasses in the approximate proportions present in normal plasma, and that no preservatives should be added.[21]

The first intravenous immunoglobulin introduced in the USA was a reduced (dithiothreitol) and alkylated (iodoacetamide) immunoglobulin solution with 5% IgG in a solution containing 10% maltose; it was low in IgG_3 and IgG_4, and did not fix complement well.[20] A number of products are now available in the USA (Table 103.1), and there is a still greater variety in other countries. In all likelihood, additional products will be licensed in the next several years.

PREPARATION AND PHARMACOLOGY OF INTRAVENOUS IMMUNOGLOBULINS

Since their introduction, immunoglobulin concentrates for intramuscular or intravenous use have been produced from pools of plasma derived from outdated blood or plasma. Plasma is obtained from whole blood donations of 1000 or more volunteer donors (called 'recovered plasma') or from an equally large number of paid plasmapheresis donors ('source plasma'). No upper limits on the number of donors contributing to a pool have been imposed, and lots have contained plasma from 100 000 to 200 000 donors. Currently, lots produced from source plasma contain plasma from up to 60 000 donors. Each donation is tested for hepatitis B surface antigen, HIV-p24 antigen, and antibodies to syphilis, HIV-1 and HIV-2, and hepatitis C. The plasma is treated with the Cohn alcohol fractionation procedure to precipitate the immunoglobulin-containing fraction. In this procedure, lipid coated viruses, including hepatitis B and HIV virus are removed, resulting in a sterile paste of concentrated immunoglobulin. After further purification, the resulting preparation, suitable for intramuscular use, is approximately 16.5% in immunoglobulin, of which 85% is IgG, 10% is IgM and 5% is IgA. Other serum proteins are present in trace amounts. Thimerosal is added as a preservative to most intramuscular Ig products made in the USA; in many other countries intramuscular immunoglobulin is preservative free.

Intravenous immunoglobulin (IVIG) is produced from these same Ig concentrates, using additional means of enriching the IgG content, while excluding other serum proteins, and adding various agents to stabilize monomeric IgG and discourage the

Current intravenous immunoglobulins

Category	Venoglobulin-S	Gammar-PIV	Gammagard S/D	Polygam S/D	Gamimune N	Iveegam EN	Sandoglobulin
Manufacturer	Alpha Therapeutic Corp	Centeon	Baxter Healthcare Corp.	Distributed by American Red Cross (ARC)	Bayer	Baxter Healthcare Corp.	Norvartis
Contraindication	Antibodies to IgA	IgA deficiency with antibodies to IgA	None (caution with IgA deficiency)	None (caution with IgA deficiency)	IgA deficiency with antibodies to IgA	IgA deficiency with antibodies to IgA	IgA deficiency with antibodies to IgA
IgA content	15.1 μg/ml	25 μg/ml	<3.7 μg/ml	<3.7 μg/ml	270 μg/ml	15–20 μg/ml	720 μg/ml
pH (after reconstitution	5.2–5.8	7.0	6.8	6.8	3.25	7.0	6.6
Plasma source	Plasmapheresis >10 000 donors	Plasmapheresis >8000 donors	Plasmapheresis >10 000 donors	>10 000 volunteer donors via the ARC	>2000 donors	Plasmapheresis >6000 donors	>16 000 volunteer donors
Half-life, days	33.5 ± 7	21	24	24	21	23–29	21
Solvent detergent treatment	Yes	No	Yes	Yes	No	No	No
Pasteurization	No	Yes	No	No	No	No	No
IgG subclass, %							
IgG_1	65.7–67.2	69	67	67	60.0	64.1	60.5
IgG_2	23.7–25.3	23	25	25	29.4	30.3	30.2
IgG_3	5.7–5.9	6	5	5	6.6	0	6.6
IgG_4	3.0–3.4	2	3	3	4.1	1.5	2.8

Table 103.1 Current intravenous immunoglobulins.

Comparison of intramuscular and intravenous human serum globulins

	Intramuscular	Intravenous
Strength	16.5% (165 mg/ml)	3%, 6%, 12% for one brand, 5% and 10% for others
Other components	0.1 M glycine	Various sugars and other stabilizers[a]
Preservative	Thimerosal, or none	None
How supplied	2 and 10 ml vials	Powder for reconstitution, or as 5–10% premixed solution.
Major advantages	Convenience of administration; infrequent side-effects	Predictable blood levels; high dosage feasible
Major disadvantages	Unreliable blood levels; discomfort at injection sites; large doses not feasible	Longer duration of treatment administration: frequent side-effects; higher cost
Frequency of side-effects	1% of injections	6–12% of infusions
Most frequent side-effects	Pain at injection site	Flushing, nausea, back ache, myalgias, rash, etc.
Other side-effects	Very uncommon	Severe headache, rare renal impairment
Dose	100 mg/kg (0.7 ml/kg)	200–500 mg/kg per month
Cost per gram	$60	$60–95

[a] Sucrose, maltose, glucose, glycine, D-mannitol, D-sorbitol, albumin, polyethylene glycol.

Table 103.2 Comparison of intramuscular and intravenous human serum globulins.

formation of aggregates (Table 103.2). The resulting intravenous solutions contain sodium in various amounts as well as one or more stabilizing agents, maltose, albumin, polyethylene glycol, D-mannitol, D-sorbitol, sucrose, glucose, or albumin. Intravenous immunoglobulin is supplied as lyophilized powder or as a premixed solution, with a final concentration of IgG in the final solution of 3, 5, 6, 10 or 12%, depending on the product. The final osmolarity of the reconstituted IgG solutions lies between 253 mOsm/l for a 5% IgG product, and 1250 mOsm/l for another product at a 10% concentration (Table 103.3).[22] The IgA content of the different brands varies between <0.4 μg/ml and 720 μg/ml (Table 103.1).[2]

INDICATIONS AND ADMINISTRATION

The primary immune diseases in which antibody deficiency occurs are the combined T and B cell defects, diseases in which severe T-cell dysfunction precludes adequate antibody production, and diseases with prominent B-cell defects. When the use of IVIG is considered, serum immunoglobulins should be tested and verified as being subnormal on at least two separate occasions. This therapy is suitable for those patients who have a significant lack of antibodies, and is thus not based on the exact level of serum IgG; on the other hand, a serum level of IgG of 400 mg/dl or less generally coincides with significant antibody deficiency. Occasionally, a subject who has a modestly reduced serum IgG and IgA but quite normal antibody production will be encountered; depending on the clinical picture, IVIG may not be necessary. Figure 103.1 illustrates the antibody response to pneumococcal vaccine for 18 patients with history of severe infections, some of whom had reduced levels of serum IgG; as the figure shows, there was no correlation between the antibody response to the vaccine and the level of serum IgG.

The diagnosis for which IVIG is most frequently required is common variable immunodeficiency, due to the relative frequency of this disorder which has an estimated incidence of 1:20 000 to 1:60 000.[23] The diagnosis of common variable immunodeficiency is based upon significantly reduced levels of serum IgG and IgA, with or without reduced levels of serum IgM, and should be verified (especially for patients with serum IgG levels of greater than 400 mg/dl) by testing for a lack of specific antibodies.[23]

The use of IVIG in IgG subclass deficiency can be controversial; it is true that subjects with IgG_2 subclass deficiency may have deficient antibody responses to bacterial polysaccharides (as for example, to pneumococcal vaccine), but others have normal responses, due to increased IgG_1 specific antibody.[24] When immunoglobulin treatment is being considered for a patient with IgG_1 or IgG_2 subclass deficiency, antibody production to a variety of protein and polysaccharide vaccines should be tested. Clearly subnormal antibody responses to more than one immunogen are the only true indications for immunoglobulin treatment. Most infants with transient hypogammaglobulinemia of infancy have normal amounts of specific antibodies, despite low levels of serum immunoglobulins, and do not need exogenous immunoglobulin.[25]

When IVIG is to be used, most physicians supervise the first few infusions in a controlled setting, since adverse reactions are

THERAPEUTIC PRINCIPLES

Uses of intravenous immunoglobulin in humoral immunodeficiencies

Combined T and B cell defects
Severe combined immunodeficiency (all types)
Wiskott–Aldrich syndrome
Hyper-IgM syndrome
Ataxia-telangiectasia with IgG_2 deficiency
Short-limbed dwarfism
X-linked lymphoproliferative syndrome

T-cell defects
Complete DiGeorge syndrome

B-cell defects
X-linked agammaglobulinemia
Common variable immunodeficiency
IgA deficiency with IgG_2 and antibody deficiency
IgG subclass deficiency with proven antibody deficiency
Antibody deficiency with normal immunoglobulins
Transient hypogammaglobulinemia (rarely)

Unknown defects
Hyper-IgE syndrome, with proven antibody deficiency

IVIG composition comparison					
IVIG	Concentration (%)	Diluent[a]	Sodium concentration	Sugar concentration	Osmolarity (mOsm/l)
Gamimune N	5	–	Trace	10% maltose	305
Gamimune N	10	–	Trace	10% maltose	278
Sandoglobulin	3	0.9% NaCl, 5% dextrose, or sterile water	0.9%	2.5% sucrose	498 444 192
Sandoglobulin	6	0.9% NaCl, 5% dextrose, or sterile water	0.9%	5% sucrose	690 636 384
Sandoglobulin	12	0.9% NaCl, 5% dextrose, or sterile water	0.9%	10% sucrose	1074 1020 768
Gammagard/Polygam	5	Sterile water	8.5 mg/ml	2% glucose	636
Gammagard/Polygam	10	Sterile water	8.5 mg/ml	4% glucose	1250
Venoglobulin-S 5%	5	–	1.3 mEq/l	5% D-sorbitol	300
Venoglobulin-S 10%	10	–	<1.0 mEq/l	5% D-sorbitol	330
Iveegam	5	Sterile water	0.3%	5% glucose	373
Gammar-PIV	5	Sterile water	0.5%	5% sucrose	330
Gammar-PIV	10	Sterile water	0.5%	10% sucrose	699

[a] Supplied as lyophilized powder or for dilution with indicated diluent.

Table 103.3 IVIG composition comparison. From Siegel J. Viral safety issues in IVIG products. *Pharmacy and Therapeutics* 1996;21S.

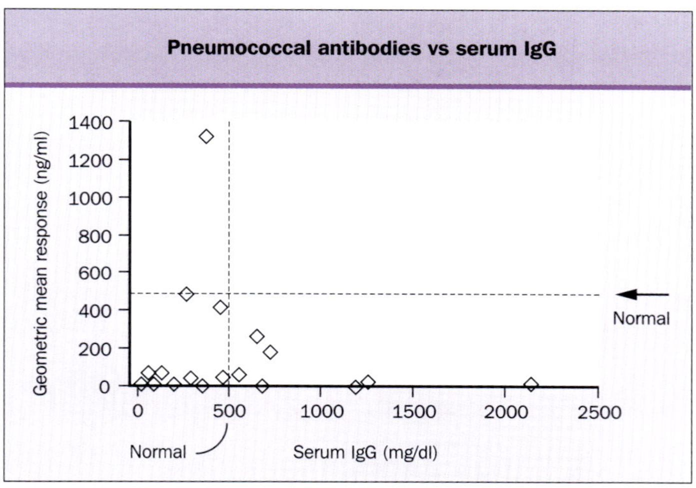

Figure 103.1 Lack of correlation between baseline serum IgG level and antibody response to pneumococcal vaccine. Eighteen adult patients referred for severe bacterial infections and/or a reduced level of serum IgG, were given a pneumococcal vaccine; one month later the serum antibody response, measured as the geometric mean response to 12 pneumococcal serotypes (Types 1, 3, 4, 6B, 7F, 8, 9N, 12F, 14, 18C, 19F, and 23F) was determined. The figure shows this geometric mean response (on the y axis) as related to the serum IgG level (on the x axis); no correlation was found. The normal serum IgG level would be 500 mg/dl or greater, as shown. The normal vaccine response for adults would be greater than 500 ng/ml of antibody, as indicated.

more likely in the first infusions. Considerations of dose are discussed below, but the more commonly used doses lie between 300 and 400 mg/kg body weight, given every three or four weeks. The recommended rate of infusion is generally 0.01–0.02 ml/kg per minute, to start with, but the rate is best individualized. Even up to 30 mg/kg per minute is tolerated in some patients.[24]

METABOLISM OF IMMUNOGLOBULIN

Of the total amount of IgG in the body, part is in the intravascular space and the rest is in the extravascular compartment.[8] IgG is in constant circulation between these two compartments. In the steady state it has been estimated that a healthy 70 kg man synthesizes 2.5 g of IgG every day (35 mg/kg per day).[8] In contrast, in common variable immunodeficiency, the synthetic rate has been estimated at 1–5 mg/kg per day and the fractional turnover rate in antibody deficiency has been estimated at 4% per day.[8] This delayed catabolism results in an extended half-life for total IgG in immunodeficiency, ranging between 30 and 70 days.[8,11] The catabolic rate of serum IgG in general seems to depend on the serum IgG concentration.[11] After an injection of ^{131}I-labeled gammaglobulin in normal controls, about one half of the total disappears from the plasma and enters the extravascular space in 48 hours. After this time, the disappearance of injected IgG is due to catabolism; the amount of IgG that is catabolized has been calculated at approximately 7% of the total per day.

The amount of IgG in the serum just after administration of IVIG depends on the starting level of IgG, and the dose given. Infusing 100 mg of IVIG/kg body weight will raise the serum IgG level by about 200 mg/dl; a dose of 500 mg/dl will increase the serum level by about 1000 mg/dl.[26–28] Some of these immunoglobulin molecules become denatured, and others become bound to antigens and removed as immune complexes. On a practical level, the half-life of infused total IgG in immunodeficient individuals is quite varied, depending on both the product and the recipient; in general it lies between 18 and 32 days. Giving consecutive doses of IVIG to a patient who has not previously received this therapy results in a gradual increase in the 'trough' level of serum IgG, this being the level of IgG found in the serum just prior to a subsequent infusion. This serum level stabilizes after giving 5 or 6 infusions at regular intervals (Fig. 103.2). On a practical level, the serum IgG level should be measured periodically prior to an immunoglobulin infusion to ascertain if the amount is at least 400–500 mg/dl, a level at the lowest limit of the normal range.

As for IgG subclasses and specific antibodies, the situation is more complex; in one group of previously immunoglobulin treated immunodeficient subjects, infused IgG had a half life of 25.8 days, IgG_1 had a half-life of about 29.7 days, IgG_2 26.9 days, and IgG_3 15.7 days. Antibodies to specific pathogens had a half life similar to that of total IgG.[29]

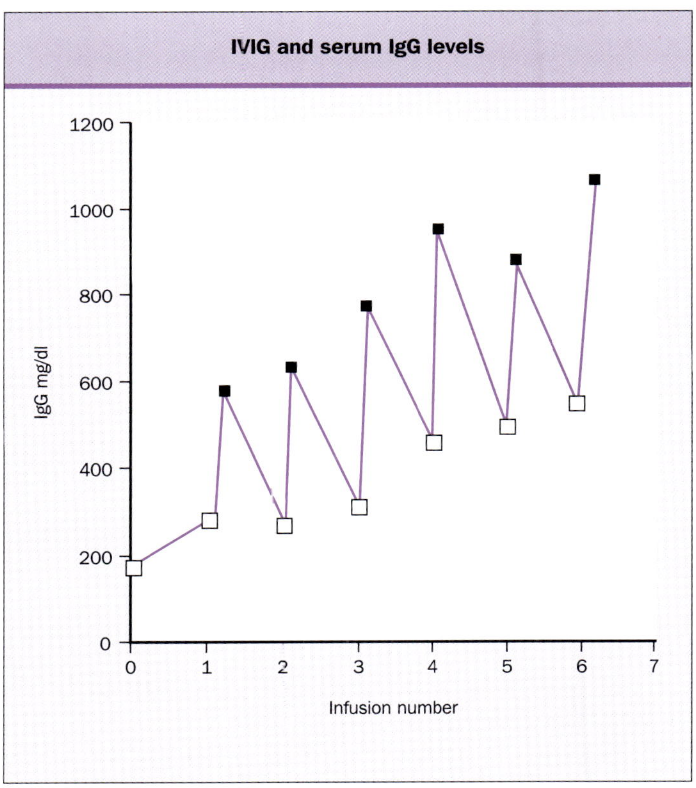

Figure 103.2 Staircase effect of constant dose of IVIG on trough and peak levels of serum IgG. A patient with common variable immunodeficiency was started on IVIG at a dose of 300 mg/kg given every 3 weeks. The level of serum IgG was measured just before (□) and just after (■) each infusion, for 6 infusions. The trough level of IgG slowly increased to become stabilized in about 6 months.

SUBCUTANEOUS INFUSION OF IMMUNOGLOBULIN

An additional method of administering immunoglobulin is by subcutaneous infusion. This method delivers immunoglobulin via a small-gauge needle into the subcutaneous tissues of the abdomen, using a portable pump. In the original studies, 0.05–0.2 ml of the intramuscular immunoglobulin concentrate was given per kg/h.[30] The maintenance dose is usually 100 mg/kg per week. The level of serum IgG can be raised to normal, the infusion is well accepted by patients, and the risk of infusion reactions is less than that of intravenous infusions. In some parts of Europe, subcutaneous infusion has been a preferred method of immunoglobulin delivery, partly because the much less expensive immunoglobulin concentrates intended for intramuscular use can be used, and partly because it is quite safe and easily applied in the home.[31] This method has also been used successfully in patients in whom anaphylactoid reactions occur when the intravenous route is used. In the USA, a mercury-free immunoglobulin concentrate for intramuscular use is available but it is nearly as expensive as the intravenous formulations. Thus, this otherwise quite satisfactory method is less used in the USA than elsewhere. Subcutaneous infusion of the intravenous products is, however, possible, and is applicable in patients who have not tolerated the intravenous route, or who have limited venous access. In this case the more concentrated immunoglobulin products (10 or 12%) can be used. Certainly this plan is preferred over the implantation of an indwelling catheter to infuse such patients.

HOME CARE AND SELF-INFUSION

Replacement therapy with IVIG is often performed in a hospital or clinic under direct medical supervision. However, intravenous infusion using a home care service is also widely practiced.[32,33] It is very convenient, less disruptive, and may cost less than infusion in a hospital setting. Home care infusion is generally done at the convenience of the patient, which may mean evening or weekend infusions. The first few infusions are performed in a clinic or hospital to observe for adverse events; afterward, using the same product and infusion scheme, infusions can be carried out in the home. Self-infusion, when performed by a trained patient or family member, can be a safe procedure for children and adults and eliminates both infusion and nursing charges. In any kind of home care arrangement, close supervision by and contact with the physician is imperative.

EFFICACY

The standard dose for intramuscular immunoglobulin in immunodeficiency is 100 mg/kg per month, given in a divided dose, every week or every two weeks. It was observed empirically that a level of serum IgG of 100–150 mg/dl, was the minimum necessary level to prevent sepsis[12] and that raising the serum IgG by 200 mg/dl, using the intramuscular preparations, provided protection from invasive bacterial infections.[8,12] However, the intramuscular route was not the optimal one. Larger patients, most male adults and patients with poor musculature could not be given adequate doses because of the volume of solution required. The simple pain of the injection at the recommended dose could deter both the patient and the physician from giving adequate therapy. Various attempts to produce a more suitable IVIG preparation resulted in a group of products that could be infused safely. The goal of the first studies using these intravenous concentrates was to establish that the intravenous forms compared favorably with intramuscular treatment in the prevention of infection in patients with humoral immunodeficiency. One report of a crossover trial of 34 patients compared the standard intramuscular dose of 100 mg/kg per month with the same dose of a reduced and alkylated preparation given intravenously.[34] Somewhat disconcertingly, the results showed that IVIG treatment was associated with a higher incidence of infections (Table 103.4A). While this might have been caused by reporting artifacts stemming from the increased number of visits made to the major medical centers by the intravenously-infused patients, it still did not appear that intravenous treatment with the product used at the given dose was clearly preferable. However, a significant reduction in rate of infection had been demonstrated for hypogammaglobulinemic patients receiving a higher dose (150 mg/kg) (Table 103.4B).[35] Since the patients in both studies had been treated with the reduced and alkylated immunoglobulin, it seems plausible that a dose of 150 mg/kg of this product may have been the minimum dose at which efficacy over intramuscular immunoglobulin could be shown.

Other investigators have analyzed the effects of IVIG given at even higher doses. Comparing 300 mg/kg of an intact immunoglobulin given at 3-week intervals to prior therapy with intramuscular immunoglobulin at standard dosage, a highly significant overall improvement was observed for the IV-treated group (Table 103.4C).[36] Although not all patients showed improvement, and several were subsequently treated with even higher doses, a dose of 300 mg/kg per 3 weeks (or 400 mg/kg per 4 weeks) benefits most patients. Another study, involving 29 subjects with X-linked agammaglobulinemia, compared the effects of administering >400 mg/kg to doses of <200 mg/kg every 3 weeks. The conclusion was that the higher dose resulted in fewer episodes of pneumonia and days spent in the hospital. Both doses demonstrated benefit when compared to intramuscular immunoglobulin.[37] In other studies, 500 mg/kg given at intervals determined by serum IgG levels, and 600 mg/kg per month, have been infused without ill effect, and produced benefit.[38] In general, postinfusion serum IgG level increases by approximately 250 mg/dl of serum for each 100 mg of immunoglobulin per kg infused. However, individual patients can display marked differences in the apparent catabolic rate of IgG, and some investigators have sought to individualize doses in order to establish a minimum trough value.[39]

Comparison of low-dose intravenous versus standard-dose intramuscular immunoglobulins

	Intravenous immunoglobulin[a]	Intramuscular immunoglobulin[b]
Number of patients	34	34
Percentage of patients with acute infections:		
Upper respiratory tract	85.3	50.0
Gastrointestinal tract	55.9	38.2
Otitis media	52.9	47.1
Bronchitis	50.0	41.2
Sinusitis	20.6	17.6
Oral	17.6	8.8
Conjunctivitis	29.4	26.5
Skin	29.4	32.4

[a] Dose 100 mg/kg per month, reduced and alkylated immunoglobulin.
[b] Dose 100 mg/kg per month, standard solution for intramuscular use.

Table 103.4A Comparison of low-dose intravenous versus standard-dose intramuscular immunoglobulins. From Ammann AJ, Ashman HF, Buckley RH, et al. Use of intravenous g-globulin in antibody immunodeficiency: Results of a multi-center controlled trial. From Ammann AJ, Ashman HF, Buckley RH, et al. Use of intravenous γ-globulin in antibody immunodeficiency: Results of a multi-center controlled trial. *Clin Immunol Immunopathol* 1982;22:60.

Comparison of intermediate-dose intravenous versus standard-dose intramuscular immunoglobulin

	Intravenous treatment[a]	Intramuscular treatment[b]
Number of patients	13	13
Number of acute infections	15	57
Acute infections/months therapy	0.067	0.295

[a] Dose 150 mg/kg per month, reducec and alkylated immunoglobulin.
[b] Dose 100 mg/kg per month, standard solution.

Table 103.4B Comparison of intermediate-dose intravenous versus standard-dose intramuscular immunoglobulin. Nolte MT, Pirofsky B, Gerritz GA, et al. Intravenous immunoglobulin therapy for antibody deficiency. *Clin Exp Immunol* 1979;36:337.

Comparison of high-dose intravenous versus standard-dose intramuscular immunoglobulin

	intravenous treatment[a]	Intramuscular treatment[b]
Number of patients	18	18
Days sick	258	834
Days on antibiotics	1820	3249

[a] Dose 300 mg/kg every 3 weeks, chemically intact, pH 4.0 immunoglobulin.
[b] Dose 40–80 mg/kg every 2 weeks, standard solution for intramuscular use.

Table 103.4C Comparison of high-dose intravenous versus standard-dose intramuscular immunoglobulin. Cunningham-Rundles C, Siegal FP, Smithwick EM, et al. Efficacy of intravenous gammaglobulin in humoral immunodeficiency disease. Ann Intern Med 1984;101:435.

THERAPEUTIC PRINCIPLES

IVIG replacement therapy: recipe for success

- Antibody deficiency has been demonstrated.
- Correct individualized dose is given (approximately 300–400 mg/kg, sometimes more).
- Wait several months for trough IgG level to stabilize.
- Patient is compliant with regular visits.
- Patient maintains close contact with physician.
- Early intervention with antibiotics at time of infection.

Patients treated adequately with immunoglobulin concentrates show significant improvement as evidenced by reduced frequency of respiratory tract infections and episodes of otitis, sinusitis, and conjunctivitis. For children, growth rates can improve perceptibly after starting IVIG treatment (Fig. 103.3). Patients with more severe tissue damage, particularly chronic pulmonary disease, do not show as much benefit. The use of higher than usual doses of IVIG in such patients may result in clinical benefit.[40] On the other hand, pulmonary complications are common in the primary immunodeficiencies, and silent progression of pulmonary changes such as bronchiectasis can occur, even in patients who have achieved apparently adequate trough levels of serum IgG (500 mg/dl or more), suggesting that IVIG replacement in these cases could not halt the progression of lung damage.[41] Patients with chronic diarrhea are not likely to have abatement of this symptom. In contrast, patients with rheumatologic disease and

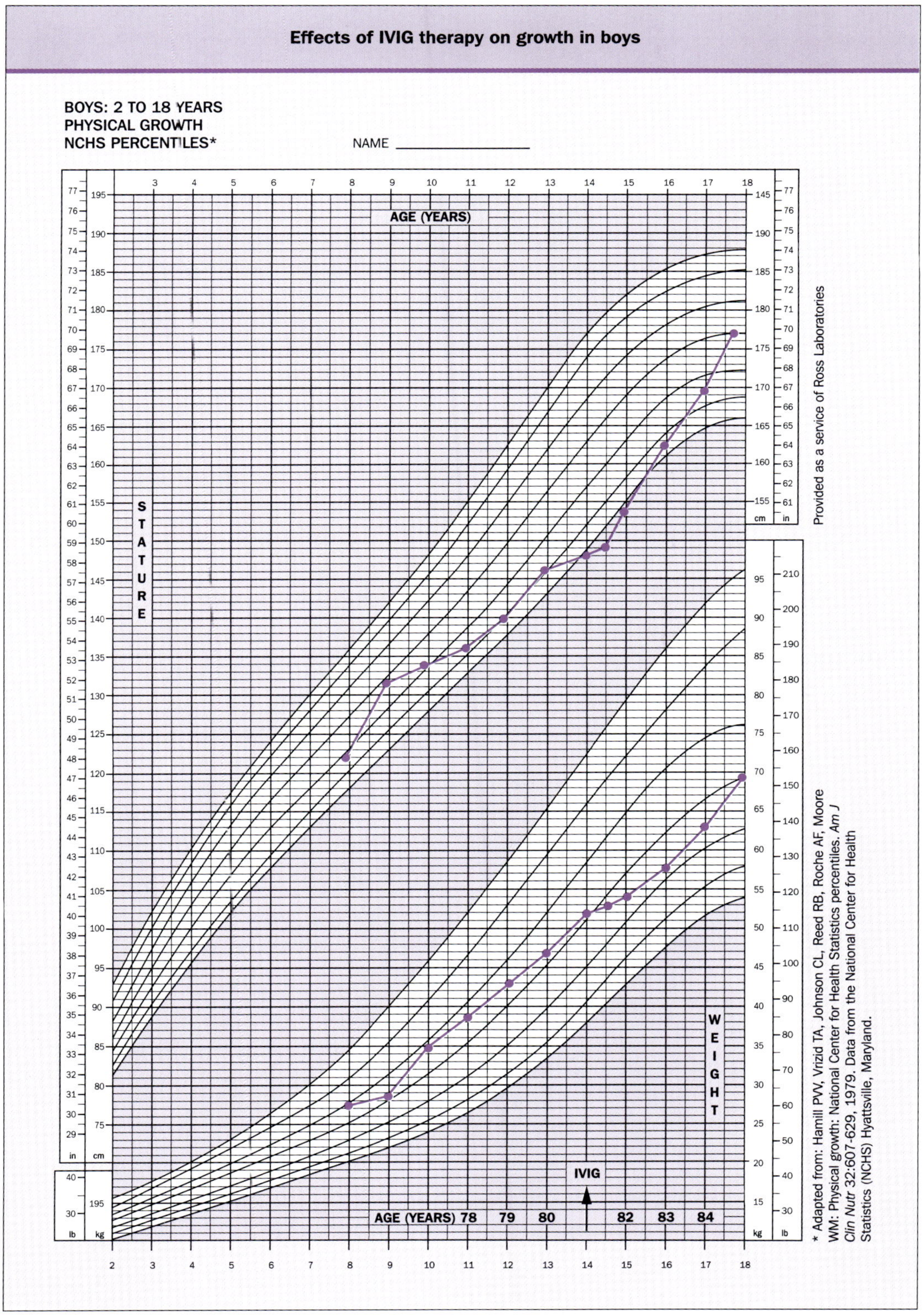

Figure 103.3 Effect of IVIG therapy on growth in an immunodeficient boy with CVID. After a male patient of 11 years old was started on IVIG, there was accelerated growth as measured by height and weight increases.

even objective joint swelling prior to therapy may experience dramatic improvement after even one or two treatments.[1–3,34–36]

SAFETY

Early studies on immunoglobulin infusions

Intramuscular injections of immunoglobulin in immunodeficiency resulted in adverse reactions in about 10% of injections.[8,12,42] The major complaint among patients was pain at the site of the injection.[8,12,42] Other reactions were mild and include muscle aches, back pain, or chills. More rarely, nausea, hives, angioedema, vomiting, flushing, chest pain, or fever were reported. In one large study one patient died after an injection.[42] Because of the side-effects to intramuscular injection and the evidence that immunoglobulin given intramuscularly or subcutaneously was only slowly absorbed into the systemic circulation, a number of early attempts were made to give the standard intramuscular solutions to immunodeficient subjects by the intravenous route. In 1962, Barandun and colleagues administered 110 ml of a 1.45% gammaglobulin solution intended for intramuscular injection to 70 individuals.[16] Ninety three percent of the antibody-deficient subjects had an adverse reaction, while only 13% of the other subjects had untoward reactions. The adverse effects occurred immediately, within minutes of starting the infusion, or were delayed 1–2 hours after the infusion was completed. The immediate reactions consisted of facial flushing, a feeling of oppression in the chest, lumbar pain, tachycardia, tachypnea, and shortness of breath. The delayed reactions included chills, slight increases in temperature, and the manifestations of the immediate reactions. Severe reactions were almost exclusively limited to the antibody-deficient group. Here the course was found to resemble anaphylaxis and included chills, dyspnea, a sense of oppression, nausea, vomiting, lumbar pain, fever of 39–40°C, circulatory collapse, and loss of consciousness. Such reactions, even very severe ones, were generally concluded in 3–4 hours. These reactions have been generally believed to be caused by complement activation arising from the infusion of aggregates,[16] although, strangely, after experiencing a reaction, patients were refractory to subsequent reactions for a period of 4–5 days. In fact, the more pronounced the reaction, the longer-lasting was the refractory period. Barandun and colleagues showed that ultracentrifuged immunoglobulin concentrates also produced reactions in antibody-deficient patients. They proposed that the retention of microbial antigens in the blood of hypogammaglobulinemic patients could lead to the formation of antigen–antibody complexes with the infused antibody.[16] Infusion of immunoglobulin concentrates can activate complement[43] and circulating immune complexes may appear after immunoglobulin infusions,[44] but these are not usually associated with clinical reactions.

Adverse reactions to commercial intravenous immunoglobulins

Infusing currently available intravenous immunoglobulins can also lead to adverse reactions. Most of these are nonanaphylactic in type, and are characterized by back or abdominal aching or pain, chills, low-grade fever, myalgias and/or headache. Slowing or stopping the infusion for 15–30 minutes will reverse most reactions. Diphenhydramine, aspirin, or ibuprofen may be helpful. More severe reactions can be treated with 50 mg hydrocortisone given intravenously, and for patients who seem predisposed to reactions, pretreatment with diphenhydramine or hydrocortisone can be helpful. Reactions of this kind are particularly likely in a patient who has not received IVIG previously, and who has had a recent bacterial infection. After two or three immunoglobulin treatments, additional infusion reactions become unlikely. The reasons for these adverse reactions are very poorly understood; they seem to diminish over time and many investigators have hypothesized that the infused immunoglobulin may complex bacterial or viral fragments, leading to immune complexes that must be slowly eliminated. Additional potential causes of infusion reactions include prekallikrein activator[45] or other contaminants of blood processing. Some of these factors could lead to the leukopenia often observed after infusion. IgE in the infused immunoglobulin is another possible cause, since IgE may be present in these concentrates and serum IgE levels are found to increase after infusion.[40]

> **CLINICAL PEARLS**
>
> **Adverse reactions of IVIG therapy: how to control**
> - Slow rate of infusion of IVIG initially.
> - Treatment with antihistamines and antipyretics/analgesics usually suffices; corticosteroids occasionally necessary. Pretreatment necessary in some patients.
> - Patients with repeated significant adverse reactions require direct medical supervision during IVIG infusions.

Antibodies to IgA

Autologous antibodies to IgA were first recognized in human sera in 1968.[46] These antibodies are present in up to 40% of sera of IgA-deficient donors,[47] and in 20% of patients with common variable immunodeficiency.[48] Infusion of blood or blood products containing IgA into a recipient who has anti-IgA antibodies can result in severe, anaphylactic infusion reactions, consisting of flushing, facial swelling, dyspnea, anxiety, cyanosis, hypotension, nausea, vomiting, circulatory collapse and, rarely, death. An occasional hypogammaglobulinemic individual may also experience adverse reactions after injection or infusion of immunoglobulin. Such reactions following IVIG can result in dramatic complement activation, and long-term persistence of C3a in the serum.[49] Anti-IgA antibodies are usually of the IgG isotype, but anti-IgA antibodies of the IgE isotype have also been identified.[50] Several immunoglobulin products intended for intravenous infusion are depleted of IgA in the course of manufacturing. These have been used successfully for hypogammaglobulinemic patients who require antibody treatment and have known or suspected anti-IgA antibodies.[51,52] Intravenous immunoglobulin may also be required for the 12–18% of IgA-deficient individuals who are IgG_2 subclass deficient and subject to recurrent infections; an IgA-depleted immunoglobulin is a good choice for these patients as well.

Transmission of virus

A major concern surrounding the infusion of blood and blood products is the ever present potential for the transmission of virus. In 1982, Gerety and Aronson evaluated the risk that plasma products would transmit hepatitis.[53] Low-risk products included albumin obtained by cold ethanol fractionation and heated at 60°C for 10 hours, and immunoglobulin concentrates produced by cold ethanol fractionation. High-risk products included the coagulation factors, antithrombin III, fibronectin, and α_1-antitrypsin. However, the following year, Lane reported that 12 of 12 patients with primary immunodeficiency given an experimental IVIG had developed non-A, non-B hepatitis.[54] Ochs et al reported in 1985 that 7 of 16 patients given an experimental IVIG developed elevated liver enzymes;[55] Bjorkander et al reported the following year that 16 of 77 subjects in another study developed non-A, non-B hepatitis after receiving another product.[56] In February 1994, two IVIG products were withdrawn after reports of hepatitis C in infused patients in Spain, Sweden, England, and the USA.[57] Ultimately, 247 cases of hepatitis were reported from 10 different countries. Since in each case the starting immunoglobulin solution was derived from plasma by cold ethanol fractionation, which had a long history of viral safety, it has remained unclear how these immunoglobulin fractions could acquire infectivity during manufacturing. The most likely reason is the removal of hepatitis C antibody-containing plasma lots after 1990, when the first tests for this antiviral antibody became available.[58]

An initial concern was the possibility that immunoglobulin concentrates could transmit the HIV virus, but even with widespread surveillance, no cases of HIV in recipients of IVIG have been reported. In fact, purposeful contamination of plasma with HIV virus and subsequent testing of residual infectivity at various points along the preparation cycle have demonstrated that several steps in the scheme remove infectivity.[59] Other viruses that have received consideration are hepatitis A and the B19 parvovirus, both non-lipid-enveloped viruses; on the other hand, transmission of these viruses via immunoglobulin products has not been reported.

Viral inactivation procedures

A number of processes – physical, enzymatic, and chemical – have been designed to inactivate viruses in blood and blood products, none of them specific for individual viruses. The cold ethanol fractionation process itself greatly reduces or eliminates transmission of hepatitis B. The first procedure specifically used to activate viruses in plasma was heating of albumin concentrates for 10 hours at 60°C; this method is suitable for albumin, but other blood proteins can become inactivated by heating. Treatment of immunoglobulin concentrates with pepsin at pH 4[16] (included to diminish complement activation), inactivates some viruses. Other compounds, β-propriolactone[60] or sulfonation used in the production of certain products to discourage complement activation, also add antiviral activity. Filters with small pore size are also used to remove viruses, but filtering large volumes of protein concentrates with reasonable flow rates has been cumbersome. Additionally the viruses that it may be desirable to remove are the small viruses such as parvovirus (18–24 nm), and hepatitis A virus (27–32 nm), not easily removed by the practical filter pore size of 35 nm. One of the more widely used viral inactivation methods in the preparation of plasma proteins, is a solvent detergent treatment, first approved in 1985.[61] In this method, the solvent, tri (n-butyl) phosphate, at 0.3% (w/v) and detergent, Triton X-100 at 1%, are added to IgG concentrates for 4 hours at 60°C, followed by removal of the solvent and detergent by oil extraction and chromatography through a hydrophobic column. Lipid-enveloped viruses, including HIV and hepatitis C, are thoroughly disrupted by these procedures.

> **CLINICAL PEARLS**
>
> **Reasons for delivery or withdrawal of product**
> - Severe headaches are a sign of CNS influx of white blood cells (aseptic meningitis). Change of IVIG product or alternative delivery route (subcutaneous) of IgG may be necessary.
> - Larger doses of IVIG (1–2 g/kg) are sometimes associated with renal failure, pulmonary insufficiency, hemolytic anemia, or thrombotic events. Cessation of treatment or initiation of alternative mode of therapy with lower doses may be necessary.
> - Virus contamination of plasma pool (e.g. hepatitis C in past; unknown virus in future).
> - Prion contamination of plasma pool (e.g. Creutzfeld–Jakob disease)?

Additional adverse reactions

Severe headaches may occur after the administration of IVIG; in a number of cases in which a lumbar puncture has been performed, spinal fluid pleocytosis with a predominance of lymphocytes has been noted, leading to the diagnosis of aseptic meningitis. This complication has been most often associated with high-dose IVIG given for autoimmune or neurologic disease, but it has been found in a few subjects with primary immunodeficiency who were given smaller doses.[62] There have also been sporadic reports of renal dysfunction and/or acute renal failure occurring in infused patients. Worldwide, 17 deaths have been reported. Current evidence suggests that IVIG products that contain sucrose are involved, perhaps causing osmotic injury to the proximal renal tubules.[63] About 55% of cases occurred in patients being treated for idiopathic thrombocytopenia purpura; fewer than 5% have occurred in subjects with primary immunodeficiency, suggesting that the larger doses used in the autoimmune diseases in comparison to those used in immunodeficiency present a greater osmotic challenge. Other potentially more serious side-effects include pulmonary insufficiency, hemolytic anemia, and thrombotic events.

Other issues in plasma manufacture need to be considered if blood derivatives could contain as yet unidentified infectious agents, one example being prions capable of transmitting a slow virus disease, Creutzfeld–Jakob disease. The bovine spongiform encephalopathy epidemic, and the appearance of new variant CJD in humans in the United Kingdom focused attention on this possibility. Disease-specific prions for new variant CJD (PrP^{vCJD}) have been detected in lymphocytes of affected subjects, leading to the decision of the UK Government not to use UK-derived plasma for production of plasma concentrates. On the other hand, the number of cases of new variant CJD has remained low for the last three years and there has been no evidence of transmission of traditional CJD or the new variant, via blood or plasma.[64]

SUMMARY

In the years prior to immunoglobulin prophylaxis, patients with substantial defects of antibody production died of sepsis or other overwhelming infections. The introduction of intramuscular immunoglobulin permitted these patients to live longer and to suffer fewer infections. However, the therapeutic dose of intramuscular immunoglobulin was dictated more by the amount of the solution that could be given by injection than by considerations of maximum efficacy. In the past decade, the development and nearly universal use of IVIG products has demonstrated the efficacy of these preparations. The infusion of these products is accompanied by a low but continued rate of adverse reactions, most of which occur for reasons that are unclear.

REFERENCES

1. National Institutes of Health Consensus Conference. Intravenous immune globulin: prevention and treatment of disease. JAMA 1990;264:3189.
2. Buckley RH, Schiff RI. The use of intravenous immune globulin in immunodeficiency disease. N Engl J Med 1991;325:110.
3. Stiehm ER. Human intravenous immunoglobulin in primary and secondary antibody deficiencies. Pediatr Infect Dis J 1997;16:696.
4. Von Behring B, Kitasato S. Uber das zustandekommen der diphtherie immunitat und der der tetanus-immunitat bei thieren. Dtsch Med Wochenschr 1890;16:1113.
5. Ehrlich P. Die Wertbemessung des diphtherie-heilserums und deren theoretische grundlagen. Klin Jahrbuch 1897;6:299.
6. Cohn EJ, Strong LB, Hughes WL Jr, et al. Preparation and properties of serum and plasma proteins. IV: A system for the separation into fractions of protein and lipoprotein components from biological tissues and fluids. J Am Chem Soc 1946;68:459.
7. Kistler P, Nitschmann HS. Large scale production of human plasma fractions. Eight years experience with the alcohol fractionation procedure of Nitschmann Kistler and Lergier. Vox Sang 1962;7:414.
8. Janeway CA, Rosen FS. The gamma globulins. IV. Therapeutic uses of gamma globulin. N Engl J Med 1966;275:826.
9. Bruton OC. Agammaglobulinemia. Pediatrics 1952;9:722.
10. Dixon FJ, Talmage DW, Maurer PH, et al. The half life of homologous gammaglobulin (antibody) in several species. J Exp Med 1952;96:313.
11. Waldman TA, Schwab PJ. (7S gammaglobulin) metabolism in hypogammaglobulinemia: Studies in patients with defective gammaglobulin synthesis. J Clin Invest 1965;44:1523.
12. Hill LB. Clinical features of hypogammaglobulinemia. Medical Research Council Special Report Series 1971;310:106.
13. Stiehm BR, Vaerman JP, Fudenberg HH. Plasma infusions in immunologic deficiency states: Metabolic and therapeutic studies. Blood 1966;28:918.
14. Schultze MB, Schwick C. Uber neue moglichkeiten intravenoser gammaglobulin-applikation. Dtsch Med Wochenschr 1962;87:1643.
15. Sgouris JT. The preparation of plasmin-treated immune gammaglobulin for intravenous use. Vox Sang 1967;13:71.
16. Barandun S, Kistler P, Jeunet F, et al. Intravenous administration of human γ-globulin. Vox Sang 1962;7:157.
17. Romer J, Moganthale JJ, Scherz B, Skvaril F. Characterization of various immunoglobulin preparations for intravenous application. Vox Sang 1982;42:62.
18. Hetherington SV, Gienbnick GS. Opsonic activity of immunoglobulin prepared for intravenous use. J Lab Clin Med 1984;104:977.
19. Bing DH. Complement interaction with immune serum globulin and immune globulin intravenous. Am J Med 1984;76(3A):19.
20. Cunningham Rundles C. Normalization of serum Clq after intravenous immunoglobulin infusion in hypogammaglobulinemia: Dependence upon methods of immunoglobulin preparation. Clin Immunol Immunopathol 1984;33:176.
21. Appropriate uses of human immunoglobulin in clinical practice: Memorandum of an IUIS/WHO meeting. Bull WHO (Geneva) 1982;60:45.
22. Siegel J. Viral safety issues in IVIG products. Pharmacy and Therapeutics 1996;21S.
23. IUIS Scientific Group. Primary Immunodeficiency Diseases. Clin Exp Immunol 1999; 118:Suppl 1:1.
24. Shackelford PG. IgG subclasses: importance in pediatric practice. Pediatr Rev 1993; 14:291.
25. Tiller TL, Buckley RH. Transient hypogammaglobulinemia of infancy: Review of the literature, clinical and immunologic feature of 11 new cases, and long term follow-up. Pediatrics 1978;92:347.
26. Buckley RH. Long term use of intravenous immune globulin in patients with primary immunodeficiency disease: inadequacy of current dosage practices and approaches to the problem. J Clin Immunol 1982;2:15S.
27. Ochs HD, Fischer SH, Wedgwood RJ. Modified immune globulin: its use in the prophylactic treatment with immune deficiency. J Clin Immunol 1982;2:22S.
28. Montanaro A, Pirofsky B. Prolonged high dose intravenous immunoglobulin in patients with primary immunodeficiency states. Am J Med 1984;76:67.
29. Mankarious S, Lee M, Fischer S, et al. The half lives of IgG subclasses and specific antibodies in patients with primary immunodeficiency who are receiving intravenous immunoglobulin. J Lab Clin Med 1988;112:634.
30. Berger M, Cupps TR, Fauci AS. Immunoglobulin replacement therapy by slow subcutaneous infusion. Ann Intern Med 1980;93:55.
31. Gardulf A, Hammarstrom L, Smith CIB. Home treatment of hypogammaglobulinemia with subcutaneous gammaglobulin for rapid infusion. Lancet 1991;338:162.
32. Ochs HD, Fisher SH, Lee ML, Delson ES, Kingdon HS, Wedgwood RJ. Intravenous immunoglobulin home treatment for patients with primary immunodeficiency diseases. Lancet 1986;1:610.
33. Ashida BR, Saxon A. Home intravenous immunoglobulin therapy by self-administration. J Clin Immunol 1986;6:306.
34. Ammann AJ, Ashman HF, Buckley RH, et al. Use of intravenous γ-globulin in antibody immunodeficiency: Results of a multi-center controlled trial. Clin Immunol Immunopathol 1982;22:60.
35. Nolte MT, Pirofsky B, Gerritz GA, et al. Intravenous immunoglobulin therapy for antibody deficiency. Clin Exp Immunol 1979;36:337.
36. Cunningham-Rundles C, Siegal FP, Smithwick EM, et al. Efficacy of intravenous gammaglobulin in humoral immunodeficiency disease. Ann Intern Med 1984;101:435.
37. Liese JG, Wintergerst U, Tympaer KD, Belohraadsky BH. High vs low dose immunoglobulin therapy in the long term treatment of X-linked agammaglobulinemia. Am J Dis Child 1995;146:325.
38. Roifman CM, Levison H, Gelfand EW. High dose versus low dose intravenous immunoglobulin in hypogammaglobulinemia and chronic lung disease. Lancet 1987;i:1075.
39. Schiff RI, Rudd C, Johnson R, Buckley RH. Use of a new chemically modified intravenous IgG – efficacy and attempts to individualize dosage. Clin Immunol Immunopathol 1984;31:13.
40. Newland AC, Macey MG, Rubel M. IgE in intravenous IgG [Letter]. Lancet 1984;1:1406.
41. Kainulainen L, Varpula M, Liippo K, Svedström E, Nikoskelainen J, Ruuskanen O. Pulmonary abnormalities in patients with primary hypogammaglobulinaemia. J Allergy Clin Immunol 1999;104:1031.
42. Soothill JF. Reactions to immunoglobulin. Medical Research Council Special Report Series 1971;310:106.
43. Frank MM, Basta M, Fries LF. The effects of intravenous immune globulin on complement-dependent immune damage of cells and tissues. Clin Immunol Immunopathol 1992;62:S82.
44. Cunningham Rundles C, Carr RI. Dietary bovine antigens and immune complex formation after intravenous immunoglobulin in common varied immunodeficiency. J Clin Immunol 1986;6381.
45. Alving BM, Tankersley DL, Mason BL, et al. Vasoactive enzymes in immunoglobulin preparations. In: Alving BM, Finlayson JS (eds) Immunoglobulins: Characteristics and uses of intravenous preparations. DHHS Publication No. (FDA) 80–9005. Washington, US Department of Health and Human Services, 1979, p. 167.

46. Vyas GN, Perkins HA, Fudenberg HH. Anaphylactoid transfusion reactions associated with anti-IgA. Lancet 1968;2:3.
47. Hammarstrom L, Person MAA, Smith CIB. Anti-IgA in selective IgA deficiency. Scand J Immunol 1983;18:5.
48. Wells JV, Buckley RH, Schanfield MS, et al. Anaphylactic reactions to plasma infusions in patients with hypogammaglobulinemia and anti-IgA bodies. Clin Immunol Immunopathol 1971;8:265.
49. Good RA, Gupta S, Pahwa S, et al. Evidence of persistent IgA/IgG circulating immune complexes associated with activation of the complement system in serum of a patient with common variable immune deficiency: Anaphylactic reactions to intravenous gammaglobulin. Acta Pathol Microbiol Immunol Scand Suppl 1984;284:49.
50. Burks AW, Sampson HA, Buckley RH. Anaphylactic reactions after gammaglobulin administration in patients with hypogammaglobulinemia. N Engl J Med 1986;314:560.
51. Bjorkander J, Hammarstrom L, Smith CIB, Buckley RH, Cunningham-Rundles C, Hanson LA. Immunoglobulin prophylaxis in patients with antibody deficiency syndromes and anti-IgA antibodies. J Clin Immunol 1987;7:8.
52. Cunningham-Rundles C, Zhou Z, Mankarious S, Courter S. Long term use of intravenous immunoglobulin subjects with anti-IgA antibodies. J Clin Immunol 1993;13:272.
53. Gerety RJ, Aronson DL. Plasma derivatives and viral hepatitis. Transfusion 1982;22:347.
54. Lane RS. Non-A, non-B hepatitis from intravenous gammaglobulin. Lancet 1983;1:974.
55. Ochs HD, Fischer SH, Virant FS, et al. Non-A, non-B hepatitis and intravenous immunoglobulin. Lancet 1985;1:404.
56. Bjorkander J, Cunningham-Rundles C, Lundin P, et al. Intravenous immunoglobulin prophylaxis in hypogammaglobulinemia causing liver damage. Am J Med 1988;84:107.
57. Centers for Disease Control. Outbreak of hepatitis C associated with intravenous immunoglobulin administration United States. MMWR 1994;43:505.
58. Finlayson J, Tankersley DL. Anti-HCV screening and plasma fractionation: the case against. Lancet 1990;335:1274.
59. Centers for Disease Control. Safety of therapeutic immunoglobulin preparations with respect to transmission of human T-lymphotropic virus type 111/lymphadenopathy associated virus infection. MMWR 1986;35:231.
60. Prince AM, Brotman SW. β-propriolactone/ultraviolet/irradiation: a review of effectiveness for inactivation of viruses in blood derivatives. Rev Infect Dis 1983;5:92.
61. Horowitz B, Wiebe ME, Lippin A, Stryker MH. Inactivation of viruses in labile blood derivatives I: Disruption of lipid-enveloped viruses by tri n (n-butyl) phosphate detergent combinations. Transfusion 1985;25:516.
62. Sekull BA, Cupler BJ, Dalakas MC. Aseptic meningitis associated with high-dose intravenous immune globulin therapy: frequency and risk factors. Ann Intern Med 1994;121:259.
63. Centers for Disease Control. Renal insufficiency and failure associated with immune globulin intravenous therapy – United States 1985–1998. MMWR Weekly 1999, 48:518.
64. Chapel HM. Safety and availability of immunoglobulin replacement therapy in relation to potentially transmissible agents. Clin Exp Immunol 1999;118(Suppl 1): 29.

Chapter 104

Intravenous Immunoglobulin in Autoimmune and Inflammatory Diseases

Mark Ballow and Mark Boguniewicz

This chapter examines the uses of intravenous immunoglobulin (IVIG) in a number of autoimmune and inflammatory diseases, and discusses the mechanisms by which IVIG exerts its immunoregulatory and anti-inflammatory actions. Although all the mechanisms by which IVIG has immunomodulatory effects are not understood, knowledge of how IVIG exerts its actions in these diseases will allow us to define appropriate indications and schedules of administration of IVIG in these diseases, and to design second-generation IVIG preparations that are better able to target the immune perturbations in these autoimmune and inflammatory processes. For many of these disorders we still have to define the exact optimal dosages for treatment. Furthermore, for many of these diseases, additional multicenter placebo-controlled clinical trials are needed to confirm clinical efficacy.

AUTOIMMUNE CYTOPENIAS

Idiopathic thrombocytopenic purpura

Idiopathic thrombocytopenic purpura (ITP) (Chapter 74) results from accelerated platelet destruction attributable to an immunologic process (Fig. 104.1). Imbach et al[1] first treated a group of children with both acute and chronic ITP using IVIG, 400 mg/kg per day for 5 days. All of them had an initial increase in platelet counts, but 2 patients with acute and 5 with chronic ITP required additional IVIG. In randomized studies of acute childhood ITP, patients responded equally well to both corticosteroids and IVIG.[2,3] However, of the patients who required more prolonged therapy, those randomized to the IVIG group did better.[3] Blanchette et al[2] showed that the number of days required to achieve a platelet count of $\geq 50 \times 10^9$/l was significantly fewer in the children given IVIG than in those receiving prednisone or no therapy. IVIG as a single dose at 0.8 g/kg was similar to 1 g/kg on 2 consecutive days, but was more rapid than intravenous anti-D or oral corticosteroids.[4] However, IVIG showed no advantages compared to corticosteroids in adults with ITP.[5] A recent retrospective study found that anti-D was as effective as IVIG in acute childhood ITP,[6] pointing out the need for larger prospective multicenter comparative trials. It is of note that a recent study found that only a minority of patients with major hemorrhage had an immediate response in platelet count to IVIG, corticosteroids, or both.[7]

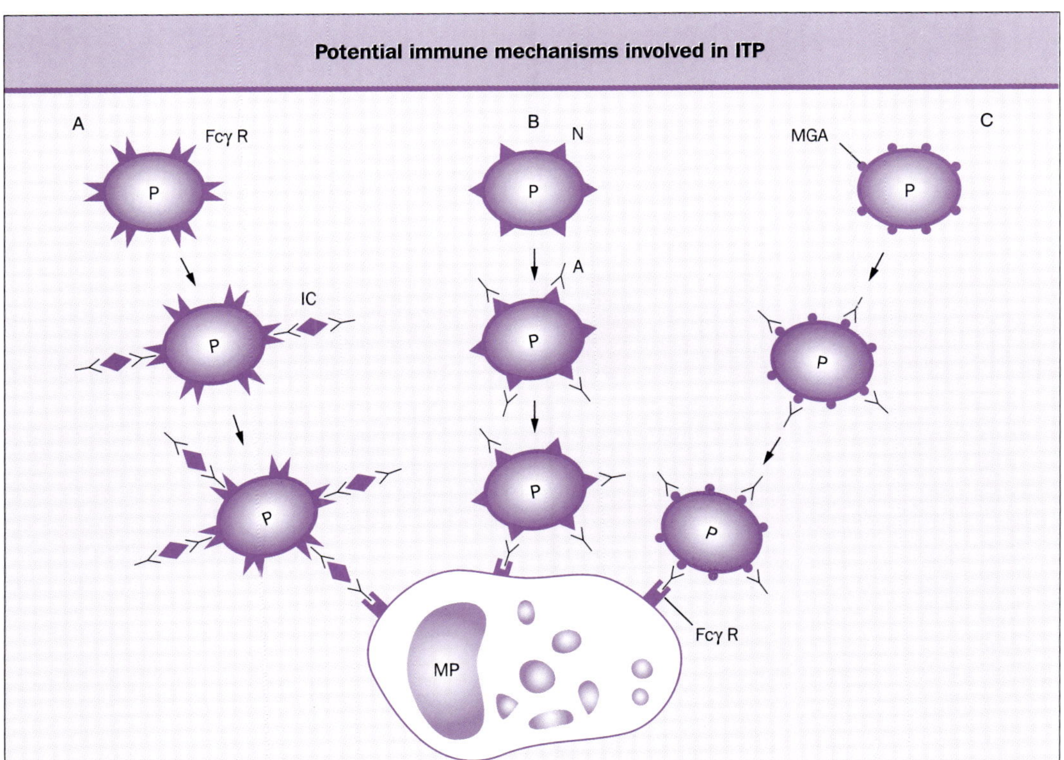

Figure 104.1 Potential immune mechanisms involved in the pathophysiology of idiopathic thrombocytopenic purpura. (**A**) Immune complexes associated with clearing of putative infectious agents bind to Fcγ receptors on the platelet surface. (**B**) Antibodies directed at neoantigens on the platelet membrane formed during recovery from infection. (**C**) Induction of cross-reacting autoantibodies directed at platelet glycoproteins (IIb/IIIa, Ib/IX). All three mechanisms lead to increased clearance or destruction of platelets by the reticuloendothelial system. P = platelet; A = antibody; N = neoantigen; FcγR = Fcγ receptor; IC = immune complex; MP = mononuclear phagocyte; MGA = membrane glycoprotein antigens.

The practice guidelines of the American Society of Hematology recommend IVIG, as initial therapy for children with ITP with serious bleeding regardless of the platelet count, and for those with platelet counts $< 10 \times 10^9/l$, those with minor purpura, or $<20 \times 10^9/l$ and mucosal bleeding.[8] IVIG is also recommended for adults with platelet counts $<50 \times 10^9/l$ with life-threatening bleeding, but the expert panel disagreed about the use of IVIG in asymptomatic adults with platelet counts $<20 \times 10^9/l$ or for those with risk factors for bleeding. Unfortunately, the efficacy of IVIG in reducing the risk of intracranial hemorrhage remains unknown. Studies in children with chronic ITP have shown that treatment with IVIG can defer the need for splenectomy.[9] Adults with chronic ITP have had substantial but transient increases in platelet counts.[10] More recently, the response of the platelet count to IVIG has been shown to correlate with the response to splenectomy, suggesting that an infusion of IVIG could help identify appropriate candidates for this surgical procedure in chronic ITP.[11] Dosages used for initial therapy of childhood ITP include single doses of 0.8–1.0 g/kg and multiple doses administered as 1 g/kg for 2 days or 0.4 g/kg for 5 days. In a small randomized trial, low-dose IVIG in a 2-day regimen of 250, 400 or 500 mg/kg per day reversed thrombocytopenia as effectively as 1 g/kg per day and may have the advantage of fewer adverse effects and lower cost.[12] However, these results need to be confirmed in a larger study before this dosing regimen can be recommended.

Fehr and colleagues[13] suggested that the IVIG treatment response in ITP was caused by a blockade of the reticuloendothelial system (RES). Sequential clearance studies of autologous radiolabeled anti-Rh(D)-sensitized erythrocytes in adults with ITP treated with IVIG showed that the increase in platelet count was accompanied by a prolonged immune clearance rate. Subsequently, Clarkson et al[14] demonstrated a marked increase in platelet count using a monoclonal antibody directed against the low-affinity Fcγ receptor found on neutrophils, NK cells, and macrophages, suggesting that this effect might be related to specific blockade of low-affinity Fcγ receptors on macrophages in the liver and in other parts of the reticuloendothelial system. In a different approach, children with acute ITP treated with intravenous Fcγ fragments showed a rapid increase in platelet counts.[15] Responders with detectable platelet-associated IgG before treatment had a significant drop in platelet IgG after this therapy. Serum soluble FcγRIII (CD16) concentrations increased with the platelet count. No soluble CD16 was detected in the Fcγ preparation used. Thus, the efficacy of Fcγ fragment therapy strengthens the hypothesis that Fcγ receptor blockade is a principal mechanism of action of IVIG in ITP, although other immunoregulatory mechanisms triggered by the presence of increased soluble CD16 concentrations in serum could be involved.

The possibility of mechanisms other than RES blockade is also suggested by a study comparing intact IVIG and Fc-depleted IVIG in patients with chronic ITP.[16] Although the group treated with intact IVIG achieved a better response than the group treated with Fc-depleted IVIG, 2 patients in the latter group had complete responses, suggesting a mechanism other than Fc receptor blockade. Fcγ receptor down-regulation or change in receptor affinity may also be involved.[17] In addition, the effects of IVIG on T and B cell function with associated decrease in antiplatelet antibodies remains to be elucidated. Idiotype–anti-idiotype interactions between antiplatelet GPIIb/IIIa autoantibodies and IVIG could affect autoantibody production in ITP.[18] An important question that remains unresolved is whether all antiplatelet autoantibodies or only some fraction are bound by anti-idiotypes in IVIG, since this would address the issue of a specificity of the immune-modulating effects of IVIG or general suppression.

Autoimmune hemolytic anemia

Autoimmune hemolytic anemia (AIHA) occurs when autoantibodies bind to determinants on the surface of red blood cell (RBC) membranes and cause the premature clearance and destruction of erythrocytes (Chapter 72). There is controversy regarding the efficacy of IVIG therapy in patients with AIHA and responses appear to be limited to patients with warm (IgG) hemolytic anemia. Patients with AIHA respond less frequently than patients with either ITP or autoimmune neutropenia. In addition, the dose of IVIG necessary to obtain a response is higher (up to 5 g/kg).[19]

Autoimmune neutropenia (Chapter 73)

The largest experience with IVIG therapy in neutropenic states has been reported in autoimmune neutropenia of infancy. This acquired condition typically occurs in the first year of life and is characterized by an absolute neutrophil count of 0–500/μl, monocytosis, and eosinophilia (Chapter 73). In general, children with this disorder tolerate well the symptoms of recurrent fever and non-life-threatening infections (gingivitis, otitis media, gastroenteritis), with recovery occurring by 4 years of age. Treatment is usually limited to antibiotic therapy. However, in children with serious infections. IVIG therapy should be considered. Bussel et al[20] reported a response rate of 88% using 1 g/kg per day of IVIG until the absolute neutrophil count was ≥ 1000/μl. Therapy should be reserved for those patients with severe infections who are responding poorly or not at all to appropriate intravenous broad-spectrum antibiotic therapy.

AUTOIMMUNE COAGULOPATHIES

Autoantibodies against factor VIII coagulant protein can cause an acquired hemophilia resulting in a spectrum of bleeding complications.[21] These acquired antibodies can be idiopathic, but are often found in patients with autoimmune disorders, inflammatory bowel disease, pemphigus, and malignancy, and in postpartum women (Chapter 74). Sultan et al[22] first reported on the use of high-dose IVIG in 2 patients with anti-factor VIII autoantibodies, showing rapid and prolonged, although incomplete, suppression of inhibitor. Subsequent studies by these investigators showed that a $F(ab')_2$ fragment prepared from IVIG inhibited autoantibody activity to factor VIIIc, suggesting an idiotypic–anti-idiotypic interaction between the IVIG and the autoantibodies.[23] In a prospective study, patients were treated with 1 g/kg of IVIG for 2 days or 400 mg/kg for 5 days followed by maintenance doses at intervals as clinically indicated.[21]

KAWASAKI SYNDROME

Kawasaki syndrome (KS) is an acute multisystem disease of unknown etiology that primarily affects infants and young children (Chapter 67).[24] KS occurs worldwide in children of all racial groups but is most prevalent in Japan and in children of Japanese ancestry.[25] Although the acute illness is generally self-limited, coronary artery abnormalities related to a generalized inflammation and immune activation of small and medium sized blood vessels develop in up to 25% of untreated patients.

In a multicenter randomized trial in the USA, the effects of IVIG 400 mg/kg per day for 4 consecutive days plus aspirin were compared to aspirin alone.[26] The results showed that 2 weeks after onset of therapy, coronary artery abnormalities were present in 23% (18 of 78) of children in the aspirin group, as compared with 8% (6 of 75) in the IVIG plus aspirin group. Seven weeks after enrolment, coronary abnormalities were present in 18% (14 of 79) of children in the aspirin group and in 4% (3 of 79) of the IVIG plus aspirin group. In a follow-up study, the efficacy of a single infusion of IVIG 2 g/kg was compared with 400 mg/kg for 4 consecutive days.[27] The relative prevalence of coronary artery lesions, adjusted for age and sex, among patients treated with the 4-day regimen, was almost twice as great as in those patients treated with the single-infusion regimen. Laboratory parameters of acute inflammation in the single-infusion group showed a more rapid trend toward normal. Lower serum IgG levels on day 4 were associated with a greater degree of systemic inflammation and with a higher prevalence of coronary abnormalities. A meta-analysis of published studies on the treatment of KS showed a dose response for IVIG with a threshold for decreased incidence of coronary artery aneurysm >1 g/kg.[28] More recently, a retrospective analysis of re-treatment of patients who remained febrile after IVIG suggested improved outcome with 2 g/kg compared with 1 g/kg of IVIG, although these findings need to be confirmed prospectively.[29]

The reason for the efficacy of IVIG treatment in KS is not well understood. Geographical clustering, epidemics and even pandemics in Japan, and seasonal variations, e.g. late winter and spring, suggest infection as an etiology. The observation that children less than 6 months or greater than 8 years of age are rarely affected suggests that the lack of a protective antibody against the putative KS agent may be an important risk factor for development of KS. Finally, in support of its infectious etiology, the acute onset of disease has clinical features that are strongly suggestive of infection.

KS is associated with marked activation of T cells and monocyte-macrophages.[30] Based on the immunologic and clinical features overlapping with a bacterial toxic shock-like syndrome, studies were carried out to determine if KS is associated with exposure to a superantigen such as a bacterial toxin.[31] In this regard, the findings that patients with acute KS have significantly elevated levels of circulating Vβ2$^+$ T cells and, to a lesser extent, Vβ8.1$^+$ T cells, supports the hypothesis that the T-cell activation associated with KS is due to a superantigen.[31] The observation that a Vβ2 (and, to a lesser extent, Vβ8) stimulating superantigen or bacterial toxin may be involved has provided a new approach to uncovering the infectious etiology of KS. Leung et al[32] cultured *S. aureus* and group A streptococci from the throat, rectum, axillae and/or groin of KS patients and tested for production of toxins, including TSST-1 and SPE-C, which are known to have marked Vβ2-stimulatory activity. TSST-1-secreting *S. aureus* was isolated in 11 cases, whereas streoptococcal toxins SPE-B and SPE-C were found in the other 2. The toxin-producing *S. aureus* isolated from these patients had a highly unusual appearance and could easily have been mistaken for coagulase-negative staphylococci.

KEY CONCEPTS

Immunoregulatory abnormalities associated with acute Kawasaki syndrome
- Increased T-cell and monocyte-macrophage activation
- Selective expansion of Vβ2$^+$ and Vβ8$^+$ T cells
- Increased serum levels of soluble CD25, CD4, and CD8
- Polyclonal B-cell activation
- Antibodies against vascular endothelial cell antigens and neutrophil cytoplasmic antigens
- Increased cytokine production (interferon, IL-1, TNF-α, IL-6)

The mechanism by which a superantigen can lead to the clinical manifestations of KS remains to be elucidated. However, acute KS is associated with marked immune activation and increased circulating cytokine levels including IL-1, IL-6, IL-8, IL-4, IL-10, and TNF-α.[31] Some of these cytokines elicit pro-inflammatory and prothrombotic responses by inducing the expression of leukocyte adhesion molecules, which localize inflammatory cells to vascular endothelial cells. The expression of endothelial–leukocyte adhesion molecules has been demonstrated in acute KS, and its down-regulation correlates with a favorable response to IVIG treatment.[30] In contrast, patients treated with aspirin alone show prolonged T and B cell activation. The magnitude and persistence of pro-inflammatory cytokine synthesis have been reported to constitute a risk for the development of coronary artery abnormalities.

IVIG has been shown to contain high titers of specific antibodies inhibitory to the activation of T cells by staphylococcal and streptococcal superantigens.[33] These findings may account for the observation that treatment of acute KS with IVIG results in a marked reduction of macrophage and T-cell activation.[34] In this regard, the efficacy of IVIG in suppressing the immune activation associated with KS, and, more importantly, its ability to prevent the development of coronary artery abnormalities in this illness, may relate to the neutralizing antibody activity of IVIG against these bacterial toxins. The findings that a threshold dose of IVIG is needed to decrease signs of acute inflammation in KS and that some patients require re-treatment suggest that IVIG contains variable antitoxin titers.[35] Finally, toxin neutralization is likely not the only beneficial effect of IVIG in KS. Other potential mechanisms of IVIG discussed in this chapter include immunomodulation of cytokine production or cytokine effects, thus inhibiting endothelial cell activation. IVIG could also inhibit vascular endothelial cell activation indirectly by its action on immune effector cells. New insights into the pathogenesis of KS will likely help to elucidate the mechanisms by which IVIG reduces coronary artery vasculitis.

NEUROMUSCULAR DISEASES

Demyelinating polyneuropathies

The inflammatory demyelinating polyneuropathies are subdivided into the acute type or Guillain–Barré syndrome (GBS), and a chronic progressive or relapsing-remitting inflammatory demyelinating polyneuropathy (CIDP)[36] (Chapter 78). Although the etiology of GBS is not known, the pathogenesis of GBS is thought to be an autoimmune process with destruction of peripheral nerve myelin. Most cases are preceded by an upper respiratory or diarrheal illness. *Campylobacter jejuni* is the most common bacterial pathogen isolated from the gastrointestinal tract.

About 80% of GBS patients recover satisfactorily. The principal approach to the treatment of these patients has been supportive therapy. In 1992, a Dutch group reported on a randomized trial comparing IVIG (0.4 g/kg per day for 5 days) and plasma exchange (PE).[37] Muscle strength improved by one grade in 34% of those treated with PE compared to 53% of those receiving IVIG; median time to improvement was 41 and 27 days, respectively. The IVIG group had fewer complications, but there had been some concerns about a high relapse rate with IVIG. In a large European multicenter randomized trial of 379 adult patients with GBS,[38] the efficacy of PE (50 ml/kg for 5 exchanges) was compared with IVIG (0.4 g/kg for 5 days), and with a combination regimen of PE followed by IVIG. There were no differences between any of the treatment groups for the major and secondary outcome measures.

It appears that PE in GBS is most effective when carried out early in the course of the disease.[39] Early recognition and treatment may thus be important for the long-term prognosis of patients who have severe disease and rapid progression. IVIG treatment is more readily available, easier, and has fever side-effects than PE, and this modality of treatment might be more useful in GBS patients at the early stage of disease, especially in patients who have evidence of rapid progression, who are older, or who have a history of diarrhea. In children with GBS, IVIG therapy was equally as effective as plasmapheresis, and was associated with fewer complications.[40]

Chronic inflammatory demyelinating polyradiculoneuropathy (CIDP) is an inflammatory neurologic disease resembling GBS that can cause prolonged disability. As for GBS, an immune-mediated mechanism for myelin destruction has been postulated in CIDP. A double-blind placebo-controlled crossover study of IVIG was performed by van Doorn and colleagues[41] for patients with CIDP. All IVIG-treated patients (0.4 g/kg IVIG per day for 5 consecutive days) improved on day 8 after therapy; in contrast, none of the patients receiving placebo improved and 2 patients underwent further deterioration. However, not all patients respond to IVIG and certainly not all patients respond to the same extent. Improvement is usually noticed within the first week of treatment and may last for 6–8 weeks. Many patients can be maintained with IVIG pulse-therapy of 1 g/kg body weight prior to the expected relapse. A beneficial response to IVIG was found to be more likely in patients with acute relapse or with disease of one year or less. Patients with sensory signs responded less well. Children with CIDP also respond well to IVIG.[42] Patients with an IgM monoclonal paraprotein associated with a demyelinating peripheral neuropathy may also respond to IVIG treatment.[43] In contrast, patients with a paraneoplastic neurological syndrome and antineuronal autoantibodies (anti-Hu and anti-Yo) did not respond to IVIG therapy.[44] Multifocal motor neuropathy shares some similarities with GBS and CIDP. This disorder is characterized by progressive distal, asymmetric limb weakness with a conduction block of motor but not sensory nerves. However, several open label studies and a control trial showed that multifocal motor neuropathy responds to IVIG therapy.[40] The beneficial effects of IVIG are, however, often not long-lasting.

These autoimmune demyelinating polyneuropathies are considered to be immunologically mediated disorders of the peripheral nervous system.[45] An initial lymphocytic infiltration, and, later on, an influx of macrophages, leads to demyelination. A variety of cellular and humoral immune perturbations has been described in patients with GBS. Elevated serum levels of several pro-inflammatory cytokines, including TNF-α and IFN-γ, have been reported. Other cytokines have been reported to be elevated in the CSF of GBS patients, including IL-1β and IL-6. Antibodies reactive against myelin components, e.g. ganglioside-specific antibodies such as GM_1, GD_{1b} and GQ_{1b}, are found in the sera of many patients with GBS. Anti GM_1 antibodies are also found in patients with motor neuropathies and motor neuron disease. Anti-GM_1 antibodies are more prominent in GBS patients lacking sensory symptoms and in those patients who have a prodromal diarrheal disease.

The association of certain viruses and bacteria and their serologies with GBS suggests that these microbial agents are involved in the pathogenesis of GBS. Van der Meché and colleagues[46] reported that sera of GBS patients have antibodies to the ganglioside GM_1 which shares epitopes on *Campylobacter* bacteria. Interestingly, the lipopolysaccharides (LPS) in the capsule of *C. jejuni*, a frequent cause of diarrheal disease preceding GBS, have epitopes related to the ganglioside GM_1 and GQ_{1b}. This has led to the hypothesis that molecular mimicry is involved in the pathogenesis of GBS, wherein immune responses against *C. jejuni* LPS produce cross-reactive antibodies to myelin with subsequent demyelination. Another possible mechanism leading to demyelination is complement deposition on the surface of Schwann cells and the myelin sheath, which leads to the recruitment of macrophages and complement-mediated damage.[47]

THERAPEUTIC PRINCIPLES

Guillain–Bauré syndrome

- Plasmapheresis and IVIG treatment are equally effective.
- There are fewer side-effects with IVIG therapy.
- Plasmapheresis is most effective when carried out early in the course of the disease.
- Because of fewer side-effects, IVIG is the therapy of choice in GBS patients with rapid progression, older age, or history of preceding diarrhea.

KEY CONCEPTS

Immune pathogenesis of GBS and CIDP

- Molecular mimicry between epitopes on capsule of *Campylobacter jejuni* and myelin
  - —Preceding history of diarrhea
  - —Positive stool culture for *C. jejuni*
- Autoantibodies to myelin components, i.e. ganglioside-specific antibodies (GM_1, GD_{1b}, GQ_{1b})
- Macrophage influx into lesions
- Complement deposition on Schwann cell and myelin sheath

Myasthenia gravis

Myasthenia gravis (MG) is an antibody-mediated autoimmune disease directed against the acetylcholine nicotinic receptor (AChR) which results in abnormalities of neuromuscular transmission leading to fluctuating weakness and fatigability (Chapter 76). A number of case reports and small, uncontrolled clinical trials have been reported in which over 100 patients were treated with IVIG.[40] A number of different preparations and dosage regimens have been employed. The overall response rate is about 74%, with improvement occurring within 3 weeks from the start of therapy. The duration of the response is variable and seems to be longer if patients are receiving steroids. AChR antibody titers declined in four trials but remained unchanged in three others. Overall, the clinical response does not appear to correlate with AChR antibody levels. Repeated courses of IVIG may be needed to maintain improvement. A recent controlled trial comparing the efficacy and side-effects of IVIG (using two IVIG dosages) to PE in MG patients undergoing exacerbation showed similar efficacy but fewer side-effects in the IVIG group.[48]

Inflammatory myopathies

Polymyositis, dermatomyositis, and inclusion body myositis are inflammatory muscle disorders characterized by muscle weakness and cellular infiltrates within the skeletal muscles (Chapter 65). These diseases are thought to have a similar pathogenesis, but each inflammatory myopathy group has characteristic clinical and immunopathologic features which sets them apart.[49] Dermatomyositis affects the proximal muscles and is associated with a violaceous rash on the face and extremities.

Dalakas and coworkers[50] conducted a double-blind, placebo-controlled study of 15 patients (age 18–55 years) with treatment-resistant dermatomyositis. Patients were randomly assigned to receive IVIG therapy (2 g/kg) or placebo every month for 3 months. The patients receiving IVIG had significant improvements in muscle strength, neuromuscular symptoms related to daily living, and skin rash. Clinical improvement became noticeable about 15 days after the first IVIG infusion. Serum creatine kinase fell by 50% after the first infusion, with further decreases toward normalization in subsequent infusions. Unfortunately, continued improvement of these patients was variable. Some patients continued to get IVIG less frequently and were able to maintain improvement along with low-dose steroids. Some patients who were unresponsive to steroids during their initial treatment regimen became steroid-responsive following IVIG infusion. Muscle biopsy studies showed marked improvement in muscle histology after IVIG treatment.[50] The mean muscle fiber diameter and the mean number of capillaries increased. Immunological activation markers, such as MHC Class I determinants and ICAM-1 expression, became diminished after IVIG therapy. TGF-β, which is up-regulated in the muscle tissues of patients with dermatomyositis, was markedly down-regulated. Finally, in muscle biopsies after therapy, the complement-mediated damage was diminished after IVIG therapy.

Inclusion body myositis (IBM) is the most common inflammatory muscle disorder in individuals above the age of 50 and is characterized by a slowly progressive muscle weakness and atrophy affecting the proximal and distal muscle groups. Dysphagia is also frequent, occurring in 60% of patients. In polymyositis and inclusion body myositis, sensitized $CD8^+$ cytotoxic T cells recognize unidentified muscle antigens, leading to phagocytosis and muscle fiber necrosis.

Initial open-label small trials suggested that IVIG was helpful in some patients with IBM, particularly with activities related to daily living. Other uncontrolled studies showed no benefit of IVIG. Dalakas and coworkers[51] conducted a double-blind placebo-controlled crossover study in 19 patients with IBM using monthly IVIG infusions of 2 g/kg or placebo for 3 months. Although there was mild statistical improvement in the IVIG group (6 of 19 patients), the study did not establish efficacy for IVIG treatment. In a follow-up study, Dalakas and coworkers[52] conducted a larger study combining IVIG therapy with prednisone. When the control group was compared with the IVIG treatment group, there appeared to be no clear benefit in either group. There were minor gains in strengths in the IVIG randomized patients, but this was not significant.

Mechanisms of action of IVIG in neuromuscular diseases

The autoimmune neurologic diseases and inflammatory myopathies provide a broad group of immunologically-mediated diseases in which many inflammatory and immune-mediated effector pathways lead to tissue destruction. These neurologic and myopathic diseases provide models for the study of the mechanisms of action by which IVIG modulates autoimmune and inflammatory processes. Several mechanisms have been proposed for the immune-modulating effects of IVIG. IVIG may modulate the inflammatory response by the suppression of cytokine production. Sharief and colleagues[53] showed that several pro-inflammatory cytokines, e.g. TNF-α and IL-1β, in GBS patients decreased with IVIG therapy. Dalakas and coworkers[54] documented reduction in tissue levels of TGF-β and TGF-β mRNA in patients with inflammatory myopathies with IVIG treatment. Although IVIG may contain antibodies to certain cytokines,[55] other work suggested that IVIG was down-regulating cytokine production by inhibiting gene expression.[56] It is of interest that PE was not associated with a decrease in these pro-inflammatory cytokines, suggesting that the mechanisms of action of PE and IVIG in GBS may be quite different.

A number of studies have shown that IVIG contains antibodies with idiotypic specificities that can bind and neutralize potentially pathogenic autoantibodies such as anti-GM_1 antibodies in GBS and CIDP and anti-AchR in MG.[57] Malik and coworkers[58] showed that anti-idiotypic antibodies in the IVIG directed against idiotypes located on the anti-GM_1 immunoglobulin molecule blocked the binding of the anti-GM_1 antibodies to their target antigen. Van Doorn et al,[59] using an immunofluorescence assay, showed that the sera of patients with GBS and CIDP contained antibodies to a cell membrane constituent of a neuroblastoma cell line. Intact IVIG or $F(ab')_2$ fragments blocked these antibodies from binding to the cell membrane of this neuroblastoma cell line. These studies again suggest an idiotype–anti-idiotype interaction as a possible mechanism by which IVIG could modulate the immune-mediated disease process and contribute to the remyelination in patients with GBS and CIDP. Support for a similar mechanism in MG comes from the fact that IgG or $F(ab')_2$ fragments in the IVIG preparations are capable of binding to AChR antibodies in vitro.[60] Vassilev et al[61] showed that normal human IVIG could suppress experimental MG in SCID mice. Further studies are necessary to determine the significance of these anti-idiotypic antibodies in IVIG as immune modulators in the pathogenesis of these autoimmune neurological diseases.

The principal inflammatory mechanism in dermatomyositis is complement (C)-dependent microangiopathy with activation of C3 and deposition of the complement C5b-9 membranolytic attack complex (MAC) on the endomysial capillaries.[49] It has been shown that IVIG can inhibit the uptake of C components on target tissues.[62] In dermatomyositis patients treated with IVIG, C3 deposition was reduced, with corresponding decreases in MAC expression on endomysial capillaries. Dalakas[63] postulated that the IVIG prevented the uptake of complement components and formation of the MAC on the endomysial capillaries in the muscle tissues of patients with dermatomyositis. Consequently, IVIG allowed neovascularization to occur and reversal of the ischemic process, resulting in muscle tissue healing. This effect of IVIG on complement deposition may be relevant to other autoimmune neurological diseases, such as MG, in which complement may be playing a role in the tissue damage at the postsynaptic junctional membrane.

Other neurological diseases

Multiple sclerosis is the most common demyelinating disorder of the central nervous system, and its pathogenesis is thought to reflect an autoimmune process (Chapter 77). Several uncontrolled and open-label studies have shown a beneficial effect of long-term IVIG therapy in the treatment of acute exacerbations in patients with multiple sclerosis. In a randomized placebo-controlled trial of monthly infusions of IVIG therapy, Fazekas and the Austrian Immunoglobulin Multiple Sclerosis Study Group[64] reported beneficial effects of IVIG in patients with relapsing-remitting multiple sclerosis. Seventy five of 150 patients received monthly doses of IVIG (0.15–0.2 g/kg). The number of patients who improved in the IVIG group was 31%, while in the placebo group only 14% of patients improved. Side-effects were minimal. Future studies need to correlate changes in disease activity with changes in multiple sclerosis lesions as measured by magnetic resonance imaging. Finally, a low dose of IVIG was utilized in this study (0.15–0.2 g/kg) in contrast to a much higher dose of monthly IVIG (1–2 g/kg) usually employed in other autoimmune diseases.

Ten to 20% of childhood epilepsies are intractable, i.e. not controlled adequately with first-line conventional antiepileptic drug therapy. Epileptic children treated with IVIG for recurrent respiratory tract infections, were said to demonstrate a decrease in the frequency and severity of their seizures. A number of investigators have suggested that immune mechanisms are important in the pathogenesis of epilepsy, particularly in cases associated with infections or vaccination. A number of reports have appeared on the responsiveness of certain patients with childhood epilepsy to IVIG therapy. The favorable effects of IVIG treatment were especially seen in children with West syndrome and Lennox–Gastaut syndrome. Two placebo-controlled studies[65,66] showed significant reductions in seizure episodes with IVIG treatment. Additional multicenter placebo-controlled trials are needed to further define the subpopulation of children with intractable seizures who would benefit from IVIG treatment, although the best candidates appear to be those patients with West syndrome and Lennox–Gastaut syndrome and those patients who have postinfectious epileptic encephalopathies. Perlmutter and coworkers[67] reported a placebo-controlled study with PE and IVIG in patients with obsessive-compulsive disorder and tic disorders (Tourette syndrome). At 1 month the PE and IVIG groups showed striking improvements on several neuropsychiatric functioning scales. Tic symptoms also significantly improved. Improvement was maintained at 1 year by 82% of the children in both the PE and IVIG groups.

SYSTEMIC VASCULITIS

Churg–Strauss vasculitis and Wegener's granulomatosis are systemic vasculitides associated with granuloma formation (Chapter 67). In 1991, Jayne et al[68] examined the therapeutic effects of high-dose IVIG on the disease activity and circulating antineutrophil cytoplasmic antibody (ANCA) levels in 7 patients with systemic vasculitis. IVIG was infused at 400 mg/kg per dose over 5 consecutive days. All 7 patients had clinical improvement that was sustained in 6 but transient in 1 patient. ANCA levels decreased by 51% of pretreatment values, and improvement started 2 days to 3 weeks after IVIG therapy; 5 patients went into full remission. Other investigators also reported beneficial clinical responses following high-dose IVIG treatment (400 mg/kg for 5 days).[69,70] Response rates vary between 60% and 100%, and may be related in some patients to a chronic parvovirus B19 infection. Further placebo-controlled studies are necessary.

RHEUMATIC DISEASES

The clinical studies of IVIG therapy in patients with rheumatoid arthritis (RA) have been small and uncontrolled; efficacy has been variable. Several open-label trials have reported benefits of IVIG therapy in patients with RA. A randomized placebo-controlled study by Silverman and coworkers[71] did not find any efficacy for IVIG in children with systemic juvenile RA.

Several studies have examined the use of IVIG in patients with systemic lupus erythematosus (SLE). In a pilot study of 12 patients with SLE, Schroeder et al[72] reported a partial transient clinical response with IVIG treatment and a decrease in anti-DNA antibody levels. Skin biopsies showed a marked reduction in the deposition of complement components and IgM. Responses could be maintained in some patients by monthly IVIG infusions. While some of these isolated clinical reports are encouraging, others indicating worsening or exacerbation of the renal disease in SLE are of concern.[73] Those SLE patients with major clinical manifestations of cutaneous vasculitis and/or cytopenias, particularly thrombocytopenia, may benefit from IVIG therapy.

Mechanisms of action of IVIG in rheumatic diseases and vasculitides

A number of mechanisms of action have been proposed to explain the immunoregulatory effects of IVIG in patients with vasculitis. Immune complexes are felt to be a major component in the pathophysiology of SLE. Several studies have suggested that IVIG can solubilize immune complexes, making them less nephritogenic.[74] This is supported by observations of decreases in circulating immune complexes in SLE patients treated with IVIG.[71]

Using adsorption columns, Williams and colleagues[75] showed that commercial IVIG contains anti-idiotypic anti-DNA antibodies and was capable of blocking the combining sites of a broad range of SLE IgG anti-DNA antibodies. IVIG contains anti-idiotypic antibodies against a number of autoantibodies such as anti-DNA, anti-factor VIII, ANCA autoantibodies, antithyroid autoantibodies and others.[76] The proposed mechanism of action of IVIG in ANCA-positive vasculitis is binding or neutralization of the ANCA autoantibodies by anti-idiotypic antibodies in the IVIG. These anti-idiotypic antibodies may also act in concert with their effects on the FcγRIIb receptor on B-cells to produce a negative 'off signal' to the B cells synthesizing these autoimmune antibodies.[77] Thus, the anti-idiotypic antibodies in IVIG may be beneficial by restoring the idiotypic control network in these autoimmune diseases.

ANTIPHOSPHOLIPID ANTIBODY SYNDROME AND RECURRENT SPONTANEOUS ABORTION

An SLE-related disorder in which IVIG has been used as treatment is the anti-phospholipid antibody syndrome that is associated with recurrent spontaneous abortion (RSA) (Chapters 60, 83). In this condition autoantibodies are present to certain phospholipids such as cardiolipin. Clinical manifestations include a thrombotic diathesis often associated with recurrent fetal loss or fetal wastage that is considered to be secondary to placental infarcts resulting in placental insufficiency. RSA, defined as two or more consecutive pregnancy losses before 20 weeks of gestation, occurs in approximately 5% of couples. Laboratory tests in these patients include false-positive tests for syphilis (VDRL) and the presence of a lupus anticoagulant (LAC). Therapy with corticosteroids, low-dose aspirin, and heparin has been directed at suppressing the production of these autoantibodies and controlling the thrombotic diathesis. Several randomized controlled trials of IVIG therapy in Europe, Canada, and the USA have been completed using dosages ranging from 25 to 30 g biweekly or 500 mg/kg monthly from early pregnancy to 28–32 weeks' gestation. Daya et al[78] performed a meta-analysis of four randomized double-blind placebo-controlled trials of IVIG in women with RSA. Two studies[79,80] showed an increase in successful pregnancy outcome with IVIG treatment, whereas two other studies[81,82] did not show positive results. The overall odds ratio was 1.48 in favor of IVIG, with a treatment effect of approximately 10%. The meta-analysis results of these four controlled studies suggest that the issue is still open. Nevertheless, IVIG may have a role in the treatment of patients with RSA.

Some investigators have suggested that the cytotoxicity of peripheral blood natural killer cells against fetal antigens may play a role in RSA.[80] Interestingly, normal pregnancy appears to be characterized by a predominantly Th2 response against trophoblast antigens, while a Th1 response characterizes patients with RSA. The increased prevalence of autoantibodies such as antiphospholipid antibodies and antinuclear antibodies may not be related to the pathogenesis of RSA but might result from an imbalance between the Th1 and Th2 immune responses. Elevated levels of natural killer cells have been found in the blood and in the uterus of women who have spontaneous abortions. It has been reported that elevated levels of NK cells in the peripheral blood are decreased in women with RSA after treatment with IVIG.[83] The effects of IVIG on cytokine synthesis may help to restore the Th1–Th2 balance during pregnancy to preserve the fetus against rejection processes.[84]

TOXIC SHOCK SYNDROME

IVIG may have therapeutic value in the treatment of patients with toxic shock syndrome secondary to *Staphylococcus aureus* or *Streptococcus pyogenes* exotoxin. An experimental toxic shock rabbit model showed that IVIG was protective when administered as long as 29 hours after the induction of toxic shock with staphylococcal exotoxin.[85] IVIG can be beneficial in patients with toxic shock syndrome. Studies by Takei et al[33] showed that IVIG inhibited *Staphylococcus* exotoxin-induced T-cell activation, and contained antibodies against exotoxins responsible for toxic shock syndromes. Norrby-Tetlund et al[35] studied various IVIG preparations and different lots of the same IVIG brand for specific neutralizing activity against streptococcal pyrogenic exotoxins and a mixture of superantigens present in the culture supernatants of group A streptococcal isolates. Great variations in the neutralizing activity of different brands and even among different lots of IVIG preparations were found. However, these findings suggest that it is possible to select one IVIG preparation that contains high levels of neutralizing activity against a wide variety of group A streptococcal superantigens and use it in the treatment of streptococcal toxic shock syndrome. The neutralizing capacity of IVIG for these bacterial superantigens is important because of their potential to stimulate the production of proinflammatory cytokines that lead to clinical disease.

SKIN DISEASES

Toxic epidermal necrolysis (TEN) or Lyell syndrome is a severe drug-induced skin disease in which apoptotic epidermal cell death results in the separation of large areas of the skin at the epidermal junction, producing the appearance of scalded skin. Keratinocyte apoptosis that precedes epidermal detachment is an early event in TEN. A number of drugs can cause TEN, including sulfonamides, anticonvulsants, and nonsteroidal anti-inflammatory medications. The mortality rate can be as high as 30%. Viard et al[86] studied serum samples from patients who had TEN and found that the serum of these patients contained very high levels of soluble Fas ligand (sFasL). Keratinocytes normally express the cell death receptor Fas. The keratinocytes of patients with TEN also express very high levels of active Fas ligand. In this small pilot study, IVIG was administered (0.2–0.75 g/kg for 4 consecutive days) to 10 patients with TEN. In all 10 patients, the progression of skin disease was rapidly interrupted within 24–48 hours with rapid skin healing and no adverse effects. In in vitro studies, IVIG was added to keratinocyte cell cultures to determine whether IVIG could interfere with Fas-mediated cell death. IVIG completely inhibited Fas-mediated keratinocyte apoptosis. This effect was related to the presence of Fas-blocking antibodies in the IVIG. In a related study, Prasad et al[87] also demonstrated that IVIG contained anti-Fas antibodies. Thus, the mechanisms by which IVIG leads to clinical improvement in patients with TEN is likely related to the inhibition of Fas-mediated keratinocyte cell death by naturally occurring Fas-blocking antibodies in the IVIG preparation. This mechanism of action of IVIG may be useful in other diseases in which tissue injury is mediated by Fas-mediated apoptosis.

Atopic diseases

Atopic dermatitis

Treatment of severe refractory atopic dermatitis (AD) with IVIG has yielded conflicting results. A recent study of high-dose IVIG (2 g/kg) concluded that IVIG had no clear clinical benefit in AD.[88]

Chronic urticaria

A subset of patients with chronic urticaria have IgG autoantibodies directed against the α chain of the high-affinity receptor for IgE,[89] suggesting an autoimmune etiology. Although IgG anti-FcεRI autoantibodies have been reported in a number of autoimmune diseases, a functional role in causing histamine release appears to be unique to chronic urticaria and is complement mediated.[90] O'Donnell et al[91] treated 10 patients with chronic severe urticaria poorly responsive to conventional therapy with IVIG 0.4 g/kg per day for 5 days. Clinical benefit was noted in 9 of these patients, including 3 who had prolonged remission over a 3-year follow-up period. The majority of responders had a decreased wheal-and-flare response to intradermal autologous serum compared with their pre-IVIG response.

ASTHMA

A number of advances and new drugs have been introduced over the past 10 years for the treatment of asthma (Chapter 50). Nevertheless, a subset of asthmatic patients continues to have frequent exacerbations of asthma and requires high doses of inhaled corticosteroids or oral systemic steroids to control their asthma. In 1991, Mazer and Gelfand[92] published an open-label study of IVIG (2 g/kg at monthly intervals) in 8 children (ages 6–17) who had severe steroid-dependent asthma. The average alternate-day steroid dose decreased, with improvements in peak-flow rates and symptom scores. The serum IgE levels decreased from 324 IU prior to therapy to 133 IU after 6 months on IVIG. Immediate hypersensitivity skin testing to inhalant allergens decreased 100-fold. Several other preliminary clinical trials suggested that IVIG was helpful in severe corticosteroid-dependent asthmatics, in whom the IVIG had a steroid-sparing effect. These clinical observations prompted other investigators to initiate randomized double-blind placebo-controlled multicenter studies. A multicenter randomized placebo-controlled study of high-dose IVIG in oral corticosteroid-dependent asthmatics was performed by Kishiyama et al.[93] There were two IVIG treatment groups, i.e. 1 and 2 g/kg at monthly intervals for 7 months. No differences were observed between the placebo (albumin 2 g/kg per month) and the two IVIG-treatment groups for FEV_1, emergency room visits, or days missed from work or school. Adverse events were common in the IVIG groups, especially in the high-dose treatment group. Subsequently, Salmun et al[94] published results of a double-blind placebo-controlled randomized trial of IVIG in children with severe asthma. Of 28 patients who completed the study, a significant reduction in oral steroid requirement occurred in both the IVIG and placebo treatment groups. In a subgroup of patients requiring extremely high doses of oral steroids (>2000 mg in the year before the study), there was a significant steroid-sparing effect by the IVIG. These authors concluded that IVIG was useful in a subgroup of severe asthmatic patients who required high doses of oral steroids. A larger placebo-controlled trial is needed to determine the efficacy of IVIG therapy in oral steroid-dependent asthmatics.

> **KEY CONCEPTS**
>
> **Postulated mechanisms of action of IVIG**
> - Neutralization of autoimmune antibodies by anti-idiotypic antibodies in the IVIG
> - Modulation of cytokine synthesis
> - Inhibit complement uptake on target tissues
> - Neutralization of staphylococcal and streptococcal exotoxins
> - Inhibition of Fas-mediated cell death by Fas-blocking antibodies in the IVIG
> - Enhance glucocorticoid receptor binding affinity
> - Inhibit B-cell function through the low-affinity FcγRIIb1 receptor.
> - Neutralizing antibodies to cytokines
> - Fc receptor blockade of reticuloendothelial system
> - Solubilization of immune complexes

A number of mechanisms have been proposed for the effects of IVIG in asthma. IVIG can modulate the synthesis of cytokines.[95] Spahn et al[96] showed that the addition of IVIG to PHA-stimulated lymphocytes shifted the dexamethasone dose–response curve rendering the cells more sensitive to the suppressive effects of steroids in patients with glucocorticoid-insensitive asthma. In addition, IVIG significantly improved glucocorticoid receptor binding affinity, which may be responsible for the steroid-sparing effects of IVIG.

The mechanisms by which IVIG suppresses immunoglobulin synthesis of B-cells have been postulated to be the inhibition of cytokine production and the direct suppression of B-cell function through the low-affinity Fcγ receptor. FcγRIIb1 receptor on B cells can provide a negative signal through protein tyrosine phosphatases (SHP-1) to inhibit B-cell proliferation and decrease antibody synthesis. The mechanism for this negative signaling in B cells is thought to be the immunoreceptor tyrosine-based inhibition motif (ITIM) that is known to be associated with the intracytoplasmic domain of the FcγRIIb1 receptor.[77] Coligation of the B-cell receptor and the FcγRIIb1 receptor could occur by the binding of IgG in IVIG through its Fc moiety. Binding could involve the FcγRIIb1 receptor and the $F(ab')_2$ moiety with anti-idiotypic antibody specificity to the B-cell antigen receptor. Thus, through pathways that modulate cytokine production and decrease B-cell Ig synthesis, with resultant diminished serum levels of IgE antibodies, IVIG may have both anti-inflammatory and immunodulating effects that modulate the immunopathogenesis of asthma.

SIDE-EFFECTS

The frequency of side-effects due to IVIG is low, even at doses of up to 2 g/kg as used for the disease conditions described in this chapter, although the true incidence remains unknown because of the voluntary nature of reporting side-effects. Most patients with side-effects attributable to high-dose IVIG experience mild symptoms such as headache, fever, chills, and nausea. These adverse events can be alleviated by slowing down the infusion rate, or by pretreatment with acetaminophen or diphenhydramine or, if necessary, with corticosteroids. Cutaneous reactions reported with IVIG infusion include urticaria, lichenoid eruptions, pruritus, and petechiae.[97] Patients with IgA deficiency may experience IgG- or IgE-mediated anti-IgA reactions during IVIG infusion. Despite the higher incidence of IgA deficiency found in patients with autoimmune diseases, severe anaphylactic/anaphylactoid reactions with IVIG infusions are extremely rare. Gammagard-SD (Baxter Healthcare) contains the least amount of IgA among currently available IVIG preparations and can be used cautiously in patients with IgA deficiency.

Aseptic meningitis has been reported in patients receiving high doses of IVIG.[98] This adverse effect appears to be unrelated to the IVIG product used, infusion rate, or underlying illness. Sekul et al[99] found that aseptic meningitis occurred in 50% of a subgroup of patients treated with high-dose IVIG who had a history of migraine headaches compared with only 4% of patients without such a history. Prophylaxis with intravenous corticosteroids is often ineffective. Symptoms may require narcotic analgesics and resolve over several days without sequelae.

Congestive heart failure following treatment with IVIG has also been reported in a small number of children with acute KS complicated by myocarditis. However, this can also be seen in children with KS treated with aspirin alone. Thromboembolic events, likely due to increased serum viscosity, have also been described in patients treated with IVIG.[100]

Deterioration of pre-existing renal disease has been reported in several SLE patients treated with IVIG[101] and transient elevation of serum creatinine has been observed in nephrotic patients receiving high-dose IVIG.[102] The US Food and Drug Administration recently summarized the epidemiology of IVIG-associated renal insufficiency and failure reported between 1985 and 1998.[103] It appears that approximately 88% of cases of IVIG-related acute renal failure reported in the USA have been associated with sucrose-containing products. Histopathologic results in a few cases have been consistent with osmotic injury. Most cases have occurred in patients treated for ITP, with fewer than 5% involving patients with primary immunodeficiencies.

IVIG preparations available in the USA are safe with respect to transmission of known viral or other infectious agents: donors are screened for HIV, HTLV-1, hepatitis A, B, and C viruses; HIV and hepatitis B are inactivated by the fractionation process; and the use of detergents, solvents, enzymes and low pH inactivates hepatitis C and other viruses. HIV has never been transmitted through IVIG infusion. Unfortunately, a number of cases of hepatitis C were associated with the use of Gammagard;[104] this product has since been replaced by Gammagard-SD, a product treated with both solvent and detergent. No convincing evidence exists for the transmission of prions through IVIG.

Overall, serious side-effects directly attributable to IVIG remain rare and, when reported, may be difficult to distinguish from clinical events that might have occurred during the natural course of the underlying illness. Suspected adverse events should be reported to the manufacturer/distributor or, in the USA, to the MEDWATCH program (800 FDA-1088).

CLINICAL PEARLS

Adverse effects of IVIG

- Most side-effects due to rate of infusion and/or high dose (2 g/kg)
- Headache, fever, chills, nausea, myalgia, arthralgia, urticaria – pretreat with acetaminophen, nonsteroidal anti-inflammatory or corticosteroids (100 mg Solucortef)
- Aseptic meningitis – history of migraine a risk factor
- Thromboembolic – older patients, dehydrated state
- Renal insufficiency:
  - — Pre-existing renal disease (SLE)
  - — Sucrose-containing IVIG products
- Transmission of infectious agents such as hepatitis C – prior to 1995
- Risk of anaphylaxis in IgA-deficient patient

CONCLUSIONS

IVIG has been found to be an effective treatment for a wide spectrum of autoimmune and inflammatory diseases. At present, it is approved by the FDA for use in ITP and KS. However, even in ITP and KS, the exact mechanism of action of IVIG remains to be fully elucidated. Although numerous mechanisms have been proposed to explain the beneficial effects of high-dose IVIG (Fig. 104.2), none can satisfactorily explain its effects in the many clinical conditions for which it has been used. It is important to recognize that IVIG contains not only a broad spectrum of IgG antibodies, but also small amounts of other immunoglobulin isotypes, as well as soluble cell membrane products and HLA determinants. These 'contaminants' may in fact play an important immunomodulatory role in autoimmune and inflammatory diseases. Better understanding of the pathogenetic mechanisms involved in these diseases will undoubtedly lead to more effective therapy with IVIG or more specific, modified forms of this product.

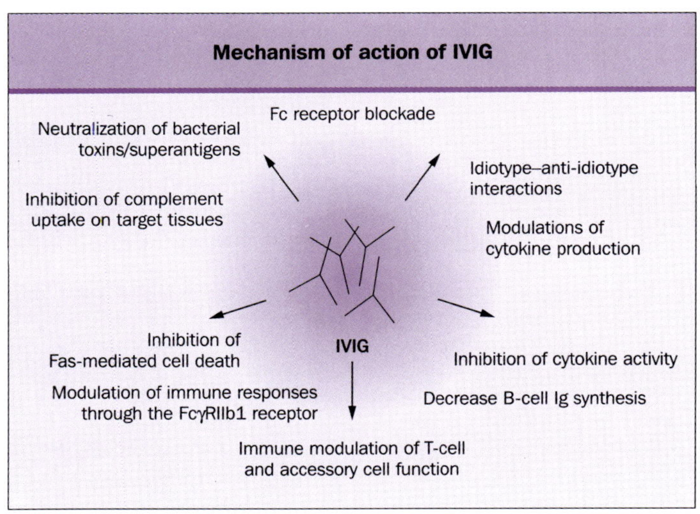

Figure 104.2 Possible mechanisms of action of IVIG. Probably no single mechanism is responsible for the immunological effects of IVIG. Several mechanisms undoubtedly work together to produce immune modulation or the anti-inflammatory effects of IVIG.

THERAPEUTIC PRINCIPLES

Treatment efficacy of IVIG in patients with autoimmune and inflammatory diseases

Proven efficacy by controlled studies
- Idiopathic thrombocytopenic purpura
- Autoimmune neutropenia
- Kawasaki syndrome
- Guillain–Barré syndrome
- Chronic inflammatory demyelinating polyradiculoneuropathy
- Multifocal motor neuropathy
- Myasthenia gravis
- Dermatomyositis (adult)

Probable treatment efficacy[a]
- Demyelinating peripheral neuropathy with IgM monoclonal paraproteins
- Multiple sclerosis
- Obsessive-compulsive and tic disorders
- Recurrent spontaneous abortion
- Toxic shock syndrome
- Toxic epidermal necrolysis
- Asthma (subset of high-dose-requiring oral corticosteroids)

Possible treatment efficacy[b]
- Autoimmune hemolytic anemia
- Autoimmune coagulopathies
- Polymyositis
- Rheumatoid arthritis (adult)
- Systemic vasculitis (ANCA positive or related to parvovirus B19 disease)
- Postinfectious or vaccine-related childhood seizure disorders (West syndrome; Lennox–Gastaut syndrome)
- Chronic urticaria with autoantibodies to FcεRI

Little or no treatment efficacy
- Inclusion body myositis
- Paraneoplastic neurological syndrome
- Juvenile rheumatoid arthritis
- Systemic lupus erythematosus
- Atopic dermatitis

[a] Few placebo-controlled trials, or supported by strong open-label clinical trials.
[b] Supported by open-label studies and anecdotal reports.

REFERENCES

1. Imbach P, d'Appuzo V, Hirt A, et al. High dose intravenous gammaglobulin for idiopathic thrombocytopenic purpura in childhood. Lancet 1981;1:1228.
2. Blanchette VS, Luke B, Andrew M, et al. A prospective, randomized trial of high-dose intravenous immune globulin G therapy, oral prednisone therapy, and no therapy in childhood acute immune thrombocytopenic purpura. J Pediatr 1993;123:989.
3. Imbach P, Wagner H, Berchtold W, et al. Intravenous immunoglobulin versus oral corticosteroids in acute immune thrombocytopenic purpura in childhood. Lancet 1985;2:464.
4. Blanchette V, Imbach P, Andrew M, et al. Randomised trial of intravenous immunoglobulin G, intravenous anti-D, and oral prednisone in childhood acute immune thrombocytopenic purpura. Lancet 1994;344:703.
5. Jacobs P, Wood L, Novitzky N. Intravenous gammaglobulin has no advantages over oral corticosteroids as primary therapy for adults with immune thrombocytopenia: a prospective randomized clinical trial. Am J Med 1994;97:55.
6. Tarantino MD, Madden RM, Fennewald DL, Patel CC, Bertolone SJ. Treatment of childhood acute immune thrombocytopenic purpura with anti-D immune globulin or pooled immune globulin. J Pediatr 1999;134:21.
7. Medeiros D, Buchanan GR. Major hemorrhage in children with idiopathic thrombocytopenic purpura: immediate response to therapy and long-term outcome. J Pediatr 1998;133:334.
8. George JN, Woolf SH, Raskob GE, et al. Idiopathic thrombocytopenic purpura: a practice guideline developed by explicit methods for the American Society of Hematology. Blood 1996;88:3.
9. Bussel J, Schulman I, Hilgartner M. Intravenous use of gammaglobulin in the treatment of chronic immune thrombocytopenic purpura as a means to defer splenectomy. J Pediatr 1983; 103:651.
10. Bussel JB, Pham LC. Intravenous treatment with gammaglobulin in adults with immune thrombocytopenic purpura: Review of the literature. Vox Sang 1987;52:206.
11. Law C, Marcaccio M, Tam P, Heddle N, Kelton JG. High-dose intravenous immune globulin and the response to splenectomy in patients with idiopathic thrombocytopenic purpura. N Engl J Med 1997;336:1494.
12. Warrier I, Bussel JB, Valdez L, Barbosa J, Beardsley DS, Group L-DIS. Safety and efficacy of low-dose intravenous immune globulin (IVIG) treatment for infants and children with immune thrombocytopenic purpura. J Pediatr Hematol Oncol 1997;19:197.
13. Fehr J, Hofmann V, Kappeler U. Transient reversal of thrombocytopenia in idiopathic thrombocytopenic purpura by high-dose intravenous gammaglobulin. N Engl J Med 1982; 306:1254.
14. Clarkson SB, Bussel JB, Kimberly RP, Valinsky JE, Nachman RL, Unkeless JC. Treatment of refractory immune thrombocytopenic purpura with an anti-Fcγ receptor antibody. N Engl J Med 1986;314:1236.
15. Debre M, Bonnet MC, Fridman WH, et al. Infusion of Fc gamma fragments for treatment of children with acute immune thrombocytopenic purpura. Lancet 1993;342:945.
16. Tovo P, Miniero R, Fiandino G, Saracco P, Messina M. Fc-depleted vs intact intravenous immunoglobulin in chronic ITP. J Pediatr 1984;105:676.
17. Kimberly K, Salmon J, Bussel J, Crow M, Hilgartner M. Modulation of mononuclear phagocyte functions by intravenous gamma globulin. J Immunol 1984;132:745.
18. Berchtold P, Dale GL, Tani P, McMillan R. Inhibition of autoantibody binding to platelet glycoprotein IIb/IIIa by antiidiotypic antibodies in intravenous gammaglobulin. Blood 1989; 74:2414.
19. Hilgartner MW, Bussel J. Use of intravenous gammaglobulin for the treatment of autoimmune neutropenia of childhood and autoimmune hemolytic anemia. Am J Med 1987; 83:25.
20. Bussel J, Lalezari P, Fikrig S. Intravenous treatment with gamma-globulin of autoimmune neutropenia of infancy. J Pediatr 1988;112:298.
21. Schwartz RS, Gabriel DA, Aledort LM, Green D, Kessler CM. A prospective study of treatment of acquired (autoimmune) factor VIII inhibitors with high-dose intravenous gammaglobulin. Blood 1995;86:797.
22. Sultan Y, Kazatchkine MD, Maisonneuve P, Nydegger UE. Anti-idiotypic suppression of autoantibodies to factor VIII (antihaemophilic factor) by high-dose intravenous gammaglobulin. Lancet 1984;2:765.

23. Sultan Y, Rossi F, Kazatchkine MD. Recovery from anti-VIIIc (antihemophilic factor) autoimmune disease is dependent on generation of anti-idiotypes against anti VIIIc autoantibodies. Proc Natl Acad Sci USA 1987;84:828.
24. Laupland KB, Dele Davies H. Epidemiology, etiology, and management of Kawasaki disease: state of the art. Pediatr Cardiol 1999;20:177.
25. Yanagawa H, Yashiro M, Nakamura Y, Kawasaki T, Kato H. Results of 12 nationwide epidemiological incidence surveys of Kawasaki disease in Japan. Arch Pediatr Adolescent Med 1995;149:779.
26. Newburger JW, Takahashi M, Burns JC, et al. The treatment of Kawasaki syndrome with intravenous gamma globulin. N Engl J Med 1986;315:341.
27. Newburger JW, Takahashi M, Beiser AS, et al. A single intravenous infusion of gamma globulin as compared with four infusions in the treatment of acute Kawasaki syndrome. N Engl J Med 1991;324:1633.
28. Durongpisitkul K, Gururaj VJ, Park JM, Martin CF. The prevention of coronary artery aneurysm in Kawasaki disease: a meta-analysis on the efficacy of aspirin and immunoglobulin treatment. Pediatrics 1995;96:1057.
29. Burns JC, Capparelli EV, Brown JA, Newburger JW, Glode MP. Intravenous gamma-globulin treatment and retreatment in Kawasaki disease. US/Canadian Kawasaki Syndrome Study Group. Pediatr Infect Dis J 1998;17:1144.
30. Leung DYM. Immunologic aspects of Kawasaki syndrome. J Rheumatol 1990;Suppl 24:15.
31. Leung DY. Kawasaki syndrome: immunomodulatory benefit and potential toxin neutralization by intravenous immune globulin. Clin Exp Immunol 1996;104:49.
32. Leung DYM, Meissner HC, Fulton DR, et al. Toxic shock syndrome toxin-secreting *Staphylococcus aureus* in Kawasaki syndrome. Lancet 1993;342:1385.
33. Takei S, Arora YK, Walker SM. Intravenous immunoglobulin contains specific antibodies inhibitory to activation of T cells by Staphylococcal toxin superantigens. J Clin Invest 1993;91:602.
34. Leung DYM, Burns J, Newburger J, et al. Reversal of immunoregulatory abnormalities in Kawasaki syndrome by intravenous gammaglobulin. J Clin Invest 1987;79:468.
35. Norrby-Teglund A, Basma H, Andersson J, McGeer A. Varying titers of neutralizing antibodies to streptococcal superantigens in different preparations of normal polyspecific immunoglobulin G: implications for therapeutic efficacy. Clin Infect Dis 1998;26:631.
36. Rostami AM. Pathogenesis of immune-mediated neuropathies. Pediatr Res 1993;33:S90.
37. van der Meché FGA, Schmitz PI, The Dutch Guillain–Barré Study Group. A randomized trial comparing intravenous immune globulin and plasma exchange in Guillain–Barré syndrome. N Engl J Med 1992;326:1123.
38. Plasma Exchange/Sandoglobulin Guillain–Barré Syndrome Trial Group. Randomised trial of plasma exchange, intravenous immunoglobulin, and combined treatments in Guillain–Barré syndrome. Lancet 1997;349:225.
39. Group. TG-BSS. Plasmapheresis and acute Guillain–Barré syndrome. Neurology 1985;35:1096.
40. Bril V, Allenby K, Midroni G, O'Connor PW, Vajsar J. IGIV in neurology – evidence and recommendations. Can J Neurol Sci 1999;26:139.
41. van Doorn PA, Brand A, Strengers PFW, Meulstee J, Vermeulen M. High-dose intravenous immunoglobulin treatment in chronic inflammatory demyelinating polyneuropathy: A double-blind, placebo-controlled, crossover study. Neurology 1990;40:209.
42. Simmons Z, Wald JJ, Albers JW. Chronic inflammatory demyelinating polyradiculoneuropathy. Muscle Nerve 1997;20:1569.
43. Cook D, Dalakas M, Galdi A, Biondi D, Porter H. High-dose intravenous immunoglobulin in the treatment of demyelinating neuropathy associated with monoclonal gammopathy. Neurology 1990;40:212.
44. Uchuya M, Graus F, Vega F, Rene R, Delattre J-Y. Intravenous immunoglobulin treatment in paraneoplastic neurological syndromes with antineuronal autoantibodies. J Neurol Neurosurg Psychiatry 1996;60:388.
45. Sater RA, Rostami A. Treatment of Guillain–Barré syndrome with intravenous immunoglobulin. Neurology 1998;51:S9.
46. van der Meché FGA, Visser LH, Jacobs BC, Endtz HP, Meuistee J, van Doorn PA. Guillain–Barré syndrome: Multifactorial mechanisms versus defined subgroups. J Infect Dis 1997;176:S99.
47. Hafer-Macko C, Sheikh K, Li CY. Immune attack on the Schwann cell surface in acute inflammatory demyelinating polyneuropathy. Ann Neurol 1996;39:625.
48. Gajdos P, Chevret S, Clair B, Tranchant C, Chastang C. Plasma exchange and intravenous immunoglobulin in autoimmune myasthenia gravis. Ann NY Acad Sci 1998; 841:720.
49. Dalakas MC. Polymyositis, dermatomyositis, and inclusion-body myositis. New Engl J Med 1991;325:1487.
50. Dalakas MC, Illa I, Dambrosia JM, Soueidan SA, et al. A controlled trial of high-dose intravenous immunoglobulin infusions as treatment for dermatomyositis. N Engl J Med 1993; 329:1993.
51. Dalakas MC, Sonies B, Dambrosia J, Sekul E, Cupler E, Sivakumar K. Treatment of inclusion-body myositis with IVIg: A double-blind, placebo-controlled study. Neurology 1997;48:712.
52. Dalakas MC, Sonies B, Koffman B, et al. High-dose intravenous immunoglobulin (IVig) combined with prednisone in the treatment of patients with inclusion-body myositis (IBM): a double blind, randomised controlled trial (Abstract). Neurology 1997;48:332.
53. Sharief MK, Ingram DA, Swash M, Thompson EJ. IV immunoglobulin reduces circulating proinflammatory cytokines in Guillain–Barré syndrome. Neurology 1999;52:1883.
54. Dalakas MC. Molecular immunology and genetics of inflammatory muscle diseases. Arch Neurol 1998;55:1509.
55. Ross C, Svenson M, Hansen M, Vejlsgaard GL, Bendtzen K. High avidity IFN-neutralizing antibodies in pharmaceutically prepared human IgG. J Clin Invest 1995;95:1974.
56. Campbell DE, Georgiou GM, Kemp AS. Pooled human immunoglobulin inhibits IL-4 but not IFN-gamma or TNF-alpha secretion following in vitro stimulation of mononuclear cells with Staphylococcal superantigen. Cytokine 1999;11:359.
57. Yuki N, Miyagi F. Possible mechanism of intravenous immunoglobulin treatment on anti-GM1 antibody-mediated neuropathies. J Neurol Sci 1996;139:160.
58. Malik U, Oleksowicz L, Latov N, Cardo LJ. Intravenous γ-globulin inhibits binding of anti-GM1 to its target antigen. Ann Neurol 1996;39:136.
59. van Doorn PA, Brand A, Vermeulen M. Anti-neuroblastoma cell line antibodies in inflammatory demyelinating polyneuropathy: Inhibition in vitro and in vivo by IV immunoglobulin. Neurology 1988;38:1592.
60. Liblau R, Gajdos P, Bustarret FA, El Habib R, Bach JF, Morel E. Intravenous γ-globulin in myasthenia gravis: interaction with antiacetylcholine receptor autoantibodies. J Clin Immunol 1991;11:128.
61. Vassilev T, Yamamoto M, Aissaoui A, et al. Normal human immunoglobulin suppresses experimental myasthenia gravis in SCID mice. Eur J Immunol 1999;29:2436.
62. Basta M, Dalakas MD. High-dose intravenous immunoglobulin exerts its beneficial effect in patients with dermatomyositis by blocking endomysial deposition of activated complement fragments. J Clin Invest 1994;94:1729.
63. Dalakas MC. Clinical relevance of IVIg in the modulation of the complement-mediated tissue damage: implications in dermatomyositis, Guillain-Barré syndrome and myasthenia gravis. In: Kazatchkine M (ed.) Intravenous immunoglobulin research and therapy. London, Parthenon Publishing, 1996, p 89.
64. Fazekas F, Deisenhammer F, Strasser-Fuchs S, Nahler G, Mamoli B, Austrian Immunoglobulin in Multiple Sclerosis Study Group. Randomised placebo-controlled trial of monthly intravenous immunoglobulin therapy in relapsing-remitting multiple sclerosis. Lancet 1997;349:589.
65. Illum N, Taudorf K, Heilmann C, et al. Intravenous immunoglobulin: a single-blind trial in children with Lennox–Gastaut syndrome. Neuropediatrics 1990;21:87.

66. Van Rijckeforsel-Harmant K, Delire M, Schmitz-Moorman W, Wieser HG. Treatment of refractory epilepsy with intravenous immunoglobulins. Results of the first double-blind/dose finding clinical study. Int J Clin Lab Res 1994;24:162.
67. Perlmutter SJ, Leitman SF, Garvey MA, et al. Therapeutic plasma exchange and intravenous immunoglobulin for obsessive-compulsive disorder and tic disorders in childhood. Lancet 1999;354:1153.
68. Jayne DRW, Davies MJ, Fox CJV, Black CM, Lockwood CM. Treatment of systemic vasculitis with pooled intravenous immunoglobulin. Lancet 1991;337:1137.
69. Levy Y, Sherer Y, George J, et al. Serologic and clinical response to treatment of systemic vasculitis and associated autoimmune disease with intravenous immunoglobulin. Int Arch Allergy Immunol 1999;119:231.
70. Finkel TH, Torok JJ, Ferguson PJ, et al. Chronic parvovirus B19 infection and systemic necrotising vasculitis: opportunistic infection or aetiological agent? Lancet 1994;343:1255.
71. Silverman E, Cawkwell G, Lovell D, et al. Intravenous immunoglobulin in the treatment of systemic juvenile rheumatoid arthritis: a randomized placebo controlled trial. J Rheumatol 1994;21:2353.
72. Schroeder JO, Zeuner RA, Euler HH, Loffler H. High dose intravenous immunoglobulins in systemic lupus erythematosus: Clinical and serological results of a pilot study. J Rheumatol 1996;23:71.
73. Jordan SC. Intravenous γ-globulin therapy in systemic lupus erythematosus and immune complex disease. Clin Immunol Immunopathol 1989;53:S164.
74. Lin CY, Hsu HC, Chiang H. Improvement of histological and immunological change in steroid and immunosuppressive drug-resistant lupus nephritis by high-dose intravenous gamma globulin. Nephron 1989;53:303.
75. Williams RC, Malone CC, Fry G, Silvestris F. Affinity columns containing anti-DNA Id+ human myeloma proteins adsorb human epibodies from intravenous gamma globulin. Arthritis Rheum 1997;40:683.
76. Dietrich G, Kazatchkine MD. Normal immunoglobulin G (IgG) for therapeutic use (intravenous Ig) contain antiidiotypic specificities against an immunodominant, disease-associated, cross-reactive idiotype of human anti-thyroglobulin autoantibodies. J Clin Invest 1990;85:620.
77. Gergely J, Sarmay G. Fc gamma RII-mediated regulation of human B cells. Scand J Immunol 1996;44:1.
78. Daya S, Gunby J, Clark DA. Intravenous immunoglobulin therapy for recurrent spontaneous abortion: A meta-analysis. Am J Reprod Immunol 1998;39:69.
79. Christiansen OB, Mathiesen O, Husth M, et al. Placebo controlled trial of treatment of unexplained secondary recurrent spontaneous abortions with I.V. immunoglobulin. Hum Reprod 1995;10:2690.
80. Coulam CB, Krysa L, Stern J, Bustillo M. Intravenous immunoglobulin for treatment of recurrent pregnancy loss. Am J Reprod Immunol 1995;34:333.
81. The German RSA/IVIG Group. Intravenous immunoglobulin in the prevention of recurrent miscarriage. Br J Obstet Gynaecol 1994;101:1072.
82. Stephenson MD, Dreher K, Houlihan E, Wu V. Prevention of unexplained recurrent spontaneous abortion using intravenous immunoglobulin: a prospective, randomized, double blinded, placebo controlled trial. Am J Reprod Immunol 1998;39:82.
83. Ruiz JE, Kwak JYH, Baum L, et al. Effects of intravenous immunoglobulin G on natural killer cell cytoxicity *in vitro* in women with recurrent spontaneous abortion. J Reprod Immunol 1996;31:125.
84. Hill JA, Polgar K, Anderson DJ. T-helper 1-type immunity to trophoblast in women with recurrent spontaneous abortion. JAMA 1995;273:1933.
85. Barry W, Hudgins L, Donta ST, Pesanti EL. Intravenous immunoglobulin therapy for toxic shock syndrome. JAMA 1992;267:3315.
86. Viard I, Wehrli P, Bullani R, Schneider P, Holler N, Salomon D. Inhibition of toxic epidermal necrolysis by blockade of CD95 with human intravenous immunoglobulin. Science 1998;282:490.
87. Prasad NKA, Papoff G, Zeuner A, et al. Therapeutic preparations of normal polyspecific IgG (IVIg) induce apoptosis in human lymphocytes and monocytes: A novel mechanism of action of IVIg involving the fas apoptotic pathway. J Immunol 1998;161:3781.
88. Wakim M, Alazard M, Yajima A, Speights D, Saxon A, Stiehm ER. High dose intravenous immunoglobulin in atopic dermatitis and hyper-IgE syndrome. Ann Allergy Asthma Immunol 1998;81:153.
89. Grattan C, Francis D, Hide M, Greaves M. Detection of circulating histamine releasing autoantibodies with functional properties of anti-IgE in chronic urticaria. Clin Exp Allergy 1991;21:695.
90. Fiebiger E, Hammerschmid F, Stingl G, Maurer D. Anti-FcεRIα autoantibodies in autoimmune-mediated disorders: identification of a structure–function relationship. J Clin Invest 1998;101:243.
91. O'Donnell BF, Barr RM, Black AK, et al. Intravenous immunoglobulin in autoimmune chronic urticaria. Br J Dermatol 1998;138:101.
92. Mazer BD, Gelfand EW. An open-label study of high-dose intravenous immunoglobulin in severe childhood asthma. J Allergy Clin Immunol 1991;87:976.
93. Kishiyama JL, Valacer D, Cunningham-Rundles C, et al. A multicenter, randomized, double-blind, placebo-controlled trial of high-dose intravenous immunoglobulin for oral corticosteroid-dependent asthma. Clin Immunol 1999;91:126.
94. Salmun LM, Barlan I, Wolf M, et al. Effect of intravenous immunoglobulin on steroid consumption in patients with severe asthma: A double-blind, placebo-controlled, randomized trial. J Allergy Clin Immunol 1999;103:810.
95. Modiano JF, Amran D, Lack G. Post transcriptional regulation of T cell IL-2 production by human pooled immunoglobulin. Clin Immunol Immunopathol 1997;83:75.
96. Spahn JD, Leung DYM, Chan MTS, Szefler SJ, Gelfand EW. Mechanisms of glucocorticoid reduction in asthmatic subjects treated with intravenous immunoglobulin. J Allergy Clin Immunol 1999;103:421.
97. Dalakas MC. Intravenous immune globulin therapy for neurologic diseases. Ann Intern Med 1997;126:721.
98. Casteels-Van Daele M, Winjndaele L, Hunninck K, et al. Intravenous immune globulin and acute aseptic meningitis. N Eng J Med 1990;323:614.
99. Sekul E, Cupler E, Dalakas M. Aseptic meningitis associated with high-dose intravenous immunoglobulin therapy: frequency and risk factors. Ann Intern Med 1994;121:259.
100. Silbert P, Knezevic W, Bridge D. Cerebral infarction complicating intravenous immunoglobulin therapy for polyneuritis cranialis. Neurology 1992;42:257.
101. Corvetta A, Della Bitta R, Gabrielli A, Spaeth PJ, Daniel G. Use of high-dose intravenous immunoglobulin in systemic lupus erythematosus: report of three cases. Clin Exp Rheum 1989;7:295.
102. Schifferli J, Leski M, Favre H, Imbach P, Nydegger U, Davies K. High-dose intravenous IgG treatment and renal function. Lancet 1991;337:457.
103. Anonymous. Renal insufficiency and failure associated with immune globulin intravenous therapy – United States, 1985–1998. MMWR Morb Mortal Wkly Rep 1999;48:518.
104. Schiff R. Transmission of viral infections through intravenous immune globulin. N Engl J Med 1994;331:1649.

Chapter 105 Gene Transfer for the Treatment of Immunodeficiency and for the Immunotherapy of Cancer

Malcolm K. Brenner and Richard E. Sutton

INTRODUCTION

Somatic cell gene transfer may be used to correct a deficit in a cell, to enhance or inhibit its pre-existing function, or to provide the cell with an entirely new capacity. This broad range of actions means that gene transfer may in principle contribute to the therapy of almost every disease, including immunodeficiency states and cancer. However, a number of criteria need to be met in order for these benefits to be produced. First, the gene's function should be understood. If, for example, a gene is active only during fetal development, there may be little purpose in attempting gene therapy for an adult. Similarly, genetic disorders in which the abnormal gene produces a transdominant effect (for example, sickle cell anemia) cannot be corrected simply by transferring a normal gene. Second, it will be necessary to transfer the genes efficiently, safely, and (ideally) in a targeted fashion, so that the correct cells are transduced. Moreover, for many applications the products of the transgenes need to be regulated, in terms of the quantity and timing of the material produced. While many gene transfer vectors are available, none meets these needs in full, and many fall far short of the desired goals. Hence, the practice of gene therapy has to a very large extent consisted of a careful selection of disease entities and treatment strategies that can exploit the limited strengths of current vectors, while avoiding their very substantial weaknesses. Undoubtedly, as our capacity to prepare safe, efficient, targeted and regulatable gene transfer vectors improves, the range of disorders that will be amenable to such treatment will grow. But for the moment, ambition must be tempered by ability. Fortunately, in both cancer and immunodeficiency diseases, even current vectors provide us with opportunities to explore worthwhile clinical applications.

CURRENT VECTORS

Since no single vector has all the characteristics desired for effective gene transfer, the choice of a gene transfer agent requires the demands of the specific application to be matched as closely as possible with the characteristics of the vector. This section outlines the structure and function of the gene transfer methodologies currently most widely used in clinical practice: retroviruses,[1] adenoviruses,[2] adeno-associated virus,[3] and liposomes.[4]

Retroviruses

Figure 105.1A shows the structure of a classic retroviral vector.[5] The structural and replicative genes (*gag*, *pol*, and *env*) of a murine retrovirus are replaced by one or more genes of interest, driven either by the retroviral promoter in the 5′ long-terminal repeat (LTR) or by an internal promoter. The retroviral constructs are made in cell lines in which the missing retroviral genes are present in *trans* and thus reproduce and package a vector that is not replication competent. Retroviral vectors have a wide target cell range, and the genetic information they convey is integrated into the host cell DNA. Thus, the transferred gene not only survives for the entire life span of the transduced cell, but is also present in that cell's progeny. Hence, these vectors are ideal for transferring genes into rapidly dividing cell populations, such as hemopoietic stem cells or lymphocytes. Provided that replication-competent virus is absent, the vector preparations appear to be nontoxic. However, retroviral vectors have several disadvantages. Because expression of the transferred gene requires viral integration of the genome, and hence a population

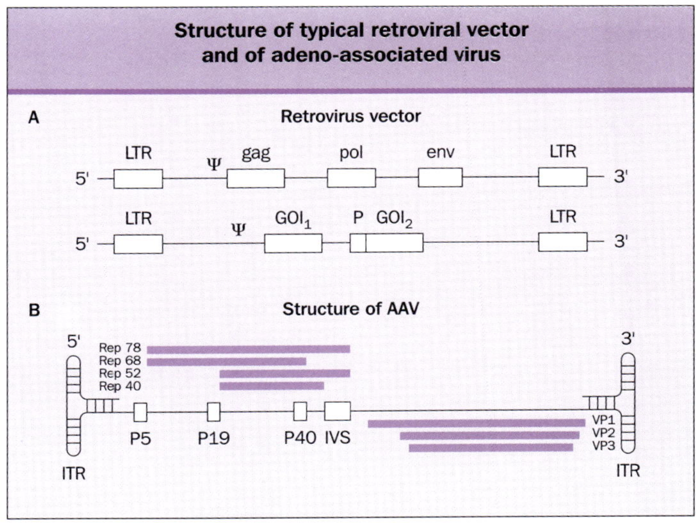

Figure 105.1 Structure of retroviral vector and adeno-associated virus (AAV). (A) Retrovirus and retroviral vector. The *gag* (reverse transcriptase), polymerase, and envelope coding sequences are removed, and supplied in *trans* by a producer cell. One or more genes of interest (GO1) are inserted, driven from the viral long-terminal repeat (LTR) promoter, or from an internal promoter (P). The viral packaging signal (Ψ) remains in the vector, so that it is appropriately packaged by the producer cell. **(B)** Structure of AAV. The AAV genome is a linear single-stranded DNA molecule. The viral genome is transcribed within three overlapping regions that produce seven primary transcripts. The transcripts obtained from each gene are shown as black lines. The virus has two palindromic inverted terminal repeats (designated ITR) which, in combination with products of the rep region, are responsible for site-specific integration. The rep products are also required for replication during coinfection with adenovirus. Genes labeled VP1–3 encode the viral capsid proteins. Promoter regions for these genes are boxed (P5, P19, P40, IVS).

Vector type	Potential advantages
HIV VISNA D-type viruses	Integrate in nondividing cells
Pseudotyped retroviruses incorporating novel proteins in viral envelope	1. Increased stability for purification 2. Increased resistance to primate complement 3. Altered target cell specificity/efficiency of transfection
Hybrid vectors Virosomes (virus coats containing plasmid DNA) Liposomes + ligands Liposomes + viral components/ DNA sequences	1. High-efficiency transfer by avoidance of endosomal degradation 2. Specific targeting 3. Integration of transferred DNA

Table 105.1 Novel vectors for gene therapy.

of dividing cells, the efficiency of transfer to many types of cell may be low.[1] It is possible to increase efficiency by bringing vector particle and target cell into close physical apposition, for example, by performing transduction on substances like fibronectin, but even then, overall levels of transfer leave much to be desired. Further, because the integration events themselves occur largely at random in the host cell DNA, regulatory genes could conceivably be damaged, contributing to oncogenesis.[6] Finally, retroviral vectors are not well suited for use in vivo, since they are generally unstable in primates and as yet they cannot be targeted to specific cell types. The development of pseudotyped particles (Table 105.1), in which a retroviral vector genome is incorporated into an envelope derived all or in part from a different virus, may improve the in vivo stability of retroviral vectors and alter their target cell range.

Adenoviruses

First-generation adenoviral vectors are El (early protein) deletion mutants and therefore are not replication competent.[2] These vectors infect a wide range of cell types and, unlike retroviruses, can transfer genes into nondividing cells. The vectors are reasonably stable in vivo and can be used to infect cells in situ. Examples include gene transfer into respiratory epithelium (the *CFTR* gene in cystic fibrosis)[2] or liver (genes encoding factor VIII and factor IX in hemophilia A or B).[7] However, adenoviral vectors are generally nonintegrating, so that the gene products are expressed from episomal DNA.[8] The episome is often lost after cell division and can be inactivated or lost even in a nondividing cell.[7] Thus, adenoviral vectors are unsuited for any application that requires long-term expression in a rapidly turning-over cell population or transfer into a stem cell and expression in that cell's progeny. A more important limitation is that most adenoviral vectors are immunogenic. Immune responses are generated against the vector proteins themselves (often preventing readministration of the vector), as well as against low levels of adenoviral proteins, expressed even when cells are transduced by defective viruses.[7] Moreover, concurrent expression of adenoviral genes appears to increase the probability of developing an immune response to the transgene product. The mechanism for this effect is unclear, but it is likely related to the ability of adenoviral entry into many cell types to trigger the release of cytokines, such as interleukins 6 and 8, which also induce a potentially highly destructive local inflammatory response.[8] Finally, adenoviral damage to vascular endothelium and to other organ systems may cause a potentially lethal disseminated intravascular coagulopathy, or a more chronic hepatocyte hypertrophy and hepatic fibrosis.[9] Since deletion of the El region alone does not prevent these toxicities, subsequent generations of adenovectors have been prepared that lack more than one set of adenoviral genes, for example, *E1* and *E4*, *E2a* and *E4*, or *E1* and *E3* and so on (reviewed in Hitt et al[10]). Although they showed less immunogenicity and toxicity and more durable transgene expression in some studies, such modified vectors produced little or no benefit in others. Indeed, administration of an *E1/E4*-deleted vector has been linked to a human death.[11] The quintessential attenuated adenovector is the so-called helper-dependent or 'gutless' vector, in which virtually all of the adenoviral genes have been removed and replaced with the gene of interest and its promoter, together with irrelevant DNA to allow packaging in the viral envelope.[12]

Adeno-associated vector

Adeno-associated virus (AAV[3] Fig. 105.1B) is a 'dependovirus' that can replicate only when an AAV-infected cell is coinfected with adenovirus or herpesvirus. Structurally, AAV is a DNA parvovirus, containing two palindromic inverted terminal repeats (ITR). When linked with two gene products from the *rep* gene region, these repeats favor site-specific integration of chromosome 19[13] by the AAV. Thus, AAV, like retroviruses, should persist for the entire life of the host cell and its progeny. Because genomic integration by AAV is relatively site-specific, the risk of oncogenesis is low. Although, in contrast to retroviruses, AAV may integrate the genomes of nondividing cells and become permanently expressed even in resting or postmitotic cells, this and other putative advantages have proved hard to exploit in clinical practice. Although the introduction of AAV into clinical use has been slow, preliminary studies in which AAV vectors encoding factor IX are injected into postmitotic tissues, such as muscle, are already producing encouraging results.[14]

Liposomes and other physical methods

Clinical experience with the available physical methods of gene transfer has primarily involved cationic liposome/DNA complexes[4] which fuse with the cell membrane and enter the endosomal uptake pathway. DNA released from these endosomes may then pass through the nuclear membrane and be expressed. The main advantage of liposomes is that they are nontoxic and can be given repeatedly. In some cell types, high levels of gene transfer have been obtained by this method. However, the DNA transferred by liposomes does not integrate the genome, and despite the incorporation of a variety of ligands into the liposome–DNA complex, the ability to target these vectors is still quite limited. More recently, successful gene transfer in vivo has been reported with use of a bio-ballistic ('gene gun') technique in which DNA coated onto colloidal gold particles is driven at high velocity by gas pressure into the cell. It is not yet clear whether this approach can be used to transduce normal or malignant hemopoietic progenitor cells with sufficient efficiency to allow therapeutic application.

Other vectors

Other vectors, including herpesviruses and lentiviruses, have been proposed as high-efficiency transducers of many cell types, and herpesviruses have recently entered clinical trials.[15] However, although these viruses many in future become substitutes for currently available vector systems, most investigators now accept that no naturally occurring virus and no simple physical vector will ever prove suitable for all gene therapy purposes. Ultimately, therefore, entirely new synthetic or semisynthetic vectors will have to be developed.[16] Alternative, fully synthetic vectors will be developed by combining components from multiple different vectors, allowing safe, efficient, and specific gene transfer and regulation (Table 105.1). In the meantime, gene therapy protocols for immunodeficiency and for cancer will require investigators to circumvent the limitations of current vectors and to choose their agents on the basis of the most important feature required.

IMPROVING VECTOR SYSTEMS

Targeting

To target viral vectors to specific cells or organ systems, it is usually necessary not only to add a targeting ligand to provide the new specificity, but also to disrupt pre-existing ligands so that the new specificity replaces, rather than adds to, the old. Moreover, the new ligands should allow the virus to enter the cells by membrane fusion or active transport, through the same intracellular pathway as the native vector. For adenoviruses in particular, retargeting may also be an important means of limiting virus-induced toxicity to vulnerable organs. Most adenoviruses bind to at least two molecules on their target cells – the coxsackie adenovirus receptor (CAR) and cell surface integrins (usually $\alpha v\beta_3$ or $\alpha v\beta_5$).[10,17] Binding is mediated by domains on the adenoviral knob protein. However, the complexity of the process has hampered efforts to effectively retarget viral vectors. Retargeting may be much simpler with liposomal vectors, whose intrinsic targeting capabilities are limited, so that simple addition of a ligand could secure the desired effect. Despite the appeal of these retargeting strategies, the only success reported to date has been infection of liver cells through directed binding to the asialoglycoprotein receptor.[18]

Regulation of transgene expression

Most effective gene therapies will require regulation of the transgene. Two approaches are available. The first relies on endogenous regulatory elements, by replacing the defective sequence with an inserted wild-type sequence – the process of homologous recombination. One promising technique for achieving this effect is the so-called 'chimeroplast' technology which utilizes a partial sequence of the gene of interest incorporating the corrected base pair, attached by hair pin structures at each end to RNA complementary to the complementary DNA strand sequence.[19] This chimeric molecule is resistant for 48 hours to intracellular exonucleases or RNAses. In animal models of several diseases (Crigler–Najjar or UDP-glucuronysyl transferase deficiency, α_1-antitrypsin inhibitor deficiency and the factor IX deficiency of hemophilia B), as many as 40% of the hepatic cells can be repaired in vivo, and clinical trials of this approach are imminent.[20]

For most disorders, regulatory elements may need to be introduced with the transgene. Thus, several regulatory structures are being developed with the intention of using orally absorbed small molecules to control transgene expression. The three systems closest to clinical use are regulated by rapamycin or tetracycline and their analogs,[21] or by the antiprogestin agent RU486.[22]

GENE THERAPY FOR IMMUNODEFICIENCY DISORDERS

Immune system cells arise from hemopoietic stem cells (HSC), and attempts to exploit gene transfer procedures in the treatment of immunodeficiency disorders might therefore profitably target these more primitive cells. The strategy would have the advantage of targeting readily obtainable cells that could be returned to the host and, in principle, repopulate the patient's body for life. Current limitations are the lack of reliable phenotypic definitions of HSC and of ex vivo assays to establish their function. Also, because the transferred gene must be passed to all HSC progeny, integrating vectors would be needed. Murine retroviruses are poorly suited for this purpose as they integrate only the genomes of dividing cells, and most stem cells are not cycling at any given time. The availability of improved transduction techniques, based on hemopoietic growth factors and colocalizing proteins such as fibronectin, has begun to overcome this obstacle.[23] The introduction of lentiviral vectors that may integrate genomic DNA in nondividing cells could improve this situation further.[24] For the moment, however, gene transfer to HSC is extremely inefficient. Hence, conditions suitable for gene therapy are those in which low levels of transgene expression would be predicted to produce benefit, and in which the minority population of gene-modified cells would have a growth advantage over the uncorrected majority. Since the gene products expressed after vector integration cannot as yet be regulated, it is advisable to choose conditions in which constitutive expression of the transgene is both safe and effective. Even with these constraints, gene therapy of the immunodeficiency disorders provides an ideal model for testing the principles outlined here.

Hereditary immunodeficiencies

Human severe combined immunodeficiency (SCID) is caused by a variety of molecular defects, including adenosine deaminase (ADA) deficiency, mutations in the cytokine receptor common γ chain, and Janus kinase-3 (JAK3) deficiency (Chapter 35). Common clinical characteristics include susceptibility to opportunistic infections, lymphopenia, and functionally inactive B and T cells.[25] The most common treatment for these patients is allogeneic bone marrow transplantation, a procedure with significant mortality, particularly if the patient lacks a sibling donor matched at the major histocompatibility complex (MHC) locus (Chapter 101). Taken together, the molecular and clinical features of SCID provide an incentive to test gene therapy strategies based on autologous hemopoietic cells.

> **KEY CONCEPTS**
>
> **Features of immunodeficiency diseases as initial candidates for gene therapy**
> - Low-level expression of gene product could be beneficial.
> - Regulation of gene expression is unnecessary.
> - Transduced cells have a survival advantage.

ADA deficiency

ADA deficiency was the first disease to be treated by gene therapy, largely because it met the criteria mandated by the limitations of then-current vectors. Studies of carriers revealed that the production of even a small amount of the gene product could be beneficial; regulation of the transgene product is unnecessary, since there is a wide range seen in normal individuals; and the transduced cells should have a survival advantage. As gene therapy for this disease was under consideration, an alternative therapy became available, namely replacement of the defective deaminase with recombinant ADA enzyme (PEG-ADA; Chapter 35). While such replacement was reasonably effective clinically, it was expensive and tedious for the patients. Paradoxically, its very accessibility encouraged experimental efforts with gene therapy: the availability of a proven treatment meant that patients could receive an additional experimental therapy without compromising their health. In addition, the increase in T lymphocytes following the replacement treatment meant that these cells, rather than HSC, could be the target for gene transfer. T cells are transduced far more readily than human HSC by the retroviral vectors that were available when these protocols were proposed.

In September 1990,[26] T cells were harvested by apheresis from two children receiving PEG-ADA and exposed to a Moloney-based retroviral vector incorporating the ADA and neomycin resistance genes. After 9–12 days of culture and expansion, the cells were administered to the patients over 18–23 months. PEG-ADA could not be completely withdrawn, and it was therefore not possible to determine whether the corrected cells had increased in number under selective pressure. Nonetheless, the proportion of circulating gene-modified T cells was 50% in one patient and <1% in the other. The transgene was clearly expressed in these cells, as shown by RNA and protein measurements, and clinically both children remained well at their 3-year follow-up examination. Skin tests to common antigens were positive, influenza-specific T cells and antibodies were detected, and there was a rising titer of isohemagglutinins. Despite this partial success, it was felt that optimal results would require transduction of stem cells rather than T cells, and gradual withdrawal of PEG-ADA to increase the selective advantage predicted for the modified cells. Initial studies in The Netherlands to test this hypothesis were not successful, but an Italian study, begun in 1992, yielded more promising results. Briefly, lymphocytes and marrow cells from two patients were transduced with two distinguishable retroviral vectors and administered over 9–24 months while the PEG-ADA dose was progressively decreased. There was persistence of gene-modified cells, particularly those originating from marrow, an increase in T-cell numbers, and the development of antigen-specific T-cell responses. In 1993, a further revision of the basic gene therapy method was tried at Los Angeles Children's Hospital with three patients diagnosed with the disease in utero.[27] Their cord blood was harvested and transduced with a Moloney vector, in the presence of hemopoietic growth factors. (Cord blood contains substantial numbers of hemopoietic stem cells, and they appear to be more responsive to growth factors and more readily transduced than stem cells from marrow or peripheral blood.) There was multilineage engraftment of the gene-modified cells, followed by the generation of ADA-expressing T lymphocytes. Importantly, as the dose of PEG-ADA was reduced, the proportion of these modified T cells progressively increased, but plateaued at levels that were considered too low to be of clinical benefit,[28] and full-dose PEG-ADA was restarted.

Common γ chain deficiency

As the technology for transducing HSC has slowly improved, gene therapists have turned their attention to other immunodeficiency states, with recent success reported for children with X-linked severe combined immunodeficiency (SCID-XL).[29] This disease accounts for 50–60% of cases of SCID and is characterized by an absence of mature T and NK lymphocytes with increased numbers of B cells. It results from abnormalities in a peptide chain (γc) shared by the receptors for IL-2, IL-4, IL-7, IL-9, and IL-15 (Chapter 12). In preclinical studies, γc-transduced $CD34^+$ cells from SCID-XL patients matured into T cells ex vivo as well as NK cells, leading to the therapeutic study in France in 1999.[29] The first two patients to be treated had a missense mutation in exon 7 (C879 → T) in the intracellular region of the molecule or a missense mutation in intron 7 (G868 (+5) → C), both resulting in loss of the transmembrane region. Before treatment, both patients had the low T-cell counts (<100/ml) typically associated with this condition, with a high B-cell count. $CD34^+$ stem cells, derived from bone marrow samples, were exposed to three cycles of infection with a MFG-γc retroviral vector, during which they were stimulated with recombinant hemopoietic growth factors (SCF, M-GSF, FLT-3 ligand, and IL-3), in the presence of human recombinant fibronectin fragments, to improve gene transfer (see Retroviral vectors above). After transduction, 40% and 20% of the $CD34^+$ cells expressed the transgene. Lymphocyte counts rose in both patients between days 75 and 90 after infusion of the transduced cells (30×10^6/kg or 13.5×10^6/kg). At day 150, one of the patients had 1800 $CD3^+$ cells/μl, including 1250 $CD4^+$ cells and 500 $CD8^+$ cells The T lymphocytes were shown to be polyclonal, to express the γc transgene, and to proliferate in vitro in the presence of mitogens, IL-2, and antigens after immunization. At day 120, the other patient had 450 $CD3^+$ $γc^+$ cells/μl, as well as T cells that proliferated in vitro after stimulation with mitogens or IL-2. Both patients have remained well since the completion of therapy and 3 additional patients have now been treated. Hence, the progeny of transduced $CD34^+$ stem cells expressing the γc gene have sufficient function to gain a selective advantage over cells not expressing the transgene, and therefore to increase to numbers compatible with normal immune function.[29]

Immunodeficiencies associated with defects in highly regulated genes

Both ADA and common γ chain deficiency are examples of gene defects in which constitutive expression of a transgene should not produce adverse effects. However, many other genes that have been implicated in immunodeficiency states may normally be tightly regulated. Efforts to repair these defects with transgenes that are constitutively or ectopically expressed could produce unexpected problems, as well as clinical benefits.

JAK3 kinase deficiency

Ligand binding to the receptors for IL-2, IL-4, IL-7, IL-9 or IL-15, which share a common γ chain, normally triggers activation of the JAK3 protein tyrosine kinase by protein phosphorylation. However, some SCID patients with characteristics similar to those of patients with X-linked SCID were recently found to have a JAK3 deficiency. The critical role of JAK3 activation in normal lymphoid development and function has been extensively defined in mutant mice in which the *Jak3* gene has been disrupted by gene targeting.[30] These mice display a SCID phenotype with severe defects in both B-lymphocyte maturation and T-lymphocyte activation, due to interruption of the cytokine-signaling pathways essential for lymphoid development and proliferation. If bone marrow from these mice is transduced with the pM5neo/Jak3 retroviral vector, and $2–5 \times 10^6$ total nucleated cells injected into individual lethally irradiated *Jak3* $^{-/-}$ recipient mice, there is a rapid and marked increase in the absolute lymphocyte count, compared with that in mice receiving transplants with uncorrected cells (3471 ± 1294 cells/μl vs. 166 ± 131 cells/μl), representing approximately half the lymphocytes seen in normal animals.[31] Flow cytometric analysis of the resurgent lymphocyte population revealed $CD4^+$ and $CD8^+$ T cells with essentially normal mitogen and IL-2 responsiveness, demonstrating restoration of the IL-2 signaling pathway after *Jak3* gene replacement. The animals also developed the ability to respond to a T-cell-dependent priming antigen, chicken γ-globulin.[32] Most significantly, from the point of view of human translation, there was evidence for in vivo selection of the transduced minority of cells, since the transgene copy number rose in the recipients' lymphoid cells but not in cells of the myeloid series, where no selective pressure would be expected. JAK3 is part of a mitogenic signal transduction pathway, and constitutive expression of the gene, as described here, might be expected to cause abnormal lymphoproliferation or even leukemia, although these problems were not seen.

CD40L (CD154) deficiency (X-linked hyper IgM)

The CD40 molecule has a central role in the induction and regulation of immune responses.[33] It is expressed by B cells, hematopoietic progenitors, endothelial cells, professional antigen-presenting cells, and epithelial cells (including those in the thymus), as well as a subset of mature T cells. Interaction of this molecule with the trimeric CD40 ligand (CD40L or CD154) usually leads to cell activation, differentiation, or both. In contrast to its receptor, CD40L is expressed predominantly by activated T cells. Its production is exquisitely regulated, occurring after T-cell activation and in concert with other receptor/counter-receptor pairs while the T cells and their targets are in intimate contact, usually within a specialized microenvironment. Inherited deficiency of the CD40L molecule, so-called 'X-linked hyper-IgM syndrome' (HIGM1), is associated with severe immune impairment, marked by failure of immunoglobulin isotype switching and defects of cell-mediated immunity.[34] Because expression of CD40L is normally closely synchronized with T-cell activation, fewer than 1% of circulating mononuclear cells are estimated to be CD40L positive at any given time. Several clinical studies with other transgenes have shown that equivalent levels of expression can be attained in vivo after transduction of human hemopoietic progenitor cells, suggesting that CD40L deficiency might be amenable to correction by gene transfer, even with currently available vectors. The $CD40L^{-/-}$ murine model has features that closely mimic the human disease.[35] These mice received marrow corrected with a retroviral vector, and constitutive expression of the CD40L transgene was confirmed by flow cytometric analysis. In one group of mice, approximately 15% of nucleated cells in bone marrow, thymus, and spleen were transgene positive, while in the second group the mean percentage of transduced cells was approximately 0.25%. A third group were given corrected thymocytes, rather than bone marrow, and in these animals the mean percentages of mCD40L-positive cells in bone marrow, thymus, or spleen were within the 0.01–0.1% range.

Despite this wide variation in the percentage of cells that were constitutively expressing the corrected gene, all mouse groups behaved identically. All developed near-complete immune reconstitution as measured by humoral and cell-mediated responses to the HK×31 attenuated strain of influenza A virus assay or by a normal T-cell-dependent response to the priming antigen DNP-KLH. Although constitutive expression of CD40L can restore immunocompetence in animals with a deficiency of this ligand, the mice went on to develop increased numbers of lymphoblasts in the thymic medulla, with progression to T-lymphoblastic lymphomas involving the thymus, spleen, and other organs by 7–9 months post-transplantation.[35] Of 19 $CD40L^{-/-}$ mice transduced with the mCD40L gene, 12 developed lymphoproliferative disease. Immunohistochemical and molecular analysis of the diseased tissue indicated expansion of a primitive $CD40^+$ thymic lymphocyte population, with progression from small polyclonal lesions to large predominantly monoclonal tumors. The implication is that constitutive expression of CD40L in a CD40L-null background causes unremitting stimulation of immature thymocytes, analogous to the uncontrolled EBV-induced stimulation of B cells that results in polyclonal lymphoproliferation progressing to monoclonal lymphoma. If this is indeed the mechanism, then safe treatment of this and perhaps of other 'regulated' immunodeficiencies will require the introduction of regulatable vectors of the type described above.

Other immunodeficiencies and their suitability for correction by gene transfer are included in Table 105.2.

Acquired immune deficiency syndrome

The use of gene transfer to correct genetic abnormalities underlying inherited immunodeficiencies has great scientific appeal, but in public health terms the most important potential application of this technology is in the treatment of HIV-induced acquired immunodeficiency.

Human immunodeficiency virus type 1 (HIV) is the causative agent of AIDS, the acquired immune deficiency syndrome. In addition to the usual structural and enzymatic retroviral gene products (Gag, Pol, and Env), this lentivirus has a number of accessory genes. It also infects nondividing cells, and the clinical illness it causes is slowly progressive in nature. HIV selectively infects $CD4^+$ helper T cells and macrophages, thus destroying the cellular arm of the immune system (Chapter 38). Unless viral replication is suppressed by successful treatment, AIDS patients have an inexorable decline in $CD4^+$ T cells and become increasingly susceptible to many well-characterized opportunistic infections, malignant diseases, and other systemic illnesses.

Until 6 years ago, the treatment of HIV infection included only a few nucleoside analog drugs with limited efficacy (e.g. AZT), resulting in therapeutic approaches that focused largely on secondary effects of the virus. With the advent of the protease inhibitors and non-nucleoside reverse transcriptase inhibitors, highly active antiretroviral therapy (HAART) was broadly instituted and has transformed HIV seropositivity into a chronic disease treated in outpatient settings, much like diabetes.

Immunodeficiency disease	Gene affected[36,37]	Gene regulation required	In vivo selection likely	Suitability for gene transfer	Clinical trials	Major problems to be overcome
Severe combined immunodeficiency	ADA deficiency	No	Yes	High	See text	Low levels of gene transfer
	TcR common Y chain	No	Yes	High	See text	Low levels of gene transfer
	Janus kinase 3	Yes (probably)	Yes	Moderate	Proposed	Adverse effects of ectopic/constitutive expression
	ZAP-70 protein tyrosine kinase	Yes	Yes (but? for CD8 T cells alone)	High	Proposed	Adverse effects of ectopic/ constitutive expression
	Purine nucleoside deficiency	No	Yes	High	In progress	Repair damage to multiple organs
MHC molecule deficiency Class I	Protein transporter TAP2	No	No	Low	None	Low levels of expression. Multiple non-marrow-derived lineages to be considered
MHC molecule deficiency Class II	Trans-activator genes: CII TA RFX5 binding protein RFXAP protein	Yes	No	Low	None	Adverse effects of constitutive expression in T-cells, fibroblasts, endothelium. Multiple non-marrow-derived lineages to be considered
Leukocyte adhesion defects	B_2 integrin common subunit (CD18)	Probably not in lymphocytes and neutrophils	No	Moderate	In progress	?Adverse effects of ectopic expression. Lack of positive selection
Wiskott–Aldrich syndrome	WASP	?	No	Moderate/Low	None	Function of gene unknown. Need for regulation unknown
Ataxia telangiectasia		Yes	No	Poor	None	Multiple organ systems involved. Gene function poorly understood
Chediak–Higashi syndrome	CHS1	Yes	No	Poor	None	Gene function poorly understood ?Adverse effects of ectopic/constitutive expression
X-linked hyper-IgM syndrome	CD40L	Yes	No	Poor	None	Adverse effects of ectopic and constitutive expression. Lack of positive selection
X-linked agammaglobulinemia	Bruton tyrosine kinase	Yes	Yes	Moderate	None	?Adverse effects of ectopic and constitutive expression

ADA = adenosine deaminase; TCR = T-cell receptor; TAP = transporter associated with antigen processing; TA = trans-activator; WASP = Wiskott–Aldrich syndrome protein; CHS = Chediak–Higashi syndrome.

Table 105.2 Candidate genes for therapy in primary immunodeficiencies.

Successfully treated patients have undetectable viral loads, increased CD4+ counts, and few opportunistic infections or other complications of AIDS. Most importantly; both the quality and duration of their lives are improved.

Despite its antiviral efficacy, HAART has serious limitations. Some regimens require more than 30 pills a day, making compliance a major issue. Increasing numbers of side-effects are being observed, especially with the protease inhibitors,[38] and adverse drug interactions abound.[39] Patients often take drug holidays (scheduled treatment interruptions) because of the improved quality of life they enjoy while off therapy. Multidrug-resistant HIV is being noted with greater frequency, both by phenotyping and genotyping, suggesting that the effectiveness of HAART will diminish over the next several years.[40] It is now clear that long-term anti-HIV therapy is required, since viral replication rebounds quickly during discontinuations of HAART (with concomitant decreases in CD4+ counts).[41] There also may be more than a single latent pool of infected T cells (memory compartment), with half-lives estimated at 6 months to half a decade.[42] Whether HAART or immunotherapy (e.g. IL-2) can substantially reduce the size of these pools is uncertain at best. Finally, there may be privileged sites of HIV replication, such as brain and testis, where the effects of HAART are unknown or limited at best. These and other reasons have compelled the development of novel antiretroviral therapies, including gene therapy.

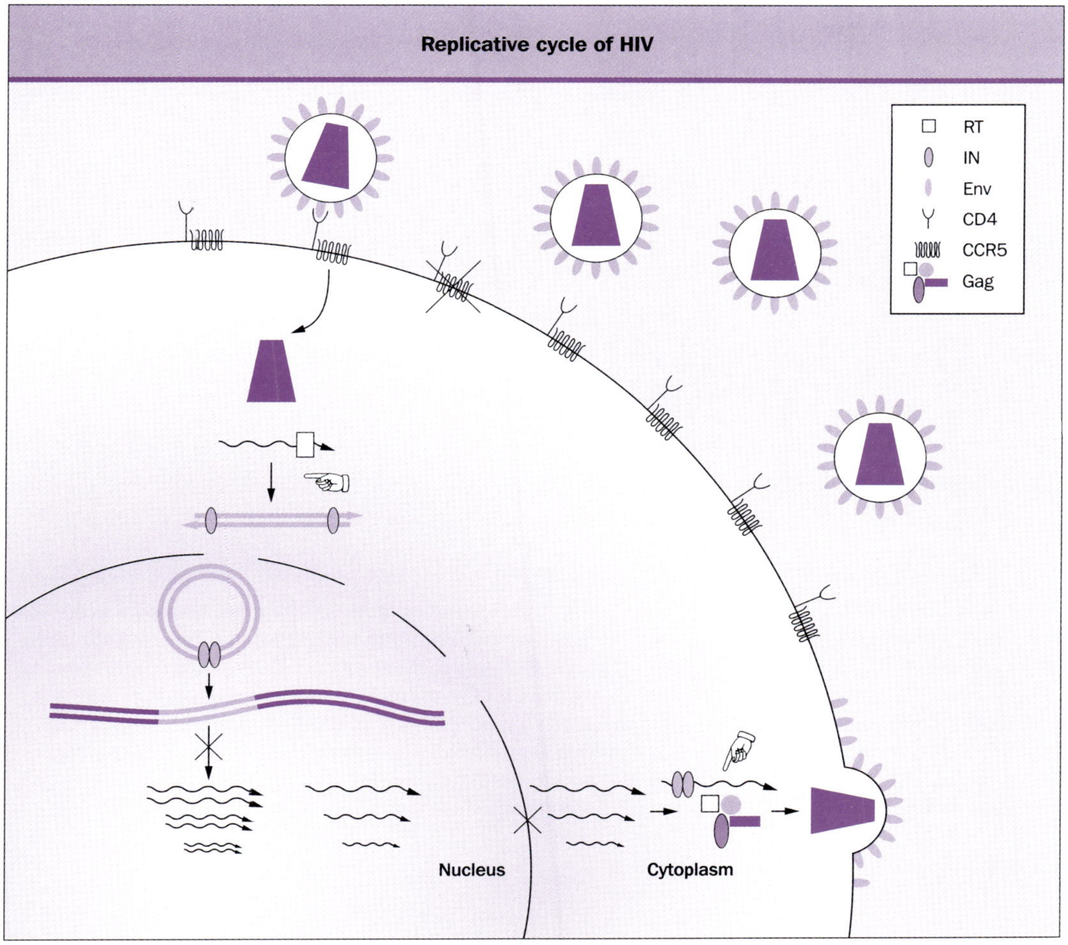

Figure 105.2 Replicative cycle of HIV. At the top are HIV particles, with one about to engage CD4. The viral core (trapezoid) enters the cell and reverse transcriptase converts the proviral RNA into ds cDNA. Multimeric integrase integrates the viral DNA into the host genome. Different classes of viral mRNA are produced and exported from the nucleus. Proviral RNA is packaged into a viral particle, which buds from the cellular plasma membrane, incorporating Env. Hands represent the sites of action of currently available anti-HIV therapeutics (RT and protease), and ×s the sites of action of gene therapeutic approaches (CCR5, Tat, and Rev).

Although many details remain uncertain, the major phases of the HIV lifecycle are relatively clear (Fig. 105.2) and offer several attractive targets for gene therapy.

HIV lifecycle: viral entry

HIV requires both CD4 and a co-receptor on the cell surface for productive infection. More than a dozen chemokine receptors function as HIV co-receptors in vitro, but the two most critical for the replication of T-cell-tropic and macrophage-tropic isolates in vivo are CXCR4 and CCR5, respectively.[43] The latter is an attractive target because individuals who are homozygous null (the so-called 'Δ32' mutation) are phenotypically normal but relatively resistant to HIV infection,[44] suggesting that CCR5 may be essential for the establishment of HIV infection and that its function may be duplicated by other chemokine receptors. Chemokine genes have been modified to contain a KDEL sequence, so the resultant proteins do not leave cytoplasm but sequester their receptors in the rough endoplasmic reticulum.[45] This 'intrakine' strategy increased the resistance of cells to HIV infection (both M- and T-tropic strains) while preserving cell function. The difficulty with this approach is that down-regulation of CCR5 may simply force HIV to use a different coreceptor, possibly CXCR4, which is essential for hemopoietic stem cell homing.

Viral transcription

Another major target for gene therapy is viral transcription. HIV encodes a transcriptional transactivator (Tat) that acts at the level of RNA elongation in conjunction with cellular factors (Fig. 105.3).[46] A stem-loop RNA element, TAR, is present at the very 5′ end at the viral mRNA, and is recognized by Tat as well as cyclin T1. This complex recruits or activates the cyclin-dependent kinase CDK9 to hyperphosphorylate the carboxy-terminal domain of RNA polymerase II to increase processivity of the enzyme. Some of these features may be unique to HIV RNA, although cyclin T1 and CDK9 undoubtedly have physiologic functions. Because of Tat's central role in viral replication, gene therapists have rightly focused their efforts on both Tat and TAR. Anti-Tat single-chain variable fragment antibodies (intrabodies) interfere with Tat function intracellularly,[47] anti-TAR ribozymes cleave TAR,[48] and polymeric TAR decoys compete with TAR for Tat binding.[49] TAR decoys, however, may also bind essential cellular co-factors and thus cause cytotoxicity. Transdominant mutants of Tat that inhibit HIV replication generally fall into two classes.[50] Activation domain mutants presumably act by outcompeting the cellular cofactor cyclin T1 for TAR recognition. ARM/NLS transdominant proteins likely function by sequestering cellular cofactors, including cyclin T1 and CDK9. In general, Tat transdominant genes only transiently or poorly inhibit HIV replication, and remain to be evaluated in clinical trials.

Viral RNA transport

Rev, the other HIV regulatory gene, directs the export of intron-containing viral messenger RNAs from the nucleus to the cytoplasm (Fig. 105.4).[47] Rev interacts specifically with the

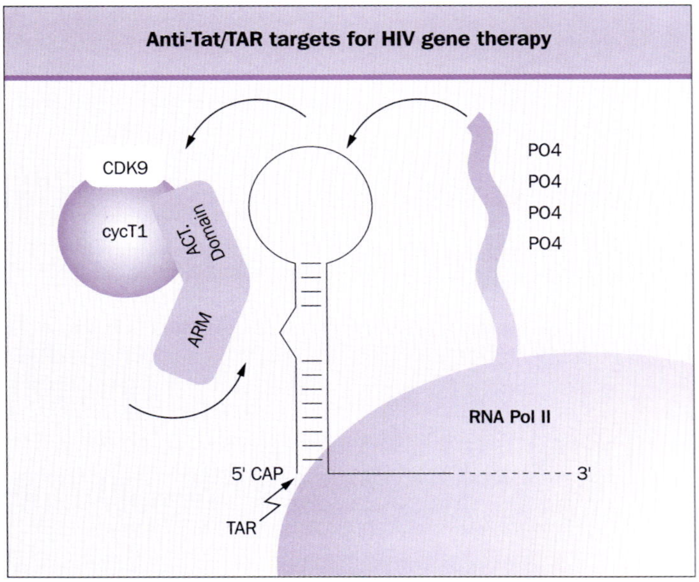

Figure 105.3 Anti-Tat/TAR targets for HIV gene therapy. TAR (lightning arrow) is illustrated as a stem loop/bulge structure. Both the arginine-rich motif (ARM) and the activation domain of Tat are shown, along with interactions with cellular factors cyclin T1 and CDK9. The carboxy-terminal domain (CTD) of RNA polymerase II is illustrated as a wavy tail. Recruitment of CDK9 to the cyclin T1–Tat–TAR complex is thought to hyperphosphorylate the CTD and increase the processivity of polymerase. Potential gene therapeutic approaches (all aimed at reducing viral transcription) are illustrated by curved arrows and include various dominant-negative forms of Tat and also TAR decoys and ribozymes.

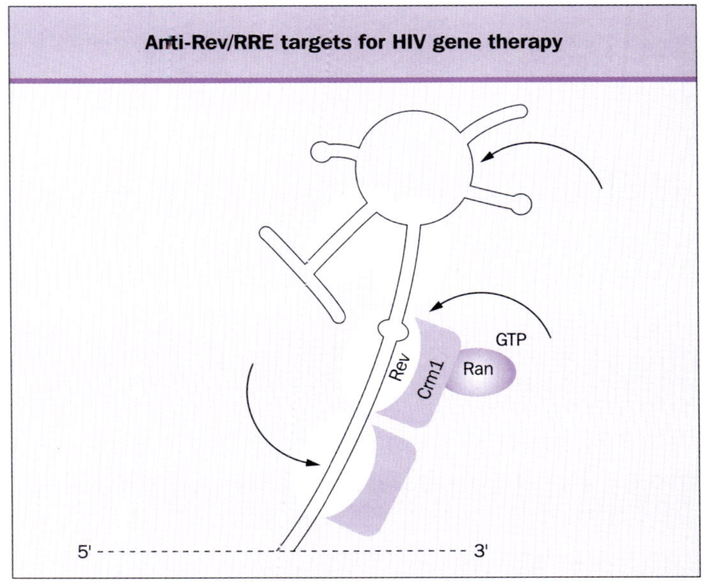

Figure 105.4 Anti-Rev/RRE targets for HIV gene therapy. A schematic of the Rev-response-element (RRE) of HIV. Note that it has multiple stem-loop structures. Rev (light ovals) specifically binds to and multimerizes on the RRE. The binding of host factor Crm1 (smoothed rectangle) to Rev is dependent upon the GTP-bound form of Ran (dark oval), another host factor involved in nuclear transport. Gene therapeutic targets are illustrated by curved arrows and include Rev trans-dominant proteins (which interfere with RRE binding, multimerization, Crm1 binding) and ribozymes which cleave the RRE.

Rev-response-element (RRE), a complex RNA stem-loop structure found within the *tat-rev* intron. In the presence of both Rev and the RRE, competition between the host's splicing apparatus and Rev allows export of intron-containing viral mRNAs, including proviral RNA, which can then be packaged, assembled, and released as infectious particles.[51] Since Rev is a shuttle protein, it has a nuclear localization signal, an RRE-binding domain, and a nuclear export domain, which interacts with components of the nuclear export machinery, such as Crm1.

Rev is essential for viral replication and thus has become a target for anti-HIV gene therapy efforts. Anti-Rev intrabodies, similar to those against Tat, have been tested,[52] as have RRE decoys,[53] which have the same theoretical disadvantage of cytotoxicity as TAR decoys. Malim et al created dominant-negative forms of Rev by site-directed mutagenesis of the NES.[54] These mutants, of which Rev M10 has been most intensely studied, bind to the RRE but not to Crm1, and thus interfere with wild-type Rev RNA export. Rev M10 has been used to inhibit HIV replication, not only in established and primary T cells in vitro, but also in two recent clinical trials[55,56] (see below). Moreover, HIV replication appears to be inversely correlated with the level of expression of Rev M10, and escape mutants have rarely, if ever, been observed.[57] Thus, strategies that are directed against the interaction of viral and cellular proteins may be more successful than those that simply target viral genes or intraviral interactions.

Combination therapy

Two or more anti-HIV genes have been used in combination, analogous to HAART. When delivered to CD4$^+$ T cells in an adenoviral vector, multimeric TAR decoys bearing a transdominant or antisense Gag sequence synergistically inhibited HIV replication, and vectors expressing double and triple copies of ribozyme–RRE decoy fusion genes increased transcript levels over those seen with single copy vectors, and inhibited diverse clades of HIV.[58] Another example is the expression of dominant-negative Tat22/37 5′ to an RRE decoy, which effectively inhibited HIV infection in Jurkat cells[59] and potently inhibited HIV replication in established and primary T cells. Finally, expression of an anti-Rev intrabody with a RRE ribozyme,[60] and the use of retroviral vectors encoding a multimeric TAR and either antisense Tat or a *gag*-specific ribozyme blocked all HIV replication in established T cells for prolonged periods of time.[49] Although untested in vivo, this last strategy is among the more promising for effective inhibition of HIV infection. As an alternative to using two separate anti-HIV genes, Belmont and colleagues designed an effective dominant-negative fusion protein called Trev (combination of Tat and Rev.[61]

Clinical trials

Two clinical trials of anti-HIV gene therapy have been published. In the first, enriched autologous CD4$^+$ T cells were transfected by microballistics with constructs expressing Rev M10 or a mutant, nonfunctional form of this protein (ΔRev M10), and returned to each of three patients.[56] As expected, cells expressing Rev M10 were more resistant to HIV in vitro and showed a survival advantage compared to cells expressing the nonfunctional protein. However, the transfection efficiency was low, the study did not extend beyond 1 week, and there was no attempt to document transgene expression by the reinfused cells.

In the second trial, peripheral CD4+ T cells were again isolated from three HIV-infected patients with early-stage disease.[55] T cells were transduced ex vivo with separate retroviral constructs encoding Rev M10 or ΔRev M10 (nonfunctional), and returned to the patients. By DNA-PCR analyses, T cells modified with Rev M10 survived longer than those transduced with ΔRev M10. RT-PCR analyses confirmed the presence of Rev M10 transcripts in cells for up to 140 days after engraftment. Immune response against Rev M10 or the vector was not detected, nor were there changes in a variety of serum biochemical, hematologic, or immunological end points. As might be expected from the small number of T cells infused, there were no consistent changes in the viral load or number of CD4+ T cells. These small, phase I clinical trials thus established the safety and feasibility of this gene transfer strategy.

Cellular targets

Although mature peripheral T cells have been utilized,[62,63] a more productive avenue may be to target the HSC that serve as T-cell and macrophage progenitors. These cells could be transduced ex vivo and transplanted into patients, where they could be expected to generate both T cells and macrophages resistant to HIV infection. As discussed for the inherited immunodeficiencies, this approach introduces several practical problems. It is extremely difficult, for example, to transduce the progenitor cells (usually defined phenotypically), and gene marking studies have shown only limited transgene expression, even though cell survival is prolonged. Moreover, limited bone marrow conditioning is likely to be required for adequate repopulation of the T-cell and macrophage compartments. A broader issue is whether the T cells derived from these HSC will be properly educated and functional, since thymic architecture is progressively destroyed during HIV infection.

Prospects

It is uncertain whether gene therapy will ever be used successfully against HIV in patients. Seventeen small-molecule antiretroviral agents are currently approved by the FDA, and an equal number will likely be approved in the coming years. In development are agents that target aspects of the viral lifecycle other than RT and protease, including viral fusion and entry, integration, transcription, and packaging, although their future availability is unclear. A safe and efficacious HIV vaccine remains a formidable challenge and may be many years from clinical use.

A number of technological barriers will have to be overcome before gene therapy is put into clinical practice. These include the identification of genes that will protect against HIV at high multiplicities of infection and the development of vectors able to efficiently transduce quiescent T cells, macrophages, and HSCs. Lentiviral vectors hold considerable promise in this regard. Careful examination of the HIV lifecycle suggests that current approaches to gene delivery have the potential of working additively, if not synergistically, with traditional pharmacotherapeutics. Vectors based upon HIV may be particularly advantageous since the vector reduces the replication of wild-type HIV by interfering with either packaging or reverse transcription. Inducible HIV vectors encoding suicide genes dependent upon both Tat and Rev may also be designed. Whether these or non-HIV-1 lentiviral vectors will ever be approved by the FDA for use in HIV-infected patients remains to be seen.

GENE THERAPY FOR MALIGNANT DISEASES

To date, the widest use of gene transfer has been in patients with cancer. There are three major routes by which gene transfer can be used to treat malignant disease. First, the tumor cell itself can be corrected by 'repairing' one or more of the genetic defects associated with the malignant process or by delivering a pro-drug-metabolizing enzyme that will render the tumor sensitive to the corresponding cytotoxic agent. This approach has an attractive elegance, but is handicapped by the inefficiency of current vectors and their lack of targeting. Second, the drug sensitivity of normal host tissues can be decreased by delivering cytotoxic drug-resistance genes to marrow precursor cells, thereby increasing the therapeutic index of chemotherapy. This approach is also hampered by the inefficiency of the gene transfer technology, which makes it difficult to protect sufficient cells in all organ systems that are damaged by conventional cytotoxic drugs. Third, the immune response to the tumor can be modified by altering the specificity or effector function of immune system cells, or by transducing a small proportion of the tumor cells with immunostimulatory genes, thereby generating an immune response to tumor-associated or tumor-specific antigens. This last approach makes use of the efficiency of the immune system and its capacity to target specific cell types to compensate for the limitations of current vectors. For that reason it has been the most popular approach clinically, and it is this 'genetic immunotherapy' approach that will be considered here. Nonimmunologic approaches to cancer gene therapy are reviewed elsewhere.[64]

Generation of tumor vaccines

Increasing evidence that human tumors may express tumor-specific or tumor-associated antigens, and that these antigens may be processed and presented on the cell surface,[65] has led to a resurgence of interest in immunologic approaches to cancer treatment, and in coupling immunotherapy with techniques to genetically modify cells. It is now possible to transfer genes that make tumors more immunogenic and effector lymphocytes more functional, leading to clinical protocols in which the immune response is exploited to destroy cancer cells. Infused T cells can also be altered by changing their effector function or modifying their receptor specificity. For example, the antitumor activity of immunocytes can be enhanced by increasing the levels of cytotoxic cytokines they produce at local tumor sites. Preclinical studies are evaluating whether tumor cell recognition can be improved by transfection of T cells with the appropriate antigen-specific T-cell receptors.[66] Many tumors express surface antigens that may be recognized by specific antibodies. In the T-body or universal receptor approach, T cells are transduced with a construct encoding a chimeric gene that contains an antibody-derived single-chain variable region linked with the T-cell receptor constant region or a T-cell signaling molecule.

KEY CONCEPTS

Alternative strategies for gene therapy of malignant diseases
- Repair of gene defects in malignant cells themselves
- Enhancement of therapeutic index of chemotherapy drugs
- Stimulation of antitumor immune response

In an attempt to enhance the immune recognition of poorly immunogenic tumors, investigators have evaluated the effect of transducing tumor cells with lymphotactic chemokines,[67] cytokine genes,[68] allogeneic MHC molecules,[4] or costimulatory molecules such as B7.1 or CD40 ligand[69] that activate cytotoxic T cells after engaging their surface ligands or counter receptors. In murine model systems, the transfection of tumor cell lines with these molecules has augmented immunogenicity. Thus, injection of neoplastic cells (including those derived from lymphoid and myeloid malignancies) in otherwise tumorigenic doses recruits immune system effector cells and eradicates injected tumor cells.[70] Often the animal is then resistant to challenges by further local injections of nontransduced parental tumor. The transduced tumor has therefore acted like a vaccine.

As of late 1999, tumor vaccines were being evaluated in more than 100 different clinical trials. Preliminary results in patients with melanoma, renal cell carcinoma, or neuroblastoma suggest that tumor cells transduced with the IL-2, *GM-CSF*, or *HLA-B7* gene can be given safely and will produce immunomodulatory effects in a substantial proportion of cases, including peripheral blood eosinophilia, a rise in NK and AK cell numbers and activity, and an increase in tumor-specific cytotoxic T-lymphocyte precursor frequencies.[68,71,72]

The clinical results of augmenting immune responses to otherwise weakly immunogenic tumors have been broadly comparable. A representative study of 10 children with advanced, relapsed neuroblastoma[71,73] can be used to illustrate progress in the field as a whole. Patients received 2–4 doses of autologous unirradiated tumor cells transduced with an adenovirus IL-2 vector as subcutaneous injections. This tumor immunogen induced a moderate local inflammatory response consisting predominantly of $CD4^+$ T lymphocytes, and a systemic response with a rise in circulating $CD25^+$ and DR^+ $CD3^+$ T cells. A specific antitumor response, manifest by an IgG antitumor antibody and increased cytotoxic T-cell killing of autologous tumor cells was also noted. Clinically, one patient had a complete tumor response, one had a partial response and three had stable disease following injection of the tumor immunogen alone. After treatment with oral etoposide, an additional patient developed a complete response, and two had very good partial responses (>90% regression). Four of the five patients with tumor responses had coexisting antitumor immune activity, as opposed to only one of the patients with nonresponsive disease. By using phage display technology, it has been possible to isolate Ig variable regions from B lymphocytes of the responder patients and thereby to prepare neuroblastoma-specific single-chain antibodies with novel specificities that may have therapeutic value in later protocols. Related results have been obtained in renal cell carcinoma and melanoma, supporting further exploration of this strategy.

Ultimately, tumor immunogens are likely to produce their greatest activity when several different immunostimulatory genes are introduced into the tumor. The immune response has at least three distinct components: (1) attraction of lymphocytes to the site of antigen presentation; (2) engagement of the antigen-specific receptor and of costimulatory molecules; and (3) amplification of the attracted, stimulated cells by growth factors. Immunotherapy that combines two or more of these separate classes of stimulatory agents should prove more effective than treatment based on single immunogens alone. In studies with murine models, for example, combinations of the T-cell-attracting chemokine lymphotactin and the T-cell growth factor IL-2 caused regression of pre-established leukemia and neuroblastoma when either agent alone was inadequate.[67] Preliminary results of clinical studies using the combination are consistent with this proposition.

THERAPEUTIC PRINCIPLES

Progress in the modification of the host immune response in gene therapy of malignant disease

- Immunize with adenovirus-IL-2 vector transduced tumor cells.
- $CD4^+$ T-cell infiltration of injection site observed.
- Specific antitumor antibody response engendered.
- T-cell killing of autologous tumor cells noted.
- Clinical responses obtained.

Modification of the host immune system

Gene-modified cytotoxic T cells

A considerable body of evidence indicates that the immune system has the potential to eradicate leukemia and perhaps lymphoma.[74] This capability is clearest in patients who have received bone marrow allografts for the treatment of a hematologic malignancy. In those cases, the presence of graft-versus-host disease (GVHD) lowers the risk of subsequent relapse, while measures that prevent GVHD, such as T-cell depletion or the use of an identical twin allograft, are associated with an increased risk of disease recurrence.[75] This so-called 'graft-versus-leukemia effect' may simply be another manifestation of GVHD, in which both normal and malignant host cells share the same host-specific polymorphisms, which can serve as targets for alloreactive T lymphocytes. It is also possible that some of the host's normal T cells are able to detect discrete antigens on tumor cells. Cytotoxic T lymphocytes (CTL) recognize processed intracellular proteins presented as short peptide fragments together with MHC molecules on the cell surface. Hence, internal proteins unique to the malignant clone may act as tumor-specific antigens for CTL. Several human malignancies contain novel proteins, such as mutated oncogenes or fusion proteins generated by chromosomal translocations.[76] Some lymphomas may express immunogenic proteins encoded by Epstein–Barr viral genes.[77] Finally, even normal proteins can elicit CTL responses if they are expressed in higher-than-usual quantities; tyrosinase and the MAGE series of proteins in melanoma cells are two good examples.[78]

If tumor cells are able to process and present these tumor-specific peptides, then it is possible that a malignancy-specific response could be generated in the absence of any other host reactivity. Immunoblastic lymphoma generated by Epstein–Barr virus (EBV) affords a useful model for evaluating this strategy, since the target antigens are well defined. EBV is a herpesvirus that infects most people. It persists in an asymptomatic state by a combination of chronic replication in the mucosa and latency in peripheral blood B cells.[79] These EBV-infected B cells are highly immunogenic and normally susceptible to killing by CTL. In immunocompromised patients, however, the infected B cells may grow unchecked, producing a rapidly progressive lymphoproliferative disease (LPD) that usually appears histologically as an immunoblastic lymphoma. This complication occurs in 1–30%

of patients who have received immunosuppressive therapy after allografting and is associated with high mortality rates.[80] EBV-specific T-cell lines can be generated ex vivo by stimulating donor T cells with EBV-transformed B cells and adoptively transferring the virus-specific T-cell lines to the marrow recipients to learn if they behave as safe and effective prophylaxis and treatment for EBV-related LPD.[81,82] To assess the survival, distribution, and activity of these cells after administration, one can mark them genetically with a retroviral vector that transfers the neomycin resistance gene (*neo*). Study of the patients treated in this manner showed that the infused CTL produced no adverse effects and were long-lived; the *neo* gene has been detected in EBV-specific CTL for up to 66 months.[80,82] In patients with EBV disease, administration of EBV-specific CTL was rapidly followed by a 1000-fold decrease in EBV DNA levels and the resolution of biopsy-proven immunoblastic lymphoma.

Gene transfer can also be used to increase the safety of CTL activity. Infusing donor-derived T cells after bone marrow transplantation (BMT) can lead to GVHD initiated by alloreactive T cells. Even if CTL clones are used, cross-reaction with MHC polymorphisms may cause GVHD in an allogeneic setting. Furthermore, therapy of established disease with T cells can result in tissue damage from inflammatory reactions. Transduction of T cells with a 'suicide gene', so that cell death can be induced if adverse effects occur, is one solution to this problem.[83] The gene most commonly used for this purpose is the thymidine kinase gene, which transfers sensitivity to the cytotoxic effects of nucleotide analogs such as ganciclovir. For this approach to be successful, all cells must contain the suicide gene, and its expression must be maintained in vivo. Suicide gene constructs have included a selectable marker such as *neo*, or a cell surface marker such as nerve growth factor gene (*NGFR*), to allow selection of the transduced cells before infusion. Suicide genes are currently being evaluated in several clinical trials of adoptive immunotherapy after transplantation. Bonini and colleagues, who are using donor T cells to treat relapse of EBV lymphoma following BMT, transfect lymphocytes after a brief (24–48 hours) primary stimulation with antigen, using a construct that contains a suicide gene and a truncated version of *NGFR* to serve as a selectable marker.[83] More than 15 patients have been treated, and in the five who developed GVHD, signs and symptoms resolved after ganciclovir therapy. Riddell and colleagues administered HIV-gag-specific CTL transduced with a construct encoding the thymidine kinase and hygromycin-resistance genes to HIV-infected patients.[84] In this study, five of six patients unexpectedly developed CTL responses specific for the transgenes, resulting in destruction of the infused cells. Several patients in the Italian study also developed thymidine kinase-specific CTL,[83] suggesting that future attempts to exploit cell suicide genes may be restricted by the immunogenicity of the transgenes. For this reason there is growing interest in alternative suicide systems that are activated after administration of a small-molecule inducer. Probably the most advanced use of these is the fas-ligand/caspase system, regulated by analogs of rapamycin.[21]

THERAPEUTIC PRINCIPLES

Gene modification of autologous cytotoxic T-cells shows promise of clinical use
- EBV-specific cytotoxic T cells marked by neomycin resistance gene.
- Proliferation of clones of EBV-specific cytotoxic T cells is produced in vitro.
- EBV-specific T cell clones infused into patient cause regression of EBV-driven proliferations.
- Clinical responses obtained.
- Neomycin gene detected in T cells up to 5 years later, documenting persistence of cell clones.

THERAPEUTIC PRINCIPLES

Use of thymidine kinase gene to induce suicide in harmful cytotoxic T-cells
- T cells transduced with thymidine kinase are destroyed by ganciclovir.
- Marker neomycin or nerve growth factor genes permit tracing of cells.
- Transfected donor cells that participate in GVH disease are killed when the patient takes ganciclovir.
- Clinical responses obtained.
- Extension of these studies to fas-ligand/caspase system regulated by rapamycin may be future modification.

Genetic modification to enhance antitumor immunity

An alternative way to enhance the antitumor activity of immunocytes is to increase the levels of the cytotoxic cytokines (such as tumor necrosis factor, or TNF) they produce at local tumor sites. This approach is being evaluated in studies with tumor-infiltrating lymphocytes (TIL).[85] The problems with this strategy are that it has been difficult to persuade TIL to secrete high levels of cytokines, and only scanty data support the belief that reinfused human TIL selectively home to tumor sites. The first six patients treated with TNF-secreting TIL have shown few side-effects, and one patient has had a sustained response.[85]

SAFETY

Several thousand patients have now received vectors or genetically modified cells in clinical trials, and only one patient – a young man with ornithine transcarbamylase deficiency who received a high dose of adenovector directly into his intrahepatic artery[11] – has died as a direct result of this procedure, possibly as the result of an acute inflammatory reaction mediated by extremely high levels of IL-6. No major toxicities have been

CLINICAL PEARLS

At the beginning of the 21st century gene therapy offers:
- Correction of some forms of primary immunodeficiency
- Possible correction of inherited metabolic diseases
- Development of novel strategies for possible treatment of HIV infection
- Rapid deployment of tumor vaccines for experimental treatment of cancer

observed among patients with cancer or an immunodeficiency disease, but as vector and expression systems become more effective, we can anticipate the induction of some adverse events.

CONCLUSIONS

Gene transfer clearly offers the prospect of a permanent cure for rare, inherited monogenic immunodeficiencies. For the much more common acquired immunodeficiency syndrome, and for the treatment of cancer, it is likely that the approach will come to represent another therapeutic modality that can contribute to the cure of these more complex and heterogeneous disorders. Fully achieving even this more modest objective will nonetheless require substantial improvements in currently available gene transfer technologies and in our understanding of the pathobiology of specific candidate diseases.

REFERENCES

1. Brenner MK, Rill DR, Moen RC, Krance RA, Mirro J Jr, Anderson WF, Ihle JN. Gene-marking to trace origin of relapse after autologous bone marrow transplantation. Lancet 1993;341:85.
2. Engelhardt JF, Yang Y, Stratford-Perricaudet LD, et al. Direct gene transfer of human CFTR into human bronchial epithelia of xenografts with E1-deleted adenoviruses. Nat Genet 1993;4:27.
3. Russell DW, Kay MA. Adeno-associated virus vectors and hematology. Blood 1999;94:864.
4. Nabel GJ, Nabel EG, Yang ZY, et al. Direct gene transfer with DNA–liposome complexes in melanoma: expression, biologic activity, and lack of toxicity in humans. Proc Natl Acad Sci USA 1993;90(23):11307.
5. Bender MA, Palmer TD, Gelinas RE, Miller AD. Evidence that the packaging signal of Moloney Murine Leukemia Virus extends into the gag region. J Virol 1987;61:1639.
6. Donahue RE, Kessler SW, Bodine D, et al. Helper virus induced T cell lymphoma in nonhuman primates after retroviral mediated gene transfer. J Exp Med 1992;176:1125.
7. Smith TA, Mehaffey MG, Kayda DB, et al. Adenovirus mediated expression of therapeutic plasma levels in human factor IX in mice. Nat Genet 1993;5:397.
8. Amin R, Wilmott R, Schwarz Y, Trapnell B, Stark J. Replication-deficient adenovirus induces expression of interleukin-8 by airway epithelial cells *in vivo*. Hum Gene Ther 1995;6:145.
9. Dai Y, Schwarz EM, Gu D, Zhang WW, Sarvetnick N, Verma IM. Cellular and humoral immune responses to adenoviral vectors containing factor IX gene: tolerization of factor IX and vector antigens allows for long-term expression. Proc Natl Acad Sci U S A 1995;92:1401.
10. Hitt MH, Parks RJ, Graham FL. Structure and genetic organization of adenovirus vectors. In: Friedmann T (ed.) The development of human gene therapy. New York, Cold Spring Harbor Laboratory Press, 1999, p 61.
11. Knorr, D. Serious adverse event on NIH Human Gene Transfer Protocol #9512–139. A phase I study of adenovector mediated gene transfer to liver in adults with partial ornithine transcarbamylase deficiency. Memorandum of 21 September 1999, Office of Recombinant DNA Activities at NIH, 1999.
12. Schiedner G, Morral N, Parks RJ, et al. Genomic DNA transfer with a high-capacity adenovirus vector results in improved in vivo gene expression and decreased toxicity [published erratum appears in Nat Genet 1998;18(3):298]. Nat Genet 1998;18:180.
13. Weitzman MD, Kyostio SRM, Kotin RM, Owens RA. Adeno-associated virus (AAV) rep proteins mediated complex formation between AAV DNA and its integration site in human DNA. Proc Natl Acad Sci 1994;91:5802.
14. Manno CS, Herzog RG, Arruda VR, et al. A phase I trial of AAV-mediated muscle-directed gene therapy for hemophilia B. Blood 1999;94:642a. (Abstract).
15. Dilloo D, Rill D, Entwistle C, et al. A novel herpes vector for the high efficiency transduction of normal and malignant human hemopoietic cells. Blood 1997;89:119.
16. Schofield JP, Caskey CT. Non-viral approaches to gene therapy. Br Med Bull 1995;51:56.
17. Barry MA, Dower WJ, Johnston SA. Toward cell-targeting gene therapy vectors: selection of cell-binding peptides from random peptide-presenting phage libraries. Nat Med 1996;2:299.
18. Templeton NS, Lasic DD. New directions in liposome gene delivery. Mol Biotechnol 1999;11:175.
19. Cole-Strauss A, Yoon K, Xiang Y, et al. Correction of the mutation responsible for sickle cell anemia by an RNA–DNA oligonucleotide. Science 1996;273:1386.
20. Kren BT, Bandyopadhyay P, Steer CJ. In vivo site-directed mutagenesis of the factor IX gene by chimeric RNA/DNA oligonucleotides. Nat Med 1998; 4:285.
21. Rossi FM, Blau HM. Recent advances in inducible gene expression systems. Curr Opin Biotechnol 1998;9:451.
22. Wang Y, O'Malley BWJ, Tsai SY, O'Malley BW. A regulatory system for use in gene transfer. Proc Natl Acad Aci USA 1994;91:8180.
23. Hanenberg H, Xiao XL, Dilloo D, Hashino K, Kato I, Williams DA. Co-localization of retrovirus and target cells on specific fibronectin adhesion domains for increased genetic transduction of mammalian cells. Nat Med 1996;2:876.
24. Naldini L. Lentiviruses as gene transfer agents for delivery to non-dividing cells. Curr Opin Biotechnol 1998;9:457.
25. Fischer A, Cavazzana-Calvo M, De Saint B, et al. Naturally occurring primary deficiencies of the immune system. Annu Rev Immunol 1997;15:93.
26. Blaese RM, Culver KW, Miller AD, et al. T lymphocyte-directed gene therapy for ADA-SCID: Initial trial results after 4 years. Science 1995;270:475.
27. Kohn DB, Hershfield MS, Carbonaro D, et al. T lymphocytes with a normal ADA gene accumulate after transplantation of transduced autologous umbilical cord blood CD34⁺ cells in ADA-deficient SCID neonates. Nat Med 1998;4:775.
28. Wimperis JZ, Brenner MK, Prentice HG, et al. Transfer of a functioning humoral immune system in transplantation of T lymphocyte depleted bone marrow. Lancet 1986;i:339.
29. Cavazzana-Calvo M, Hacien-Bey S, de Saint G, et al. Correction of SCID-X1 disease phenotype following gamma-c gene transfer by a retroviral vector into CD34+ cells in two children. Blood 1999;94:367a (Abstract).
30. Nosaka T, van Deursen JM, Tripp RA, et al. Defective lymphoid development in mice lacking Jak3 [published erratum appears in Science 1996;271(5245):17]. Science 1995;270: 800.
31. Bunting KD, Sangster MY, Ihle JN, Sorrentino BP. Restoration of lymphocyte function in Janus kinase 3-deficient mice by retroviral-mediated gene transfer. Nat Med 1998;4:58.
32. Bunting KD, Flynn KJ, Riberdy JM, Doherty PC, Sorrentino BP. Virus-specific immunity after gene therapy in a murine model of severe combined immunodeficiency. Proc Natl Acad Sci USA 1999;96:232.
33. Noelle RJ. CD40 and its ligand in host defense. Immunity 1996;4:415.
34. Kroczek RA, Graf D, Brugnoni D, et al. Defective expression of CD40 ligand on T cells causes 'X-linked immunodeficiency with hyper-IgM (HIGM1)'. Immunol Rev 1994;138:39.
35. Brown MP, Topham D, Sangster MY, et al. Thymic lymphoproliferative disease after successful correction of CD40 ligand deficiency by gene transfer in mice. Nat Med 1998;4:1253.
36. Candotti F, Blaese RM. Gene therapy of primary immunodeficiencies. Springer Semin Immunopathol 1998;19:493.
37. Minegishi Y, Rohrer J, Conley ME. Recent progress in the diagnosis and treatment of patients with defects in early B-cell development. Curr Opin Pediatr 1999;11:528.

38. Carr A, Samaras K, Chisholm DJ, Cooper DA. Abnormal fat distribution and use of protease inhibitors. Lancet 1998;351:1736.
39. Burman WJ, Gallicano K, Peloquin C. Therapeutic implications of drug interactions in the treatment of human immunodeficiency virus-related tuberculosis. Clin Infect Dis 1999;28:419.
40. Hecht FM, Grant RM, Petropoulos CJ, et al. Sexual transmission of an HIV-1 variant resistant to multiple reverse-transcriptase and protease inhibitors. N Engl J Med 1998;339:307.
41. Chun TW, Fauci AS. Latent reservoirs of HIV: obstacles to the eradication of virus. Proc Natl Acad Sci USA 1999;96:10958.
42. Finzi D, Blankson J, Siliciano JD, et al. Latent infection of CD4+ T cells provides a mechanism for lifelong persistence of HIV-1, even in patients on effective combination therapy. Nat Med 1999;5:512.
43. Littman DR. Chemokine receptors: keys to AIDS pathogenesis? Cell 1998;93:677.
44. Liu R, Paxton WA, Choe S, et al. Homozygous defect in HIV-1 coreceptor accounts for resistance of some multiply-exposed individuals to HIV-1 infection. Cell 1996;86:367.
45. Yang AG, Bai X, Huang XF, Yao C, Chen S. Phenotypic knockout of HIV type 1 chemokine coreceptor CCR-5 by intrakines as potential therapeutic approach for HIV-1 infection. Proc Natl Acad Sci USA 1997;94:11567.
46. Cullen BR. HIV-1 auxiliary proteins: making connections in a dying cell. Cell 1998;93:685.
47. Mhashilkar AM, Bagley J, Chen SY, Szilvay AM, Helland DG, Marasco WA. Inhibition of HIV-1 Tat-mediated LTR transactivation and HIV-1 infection by anti-Tat single chain intrabodies. EMBO J 1995;14:1542.
48. Sun LQ, Pyati J, Smythe J, Wang L, Macpherson J, Gerlach W, Symonds G. Resistance to human immunodeficiency virus type 1 infection conferred by transduction of human peripheral blood lymphocytes with ribozyme, antisense, or polymeric transactivation response element constructs. Proc Natl Acad Sci USA 1995;92:7272.
49. Chang HK, Gendelman R, Lisziewicz J, Gallo RC, Ensoli B. Block of HIV-1 infection by a combination of antisense tat RNA and TAR decoys: a strategy for control of HIV-1. Gene Ther 1994;1:208.
50. Ulich C, Harrich D, Estes P, Gaynor RB. Inhibition of human immunodeficiency virus type 1 replication is enhanced by a combination of transdominant Tat and Rev proteins. J Virol 1996;70:4871.
51. Malim MH, Tiley LS, McCarn DF, Rusche JR, Hauber J, Cullen BR. HIV-1 structural gene expression requires binding of the Rev trans-activator to its RNA target sequence. Cell 1990;60:675.
52. Duan L, Zhu M, Bagasra O, Pomerantz RJ. Intracellular immunization against HIV-1 infection of human T lymphocytes: utility of anti-rev single-chain variable fragments [published erratum appears in Hum Gene Ther 1998;9(5):765]. Hum Gene Ther 1995;6:1561.
53. Bahner I, Kearns K, Hao QL, Smogorzewska EM, Kohn DB. Transduction of human CD34+ hematopoietic progenitor cells by a retroviral vector expressing an RRE decoy inhibits human immunodeficiency virus type 1 replication in myelomonocytic cells produced in long-term culture. J Virol 1996;70:4352.
54. Malim MH, Bohnlein S, Hauber J, Cullen BR. Functional dissection of the HIV-1 Rev trans-activator – derivation of a trans-dominant repressor of Rev function. Cell 1989;58:205.
55. Ranga U, Woffendin C, Verma S, Xu L, June CH, Bishop DK, Nabel GJ. Enhanced T cell engraftment after retroviral delivery of an antiviral gene in HIV-infected individuals. Proc Natl Acad Sci USA 1998;95:1201.
56. Woffendin C, Ranga U, Yang Z, Xu L, Nabel GJ. Expression of a protective gene prolongs survival of T cells in human immunodeficiency virus-infected patients. Proc Natl Acad Sci USA 1996;93:2889.
57. Hamm TE, Rekosh D, Hammarskjold ML. Selection and characterization of human immunodeficiency virus type 1 mutants that are resistant to inhibition by the transdominant negative RevM10 protein. J Virol 1999;73:5741.
58. Gervaix A, Li X, Kraus G, Wong-Staal F. Multigene antiviral vectors inhibit diverse human immunodeficiency virus type 1 caldes. J Virol 1997;71:3048.
59. Caputo A, Rossi C, Bozzini R, Betti M, Grossi MP, Barbanti-Brodano G, Balboni PG. Studies on the effect of the combined expression of anti-tat and anti-rev genes on HIV-1 replication. Gene Ther 1997;4:288.
60. Duan L, Zhu M, Ozaki I, Zhang H, Wei DL, Pomerantz RJ. Intracellular inhibition of HIV-1 replication using a dual protein- and RNA-based strategy [published erratum appears in Gene Ther 1998;5(4):570]. Gene Ther 1997;4:533.
61. Aguilar-Cordova E, Chinen J, Donehower LA, Harper JW, Rice AP, Butel JS, Belmont JW. Inhibition of HIV-1 by a double transdominant fusion gene. Gene Ther 1995; 2:181.
62. Walker RE, Carter CS, Muul L, et al. Peripheral expansion of pre-existing mature T cells is an important means of CD4+ T-cell regeneration HIV-infected adults. Nat Med 1998;4:852.
63. Brodie SJ, Lewinsohn DA, Patterson BK, et al. In vivo migration and function of transferred HIV-1-specific cytotoxic T cells. Nat Med 1999;5:34.
64. Brenner MK. The applications of gene transfer of pediatric malignant disease. In: Pizzo PA, Poplack DG (eds) Principles and practice of pediatric oncology. Philadelphia, J.B. Lippincott, 1997, 375.
65. Cheever MA, Disis ML, Bernhard H, et al. Immunity to oncogenic proteins. Immunol Rev 1995;145:33.
66. Eshhar Z. Tumor specific T bodies: towards clinical application. Cancer Immunol Immunother 1997;45:131.
67. Dilloo D, Bacon K, Holden W, Zhong W, Burdach S, Zlotnik A, Brenner M. Combined chemokine and cytokine gene transfer enhances antitumor immunity. Nat Med 1996;2:1090.
68. Soiffer R, Lynch T, Mihm M, et al. Vaccination with irradiated autologous melanoma cells engineered to secrete human granulocyte-macrophage colony-stimulating factor generates potent antitumor immunity in patients with metastatic melanoma. Proc Natl Acad Sci USA 1998;95:13141.
69. Townsend SE, Allison JP. Tumor rejection after direct costimulation of CD8+ T-cells by B7 transfected melanoma cells. Science 1993;259:368–370.
70. Fearon ER, Pardoll DM, Itaya T, et al. Interleukin-2 production by tumor cells bypasses T helper function in the generation of an antitumor response. Cell 1990;60:397.
71. Bowman L, Grossmann M, Rill D, et al. IL-2 adenovector-transduced autologous tumor cells induce antitumor immune responses in patients with neuroblastoma. Blood 1998;92:1941.
72. Simons JW, Jaffe EM, Weber CE, et al. Bioactivity of autologous irradiated renal cell carcinoma vaccines generated by ex-vivo granulocyte-macrophage colony-stimulating factor gene transfer. Cancer Res 1997;57:1537.
73. Bowman LC, Grossmann M, Rill D, et al. IL-2 gene-modified allogeneic tumor cells for treatment of relapsed neuroblastoma. Hum Gene Ther 1998;9:1303.
74. Kolb H-J, Schattenberg A, Goldman JM, et al. Graft-versus-leukemia effect of donor lymphocyte infusions in marrow grafted patients. Blood 1995;86:2041.
75. Horowitz MM, Gale RP, Sondel PM, et al. Graft-versus-leukemia reactions after bone marrow transplantation. Blood 1990;75:555.
76. Brenner MK, Heslop HE. Graft-versus-host reactions and bone marrow transplantation. Curr Opin Immunol 1991;3:752.
77. Heslop HE, Rooney CM. Adoptive immunotherapy of EBV lymphoproliferative diseases. Immunol Rev 1997;157:217.
78. van Der Bruggen P, Traversari C, Chomez P, et al. A gene encoding an antigen recognized by cytolytic T lymphocytes on a human melanoma. Science 1991;254:1643.
79. Rickinson AB, Moss DJ. Human cytotoxic T lymphocyte responses to Epstein–Barr virus infection. Annu Rev Immunol 1997;15:405.
80. Aguilar LK, Rooney CM, Heslop HE. Lymphoproliferative disorders involving Epstein–Barr virus after hemopoietic stem cell transplantation. Curr Opin Oncol 1999;11:96.
81. Heslop HE, Ng CYC, Li C, et al. Long-term restoration of immunity against Epstein–Barr virus infection by adoptive transfer of gene-modified virus-specific T lymphocytes. Nat Med 1996;2:551.
82. Rooney CM, Smith CA, Ng CYC, et al. Infusion of cytotoxic T cells for the prevention and treatment of Epstein–Barr virus-induced lymphoma in allogeneic transplant recipients. Blood 1998;92:1549.
83. Bonini C, Ferrari G, Verzeletti S, et al. HSV-TK gene transfer into donor lymphocytes for control of allogeneic graft versus leukemia. Science 1997;276:1719.

84. Riddell SR, Elliot M, Lewinsohn DA, et al. T-cell mediated rejection of gene-modified HIV-specific cytotoxic T lymphocytes in HIV-infected patients. Nat Med 1996;2:216.

85. Hwu P, Rosenberg SA. The use of gene-modified tumor infiltrating lymphocytes for cancer therapy. Ann NY Acad Sci 1994;716:188.

Section 10 Prevention and Therapy of Immunologic Diseases
D Anti-Inflammatory Medications

Chapter 106 Glucocorticoids

Joseph D. Spahn, Donald Y.M. Leung and Stanley J. Szefler

Their potent anti-inflammatory and immunosuppressive effects have led to glucocorticoids (GCs) being widely used in a number of immune-mediated diseases including autoimmune (e.g. inflammatory bowel disease, multiple sclerosis), rheumatologic (systemic lupus erythematous, rheumatoid arthritis) and allergic (asthma, atopic dermatitis, allergic rhinitis) disorders and transplant rejection. A huge body of clinical experience has accumulated in the half century since their initial use, with great strides made in our understanding of how GCs act at the molecular and cellular level. In addition, we are acutely aware of both their clinical efficacy and their potential for significant morbidity with long-term administration. This chapter provides a brief overview of the structure, mechanisms of action, pharmacokinetics, efficacy, and adverse effects of systemically administered GCs, using asthma as the prototypic immune-mediated disease for which oral GCs are administered.

KEY CONCEPTS

Glucocorticoids

- By virtue of their ability to inhibit multiple facets of the immune response, glucocorticoids are an effective treatment for allergic, autoimmune, and rheumatologic diseases.
- As all nucleated cells contain glucocorticoid receptors, it is, at this time, impossible to separate the anti-inflammatory from the metabolic effects of glucocorticoids.
- Long-term use of systemic glucocorticoids results in a multitude of adverse effects including growth suppression in children, osteoporosis, cataracts, myopathy, and the development of cushingoid body habitus.
- Persistent immune activation can reduce GC sensitivity.

MECHANISMS OF ACTION

Actions at the molecular level

A great deal of research over the past 20 years has improved our understanding of how GCs act, yet the precise mechanism(s) by which they suppress inflammation is at present incompletely understood. We know that GCs act directly and indirectly by influencing gene transcription. With up- or down-regulation of gene transcription comes modulation of immune/inflammatory response (Table 106.1). GCs are highly lipid soluble and consequently they easily diffuse across cell membranes (Fig. 106.1). Once within the cytoplasm, they bind with high affinity to a specific cytoplasmic receptor, termed the GC receptor (GCR). This 'inactive' cytosolic GCR is a hetero-oligomer noncovalently associated with heat-shock proteins and immunophilin. Upon ligand (GC) binding, a confirmational change results in the dissociation of the accessory proteins from the receptor complex. The GC–GCR complex is then transported from the cytoplasm into the nucleus through nuclear pores. Once in the nucleus, dimers of the receptor complex form with subsequent binding to specific regions of DNA, termed GC response elements or GRE, upstream from the promoter sites of steroid-responsive genes. Binding of the GC–GCR complex to the GRE results in either up- or down-regulation of gene products. It has been estimated that there are 10–100 genes that have GRE sites. These genes are steroid responsive in that they can be directly influenced by GCs.[1] Many genes encoding pro-inflammatory cytokines do not have GREs, therefore GC must also indirectly influence gene transcription. Insight into this mechanism of action comes from studies that have focused on GC–GCR complex–transcription factor interactions (Fig. 106.1). Transcription factors such as activator protein-1 (AP-1) and nuclear factor κB (NF-κB) are proteins involved in the up-regulation of cytokine gene transcription. By binding to these transcription factors, the GCR complex inhibits binding of the transcription factor to its DNA binding site with the end result being inhibition of pro-inflammatory gene transcription.[2,3]

GCs can also influence gene transcription by stimulating the production of IκBα. This protein 'inactivates' NF-κB by binding to it before it can enter the nucleus (Fig. 106.1). Since NF-κB must bind to DNA sites within the nucleus for gene transcription of pro-inflammatory cytokines to occur, cytokine gene transcription is inhibited.[4,5] In addition to inhibiting gene transcription,

Mechanisms of GC action in asthma

'Positive effects'

A. Potentiation of β-adrenergic receptors
B. Vasoconstrictive properties
C. Up-regulation of IκB
D. Up-regulation of lipocortin expression

'Inhibitory effects'

A. Inhibition of the cytokines involved in the allergic inflammatory response
B. Inhibition of leukocyte activation, function, and survival:
  1. T lymphocytes
  2. Eosinophils
  3. Monocyte/macrophages
C. Inhibition of leukocyte adhesion/migration
D. Inhibition of the production and/or release of inflammatory mediators:
  1. Lipid mediators (platelet-activating factor, leukotrienes, prostaglandins)
  2. Eosinophil-derived cytotoxic proteins (eosinophil cationic protein, major basic protein).

Table 106.1 Mechanisms of GC action in asthma.

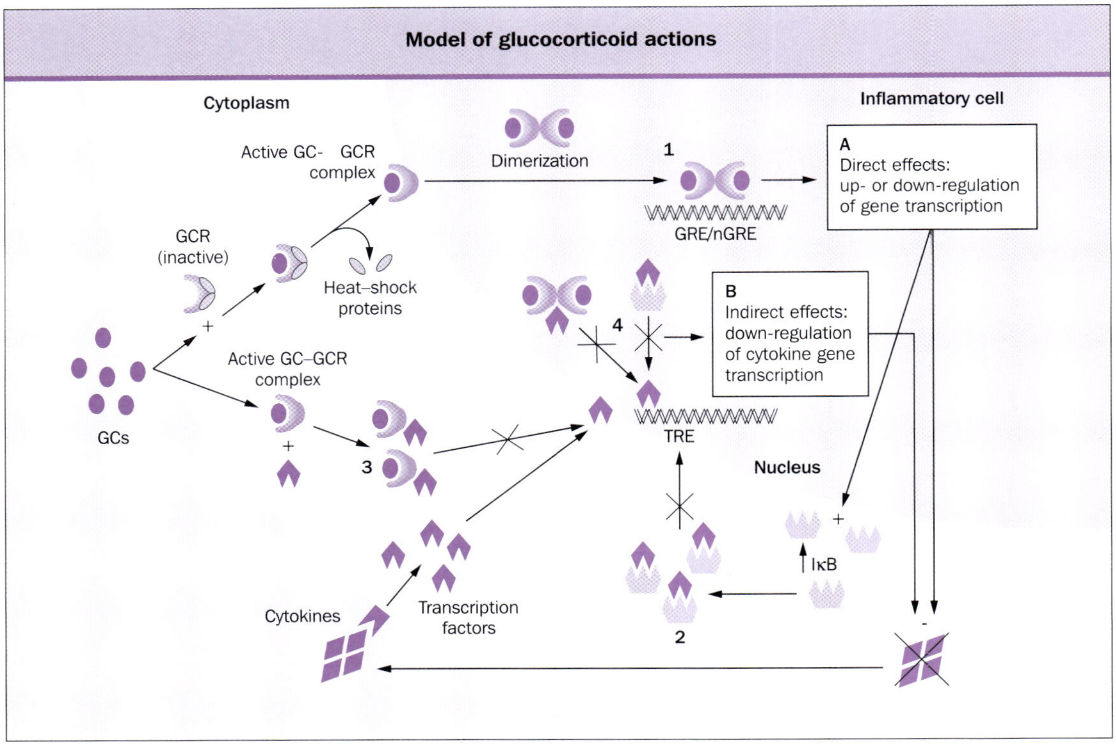

Figure 106.1 Model of GC actions. Glucocorticoids (GC) easily diffuse across the plasma membrane of inflammatory cells where they then bind to a cytoplasmic receptor termed the GC receptor (GCR). The GC–GCR complex is then transported to the nucleus where it dimerizes before binding to sites on the DNA (GC response elements or GREs) of GC-responsive genes (outlined at step 1). In this way, GCs either up-regulate or down-regulate gene transcription. GCs can also inhibit the transcription of pro-inflammatory cytokines indirectly, either by stimulating the production of Iκb which then interferes with the ability of transcription factor function (step 2), or by binding to transcription factors directly (outlined at step 3). Transcription factors are essential in the transcription of pro-inflammatory cytokine genes. By interfering with the ability of transcription factors to bind to their binding sites, termed transcription factor response elements or TREs, GCs prevent transcription factor-induced gene transcription from occurring (outlined at step 4).

GCs can alter post-transcriptional events such as mRNA translation, protein synthesis, and protein secretion. As an example, GCs have been shown to decrease the stability of interferon mRNA by activation of a ribonuclease that degrades the AU-rich sequences in the untranslated region of this gene.[6] The decrease in mRNA stability leads to a shorter half-life and, ultimately, less protein synthesized.

Actions at the cellular level

Studies evaluating the effect of GCs on cytokine production have uniformly shown them to display inhibitory properties. Specifically, GCs have been shown to inhibit interleukin-1 (IL-1), IL-2, IL-3, IL-4, IL-5, IL-6, IL-13, GM-CSF, and tumor necrosis factor alpha. Many of these cytokines are believed to play significant roles in the allergic inflammatory response. Leukocyte adhesion to the vascular endothelium and eventual migration to airway epithelium comprises an essential component of the airway inflammatory response. GCs have been shown to decrease neutrophil influx in injury-induced inflammation,[7,8] inhibit the influx of eosinophils in experimentally induced cutaneous late-phase allergic responses,[9] and to decrease the numbers of cells infiltrating into the bronchial mucosa of asthmatics.[10] Up-regulation of adhesion molecules involved in this process such as E-selectin, vascular cell adhesion molecule-1 (VCAM-1), and intercellular adhesion molecule-1 (ICAM-1) on endothelial cells has been demonstrated in vitro by exposure to pro-inflammatory cytokines.[11–13] GCs are not thought to decrease directly the expression of adhesion molecules; rather they act indirectly by inhibiting the production of pro-inflammatory cytokines and mediators that are essential for the up-regulation of these molecules.

In addition to inhibiting cytokine production and leukocyte trafficking, GCs can also inhibit lipid mediators of allergic inflammation under certain conditions. The eicosanoids comprise a group of oxygenated metabolites of arachidonic acid and include the cyclooxygenase metabolites prostaglandin D_2, thromboxane B_2, and prostaglandin $F_{2\alpha}$ and the products of the 5-lipoxygenase pathway leukotrienes (LT) LTC_4, LTD_4 and LTE_4 (LT) LTC_4, LTD_4 and LTE_4. These compounds are major mediators of bronchoconstriction and increased vascular permeability and are found in elevated concentrations in chronic asthma[14] (Chapter 45). In addition, LTB_4 has profound chemotactic activity for inflammatory cells including eosinophils, monocytes, and neutrophils. Although in vitro studies have clearly demonstrated the efficacy of GC in suppressing eicosanoid production,[15] in vivo studies have not uniformly confirmed these findings.[16,17] Of importance, ex vivo studies of macrophage-enriched bronchoalveolar lavage (BAL) cells have shown oral GC therapy to reduce significantly the ability of these cells to spontaneously release eicosanoids,[16] and pretreatment of these cells with methylprednisolone (MPn) prior to stimulation with the calcium ionophore A23187 resulted in significant inhibition of both prostaglandins and leukotrienes.[15]

It remains to be determined what role GC have in suppressing airway eosinophil eicosanoid production.

Increased vascular permeability with subsequent leakage of plasma proteins into the airway interstitium constitutes a major component of the inflammatory response noted in asthma. Significant airway edema has long been noted in fatal asthma[18] and recently in stable chronic asthma.[18] GCs display potent vasoconstrictive properties. GC inhibition of plasma leakage and edema most likely occurs by inhibiting mediator-induced capillary leakage.[19] This is a potentially important property of GCs in the treatment of asthma. By decreasing capillary permeability at sites of inflammation, GCs reduce the degree of airway edema, and thus results in less airway constriction. In addition, with less plasma exudation comes a reduction in the concentration of inflammatory and chemotactic factors, with subsequent modulation of the inflammatory response.

Another important and unique mechanism by which GCs act in asthma derives from their ability to potentiate the effect of adrenergic stimulation. GCs have been shown to up-regulate the number of β-adrenoceptors in lymphocytes of individuals who have developed β-agonist-induced desensitization.[20] In vivo studies evaluating the additive effects of GC on β-agonist response have yielded conflicting results. Ellul-Micallef and Fenech[21] reported that a single dose of prednisolone significantly improved the responsiveness to inhaled isoprenaline in 8 out of 10 severe asthmatics who were previously documented to be poorly responsive to β-agonists. Shenfield et al also found a positive interaction between oral prednisone and inhaled isoprenaline in 6 of 9 asthmatics.[22] The patients who demonstrated a favorable response were noted to have significant improvements in their baseline FEV_1 over the course of the study and were noted to display a potentiation of isoprenaline on FEV_1 during prednisone treatment. Finally, a recent study by Wempe et al further clarified the effects of GCs on inhaled β-agonists.[23] GC therapy resulted in improved baseline lung function and diminished bronchial hyperresponsiveness (BHR), but no difference in the degree of post-albuterol bronchodilation was noted between those on placebo and those on GCs. In summary, these investigators demonstrated improvements in pre-bronchodilator FEV_1 values following a course of GC therapy, but failed to demonstrate an additive effect of GCs on β-agonist responsiveness. The authors attributed this lack of added bronchodilation to a 'ceiling' effect in that post-β-agonist FEV_1 values were almost normal in all three groups, and thus no further effect could be demonstrated.

CHEMISTRY

Synthetic GCs are cortisone-based molecules that have undergone structural modifications designed to enhance their potencies and prolong their durations of action. Anti-inflammatory GCs have a 17-hydroxyl group at the 17-position and methyl groups at carbons 18 and 19 (Fig. 106.2). Other features necessary for activity are a ketone at carbons 3 and 20, a double bond between carbons 4 and 5 of the A-ring, and a hydroxyl group at the 11-position of the C-ring. Modifications to the basic steroid structure have increased anti-inflammatory effects while decreasing mineralocorticoid effects; however it has not been possible to eliminate the unwanted metabolic effects while retaining the desired anti-inflammatory properties of the synthetic GCs that are systemically administered.[24] Specific examples of structural changes that have resulted in increased anti-inflammatory potency include the 1,2 double bond in the A-rings of prednisone, prednisolone, methylprednisolone (MPn) and dexamethasone, and the methyl group at the 6-position in the B-ring of MPn. Dexamethasone has a fluorine group at the 9 carbon position. Cortisone and prednisone are pro-drugs; they are inactive moieties that require biotransformation of their 11-ketone groups via metabolic pathways to 11-hydroxy molecules. This conversion results in their active forms, cortisol and prednisolone.[24]

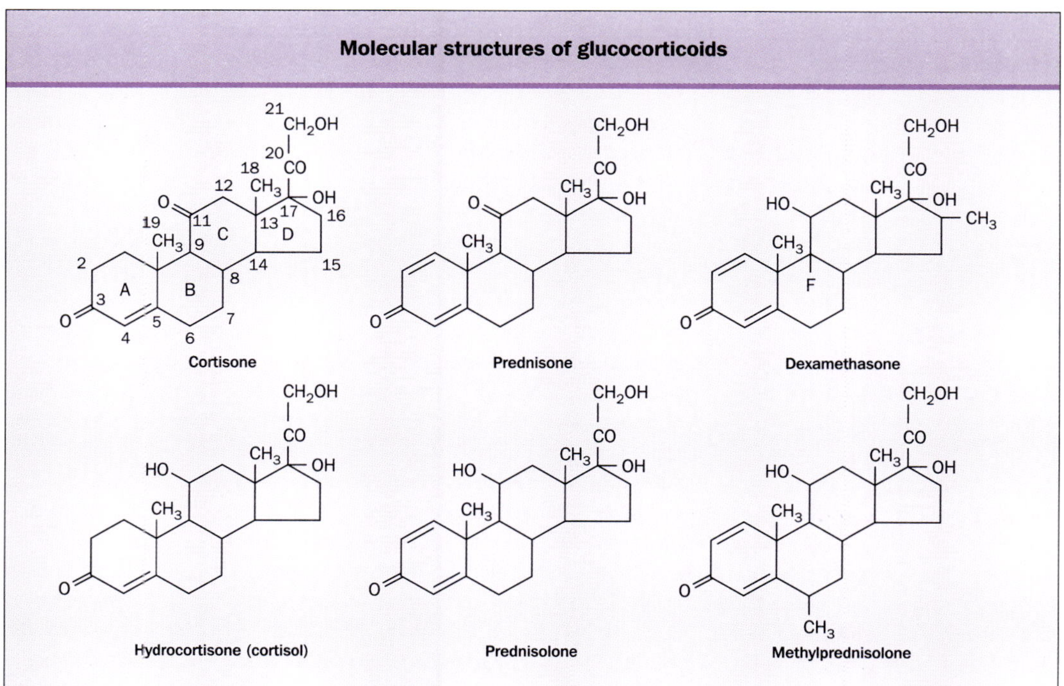

Figure 106.2 Molecular structures of commonly administered systemic GCs and available inhaled GCs used in the treatment of asthma. Carbon and ring nomenclature is noted for cortisone.

PHARMACOKINETICS/PHARMACODYNAMICS

The pharmacokinetics of GCs, i.e. their absorption, distribution, and elimination characteristics, are important determinants of their magnitude and duration of action.[25] These factors can also influence dosing strategies; however, in general GC dosing regimens are not dependent upon pharmacokinetic parameters. Some drug interactions result in a clinically significant reduction of systemic GC exposure. In this scenario, clinical response to treatment would be expected to be diminished.

GCs are highly lipophilic and are rapidly absorbed from the gastrointestinal tract following oral administration. Absorption is relatively complete and bioavailability is generally high. Prednisone and prednisolone are both rapidly absorbed following administration via oral (swallowed) liquid and tablet formulations with peak plasma concentrations occurring at 1 and 2 hours respectively. Oral absorption of GCs is, in general, not affected by age or disease states, but can be diminished by concomitant antacid administration. Relative bioavailability in normals following administration with antacids was only 57–75% compared to that observed without antacids. In theory, inflammatory bowel disease might also affect absorption; however, only initial delays with no alterations of bioavailability have been reported.[26] Once absorbed, prednisone is rapidly transformed to prednisolone via first-pass metabolism, a process that is relatively complete. Ratios of prednisone to prednisolone achieved are approximately 1:5–10.[24] MPn is more slowly absorbed than prednisone and prednisolone. Its binding to transcortin, a GC-binding protein, is reduced; this is thought to be a result of its 6-methyl group.[27] This modification also changes the susceptibility of MPn to alterations of its metabolism by other medication.

Metabolism of GCs occurs by reduction of the 4,5 double bond and 3-ketone and 20-ketone groups, hydroxylation at the 2-position of the A-ring and the 6-position of the B-ring, and conversion of the 11-hydroxyl group to a ketone group.[24] As mixed function oxidases and glucuronyl transferases are important in the biotransformation of GCs, there is the potential for hepatic dysfunction to reduce metabolism.[24] Despite this, liver disease is not a significant factor in individualizing doses because glucuronidation is largely maintained in patients with advanced liver failure and metabolism occurs in other body tissues.[28] If plasma proteins are significantly altered, efficacy can be affected since the free (unbound) drug is responsible for biochemical and physiologic effects.[24] GC clearance can be altered by disease states. Hyperthyroid patients require higher GC doses because there is enhanced nonrenal clearance. With hypothyroid patients, slowed elimination is a concern; however this has not been well studied.[28] Cystic fibrosis results in enhanced clearance of prednisolone.[29] Asthma is not thought to affect metabolism of GCs, although conflicting data have been reported.[30,31] Likewise, age and obesity do not appear to significantly affect the disposition of GCs.[28]

GC elimination may also be altered by numerous concomitant medications (Table 106.2). Drug interactions can result in either reduced or enhanced clearance, and consequently an increased risk for adverse effects or a diminished therapeutic response. The anticonvulsants phenytion, phenobarbital, and carbamazepine cause an increased rate of elimination for prednisolone and MPn.[32] In one study, concomitant treatment with phenobarbital, carbamazepine, and phenytoin, increased elimination of prednisolone by 41%, 79%, and 76%, respectively whereas, MPn clearance was increased by 208%, 341%, and 478%.[32] Rifampin also enhances the clearance of GCs and can result in a diminished therapeutic effect with breakthrough asthma symptoms in steroid-dependent patients.[33]

Drugs that interfere with GCs

GC	Drugs that increase clearance	Drugs that decrease clearance
Methylprednisolone	Carbamazepine Phenobarbital Phenytoin Rifampin	Ketoconazole Troleandomycin Erythromycin Clarithromycin Oral contraceptives
Prednisolone	Rifampin Antacids (reduced bioavailability) Carbamazepine Phenobarbital Phenytoin	Ketoconazole Oral contraceptives

Table 106.2 Drugs that interfere with GCs.

In contrast, other medications can reduce GC elimination. Reductions of clearance by 27% and 60% have been described for prednisolone and MPn, respectively, with concomitant ketoconazole.[34] The macrolide antibiotics erythromycin, troleandomycin, and clarithromycin can also delay GC clearance; however, this effect is limited to MPn.[35] MPn clearance can be reduced from 50% to 70% with concomitant administration of the above compounds. Lastly, oral contraceptives can cause a reduction in prednisolone elimination of approximately 50%.[36]

If one of the above drug interactions that increases clearance is present, one might initially consider addressing the problem by simply increasing the dose. This strategy may not always result in therapeutic benefit, however. The most obvious step in optimizing response to GC therapy is to discontinue the interacting medication. Often this may not be feasible and other interventions are required. One such option would be to change to a GC that is less susceptible to the interaction. In the case of interacting anticonvulsants, this would constitute switching from MPn to prednisone. As MPn is more susceptible to anticonvulsant interactions, a switch from prednisone to MPn would not be advisable.

GC pharmacokinetics studies have been performed in asthmatic patients who respond poorly to therapy and/or patients who have failed to develop overt GC-associated adverse effects despite a long history of oral GC therapy to assess whether an abnormality in absorption and clearance of GCs may be contributing to their poor response. Subsets of patients have been noted to have inherently rapid clearance of prednisolone or MPn, which likely contributed to the lack of benefit observed.[37] Although studies to assess GC pharmacokinetics are not readily available, a pharmacokinetic abnormality might be suspected in patients with a clinical presentation of poor responsiveness with a lack of adverse effects. In these patients, a simple change in GC. may elicit an improved response. In others a 'split' dosing regimen consisting of two thirds of the total daily GC dose in the morning with the remaining one third administered in the afternoon would provide for a more normal plasma concentration vs. time curve and could result in better responsiveness. This strategy might also be beneficial in patients in whom an interacting medication (anticonvulsants, rifampin) might be present. If these changes offer no benefit, a change to a GC with a prolonged half-life would be another option.

Pharmacodynamics can be measured with regard to onset of action, peak effect, duration of effect, and offset of action. In the event that GCs are not hindered by abnormally influenced pharmacokinetics and reach the target tissues in adequate concentrations, a number of steps previously discussed that involve the GCR are still required for them to exert their biological effects. These likely contribute to the slow onset and slow dissipation of effects that characterize GC actions. This principle is consistent with observed responses of patients with asthma following systemic administration of GCs. In stable asthmatics given a single dose of 40 mg of prednisolone, onset of improved pulmonary function was observed 3 hours after administration with a maximal effect at 9–12 hours, followed by a gradual return to near baseline values at 36 hours after administration.[38]

EFFICACY OF GCS IN ASTHMA

Effect on bronchial hyperresponsiveness

A sentinel feature of asthma is heightened bronchial responsiveness (termed bronchial hyperresponsiveness or BHR) to nonspecific stimuli. Several studies have shown significant correlations between the degree of BHR and disease severity, frequency of symptoms, and need for treatment.[39] Although the precise relationship remains elusive, airway inflammation appears to contribute to BHR, but the two conditions are not necessarily directly linked. Oral GCs have been demonstrated to abolish the heightened BHR associated with in vivo allergen exposure, and to diminish nonspecific BHR caused by methacholine when given in large doses. Bhagat and Grunstein[40] evaluated the effect of either prednisone (60 mg/day) or placebo for 7 days in 10 children with atopic asthma and found significant improvements in the mean baseline FEV_1 and log PD_{20}-FEV_1 following prednisone compared to baseline and placebo therapy. Although all subjects increased their PD_{20} values after prednisone, none of the values was even close to normal. Those who demonstrated the greatest improvement in BHR were those with FEV_1 values below 75% of predicted. Robinson et al[41] found similar results in a group of adults with moderate asthma. Methacholine challenges with bronchoscopy with bronchoalveolar lavage were performed in 18 asthmatics before and after a 2-week course of prednisolone or matched placebo. A significant decrease in BHR was noted in those given prednisolone, compared to the placebo-treated group. This improvement in BHR was associated with a reduction in the number of BAL eosinophils, and numbers of BAL cells expressing mRNA for IL-4 and IL-5. These data suggest that GCs, by inhibiting cytokine synthesis, inhibit airway eosinophilia, which in turn results in reduced BHR.

Thus, GCs have beneficial effects on reducing the degree of BHR in patients with asthma. It has been suggested that, by decreasing BHR, GC therapy can decrease both the onset and severity of asthma attacks and thereby potentially reduce the potential morbidity and mortality of asthma.[42] GC therapy can not, however, completely abolish BHR. If BHR were a direct result of airway inflammation, one would expect GC therapy to completely ameliorate it. The fact that this is not the case argues against inflammation being solely responsible for BHR. It is likely that BHR may, in part, be an intrinsic property of the lung in asthma, and thus incompletely sensitive to the effects of GCs.[43] An alternative explanation would be that GCs inadequately suppress airway inflammation–either by the administration of an insufficient dose, or failure to administer the GC for an adequate period of time. In one of the few studies in which long-term administration of GC therapy was evaluated, Lundgren et al[44] found 10 years of inhaled GC therapy to result in nearly complete suppression of airway inflammation in 6 patients with severe asthma. Despite the resolution of airway inflammation and epithelial damage, all subjects continued to display a significant degree of BHR, with PC_{20} values ranging from 0.06 to 1.5 mg/ml methacholine. Thus, inflammation is most likely just one of a number of factors involved in the pathogenesis of BHR, with genetic and environmental factors also contributing to an asthmatic's baseline or intrinsic BHR.

> **CLINICAL PEARLS**
>
> **Efficacy of GCs in asthma**
>
> **Chronic asthma**
> - Improvement in baseline lung function in patients with airflow obstruction
> - Reduction in nonspecific bronchial hyperresponsiveness
> - Reduction in airway inflammation
>
> **Acute asthma**
> - Reduction in symptoms
> - Improvement in lung function (PEF, FEV_1)
> - Improvement in PaO_2
> - Reductions in rate of urgent care visits and hospitalization if treated early
> - Reduction in rate of relapse following emergency room visit and/or hospitalization

Effects on acute asthma

The first placebo-controlled study evaluating the effect of cortisone acetate (the available GC at the time) in acute asthma was published in 1956.[45] In this study, the effect of a 9-day course of cortisone or matched placebo plus standard therapy was studied in 32 patients admitted to the hospital with status asthmaticus. Patients randomized to receive cortisone displayed a significant improvement in their clinical status within the first 24 hours, and a significant reduction in their respiratory rate within 48 hours compared to those on placebo. By day 4, 67% of the patients on cortisone no longer had 'disabling bronchial obstruction' compared to only 24% of control patients. In addition, 29% of control patients required hydrocortisone (HC) therapy due to worsening asthma status, with all of these patients subsequently improving. The investigators concluded that GC therapy was effective in those individuals unresponsive to a 24-hour course of conventional therapy, and recommended using HC in patients refractory to standard treatment.[45] This classic study set the stage for the multitude of studies that have subsequently evaluated GCs in acute asthma, as outlined below.

Acute asthma in adults

Fanta et al,[46] in a double-blind placebo-controlled study, evaluated the effect of HC (2 mg/kg bolus followed by

0.5 mg/kg/h × 24 h) vs. saline in patients hospitalized with acute severe asthma. HC was superior to placebo in improving lung function, with HC resulting in an increase in the FEV_1 of 118 ± 25% vs. 35 ± 22% in the placebo-treated group. Littenberg and Gluck evaluated the effect of a single dose of intravenous MPn in the emergency room (ER) treatment of acute asthma.[47] Nearly 100 patients who presented to the ER with acute asthma were enrolled to receive either intravenous MPn (125 mg) or saline; both groups received standard emergency treatment (subcutaneous epinephrine or terbutaline, supplemental oxygen, inhaled metaproteranol and IV aminophylline as indicated for an average of 4 hours). Both groups had similar subjective and spirometric indices upon entry but, after 4 hours, only 19% of MPn-treated patients required hospitalization compared to 47% of placebo-treated patients. In addition, those who received MPn had a larger improvement in their mean FEV_1 compared to those who received placebo, although the difference did not reach statistical significance. The authors concluded that prompt use of GCs in the ER treatment of asthma could reduce the number of hospitalizations and effect substantial savings in health care costs.

Chapman et al[48] evaluated the effect of a short course of oral prednisone vs. placebo in a group of asthmatics discharged from the ER for an acute exacerbation with the rate of relapse as their primary outcome variable. Ninety-three patients were randomized to prednisone (40 mg tapering to 0 mg) or placebo for 8 days with follow-up spirometry, and symptom evaluations 1, 7, and 14 days after discharge from the emergency room. A relapse was defined as any unscheduled medical visit for asthma symptoms. A significant decrease in the rate of relapse during the first 10 days of follow-up was noted in the group receiving prednisone compared to those receiving placebo. In addition, those on prednisone reported fewer symptoms and decreased β-agonist use during the first week of the trial. The relapse-reducing effect of prednisone was greatest in the group of patients discharged from the emergency room with the most severe airflow obstruction (FEV_1 <60%).

Other studies have sought to determine the optimal GC dose in acute asthma. Haskell et al[49] evaluated the effect of MPn administered in low (15 mg), medium (40 mg), or high (125 mg) dose every 6 hours in hospitalized patients with acute asthma and found favorable responses in all groups, with the medium- and high-dose courses showing the greatest effect on FEV_1. No difference in FEV_1 values was noted between the medium- and high-dose groups at 3 days, suggesting that both were equally effective upon conclusion of the study. In contrast, Marquette et al[50] found no difference in efficacy between low- and high-dose MPn in the treatment of acute severe asthma. These investigators evaluated 1 mg vs. 6 mg/kg/day administered in 4 divided doses, using FEV_1 as the primary outcome variable. Both groups had similar baseline FEV_1 values (low-dose 32%, high-dose 27%) and both improved markedly over time. Upon completion of the study, the mean FEV_1 values were not significantly different between the two groups, with mean values of 53% and 45% of predicted in the low-dose and the high-dose group, respectively. In one of the few studies evaluating dose–response relationships in asthmatics who required an oral GC burst, Webb evaluated 3 doses of prednisolone – 0.2, 0.4, and 0.6 mg/kg/day – for 2 weeks in 10 asthmatics during 3 separate exacerbations.[51] Significant differences in peak expiratory flow rare (PEFR) were noted between the 3 doses, the largest improvement being seen with high-dose prednisolone. Webb also noted that a plateau effect was noted at 8 days for all 3 doses, suggesting that the time course of response in not dose-dependent.

Just as there is no clear consensus concerning the dose of GC to be used in acute asthma, controversy exists regarding the duration of treatment. Because the duration of treatment is in part related to the severity of the initial episode, recommendations for the length of treatment must be tailored to the individual case. With that in mind, it has recently been recommended that patients admitted in status asthmaticus should be treated with at least 36–48 h of IV therapy, with a switch to oral GC therapy when tolerated.[52] The duration of the oral GC taper again will depend on the individual's response but should span 4–12 days. An intriguing article by Hatton et al sought to determine whether a prolonged oral GC taper was superior to an abrupt cessation of GC therapy following recovery from an acute asthma exacerbation.[53] Thirty-five patients admitted to the hospital for an acute exacerbation of asthma were enrolled into the study after they had successfully responded to oral prednisolone and aggressive bronchodilator therapy. All subjects had PEFRs within 15% of their best or predicted PEFR and had stable PEFRs (<15% variability) for 48 h at the time of entry into the study. The patients were then discharged to home on inhaled budesonide and a tapering course of prednisolone (40 mg on the first day with a decrease in dose by 5 mg every second day) or placebo for 2 weeks. No difference was found between the two groups at all follow-up periods, and no relapses were noted in either group during the 28-day follow-up period. The authors concluded that a prolonged prednisolone taper was not required following recovery from an acute asthma exacerbation if GC treatment was continued until a satisfactory and stable PEFR was achieved. It should be noted that all subjects were on budesonide, a potent inhaled GC, which may have prevented deterioration in lung function in the patients treated with placebo.

In summary, although multiple studies have documented the effectiveness of systemic GC therapy in acute asthma, a clear consensus on the optimal dose, route of administration (oral vs. intravenous), and duration of treatment has yet to be determined. McFadden has recommended administering MPn 40 mg intravenously every 6 h or prednisone 60 mg orally every 6–8 h for 36–48 h with a taper to 60 mg prednisone per day when the FEV_1 approaches 50% of predicted.[52] This dose is held for the next 4 days before instituting a taper in 4-day intervals, reaching 0 mg in 12 days. The National Heart Lung and Blood Institute (NHLBI) guidelines recommend prednisone, MPn, or prednisolone 120–180 mg/day in 3 or 4 doses for 48 hours, then 60–80 mg/day until PEF reaches 70% of predicted or personal best. Therapy following hospitalization or an ER visit may last from 3 to 10 days.[54]

Efficacy studies of acute asthma in children

Several studies have evaluated systemic GC therapy in children with acute asthma. The majority have demonstrated GC therapy to result in improved lung function and PaO_2, and diminished wheezing and fewer relapses. At least three studies have evaluated the effect of intravenous GC therapy in status asthmaticus. In two studies, GCs were shown to have beneficial effects, while the third study failed to demonstrate benefit. Younger et al[55] evaluated the effect of intravenous MPn (1 mg/kg every 6 h) vs. placebo in 49 children admitted with status asthmaticus and found improvements in clinical symptom scores at 24 h, PEFR, and FEF_{25-75} by 36 h in the group of patients on MPn. However, no differences with regard to duration of hospitalization, FEV_1 and FVC values were noted between the two groups. Of greater significance, those patients who received MPn were noted to have fewer relapses in the 4-week follow-up period following discharge from the hospital.

Studies evaluating the effect of a single dose of GC in the ER setting have uniformly shown this therapy to be superior to placebo in decreasing the number of children who ultimately require admission. A large study by Scarfone et al[56] illustrates this point. They studied the effect of 2 mg/kg of orally administered prednisone or placebo in 75 children aged 1–17 years who presented to the ER with an acute asthma exacerbation. Each group then received an identical regimen of nebulized albuterol for up to 4 hours. Fewer patients who received prednisone required subsequent hospitalization (31%) compared to those who had received placebo (49%). When only the most acutely ill patients were evaluated, the effect of prednisone was even greater: only 32% of those treated with prednisone were hospitalized compared to 72% of placebo-treated patients. This is one of many studies that have demonstrated oral GC therapy to be as effective as intravenous GC therapy in acute childhood asthma.[57,58]

Harris et al, in an important study published over 10 years ago, evaluated whether early intervention with oral GC therapy during an acute asthma exacerbation would prevent further progression of asthma symptoms.[59] In this study, prednisone (30–40 mg twice daily for 7 days) or matching placebo was administered in 41 children who presented to the clinic with an acute asthma exacerbation that was inadequately responsive to inhaled β-agonist therapy. During the 7-day course of prednisone therapy, every patient improved and only one relapse occurred following discontinuation of prednisone therapy. In contrast, 42% of those on placebo required rescue intervention secondary to continued symptoms, worsening pulmonary function, and increased need for bronchodilator therapy. As continued symptoms often lead to emergency care and/or hospitalization, the above study supports the use of oral steroid therapy early in the course of an acute exacerbation not completely responsive to bronchodilators.

As is the case for adult asthma, the optimal dose, duration of treatment, and the route of GC administration remain largely empiric and depend largely on the severity of the acute exacerbation. Orally administered GCs are rapidly absorbed and have been found to be as effective as intravenous GCs, and oral therapy can therefore be used in many cases.[57,58] With that said, children in severe respiratory distress and those who require high flow rates of oxygen for adequate treatment of hypoxemia are obvious candidates for intravenous GC therapy. If intravenous therapy is required, MPn (1 mg/kg administered every 6 h) is the drug of choice as it has less mineralocorticoid activity and thus fewer potential adverse effects than HC. Once oral medications are tolerated, a switch to oral prednisone can be made at a dose of 2 mg/kg/day in 2 divided doses for an additional 2–4 days, followed by a taper to 1 mg/kg/day administered in a single morning dose for an additional 2–4 days prior to stopping. The NHLBI guidelines recommend administering either prednisone, prednisolone, or MPn, 1 mg/kg/dose every 6 h for 48 h then 1–2 mg/kg/day (maximum dose 60 mg/day) in 2 divided doses until PEF is 70% of predicted or personal best.[54]

Efficacy of oral GC therapy in severe persistent asthma

With the advent of high-potency inhaled GC therapy, the number of patients who continue to require chronic oral GC therapy to control their disease has greatly diminished. Unfortunately, a subset of patients with severe persistent asthma requires chronic oral GC therapy; these patients are often referred to as steroid-dependent asthmatics. Although chronic oral GC therapy in this group is recommended, there is very little in the published literature on this group of challenging patients. One of the first studies evaluating long-term oral GC therapy in asthma was published in 1956.[60] Ninety-six patients received cortisone or placebo for 6 months. The study drugs were administered 3 times daily with an initial cortisone dose of 300 mg/day, and the dose was then tapered as clinically indicated. Upon completion of the study period, the medications were withdrawn, if tolerated, over a 12-week period. A significant improvement in physical exam findings was found in the cortisone-treated patients after 2 weeks and was sustained for the next 8 weeks. In addition, cortisone therapy resulted in a significant improvement in exercise tolerance at 2 weeks, which was sustained throughout the trial. Of importance, only 22% of cortisone-treated patients who withdrew from the study did so secondary to worsening asthma compared to 50% of the placebo patients. As expected, all 27 of the patients on cortisone developed at least one steroid-associated side-effect. In summary, this study showed cortisone to be effective, both subjectively and objectively, during the first 2 months of therapy. In addition, patients receiving placebo were more likely to be withdrawn from the study as a result of worsening asthma control compared to those on cortisone. This study was one of the first to describe many of the adverse effects associated with chronic oral GC use.

Given that daily administration of oral GC therapy was associated with multiple adverse effects, Harter et al[61] evaluated the effectiveness and adverse effects profile of intermittently administered oral GC therapy, the results of which were published in the *New England Journal of Medicine* in 1963. These investigators made the important observation that the therapeutic effects of steroids appeared to persist longer than their metabolic effects. Consequently, they sought to determine the effectiveness of intermittently administered GC therapy. In particular, they wanted to find a dosage schedule sufficiently short that the anti-allergic properties of the GC would remain, but long enough to allow for metabolic equilibrium to be established. Several dosage schedules were studied and a single morning dose of oral steroid administered every 48 hours was found to be the most effective in optimizing asthma care while minimizing the potential for adverse effects. This is an important study, not only from a historical perspective but also because this article set the standard for using alternate-day GC therapy in the severe asthmatic.

GC-insensitive asthma

The vast majority of asthmatics respond well to GC therapy, but a minority continue to have evidence of ongoing disease despite high-dose daily therapy. These patients are termed GC insensitive. The diagnosis of GC-insensitive asthma is a clinical one, in which the following features are often identified: difficult-to-control asthma with chronic airflow limitation ($FEV_1 < 70\%$), a significant nocturnal component as reflected by AM dipping of pulmonary function, and most important, a poor clinical and spirometric response to oral GC therapy, generally less than a 15%

CLINICAL PEARLS

Features of GC-insensitive asthma
- Chronic airflow limitation ($FEV_1 < 70\%$)
- Nocturnal asthma accompanied by morning dip in pulmonary function
- Less than 15% improvement in FEV_1 following GC trial

improvement in pre-bronchodilator FEV_1 following at least one week of oral GC therapy at approximately 40 mg per day of prednisone.

Several immunologic abnormalities that may contribute to GC insensitivity have been described. Among these are a reduced ability of GCs to inhibit phytohemagglutinin-stimulated peripheral blood mononuclear cell (PBMC) proliferation in GC-insensitive, compared to GC-responsive, asthmatics and normal controls.[62] GC-insensitive asthmatics also have elevated percentages of T lymphocytes bearing the activation markers IL-2R and HLA-DR compared to GC-responsive asthmatics and normal controls.[63] Furthermore, GCs fail to suppress IL-2 and IFN-γ production in mitogen-stimulated PBMCs isolated from patients with GC-insensitive asthma.[63] The above data suggest that T cells from GC-insensitive asthmatics are in an activated state at baseline compared to those from GC-sensitive asthmatics and nonasthmatic controls. This state may render them less susceptible to the suppressive effects of glucocorticoids.

Chemical mutational analysis of GCRs from GC-insensitive asthmatics has failed to reveal mutations that would explain the phenomenon.[64] Recent studies have identified two GCR abnormalities in PBMCs from patients with GC-insensitive asthma.[65] The first abnormality (type 1) involves a significant reduction in GCR binding affinity, while the second abnormality (type 2) manifests as a relative deficiency of GC receptor sites per cell. The type 1 GCR defect is most commonly identified and it appears to be confined to T cells. It is felt to be an acquired, reversible, and inflammation-driven phenomenon. The type 2 defect is much less common, and appears to be a genetic abnormality affecting all cell types. Individuals with the type 1 defect manifest many of the GC-induced adverse effects of chronic oral steroid use but derive little, if any, therapeutic benefit from GC treatment. Those with the type 2 defect often display fewer than expected GC-associated adverse effects despite long histories of chronic oral GC use. As is the case for the type 1 defect, these individuals fail to demonstrate significant benefit from GC therapy.

In addition to ligand-binding defects, abnormalities in DNA binding have also been described.[66,67] Adcock et al evaluated the ability of dexamethasone to increase GCR–GRE binding[66] and found dexamethasone to induce a rapid increase in GRE binding in PBMCs from GC-sensitive and nonasthmatic controls, while it failed to induce binding in the GC-insensitive asthmatics. A follow-up article found GC-insensitive asthmatics to have increased basal expression of AP-1 DNA binding, suggesting that increased levels of AP-1 prevented GCR-DNA binding.[67] A recent study also found increased expression of an alternatively spliced form of the GCR, termed GCRβ, in the peripheral blood and BAL cells of GC-insensitive asthmatics.[68] The expression of this 'inactive' form of the GCR was up-regulated following exposure to the combination of IL-2 and IL-4 in vitro. It is of note that this form of the receptor has both poor ligand and poor DNA binding.[69]

THERAPEUTIC PRINCIPLES

Glucocorticoids
- The pharmacokinetics of glucocorticoids are dissociated from their pharmacodynamics.
  - —Onset of action occurs long after peak levels have been achieved.
  - —Duration of effect continues long after the glucocorticoid has been cleared from the systemic circulation.
- Clear dose–response relationships are difficult to determine in terms of measures of efficacy, while dose–response relationships have been documented for adverse effects.
- To minimize the potential for adverse effects, use the smallest amount of GC for the shortest period of time that safely controls the disease.
- If chronic GC therapy is required, every attempt should be made to taper the dose to an alternate-day schedule. A dose of prednisone 20 mg administered on alternate days is preferable to 10 mg administered daily, even though the daily dose is the same.
- If long-term glucocorticoid therapy is expected, monitoring for adverse effects is essential and includes frequent monitoring of linear growth (in children), along with yearly bone mineral density determinations and ophthalmologic exams.

GLUCOCORTICOIDS IN OTHER DISEASES

Rheumatoid arthritis was the first disease to be treated with GCs over 50 years ago. Since then, GCs have become a cornerstone of the treatment for rheumatologic and autoimmune diseases. No other class of medications has been shown to be as effective in suppressing the acute manifestations of these diseases.[70] Due to their propensity for adverse effects, many of which can be debilitating (see below), GCs are primarily used for the treatment of acute manifestations of rheumatoid arthritis (RA), systemic lupus erythematosus (SLE), and other vasculitides. Unlike the situation in severe asthma, many alternative immunomodulatory agents are effective in the treatment of diseases such as RA; as a result, many patients with RA can be successfully treated without the use of chronic oral GC therapy.

Glucocorticoids are the most effective therapy for the management of the acute manifestations of SLE.[71] Depending on the severity, either high-dose oral prednisone (60 mg per day in 1 or 2 divided doses) or intermittent pulse therapy (IV methylprednisolone 1 g) repeated for 3 days can be used. Intermittent pulse therapy is often used in life-threatening situations such as acute glomerulonephritis or vasculitis in RA. Its duration of action can extend from weeks to months and it is devoid of many of the adverse effects of chronically administered oral GC therapy. With that said, several acute and potentially life-threatening effects have been associated with pulse therapy; these include cardiovascular collapse, myocardial infarction, and severe infection.[72] If oral GCs are used, and successful, attempts should be made to slowly taper the dose to the lowest tolerated dose, alternate-day therapy being the objective.

Glucocorticoids are used for many manifestations of RA: in acute flares, as a bridging therapy from nonsteroidal anti-inflammatory agents to immunomodulatory agents early in the course of the disease, and in patients with established disease, as a chronic therapy. In cases of acute severe RA, pulse IV methylprednisolone therapy (200 mg to 1 g) is effective. As noted with SLE, the response to pulse therapy is often rapid and sustained. Unfortunately, pulse therapy has not been shown to induce disease remission.[73] A recently published randomized placebo study compared the effectiveness of daily low-dose prednisone (7.5 mg) to existing standard therapy in patients with active disease of short duration (<2 years) and found that prednisone significantly diminished the progression of joint erosion of the hands.[74] This study was somewhat controversial; suggested problems included the statistics used, overinterpretation of the data, and concern regarding the potential for bone mineral loss with the dose used over time. Thus, chronic prednisone therapy may or may not result in long-term disease modification, yet it is likely to result in adverse effects over time. As in the case of all other diseases, every attempt should be made to use the lowest tolerated dose, and if possible to use a combination of therapies or other antirheumatic disease therapies with less potential for toxicity.

Oral GC burst therapy has also been shown to be effective for the treatment of severe and extensive contact dermatitis. Doses of 0.5–1 mg/kg per day of prednisone with a slow taper over 2–3 weeks are usually sufficient. Other allergic disorders where short-course systemic GC therapy can be used include severe atopic dermatitis refractory to topical GC therapy, and severe urticaria flares. In both cases, systemic GCs should be used when all other attempts at treatment have failed, and they should only be used as rescue therapy for a short duration of time. In both cases, the dose should be slowly tapered as the diseases are likely to flare if the dose is abruptly stopped.

Adverse effects associated with systemic GC use

1. Endocrinologic effects
   - Adrenal suppression
   - Growth suppression and delayed sexual maturation in children
   - Weight gain, cushingoid stigmata
   - Diabetes mellitus
2. Metabolic effects:
   - Hypokalemia, hyperglycemia, hyperlipidemia
3. Musculoskeletal effects
   - Osteoporosis/vertebral compression fractures
   - Aseptic necrosis of bone (hips, shoulders, knees)
   - Myopathy (acute and chronic)
4. Dermatolic effects
   - Dermal thinning/increased skin fragility
   - Striae
   - Acne
   - Hirsutism
5. Ophthalmologic effects
   - Cataracts
   - Glaucoma
6. Immunologic effects:
   - Diminished immunoglobulin G (IgG) levels
   - Loss of delayed-type hypersensitivity (DTH)
   - Increased risk of opportunistic infection/severe varicella infection
7. Cardiovascular effects
   - Hypertension
   - Atherosclerosis
8. Hematologic effects
   - Lymphopenia
   - Eosinopenia
   - Neutrophilia
9. Psychologic/neurologic effects:
   - Mood swings, psychosis
   - Steroid withdrawal syndrome
   - Psendotumor cerebri

Table 106.3 Adverse effects associated with systemic GC use.

ADVERSE EFFECTS OF GC THERAPY

Associated with the anti-inflammatory effects of GCs are a multitude of potential adverse effects that severely limit their long-term use. All nucleated cells have a common GC receptor, all are affected by GC therapy, and all are thus susceptible to the development of untoward effects. These effects can occur immediately (i.e. metabolic effects) or can develop insidiously over several months to years (i.e. growth suppression, osteoporosis, and cataracts). In addition, some adverse effects are limited to children (growth suppression), some appear to be disease specific (vascular necrosis of bone and systemic lupus erythematosus), while others require interaction with other drugs (nonsteroidal drugs and the development of peptic ulcer disease). It is widely held that adverse effects occur in both a dose-dependent and duration-of-treatment manner, although this has not been extensively studied. Table 106.3 lists many of the common adverse effects associated with chronic GC use. The following discussion focuses on those adverse effects that are especially important for the clinician caring for the chronically GC-dependent asthmatic, but is also applicable to other diseases in which GCs are regularly administered. Failure to recognize and adequately treat these problems could result in severe morbidity. It has recently been suggested that the adverse effects of GCs may be separable from their anti-inflammatory effects by exploiting the fact that the metabolic effects of GCs are mediated primarily by DNA binding to GREs, whereas their anti-inflammatory effects are mediated primarily by transcription factor inhibition. Thus, if one could develop a novel GC that failed to bind to GREs yet inhibited transcription factor function, one would have an effective anti-inflammatory agent without the myriad adverse effects described below.

Adrenal suppression

Patients on chronic oral GC therapy will likely have significant adrenal suppression. Patients with adrenal suppression are at risk of developing acute adrenal insufficiency at times of acute stress such as acute trauma, during surgical procedures, or with gastroenteritis associated with diarrhea and/or emesis. Acute adrenal insufficiency is a medical emergency requiring prompt diagnosis and rapid treatment with intravenous HC (2 mg/kg initially followed by 1.5 mg/kg every 6 hours until stabilization is achieved and oral therapy is tolerated) and vigorous fluid replacement with normal saline if dehydration and hypotension are present. All patients on chronic high-dose GC therapy should be considered to be adrenally suppressed and should wear a medical alert bracelet that identifies them as being at risk for developing acute adrenal insufficiency. All adrenally suppressed individuals should be given HC at the time of any surgical procedure (1–2 mg/kg) and every 6 hours thereafter for the next 24–48 hours, with a switch to their usual oral GC dose when oral medications are tolerated.[75] The same recommendations are to be followed at other times of acute stress. Complete recovery from adrenal suppression can take from 6 months to 1 year after cessation of long-term GC use.

Growth suppression

Growth suppression is arguably the GC-associated adverse effect that causes the greatest amount of concern for those who care for children. The mechanism(s) involved in GC-associated growth suppression remain poorly understood but may involve suppression of growth hormone production, somatomedin activity, and/or direct inhibitory effects on bone and connective tissue.[76] Chronic daily therapy, frequent short courses, or high-dose alternate-day GC therapy all can result in inhibition of linear growth. Alternate-day GC administration is thought to produce less suppression of linear growth, although significant growth suppression can still occur on alternate-day regimens.[77] Complicating the issue of GC-induced linear growth suppression in asthma is the finding that the disease itself can impair growth.[78] This is a long-known and somewhat controversial area, especially as it pertains to whether chronic inhaled GC therapy can also result in growth suppression. As daily or high-dose alternate-day GC therapy for extended periods of time can result in permanent growth retardation, every effort should be made to decrease the amount of oral GC to less than 10 mg on alternate days. Doses at or below this value do not appear to significantly impede growth velocity.[77] If the oral GC dose can not be tapered and/or the child remains significantly growth impaired, a trial of recombinant growth hormone therapy can be initiated. Growth hormone therapy has been shown to increase linear growth in children on chronic oral GC therapy[79] as long as the GC dose is less than 0.35 mg/kg per day.

Osteoporosis

Osteoporosis is the one GC-associated adverse effect that, if unrecognized and untreated, can produce significant morbidity. Unfortunately, GC-induced osteoporosis is often overlooked due to its insidious onset and the insensitivity of conventional diagnostic methods. Although the etiology of GC-induced osteoporosis is complex, the mechanisms involved include decreased calcium absorption from the intenstinal tract and decreased renal reabsorption.[76] As a result, a negative calcium balance ensues that leads to secondary hyperparathyroidism and subsequent enhanced bone resorption. Osteoblast function is also inhibited, resulting in decreased bone growth, while osteoclast activity is stimulated, which further contributes to bone resorption. Trabecular bone such as the ribs and vertebrae are more sensitive to the effect of GCs than cortical bone.[80] Factors that increase the likelihood of the development of osteoporosis include inactivity, sex hormone deficiency, a diet deficient in calcium, and concurrent use of certain drugs (e.g. furosemide, anticonvulsants, and excessive thyroid hormone replacement).[81]

Demineralization of bone is not detectable on conventional radiographs until a significant amount of bone mineral density is lost, and the diagnosis of osteoporosis therefore is best made utilizing a densitometer.[82] Further assessment of the steroid-dependent asthmatic may include a 24-hour urine calcium measurement, which can provide information regarding the extent of GC-induced calcium loss. Biochemical markers to measure osteoblast and osteoclast activity have recently been developed[76], but at present their use is confined primarily to research protocols. These biochemical markers may eventually be routinely available, but at present insufficient information is available to apply them to general clinical practice.

Treatment of osteoporosis, as is the case for all steroid-induced adverse effects, consists of attempting to decrease the oral GC dose and/or frequency of dosing, increasing calcium intake to 1000–1500 mg of elemental calcium per day supplemented with at least 400 IU/day of vitamin D, and increasing physical activity, especially gravity-dependent activities such as walking. Activities such as high-impact aerobics, contract sports (football, wrestling), and heavy lifting should be avoided as these activities can result in compression fractures of the vertebral bodies (bending, lifting, contact sports) in addition to fractures of the long bones (contact sports). If hypercalcuria is present, hydrochlorothiazide can be used alone or in combination with a potassium-sparing diuretic. Patients with severe osteoporosis may require treatment with a remittive medication. Alendronate, a 'second generation' bisphosphonate, has recently been shown to be effective in not only preventing but also treating GC-induced osteoporosis.[83] Alendronate appears to be somewhat more effective than etidronate, and it is easier to administer.[84] Alendronate is administered once daily, while etidronate must be given cyclically alternating with calcium.

Cataracts

Posterior subcapsular cataracts (PSC) are a well-described complication of chronic GC therapy with prevalence rates of up to 29%. Rooklin et al[85] found posterior subcapsular cataracts in 7 of 24 children with asthma who required maintenance oral steroid therapy for at least 1 year. Those children with cataracts were on >10 mg per day of prednisone and had a duration of prednisone use of over 1 year. Toogood et al[86] recently evaluated the association between the development of PSC and inhaled and oral GC therapy in adult asthmatics. These investigators found significant positive correlations between both the daily dose and the duration of prednisone use, but not with dose/duration of inhaled GC therapy. GC-associated cataracts are often small, but can at times significantly affect visual acuity and can require surgical intervention. Although the development of cataracts appears to be related to the daily dose, cumulative dose, and the duration of treatment, there is a significant degree of variability with respect to individual susceptibility to cataract formation. It is unknown whether GC dose reduction will result in regression or disappearance of the cataract, although some studies suggest that, if cataract is recognized early, regression can occur.[85,87] A yearly ophthalmologic evaluation for the presence of cataracts is recommended for all patients receiving maintenance oral GC therapy.

Myopathy

GC therapy can result in two distinct types of myopathy.[88] An acute, severe myopathy has been described in patients admitted to the intensive care unit with acute asthma who require incubation, mechanical ventilation, concurrent use of muscle relaxant therapy, and short-term high-dose parenteral GC therapy. This presentation is rare, and apparently requires an undetermined interaction between systemic GCs and paralytic agents.[89] Affected patients often have markedly elevated serum creatine phosphokinase (CPK) levels and diffuse necrosis of skeletal muscle on biopsy specimens.[89] Recovery begins after GC withdrawal, but more than 6 months may be required for complete resolution of muscle weakness.

More common is the insidious development of proximal muscle atrophy in patients who require chronically administered GCs.[76,90] As with the other GC-associated adverse effects, those patients receiving daily GCs or large alternate-day doses are at greatest risk. Isokinetic muscle testing of hip flexor strength appears to be the most sensitive and objective measure of proximal muscle weakness.[90] Enzymes of muscle origin such as CPK, aldolase, and lactate dehydrogenase are typically not elevated, and biopsy of affected muscle reveals atrophy rather than necrosis of muscle fibers. To correct and/or prevent GC-induced myopathy, every attempt should be made to taper the GC dose, together with implementation of a program designed to improve muscle strength.[91] As was noted with the acute form, more than 6 months of rehabilitation may be required before normal muscle strength develops in those children with chronic GC-induced myopathy.

Other adverse effects

Other common adverse effects of chronic GC therapy include increased appetite with weight gain and the development of a cushingoid habitus consisting of a moon facies, buffalo hump, central obesity with wasting of the extremities, atrophy of the skin with the development of striae, and hirsutism. Psychologic disturbances from increased emotional lability to frank psychosis can occur, as well as hypertension, peptic ulcer disease, atherosclerosis, aseptic necrosis of bone, and diabetes mellitus. Chronic GC use can also result in immunologic attenuation with loss of delayed-type hypersensitivity, diminished IgG levels without change in functional antibody response, potential for reactivation of latent tuberculosis infection, and possible increased risk for infection, especially the development of severe varicella.

In summary, chronic GC use is associated with multiple adverse effects. Since the magnitude of adverse effects is often related to the dose, the frequency of administration, and the duration of GC use, every consideration should be given to minimize GC doses and maximize other modes of therapy. Unfortunately, patients with severe disease can not be successfully tapered off oral GCs without putting them at even greater risk for morbidity or mortality associated with disease exacerbations. It is therefore incumbent upon the clinician to monitor for the development and progression of adverse effects and to take appropriate steps to minimize the risk and impact of adverse GC effects.

REFERENCES

1. Barnes PJ, Greening AP, Crompton GK. Glucocorticoid resistance in asthma. Am J Respir Crit Care Med 1995;152:S125.
2. Adcock IM, Brown CR, Gelder CM, Shirasaki H, Peters MJ, Barnes PJ. The effects of glucocorticoids on transcription factor activation in human peripheral blood mononuclear cells. Am J Physiol 1995;37:C331.
3. Ray A, Prefontaine KE. Physical association and functional antagonism between the p65 subunit of transcription factor NF-kappa B and the glucocorticoid receptor. Proc Natl Acad Sci USA 1994;91:752.
4. Scheinman RI, Cogswell PC, Lofquist AK, Baldwin AS. Role of transcriptional activation of IκBα in mediation of immunosuppression by glucocorticoids. Science 1995;270:283.
5. Auphan N, DiDonato JA, Rosette C, Helmberg A, Karin M. Immunosuppression by glucocorticoids: Inhibition of NF-κB activity through induction of IkB synthesis. Science 1995;270:286.
6. Peppel K, Vinci JM, Baglioni C. The AU-rich sequences in the 3′ untranslated region mediate the increased turnover of interferon mRNA induced by glucocorticoids. J Exp Med 1991;173:349.
7. Rebuck JW, Smith RW, Margulis RR. The modification of leukocyte function in human windows by ACTH. Gastroenterol 1951;19:644.
8. Bishop CR, Athens JW, Boggs DR, Warner HR, Cartwright GE, Wintrobe MM. Leukokinetic studies XIII. A non-steady-state kinetic evaluation of the mechanism of cortisone-induced granulocytosis. J Clin Invest 1968;47:249.
9. Charlesworth EN, Kagey-Sobotka A, Schleimer RP, Norman PS, Lichtenstein LM. Prednisone inhibits the appearance of inflammatory mediators and the influx of eosinophils and basophils associated with the cutaneous late-phase response to allergen. J Immunol 1991;146:671.
10. Laitinen LA, Laitinen A, Haahtela T. A comparative study of the effects of an inhaled corticosteroid, budesonide, and a β_2-agonist, terbutaline, on airway inflammation in newly diagnosed asthma: a randomized double-blind, parallel-group controlled trial. J Allergy Clin Immunol 1992;90:32.
11. Bochner BS, Luscinskas FW, Gimbrone MA, et al. Adhesion of human basophils, eosinophils, and neutrophils to interleukin 1-activated human vascular endothelial cells: contributions of endothelial cell adhesion molecules. J Exp Med 1991;173:1553.
12. Thornhill MH, Kyan-Aung U, Haskard DO. IL-4 increases human endothelial cell adhesiveness for T cells but not neutrophils. J Immunol 1990;144:3060.
13. Bochner BS, Peachell PT, Brown KE, Schleimer RP. Adherence of human basophils to cultured umbilical vein endothelial cells. J Clin Invest 1988;81:1355.
14. Lam S, Chan H, LeRichie JC, Chan-Yeung M, Salari H. Release of leukotrienes in patients with bronchial asthma. J Allergy Clin Immunol 1988;81:711.
15. Balter MS, Eschenbacher WL, Peters-Golden M. Arachidonic acid metabolism in cultured alveolar macrophages from normal, atopic, and asthmatic subjects. Am Rev Respir Med 1988;138:1134.
16. Sebaldt RJ, Sheller JR, Oates JA, Roberts LJ, Fitzgerald GA. Inhibition of eicosanoid biosynthesis by glucocorticoids in humans. Proc Natl Acad Sci USA 1990;87:6974.
17. Dworski R, Fitgerald GA, Oates JA, Sheller JR. Effect of oral prednisone on airway inflammatory mediators in atopic asthma. Am J Respir Crit Care Med 1994;149:953.
18. Laitinen LA, Heino M, Laitinen A, Kava T, Haahtela T. Damage of the airway epithelium and bronchial reactivity in patients with asthma. Am Rev Respir Dis 1985;131:599.
19. Boschetto P, Rogers DF, Fabbri M, Barnes PJ. Corticosteroid inhibition of airway microvascular leakage. Am Rev Respir Dis 1991;143:605.
20. Hui KKP, Conolly ME, Tashkin DP. Reversal of human lymphocyte β-adrenoceptor desensitization by glucocorticoids. Clin Pharmacol Ther 1982;32:566.
21. Ellul-Michallef R, Fenech FF. Effect of intravenous prednisolone in asthmatics with diminished adrenergic responsiveness. Lancet 1975;ii:1269.
22. Shenfield GM, Hodson ME, Clarke SW, Paterson JW. Interaction of corticosteroids and catecholamines in the treatment of asthma. Thorax 1975;30:430.
23. Wempe JB, Postma DS, Breederveld N, Alting-Hebing D, van der Mark, Koeter GH. Separate and combined effects of corticosteroids and bronchodilators on airflow obstruction and airway hyperresponsiveness in asthma. J Allergy Clin Immunol 1992;89:679.
24. Kamada AK, Szefler SJ. Mechanism of action of glucocorticoids in asthma and rhinitis. In: Busse W, Holgate S (eds) Asthma and rhinitis. Cambridge, MA, Blackwell Scientific, 1994, 1255.
25. Boudinot FD, D'Ambrosio R, Jusko WJ. Receptor-mediated pharmacodynamics of prednisolone in the rat. J Pharmacokinet Biopharm 1989;17:209.

26. Milsap RL, George DE, Szefler SJ, Murray KA, Lebenthal E, Jusko WJ. Effect of inflammatory bowel disease on absorption and disposition of prednisolone. Dig Dis Sci 1983;28:161.
27. Khalafallah N, Jusko WJ. Tissue distribution of prednisolone in the rabbit. J Pharmacol Exp Ther 1984;229:719.
28. Frey BM, Frey FJ. Clinical pharmacokinetics of prednisone and prednisolone. Clin Pharmacokinet 1990;19:126.
29. Dove AM, Szefler SJ, Hill MR, Jusko WJ, Larsen GL, Acurso FJ. Altered prednisolone pharmacokinetics in patients with cystic fibrosis. J Pediatr 1992;120:789.
30. May CS, Caffin JA, Halliday JW, Bochner F. Prednisolone pharmacokinetics in asthmatic patients. Br J Dis Chest 1980;74:91.
31. McAllister WAC, Mitchell DM, Collins JV. Prednisolone pharmacokinetics compared between night and day in asthmatic and normal subjects. Br J Clin Pharmacol 1981;11:303.
32. Bartoszek M, Brenner AM, Szefler SJ. Prednisolone and methylprednisolone elimination in children receiving anticonvulsant therapy. Clin Pharmacol Ther 1987;42:424.
33. Udwadia ZF, Sridhar G, Beveridge CJ, Soutar C, McHardy GJR, Leitch AG. Catastrophic deterioration in asthma induced by rifampicin in steroid-dependent asthma. Respir Med 1993;87:629.
34. Zurcher RM, Frey BM, Frey FJ. Impact of ketoconazole on the metabolism of prednisolone. Clin Pharmacol Ther 1989;45:366.
35. Fost DA, Leung DYM, Martin RJ, Brown EE, Szefler SJ, Spahn JD. Inhibition of methylprednisolone elimination in the presence and absence of clarithromycin therapy. J Allergy Clin Immunol 1999;103:1031.
36. Boekenoogen SJ, Szefler SJ, Jusko WJ. Prednisolone disposition and protein binding in oral contraceptive users. J Clin Endocrinol Metab 1983;56:702.
37. Hill MR, Szefler SJ, Ball BD, Bartoszek M, Brenner AM. Monitoring glucocorticoid therapy: a pharmacokinetic approach. Clin Pharmacol Ther 1990;48:390.
38. Ellul-Micallef R, Borthwick RC, McHardy GJR. The time-course of response to prednisolone in chronic bronchial asthma. Clin Sci Mol Med 1974;47:105.
39. Hargreave FE, Ryan G, Thomson NC, et al. Bronchial responsiveness to histamine or methacholine in asthma: measurement and clinical significance. J Allergy Clin Immunol 1981;68:347.
40. Bhagat RG, Grunstein MM. Effect of corticosteroids on bronchial responsiveness to methacholine in asthmatic children. Am Rev Respir Dis 1985;131:902.
41. Robinson D, Hamid Q, Ying S, Bentley A, Assoufi B, Durham, Kay AB. Prednisolone treatment in asthma is associated with modulation of bronchoalveolar lavage cell interleukin-4, interleukin-5, and interferon-γ cytokine gene expression. Am Rev Respir Dis 1993;148:40.
42. Israel RH, Poe RH, Wicks CM, Greenblatt DW, Kallay MC. The protective effect of methylprednisolone on carbachol-induced bronchospasm. Am Rev Respir Dis 1984;130:1019.
43. Rogers DF, O'Connor BJ. Airway hyperresponsiveness: relation to asthma and inflammation? Thorax 1993;48:1095.
44. Lundgren R, Soderberg M, Horstedt P, Stenling R. Morphological studies of bronchial mucosal biopsies from asthmatics before and after ten years of treatment with inhaled steroids. Eur Respir J 1988;1:883.
45. Medical Research Council. Controlled trial of the effect of cortisone acetate in status asthmaticus. Lancet 1956;ii:803.
46. Fanta CH, Rossing TH, McFadden ER. Glucocorticoids in acute asthma: a critical controlled study. Am J Med 1983;74:845.
47. Littenberg B, Gluck EH. A controlled trial of methylprednisolone in the emergency treatment of acute asthma. N Engl J Med 1986;314:150.
48. Chapman KR, Verbeek RP, White JG, Rebuck AS. Effect of a short course of prednisone in the prevention of early relapse after the emergency room treatment of acute asthma. N Engl J Med 1991;324:788.
49. Haskell RJ, Wong BM, Hansen JE. A double-blind, randomized clinical trial of methylprednisolone in status asthmaticus. Arch Intern Med 1983;143:1324.
50. Marquette C-H, Stach B, Cardot E, et al. High-dose and low-dose systemic corticosteroids are equally efficient in acute severe asthma. Eur Respir J 1995;8:22.
51. Webb JR. Dose response of patients to oral corticosteroid treatment during exacerbations of asthma. Br J Med 1986;292:1045.
52. McFadden Jr ER. Dosages of corticosteroids in asthma. Am Rev Respir Dis 1993;147:1306.
53. Hatton MQF, Vathenen AS, Allen MJ, Davies S, Cooke NJ. A comparison of 'abruptly stopping' with 'tailing off' oral corticosteroids in acute asthma. Respir Med 1995;89:101.
54. Expert Panel Report 2: Guidelines for the diagnosis and management of asthma. National Institutes of Health, National Heart Lung and Blood Institute. NIH publication No. 1997;97–4051.
55. Younger RE, Gerber PS, Herrod HG, Cohen RM, Crawford LV. Intravenous methylprednisolone efficacy in status asthmaticus of childhood. Pediatrics 1987;80:225.
56. Scarfone RJ, Fuchs SM, Nager AL, Shane SA. Controlled trial of oral prednisone in the emergency department treatment of children with acute asthma. Pediatrics 1993;92:513.
57. Becker JM, Arora A, Scarfone RJ, et al. Oral versus intravenous corticosteroids in children hospitalized with asthma. J Allergy Clin Immunol 1999;103:586.
58. Ratto D, Alfaro C, Sipsey J, et al. Are intravenous corticosteroids required in status asthmaticus? JAMA 1988;260:527.
59. Harris JB, Weinberger MM, Nassif E, Smith G, Milavetz G, Stillerman A. Early intervention with short courses of prednisone to prevent progression of asthma in ambulatory patients incompletely responsive to bronchodilators. J Pediatr 1987;110:627.
60. Medical Research Council. Controlled trial of the effects of cortisone acetate in chronic asthma. Report to the Medical Research Council by the subcommittee on clinical trials in asthma. Lancet 1956;ii:798.
61. Harter JG, Reddy WJ, Thorn GW. Studies on an intermittent corticosteroid dosage regimen. N Engl J Med 1963;269:591.
62. Alvarez J, Surs WK, Leung DYM, Ikle D, Gelfand EW, Szefler SJ. Steroid-resistant asthma: Immunologic and pharmacologic features. J Allergy Clin Immunol 1992;89:714.
63. Corrigan CJ, Brown PH, Barnes NC, Tsai J-J, Frew AJ, Kay AB. Glucocorticoid resistance in chronic asthma. Peripheral blood T lymphocyte activation and comparison of the T lymphocyte inhibitory effects of glucocorticoids and cyclosporin A. Am Rev Respir Dis 1991;144:1026.
64. Lane SJ, Arm JP, Staynov DZ, Lee TH. Chemical mutational analysis of the human glucocorticoid receptor cDNA in glucocorticoid-resistant bronchial asthma. Am J Respir Cell Mol Biol 1994;11:42.
65. Sher ER, Leung DYM, Surs W, Kam JC, Zieg G, Kamada AK, Szefler SJ. Steroid resistant asthma. Cellular mechanisms contributing to inadequate response to glucocorticoid therapy. J Clin Invest 1994;93:33.
66. Adcock IA, Lane SJ, Brown CR, Peters MJ, Lee TH, Barnes PJ. Differences in binding of glucocorticoid receptor to DNA in steroid-resistant asthma. J Immunol 1995;154:3500.
67. Adcock IM, Lane SJ, Brown CR, Lee TH, Barnes PJ. Abnormal glucocorticoid receptor-activator protein 1 interaction in steroid-resistant asthma. J Exp Med 1995;182:1951.
68. Leung DYM, Hamid Q, Vottero A, et al. Association of glucocorticoid insensitivity with increased expression of glucocorticoid receptor β. J Exp Med 1997;186:1567.
69. Bamberger CM, Bamberger A-M, de Castro M, Chrousos GP. Glucocorticoid receptor β, a potential inhibitor of glucocorticoid action in humans. J Clin Invest 1995;95:2435.
70. Wilder RL. Corticosteroids. In: Klippel JH, Weyland CM, Wortmann RL (eds) Primer on the rheumatic diseases, 11th edn. Atlanta Georgia, Arthritis Foundation, 1997, chapter 53, p. 427.
71. Gladman DD, Urowitz MB. Connective tissue disorders: Management of systemic lupus erythematosus. In: Klippel JH, Dieppe PA (eds) Practical rheumatology. London, Mosby/Times Mirror International, 1995, chapter 32, p. 321.
72. Kirwan JR. Systemic corticosteroids in rheumatology. In: Klippel JH, Dieppe PA (eds) Rheumatology, 2nd edn. London, Mosby International, 1998, chapter 6, p. 6.1.
73. Hilliquin P, Menkes C-J. Rheumatoid arthritis: Evaluation and management of early and established rheumatoid arthritis. In: Klippel JH, Dieppe PA (eds) Practical rheumatology. London, Mosby/Times Mirror International, 1995, chapter 17, p. 191.

74. Kirwan JR and the Arthritis and Rheumatism Council Low-Dose Glucocorticoid Study Group. The effect of glucocorticoids on joint destruction in rheumatoid arthritis. N Engl J Med 1995;333:142.
75. Muller BA, Fieselmann JF, Richerson HB. Minimizing surgical risk for your asthmatic patient. J Respir Dis 1993;14:402.
76. Lukert BP, Raisz LG. Glucocorticoid-induced osteoporosis: pathogenesis and management. Ann Int Med 1990;112:352.
77. Reimer LG, Morris HG, Ellis FE. Growth of asthmatic children during treatment with alternate-day steroids. J Allergy Clin Immunol 1975;55:224.
78. Russell G. Asthma and growth. Arch Dis Child 1993;69:695.
79. Rivkees SA, Danon M, Herrin J. Prednisone dose limitation of growth hormone treatment of steroid-induced growth failure. J Pediatr 1994;125:322.
80. Adinoff AD, Hollister JR. Steroid-induced fractures and bone loss in patients with asthma. N Engl J Med 1983;309:265.
81. Hamilos DL. Glucocorticoid osteoporosis: a need for greater awareness and action. J Asthma 1994;31:1.
82. Johnston CC, Slemenda CW, Melton LJ. Clinical use of bone densitometry. N Engl J Med 1991;324:1105.
83. Saag KG, Emkey R, Schnitzer TJ, et al. Alendronate for the prevention and treatment of glucocorticoid-induced osteoporosis. N Engl J Med 1998;339:292.
84. Adachi JD, Benson WG, Brown J, et al. Intermittent etidronate therapy to prevent corticosteroid-induced osteoporosis. N Engl J Med 1997;337:382.
85. Rooklin AR, Lampert SI, Jaeger EA, McGeady SJ, Mansmann HC. Posterior subcapsular cataracts in steroid-requiring asthmatic children. J Allergy Clin Immunol 1979;63:383.
86. Toogood JH, Markov AE, Baskerville J, Dyson C. Association of ocular cataracts with inhaled and oral steroid therapy during long-term treatment of asthma. J Allergy Clin Immunol 1993;91:571.
87. Forman AR, Loreto JA, Tina LU. Reversibility of corticosteroid associated cataracts in children with the nephrotic syndrome. Am J Ophthalmol 1977;84:75.
88. Dekhuijzen PNR, Decramer M. Steroid-induced myopathy and its significance to respiratory disease: a known disease rediscovered. Eur Respir J 1992;5:997.
89. Douglas JA, Tuxen DV, Horne M, Scheinkestel CD, Weinmann M, Czarny D, Bowes G. Myopathy in severe asthma. Am Rev Respir Dis 1992;146:517.
90. Bowyer SL, LaMothe MP, Hollister JR. Steroid myopathy: incidence and detection in a population with asthma. J Allergy Clin Immunol 1985;76:234.
91. Hickson RC, Davis JR. Partial prevention of glucocorticoid-induced muscle atrophy by endurance training. Am J Physiol 1981;241:E226.

Chapter 107 Nonsteroidal Anti-inflammatory Drugs

Laurel J. Mengle-Gaw and Benjamin D. Schwartz

The use of anti-inflammatory substances for therapeutic purposes dates back approximately 3500 years when the Ebers papyrus of Egypt suggested that a preparation of dried myrtle leaves be applied to the abdomen and back to expel rheumatic pains from the womb.[1] Around 400 BC, Hippocrates discovered that chewing on willow bark could relieve pain and fever, and in the second century AD, Pliny the Elder and Galen recommended willow leaves for pain. Extracts of willow bark were drunk by Native Americans in the New World to reduce fever, and salicylate-containing plants were applied topically in China and other parts of Asia. In 1763, Reverend Edward Stone presented his *Account of the Success of the Bark of the Willow in the Cure of the Agues* to the Royal Society of London, in which he described the use of powdered willow bark to relieve fever in 50 patients.

In 1828, German chemists isolated the active ingredient of willow bark, salicin. Crystalline salicin served as the basis for the synthesis of salicylic acid, which was used to treat fever and rheumatism. Felix Hoffman, a young chemist working at Bayer Company, synthesized acetylsalicylic acid – allegedly to meet his father's request for a salicylate preparation that would treat his rheumatism but would be milder on his stomach.[1] Bayer named this compound Aspirin: 'a' from acetyl, 'spir' from *Spirea*, the genus containing meadowsweet from which the salicylate was derived, and 'in' as a common ending for medications. Aspirin is a Bayer trademark in many countries, but not in the USA.

By the 1950s, high-dose aspirin was being prescribed for rheumatoid arthritis. In 1971, Sir John Vane discovered that aspirin worked by inhibiting the action of cyclooxygenase (COX, also termed prostaglandin endoperoxide synthetase) in synthesizing prostaglandins, for which he received the Nobel Prize.[2] Later in the 1970s, several new drugs with anti-inflammatory properties were synthesized. To distinguish these from anti-inflammatory glucocorticoids, these drugs, including aspirin and other salicylates, were collectively termed nonsteroidal anti-inflammatory drugs, or NSAIDs.

In the late 1980s and early 1990s, a series of discoveries were made which led to the identification of two COX enzymes – COX-1, which is a constitutively expressed isoform involved in physiologic maintenance functions, and COX-2, which is predominantly synthesized in response to inflammatory stimuli.[3,4] This recognition rather quickly resulted in the synthesis of compounds that specifically inhibit COX-2, while sparing COX-1.

NSAIDs represent many different chemical classes, but can be placed into three categories with respect to inhibition of COX-1 and COX-2: *nonselective* NSAIDs, indicating that they either preferentially inhibit COX-1, or inhibit COX-1 and COX-2 at about the same concentration; COX-2-*selective* NSAIDs, indicating that they preferentially inhibit COX-2, but at higher therapeutic concentrations can also inhibit COX-1; and COX-2-*specific* NSAIDs, indicating that, even at higher therapeutic concentrations, these compounds inhibit COX-2 and spare COX-1. While NSAIDs largely share the same therapeutic properties, the adverse effect profile of each NSAID depends in part on its behavior with respect to COX-1 and COX-2 inhibition.

BIOCHEMISTRY AND PHARMACOLOGY OF NSAIDS

Mechanism of action of NSAIDs

The finding of John Vane that aspirin and other NSAIDs he tested inhibited the production of prostaglandins strongly suggested that NSAIDs work by inhibiting the enzymatic action of COX.[2] This concept received support from the observation that as new and different chemical classes of NSAIDs were synthesized, they all could be shown to inhibit COX. The COX enzyme has two distinct active sites, termed the cyclooxygenase active site and the peroxidase active site. Physiologically, the cyclooxygenase active site cyclizes arachidonic acid and adds a hydroperoxy group to carbon 15 to form prostaglandin G_2 (PGG_2). The separate peroxidase active site of the same COX molecule then reduces this hydroperoxy group to the hydroxy group to form PGH_2. NSAIDs inhibit the cyclooxygenase active site of COX, but have no effect on the peroxidase active site, a finding confirmed by recent X-ray crystallographic evidence of COX incubated with selected NSAIDs.[5]

The demonstration of two COX isoenzymes, COX-1 and COX-2, prompted numerous investigations to define the structure–function relationship of each isoform. COX-1 and COX-2 are encoded by two different genes. The amino acid sequences of human COX-1 and human COX-2 are 78% similar and 63% identical. The cyclooxygenase active sites (and the NSAID binding sites) of human COX-1 and human COX-2 are highly conserved, differing by only a single amino acid at residue 523, which is an isoleucine in COX-1 and a valine in COX-2 (Fig. 107.1). The

> **KEY CONCEPTS**
>
> **COX-2 specific NSAIDs are specific because of two different mechanisms**
>
> - COX-2 specific inhibitors fit into the active site side pocket of COX-2, which is absent from COX-1.
> - COX-2 specific inhibitors exhibit a time-dependent irreversible inhibition of COX-2, which appears to alter the conformation of the active site.

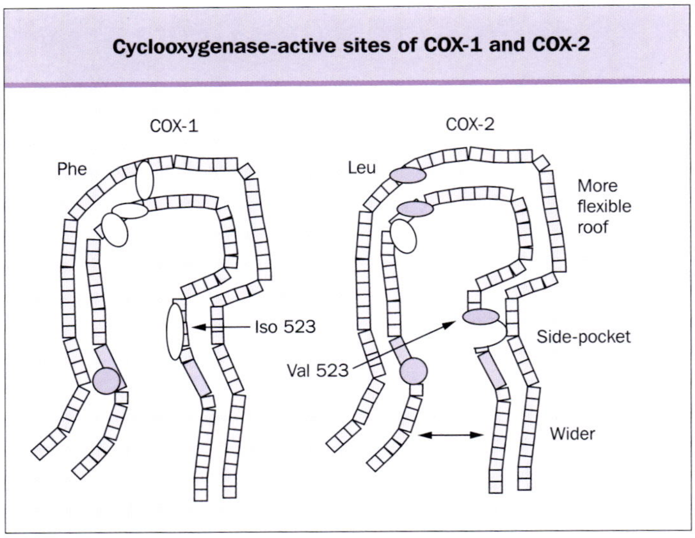

Figure 107.1 Differences between the cyclooxygenase active sites of COX-1 and COX-2. The isoleucine at position 523 in COX-1 is replaced by a valine in COX-2. This substitution creates a side pocket in the active binding site of COX-2, not present in COX-1, and a somewhat wider binding site in COX-2.

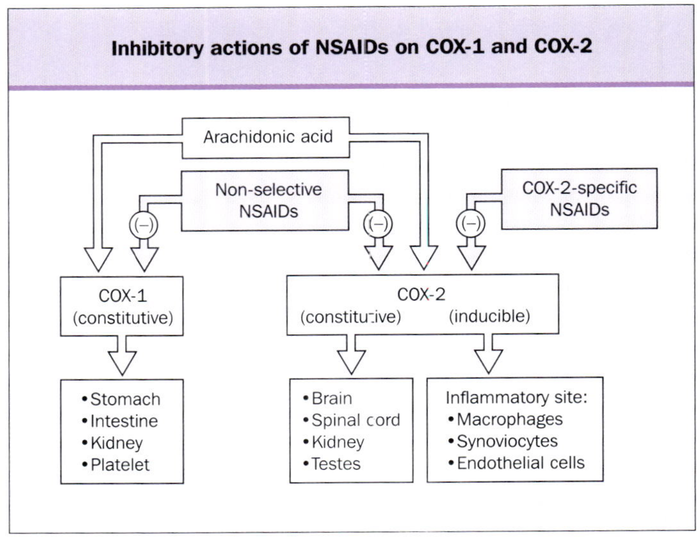

Figure 107.2 The tissues in which COX-1 and COX-2 are constitutively expressed, and COX-2 is inducibly expressed, and where NSAIDs may exhibit clinical effects. The inhibitory actions of nonselective NSAIDs on COX-1 and COX-2, and the inhibitory actions of COX-2-specific NSAIDs on constitutive and inducible COX-2 are schematically illustrated.

absence of the additional methyl group on the valine in COX-2 compared to the isoleucine in COX-1 creates a side pocket as part of the COX-2 NSAID binding site that is not present in that of COX-1, and increases the overall size of the binding site.[6] Conventional NSAIDs for the most part can fit the NSAID binding site of either COX-1 or COX-2. With the exception of aspirin, most conventional NSAIDs act as reversible competitive inhibitors of both COX-1 and COX-2. Aspirin acetylates the active cyclooxygenase site, forming a covalent bond, and thus acts as an irreversible inhibitor of both COX-1 and COX-2.

In contrast, COX-2-specific inhibitors such as celecoxib and rofecoxib are larger than conventional NSAIDs and have a conformation that precludes them from readily fitting into the NSAID binding site of COX-1, but allows them to easily fit into the side pocket of the NSAID binding site of COX-2. This difference in part explains the COX-2 selectivity of these newer NSAIDs. In addition, however, kinetic studies have established two distinct mechanisms by which COX-2-specific NSAIDs inhibit COX-1 and COX-2. Specific COX-2 inhibitors such as celecoxib and rofecoxib exhibit a time-dependent irreversible inhibition of COX-2, whereby the drug appears to alter the active cyclooxygenase site following binding. In contrast, at very high doses, these same compounds can act as time-independent reversible inhibitors of COX-1, with the degree of inhibition of COX-1 being dependent on drug concentration, arachidonic acid concentration, and affinity for the active site.[7,8]

Distribution of COX-1 and COX-2

COX-1 is constitutively expressed in most tissues, and appears to act in a homeostatic or cytoprotective manner. The tissues expressing COX-1 that exhibit the most clinically relevant NSAID effects are the gastrointestinal mucosa, the kidneys, and platelets (Fig. 107.2). (While the gastrointestinal mucosa and the kidney can also express COX-2, platelets only express COX-1, and cannot be induced to express COX-2). In contrast, COX-2 is absent from most tissues (it does appear to be constitutively expressed in brain, testes, and the kidney),[9] but can be induced in most tissues by cytokines, endotoxin, tumor promoters, growth factors, and gonadotropins.[3,10] After induction, COX-2 can be found in macrophages, monocytes, synoviocytes, ovarian follicles, colonic adenomas and cancer cells, vascular smooth muscle cells, bone, and amnion, and in increased amounts in brain, spinal cord, and the kidney. At least one report suggests that COX-2 mRNA and protein induction occurs in T cells following T-cell receptor/CD3 or PMA stimulation, is blocked by cyclosporin A, and plays a role in immune activation;[11] at the time of this writing, there are no reports of the presence of COX-2 in B cells.

COX-1 and COX-2 have identical enzymatic actions, and synthesize PGH_2. Depending on the tissue where it is synthesized, PGH_2 can be converted to prostaglandins PGD_2, PGE_2, $PGF_{2\alpha}$, and PGI_2 (prostacyclin), and thromboxane. In turn, the physiologic or pathophysiologic actions of each of these prostanoids are dependent on the microenvironment where it is made. PGE_2

> **KEY CONCEPTS**
>
> **Two distinct cyclooxygenase (COX) enzymes exist**
> - COX-1 is generally constitutively expressed in most tissues, and is involved in homeostasis and 'housekeeping' functions.
> - COX-2 is absent from most tissues, but its expression can be induced by cytokines, endotoxin, tumor promoters, growth factors, and gonadotropins.
> - COX-2 is constitutively expressed in brain, testes, and kidney.
> - The cyclooxygenase active site (i.e the NSAID-binding site) of COX-2 contains a side pocket absent from COX-1, and is wider than that of COX-1.

synthesized by the cells of the gastric mucosa serves a cytoprotective role, while PGE_2 synthesized by the synovial lining of a rheumatoid arthritis joint is pro-inflammatory. Thromboxane A_2 (TxA_2) is synthesized by platelets and promotes their aggregation. PGI_2 is synthesized within arterial walls, inhibits the aggregation of platelets, is a potent vasodilator, and therefore opposes the actions of TxA_2. In addition, prostaglandins can act in an autocrine, paracrine, or endocrine manner. Actions promoted by selected prostaglandins and thromboxanes are summarized in Table 107.1.[10] Inhibition of COX-1-synthesized prostaglandins or thromboxanes by NSAIDs appears to be responsible for many of the common adverse effects of NSAIDs such as stomach ulcers, renal effects, and inhibition of platelet aggregation. When prostaglandins are synthesized by induced COX-2 at particular tissue sites, their pro-inflammatory actions can result in erythema, edema, tenderness, pain, and fever. Inhibition of COX-2 by NSAIDs thus largely explains their anti-inflammatory, analgesic, and antipyretic actions. In addition, COX-2-specific inhibitors may be immunosuppressive. COX-2 inhibitors, but not conventional NSAIDs, appear to diminish early and late events of T-cell activation, including CD25 and CD71 cell surface expression, IL-2, TNF-α, and IFN-γ production, and cell proliferation.[11]

Chemical properties of NSAIDs

NSAIDs as a class are weak organic acids, and lipophilic. Thus, the lower the pH, the greater is the lipophilicity of the NSAID.

Actions of prostaglandins and thromboxane

COX product	Cells/tissues where COX product predominates	Actions of COX product
PGE_2	Renal medulla Gastric mucosa Platelets Microvascular endothelium	Vasodilation Inhibition of tubular sodium reabsorption Bronchodilation Contraction of gravid uterine smooth muscle Modulation of lymphocyte function Modulation of neurotransmission Sensitizing nociceptor nerve endings to chemical and mechanical stimuli, thus lowering threshold to pain Stimulation of osteoclastic bone resorption
$PGF_{2\alpha}$		Bronchoconstriction Contraction of uterine smooth muscle Vasoconstriction of uterine vessels and veins
PGI_2	Vascular endothelium and subendothelium	Inhibition of platelet aggregation Promotes platelet disaggregation Inhibition of platelet and neutrophil adherence to damaged endothelium Vasodilation Bronchodilation
PGD_2	Mast cells	Vasodilation Increased vascular permeability Bronchoconstriction Stimulation of random migration of neutrophils and eosinophils
TxA_2	Platelets Human monocytes	Promotion of platelet aggregation Bronchoconstriction Vasoconstriction

Table 107.1 Actions of prostaglandins and thromboxane.

KEY CONCEPTS

The actions of prostanoids depend on the microenvironment where they are made

- COX-1 and COX-2 both synthesize PGG_2, which serves as a precursor to other prostanoids and thromboxane.
- PGE_2 synthesized by the cells of the gastric mucosa serves a cytoprotective role.
- PGE_2 synthesized by the synovial lining of a rheumatoid arthritis joint is pro-inflammatory.
- Thromboxane A_2 (TxA_2) synthesized by platelets promotes their aggregation.
- PGI_2 synthesized within arterial walls inhibits platelet aggregation and is a potent vasodilator.
- Prostaglandins can act in an autocrine, paracrine, or endocrine manner.

This combination of chemical properties allows NSAIDs to cross lipid membranes, including the blood–brain barrier, and accumulate in acidic tissues such as the stomach, renal medulla, and sites of inflammation.[12]

Classes of NSAIDs

NSAIDs can currently be categorized by chemical class and by COX-2 selectivity. The chemical classification of selected NSAIDs with half-lives and usual dosages is given in Table 107.2.[13,14] The COX-2 selectivity of NSAIDs has been defined by the COX-1/COX-2 ratio. The larger this ratio, the greater is the selectivity of the compound for COX-2 (i.e. the greater the COX-1 inhibitor dose required for a comparable effect by a COX-2 inhibitor). However, this ratio can be determined from a number of different in vitro and in vivo assays, each of which can generate different results. It is important to realize that, particularly for the in vitro assays, the assay conditions can vary from laboratory to laboratory, and as a result, the ratio for a given drug can vary over a wide numerical range depending on the laboratory reporting the result.

The most direct in vitro assay is that which determines the concentrations required to inhibit 50% of the activities (the IC_{50}s) of purified recombinant human COX-1 and purified recombinant human COX-2, respectively. This assay, however, does not account for factors that occur in vivo, such as intracellular location of COX-1 and COX-2, and potential differences in local intracellular NSAID concentrations. A second in vitro assay is the whole blood assay, which examines the IC_{50}s needed to inhibit the synthesis of thromboxane (a purely COX-1-initiated event) synthesized by platelets during aggregation, and of PGE_2 elaborated following lipopolysaccharide stimulation of monocytes (a purely COX-2-mediated event).[15] However, the results of this assay can be affected by the particular assay conditions. The most relevant COX-1/COX-2 ratio is that which can be determined by in vivo assays. Such assays were developed in the rat, and were used to determine the dose required to inhibit 50% of the activities (the ED_{50}s) of COX-1 (as determined by synthesis of gastric prostaglandins) and of COX-2 (as determined by synthesis of prostaglandins induced in response to carrageenan injected into an air pouch), respectively.[16] The COX-1/COX-2 ratios as determined by various assays are given in Table 107.3.[17–20]

Chemical classification of NSAIDs			
Drug generic name (brand name in USA)	**Dose range (mg/day)**	**Half-life (hours)**	**Doses per day**
Salicylic acid derivatives			
Aspirin	1000–6000	4–15	2–4
Magnesium choline salicylate (Trilisate)	1500–4000	9–17	2–4
Salsalate (Disalcid)	1000–3000	4–16	2–3
Diflunisal (Dolobid)	500–1500	8–12	2–3
Indole and indene acetic acids			
Indomethacin (Indocin)	50–200	4.5	2–4
Sulindac (Clinoril)	300–400	16[a]	2
Etodolac (Lodine)	600–1200	7	3–4
Heteroaryl acetic acids			
Tolmetin (Tolectin)	800–1800	1–5	4–6
Diclofenac (Voltaren; Cataflam)	75–150	1–2	2–3
Ketorolac (Toradol)[b]	15–120	2.5–6	4
Arylpropionic acids			
Ibuprofen (Motrin)	1200–3200	2	3–6
Naproxen (Naprosyn)	250–1500	12–17	2
Flurbiprofen (Ansaid)	100–300	3–4	2–4
Ketoprofen (Orudis)	200–225	2	3–4
Fenoprofen (Nalfon)	900–3200	3	3–4
Oxaprozin (Daypro)	600–1200	49–60	1
Anthranilic acids (fenamates)			
Mefenamic acid (Ponstel)[c]	500–1000	2–3	2–4
Meclofenamic acid (Meclomen)	200–400	2–3	4
Enolic acids			
Piroxicam (Feldene)	20	50	1
Meloxicam (Mobic)[d]	7.5–15	20	1
Phenylbutazone (Butazolidine)	200–800	40–80	1–4
Alkanones			
Nabumetone (Relafen)	1000–2000	22–30[a]	1–2
Pyrazoles			
Celecoxib (Celebrex)	200–400	11	1–2
Furanones			
Rofecoxib (Vioxx)	12.5–25	17	1
Sulfonanilides			
Nimesulide[d]	100	3	2

[a]Half-life of active metabolite.
[b]Use not to exceed 5 days.
[c]Use not to exceed 1 week.
[d]Not available in the USA at the time of this writing.

Table 107.2 Chemical classification of NSAIDs.

COX-1/COX-2 ratios[a] for selected NSAIDs by various assays			
Drug	**Human recombinant enzymes[b] COX-1 IC_{50}/ COX-2 IC_{50}**	**Whole blood assay[c] COX-1 IC_{50}/ COX-2 IC_{50}**	**In vivo[d] COX-1 ED_{50}/ COX-2 ED_{50}**
Nonselective (conventional) NSAIDs[e]			
Flurbiprofen	—[f]	0.097	—
Ketoprofen	—	0.123	—
Tolmetin	—	0.254	—
Aspirin	—	0.321	—
Oxaprozen	—	0.397	—
Naproxen	0.136	0.559	5
Indomethacin	0.1	0.562	2
Ibuprofen	0.215	0.592	0.1
Ketorolac	—	0.610	—
Piroxicam	1.026	1.266	0.1
Diclofenac	3	20	5
Mefenamic acid	—	12.5	—
Selective COX-2 inhibitors			
6-MNA	—	1.563	0.01
Etodolac	>1.852	9.09	0.2
Meloxicam	0.765	11.1	0.5
Nimesulide	—	25	—
Specific COX-2 inhibitors			
Celecoxib	375	9.09	>33
Rofecoxib	1000[a]	20	—

[a]Expressed as the ratio of the 50% inhibitory concentration or inhibitory dose for COX-1 to the 50% inhibitory concentration or inhibitory dose for COX-2. Ratios <1 indicate preferential inhibition of COX-1. Ratios >1 indicate preferential inhibition of COX-2. The larger the ratio, the more selective the drug. These ratios may vary by 10-fold depending on assay conditions.
[b]Data from reference 18.
[c]Data from reference 19.
[d]Data from reference 20.
[e]Designations of COX-2 nonselective, selective, and specific are based on presence or absence of inhibition of COX-1-mediated events at therapeutic levels of NSAID which inhibit COX-2-mediated events in vivo
[f] – indicates information not available.

Table 107.3 COX-1/COX-2 ratios[a] for selected NSAIDs by various assays. Chan C-C, Boyce S, Brideau C, et al. Rofecoxib [Vioxx, MK-0966; 4-(4′-methylsulfonylphenyl)-3-phenyl-2-(5H)-furanone]: A potent and orally active cyclooxygenase-2 inhibitor. Pharmacological and biochemical profiles. *J Pharm Exp Ther* 1999;290:551.

Ultimately, the most meaningful classification of an NSAID with respect to COX-2 selectivity is that based on clinical criteria. On this basis, NSAIDs can be categorized: (1) as 'COX-2 non-selective', whereby at clinically relevant therapeutic doses the NSAID inhibits COX-1-mediated events preferentially or inhibits COX-1 and COX-2-mediated events approximately equally; (2) as 'COX-2-selective' or 'COX-2-preferential', whereby the NSAID inhibits COX-2-mediated events at low thereapeutic doses, but inhibits COX-1-mediated events at higher clinically therapeutic doses; and (3) as 'COX-2-specific', whereby the NSAID inhibits only COX-2-mediated events even at high therapeutic doses. Clinical data suggest that at least two currently available NSAIDs, celecoxib and rofecoxib, are truly 'COX-2-specific' (see below).

CLINICAL EXPERIENCE – EFFICACY OF NSAIDS

Analgesic and antipyretic efficacy of NSAIDs

Local tissue injury and inflammatory diseases such as rheumatoid arthritis and osteoarthritis are associated with increased prostaglandin synthesis, which sensitizes pain receptors to lower levels of stimuli.[21] NSAIDs exert their analgesic effects by interfering with the hyperalgesia induced by local synthesis of prostaglandins at the site of injury or inflammation. In addition, prostaglandins are thought to act centrally to facilitate transmission of pain responses,[22] and NSAIDs can cross the blood–brain barrier to act at these central sites[23] Studies in animal models have implicated both COX-1 and COX-2 in the release of centrally and peripherally acting prostaglandins, and have suggested that inhibition of both COX-1 and COX-2 may contribute to the spinal analgesic and antihyperalgesic actions of NSAIDs.[24] However, the relative roles of the two COX isoforms have not yet been completely defined. COX-2 expression is increased locally at sites of injury and inflammation,[25] as well as in spinal cord neurons following peripheral inflammation.[26] At doses that maintain selectivity for COX-2, COX-2 inhibitors have shown equal analgesic efficacy to nonselective NSAIDs for treatment of pain associated with several conditions such as dental surgery, osteoarthritis, and dysmenorrhea.[22,27]

Exogenous pyrogens (e.g. bacterial endotoxin and viruses) induce fever via a cascade of molecular interactions that includes induction of the synthesis and release of the endogenous pyrogenic cytokines IL-1 and IL-6, which in turn induce COX-mediated prostaglandin synthesis in the central nervous system. Nonselective NSAIDs are effective antipyretics in both animal models and humans by inhibiting synthesis of fever-mediating prostaglandins. Recent biochemical and clinical data implicate the COX-2 isoform in the pathogenesis of fever in humans. COX-2 expression is induced in the brain vasculature, with temporal correlation to the development of fever,[28] and COX-2 knockout mice fail to develop fever in response to inflammatory stimuli.[29] COX-2-specific inhibitors reduce naturally occurring fever in humans with an efficacy similar to that of nonselective NSAIDs.[30]

Anti-inflammatory efficacy of NSAIDs

NSAIDs are widely prescribed for and provide effective treatment of a variety of inflammatory conditions, including osteoarthritis, rheumatoid arthritis, acute gout, acute bursitis, and spondylarthropathies. Substantial individual variability exists with respect to the pharmacology and pharmacokinetics of these drugs, necessitating individualization of treatment to the patient and disease. Often, patients who do not tolerate or do not respond to a particular NSAID will respond favorably to another NSAID. Furthermore, the optimal dosage varies from one disorder to the next. Moderate doses are often sufficient to treat osteoarthritis, whereas rheumatoid arthritis or other types of chronic inflammatory arthritis usually require sustained therapy with maximum tolerated doses. Combinations of salicylate and NSAIDs or two NSAIDs appear to provide no greater therapeutic benefit than single-drug therapy, and probably result in additive toxicity.

Experimental evidence suggests that local PGE_2 production is central to the pathogenesis of inflammation. Results obtained in animal models of inflammatory arthritis associate increased expression of COX-2 with increased prostaglandin production in inflamed joint tissues[31] COX-2 is greatly up-regulated at sites of inflammation in humans; induction of COX-2 expression has been observed in cartilage from osteoarthritis patients and synovial tissue from rheumatoid arthritis patients.[32] COX-2 expression in primary cultures of human synovial tissue or inflammatory cells (e.g. monocytes) is induced by the pro-inflammatory cytokines IL-1 and TNF-α, while the anti-inflammatory cytokines IL-4 and IL-13 and immunosuppressive glucocorticoids decrease COX-2 levels.[33] Clinical trials comparing COX-2-specific inhibitors with nonselective NSAIDs in osteoarthritis and rheumatoid arthritis have shown that the same therapeutic endpoints are reached with both types of drugs, suggesting that nonselective NSAIDs probably reduce inflammation through inhibition of COX-2.[34]

Efficacy of NSAIDs in cancer

Epidemiological data have shown an association between regular use of aspirin or other NSAIDs and decreased incidence of and mortality from colorectal cancer.[35] Regular aspirin use has been shown to decrease both colorectal cancer incidence and mortality by approximately 40%. Sulindac administration has been shown to reduce the size and number of adenomas in patients with familial adenomatous polyposis (FAP), a hereditary disease that leads to colorectal cancer by the fifth decade of life in virtually all patients.[36] COX-2 has been implicated in carcinogenesis in animal models of the disease,[37] and COX-2 has been shown to be highly up-regulated in human colorectal adenomas and adenocarcinomas compared with normal mucosa,[38] suggesting a role for COX-2 in transformation. However, no data are yet available to demonstrate an association between NSAID administration and decrease in cancer incidence in patients with FAP. The COX-2-specific inhibitor celecoxib has been shown to reduce significantly the size and number of colorectal polyps in patients with FAP, and has been approved by the Food and Drug Administration as an adjunct to usual care for patients with FAP.[39] Increased prostaglandin synthesis via COX-2 up-regulation in bladder cancer,[40] and GI cancers[41] suggests that COX-2-specific inhibitors may also be useful in the prevention or treatment of these cancers.

Effects of NSAIDs in Alzheimer's disease

Nonselective NSAIDs have been evaluated for the treatment and prevention of Alzheimer's disease, with promising results. Studies have shown slower disease progression and cognitive decline in NSAID-treated patients compared with matched control populations.[42] Longitudinal studies have demonstrated that the relative risk of developing Alzheimer's disease is decreased in patients using NSAIDs and is associated with the duration of use.[43] Animal studies have shown that COX-2 is localized during development to areas of the brain related to memory (e.g. hippocampus, cortex), and that COX-2 appears to be involved in postsynaptic signaling of cortical and other excitatory neurons in the adult brain.[44] COX-2 expression in the brain can be up-regulated by a variety of stressful stimuli, including seizure. Other animal studies have shown up-regulation of COX-2 in activated microglia in cerebral inflammatory processes which are thought to parallel the inflammatory cascade of events in the human brain that lead to deposition of β-amyloid protein, the hallmark histologic manifestation of Alzheimer's disease.[45] These clinical and biochemical data suggest a potential for COX-2-specific NSAIDs in the future treatment and prevention of Alzheimer's disease.

CLINICAL EXPERIENCE – TOXICITIES OF NSAIDS

Although NSAIDs are generally well tolerated, they are associated with a wide spectrum of potential clinical toxicities. Many of the side-effects are attributed to inhibition of the constitutively expressed COX-1 enzyme, and appear to be significantly reduced through the use of COX-2-specific inhibitors. In general, side-effects tend to be dose-related.

Gastrointestinal toxicity

The chief clinical limitation of nonselective NSAIDs is undoubtedly their toxic effect on the upper gastrointestinal (GI) tract,

CLINICAL PEARLS

The net effects of each NSAID depend on relative inhibition of COX-1 and COX-2

- The clinical benefits of NSAIDs result from their inhibition of COX-2.
- The major toxicities of NSAIDs result from inhibition of COX-1.
- In general, the more selective an NSAID is for COX-2, the greater its safety profile.

including ulceration, bleeding, and perforation. Nonselective NSAIDs are thought to exert a direct toxic effect on the gastroduodenal mucosa, as well as an indirect effect via inhibition of COX-1-induced cytoprotective prostaglandins. Prostanoids PGE_2 and PGI_2, synthesized in the gastrointestinal mucosa, protect the mucosa and limit gastric acid output. Central mucosal defense mechanisms are compromised by the decreased prostaglandin production caused by chronic NSAID-induced COX-1 inhibition, leading to ulceration and bleeding diathesis. NSAID-induced inhibition of COX-1 leads to increased gastric acid production, decreased production of bicarbonate, and a decreased rate of cellular proliferation of the gastric mucosa, all of which impair the normal protective mechanisms of the stomach. NSAIDs cause or aggravate gastrointestinal bleeding, both by increasing acid production in the stomach and by decreasing platelet adhesiveness (see below). Some NSAIDs may also elicit immune responses, with the generation of antibodies to mucosal prostaglandins.[46] Indomethacin, sulindac, and meclofenamate sodium all undergo enterohepatic recirculation; thus, the gastrointestinal exposure to these drugs is increased, and their gastrointestinal toxicity is enhanced. Slow dissolution of firmly compressed aspirin tablets may cause irritation and superficial ulceration of gastric mucosa. Additionally, mucosal damage may result from back diffusion of hydrogen ions caused by ion-trapping of weak organic acids like NSAIDs within mucosal cells.[47]

The US Food and Drug Administration estimates that gastrointestinal ulcers, bleeding, and perforation occur in approximately 1–2% of patients using nonselective NSAIDs for 3 months, and approximately 2–5% of those using them for 1 year. Two to four per cent of patients on long-term therapy are hospitalized each year because of GI complications.[48] Prior peptic ulcer disease, advanced age, high NSAID doses or therapy with multiple NSAIDs, and concomitant therapy with either corticosteroids or anticoagulants all increase the risk of a GI complication in patients taking nonselective NSAIDs chronically. There are some data to indicate that comorbidities such as cardiovascular disease and rheumatoid arthritis increase the risk of NSAID-induced GI complications. The role of *Helicobacter pylori* in increasing risk for NSAID-associated ulcers has not been systematically evaluated in epidemiological studies.

Strategies to minimize NSAID gastropathy include using the lowest NSAID dose possible to control the patient's symptoms, the substitution of a nonacetylated salicylate, and administration of supplemental gastroprotective agents such as proton pump inhibitors, H_2-receptor antagonists, and the synthetic prostaglandin misoprostol. Postmarketing surveillance and endoscopic studies have confirmed that the incidence of gastroduodenal mucosal injury is reduced with the use of nabumatone, etodolac, and meloxicam, in part due to their selectivity for COX-2 inhibition, with a minimal effect on COX-1, at least at lower therapeutic doses. In addition, etodolac and nabumatone have little or no enterohepatic recirculation.[49,50] Specific COX-2 inhibitors have been shown to markedly reduce injury to the gastroduodenal mucosa. Two of the compounds, celecoxib and rofecoxib, have been studied extensively and appear to maintain their selectivity for COX-2 at doses substantially higher than those required to affect inflammation. The incidence of gastroduodenal ulcers attributable to specific COX-2 inhibitors is not significantly different from that found with placebo.[51]

Platelet effects

COX-1 is the only cyclooxygenase isoform in platelets, and platelets use COX-1-derived PGH_2 to generate thromboxane A_2, a key autocrine stimulator of platelet aggregation and vasoconstriction. Nonselective NSAIDs, by inhibiting COX-1 and thus platelet thromboxane A_2 synthesis, inhibit platelet function and predispose patients to bleeding. Platelets lack mitochondria and are unable to synthesize additional cyclooxygenase, thus acetylation of this enzyme by aspirin irreversibly inhibits platelet activation in response to a variety of stimuli. This effect persists for 10–12 days until the acetylated platelets are replaced by newly produced platelets that have not been exposed to aspirin.[52] This property has led to the use of aspirin in doses as low as 80 mg daily in cardioprophylaxis to prevent platelet aggregation and emboli in patients prone to transient ischemic attacks, but it also increases the risk of gastrointestinal and other bleeding events. In contrast to aspirin, other nonselective NSAIDs exert reversible cyclooxygenase inhibition, and their platelet effects correlate roughly with the half-life of the drug, lasting only as long as the drug is present.

Aspirin and other nonselective NSAIDs do not cause major bleeding events in the vast majority of patients who use them. The clinical manifestations induced by exposure to nonselective NSAIDs are mild, in part because thromboxane A_2 is only one of several mediators of platelet activation. Thrombin and other strong platelet agonists can induce platelet aggregation even in the presence of concomitant exposure to nonselective NSAIDs.[53] However, in patients with impaired hemostasis, the decreases in platelet thromboxane A_2 resulting from COX-1 inhibition can pose significant clinical risk. Gastrointestinal bleeding is the most common spontaneous bleeding event associated with the use of aspirin and nonselective NSAIDs. Other clinical bleeding prob-

THERAPEUTIC PRINCIPLES

Efficacy and toxicities of NSAIDs

- NSAIDs are anti-inflammatory, analgesic, and antipyretic.
- Nonselective NSAIDs: cause gastrointestinal ulceration, leading to bleeding, performation, or obstruction in a small percentage but large number of patients; prevent platelet aggregation; and alter renal physiology leading to salt and water retention.
- Because COX-2 is constitutively expressed in the kidney, COX-2-specific inhibitors may also alter renal physiology, leading to edema and hypertension in some patients.

lems associated with the use of nonselective NSAIDs are increased risk of intracerebral hemorrhage, fetal and neonatal bleeding abnormalities caused by maternal ingestion of NSAIDs in the peripartum period, and increased risk of postoperative bleeding following cardiac and other surgeries in patients taking aspirin and other NSAIDs preoperatively.[54] COX-2-specific NSAIDs, which have been shown to preserve platelet function at therapeutic doses, should obviate these bleeding problems and their use should not need to be restricted perioperatively.[55]

Renal toxicity

NSAIDs can adversely affect renal function by inhibiting synthesis of renal prostaglandins important for solute homeostasis and for maintenance of renal blood flow. The most significant clinical effects of NSAIDs are decreased sodium and potassium excretion and decreased renal perfusion. NSAIDs, by decreasing renal PGE_2 levels, increase sodium reabsorption, causing weight gain and edema in some patients and, in rare cases, congestive heart failure. In addition, the effect of NSAIDs on sodium retention can decrease the response to antihypertensive drugs, particularly diuretics and ACE inhibitors. Inhibition of renal prostaglandin I_2 (PGI_2) by NSAIDs decreases potassium excretion and can cause hyperkalemia, usually mild but in rare cases sufficiently severe to cause cardiac arrest. Patients at risk for hyperkalemia (e.g. those with renal insufficiency or on potassium-sparing diuretics) should have their serum potassium levels monitored at the onset of NSAID therapy, since decreases in potassium secretion can occur with the first dose of NSAID. Although maintenance of renal blood flow is independent of renal prostaglandin synthesis in healthy individuals, in clinical conditions where actual or circulating volume is decreased (congestive heart failure, cirrhosis, and renal insufficiency), renal perfusion is maintained by vasodilating renal prostaglandins. NSAID administration to at-risk patients can result in decreases in renal blood flow sufficient to cause acute renal failure. Since acute renal failure can develop with the first dose of NSAID, careful monitoring of at-risk patients is important. It is likely that the risk of developing acute renal failure from NSAID therapy is related to both dose and half-life, higher doses of longer-acting NSAIDs being associated with greater risk.[56] Because both COX-1 and COX-2 are expressed in the kidney,[57] and the relative physiological roles of each enzyme in the kidney have not been fully elucidated, the extent to which these adverse clinical effects might be obviated by COX-2-specific inhibitors has not been fully determined. COX-2-specific inhibitors have been shown to inhibit some renal prostaglandins,[58] and cause edema in 2–4% of patients in controlled clinical trials,[14] indicating that both nonselective and COX-2-specific inhibitors may have similar effects on sodium homeostasis. Whether there are differences among NSAIDs for risk of acute renal failure is unclear. Both nonselective and COX-2-specific NSAIDs should be used with appropriate monitoring in patients at risk for NSAID-induced adverse renal events.

Hepatic toxicity

Hepatic toxicity has been reported with virtually all NSAIDs in current use. Most of this toxicity is clinically mild and seems to be unrelated to the inhibition of COX. Reversible hepatocellular toxicity, characterized by elevation of aminotransaminases, has been observed in up to 15% of patients treated with NSAIDs.[59] High anti-inflammatory doses of aspirin may cause this effect in up to 50% of patients, and even more frequently in patients with Still's disease and SLE. Transaminase elevations can occur at any time after initiation of treatment, and usually revert to normal with dosage adjustment or discontinuation of the drug. In rare cases, NSAIDs may induce more severe hepatic dysfunction, causing elevated bilirubin or prolonged prothrombin times, in which case the drug must be discontinued.

Clinically significant events reflecting NSAID hepatotoxicity are uncommon. It has been estimated from case–control studies that NSAID therapy increases the risk of hospitalization for acute symptomatic hepatitis by approximately two-fold.[60] Hepatocellular cholestasis and granulomatous hepatitis induced by phenylbutazone may be fatal in some patients. The most commonly reported hepatotoxicity of clinical significance occurs with sulindac. This drug is associated with a syndrome that appears to be allergic in nature, characterized by fever, rash, eosinophilia, and liver enzyme elevations. The hepatic toxicities observed with NSAIDs do not seem to result from inhibition of COX, therefore they would not be expected to be more or less likely with the use of COX-2-specific inhibitors. COX-2-specific inhibitors have not been fully evaluated in patients with severe hepatic disease and should therefore be used with the same caution as the nonselective NSAIDs.

CNS effects

Both COX isoforms are present in the central nervous system, in neurons as well as in vascular and glial cells. NSAIDs have been associated with central nervous system side-effects. Salicylates can cause dose-dependent tinnitus and hearing loss, and overdoses can severely affect the central nervous system, culminating in coma and death; overdoses of other NSAIDs are much less toxic. Occasionally, some patients experience severe headaches upon initiation of NSAID therapy; this effect may be more common with indomethacin than with other NSAIDs. Confusion may appear in elderly patients treated with indomethacin, naproxen, or ibuprofen. Aseptic meningitis has occurred rarely in patients treated with NSAIDs, most commonly ibuprofen.[61] It has been reported primarily in patients who have an underlying autoimmune disease, such as SLE or mixed connective tissue disease, and recurs with rechallenge using the same medication but not with alternative NSAIDs, indicating that this is an idiopathic response to an individual drug, not a mechanism-based effect.

Effects of NSAIDs on cartilage and bone

Studies using nonselective NSAIDs have shown that these drugs may accelerate the process of cartilage destruction in osteoarthritis, largely by inhibiting proteoglycan biosynthesis in cartilage.[62] Potent inhibitors of prostaglandin synthesis, such as indomethacin and aspirin, have been shown to reduce proteoglycan synthesis in cartilage and promote the acceleration of joint space narrowing observed radiologically in patients with osteoarthritis. Interestingly, indomethacin is one of several NSAIDs shown to lack collagenase inhibitory activity, and it may be that the combined inhibition of proteoglycan biosynthesis and lack of inhibition of collagenase activity allow for acceleration of cartilage destruction by indomethacin. Interestingly, the COX-2-selective inhibitor, meloxicam, shows no inhibitory effects on proteoglycan biosynthesis, but does inhibit collagenase activity, so would be predicted to be cartilage sparing; however, the effects of meloxicam on the progression of joint changes in osteoarthritis have not yet been definitively tested.[63]

The effects of NSAID therapy on bone proliferation and remodelling are complex and often contradictory. Prostaglandins can stimulate collagen synthesis and bone formation, as well as promoting bone resorption.[64] It has been reported that NSAIDs suppress bone repair and remodeling and also slow the process of bone loss associated with some inflammatory conditions.[65] Studies on the effects of nonselective NSAIDs in animal models of osteoporosis have given conflicting results, showing both protection against and acceleration of bone loss.[66,67] The effects of COX-2-specific inhibitors on cartilage and bone structure have not yet been examined and are difficult to predict; COX-1 is expressed in osteoarthritic cartilage and appears to be important in the repair of both cartilage and bone.[68] Thus, the net observed effect of a particular NSAID on bone and cartilage structure results from a complicated interplay of COX-1 and COX-2-controlled prostaglandin-mediated resorptive and formative processes.

Drug interactions of NSAIDs

Individual NSAIDs vary in their interactions with other classes of drugs, but many of these interactions have their basis in the mechanism of action of NSAIDs and are common to many, if not all, NSAIDs.[13,14] Aspirin, in other than cardiovascular protective doses, and other NSAIDs should not be used together, as they increase the potential for adverse effects common to this class. In addition, aspirin and NSAIDs may share the same protein-binding sites: either aspirin can displace the NSAID, resulting in increased clearance and decreased plasma levels of the NSAID, or the NSAID can displace aspirin. Some NSAIDs, including aspirin, can cause displacement of other drugs from their protein-binding sites, so caution is necessary with patients on sulfonylurea hypoglycemics, phenytoin, valproic acid, and carbonic anhydrase inhibitors. Some, but not all, NSAIDs can also displace warfarin. Even with NSAIDs that do not displace warfarin, patients on warfarin and an NSAID need to have their prothrombin times and/or INRs monitored. The interference of NSAIDs with synthesis of renal prostaglandins can blunt the natriuretic effects of loop and thiazide diuretics, and diminish the antihypertensive effects of ACE inhibitors and β-blockers. Many, but not all, NSAIDs can cause decreased renal clearance and increased plasma levels of lithium, digoxin, cyclosporin A, and methotrexate. Patients on these drugs, and also on an NSAID should be monitored closely for toxicity. Antacids may interfere with absorption and therefore decrease plasma concentrations of some NSAIDs. Probenecid may decrease renal clearance and increase blood levels of some NSAIDs.

The COX-2-specific NSAIDs share most of the same concerns regarding drug interactions. In addition, it is known that celecoxib is metabolized by cytochrome P450 2C9, so any inhibitor of this enzyme should be used with caution in patients on celecoxib. In particular, administration of fluconazole at 200 mg per day resulted in a two-fold increase in the plasma concentration of celecoxib. In contrast to most NSAIDs, co-administration of celecoxib and methotrexate does not appear to increase methotrexate levels. Rofecoxib is metabolized primarily by cytosolic enzymes, and not by the P450 system. However, coadministration of rifampin with rofecoxib results in a 50% decrease in rofecoxib plasma concentrations, primarily through induction by rifampin of general hepatic metabolic activity.

CONCLUSIONS

NSAIDs are the most widely prescribed class of drugs. They are effective as analgesics and anti-inflammatories for a wide variety of clinical indications, but are accompanied by a wide spectrum of mechanism-based side-effects. The identification of two isoforms of cyclooxygenase, COX-1 and COX-2, has led to the demonstration that COX-1 is constitutively expressed in most tissues, and is homeostatic, and that COX-2 can be induced by a number of stimuli and is largely responsible for inflammation, increased pain, and fever. Recent advances by pharmaceutical companies have led to the development of COX-2-specific inhibitors, which should provide access to the efficacy of NSAIDs in a broader patient population for two reasons: first, COX-2-specific inhibitors are better tolerated, so they can be used for existing indications by patients previously limited in their use of conventional NSAIDs because of adverse effects; and, second, COX-2-specific inhibitors, owing to their better safety profile, can be tested for efficacy in more chronic conditions, including the prevention of certain cancers and Alzheimer's disease.

REFERENCES

1. Vane JR, Botting RM. The history of anti-inflammatory drugs and their mechanism of action. In: Bazan N, Botting J, Vane J (eds) New targets in inflammation. Inhibitors of COX-2 or adhesion molecules. London, Kluwer Academic William Harvey 1996, p 1.
2. Vane JR. Inhibition of prostaglandin synthesis as a mechanism of action for aspirin-like drugs. Nature New Biology 1971;231:232.
3. Fu J-Y, Masferrer JL, Seibert K, Raz A, Needleman P. The induction and suppression of prostaglandin H_2 synthase (cyclooxygenase) in human monocytes. J Biol Chem 1990;265:16737.
4. Xie W, Robertson DL, Simmons DL. Mitogen-inducible prostaglandin G/H synthase: a new target for nonsteroidal anti-inflammatory drugs. Drug Dev Res 1992;25:249.
5. Loll PJ, Picot D, Garavito RM. The structural basis of aspirin activity inferred from the crystal structure of inactivated prostaglandin H_2 synthase. Nature Struct Biol 1995;2:637.
6. Luong C, Miller A, Barnett J, Chow J, Ramesha C, Browner MF. Flexibility of the NSAID binding site in the structure of human cyclooxygenase-2. Nature Struct Biol 1996;3:927.
7. Chan C-C, Boyce S, Brideau C, et al. Rofecoxib [Vioxx, MK-0966; 4-(4'-methylsulfonylphenyl)-3-phenyl-2-(5H)-furanone]: A potent and orally active cyclooxygenase-2 inhibitor. Pharmacological and biochemical profiles. J Pharm Exp Ther 1999;290:551.
8. Gierse JK, Koboldt CM, Walker MC, Seibert K, Isakson PC. Kinetic basis for selective inhibition of cyclo-oxygenases. Biochem J 1999;339:607.
9. Komhoff M, Grone HJ, Klein T, Seyberth HW, Nusing RM. Localization of cyclooxygenase-1 and -2 in adult and fetal human kidney: implication for renal function. Am J Physiol 1997;272:460.
10. Halushka PV. Prostaglandins and related compounds. In: Goldman L, Bennett JC (eds). Cecil Textbook of medicine, 21st edn. Philadelphia, W.B. Saunders, 2000, p 1189.
11. Iniguez MA, Punson C, Fresno M. Induction of cyclooxygenase-2 activated T lymphocytes: regulation of T cell activation by cyclooxygenase-2 inhibitors. J Immunol 1999;163:111.
12. Brune K, Graft P. Non-steroid anti-inflammatory drugs: influence of extracellular pH on biodistribution and pharmacological effects. Biochem Pharmacol 1978;27:525.

13. Insel PA. Analgesic-antipyretic and anti-inflammatory agents and drugs employed in the treatment of gout. In: Hardman JG, Limbird LE (eds) Goodman and Gilman's The pharmacological basis of therapeutics, 9th edn. New York, McGraw-Hill, 1996, p 617.
14. Physician's Desk Reference, 54th edition. Montvale, NJ, Medical Economics Co., 2000.
15. Brideau C, Kargman S, Liu S, et al. A human whole blood assay for clinical evaluation of biochemical efficacy of cyclooxygenase inhibitors. Inflamm Res 1996;45:68.
16. Masferrer JL, Zweibel BS, Manning PT, et al. Selective inhibition of inducible cyclooxygenase 2 *in vivo* is anti-inflammatory and non-ulcerogenic. Proc Natl Acad Sci USA 1994;91:3228.
17. Masferrer JL, Isakson PC, Seibert K. Cyclooxygenase-2 inhibitors. A new class of anti-inflammatory agents that spare the gastrointestinal tract. Gastroenterol Clin North Am 1996;25:363.
18. Schwartz BD. COX-2 inhibitors: A safer class of drugs for inflammatory pain. Novel targets in the treatment of pain. Southborough, MASS, International Business Communications Compendium, 1997.
19. Feldman M, McMahon AT. Do cyclooxygenase-2 inhibitors provide benefits similar to those of traditional nonsteroidal anti-inflammatory drugs, with less gastrointestinal toxicity? Ann Int Med 2000;132:134.
20. Masferrer JL, Zweifel BS, Seibert K, Needleman P. Selective regulation of cellular cyclooxygenase by dexamethasone and endotoxin in mice. J Clin Invest 1990;86:1375.
21. Dray A, Urban L. New pharmacological strategies for pain relief. Ann Rev Pharmacol Toxicol 1996;36:253.
22. Yamamoto T, Nozaki-Taguchi N. Analysis of the effects of cyclooxygenase (COX-1 and COX-2) in spinal nociceptive transmission using indomethacin, a non-selective COX inhibitor, and NS-398, a COX-2-selective inhibitor. Brain Res 1996;739:104.
23. Cashman JN. The mechanism of action of NSAIDs in analgesia. Drugs 1996;52:13.
24. Willingale HL, Gardiner NJ, McLymont N, Giblett S, Grubb B. Prostanoids synthesized by cyclooxygenase isoforms in rat spinal cord and their contribution to the development of neuronal hyper-excitability. Br J Pharmacol 1997;122:1593.
25. Seibert K, Zhang Y, Leahy K, et al. Pharmacological and biomedical demonstration of the role of cyclooxygenase 2 in inflammation and pain. Proc Natl Acad Sci USA 1994;91:12013.
26. Beiche F, Scheuerer S, Brune K, Geisslinger G, Goppelt-Struebe M. Up-regulation of cyclooxygenase-2 mRNA in the rat spinal cord following peripheral inflammation. FEBS Lett 1996;390:165.
27. Morrison BW, Daniels SE, Kotey P, Cantu N, Seidenberg B. Rofecoxib, a specific cyclooxygenase-2 inhibitor, in primary dysmenorrhea: a randomized controlled trial. Obstet Gynecol 1999;94:504.
28. Cao C, Matsumura K, Yamagata K, Watanabe Y. Induction by lipopolysaccharide of cyclooxygenase-2 mRNA in rat brain: Its possible role in the febrile response. Brain Res 1995;697:187.
29. Li S, Wang Y, Matsumura K, Ballou LR, Morhan SG, Blatteis CM. The febrile response to lipopolysaccharide is blocked in cyclooxygenase-2 (–/–) but not cyclooxygenase-1 (–/–) mice. Brain Res 1996;825:86.
30. Schwartz JI, Chan CC, Mukhopadhyay S, et al. Cyclooxygenase-2 inhibition by rofecoxib reverses naturally occurring fever in humans. Clin Pharmacol Ther 1999;65:653.
31. Anderson GD, Hauser SD, McGarity KL, Bremer ME, Isakson PC, Gregory SA. Selective inhibition of cyclooxygenase (COX)-2 reverses inflammation and expression of COX-2 and interleukin 6 in rat adjuvant arthritis. J Clin Invest 1996;97:2672.
32. Amin AR, Attur M, Patel RN, et al. Superinduction of cyclooxygenase-2 in human osteoarthritis-affected cartilage: influence of nitric oxide. J Clin Invest 1997;99:123.
33. Crofford LJ. COX-1 and COX-2 tissue expression: implications and predictions. J Rheum 1997;24:15.
34. Hubbard R, Geis GS, Woods E, Yu S, Zhao W. Efficacy, tolerability, and safety of celecoxib, a specific COX-2 inhibitor, in osteoathritis. Arthritis Rheum 1998;41 Suppl 9:S196.
35. Smalley WE, DuBois RN. Colorectal cancer and nonsteroidal anti-inflammatory drugs. Adv Pharmacol 1997;39:1.
36. Waddell WR, Ganser GF, Cerise EJ, Loughry RW. Sulindac for polyposis of the colon. Am J Surg 1989;157:175.
37. Oshima M, Dinchuk JE, Kargman SL, et al. Suppression of intestinal polyposis in $Apc^{716\Delta}$ knockout mice by inhibition of cyclooxygenase-2 (COX-2). Cell 1996;87:803.
38. Eberhart CE, Coffrey RJ, Radhika A, Giardiello FM, Ferrenbach S, Dubois RN. Up-regulation of cyclooxygenase-2 gene expression in human colorectal adenomas and adenocarcinomas. Gastroenterology 1994;107:1183.
39. Federal Drug Administration Oncologic Drugs Advisory Committee Meeting on Celecoxib, proceedings, December 14, 1999.
40. Dubois RN, Abramson SB, Crofford L, et al. Cyclooxygenase in biology and disease. FASEB J 1998;12:1063.
41. Thun MJ, Namboodiri MM, Heath CW Jr. Aspirin use and reduced risk of fatal colon cancer. N Engl J Med 1991;325:1593.
42. Rich JB, Rasmussen DX, Folstein MF, Carson KA, Kawas C, Brandt J. Nonsteroidal anti-inflammatory drugs in Alzheimer's disease. Neurology 1995;45:51.
43. Stewart WF, Kawas C, Corrada M, Metter J. Risk of Alzheimer's disease and NSAID use. Neurology 1997;48:626.
44. Kaufman WE, Worley PF, Pegg J, Bremer M, Isakson P. COX-2, a synaptically-induced enzyme, is expressed by excitatory neurons at postsynaptic sites in rat cerebral cortex. Proc Natl Acad Sci USA 1996;93:2317.
45. Bauer MKA, Lieb K, Schulze-Osthuff K, et al. Expression and regulation of cyclooxygenase-2 in rat microglia. Eur J Biochem 1997;243:726.
46. Redfern JS, Feldman M. Role of endogenous prostaglandins in preventing gastrointestinal ulceration: induction of ulcers by antibodies to prostaglandins. Gastroenterology 1989;96(suppl):596.
47. Schoen RT, Vender RJ. Mechanisms of non-steroidal anti-inflammatory drug-induced gastric damage. Am J Med 1989;86:449.
48. McCarthy DM. Non-steroidal anti-inflammatory drug-related gastrointestinal toxicity: definitions and epidemiology. Am J Med 1998;105(suppl 5A):35.
49. Schattenkirchner M. An updated safety profile of etodolac in several thousand patients. Eur J Rheumatol Inflamm 1990;10:56.
50. Distel M, Mueller C, Bluhmki E, Fries J. Safety of meloxicam: a global analysis of clinical trials. Br J Rheumatol 1996;35 Suppl 1:68.
51. Lanza FL, Rack MF, Callison DA, et al. A pilot endoscopic study of the gastroduodenal effects of SC-58635, a novel COX-2-selective inhibitor. Gastroenterology 1997;112 (suppl):A194.
52. Clements PJ, Paulus HE. Non-steroidal antirheumatic drugs. In: Kelley WN, et al (eds) Textbook of rheumatology, 5th edn. Philadelphia, WB Saunders, 1997, p 707.
53. Kroll MH, Hellums JD, McIntire LV, Schafer AI, Moake JL. Platelets and shear stress. Blood 1996;88:1525.
54. Schafer AI. Effects of nonsteroidal anti-inflammatory therapy on platelets. Am J Med 1999;106(5B):25S.
55. Mengle-Gaw L, Hubbard RC, Karim A, et al. A study of the platelet effects of SC-58635, a novel COX-2-selective inhibitor. Arthritis Rheum 1997;40 Suppl 9:S93.
56. Henry D, Page J, Whyte I, Nanra R, Hall C. Consumption of nonsteroidal anti-inflammatory drugs and the development of functional renal impairment in elderly subjects: results of a case-control study. Br J Clin Pharmacol 1997;44:85.
57. Cheng HF, Wang JL, Zhang MZ, et al. Angiotensin II attenuates renal cortical cyclooxygenase-2 expression. J Clin Invest 1999;103:653.
58. McAdam BF, Catella-Lawson F, Mardini IA, Kapoor S, Lawson JA, Fitzgerald GA. Systemic biosynthesis of prostacyclin by cyclooxygenase (COX)-2: the human pharmacology of a selective inhibitor of COX-2. Proc Natl Acad Sci USA 1999;96:272.
59. Katz LM, Love PY. NSAIDs and the liver. In: Famaey JP, Paulus HE (eds) Clinical applications of NSAIDs: Subpopulation therapy and new formulations. New York, Marcel Dekker, 1992, p 247.
60. Garcia Rodriguez LA, Williams R, Debry LE, et al. Acute liver injury associated with nonsteroidal anti-inflammatory drugs and the role of risk factors. Arch Intern Med 1994;154:311.

61. Schlegel SI. General characteristics of nonsteroidal anti-inflammatory drugs. In: Paulus HE, Furst DE, Dromgoole S (eds) Drugs for rheumatic disease. New York, Churchill Livingstone, 1987, p 203.
62. Jones AC, Doherty M. The treatment of osteoarthritis. Br J Clin Pharmacol 1992;33:357.
63. Rainsford KD, Ying C, Smith FC. Effects of meloxicam, compared with other NSAIDs, on cartilage proteoglycan metabolism, synovial prostaglandin E2, and production of interleukins 1, 6 and 8 in human and porcine explants in organ culture. J Pharm Pharmacol 1997;49:991.
64. Kawaguchi H, Pilbeam CC, Harrison JR, Raisz LG. The role of prostaglandins in the regulation of bone metabolism. Clin Orthop Relat Res 1995;313:36.
65. Ho ML, Chang JK, Chuang LY, Hsu HK, Wang GJ. Effects of nonsteroidal anti-inflammatory drugs and prostaglandins on osteoblastic function. Biochem Pharmacol 1999;58:983.
66. Jiang Y, Zhao J, Genant HK, Dequeker J, Geusens P. Bone mineral density and biomechanical properties of spine and femur in ovariectomized rats treated with naproxen. Bone 1998;22:509.
67. Saino H, Matsuyama T, Takada J, Kaku T, Ishi S. Long-term treatment with indomethacin reduces vertebral bone mass and strength. J Bone Miner Res 1997;12:1844.
68. Dubois RN, Abramson SB, Crofford L, et al. Cyclooxygenase in biology and disease. FASEB J 1998;12:1063.

Chapter 108

Leukotriene Inhibitors

Sally E. Wenzel

Inflammation is likely the most significant contributing factor to the symptoms and physiologic changes of asthma. As part of this inflammatory process, activation of the arachidonic acid cascade leads to production of lipid mediators known as leukotrienes (LTs). These LTs are thought to play a central role in the bronchoconstriction, edema formation, and increase in mucus associated with the symptoms of asthma. In the last several years, new drugs have become available that were specifically developed to interfere with that pathway, namely, leukotriene receptor antagonists (LTRAs) and 5-lipoxygenase (5-LO) inhibitors. This is the first time that such 'designer drugs' have become available as a new option to manage chronic asthma.

THE LEUKOTRIENE PATHWAY

LTs are potent lipid mediators that have long been implicated in the pathogenesis of asthma. They are products of the metabolism of arachidonic acid, formed from phospholipids which are ubiquitous elements of cellular membranes. Phospholipids in the cell or nuclear membrane can be metabolized by enzymes, known as phospholipases, leading to the production of arachidonic acid. This arachidonic acid can then be further metabolized by a variety of pathways, including the cyclooxygenase pathway which leads to production of prostaglandins and thromboxane (and is inhibited by aspirin and other nonsteroidal anti-inflammatory compounds), and the 5-LO pathway which leads to the production of LTs[1] (Fig. 108.1). Activation of 5-LO is thought to require generalized cellular activation and the availability of arachidonic acid as substrate. It is presumed to require interactions with a protein known as 5-LO activating protein (FLAP), which is thought to channel arachidonic acid to the enzyme 5-LO.[1] In certain inflammatory cells (macrophages, neutrophils, and likely mast cells) this process is felt to occur at the nuclear (rather than the cytoplasmic) membrane.[2] 5-LO activation then leads to the production of an intermediate known as LTA_4, which can be further metabolized, depending on cell type, to LTB_4 or the cysteinyl-LTs, LTC_4, D_4 and E_4 (formerly known as slow-reacting substance of anaphylaxis).

LTs are produced almost exclusively by cells of the myeloid lineage. LTC_4 is produced primarily by mast cells, basophils, and eosinophils, cells commonly associated with asthma.[1] LTB_4 is produced primarily by neutrophils and monocyte-macrophages, and its role in asthma has been less clear. Cysteinyl-LTs are potent bronchoconstrictors (100–1000 times more potent than histamine) that enhance membrane permeability and decrease mucociliary clearance[3] (Table 108.1). In addition, inhalation of LTE_4 has recently been shown to lead to the chemoattraction of eosinophils into the lungs of asthmatics.[4] Some of this chemoattractant activity may occur through secondary activation of the eosinophil chemoattractant and activator, interleukin-5.[5] LTB_4 is a potent chemoattractant for neutrophils and eosinophils, as well as an activator of neutrophils which appears to enhance adhesion and migration of the cells through the endothelium.[3] Recently, both LTRAs and 5-LO inhibitors have been shown to decrease airway eosinophils, supporting the chemoattractant qualities of these leukotrienes.[6–8] Both cysteinyl-LTs and LTB_4 have been measured in body fluids of asthmatics, including bronchoalveolar lavage (BAL) fluid, urine, and blood.[6,9–11] The cysteinyl-LTs are increased in asthmatic BAL fluid after allergen and aspirin challenges, and at night in nocturnal asthmatics (along with LTB_4).[6,11,12] It is interesting that BAL levels of LTB4 in

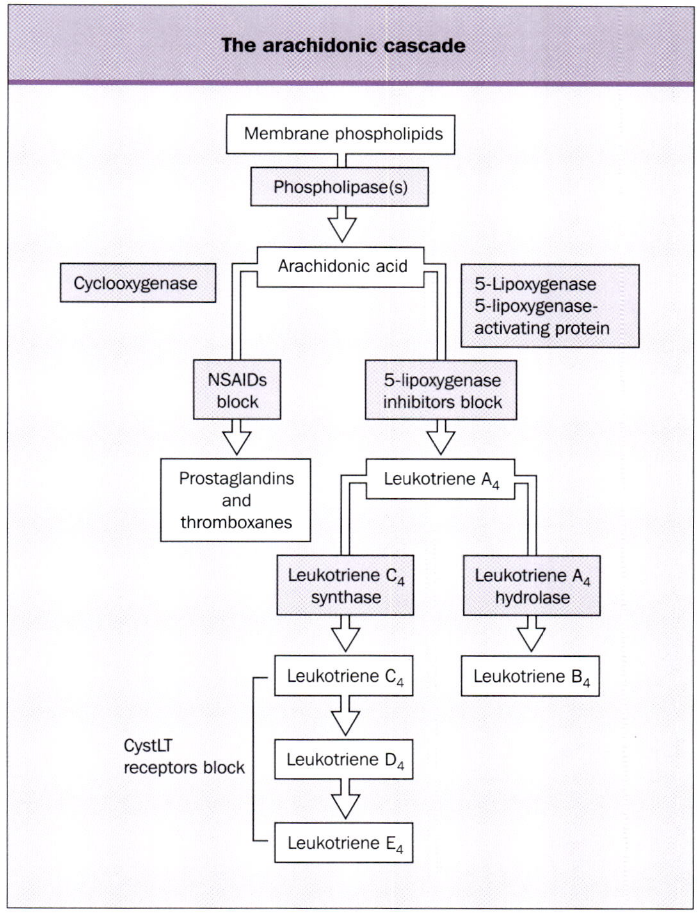

Figure 108.1 The arachidonic cascade. CystLT=cysteinyl-leukotriene receptor; NSAID=nonsteroidal anti-inflammatory drug.

Biologic properties of the leukotrienes
Cysteinyl-LTs
Bronchoconstriction
Mucus production
Decreased mucus
Decreased clearance
Vasodilation
Edema
Eosinophil chemotaxis
LTB_4
Neutrophil chemotaxis
Neutrophil migration
Neutrophil activation
Eosinophil chemotaxis

Table 108.1 Biologic properties of the leukotrienes.

nocturnal asthmatics correlate with both the eosinophil influx and fall in forced expiratory volume in 1 minute (FEV_1). The cysteinyl-LTs are also increased in urine from patients in status asthmaticus, decreasing with treatment.[9,13] Cysteinyl-LTs in humans appear to activate cells predominantly through a single receptor, known as the cysLT1 receptor. This receptor has recently been cloned, and mRNA for the receptor has been localized in airway smooth muscle cells and alveolar macrophages.[14] It is not yet known whether there are differences in the distribution or amounts of the receptor in different disease states, or whether the second LT receptor, the cysLT2 receptor, will prove to be important in human diseases. LTB_4 functions solely through the LTB_4 receptor, which was also recently cloned.[15] An extensive overview of the location of this receptor in the airways has also not been performed.

Modulation of LT activity has centered on two components of the pathway. Antagonists of the cysLT1 receptor and inhibitors of 5-LO have both undergone large-scale clinical trials (Table 108.2). The chief biologic difference between the LTRAs and the 5-LO inhibitors is that LTRAs inhibit the activity of the cysteinyl-LTs only, while 5-LO inhibitors block the production of both LTB_4 and the cysteinyl-LTs. Whether this difference has clinical applications for asthma therapy remains unclear. Both LTRAs and 5-LO inhibitors have been investigated in 'proof of concept' studies, such as allergen challenge, and in 'day-to-day' or 'chronic' asthma. To date, these agents have largely been studied in mild to moderate asthmatics, but recently data are emerging from patients with more severe illness as well.

Leukotriene antagonists and pathway inhibitors
Receptor antagonists
Block the actions of cysteinyl-leukotrienes
• Zafirlukast (Accolate®)
• Montelukast (Singulair®)
• Pranlukast (Onon®)
Pathway inhibitors
Block the production of LTB4 *and* cysteinyl-leukotrienes
• Zileuton (Zyflo®)

Table 108.2 Leukotriene antagonists and pathway inhibitors.

CLINICAL RELEVANCE

Leukotrienes

- Cysteinyl leukotrienes are produced in the lungs of asthmatics by mast cells, eosinophils, and basophils.
- Cysteinyl leukotrienes are potent bronchoconstrictors that also increase edema formation.
- Leukotrienes may contribute to the eosinophil influx in the airways of asthmatics.
- Leukotriene receptor antagonists and inhibitors improve asthma symptoms and airflow limitation.

EFFICACY IN 'PROOF OF CONCEPT' STUDIES (CHALLENGE AND BRONCHOSCOPIC STUDIES)

In recent years, LTRAs have been developed that shift the dose–response curve to inhaled LTD_4 by 30–100-fold, indicating almost complete blockade of the LT receptor.[16] 5-LO inhibitors have been developed which demonstrate greater than 80% inhibition of the 5-LO enzyme in vitro (ionophore-stimulated LTB_4 production), although the in vivo level of inhibition may be lower.[6,17] As noted previously, the clinical relevance of these different modes of action is unclear.

LT modulators effectively inhibit allergen- and aspirin-induced asthma, with modest reductions in exercise-induced bronchoconstriction (EIB) as well. While the inhibition of the late bronchoconstriction associated with allergen challenge is approximately 50%, the early phase of bronchoconstriction, which is felt to be predominantly mast cell driven, is almost completely abolished[9] (Fig. 108.2). In addition to the improvement in obstruction, the LTRA zafirlukast has demonstrated a small but significant ability

Inhibition of allergen-induced bronchoconstriction

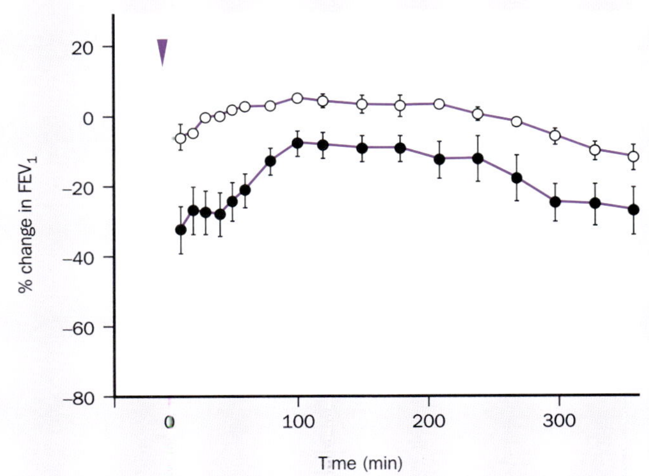

Figure 108.2 Inhibition of allergen-induced bronchoconstriction by the LTRA, zafirlukast. ● =placebo; ○=zafirlukast. (By permission from Taylor IK, Fuller RW, Dollery CT. Effect of cysteinyl-leukotriene receptor antagonist ICI 204,219 on allergen-induced bronchoconstriction and airway hyperreactivity in atopic subjects. Lancet 1991;337:690.)

to limit the increase in airway reactivity that normally occurs after allergen exposure.[9] Although there is a report of a small improvement in bronchial hyperreactivity, it is not of the same magnitude as would be seen with inhaled corticosteroids.[18,19] Of note, eosinophil numbers in sputum during the time of the late-phase response have not been reported to decrease (from placebo) following treatment with the receptor antagonist montelukast, despite 50% inhibition of the airflow limitation associated with the late phase.[20] Therefore, the mechanism behind the improvement in the late-phase response with this class of drugs is not clear.

Bronchoconstriction associated with aspirin challenge has also been almost completely prevented by LTRAs and 5-LO inhibitors, confirming the importance of LTs in the bronchospasm associated with the aspirin reaction.[21,22] Studies utilizing 5-LO inhibitors in this population have demonstrated an associated reduction in urinary LTE_4 excretion, and, intriguingly, a reduction in nasal tryptase levels as well.[22] Longer-term studies of aspirin-sensitive asthmatics also support the efficacy of chronic dosing in this population.[23] These populations of more severe asthmatics had incremental improvements in FEV_1 and symptoms with the further addition of a 5-LO inhibitor or a cysteinyl-LT receptor antagonist, despite treatment with inhaled, as well as oral, corticosteroids. Studies with the 5-LO inhibitor zileuton demonstrated improvement in nasal/sinus symptoms as well.[23]

The bronchoconstriction associated with exercise is inhibited consistently by LTRAs, in the range of 30–50%. This inhibition appears to compare favorably to pretreatment with cromolyn.[24] A long-term study with montelukast demonstrated sustained protection against exercise-induced bronchospasm (EIB) over the 12 weeks of the study, when montelukast was taken 16–18 hours prior to exercise.[25] These results compared favorably and significantly to outcomes with salmeterol in a recent long-term study of protection against EIB. Long-term use of salmeterol, as suggested by previously published studies, led to a reduction in protection against EIB over time, while the protection afforded by the LTRA montelukast was maintained throughout the course of the study.[26,27]

The effect of leukotriene inhibitors on inflammation in the airways has only recently been described, with the first published biopsy study and an additional report in abstract form.[28,29] Both LTRAs and 5-LO inhibitors may decrease the inflammatory cell influx into the airways after instillation of allergen. Administration of zafirlukast for one week before instillation of allergen directly into the airways of asthmatics significantly decreased the influx of basophils and lymphocytes into the airways 48 hours after allergen exposure, when compared to placebo. Zafirlukast also tended to decrease the numbers of eosinophils migrating into the airways.[30] There was an associated decrease in airway histamine and tumor necrosis factor-α levels, although the mechanisms behind these reductions are not clear. Similar findings were seen with the 5-LO inhibitor, zileuton.[28] In contrast, however, in an *inhaled* allergen challenge model no effect on the late-phase sputum eosinophilia was seen with the LTRA montelukast.[20]

Using a nocturnal asthma model, the 5-LO inhibitor zileuton was found to decrease urinary and BAL LT levels, while improving pulmonary function and symptoms in patients with nocturnal asthma. The improvement in FEV_1 correlated with the levels of LTB_4 in the airways. Additionally, the eosinophils in the BAL and peripheral blood decreased significantly, supporting a cellular level anti-inflammatory effect.[6]

Studies of the anti-inflammatory effect in chronic asthma are also beginning to emerge. The LTRA pranlukast (available in Asia since 1995) was shown to decrease airway eosinophils in endobronchial biopsy samples after 6 weeks of therapy. However, there was no significant improvement in FEV_1 during the course of therapy.[8] A second study, utilizing sputum analysis, demonstrated a significant decrease in sputum eosinophils, following 6 weeks of therapy with montelukast.[7] Of note, subjects were screened for inclusion into the study based on a baseline elevation in sputum eosinophils. In those subjects with baseline eosinophilia, the improvement in FEV_1 with montelukast therapy was greater than in randomly selected patients. Finally, virtually all published studies of LT-modulating drugs have demonstrated a significant decrease in circulating eosinophil numbers.[6,31,32]

EFFICACY IN CHRONIC ASTHMA

Some LT modulators induce a rapid and significant immediate bronchodilating effect of between 15% and 30%.[33] With intravenous formulations (currently not available), this can occur within 20 minutes of dosing. This effect has also been seen with zileuton and high doses of zafirlukast.[34,35] These results imply that LTs are continuously present in the airways of asthmatics and are playing an important role in maintaining baseline asthmatic bronchoconstriction. In addition, concomitant treatment of these individuals with a β-agonist induces an additive effect on the bronchodilation, suggesting that the two types of compounds are working through different bronchodilating pathways.[33] Clinical trials are under way to assess the implications of this effect for treatment of status asthmaticus. Multiple long-term (3–6-month) placebo-controlled trials have been published with the LTRAs and the 5-LO inhibitor zileuton. The asthma in the patients studied has generally been mild to moderate as judged by FEV_1, medication needs, and symptom scores. In this population of asthmatics, these compounds have consistently shown both statistical and clinical efficacy, with sustained and significant improvements in FEV_1, symptom scores, and β-agonist use for the duration of the trials as compared to placebo[32,36,37] (Fig. 108.3) Nocturnal asthma symptoms also appear to be improved by these compounds. Asthma quality of life scores have been clinically and significantly improved with both montelukast and zileuton.[38] LTRAs significantly decreased the number of occasions on which study subjects needed a steroid burst.[32,39] From a health economic perspective, there were statistically significant improvements in days missed from work and school, as well as significantly decreased rates of asthma exacerbation.[31,32,37] A recent year-long study showed that the addition of zileuton to 'usual care' (inhaled steroids, theophylline, cromones) reduced the need for steroid bursts, ER visits, and hospitalizations when compared to the 'usual care' alone group.[40]

An 8-week study with montelukast (5 mg given orally in the evening) recently demonstrated safety and efficacy compared to placebo in children 6–14 years of age. Forty-three per cent of these children were already on concurrent treatment with inhaled corticosteroids (ICS).[41] The improvement in FEV_1 was in the range seen in the adult studies and was no different between those treated (or not) with ICS.

In all of the studies of the leukotriene-modulating drugs it has become clear that not all patients respond to this class of drugs, but that 50–60% of patients have a 'significant' clinical response.[31]

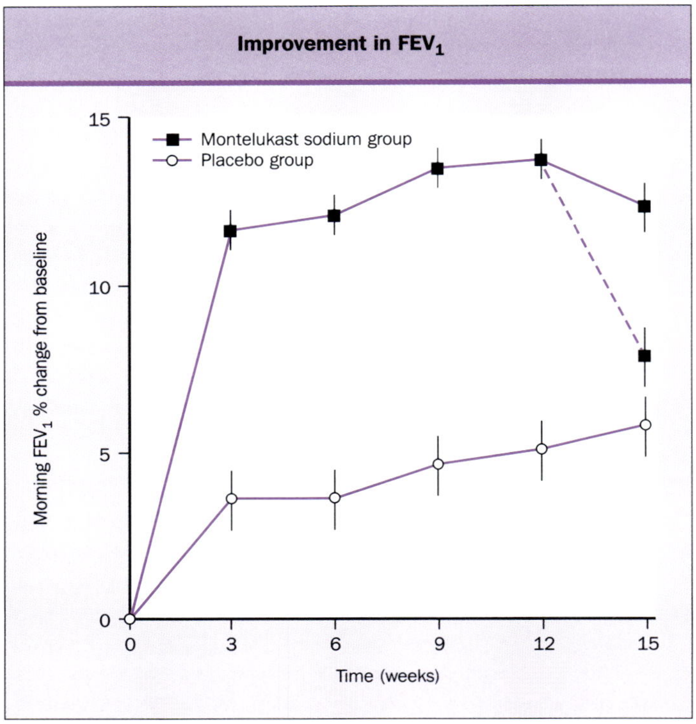

Figure 108.3 Improvement in FEV_1 with the LTRA antagonist, montelukast, as compared to placebo. (Adapted by permission from Reiss TF, Chervinsky P, Dockhorn RJ, et al. *Arch Intern Med* 1998;158:1213.)

This percentage is likely somewhat less than the percentage of responders seen for ICS. However, the reasons for this selective response pattern are not known. Recent studies suggest that certain mutations in the promoter region of the 5-LO enzyme may contribute to the level of responsiveness.[42,43] However, it is likely that a variety of other factors, including the heterogeneity of the disease of asthma, are also involved in the range of responses seen. There are currently no clinical or biomarkers available that predict which patients will respond to anti-LT therapy.

Efficacy in comparison with inhaled corticosteroids

Comparison studies to ICS have now been carried out with the LTRAs zafirlukast, montelukast, and pranlukast with remarkably similar results. All of these studies suggest that LTRAs are not as effective as low-dose beclomethasone in improving FEV_1. Generally, the improvement in FEV_1 with low-dose (400 μg) beclomethasone has been twice that seen with the LTRAs. However, less consistent differences have been seen between the two types of drugs when evaluating other outcomes, such as symptoms, β-agonist use and exacerbations.[31,44] It is interesting that the effect of both of these classes of drugs on circulating eosinophils was similar.[31] The reasons for these differing levels of effect on physiologic and clinical outcomes are not certain, but this suggests that longer-term studies are necessary to evaluate clinical differences between the two classes of drugs. It should be noted that these studies were all done in patients whose asthma could generally be classified as moderate persistent by the most recent National Heart, Lung and Blood Institute/National Asthma Education and Prevention Program (NHLBI/NAEPP) guidelines.[45] Comparisons in truly mild persistent asthmatics have not been published and are likely to be more difficult to carry out due to the normal FEV_1 at baseline. However, it is not clear whether results from moderate persistent asthma should be extrapolated to these patients with milder disease.

Efficacy as steroid-sparing or tapering agents

Finally, from a clinical efficacy perspective, recent studies with all of the LT-modulating drugs suggest that there are additional benefits to the use of these drugs in patients currently treated with inhaled corticosteroids. There is some scientific rationale to this combination, as several studies of corticosteroid use in vivo have failed to demonstrate substantial reductions in LT production.[46,47] Two published studies have confirmed the ability of LTRAs to allow clinically successful reduction in high ICS doses beyond that seen with placebo. The first study demonstrated that the concomitant use of pranlukast allowed the inhaled corticosteroid dose (1600 μg/day) to be cut to 800 μg/day in moderate asthmatics without compromising asthma control.[48] The addition of pranlukast maintained morning and evening peak flows, despite the reduced beclomethasone dose. Similarly, while patients receiving the reduced dose of beclomethasone (with placebo) had increases in peripheral blood eosinophils and exhaled nitric oxide, there were no increases in these parameters in those patients in whom pranlukast was added to the reduced ICS dose. The second study was done with montelukast. In that study, ICS were tapered from ~1600 μg/day to 1000 μg/day in a single-blind placebo run-in period. At that point, subjects were treated with montelukast or placebo. The group treated with montelukast was able to reduce ICS by another 47%, while the group on placebo reduced 30%.[49]

Questions are also beginning to emerge as to what is the best 'add-on' therapy for patients who are still symptomatic on low to moderate doses of ICS. Studies have supported the ability of long-acting β-agonists to improve both FEV_1 and exacerbation rates to a degree greater than doubling the dose of the ICS.[50,51] Similarly, a recent study with montelukast suggested that the addition of montelukast to low-dose beclomethasone improved FEV_1 to a greater degree than either agent alone.[52] Unfortunately, no comparison to either doubling the dose of the beclomethasone or to a long-acting β-agonist was included. A recent short-term (4-week) study of the addition of zafirlukast or salmeterol to patients on low-dose ICS (who remain uncontrolled) demonstrated superior efficacy of salmeterol on both symptoms and FEV_1.[53] There were no differences in exacerbations in this short-term study. Although there are some continuing concerns over an increase in inflammation following long-term ICS tapering (when done in the setting of concomitant treatment with a long-acting β-agonist), studies of larger scale and longer duration are needed to determine the best 'add-on' therapy to ICS.[54]

Long-term 'effectiveness'

Development of asthma therapies has generally centered around 'classic efficacy' studies: double-blind, placebo-controlled studies in controlled populations. ICS have performed very well in these controlled trials, yet there has been slow patient and physician buy-in to their use, and mortality and morbidity figures (especially in the USA) have not dropped concurrent with their increased use and acceptance.[55] Although longer-term, nonpharmaceutical-sponsored trials are needed, emerging data support an equal level of benefit of open-label (rather than controlled) low-dose beclomethasone as compared with that of an LTRA over a 2-year period.[41] This is in stark contrast to the superiority of ICS seen in controlled clinical trials.[31] The reasons for this difference in open-label versus double-blind controlled effect on FEV_1 and symptoms are not known, but it is likely that at least some of the effect is due to the better 'compliance/adherence' with oral as opposed to inhaled medications.[56] This preference for the oral form of the LTRA has been seen in two studies (published only in abstract form). In the first, open-label zafirlukast was preferred to inhaled beclomethasone by a 2:1 margin,[57] while in the second, the level of compliance to montelukast (vs. inhaled cromolyn) therapy in a pediatric population was also nearly twice as good.[58] Further studies in this area are needed before adequate conclusions can be drawn.

USE IN DISEASES OTHER THAN ASTHMA

None of the LT-modulating drugs is currently approved for treatment of any illness except asthma. It is possible that these drugs may have some efficacy in allergic rhinitis.[59,60] However, the results have been inconsistent. These drugs have not been formally investigated in general chronic sinusitis, but there is some indication that they may help nasal and sinus symptoms in aspirin-associated disease.[23] Anecdotal reports also exist for use in chronic urticaria and atopic dermatitis, but formal studies are lacking.

GENERAL USAGE INFORMATION

LT-modulating drugs are given orally from one to four times per day. This oral dosing may lead to better patient compliance. Zafirlukast is dosed as 20 mg orally b.i.d. (without food), montelukast 10 mg once in the evening (adults) and zileuton 600 mg q.i.d. All the clinical trials with montelukast were done with bedtime dosing. Nothing is known regarding dosing at other times of the day.

SAFETY

In general, leukotriene inhibitors appear to be well tolerated. Zileuton has a 3% incidence of elevations in ALT as compared to placebo.[32] Higher doses of zafirlukast (80 mg b.i.d.) likely have a similar effect on transaminases. No effect has been seen with montelukast.

THERAPEUTIC PRINCIPLES

Leukotriene inhibitors

- Leukotriene modulators consist of both cysteinyl leukotriene receptor antagonists and 5-lipoxygenase inhibitors.
- Approximately 50–60% of patients treated with leukotriene modulators have a good clinical response.
- Can be used with inhaled corticosteroids for added benefit.
- Side-effects are minimal:
  - — Increased liver function tests with zileuton and high-dose zafirlukast.
  - — Risk for Churg–Strauss syndrome with receptor antagonists.

All of these compounds are metabolized by the liver. Thus, the possibility for significant drug interactions with other drugs metabolized by the P450 enzyme system clearly exists, but many such interactions (e.g. with antiepileptic drugs) have not yet been reported. Zafirlukast (and to a smaller extent, zileuton) has considerable interaction with warfarin, such that the dose of warfarin will likely have to be cut by up to 50%. Zileuton is also metabolized via the specific cytochrome P450 system that metabolizes theophylline, and recommendations for concurrent use suggest decreasing the dose of theophylline by 50% and then checking a theophylline level. In addition, food appears to interfere with the absorption of zafirlukast, and the drug must be administered one hour before or after meals.

Of perhaps greatest concern is the possible association of zafirlukast with Churg–Strauss syndrome, a rare eosinophilic vasculitis. Eight patients, previously treated with a tapered regime of oral steroids, who were treated with zafirlukast were reported to present with Churg–Strauss syndrome. Since that report, further reports of Churg–Strauss syndrome have been received with both montelukast and pranlukast.[61] It is currently unclear whether this was a direct causal effect, or whether the Churg–Strauss syndrome was present previously and was unmasked when oral steroids were tapered. In fact, the majority of the patients who developed Churg–Strauss syndrome were on oral corticosteroids. More information is needed before definite conclusions can be drawn, but physicians should seriously consider complaints regarding new rashes or neurologic or worsening respiratory symptoms.[62] All of these symptoms would deserve assessment, with a minimum of a chest X-ray and eosinophil count.

HOW WILL THESE COMPOUNDS BE USED IN THE TREATMENT OF ASTHMA?

As the understanding of the long-term efficacy and safety of these LT modulators improves, our ability to place these drugs into the treatment guidelines will also improve. The initial evaluation of these drugs by the most recent (1997) NHLBI/NAEPP guidelines suggested that LT-modulating drugs could be used as alternatives to ICS in the treatment of mild persistent asthma.[45] In these particular patients, who have few symptoms and normal FEV_1, a distinct advantage of these compounds could be the oral dosing, which may lead to better compliance/adherence. Their use as single agents in moderate persistent asthma cannot be recommended at this time, due to the superiority of the effect of ICS on FEV_1 and the more complete data on long-term outcomes and anti-inflammatory effect that exist with the ICS. However, emerging data support their use as 'add-on therapy' in patients still symptomatic on ICS, or in those patients on high-dose ICS, in an attempt to taper the ICS dose. Long-term comparison studies with long-acting β-agonists are needed to determine the 'best' additional therapy, but the selection may still need to be individualized to the particular patient. These drugs should continue to be very helpful in the treatment of aspirin-sensitive asthmatics. Determination of whether any clinically significant differences exist between the LTRAs and the 5-LO inhibitors will likely require the development of better 5-LO inhibitors than the currently available drug, zileuton. Further clinical experience with the long-term disease-modifying effects of these drugs is necessary before their final place in asthma treatment guidelines is known.

KEY CONCEPTS

Leukotriene inhibitors

- Leukotrienes are inflammatory mediators involved in the pathogenesis of asthma.
- Leukotriene-modulating drugs inhibit bronchospasm caused by exercise, allergen, and aspirin challenges and may have anti-inflammatory effects.
- Leukotriene-modulating drugs improve FEV_1 and symptoms and decrease exacerbations with chronic use.
- Efficacy and effectiveness studies of long-term treatment with leukotriene-modulating drugs as compared to traditional forms of therapy are needed.

SUMMARY

LTs, lipid mediators of inflammation, have proven to be important biochemicals involved in the symptoms and physiologic changes of asthma. In the last three years, three new drugs that modulate the leukotriene pathway have completed development and are now available. The first subclass of these drugs, LTRA (zafirlukast and montelukast), block the interaction of the cysteinyl form of the leukotrienes with the cell type bearing the receptor. The second subclass, the 5-LOI (zileuton) inhibit the 5-LO enzyme and prevent the formation of both cysteinyl LTs and LTB_4. The LT modulators have shown efficacy in inhibiting the physiologic changes occurring after allergen, aspirin, and exercise challenge in asthmatics. In addition, they have shown efficacy in improving symptoms, β-agonist use and FEV_1 in chronic, 'day-to-day' asthma in patients with mild disease. Comparison studies with low doses of inhaled corticosteroids suggest that LTs have lesser effects on FEV_1, although symptom scores and exacerbation rates are similar. Finally, emerging data suggest that these drugs are beneficial in decreasing the dose of inhaled corticosteroids necessary to control more moderate to severe asthma. While long-term studies will be helpful in determining the 'disease-modifying' effects of these drugs, current data suggest that they will be useful in the treatment of a broad range of asthmatic patients.

REFERENCES

1. Henderson WR Jr. The role of leukotrienes in inflammation. Ann Intern Med 1994;121:684.
2. Brock TG, McNish RW, Bailie MB, Peters-Golden M. Rapid import of cytosolic 5-lipoxygenase into the nucleus of neutrophils after in vivo recruitment and in vitro adherence. Am Soc Biochem Mol Biol 1997;272:8276.
3. Lewis RA, Austen F, Soberman RJ. Leukotrienes and other products of the 5-lipoxygenase pathway. N Engl J Med 1990;323(10):645.
4. Laitinen LA, Laitinen A, Haahtela T, et al. Leukotriene E4 and granulocytic infiltration into asthmatic airways. Lancet 1993;341:989.
5. Underwood DC, Osborn RR, Newsholme SJ, Torphy TJ, Hay DWP. Persistent airway eosinophilia after leukotriene (LT) D4 administration in the guinea pig. Am J Respir Crit Care Med 1996;154:850.
6. Wenzel S, Trudeau J, Kaminsky D, et al. Effect of 5-lipoxygenase inhibition on bronchocontraction and airway inflammation in nocturnal asthma. Am J Respir Crit Care Med 1995;152:897.
7. Pizzichini E, Leff JA, Reiss TF, et al. Montelukast reduces airway eosinophilic inflammation in asthma: a randomized, controlled trial. Eur Respir J 1999;14:12.
8. Nakamura Y, Hoshino M, Sim JJ, et al. Effect of the leukotriene receptor antagonist pranlukast on cellular infiltration in the bronchial mucosa of patients with asthma. Thorax 1998;53:835.
9. Taylor IK, Fuller RW, Dollery CT. Effect of cysteinyl-leukotriene receptor antagonist ICI 204,219 on allergen-induced bronchoconstriction and airway hyperreactivity in atopic subjects. Lancet 1991;337:690.
10. Westcott JY, Smith HR, Wenzel SE, et al. Urinary leukotriene E4 in patients with asthma. Am Rev Respir Dis 1991;143:1322.
11. Wenzel SE, Larsen GL, Johnston K, Voelkel NF, Westcott JY. Elevated levels of leukotriene C4 in bronchoalveolar lavage fluid from atopic asthmatics after endobronchial allergen challenge. Am Rev Respir Dis 1990;142:112.
12. Szczeklik A, Sladek K, Dworski R, et al. Bronchial aspirin challenge causes specific eicosanoid response in aspirin-sensitive asthmatics. Am J Respir Crit Care Med 1996;154:1608.
13. Westcott JY, Johnston K, Batt RA, Wenzel SE, Voelkel NF. Measurement of peptidoleukotrienes in biologic fluid. J Appl Physiol 1990;68:2640.
14. Lynch KR, O'Neill GP, Liu Q, et al. Characterization of the human cysteinyl leukotriene CysLT1 receptor. Nature 1999;399:789.
15. Yokomizo T, Izumi T, Chang K, Takuwa Y, Shimizu T. A G-protein-coupled receptor for leukotriene B4 that mediates chemotaxis. Nature 1997;387:620.
16. Smith LJ, Glass M, Minkwitz MC. Inhibition of leukotriene D4-induced bronchoconstriction in subjects with asthma: A concentration-effect study of ICI 204,219. Clin Pharmacol Ther 1993;54:430.
17. McGill KA, Busse WW. Zileuton. Lancet 1996;348:519.
18. Fujimura M, Sakamoto S, Kamio Y, Matsuda T. Effect of a leukotriene antagonist, ONO-1078, on bronchial hyperresponsiveness in patients with asthma. Respir Med 1993;87:133.
19. Bel EH, Timmers MC, Hermans J, Dijkman JH, Sterk PJ. The long-term effects of nedocromil sodium and beclomethasone dipropionate on bronchial responsiveness to methacholine in nonatopic asthmatic subjects. Am Rev Respir Dis 1990;141:21.
20. Diamant Z, Hiltermann JT, Van Resen ELJ, et al. The effect of inhaled leukotriene D4 and methacholine on cell differentials in sputum from patients with asthma. Am J Respir Crit Care Med 1997;155:1247.
21. Christie P, Smith C, Lee TH. The potent and selective sulfidopeptide leukotriene antagonist, SK&F 104353 inhibits aspirin induced asthma. Am Rev Respir Dis 1991;144:957.
22. Fischer AR, Rosenberg MA, Lilly CM, et al. Direct evidence for a role of the mast cell in the nasal response to aspirin in aspirin-sensitive asthma. J Allergy Clin Immunol 1994;94:1046.
23. Dahlen B, Nizankowska E, Szczeklik A, et al. Benefits from adding the 5-lipoxygenase inhibitor Zileuton to conventional therapy in aspirin-intolerant asthmatics. Am J Respir Crit Care Med 1998;157:1187.
24. Robuschi M, Riva E, Fuccella L, et al. Prevention of exercise-induced bronchoconstriction by a new leukotriene antagonist (SK&F 104353). Am Rev Respir Dis 1992;145:1285.
25. Leff JA, Busse WW, Pearlman D, et al. Montelukast, a leukotriene-receptor antagonist, for the treatment of mild asthma and exercise-induced bronchoconstriction. N Engl J Med 1998;339:147.
26. Nelson JA, Strauss L, Skowronski M, et al. Effect of long term salmeterol treatment on exercise-induced asthma. N Engl J Med 1998;339:141.

27. Villaran C, O'Neill SJ, Helbling A, et al. Montelukast versus salmeterol in patients with asthma and exercise-induced bronchoconstriction. J Allergy Clin Immunol 1999;104:547.
28. Kane GC, Tollino M, Pollice M, et al. Insights into IgE-mediated lung inflammation derived from a study employing a 5-lipoxygenase inhibitor. Prostaglandins 1995;50:1.
29. Calhoun WJ, Lavins BJ, Minkwitz MC, et al. Effect of zafirlukast (Accolate) on cellular mediators of inflammation. Am J Respir Crit Care Med 1998;157:1381.
30. Calhoun WJ, Lavins BJ, Glass M. Effect of Accolate® (Zafirlukast) on bronchoalveolar lavage fluid (BAL) after segmental antigen bronchoprovocation (SBP) in patients with mild to moderate asthma. Am J Respir Crit Care Med 1995;151:Abstract 42.
31. Malmstrom K, Rodriguez-Gomez G, Guerra J, et al. Oral montelukast, inhaled beclomethasone, and placebo for chronic asthma. Ann Intern Med 1999;130:487.
32. Liu MC, Dube LM, Lancaster J, Group ZS. Acute and chronic effects of a 5-lipoxygenase inhibitor in asthma: a 6-month randomized multicenter trial. J Allergy Clin Immunol 1996;98:859.
33. Gaddy J, Margolskee D, Bush R, Williams VC, Busse WW. Bronchodilation with a potent and selective leukotriene D4 (LTD4) receptor antagonist (MK-571) in patients with asthma. Am Rev Respir Dis 1992;146:303.
34. Israel E, Rubin P, Kemp J, et al. The effect of inhibition of 5-lipoxygenase by Zileuton in mild-to-moderate asthma. Ann Intern Med 1993;119(11):1059.
35. Bateman ED, Aitchison JA, Summerton L, Harris A. The early onset of action of zafirlukast (Accolate®) in patients with asthma. Am J Respir Crit Care Med 1997;155:Abstract 663.
36. Spector SL, Smith LJ, Glass M. Effects of 6 weeks of therapy with oral doses of ICI 204,219, a leukotriene D4 receptor antagonist, in subjects with bronchial asthma. Am J Respir Crit Care Med 1994;150:618.
37. Suissa S, Dennis R, Ernst P, Sheehy O, Wood-Dauphinee S. Effectiveness of the leukotriene receptor antagonist zafirlukast for mild-to-moderate asthma. A randomized, double-blind, placebo-controlled trial. Ann Intern Med 1997;126(3):177.
38. Reiss TF, Chervinsky P, Edwards T, et al. Montelukast (MK-0476), a cysLT, receptor antagonist, improves asthma outcomes over a 3-month treatment period. Am J Respir Crit Care Med 1997;155:A662.
39. Barnes NC, Black B, Syrett N, Cohn J. Reduction of exacerbations of asthma in multinational clinical trials of zafirlukast (Accolate™). Am J Respir Crit Care Med 1996;153 part 2:Abstract 802.
40. Lazarus SC, Lee TM, Wright S, et al. Secondary outcomes analysis of zileuton plus usual care vs. usual care alone in the treatment of patients with asthma. Ann Allergy Asthma Immunol 1997;78(1):94.
41. Knorr B. Evaluation of long-term effect of montelukast in adult and pediatric patients. Eur Respir J 1999;14:290s.
42. In KH, Asano K, Beier D, et al. Naturally occurring mutations in the human 5-lipoxygenase gene promoter that modify transcription factor binding and reporter gene transcription. J Clin Invest 1997;99:1130.
43. Drazen JM, Yandava CN, Dube L, et al. Pharmacogenetic association between ALOX5 promoter genotype and the response to anti-asthma treatment. Nat Genet 1999;22:168.
44. Wenzel S, Chervinsky P, Kerwin E, et al. Oral Pranlukast (Ultair®) vs inhaled beclomethasone: results of a 12-week trial in patients with asthma. Am J Respir Crit Care Med 1997;155:Abstract 203.
45. National Asthma Education and Prevention Program Expert Panel Report 2: Guidelines for the Diagnosis and Management of Asthma, 1997. Publication No. 97–4051.
46. Dworski R, Fitzgerald GA, Oates JA, Sheller JR. Effect of oral prednisone on airway inflammatory mediators in atopic asthma. Am J Respir Crit Care Med 1994;149:953.
47. O'Shaughnessy KM, Wellings R, Gillies B, Fuller RW. Differential effects of fluticasone propionate on allergen-evoked bronchoconstriction and increased urinary leukotriene E4 excretion. Am Rev Respir Dis 1993;147:1472.
48. Tamaoki J, Kondo M, Sakai N. Leukotriene antagonist prevents exacerbation of asthma during reduction of high-dose inhaled corticosteroid. Am J Respir Crit Care Med 1997;155:1235.
49. Lofdahl C-G, Reiss TF, Leff JA, et al. Randomised, placebo controlled trial of effect of a leukotriene receptor antagonist, montelukast, on tapering inhaled corticosteroids in asthmatic patients. BMJ 1999;319:87.
50. Pauwels RA, Lofdahl C-G, Postma DS, et al. Effect of inhaled formoterol and budesonide on exacerbations of asthma. N Engl J Med 1997;337:1405.
51. Greening AP, Ind PW, Northfield M, Shaw G. Added salmeterol versus higher-dose corticosteroid in asthma patients with symptoms on existing inhaled corticosteroid. Lancet 1994;344:219.
52. Laviolette M, Malmstrom K, Lu S, et al. Montelukast added to inhaled beclomethasone in treatment of asthma. Am J Respir Crit Care Med 1999;160:1.
53. Busse W, Nelson H, Wolfe J, et al. Comparison of inhaled salmeterol and oral zafirlukast in patients with asthma. J Allergy Clin Immunol 1999;103:1075.
54. McIvor RA, Pizzichini E, Turner MO, et al. Potential masking effects of salmeterol on airway inflammation in asthma. Am J Respir Crit Care Med 1998;158:924.
55. Sly RM, O'Donnell R. Stabilization of asthma mortality. Ann Allergy Asthma Immunol 1997;78:347.
56. Kelloway JS, Wyatt RA, Adlis SA. Comparison of patients' compliance with prescribed oral and inhaled asthma medications. Arch Intern Med 1994;154:1349.
57. Ringdal N, Whitney JG, Summerton L. Problems with inhaler technique and patient preference for oral therapy – tablet zafirlukast vs inhaled beclomethasone. Am J Respir Crit Care Med 1998;157:A416.
58. Volovitz B, Duenas-Meza E, Chmielewska-Szewczyk D, et al. Montelukast vs cromolyn for treatment of 6–11 year old children with asthma. Am J Respir Crit Care Med 1999;159:A140.
59. Knapp HR. Reduced allergen-induced nasal congestion and leukotriene synthesis with an orally active 5-lipoxygenase inhibitor. N Engl J Med 1990;323:1745.
60. Donnelly AL, Glass M, Minkwitz MC, Casale TB. The leukotriene D4-receptor antagonist, ICI 204,219, relieves symptoms of acute seasonal allergic rhinitis. Am J Respir Crit Care Med 1995;151:1734.
61. Wechsler ME, Pauwels R, Drazen JM. Leukotriene modifiers and Churg–Strauss syndrome. Drug Safety 1999;21:241.
62. Wechsler ME, Garpestad E, Flier SR, et al. Pulmonary infiltrates, eosinophilia, and cardiomyopathy following corticosteroid withdrawal in patients with asthma receiving zafirlukast. JAMA 1998;279:455.

Chapter 109 Antihistamines

Philip Lieberman

INTRODUCTION

Since the last edition of this text there have been dynamic changes in the employment of the 'second-generation' antihistamines. Two of these, terfenadine and astemizole, have been withdrawn from the American market. In their place three new antihistamines – cetirizine, fexofenadine, and azelastine – have appeared for the therapy of rhinitis. Three new antihistamines approved for ocular use in the therapy of allergic conjunctivitis have been released: levocabastine, olopatadine, and ketotifen. In addition, over the last several years, a body of knowledge concerning potentially beneficial nonantihistaminic activities ('antiallergic activities') of antihistamines has been developed and further strides in our knowledge of the binding kinetics and bindings sites of the antihistamines on the histamine receptor has accumulated. This chapter will features a discussion of these newer 'second-generation' antihistamines, the 'antiallergic activity' of antihistamines, and to some extent the nature of the binding of antihistamines to the H_1 receptor.

HISTORICAL PERSPECTIVE

Histamine (β-imidazolethylamine) was first found in an extract of ergot, where it appeared as a result of bacterial activity. Shortly after the turn of the century, Dale and Laidlaw[1] defined its pharmacologic activity as a smooth muscle stimulant and a vasodepressor agent. They made the observation that the activities of histamine were similar to those observed in experimental anaphylaxis in animals. In 1927, Best, Dale, Dudley, and Thorpe established histamine as a naturally occurring chemical in tissue by isolating it from lung and liver.[2] At about the same time Lewis et al[3] identified a substance they named 'H-substance' that produced a wheal-and-flare reaction in skin. It was soon recognized that H-substance was identical to histamine. In 1932, Weiss et al[4] first described the pharmacologic effects of histamine infusion in humans. These observations established histamine as a mediator of immediate hypersensitivity reactions and the need to develop therapeutic agents capable of antagonizing its effects. The first such agent was synthesized in 1937 by Staub and Bovet, but this drug, 929-F, was too toxic for human use.[5] Further efforts to synthesize antihistamines resulted in the first clinically applicable drug, phenbenzamine (Antergan) in 1942, which was rapidly followed by the production of pyrilamine (Neo-antergan) which is still in use today.[6] In the late 1970s and early 1980s, the development of nonsedating antihistamines ensued, and the first nonsedating antihistamine, terfenadine, became available in the USA in 1985.

In 1966, Ash and Schild made the observation that antihistamines did not block all the activities of histamine, especially gastric acid secretion, and postulated the existence of a second histamine (H_2) receptor.[7] In 1972, Black et al[8] experimentally confirmed Ash and Schild's postulations by establishing the existence of the H_2 receptor.

HISTAMINE

Histamine is found widely distributed through the body, with highest concentrations in the lung, skin, and gastrointestinal tract. The vast majority of histamine is found in mast cells and basophils. However, histamine formation and storage also occurs in the central nervous system, epidermal cells, gastric mucosa, and rapidly growing tissue.

Histamine is involved in several physiologic and pathologic processes. It is a chemical neurotransmitter of the central nervous system, it regulates the microcirculation, and it stimulates gastric acid secretion. Most of the actions of histamine are mediated by three receptor types (H_1, H_2, H_3). Other, less well defined histamine receptors (non-H_1, non-H_2, non-H_3) also exist and these may play a role in transfer of intracellular messages.[9]

H_1 receptors are most important in the production of the symptoms of immediate hypersensitivity reactions. The major effects produced by stimulation of H_1 receptors include contraction of bronchial smooth muscle, stimulation of peripheral nerve endings to produce pruritus and pain, stimulation of the vagus nerve endings with the production of reflex bronchoconstriction and cough, and induction of increased vascular permeability.

The most important actions mediated through the H_2 receptor are an increase in gastric acid production, a down-regulation of a number of immunologic and pro-inflammatory responses, and a direct effect on the heart. The combination of H_1 and H_2 receptor stimulation is necessary for the maximal expression of effects such as peripheral vasodilatation (producing flushing, headaches, hypotension) and the induction of mucus secretion.

The H_3 receptor is a presynaptic receptor that, upon stimulation with histamine, exerts a negative feedback on histamine synthesis and release from nerve endings. As such, it plays a role in the inhibition of histamine synthesis in the central nervous system, lung, and skin. Stimulation of this receptor can reduce peptide release from nonadrenergic, noncholinergic nerves in the airway and may also modulate cholinergic neurotransmission.[10]

Activity of histamine on target organs

It is important to understand the activity of histamine on target organ sites, especially in regard to the contribution of H_1 and H_2 receptors in the production of these responses. The rational therapy of histamine-induced disease depends on such an understanding, most notably in the treatment of symptoms related to the heart and peripheral vasculature. This is especially true regarding the therapy and prevention of anaphylactic episodes.

Vascular bed

The overall effect of histamine on the vascular bed is dilatation, which results in flushing, lowering of peripheral resistance, and a fall in systolic blood pressure. In addition there is an increase in capillary permeability, mainly caused by a separation of the endothelial cells of the postcapillary venules, exposing the permeable basement membrane. Vasodilatation is mediated by both H_1 and H_2 receptors, with maximal vasodilatation achieved by stimulation of both.

H_2 receptors exert their effect via a direct action on the vascular smooth muscle, whereas H_1 receptors exert their effect not only directly on smooth muscle but also indirectly by stimulation of endothelial cells. Endothelial cell stimulation results in the production of smooth muscle relaxing factors, which include nitric oxide and possibly prostaglandins. This indirect vasodilatory action plays an important role in the cumulative vasodilatory response mediated by H_1 receptors, and is mediated solely by the H_1 receptor.

Heart

The effect of histamine on the heart is mainly mediated through the H_2 receptor; however, the H_1 receptor also plays a significant role. The vasodilatory response to histamine results in a reflex tachycardia. In addition, histamine exerts a direct effect on the heart that is both inotropic and chronotropic. H_2 receptor stimulation increases the rate and force of both atrial and ventricular contraction, probably by enhancing calcium influx. H_1 receptor activation speeds the heart rate by hastening diastolic depolarization of the sinoatrial node. Contraction of the coronary arteries is mediated through the activity of the H_1 receptor.[11]

Extravascular smooth muscle

Histamine produces varying effects on extravascular smooth muscle, including smooth muscle contraction in the bronchial tree, mediated via the H_1 receptor. The H_1 receptor also produces modest contraction of the smooth muscle of the human uterus, whereas the H_2 receptor can produce uterine relaxation. The gastrointestinal smooth muscle response varies from species to species, but the predominant effect is contraction, which is mediated through the H_1 receptor.

Glandular secretion

An important biologic effect of histamine in hypersensitivity reactions is the excess production of mucus, which appears to be mediated through both H_1 and H_2 receptors. The H_2 receptor increases the amount of mucus glycoprotein secretion from goblet cells and bronchial glands, whereas the H_1 receptor increases the viscosity of the mucus.[10]

Immune regulation

Histamine regulation of immune and inflammatory responses is mediated through the H_2 receptor and appears to be directly related to an increase in intracellular cAMP. This results in a negative feedback on basophil (but not mast cell) histamine release.

H_1 ANTAGONISTS

For the purpose of this chapter the H_1 antagonists are divided into older, 'classical' or 'first-generation' agents, which pass the blood–brain barrier, and newer, 'second-generation', nonsedating agents, which generally do not. This classification is imperfect because some 'nonsedating' agents, which generally do not. This classification is imperfect because some 'nonsedating' agents in larger doses can produce sedation; however, in the recommended doses, there is a distinct difference between these two groups.

Classical, first-generation H_1 antagonists

Structure–function relationships and chemical classification

Although it is clear that classification schemes dependent on chemical structure are imperfect, such classification still has merit since it provides insight into mechanisms of action. This traditional classification scheme is outlined in Figures 109.1 and 109.2.

All H_1 antagonists are competitive or noncompetitive inhibitors of histamine at the target site (discussed later in this chapter). That is, their pharmacologic activity depends on preventing the binding of histamine to tissue receptors. Most, but not all, first-generation H_1 antagonists have a structural resemblance to histamine in that they contain a substituted ethylamine moiety. It was previously felt that this moiety was responsible for the competitive (or noncompetitive) binding of tissue receptor sites between the antihistamine molecule and histamine itself. However, with the development of newer agents that do not

KEY CONCEPTS

Importance of subclasses of histamine receptors

Major effects mediated by H_1 receptor
- Bronchospasm
- Pruritus
- Vascular permeability

Major effects mediated by H_2 receptors
- Gastric acid secretion
- Inotropic and chronotropic cardiac stimulation
- Immune down-regulation

Major effects mediated by both H_1 and H_2 receptors
- Vasodilation
- Mucus secretion

Structure of histamine and the basic formula of classic H_1 antagonists

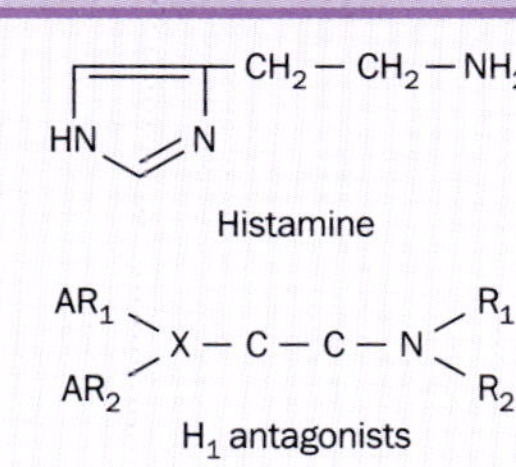

Figure 109.1 Structure of histamine and the basic formula of classic H_1 antagonists.

Structural classification of classic H_1 antagonists

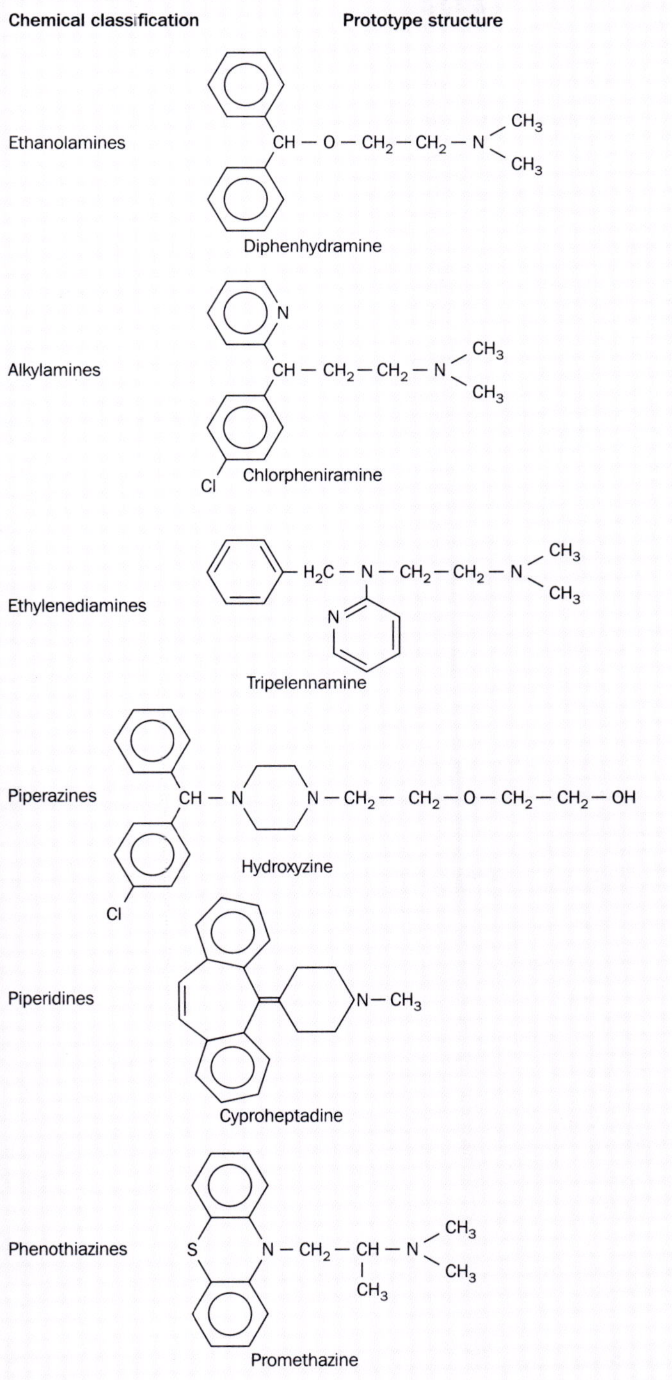

Figure 109.2 Structural classification of classic H_1 antagonists.

have an ethylamine moiety, it has become evident that antihistaminic activity does not require this shared structure.

The prototype basic structure of the ethylamine-containing first-generation H_1 antagonists (which represent the majority of drugs) is seen compared to histamine in Figure 109.1. These drugs contain the ethylamine moiety attached to aromatic substituents (AR_1, AR_2) by a nitrogen, carbon, or oxygen linkage (X). The two aromatic rings may be bridged, as in tricyclic antihistamines, or the ethylamine may actually be part of a ring structure. The aromatic substituents in these compounds make them lipid soluble, so they pass through the blood–brain barrier.

The classification of first-generation H_1 antagonists traditionally has been based on the atom linking the ethylamine grouping to the aromatic substituents (Figure 109.2). If the link is via oxygen, the drugs are ethanolamines; if via carbon, they are termed alkylamines; and if via nitrogen, they are ethylenediamines. This structural classification does not apply to piperazines, piperidines, and phenothiazines. Most authors do not include nonsedating drugs such as terfenadine and astemizole within the classification. However, both drugs have aromatic ring structures on either side of the carbon chain and from a theoretical standpoint still fall within this classification (Fig. 109.3).[2]

Drugs in each class have been said to have clinically unique and pertinent activities that distinguish their therapeutic application (Table 109.1). Ethanolamines as a group appear to have significant antimuscarinic activity and are relatively potent sedatives. The alkylamines are thought to produce the least drowsiness of any of the classical antihistamines and may induce a paradoxical central nervous system stimulation, especially in children. Those in the ethylenediamine group as a rule have less sedative activity than ethanolamines and are said to produce more gastrointestinal side-effects. The piperazines are a heterogeneous group of drugs. Some are highly sedating, and others such as cyclizine and meclizine have antiemetic and anti-motion sickness properties. As a rule, the piperidine group has low sedating potential. Cyproheptadine, a member of this group, has significant antiserotonin activity.[12] The phenothiazines have considerable anticholinergic and sedative activity, and some are antiemetics.

The existence of these unique features must be viewed with some reserve since they are not shared by all drugs within the class, and there is great patient-to-patient variability in response to these agents. The other clinical observation that has been based on this classification is the suggestion that a switch from one class to another may overcome apparent 'tolerance' after long-term administration. However the actual existence of drug tolerance has been called into question and is doubtful,[10,13] and adjustments in therapy based upon this chemical classification do not appear to be warranted.

Pharmacokinetics

The pharmacokinetic and pharmacodynamic properties of selected first-generation antagonists are compared in Table 109 2.

All first-generation H_1 receptor antagonists are rapidly absorbed after oral administration and reach peak serum

KEY CONCEPTS

Pharmacokinetics and pharmacodynamics of H_1 antagonists

- All presently available drugs are metabolized by the cytochrome P450 system in liver.
- Pharmacodynamic effects are delayed in onset when compared to serum levels.
- Pharmacodynamic effects persist for a significant period of time after serum levels decline.

Table 109.1 **Characteristics of representative first-generation H_1 antagonists based upon chemical classification.**

Characteristics of representative first-generation H_1 antagonists based upon chemical classification

Chemical class	Examples	Comments
Ethanolamines	Diphenhydramine Clemastine Carbinoxamine	Significant antimuscarinic effects. Can be potent sedatives, but sedative potential varies, with clemastine producing the least amount. Low incidence of gastrointestinal side-effects. Can have some anti-motion sickness activity. Diphenhydramine and clemastine both available over the counter
Alkylamines	Chlorpheniramine Brompheniramine Dexchlorpheniramine Triprolidine	Relatively moderate incidence of drowsiness. Moderate anticholinergic effect. No antiemetic or anti-motion sickness activity. Little gastrointestinal side-effect. All available over the counter. Occasional paradoxical central nervous system stimulation, especially in children
Ethylenediamines	Tripelennamine Pyrilamine Antazoline	Mild to moderate sedation. Slight anticholinergic effect. Some local anesthetic effect. Pyrilamine is sold over the counter and is the oldest antihistamine preparation available today. As a group, may have more frequent gastrointestinal side-effects
Piperazines	Hydroxyzine Meclizine Cyclizine	Hydroxyzine has highest sedative activity in group. Meclizine and cyclizine relatively low sedative activity with main use being for vertigo, anti-motion sickness, and antiemetic activity. Hydroxyzine has significant anticholinergic activity
Piperidines	Cyproheptadine Phenindamine Azatadine	Mild to moderate sedation. Little anticholinergic activity, antiemetic activity, and anti-motion sickness activity. Cyproheptadine has potent antiserotonin effect. As a class has relatively high incidence of paradoxical central nervous system stimulatory activity
Phenothiazines	Promethazine Methdilazine Trimeprazine	Usually highly sedating. Strong antiemetic, anticholinergic activity. Main clinical use is as antiemetics

Table 109.2 **Pharmacokinetic and pharmacodynamic characteristics of selected first-generation H_1 antagonists.** Data based on studies in healthy adults and children. Compiled from Garrison & Rall[2] and Simons & Simons.[10,15]

Pharmacokinetic and pharmacodynamic characteristics of selected first-generation H_1 antagonists

Drug	Approximate time at which peak serum concentration is reached after oral dose (hours)	Approximate half-life (hours)	Approximate duration of biologic activity (suppression wheal and flare) (hours)
Diphenhydramine	$\frac{3}{4}$–$2\frac{1}{2}$	8–9	6–10
Chlorpheniramine	$1\frac{1}{2}$–$2\frac{1}{2}$	20–24	24
Hydroxyzine	1–$2\frac{1}{2}$	20	36
Brompheniramine	2–3	24	9

concentrations in 2–3 hours when given in liquid form. Most have a duration of action of 4–6 hours, but some have longer durations of action (discussed later in this chapter). Studies of diphenhydramine suggest that H_1 antagonists are disseminated throughout the body including the central nervous system.[2] Antihistamines are secreted in breast milk, and the concentration is dependent upon serum concentration.

All first-generation H_1 antagonists are extensively metabolized in the liver, and little, if any, of these drugs is excreted unchanged in the urine. All of these agents are metabolized by the hepatic cytochrome P450 system. Clearance rates are variable and half-lives differ according to the metabolic potential of the patient; children have shorter and the elderly have longer elimination half-lives. Severe hepatic dysfunction can prolong the half-life, and suggested dosage regimens must be altered accordingly.

Pharmacodynamics

An important principle of the pharmacodynamic activity of these drugs is that their tissue effect is somewhat delayed compared to serum levels and can extend far beyond the life of the drug in the serum.[14,15] For example, a single dose of hydroxyzine significantly suppresses histamine-induced wheal and flare for 36 hours, reducing the mean flare size for as long as 60 hours despite a negligible serum concentration. Meclizine is another first-generation antihistamine that has a duration of action extending far beyond significant serum levels.[2]

Therapeutic effects can occur in doses that do not produce sedation. For example, diphenhydramine may be effective with serum concentrations as low as 25 ng/ml, whereas sedation does not seem to occur in most patients until a serum level of 50 ng/ml is reached.[16]

As noted, the tissue effect of antihistamines is delayed relative to peak serum concentrations. For hydroxyzine, maximal suppression of wheal and flare does not occur until 7 hours after mean peak serum concentrations have been reached.[15] These observations indicate that it is best to administer H_1 antagonists before allergen exposure. In addition, because of the prolonged tissue activity, the recommended 6-hour frequency for dosing many of these drugs may not be required. Finally, dosage adjustments should be considered based on clearance differences associated with extremes in age, and in the presence of liver disease.

Other pharmacologic actions

First-generation antihistamines have a number of different pharmacologic activities not related to their antihistaminic properties. One of the most prominent of these is their antimuscarinic activity. Although this can produce side-effects, it may also have a beneficial effect in drying secretions in patients suffering from rhinorrhea. They also produce α-adrenergic blocking activity, antidopaminergic (dopamine-2 receptor) activity, antiserotonergic activity, mild calcium channel blocking activity, local anesthetic properties, antiemetic and anti-motion sickness activity, and, with certain agents, the ability to prevent both in vitro and in vivo histamine release.[17,18] For example, promethazine and pyrilamine have especially prominent local anesthetic effects, and promethazine is an effective antiemetic agent.[2] Promethazine, diphenhydramine, and cyclizine can exert effects on antigen-induced histamine release.[19] The actual effect of these pharmacologic activities on the final therapeutic response is not known but may be of clinical importance.

Side-effects

By far the most common and significant side-effect of first-generation antihistamines is drowsiness. Their soporific activity can clearly be attributed to the fact that these drugs pass through the blood–brain barrier and exert their effect on the central nervous system. The exact mechanism(s) by which these drugs produce drowsiness is unknown but may include the antihistaminic, anticholinergic, anti-α-adrenergic, antiserotonergic, and/or calcium channel blocking activities. It should be noted that the antihistaminic activity does not necessarily correlate with the sedative potential, suggesting that this is not the sole mechanism producing this side-effect. The degree of sedation depends on many factors, including age, the pattern and quality of nocturnal sleep, and concurrent medication. First-generation antihistamines clearly potentiate the activity of other sedative drugs such as alcohol[20] and tranquilizers.[6] The frequency of sedation ranges between 10% and 20% and can be severe enough to limit the drug's administration.[6]

Of great importance is the fact that the *subjective degree of drowsiness does not necessarily correlate with the objective assessment of central nervous system impairment*.[21] This important concept means that patients may not notice drowsiness but still have impaired function measured objectively and, therefore, may be in danger if operating machinery or driving for example. It also places in question clinical reports that rely only on the self-awareness of drowsiness to assess the sedative effect of antihistamines. Although drowsiness can be overcome by the exertion of will, impairment of cognitive function and psychomotor performance cannot and will persist until the effect of the drug abates.[22] Since these drugs can produce impairment without sedation and inhibit performance on tests of psychomotor reflexes and driving skills, civilian and military aircraft pilots are prohibited from taking these drugs while flying.[6]

Paradoxical central nervous system stimulation can be encountered in some patients, especially children. Other less common central nervous system side-effects include dizziness, tinnitus, blurred vision, and tremors. The next most frequent group of side-effects is those produced by the antimuscarinic actions of first-generation antihistamines. These include dryness of the mouth, urinary retention and dysuria, blurring of vision, and constipation. Other side-effects are uncommon and include loss of appetite, nausea, abdominal pain, and diarrhea. Drug allergy to antihistamines has been reported. Leukopenia, agranulocytosis, and hemolytic anemia are extremely rare. Although teratogenic effects have been noted in animals, there has been no documentation of these in humans.

Acute toxicity resulting from overdose can produce central nervous system effects, including hallucinations, central nervous system excitement, profound sedation, ataxia, incoordination, and convulsions. Other findings are fixed and dilated pupils, as well as the frequent finding of sinus tachycardia and, less commonly, ventricular arrhythmias. The anticholinergic effects of dry mouth and urinary retention are usually observed and fever may be present. Fatal overdose reactions have occurred with profound coma and respiratory collapse.

> **CLINICAL PEARLS**
>
> **Side-effects of first-generation H_1 antagonists**
> - Drowsiness
> - Potentiates effects of alcohol, tranquilizers
> - Impaired motor skills – driving, flying
> - Paradoxical hyperactivity in some children
> - Dryness of mouth
> - Urinary retention, constipation

Nonsedating, second-generation antihistamines

This discussion will be limited to the second-generation antihistamines presently available in the USA. These include loratadine, cetirizine, and fexofenadine which are administered orally for the treatment of allergic rhinitis and allergic skin disease, azelastine which is administered by nasal spray for the treatment of allergic and nonallergic rhinitis, and three drugs – levocabastine, olopatadine, and ketotifen – which are available for intraocular administration to treat allergic conjunctivitis. The term 'nonsedating' is actually somewhat of a misnomer since some of these drugs (cetirizine and azelastine) do not have an FDA nonsedating label, and others such as loratadine can be sedating when given in amounts exceeding the recommended dose.[17]

These drugs are not as easily classified by structure as are the first-generation antihistamines because they do not always contain an ethylamine side chain. Therefore, the postulated structure–function relationships for first-generation antihistamines do not, in general, apply to this group of drugs. Nonsedating antihistamines are of diverse chemical structure, and many can be considered drugs with multiple pharmacologic effects in addition to their antihistaminic activity.

In fact, these drugs are not all competitive antagonists of histamine. For example, ketotifen is a noncompetitive histamine (H_1) receptor antagonist that binds to a site separate from that to which histamine binds on the H_1 receptor and therefore sterically hinders the binding of histamine. This is an important concept since a noncompetitive inhibitor cannot be displaced by histamine. Although the exact binding site of azelastine has not been demonstrated, on the basis of its structure and other activities it is also most likely a noncompetitive histamine antagonist.

Even though cetirizine and azelastine do not have FDA approval as nonsedating, they clearly appear to be less sedating than 'classical' antihistamines. Numerous studies have demonstrated that all of the second-generation drugs produce less significant subjective sedation or objectively assessed impairment of function.[23] Many factors may account for the lack of sedation of these agents, but the most important seems to be the fact that they do not pass through the blood–brain barrier.

Another postulated mechanism for the lack of sedation in this class of drugs is their relative specificity for the H_1 receptor. In general, compared to first-generation antihistamines, they are highly specific for the H_1 receptor and show little or no binding to muscarinic, 5-hydroxytryptaminergic, and α-adrenergic receptors. In addition, it has been suggested that they have a greater affinity for peripheral rather than central H_1 receptors.[17]

Pharmacokinetics for second-generation antihistamines

There are certain nuances that distinguish the pharmacokinetic profiles of these drugs. However, for the most part, generalizations can be made about the pharmacokinetics of these agents.[23–26]

The second-generation antihistamines can be viewed from one perspective as having similar, ring-structure, core moieties (Fig. 109.3) and therefore it appears to be the side chains joining the cores that may determine the absorption, elimination, and distribution of each agent.[27] The distinctive pharmacokinetic profiles are summarized in Table 109.3.

All second-generation H_1 antagonists are well absorbed, and peak plasma concentrations are reached within a few hours after administration. They all appear to be well distributed into body tissues. Most are highly protein bound in both circulation and tissue. Terminal elimination half-lives range from approximately 7 to 22 hours for the drugs under discussion.

Loratadine and azelastine undergo extensive first-pass metabolism by the cytochrome P450 system in the liver. Shortly after single doses of these drugs the concentration of the metabolites is greater than that of the parent drug. In both instances the metabolites have antihistamine activity.[26] On the other hand, neither cetirizine nor fexofenadine undergoes extensive liver metabolism and neither has active metabolites. The majority of these drugs are excreted unchanged in the feces and urine.

The P450 isoforms responsible for the metabolism of loratadine are known (CYP3A4 and CYP2D6) whereas the isoform responsible for the metabolism of azelastine has not been established.

Structures of selected second generation antihistamines

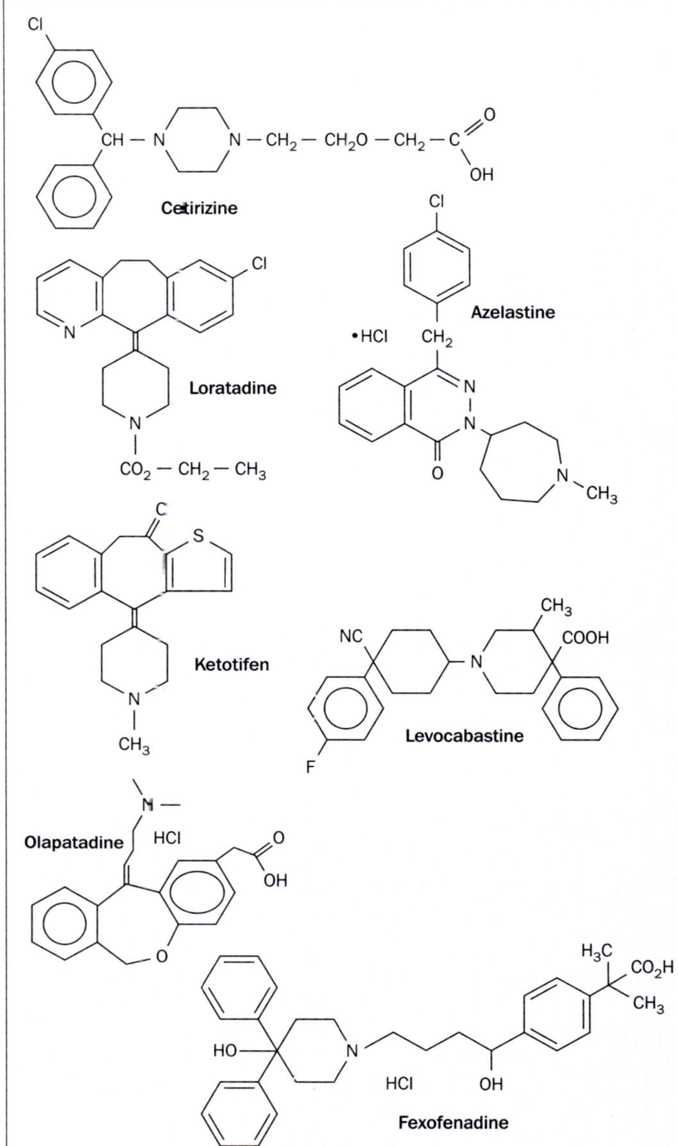

Figure 109.3 Structures of selected 'second-generation' antihistamines.

Single dose pharmacokinetics of selected second-generation antihistamines in healthy adults

Drug	Major metabolite	Activity of metabolite	Dose (mg)	T_{max} (h)	Effect of food on absorption	T 1/2 (h)	Plasma protein bound %	Excretion % feces	Excretion % urine	Hepatic metabolism
Loratadine	Descarboethoxy	4 × parent	10 q.d.	1.2 ± 0.3 (1.5 ± 0.7)	Increase	7.8 ± 4.2 (24 ± 9.8)	97–99	40	40	CYP3A4 (P450) CYP2D6 (P450)
Cetirizine	None	NA	10 q.d.	1.0 ± 0.5	None	7–10	93	10	70	Not significant
Fexofenadine	None	NA	60 b.i.d.	1.3–2.6	Decrease	14.4	60–70	80	11	Not significant
Azelastine	Desmethyl	Relative potency unknown	0.55 b.i.d.	2–3	Not applicable	22 (54)	78–88	75	24	P450 (isoform unknown)

Table 109.3 Single dose pharmacokinetics of selected second-generation antihistamines in healthy adults.

Of recent interest regarding the pharmacokinetics of antihistamines is the multidrug resistance transporter system, P-glycoprotein. This system is responsible for active transport of medications, limiting their absorption from the gastrointestinal tract and entrance into the central nervous system. In the intestine, the system transports molecules from the cell into the lumen, and in the CNS it prevents drugs from entering the central nervous system. P-glycoprotein regulation of drug plasma levels appears to be linked to the CYP3A4-P450 isoform. It appears to be responsible for transport of drugs that are metabolized by this P450 isoform; these include erythromycin, ketoconazole, quinidine, and verapamil. Thus far this system has not been shown to exert clinically important effects on the metabolism of second-generation antihistamines, however it appears to be responsible for the increase in plasma levels of fexofenadine when this drug is administered in conjunction with ketoconazole or erythromycin. Erythromycin increases the bioavailability of fexofenadine by 103% and ketoconazole increases it by 159%. Both erythromycin and ketoconazole appear to interfere with the external transport of fexofenadine via the P-glycoprotein system of the gut.[26,28]

Pharmacodynamics

The pharmacodynamic principles for second-generation antihistamines are similar to those for first-generation drugs. The pharmacodynamic profiles of selected second-generation antihistamines are seen in Table 109.4. Tissue activity is slightly delayed compared to serum levels, but, as a rule, tissue concentrations reach maximum level rapidly after oral administration, with cutaneous wheal-and-flare suppression occurring within two hours.[29,30] In addition, activity in tissue may extend beyond the presence of detectable blood levels.[26] Peak tissue activity usually occurs 5–8 hours after oral administration of a single dose. The maximum activity can last for several hours, even, as noted, when plasma concentrations have declined significantly. This indicates either the presence of active metabolites in the tissue or perhaps high tissue-binding affinity and/or avidity. This accounts for an important clinical phenomenon, the persistence of tissue activity after the discontinuation of the drug. This is of note for allergy evaluation by cutaneous testing. In most instances there is some suppression of wheal and flare for at least 24 hours after the drug is discontinued. Of the agents considered in this chapter, loratadine seems to account for the longest duration of suppression (7 days).[26]

One notable fact is that, using histamine-induced wheal and flare suppression as a model, there appears to be no tachyphylaxis or tolerance resulting from the long-term administration of second-generation H_1 antagonists.[31,32]

Pharmacodynamics of selected second-generation antihistamines based on suppression of histamine-induced wheal and flare

	Onset (h)	Duration of action (h)	Persistence of tissue activity after cessation of regular administration (days)
Loratadine	3	24	7
Cetirizine	0.7	>24	3
Fexofenadine	2	24	2
Azelastine	1	12	2

Table 109.4 Pharmacodynamics of selected second-generation antihistamines based on suppression of histamine-induced wheal and flare.

Antiallergic, anti-inflammatory effects

There has been recent interest in the potentially beneficial effects of second-generation antihistamines that are unrelated to their antihistaminic activity. In fact, three agents, azelastine, ketotifen, and oxatomide, have been classified specifically as 'H_1 receptor antagonists used primarily for their antiallergic effects'.[33] Azelastine and ketotifen were originally employed as agents for the therapy of asthma and have been shown to exert significant, albeit modest, beneficial effects and anti-inflammatory activity when employed for the treatment of this condition.[33] Second-generation antihistamines have demonstrated 'antiallergic-anti-inflammatory' activity in numerous spheres.[34–39] Perhaps the best known of these activities relates to the ability of antihistamines to inhibit mediator release from both mast cells and basophils. This has been demonstrated for a number of agents, both in vitro[34] and in vivo.[40] Suppression of mast cell degranulation has been demonstrated for both immunologic and nonimmunologic stimuli including allergen, anti-IgE, 4880, substance P, calcium ionophore A23187, and concanavalin A. There is some variation regarding the effects of individual antihistamines in each system. For example, in human lung mast cells, ketotifen has been reported to be an effective inhibitor of the release of leukotrienes but a poor inhibitor of histamine release, whereas azelastine has been reported to inhibit the release of both mediators.[34] Studies of the prevention of mediator release after allergen nasal challenge also demonstrate similar selective effects.[40]

Antihistamines can also regulate the migration and activation of inflammatory cells. They have been shown, in several systems, to prevent both influx of eosinophils and neutrophils to sites of inflammation. The accumulation of these cells may be inhibited by a down-regulation of the expression of adhesion molecules[36] or by a direct antichemotactic effect.[34] In addition they can prevent cell activation and cytokine secretion as well as the production of superoxide radicals and the generation of leukotrienes.[34]

The exact mechanism of production of these antiallergic-anti-inflammatory effects is unknown. Of particular interest, however, is the effect of azelastine on the expression of mRNAs for IL-1β IL-6, GM-CSF, and TNF-α in human peripheral blood leukocytes and monocytes. Azelastine can suppress the production of these agents by blocking the activation of NF-KB.[41] Other postulated mechanisms include suppression of signal transduction and interference with calcium channels. However at this time the exact mechanism of action of these anti-inflammatory effects remains undetermined.

In addition, their clinical significance has not been established. In most of the in vitro studies the concentrations of the agents used are above those achieved clinically. However, based on at least one study of azelastine, demonstrating the effectiveness of this drug in chronic nonallergic rhinitis,[42] a condition probably not mediated by histamine in most instances, it can be assumed that some of the nonantihistamine antiallergic effects of this drug are of clinical importance.

THERAPEUTIC PRINCIPLES

Second-generation antihistamines having anti-inflammatory, antiallergic effects may be of clinical significance due to:
- Prevention of mast cell degranulation
- Down-regulation of adhesion molecules
- Decreased chemotaxis
- Reduction in cytokine secretion
- Reduction in superoxide radicals
- Decreased synthesis of leukotrienes

Specific agents available in the USA at this time

Loratadine

Loratadine is a derivative of azatadine. Its structure resembles that of the tricyclic antidepressants. It is more polar and less basic than the parent compound because of the addition of a carboxyethyl ester moiety. This modification decreases the central nervous system penetration of the drug. Loratadine does not contain an ethylamine grouping and therefore has no structural resemblance to histamine. It acts via competitive inhibition despite the fact that it does not have the ethylamine group, which calls into question the functional role of this structure and suggests that it is not a sine qua non for antihistamine activity. However, the nature of the interaction between loratadine and the receptor site is unknown. Loratadine is well absorbed, with a mean peak concentration after a 10 mg dose of 4.7 ng/ml. It is extensively metabolized by first-pass mechanism in the liver generating descarbethoxyloratadine, an active antihistamine that is four times more potent than loratadine itself. Peak serum concentrations of loratadine appear 1–2 hours after dosing, and peak serum concentrations of descarbethoxyloratadine appear $1\frac{1}{2}$ to $3\frac{1}{2}$ hours after dosing. The elimination half-life of loratadine is 8–14 hours and that of its metabolite is 17–24 hours, which accounts for the 24-hour duration of action of the drug. Wheal inhibition is detected at $1\frac{1}{2}$ hours after administration, reaches a peak at 4–6 hours, and may last 36–48 hours. There is an approximate 50% diminution in wheal and flare after a single 10 mg dose. Loratadine is relatively specific for the H_1 receptor; however, at higher doses there may be some antimuscarinic, anti-α-adrenergic, antiserotenergic, and antileukotriene activity.[17]

Cetirizine

Cetirizine is a carboxylic acid metabolite of hydroxyzine with the carboxyl group having a negative charge at physiologic pH. Absorption from the gastrointestinal tract is rapid, with a 10 mg dose producing maximum serum concentrations of 300 ng/ml 1 hour after oral administration. Cetirizine has a mean plasma half-life of approximately 8 hours and its terminal elimination half-life is nearly 25 hours. Its time course in the plasma closely parallels its wheal inhibition activity, with maximum inhibition achieved between 4 and 8 hours. The mean percentage inhibition of the histamine-induced wheal reaction is approximately 73%, and some inhibition is still detectable at 36 hours. Cetirizine is highly specific for the H_1 receptor, demonstrating no anticholinergic, antiserotonergic, or calcium channel blocking activity.

Cetirizine is not significantly metabolized in the liver. Sixty to seventy per cent of a cetirizine dose appears unchanged in the urine. Only approximately 8–10% is metabolized by the P450 cytochrome oxidase pathway.[43] This may make it the drug of choice in patients with liver disease or who are taking other drugs affecting the cytochrome P450 enzyme system. The serum elimination half-life of cetirizine is less in children than in the elderly and is markedly prolonged (19 hours) in adults with renal insufficiency.[44]

Cetirizine can reduce both the early- and late-phase cutaneous reactions to allergen injection.[45] Presumably this is due to its modulation of the migration of inflammatory cells, especially eosinophils, to the site of the reaction.[27] This anti-inflammatory activity appears to account for its ability to diminish the lesions of delayed pressure urticaria, whereas other antihistamines are normally ineffective in this regard.[46]

Fexofenadine

Fexofenadine, like cetirizine, undergoes no significant hepatic biotransformation. Approximately 80% of the dose of the drug is recovered in unchanged form in the feces, and approximately 12% in the urine. The half-life of fexofenadine in healthy adults ranges from 11 to 15 hours. The half-life in children is similar. Renal disease results in somewhat slower elimination. However this is of no clinical significance unless impairment is marked. Hepatic impairment does not affect absorption or elimination to any significant extent.

Of note is the effect of the concomitant administration of erythromycin and ketoconazole on blood levels. As noted earlier, both erythromycin and ketoconazole increase plasma levels of fexofenadine, probably because fexofenadine shares the same P-glycoprotein elimination system. However, the increase results in levels well within the tolerated range in clinical trials and therefore it is doubtful that these drug interactions are of clinical importance.[26,29]

Fexofenadine causes peak suppression of histamine-induced wheal and flare somewhere between 3 and 12 hours after its single dose administration. There is still significant suppression at 24 hours. When given for a week it can produce residual effects on histamine suppression for two days after cessation of administration.

Azelastine

Azelastine is unique among presently available antihistamines in the USA because it is administered by nasal spray. After intranasal administration systemic bioavailability of azelastine is approximately 40%. The recommended dose is two sprays each nostril b.i.d. (a total dose of approximately 1 mg per day). Intranasal administration results in maximal plasma concentrations that are achieved in 2–3 hours. At this dose the maximum blood level is approximately 1.09 ng/ml. Azelastine has an active metabolite, desmethylazelastine, which probably extends the duration of action of the drug. The half-life of the parent compound is 22 hours and that of the active metabolite 54 hours. Ten days after oral administration of a 4 mg dose of radiolabeled azelastine, approximately 24% of the radioactivity was recovered in the urine and 75% in the feces.

Azelastine has an onset of action within the first hour of administration and reaches peak activity at approximately 1–3 hours after administration. It has a duration of activity of about 12 hours.

Some suppression of histamine-induced skin wheal and flare has been seen after the intranasal administration of azelastine but this effect is probably of little clinical significance and appears to abate within 48 hours of cessation of the drug.

Azelastine is also somewhat unusual in terms of its clinical effect in that it seems to reduce nasal obstruction and appears to be effective in chronic nonallergic rhinitis.[42,47]

Although this drug is not approved by the FDA as a non-sedating agent, the incidence of sedation in clinical trials appears to be low (approximately 2–3%).[47]

Choice of agent

There is no clear-cut 'drug of choice' regarding the use of second-generation antihistamines. There are, however, some clinically distinguishing features as summarized in Table 109.5.

At the time of the preparation of this manuscript loratadine and cetirizine were both approved for use in children whereas fexofenadine and azelastine were not. However, approval for both of these drugs for use in children was under review.

Loratadine is available in three forms – a tablet, a syrup, and a dissolvable wafer. Cetirizine is available in a tablet and syrup. Fexofenadine is only available at this time in a capsule. As noted, azelastine is administered by nasal spray. Both loratadine and fexofenadine are available in a combined form with pseudoephedrine as a decongestant. Fexofenadine and loratadine are clearly non-sedating at recommended doses whereas azelastine and cetirizine have shown some sedating potential. Loratadine and cetirizine are pregnancy category B whereas fexofenadine and azelastine are pregnancy category C. Food intake actually increases loratadine bioavailability whereas it decreases that of fexofenadine. It has no effect on cetirizine. Both cetirizine and loratadine are administered once daily whereas fexofenadine, at the time of this writing, required twice-daily administration. However, it should be noted that a once-daily form of fexofenadine was being evaluated by the FDA during the preparation of this chapter. Azelastine requires twice-daily administration.

Azelastine seems to differ from the other agents in that it is effective as monotherapy in the treatment of nonallergic rhinitis and has some beneficial effect on nasal congestion.

Age, liver disease, and renal disease usually do not require the dose of any of these agents to be altered; however, severe renal impairment might require dosage adjustments for cetirizine and fexofenadine, and possibly even for loratadine. Severe liver impairment might require dosage adjustments for loratadine and cetirizine. No hepatic drug interaction has been described for any of these agents, but the co-administration, as noted, of erythromycin and ketoconazole with fexofenadine results in increased bioavailability of this antihistamine. However, this is probably of no clinical significance.

Antihistamines available only for intraocular use

In the USA, three antihistamines are available only for intraocular administration for the treatment of allergic conjunctivitis. These are ketotifen, levocabastine, and olopatadine.

Ketotifen

Ketotifen, like azelastine, has potent nonantihistamine anti-inflammatory activity. It inhibits mediator release from mast cells and basophils, degranulation of eosinophils and neutrophils, chemotaxis of eosinophils, leukotriene generation, and the generation of platelet-activating factor.[48,49]

After oral administration, ketotifen is completely absorbed with peak concentrations occurring at about 3 hours. The absorption half-life is about 1 hour. The absorbed drug is distributed extensively to circulating cells and 16–18% is bound to plasma proteins. Sixty to seventy per cent of the dose is excreted as metabolites. Both ketotifen and its metabolites appear to be largely excreted in the urine, with fecal elimination found only after the first 24 hours. Based on the above pharmacokinetic data, it is assumed that any systemically absorbed ketotifen administered by ophthalmic application would be extensively metabolized and eliminated via the urine. The recommended dosage is 1 drop every 8–12 hours. It is classified as pregnancy category C.

Clinical Profiles of Selected Second-Generation Antihistamines

Drug	Preparations available	Available with decongestant	FDA approved non-sedating	Pregnancy category	Food effect on bioavailability	Dosing frequency	Pediatric uses approved by FDA	Effect as single agent in nonallergic rhinitis	Effect on nasal congestion	Need to alter dose[a] elderly	Need to alter dose[a] liver disease	Need to alter dose[a] renal disease	Drug interaction
Loratadine	Tablet, syrup, dissolvable wafer	Yes	Yes	B	Increase	q.d.	Yes	No	Little to none	–	Possible decrease	Possibly decrease	–
Cetirizine	Tablet, syrup	No	No	B	None	q.d.	Yes	No	Little to none	–	Possibly decrease	Possibly decrease	–
Fexofenadine	Capsule	Yes	Yes	C	Decrease	b.i.d.[a]	Pending	No	Little to none	–	–	Possibly decrease	Coadministration of erythromycin or ketoconazole increases plasma level of fexofenadine (see text)
Azelastine	Nasal spray	No	No	C	None	b.i.d.	Pending	Effective	Most studies indicate beneficial effect	–	–	–	–

[a]Adjustment only suggested for moderate to severe liver or renal impairment.

Table 109.5 Clinical profiles of selected second-generation antihistamines.

Levocabastine

Levocabastine absorption from the eye occurs within 1–2 hours. The bioavailability from topical ocular administration ranges from 30% to 60%. Steady-state plasma levels after the application of a 0.05% ophthalmic suspension 1 drop 3 times a day are 1.6 μg/l. The drug has a plasma protein binding of approximately 65%.

There is very little hepatic metabolism, with about 75% of the drug being excreted unchanged in the urine and 10–20% unchanged in the feces. The half-life of levocabastine is fairly prolonged, being between 35 and 40 hours regardless of the route of administration. Eye drops administered regularly do not suppress histamine-induced wheal and flare.[50–52]

Olopatadine

Olopatadine, like ketotifen and azelastine, appears to be an antihistamine with significant anti-inflammatory activity, at least based upon its ability to inhibit antihistamine release from mast cells. It is a selective H_1 antagonist that is devoid of effects on α-adrenergic, dopaminergic, and muscarinic receptors. The recommended dose is 1–2 drops in each affected eye b.i.d. at an interval of 6–8 hours. With this dose plasma concentrations are generally below the level of the standard quantitative assay (less than 0.5 ng/ml). The peak serum concentrations are usually reached within 2 hours of dosing and, when measurable, range from 0.5 to 1.3 ng/ml.

The half-life in plasma is approximately 3 hours and elimination is primarily through renal excretion with 60–70% of the dose recovered in the urine as the parent drug. Two metabolites are found in low concentrations in the urine: the mono-desmethyl and N-oxide moieties. Olopatadine has been classified as pregnancy category C. It has been identified in the milk of nursing rats following oral administration.[53]

Side-effects of second-generation antihistamines

As a class, the second-generation antihistamines have relatively few side-effects. As noted, some sedation can occur with the administration of azelastine and cetirizine, but its incidence seems to be lower than with the classic first-generation antihistamines.

None of the presently available drugs is known to prolong the Q–T interval, and none of them therefore carries a warning regarding the production of ventricular arrhythmias.

There is no evidence to date that any of the second-generation antihistamines are responsible for fetal abnormalities in humans. They do, however, cross the placenta. All, as noted, are classified in either FDA category C or B.

It is likely that all of the second-generation antihistamines are excreted in breast milk,[24] but there is no evidence that they exert any clinically significant side-effect in nursing infants. However there is an admonition against their use in nursing mothers because of the likelihood of their presence in breast milk.

It has been known that some antihistamines (e.g. astemizole) are associated with increase in body weight and appetite, however none of the drugs presently available for use in the USA has been known to cause significant increase in appetite or weight gain when administered in standard doses by approved routes of administration.

REFERENCES

1. Dale HH, Laidlaw PP. The physiologic action of beta-imidazole ethylamine. J Physiol (Lond) 1911;41:318.
2. Garrison JC, Rall TW. Autacoids: Drug therapy of inflammation. In: Goodman LS, Gilman A (eds). Goodman and Gilman's The pharmacological basis of therapeutics, 8th edn. New York, Pergamon Press, 1990.
3. Lewis T. The blood vessels of the human skin and their responses. London, Shaw and Sons, 1927.
4. Weiss S, Robb GP, Ellis LB. The systemic effects of histamine in man with special reference to the responses of the cardiovascular system. Arch Intern Med 1932;49:360.
5. Staub AM, Bovet D. Action de la thymoxyethyl-diethyl-amine (939F) et des ethers phenoliques sur le schoc anaphylactique du cobaye. R Soc Biol 1937;125:818.
6. Kaliner MA, Check WA. Nonsedating antihistamines. Allergy Proc 1988;9:649.
7. Ash AS, Schild HO. Receptors mediating some actions of histamine. Br J Pharmacol 1966;27:427.
8. Black JW, Duncan WAM, Durant GJ, et al. Definition and antagonism of histamine H2-receptors. Nature 1972;236:385.
9. Haqaksma EEJ, Leurs R, Timmerman H. Histamine receptors: subclasses and specific ligands. Pharmacol Ther 1990;47:73.
10. Simons FER, Simons KJ. Histamine and H1 receptor antagonists. In: Smith C, Reynard A (eds) Textbook of pharmacology. Philadelphia, W.B. Saunders, 1992.
11. Lieberman P. The use of antihistamines in the prevention and treatment of anaphylaxis and anaphylactoid reactions. J Allergy Clin Immunol 1990;86(S):684.
12. Peroutka SJ. Drugs effective in therapy of migraines. In: Goodman LS, Gillman A (eds) The pharmacological basis of therapeutics, 9th edn. New York, McGraw-Hill, 1996, p 487.
13. Kemp JP. Does tolerance develop with prolonged use of antihistamines? J Respir Disease 1990;11(4 Suppl):S27.
14. Simons FER, Frith EM, Simons KJ. The pharmacokinetics and antihistaminic effects of brompheniramine. J Allergy Clin Immunol 1982;70:458.
15. Simons FER, Simons KJ. H1 receptor antagonists: clinical pharmacology and use in allergic disease. Pediatr Clin North Am 1983;30:899.
16. Carruthers SG, Shoeman DW, Hignite CE, et al. Correlation between plasma diphenhydramine level and sedative and antihistamine effects. Clin Pharmacol Ther 1978;23:375.
17. Rimmer SJ, Church MK. The pharmacology and mechanisms of action of histamine H1 antagonists. Clin Exp Allergy 1990;20(Suppl 2):3.
18. Naclerio RM, Togias AG. The role of antihistamines in allergic rhinitis therapy. J Respir Disease 1990;11(4 Suppl):S11.
19. Simons FER. The antiallergic effect of antihistamines (H1-receptor antagonists). J Allergy Clin Immunol 1990;90:705.
20. Linnoilia M. Effects of antihistamines and alcohol on psychomotor skills related to driving. Eur J Clin Pharmacol 1973;5:247.
21. Meltzer EO. Performance effects of antihistamines. J Allergy Clin Immunol 1990;8:613.
22. Gengo FM, Gabos C. Antihistamines, drowsiness, and psychomotor impairment: central nervous system effect of cetirizine. Ann Allergy 1987;59 (part II):53 (proceedings of a symposium – cetirizine, a recent advance in selective antihistamines therapy – supplement).
23. Slater JW, Zechnich AD, Haxby DG. Second-generation antihistamines. Drugs 1999;57:31.
24. Horak F, Stubner UP. Comparative tolerability of second generation antihistamines. Drug Safety 1999;20:385.
25. Gonzalez MA, Estes KS. Pharmacokinetic overview of oral second-generation H1 antihistamines. Int J Clin Pharmacol Ther 1998;36:292.

26. Simons FER, Simons KJ. Clinical pharmacology of new histamine H1 receptor antagonists. Clin Pharmacokinet 1999;36:329.
27. Du Buske LM. Clinical comparison of histamine H1-receptor antagonist drugs. J Allergy Clin Immunol 1996;98:S307.
28. Timmerman H. Why are nonsedating antihistamines nonsedating? Clin Exp Allergy 1999;29:13.
29. Simons FER, Bergman JN, Watson WTA, et al. The clinical pharmacology of fexofenadine in children. J Allergy Clin Immunol 1996;98:1062.
30. Simons FER, Watson WTA, Simons KJ. Pharmacokinetics and pharmacodynamics of ebastine in children. J Pediatr 1993;122:641.
31. Bousquet J, Chanal I, Skassa-Brociek W, et al. Lack of subsensitivity to loratadine during long-term dosing during 12 weeks. J Allergy Clin Immunol 1990;86:248.
32. Watson WTA, Simons KJ, Chen XY, et al. Cetirizine: a pharmacokinetic and pharmacodynamic evaluation in children with seasonal allergic rhinitis. J Allergy Clin Immunol 1989;84:457.
33. Bousquet J, Campbell AM, Canonica CW. H_1-receptor antagonists: Structure and classification. In: Simons FER (ed.) Histamine and H_1-receptor antagonists in allergic disease (7). New York, Marcel Dekker, 1996, p 91.
34. Church MK, Collinson AD, Okayama Y. H_1-Receptor antagonists: anti-allergic effects in vitro. In: Simons FER (ed.) Histamine and H_1-receptor antagonists in allergic disease (7). New York, Marcel Dekker, 1996, p 1.
35. Church MK. Non-H1-receptor effects of antihistamines. Clin Exp Allergy 1999;29:39.
36. Ciprandi G, Passalacqua G, Canonica GW. Effects of H1 antihistamines on adhesion molecules: a possible rationale for long-term treatment. Clin Exp Allergy 1999;29:49.
37. Cuss FM. Beyond the histamine receptor: effect of antihistamines on mast cells. Clin Exp Allergy 1999;29:54.
38. De Vos C. H1-receptor antagonists: effects on leukocytes, myth or reality? Clin Exp Allergy 1999;29:60.
39. Devalia JL, Davies RJ. Effect of antihistamines on epithelial cells. Clin Exp Allergy 1999;29:64.
40. Naclerio RM, Baroody FM. H1-receptor antagonists: Antiallergic effects in humans. In: Simons FER (ed.) Histamine and H_1-receptor antagonists in allergic disease (7). New York, Marcel Dekker, 1996, p 145.
41. Yoneda K, Yamamato T, Veta E, Osaki T. Suppression by azelastine HCL of NF-κB activation involved in generation of cytokines and nitric oxide. Jpn J Pharmacol 1997;73:145.
42. Banov C, LaForce C, Lieberman P. Double-blind trial of Astelin nasal spray in the treatment of vasomotor rhinitis. Ann Allergy Asthma Immunol 2000: in press.
43. Sheffer AL, Samuels LL. Cetirizine: antiallergic therapy beyond traditional antihistamines. J Allergy Clin Immunol 1990;86:10409.
44. Simons FER. Comparing the new H1 receptor antagonists. J Respir Disease 1993;11(Suppl):S6.
45. Pierson WE. Cetirizine: a unique second-generation antihistamine for treatment of rhinitis and chronic urticaria. Clin Ther 1991;13:92.
46. Kontow FTK, Maniatokov G, Pateologis G, Aroni K. Cetirizine inhibits delayed pressure urticaria. Ann Allergy 1990;65:520.
47. Berger WE, Fineman SM, Lieberman P, Miles RM, and the Rhinitis Study Group. Double-blind trials of azelastine nasal spray monotherapy versus combination therapy with loratadine tablets and beclomethasone nasal spray in patients with seasonal allergic rhinitis. Ann Allergy Asthma Immunol 1999;82(6):535.
48. Nabe M, Miyagawa H, Agrawai DK, Sugiyama H, Townley RG. The effect of ketotifen on eosinophils as measured at LTC4 release and by chemotaxis. Allergy Proc 1991;12:267.
49. Podleski WK, Panaszek BA, Schmidt JL, Burns RB. Inhibition of eosinophils degranulation by ketotifen in a patient with milk allergy, manifested as bronchial asthma – an electron microscope study. Agents Actions 1984;15:177.
50. Pesco-Koplowitz L, Hassall A, Lee P, et al. Lack of effect of erythromycin and ketoconazole on the pharmacokinetics and pharmacodynamics of steady-state intranasal levocabastine. J Clin Pharmacol 1999;39:76.
51. Dechant KL, Goa KL. Levocabastine: a review of its pharmacological properties and therapeutic potential as a topical antihistamine in allergic rhinitis and conjunctivitis. Drugs 1991;41:202.
52. Heykants J, Van Peer A, Van de Velde V, et al. The pharmacokinetic properties of topical levocabastine: a review. Clin Pharmacokinet 1995;29:221.
53. Patanol (olopatadine hydrochloride ophthalmic solution) in Physicians' Desk Reference (PDR) 1998;52:484.

Chapter 110 Immunomodulating Pharmaceuticals

Keith M. Hull and Dimitrios T. Boumpas

The use of immunomodulating drugs has changed substantially in recent years. Newer drugs have emerged in the therapeutic armamentarium while others are clearly falling out of favor. Moreover, combination therapy with several of these drugs has been shown to be more effective than single agent therapy without a significant increase in toxicity. Drug-free remissions rarely occur, and consequently patients must receive continuous administration. The precise mechanism by which these drugs exert their immunomodulatory effect remains largely unknown.

This chapter reviews the pharmacology, proposed mechanisms of action, and clinical use of azathioprine, chlorambucil, cyclophosphamide, fludarabine, leflunomide, methotrexate, mycophenolate mofetil and sulfasalazine, whose chemical structures are given in Figure 110.1. Although their usage differs among diseases, the chapter discusses general principles of administration. Other immunosuppressive agents are discussed elsewhere: cyclosporine, tacrolimus, and sirolimus (Chapter 111); glucocorticoids (Chapter 106), NSAIDs (Chapter 107), leukotriene inhibitors (Chapter 108), antihistamines (Chapter 109) and biological immunomodulators (Chapters 114–117).

AZATHIOPRINE AND 6-MERCAPTOPURINE

6-Mercaptopurine (6-MP) was first utilized in 1940 but has essentially been replaced by its prodrug, azathioprine. Azathioprine was first synthesized in 1957, found to be useful in rheumatoid arthritis in 1964,[1] and received FDA approval in 1981 for the treatment of rheumatoid arthritis. The most common use of azathioprine today is as an immunomodulator for treating transplant recipients and immunoinflammatory disorders.

Mechanism of action

Azathioprine undergoes rapid intracellular conversion to its active metabolite, 6-MP, a purine analog of guanine and hypoxanthine (Table 110.1). 6-Mercaptopurine is then activated by hypoxanthine-guanine phosphoriboxyltransferase to form the active metabolites 6-thionosinic acid and 6-thioguanylic acid. These active metabolites interfere with de novo purine biosynthesis and are also incorporated into DNA by an as yet undetermined mechanism. Ultimately, 6-MP and its metabolites reduce DNA and RNA synthesis, resulting in cell death. Although the exact mechanisms are lacking, studies demonstrate that azathioprine decreases T and B lymphocytes and antibody formation[2] and decreases B lymphocytes proliferation, perhaps by decreasing nitric oxide formation.[3] Additionally, azathioprine inhibits NK cell activity and decreases neutrophil migration and endothelial cell proliferation.

THERAPEUTIC PRINCIPLES

Azathioprine
- Purine analog
- Gastrointestinal and hematologic toxicities common
- Dosage for renal transplant recipients: 3–5 mg/kg/day
- Dosage for autoimmune disorders: 1–2.5 mg/kg/day
- Coadministration of allopurinol contraindicated
- Monitoring of CBC and liver function tests
- Useful as glucocorticoid-sparing agent and/or maintenance therapy

Pharmacokinetics

Following absorption, azathioprine is distributed rapidly throughout the body with a plasma half-life of 3 hours and an oral bioavailability of 45%. It is approximately 30% bound to plasma proteins. Its major metabolites include 6-mercaptopurine, deoxythioguanine monophosphate, and thioguanine monophosphate but the majority is converted to the inactive metabolite 6-thiouric acid via the enzyme xanthine oxidase. Diminished activity of xanthine oxidase either by drugs (e.g. allopurinol) or via enzyme deficiencies (e.g. Lesch–Nyhan syndrome and thiopurine methyltransferase deficiency) greatly increases azathioprine metabolites and thus toxicity. The vast majority of azathioprine is excreted as 6-thiouric acid via the kidney and approximately 10% is excreted unchanged.

Adverse effects

Azathioprine is generally well tolerated; the adverse effects most often cited are gastrointestinal disturbances, bone marrow suppression, and infections. A study reporting adverse effects of azathioprine in 546 patients with rheumatoid arthritis demonstrated that gastrointestinal problems accounted for nearly 60% of therapy terminations.[4] Disturbances include benign symptoms such as taste alteration, nausea, vomiting, diarrhea, and abdominal pain. These symptoms can be minimized by administering azathioprine in divided doses or after meals. Hepatotoxicity occurs in less than 1% of rheumatoid arthritis patients on azathioprine but can be as high as 3–10% in other patient populations. Hepatotoxic events include hypersensitivity, cholestasis, peliosis hepatis, Disse space fibrosis, veno-occlusive disease, and nodular regenerative hyperplasia. The hypersensitivity syndrome primarily affects males and occurs 2–3 weeks after initiating azathioprine therapy, 6 months in liver transplant recipients.[5] The majority of hepatotoxicity is reversible after discontinuation of the drug. Pancreatitis has been reported rarely and is believed to be

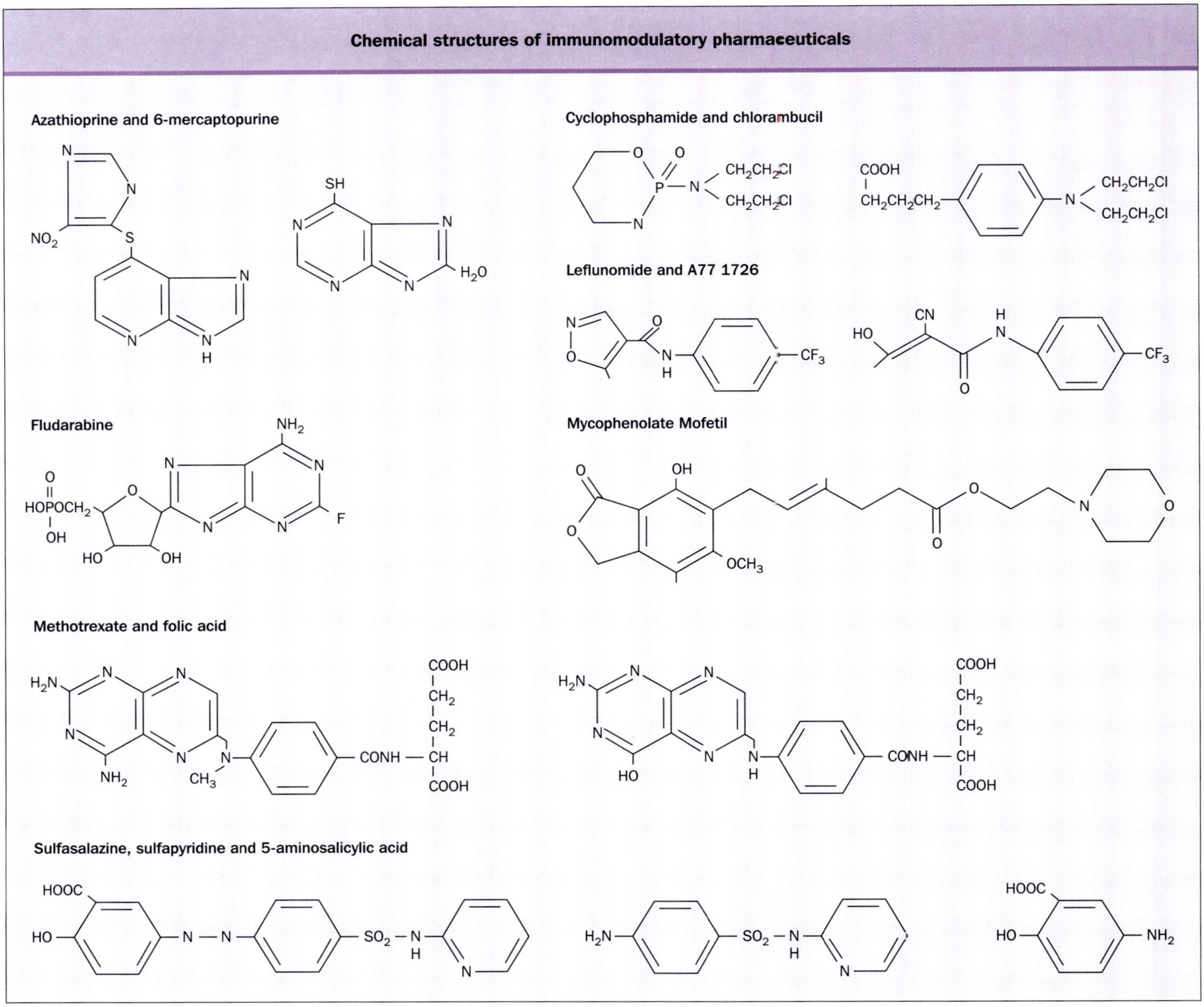

Figure 110.1 Chemical structures of immunomodulatory pharmaceuticals.

due to a hypersensitivity reaction. Symptoms can be severe and have been reported to occur 2–4 weeks after initiation of therapy. As with hepatotoxicity, patients presenting with symptoms of pancreatitis should have their azathioprine discontinued.

Bone marrow suppression can be severe and occurs commonly. The effect is dose dependent and can be reversed with either dose reduction or discontinuation. While all three cell lineages may be affected, leukopenia is more common. It is important to remember that leukopenia does not correlate with therapeutic efficacy. Eosinophilia, anemia, aplastic anemia, megaloblastic anemia, red cell aplasia, and leukocytosis have been reported. Azathioprine-induced leukopenia allows for the increased risk of opportunistic infections including the usual pathogens but also cytomegalovirus, herpes, and human papilloma virus.

The controversy of whether azathioprine treatment is linked to an increased frequency of malignancies stems from early studies from the transplant literature.[6] Several subsequent studies supported this claim,[7] but the majority of studies have failed to demonstrate a definite link between azathioprine and an increased incidence of malignancy when patients are compared to appropriate disease-matched controls.[8]

Numerous drugs can interact with azathioprine and complicate therapy. For example, angiotensin-converting enzyme inhibitors may result in leukopenia or anemia, and warfarin efficacy may be decreased. The concomitant use of allopurinol, a xanthine-oxidase inhibitor, and azathioprine should be avoided if possible; if not, then the dose of azathioprine should be decreased by 50–75% and hematologic parameters closely monitored.

Principles of administration

Azathioprine can be given either intravenously or orally. In general, the usual initiating dose of azathioprine in renal transplant recipients is 3–5 mg/kg/day starting at the time of transplantation. In patients with autoimmune disease it can be started

Table 110.1 Mechanisms of action of immunomodulating pharmaceuticals.

Mechanisms of action of immunomodulating pharmaceuticals		
Drug	**Active agent**	**Mechanism**
Azathioprine	6-Thioguanylic acid 6-Thioinosinic acid	Inhibition of de novo purine synthesis
Chlorambucil	Phenylacetic acid mustard	Cross-links DNA
Cyclophosphamide	Phosphoramide mustard	Cross-links DNA
Fludarabine	F-ara-ATP	Disrupts DNA and RNA synthesis
Leflunomide	A77 1726	Inhibits de novo pyrimidine synthesis via antagonism of dihydroorotate dehydrogenase
Methotrexate	Polyglutamated methotrexate	Increases extracellular adenosine Dihydrofolate reductase inhibitor
Mycophenolate mofetil	Mycophenolic acid	Inhibition of de novo purine synthesis via antagonism of inositol monophosphate dehydrogenase
Sulfasalazine	Sulfapyridine 5-Aminosalicylic acid	Increases extracellular adenosine Nuclear factor-κB inhibition

at 1 mg/kg/day for several days and increased by 0.5 mg/kg/day every 4 weeks to an optimally effective dose of 2.5 mg/kg/day. Patients with a glomerular filtration rate (GFR) greater than 50 ml/min do not need dose adjustment while patients with a GFR between 10 and 50 ml/min should receive 75% of the normal dose. Patients with GFR less than 10 ml/min should receive a 50% dose reduction. The combination of azathioprine with alkylating agents should be avoided if possible because of the potential for severe hematologic reactions and malignancy. Azathioprine has not been associated with increased teratogenicity although only small studies have been conducted. Therefore, considering the benefit–risk ratio, azathioprine can probably be used safely during pregnancy in selected patients.

Complete blood cell counts and liver function tests should be monitored every 2 weeks for the first 4 weeks, then every 4 weeks thereafter. If the dose is adjusted, or the white cell count falls but is greater than 3.0×10^6 cells/l then more frequent testing is recommended. If the white blood cell count falls below 3.0×10^6 cells/l then azathioprine should be discontinued and cell blood counts followed closely.

Efficacy

Azathioprine has been found to be effective in numerous disease processes where immunosuppression plays a therapeutic role. It is used most commonly, however, in the treatment of rheumatoid arthritis, prevention of organ transplant rejection, inflammatory bowel disease, autoimmune hepatitis, and rheumatoid arthritis.

Azathioprine has been found to be effective compared to placebo in improving both subjective and objective parameters of rheumatoid arthritis.[9] Azathioprine alone has rarely been used for the treatment of rheumatoid arthritis. It is less effective than methotrexate and demonstrates a worse benefit/adverse effect profile and a worse drug survival. Combining azathioprine with other disease-modifying antirheumatic drugs (DMARDs), e.g. sulfasalazine, methotrexate, hydroxychloroquine, or prednisolone, has been demonstrated to be more effective than azathioprine alone in treating active rheumatoid arthritis. Azathioprine is currently used in conjunction with other immunosuppressants as primary prophylaxis against rejection in kidney transplant recipients, although it may be less effective than the newer drug, mycophenolate mofetil, which also acts via inhibition of the purine nucleotide pathway. Despite the substantial difference in cost, some authors are supporting the use of mycophenolate mofetil over azathioprine for the primary prophylaxis of transplant rejection.[10] A recent study suggests that azathioprine may be useful as monotherapy in HLA-identical siblings receiving renal transplants.

Both azathioprine and 6-MP have been demonstrated to be useful in a number of situations for Crohn's disease, namely disease remission maintenance,[11] refractory disease, and fistulizing disease.[12] The role of azathioprine in ulcerative colitis is less clear. Data pooled from several studies suggest that azathioprine may be useful for steroid sparing and maintenance of remission. In proliferative lupus nephritis, azathioprine has been found to be no more effective than high-dose corticosteroids.[13] However, it is useful as a glucocorticoid-sparing agent and may be useful as maintenance therapy after induction therapy with cyclophosphamide. Similarly, a recent study has demonstrated azathioprine to be as effective as oral cyclophosphamide in maintaining remission in ANCA-associated systemic vasculitis following cyclophosphamide induction.[14]

CYCLOPHOSPHAMIDE/CHLORAMBUCIL

Nitrogen mustard was the first alkylating agent demonstrated to be effective in the treatment of rheumatoid arthritis. Beginning in the 1960s, cyclophosphamide and chlorambucil were used for vasculitis, rheumatoid arthritis, and systemic lupus erythematosus.[15] While their use has revolutionized the treatment of lupus nephritis and vasculitis, the associated toxicity has limited their use to the treatment of severe disease manifestations.

Mechanism of action

Cyclophosphamide and chlorambucil are alkylating agents that are actually prodrugs which rapidly metabolize to their active forms, phosphoramide mustard and phenylacetic acid mustard, respectively. Their action is largely mediated by cross-linking

THERAPEUTIC PRINCIPLES

Cyclophosphamide and chlorambucil

- Alkylating agents.
- Gastrointestinal and hematologic toxicities are common.
- Rate of gonadal failure is dependent on cumulative dose and increasing age.
- Both drugs may increase incidence of hematologic malignancies.
- Potential hemorrhagic cystitis and bladder cancer with cyclophosphamide therapy; therefore adequate hydration should be maintained while on therapy, as well as co-administration of MESNA.
- Cyclophosphamide oral dosage: 1–2 mg/kg/day.
- Cyclophosphamide pulse IV dosage: 500–1000 mg/m^2 body surface area.
- Monitoring of CBC, liver function tests, and life-long urinalysis.
- Nonglomerular hematuria requires cystoscopy for thorough evaluation.
- Chlorambucil oral dosage: 0.1–0.2 mg/kg/day.

DNA, and to a lesser extent RNA, thus disrupting transcription and translation. Both proliferating and resting cells are affected, and the degree of immunosuppression is dependent on the dose and duration of therapy. Cyclophosphamide therapy reduces both T-cell (CD4 greater than CD8) and B-cell function with subsequent decreases in both cellular and humoral immunity.[16] Cessation of monthly bolus cyclophosphamide therapy after one year results in slow recovery of CD4 T-cell and B-cell recovery over a period of months, demonstrating this drug's ability to suppress both lines of lymphocytes.[17]

Pharmacokinetics

Cyclophosphamide can be administered either intravenously or orally, where it demonstrates a bioavailability of at least 75%. Once absorbed, it is rapidly metabolized by hepatic enzymes to form the active metabolites 4-aldophosphamide, acrolein, and nitrogen mustard. Approximately 95% of cyclophosphamide is excreted by the kidney. Acrolein is also renally excreted and is thought to account for the cyclophosphamide-related bladder toxicity.

Chlorambucil is generally administered orally and demonstrates a bioavailability of over 80%. Once absorbed, it is rapidly metabolized to its active metabolite phenylacetic acid mustard, which is almost exclusively excreted by the kidney within 24 hours.

Adverse effects

Cyclophosphamide toxicities are often dose-related and the limiting factor in its use. Common adverse effects include alopecia as well as nausea and vomiting, which can often be controlled with antiemetic medications. Of more concern however is cyclophosphamide-induced bone marrow suppression, bladder toxicity, carcinogenicity, and infertility.

Bone marrow suppression is common during cyclophosphamide therapy and is dose-dependent. Leukocyte nadir occurs between 7 and 14 days following an intravenous pulse of cyclophosphamide, and dose adjustment is required for leukocyte counts less than 1.5×10^6 white blood cells/l (Table 110.2). Patients treated with daily oral cyclophosphamide need frequent monitoring of their complete blood cell counts, with dose adjustments necessary for leukocyte counts less than 3.0×10^6 white blood cells/l. As a result of bone marrow suppression patients are immunocompromised and susceptible to bacterial, fungal, and viral infections. Risk factors include multiple organ involvement, concomitant daily or split, high-dose glucocorticoid use (>0.5 mg/kg/day), and white blood cell count nadirs below 3.0×10^6 cells/l for patients on daily oral therapy. Prophylaxis with trimethoprim–sulfamethoxazole (160 mg/800 mg) orally three times weekly for *Pneumocystis carinii* pneumonia is recommended for patients being treated with continuous daily cyclophosphamide for vasculitis but not necessarily for most patients with SLE receiving intravenous bolus therapy.

Hemorrhagic cystitis and transitional cell carcinomas are potentially serious consequences of cyclophosphamide therapy and are believed to occur as a result of the toxic metabolite, acrolein. Hemorrhagic cystitis is more likely to occur in patients receiving daily oral cyclophosphamide versus intravenous pulse doses, presumably as a result of continued exposure of bladder mucosa to acrolein. Several strategies exist to minimize bladder toxicity depending on the route of administration of cyclophosphamide. Patients receiving intravenous bolus administration should receive pre- and post-transfusion intravenous hydration as well as administration of 2-mercaptoethanesulfonate (MESNA) which is reported to bind and neutralize acrolein,

National Institutes of Health pulse intravenous cyclophosphamide protocol

Dosage
Creatinine clearance >30 ml/min: initially 750 mg/m^2 body surface area (BSA) may increase to a maximum of 1000 mg/m^2 BSA if tolerated.
Creatinine clearance <30 ml/min: initially 500 mg/m^2 BSA.

Monitoring of white blood cell count (WBC; days 10 and 14)
If nadir WBC <1500/mm^3, reduce subsequent dose of cyclophosphamide by 25%.
If nadir WBC >4000/mm^3, increase subsequent doses of cyclophosphamide to a maximum of 1000 mg/m^2.

Preparation and infusion
Mix cyclophosphamide dose in 150 ml of normal saline or D5W.
Infuse over 60 minutes.

MESNA administration
Each MESNA dose is 20% of the total cyclophosphamide dose.
Infuse MESNA immediately before cyclophosphamide and every 3 hours thereafter for a total of 4 doses.

Antiemetic regimen
Dexamethasone 10 mg orally 3–4 hours after cyclophosphamide dose.
Odansetron 4–8 mg intravenously or orally starting 4 hours after cyclophosphamide dose then every 4 hours thereafter for 3 doses.
Granisetron 10 μg/kg intravenously 30 minutes prior to cyclophosphamide dose.

Diuresis
In patients with normal cardiovascular function, hydration with $D_5\frac{1}{2}$ normal saline @150–200 ml/hour for a total of 2–4 liters.
Diuretics may be utilized to enhance diuresis.
Alternatively, if patient is unable to tolerate intravenous fluids or empty bladder then bladder irrigation should be instituted.

Table 110.2 National Institutes of Health pulse intravenous cyclophosphamide protocol.

theoretically decreasing the risk of bladder toxicity. Patients receiving daily oral therapy should be instructed to take their dose in the morning with a large amount of water followed with large amounts of oral hydration throughout the day. Patients unable to empty their bladder should undergo bladder irrigation.

High cumulative doses of cyclophosphamide have been associated with a high frequency of malignancies. The risk of malignancy is dose-dependent and is substantial for patients receiving more than 80 g. Urinalysis should be performed monthly during the period patients are receiving cyclophosphamide therapy, and because the risk of cyclophosphamide-induced bladder cancer is lifelong patients should receive continued surveillance with urinalysis every 3–6 months thereafter to look for nonglomerular hematuria. It is important to note that urine cytology is not sensitive enough to detect bladder cancer; patients who develop the new onset of nonglomerular hematuria at any time during or after therapy therefore require a cystoscopy to visualize the bladder mucosa for possible carcinoma. Patients with persistent nonglomerular hematuria should receive cystoscopy every 1–2 years. Ovarian and testicular failure is a common adverse effect of cyclophosphamide therapy and its incidence rises with increasing cumulative dose and patient age. The cumulative cyclophosphamide dose needed to produce amenorrhea was as little as 5.2 g in women over the age of 40 and as much as 20.4 g in women between the ages of 20 to 29 years.[18]

Chlorambucil shares many of the same adverse effects of cyclophosphamide, including infertility, but there are two notable variations. First, chlorambucil does not produce bladder toxicity, as does cyclophosphamide. Secondly, chlorambucil is known to induce hematologic malignancies with greater frequency than cyclophosphamide, especially acute myeloblastic leukemia.

Principles of administration

Hemorrhagic cystitis is extremely rare after intermittent pulse cyclophosphamide but nausea and vomiting are more common (Table 110.3). Daily oral cyclophosphamide is well tolerated but possesses a higher risk of hemorrhagic cystitis. Dosages vary but those less than 1 mg/kg/day may be less effective and patients with Wegener granulomatosis may require up to 4 mg/kg/day. Therefore it is recommended that patients maintain adequate hydration with frequent urination while on daily therapy. Cystoscopy should be performed in response to positive microscopic or gross hematuria. Additionally, patients should have a complete blood cell count every 2–4 weeks with an adjustment of the cyclophosphamide dose for those with leukocyte counts less than 3.0×10^6 white blood cells/l.

It is recommended that patients with renal insufficiency receive reduced dosages of cyclophosphamide. In general, patients with a glomerular filtration rate between 10 and 50 ml/min should receive 75% of the normal dose while patients with a glomerular filtration rate less than 10 ml/min should receive 50% of the normal dose. Patients who are on hemodialysis and require pulse intravenous cyclophosphamide should receive a dose of 500 mg/m^2 and receive dialysis 12 hours after administration.

Chlorambucil is generally started at oral doses between 0.1 and 0.2 mg/kg/day and lowered as necessitated by either toxicity or efficacy in treating the disease. The lowest possible dose should be achieved that effectively maintains leukocyte counts between 3.0 and 4.0×10^6 white blood cells/l. Complete blood cell count should be performed weekly with initiation of therapy, and then monthly once a stable dose has been achieved.

Table 110.3 Immunomodulating drugs.[a]

	Immunomodulating drugs[a]							
Toxicity	**CPA**	**Chlor**	**AZA**	**MTX**	**D-PEN**	**SSAL**	**H_2N**	**GLUC**[b]
Liver	–	–	+	+++	–	+	–	–
Lung	+	–	+	+++	+	+	–	–
Gastrointestinal	+++	+	+++	+++	+	+++	+++	++
Mucocutaneous	++	++	+	+++	++	++	+	–
Hematologic	+++	+++	++	+	+	++	+++	–
Teratogenicity	+++	+++	++	++	++	–	+++[c]	–
Malignancy	+++	+++	+	+	–	–	+++[c]	–
Infections[d]	+++	+++	++	++	–	–	+++[c]	++
Cystitis	+++	–	–	–	–	–	–	–
Infertility	+++	+++	–	–	–	++	+++	–
Autoimmunity	–	–	–	–	++	–	–	–

[a]Relative association of individual immunomodulative drugs and toxicity. Estimations are based on available data. Definitive comparative studies are not available. (–), no association; (+) → (+ + +), weak → strong association (relative to other agents); CPA, cyclophosphamide; Chlor, chlorambucil; AZA, azathioprine; MTX, methotrexate; D-PEN, D-penicillamine; SSAL, sulfasalazine; H_2N, nitrogen mustard; GLUC, glucocorticoids.
[b]Glucocorticoids have additional unique toxicities. See Chapter 106.
[c]Estimate based on experience with other alkylating agents. Data on H_2N not available.
[d]Serious infections that require intravenous antibiotics.

Screening for hematologic malignancies is suggested for both cyclophosphamide- and chlorambucil-treated patients although no strict guidelines exist. Similarly, sperm banking may be considered for males because of the possibility of gonadal failure. Current studies may soon support the coadministration of a gonadotropin-releasing hormone agonist to prevent premature ovarian failure or testosterone to prevent azoospermia. Pregnancy and breast feeding are strictly contraindicated during cyclophosphamide or chlorambucil therapy.

Efficacy

Cyclophosphamide therapy has revolutionized the treatment of several previously life-threatening autoimmune conditions, namely systemic lupus erythematosus with major organ involvement and systemic vasculitis. Studies at the National Institutes of Health have clearly demonstrated treatment with monthly intravenous cyclophosphamide to be superior to pulse-dose methylprednisolone alone and to possess a greater therapeutic index than daily oral cyclophosphamide in patients with proliferative lupus nephritis. Indeed, intermittent intravenous cyclophosphamide has been shown to significantly induce remission, prevent progression, preserve renal function, prevent progressive renal scarring, and reduce the risk of end-stage renal failure.[19–21] The concurrent administration of pulse-dose methylprednisolone produces a more rapid response and a greater probability of renal remission. Although previously this additional benefit was thought to be at the cost of increased adverse effects, recent evidence fails to demonstrate increased toxicity with the addition of methylprednisolone 10 years after therapy.[22]

In contrast to the findings in lupus nephritis, several studies have demonstrated daily oral cyclophosphamide therapy to be much more effective than pulse intravenous cyclophosphamide for inducing and sustaining disease remission in patients with Wegener granulomatosis.[23] Patients with organ- or life-threatening disease are generally started on daily oral cyclophosphamide at 2 mg/kg/day with dose adjustment as necessary to keep leukocyte counts greater than 3.0×10^6 white blood cells/l and prednisone 1 mg/kg/day with subsequent tapering. Studies suggest that, after remission is obtained with cyclophosphamide and prednisone, weekly methotrexate, azathioprine, or mycophenolate mofetil may be useful as maintenance therapy and thereby decrease cyclophosphamide toxicity. Similarly, patients with mild disease, e.g. limited sinus disease, do not require cyclophosphamide therapy but may benefit from methotrexate for induction therapy.

Cyclophosphamide has consistently been demonstrated to be effective in the treatment of rheumatoid arthritis, using both subjective and objective criteria including bone erosions. However, because of its long-term toxicity, it has been recommended to be reserved for the treatment of severe life- or critical organ-threatening manifestations of rheumatoid arthritis such as rheumatoid arthritis-associated vasculitis or scleromalacia perforans. Daily oral or pulse intravenous cyclophosphamide has been demonstrated to be useful in treating scleroderma-induced interstitial pneumonitis, and placebo-controlled studies are currently being conducted. Additionally, cyclophosphamide has been demonstrated to be effective in patients with aplastic anemia.[24]

Chlorambucil has been demonstrated to be useful in the treatment of severe, nonocular manifestations of Behçet syndrome, as well as refractory rheumatoid arthritis, systemic lupus erythematosus, multiple sclerosis, sarcoidosis, dermatomyositis, and systemic vasculitis. However, because of the greatly increased risk of developing a hematologic malignancy, chlorambucil should probably not be used as first-line therapy.

FLUDARABINE

Fludarabine is an adenosine analog that specifically targets both resting and proliferating lymphocytes. It first entered clinical trials in 1982 and received FDA approval in November 1991 for use in patients with chronic lymphocytic leukemia who were refractory to standard alkylating agents. Cladribine is also an adenosine analog that was initially developed as an immunosuppressive agent and later found to possess antiproliferative activity against a variety of leukemia cell lines with potent immunosuppressive and myelosuppressive effects in patients.

Mechanism of action

Fludarabine is rapidly metabolized to F-ara-A that is then transported intracellularly via nucleoside transport systems. Once within the cell, F-ara-A undergoes intracellular phosphorylation by deoxycytidine to form the active metabolite F-ara-ATP that imparts its effect by incorporation into elongating nucleic acid chains resulting in the termination of DNA or RNA synthesis. F-ara-ATP inhibits DNA and DNA ligase I.

Not only is fludarabine able to inhibit the proliferation of rapidly dividing lymphocytes but it also acts on quiescent lymphocytes by inducing apoptosis.[25] Resting lymphocytes are constantly repairing breaks in DNA and if an increase in this activity is required it leads to the consumption of NAD for poly-ADP-ribose synthesis. One hypothesis is that the purine nucleoside analogs (e.g. fludarabine) may selectively induce DNA breakage in resting lymphocytes and therefore accelerate DNA repair as described above and ultimately lead to the depletion of ADP and ATP. Recently fludarabine has been shown to inhibit STAT1 signaling in proliferating and resting lymphocytes.[26]

Pharmacokinetics

Peak plasma concentrations of fludarabine occur at approximately 2–4 minutes after an intravenous infusion, with peak plasma concentrations of F-ara-A occurring shortly thereafter. Orally administered fludarabine demonstrates an approximate 75% bioavailability.

Once within the cell, F-ara-A undergoes a series of phosphorylations – first by deoxycytidine kinase to form F-ara-A monophosphate, then by adenylic kinase and nucleoside diphosphate kinase to its active form, F-ara-ATP. Peak intracellular F-ara-

THERAPEUTIC PRINCIPLES

Fludarabine

- Purine analog that acts on activated and resting lymphocytes.
- Gastrointestinal and hematologic toxicities are common.
- Use of irradiated blood products is recommended secondary to possible graft-versus-host disease.
- Monitoring of CBC.
- Drug of choice for chronic lymphocytic leukemia. Role in autoimmune disease is under investigation.

ATP concentrations are achieved within 3–4 hours after fludarabine infusion and exhibit a median half-life of 23 hours. Elimination is primarily via renal excretion, and dose adjustments are necessary in patients with renal failure.

Adverse effects

Myelosuppression is the major dose-limiting adverse effect for fludarabine. Neutropenia and thrombocytopenia occur more commonly than do leukopenia and anemia. Instances of hemolytic anemia, eosinophilia, and Evans syndrome have also been reported. Fludarabine has been reported to cause neurotoxicity even at low doses; this can present with dysarthria, weakness, seizures, and visual symptoms including cortical blindness. Nausea, vomiting, and diarrhea are common. Extreme caution needs to be exercised when administering blood products to fludarabine-treated patients as several cases of graft-versus-host disease following blood transfusion have been reported.[27] It is therefore recommended that all patients treated with fludarabine receive irradiated blood products. As with most immunosuppressants, patients treated with either fludarabine or cladribine are prone to develop opportunistic infections including cryptococcal meningitis.

Principles of administration

Fludarabine and cladribine are both generally administered as intravenous solutions but both drugs have also been administered as a subcutaneous injection. Fludarabine dosage should be adjusted in patients with renal insufficiency and use of the drug is contraindicated during pregnancy and breast feeding. Complete blood counts should be checked weekly during therapy.

Efficacy

While fludarabine is commonly used for hematological malignancies, several pilot studies have investigated its role as an immunosuppressive agent in rheumatoid arthritis and lupus nephritis.[28] A randomized, double-blind, placebo-controlled study demonstrated promising results of cladribine in the treatment of relapsing multiple sclerosis as evidenced by decreased frequency and duration of relapses.[29]

LEFLUNOMIDE

Leflunomide is a novel isoxazole derivative that is structurally unrelated to other disease-modifying antirheumatic drugs currently in use. Leflunomide has been demonstrated to be effective in animal models of arthritis, autoimmune disease, graft rejection including renal, cardiac, skin, and small bowel. Leflunomide has been approved in Europe and the USA for the treatment of patients with rheumatoid arthritis and is currently being evaluated in phase I clinical trials for use in renal transplant recipients and for the treatment of gliomas.

Mechanism of action

The active metabolite of leflunomide, A77 1726, inhibits dihydroorotate dehydrogenase (DHODH), the fourth enzyme required for de novo pyrimidine biosynthesis. In vitro, A77 1726-induced inhibition of lymphocyte proliferation occurs at the nM to low μM range and can be reversed by the addition of uridine or cytidine to cell cultures, supporting the concept that it is acting as a DHODH inhibitor. A77 1726 is also thought to inhibit protein tyrosine kinases but at much higher concentrations than that required to inhibit lymphocyte proliferation via DHODH. Tyrosine kinases play a critical role in intracellular signaling involved in mediating cell growth and transformation. The significantly lower concentrations of A77 1726 required to inhibit cell proliferation via DHODH, compared with that of tyrosine kinases, suggests to many researchers that A77 1726 derives the majority of its mechanism of action in vivo as an inhibitor of DHODH. However, the antitumor effect of leflunomide has been suggested to be mediated primarily by tyrosine kinase inhibition.

Additional proposed mechanisms for A77 1726 include enhanced production of TGF-β in lymphocytes,[30] impaired N-glycosylation of adhesion molecules via depletion of pyrimidine nucleotides,[31] inhibition of basophil histamine release,[32] cyclooxygenase-2 inhibition,[33] inhibition of T-cell dependent and independent B-cell proliferation with suppression of antibody formation inhibition,[34] inhibition of TNF-dependent nuclear factor-κB activation and gene expression.[35]

> **THERAPEUTIC PRINCIPLES**
>
> **Leflunomide**
> - Dihydroorotate dehydrogenase antagonist
> - Gastrointestinal toxicity common
> - Liver transaminase elevation common
> - Dosage: loading dose of 100 mg/day for 3 days then 20 mg/day
> - Monitoring of CBC and liver function tests
> - Synergy with methotrexate but may result in increased hepatotoxicity

Pharmacokinetics

Approximately 80% of an oral dose of leflunomide is absorbed by the gastrointestinal tract and is unaffected by food. Leflunomide is then rapidly converted to its active metabolite A77 1726. Greater than 99% of A77 1726 binds to serum proteins and has an average half-life of 11 days (range of 4–28 days). The primary sites of elimination are the kidney (43%) and liver (48%). Leflunomide does not need to be dose-adjusted in patients with renal failure. Studies in patients with hepatic insufficiency are lacking but, considering the role of the liver in leflunomide metabolism, it may affect the conversion to A77 1726 and its subsequent clearance.

The coadministration of rifampin has been demonstrated to increase levels of A77 1726 by as much as 40%, therefore caution and increased monitoring of adverse effects are recommended when these two drugs are simultaneously prescribed. It is noteworthy, however, that the coadministration of methotrexate with leflunomide has been demonstrated to increase liver enzymes by as much as 3 times the upper limit of normal.

Adverse effects

A recent 2-year trial comparing leflunomide and methotrexate in patients with rheumatoid arthritis reported similar rates of adverse reactions between the two drugs. The most common adverse effects were diarrhea, abdominal pain, nausea, oral ulcers, alopecia, rash, infections, and reversible liver enzyme elevation of greater than two times normal.[36] Leflunomide-induced elevation of liver enzymes appears to be a dose-dependent and reversible event. It is currently recommended that patients do not receive live vaccines while being treated with leflunomide, and its use is contraindicated during pregnancy and breast feeding.

Principles of administration

Leflunomide is supplied in 10 mg, 20 mg, and 100 mg coated tablets. In general, a loading dose of leflunomide is initiated at 100 mg daily for 3 days, then a maintenance dose of 20 mg daily is given. If adverse effects are intolerable a dose of 10 mg daily may be tried. No dose adjustments are necessary in geriatric patients or those with renal insufficiency. There should be increased vigilance for adverse effects in patients with hepatic insufficiency given the role of hepatic metabolism in leflunomide activation and clearance. Leflunomide can be safely administered with NSAIDs and glucocorticoids. As a result of its high serum protein binding and enterohepatic clearance it may take over 2 years to reach undetectable plasma levels of A77 1726; however, rapid reduction of serum concentrations of A77 1726 can be achieved (in approximately 1–2 days) with the oral administration of cholestyramine. In fact, since leflunomide is a Food and Drug Pregnancy Risk Category X drug, it is recommended that female patients who desire to become pregnant receive cholestyramine 8 g every 8 hours for 11 days and that an A77 1726 level be obtained to ensure that it is below 0.02 mg/l.

Liver enzyme tests (AST and ALT) should be obtained at baseline and every 4 weeks initially until stable, then at an interval determined by the individual clinical situation. A recent study analyzing the pharmacokinetics, safety, and efficacy of the combination of leflunomide and methotrexate in patients with rheumatoid arthritis found no significant pharmacokinetic interaction but did note a significantly increased incidence of liver enzyme elevation than with use of methotrexate alone.

Efficacy

Numerous studies in patients with active rheumatoid arthritis have now demonstrated the efficacy of leflunomide versus placebo in improving signs and symptoms of active rheumatoid arthritis, delaying radiographic erosions, and improving overall quality of life.[37–39] Several studies have directly compared leflunomide to conventional therapies and have concluded that it is equally effective to sulfasalazine,[37] methotrexate,[39] and cyclosporine[40]. A recent open-label study investigated the safety, efficacy, and pharmacokinetics of the combination of leflunomide and methotrexate in patients with rheumatoid arthritis who were refractory to methotrexate treatment alone. The authors concluded that the combination of methotrexate and leflunomide might be useful in patients who have an inadequate response to monotherapy with methotrexate. Although the combination was generally well tolerated, there was a noted increase in the number of patients in the combination group with elevated liver enzymes, albeit reversible. Currently, leflunomide is only approved for use in the treatment of rheumatoid arthritis although it has been demonstrated to evoke significant immunosuppressant activity in preclinical trials of organ transplantation.

METHOTREXATE

During the 1960s methotrexate was utilized for treatment of patients with psoriasis, and within a decade reports of its efficacy in rheumatoid arthritis patients were reported. Today, methotrexate is the most common DMARD prescribed for the treatment of rheumatoid arthritis in the USA and is used in numerous other autoimmune and inflammatory disorders.

THERAPEUTIC PRINCIPLES

Methotrexate

- Indirect adenosine agonist.
- Dihydrofolate reductase antagonist.
- Gastrointestinal, hematologic, and mucocutaneous toxicities common.
- Potentially serious hepatic, hematologic, and pulmonary toxicity occurs although rare.
- Dosage: 5–30 mg/week in single dose.
- Coadministration of folic acid 1–2 mg daily or leucovorin 2.5–5 mg 24 hours after methotrexate administration reduces frequency and severity of some adverse effects.
- Dose reduction necessary in patients with decreased glomerular filtration rate and alcohol use.
- Monitor CBC, liver function tests, and creatinine every 4–8 weeks.
- Obtain baseline chest radiograph.

Mechanism of action

The rationale for using methotrexate in the treatment of malignancies or psoriasis derives from its action as a potent dihydrofolate reductase (DHFR) inhibitor. This action of methotrexate is believed to account for its antiproliferative effect not only in malignancies but also in other rapidly dividing cells such as those found in the mucous membranes, epidermis, and bone marrow. Methotrexate was introduced in the treatment of rheumatoid arthritis with the reasoning that it might inhibit lymphocyte proliferation, which is thought to play a critical role in the pathogenesis of rheumatoid arthritis.

That methotrexate is acting solely as a DHFR inhibitor in rheumatoid arthritis has been called into question and a growing body of evidence suggests that methotrexate may be acting via alternative immunomodulatory mechanisms such by increasing extracellular adenosine.

Methotrexate is actively transported into cells where it is then polyglutamated and retained intracellularly for long periods while still maintaining its biologic activity. Clinically, patients with rheumatoid arthritis treated with methotrexate have been demonstrated to have accumulations of polyglutamated methotrexate in their hepatocytes. The polyglutamate derivative of methotrexate most potently inhibits the enzyme 5-aminoimidazole-4-carboxamide ribonucleotide (AICAR) transformylase that catalyzes the reaction of AICAR to formyl-AICAR. Intracellular accumulation of AICAR ultimately results in enhanced adenosine release into the extracellular compartment by several possible mechanisms: increased production, decreased metabolism, or extracellular generation. In vitro, methotrexate promoted adenosine release from endothelial cells and fibroblasts, an effect that was further enhanced in the presence of stimulated neutrophils or hydrogen peroxide.[41] Mice administered relevant doses of weekly methotrexate demonstrated a three-fold increase in AICAR accumulation in splenocytes as well as higher adenosine concentrations within inflammatory exudates versus saline-treated controls.[42] Extracellular adenosine is then proposed to suppress inflammation by stimulating adenosine receptors. Adenosine receptors mediate an anti-inflammatory effect by inhibiting production of tumor necrosis factor-alpha (TNF-α),[43] as observed following methotrexate treatment, IL-6, IL-8,[44] neutrophil-derived reactive oxygen metabolites,[45] and leukotriene B_4,[46] while increasing IL-10 release[47] and transcription of IL-1 receptor antagonist mRNA.[48] Other proposed mechanisms include methotrexate-induced inhibition of prostaglandin E_2[49] and an increase in Th2 cytokines relative to Th1 cytokines.[50]

Pharmacokinetics

Methotrexate can be administered orally, intramuscularly, subcutaneously, or intravenously. Methotrexate is well absorbed from the gastrointestinal tract at doses below 30 mg, and is completely absorbed when given via a parenteral route. It is approximately 50% bound to plasma proteins with an estimated half-life of 6–12 hours and is primarily excreted by the kidney. Therefore, in patients with a decreased glomerular filtration rate (GFR), as with the elderly, it is imperative that the dose of methotrexate be decreased to avoid adverse effects. In general, patients with a GFR between 10 and 50 ml/min are recommended to receive 50% of the normal dosage and followed closely for bone marrow suppression. Similarly, methotrexate can produce hepatotoxicity and therefore it is also recommended that a dose reduction be made for patients with hepatic insufficiency.

Adverse effects

While most patients will experience an adverse reaction to methotrexate at some point during their treatment, either reduction of the dose or temporary discontinuation of the drug can reverse most problems. In general, methotrexate is well tolerated and fewer patients withdraw from therapy with methotrexate than any other DMARD currently used. The majority of adverse effects are benign and include fatigue, malaise, nausea, and vomiting (which usually occur within 24 hours of taking the drug), alopecia, mucous membrane ulcerations, and exacerbation of rheumatoid nodules. Prescribing daily folic acid supplementation concurrently with methotrexate can significantly reduce some of these adverse effects without affecting methotrexate efficacy. Of greatest concern are the adverse effects associated with the liver, lung and bone marrow, which warrant vigilant surveillance.

The American College of Rheumatology recommends liver chemistry tests, hepatitis virus profile, and complete blood cell count prior to initiating therapy. If transminases are elevated or there is a previous history of hepatitis then a liver biopsy prior to initiation of therapy is recommended. During treatment, patients should have liver enzymes routinely monitored every 4–8 weeks; if transaminases are elevated in 5 of 9 readings over a period of 12 months or a drop in serum albumin is observed then a liver biopsy is recommended.

Pneumonitis occurs in up to 5% of patients taking methotrexate and is not related to dose or duration of therapy. The clinical spectrum varies but pneumonitis commonly presents clinically with fever, nonproductive cough, dyspnea, and infiltrates on chest radiograph. Risk factors include older age, diabetes, rheumatoid pleuropulmonary involvement, previous DMARD therapy, and hypoalbuminemia. It is imperative to rule out a bacterial or opportunistic infection, especially *Pneumocystis carinii*, in this clinical setting as patients taking methotrexate have an increased susceptibility. If the chest radiograph appears normal and clinical suspicion is high then CT scanning is warranted and may reveal diffuse abnormalities. When pneumonitis is suspected, methotrexate must be discontinued immediately, upon which the vast majority of patients improve.

Hematologic involvement is not infrequent and is generally minor. Most commonly observed is a mild macrocytosis with or without an anemia. While uncommon, pancytopenia and thrombocytopenia may occur; patients with renal insufficiency or hypoalbuminemia, or those taking sulfa drugs may be at an increased risk. Additionally, methotrexate does not appear to cause an increased incidence of lymphoproliferative disorders.

Principles of administration

Methotrexate is generally started orally at a dosage of 7.5 mg once weekly with dosages increased safely to 30 mg once weekly as necessitated. Weekly intramuscular injections of methotrexate are appropriate if poor gastrointestinal absorption is present or the patient is unable to tolerate high doses orally. If gastrointestinal adverse effects occur, giving divided doses over a 12–36-hour period may be attempted. Lower doses are recommended in the elderly and renal insufficient patient secondary to decreased glomerular filtration. Efficacy is usually noted between 3 and 8 weeks after initiating therapy. It is recommended that either daily folic acid or weekly folinic acid be given concurrently with methotrexate treatment; this aids in reducing toxicity without affecting efficacy. Prior to initiating methotrexate therapy, a complete blood count with differential, chemistry profile including serum creatinine, liver function tests, and hepatitis virus screen should be performed. Once therapy is initiated, liver enzymes, complete blood count, and serum creatinine should be monitored every 4–8 weeks, preferably as near as possible to the time of the next weekly dose. Methotrexate is contraindicated during pregnancy and breast feeding.

Efficacy

Numerous studies have now demonstrated the efficacy of methotrexate as a single agent to improve both subjective and objective findings of rheumatoid arthritis, including prevention of bone erosions. One advantage of methotrexate is that it is relatively well tolerated; consequently patients remain on the drug longer than other DMARDs. Much attention is currently being paid to combining methotrexate with other DMARDs to further prevent damage and to control symptoms in rheumatoid arthritis. Several such studies have demonstrated that triple therapy consisting of sulfasalazine, hydroxychloroquine, and methotrexate is more effective than any of the drugs alone or any combination of drugs as a double therapy.[50] The addition of a biologic anti-tumor necrosis factor-α drug acts synergistically with methotrexate to suppress symptoms and prevent bone erosions.[51]

Although not as effective as cyclophosphamide, methotrexate has also been found to be effective in inducing remission in Wegener granulomatosis. It is currently recommended as first-line therapy in non-life-threatening Wegener granulomatosis and for maintenance therapy following cyclophosphamide and prednisone induction therapy. Methotrexate is also commonly used in psoriatic arthritis, adult Still's disease, polymyositis, dermatomyositis, musculoskeletal and cutaneous manifestations of SLE, inflammatory bowel disease, and biliary cirrhosis.

MYCOPHENOLATE MOFETIL

Gosio first described mycophenolic acid (MPA) from penicillin mold cultures in 1896 but it was not until 1913, when Alsberg and Black isolated the compound from *Penicillium stoloniferum* fermentation products, that it received its name.[52] During the 1980s mycophenolate was developed and numerous studies demonstrated its ability to prevent acute rejection, as well as treat refractory rejection in liver, heart, and renal transplant recipients. Subsequently, the FDA approved mycophenolate mofetil for use in transplantation in 1995.

Mechanism of action

Mycophenolate mofetil is a prodrug that is hydrolyzed in the liver to form the biologically active parent compound MPA. MPA derives the majority of its effect as a potent, noncompetitive inhibitor of inositol monophosphate dehydrogenase (IMPDH), which is essential for de novo guanosine nucleotide synthesis (Fig. 110.2). The inhibition of IMPDH results in a depletion of intracellular guanosine nucleotides that are required for de novo purine synthesis.

In contrast to most other cells in the body that can utilize both the de novo and salvage pathways, proliferating lymphocytes appear to depend primarily on the de novo pathway for purine nucleotide formation, hence the ability of MPA to impart a selective immunosuppressive effect as proliferating lymphocytes are targeted to a much larger extent than are other cells.

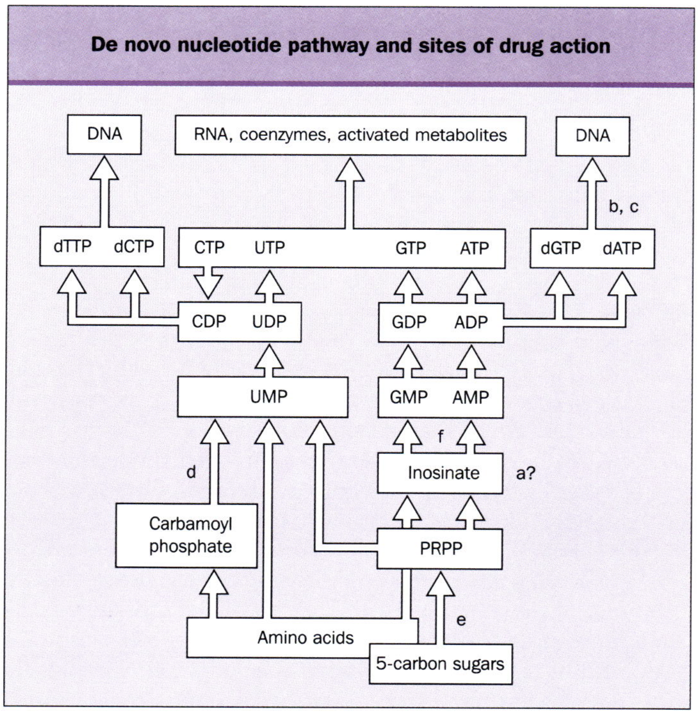

Figure 110.2 De novo nucleotide pathway and sites of drug action. (a) Azathioprine; (b) cladribine; (c) fludarabine; (d) leflunomide; (e) methotrexate; (f) mycophenolate mofetil. DNA, deoxyribonucleic acid; RNA, ribonucleic acid; dTTP, deoxythimidine triphosphate; dCTP, deoxycytidine triphosphate; CTP, cytidine triphosphate; CDP, cytidine diphosphate; UTP, uridine triphosphate; UDP, uridine diphosphate; UMP, uridine monophosphate; GTP, guanosine triphosphate; GDP, guanosine diphosphate; GMD, guanosine monophosphate; ATP, adenosine triphosphate; ADP, adenosine diphosphate; AMP, adenosine monophosphate; PRPP, phosphoribose pyrophosphate; dGTP, deoxyguanosine; dATP, deoxyadenosine.

THERAPEUTIC PRINCIPLES

Mycophenolate mofetil

- Inositol monophosphate dehydrogenase antagonist.
- Gastrointestinal and hematologic toxicities are common.
- Dosage: 2000–5000 mg/day in divided doses.
- Dose reduction necessary in patients with decreased glomerular filtration rate.
- Monitor CBC weekly for first month, then twice monthly for 2 months, then monthly for the remainder of one year.
- Marginal benefit over azathioprine in solid organ transplantation.

MPA has been demonstrated to decrease the adherence of human monocytes to endothelial cells. In vitro studies suggest that this may be mediated via MPA-induced depletion of the guanosine nucleotide pool, thereby inhibiting the guanosine-dependent incorporation of mannose and fucose into membrane glycoproteins including adhesion molecules.

MPA has also been demonstrated to inhibit proliferation of B lymphocytes to both T cell-dependent and independent mitogens, as well as inhibiting T-lymphocyte proliferation.[53] These effects can be reversed in vitro by the addition of guanosine.[54] Initial events in T-cell activation such as cytokine production and their effect on the expression of CD40 ligand do not appear to be affected. At increased concentrations, MPA inhibits fibroblast and smooth muscle cell proliferation.

Pharmacokinetics

After gastrointestinal absorption mycophenolate mofetil is rapidly and completely hydrolyzed to the biologically active form, MPA. A single dose of mycophenolate mofetil 1.5 g given orally to healthy volunteers demonstrated peak serum concentrations at 1 hour with a secondary peak at 8–12 hours, a biologic half-life of 17 hours, and approximately 94% bioavailability. MPA is almost completely bound (>99%) to serum albumin. MPA is metabolized largely by the liver via uridine diphosphate-glucuronosyl transferase to form mycophenolic acid glucuronide (MPAG), of which approximately 87% is excreted in the urine. An estimated 6% of MPAG is eliminated in the bile where it undergoes deconjugation by intestinal microflora β-glucuronidase and is subsequently reconverted to MPA and reabsorbed. This enterohepatic circulation accounts for the secondary peak seen in plasma concentrations of MPA after an oral dose of mycophenolate mofetil. MPAG is at best a weak inhibitor of IMPDH, with estimates ranging between 10 and 1000-fold higher inhibitory concentrations than that of MPA.

Adverse effects

Gastrointestinal disturbances are the most commonly reported adverse effect of mycophenolate mofetil. These effects are dose-dependent and include nausea, vomiting, diarrhea, constipation, abdominal cramping, and anorexia, each of which is reversible after either lowering of the dose or discontinuation of the drug. Rare cases of hemorrhagic gastritis and pancreatitis have been reported. Both conditions appeared to resolve after discontinuation of the drug.

Renal transplant recipients receiving mycophenolate mofetil experienced urinary tract infections, hematuria, and rarely renal tubular necrosis. Cardiac transplant patients demonstrated an increase in both blood urea nitrogen and serum creatinine. Dysuria, urinary urgency, vaginal burning, and bleeding have been reported during the treatment of psoriasis. All these symptoms decreased in severity and/or frequency after the first year of treatment. Leukopenia, anaemia, and thrombocytopenia have all been reported with the use of mycophenolate mofetil. Limited studies of mycophenolate mofetil use in patients with rheumatoid arthritis or those with renal and heart transplants have not reported an increased incidence of carcinoma.

The majority of adverse effects are attenuated with a decrease in the dose of mycophenolate mofetil, dose division, or discontinuation of the drug. Long-term safety data demonstrate that adverse effects diminish with extended use of the drug, and neurotoxicity, hepatotoxicity, and nephrotoxicity are rare occurrences with mycophenolate mofetil.

Principles of administration

Mycophenolate mofetil is available in 250 mg capsules, 500 mg tablets, an oral suspension which when constituted contains 200 mg/ml, and an intravenous preparation. In general, oral mycophenolate mofetil is usually started at 2000 mg daily given in two divided doses but may be increased to doses as high as 5000 mg daily in patients with refractory psoriasis. Dose reduction is not necessary in renal transplant patients experiencing delayed graft function postoperatively, but patients outside the immediate post-transplant period who are experiencing severe chronic renal impairment (GFR <25 ml/min/1.73 m^2) should not receive mycophenolate mofetil doses greater than 2 g daily. No dose adjustment is necessary for hepatic insufficiency. If the patient develops neutropenia, the dose of mycophenolate mofetil should either be decreased or discontinued altogether.

Efficacy

Mycophenolate mofetil has been demonstrated to be an effective rescue therapy in renal, heart, and liver transplant recipients. Trials studying the effectiveness of mycophenolate mofetil in combination with cyclosporine and glucocorticoids as primary prophylaxis in renal transplant recipients have demonstrated an increase in both renal graft and patient survival compared with cyclosporine and glucocorticoids alone.[55,56] A recent multicenter heart transplant trial comparing mycophenolate mofetil (3 g/d) versus azathioprine (1.5–3 mg/kg/day) demonstrated the ability of mycophenolate mofetil to decrease 1-year mortality (6.2% versus 11.4% in the azathioprine group) and to decrease the requirement for rejection treatment (65.7% versus 73.7%).[57] An interim report of a prospective randomized trial in liver transplant recipients studying tacrolimus and glucocorticoids with or without mycophenolate mofetil only demonstrated a slight benefit in the rate of rejection, a decrease in perioperative renal impairment, and steroid reduction.[58] A recent prospective randomized trial in orthotopic liver transplant recipients demonstrates a clear ability of mycophenolate mofetil as primary prophylaxis to help prevent rejection in conjunction with cyclosporine or tacrolimus.[59] Overall, mycophenolate appears to have an advantage over azathioprine in terms of acute rejection but long-term graft survival may be equivalent.

Although no well-designed prospective double-blind study of mycophenolate mofetil in rheumatoid arthritis patients has been performed to date, one trial in patients with refractory rheumatoid arthritis demonstrated the ability of mycophenolate mofetil to decrease significantly the number of painful and swollen joints. Mycophenolate mofetil in combination with prednisone has been reported in a small case series to significantly decrease proteinuria and serum creatinine values in patients with lupus nephritis who previously have failed cyclophosphamide therapy.[60]

SULFASALAZINE

Sulfasalazine is a two-component compound joined by an azo bond consisting of an anti-inflammatory agent, salicylic acid, and an antibiotic, sulfapyridine. It was first synthesized in the 1930s for the treatment of rheumatoid arthritis but was apathetically received by the rheumatologic community. During the 1960s it became routinely used for the treatment of inflammatory bowel disease, for which it is still utilized today. During the late 1970s interest was rekindled regarding its efficacy in rheumatoid arthritis and since that time it has become accepted as a safe and effective second-line option for treating inflammatory synovitis.

Mechanism of action

Sulfasalazine was originally synthesized with the intention that the sulfapyridine component of the molecule would treat a bacterial infection that was believed to be the underlying etiology of rheumatoid arthritis. Indeed, sulfapyridine has been demonstrated to inhibit growth of several bacterial species, primarily of the gut, which could potentially decrease the load of potential bacterial antigens. However, it seems unlikely that this is the primary mode of action. The overall number of circulating activated lymphocytes is reduced following 12 weeks of sulfasalazine therapy and, in vitro, it decreases immunoglobulin production and inhibits the release of IL-1, IL-2, TNF-α, IL-6, and IFN-γ. A recent report suggests that sulfasalazine may selectively inhibit nuclear factor-κB.[61]

The precise mechanism of action of sulfasalazine is unclear and a controversy exists regarding whether the parent compound or its metabolites are responsible for its immunomodulatory effect. Strong evidence now suggests that sulfasalazine works by a mechanism similar to that of methotrexate in elevating extracellular adenosine levels and mediating anti-inflammatory pathways via adenosine receptors (see methotrexate).[41,62]

THERAPEUTIC PRINCIPLES

Sulfasalazine

- Salicylate–sulfapyridine hybrid.
- Sulfapyridine is the active metabolite in inflammatory synovitis.
- 5-Aminosalicylic acid is the active metabolite in inflammatory bowel disease.
- Gastrointestinal, hematologic, and cutaneous toxicities are common and may be severe.
- Reversible male infertility.
- Dosage: 1500–6000 mg/day.
- Monitor CBC, liver function tests, and creatinine.

Pharmacokinetics

Sulfasalazine is 99% protein bound, demonstrates peak concentrations within 3–5 hours following administration, and has an apparent half-life of 7 hours. Sulfapyridine is also readily absorbed while 5-aminosalicylic acid is largely retained in the colon, where approximately 75% is excreted in the feces. Sulfapyridine is 70% protein bound, demonstrates a serum peak approximately 12 hours after a dose, and is largely metabolized in liver, ultimately undergoing glucuronidation. 5-aminosalicylic acid is mostly acetylated by the liver and renally excreted.

Adverse effects

In general, sulfasalazine is relatively well tolerated, with the majority of adverse effects occurring within the first several months; however, only approximately 20% of patients will remain on the drug after 5 years. Common reactions include gastrointestinal disturbances, skin rashes, and hematologic manifestations. The majority of these side-effects can be resolved following dose reduction.

Sulfasalazine should be avoided in patients with a known sulfa allergy. Even in patients without a known allergy history up to 50% will develop a maculopapular rash, pruritis, or urticaria that may be associated with fever. Frequently this occurs early after initiating therapy. Severe exfoliative dermatitis, Stevens–Johnson syndrome, and drug-induced lupus have been reported.

Patients may experience leukopenia within the first 3–6 months following the initiation of therapy. This may be severe and potentially fatal but early discontinuation of sulfasalazine can reverse the leukopenia. It is therefore recommended that the complete blood count be monitored closely. Macrocytosis, thrombocytopenia, and agranulocytosis have been reported.

Sulfasalazine is safe during breast feeding but should be avoided during pregnancy despite the reported absence of teratogenicity. Reversible male infertility as a result of decreased sperm count and motility and morphological abnormalities has been reported but is not an absolute contraindication for therapy in males. Screening for G6PD deficiency in high-prevalence populations, e.g. African-Americans, is recommended.

Principles of administration

Sulfasalazine is manufactured as 500 mg tablets and comes prepared in an enteric-coated form that is better tolerated than the noncoated form. The recommended daily dose of sulfasalazine, in equally divided doses, is between 2 and 4 g/day. Improved tolerance can be obtained by starting patients on doses of 500 mg/day to 1 g/day and increasing dosage by 500 mg/day increments weekly until the desired dose is obtained. Prior to initiating therapy a comprehensive metabolic panel and complete blood count should be obtained. Then the complete blood count should be monitored every 2–4 weeks during the first 3 months of therapy and thereafter every 6–8 weeks. Agranulocytosis occurs suddenly and may occur between monitoring; it is imperative therefore that patients understand the possibility of sulfasalazine's hematologic effects and be instructed to notify medical personnel of symptoms such as sore throat, fever, and fatigue.

Efficacy

Sulfasalazine has been known since the 1960s to be superior to placebo for the treatment of mild to moderate ulcerative colitis; however, its role in Crohn's disease is less clear. Crohn's disease limited to the colon and possibly ileocecum appears to be responsive to sulfasalazine treatment but requires daily doses of 4–6 g, resulting in substantial adverse effects. The 5-aminosalicylic acid component of sulfasalazine has since been found to be the clinically active metabolite in ulcerative colitis and, consequently, several different preparations of 5-aminosalicylic acid are now available for use in the treatment of inflammatory bowel disease.

Sulfasalazine has been demonstrated to be an effective second-line agent for the treatment of rheumatoid arthritis and is more effective than hydroxychloroquine and D-penicillamine in preventing bone erosions. Clinical benefit can be expected at approximately 4 weeks after starting therapy. Combining sulfasalazine with various other DMARDs has demonstrated a synergistic effect in treating rheumatoid arthritis. Particularly effective has been the combination of sulfasalazine, methotrexate, and hydroxychloroquine. Sulfasalazine has also been demonstrated to be effective in the treatment of psoriatic arthritis, HLA-B27 spondyloarthropathy, ankylosing spondylitis, and juvenile rheumatoid arthritis.

REFERENCES

1. Galens GJ, Bull FE, Bartholomew LE. The treatment of rheumatoid arthritis with 6-mercaptopurine and azathioprine. Arthritis Rheum 1964;7:735.
2. Yu DT, Clements PJ, Peter JB, et al. Lymphocyte characteristics in rheumatic patients and the effect of azathioprine therapy. Arthritis Rheum 1974;17:37.
3. Hortelano S, Bosca L. 6-Mercaptopurine decreased the Bcl-2/Bax ratio and induces apoptosis in activated B-lymphocytes. Mol Pharmacol 1997;51:414.
4. Singh G, Fries JF, Spitz P, Williams CA. Toxic effects of azathioprine in rheumatoid arthritis. A national postmarketing perspective. Arthritis Rheum 1989;32:837.
5. Romagnuolo J, Sadaowski DC, Lalor E, et al. Cholestatic hepatocellular injury with azathioprine: a case report and review of the mechanisms of hepatotoxicity. Can J Gastroenterol 1998;12:479.
6. Hoover R. Risk of cancer in renal-transplant recipients. Lancet 1973;2:55.
7. Matteson EL, Hickey AR, Maguire L, Tilson HH, Urowitz MB. Occurrence of neoplasia in patients with rheumatoid arthritis enrolled in a DMARD registry. J Rheumatol 1991;18:809.
8. Wessel F, Abendroth K, Wisheit M. Malignant transformation during immuno-suppressive therapy (Azathioprine) of rheumatoid arthritis and systemic lupus erythematosus. A retrospective study. Scand J Rheumatol 1987;67:S73.
9. Urowitz MB, Hunter T, Bockman AAM, Gordon DA, Smythe HA, Ogryzlo MA. Azathioprine in rheumatoid arthritis: a double-blind study comparing full dose to half dose. J Rheumatol 1974;1:274.
10. Seikaly MG. Mycophenolate mofetil – is it worth the cost? The in-favor opinion. Pediatr Transplant 1999;3:79.
11. Candy S, Wright J, Gerber M, Adams G, Gerig M, Goodman R. A controlled double blind study of azathioprine in the management of Crohn's disease. Gut 1995;37:674.
12. Sandborn WJ, Van Os EC, Zins BJ, Tremaine WJ, Mays DC, Lipsky JJ. An intravenous loading dose of azathioprine decreases the time to response in patients with Crohn's disease. Gastroenterology 1995;109:1808.
13. Austin HA III, Klippel JH, Balow JE, et al. Therapy of lupus nephritis. Controlled trial of prednisone and cytotoxic drugs. N Engl J Med 1986;314:614.

14. Luqmani R, Jayne D, EUVAS. A multi-center randomised trial of cyclophosphamide versus azathioprine during remission in ANCA-associated systemic vasculitis (Cycazarem). Presented at the Meeting of the American College of Rheumatology, 12–18 November 1999, Boston, Massachusetts, USA.
15. Thorpe P, Hassall JE, York JR. Rheumatoid arthritis treated with chlorambucil: a five-year follow-up. Med J Aust 1976;2:197.
16. Zhu LP, Cupps TR, Whalen G, Fauci AS. Selective effects of cyclophosphamide therapy on activation, proliferation, and differentiation of human B cells. J Clin Invest 1987;79:1082.
17. Moody DJ, Fahey JL, Grable E, et al. Administration of monthly pulses of cyclophosphamide in multiple sclerosis patients. Delayed recovery of several immune parameters following discontinuation of pulse-dose cyclophosphamide treatment. J Neuroimmunol 1987;14:175.
18. Boumpas DT, Austin HA III, Vaughn EM, Yarboro CH, Klippel JH, Balow JE. Risk for sustained amenorrhea in patients with systemic lupus erythematosus receiving intermittent pulse cyclophosphamide therapy. Ann Intern Med 1993;119:366.
19. Gourley MF, Austin HA, Scott D, et al. Methylprednisolone and cyclophosphamide alone or in combination, in patients with lupus nephritis. A randomized, controlled trial. Ann Intern Med 1996;125:549.
20. Balow JE, Austin HA, Muenz LR, et al. Effect of treatment on the evolution of renal abnormalities in lupus nephritides. N Engl J Med 1984;311:491.
21. Austin HA, Klippel JH, Balow JE, et al. Therapy of lupus nephritis: Controlled trial of prednisone and cytotoxic drugs. N Engl J Med 1986;314:614.
22. Illei GG, Crane M, Austin HA, et al. Long-term follow-up of patients with lupus nephritis treated with pulses of methylprednisolone and cyclophosphamide. Arthritis Rheum (in press)
23. Hoffman GS, Leavitt RY, Fleisher TA, Minor JR, Fauci AS. Treatment of Wegener's granulomatosis with intermittent high-dose intravenous cyclophosphamide. Am J Med 1990;89:403.
24. Brodsky RA. Biology and management of acquired severe aplastic anemia. Curr Opin Oncol 1998;10:95.
25. Zinzani PL, Tosi P, Visani G, et al. Apoptosis induction with three nucleoside analogs on freshly isolated B-chronic lymphocytic leukemia cells. Am J Hematol 1994;47:301.
26. Frank DA, Mahajan S, Ritz J. Fludarabine-induced immunosuppression is associated with inhibition of STAT1 signaling. Nat Med 1999;5:444.
27. Deane M, Gor D, Macmahon E, et al. Quantification of CMV viraemia in a case of transfusion-related graft-versus-host disease associated with purine analogue treatment. Br J Haematol 1997;99:162.
28. Davis JC Jr, Austin H, Boumpas D, et al. A pilot study of 2-chloro-2′-deoxyadenosine in the treatment of systemic lupus erythematosus-associated glomerulonephritis. Arthritis Rheum 1998;41:335.
29. Romine JS, Sipe JC, Koziol JA, Zyroff J, Beutler E. A double blind, placebo-controlled, randomized trial of cladribine in relapsing-remitting multiple sclerosis. Proc Assoc Am Physicians 1999;111:35.
30. Cao WW, Kao PN, Aoki Y, Xu JC, Shorthouse R, Morris RE. A novel mechanism of action of the immunomodulatory drug, leflunomide: Augmentation of the immunosuppressive cytokine, TGFβ1, and suppression of the immunostimulatory cytokine, IL-2. Transplant Proc 1996;28:3079
31. Fairbanks LD, Bofill M, Ruckerman K, Simmonds HA. Importance of ribonucleotide availability to proliferating T-lymphocytes from healthy humans. J Biol Chem 1995;270:29682.
32. Bartlett RR, Mattar T, Weithmann U, Anagnostopoulos H, Popvic S, Schleyerbach R. Leflunomide (HWA 486): A novel immunorestoring drug. Therapeutic approaches to inflammatory diseases. In: Lewis AJ, Doherty NS, Ackerman NR (eds) Proceedings of the Fourth International Conference of the Inflammation Research Association, October 23–27, Whitehaven, Elsevier, 1988, p. 215.
33. Hamilton LC, Vojnovic I, Warner TD. A77 1726, the active metabolite of leflunomide, directly inhibits the activity of cyclo-oxygenase-2 in vitro and in vivo in a substrate-sensitive manner. Br J Pharm 1999;127:1589.
34. Morris RE, Huang X, Cao W, Zheng B, Shorthouse RA. Leflunomide (HWA486) and its analog suppress T- and B-cell proliferation in vitro, acute rejection, ongoing rejection, and antidonor antibody synthesis in mouse, rat and cynomolgus monkey transplant recipients as well as arterial intimal thickening after balloon catheter injury. Transplant Proc 1995;27:161.
35. Manna SK, Aggarwal BB. Immunosuppressive Leflunomide metabolite (A77 1726) blocks TNF-dependent nuclear factor-κB activation and gene expression. J Immunol 1999;162:2095.
36. Cohen S, Weaver A, Schiff M, Strand V, for the Leflunomide Study Group. Treatment of active rheumatoid arthritis with leflunomide compared with placebo and methotrexate. Presented at the Meeting of the American College of Rheumatology, 12–18 November 1999, Boston, Massachusetts, USA.
37. Smolen JS, Kalden JR, Scott DL, et al. Efficacy and safety of leflunomide compared with placebo and sulphasalazine in active rheumatoid arthritis: a double blind, randomized, multicenter trial. Lancet 1999;353:259.
38. Schiff M, Sharp J, Smolen J, Emery P, Strand V, for the Leflunomide Investigators Study Group. Consistency of leflunomide effect for slowing the radiographic disease progression of active rheumatoid arthritis: results from three controlled trials [abstract]. Arthritis Rheum 1999;42:S81.
39. Strand V, Cohen S, Schiff M, et al. Treatment of active rheumatoid arthritis with leflunomide compared with placebo and methotrexate. Arch Intern Med 1999;159:2542.
40. Popovic M, Stefanovic D, Pejnovic N, et al. Comparative study of the clinical efficacy of four DMARDs (leflunomide, methotrexate, cyclosporin and levamisole) in patients with rheumatoid arthritis. Transplant Proc 1998;30:4135.
41. Cronstein BN, Eberle MA, Gruber HE, et al. Methotrexate inhibits neutrophil function by stimulating adenosine release from connective tissue cells. Proc Natl Acad Sci USA 1991;88:2441.
42. Cronstein BN, Naime D, Ostad E. The anti-inflammatory mechanism of methotrexate: Increased adenosine release at inflamed sites diminishes leukocyte accumulation in an in vivo model of inflammation. J Clin Invest 1993;92:2675.
43. Sajjadi FG, Takabayashi K, Foster AC, et al. Inhibition of TNFα expression by adenosine: Role of A3 adenosine receptors. J Immunol 1996;117:1639.
44. Bouma MG, Srad RK, van den Wildenberg FA, et al. Differential regulatory effects of adenosine on cytokine release by activated human monocytes. J Immunol 1994;1:4159.
45. Cronstein BN, Kramer SB, Weissmann G, et al. Adenosine: a physiological modulator of superoxide anion generation by human neutrophils. J Exp Med 1983;158:1160.
46. Krump E, Lemay G, Borgeat D. Adenosine A2 receptor-induced inhibition of leukotriene B4 synthesis in whole blood ex vivo. Br J Pharmacol 1996;117:1639.
47. Le Moine O, Stordeur P, Schandene L, et al. Adenosine enhances IL-10 secretion by human monocytes. J Immunol 1996;156:4408.
48. Vergne P, Liagre B, Bertin P, et al. Methotrexate and cyclooxygenase metabolism in cultured human rheumatoid synoviocytes. J Rheumatol 1998;25:433.
49. Constantin A, Loubet-Lescoulie P, Lambert N, et al. Anti-inflammatory and immunoregulatory action of methotrexate in the treatment of rheumatoid arthritis. Arthritis Rheum 1998;41:48.
50. O'Dell J, Leff R, Paulsen G, et al. Methotrexate (M), Hydroxychloroquine (H), Sulfasalazine (S) versus M-H or M-S for rheumatoid arthritis (RA): Results of a double-blind study. Arthritis Rheum 1999;42:S117.
51. Weinblatt ME, Kremer JM, Bankhurst AD, et al. A trial of etanercept, a recombinant tumor necrosis factor receptor: Fc fusion protein, in patients with rheumatoid arthritis receiving methotrexate. N Engl J Med 1999;340:253.
52. Gosio B. Ricerche batteriologiche e chimiche sulle alterazoni del mais. Rivista d'Igiene e Sanita Pugbblica Ann 1896;7:825.
53. Chang CC, Aversa G, Punnonen J, Yssel H, De Vries JE. Brequinar sodium, mycophenolic acid, and cyclosporin A inhibit different stages of IL-4 or IL-13-induced human IgG4 and IgE production in vitro. Ann NY Acad Sci 1993;696:424.

54. Allison AC, Lafferty KJ, Fliri H. Immunosuppressive, antiinflammatory drugs. Ann NY Acad Sci 1993;696:424.
55. Sollinger HW, for the US Renal Transplant Mycophenolate Mofetil Study Group. Mycophenolate mofetil for the prevention of acute rejection in primary cadaveric renal allograft recipients. Transplantation 1995;60:225.
56. The European Multicenter Renal Transplant Mycophenolate Mofetil Study Group. Placebo-controlled study of mycophenolate mofetil combined with cyclosporin and corticosteroids for prevention of acute rejection. Lancet 1995;345:1321.
57. Kobashigawa JA, Miller L, Renlund DG, et al. A randomized active-controlled trial of mycophenolate mofetil in heart transplant recipients. Transplantation 1998;66:507.
58. Jain AB, Hamad I, Rakela J, et al. A prospective randomized trial of tacrolimus and prednisone vs. tacrolimus, prednisone and mycophenolate mofetil in primary adult liver transplant recipients: An interim report. Transplantation 1998;66:1395.
59. Fisher RA, Ham JM, Marcos A, et al. A prospective randomized trial of mycophenolate mofetil with neoral or tacrolimus after orthotopic liver transplantation. Transplantation 1998;66:1616.
60. Jonsson CA, Svensson L, Carlston H. Beneficial effect of the inosine monophosphate dehydrogenase inhibitor mycophenolate mofetil on survival and severity of glomerulonephritis in systemic lupus erythematosus-prone MRL/lpr/lpr mice. Clin Exp Immunol 1999;116:534.
61. Wahl C, Liptay S, Adler G, Schmid RM. Sulfasalazine: a potent and specific inhibitor of nuclear factor kappa B. J Clin Invest 1998;101:1163.
62. Cronstein BN, Montesinos MC, Weissmann G. Salicylates and sulfasalazine, but not glucocorticoids inhibit leukocyte accumulation by an adenosine-dependent mechanism that is independent of inhibition of prostaglandin synthesis and p105 of NFκB. Proc Natl Acad Sci USA 1999;96:6377.

Section 10 Prevention and Therapy of Immunologic Diseases
E Immunosuppressives

Chapter 111

Immunophilins and the Immunophilin-binding Agents

Anthony D. Cristillo and Barbara E. Bierer

The immunophilins are a large family of highly conserved, ubiquitously expressed proteins that were initially characterized by their ability to bind a number of immunosuppressive agents, including cyclosporin A (CsA), tacrolimus (FK506), and sirolimus (also termed rapamycin). The immunophilins are characterized by eight antiparallel β strands that form a right-handed β barrel covered by connecting loops and α helices.[1–3] Within this structure, the amino and carboxyl termini are located at opposite ends of the molecule surrounding a large hydrophobic core pocket formed by four of the eight β strands and their connecting loops. It is within this core pocket that proline-containing proteins bind. Immunophilins share the ability to catalyze the isomerization of proline residues between their *cis* and *trans* configuration and are therefore thought to play a role in protein folding.[4] The immunophilins identified to date fall into one of three categories: (1) cyclophilins that bind CsA; (2) FK506 binding proteins (FKBPs) that bind tacrolimus and sirolimus; and (3) parvulins. Schematic representations of the cyclophilins, FKBPs, and parvulins are shown in Figure 111.1.

Studies have revealed that the immunophilins identified thus far are capable of binding not only immunosuppressive agents but also a variety of other targets including heat-shock proteins, cell-cycle regulatory factors, and the HIV-1 Gag capsid protein, as discussed below. Members of the immunophilin protein family have been identified in all species examined to date including plants; they have been found to vary in molecular weight, subcellular localization, binding agents, and suggested functions (Tables 111.1, 111.2). They are thought to play key roles in immunosuppression and protein folding, as well as the regulation of RNA splicing and Ca^{2+} homeostasis.

This chapter reviews our current understanding of cyclophilins, FKBPs, and parvulins. It summarizes our present knowledge of immunophilin-binding agents and discusses the biological roles of immunophilin/binding agent complexes as well as their therapeutic value. While much progress has been made in understanding the molecular basis for therapeutic action of the immunosuppressive drugs, a number of central questions remain and are reviewed.

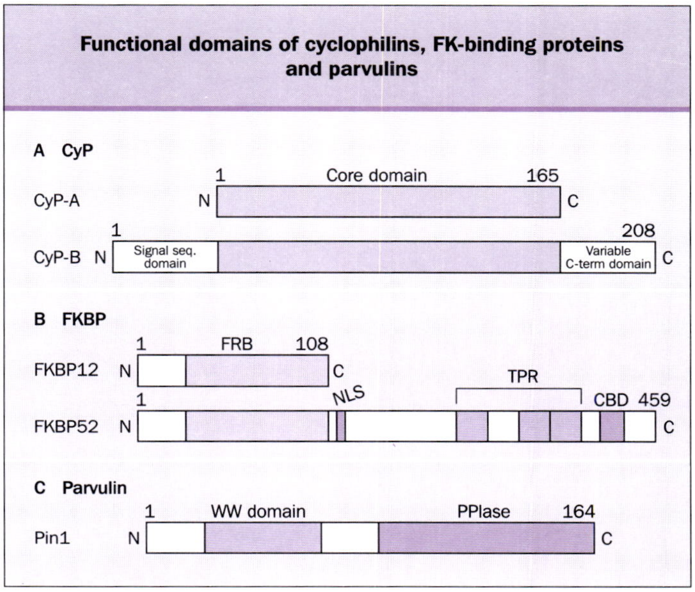

Figure 111.1 Functional domains of cyclophilins (CyPs), FK-binding proteins (FKBPs), and parvulins. (**A**) CyP-A and other members of the cyclophilin family have a highly conserved central core domain that contains both a CsA-binding region and a prolyl isomerase domain. Unlike CyP-A, CyP-B also has an N-terminal endoplasmic reticulum (ER)-directed signal sequence and a C-terminal variable domain. Other cyclophilin members differ in the amino- and carboxy-terminal extensions. (**B**) The prototype FKBP is FKBP12, a 12 kDa protein that has a characteristic FK506 and sirolimus binding (FRB) domain to which binding of FK506 and sirolimus occurs. FKBP52 also contains a nuclear localization signal (NLS), a C-terminal calmodulin-binding domain (CBD), and a tetratricopeptide repeat region (TPR) that mediates protein–protein interactions. (**C**) The parvulin Pin1 has a WW domain that contains two signature tryptophan residues and mediates protein–protein interactions. Pin1 also has a peptidyl prolyl *cis-trans* isomerase (PPIase) domain responsible for its enzymatic activity.

CALCINEURIN: THE COMMON MOLECULAR TARGET OF CSA/CYCLOPHILIN AND TACROLIMUS/FKBPs

The immunosuppressant cyclosporine (also termed cyclosporin A, CsA) was first identified in 1970 as a result of an antifungal screening procedure undertaken by Sandoz Ltd (Basel, Switzerland). Thiele and coworkers isolated new strains of fungi from soil samples obtained from the USA and Norway.[5] These fungi were found to synthesize and secrete metabolites that were later termed cyclosporins; the strains themselves were isolated and classified as *Tolypocladium inflatum*. The Norwegian soil samples were later used for large-scale production of cyclosporine by fermentation. The initial isolation of cyclosporine yielded a mixture of two homologous components, CsA and CsB; in rodent studies, the CsA isolate exhibited immunosuppressive activity. Borel and coworkers demonstrated that purified CsA from this mixture possessed immunosuppressive properties in both in vitro and in vivo studies,[5] properties that have now been extensively investigated.

Cyclophilins			
Cyclophilin	**Molecular weight (kDa)**	**Subcellular localization**	**Suggested function**
CyP-A	18	Cytosol/nucleus	Inhibits calcineurin when bound to CsA, HIV cofactor, K_d (CsA) = 6
CyP-B	21	Secreted/ER	Protein folding(?); interacts with CAML, may regulate Ca^{2+} homeostasis, K_d (CsA) = 9
CyP-C	22	Secreted/cytosolic vesicles	Interacts with CyCAP (Mac-2 binding protein); LPS response modulator, K_d (CsA) = 6
CyP-D	18	Mitochondria	Chaperone (?); involved in opening of mitochondrial pore in apoptosis
CyP-E		Cytosol	
CyP-X		Cytosol	
CyP33A		Nucleus	RNA-binding?
CyP33B		Nucleus	RNA-binding?
CyP40	40	Cytosol	Component of glucocorticoid receptor; regulator of heat-shock response
CyP60	60	Nucleus	Unknown
CARS-CyP/matrin CyP	89	Nucleus, nuclear speckles?	RNA splicing?
Hal539-CyP		Cytosol	
NK-TRCyP	150	Nucleus, cell membrane?	Tumor recognition?; RNA splicing cofactor?
Nup358/RanBP2	358	Nuclear pore, cytosolic face of nuclear pore	Chaperone?; involved in processing of opsin mRNA
PPIE	33 (predicted)	Unknown	Co-amplified with L-myc in small cell lung cancer
SnuCyp-20	20	Nucleus, nuclear speckles?	RNA splicing?
USA-CyP		Nucleus	SnRNP-associated; involved in splicing regulation

Table 111.1 Cyclophilins.

FK506 binding proteins (FKBPs)			
FKBP	**Molecular weight (kDa)**	**Subcellular localization**	**Suggested function**
FKBP12	11.8	Cytosol	Binds IP_3R, RyR1, type 1 TGF-β receptor, calcineurin when complexed with FK506, TOR when complexed with sirolimus. K_d(FK506) = 0.4 nM; K_d(sirolimus) = 0.2 nM
FKBP12.6	11.6	Cytosol	86% homology to FKBP12. Binds IP_3R, RyR1, RyR2, type 1 TGF-β receptor
FKBP13	13	ER	K_d(FK506) = 55 nmol
FKBP23	23	ER	
FKBP25	25	Nucleus	Binds to nucleolin. K_d(FK506) = 106 nmol
FKBP38	38	ND	
FKBP51	51	Cytosol	Binds hsp90, calcineurin
FKBP52	52	Nucleus/cytosol	Binds to dynein, hsp90, FAP48, FAP68, PAH, steroid receptor. K_d(FK506) = 10 nmol
FKBP65	65	Membrane(?)	Binds to hsp90, raf kinase. K_d(FK506) = 45 nmol
FKBP6		ND	
IPBP12		Membrane	

Table 111.2 FK506 binding proteins (FKBPs).

A fungal cyclic undecapeptide (Fig. 111.2), cyclosporine has been used widely in both kidney and heart transplantation for the prevention of allograft rejection,[6] in bone marrow and stem cell transplantation to prevent graft-versus-host disease (GVHD), and in the therapy of chronic autoimmune inflammatory pathologies.[7,8] Cyclosporine not only revolutionized the approach to and success of transplantation medicine but has also provided an invaluable tool for the study of T-cell signaling. Although

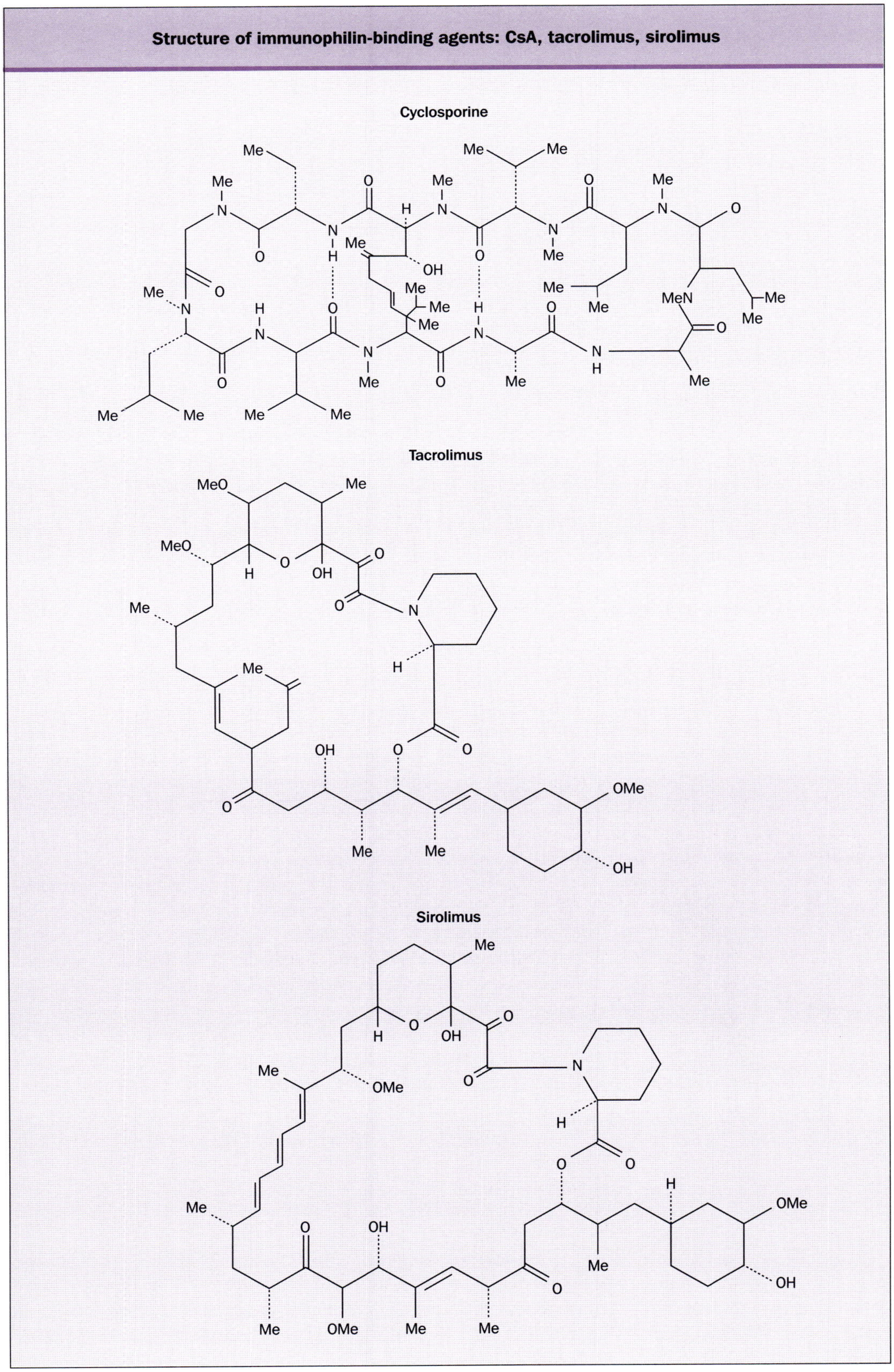

Figure 111.2 Structure of immunophilin-binding agents: CsA, tacrolimus, sirolimus. The chemical structure of the fungal cyclic undecapeptide CsA is shown (top). Isolated from *Tolypocladium inflatum*, CsA binds the immunophilin CyP-A and is used in organ and stem cell transplantation and in a variety of autoimmune disorders. The structure of the macrolide antibiotic tacrolimus (FK506) is also shown (middle). Isolated from *Streptomyces tsukubaensis*, tacrolimus binds the immunophilin FKBP12 and is approved for use in the prevention of rejection in liver and kidney transplantation. Structurally similar to FK506, the macrocyclic triene antibiotic sirolimus (sirolimus, bottom) was isolated from *Streptomyces hygroscopicus*, also binds FKBP12, and is approved fro use in renal transplantation.

cyclosporine can bind to most of the cyclophilins identified, CyP-A has been demonstrated to be the major target of CsA in T lymphocytes[2,7] (see Fig. 111.1, Table 111.1). Tacrolimus (Fig. 111.2) was also isolated from the fermentation broth of a yeast strain and was also shown to have immunosuppressive properties; the in vitro effects of tacrolimus appeared similar to those of cyclosporine.[2,7] Although tacrolimus can bind to all FKBPs identified to date, FKBP12 appears to be the predominant cytoplasmic FKBP in T cells.[2,7] Immunosuppression does not result from inhibition of rotamase activity.[9] It is now appreciated that the CsA/CyP-A and the tacrolimus/FKBP complexes bind to and inhibit the Ca^{2+}/calmodulin-dependent serine/threonine phosphatase calcineurin (Cn; also termed protein phosphatase 2B or PP2B),[10,11] an essential intermediate in T-cell signaling from the T-cell antigen receptor. Calcineurin is a heterodimer composed of CnA and CnB subunits (Fig. 111.3). CnA is the 61 kDa catalytic subunit that binds calmodulin; three isoforms, and multiple splicing variants, of this subunit exist.[12] CnB is the 19 kDa regulatory subunit that binds Ca^{2+}; two mammalian genes have been identified that encode CnB.[12] It is only the heterodimer that is active and the holoenzyme that is stable. Calcineurin activity is regulated by the intracellular concentration of calcium and of calmodulin[12] and by reactive oxygen species.[13] The influx of calcium following T-cell receptor (TCR) cross-linking leads to the calcium-bound calmodulin binding to the carboxyterminus of CnA, promoting the displacement of the autoinhibitory domain[14] and leading to enzymatic activation.[15] Calcineurin activity is required for transcriptional activation of a number of cytokine and other genes. In addition to regulation of these cytokines, calcineurin also regulates ion channel and protein transport, binds several structural proteins, modulates the enzymatic activity of various downstream targets, and plays a role in apoptosis.

The intracellular signaling pathways stimulated by ligation of the T-cell antigen receptor have been well studied (Fig. 111.4). Not a tyrosine kinase itself, TCR cross-linking induces the aggregation of a number of signaling molecules in a large molecular complex. These molecules include members of the src-related tyrosine kinases ($p56^{Lck}$, $p59^{Fyn}$), the Syk/ZAP-70 tyrosine kinase family, and a number of adaptor proteins (LAT, Grb2, GADS, among others) that then bind and activate a number of other proteins. Ligation of the TCR complex induces the phosphorylation of phospholipase C (PLCγ) that itself activates members of the protein kinase C family leading to Ras signaling and, thereby,

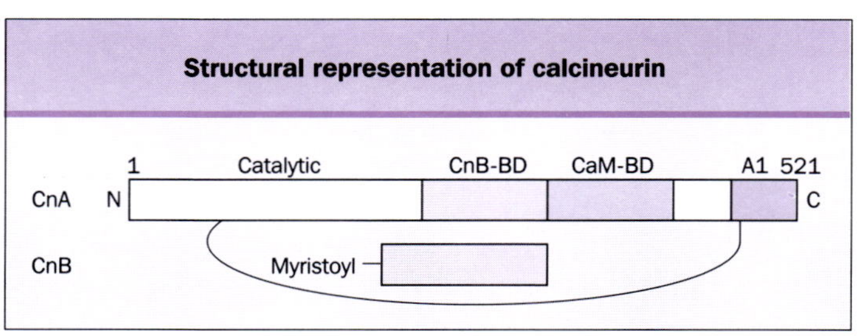

Figure 111.3 Structural representation of calcineurin. Calcineurin is a heterodimer of two subunits, with a 61 kDa catalytic subunit (CnA) and a 19 kDa regulatory subunit (CnB) that is myristylated at its aminoterminal end. CnA has a CnB-binding domain (CnB-BD), a calmodulin-binding domain (CaM-BD), and an autoinhibitory (AI) domain that, in the inactive state, appears to bind at or near, and inhibit the activity of, the phosphatase active site.

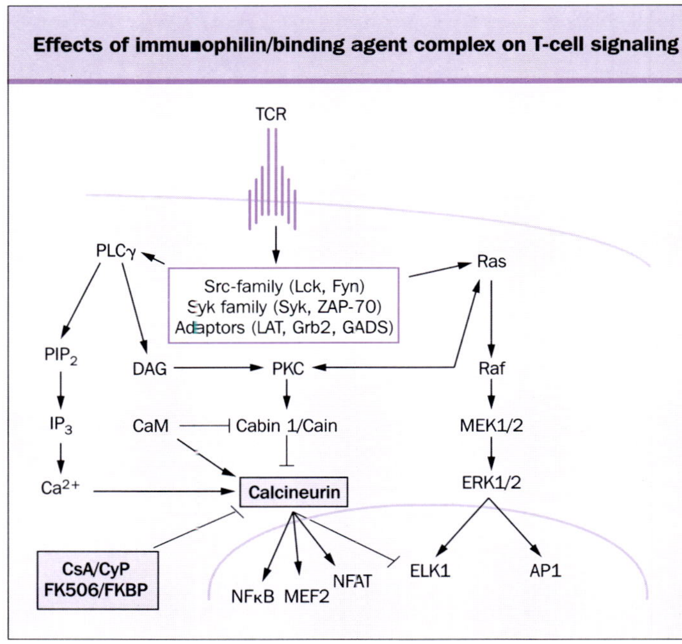

Figure 111.4 Effects of immunophilin/binding agent complex on T-cell signaling. Stimulation of T lymphocytes via the T-cell receptor (TCR) mediates intracellular signaling events that include the activation of protein kinase C as well as an increase in intracellular calcium levels. Calcium and calmodulin are recruited to activate calcineurin, a phosphatase important for activation of a number of transcription factors. The calcium/calmodulin-dependent activation of serine/threonine phosphatase calcineurin is inhibited by both CsA/CyPA and FK506/FKBP12 complexes and in vivo, by Cain/Cabin I.

transcriptional activation of AP1 (c-fos, c-jun) elements. In addition, PLCγ induces inositol 3,4,5 trisphosphate (IP_3) that in turn promotes the release of calcium from the endoplasmic reticulum (ER). In addition, T-cell activation results in the influx of calcium from the extracellular environment. Increases in intracellular calcium concentration, together with calmodulin, activate calcineurin, an enzyme that is required for the activation of a number of transcription factors.

A number of in vivo substrates of calcineurin have been identified. The serine-threonine phosphatase binds to and dephosphorylates the transcription factor NF-AT in the cytosol,[16] NF-AT dephosphorylation, in turn, results in its translocation to the nucleus.[17] Once in the nucleus, NF-AT binds to its DNA recognition sequence on the promoter of numerous target genes, most notably the cytokine genes, including interleukin (IL)-2, IL-3, IL-4, IL-12, inflammatory mediators (e.g. TNF-α), and growth factors (e.g. GM-CSF), resulting in their transactivation.[16] Inhibition of calcineurin activity by the drug/immunophilin complex inhibits the dephosphorylation of and nuclear translocation of NF-AT and thereby the transactivation of NF-AT-dependent genes. In this manner, the Ca^{2+}-dependent activation of antigen-reactive and cytokine-dependent T cells can be inhibited.[2,16]

Considerable evidence exists to suggest that NF-AT is not the only transcription factor regulated by calcineurin. Transcription of genes, expressed in cell types other than T lymphocytes in which NF-AT is not a central regulatory transcription factor, has been shown to be inhibited by cyclosporine. The transcriptional activity of Elk-1 is induced by serine phosphorylation by mitogen-activated protein (MAP) kinase activity, a site that is dephosphorylated by calcineurin; Elk-1 activity is thus negatively regulated by calcineurin.[18] Furthermore, regulation by calcineurin may not be direct: calcineurin has been shown to act cooperatively with protein kinase C (PKC) θ to activate the MAP kinase family member JNK,[19] and JNK phosphorylates not only Elk-1 but also c-Jun and ATF-2.[20] Earlier studies had identified the transcription factor NF-κB to be regulated by calcineurin;[21] NF-κB is localized to the cytoplasm by binding dephosphorylated I-κB. It was later shown that calcineurin and PKC cooperate to activate the I-κB kinase (IKK) complex and thus NF-κB activation in T lymphocytes.[22] Finally, there is considerable evidence that calcineurin regulates the cAMP- and calcium-responsive transcription factor cAMP responsive element (CRE)-binding protein (CREB) in a tissue- and cell-type specific manner.[23]

It is important to note that calcineurin may have both positive and negative effects on lymphoid and on nonimmune cells. While calcineurin appears to be required for transcriptional activation of cytokine genes, it negatively regulates gene expression in certain cell types; the effect of the drug cyclosporine and/or tacrolimus, therefore, is to induce (not inhibit) transcription of certain genes. Cyclosporine has been shown to increase *egr-1* and c-*fos* expression in a calcium-dependent and calcineurin-dependent manner.[24] Cyclosporine has also been shown to increase production of hepatocyte growth factor, a finding that correlates with the effect of this drug on rat liver regeneration.[25] Importantly, the expression of and production of transforming growth factor-beta (TGF-β) appears to be regulated by cyclosporine[26] and by calcineurin.[27] The effects on TGF-β production are complex. Cyclosporine-dependent TGF-β expression induces the cell-cycle inhibitor p21 in both lymphoid and nonlymphoid cells.[28] While increased TGF-β production correlates with immunosuppression, it also appears to correlate with renal fibrosis[29] and nephrotoxicity,[26] as well as anchorage-independent (invasive) growth and cancer progression in nude mice.[30] These effects appear to be independent of effects on the immune system or immune surveillance. Whether tacrolimus will induce a similar spectrum of effects remain to be determined.

One considerable limitation in the clinical use of cyclosporine and tacrolimus is the renal and hepatic toxicity[7,31] observed with prolonged administration. Other side-effects such as hypertension and neurotoxicity are common as well.[6,7] Although the mechanisms by which these toxicities occur are not known, the fact that many are shared between cyclosporine and tacrolimus has led to the suggestion that the side-effects of drug administration are secondary to inhibition of calcineurin, and not to drug metabolites or secondary molecular targets. To this end, the demonstration of isoform-specific expression of calcineurin in T cells (calcineurin A β_2) has led to speculation that specific inhibitors of calcineurin, targeting specific isoforms of the phosphatase, might be designed.[32] Substrate specificity may also confer an approach to the molecular design of agents with greater selectivity: peptides that specifically inhibit calcineurin-mediated dephosphorylation of NF-AT but not other targets have been identified.[33] Such peptides are hoped to provide a prototype for rational drug design. Finally, cyclosporine drug formulations have been modified to optimize and stabilize absorption.[34]

CYCLOPHILINS

The first member of the cyclophilin family to be identified was an 18 kDa soluble protein that was termed cyclophilin A (CyP-A) for its ability to bind the immunosuppressive agent cyclosporine[2,35] (Table 111.1). CyP-A forms a high-affinity, cytoplasmic molecular complex with cyclosporine and thus inhibits specific signaling pathways in T lymphocytes, resulting in immunosuppression. As with other members of this highly conserved protein family, CyP-A was shown to catalyze the *cis*- to *trans*- isomerization of peptidyl-prolyl peptide bonds.[2,35] Because all immunophilins shared the isomerase (also termed rotamase) activity, it was hypothesized that catalysis of protein folding and subcellular trafficking may be an important in vivo role for members of the immunophilin family, a concept that has been difficult to prove.

Cyclophilin homologs are present in all species examined to date; in mammalian cells, cyclophilins are expressed in all tissues. Taken together, the conserved expression suggests that the immunophilin family serves an essential biological function. A number of different mammalian cyclophilins have been identified – proteins that vary in molecular weight, in subcellular localization, and in suggested function (Table 111.1). One common characteristic of the cyclophilin family is a highly conserved core domain that contains both the isomerase active domain and the CsA-binding site (Fig. 111.1); the critical amino acids that define the isomerase-active and the drug-binding domains are identical. It is therefore not surprising that binding of CsA to CyP-A was shown to inhibit its enzymatic (isomerase) activity.[1,2] The amino

KEY CONCEPTS

Distinguishing features of immunophilin-binding immunosuppressants

Cyclosporine
- Cyclic undecapeptide
- Binds cyclophilins
- Does not bind FK506 binding proteins (FKBPs)
- Inhibitor of calcineurin phosphatase activity
- Inhibitor of cyclophilin rotamase activity
- Regulator of gene transcription

Tacrolimus
- Macrolide antibiotic
- Binds FKBPs
- Does not bind cyclophilins
- Inhibitor of calcineurin phosphatase activity
- Inhibitor of FKBP rotamase activity
- Regulator of gene transcription

Sirolimus
- Macrolide antibiotic
- Binds FKBPs
- Does not bind cyclophilins
- Does not inhibit calcineurin
- Binds and inhibits protein kinase mTOR (mammalian target of sirolimus)
- Inhibitor of FKBP rotamase activity
- Inhibitor of protein translation
- Toxicity profile distinct from cyclosporine and tacrolimus

acid sequence identity is greater than 80% among the core regions of CyP-A, CyP-B, and CyP-C.[2,35] The core region is flanked by less conserved amino- and carboxyl-terminal ends that give the different cyclophilins their distinct specificities, and confers a 65% homology when comparing the entire coding sequence of CyP-A and CyP-B, and 70% between CyP-B and CyP-C.

The subcellular localization of the cyclophilins varies: members can be found in the nucleus, cytosol, mitochondria, and endoplasmic reticulum, implying that the substrates or functions of the cyclophilins may differ among the different members of the family. Moreover, evidence exists that some of the cyclophilins, such as CyP-B and CyP-C, are encoded with a signal peptide that directs them to the secretory pathway, and cyclophilins have been found in human milk and blood plasma.[36] Enzymatically active CyP-A has been detected in the synovial fluid of patients afflicted with rheumatoid arthritis but not osteoarthritis,[37] consistent with the observation that cyclophilins appear to act as leukocyte chemotactic factors.[38]

Cyclophilins have a number of cellular binding partners. In the absence of drug, CyP-A binds to and stimulates the activity of a thiol-specific anti-oxidant protein, AOP-1.[39] In addition, CyP-A and the related CyP-B were shown to bind the HIV-1 Gag protein and are consequently thought to be important for HIV-1 infectivity and replication[40] (see below).

Cyclophilin B (CyP-B), a 21 kDa protein localized to the endoplasmic reticulum,[41] has been suggested to play a regulatory role in calcium (Ca^{2+}) homeostasis and inflammation. Using a two-hybrid screening procedure to identify CyP-B-binding partners, Bram and Crabtree[42] identified an interacting partner that was a 33 kDa ubiquitous protein termed *ca*lcium *m*odulating cyclophilin *l*igand (CAML, Fig. 111.5A). Highly conserved in human, mouse, and chicken, CAML has three putative transmembrane segments at its carboxyterminus. In model T-cell (Jurkat) lines, CAML over-expression resulted in the activation of calcium flux[43] as well as an increase in the activity of an NF-AT-luciferase reporter construct.[44] CAML has been shown to colocalize with sarcoplasmic/endoplasmic reticulum calcium/ATPase-2 and calreticulin, further defining its role in regulation of capacitative calcium influx.[43] CAML appears to be an integral membrane protein of the endoplasmic reticulum (and potentially other internal Ca^{2+} stores) and may act as a signaling adaptor protein that links cell-surface receptors (i.e. the CAML-interacting protein, TACI[44]) to internal Ca^{2+} stores (Fig. 111.5B).

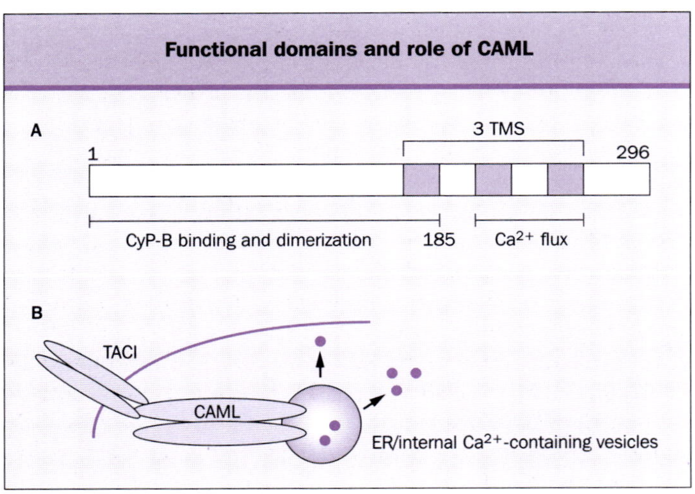

Figure 111.5 Functional domains and role of CAML. (**A**) CAML is a 33 kDa protein that has three transmembrane segments (TMS) at its carboxyl terminus, two of which are required for calcium flux. Amino acids 1–185 are required for CyPB binding and dimerization. (**B**) In the suggested model, the homodimer CAML acts at the endoplasmic reticulum (ER) as a signaling adapter protein linking cell-surface receptors (i.e. TACI) to internal calcium stores.

CyP-C is a membrane-bound, vesicle-associated 23 kDa protein that is secreted in a cyclosporine-sensitive fashion.[11] CyP-C associates with a 77 kDa glycoprotein termed cysteine-rich *C*yP-*C*-*a*ssociated *p*rotein (CyCAP), a member of the scavenger-receptor superfamily, in the absence of cyclosporine.[45] Murine CyCAP is 69% identical to the human Mac-2 binding protein (Mac-2BP), also a member of the scavenger-receptor cysteine-rich (SRCR) protein superfamily. CyCAP is normally secreted and modulates the lipopolysaccharide and endotoxin responses, specifically by modulating the production of inflammatory cytokines.[46] CyP-D, another member of this protein family, is localized to the mitochondrial matrix and is thought to regulate the opening of the mitochondrial pore during apoptosis.[47] The addition of cyclosporine inhibits the opening of the mitochondrial pore following proapoptotic stimuli, and thus prevents cytochrome c release and cell death.[48]

CyP40 is a 40 kDa cytosolic protein that has an aminoterminus that is similar to that of CyP-A and a carboxyterminus that is similar to that of FKBP12.[49] CyP40 not only possesses a prolyl isomerase domain, characteristic of immunophilins, but also three tetratricopeptide repeats (TPR), characteristic of FKBPs (see below). The TPR domains are a degenerate 34 amino acid region involved in protein–protein interactions.[50] CyP40 is thought to form a dimeric complex with heat-shock protein 90 (Hsp90) via binding of the CyP40 TPR domains to a TPR-binding pocket within Hsp90.[50,51] In association with Hsp90, CyP40 is a component of the glucocorticoid and estrogen receptors and may serve a regulatory role in the heat-shock response and in steroid receptor-mediated signaling.[51]

The immunophilin USA-CyP was originally identified by its ability to bind to several proteins involved in RNA splicing, hPrp3 and hPrp4.[52] The complex that forms by the binding of USA-CyP/hPrp3/hPrp4 constitutes the U4/U6 snRNP that plays a central role in pre-mRNA splicing.[52] Recently, the binding site for USA-CyP has been identified as a 30 amino acid region in the aminoterminus of hPrp4. USA-CyP also complexes the RNA-splicing factor hPrp18.[53] It has been suggested that hPrp18 and hPrp4 function in anchoring their respective complexes while USA-CyP acts on other sites in the spliceosome. Evidence suggests that USA-CyP may be working either during the assembly of splicing factors into larger complexes preceding splicing or during the splicing reaction. In addition to USA-CyP, several other cyclophilins including SnuCyP20, NK-TRCyP, CARS-CyP/MatrinCyP, CyP33, and Nup358/RanBP2 bind RNA and have been suggested to regulate RNA splicing or processing.[54,55] Other cyclophilins remain for which binding partners and function have not been identified.

Cyclophilin–HIV interactions

The endogenous interaction of the cyclophilins A and B with the retrovirus HIV-1 deserves special consideration secondary to its importance in the pathogenesis and potential treatment of acquired immune deficiency syndrome (AIDS). HIV-1 consists of several genes that encode all the necessary proteins for viral proliferation and survival. Included amongst these genes is *env*, which encodes the precursors of several envelope glycoproteins, and *gag*, which encodes the precursors of several virion and capsid proteins.[56,57] Two glycoproteins encoded by *env* include gp120 and gp41. gp120 is a highly glycosylated, hydrophilic protein that consists of a CD4 receptor binding domain and five hypervariable regions. It is found on the external surface of virion membranes as well as the plasma membrane of infected cells and is responsible for the recognition of cell-surface receptors. gp41 is a hydrophobic protein that traverses the lipid bilayer membranes of both virions and cells and is responsible for fusion of viral and cellular membranes. One of the proteins encoded by *gag* is the p24 capsid protein. It forms the major internal structural feature of the virion, the core shell, and is responsible for both the packaging of genomic viral RNA into virions and uncoating.

Prior to viral penetration, high-affinity binding occurs between the envelope glycoprotein gp120 and the CD4 receptor on the surface of macrophages and T lymphocytes. A conformational change then occurs and results in the interaction of gp120 with gp41. This interaction is very important for the subsequent binding of gp120 to the chemokine receptors CCR5, on macrophages, or CXCR4, on T cells. Binding results in a second conformational change that gives rise to a hairpin structure. Subsequently, integration of the virus into the cell membrane occurs.[58]

In vitro the third hypervariable loop (V3) of the envelope glycoprotein gp120 binds to members of the cyclophilin family including CyP-A and CyP-B.[40,59] In addition, a weaker interaction occurs between FKBP12 (see below) and gp120.[59] It has been suggested that the rotamase activity of the cyclophilins may mediate the conformational changes that are required for the binding of gp120 to gp41 and for subsequent chemokine receptor binding necessary for viral fusion. It is furthermore possible that the inhibition of viral fusion by CsA is mediated by blocking CyP-A binding to the V3 loop of gp120, thereby inhibiting the isomerization of gp120 that is required for binding and fusion.[40,57,59]

Cyclophilins have also been suggested to play key roles in various stages of post-entry viral replication. Nuclear translocation of viral DNA was abrogated by CsA and therefore the completion of viral reverse transcription was affected;[60] this suggests the involvement of CyP-A. The data are complicated, however, in that others have demonstrated that NF-AT activity is required for viral reverse transcription and that it can be inhibited by both CsA and FK506.[61]

In the late stages of viral maturation, there is an increase in the levels of HIV-1 proteins encoded by *gag*. This event is followed by proteolytic cleavage of the immature p24 capsid (CA) protein which yields mature p24 that can undergo oligomerization followed by capsid cone formation and encapsulation of viral RNA.[56] CyP-A is packaged into HIV-1 virions through specific interactions with the CA protein p24. At a molar ratio of 1:10 (CyP-A:CA), it has been suggested that CyP-A may function to destabilize interactions in the viral capsid and therefore promote viral uncoating. Although evidence exists for this role in facilitating in vivo core disassembly after host infection,[62,63] there is also evidence to suggest that such a role is unlikely.[64] More studies are therefore necessary to elucidate the role(s) of CyP-A during the viral lifecycle.

FKBPs

The *FK*506 *b*inding *p*roteins (FKBPs) were the second immunophilin family to be identified, the first member of which was a 12 kDa soluble protein able to bind the immunosuppressant tacrolimus (FK506) and was therefore termed FKBP12[65,66] (see Fig. 111.1). Tacrolimus was first identified by studies directed at finding less toxic immunosuppressive agents. Goto et al (1987) screened fermentation broths of *Streptomyces* for agents that inhibited specifically a murine mixed lymphocyte reaction (MLR). From this screen, a potently immunosuppressive strain was isolated from a soil sample obtained from Tsukuba, Japan;[67] the strain was therefore designated *Streptomyces tsukubaensis*. The immunosuppressant isolated from this strain is now termed tacrolimus (FK506). In vitro studies revealed that tacrolimus was more potent than CsA on a molar basis: tacrolimus and cyclosporine were found to inhibit IL-2 production in mouse MLR supernatants with an inhibitory concentration (IC_{50}) of 0.1 nmol/l and 10 nmol/l, respectively. Tacrolimus and cyclosporine also significantly reduced the generation of cytotoxic T lymphocytes (CTL); these in vitro findings correlated with inhibition of in vivo allograft responses.[67,68]

FKBPs and cyclophilins share no amino acid sequence homology. Therefore, while tacrolimus binds to FKBP members, it does not bind to cyclophilins. Similarly, CsA has no affinity for either FKBP12 or other members of the FKBP protein family. Tacrolimus is a macrolide antibiotic that bears no similarity to cyclosporine but has immunosuppressive properties similar to those of cyclosporine. We now know that the tacrolimus/FKBP complex, like CsA/CyP, also binds to and inhibits the phosphatase activity of calcineurin, a finding that explains the common biological properties of the two drugs. Bram and coworkers[69] demonstrated that the relative potency of cyclosporine and tacrolimus to function as immunosuppressants correlated with their ability to inhibit calcineurin.

The isolation and characterization of tacrolimus led to the realization that its structure resembled that of another, previously identified, macrolide termed sirolimus (rapamycin) (Fig. 111.2). Indeed, sirolimus was found to bind to FKBPs, including FKBP12, and, like tacrolimus, was found to inhibit isomerase (rotamase) activity. Sirolimus had been isolated based on its antifungal and antiproliferative properties, and was later found to have immunosuppressive actions as well. Of note, in vitro and in vivo studies suggested that the target of sirolimus action differed from that of tacrolimus or cyclosporine. Sirolimus was also found to function only when bound to an FKBP in an intracellular complex; the molecular target of sirolimus/FKBP differed from that of tacrolimus/FKBP. Unable to bind calcineurin, the sirolimus/FKBP complex was found to bind to a protein termed the mammalian target of sirolimus (TOR) (Fig. 111.6), a member of the DNA PK family, discussed further below.

Like members of the cyclophilin family, FKBPs are abundant and diverse proteins, broadly represented in all species and tissues. Comparable to CyP-A but with different substrate specificity, FKBP12 possesses peptidyl prolyl *cis/trans* isomerase (rotamase) activity.[1,49,66] The rotamase activity of FKBP12 is inhibited by binding either tacrolimus or sirolimus[1,49,66] and, as

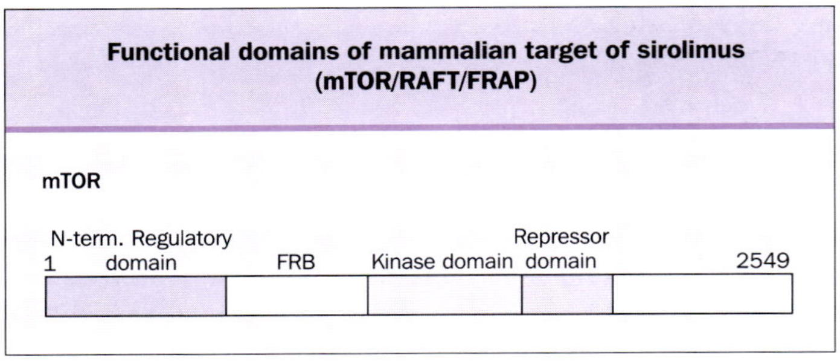

Figure 111.6 Functional domains of mammalian target of sirolimus (mTOR/RAFT/FRAP). RAFT/FRAP/mTOR is a 2549 amino acid protein with an amino-terminal regulatory domain that is responsible for intermolecular interactions and subcellular localization. mTOR also has an FRB domain to which the FKBP12/sirolimus complex binds, a PI3K-related catalytic domain (kinase domain), and a regulatory domain (repressor domain).

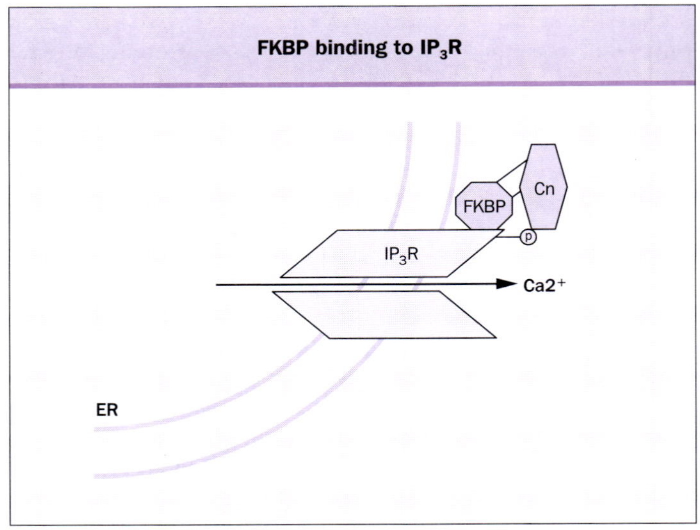

Figure 111.7 FKBP binding to IP$_3$R. Schematic of FKBP12 interacting with the calcium channel IP$_3$R found on the endoplasmic reticulum. The proposed model suggests that binding of FKBP12 to IP$_3$R brings calcineurin (Cn) in close proximity to its target, IP$_3$R. Dephosphorylation of the IP$_3$R by calcineurin results in modulation of the calcium channel.

anticipated, the drug-binding and rotamase-active sites of FKBP12 share critical amino acids. As mentioned, in the presence of tacrolimus or sirolimus, FKBP12 and a related FKBP protein, FKBP12.6, inhibit calcineurin activity.

The molecular targets of FKBPs in the absence of either tacrolimus or sirolimus are the subject of intense investigation. In the absence of drug, FKBP12 has several binding partners including the inositol-3-phosphate receptor (IP$_3$R),[70] the skeletal muscle ryanodine receptor (RyR1),[71] and the type 1 tumor growth factor-β (TGF-β) receptor.[72] FKBP12.6 binds not only to the same receptors as FKBP12, but also to the cardiac muscle ryanodine receptor 2 (RyR2).[73] These ion channels play key roles in calcium-mediated signaling that control a number of cellular functions including muscle contraction and T-cell activation. It was therefore hypothesized that FKBPs may serve a regulatory role in calcium channel function. The association of FKBP12 (and of FKBP12.6) with the IP$_3$R and the RyR stabilizes the conformation of the receptor and modulates calcium conductance.[74,75]

The IP$_3$R is a calcium channel found on the endoplasmic reticulum of almost all cell types; the interaction of FKBP12 with the IP$_3$R occurs at a binding site that resembles that of tacrolimus/FK506.[76] It was suggested that the binding region (interface) formed between FKBP12 and the IP$_3$R, mimicking that of tacrolimus/FKBP12, enables the interaction of FKBP12 with calcineurin, in the absence of drug. Several studies support a model in which the IP$_3$R/FKBP12 interaction brings calcineurin in close proximity to its target, IP$_3$R, allowing the dephosphorylation of the IP$_3$R and modulation of calcium flux (Fig. 111.7).[70]

The ryanodine receptor is a ligand-activated calcium channel present on the sarcoplasmic reticulum that controls intracellular calcium release required for striated muscle contraction. Binding FKBP12 to RyR1[71] and FKBP12.6 to both RyR1 and RyR2[73] stabilizes the calcium release channel on the sarcoplasmic reticulum. In addition, there is evidence that the phosphorylation of RyR2 by PKA mediates the dissociation of RyR2 from FKBP12.6.[74] FKBP12 provides a docking site for calcineurin that can, in turn, regulate calcium oscillations by modification of the phosphorylation state of the receptor.[74] The clinical importance of the FKBP12/IP$_3$R association was established by the generation of mice lacking expression of FKBP12; FKBP12-deficient mice demonstrate a number of cardiac defects including dilated cardiomyopathy.[77] Furthermore, RyR2 is hyperphosphorylated and the molecular complex formed between FKBP12.6, RyR2, and PKA is dysregulated in patients with heart failure.[74] Taken together, the results of these studies further support the importance of FKBPs in calcium channel function.

Other FKBP isoforms have also been described with varying molecular weights and subcellular localizations (Table 111.2).[1,49] Members of the FKBP family are distributed in the cytosol, nucleus, ER, and membrane. Another 12 kDa FKBP, termed inositol phosphate binding protein (IPBP12), binds inositol phosphates as well as tacrolimus and sirolimus, and may play a role in regulating calcium flux as well.[78] FKBP13 resides in the endoplasmic reticulum and may promote proper molecular folding and conformation. It has recently been shown to interact with the erythrocyte protein 4.1.[79] The glycoprotein FKBP23 has also been localized to the endoplasmic reticulum; FKBP23 appears to bind calcium and is found preferentially in heart, lung, and testis.[80]

Many of the FKBPs contain, in addition to prolyl-isomerase domains, domains of highly conserved tetratricopeptide repeats (TPR) that bind the heat-shock protein family. FKBP51, FKBP52 and FKBP65 all contain TPR motifs that bind Hsp90.[1,50] FKBP51 and FKBP52 are homologous to one another. FKBP52 binds to the glucocorticoid receptor and may be involved in subcellular movement within the cell. The physiological roles of these proteins remain to be identified.

PARVULINS

The immunophilin parvulin family was initially isolated from the bacterium *E. coli*[81] and its members possess the characteristic prolyl isomerase activity of other immunophilins. Parvulin family members share two characteristic functional domains. The first is an aminoterminal WW domain, consisting of two highly conserved tryptophan amino acids, a domain that is responsible for protein–protein interactions (Fig. 111.1). The second highly conserved domain is the carboxyterminal prolyl-isomerase domain, responsible for the rotamase activity. Several parvulin-binding agents have now been identified, and ongoing studies continue to elucidate the signaling pathways that are regulated by these complexes.

Eukaryotic members of the parvulin immunophilin family include human Pin1, human Par14, yeast Ptf1/Ess1, and Sspl in *Neurospora crassa* and have been shown to function in protein folding and cell-cycle regulation. Pin1 is a highly conserved parvulin that binds to a subset of mitotic phosphoproteins in a phosphorylation-dependent manner.[82] Pin1 is also essential for the G2–M transition of the cell cycle.[82] Regulation of the cell cycle is thought to occur via the interaction of Pin1 with its binding partners including Cdc25, Cdc27, Myt1, and Plk1.[83,84] Pin1 is not only required for normal progression through the cell cycle but can also inhibit entry into mitosis.[85]

Studies in yeast have also demonstrated that the Pin1 homolog Ess1 interacts with the carboxy-terminal domain of RNA pol II.[86] It is thought that this binding may play a role in the regulation of protein binding to the RNA Pol-transcriptosome complex. In turn, this could influence RNA processing at the level of chromatin opening, transcriptional initiation, elongation, termination, 3′ end processing and/or splicing.[86] The observation that Ess1 affects the mRNA levels of several mitotic regulators is consistent with the proposed model of Ess1/Pin1-dependent cell cycle regulation. It is possible that novel parvulin binding agents may represent a new class of immunosuppressive and/or antimitotic agents.

SIROLIMUS AND ITS MOLECULAR TARGET

In the search for novel antifungal agents, sirolimus (rapamycin) was identified as a macrocyclic triene antibiotic produced by *Streptomyces hygroscopicus* from a soil sample collected from the Vai Atore region of Easter Island.[87] Sirolimus was initially shown to have potent activity against the yeast *Candida albicans*[88] as well as to have activity against certain murine tumor model systems.[89] Sirolimus was found to be more effective than CsA in inhibiting mitogen-stimulated proliferation of human peripheral blood mononuclear cells, although it was not found to alter IL-2 or IL-2-receptor expression.[90] In contrast to tacrolimus and CsA, sirolimus was shown to inhibit growth factor dependent T-cell proliferation subsequent to binding of the cytokine to its receptor.[91]

As mentioned, sirolimus is structurally similar to FK506 (Fig. 111.2) and binds to the same immunophilin family as FK506.[1,2,7] Unlike the other immunophilin/immunosuppressant complexes FK506/FKBP12 and CsA/CyP-A, the sirolimus/FKBP12 complex does not target calcineurin but binds to a 289 kDa protein termed *m*ammalian homolog of the yeast target of sirolimus (mTOR)[92] (Figs 111.6, 111.8). This protein has also been termed *sirolimus* and *FKBP12 target* (RAFT) and *FKBP12* and *sirolimus associated protein* (FRAP). Although mTOR/FRAP/RAFT has a carboxyterminal domain with homology to that of the kinase domain of phosphatidylinositol-3-kinase (PI-3-kinase), the protein preferentially acts as a serine/threonine kinase on protein substrates.[93] The endogenous role of mTOR/FRAP/RAFT appears to be control of the translational machinery and amino acid transport in a wide variety of cells.

Mammalian TOR/FRAP/RAFT has been shown to be a kinase that undergoes autophosphorylation correlating with enzymatic activity and is able to phosphorylate a number of protein substrates such as the serine/threonine kinase p70 S6 kinase.[94] When phosphorylated, p70 S6 kinase, in turn, is able to phosphorylate the ribosomal protein S6;[7,91] S6 phosphorylation appears to enhance the synthesis of ribosomal proteins and polysome assembly, thus increasing the rate of protein elongation and translation. Binding of the sirolimus/FKBP12 complex to FRAP/RAFT/mTOR inhibits the phosphorylation of p70 S6 kinase, thus blocking the phosphorylation of S6 protein and subsequent translation (Fig. 111.8).

There are other important substrates of mTOR/FRAP/RAFT, some initially characterized by their sirolimus sensitivity; whether each is a direct substrate of the mTOR kinase is not clear. The phosphorylation of 4E-BP1, a repressor of translational initiation, is sirolimus-sensitive.[95] In the dephosphorylated state, 4E-BP1 blocks the interaction between the translational elongation factor, EIF-4F, and the 5′-cap structure found on all mammalian mRNAs (Fig. 111.8). In this manner, sirolimus inhibits protein translation and, for instance, the T-cell response to antigen at a time point downstream of either FK506 or CsA.

Sirolimus has also been reported to have antiproliferative effects on certain tumor cell lines including prostate, glioblastoma, lymphoma, melanoma, and small cell lung cells.[96] In several of these cell lines, mTOR has been demonstrated to be constitutively hyperphosphorylated. The anticancer effect of the sirolimus/FKBP12 complex may involve binding and inhibition of mTOR; clarification of the molecular pathways regulated by mTOR may provide novel therapeutic targets for treatment.

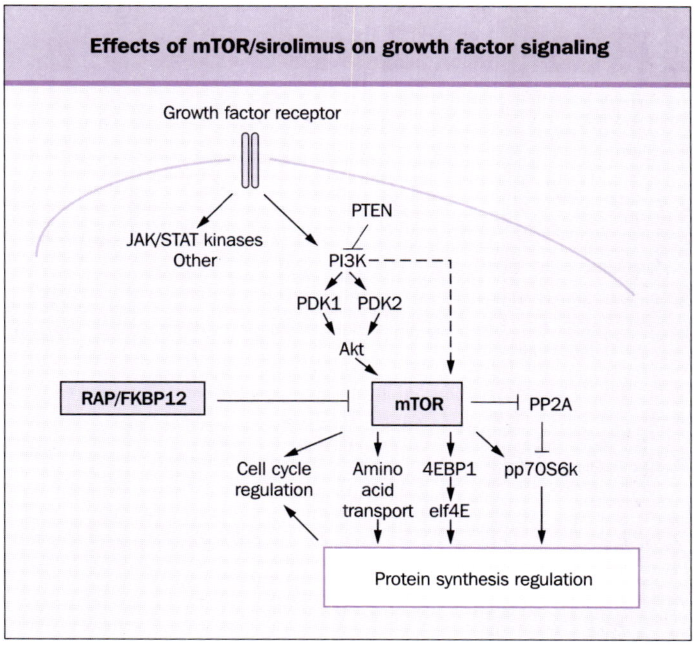

Figure 111.8 Effects of mTOR/sirolimus on growth factor signaling. mTOR plays a key role in the regulation of protein synthesis by a number of mechanisms, resulting in regulation of the cell cycle and protein synthesis. Binding of the FKBP12/sirolimus complex to mTOR inhibits the phosphorylation of p70 S6 kinase, the subsequent phosphorylation of S6 protein, and protein synthesis. Amino acid transport and the phosphorylation of 4E-BP1, a repressor of translational initiation, are both sirolimus-sensitive.

CLINICAL UTILITY OF CYCLOSPORINE, TACROLIMUS, AND SIROLIMUS

As mentioned, each of the immunophilin-binding agents has been approved by the US Food and Drug Administration for human use. Cyclosporine and tacrolimus are both approved for use in the treatment of and prevention of organ rejection following liver and kidney transplantation, and sirolimus was recently approved for use in prevention of acute renal transplant rejection. Each of these agents has been used in stem cell transplantation as well, most often for the prevention or treatment of acute graft-versus-host disease, and their utility in the treatment of a variety of autoimmune disorders is currently being explored.

Controlled, randomized, multicenter trials comparing tacrolimus and cyclosporine, each in combination with other agents, have been completed. Importantly, organ graft and patient survival has been similar. It is difficult, however, to compare either the efficacy or toxicity of these agents directly; this difficulty results from several sources. First, early studies used regimens that are not recommended today: it is now appreciated that the target therapeutic tacrolimus concentration used in the early liver and renal trials[97,98] was higher than is currently recommended. Two different tacrolimus dosing regimens were used but the results were not stratified for dose nor was efficacy correlated to dose. It is possible that the high tacrolimus target concentrations contributed to the somewhat higher incidence of neurotoxicity and renal insufficiency[97,98] observed without modifying efficacy. Second, the current availability of microemulsion formulations of cyclosporine changes the drug bioavailability and may have an impact upon the results achieved. Third, long-term follow-up, including response to later acute rejection episodes and complications from immunosuppression, have not been reported. Finally, important variables such as quality of life and cost have not been directly compared.

A limitation of both cyclosporine and tacrolimus is their narrow therapeutic window. Close monitoring of blood levels is important and critical for prevention of both organ rejection and complications. In addition, the liver metabolizes both agents: blood levels may change with administration of other medicines that affect the hepatic cytochrome P-450 enzyme system. In recipients of stem cell (e.g. bone marrow and peripheral blood stem cells) transplants, long-term immunosuppression results in increased infectious complications that often contribute to late mortality.

The side-effects of cyclosporine and tacrolimus appear to overlap but are not identical. The most common toxicities of both drugs are nephrotoxicity, neurotoxicity, and hypertension. Essentially all patients suffer a decrease in the measured glomerular filtration rate, clinically apparent and resulting in renal insufficiency in over 75% of recipients of liver transplants.[97,98] Hypertension is common, and may be controlled by calcium channel antagonists (with attention to modification of drug concentration). Neurotoxicity is manifest by a range of symptoms including headaches, tremulousness, sleep disturbance and, more seriously, by a syndrome characterized as a reversible posterior leukoencephalopathy[99] that may result in coma. These complications are often, but not always, attenuated and/or reversed by decreasing the dose or discontinuing the drug. Permanent sequelae, including azotemia, may result.

The toxicity profile shared between tacrolimus and cyclosporine is hypothesized to be secondary to an effect on calcineurin; calcineurin may be an important intermediate in, for instance, renal physiology and neural transmission. In addition, the use of molecular analogs of tacrolimus and cyclosporine that bind to immunophilins suggests that immunophilin binding and inhibition of isomerase activity do not account for nephrotoxicity. Calcineurin colocalizes with FKBPs in brain tissue sections and is downstream of glutamate and NMDA receptors. In so far as calcineurin inhibition accounts not only for therapeutic efficacy but also for toxicity, drug analogs that target calcineurin are also predicted to have a similarly narrow therapeutic window. Instead, efforts are underway to identify and develop inhibitors of the specific substrates of calcineurin important for immunosuppression.

The toxicity profile of cyclosporine does not overlap entirely with that of tacrolimus, however. Prolonged administration of cyclosporine has been reported to be associated with gingival hyperplasia, coarsening of facial features, and hirsutism; these side-effects are not evident with tacrolimus administation, at least in the collective experience to date. These side-effects, therefore, may be secondary to metabolites of cyclosporine or potentially to tissue-specific expression of, or unique members, or specific functions of cyclophilins not shared with the FKBPs.

As might be predicted from an understanding of the molecular target of sirolimus, the toxicity profile of this drug appears to differ from that of tacrolimus and cyclosporine. Nephrotoxicity is not a prominent feature of sirolimus administration, nor is hypertension or neurotoxicity. The most common side-effects of sirolimus are hyperlipidemia, including hypercholesterolemia,

CLINICAL PEARLS

Clinical utility of cyclosporine, tacrolimus, and sirolimus

	Cyclosporine	Tacrolimus	Sirolimus
Therapy			
Liver transplantation	+	+	?
Kidney transplantation	+	+	+
Bone marrow and stem cell transplantation	+	+	?
Autoimmune diseases	?	+	?
Narrow therapeutic window	+	+	?
Metabolism by hepatic cytochrome P-450	+	+	?
Side-effects			
Neurotoxicity	+	+	–
Nephrotoxicity	+	+	–
Hypertension	+	+	–
Infection/mortality	+	+	+
Gingival hyperplasia	+	–	–
Coarse facial features	+	–	–
Hirsutism	+	–	–
Hyperlipidemia	–	–	+
Hematologic effects	–	–	+
Malignancy (i.e. EBV-driven lymphoma)	+	+	?

+, yes; –, no; ?, not determined.

and hematologic toxicities including leukopenia and thrombocytopenia. This profile allows the administration of sirolimus in combination with either cyclosporine, a regimen that has been tested,[100,101] or potentially with tacrolimus. In addition, sirolimus administration has been shown to permit reduction of corticosteroid and cyclosporine dosages[102,103] and may thereby attenuate the toxicities of the immunosuppressive agents. The role of sirolimus as an adjunct to the armamentarium of immunosuppressive agents is only beginning to be explored.

IMMUNOPHILINS AND THEIR BINDING AGENTS: A LOOK AHEAD

Although much has been accomplished in the study of immunophilins and their binding agents, many questions remain unanswered. Future studies will attempt to determine what the in vivo natural ligand(s) are for these immunophilins as well as their normal physiological roles. Studies will address whether different family members of CyPs, FKBPs, and parvulins can carry out compensatory functions, and efforts will be made to isolate specific inhibitors for the different immunophilins. Future work will also address the question of a relationship between *cis-trans* prolyl isomerase activity and biological function. Moreover, studies will assess if there is a relationship between prolyl isomerase activity and cellular signaling. Further steps will be taken to determine existing immunophilin-specific pathways that are independent of immunosuppressant drugs. Continued studies will attempt to unravel the mechanisms by which the immunophilin/drug complexes lead to nephrotoxicity as well as other clinical complications. Further efforts will be made to modify existing immunosuppressants as well as to isolate new agents that can demonstrate the immunosuppressive actions of current drugs without the undesired toxic side-effects. Efforts will be made to further our understanding of the associations between immunophilins and their binding agents. To this end, the existence of immunosuppressants that are independent of immunophilin binding for their actions may be explored.

REFERENCES

1. Fruman DA, Burakoff SJ, Bierer BE. Immunophilins in protein folding and immunosuppression. FASEB J 1994;8:391.
2. Schreiber SL, Crabtree GR. The mechanism of action of cyclosporin A and FK506. Immunol Today 1992;13:136.
3. Gething MJ, Sambrook J. Protein folding in the cell. Nature 1992;355:33.
4. Takahashi N, Hayano T, Suzuki M. Peptidyl-prolyl cis-trans isomerase is the cyclosporin A-binding protein cyclophilin. Nature 1989;337:473.
5. Borel JF, Kis ZL. The discovery and development of cyclosporine (Sandimmune). Transplant Proc 1991;23:1867.
6. Kahan BD. Cyclosporine. N Engl J Med 1989;321:1725.
7. Bierer BE, Hollander G, Fruman D, Burakoff SJ. Cyclosporin A and FK506: molecular mechanisms of immunosuppression and probes for transplantation biology. Curr Opin Immunol 1993;5:763.
8. Bach JF. Cyclosporin and autoimmune disease. Lancet 1991;338:59.
9. Bierer BE, Mattila PS, Standaert RF, et al. Two distinct signal transmission pathways in T lymphocytes are inhibited by complexes formed between an immunophilin and either FK506 or rapamycin. Proc Natl Acad Sci USA 1990;87:9231.
10. Liu J, Farmer JDJ, Lane WS, et al. Calcineurin is a common target of cyclophilin-cyclosporin A and FKBP-FK506 complexes. Cell 1991;66:807.
11. Friedman J, Weissman I. Two cytoplasmic candidates for immunophilin action are revealed by affinity for a new cyclophilin: one in the presence and one in the absence of CsA. Cell 1991;66:799.
12. Klee CB, Ren H, Wang X. Regulation of the calmodulin-stimulated protein phosphatase, calcineurin. J Biol Chem 1998;273:13367.
13. Wang X, Culotta VC, Klee CB. Superoxide dismutase protects calcineurin from inactivation. Nature 1996;383:434.
14. Sagoo JK, Fruman DA, Wesselborg S, Walsh CT, Bierer BE. Competitive inhibition of calcineurin phosphatase activity by its autoinhibitory domain. Biochem J 1996;320:879.
15. Cardenas ME, Heitman J. Role of calcium in T-lymphocyte activation. Adv Second Messenger Phosphoprotein Res 1995;30:281.
16. Rao A, Luo C, Hogan PG. Transcription factors of the NFAT family: regulation and function. Annu Rev Immunol 1997;15:707.
17. Luo C, Shaw KT, Raghavan A, et al. Interaction of calcineurin with a domain of the transcription factor NFAT1 that controls nuclear import. Proc Natl Acad Sci U S A 1996;93:8907.
18. Tian J, Karin M. Stimulation of Elk1 transcriptional activity by mitogen-activated protein kinases is negatively regulated by protein phosphatase 2B (calcineurin). J Biol Chem 1999;274:15173.
19. Werlen G, Jacinto E, Xia Y, Karin M. Calcineurin preferentially synergizes with PKC-theta to activate JNK and IL-2 promoter in T lymphocytes. EMBO J 1998;17:3101.
20. Gupta S, Campbell D, Derijard B, Davis RJ. Transcription factor ATF2 regulation by the JNK signal transduction pathway. Science 1995;267:389.
21. Frantz B, Nordby EC, Bren G, et al. Calcineurin acts in synergy with PMA to inactivate I kappa B/MAD3, an inhibitor of NF-kappa B. EMBO J 1994;13:861.
22. Trushin SA, Pennington KN, Algeciras-Schimnich A, Paya CV. Protein kinase C and calcineurin synergize to activate IκB kinase and NFκB in T lymphocytes. J Biol Chem 1999;274:22923.
23. Schwaninger M, Blume R, Kruger M, et al. Involvement of the Ca(2+)-dependent phosphatase calcineurin in gene transcription that is stimulated by cAMP through cAMP response elements. J Biol Chem 1995;270:8860.
24. Schaefer A, Magocsi M, Fandrich A, Marquardt H. Stimulation of the Ca2+-mediated egr-1 and c-fos expression in murine erythroleukaemia cells by cyclosporin A. Biochem J 1998;335:505.
25. Morii Y, Kawano K, Kim YI, et al. Augmentive effect of cyclosporin A on rat liver regeneration: influence on hepatocyte growth factor and transforming growth factor-beta (1). Eur Surg Res 1999;31:399.
26. Khanna AK, Cairns VR, Becker CG, Hosenpud JD. Transforming growth factor (TGF)-beta mimics and anti-TGF-beta antibody abrogates the in vivo effects of cyclosporine: demonstration of a direct role of TGF-beta in immunosuppression and nephrotoxicity of cyclosporine. Transplantation 1999;67:882.
27. Alevizopoulos A, Dusserre Y, Ruegg U, Mermod N. Regulation of the transforming growth factor beta-responsive transcription factor CTF-1 by calcineurin and calcium/calmodulin-dependent protein kinase IV. J Biol Chem 1997;272:23597.
28. Khanna AK, Hosenpud JD. Cyclosporine induces the expression of the cyclin inhibitor p21. Transplantation 1999;67:1262.
29. Cuhaci B, Kumar MS, Bloom RD, et al. Transforming growth factor-beta levels in human allograft chronic fibrosis correlate with rate of decline in renal function. Transplantation 1999;68:785.
30. Hojo M, Morimoto T, Maluccio M, et al. Cyclosporine induces cancer progression by a cell-autonomous mechanism. Nature 1999;397:530.
31. Mason J. Pharmacology of cyclosporine (sandimmune). VII. Pathophysiology and toxicology of cyclosporine in humans and animals. Pharmacol Rev 1990;41:423.

32. Jiang H, Xiong F, Kong S, et al. Distinct tissue and cellular distribution of two major isoforms of calcineurin. Mol Immunol 1997;34:663.
33. Hogan PG, Rao A. Transcriptional regulation. Modification by nuclear export? Nature 1999;398:200.
34. Parquet N, Reigneau O, Humbert H, et al. New oral formulation of cyclosporin A (Neoral) pharmacokinetics in allogeneic bone marrow transplant recipients. Bone Marrow Transplant 2000;25:965.
35. Walsh CT, Zydowsky LD, McKeon FD. Cyclosporin A, the cyclophilin class of peptidylprolyl isomerases, and blockade of T cell signal transduction. J Biol Chem 1992;267:13115.
36. Mariller C, Allain F, Kouach M, Spik G. Evidence that human milk isolated cyclophilin B corresponds to a truncated form. Biochim Biophys Acta 1996;1293:31.
37. Billich A, Winkler G, Aschauer H, Rot A, Peichl P. Presence of cyclophilin A in synovial fluids of patients with rheumatoid arthritis. J Exp Med 1997;185:975.
38. Xu Q, Leiva MC, Fischkoff SA, Handschumacher RE, Lyttle CR. Leukocyte chemotactic activity of cyclophilin. J Biol Chem 1992;267:11968.
39. Jaschke A, Mi H, Tropschug M. Human T cell cyclophilin 18 binds to thiol-specific antioxidant protein Aop1 and stimulates its activity. J Mol Biol 1998;277:763.
40. Luban J, Bossolt KL, Franke EK, Kalpana GV, Goff SP. Human immunodeficiency virus type 1 Gag protein binds to cyclophilins A and B. Cell 1993;73:1067.
41. Price ER, Zydowsky LD, Jin MJ, et al. Human cyclophilin B: a second cyclophilin gene encodes a peptidyl-prolyl isomerase with a signal sequence. Proc Natl Acad Sci U S A 1991;88:1903.
42. Bram RJ, Crabtree GR. Calcium signalling in T cells stimulated by a cyclophilin B-binding protein. Nature 1994;371:355.
43. Holloway MP, Bram RJ. Co-localization of calcium-modulating cyclophilin ligand with intracellular calcium pools. J Biol Chem 1998;273:16346.
44. von Bulow GU, Bram RJ. NF-AT activation induced by a CAML-interacting member of the tumor necrosis factor receptor superfamily. Science 1997;278:138.
45. Friedman J, Trahey M, Weissman I. Cloning and characterization of cyclophilin C-associated protein: a candidate natural cellular ligand for cyclophilin C. Proc Natl Acad Sci USA 1993; 90:6815.
46. Trahey M, Weissman IL. Cyclophilin C-associated protein: a normal secreted glycoprotein that down-modulates endotoxin and proinflammatory responses in vivo. Proc Natl Acad Sci USA 1999;96:3006.
47. Tanveer A, Virji S, Andreeva L, et al. Involvement of cyclophilin D in the activation of a mitochondrial pore by Ca2+ and oxidant stress. Eur J Biochem 1996;38:166.
48. Scorrano L, Nicolli A, Basso E, Petronilli V, Bernardi P. Two modes of activation of the permeability transition pore: the role of mitochondrial cyclophilin. Mol Cell Biochem 1997;174:181.
49. Fretz H, Albers MW, Galat A, et al. Rapamycin and FK506 binding proteins (immunophilins). J Am Chem Soc 1991;113:1409.
50. Lamb JR, Tugendreich S, Hieter P. Tetratricopeptide repeat interactions: to TPR or not to TPR? Trends Biochem Sci 1995;20:257.
51. Kieffer LJ, Seng TW, Li W, et al. Cyclophilin-40, a protein with homology to the p59 component of the steroid receptor complex. J Biol Chem 1993;268:12303.
52. Horowitz DS, Kobayashi R, Krainer AR. A new cyclophilin and the human homologues of yeast Prp3 and Prp4 form a complex associated with U4/U6 snRNPs. RNA 1997;3:1374.
53. Horowitz DS, Lee E. The cyclophilin USA-CyP is involved in both steps of pre-mRNA splicing in humans; #108. Immunophilins: cellular functions and immunosuppressive drug targets (C6). Silverthorne, CO, Keystone Symposia, 2000.
54. Ferreira PA, Nakayama TA, Pak WL, Travis GH. Cyclophilin-related protein RanBP2 acts as chaperone for red/green opsin. Nature 1996;383:637.
55. Mortillaro MJ, Berezney R. Matrin CYP, an SR-rich cyclophilin that associates with the nuclear matrix and splicing factors. J Biol Chem 1998;273:8183.
56. Freed EO. HIV-1 gag proteins: diverse functions in the virus life cycle. Virology 1998;251:1.
57. Wyatt R, Sodroski J. The HIV-1 envelope glycoproteins: fusogens, antigens, and immunogens. Science 1998;280:1884.
58. Lu M, Ji H, Shen S. Subdomain folding and biological activity of the core structure from human immunodeficiency virus type 1 gp41: implications for viral membrane fusion. J Virol 1999;73:4433.
59. Endrich MM, Gehring H. The V3 loop of human immunodeficiency virus type-1 envelope protein is a high-affinity ligand for immunophilins present in human blood. Eur J Biochem 1998;252:441.
60. Sun Y, Pinchuk LM, Agy MB, Clark EA. Nuclear import of HIV-1 DNA in resting CD4+ T cells requires a cyclosporin A-sensitive pathway. J Immunol 1997;158:512.
61. Kinoshita S, Chen BK, Kaneshima H, Nolan GP. Host control of HIV-1 parasitism in T cells by the nuclear factor of activated T cells. Cell 1998;95:595.
62. Endrich MM, Gehrig P, Gehring H. Maturation-induced conformational changes of HIV-1 capsid protein and identification of two high affinity sites for cyclophilins in the C-terminal domain. J Biol Chem 1999;274:5326.
63. Streblow DN, Kitabwalla M, Malkovsky M, Pauza CD. Cyclophilin A modulates processing of human immunodeficiency virus type 1 p55Gag: mechanism for antiviral effects of cyclosporin A. Virology 1998;245:197.
64. Wiegers K, Rutter G, Schubert U, Grattinger M, Krausslich HG. Cyclophilin A incorporation is not required for human immunodeficiency virus type 1 particle maturation and does not destabilize the mature capsid. Virology 1999;257:261.
65. Siekierka JJ, Hung SH, Poe M, Lin CS, Sigal NH. A cytosolic binding protein for the immunosuppressant FK506 has peptidyl-prolyl isomerase activity but is distinct from cyclophilin. Nature 1989;341:755.
66. Harding MW, Galat A, Uehling DE, Schreiber SL. A receptor for the immunosuppressant FK 506 is a cis-trans peptidyl-prolyl isomerase. Nature 1989;341:758.
67. Kino T, Hatanaka H, Hashimoto M, et al. FK-506, a novel immunosuppressant isolated from a Streptomyces I. Fermentation, isolation, and physico-chemical and biological characteristics. J Antibiot 1987;40:1249.
68. Kino T, Hatanaka H, Miyata S, et al. FK-506, a novel immunosuppressant isolated from a Streptomyces II. Immunosuppressive effect of FK-506 in vitro. J Antibiot 1987;40:1256.
69. Bram RJ, Hung DT, Martin PK, Schreiber SL, Crabtree GR. Identification of the immunophilin capable of mediating inhibition of signal transduction by cyclosporin A and FK506: roles of calcineurin binding and cellular location. Mol Cell Biol 1993;13:4760.
70. Cameron AM, Steiner JP, Sabatini DM, et al. Immunophilin FK506 binding protein associated with inositol 1,4,5-triphosphate receptor modulates calcium flux. Proc Natl Acad Sci U S A 1995;92:1784.
71. Jayaraman T, Brillantes AM, Timerman AP, et al. FK506 binding protein associated with the calcium release channel (ryanodine receptor). J Biol Chem 1992;267:9474.
72. Wang T, Donahoe PK, Zervos AS. Specific interaction of type I receptors of the TGF-beta family with the immunophilin FKBP-12. Science 1994;265:674.
73. Timerman AP, Onoue H, Xin HB, et al. Selective binding of FKBP12.6 by the cardiac ryanodine receptor. J Biol Chem 1996;271:20385.
74. Marx SO, Reiken S, Hisamatsu Y, et al. PKA phosphorylation dissociates FKBP12.6 from the calcium release channel (ryanodine receptor): defective regulation in failing hearts. Cell 2000;101:365.
75. Chen L, Molinski TF, Pessah IN. Bastadin 10 stabilizes the open conformation of the ryanodine-sensitive Ca(2+) channel in an FKBP12-dependent manner. J Biol Chem 1999;274:32603.
76. Cameron AM, Nucifora FC Jr, Fung ET, et al. FKBP12 binds the inositol 1,4,5-triphosphate receptor at leucine-proline (1400–1401) and anchors calcineurin to this FK506-like domain. J Biol Chem 1997;272:27582.
77. Shou W, Aghdasi B, Armstrong DL, et al. Cardiac defects and altered ryanodine receptor function in mice lacking FKBP12. Nature 1998;391:489.
78. Cunningham EB. The human erythrocyte membrane contains a novel 12-kDa inositolphosphate-binding protein that is an immunophilin. Biochem Biophys Res Commun 1995;215:212.

79. Walensky LD, Gascard P, Fields ME, et al. The 13-kD FK506 binding protein, FKBP13, interacts with a novel homologue of the erythrocyte membrane cytoskeletal protein 4.1. J Cell Biol 1998;141:143.
80. Nakamura T, Yabe D, Kanazawa N, et al. Molecular cloning, characterization, and chromosomal localization of FKBP23, a novel FK506-binding protein with Ca2+-binding ability. Genomics 1998;54:89.
81. Rahfeld JU, Schierhorn A, Mann K, Fischer G. A novel peptidyl-prolyl cis/trans isomerase from *Escherichia coli*. FEBS Lett 1994;343:65.
82. Lu KP, Hanes SD, Hunter T. A human peptidyl-prolyl isomerase essential for regulation of mitosis. Nature 1996;380:544.
83. Shen M, Stukenberg PT, Kirschner MW, Lu KP. The essential mitotic peptidyl-prolyl isomerase Pin1 binds and regulates mitosis-specific phosphoproteins. Genes Dev 1998;12:706.
84. Crenshaw DG, Yang J, Means AR, Kornbluth S. The mitotic peptidyl-prolyl isomerase, Pin1, interacts with Cdc25 and Plx1. EMBO J 1998;17:1315.
85. Yaffe MB, Schutkowski M, Shen M, et al. Sequence-specific and phosphorylation-dependent proline isomerization: a potential mitotic regulatory mechanism. Science 1997;278:1957.
86. Morris DP, Phatnani HP, Greenleaf AL. Phospho-carboxyl-terminal domain binding and the role of a prolyl isomerase in pre-mRNA 3′-End formation. J Biol Chem 1999;274:31583.
87. Sehgal SN, Baker H, Vezina C. Rapamycin (AY-22,989), a new antifungal antibiotic. II. Fermentation, isolation and characterization. J Antibiot 1975;28:727.
88. Singh K, Sun S, Vezina C. Rapamycin (AY-22,989), a new antifungal antibiotic. IV. Mechanism of action. J Antibiot 1979;32:630.
89. Eng CP, Sehgal SN, Vezina C. Activity of rapamycin (AY-22,989) against transplanted tumors. J Antibiot 1984;37:1231.
90. Dumont FJ, Staruch MJ, Koprak SK, Melino MR, Sigal NH. Distinct mechanisms of suppression of murine T cell activation by the related macrolides FK-506 and rapamycin. J Immunol 1990;144:251.
91. Calvo V, Crews CM, Vik TA, Bierer BE. Interleukin 2 stimulation of p70 S6 kinase activity is inhibited by the immunosuppressant rapamycin. Proc Natl Acad Sci USA 1992;89:7571.
92. Heitman J, Movva NR, Hall MN. Targets for cell cycle arrest by the immunosuppressant rapamycin in yeast. Science 1991;253:905.
93. Carpenter CL, Cantley LC. Phosphoinositide kinases. Biochemistry 1990;29:11147.
94. Brown EJ, Beal PA, Keith CT, et al. Control of p70 S6 kinase by kinase activity of FRAP in vivo. Nature 1995;377:441.
95. Beretta L, Gingras AC, Svitkin YV, Hall MN, Sonenberg N. Rapamycin blocks the phosphorylation of 4E-BP1 and inhibits cap-dependent initiation of translation. EMBO J 1996;15:658.
96. Abraham RT. Mammalian target of rapamycin: immunosuppressive drugs uncover a link between mitogenic signaling and translational control; #28. Immunophilins: cellular functions and immunosuppressive drug targets (C6) Silverthorne, CO, Keystone Symposia, 2000.
97. The U.S. Multicenter FK506 Liver Study Group. A comparison of tacrolimus (FK506) and cyclosporine for immunosuppression in liver transplantation. N Engl J Med 1994;331:1110.
98. European FK506 Multicentre Liver Study Group. Randomised trial comparing tacrolimus (FK506) and cyclosporin in prevention of liver allograft rejection. Lancet 1994;344:423.
99. Gijtenbeek JM, van den Bent MJ, Vecht CJ. Cyclosporine neurotoxicity: a review. J Neurol 1999;246:339.
100. Qi S, Xu D, Peng J, Liu D, Chen H. Synergistic effect of rapamycin and cyclosporine in prevention of acute kidney allograft rejection in the mouse. Microsurgery 1999;19:344.
101. Saggi BH, Fisher RA, Naar JD, et al. Intragraft cytokine expression in tolerant rat renal allografts with rapamycin and cyclosporin immunosuppression. Clin Transplant 1999;13:90.
102. Kahan BD, Podbielski J, Napoli KL, et al. Immunosuppressive effects and safety of a sirolimus/cyclosporine combination regimen for renal transplantation. Transplantation 1998;66:1040.
103. Kahan BD, Julian BA, Pescovitz MD, Vanrentergehen Y, Neylan J. Sirolimus reduces the incidence of acute rejection episodes despite lower cyclosporine doses in caucasian recipients of mismatched primary renal allografts: a phase II trial. Rapamune Study Group. Transplantation 1999;68:1526.

Section 10 Prevention and Therapy of Immunologic Diseases
F Immune Modulation

Chapter 112

Vaccines

Barry T Rouse, Edina Moylett, I Celine Hanson

INTRODUCTION

Vaccination is one of the most powerful tools used in the control of infectious diseases. In the developed world, vaccines control disease caused by many human viral and toxin-producing bacterial pathogens. The impact of vaccination on infectious diseases is outlined in Table 112.1 which shows baseline twentieth century annual morbidity and 1998 provisional morbidity for nine vaccine-preventable conditions in children.[1] Owing to the successful development and application of vaccines, current efforts are directed at the expansion of vaccination to include prevention of cancer, pregnancy, and autoimmune disease.[2–7] However, vaccinology's victory is by no means complete. Most notably, satisfactory vaccines are lacking for all parasitic infections, especially malaria, the cause of significant mortality in the developing world.[8,9] Similarly, effective vaccines remain unavailable for pathogens such as *Mycobacterium tuberculosis*, *Vibrio cholerae*, herpes viruses, common cold agents, and human immunodeficiency virus (HIV), the cause of the AIDS pandemic.[10–12]

The development and elucidation of the immunization process for the prevention of infectious diseases contributed significantly to the discipline of immunology. Early efforts led to the recognition of two general types of immunization, those that induce an active immune response to an antigen (vaccination) and those that provide immunization passively. At present, passive immunization is restricted to the use of immune serum to provide temporary antibody-mediated immunity. Active immunization is the administration of a vaccine to induce an immune response that can prevent an infectious disease. The vaccine may consist of the microorganism in a live but attenuated (infectious) or inactive (noninfectious) form, or a molecular product or constituent of the microorganism. The immune response may be humoral, cell-mediated, or both.

The ideal vaccine should be nonreactogenic (i.e. without undesirable side-effects) easy to administer, highly immunogenic, and protective with lasting immunity. No currently available vaccine meets all these criteria. Increases in incidence of pediatric cases of intussusception following the recent introduction of the rotavirus vaccine led to its subsequent withdrawal. Other withdrawals have included the inactivated 'flu' vaccine and vaccines directed against enterobacterial infections.[13,14] Despite these adverse events, the development of new and improved vaccines remains a priority. Innovative developments in the fields of molecular biology and immunology should aid in achieving this goal.

HISTORY

The observation that following certain infectious conditions the individual either did not develop repeat infection or developed an attenuated form of the disease on re-exposure formed the

Impact of vaccination on morbidity from infections diseases

Disease	Baseline 20th century annual morbidity	1998 provisional morbidity	% Decrease
Smallpox	48 164	0	100.0%
Diphtheria	175 885	1	100.0%
Pertussis	147 271	6279	95.7%
Tetanus	1314	34	97.4%
Poliomyelitis (paralytic)	16 316	0	100.0%
Measles	503 282	89	100.0%
Mumps	152 209	606	99.6%
Rubella	47 746	345	99.3%
Congenital rubella syndrome	823	5	99.4%
Haemophilus influenzae type b	20 000	54	99.7%

Table 112.1 Baseline twentieth century annual morbidity and 1998 provisional morbidity from nine diseases with vaccines recommended before 1990 for universal use in children – USA. (From Ten great public health achievements – United States, 1900–1999. *MMWR Morb Mortal Wkly Rep* 1999;48:241.)

basis for the concept of vaccination. Undoubtedly this prompted the administration of smallpox pustular or scab material (variolation) in ancient times with the hope of providing an attenuated infection that would convey life-long immunity.[15] This procedure of variolation was introduced into England by Lady Montague Wortley in 1721, and was widely used there as well as in the American colonies among some segments of society. Jenner similarly practiced variolation and this may have contributed to his observation of immunity among milkmaids.[16] Jenner's vaccine for smallpox was safe and did not produce disease. However, were that vaccine used today, HIV-infected and other immunosuppressed individuals would be at risk of death from disseminated smallpox.

Scientific vaccinology began with Pasteur.[17] He realized the significance of early accidental experiments in which exposure to chicken cholera bacteria led to the development of an attenuated culture that could protect against subsequent exposure to the virulent agent. Using various means of attenuation, Pasteur went on to produce several vaccines. His most notable achievement was a vaccine produced from dried spinal cords of infected rabbits that protected his famous patient, Jacob Meister, against rabies. The world became excited, and this period produced many early vaccine options.[18,19] Many believed that infectious diseases would become historical curiosities.

Early successful vaccines were developed by inactivation of microorganisms or their toxins by chemical or physical means. In addition, after the discovery of antibody by Von Behring and Kitasato in 1890, complexes of toxin with antitoxins were observed to confer immunity.[20] Major developments in vaccinology came in the 1930s with the discovery that some viruses could be grown and attenuated in embryonic eggs, and in the 1950s with the development of cell cultures to propagate viruses, most notably poliovirus.[21] The successful attenuated (Albert Sabin) and inactivated (Jonas Salk) poliovirus vaccines have greatly reduced the incidence of paralytic polio worldwide.[22,23] However, the threat of vaccine-associated disease with the live vaccine in undiagnosed immunodeficient children, as well as immunosuppressed relatives of normal children, has mandated the use of the inactive vaccine (Salk) for the primary polio series.[24–26]

Vaccinology gave rise to the sciences of microbiology and immunology. Along with molecular biology, these sciences have set the stage for further triumphs in vaccine development. The first significant achievement was the development of a successful vaccine against hepatitis B using a recombinant protein derived from yeast.[27] Viral recombinant proteins are but one of the many modern approaches to vaccines (Table 112.2). Other approaches include recombinant bacterial or viral vectors, genetic mutants, nucleic acids, and synthetic peptides as discussed subsequently. Nevertheless, the challenges for vaccinologists remain substantial.[28]

In addition to their use for prophylaxis, vaccines are also considered for use as therapeutic agents, but only with hepatitis B and rabies virus infection, has this been a successful approach.[29,30] In the future, therapeutic allergy and cancer vaccines will be developed to control disease. Therapeutic vaccines are designed to increase the level and balance of immunity; they should control the manifestations of chronic or recurrent diseases such as AIDS, herpesvirus infections, cancer, and allergy.

Although prophylactic vaccines represent the most cost-effective means to prevent disease, unfortunately many of these vaccines are ineffective or unavailable for many important infectious agents. This chapter analyzes why some infections are refractory to control by vaccines and what might be done to change this.

Types of prophylactic vaccines

Type of vaccine	Comments	Example	
		Viral	Bacterial
Live attenuated organism	The organism is attenuated such that it does not produce clinical disease but still retains the ability to replicate to an extent that is sufficient to induce immunity	Polio (Sabin), measles, mumps, rubella, yellow fever, varicella, rotavirus.	Bacilus Calmette–Guérin (BCG), typhoid
Killed organism	The vaccine consists of the whole organism that has been inactivated to prevent any replication in vivo but immunogenicity is preserved	Polio (Salk), influenza, Japanese encephalitis, rabies, hepatitis A	Pertussis, cholera, typhoid
Subunit vaccines	The vaccine consists of subcomponents of the organism. These subcomponents can either be surface proteins of a virus or proteins and/or polysaccharides of bacteria	Hepatitis B	*Haemophilus influenzae* B, pneumococci, meningococci, typhoid, pertussis, anthrax
Antitoxins	The vaccine consists of inactivated toxin (toxoid) that is no longer toxic but retains immunogenicity	None	Diphtheria, tetanus
Vectored vaccines	These vaccines are currently in development. The idea is to construct recombinant viral or bacterial vectors that express the antigen of interest and to use these recombinant vectors as vaccines. See Table 112.7 for list of promising viral and bacterial vectors	None licensed, but several in phase I and II clinical trials	
Nucleic acid (DNA) vaccines	Currently a very popular approach but still at the experimental/developmental stage. The vaccine consists of plasmid DNA expressing the antigen of interest	None licensed, but several in phase I and II clinical trials	

Table 112.2 Types of prophylactic vaccines.

CLASSIFICATION OF VACCINES

A complete list of vaccines licensed for use in the USA is provided in Table 112.3[31] Included are live and killed preparations, whole organisms, subunits of an organism, and rDNA-produced protein. To be effective, inactivated nonreplicating vaccines usually require repeated administration. In general, live attenuated vaccines achieve better levels of immunity and sometimes require only a single administration. New-generation inactivated vaccines are usually composed of minimally reactogenic pathogen subcomponents, but invariably are less immunogenic and require coadministration with facilitators called adjuvants. Most preparations are administered parentally, few are oral.

As mentioned previously, several infectious agents are refractory to control by prophylactic vaccines. Most commonly the fault lies with induction of an inadequate or imbalanced immune response similar to that seen with natural infection, and the response is inadequate to contain reinfection and disease expression. In such circumstances, effective vaccines will need to improve upon nature. A similar demand holds true for vaccines designed for therapeutic use. Here the scenario is that the host is already infected or is suffering from a pathologic lesion such as cancer or allergy. Lesions may exist because of a misguided or imbalanced immune response. To correct immune inadequacies with therapeutic vaccines represents a major challenge, but substantial progress is expected in the near future. Vaccines based on immunoprotective epitopes and potent yet nonreactogenic adjuvants are likely to form part of the therapeutic vaccine arsenal.

Live attenuated vaccines

Live attenuated vaccines provide the most effective and long-lasting immune response against organisms that, following natural infection, induce effective immunity. Replication of the microbe in the host provides amplification of the inoculated dose and in the process presents the protective antigens to the host's immune system in a more natural fashion. The expected result is the induction of an immune response that is comparable to natural infection. However, safety of live vaccines is a greater concern than with inactivated vaccines since inadequate attenuation may result in reversal to the naturally virulent form of the organism.[24] In addition, since potency depends on maintenance of infectivity, proper storage, including maintenance of a cold chain for transport, is essential.[31]

Attenuated viral vaccines were formerly prepared by frequent passage in embryonated eggs, cell cultures, or heterologous hosts. During such passage, mutations occurred and surviving viruses became less virulent in the natural host. The process of mutation could be accelerated by the use of chemical mutagens selecting for phenotypes such as temperature sensitivity and change in protease susceptibility. Attenuated vaccines retain their best immunogenicity if they have few mutations. However, few mutations can result in reversion to virulence, such as occurs with type III poliovirus vaccine where the principal mutation at position 472 responsible for avirulence can revert to the wild-type genotype.[1] The latter explains in part why inactive polio vaccine is now recommended.[24]

Live attenuated vaccines are particularly effective against viral agents which have a complex pathogenesis that includes systemic spread to target organs. Examples include mumps, measles, rubella, yellow fever, and polioviruses. Vaccines against these agents are among 16 of the currently licensed products in the USA (Table 112.4). The five vaccines previously mentioned were all produced by blind passage in embryonated eggs or cell culture relying on genetic roulette to generate mutations that confer the attenuation phenotype. In most instances, the genes involved in attenuation remain unknown. Although passage of virus in heterologous tissues, usually at low temperature and in the presence of chemical mutagens, is still used to develop live virus vaccines (e.g. respiratory syncytial virus, paramyxoviruses, and alphaviruses) the modern trend is to exploit our increasing knowledge of genome sequences (Table 112.5).[32] One favored approach is to introduce mis-sense mutations that specify an amino acid substitution into a coding region important for viral function. Mis-sense mutants with easily definable phenotypes such as temperature-sensitive (ts) mutants, protease activation and receptor binding are often employed.[28] The incorporation of multiple ts mutations into the same gene using recombinant cDNA technology is a favored approach since it is easy to select for mutants that grow only at low temperatures. The approach applies particularly well to respiratory viruses since mutants can be produced that replicate in the colder upper respiratory tract but not in the warmer lower tract, the major site of disease. A live influenza virus vaccine, to be administered intransally, based on this concept is currently being developed in the USA.[33] Changes in the surface binding proteins could also be selected for by growing mutants in the presence of neutralizing monoclonal antibodies. The resistant mutants are referred to as *m*onoclonal *a*ntibody *r*esistant (mar) mutants. The approach has been used to produce mutants in the G glycoprotein of rabies virus.[29]

A more practical genetic approach to produce new attenuated vaccines is to generate deletion mutants. These can be produced in one or more genes that are not required for replication in vitro, but nonetheless are needed in vivo for replication and/or virulence. This approach works well for poxviruses, herpesviruses, and adenoviruses, whose large genomes contain many nonessential genes for in vitro replication. It is more safe, however, to delete essential proteins and grow up the mutant in cell lines that complement missing genes. This approach was used to produce the gH deletion mutant for herpes simplex virus (HSV) currently under phase III trial as a vaccine candidate.[34] Alternative methods of attenuation include gene insertions into the virulence proteins. Such a procedure could result not only in attenuation, but the inserted gene could encode a regulatory molecule such as a cytokine that may serve to guide the nature of the immune response induced.[35]

Two final methods of attenuation also employ an expanding knowledge of viral genetics. First, the approach of gene incompatibility is being used to generate attenuated influenza virus vaccines. These vaccines are made by constructing viruses whose genomes contain one or more gene segments from a heterologous species of influenza or a mutated cold-adapted segment phenotype, along with segments from the wild-type virus. The mutants are referred to as reassortants. The influenza virus vaccine developed initially at NIH (pending licensure) relies on this concept.[33] A second reassortant approach was used to produce the highly effective (recently withdrawn) rotavirus vaccine.[36] Rotavirus has a genome that consists of ten segments. The vaccine strain has nine segments of simian origin but one segment encoding the human VP7 protective antigen. There are four types of human rotaviruses and the quadrivalent vaccine includes four separate

Currently licensed vaccines in the USA			
Vaccine	**Type**	**Indication**	**Route**
Adenovirus	Live virus	Military recruits	Oral
Anthrax	Inactivated bacteria	Exposure risk	SC
BCG	Live bacteria	Exposure risk, continuous childhood exposure to infectious source	ID (preferred) or SC
Cholera	Inactivated bacteria	Travel risk	SC, IM, or ID
DTaP	Toxoids with inactivated bacterial components	Childhood series	IM
DT, DT	Toxoids	Booster vaccine	IM
Hepatitis A	Inactivated viral antigen	Exposure risk	IM
Hepatitis B	Inactivated viral antigen	Newborn series, exposure risk	IM
Hib conjugates	Polysaccharide–protein conjugate	Childhood series	IM
Influenza	Inactivated virus (whole virus), viral components	Elderly, occupational risk, underlying disease state	IM
Japanese encephalitis	Inactivated virus	Prolonged exposure risk	SC
Lyme disease	Inactivated protein	Prolonged exposure in moderate – high risk area	IM
Measles	Live virus	Childhood series	SC
Meningococcal	Polysaccharide vaccine	Asplenia, complement deficiency, college students, military recruits, travel risk, outbreak risk	SC
MMR	Live viruses	Childhood series	SC
Mumps	Live virus	Childhood series	SC
Pertussis	Inactivated bacteria	Childhood series	IM
Plague	Inactivated bacteria	Occupational exposure	IM
Pneumococcal	Polysaccharide	Asplenia, complement deficiency, elderly	IM or SC
Pneumococcal	Protein-conjugate	Childhood series, abnormal humoral response to polysaccharide antigen in high-risk patient	IM
Inactivated poliovirus (IPV)	Inactivated virus	Childhood series, travelers, occupational exposure	SC
Oral poliovirus (OPV)	Live virus	Developing countries, recent or ongoing wild-type poliovirus exposure	Oral
Rabies	Inactivated virus	Postexposure prophylaxis	IM or ID
Rubella	Live virus	Childhood series, postexposure prophylaxis, nonimmune postpubertal females	SC
Tetanus	Toxoid	Childhood series, postexposure prophylaxis	IM
Typhoid	Inactivated bacteria Capsular polysaccharide Live bacteria	Travel risk, household contact, occupational risk	SC SC Oral
Varicella	Live virus	Childhood series, nonimmunized adults	SC
Yellow fever	Live virus	Travel exposure to endemic area	SC

Table 112.3 Currently licensed vaccines in the USA. (Modified from American Academy of Pediatrics 2000 Active and passive immunization vaccine handling and storage. In: Pickering LK (ed.) *Redbook: Report of the Committee of Infectious Diseases*, 25th edn. Elk Grove Village, IL, American Academy of Pediatrics, 2000, p 1 with permission.)

Viral vaccines licensed in the USA					
Virus vaccine	Number of serotypes covered by vaccine	Type of vaccine		Target population	Comments
		Live	Nonliving		
Adenovirus	2	+		Military recruits	Wild-type virus in enteric-coated capsules for oral administration to selectively infect the gut Lapse in manufacturing
Hepatitis A	1		+	Travelers, health care workers	Parenteral immunization with whole inactivated virus vaccine, 2 doses
Hepatitis B	1		+	Universal childhood	Parenteral immunization with recombinant VLP, 3 doses
Influenza A and B	3 (H1N1 and H3N2 and type B)		+	Elderly, patients with cardiopulmonary disease, others	Repeat annual parenteral immunization with disrupted virus vaccine
Japanese encephalitis virus	1		+	Travelers to endemic region	Parenteral immunization whole inactivated virus vaccine
Measles	1	+		Universal childhood	Parenteral immunization booster dose recommended at 4–6 years of age
Mumps	1	+		Universal childhood	Parenteral immunization booster dose recommended at 4–6 years of age
Poliovirus	3	+	+	Universal childhood	Two doses of inactivated whole virus vaccine followed by two doses of oral live attenuated virus
Rabies	1		+	High-risk persons	Prophylactic and therapeutic uses
Rubella	1	+		Universal childhood	Parenteral immunization
Smallpox	1	+		No longer used	Intradermal vaccine used to eradicate smallpox
Yellow fever	1	+		Travelers to endemic region	Parenteral immunization

Table 112.4 Viral vaccines licensed in the USA. (Modified from Murphy BR, Chanock M. Immunization against viral disease. In: Fields BN, Knipe DM, Howley PM, et al (eds) *Fields Virology*. Philadelphia, Lippincott Williams and Wilkins, 2001.)

Genetic approaches being used to develop live attenuated vaccines
Attenuation mutations introduced into the coding or noncoding regions • missense – respiratory syncytial virus • insertions – poxviruses, RSV, dengue
Deletion mutants – herpes simplex virus, HIV
Attenuation produced by gene incompatibility, e.g. influenza
Antigenic chimeric viruses (reassortants), e.g. rotavirus

Table 112.5 Genetic approaches being used to develop live attenuated vaccines.

reassortants each containing one of the four types of human VP7 gene segments.[36]

Nonconjugated attenuated vaccines have been far less successful for use against nonviral pathogens, particularly in children.[37] Attenuated vaccines against typhoid are available, but these are barely effective and highly reactogenic.[38] In addition, attenuated vaccines against other agents such as parasites are under development. In some countries, antiparasite attenuated vaccines have been used from time to time in veterinary medicine, but their expense and short half-lives have led to their discontinuation.

Nonliving (killed) vaccines

The early vaccines developed in the Pasteur era and in the first part of this century were all nonliving, consisting either of inactivated whole organisms or chemically inactivated bacterial products. Some of the whole-organism preparations continue to be effective vaccines: pertussis vaccine, the Salk poliovirus vaccine, and hepatitis A vaccine are examples. However, when direct comparisons have been possible, inactivated vaccines appear less effective than attenuated alternatives. Moreover, except for whole-cell pertussis vaccine, which has excellent efficacy, whole-organism vaccines against bacteria are only marginally effective and usually highly reactogenic.[39] Vaccines that use bacterial products may be very effective if immunity depends on the induction of IgG antibody to prevent toxin or pathogen attachment to cells. Examples of this include vaccines against exotoxin-producing bacteria (e.g. tetanus). In addition, vaccines

KEY CONCEPTS

Advantages and disadvantages of live attenuated vaccines

Advantages
- Preserve immunogenicity of virulent agent, especially the largely conformational antigens involved in antibody induction
- Mimic natural infection more effectively than inactive vaccines
- Usually stimulate multiple components of the immune system including T-cell immunity and mucosal immunity mediated by IgA
- Herd immunity

Disadvantages
- Cannot vaccinate in early infancy because of interference by maternal antibody, although less problematic if vaccine is administered mucosally
- May contain adventitious agents
- Can revert to virulence by mutation or interserotypic recombination
- Can cause serious illness in immunosuppressed individuals
- Naturally occurring wild-type viruses may interfere with vaccine potency, but multiple doses can overcome this problem
- Stringent storage instructions to maintain vaccine efficacy and safety

composed of component carbohydrates may be effective against some encapsulated bacteria. Protection against endotoxin-producing bacteria by vaccines is far more difficult to achieve.

Simple polysaccharide (e.g. polyribosylribitalphosphate, PRP), such as is contained within the original *H. influenzae* type B (Hib), fails to induce an adequate immune response in selective older children and children younger than 24 months of age. To overcome this problem, investigators coupled PRP to carrier proteins and demonstrated improved antigenicity in primary and secondary immunization.[40] This conjugation converted the immune response from thymus-independent to thymus-dependent. Three specific Hib-conjugate vaccines are currently licensed for use in the USA: one consists of polysaccharide coupled to diphtheria toxoid, a second oligosaccharide coupled to a nontoxic variant of diphtheria toxin, and a third polysaccharide coupled to a protein complex from *Neisseria meningitidis*. A further example of polysaccharide-conjugate vaccine is the recently licensed heptavalent pneumococcal vaccine, PCV7 (Prevnar, Lederle Laboratories/Wyeth-Ayerst Pharmaceuticals).[41] Several protein conjugate oligosaccharide and polysaccharide pneumococcal vaccines linked with proteins, such as meningococcal outer membrane protein, tetanus toxoid, a mutant nontoxic diphtheria toxin, CRM_{197}, and diphtheria toxoids have been evaluated for safety and immunogenicity in infants and children. Each of these polysaccharide conjugate pneumococcal vaccines has been found to induce good immune responses in infants younger than 1 year, and amnestic (i.e. memory) responses have been observed after booster doses. PCV7 is composed of seven pneumococcal antigens (polysaccharide serotypes 4, 6B, 9V, 14, 19F, and 23F and an oligosaccharide serotype 18C) conjugated to 20μg of CRM_{197} by reductive amination.[42]

Inactivated vaccines require repetitive immunization to achieve an acceptable immune response. Furthermore, periodic boosting is also required. Even with this approach, inactivated vaccines often represent poor vaccines. For example, the process of inactivation may impair the immunogenicity of protective antigens. The result may be inferior antibody production and/or the induction of an imbalanced T-cell response. There are several instances of unexpected adverse effects of inactivated vaccines. Most notable are examples of potentiated disease in recipients of inactivated measles and respiratory syncytial virus vaccines that occur upon subsequent exposure to the virulent virus.[43,44]

Inactivated vaccines also fall short in inducing mucosal immunity and CD8 T cell-mediated immune responses. This, and other disadvantages, however, must be balanced against higher safety, cheaper cost to produce and store, and the usual resistance to interference by pre-existing antibody. Since inactivated vaccines are *never* disease-producing, there are many ongoing attempts to produce formulations which exploit the advantages of nonliving vaccines (Table 112.6). These approaches include the use of purified proteins produced by recombinant DNA technology, synthetic peptides, anti-idiotype vaccines and nucleic acids (i.e. DNA vaccines). The latter are particularly attractive alternatives for infectious agents (parasites, etc.) for which no effective vaccine currently exists.

Hepatitis B vaccine is an example of a licensed and actively used vaccine that employs recombinant DNA technology.[27] This remarkably effective vaccine consists of a surface protein of the virus produced by recombinant DNA technology in yeast. The recombinant protein assembles spontaneously into 22 nm virus-like proteins which likely account for the high immunogenicity. This vaccine is effective without the need for an adjuvant. All other forms of protein, carbohydrate, or synthetic peptide vaccines require adjuvants to enhance immunogenicity.

Synthetic peptides as vaccines aroused considerable interest, especially as it was theorized that such vaccines should be cheap to manufacture, nonreactogenic, and capable of producing an immune response targeting immunoprotective determinants alone. Experimentally, various formulations of synthetic peptides

New approaches for better vaccines
Inactivated vaccines
Recombinant proteins produced in yeast, bacteria, cell culture, or plants
Synthetic peptides
Anti-idiotypic vaccines
Nucleic acid vaccines
Adjuvants and novel products • Aluminum salts • Emulsification in oils • ISCOMS and liposomes to encapsulate antigen • CpG containing oligodinucleotides • Antigen polymerization • Cholera toxin B • C3d • Cytokines and chemokine co-administration • Targeting antigens to dendritic cells • Use of heat-shock protein carriers

Table 112.6 New approaches for better vaccines.

conferred immunity, but almost uniformly they were inferior in potency to other vaccine forms. Formulation with powerful adjuvants did not significantly enhance immunogenicity. In addition, major histocompatibility complex restricted responses against single epitopes provide inadequate protection. Synthetic peptides appear to have been almost uniformly abandoned. The same fate has befallen anti-idiotypic antibody vaccines.

In contrast, immunization with nucleic acids that encode protective antigens is an exciting and viable field in present-day vaccinology.[45] Clinical trials are currently underway with at least two DNA vaccine candidates. The unexpected immunogenicity of plasmid DNA encoding a group protein was first observed in 1992.[32] Soon afterwards, groups showed that plasmid DNA encoding viral proteins induced a range of immune responses, most notably cytotoxic T-lymphocyte (CTL) responses, and conferred protection against viral challenge.[46] Indeed, the pattern of immunity engendered resembled that induced by conventional attenuated live vaccines. Since 1993, the nucleic acid vaccine approach has been extended with various levels of success to a wide range of pathogens, including viruses, bacteria, and parasites.[47]

Nucleic acid vaccines have several attractive features including apparent lack of reactivity/adverse events and minimal expense. Although the nucleic acid vaccines do not multiply, they do remain in the body for some time and encode the synthesis of authentic proteins. In murine models, these vaccines induce potent CTL responses. Since nucleic acid vaccines are less efficient at antibody induction, it is unlikely that they will replace many existing vaccines whose efficacy is related to antibody-mediated protection. Nucleic acid vaccines induce immunity slowly and antibody levels rarely reach the potency of other vaccine formulations (e.g. attenuated vaccines). The future role of nucleic acid vaccines will likely be related to the following: (a) efficacy in the presence of passive maternal antibody will allow for their use in vaccinating infants at earlier ages than with conventional vaccines; (b) nucleic acid vaccines offer options for protection against infectious agents like tuberculosis and malaria, which have no effective vaccine; and (c) recent observations suggest that immunogenicity is enhanced when a host is first primed with DNA vaccine and then boosted with another formulation.[48,49] A final potential advantage of nucleic acid vaccines is that concomitant administration of immune costimulator DNA can be conveniently performed and produce a customized immune response. This latter approach is being evaluated against many agents, in particular HIV.[49]

Recombinant vectors

Since the introduction 15 years ago of vaccinia virus as a vector, the recombinant vector approach has been carefully studied by vaccinologists.[50] Using a recombinant vector design offers the advantages of a live attenuated vaccine with the selectivity of a subunit vaccine. Vector vaccines use engineered genes encoding protective antigens from one or even many organisms. Immune costimulator molecules such as cytokines can also be included in such vaccines.[51] Historically, the vaccinia vector was first used, and its advantages included stability at room temperature, ease of administration, and potency as a T-cell immunogen. However, in an era of HIV, vaccinia virus is considered as potentially too dangerous for use as a vector in human subjects. Several other vectors, both viral and bacterial, have since been evaluated and these include a number of other poxvirus types. A partial list of vectors under investigation includes herpes simplex virus, adenovirus, rhabdoviruses, alphaviruses, flaviviruses, polioviruses, salmonella, shigella, listeria, and BCG (Table 112.7). As yet, none has been developed to the point of producing a commercially viable vaccine for humans. However, recombinant vectors that successfully achieve immunity upon enteric administration could represent a valuable addition to the vaccine arsenal and, hence, their evaluation continues.

Recombinant delivery systems for future vaccines
Plasmid 'naked' DNA
Bacterial vectors • Listeria • Mycobacteria • Salmonella • Shigella
Viral vectors • Adenoviruses • Alphaviruses • Lentiviruses • Poxviruses • Retroviruses
This is a partial list of the many bacterial and viral vectors currently being tested.

Table 112.7 Recombinant delivery systems for future vaccines.

Adjuvants

Microbes themselves are often potent immunogens because they act as nonspecific adjuvants as well as sources of specific antigens. For example, Freund's complete adjuvant contains killed mycobacteria which themselves act as immune stimulators. Most isolated proteins, as well as some inactivated whole organisms, are poorly immunogenic unless administered along with an adjuvant. In the USA, only the weak adjuvant aluminum hydroxide is licensed for use. Evolution of other adjuvants is likely in the future. Adjuvants likely function to enhance immunity in several ways: (a) by producing an antigen depot that is slowly released over time; (b) through recruitment of cells involved in antigen

KEY CONCEPTS

Advantages and disadvantages of inactivated vaccines

Advantages

- Safety – no risk of infection in immunosuppressed or reversion to virulence
- Easy to produce and store
- Less affected by pre-existing antibody

Disadvantages

- Must be repeatedly administered
- May not preserve immunoprotective antigens
- Poor inducers of T-cell immunity, especially CD8 T cells
- Poor inducers of mucosal immunity
- May potentiate disease because of imbalanced immune response induction
- May generate immune response to tissue antigens derived from producer cells – this could be allergenic

presentation; and (c) by stimulating the production of costimulator molecules (cytokines) important for immune induction. The most potent adjuvants are not acceptable for use since they have unacceptable reactogenicity and may have potential carcinogenicity. Promising adjuvants, specifically oil in water, MF59, and immune stimulator compounds (ISCOMS), may soon find use in human vaccines. ISCOMS are cage-like structures that consist mainly of plant-derived saponins and various phospholipids.[52] They are nontoxic and have been shown to enhance antibody and T-cell responses to many antigens. Their use is currently confined to veterinary medicine. Other adjuvants that may find a use in the near future are cholera toxin B, a potent adjuvant for mucosal responses, and CpG containing oligodinucleotides.[53,54]

PRACTICES OF IMMUNIZATION

The Red Book (Committee on Infectious Diseases, American Academy of Pediatrics and the Center for Disease Control and Prevention) publishes current guidelines and immunization practices for all vaccines listed in Table 112.3.[31] The clinical expression of an individual vaccine-preventable disease and the quality of the protective vaccine determine the recommendation for specific use of any individual vaccine. For example, universal immunization starting at an early age is recommended for hepatitis B, measles, polio, diphtheria, tetanus and *H. influenzae* type b since effective long-lasting vaccines are available for these life-threatening infections.

In circumstances of limited disease exposure but availability of a potent vaccine, immunization recommendations may be determined by exposure risk. Examples include recommendations for the meningococcal vaccine that target military personnel and college entry students, as well as civilians with documented exposure to serotypes A or C contained within the vaccine. In addition, immunization with yellow fever vaccine, hepatitis A vaccine, rabies vaccine as well as the newly licensed Lyme disease vaccine is limited to exposure risk.

Influenza vaccine is prepared annually based on expected prevalent influenza strains. This vaccine is designed to have an impact on both frequency and severity of influenza disease burden, but not to prevent annual epidemics. Owing to sub-optimal vaccine efficacy but large disease burden, influenza immunization recommendations are focused on suppression rather than eradication of disease. Influenza immunization is recommended for all patients at risk for severe disease. Vaccine-induced protection is 70–80%. In addition, only the subvirion or purified surface-antigen vaccines, i.e. 'split-virus' vaccines, should be administered to children younger than 13 years to minimize adverse effects.

A complex and ever-increasing list of vaccines is recommended in the early childhood to adolescent period. In an attempt to simplify the schedule (Fig. 112.1), vaccines are co-administered at different sites simultaneously.[55] This process of antigen mixing has been thoroughly studied and no contraindications to simultaneous administration of multiple vaccines have been documented. Evaluation of the immune response following multiple immunizations is important. In general, the response to one vaccine does not interfere with another. Exceptions to this include interference among the three oral poliovirus serotypes in

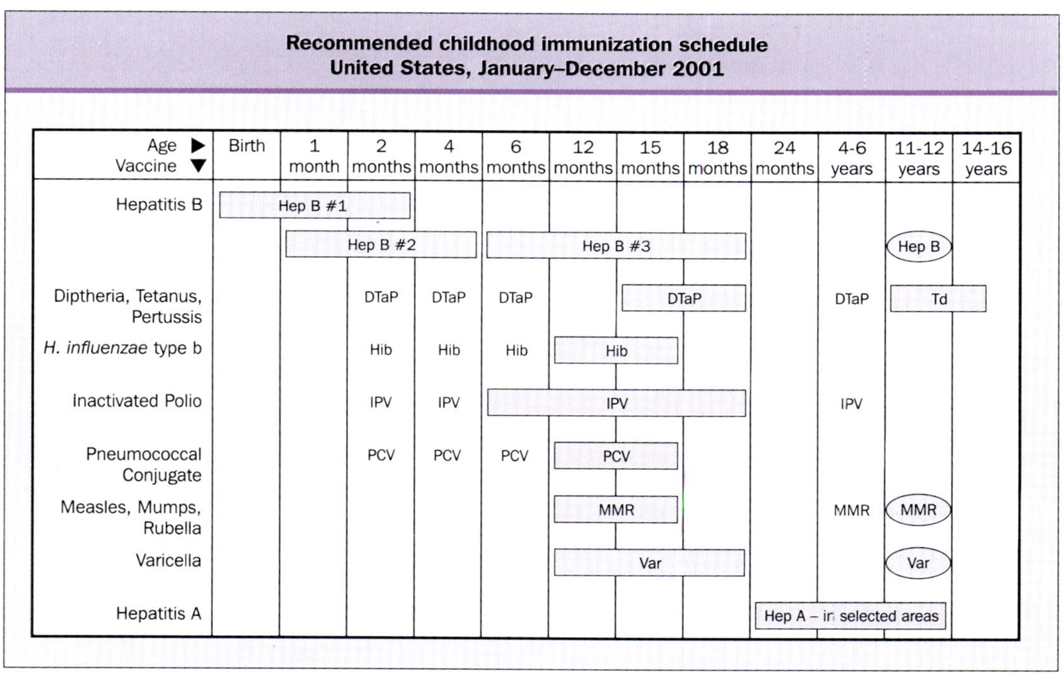

Figure 112.1 Recommended childhood immunization schedule for the USA January–December 2000. Vaccines are listed under routinely recommended ages. Bars indicate range of recommended ages for immunization. Any dose not given at the recommended age should be given as a 'catch-up' immunization at any subsequent visit when indicated and feasible. Ovals indicate vaccines to be given if previously recommended doses were missed or given earlier than the recommended minimum age. Approved by the Advisory Committee on Immunization Practices (ACIP), the American Academy of Pediatrics (AAP), and the American Academy of Family Physicians (AAFP). (With permission from the American Academy of Pediatrics 2000 Active and passive immunization vaccine handling and storage. In: Pickering LK (ed.) *Redbook: Report of the Committee of Infectious Diseases*, 25th edn. Elk Grove Village, IL, American Academy of Pediatrics, 2000, p 1.)

trivalent OPV and concurrent administration of cholera and yellow fever vaccines. As a result of the increasing number of vaccines approved for use or under development, other combinations of products are under evaluation to simplify schedules further. For those in whom early or rapid immunization is urgent, or those not immunized on schedule, simultaneous vaccination with multiple products allows for more rapid protection. In addition, simultaneous administration of multiple vaccines can raise immunization rates considerably.

Recommended vaccines for adult patients are few and include: (a) meningococcal and adenovirus vaccines for military recruits; (b) annual influenza and pneumococcal vaccines for elderly persons; and (c) bivalent diphtheria and tetanus toxoid vaccine at 10-year intervals. Hepatitis B vaccine, previously administered based on exposure risk, is now universally administered as part of the childhood immunization schedule. This recommendation resulted from the conclusion that effective and cost-efficient prevention among adults required the vaccination to be given during childhood.

For patients receiving intravenous immunoglobulin (IVIG) as passive immunization or as a modality of therapy, recommendations exist concerning administration of live viral vaccines. High doses of immunoglobulin have been shown to inhibit the response to measles vaccine for a prolonged period of time. The duration of inhibition varies with the dose and route of immunoglobulin delivery. If an immunoglobulin preparation must be administered within 14 days of receipt of a live viral vaccine, it is generally accepted that the individual should be reimmunized at a later time or tested for seroconversion.

ADVERSE EVENTS

The goal of vaccine development is to maintain the highest level of protection with the lowest rate of adverse events. Recommendations for vaccination practice are designed to maximize disease prevention and minimize risk by providing advice on vaccine dose, timing and site of administration, and by highlighting situations that suggest that added protection is necessary or, in contrast, where immunizations are contraindicated. Owing to the importance of possible adverse events associated with the currently recommended adult and pediatric immunization schedule, a number of sophisticated reporting mechanisms exist. Serious adverse events following certain vaccines demand mandatory reporting as proposed in the US National Childhood Vaccine Injury Act of 1986. However, for the majority of adverse events a primarily passive surveillance system is in existence, the Vaccine Adverse Event Reporting System (VAERS). To supplement the VAERS program, the Centers for Disease Control and Prevention (CDC) formed partnerships with four large health maintenance organizations to establish the Vaccine Safety Data Link (VSD) project, an active surveillance system designed to monitor continually vaccine safety. The VSD has been instrumental in the investigation and affirmation of vaccine safety in many clinical situations. An example of the utility of VAERS and VSD systems was the rapid evaluation of intussusception and rotavirus vaccine, resulting in rapid removal of the vaccine from the US market.

The most frequently reported side-effects of parenterally administered vaccines include swelling and pain at the injection site.[31] The reaction, an inflammatory response to foreign material, is encountered more often following intradermal than intramuscular injections. The majority of these adverse events are short-lived and do not warrant specific intervention. Local reactions increase in frequency and severity if alum adjuvant is present, owing to delayed clearance of the foreign material. Other commonly reported but transient side-effects of immunization include systemic events such as fever, headache, malaise, and myalgias. Not unlike local reactions, systemic reactions are primarily a consequence of inflammatory responses and usually associated with a local reaction.

An adverse reaction attributable to hypersensitivity to a component of the vaccine is a risk for all vaccines. Described reactions include IgE antibody-mediated wheal and flare, urticaria, angioedema, and full-blown anaphylaxis as well as a variety of Arthus-type reactions and immune complex-mediated serum sickness. Severe reactions are rare and are largely attributed to an unknown sensitivity to a preservative or a component of the system used to prepare the vaccine antigen.

Whole-cell pertussis vaccine was suspected to be associated with adverse neurological events. Despite failure to confirm causality scientifically, there was adequate concern to prompt the development of a safe and less reactogenic vaccine. The currently licensed acellular pertussis products produce significantly less fever, local and systemic events.

Live attenuated vaccines carry the risk of producing infection, particularly in the immunocompromised host. Live poliovirus vaccine is no longer recommended as part of the early childhood vaccination schedule owing to the risk of vaccine-associated paralytic polio in the immunocompromised recipient or household contacts.[55] Similarly, universal administration of BCG (bacille Calmette–Guérin) is not recommended owing to the prevalence of HIV infection throughout the world.

More recent controversial issues regarding vaccine safety include hepatitis B immunization and multiple sclerosis (MS), measles, mumps and rubella (MMR) immunization and autism, and more recently MMR and inflammatory bowel disease. Following isolated reports by French neurologists of hepatitis B vaccines being associated with onset or relapse of MS, the perception that the vaccine causes MS developed. In the wake of adverse publicity a dramatic decline in vaccine utilization ensued. Subsequently, a group of international experts convened in 1998 to discuss this concern and concluded that the available data did not support a causal link between hepatitis B vaccination and MS.[56] Owing to a change in hepatitis B vaccination practices in France, with the exclusion of mandatory vaccination of pre-adolescents, a number of clinical trials were initiated to evaluate the claim of a link between MS and hepatitis B immunization. To date the available epidemiology data from France and elsewhere do not uphold this claim.

A variety of factors are associated with increased incidence of certain forms of autism, including infectious, metabolic, genetic, neurological, and environmental factors. An initial observation linking chronic enterocolitis and a regressive neurological disorder with the MMR vaccine was proposed by Dr Andrew Wakefield, United Kingdom.[57] This hypothesis was based on a case series from 12 children, with limited control data. Subsequent to this report, a British epidemiological study conducted by Taylor et al to examine children born with autism since 1979 failed to identify a link between MMR and autism.[58] Follow-up histological data from the initial study failed to identify any MMR-related material in the colonic biopsy material. At the current time, the best

THERAPEUTIC PRINCIPLES

Administration of vaccines

- The majority of live viruses are administered via the subcutaneous route.
- The majority of inactivated vaccines are administered via the intramuscular route.
- The following are absolute contraindications to vaccine administration:
  - Anaphylactic reaction to any prior vaccine contraindicates further doses of that vaccine.
  - Encephalopathy within 7 days of receipt of DTaP/DTP.
  - Anaphylaxis to neomycin or streptomycin contraindicates the use of IPV.
  - Anaphylaxis to neomycin/gelatin contraindicates the use of MMR and varicella.
  - Anaphylaxis to baker's yeast contraindicates the use of hepatitis B.
  - Live virus vaccines should not be administered to persons with underlying immunodeficiency, e.g. hematologic and solid tumors, congenital immunodeficiency, and long-term immunosuppressive therapy.
  - Varicella and OPV are contraindicated for HIV-infected patients; MMR is recommended at the usual ages for persons with asymptomatic HIV infection and for those with symptomatic infection who are not severely immunocompromised; MMR is contraindicated for severely immunocompromised HIV-infected patients.
  - All live virus vaccines are contraindicated in pregnancy.
- An anaphylactic reaction to egg ingestion was previously considered a contraindication to MMR administration unless skin testing, and if indicated, desensitization was performed; however, as of 1997, skin testing is no longer recommended as it does not accurately predict anaphylaxis to the MMR vaccine.

available scientific data do not support an association between autism or other behavioral disorders and the MMR vaccine.

Thimerosal has been used as an additive to biologics and vaccines since the 1930s because it is very effective for killing bacteria used in several vaccines and for preventing bacterial contamination, particularly in opened multidose containers. The thimerosal content of vaccines varies from 0 to 0.01%, which is equivalent to 0–25 μg/ml of mercury. Owing to the recognized adverse health effects of mercury exposure, the American Academy of Pediatrics published recommendations concerning the use of thimerosal-containing vaccines. The AAP believes that physicians should minimize children's exposure to thimerosal, but they should not compromise the health of children by withholding routinely recommended immunizations.[59]

NEW APPROACHES TO IMMUNIZATION

Mucosal vaccines

Mucosal surfaces are prevalent throughout the body and serve as a portal of entry for many existing and emerging pathogens such as influenza virus and HIV. Mucosal immunity, which is important for long-term protection, forms a first line of defense against mucosally transmitted pathogens. Adaptive host immunity at the mucosal surface consists primarily of CD4 T cells, secretory immunoglobulin A, and antigen-specific CTL. The common mucosal immune system involves homing of antigen-specific lymphocytes to mucosal effector sites other than that at which the initial antigen exposure occurred. Different immunization routes, such as oral, rectal, or intranasal, can induce a generalized mucosal immune response. CTL responses at mucosal surfaces are dictated locally and are not the result of systemic extension. Only a few mucosal vaccines, mostly oral, have been licensed for human use, including oral poliovirus, *Salmonella typhi*, and the recently withdrawn rotavirus vaccine. The cold-adapted influenza virus, currently in advanced clinical trials, is the first mucosal vaccine given intranasally to humans and has been shown to generate protective immune responses.[60] Another potential area of development for mucosal vaccines is the use of bacterial adhesins. Mucosal antibodies to these proteins block the pathogen's ability to penetrate mucosal barriers. The pilus-associated FimH from uropathogenic *E. coli* binding to mannose-oligosaccharides is a vaccine target currently undergoing clinical trials.[61]

Maternal immunization

The concept of maternal immunization is not a new approach, but it is an additional method for vaccine delivery that can have great impact upon the wellbeing of full-term newborn infants. Women in the later stages of pregnancy are capable of producing adequate amounts of antibodies in response to vaccines. IgG antibodies, especially of the IgG_1 subtype, have been demonstrated to cross the placenta readily, particularly during the latter weeks of gestation. Additionally, low levels of protective maternal antibodies against certain pathogens are associated with adverse outcome in infected newborns. In the USA a number of vaccines are currently indicated during the last trimester of pregnancy, including inactive influenza virus vaccine and tetanus–diphtheria toxoid. In addition, a number of vaccines are recommended in special circumstances (women at high risk because of underlying conditions or probable exposure during epidemics or travel to endemic areas); these include poliovirus (live or inactivated), pneumococcal polysaccharide, meningococcal polysaccharide, hepatitis A and B, and yellow fever vaccine.[62] Vaccines currently undergoing research and development include, group B streptococcus, pneumococcal conjugate, meningococcal conjugate, RSV-subunit vaccine (purified fusion protein), parainfluenza-3, acellular pertussis and attenuated influenza virus vaccine. Of primary concern when developing and implementing vaccines for use during pregnancy is the safety of the mother, fetus, and newborn child. Vaccination of pregnant women has been practiced extensively in the USA since 1957. A large collaborative study examining 50 000 women over 7 years failed to identify increased risk for adverse outcome in the infants of vaccinees.[63] As well as safety issues, the effect of passively administered antibodies on the developing immune system of the newborn is another area for concern; however, this has not been a problem when immunoglobulin or monoclonal antibody products are exogenously administered to infants.

SUMMARY

Since the development of Jenner's first 'vaccine' considerable advances have been made in the field of vaccinology. New and

CLINICAL PEARLS

Vaccination in children

- Childhood vaccinations have a major impact on the reduction and elimination of many causes of morbidity and mortality among children.
- Vaccine-preventable diseases have a costly impact, resulting in doctor's visits, hospitalizations, and premature deaths.
- The Americas were certified polio-free in 1994. Intensified efforts are on track to eradicate wild poliovirus worldwide by 2005.

improved techniques in molecular biology, especially in the field of DNA vaccines, will help in the development of vaccines that mimic natural infection as well as being safe to administer. However, safety issues remain of paramount importance. We recently experienced the harmful effects of adverse publicity on MMR immunization utilization. In order for the World Health Organization to meet its goals of global polio eradication, it is necessary to maintain maximal vaccine delivery. Vaccination programs may begin with vaccine development, but in order to be successful they require ongoing education and comprehensive participation.

REFERENCES

1. Ten great public health achievements – United States, 1900–1999. MMWR Morb Mortal Wkly Rep 1999;48:241.
2. Pinilla-Ibarz J, Cathcart K, Scheinbert DA. CML vaccines as a paradigm of the specific immunotherapy of cancer. Blood Rev 2000;14:111.
3. Basak S, Eck S, Gutzmer R, et al. Colorectal cancer vaccines: antiidiotypic antibody, recombinant protein, and viral vector. Ann NY Acad Sci 2000;910:237.
4. Naz RK. Vaccine for contraception targeting sperm. Immunol Rev 1999;171:193.
5. Weissert R, Lobell A, de Graaf KL, et al. Protective DNA vaccination against organ-specific autoimmunity is highly specific and discriminates between single amino acid substitutions in the peptide autoantigen. Proc Natl Acad Sci USA 2000;97:1689.
6. Matsumoto Y, Jee Y, Sugisaki M. Successful TCR-based immunotherapy for autoimmune myocarditis with DNA vaccines after rapid identification of pathogenic TCR. J Immunol 2000;164:2248.
7. Araga S, Xu L, Nakashima K, Villain M, Blalock JE. A peptide vaccine that prevents experimental autoimmune myasthenia gravis by specifically blocking T cell help. FASEB J 2000;14:185.
8. Abath FG. Development of vaccines against human parasitic diseases: tools, current status and perspectives. Expert Opin Investig Drugs 2000;9:301.
9. Galindo CM, Acosta CJ, Schellenbert D, et al. Humoral immune responses during a malaria vaccine trial in tanzanian infants. Parasite Immunol 2000;22:437.
10. Kahn JS. Respiratory syncytial virus vaccine development. Curr Opin Pediatr 2000;12:257.
11. Nathanson N, Mathieson BJ. Biological considerations in the development of a human immunodeficiency virus vaccine. J Infect Dis 2000;182:579.
12. Mills J, Desrosiers R, Rud E, et al. Live attenuated HIV vaccines: a proposal for further research and development. AIDS Res Hum Retroviruses 2000;16:1453.
13. Withdrawal of rotavirus vaccine recommendation. MMWR Morb Mortal Wkly Rep 1999;48:1007.
14. Safranek TJ, Lawrence DN, Kurland LT, et al. Reassessment of the association between Guillain–Barre syndrome and receipt of swine influenza vaccine in 1976–1977: results of a two-state study. Expert Neurology Group. Am J Epidemiol 1991;133:940.
15. Rabasa R. George Washington and variolation; Edward Jenner and vaccination. JAMA 1986;255:1881.
16. Bloch H. Edward Jenner (1749–1823). The history and effects of smallpox, inoculation, and vaccination. Am J Dis Child 1993;147:772.
17. Pasteur L. De l'attenuation du virus du cholera des poules. C R Acad Sci 1880;91:637.
18. Roux E, Yersin A. Contribution a l'etude de la diphtherie. Annals de L'Institut Pasteur (Paris) 1888;2:629.
19. Salmon DE, Smith T. On a new method of producing immunity from contagious diseases. Am Vet Rev 1886;10:63.
20. Von Behring E, Kitasato S. The mechanisms of diphtheria immunity and tetanus immunity in animals. 1890 (classical article). Mol Immunol 1991;28:1317,1319.
21. Merchant DJ. Cell cultures for virus vaccine production. General conclusions from the conference. Natl Cancer Inst Monogr 1968;29:583.
22. Salk J, Salk D. Control of influenza and poliomyelitis with killed virus vaccines. Science 1977;195:834.
23. Sabin AB. Oral poliovirus vaccine. History of its development and prospects for eradication of poliomyelitis. JAMA 1965;194:872.
24. Georgescu MM, Balanant J, Macadam A, et al. Evolution of the Sabin type 1 poliovirus in humans: characterization of strains isolated from patients with vaccine-associated paralytic poliomyelitis. J Virol 1997;71:7758.
25. Prolonged poliovirus excretion in an immunodeficient person with vaccine-associated paralytic poliomyelitis. MMWR Morb Mortal Wkly Rep 1997;46:641.
26. Sutter RW, Prevots DR, Cochi SL. Poliovirus vaccines. Progress toward global poliomyelitis eradication and changing routine immunization recommendations in the United States. Pediatr Clin North Am 2000;47:287.
27. Valenzuela P, Medina A, Rutter WJ, et al. Synthesis and assembly of hepatitis B virus surface antigen particles in yeast. Nature 1982;298:347.
28. Murphy BR, Chanock M. Immunization against viral disease. In: Fields BN, Knipe DM, Howley PM, et al. (eds) Fields Virology. Philadelphia, Lippincott Williams and Wilkins, 2001.
29. Coulon P, Ternaux JP, Flamand A, et al. An avirulent mutant of rabies virus is unable to infect motoneurons in vivo and in vitro. J Virol 1998;15:248.
30. Zoulim F, Trepo C. New antiviral agents for the therapy of chronic hepatitis B virus infection. Intervirology 1999;42:125.
31. American Academy of Pediatrics 2000 Active and passive immunization vaccine handling and storage. In: Pickering LK (ed.) Redbook: Report of the Committee of Infectious Diseases, 25th edn. Elk Grove Village, IL, American Academy of Pediatrics, 2000, p 1.
32. Tang DC, DeVit M, Johnston SA. Genetic immunization is a simple method for eliciting an immune response. Nature 1992;356:152.
33. Maassab HF, La Montagne JR, DeBorde DC. Live influenza virus vaccines. In: Plotkin SA, Mortimer EA (eds) Vaccines. Philadelphia, Saunders, 1998, p 435.
34. Forrester A, Farrell H, Wilkinson G, et al. Construction and properties of a mutant herpes simplex virus type 1 with glycoprotein H coding sequences deleted. J Virol 1992;66:341.
35. Kuklin NA, Daheshia M, Marconi PC, et al. Modulation of mucosal and systemic immunity by enteric administration of nonreplicating herpes simplex virus expressing cytokine genes. Virology 1998;240:245.
36. Perez-Schael I, Guntinas MJ, Perez M, et al. Efficacy of the rhesus rotavirus-based quadrivalent vaccine in infants and young children in Venezuela. N Engl J Med 1997;337:1181.
37. Anderson P. Antibody responses to *Haemophilus influenzae* type b and diphtheria toxin induced by conjugates of oligosaccharides of

the type b capsule with the non-toxic protein CRM_{197}. Infect Immun 1983;39:233.
38. Klugman KP, Koornhof JH, Robbins JB, et al. Immunogenicity, efficacy and serological correlate of protection of *Salmonella typhi* Vi capsular polysaccharide vaccine three years after immunization. Vaccine 1996;14:435.
39. Pichichero ME, Edwards KM, Anderson EL, et al. Safety and immunogenicity of six acellular pertussis vaccines and one whole-cell pertussis vaccine given as a fifth dose in four- to six-year-old children. Pediatrics 2000;105:e11.
40. Adams WG, Deaver KA, Cochi SL, et al. Decline of childhood *Haemophilus influenzae* type b (Hib) disease in the Hib vaccine era. JAMA 1993;269:221.
41. Overturf GD. American Academy of Pediatrics. Committee on Infectious Diseases. Technical report: prevention of pneumococcal infections, including the use of pneumococcal conjugate and polysaccharide vaccines and antibiotic prophylaxis. Pediatrics 2000;106:367.
42. Shinefield HR, Black S, Ray P, et al. Safety and immunogenicity of heptavalent pneumococcal CRM197 conjugate vaccine in infants and toddlers. Pediatr Infect Dis J 1999;18:757.
43. Fulginiti VA, Eller JJ, Downie AW, et al. Altered reactivity to measles virus. Atypical measles in children previously immunized with inactivated measles virus vaccines. JAMA 1967;202:1075.
44. Kim HW, Canchola JG, Brandt CD, et al. Respiratory syncytial virus disease in infants despite prior administration of antigenic inactivated vaccine. Am J Epidemiol 1969;89:422.
45. Donnelly JJ, Ulmer JB, Shiver JW, et al. DNA vaccines. Annu Rev Immunol 1997;15:617.
46. Ulmer JB, Donnelly JJ, Parker SE, et al. Heterologous protection against influenza by injection of DNA encoding a viral protein. Science 1993;259:1745.
47. Manickan E, Karem K, Rouse BT. DNA vaccines, a modern gimmick or a boon to vaccinology? Crit Rev Immunol 1997;17:139.
48. Manickan E, Yu Z, Rouse BT. DNA immunization of neonates induces immunity despite the presence of maternal antibody. J Clin Invest 1997;100:237.
49. Letvin NL, Montefiori DC, Yasutomi Y, et al. Potent, protective anti-HIV immune responses generated by bimodal HIV DNA protein vaccination. Proc Natl Acad Sci USA 1997;94:9378.
50. Moss B, Flexner C. Vaccinia virus expression vectors. Annu Rev Immunol 1987;5:305.
51. Lin R, Tarr PE, Jones TC. Present status of the use of cytokines as adjuvants with vaccines to protect against infectious diseases. Clin Infect Dis 1995;21:1439.
52. Villacres MC, Behdoudi S, Mikkila T, et al. Internalization of iscom-borne antigens and presentation under MHC class I or class II restriction. Cell Immunol 1998;185:30.
53. Sun J-B, Holmgren J, Czerkinsky C. Cholera toxin B subunit: an efficient transmucosal carrier-delivery system for induction of peripheral immunological tolerance. Proc Natl Acad Sci USA 1994;91:10795.
54. Davis HL, Weeranta R, Waldschmidt TJ, et al. CpG DNA is a potent enhancer of specific immunity in mice immunized with recombinant hepatitis B surface antigen. J Immunol 1998;160:870.
55. Recommended childhood immunization schedule – United States, 2000. MMWR Morb Mortal Wkly Rep 2000;49:35,47.
56. Monteyne P, Andre FE. Is there a causal link between hepatitis B vaccination and multiple sclerosis? Vaccine 2000;18:1994.
57. Wakefield AJ, Murch SH, Anthony A, et al. Ileal-lymphoid-nodular hyperplasia, non-specific colitis, and pervasive developmental disorder in children. Lancet 1998;351:637.
58. Taylor B, Miller E, Farrington CP, et al. Autism and measles, mumps, and rubella vaccine: no epidemiological evidence for a causal association. Lancet 1999;353:2026.
59. Summary of the joint statement on thimerosal in vaccines. American Academy of Family Physicians, American Academy of Pediatrics, Advisory Committee on Immunization Practices, Public Health Service. MMWR Morb Mortal Wkly Rep 2000;49:622,631.
60. Longini IM, Halloran ME, Nizam A, et al. Estimation of the efficacy of live, attenuated influenza vaccine from a two-year, multi-center vaccine trial: implications for influenza epidemic control. Vaccine 2000;18:1902.
61. Langermann S, Mollby R, Burlein JE, et al. Vaccination with FimH adhesin protects cynomolgus monkeys from colonization and infection by uropathogenic *Escherichia coli*. J Infect Dis 2000;181:774.
62. Greby SM, Singleton JS, Walker FJ, Strikas RA. Observations from the CDC: promoting women's health through age-appropriate vaccination. J Womens Health Gend Based Med 1999;8:1225.
63. Heinonen OP, Slone D, Shapiro S. Immunizing agents. In: Kaufman DW (ed.) Birth defects and drugs in pregnancy. Littleton, MA, Publishing Sciences Group, 1977, p 314.

Chapter 113

Immunotherapy of Allergic Disease

Anthony J Frew

INTRODUCTION

Specific allergen immunotherapy (SIT) involves the administration of allergen extracts to modify or abolish symptoms associated with atopic allergy. The process is specific, in that the treatment is targeted at those allergens recognized by the patient and physician as responsible for symptoms. A decision to use SIT therefore demands a careful assessment of the patient's condition and the role of allergic triggers. This form of therapy was first attempted at the end of the nineteenth century and then reported in the second decade of the twentieth century by Noon and Freeman at St Mary's Hospital, London.[1] Immunotherapy then became popular in North America and in Europe but some differences in practice have gradually developed either side of the Atlantic. Typically, patients are started on a very low dose of allergen, given by subcutaneous injection. The dose is then increased in a series of weekly injections until a plateau or maintenance dose is achieved. The maintenance dose is then given at 4–6 weekly intervals for 3–5 years. Alternative induction regimens may give several doses on each day, or may give the whole series of incremental injections in a single day (rush protocols). The main drawback to rush and semi-rush protocols is the risk of adverse reactions, which are much more common than in conventional protocols. On the other hand, full protection can be attained in a few days as compared to the three months required in the conventional regimen.

With the increasing trend towards evidence-based practice, allergists have been challenged to provide data to support their use of SIT. While many older studies were of doubtful quality, recent clinical trials have confirmed the usefulness of SIT as a treatment for allergic rhinitis and hypersensitivity to wasp and bee venom. The value of SIT as a primary treatment for asthma has, however, been more controversial.

CLINICAL PEARLS

Justification of the use of SIT in allergic diseases

- Molecular science is beginning to substantiate the nearly 100-year history of giving SIT to patients with inhaled allergies.
- Despite the in vitro evidence of benefit of SIT, the most important endpoints are the relief of symptoms in patients and improvement in the quality of life.
- Healthcare maintenance organizations are demanding cost–benefit analysis of SIT to justify its expense.
- Modulation of the natural history of allergic diseases (e.g. asthma) must be carefully explored.

MECHANISMS

Several mechanisms have been proposed to explain the beneficial effects of immunotherapy (Table 113.1). Early studies showed that SIT induces allergen-specific IgG antibodies. This led to suggestions that SIT might work by inducing antibodies that would intercept the allergen and 'block' the allergic response. In patients treated for venom anaphylaxis, the development of allergen-specific IgG antibody correlates with clinical efficacy, but for other allergens the magnitude of the IgG response is not closely related to the degree of efficacy. Moreover, the rise in IgG follows rather than precedes the onset of clinical benefit. Allergen-specific IgE levels rise temporarily during the initial phase of SIT, but fall back to pretreatment levels during maintenance therapy.[2] The immediate skin test response can be reduced after SIT but this effect is relatively small compared to the degree of clinical benefit. In contrast, the late-phase skin test response is virtually abolished after successful SIT. Similar patterns are observed for late-phase nasal and airway responses.[3]

With the recognition of the role of T cells as orchestrators of the allergic response, investigators have focused on the effects of SIT on cellular responses to allergen. Both in the skin and in the nose, successful SIT is accompanied by a reduction in T-cell and

Possible mechanisms of immunotherapy
• Induction of IgG (blocking) antibodies
• Reduction in specific IgE (long-term)
• Reduced recruitment of effector cells
• Altered T-cell cytokine balance (shift to Th1 from Th2)
• T-cell anergy

Table 113.1 Possible mechanisms of immunotherapy.

KEY CONCEPTS

Immunological events observed in systemic and nasal immunotherapy of allergic disease

- Allergen taken up by subcutaneous or mucosal dendritic cells
- Dendritic cells present allergen to T cells in presence of IL-12 causing Th1 shift
- Increased proportion of IL-2, IFN-γ, IL-12 expressing (Th1) T cells is observed locally
- Decreased recruitment of T cells and eosinophils
- Increased concentrations of allergen-specific IgG antibodies

eosinophil recruitment in response to allergen challenge. In parallel, there is a shift in the balance of Th1 and Th2 cytokine expression in the allergen-challenged site. Th2 cytokine expression is not affected but there is an increased proportion of T cells expressing the Th1 cytokines IL-2, IFN-γ, and IL-12.[4–6] These findings suggest that SIT has a modulatory effect on allergen-specific T cells, which would explain why the clinical and late-phase responses are attenuated without such a large effect on allergen-specific antibody levels.

SIT FOR VENOM HYPERSENSITIVITY

Anaphylaxis to hymenoptera venom is relatively rare, but can be fatal (Chapter 47). Venom-specific IgE antibodies can be found in 30–40% of adults for a few months following a sting, but these usually disappear in a few months. Some individuals react more vigorously with high concentrations of venom-specific antibodies, which may persist for many years without further exposure to stings. These patients are at risk of anaphylaxis to subsequent stings and a small number die from anaphylaxis each year. Estimates are hard to come by, but a figure of 10–20 deaths per year in the USA has been cited. This problem should not be confused with deaths from 'killer bees' which are behaviorally inclined to cause multiple stings, and hence cause death by massive envenomation. A decision to embark on venom immunotherapy requires careful assessment of the patient as well as an understanding of the natural history of venom allergy.[7] Patients who have experienced systemic symptoms after a sting are at much greater risk of anaphylaxis on subsequent stings, as compared to patients who have only had large local reactions. The frequency of systemic reactions to stings in children and adults with a history of large local reactions is about 5–10%, whereas the risk in patients with a previous systemic reaction is between 30% and 70%. In general, children are less at risk of repeated systemic reactions, as are those with a history of milder reactions. With time, the risk of a systemic reaction decreases: by 10 years after a previous systemic response, the risk is about 15%, compared to the general population risk of 2–3%. In making a decision about venom SIT, one should also take account of occupational and geographic factors that may affect the likelihood of future stings. Bee stings are much commoner in beekeepers, their families and neighbors, while wasp stings tend to be sporadic but are an occupational hazard for bakers and greengrocers. Other factors to be considered are the potential risks of emergency treatment with epinephrine and the various medical contraindications to SIT (see below).

The introduction of pure venom SIT preparations has led to a substantial improvement in the effectiveness of SIT for venom allergy. Desensitization with venom extracts accelerates the rate at which the risk decreases and has been shown to provide protection against field and laboratory stings. After completing venom SIT, there is a residual risk of systemic reactions of about 10%, but these are typically mild. Consideration should also be given to providing injectable epinephrine and other anti-allergic medication for use in the event of a sting during therapy.

SIT FOR ALLERGIC RHINITIS

SIT has been widely used to treat allergic rhinitis. As with other uses of SIT, it is important to select patients appropriately. The allergic basis of the rhinitis should be carefully assessed both on history and on skin tests or blood tests, and other causes should be excluded. Tests of nasal sensitivity are not used in routine clinical practice but may be useful for assessing effectiveness in clinical trials.

The effectiveness of SIT in seasonal allergic rhinitis has been confirmed in many trials, using grass, ragweed and birch pollen. Moreover, SIT has been shown to be clinically effective even in patients with severe seasonal rhinitis that is resistant to conventional drug therapy.[8] In this landmark study, SIT was used to treat a group of patients with grass pollen rhinitis that was resistant to standard therapy. The active group showed a highly significant decrease in symptoms and medication use in the first year of treatment, which was accompanied by reduced nasal and conjunctival sensitivity to allergen (Fig. 113.1). On maintenance

Reduction in symptom and drug scores in patients with allergic rhinitis treated with grass pollen extract

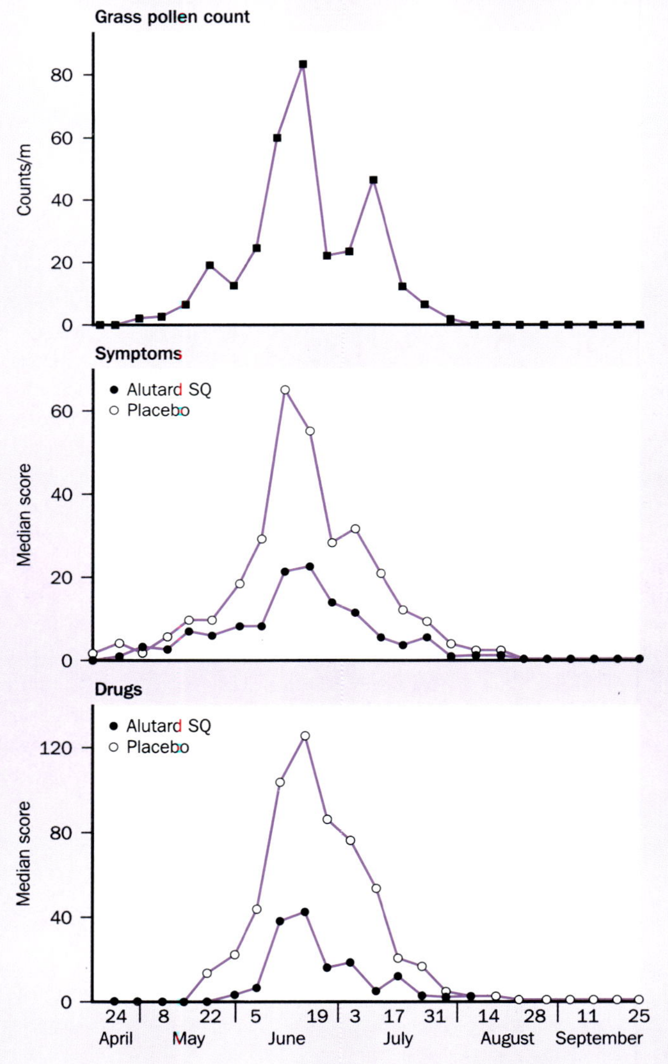

Figure 113.1 Effect of grass pollen extract (Alutard SQ) SIT on symptom and drug scores. Average weekly grass pollen counts (1989), and symptom and drug scores for (Alutard SQ) and placebo groups. Arrows represent the beginning (15 May) and end (25 July) of the pollen season. (From Varney VA, Gaga M, Frew AJ, Aber VR, Kay AB, Durham SR. Usefulness of immunotherapy in patients with severe summer hay fever uncontrolled by antiallergic drugs. *BMJ* 1991;302:265, with permission.)

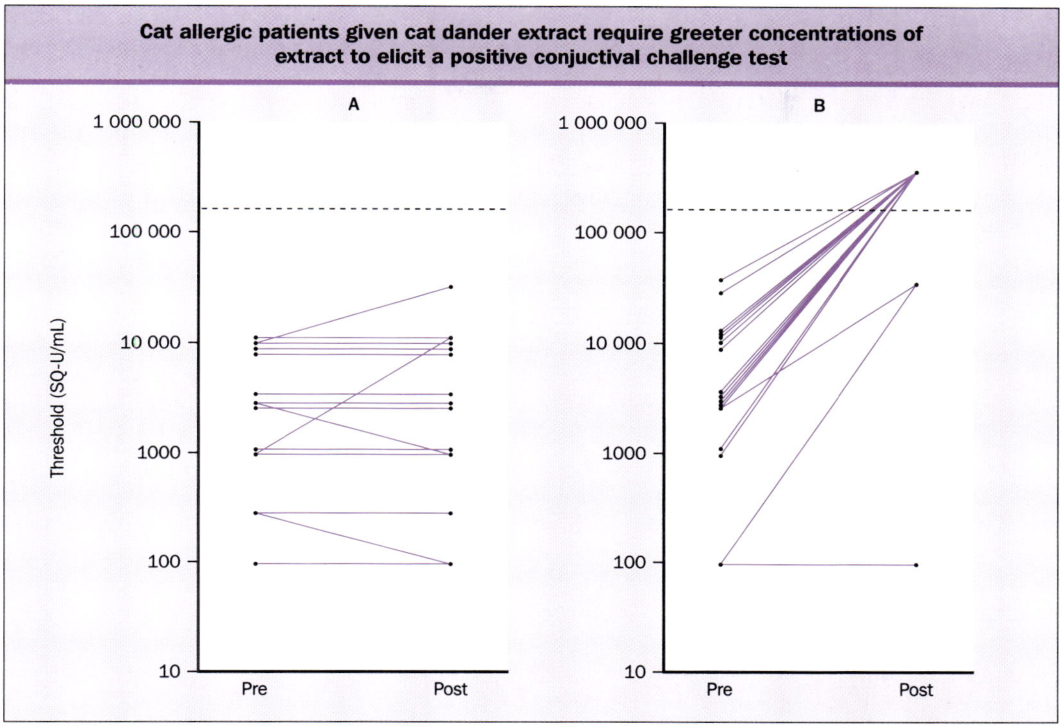

Figure 113.2 Effect of SIT with cat dander extract on conjunctival provocation threshold. (A) placebo; (B) cat dauder extract. Patients given cat dauder required more concentrated extract to elicit a positive vedation than did patients given placebo (From Varney VA, Edwards J, Tabbah K, Brewster H, Mavroleon G, Frew AJ. Clinical efficacy of specific immunotherapy to cat dander: a double-blind placebo-controlled trial. *Clin Exp Allergy* 1997;27:860, with permission.)

therapy, symptoms and rescue medication usage were further reduced. Limited data are available regarding the long term efficacy in rhinitis, but a recent study demonstrate that the effects last for at least 6 years after discontinuing therapy.[9] The benefits of SIT for perennial rhinitis are less than for seasonal rhinitis. In part this reflects the difficulty in determining the extent to which allergy is responsible for perennial symptoms. Allergy to house dust mite is common and does not always cause symptoms. Conversely, there are other causes of perennial rhinitis including vasomotor instability, infection, aspirin sensitivity, etc. Nevertheless, clinical trials have shown a definite benefit in appropriately selected subjects. Clearer evidence has been obtained in rhinitis due to pet allergy. Several studies have shown a marked improvement in tolerance of cat exposure after SIT, confirmed both on challenge tests (Fig. 113.2) and simulated natural exposure.[10]

As with any therapy, the risks and cost-effectiveness of SIT need to be assessed on a case-by-case basis. Current drug therapy for rhinitis can be very effective, but a significant proportion of rhinitis patients experience nose bleeds from intranasal steroids and drowsiness from antihistamines. Others find pharmacotherapy inconvenient or ineffective. Moreover, we are now more aware of the adverse effects of rhinitis on quality of life. SIT offers a useful option for these patients as well as a logical approach to dealing with the underlying problem.

SIT FOR ASTHMA

Immunotherapy was widely used to treat allergic asthma in the UK prior to 1986 but evidence of severe adverse reactions, including a small number of fatalities has led to SIT being abandoned for asthma treatment in the UK, although asthma remains a common indication for SIT in North America and continental Europe.[11,12]

Current drug therapies for asthma are aimed at suppressing the airways inflammation that is a characteristic feature of asthma. None of these treatments is curative and asthma recurs rapidly on cessation of treatment. Moreover, none of the current drug therapies is directed against agents that might cause asthma. Allergen avoidance has been proposed as a potentially useful maneuver in those with allergic asthma, but while extreme forms of allergen avoidance (e.g. admission to hospital, sending children to holiday homes at altitude), can improve the control of asthma, there is little evidence that such benefit can be achieved by the degree of allergen avoidance achievable in suburban homes. There is, therefore, scope for improving asthma care and for identifying allergen-specific therapies. SIT offers the possibility of deviating the immune response away from the allergic pattern and towards a more protective or less damaging response. However, SIT remains controversial as a treatment for asthma because of the potential side-effects.

Assessing effectiveness in asthma trials

The two main keys to success in designing any clinical trial are the application of appropriate criteria for subject recruitment and the selection of appropriate clinical endpoints (Table 113.2). When assessing improvement in asthma, it is important to remember that the majority of patients with atopic asthma have relatively mild disease that is usually easy to control with standard doses of conventional antiasthma drugs. Cases of severe disease are relatively few in number and the role of allergy in their disease is often less obvious than in mild cases. In mild cases, resting spirometry is often close to predicted values so there is little scope for improvement in simple spirometric measures such as FEV_1. Peak expiratory flow rates (PEFR) may show improvement, especially the early morning values, which are most likely to be reduced below the patient's best possible value. Objective measures of bronchial irritability are more useful markers and a

Endpoints for trials of specific immunotherapy in asthma	
Spirometry	airflow obstruction – FEV_1, PEFR bronchial irritability – histamine/methacholine PC_{20}
Symptoms	Wheeze, nocturnal waking, cough, breathlessness, time off work/school (diary cards or visual analog scales)
Drug use	Bronchodilator use as surrogate for symptoms
Cost–benefit	Reduction in other drugs, lost work, etc., compared to costs of SIT and time lost due to SIT
Safety	Standard toxicity tables
Immunology	Allergen-specific IgG_4 Skin test responses Nasal allergen challenge responses Inhalation allergen challenge responses

Table 113.2 Endpoints for trials of specific immunotherapy in asthma.

shift in the concentration of histamine or methacholine needed to induce a 20% fall in FEV_1 (PC_{20}) is commonly used. This measurement can be quite variable within individuals, so the minimum change that would be clinically significant is a change of at least one doubling dilution in the PC_{20}. Other bronchial challenge tests such as exercise challenge or adenosine inhalation may provide additional insights into the ability of an antiasthma treatment to prevent acute attacks. Both these parameters depend indirectly on the PC_{20} so again it is important to consider statistical and biological significance separately.

Although these challenge models are useful surrogates for evaluating antiasthma treatment, more credence is placed on improvements in the symptoms or progression of the disease than on protection against laboratory challenges. Lately there has been a move to assess efficacy in terms of improvements in quality of life or as health gain per unit cost. These analyses are relatively unsophisticated at present and require careful validation to ensure that the quality of life instrument is sensitive to the illness being studied and that the economic model is realistic.

Finally, many trials of SIT have studied laboratory surrogate markers of efficacy such as changes in IgG subclasses, in vivo challenges of the nose or skin test responses. While such measures undoubtedly do change during SIT, and may shed light on the mechanism of successful SIT, they cannot be used to provide direct evidence of clinical effectiveness in asthma.

Trials of SIT in asthma

The efficacy of SIT in adult asthma has been assessed in many trials over the last 50 years. The results of these studies have often been difficult to interpret, either because poor-quality allergen extracts were used or because of poor study design. Many trials were not placebo-controlled; they were either open or single-blind, and in most cases, only small numbers of patients were treated. A recently published meta-analysis identified 62 randomized controlled trials, reported in 67 papers published between 1954 and 1998. 28 of these were for mite allergy, 15 for pollen allergy, 9 for animal dander allergy, and 2 for mold allergy while the remainder used combinations of allergens, or extracts that have subsequently fallen out of favor.[12] A wide variety of different measurements were made, which makes it difficult to reach a formed view on the overall effectiveness of SIT. Symptom scores were reported in 22 trials and overall there was a small but definite improvement in those groups treated with mite SIT or pollen SIT, compared to the placebo-treated groups (Table 113.3). There was a parallel reduction in asthma medication usage but no improvement in lung function measurements. However, SIT did reduce the airways response to inhalation of specific allergen (Table 113.4).

Three double-blind placebo-controlled (DBPC) studies have found that SIT has a beneficial effect in patients with grass pollen asthma as assessed by a reduction in asthma symptom and treatment scores. Active treatment led to a 60–75% reduction in

Effect of SIT in asthma – meta-analysis of effect on symptom scores

Comparison: allergen immunotherapy vs placebo
Outcome: asthma symptom scores

Study	Weight %	SMD* (95% CI random)
Mite immunotherapy		
Armentia Medina, et al. *Allergol Immunopathol (Madr)* 1995;23:211	4.7	–2.083 [–2.942,–1.224]
Torres Costa, et al. *Allergy* 1996;51:238	4.7	–0.768 [–1.640,0.105]
Machiels, et al. *J Clin Invest* 1990;85:1024	5.2	–0.461 [–1.184,0.262]
Pichler, et al. *Allergy* 1997;52:274	5.2	–0.438 [–1.165,0.289]
Franco, et al. *Allergol Immunopathol (Madr)* 1995;23:58	5.7	0.000 [–0.560,0.560]
Subtotal (95% CI) Chi-square 16.30 (df=4) Z=2.09	25.5	–0.709 [–1.373,–0.045]
Other immunotherapy		
Alvarez Cuesta, et al. *J Allergy Clin Immunol* 1994;93:556	4.3	–2.271 [–3.251,–1.291]
Varney, et al. *Clin Exp Allergy* 1997;27:860	4.8	–1.286 [–2.113,–0.459]
Valovirta, et al. *Ann Allergy* 1984;53:85 and 1986;57:173	5.0	–0.246 [–1.008,0.517]
Adkinson, et al. *N Engl J Med* 1997;336–324–331	6.3	0.260 [–0.098,0.618]
Subtotal (95%CI) Chi-square 30.12 (df=3) Z=1.4	20.5	–0.828 [–1.921,0.264]

*Standardized mean difference (SMD) ≤ 0 (favors immunotherapy); SMD ≥ 0 (favors placebo)

Table 113.3 Effect of SIT in asthma – meta-analysis of effect on symptom scores. (Adapted from Abramson M, Puy R, Weiner J. Immunotherapy in asthma: an updated systematic review. *Allergy* 1999;54:1022, with permission.)

Effect of SIT in asthma – meta-analysis on specific airway responses to allergen

Comparison: allergen immunotherapy vs placebo
Outcome: allergen-specific BHR indices

Study	Weight %	SMD* (95% CI random)
Log PD_{20} mite		
Machiels, et al. *J Clin Invest* 1990;85:1024–1035	4.3	–1.429 [–2.473,–0.385]
Bousquet J, et al. *J Allergy Clin Immunol* 1985;76:734–744	6.9	–1.146 [–1.967,–0.326]
Van Bever and Stevens. *Eur Respir J* 1992;5:318–322.	4.6	–1.071 [–2.077,–0.066]
Newton, et al. *Br J Dis Chest* 1978;72:21–28	3.7	–0.862 [–1.975,0.252]
Subtotal (95% CI)	19.5	–1.136 [–1.624,–0.648]
Chi-square 10.55 (df=3) Z=4.56		
Log PD_{20} animal dander		
Alvarez Cuesta, et al. *J Allergy Clin Immunol* 1994;93:556–566	4.6	–1.080 [–2.088,–0.071]
Varney, et al. *Clin Exp Allergy* 1997;27:860–867	7.7	–0.793 [–1.569,–0.017]
Van Metre, et al. *J Allergy Clin Immunol* 1988;82:1055–1068	5.8	–0.737 [–1.628,0.155]
Sundin, et al. *J Allergy Clin Immunol* 1986;77:478–487	10.1	–0.674 [–1.350,0.002]
Ohman, et al. *J Allergy Clin Immunol* 1984;74:230–239	5.0	–0.295 [–1.254,0.664]
Subtotal (95% CI)	33.3	–0.711 [–1.084,–0.337]
Chi-square 1.29 (df=4) Z=3.73		
Total (95% CI)		
Chi-square 12.63 (df=12) Z=6.33	100.0	–0.695 [–0.911,–0.480]

*Standardized mean difference (SMD) ≤ 0 (favors immunotherapy); SMD ≥ 0 (favors placebo)

Table 113.4 Effect of SIT in asthma – meta-analysis on specific airway responses to allergen. (Adapted from Abramson M, Puy R, Weiner J. Immunotherapy in asthma: an updated systematic review. *Allergy* 1999;54: 1022–1041, with permission.)

symptom scores as compared to placebo-treated patients. An important recent study of SIT for ragweed allergy found that patients who received active injections had an improvement in peak flow rates during the pollen season as well as reduced hay fever symptoms and reduced sensitivity to laboratory challenge with ragweed pollen extracts.[13] In addition, the active group required much less anti-asthma medication. However, the economic analysis indicated that the cost-saving in asthma drugs was less than the costs of SIT (Fig. 113.3).

In asthmatic patients sensitive to cats, SIT with standardized aqueous extracts reduces the early asthmatic response to inhaled allergen and attenuates responses to cat room exposure.

Cost-benefit analysis of SIT in asthma

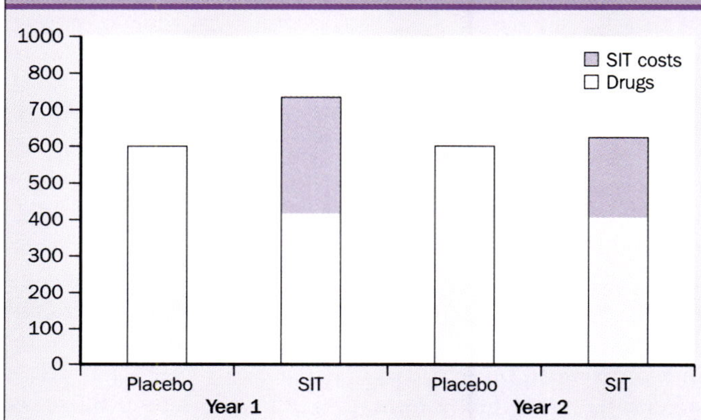

Figure 113.3 Cost–benefit analysis of SIT in asthma. No total cost savings were achieved in patients given SIT and asthma drugs. (Adapted from Creticos PS, Reed CE, Norman PS, et al. Ragweed immunotherapy in adult asthma. *N Engl J Med* 1996;334:501, with permission.)

Interestingly these studies showed a clear delay in onset of symptoms and an overall reduction in symptoms and peak flow recordings after exposure to cats in a 'cat room', but there was no protection against allergen-induced increases in nonspecific bronchial hyperresponsiveness. Another study of cat IT for asthma used a depot preparation and found a reduction in both specific and nonspecific bronchial reactivity (to cat extract and histamine respectively).[14] In contrast, SIT with a dog dander extract was unsuccessful.

Several DBPC studies have examined the effects of SIT in asthmatic patients sensitive to house dust mite. The initial series of studies dates from 1975 to 1985 and used tyrosine-adsorbed or depot preparations. In some respects these studies produced conflicting results. A total of 118 subjects received active treatment in 6 well designed studies. Two of these were in asthmatic children aged 5–15 years (total 40 children). In this age band, substantial reductions in drug requirements were reported, but no such improvement in asthma control was found in the four adult studies (total 78 subjects aged 15–68 years). Subsequent studies using more modern extracts have found beneficial effects on symptoms, antiasthma drug use, and bronchial hyperresponsiveness.[12]

Comparison of SIT with other types of treatment for asthma

The majority of clinical trials of SIT for asthma have compared SIT either with historical controls or with a matched placebo-treated group. To date, the effectiveness of specific SIT in asthma has rarely been compared with conventional management (with avoidance measures and conventional inhaled or oral drugs). One recent study assessed SIT in asthmatic children receiving conventional drug therapy and found no additional benefit in patients who were already receiving optimal drug therapy.[15] There are some significant criticisms of this study and further work of this type is urgently needed. It is also important that trials include analysis of cost–benefit and cost-effectiveness since purchasers of health care are increasingly demanding this evidence before agreeing to fund therapies.

Effects on natural history of allergic disease

A proportion of patients with allergic rhinitis go on to develop asthma each year. It has been suggested that SIT may modify the natural history of asthma in children who are known to be atopic but have not yet developed asthma. This annual rate of progression has been estimated at 5% in college students[16] but this is, perhaps surprisingly, an area of considerable ignorance. A number of long term epidemiological studies are now in progress, under the auspices of the ISAAC programe and should soon shed light on the rate of progression at different ages and the extent of regional and international variation. Only limited data are available to support the proposition that SIT may alter the natural rate of progression. An early open study using uncharacterized mixed allergen extracts supported this view, but among other problems, this study failed to allow for the spontaneous improvement that often occurs in asthmatic patients.[17] New evidence is now emerging to indicate that SIT can modify the natural history of allergic disease through childhood and into adult life.[18] If this is confirmed, it will have a major bearing on the economic and clinical arguments surrounding SIT and asthma. There is as yet no evidence to support claims that SIT is different from drug therapy in terms of influencing the evolution of established asthma. Studies that have investigated withdrawal of therapy have found rapid recurrence of asthma symptoms although rhinitis symptoms seem to show much more sustained relief after SIT.

In summary, SIT is a controversial type of treatment for asthma. While it seems entirely logical to try to treat allergic disorders by specifically suppressing the immune response to the triggering agents, the critical issue is whether SIT in its present form is the best option for managing patients with asthma. To assess this requires proper comparisons of best current SIT versus best current drug therapy, with robust endpoints including symptoms, objective measures of lung function, evaluation of cost–benefit ratios, safety, and quality of life. In vitro and in vivo measures such as skin test responses or allergen-specific IgG_4 measurements are not sufficiently specific or sensitive to serve as surrogates for clinical efficacy. To date there have been relatively few well controlled studies of SIT in asthma, but there is increasing evidence that SIT is beneficial in mite-induced and pollen-induced asthma. The clinical efficacy of SIT in adult asthmatic patients sensitive to cats or molds is less certain, and no comparative studies with conventional treatment have been performed. Further clinical trials are indicated, particularly in mild to moderate childhood asthma and also in patients with atopic disease who have not yet developed asthma but are at high risk of progression to asthma.

SAFETY

The main factor cited against the widespread adoption of SIT for asthma is the risk of serious adverse reactions. In the UK, between 1957 and 1986, 26 fatal reactions due to SIT were reported to the Committee on Safety of Medicines.[19] In 17 of the fatal cases, the indication for SIT was documented: 16 of these 17 patients were receiving SIT to treat asthma. Similarly, in the American Academy of Allergy, Asthma and Immunology confidential inquiry into SIT-associated deaths, asthma appeared to be in virtually all the fatal cases.[20] In those where asthma was not cited as a contributory factor, documentation of asthma status was missing, and certainly bronchospasm was a cardinal feature of the clinical course of the anaphylactic reactions. The incidence of systemic reactions in patients receiving SIT for asthma varies between series and has been reported to range from 5% to 35%. The central issue in using safety as an endpoint is to recognize that all treatments carry risks. Where differential risks exist between therapies, a more risky therapy can only be justified if that therapy offers substantial additional benefit over the safer therapy. The science of assessing risk–benefit ratios is still in its infancy and we have to recognize that even when faced with the same facts, different patients and agencies can come to widely varying risk assessments.

Separately, it is generally agreed that immunomodulatory treatments should not be used in patients with autoimmune disorders or malignant disease. While there is no hard evidence that SIT is actually harmful in these groups, it seems unwise to attempt manipulation of the immune system in such patients, not least because of the risk that spontaneous and unrelated variations in the autoimmune disorder or cancer may be blamed on SIT. Other medical contraindications to SIT include the coexistence of significant cardiac disease which may be exacerbated by any adverse reactions to SIT. Patients on β-blockers should also not receive SIT. Although they are not at increased risk of adverse reactions, they will not respond to the epinephrine which would be needed to treat adverse reactions to SIT.

ALTERNATIVE FORMS OF IMMUNOTHERAPY

Allergic disorders have attracted more than their fair share of attention from alternative medical practitioners. Alternative allergy practice covers three principal themes: the use of unconventional diagnostic tests to seek causative agents for diseases that are clearly allergic in origin; the use of unconventional therapies to treat allergic disease; and the diagnosis and therapy of diseases that are not conventionally considered to involve allergic mechanisms.

Unconventional forms of immunotherapy include the use of topical immunotherapy, enzyme-potentiated desensitization and homeopathic desensitization.

Topical immunotherapy

High-dose topical immunotherapy regimens were used in the first half of the twentieth century, but then lost ground to injection immunotherapy in conventional medical practice. Sublingual immunotherapy (SLIT) is based on the concept that allergens given via the mucosal surface are handled differently from allergens given by injection, leading to a form of immunological tolerance. It has been shown in animal models that IgE responses to allergens can be reduced or prevented by oral administration of allergen. The precise mechanisms by which this 'oral tolerance' is induced remain unclear, but it seems likely that the route of allergen processing and presentation is a critical determinant of the subsequent T-cell response. In mice, locally administered allergen is taken up by mucosal dendritic cells and then presented to T cells together with IL-12, biasing the response towards a Th1 profile and away from the pro-IgE Th2 profile. It is less clear whether this mechanism can suppress established allergic responses. In contrast to animal models, the immunological response to SLIT in human studies has been relatively modest. Some changes have been found in skin sensitivity but most studies have not found any change in systemic parameters such as specific IgE, specific IgG or T-cell cytokine balance.

The 1998, a European Academy of Allergology and Clinical Immunology position paper[21] identified 31 studies of local immunotherapy, of which 14 used nasal immunotherapy, 2 gave the allergen direct into the airways, 9 used the oral route and 6 the sublingual route. Most of these studies were quite small, and various different methodologies had been used, but by careful meta-analysis, some conclusions could be drawn. First, it was apparent that nasal immunotherapy was effective, with a benefit found in 13 out of 14 studies. The benefit appeared to be sustained only while the therapy was continued: after 2 years of successful therapy, the level of symptoms in the subsequent season was similar to that in untreated patients. Local side-effects were common, and it is arguable that nasal immunotherapy might be working by causing repeated degranulation of local mast cells, and subsequent local tolerance of allergic inflammation, rather than through a true immunological effect. Oral immunotherapy seemed to be ineffective, with 7 of 9 eligible studies showing no benefit. Only 6 eligible studies of SLIT were identified, 4 in adults and 2 in children. A total of 117 patients received active therapy in these studies. All of these found a benefit for active therapy. All 6 of these studies used the sublingual–swallow method, i.e. the extract was placed under the tongue, held there for a period of minutes, and then swallowed. Systemic side-effects were relatively rare, and none of the side-effects were judged to be life-threatening. A significant reduction in skin test reactivity was found in one study but there were no measurable changes in bronchial responsiveness to allergen or to methacholine. The EAACI position paper concluded that sublingual immunotherapy has been shown to be efficacious in patients with rhinitis, but insufficient information was available to draw any conclusions for its use in asthma. Since 1998, a number of further studies have been published that have added to the evidence base, but it is still too early to recommend SLIT as a viable alternative to conventional injection SIT.

Enzyme-potentiated desensitization (EPD)

EPD uses very small doses of allergens, given together with the enzyme β-glucuronidase. The allergen doses are approximately 0.1% of the doses used in conventional SIT, and side-effects are apparently not encountered. The theory behind EPD is that the β-glucuronidase enables the allergen to gain access to the immune system more efficiently than is possible with conventional SIT. No convincing evidence to support the efficacy of EPD has been forthcoming.

Homeopathic desensitization

A detailed discussion of the principles underlying homeopathy lies outside the scope of this chapter. However, homeopathy espouses the concept that diseases may be treated by very small doses of substances that cause similar symptoms. Some homeopathic remedies are mimics of the disorder, while others use the actual material that triggers the disorder. Thus, homeopathic remedies for hay fever bear some superficial similarity to SIT,[22] although the scientific validity of homeopathic treatment generally is very dubious.

FUTURE DIRECTIONS

Developments in molecular biology should lead to improvements in conventional SIT (Table 113.5). Possible avenues include the use of recombinant allergens, which would allow much better standardization of allergen vaccines, as well as some fine tuning of vaccines for patients with unusual patterns of reactivity. Most allergic patients react to the same components of an allergen extract, the so-called 'major allergens', which are defined as those allergens recognized by over 50% of sera from a pool of patients with clinically significant allergy to the material in question. However, not all patients recognize all major allergens and some patients only recognize allergens that are not recognized by the majority of allergic patient sera. This latter group may not respond to standard extracts, but might be better treated by a combination of allergens to which they are sensitive. Until the advent of molecular cloning, this was impossible to achieve. The availability of recombinant allergens for SIT should thus lead to better characterization of the range of sensitivities, and ultimately to better vaccine products.

Since the epitopes recognized by IgE molecules are usually three dimensional whereas the epitopes recognized by T cells are short linear peptide fragments of the antigen, it should be possible to use peptide fragments of allergens to modulate T cells without risking anaphylaxis. Two distinct approaches have been tested. Either large doses of natural sequence peptides are given, deceiving the T-cell into high dose tolerance,[23] or else an altered peptide ligand can be given. Both approaches require consideration of the MHC type of the individual undergoing treatment. By sequential alteration of Der p peptides, it is possible to suppress proliferation of T-cell clones recognizing native Der p peptides, as well as suppressing their expression of CD40 ligand and their production of IL-4, IL-5 and IFN-γ. These anergic T cells do not provide help for B cells class switching to IgE, and importantly this anergy cannot be reversed by providing exogenous IL-4.[24]

From epidemiological and experimental studies, we know that vaccination with mycobacteria has antiallergic properties. In Japan, early vaccination with BCG was associated with a substantial reduction in the risk of developing allergy[25] although similar associations were not evident in Sweden.[26] In the laboratory, it has been shown that administration of BCG before or during sensitization to ovalbumin reduces the degree of airway eosinophilia that follows subsequent challenge with ovalbumin (Fig. 113.4). This effect is not mediated through any direct effect on IgE production, or blood eosinophil numbers, but is mediated through IFN-γ and can be reversed by exogenous IL-5 (Fig. 113.5).[27]

Possible new technologies for immunotherapy
Recombinant allergens
T-cell peptide vaccines
Th1 immunostimulants (e.g. mycobacteria, CpG)
Allergen-immunostimulant complexes
Anti-IgE

Table 113.5 Possible new technologies for immunotherapy.

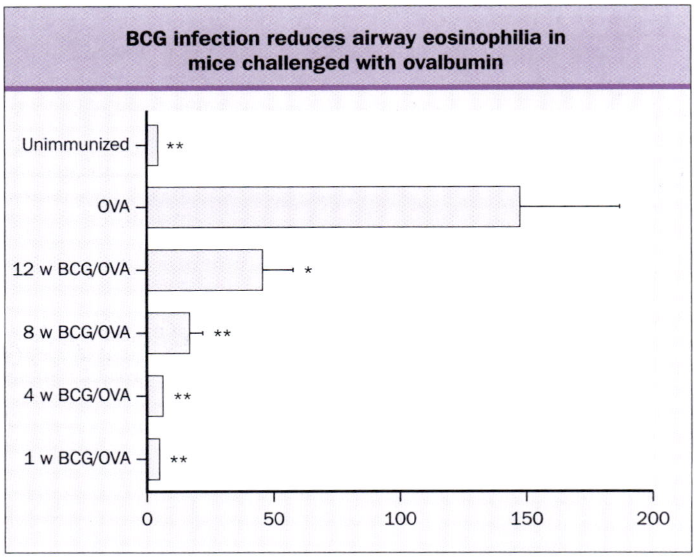

Figure 113.4 Effect of BCG on animal model of allergic sensitization. The inhibition of airway eosinophilia reduced by ovalbumin (OVA) is dependent upon the time in weeks (w) between infection by BCG abd challenge. (From Erb KJ, Holloway JW, Sobeck A, Moll H, Le Gros G. Infection of mice with Mycobacterium bovis–Bacillus Calmette-Guerin (BCG) suppresses allergen-induced airway eosinophilia. *J Exp Med* 1998;187:561, with permission.)

Two new approaches using DNA vaccines are also undergoing serious consideration. The first of these is a general approach, using CpG oligodeoxynucleotides (ODN). This technology is essentially a refinement of vaccination adjuvant technology, since CpG ODN have been shown to be the principal activity in complete Freund's adjuvant. Pre-administration of CpG ODN prevented both airways eosinophilia and bronchial hyperresponsiveness in a mouse model of asthma.[28] Moreover, these effects were sustained for at least 6 weeks after CpG ODN administration.[29] Experiments are also being conducted with CpG ODN coupled to ragweed allergen, which enhances immunogenicity in terms of eliciting a Th1-type response to the ragweed allergen, but reduces its allergenicity.[30] Antisense DNA vaccines could also be used to down-regulate airway adenosine receptors. In animal models of asthma this leads to a reduction in allergen-induced airway responses.[31] A contrasting approach is to use allergen-specific naked DNA sequences as vaccines. This technology is still in its infancy, but preliminary data suggest that giving naked DNA leads to production of allergens from within the airways epithelial cells.[32,33] Due to the different handling pathways for endogenous and exogenous allergens, it seems that the endogenously produced allergen elicits a Th1-type response and, if this can be reproduced in allergic humans, it is hoped that this may overcome the existing Th2-pattern response and eliminate the allergy. However, the potential for generating a powerful Th1-type response to ubiquitous agents means that this approach will need careful evaluation in animal models before it can be pursued in man.

Another approach that has reached clinical trials is to use a monoclonal antibody directed against IgE. By raising antibodies against the portion of IgE which is recognized by the high-affinity Fc_{ε} receptor, it is possible to derive anti-IgE antibodies that bind free IgE molecules but do not cross-link IgE bound to the mast cell or basophil surface. Treatment with humanized monoclonal anti-IgE antibodies is extremely effective in reducing the serum concentration of free IgE, although the IgE seems to remain in the circulation in the form of immune complexes. Treatment with anti-IgE reduces immediate and late-phase responses to inhaled allergen.[34,35] When given over a 12 week period to patients with steroid-dependent asthma, it was possible to achieve substantial reductions in the dosage of oral and inhaled steroids (Fig. 113.6).[36] Anti-IgE should also work in patients with milder asthma, who are generally more likely to be atopic. However, the costs and inconvenience of anti-IgE may preclude its use in patients with milder disease. On the other hand, anti-IgE has the advantage over SIT of being a general therapy, and may work in patients with multiple allergic sensitization who are more difficult to treat with conventional SIT. Further work is needed to define the groups of patients who will benefit most from this approach.

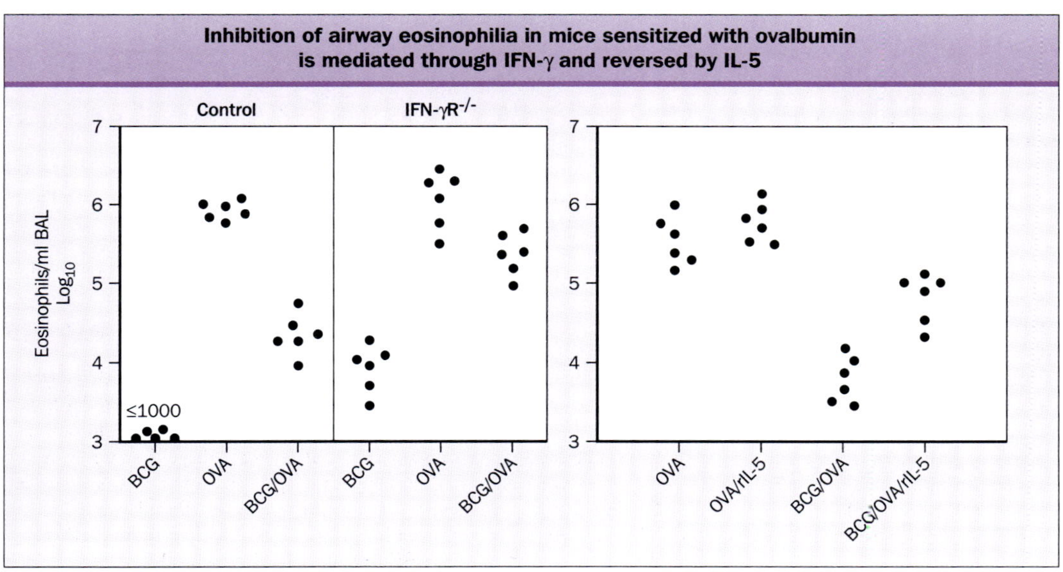

Figure 113.5 Effect of BCG mediated through IFN-γ and reversed by IL-5 etc. in animal model of allergic sensitization. Left panels: BCG reduces the airway eosinophilia in mice, but IFN-γ knockout mice (R–/–) do not demonstrate the BCG effect as clearly. Right panel: administration at IL-5 reverses the BCG-induced IFN-γ effect (From Erb KJ, Holloway JW, Sobeck A, Moll H, Le Gros G. Infection of mice with ycobacterium bovis–Bacillus Calmette-Guerin (BCG) suppresses allergen-induced airway eosinophilia. *J Exp Med* 1998;187:561, with permission.)

Anti-IgE monoclonal antibody treatment reduces the need for steroids in asthmatic patients

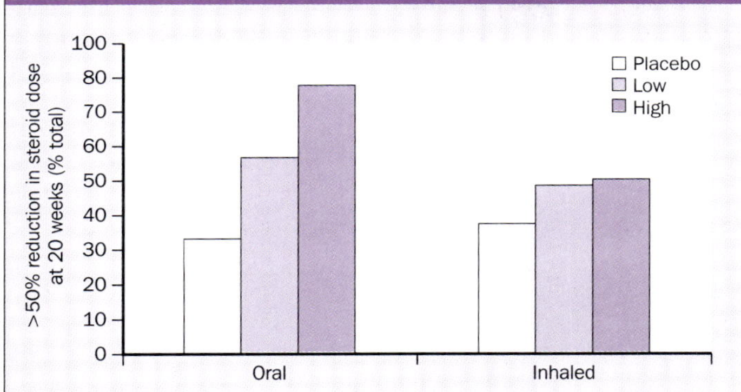

Figure 113.6 Effect of anti-IgE on steroid requirement. (Adapted from Milgrom H, Fick RB Jr, Su JQ, Reimann JD, Bush RK, Watrous ML, Metzger WJ. Treatment of allergic asthma with monoclonal anti-IgE antibody. rhuMAb-E25 Study Group. *N Engl J Med* 1999;341:1966, with permission.)

CONCLUSIONS

Despite a century of use, the precise mechanisms of action of SIT remain uncertain. SIT is established as a treatment for allergic rhinitis and for venom hypersensitivity, but is more controversial when used to treat allergic asthma. When used in appropriately selected patients, SIT is effective and acceptably safe, but care is needed to recognize and treat adverse reactions. Appropriate training of allergists and SIT clinic support staff is essential. Future directions in SIT include the development of better standardized vaccines, and the use of recombinant allergens, both of which should improve the safety profile of SIT. In parallel, the development of more general immunomodulatory therapies may allow a more general approach to be taken, which would be particularly advantageous for those patients with sensitization to multiple allergens.

THERAPEUTIC PRINCIPLES

Use of SIT in patients with suspected allergy

- Disease must be allergic in nature.
- Objective IgE-mediated positive tests:
  - skin tests
  - in vitro tests in certain cases.
- The risk of serious reactions or a poor quality of life must be sufficiently impaired:
  - conventional medications do not work
  - antihistamines create daytime drowsiness
  - avoidance of allergen is not possible.
- Systemic reactions to SIT itself are held to a minimum:
  - correct build-up doses are given
  - direct medical observation after injections
  - patient adherence to schedule is essential.
- Complete relief of symptoms is not possible.
- Length of treatment with SIT:
  - 3–5 years and re-evaluate patient.

REFERENCES

1. Freeman J. Vaccination against hay fever: report of results during the first three years. Lancet 1914;1:1178.
2. Creticos PS, Van Metre TE, Mardiney MR, Rosenberg GL, Norman PS, Adkinson NF Jr. Dose response of IgE and IgG antibodies during ragweed immunotherapy. J Allergy Clin Immunol 1984;73:94.
3. Iliopoulos O, Proud D, Adkinson NF Jr, et al. Effects of immunotherapy on the early, late, and rechallenge nasal reaction to provocation with allergen: changes in inflammatory mediators and cells. J Allergy Clin Immunol 1991;87:855.
4. Durham SR, Ying S, Varney VA, et al. Grass pollen immunotherapy inhibits allergen-induced infiltration of CD4+ T lymphocytes and eosinophils in the nasal mucosa and increases the number of cells expressing messenger RNA for interferon-gamma. J Allergy Clin Immunol 1996;97:1356.
5. McHugh SM, Deighton J, Stewart AG, Lachmann PJ, Ewan PW. Bee venom immunotherapy induces a shift in cytokine responses from a TH-2 to a TH-1 dominant pattern: comparison of rush and conventional immunotherapy. Clin Exp Allergy 1995;25:828.
6. Ebner C, Siemann U, Bohle B, et al. Immunological changes during specific immunotherapy of grass pollen allergy: reduced lymphoproliferative responses to allergen and shift from TH2 to TH1 in T-cell clones specific for Phl p 1, a major grass pollen allergen. Clin Exp Allergy 1997;27:1007.
7. Golden DBK, Marsh DG, Freidhoff LR, Kwiterovich KA, Addison B, Kagey-Sobotka A, Lichtenstein LM. Natural history of Hymenoptera venom sensitivity in adults. J Allergy Clin Immunol 1997;100:760.
8. Varney VA, Gaga M, Frew AJ, Aber VR, Kay AB, Durham SR. Usefulness of immunotherapy in patients with severe summer hay fever uncontrolled by antiallergic drugs. BMJ 1991;302:265.
9. Durham SR, Walker SM, Varga EM, et al. Long-term clinical efficacy of grass-pollen immunotherapy. N Engl J Med 1999;341:468.
10. Varney VA, Edwards J, Tabbah K, Brewster H, Mavroleon G, Frew AJ. Clinical efficacy of specific immunotherapy to cat dander: a double-blind placebo-controlled trial. Clin Exp Allergy 1997;27:860.
11. Bousquet J, Lockey R, Malling HJ, et al. Allergen immunotherapy: therapeutic vaccines for allergic diseases. World Health Organization. American Academy of Allergy, Asthma and Immunology. Ann Allergy Asthma Immunol 1998;81:401.
12. Abramson M, Puy R, Weiner J. Immunotherapy in asthma: an updated systematic review. Allergy 1999;54:1022.
13. Creticos PS, Reed CE, Norman PS, et al. Ragweed immunotherapy in adult asthma. N Engl J Med 1996;334:501.
14. Lilja G, Sundin B, Graff-Lonnevig V, et al. Immunotherapy with cat- and dog-dander extracts. IV. Effects of 2 years of treatment. J Allergy Clin Immunol 1989;83:37.
15. Adkinson NF Jr, Eggleston PA, Eney D, et al. A controlled trial of immunotherapy for asthma in allergic children. N Engl J Med 1997;336:324.
16. Horak F. Manifestation of allergic rhinitis in latent-sensitized patients. A prospective study. Arch Otorhinolaryngol 1985;242:239.
17. Johnstone DE, Dutton A. The value of hyposensitization therapy for bronchial asthma in children-a 14-year study. Pediatrics 1968;42:793.
18. Des Roches A, Paradis L, Menardo JL, Bouges S, Daures JP, Bousquet J. Immunotherapy with a standardized Dermatophagoides pteronyssinus extract. VI. Specific immunotherapy prevents the onset of new sensitizations in children. J Allergy Clin Immunol 1997;99:450.
19. Committee on the Safety of Medicines. CSM update: immunotherapy. Br Med J 1986; 293:948.

20. Stewart GE 2d, Lockey RF. Systemic reactions from allergen immunotherapy. J Allergy Clin Immunol 1992;90:567.
21. Malling HJ, Abreu-Nogueira J, Alvarez-Cuesta E, et al. Local immunotherapy. Allergy 1998;53:933.
22. Reilly DT, Taylor MA, McSharry C, Aitchison T. Is homoeopathy a placebo response? Controlled trial of homoeopathic potency, with pollen in hayfever as model. Lancet 1986;2:881.
23. O'Hehir RE, Yssel H, Verma S, de Vries JE, Spits H, Lamb JR. Clonal analysis of differential lymphokine production in peptide and superantigen induced T cell anergy. Int Immunol 1991;3:819.
24. Fasler S, Aversa G, de Vries JE, Yssel H. Antagonistic peptides specifically inhibit proliferation, cytokine production, CD40L expression, and help for IgE synthesis by Der p 1-specific human T-cell clones. J Allergy Clin Immunol 1998;101:521.
25. Shirakawa T, Enomoto T, Shimazu S, Hopkin JM. The inverse association between tuberculin responses and atopic disorder. Science 1997;275:77.
26. Strannegard IL, Larsson LO, Wennergren G, Strannegård O. Prevalence of allergy in children in relation to prior BCG vaccination and infection with atypical mycobacteria. Allergy 1998;53:249.
27. Erb KJ, Holloway JW, Sobeck A, Moll H, Le Gros G. Infection of mice with *Mycobacterium bovis*–Bacillus Calmette-Guerin (BCG) suppresses allergen-induced airway eosinophilia. J Exp Med 1998;187:561.
28. Kline JN, Waldschmidt TJ, Businga TR, Lemish JE, Weinstock JV, Thorne PS, Krieg AM. Modulation of airway inflammation by CpG oligodeoxynucleotides in a murine model of asthma. J Immunol 1998;160:2555.
29. Sur S, Wild JS, Choudhury BK, Sur N, Alam R, Klinman DM. Long term prevention of allergic lung inflammation in a mouse model of asthma by CpG oligodeoxynucleotides. J Immunol 1999;162:6284.
30. Tighe H, Takabayashi K, Schwartz D, et al. Conjugation of immunostimulatory DNA to the short ragweed allergen amb a 1 enhances its immunogenicity and reduces its allergenicity. J Allergy Clin Immunol 2000;106:124.
31. Metzger WJ, Nyce JW. Oligonucleotide therapy of allergic asthma. J Allergy Clin Immunol 1999;104:260.
32. Hsu CH, Chua KY, Tao MH, Lai YL, Wu HD, Huang SK, Hsieh KH. Immunoprophylaxis of allergen-induced immunoglobulin E synthesis and airway hyperresponsiveness in vivo by genetic immunization. Nat Med 1996;2:540.
33. Hartl A, Kiesslich J, Weiss R, et al. Immune responses after immunization with plasmid DNA encoding Bet v 1, the major allergen of birch pollen. J Allergy Clin Immunol 1999;103:107.
34. Boulet LP, Chapman KR, Côté J, et al. Inhibitory effects of an anti-IgE antibody E25 on allergen-induced early asthmatic response. Am J Respir Crit Care Med 1997;155:1835.
35. Fahy JV, Fleming HE, Wong HH, et al. The effect of an anti-IgE monoclonal antibody on the early- and late-phase responses to allergen inhalation in asthmatic subjects. Am J Respir Crit Care Med 1997;155:1828.
36. Milgrom H, Fick RB Jr, Su JQ, Reimann JD, Bush RK, Watrous ML, Metzger WJ. Treatment of allergic asthma with monoclonal anti-IgE antibody. rhuMAb-E25 Study Group. N Engl J Med 1999;341:1966.

Chapter 114 Colony-stimulating Factors

Malcolm A.S. Moore

The hematopoietic system is regulated by a complex interplay of hematopoietic growth factors with pleiotropic and frequently overlapping activities that orchestrate steady-state as well as acute responses involving specific cell lineages. For historical reasons, hematopoietic growth factors have been named after the lineage they regulate (e.g. erythropoietin), after their cellular origins (e.g. interleukins), or after assays that permitted their detection (e.g. colony-stimulating factor). Colony stimulating factors (CSFs) regulate the daily production of $>10^{11}$ granulocytes and monocytes and are able to increase production upon demand by up to 30-fold within a few days. CSFs were first identified as factors capable of stimulating hematopoietic colony formation in semisolid culture assays. Three species are identified by the pattern of clonogenic differentiation induced: granulocyte CSF (G-CSF), stimulating exclusively neutrophil differentiation; macrophage CSF (M-CSF or CSF-1), stimulating monocyte/macrophage differentiation; and oligostimulatory granulocyte/macrophage CSF (GM-CSF), inducing colonies of variable mixtures of neutrophils, eosinophils, and macrophages. Interleukin-3, also named multi-CSF, shares some functional similarity with GM-CSF including signaling through a shared receptor. G- and GM-CSF have found extensive clinical applications, and this chapter focuses on these factors.

CHARACTERISTICS OF G-CSF AND GM-CSF AND THEIR RECEPTORS

Granulocyte CSF

The purification and molecular cloning of G-CSF was accomplished between 1984 and 1986[1,2] and clinical development commenced in 1986, with approval for clinical use in cancer patients treated with chemotherapy. Human G-CSF is an O-glycosylated protein of 19.6 kDa consisting of four antiparallel α helices arranged to form a helical bundle.[3,4] It is biologically active in picomolar concentrations (Table 114.1). Isolation of cDNA clones containing the full coding sequences of the mature protein revealed two molecules of 174 and 178 amino acids, derived by alternative splicing. Recombinant *E. coli*-derived human G-CSF, lacking glycosylation and with an additional amino-terminal methionine, has the generic name filgrastim and the trade name Neupogen® in North America and Europe. Endogenous levels of circulating G-CSF in normal individuals are generally below levels of detection by immunoassay (<30 pg/ml), but during infectious episodes or following cytotoxic chemotherapy or marrow transplantation serum levels rise, tending to peak just before recovery from the neutrophil nadir.

Both transcriptional activation and post-transcriptional mechanisms are important in regulating G-CSF gene expression. G-CSF is constitutively transcribed by a variety of cell types, including fibroblasts, endothelial cells, and macrophages. G-CSF mRNA has a half-life of less than 15 minutes, and on induction by lipopolysaccharide (LPS) or cytokines such as IL-1 or tumor necrosis factor (TNF), the half-life of mRNA increases transiently, with a gradual diminution of gene expression within 8–12 hours of the peak.[3,4] The G-CSF receptor (G-CSF-R) is encoded by a single gene on chromosome 1p32–p34[5] (Table 114.2). High-affinity (K_D of 900 pmol/l) receptors are expressed on mature neutrophils (500–3000 per cell), as well as on myeloblasts, promyelocytes, myeloid progenitors, and pluripotent stem cells. G-CSF-Rs are rapidly down-modulated upon G-CSF binding and are also rapidly 'trans-down-modulated' at 37°C on exposure of the cells to GM-CSF, TNF, LPS, and the chemotactic peptide f-Met-Leu-Phe ($t_{1/2}$ 15 min).[3,4] The human G-CSFR cDNA encodes integral membrane proteins, 759 and 812 amino acids in length, with identical extracellular and membrane-spanning sequences[5] (Table 114.2). Different COOH termini of 34 and 87 residues arise by alternative splicing. Human neutrophils express predominantly transcripts of the long form, whereas the shorter

Table 114.1 Molecular characteristics of human CSFs[a].

Molecular characteristics of CSFs					
CSF mass	**Molecular (kDa)[b]**	**Amino acid length**	**Carbohydrate[c]**	**No. of exons**	**Chromosome**
G-CSF	19.6	174/177	10	5	17q21–22
M-CSF	44/86	224/554	2–4N+0	10	1p13–21
GM-CSF	14–32	124/127	2N	4	5q21–22

[a]Distinguishes alternatively spliced forms.
[b]Mature post-translationally processed polypeptides.
[c]Carbohydrate chains linked to asparagine; N or O indicates carbohydrate linkage points.

Table 114.2 Molecular characteristics of the human CSF receptors[a].

Molecular characteristics of CSF receptors

Receptor	Affinity (K_D nM)	No. per cell × 10^3	Molecular mass (kDa)[b]	Amino acid length	Chromosome
G-CSF-R	0–1	0.05–1.5	130/150	795/812	1p35–34.3
M-CSF-R	0.0002	2–120	150	953	5q33.3
GM-CSF α chain	0.9–2.0	0.3–2.4	80–100	400/410	X-Y
GM-CSF β chain	—	?	100–135	881	22q31
GM-CSF αβ chain	0.01–0.1	<10			

[a]Distinguishes alternatively spliced forms.
[b]Mature post-translationally processed polypeptides.

form is specifically expressed in nonhematopoietic cells such as placenta. The alternative cytoplasmic domains may confer functional differences, and it has been proposed that the smaller form functions in ligand transport or sequestration in placental tissue. Alternatively, the two isoforms may differ in signal transduction properties, because the long form of the receptor contains one potential C kinase phosphorylation site. The extracellular region of the G-CSF-R is composed of four distinct types of structural domains. Two domains are identified by the presence of highly conserved cystine residues and a WSXWS (Trp-Ser-X-Trp-Ser) motif within a less well-conserved 100-amino acid stretch that characterizes a hematopoietic receptor superfamily.[3] This family also includes the erythropoietin-R, IL-7R, IL-9R, IL-2Rα, IL-2Rβ, IL-5R, GM-CSF-R, IL-3Rα, IL-3Rβ, IL-6R, oncostatin M-R, leukemia inhibitory factor-R (LIF-R), and the signal-transducing transmembrane glycoprotein gp130.[6] The receptor also incorporates one NH_2-terminal immunoglobulin-like domain characteristic of the Ig superfamily of receptors. Three additional repeats of fibronectin type III domains are also present and are found in LIF-R, gp130, and the α chains of IL-3, IL-5, and GM-CSF-R. Two G-CSF-R domains make direct contact with one G-CSF molecule, leading to dimerization and signal transduction.

The primary action of G-CSF is on cells of the neutrophil lineage, including myeloid progenitors (colony-forming units, CFU-GM) and on morphologically identifiable myeloid precursors.[3] G-CSF gene knockout (–/–) mice have overtly normal postnatal development, but have a 70–90% reduction in neutrophils, a reduction in CFU-GM, and a reduced capacity to mobilize neutrophils on challenge with infectious agents.[7] G-GSF has no direct proliferative action on primitive progenitors, for example CD34⁺ lineage-negative (Lin⁻) cells, although it will stimulate more committed CD34⁺ and CD33⁺ cells.[8] Human CD34⁺ Lin⁻ cells also proliferate and generate committed progenitors in the presence of c-kit ligand (KL) + IL-3, and a six-factor combination of KL + IL-3 + IL-1 + IL-6 + GM-CSF + G-CSF gave maximum expansion of CD34⁺ cells.[8,9] Current evidence supports a mostly stochastic model of hematopoiesis, in which cytokines provide important growth and survival signals, but do not direct terminal differentiation. Ecotropic expression of the G-CSF-R in normal hematopoietic progenitors results in G-CSF-dependent differentiation of these cells into mature granulocytes, macrophages, megakaryocytes, and erythroid cells.[10] The stochastic view is also supported by studies in which a chimeric receptor consisting of the extracellular G-CSF-binding domain was fused to the cytoplasmic domain of the erythropoietin-R, since, upon expression in cells, G-CSF induced mature neutrophils.[11] The action of G-CSF on mature neutrophils is summarized in Table 114.3.

KEY CONCEPTS

Characteristics of the CSFs

- Glycoproteins with overlapping function but no structural homology
- Interact with specific high-affinity receptors on myeloid cells
- Required continuously throughout myeloid differentiation
- Stimulate proliferation of myeloid progenitors
- Enhance effector functions of mature myeloid cells
- Present in serum and produced by many cell types upon activation

Granulocyte-macrophage CSF

Human GM-CSF cDNA encodes a polypeptide of 144 amino acids, with a 17-amino acid leader sequence, two *N*-glycosylation sites, and two intrachain disulfide bonds.[12] Variations in the molecular mass of GM-CSF from 14 to 30 kDa are due to variable glycosylation, with up to 50% of the molecule being carbohydrate (Table 114.1). Recombinant GM-CSF produced by COS cells (regramostim) or by yeast cells (sargramostim) is glycosylated, the latter to a lesser degree than the endogenous GM-CSF, from which it also differs by containing a leucine instead of proline at position 23. The degree of glycosylation is important since it can affect pharmacokinetics, biological activity, antigenicity, and toxicity. Sargramostim, for example, has a substantially reduced receptor-binding affinity as compared to nonglycosylated material produced in *Escherichia coli* (molgramostim).

The chromosomal gene for GM-CSF has been mapped to the long arm of human chromosome 5 (5q21–q32), 9 kb downstream from the IL-3 gene[13] (Table 114.1). This arm is also the location of the genes for IL-4, IL-5, IL-9, IL-13, the receptors for platelet-derived growth factor, c-fms (M-CSF-R), an early growth

Action of G-CSF, GM-CSF, and M-CSF on the function of mature hematopoietic cells

Cell type	Function	GM-CSF	G-CSF	M-CSF
Neutrophils	Survival	+	+	–
	Migration inhibition (LAM-1 ↓)	+	–	–
	Adhesion (CD11b ↑)	+	+	–
	Phagocytosis, degranulation	+	–	–
	C3biR, FcγR, FMLPR ↑	+	+	–
	Superoxide generation[a]	+	+	–
	Arachidonic acid, leukotriene release	+	–	–
	Cytokine secretion	+	–	–
	ADCC ↑	+	+	–
	Uptake, destruction of bacteria, parasites	+	+	–
Monocyte/macrophages	Survival, proliferation	+	–	+
	Superoxide, NO generation[a]	+	–	+
	Class II MHC, CD1a, b, c ↑	+	–	±
	Uptake, destruction of bacteria, parasites, fungi	+	–	+
	ADCC ↑	+	–	+
	Cytokine,[a] plasminogen activator production	+	–	+
Eosinophils	Survival	+	–	–
	ADCC↑	+	–	–
	Anti-*Schistosomula* activity	+	–	–
	Leukotriene synthesis	+	–	–
Basophils	Histamine release	+	–	–
Langerhans/dendritic cells	Maturation viability, function	+	–	–
	CD1a, Class II MHC ↑	+	–	–
Osteoclasts	Bone resorption	–	+	+

[a]With priming, e.g. by fMLP (neutrophils) or with adhesion or cytokines (monocytes).

Table 114.3 Action of GM-CSF, G-CSF, and M-CSF on the function of mature hematopoietic cells.

response gene (EGR-1), and the interferon regulatory factor-1 gene. The long arm of chromosome 5 is frequently involved in deletion or rearrangement in acute myeloid leukemia, and a refractory anemia/preleukemia 5q-syndrome is associated with deletion of the long arm that could lead to expression of aberrant or recessive alleles.[14]

GM-CSF is an inducible product of a variety of cell types. It is produced by antigen, lectin or IL-2-stimulated T lymphocytes; antigen, LPS or IL-1 stimulated B lymphocytes; macrophages activated by LPS, phagocytosis or adherence and IL-1; or TNF-stimulated fibroblasts and endothelial cells.[13] In these various inducible cells, the accumulation of GM-CSF mRNA is due to both increased transcription rate and post-transcriptional stabilization of the mRNA. GM-CSF has been proposed as an important component of leukemic transformation since GM-CSF transcripts are found in a high percentage of acute myelogenous leukemia (AML) cases.

The receptor for GM-CSF (GM-CSF-R), like that for IL-3 and IL-5, is a heterodimer composed of a ligand-specific α chain and a common β chain.[6,13,14] The GM-CSF-R α chain is encoded by a gene situated within the pseudo-autonomous region, an area of homology between the ends of the human sex chromosomes that undergoes obligatory exchange between the X and Y chromosomes during meiosis, thereby behaving 'pseudo-autosomally'[14] (Table 114.2). The common β subunit of GM-CSF-R is shared with IL-3 and IL-5 receptors and is encoded by a gene located on chromosome 22q12–13. The α and β chains belong to the hematopoietin receptor superfamily, with the presence of a 200-amino acid module in the extracellular region, conserved cysteines, and a WSXWS motif.[6,13] The α chain also has a fibronectin type III domain. In humans, only one β chain exists. Three isoforms of the α chain have been described and are generated by alternative splicing. Two forms, 400 and 410 amino acids, are identical in the extracellular transmembrane and proximal cytoplasmic domain but show complete lack of identity in the terminal 54 and 64 amino acids (Table 114.2). The third form has a transmembrane deletion and so may occur in soluble form. The differential expression of the isoforms on different cell types or at different stages of differentiation may result in different types of GM-CSF response. The receptor is expressed at levels of 50–500 receptors per cell on myeloid progenitors, neutrophils, monocytes, eosinophils and dendritic cells, but not lymphoid or erythroid populations.[13] The signal transduction pathway involves physical association of β chain (βc) with JAK2 with subsequent activation of STAT1, STAT2 and STAT5. A second pathway involves activation of *ras* and MAP kinases with consequent activation of *c-fos* and *c-jun*.[15]

The biological effects of GM-CSF were initially related to its ability to stimulate proliferation and differentiation of myeloid-committed progenitors (CFU-GM). GM-CSF can promote proliferation and differentiation of eosinophils, basophils, megakaryocytes, erythroid, and dendritic cells in synergy with other factors (e.g. with erythropoietin for erythropoiesis, with TNF or IL-4 for dendritic differentiation).[13] In synergy with KL or FL it stimulates multipotent progenitors and stem cells, including high proliferative potential-CFU.[16]

$CD34^+$ cells in marrow and CSF-mobilized peripheral blood generated colonies of dendritic cells (DC) in semisolid culture with GM-CSF and TNF, and large numbers of functionally mature DC can be generated over 12–14 days in suspension culture with these same cytokines.[17] Development of DC from $CD34^+$ progenitors occurs via the development of an intermediate $CD14^+$ $HLA\text{-}DR^+$, cfms $(M\text{-}CSF\text{-}R)^+$ cell that lacks myeloperoxidase and nonspecific esterase. These cells possess substantial phagocytic capacity and are bipotential, generating typical adherent $CD14^+$ phagocytic macrophages in the presence of M-CSF, and of $CD14^-$, $cfms^-$, $CD1a^+$, $CD83^+$, $HLA\text{-}DR^{+++}$ dendritic cells in the presence of GM-CSF and TNF.[18] Blood monocytes also differentiate into DC without proliferation; in the presence of GM-CSF, this pathway is reversible, but exposure to TNF induces an apparently irreversible maturation of DC with down-modulation of cfms. Physiological conditions inducing monocyte differentiation to DC involve transendothelial egress of monocytes to extravascular sites, e.g. of inflammation, phagocytosis, and reverse transendothelial migration of a portion of the cells which re-enter the circulation as DC.[19] The phagocytosis process provides a strong stimulus for DC maturation and the endothelium may be a source of GM-CSF and proinflammatory cytokines.

GM-CSF promotes survival of myeloid cells, including mature neutrophils, by suppressing apoptosis. At low concentrations GM-CSF enhances neutrophil motility, but at high concentrations it inhibits motility, thus providing a concentration gradient effect, first attracting and then maintaining these cells at sites of inflammation. The pleiotropic functions of GM-CSF extend to enhancement of innate as well as specific immune responses, which can be initiated alone or in synergy with other cytokines such as TNF (Table 114.3).[13] Actions on mature neutrophils include up-regulation of surface adhesion molecules CD11b and LAM-1, enhanced phagocytosis, priming for respiratory burst with resultant increased superoxide anion generation, increased antibody-dependent cellular cytotoxicity, and inhibition of apoptosis. GM-CSF enhances monocyte and macrophage fungistatic and antimycobacterial activity. GM-CSF enhances macrophage antigen presentation by increasing expression of MHC Class I and II molecules, B-7 (CD80) accessory molecules and CDI_b nonpolymorphic molecules important for presentation of nonpeptide mycobacterial antigens. Macrophage G-CSF, IL-1, and TNF production, and to a lesser extent IL-12 production are enhanced by GM-CSF treatment.[20]

Mice in which the GM-CSF gene is knocked out exhibit normal steady-state hematopoiesis, suggesting either functional redundancy of the myeloid regulatory factors or lack of a role for the factor in normal hematopoiesis.[21] A universal abnormality in these mice is a pulmonary pathology with similarities to human alveolar proteinosis, that involves accumulation of pulmonary surfactant protein and associated opportunistic infection. Mice lacking both GM-CSF and G-CSF have a greater degree of neutropenia at birth and higher mortality than those lacking G-CSF only, but in the adult neutrophil levels were comparable.[21] More surprising is the normality of hematopoiesis in βc/IL-3 double-mutant mice that lack the entire GM-CSF, IL-3, and IL-5 function.[22] The mice showed normal hematopoietic parameters except for reduced numbers of eosinophils and lack of an eosinophil response to *Listeria monocytogenes*. Hematopoietic recovery after administration of the myelosuppressive drug 5-fluorouracil was unimpaired, indicating that these three cytokines were dispensable for hematopoiesis in an emergency as well as in steady state.

IN VIVO ACTION OF COLONY-STIMULATING FACTORS

Granulocyte CSF

The subcutaneous or intravenous administration of recombinant *E. coli*-derived G-CSF results in an acute decrease in circulating monocytes and neutrophils within the first hour, followed by a dose-dependent increase in mature segmented polymorphonuclear granulocytes and some band forms, reaching 100 000/mm^3 within 7 days with doses of >10 μg/kg/day.[3,23] Marrow cellularity increases, with a major increase in the postmitotic neutrophil compartment and amplification of the mitotic compartment at doses of >3 μg/kg/day. Bone marrow progenitors (CFU-GM, CFU-E, CFU-MK) remain unchanged or slightly decreased in frequency in the marrow, but the fraction in S phase increases significantly, and circulating progenitors increase up to 100-fold. Labeling studies demonstrate that G-CSF promotes an average of 3.2 extra amplification divisions during neutrophil development, with labeled cells appearing in the circulation within 24 hours compared to the normal 4–5 days.[24] Upon cessation of CSF administration, the number of circulating neutrophils falls rapidly and the marrow *S*-phase fraction falls below pretreatment levels. Such quiescence can be exploited to protect myeloid progenitors from cycle-specific chemotherapy.

Granulocyte-macrophage CSF

Infusion of GM-CSF results in a dose-dependent rise of up to 7 to 10-fold in neutrophils, monocytes, and eosinophils, beginning within a week and resulting from increased proliferation and differentiation within the marrow.[25] The cycle status of marrow progenitors increases markedly, the birth rate of cycling myeloid cells increases 3-fold, the duration of S phase decreases from 14.2 to 9.1 hours and the cell-cycle time from 86 to 24 hours.[26] Following cessation of GM-CSF treatment, the myeloid lineage enters a phase of rebound quiescence. Circulating progenitors of all lineages increase 3 to 20-fold following prolonged CSF administration and may be harvested for autologous transplantation. The neutrophils show increased functional activity, as measured by phagocytosis, degranulation, superoxide anion generation, and antibody-dependent cellular cytotoxicity (ADCC).[27] Eosinophils exhibit increased ADCC and anti-*Schistosomula* activity, and monocytes exhibited increased ADCC and antifungal activity. Dose-dependent neutrophil migration inhibition occurs, with a marked impairment of migration into sterile skin abrasions seen when GM-CSF is given by continuous infusion.[28]

CLINICAL APPLICATIONS OF CSF THERAPY ADJUNCTS TO THE CHEMOTHERAPY OF SOLID TUMORS

The use of G- and GM-CSFs can be divided into primary prophylaxis (initiation of CSF before the occurrence of neutropenia), secondary prophylaxis (initiation of a CSF in cycles of chemotherapy subsequent to the occurrence of chemotherapy-induced prolonged neutropenia or neutropenic fever), and therapeutic use (initiation of a CSF in the setting of established neutropenia with or without fever). The first clinical trials of G-CSF involved administration to patients receiving multiagent chemotherapy for bladder cancer[23] and small-cell lung cancer.[29] G-CSF accelerated neutrophil recovery and resulted in higher neutrophil nadir counts. This, in turn, led to fewer episodes of fever, infection, and severe mucositis, permitting more patients to receive their chemotherapy on schedule.[3] A randomized, placebo-controlled, double-blind trial of G-CSF in small-cell lung cancer patients receiving cyclophosphamide, adriamycin, and etoposide chemotherapy conclusively demonstrated its efficacy in ameliorating chemotherapy-induced neutropenias.[30] During the initial cycle of chemotherapy, G-CSF reduced the depth of the neutrophil nadir and the duration of severe neutropenia, defined as circulating neutrophil counts $<0.5 \times 10^9$ cells/l (3 vs. 6 days) (Fig. 114.1). During all cycles, the number of days of hospitalization, days with intravenous antibiotics, and incidence of confirmed infections were all reduced approximately 50% when compared to cycles with placebo (Fig. 114.2).

In nine representative phase III trials of G- or GM-CSF in chemotherapy of solid or hematological malignancies with established febrile neutropenia, the impact on duration of fever or hospitalization was much less affected than was the impact on duration of neutropenia.[31] Indeed, with GM-CSF only 2 of 5 trials showed reduction in neutropenia, with only one showing reduction in hospitalization and none with reduced duration of fever. Better results were seen with G-CSF, with 4 out of 4 trials showing reduced duration of neutropenia, 2 of 4 reduced hospitalization, and 1 of 4 reduced duration of fever.

The primary use of G-CSF is in patients receiving chemotherapy with an expected rate of neutropenia exceeding 40% in the absence of growth factor. The resulting reduction in neutropenia and its complications has led to this therapy being the standard of care as defined by an American Society for Clinical Oncology panel of experts.[32] Recent cost analysis incorporating both direct and indirect costs of care of hospitalization for febrile neutropenia suggests that a lower threshold, such as 20%, might be cost-effective for the use of G-CSF.[32] Chemotherapy often results in clinically significant mucositis, manifested by pain and oral ulceration. Neutropenia contributes to the pathogenesis of mucositis by enhancing secondary infection and ulceration. A number of studies have demonstrated a decrease in mucositis incidence in patients receiving chemotherapy with G-CSF as opposed to those receiving chemotherapy alone.[31] The recommended subcutaneous doses of G-CSF and GM-CSF are 5 μg/kg/d and 250 μg/m²/d, respectively, beginning 1 day after chemotherapy, although later trials suggest a delay of CSF until 72 h after chemotherapy may be equally efficacious. The development and clinical application of pegylated (polyethylene glycol-conjugated) G-CSF with a

CLINICAL PEARLS

Administration of G-CSF and GM-CSF

- Stimulate granulocyte production.
- Enhance granulocyte function.
- Peripheralize hematopoietic progenitors that can be used in transplantation.

G-CSF stimulation of neutrophil recovery in a lung cancer patient following chemotherapy

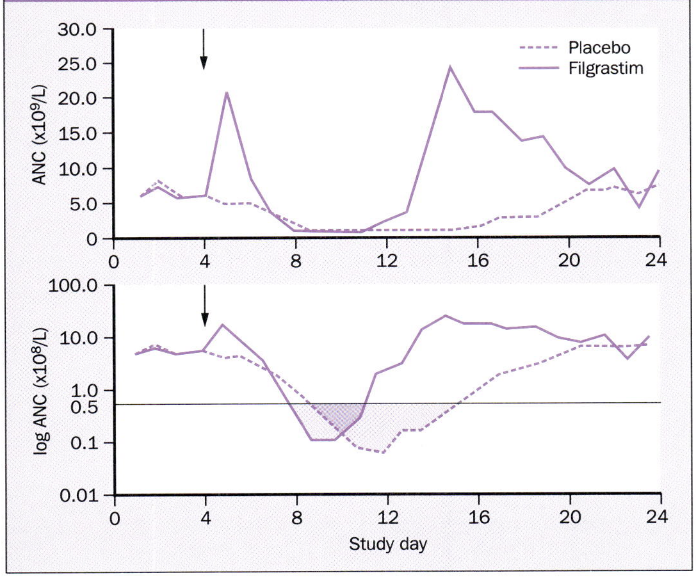

Figure 114.1 G-CSF stimulation of neutrophil recovery in a lung cancer patient following chemotherapy. Mean absolute neutrophil count (ANC) in patients with small-cell lung cancer treated with G-CSF (filgrastim) in the first cycle of chemotherapy. The counts are shown on a linear scale (top) and log scale (bottom). The arrow denotes the start of placebo or G-CSF administration. The hatching highlights the degree and duration of neutropenia (counts $<0.5 \times 10^9$ per liter). (From Crawford J, Ozer H, Stoller R, et al. Reduction by granulocyte colony-stimulating factor of fever and neutropenia induced by chemotherapy in patients with small-cell lung cancer. *N Engl J Med* 1991;315:164.)

Improvement in clinical end-points following G-CSF therapy in lung cancer

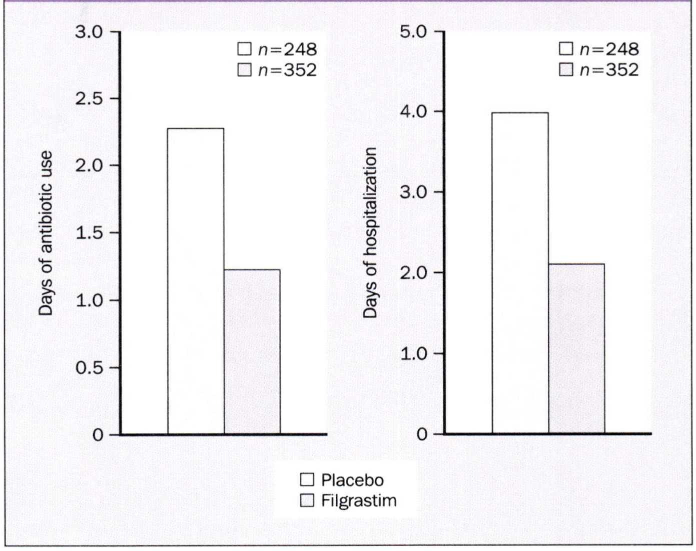

Figure 114.2 Improvement in clinical end-points following G-CSF therapy in lung cancer. Secondary clinical end-points in patients with small-cell lung cancer treated with G-CSF (filgrastim). The mean duration of use of intravenous antibiotic drugs is expressed as the number of days per cycle in which the study drug was given in blinded fashion, as is the mean duration of hospital stay. (From Crawford J, Ozer H, Stoller R, et al. Reduction by granulocyte colony-stimulating factor of fever and neutropenia induced by chemotherapy in patients with small-cell lung cancer. *N Engl J Med* 1991;315:164.)

prolonged in vivo survival will alter G-CSF scheduling recommendations, since a single injection mobilized CD34+ cells and elevated neutrophils for up to 10 days.[33]

Since the first use of CSFs to deliver dose-dense therapy in 1989 in advanced breast cancer, a multitude of phase I and II and some randomized trials have taken place evaluating dose intensification with CSFs. CSFs can be used to increase the dose of chemotherapy as well as reducing the dosing interval between cycles, or both ('dose-dense' therapy). With this latter strategy in some studies complete remissions (CRs) of 48–78% were reported.[34] Dose intensity can be increased 1.5 to 2.5-fold with CSFs, but while many of these studies showed an increase in response rate to 80% or more, randomized trials did not show an advantage for either duration of response or overall survival. The potential benefits of intensification may be reduced by the emergence of dose-limiting nonhematopoietic toxicities. Despite the apparent lack of impact on survival, intensive treatment is short and may be used as a first-line treatment in order to obtain a major response as quickly as possible and to minimize impairment of quality of life.

CLINICAL APPLICATIONS OF CSF THERAPY IN HEMATOLOGIC MALIGNANCIES

G- and GM-CSFs have therapeutic applications for treatment of the neutropenia associated with the clinical presentation of acute leukemias and myelodysplastic syndromes (MDS), as well as the leukopenia associated with high-dose chemotherapy. The proliferative and differentiative actions of CSFs on myeloid cells also provide a rationale for their use in acute myeloid leukemia (AML) and MDS. The use of G- and GM-CSF to accelerate recovery after myelosuppressive chemotherapy of AML has been controversial in view of in vitro studies suggesting that it could be a growth-stimulatory factor in cultures of some leukemias.[35]

Many randomized trials have appraised the value of G-CSF or GM-CSF in combination with intensive induction and consolidation chemotherapy in AML patients. The aim is two-fold: (1) to reduce the length of chemotherapy-induced grade 4 neutropenia, and (2) to improve the effects of chemotherapy by a direct or indirect action on leukemic cells involving modification of the cell-cycle status or induction of differentiation/apoptosis. The results of 16 randomized trials of G-CSF in AML and high-risk MDS showed a significant reduction in neutropenia which translated into reduced duration of hospitalization and antibiotic usage.[36] There was, however, no improvement in incidence of severe infection or in resulting induction death rate in all trials testing these criteria. Yeast-derived glycosylated GM-CSF, but not *E. coli*-derived nonglycosylated GM-CSF, accelerated neutrophil recovery after intensive induction chemotherapy and decreased incidence and severity of infection. This resulted in improved complete remission (CR) rate, but had no beneficial effect on survival.[36] An antileukemic effect of G-CSF has been indicated in some trials where a significant increase in CR rate was reported. Taken together, the results indicate that patients with a poor prognosis, such as the elderly (>60 years) and those with unfavorable cytogenetics or post-MDS AML, may achieve a CR more frequently following G-CSF treatment. However, in a large 800 patient MRC trial, age subgroup analysis showed that CR rate was significantly reduced in younger patients (<40 years) in the G-CSF treated arm (79% vs. 93%, $P = 0.003$), resulting in a lower survival rate at 2 years.[36,37] There may be detrimental effects of G-CSF after completion of intensive induction chemotherapy in younger AML patients, as has been reported with GM-CSF.[38] Debate continues as to the efficacy of CSF treatment as far as morbidity and mortality is concerned even in elderly patients, possibly reflecting the heterogeneity of the disease as well as differences in dosing and scheduling of CSF administration.[39]

Adult acute lymphoblastic leukemia (ALL) patients appear to benefit from the simultaneous administration of G-CSF with induction chemotherapy because of a significant reduction of neutropenia, a trend to fewer infections, and a more rapid completion of chemotherapy. In high-risk pediatric ALL patients, G-CSF administered prophylactically in the interval between chemotherapy courses significantly reduced febrile episodes, infectious episodes, and duration of intravenous antibiotic usage, and allowed for a tighter adherence to treatment schedule.[37] Japanese investigators conducted a double-blind controlled study to assess whether G-CSF given before and during chemotherapy stimulated AML cell proliferation. In 58 adult patients there was a trend to higher remission in the G-CSF group (50% vs. 37%) but no difference in event-free survival nor in disease-free survival once CR was achieved.[37] Administration of GM-CSF prior to or during chemotherapy in an attempt to sensitize blast cells to chemotherapy was reported to lead to longer remissions in younger (but not older) patients in one study,[40] but other studies have shown either no difference or a lower CR rate with no effect of remission duration or survival.[39]

G-CSF has also been found to have antileukemic activity in AML that has recurred after allogeneic transplantation, suggesting that CSF modulation of the immune system has antileukemic potential.[41] In MDS, both G-CSF and GM-CSF increase circulating neutrophils in the majority of patients, with a minority of patients treated with GM-CSF showing an increase in platelets and/or reticulocytes.[42] A substantial number of patients had both an erythroid and myeloid response when treated with a combination of G-CSF and erythropoietin.[43] In 6 trials of G-CSF in MDS patients, absolute neutrophil counts rose to normal levels in 90% of patients, with improved neutrophil function and with a decrease in infectious episodes.[42] In a randomized phase III trial of 102 patients with RAEB and RAEB-T median survival was shorter in the G-CSF treatment group due to a higher rate of death due to bleeding, but retrospective analysis revealed a skewed distribution with more than twice as many patients with pronounced thrombocytopenia entered onto the G-CSF limb.[42] Combinations of G-CSF with all-*trans* retinoic acid did not reveal any superiority over G-CSF alone. A review of over 324 MDS patients treated with GM-CSF in a number of trials has

THERAPEUTIC PRINCIPLES

Clinical uses of G-CSF and GM-CSF

G-CSF and GM-CSF are used for the treatment of:

- Chemotherapy-induced myelosuppression
- Febrile neutropenia or sepsis
- Congenital and idiopathic neutropenia
- Myelodysplastic syndromes
- Post-marrow transplant recovery
- HIV infection and its complications
- Antitumor therapy: vaccine adjuvant

shown that >80% of patients had increases in absolute neutrophil counts (ANC) and decreased infection. In one large randomized trial of GM-CSF with treatment periods in excess of 6 months, there was a sustained increase in neutrophil, monocyte, eosinophil, and lymphocyte counts but a decrease in platelets.[42] Advanced MDS treated with cytosine–arabinoside in the presence of GM-CSF in two trials gave remission rates comparable to cytosine–arabinoside alone (15–17%). Treatment-related hematotoxicity with pronounced thrombocytopenia was responsible for a considerable early death rate in both studies.[42]

USE OF CSFS IN BONE MARROW TRANSPLANTATION

The first multicenter, randomized, double-blind trial of GM-CSF was with 128 patients with lymphoid malignancies.[43] Both placebo and treated patients had identical numbers of days of severe neutropenia post bone marrow transplantation (BMT); however, patients given GM-CSF achieved a neutrophil count of 500/μl at 19 days, as compared to 26 days for controls. This resulted in a median of 6 fewer days of hospitalization and a reduced frequency of infectious episodes. In a subsequent double-blind, placebo-controlled trial, in acute lymphoblastic leukemia patients receiving autologous BMT following total body irradiation and high-dose chemotherapy, GM-CSF accelerated granulocyte recovery by 1 week, with half as many infectious episodes but no statistically significant difference in survival or platelet recovery.

G-CSF also proved effective at doses of 16–64 μg/kg/day for up to 28 days following autologous BMT in a number of phase I and II trials. In a randomized, dose-ranging trial of G-CSF in 121 patients with nonmyeloid malignancy, a median neutrophil count of 550/μl was achieved at 13 days vs. 19 days in the control arm.[44] In contrast to the GM-CSF trials, there was no toxicity associated with G-CSF usage, and hospitalization was reduced by 11–15 days.

In a prospective randomized study of GM-CSF in 57 patients receiving T-cell-depleted allogeneic BMT, the GM-CSF group showed a significantly faster recovery of granulocytes and monocytes, a reduced incidence of pneumonia, and no influence on the incidence and severity of graft-versus-host disease.[45]

USE OF CSFs TO PERIPHERALIZE PROGENITOR CELLS FOR AUTOLOGOUS PERIPHERAL BLOOD TRANSPLANTATION

Autologous peripheral blood stem cell (PBSC) transplantation as a supplement or an alternative to BMT results in a more rapid restoration of platelets and neutrophils than does BMT alone, provided that cells are harvested after circulating numbers of progenitors are expanded. Harvesting during the regeneration phase following chemotherapy administration, e.g. with 2–7 g/m^2 cyclophosphamide, results in an increase in circulating CFU-GM as much as 100-fold over baseline. Mobilization, with or without chemotherapy, can be achieved with G- or GM-CSF. A more than 1000-fold increase in circulating CFU-GM can be obtained following GM-CSF and cytoxan treatment.[46] A highly significant correlation exists between circulating CFU-GM and CD34$^+$ cells, and following GM-CSF plus cytoxan treatment, 0.5×10^9 CD34$^+$ cells can readily be harvested by leukapheresis.[47] In general, $\geq 5 \times 10^6$ CD34$^+$ cells/kg result in prompt and durable platelet engraftment. Patients receiving $<1\text{–}2 \times 10^6$ CD34$^+$ cells are at risk for delayed platelet recovery or engraftment failure. When using G-CSF alone, 20% of patients required ≥ 4 aphereses to reach 1×10^6 CD34$^+$ cells/kg, and 60% of patients required ≥ 4 aphereses to reach 5×10^6 CD34$^+$ cells per kg.[48] One strategy to improve peripheral blood progenitor cell (PBPC) yield is to use G-CSF in combination with chemotherapy or in combination with other growth factors. The most extensively studied combination is G-CSF with the c-kit ligand, also termed stem cell factor (SCF). A multicenter phase III trial was undertaken in 203 patients with high-risk stage I–IV breast cancer who had received a median of five cycles of prior chemotherapy randomized to receive G-CSF alone (10 μg/kg/day) or G-CSF plus SCF (20 μg/kg/day) for 9 days. Patients in the SCF + G-CSF group reached the target number of $\geq 5 \times 10^6$ CD34$^+$ cells after 4 apheresis procedures, whereas patients in the G-CSF alone group required a median of ≥ 6 apheresis procedures.[49] G-CSF was reported to be more effective than GM-CSF in mobilizing PBPC, because it was necessary to increase GM-CSF near to its dose-limiting toxicity to achieve comparable peripheralization.

Autologous rescue in metastatic breast cancer using GM-CSF-mobilized PBPC accelerated neutrophil recovery (by 9 days) and platelet recovery (by 10 days), reducing both morbidity and platelet transfusion requirements.[50] Similar results were obtained using G-CSF-mobilized PBPC, which accelerated neutrophil recovery by 2 days and platelet recovery by 17 days, when compared to recipients of nonmobilized PBPC.[51] In a comparison of G-CSF-mobilized and GM-CSF-mobilized PBPC, both led to accelerated neutrophil recovery as compared to BMT, with reduced antibiotic usage and shorter stay in intensive care.[52] Patients receiving G-CSF-primed PBPC also experienced a reduction in median days in hospital and in numbers of red cell and platelet transfusions.

G-CSF-mobilized PBPC are being used increasingly in allogeneic transplantation, with faster platelet and neutrophil recovery than with marrow. Early studies reported less acute graft-versus-host disease (GVHD) and decreased hospital stay and overall morbidity than traditionally observed with allogeneic marrow. However, later studies observed a high rate of chronic GVHD, with 90% of patients in one study remaining on some form of GVHD therapy at more than 18 months after transplant.[53] It appears that the infusion of large numbers of peripheral blood T cells is responsible for the GVHD. In order to overcome this problem a number of investigators are utilizing CD34$^+$ selection to reduce contaminating T cells by 2–3 logarithms. Secondary strategies to add back certain T-cell subsets at day 30 or later to maintain antitumor effects while avoiding the period of highest risk of acute GVHD are also underway. A strategy for overcoming HLA mismatch has been developed and involves infusion of up to 10-fold greater numbers of G-CSF-mobilized CD34$^+$ cells compared to bone marrow transplants. This strategy has been successful in engrafting patients who lack a five or six antigen HLA-matched donor and has also been used in HLA-matched unrelated donor transplants with excellent engraftment and no apparent increase in acute GVHD.[54]

CSF TREATMENT OF CHRONIC NEUTROPENIA

Hematologic disorders associated with severe, chronic neutropenia can be categorized into congenital forms, including Kostmann syndrome, Shwachman–Diamond syndrome, myelocathexis,

G-CSF response of patients with congenital neutropenia

Diagnosis	Number of patients	Months on G-CSF	Dose G-CSF (μg/kg/day)	Absolute neutrophil count Baseline	Absolute neutrophil count Median post treatment
Kostmann	17	35 ± 3	15 ± 3	50 ± 23	1534 ± 163
G-CSF nonresponders	2	3	60	0	100
Shwachman–Diamond	2	26	15	154	1960
Myelocathexis	1	13	1	56	1008

Table 114.4 G-CSF response of patients with congenital neutropenia.

cyclic neutropenia, and a heterogeneous group of idiopathic neutropenias, some of which may have an immunologic basis.[3,55]

Cyclic neutropenia is an inherited disorder of humans and gray collie dogs, characterized by regular (21 or 14 days, respectively) fluctuations in peripheral neutrophils, monocytes, and eosinophils, and marrow progenitor cells. In human cyclic neutropenia, G-CSF shortened the neutropenia cycles, increased their amplitude, and reduced the severity of the nadirs.[3,55] GM-CSF was ineffective. Kostmann syndrome is characterized by severe neutropenia, maturation arrest of the myeloid lineage, and infant onset of severe, recurrent bacterial infections. In this syndrome, as in cyclic neutropenia, the neutrophil defect is frequently compensated by a monocytosis and eosinophilia. In vitro and in vivo, maturation arrest can be overcome with G-CSF, with normal neutrophil differentiation in colony assay with 1–10 ng/ml of G-CSF, and normal peripheral neutrophil counts obtained upon daily administration of 5–20 μg of G-CSF per kilogram body weight per day (Table 114.4).[3,56] Some patients have a more refractory neutropenia and require higher doses of G-CSF, up to 40 μg/kg/day, to produce normal neutrophil numbers. GM-CSF has not proved effective in correcting the neutropenic defect. A rare subgroup of congenital neutropenias has proved completely refractory to G-CSF, both in vivo and in vitro, and may represent a different genetic disorder.[3] In one such patient a mutation has been reported in the extracellular domain of the G-CSF receptor which affected ligand–receptor complex formation with severe consequences for intracellular signal transduction.[57] No genomic defect or defect in transcription or translation of the G-CSF gene in marrow stromal cells or monocytes has been seen in any patient with congenital neutropenia; serum levels of G-CSF are frequently elevated in these patients.[58] Normal to elevated numbers of high-affinity G-CSF receptors are found on all neutrophils, monocytes, and marrow cells of G-CSF-responsive patients before and after G-CSF therapy, and normal receptor down-modulation and ligand internalization occurs.[10] A multicenter, randomized, controlled trial of G-CSF in 123 patients with severe, chronic neutropenia (60 congenital neutropenia, 21 cyclic neutropenia, and 42 idiopathic neutropenias) has been undertaken. Of 120 evaluable patients, 108 showed a response, either partial (with median neutrophils $>0.5 \times 10^9$/l) or complete (with neutrophils $>1.5 \times 10^9$/l).[58] Overall, there was a 16-fold increase of neutrophil counts over control, and a response was seen in a few days in most patients. The incidence and duration of infection-related events was significantly reduced. Patients with chronic idiopathic neutropenia of adults (CINA) exhibit qualitatively normal but quantitatively deficient neutrophil differentiation in vitro in marrow colony assay with G-CSF, and patients show restoration to normal neutrophil counts upon G-CSF treatment.[56,58] Increased serum levels of inflammatory cytokines such as IL-1 and TNF have been reported in CINA patients, and approximately 82% of these patients had TGF-β1 levels higher than the upper limit of normal.[59] These levels correlated inversely with the number of neutrophils and the frequency of marrow $CD34^+/CD33^+$ cells. It is possible that increased TGF-β1 production by the bone marrow stromal cells of these patients inhibits myelopoiesis.

In an analysis of 420 patients in the Severe Chronic Neutropenia International Registry, 16/220 patients treated with G-CSF for as many as 8 years developed AML or MDS.[3] None of the patients with cyclic or idiopathic neutropenia developed AML/MDS and no relationship was seen with dose or duration of dosing of G-CSF. In one study, all patients tested with severe congenital neutropenia associated with progression to AML or MDS showed G-CSF receptor nonsense mutations leading to truncation of the C-terminal region critical for maturation signaling.[3]

Drug-induced neutropenias occur with unpredictable frequency (e.g. following treatment with phenothiazines and aminopyrine) and G-CSF has been used extensively to hasten neutrophil recovery in such cases.[3] Neutropenia is sometimes associated with rheumatoid arthritis as part of the Felty syndrome and systemic lupus erythematosus. The neutropenia of Felty syndrome has been attributed to serum inhibitory factors or T-cell suppressor mechanisms directed against myeloid progenitors, antigranulocyte antibodies, and circulating immune complexes.[3,60] Some patients exhibit a neutrophil response to G-CSF, although in some patients there is exacerbation of arthritis during neutrophil recovery.

G- AND GM-CSF FOR HIV TREATMENT AND IMMUNE RECONSTITUTION

There are a number of emerging applications for G- and GM-CSF beyond their initial indications as stimulators of neutrophil recovery in acquired neutropenia[3,61–68] (Table 114.5). GM-CSF knockout mice have significant abnormalities in T-cell function, including diminished CD4 proliferative response, impaired T-cell help for IgG production, and reduced cytotoxic T-cell response.[69] Although the GM-CSF cognate receptor is reportedly absent on T cells, GM-CSF-R mRNA has been reported, sug-

Table 114.5 Emerging applications of GM-CSF.

Emerging applications of GM-CSF		
		References
Fungal infections	Decreases incidence of fungal infections versus placebo in AuBMT patients. Reduces mortality due to fungal infection in elderly AML patients. Improves recovery from *Candida* and *Aspergillus* infections as an adjuvant to amphotericin B. Improves oropharyngeal candidiasis refractory to fluconazole in HIV-infected patients.	61, 62
HIV infection and its complications	Increases CD4 count. Decreases viral load. As adjuvant treatment of *Mycobacterium avium* reduces viable intracellular *mycobacteria*.	61
Vaccine adjuvant	Enhances antibody response to hepatitis B vaccine. Increases the percentage of patients who seroconvert to all three strains of flu vaccine.	61, 63, 64
Antitumor therapy	Prolongs disease-free survival and overall survival compared with historical controls in patients with advanced melanoma. Of 20 stage IV melanoma patients who received GM-CSF as an adjuvant to a melanoma vaccine, 4 had partial to complete response.	61, 65
Immunotherapy for AML	Decreases risk of relapse compared with controls (37.4% vs 49.5%).	66
Mucositis stomatitis, diarrhea	Reduces incidence and severity of mucositis in patients with sarcoma, advanced head and neck cancer, and those undergoing allogeneic BMT. Shortens the duration of mucositis in children undergoing stem cell transplant. Decreases rates of diarrhea in colorectal cancer patients receiving 5-FU.	61
Wound healing	Intradermal injections of rHuGM-CSF result in enlarged keratinocytes. keratinocyte proliferation, thickening of the epidermis, accumulation of Langerhans cells, and enhanced healing. Reduces mean ulcer surface area versus saline in patients with chronic leg ulcers.	67, 68

Modified from Armitage JO. Emerging applications of recombinant human granulocyte-macrophage colony-stimulating factor. Blood 1998;92:4491.

gesting possible low-level expression. This would explain reports of GM-CSF augmentation of IL-2 induction of lymphokine-activated killer (LAK) cells, and amplification of IL-2-induced human T-cell proliferation in vitro.[70] Administration of GM-CSF to lymphoma patients increased CD8 and CD4 counts and CD25 expression, and accelerated recovery of CD4 cells after autologous bone marrow transplantation.[71]

HIV-infected monocytes and CD4 T cells exhibit diminished secretion of GM-CSF. GM-CSF diminishes the HIV-infectibility of macrophages, probably as a result of down-regulation of the CCR-5 and CXCR4 chemokine receptors which serve, respectively, as coreceptors for M-tropic and dual-tropic strains of HIV-1.[70] GM-CSF enhances the antiviral effect of zidovudine against HIV-1-infected macrophages, probably as a result of increased thymidine kinase activity resulting in increased concentration of azidothymidine-5′-triphosphate.[70] With long-term GM-CSF treatment of leukopenic HIV-infected patients there was a reduction in opportunistic infection and a significant increase in CD4 and CD8 T-cell counts.[72] The ability of GM-CSF to prevent HIV infection of macrophages and CD4 T cells could potentially accelerate viral eradication, particularly if administered with antiretroviral therapy. A placebo-controlled randomized trial of twice-weekly GM-CSF for 6 months in HIV-infected patients with baseline CD4 counts of $<333/mm^3$ receiving zidovudine, revealed a greater reduction of viral load and a significant increase in CD4 counts in the GM-CSF treated group.[70]

Although the incidence of severe bacterial infections in neutropenic HIV-infected patients is lower than in cancer patients receiving chemotherapy, the relative risk is comparable and there is an exponentially increasing incidence of severe bacterial infections in HIV-infected patients as neutropenia develops, particularly when the ANC falls below $0.5 \times 10^9/l$.[73] In a case-control study of a cohort of 1403 HIV-infected patients, the occurrence of severe bacterial and fungal infections was significantly higher in the neutropenic patients than in the control patients, and risk of severe infection was strongly associated with neutrophil count.[74] Thus prevention of neutropenia that may be achievable with G-CSF treatment may be expected to have a major impact on hospitalization, mortality, and quality of life of AIDS patients. G-CSF was also evaluated in HIV patients in order to prevent or ameliorate zidovudine or ganciclovir-induced neutropenia. In six published trials, neutropenia was decreased and continuation of ganciclovir or AZT treatment permitted, without dose-limiting toxicity.[75] In a phase III study to assess the effect of G-CSF in patients with advanced HIV infection, 258 patients were enrolled and G-CSF dosage adjusted to maintain an ANC of $2–10 \times 10^9/l$.[76] Overall, G-CSF-treated patients developed 31% fewer bacterial infections than the control group and had fewer days of hospitalization and more prolonged survival.[74] In a study of 152 patients with HIV and an ANC $<1 \times 10^9/l$, randomized to receive G-CSF or not, the treated patients had a significantly longer survival than the controls (397 days vs. 165 days).[77]

Addition of G-CSF to a regimen of clarithromycin and ethambutol in *Mycobacterium avium*-infected HIV patients improved survival and promoted more rapid clearance of *M. avium* from the blood.[74] Administration of G-CSF to pediatric HIV-infected patients has been well tolerated, resulting in fewer hospitalizations, fewer febrile episodes, higher leukocyte counts, and better tolerance of potentially myelotoxic agents such as ganciclovir.[78]

Pro-inflammatory cytokines may increase CD4 T-cell HIV replication, and G-CSF, by inducing an anti-inflammatory cytokine pattern, may thus be able to decrease HIV replication. TNF-α and IFN-γ release from LPS-stimulated blood was suppressed by G-CSF treatment in high-risk HIV-infected patients. Patients with advanced HIV infection had reduced release of IL-2 and IL-4 by their lymphocytes following in vitro staphylococcal endotoxin B exposure.[79] G-CSF could restore IL-2 production in the blood of such patients.[79] IL-2 production by CD4 T cells is required to maintain CD8 T-cell control of HIV replication, and studies have suggested clinical benefit from administration of rHuIL-2 to HIV-infected patients. However, IL-2 therapy is associated with flu-like symptoms, whereas restoration of endogenous IL-2 production with G-CSF did not have this side-effect.[79]

ROLE OF G- AND GM-CSF IN SYSTEMIC INFLAMMATORY RESPONSE SYNDROME AND SEPSIS

G-CSF has been shown to be a biological response modifier with anti-inflammatory characteristics beyond those of a simple hematopoietic growth factor.[79] In a study of normal volunteers receiving G-CSF, the subsequent response of their blood to in vitro stimulation with various bacterial stimuli, such as endotoxin lipopolysaccharide (LPS), revealed increased levels of IL-1 receptor antagonist (IL-1Ra), and both p55 and p75-soluble tumor necrosis factor receptors.[80] Concomitantly there were reduced levels of LPS-induced TNF-α and IFN-γ. These observations were duplicated in vivo when G-CSF-treated volunteers were challenged with LPS.[79]

Systemic inflammatory response syndrome (SIRS) is a primary host response to a variety of severe insults such as trauma, burns, pancreatitis, or major surgery. It is associated with overproduction of TNF-α and IL-1. Sepsis is a clinical state caused when bacterial infection leads to an exaggerated host inflammatory response involving macrophage and T-cell activation and release of cytokines including TNF-α, IL-1, IFN-γ, and IL-12. In turn these cytokines may synergize with lipopolysaccharides to stimulate release of nitrous oxide in a variety of cell types. G-CSF represents an important survival factor for neutrophils, inhibiting their apoptosis during both SIRS and sepsis. G-CSF stimulates anti-inflammatory type-2 cytokine production (IL-4 and IL-10); increases IL-1 receptor antagonist (IL-1Ra) production to counteract the IL-1-mediated inflammatory cascade; increases expression and shedding of IL-6 receptor to accelerate IL-6 clearance; increases expression of soluble p55 and p75 TNF receptors; and reduces circulating IL-8 levels.[81] Thus, while G-CSF is a member of the inflammatory cytokine cascade, it displays important regulatory properties by attenuating the pro-inflammatory cytokine response that would otherwise predominate. This is the rationale for administering G-CSF to critically ill patients at risk of or with sepsis/SIRS to improve neutrophil function and to modulate the otherwise predestined release of inflammatory mediators. Ischemia/reperfusion injury is a frequent consequence of surgical or hemorrhagic shock and trauma. G-CSF has proved therapeutic in this condition by improving endotoxin clearance[82] and protecting endothelial cells by immediate induction of IL-1Ra. G-CSF also stimulates hemoxygenase-1 expression in endothelium, thus protecting against oxidative damage. In placebo-controlled trials of G-CSF in patients with bacterial pneumonia, the development of sepsis-related organ failure and disseminated intravascular coagulopathy was significantly reduced in G-CSF recipients, and clinical benefits were more pronounced in patients with multilobar pneumonia.[83] G-CSF has proven effective as an adjunct to antibiotics and surgical treatment of foot infections in diabetic patients, resulting in earlier eradication of the pathogens, quicker resolution of the cellulitis, shorter hospital stay, and shorter duration of antibiotic treatment.[84] Studies of G-CSF in premature or low-birthweight neonates with bacterial sepsis have shown that neutrophil numbers and functions were enhanced and that treatment was well tolerated. Larger randomized studies are underway to ascertain effects on infectious morbidity and mortality.[85]

Exposure of macrophages to GM-CSF primes them for enhanced release of inflammatory cytokines including TNF, IL-1, and IL-6 when triggered by LPS. After intravenous challenge with endotoxin, animals pretreated with GM-CSF exhibited a significant increase in circulating TNF, and nonlethal doses of endotoxin became lethal.[86] While GM-CSF may decrease the bacterial burden in acute bacterial infection, its protective action may be counterbalanced by an exaggerated systemic cytokine response. In contrast, G-CSF diminished endotoxin-induced lung injury, and was protective against organ failure caused by a near-lethal dose of endotoxin in mice.[85]

TOXICITIES OF CSFs

GM-CSF toxicities reported in the various clinical trials reviewed include bone pain, myalgia/arthralgia, fever, and chills, with dose-limiting toxicity being pericarditis and pleural and peritoneal effusions (capillary leak syndrome). Many of these may be attributed to the ability of GM-CSF to induce prostaglandin production and various cytokine cascades via monocyte, neutrophil, and eosinophil activation. GM-CSF at doses of $\geq 3\ \mu g/kg$, particularly when administered by an intravenous route, may elicit a first-dose reaction of transient hypoxia, hypotension, tachycardia, flushing, musculoskeletal pain, vomiting, rigors, and syncope.[87] The cause may be the release of vasoactive mediators inducing regional intrapulmonary ventilation–perfusion mismatching. Yeast-derived GM-CSF has a slower rate of distribution and a higher rate of leukotriene metabolism than the *E. coli*-derived GM-CSF. Increased leukotriene production is thought to relate to clinical toxicities such as fluid retention, fever, myalgia, and respiratory toxicity. G-CSF is well tolerated, with mild to moderate bone pain being the most frequent and significant side-effect. Additional toxicities include chest tightness, mild headache, and, rarely, flushing.[3]

FUTURE DIRECTIONS

The CSFs are not simply congeners, and the creation and conservation of these distinct genes implies distinct functions in addition to their overlapping properties. Thus, the question is not whether one factor is 'better' than the others in the clinic, but whether we have discovered the most appropriate use for each factor based upon full knowledge of its unique biologic role. One example is the ability of GM-CSF to lower serum cholesterol concentrations.[88] In a rabbit model, GM-CSF-induced lowering of serum cholesterol may be mediated by enhancement of macrophage functions in lipid metabolism and an increase in the levels of mRNA for the very low density lipoprotein (VLDL) receptor.[89]

GM-CSF augments antigen presentation by a variety of cells, and this property may be used to promote specific antitumor immunity (Table 114.5). Tumor cells transduced with GM-CSF are highly effective in stimulating long-lasting and specific immunity. In malignant B cells, the idiotype of the surface immunoglobulin serves as a weak tumor-specific antigen, but fusion of the idiotype region with GM-CSF converts it into a strong immunogen capable of inducing an immune response and protecting mice from challenge with an otherwise lethal dose of tumor cells.[90] GM-CSF as a vaccine adjuvant when mixed with a soluble antigen induces both an antibody and T-cell antigen-specific immune response in a rodent model.[91] Others have transfected GM-CSF into established tumors with DNA encoding GM-CSF, or directly injected GM-CSF into established tumors, and have shown induction of antitumor immune response in several murine systems.[92] These results have led to phase I human clinical trials using autologous GM-CSF gene-transduced, irradiated tumors as vaccines in patients with metastatic renal cell carcinoma[93] and melanoma.[94] Others have used GM-CSF antigen fusion proteins as immunogens and shown enhanced immunity to the antigen.[95] A complication to the preceding strategies is provided by a report that yeast-derived GM-CSF when used as a vaccine adjuvant in patients led to the development of a T-cell (17% of patients) and antibody response (72% of patients) to recombinant GM-CSF, however no adverse hematological consequences were observed.[96]

Further uses of CSFs will undoubtedly involve a combination biotherapy approach based on knowledge of additive or synergistic interactions with other hematopoietic growth factors, most notably c-kit ligand, flk-2/fit3 ligands, and the family of interleukins. Cytokines may be used in combinations appropriate to eliciting specific biologic responses seemingly as distinct as stimulating pluripotential stem cells or enhancing antitumor, antifungal, or antibacterial activity of mature granulocytes, phagocytic mononuclear cells, and dendritic cells.

REFERENCES

1. Welte K, Platzer E, Lu L, et al. Purification and biochemical characterization of human pluripotent hematopoietic colony-stimulating factor. Proc Natl Acad Sci USA 1985;82:1526.
2. Souza LM, Boone TC, Gabrilove JL, et al. Recombinant human granulocyte colony-stimulating factor: effects on normal and leukemic myeloid cells. Science 1986;232:61.
3. Welte K, Gabrilove J, Bronchud MH, et al. Filgrastim (r-metHuG-CSF): the first 10 years. Blood 1996;88:1907.
4. Roberts WR, Nicola NA. Granulocyte colony-stimulating factor. In: Garland JM, Quesenberry PJ, Hilton DJ (eds) Colony stimulating factors: molecular and cellular biology, 2nd edn. New York, Marcel Dekker, 1997, p 203.
5. Tweardy DJ, Anderson K, Cannizzaro LA, et al. Molecular cloning of cDNAs for the human granulocyte colony-stimulating factor receptor from HL-60 and mapping of the gene to chromosome region 1p32–34. Blood 1992;79:1148.
6. Hilton DJ. Receptors for hematopoietic regulators. In: Garland JM, Quesenberry PJ, Hilton DJ (eds) Colony stimulating factors: molecular and cellular biology, 2nd edn. New York, Marcel Dekker, 1997, p 49.
7. Metcalf D. The granulocyte-macrophage regulators: Reappraisal by gene inactivation. Exp Hematol 1995;23:569.
8. Moore MAS, Hoskins I. Ex vivo expansion of cord blood derived stem cells and progenitors. Blood Cells 1994;20:468.
9. Engelhardt M, Kumar R, Albanell J, et al. Telomerase regulation, cell cycle, and telomere stability in primitive hematopoietic cells. Blood 1997;90:182.
10. Jacob J, Haug JS, Raptis S, Link DC. Specific signals generated by the cytoplasmic domain of the granulocyte colony-stimulating factor (G-CSF) receptor are not required for G-CSF-dependent granulocytic differentiation. Blood 1998;92:353.
11. Semerad CL, Poursine-Laurent J, Liu F, Link DC. A role for G-CSF receptor signaling in the regulation of hematopoietic cell function but not lineage commitment or differentiation. Immunity 1999;11:153.
12. Gasson JC, Weisbart RH, Kaufman SE, et al. Purified human granulocyte-macrophage colony-stimulating factor: direct action on neutrophils. Science 1984;226:1339.
13. Rasko JEJ. Granulocyte-macrophage colony stimulating factor and its receptor. In: Garland JM, Quesenberry PJ, Hilton DJ (eds) Colony stimulating factors: molecular and cellular biology, 2nd edn. New York, Marcel Dekker, 1997, p 163.
14. Willman CL, Sever CE, Pallavicini MG, et al. Deletion of IRF-1 mapping to chromosome 5q31.1, in human leukemia and preleukemic myelodysplasia. Science 1993;259:968.
15. Ihle NJ. Cytokine receptor signalling. Nature 1995;377:591.
16. Muench MO, Schneider JG, Moore MAS. Interactions among colony stimulating factors, IL-1β, IL-6 and Kit-Ligand (KL) in the regulation of primitive murine hematopoietic cells. Exp Hematol 1992;20:339.
17. Young JW, Szabolcs P, Moore MAS. Identification of dendritic cell colony-forming units among normal human $CD34^+$ bone marrow progenitors that are expanded by c-kit-ligand and yield pure dendritic cell colonies in the presence of granulocyte/macrophage colony-stimulating factor and tumor necrosis factor α. J Exp Med 1995;182:1111.
18. Szabolcs P, Avigan D, Gezelter S, et al. Dendritic cells and macrophages can mature independently from a human bone marrow-derived, post-colony-forming unit intermediate. Blood 1996;87:4520.
19. Randolph GJ, Beaulieu S, Lebecque S, Steinman RM, Muller WA. Differentiation of monocytes into dendritic cells in a model of transendothelial trafficking. Science 1998;282:480.
20. Deresinski SC. Granulocyte-macrophage colony-stimulating factor: potential therapeutic, immunological and antiretroviral effects in HIV infection. AIDS 1999;13:633.
21. Metcalf D. The granulocyte-macrophage regulators: Reappraisal by gene inactivation. Exp Hematol 1995;23:569.
22. Nishinakamura R, Miyajima A, Mee PJ, et al. Hematopoiesis in mice lacking the entire granulocyte-macrophage colony-stimulating factor/Interleukin-3/Interleukin-5 functions. Blood 1996;88:2458.
23. Gabrilove JL, Jakubowski A, Fain K, et al. Phase I study of granulocyte colony-stimulating factor in patients with transitional cell carcinoma of the urothelium. J Clin Invest 1988;82:1454.
24. Lord BI, Bronchud MH, Owens S, et al. The kinetics of human granulopoiesis following treatment with granulocyte colony-stimulating factor in vivo. Proc Natl Acad Sci USA 1989;86:9499.
25. Herrmann F, Schultz G, Lindemann A, et al. Hematopoietic responses in patients with advanced malignancy treated with recombinant human granulocyte-macrophage colony-stimulating factor. J Clin Oncol 1989;7:159.
26. Aglietta M, Piacibello W, Sanavio F, et al. Kinetics of human hemopoietic cells after in vivo administration of granulocyte-macrophage colony-stimulating factor. J Clin Invest 1989;83:551.

27. Kaplan SS, Basford RE, Wing E, et al. The effect of recombinant human granulocyte-macrophage colony-stimulating factor on neutrophil activation in patients with refractory carcinoma. Blood 1989;73:636.
28. Addison IE, Johnson B, Devereux S, et al. Granulocyte-macrophage colony-stimulating factor may inhibit neutrophil migration in vivo. Clin Exp Immunol 1989;76:149.
29. Branchud MH, Scarffe JH, Thatcher N, et al. Phase I/II study of recombinant human granulocyte colony-stimulating factor in patients receiving intensive chemotherapy for small cell lung cancer. Br J Cancer 1987;56:908.
30. Crawford J, Ozer H, Stoller R, et al. Reduction by granulocyte colony-stimulating factor of fever and neutropenia induced by chemotherapy in patients with small-cell lung cancer. N Engl J Med 1991;315:164.
31. Johnston EM, Crawford J. Hematopoietic growth factors in the reduction of chemotherapeutic toxicity. Semin Oncol 1998;25:552.
32. American Society for Clinical Oncology Ad Hoc Colony-Stimulating Factor Guidelines Expert Panel. Update of recommendations for the use of hematopoietic colony stimulating factors: Evidence-based clinical practice guidelines. J Clin Oncol 1996;14:1957.
33. Molineaux G, Kinstler O, Briddle B, et al. A new form of Filgrastim with sustained duration in vivo and enhanced ability to mobilize PBPC in both mice and humans. Exp Hematol 1999;27:1724.
34. Clemons M, Gharif R, Howell A. The value of dose intensification of standard chemotherapy for advanced breast cancer using colony-stimulating factors alone. Cancer Treat Rev 1998;24:173.
35. Miyauchi J, Kelleher CA, Yang TC, et al. The effects of three recombinant growth factors, IL-3, GM-CSF, and G-CSF, on the blast cells of acute myeloblastic leukemia maintained in short-term suspension culture. Blood 1987;70:657.
36. Dombert H. Granulocyte colony-stimulating factor in combination with intensive chemotherapy in the treatment of acute myeloid leukemia. Leuk Res 1998;22:1137.
37. Ohno R. Granulocyte colony-stimulating factor, granulocyte-macrophage colony-stimulating factor and macrophage colony-stimulating factor in the treatment of acute myeloid leukemia and acute lymphoblastic leukemia. Leuk Res 1998;22:1143.
38. Zittoun R, Suciu S, Mandelli F, et al. Granulocyte-macrophage colony-stimulating factor associated with induction treatment of acute myelogenous leukemia: a randomized trial by the European Organization for Research and Treatment of Cancer Leukemia Cooperative Group. J Clin Oncol 1996;14:2150.
39. Estey E. Hematopoietic growth factors in the treatment of acute leukemia. Curr Opin Oncol 1998;10:23.
40. Buchner T, Hiddemann W, Wormann B, et al, for the AML Cooperative Group. Hematopoietic growth factors in acute myeloid leukemia. Hematol Blood Transfusion 1996;38:445.
41. Giralt S, Escudier S, Kantarjian H, et al. Treatment with filgrastim for relapse of leukemia and myelodysplasia after allogeneic bone marrow transplantation: preliminary observations. N Engl J Med 1993;329:757.
42. Ganser A, Karthaus M. Clinical use of hematopoietic growth factors in the myelodysplastic syndromes. Leuk Lymphoma 1997;26 (Suppl 1):13.
43. Brandt SJ, Peters WP, Atwater SK, et al. Effect of recombinant human granulocyte-macrophage colony-stimulating factor on hematopoietic reconstitution after high-dose chemotherapy and autologous bone marrow transplantation. N Engl J Med 1988;318:896.
44. Linch DC, Scarffe H, Proctor S, et al. Randomized vehicle-controlled dose-finding study of glycosylated recombinant human granulocyte colony-stimulating factor after bone marrow transplantation. Bone Marrow Transplant 1993;11:307.
45. De Witte T, Gratwhol A, Van Der Lely N, et al. Recombinant human granulocyte-macrophage colony-stimulating factor accelerates neutrophil and monocyte recovery after allogeneic T-cell-depleted bone marrow transplantation. Blood 1992;79:1359.
46. Gianni AM, Sienna S, Bregni M, et al. Granulocyte-macrophage colony-stimulating factor to harvest circulating haemopoietic stem cells for autotransplantation. Lancet 1989;2:580.
47. Sienna S, Bregni M, Brando B, et al. Circulation of $CD34^+$ hematopoietic stem cells in the peripheral blood of high-dose cyclophosphamide-treated patients: enhancement by intravenous recombinant human granulocyte-macrophage colony-stimulating factor. Blood 1989;74:1905.
48. Shpall EJ. The utilization of cytokines in stem cell mobilization strategies. Bone Marrow Transplant 1999;23(Suppl 2):S13.
49. Shpall EJ, Wheeler CA, Turner SA, et al. A randomized Phase 3 study of peripheral blood progenitor cell mobilization with stem cell factor and filgrastim in high risk breast cancer patients. Blood 1999;8:2491.
50. Kritz A, Crown P, Motzer RJ, et al. Beneficial impact of peripheral blood progenitor cells in patients with metastatic breast cancer treated with high-dose chemotherapy plus granulocyte-macrophage colony-stimulating factor, a randomized trial. Cancer 1993;71:2515.
51. Chao NJ, Schriber JR, Grimes K, et al. Granulocyte colony-stimulating factor 'mobilized' peripheral blood progenitor cells accelerate granulocyte and platelet recovery after high-dose chemotherapy. Blood 1993;81:2031.
52. Peters WP, Rosner G, Ross M, et al. Comparative effects of granulocyte-macrophage colony-stimulating factor (GM-CSF) on priming peripheral blood progenitor cells for use with autologous bone marrow after high-dose chemotherapy. Blood 1993;81:1709.
53. Shea TC. Introduction: Current issues in high-dose chemotherapy and stem cell support. Bone Marrow Transplant 1999;23(Suppl 2) S1.
54. Beelen DW, Ottinger HD, Elmagaci A, et al. Transplantation of filgrastim-mobilized peripheral blood stem cells from HLA-identical siblings or alternative family donors in patients with hematological malignancies; a prospective comparison of clinical outcome, immune reconstitution, and hematopoietic chimerism. Blood 1997;90:3296.
55. Gillio AP, Gabrilove JL. Cytokine treatment of inherited bone marrow failure syndromes. Blood 1993;81:1669.
56. Dale DC, Bonilla MA, Davis MS, et al. The neutropenia study group: a randomized, controlled phase II trial of recombinant human G-CSF in treatment of patients with severe chronic neutropenia. Blood 1993;81:2496.
57. Ward AC, van Aesch YM, Gits J, et al. Novel point mutation in the extracellular domain of the granulocyte colony-stimulating factor (G-CSF) receptor in a case of severe congenital neutropenia hyporesponsive to G-CSF treatment. J Exp Med 1999;190:497.
58. Moore MAS. Clinical implications of positive and negative hematopoietic stem cell regulators. Review Stratton Lecture. Blood 1991;78:1.
59. Papadaki HA, Giouremou K, Eliopoulos GD. Low frequency of myeloid progenitor cells in chronic idiopathic neutropenia of adults may be related to increased production of TGF-beta1 by bone marrow stromal cells. Eur J Haematol 1999;63:154.
60. Hoshina Y, Moriuchi J, Nakamura Y, et al. CD4+ T cell mediated leukopenia of Feltys syndrome successfully treated with granulocyte-colony-stimulating factor and methotrexate. Arthritis Rheum 1994;37:298.
61. Armitage JO. Emerging applications of recombinant human granulocyte-macrophage colony-stimulating factor. Blood 1998;92:4491.
62. Swindells S, Kleinschmidt DR, Hayes FA. Pilot study of adjunctive GM-CSF (yeast-derived) for fluconazole-resistant oral candidiasis in HIV-1 infection. Infect Dis Clin Prac 1997;6:278.
63. Tarr PE, Lin R, Mueller EA, et al. Evaluation of tolerability and antibody response after recombinant human granulocyte-macrophage colony-stimulating factor (rhGM-CSF) and a single dose of recombinant hepatitis B vaccine. Vaccine 1996;14:119.
64. Hess G, Kreiter F, Kosters W, et al. The effect of granulocyte-macrophage colony-stimulating factor (GM-CSF) on hepatitis B vaccination in haemodialysis patients. J Viral Hepatitis 1996;3:149.
65. Spitler LE, Grossbard ML, Ernstoff MS, et al. Adjuvant therapy of stage III and IV malignant melanoma using yeast derived, GM-CSF. Melanoma Res 1997;7:160.
66. Richard C, Baro J, Bello-Fernandez C, et al. Recombinant human granulocyte-macrophage colony stimulating factor (rhGM-CSF) administration after autologous bone marrow transplantation for acute myeloblastic leukemia enhances activated killer cell function and may diminish leukemic relapse. Bone Marrow Transplant 1995;15:721.

67. Marques da Costa R, Jesus FM, Aniceto C, et al. Double-blind randomized placebo-controlled trial of the use of granulocyte-macrophage colony-stimulating factor I chronic leg ulcers. Am J Surg 1997;173:165.
68. Raderer M, Kornek G, Hejna M, et al. Topical granulocyte-macrophage colony-stimulating factor in patients with cancer and impaired wound healing. J Natl Cancer Inst 1997;89:263.
69. Wada H, Noguchi Y, Marino MW, et al. T cell function in granulocyte-macrophage colony-stimulating factor deficient mice. Proc Natl Acad Sci USA 1997;94:12257.
70. Deresinski SC. Granulocyte-macrophage colony-stimulating factor: potential therapeutic, immunological and antiretroviral effects in HIV infection. AIDS 1999;13:633.
71. San Miguel JF, Hernandez MD, Gonzalez M, et al. A randomized study comparing the effect of GM-CSF and G-CSF on immune reconstitution after autologous bone marrow transplantation. Br J Haematol 1996;94:140.
72. Barbaro G, Di Lorenzo G, Grisorino B, et al. Effect of recombinant human granulocyte-macrophage colony stimulating factor on HIV-related leukopenia: a randomized controlled clinical study. AIDS 1997;11:1453.
73. Jacobson MA, Liu RC, Davies D, et al. Human immunodeficiency virus disease-related neutropenia and the risk of hospitalization for bacterial infection. Arch Intern Med 1997;64:328.
74. Hermans P, Sommereijns B, Van Cutsem N, et al. Neutropenia in patients with HIV infection: A case control study in a cohort of 1403 patients between 1982 and 1993. J Hematother Stem Cell Res 1999;8(Suppl 1):S23.
75. Foote M, Welch W. Review. biopharmaceutical drug development: Filgrastin (r-metHuG-CSF) used in patients with HIV infection. J Hematother Stem Cell Res 1999;8(Suppl 1):S3.
76. Kuritzkes DR, Parenti D, Ward DJ, et al. Filgrastim prevents severe neutropenia and reduces infective morbidity in patients with advanced HIV infection: results of a randomized, multicenter, controlled trial. AIDS 1998;12:65.
77. Keiser P, Rademacher S, Smith J, et al. G-CSF association with prolonged survival in HIV-infected patients with disseminated *Mycobacterium avium* complex infection. Int J AIDS 1998;9:394.
78. Zuccotti GV, Plebani A, Biasucci G, et al. Granulocyte-colony stimulating factor and erythropoietin therapy in children with human immunodeficiency virus infection. J Int Med Res 1996;24:115.
79. Hartung T. Anti-inflammatory aspects of filgrastim and impact on IL-2 release. J Hematother Stem Cell Res 1999;8(Suppl 1):S21.
80. Pajkrt D, Manten A, van der Poll T, et al. Modulation of cytokine release and neutrophil function by granulocyte colony-stimulating factor during endotoxemia in humans. Blood 1997;90:1915.
81. Weiss M, Moldawer LL, Schneider EM. Granulocyte colony-stimulating factor to prevent the progression of systemic nonresponsiveness in systemic inflammatory response syndrome and sepsis. Blood 1999;93:425.
82. Freeman BD, Quezado M, Zeni M, et al. rG-CSF reduces endotoxemia and improves survival during *E. coli* pneumonia. J Appl Physiol 1997;83:1467.
83. Nelson S, Farkas S, Fotheringham N, et al. Filgrastim in the treatment of hospitalized patients with community-acquired pneumonia. J Infect Dis 1998;178:1075.
84. Gough A, Clapperton M, Rolando N, et al. Randomized placebo-controlled trial of granulocyte-colony stimulating factor in diabetic foot infection. Lancet 1997;350:855.
85. Root RK, Dale DC. Granulocyte colony-stimulating factor and granulocyte-macrophage colony stimulating factor: comparisons and potential for use in the treatment of infections in nonneutropenic patients. J Infect Dis 1999;179(Suppl 2):S342.
86. Tiegs G, Barsigg J, Matiba B, et al. Potentiation by granulocyte-macrophage colony-stimulating factor of lipopolysaccharide toxicity in mice. J Clin Invest 1994;93:2616.
87. Lieschke GJ, Cebon J, Morstyn G. Characterization of the clinical effects after the first dose of bacterially synthesized recombinant human granulocyte-macrophage colony-stimulating factor. Blood 1989;74:2634.
88. Nimer SD, Champlin RE, Golde DW. Serum cholesterol lowering activity of granulocyte-macrophage colony-stimulating factor. JAMA 1988;260:3297.
89. Ishibashi T, Yokoyama K, Shindo J, et al. Potent cholesterol-lowering effect by human granulocyte-macrophage colony-stimulating factor in rabbits. Possible implications of enhancement of macrophage functions and an increase in mRNA for VLDL receptor. Arterioscler Thromb 1994;14:1534.
90. Tao M-H, Levy R. Idiotype/granulocyte-macrophage colony-stimulating factor fusion protein as a vaccine for B-cell lymphoma. Nature 1993;362:755.
91. Disis ML, Bernhard H, Shiota FM, et al. An effective adjuvant for protein and peptide base vaccines. Blood 1996;88:602.
92. Kurane S, Arca MT, Aruga A, et al. Cytokines as an adjuvant to tumor vaccines: Efficacy of local methods of delivery. Ann Surg Oncol 1997;4:579.
93. Simpons JW, Jafee EM, Weber CE, et al. Bioactivity of autologous irradiated renal cell carcinoma vaccines generated by ex vivo granulocyte-macrophage colony-stimulating factor gene transfer. Cancer Res 1997;57:1537.
94. Ellem KA, O'Rourke MG, Johnson GR, et al. A case report: Immune responses and clinical course of the first use of granulocyte/macrophage colony-stimulating factor-transduced autologous melanoma cells for immunotherapy. Cancer Immunol Immunother 1997;44:10.
95. Wortham C, Grinberg L, Kaslow DC, et al. Enhanced protective antibody response to PspA after intranasal or subcutaneous injections of PspA genetically fused to granulocyte-macrophage colony-stimulating factor or interleukin-2. Infect Immun 1998;66:1513.
96. McNeel DG, Schiffman K, Disis ML. Immunization with recombinant human granulocyte-macrophage colony-stimulating factor as a vaccine adjuvant elicits both a cellular and humoral response to recombinant human granulocyte-macrophage colony-stimulating factor. Blood 1999;93:2653.

Chapter 115 Interleukins and Interferons

Dimitrios T. Boumpas, Calman Prussin, Gülbû Uzel and JoAnn M. Mican

Cytokines are soluble proteins produced by a variety of cells including those of the immune system that function in a paracrine and/or autocrine fashion. Major categories of cytokines include interleukins and interferons. These cytokines mediate many different actions depending on the target cell affected. Cytokines have been identified as playing a central role in initiating and controlling immune responses, making these proteins potential therapeutic agents for the treatment of a variety of human diseases.

Natural interferons were first studied in the treatment of human disease, primarily malignancies and viral infections, in the late 1960s and early 1970s. Limited availability of natural cytokines hindered early clinical studies. However the advent of recombinant DNA technology generating readily available purified cytokines has allowed the clinical study of cytokines in many diseases. In this chapter the status of interferons and interleukins in the treatment of infectious diseases, malignancy, immunodeficiency, allergic disease, and autoimmunity is discussed.

TREATMENT OF INFECTIOUS DISEASES

Appreciation of the critical role interferons and interleukins play in maintaining normal immune function and specifically their role in the host defense to pathogenic agents led to the investigation of their use in the treatment of various infectious diseases. Included in this section will be a discussion of their application in the treatment of hepatitis B, hepatitis C, condylomata acuminata, recurrent respiratory papillomatosis, HIV, mycobacterial infections, leprosy and leishmanial infections.

Hepatitis B

The hepatitis B virus (HBV), a hepadnavirus, is a small DNA virus that causes chronic infection in approximately 400 million people worldwide. In many of these individuals this leads to cirrhosis and hepatocellular carcinoma. Since 1981 an effective vaccine for HBV has been available and recent reductions in the prevalence of infection, development of HBV carrier state, and incidence of hepatocellular carcinoma have been reported.[1] In spite of this, there remain millions of chronically infected individuals who require treatment to decrease the progression to cirrhosis and hepatocellular carcinoma.

Several reviews of chronic HBV infection have recently been written[1,2] and should be referred to for more in-depth discussion of the disease and treatment. Chronic HBV infection is characterized by ongoing viral replication, as evidenced by the presence of HBV DNA and usually hepatitis B e antigen (HBeAg) in serum. The goal of therapy is to stop progression of liver injury by suppressing viral replication since cirrhosis is unusual in patients in whom viral replication is suppressed.[1] Remissions are diagnosed based on the loss of markers of active viral replication, and sustained loss of markers results in biochemical, clinical, and histological remission.

Interferon-α (IFN-α) was the first agent demonstrated to have a beneficial effect on chronic HBV infection and received FDA approval for this indication in 1992. A course of 4–6 months' duration in doses of 5 million units (MU) daily or 10 MU subcutaneously 3 times per week induces long-term remission in 25–40% of patients.[2] A meta-analysis of 15 randomized, controlled trials revealed that 33% of patients treated with IFN-α lost HBeAg from the serum versus 12% of controls, and 37% lost serum HBV DNA versus 17% of controls.[3] A long-term follow-up study of 103 patients treated with IFN-α revealed that clearance of HBeAg was the strongest predictor for survival with 5-year survival without complications of 95% compared to less than 50% in those patients who did not clear HBeAg.[4] Overall survival as well as survival without complications was significantly longer in those who cleared HBeAg after IFN-α treatment.

Current recommendations for therapy with IFN-α include elevations of serum aminotransferases, detectable levels of HBsAg, HBeAg, HBV DNA in serum, chronic hepatitis on liver biopsy and compensated liver disease. Factors that predict those patients who will have a favorable response include low HBV DNA level (<200 pg/dl), high serum aminotransferase levels (>100 U/l) and moderate to severe inflammation on liver biopsy.[1] Factors that predict for a poor response include immunosuppression, normal serum aminotransferase levels and decompensated cirrhosis.[1]

Hepatitis C

Hepatitis C (HCV) infection is caused by a RNA virus that is a member of the Flaviviridae family. Worldwide there are more than 100 million persons infected with HCV. Approximately 70–80% of infected individuals will become chronic carriers of HCV, most having mild disease with slow progression, however 15–20% will progress over decades to develop cirrhosis, end-stage liver disease, and in some, liver cancer. Several reviews of HCV infection have recently been written[5,6] and should be referred to for more detailed discussion of the disease and treatment.

IFN-α was the first agent shown to be effective in the treatment of chronic HCV infection. In the late 1980s, several randomized studies were published demonstrating temporary remissions in approximately 40% of patients treated with a regimen of 2–3 MU of recombinant IFN-α, three times weekly for 24 weeks.[7,8] However, relapses were common, occurring in greater than 50% of those treated.

In March 1997, a consensus conference sponsored by the NIH recommended that patients who have persistently abnormal alanine aminotransferase levels, HCV RNA in serum, and evidence on liver biopsy of either fibrosis or moderate degrees of inflammation, be treated with IFN-α 3 MU three times weekly for 12 months. Patients with persistently normal aminotransferase levels and mild hepatitis as well as those with decompensated cirrhosis should not be treated outside of a clinical trial.[9]

Since the consensus conference there have been important advances in the management of HCV infection. Several large multicenter, prospective controlled trials have shown that the combination of IFN-α with ribavirin (a nucleoside analog) provides higher sustained responses than IFN-α alone,[10,11] including select patients who relapsed following IFN-α monotherapy.[12] Although long-term follow-up is not available for the combination IFN-α/ribavirin studies, it has been found that the majority of patients who remain in remission at 6 months post IFN-α monotherapy continue to be HCV RNA negative and show improvement in liver inflammation and fibrosis 10 years later.[13,14]

Clearly, more effective therapies are needed for the treatment of HCV infection. Interleukin 10 (IL-10) is an anti-inflammatory cytokine that modulates hepatic fibrogenesis. Recently, in a randomized, double-blinded study, IL-10 was shown to normalize alanine aminotransferase levels, improve liver histology, and reduce liver fibrosis in greater than 50% of those treated.[15] Similar to ribavirin monotherapy studies, reductions in serum HCV RNA levels were not seen. These results are encouraging and suggest that IL-10 may be a therapeutic option in patients chronically infected with hepatitis C. However the most exciting new treatment is polyethylene glycol-conjugated IFN-α, with preliminary response rates approximately double that seen utilizing standard IFN-α preparations.

Diseases caused by human papilloma viruses – condylomata acuminata and recurrent respiratory papillomatosis

Condylomata acuminata (genital warts) is a sexually transmitted disease caused by papillomaviruses, usually types 6 and 11. Studies of IFN effectiveness in the treatment of diseases caused by papillomaviruses date back to 1974, when leukocyte IFN was injected into a patient's plantar warts, causing the warts to disappear and reappear with discontinuation of the IFN injections.[16] Numerous studies have followed, demonstrating effectiveness of local injections of IFN-β in treating common warts,[17] subcutaneous injections of IFN-γ or IFN-α for treating condylomata acuminata, and local injections of IFN-α for treating condylomata acuminata.[18] Intralesional injection of IFN-α has gained FDA approval for the treatment of condylomata acuminata.

Recurrent respiratory papillomatosis (RRP) is a disease characterized by recurrent growth of benign papillomas throughout the respiratory tract. The causative agent of RRP is believed to be human papillomavirus (HPV). HPV types 6 and 11 have consistently been identified in the excised papilloma of patients with respiratory papillomatosis. RRP occurs in both children (juvenile onset, <5 years) and adults (adult onset, >20 years) and most patients are treated successfully with a limited number of endoscopic laser excisions or surgery. In other patients the papillomas regrow rapidly, spread to uninvolved sites, require numerous excisions, and can result in airway obstruction. For patients with aggressive RRP, several adjuvant drug therapies have been studied.

> **KEY CONCEPTS**
>
> **Cytokine applications for infectious diseases**
> - IFN-α induces long-term remissions in 25–40% of patients with chronic hepatitis B infection.
> - Combination treatment with IFN-α and ribavirin induces long-term remissions in 41% of patients with chronic hepatitis C infection.
> - IFN is effective for the treatment of condylomata acuminata and recurrent respiratory papillomatosis.
> - IL-2 combined with antiretroviral medications increases CD4 counts in HIV-infected patients.
> - There is encouraging early experience with IFN-γ in treatment of nontuberculous mycobacteria, leprosy, and leishmanial infections.

In 1981, Haglund et al reported the open-label use of IFN-α administered subcutaneously in 7 patients with severe juvenile onset RRP.[19] While on treatment the papillomas decreased in size. Progression was seen when IFN-α was discontinued, however regression again occurred with the reinstitution of IFN-α. Several open-label studies followed that displayed similar results.

In 1988, Leventhal et al reported the results of a randomized, crossover IFN-α trial in 66 patients with juvenile onset RRP.[20] Half of the patients received IFN-α-n1 intramuscularly 5 MU/m^2 daily for 28 days and then 3 times weekly for 5 months, followed by 6 months of observation. The other half were observed for 6 months and then treated. During periods of drug administration there was a statistically significant decrease in extent and severity of disease. Nine of 57 patients with assessable airway disease achieved complete remission while no patients achieved complete remission during 6 months of observation alone. As was seen in prior reports, the patients who discontinued drug therapy showed a significant rise in score within 4 months.

A long-term follow-up of this study was published in 1991, revealed approximately a 40% complete remission and a 40% partial remission rate over a 5-year period.[21] Based on the results of this study it has been recommended that patients with RRP who require surgery every 2–3 months be given a 6 month trial of IFN-α. To date, a clinical trial establishing the optimal dose and duration of treatment with IFN-α for RRP has not been published.

Human immunodeficiency virus (HIV)

HIV infection results in a severe cellular immunodeficiency disease, characterized by decreased CD4 cells, that results in the development of opportunistic infections and other complications (Chapter 38, 39). Treatment of HIV-infected patients consists of antimicrobial prophylaxis and combination antiretroviral therapy to suppress HIV replication. Although much success has been achieved with these therapies, complete suppression of virus replication is not possible with current antiretroviral medications. In addition, maximal suppression of HIV replication is often difficult to achieve and/or maintain in many HIV-infected patients. One complementary treatment approach that has been evaluated is the use of interleukin 2 (IL-2).

IL-2 is a T-cell-derived cytokine with many effects on the immune system including activation, proliferation, and differentiation of both T and B lymphocytes and natural killer (NK) cells (Chapter 12). Early in vitro studies culturing peripheral blood mononuclear cells from patients with AIDS in IL-2 demonstrated improvement in defective T-cell proliferative responses to antigen and mitogen, NK-cell activity, antigen-specific cytotoxic lymphocyte activity, and production of IFN-γ.[22]

In 1995, Kovacs et al published an open-label study of 10 HIV-infected patients who received IL-2, 18 million IU/day intravenously, for 5 days, every 8 weeks.[23] Six of 10 patients with baseline CD4 cell counts above 200 cells/mm³ experienced sustained increases in CD4 cell counts. In 1996, a randomized controlled study of IL-2 therapy in HIV-infected patients corroborated the earlier observations.[24] In this study, 60 patients with CD4 cell counts above 200 cells/mm³ were randomized to receive either nucleoside analog antiretrovirals alone or in combination with 6 cycles of intravenous IL-2 administered every 2 months, for 5 days, starting at a dose of 18 million IU/day. At the end of 12 months, the mean CD4 count increased from 428+/–25 cells/mm³ at baseline to 916+/–128 cells/mm³ in the IL-2 group, compared to a decrease in the mean CD4 count from 404+/–29 cells/mm³ to 349+/–41 cells/mm³ in the control group ($P<0.001$) (Fig. 115.1).

Adverse effects commonly seen in these studies include constitutional symptoms of a 'flu-like' illness (fever, chills, fatigue, myalgias and arthralgias), nausea, vomiting, diarrhea, sinus congestion, rash, pruritus, and local erythematous reactions at the sites of subcutaneous injections. Laboratory abnormalities include: low serum levels of calcium, magnesium, albumin and sodium; elevated hepatic aminotransferases and bilirubin; and anemia and thrombocytopenia. Additional studies have followed, including studies of intermittent subcutaneous administration of IL-2,[25] that continue to demonstrate increases in CD4 cell counts and also demonstrated that the severity of adverse effects is generally dose related and that subcutaneously administered IL-2 appears better tolerated than intravenously administered IL-2. In addition, a recent pooled analysis of three randomized controlled studies of IL-2 revealed not only a higher mean change from baseline CD4 cell count (368 vs 153 cells/l; $P = 0.003$) but also demonstrated a significantly lower mean change from baseline plasma HIV RNA (–0.98 vs –0.63 log copies/ml; $P = 0.004$) in patients randomized to receive IL-2.[26]

The above cited studies were all performed before the use of potent antiretroviral therapy (ART). Recently, a randomized controlled multicenter trial of subcutaneous IL-2 therapy in combination with ART demonstrated that in the IL-2 group the mean percentage increase in CD4 cell counts at 1 year was 112% compared with 18% in recipients of ART alone ($P <0.001$).[27] Again, a significant decrease in HIV viral RNA level was seen in the group receiving IL-2 (–0.28 vs 0.09 log(10) copies; $P = 0.03$). Whether the findings in these studies will translate into improved clinical outcomes in HIV-infected patients is still not known, however, phase III clinical end-point trials are currently underway to address this question. IL-2 therapy of patients with HIV-1 infection is not FDA-approved and should be administered as part of clinical trials designed to help further elucidate the role of IL-2 in the management of patients who are infected with HIV.

IFN-α, known to inhibit HIV-1 replication in cell culture, has been studied since the 1980s for the treatment of patients infected with HIV-1. Results of these studies have yielded variable results, however some did reveal significantly lower mean changes from baseline plasma HIV RNA levels in the groups randomized to receive IFN-α.[28] The decreases in HIV-1 RNA levels have been modest at best and these studies were conducted prior to the use of potent antiretroviral therapy.

Mycobacterial infections

Nontuberculous mycobacteria (NTM) are ubiquitous organisms that have low intrinsic virulence. Infections caused by NTM in

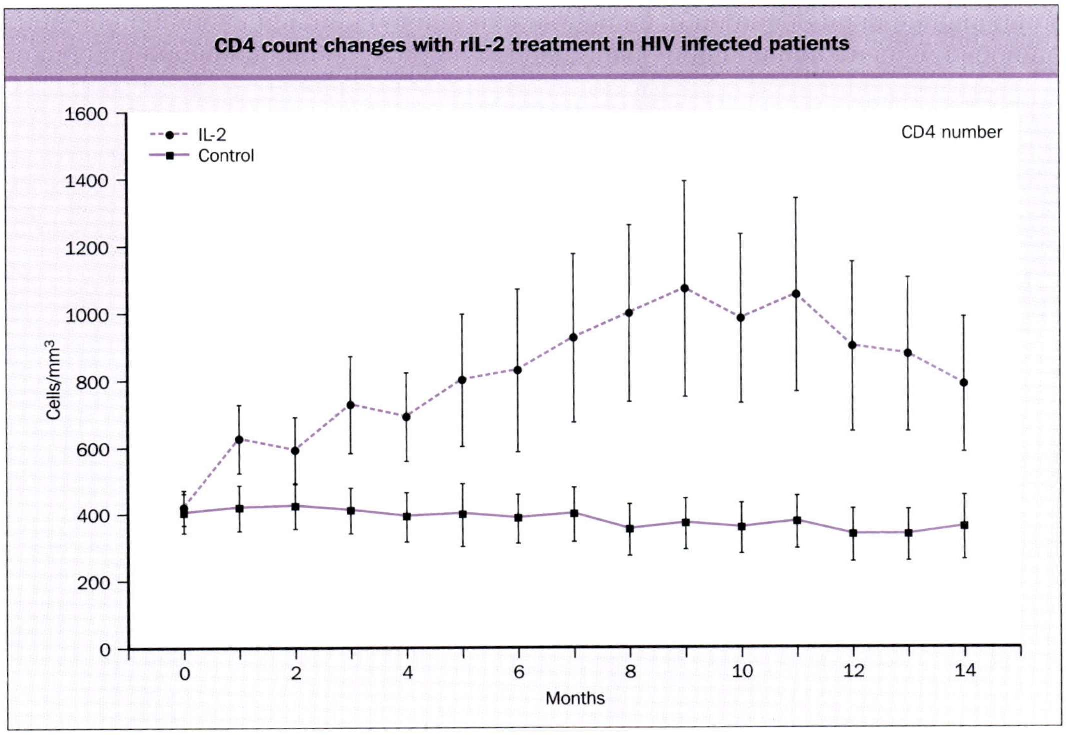

Figure 115.1 CD4 count changes with rIL-2. Change in CD4 lymphocyte counts during a randomized trial of intravenously administered IL-2 and antiretroviral drugs or antiretroviral drugs alone. (Reprinted in modified form from Kovacs JA, Vogel S, Albert JM, et al. Controlled trial of interleukin-2 infusions in patients infected with the human immunodeficiency virus. *N Engl J Med* 1996;335:1350.)

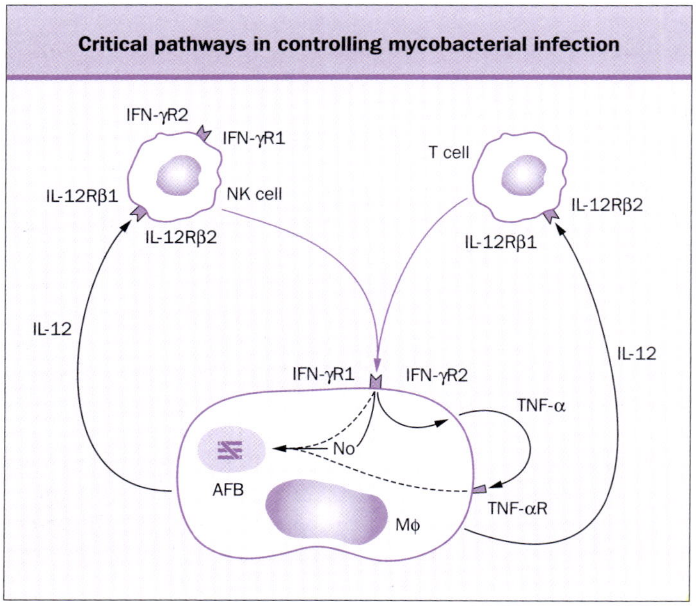

Figure 115.2 Critical pathways in controlling mycobacterial infection.

otherwise low-risk patients have helped us understand the host factors involved in immunity against mycobacteria. Signaling pathways in monocytes and macrophages via cytokines and their receptors have been shown to be critically important in the containment of mycobacterial disease (Fig. 115.2). In 1994, Holland et al reported that IFN-γ, when used in combination with conventional antimycobacterial therapy, could be useful in the treatment of refractory disseminated NTM infections.[29] Recently, disseminated infections with NTM or BCG have been linked to defined genetic defects in the IFN-γ/IL-12 pathways as well as to familial or sporadic cases with unknown molecular defects, patients with isolated CD4 lymphopenia, and those with HIV infection or immunosuppression. A number of these patient groups have been the focal point for exploring cytokine therapy, mainly involving IFN-γ.[30–37]

Patients with abnormal IL-12 and/or IFN-γ production or idiopathic CD4 lymphocytopenia in the absence of HIV infection form the main group affected by NTM. Among this cohort, those who have an intact IFN-γ receptor (R) have distinct mitogen responses with typically low IFN-γ production in response to phytohemagglutinin, yet their genetic defect remains unknown.[35] A combination of antimycobacterial agents and IFN-γ administered subcutaneously at a dose of 50 μg/m² body surface area three times per week in patients with disseminated NTM infection cleared the infection and blood cultures while improving clinical condition in most patients.[29,38] Treatment should be extended until the disease is eradicated or significant clinical improvement is achieved; IFN-γ therapy may be required for one year or longer. Side-effects related to IFN-γ include low-grade fever, headache, and joint and muscle pain, all of which are easily managed with oral acetaminophen prior to the dose. Relapse of infection is not uncommon when IFN-γ is discontinued despite continuation of the antibiotics. This is likely due to the fact that the underlying immunologic problem persists.[38]

In complete IFN-γ R1 and complete IFN-γ R2 deficiencies, the cells do not respond to IFN-γ. In partial IFN-γ R1 deficiency, patients have an intermediate phenotype between normal and complete IFN-γ R1 deficiency, and a response to IFN-γ can be achieved in vitro at higher than normal concentrations.[30]

Localized pulmonary disease secondary to NTM infection is a separate entity from disseminated disease. This is commonly seen in patients with underlying structural lung problems (i.e. bronchiectasis, cystic fibrosis, smoking) or elderly women with slight body habitus. The underlying predisposition at the genetic or cellular level remains unknown but treatment of this cohort of patients with systemic administration of IFN-γ is being studied. The best results with IFN-γ have been achieved in those with non cavitary lung disease (Holland SM, unpublished data). There is one case report of a partial response to aerosolized IFN-γ in a cavitary pulmonary NTM infection.[39]

Studies of IFN-γ use in AIDS-related NTM infection are limited but it is clear that IFN-γ works as an adjuvant only in combination with anti-mycobacterials in this setting. IFN-γ effects were observed in the presence of low CD4⁺ T-cell counts, suggesting some T cell-independent effect.[40]

Open-label, intradermal IL-2 has been studied in conjunction with conventional antituberculous therapy in small numbers of patients infected with multidrug resistant tuberculosis (MDRTB). Some patients appeared to demonstrate improved bacillary clearance from sputum along with improvement in radiographs and enhanced immunity to *Mycobacterium tuberculosis* in vitro.[41]

Lepromatous leprosy

Nathan et al first used IFN-γ in the treatment of lepromatous leprosy at a dose of 1–10 μg/day injected directly into the cutaneous lesion daily for three days in addition to antimicrobials.[42] IFN-γ was shown to enhance granuloma formation and markers of local inflammation, and decrease cutaneous bacterial burden. In long-term studies of IFN-γ in leprosy, erythema nodosum leprosum (ENL), a toxic immune response leading to nerve damage, was a complicating phenomenon, but was readily suppressible with thalidomide. Sixty per cent of patients treated with the combination of IFN-γ and antimycobacterial drugs developed ENL compared to 17% of those treated with anti mycobacterial drugs alone.[43] It is not clear if this effect is truly related to long-term IFN-γ therapy in leprosy since it is not seen in any other disease entity for which IFN-γ is used.

Low-dose IL-2, given intradermally, has been shown to reduce numbers of *Mycobacterium leprae* both at the injection site and at remote skin sites.[44] In addition, cutaneous infiltration of CD4⁺ lymphocytes, monocytes, and Langerhans cells occurred and increased levels of circulating antibody to *M. leprae* antigens were observed.

Leishmanial infections

Leishmaniasis is a protozoal infection caused by intracellular parasites of the *Leishmania* species. It has various clinical presentations including localized cutaneous, mucocutaneous, or visceral forms (kala-azar) of the disease. There are case reports of patients with refractory mucocutaneous leishmaniasis in whom the disease remitted when IFN-γ was combined with pentavalent antimony treatment.[45] Addition of IFN-γ has also been demonstrated to decrease the duration of antimony compound treatment (10 vs 20 days) needed to successfully treat the infection. In visceral leishmaniasis, patient lymphocytes are unable to produce IL-2 and IFN-γ in response to leishmanial antigens,[46] leading to defective macrophage killing of the parasite. IFN-γ, when used in combination with the standard chemotherapeutic agents, appears to fill in this gap in the cellular response at the same time as increasing the intracellular concentration of the therapeutic agents.

A single study of three patients with disseminated cutaneous leishmaniasis treated with intradermal IL-2 demonstrated findings analogous to those reported in leprosy: reductions in numbers of organisms in nodular lesions that were injected with IL-2, along with infiltration by $CD4^+$ lymphocytes and plasma cells.[47]

TREATMENT OF MALIGNANCIES

Appreciation of the critical role interferons and interleukins play in maintaining normal immune function, as well as their antiproliferative and cytolytic activity against tumor cells, led to the investigation of their use in the treatment of various malignancies. Included in this section is a discussion of their use in the treatment of Kaposi sarcoma, hairy cell leukemia, chronic myelogenous leukemia, multiple myeloma, and follicular lymphoma. In addition, the use of interleukin 11 in the treatment of chemotherapy-induced thrombocytopenia is discussed. Cytokine-based treatment of melanoma and renal cell carcinoma is discussed in Chapter 100.

AIDS-associated Kaposi sarcoma

Kaposi sarcoma (KS) is a tumor of vascular origin; there are four clinical variants including classic KS, endemic KS, immunosuppression-associated or transplantation-associated KS, and AIDS-associated KS. These variants have identical histologic features (spindle-shaped tumor cells surrounding vascular slits), but differ in the specific populations of patients affected, the sites involved, and the clinical course. In 1994, herpesvirus-like DNA sequences were identified in tissues from patients with AIDS-associated KS.[48] These identical viral sequences, called either Kaposi sarcoma-associated herpesvirus (KSHV) or herpesvirus-8 (HHV-8), have since been identified in all variants of KS (Chapter 95). Although it appears that HHV-8 is important in pathogenesis of KS, the exact role it plays in tumor formation is an area of ongoing research.

The AIDS-associated variant was one of the first recognized manifestations of AIDS. In these individuals the tumor was disseminated and had an aggressive, frequently fatal course.[49] In 1983, in an open-label study, IFN-α was found to be effective in the treatment of patients with KS.[50] High doses of IFN-α were used and dramatic tumor regression of lesions in the skin, lymph nodes, oral cavity, and gastrointestinal tract was observed, with up to 40% response rate.

Numerous studies since have corroborated these findings and shown that intralesional IFN-α is effective for cutaneous disease. In addition, lower doses of IFN-α in combination with nucleoside analog antiretroviral medications have been shown to induce tumor regression. IFN-α dosage usually starts at 5–10 MU per day given subcutaneously and is titrated based on tumor response and side-effects.[51] When IFN-α is used in combination with potent antiretroviral medications, doses as low as 1 MU per day have been found to be effective.

Hairy cell leukemia

Hairy cell leukemia (HCL) is a chronic lymphoproliferative disease characterized by splenomegaly, pancytopenia, recurrent infections, and infiltration of the bone marrow with malignant B cells that have fine, irregular cytoplasmic projections (hairy cells). Splenectomy was the first successful treatment for HCL and although most patients respond initially, nearly all patients relapse at some point following the procedure.

In 1984, Quesada first reported that IFN-α was a highly effective treatment for HCL, treating 7 patients with 3 MU intramuscularly, daily.[52] Over 2–3 months complete remissions occurred in 3 of 7 patients and partial remissions in the remaining 4 patients. Numerous studies since have confirmed the efficacy of recombinant IFN, with improvement seen in nearly all patients treated.[53,54] Administered doses are usually 2–3 MU/m^2 given subcutaneously three times a week for up to 18 months. Normalization of peripheral blood counts has occurred in 50–80% of patients treated, associated with a reduction in the incidence of serious infections and the need for transfusions.[53]

Long-term follow-up studies reveal that remissions occur in only 20–30% of patients after the initial course of treatment.[54,55] however, in patients who have relapsed, retreatment has been shown to reinduce remission.[56] Continued (maintenance) therapy for longer than 12 months has been shown to result in increased progression-free survival.[57]

The purine analogs, 2′-deoxycoformycin and 2-chlorodeoxyadenosine, result in initial remissions in greater than 90% of HCL patients treated. Long-term results reveal a relapse rate of only 20–30%.[54] Although IFN-α remains a therapeutic option for the treatment of patients with HCL, purine analogs are considered by many to be first-line treatment.

Chronic myelogenous leukemia

Chronic myelogenous leukemia (CML) is a myeloproliferative disorder characterized by increased granulocytes, the Philadelphia (Ph) chromosome, and a characteristic triphasic clinical course. It begins with a benign chronic phase, proceeds to an accelerated phase, and ends with a blastic phase, which is generally fatal. The Ph chromosome, a shortened chromosome 22, results from a reciprocal translocation between chromosomes 9 and 22 resulting in *BCR–ABL* fusion genes (Chapter 93).

Recently, several updates of the biology and treatment of CML have been published.[58,59] Allogeneic stem-cell transplantation from HLA-matched sibling donors achieves survival rates of 50–70% at 10 years; although this procedure is considered curative, only 15–20% of patients with CML are eligible because of donor availability and age restrictions. An effective alternative first-line therapy for CML patients is IFN-α.

In 1983, Talpaz et al reported hematologic remissions in 5 of 7 patients treated with IFN-α.[60] Since then, numerous studies have revealed high complete hematologic remission rates (46–80%) and complete cytogenetic response rates of 13–32% (partial of 11–16%) utilizing doses of IFN-α that ranged from 2 to 5 MU/m^2 daily. These studies also revealed that increased doses of IFN-α correlated with increased response rates, and the ability to achieve a complete cytogenetic response was an independent predictor of survival.[59]

Several randomized studies, as well as a meta-analysis of seven randomized studies of IFN-α treatment have demonstrated increased complete and partial cytogenetic responses as well as increased survival compared to chemotherapy.[59] In the meta-analysis, the 5-year survival rates were 57% with IFN-α compared to 42% with chemotherapy. More recently, several studies of

KEY CONCEPTS

Cytokine applications for malignant disease

- IFN-α is effective treatment for AIDS-associated Kaposi sarcoma.
- IFN-α induces remissions in patients with hairy cell leukemia.
- IFN-α alone or in combination with cytosine arabinoside induces hematologic and cytogenetic remissions in patients with CML.
- A meta-analysis of IFN-α therapy in patients with multiple myeloma has demonstrated increased response rates and survival benefit but its therapeutic role is unresolved.
- IFN-α in conjunction with chemotherapy delays disease progression and increases survival in patients with follicular lymphoma.
- IL-11 decreases platelet transfusion requirement and time to platelet recovery in patients receiving chemotherapy.

combination therapy with IFN-α and cytosine arabinoside have demonstrated increased complete hematologic and cytogenetic remissions and increased survival as compared to IFN-α therapy alone.[59]

IFN-α has been studied in patients with cytogenetic relapses following transplantation, resulting in 20–40% cytogenetic responses. Polyethylene glycol (PEG) conjugated IFN-α has been studied in the treatment of CML. PEG IFN-α has a longer half-life than standard IFN-α and was administered once a week. Treatment of 21 patients resulted in a 50% response rate, including 4 of 13 patients who had not responded to standard IFN-α.[61]

Although it is clear that IFN-α (along with allogeneic stem-cell transplantation) is considered a first-line therapy for CML, many questions remain. Should IFN-α be given with or without cytosine arabinoside? Will PEG IFN-α be a better tolerated and more effective form of therapy? What dose of IFN-α should be used and how long should therapy continue?

Multiple myeloma

Multiple myeloma is a disease characterized by bone marrow infiltration with malignant plasma cells that produce monoclonal immunoglobulins – usually IgG or IgA (Chapter 97). Clinically, patients develop anemia, osteolytic bone lesions, renal insufficiency, and recurrent bacterial infections. Treatment modalities include chemotherapy alone, high-dose chemotherapy with autologous stem-cell transplantation, allogeneic transplantation and IFN-α.

IFN-α treatment of patients with multiple myeloma has been studied for many years. Several early encouraging open-label studies were followed by randomized studies of maintenance therapy with IFN-α (2–3 MU/m^2, 3 times per week) versus placebo following chemotherapy induction. Significantly prolonged duration of remission and survival benefit were observed in several studies but not all.[62] A recent meta-analysis including 12 IFN-α maintenance trials (1543 patients) reported significantly prolonged progression-free survival and overall survival in the IFN-α maintenance group.[63] Studies of maintenance therapy with IFN-α and steroids (dexamethasone or prednisone) are encouraging, with early results revealing increased duration of remissions and survival.[62]

Randomized trials combining IFN-α and induction chemotherapy have also had mixed results. The recent meta-analysis[63] included 12 IFN-α trials (2469 patients) and reported significantly increased response rate, remission duration, and survival (P=0.05). The role of IFN-α is currently not settled but continues to be studied as part of induction therapy together with chemotherapy or as maintenance therapy in patients who have responded to induction therapy.

Follicular lymphoma

Follicular lymphoma is the most common subtype of non-Hodgkin lymphoma and is characterized by an indolent course with relatively long median survival (7–10 years) despite disseminated disease being present in most patients at presentation (Chapter 96). This low-grade lymphoma responds very well to most therapeutic interventions, however multiple remissions and relapses usually characterize the clinical course, even after complete initial remissions. Regardless of the initial treatment chosen, most patients eventually die from the lymphoma.[64]

IFN-α has been studied in several randomized trials of patients with follicular lymphoma and several authors recently reviewed these studies.[64–66] Delays in disease progression and survival benefit have been demonstrated in some but not all of these trials, specifically those that used an anthracycline-based combination chemotherapy induction regimen. In addition, IFN-α maintenance therapy has been shown to delay disease progression when administered after induction chemotherapy. In 1997, the FDA approved the use of IFN-α-2b in conjunction with chemotherapy for the treatment of follicular lymphoma.

Interleukin 11 for chemotherapy-induced thrombocytopenia

Interleukin 11 is a pleiotropic cytokine that stimulates the proliferation of hematopoietic stem cells and megakaryocyte progenitors and induces megakaryocyte maturation. In a multicenter trial of recombinant human IL-11 (rhIL-11) in patients with cancer who had already required platelet transfusions secondary to chemotherapy, patients were randomized to receive placebo or rhIL-11 at 50 or 25 μg/kg subcutaneously daily for 14–21 days, beginning 1 day after chemotherapy. A significant decrease in the requirement for platelet transfusions occurred in the patients receiving 50 μg/kg per day as compared to those receiving placebo.[67] In a clinical study of women with advanced breast cancer receiving cyclophosphamide, doxorubicin, and G-CSF, it was found that those who received rhIL-11 had a significant reduction in the total number of platelet transfusions required and the time to platelet recovery.[68] Adverse effects included fatigue and occasional atrial arrhythmias and syncope. In 1997 the FDA approved the use of IL-11 (Oprelvekin) for the prevention of severe thrombocytopenia following myelosuppressive chemotherapy in patients with nonmyeloid malignancies.

TREATMENT OF IMMUNODEFICIENCY DISEASES

Interferons and interleukins are integral components of the immune system. They have wide-ranging effects including the induction of cell development, differentiation, and proliferation. As such, these cytokines play critical roles in both the innate and adaptive immune responses which suggests a possible therapeutic role for managing selected immune deficiencies. Included in this section is a discussion of IFN-γ treatment of patients with chronic granulomatous disease and osteopetrosis, and IL-2 therapy of patients with common variable immunodeficiency.

Chronic granulomatous disease

Chronic granulomatous disease (CGD) of childhood is an uncommon disease characterized by disorders of phagocyte oxidative metabolism resulting in recurrent infections caused by catalase-positive microorganisms and granuloma formation secondary to severe chronic inflammation (Chapter 37). IFN-γ has been shown to reduce the number of severe infections and hospitalizations by 70% when administered subcutaneously at a dose of 50 μg/m², 3 times weekly, to patients with CGD.[69,70] It does not, however, prevent the formation, or reduce the size, of granulomas. Long-term follow-up (up to 10 years) of these patients has not revealed any unexpected toxicities or interference with growth or development related to long-term use of IFN-γ.[71,72] IFN-γ was approved by the FDA for the prophylactic treatment of CGD in 1991.

Osteopetrosis

Congenital, malignant osteopetrosis is a disease characterized by reduced leukocyte superoxide formation, an increased incidence of infections, and defective osteoclast function with decreased bone reabsorption. Most children die within the first decade of life from severe infections, neurologic deficits, or bone marrow failure. Bone marrow transplantation is curative, however only about 40% of these patients have a suitable donor.

Based on the success seen with IFN-γ treatment of patients with chronic granulomatous disease, a 6-month trial of IFN-γ 1.5 μg/kg 3 times a week, subcutaneously, was undertaken in 8 patients with osteopetrosis.[73] A significant decrease in trabecular bone volume was observed as well as an increase in hemoglobin concentration, platelet count, and superoxide leukocyte production. A follow-up study of 14 patients treated with the same regimen for 18 months revealed findings similar to the prior study. Additionally, in 6 patients for whom pretreatment data were available, a 96% decrease in the frequency of infections requiring antibiotic therapy was observed. Long-term IFN-γ therapy increases bone resorption and hematopoiesis and improves leukocyte function.[74] In 2000, the FDA approved IFN-γ1b for the treatment of malignant osteopetrosis.

Common variable immunodeficiency

Common variable immunodeficiency (CVI) is a heterogeneous syndrome characterized by hypogammaglobulinemia and recurrent bacterial infections (Chapter 34). Treatment of CVI involves aggressive treatment of infections with antibiotics and regular infusions of intravenous immunoglobulin. Many patients with CVI have abnormalities of T-cell activation and deficient secretion of cytokines including IL-2.[75] Because of this and the knowledge that IL-2 can promote the secretion of immunoglobulins in vitro, trials using IL-2 therapy have been undertaken. In a patient who received open-label polyethylene glycol-conjugated (PEG) interleukin 2, 250 000 IU/m², weekly by subcutaneous injection, increased in vitro immunoglobulin secretion, increased serum IgA and IgM levels, increased lymphocyte proliferative responses, increased mononuclear cell production of IL-2 and IL-6, and clinical improvement were demonstrated.[76] In a small, placebo-controlled, double-blind, crossover study of 10 patients, a significant reduction in severe infections was observed; however, this decrease occurred not while the patients were receiving IL-2 but during the 6 months following while receiving placebo.[77] The question of whether clinical benefit will occur in CVI patients with IL-2 treatment should be answered when the results of a large placebo-controlled study become available.

> **KEY CONCEPTS**
>
> **Cytokine applications in immunodeficiency**
> - IFN-γ reduces the number of infections and hospitalizations in patients with chronic granulomatous disease.
> - IFN-γ therapy decreases trabecular bone volume and frequency of infections and increases hemoglobin and platelet counts in patients with osteopetrosis.
> - Preliminary results suggest that IL-2 may decrease the number of infections in some patients with common variable immunodeficiency.

TREATMENT OF ALLERGIC DISEASES

Cytokines play a major role in the establishment and maintenance of allergic diseases. In particular, the presence of allergen-specific T cells of the Th2 cytokine phenotype has been associated with allergy, asthma, atopic dermatitis, and eosinophilia.[78] The cytokines expressed by Th2 cells – IL-4, 5, 9 and 13 – have distinct biological activities which account for many of the pathological features of these diseases. Conversely, pro-inflammatory cytokines such as IFN-γ as well as IFN-α antagonize some of the activities of the Th2 cytokines. With this increased understanding of the role of cytokines in allergic diseases, attempts have been made to treat allergic disease using recombinant cytokines and cytokine inhibitors.

Asthma

IFN-α and IFN-γ have both been studied in the treatment of asthma. No improvement in pulmonary function was demonstrated in a small placebo-controlled trial of IFN-α2a given to asthmatic children. However a recent case report notes a clinical response to IFN-α including improvement in airflow and decreases in corticosteroid dosage in a patient with severe corticosteroid-unresponsive asthma. Interestingly, there is a case report of 2 patients with hepatitis C and pre-existing mild asthma receiving IFN-α2b with subsequent exacerbations of their asthma.[79] In both cases the asthma was exacerbated for a second time when IFN-α therapy was resumed. In summary, it is still unclear whether IFN-α has any role in cases of severe asthma unresponsive to conventional therapy.

IFN-γ antagonizes many of the activities of Th2 cytokines and as such would appear to be a good candidate for an antiallergic cytokine therapy. There have been two trials of IFN-γ in asthma. In a blinded placebo-controlled study of 20 subjects with severe corticosteroid-dependent asthma treated with subcutaneous IFN-γ 50 μg/m²/day for 90 days no significant changes were found in either FEV_1 or peak flow.[80] A later open-label study of 5 mild asthmatics examined nebulized IFN-γ administered in an escalating dose, culminating in a dose of 500 μg given 3 times over the last week of the study.[81] No change was noted in FEV_1, morning peak expiratory flow, methacholine PC_{20}, or clinical symptom scores. Four of 5 subjects had a decrease in the percentage of bronchoalveolor lavage eosinophils. These limited studies suggest that IFN-γ is not an effective treatment for asthma.

IL-4 plays a central role in driving Th2 responses, as it has the unique activity of priming naive T cells to become Th2 cells. Additionally, IL-4 and IL-13 share a number of activities such as induction of IgE class switching and up-regulation of VLA-4, eotaxin and mucin. As such, IL-4 is an attractive target for inhibition. A soluble recombinant form of the IL-4 receptor α chain (rIL-4R) binds IL-4 and blocks its biological activity both in vitro and in vivo. Despite the fact that IL-4 and IL-13 share some of the same receptor components, IL-4R has no blocking activity against IL-13.

In a phase I/II blinded placebo-controlled study, 25 moderate allergic asthmatic subjects received a single dose of inhaled rIL-4R 1500 μg, rIL-4R 500 μg or placebo after stopping inhaled corticosteroids and were followed for 14 days.[82] The high-dose rIL-4R group had significantly greater FEV_1, lower symptom scores, and decreased need for β-agonist rescue than the placebo group. In a preliminary analysis of a phase II study in which 181 moderate to severe asthmatics were treated with weekly inhaled IL-4R (1800 μg or 900 μg) or placebo, subjects treated with rIL-4R demonstrated significant improvements in FEV_1 when compared to placebo. Subjects with more severe asthma also demonstrated significant improvements in peak flow and asthma symptom scores relative to placebo. Although these results are encouraging, further clinical studies of rIL-4R are required to establish its clinical efficacy.

IL-5 plays a key role in the generation of eosinophilic inflammation that is characteristic of asthma. Antibodies to IL-5 have been shown to inhibit allergen-induced airway inflammation in animal models of mice. Humanized monoclonal antibodies to IL-5 have been developed that reduce peripheral blood eosinophilia and inhibit eosinophil trafficking to the airway after allergen challenge in asthmatic subjects. Despite this clear bioactivity in vivo, this treatment did not affect either the early or late phase drop in airflow after allergen challenge.[83] Further studies are now underway to examine the activity of anti-IL-5 in chronic asthma.

IL-12 is the key regulator promoting Th1 cell development. Additionally, IL-12 increases IFN-γ production by T and NK cells. In a phase I study, IL-12 administered to asthmatic subjects was associated with a reduction in the number of circulating eosinophils but no effect on allergen-induced bronchospasm or bronchial hyperresponsiveness.[84] Further studies are needed to determine if IL-12 has any role in the treatment of asthma.

KEY CONCEPTS

Cytokine applications in allergic disease

- Neither IFN-α nor IFN-γ has clear therapeutic efficacy in asthma.
- Soluble IL-4 receptor by inhalation shows promising results in asthma.
- IFN-γ is an effective treatment in atopic dermatitis refractory to standard therapies.
- IFN-α is an effective treatment for hypereosinophilic syndrome which is unresponsive to standard therapy.

Atopic dermatitis

In two small open-label studies in severe atopic dermatitis, IFN-α2b at doses of 3 MU, 3–7 times per week, showed clinical efficacy in improving skin lesions.[85,86] Few additional studies have been performed due to the better side-effect profile and generally favorable results obtained with IFN-γ.

In placebo-controlled, blinded studies, subcutaneous injections of IFN-γ at doses of 50 $\mu g/m^2$/day have repeatedly been shown to be effective in the treatment of atopic dermatitis.[87] In a 12-week placebo-controlled trial, recombinant IFN-γ demonstrated significant improvements in physician and patient evaluations of clinical response, and erythema and excoriation scores. There was also a trend towards less use of topical corticosteroid in the IFN-γ treated group. IFN-γ treatment caused a greater than 50% reduction in blood eosinophilia, which has been similarly noted in other studies of IFN-γ. A corresponding drop in lesional skin eosinophilia has been noted in a more recent study. No reductions in serum IgE or in allergen-specific IgE have been noted in any studies of IFN-γ. These results suggest that IFN-γ may act by inhibiting allergic inflammation rather than by inhibition of the IgE response itself. Thus, IFN-γ may have a role in the treatment of atopic dermatitis in patients who are unresponsive to traditional therapies. However, with the advent of topical tacrolimus therapy, the need for IFN as a salvage therapy in atopic dermatitis is limited.

Hypereosinophilic syndrome

IFN-α2b has been shown to lower peripheral blood eosinophil counts in multiple studies and has been used to treat idiopathic hypereosinophilic syndrome.[88] IFN-α2b yielded a greater than 90% reduction in the number of circulating eosinophils in 4 of 6 subjects treated with 1.5 MU/day. This reduction was reversible upon discontinuation. Two subjects with severe mucosal ulcers, which are typically resistant to all forms of treatment, had complete resolution of ulcers during the course of therapy. Thus, IFN-α may have a role in the treatment of hypereosinophilic syndrome that is unresponsive to standard therapy.

TREATMENT OF AUTOIMMUNE DISEASES

Cytokines mediate a wide variety of biological activities that are relevant to autoimmune diseases including immune response, inflammation, and tissue repair and remodeling. Excessive production of pro-inflammatory cytokines and/or the relative paucity of anti-inflammatory/regulatory cytokines contribute to tissue injury. Restoring cytokine balance can be achieved for therapeutic purposes either by blocking inflammatory cytokines such TNF-α or IL-1 (Chapters 116, 117) or by inducing or administering exogenously anti-inflammatory/immunoregulatory cytokines. Since most autoimmune diseases share common effector pathways, cytokine therapy may be of benefit in a variety of such diseases.

Multiple sclerosis

Therapy with IFN-β has emerged in recent years as a major advance in the management of multiple sclerosis (MS). MS is thought to be due to a cell-mediated autoimmune response directed against CNS myelin components. There are at least four clinical subtypes of this disease. The relapsing-remitting form (RR-MS) is the most common (80–85%) and is characterized

KEY CONCEPTS

Cytokine applications in autoimmune disease

- Therapy involves anti-inflammatory (IL-4, IL-10, IL-11) and immunoregulatory (IFN-α,β,γ) cytokines.
- IFN-β reduces relapses and progression of sustained clinical disability in patients with relapsing-remitting multiple sclerosis.
- Minimal clinical benefit has been observed with IFN-α in primary Sjögren syndrome and cryoglobulinemic vasculitis, and with IFN-γ in scleroderma and idiopathic pulmonary fibrosis.
- Initial clinical experience with IL-10 has been encouraging in Crohn's disease and psoriasis but not in rheumatoid or psoriatic arthritis.

by acute attacks (relapses) followed by remissions and a steady baseline. Failure to recover from relapse is a major cause of disability but up to 30–50% of these patients accrue additional disability with subclinical relapses (secondary progressive phase MS).

Three large placebo-controlled, double-blind studies and several smaller studies have demonstrated the efficacy of various forms of IFN-β administered either subcutaneously or intramuscularly in patients with RR-MS.[89–91] The aggregate results of these trials showed:(1) a decrease in the cumulative burden of disease, the number of active lesions on MRI, and MS-related brain atrophy;(2) an approximately 30% decrease in number of relapses; and (3) a decrease in progression of sustained clinical disability. Although the beneficial effects of IFN-β were initially only shown for patients with RR-MS, a subsequent study demonstrated a delay in sustained neurological deterioration even in patients with the secondary progressive phase of the disease.[92] The most common side-effects of IFN-β are flu-like symptoms, headache, mild elevations in liver-associated enzymes, and anemia. Although depression is a possible adverse effect with IFN therapy, in these studies no significant relationship was observed with IFN-β.

Fibrosing diseases

IFN-γ is a potent inhibitor of collagen synthesis and of the migration and proliferation of dermal fibroblasts. Several studies (most of them small and open-label) in patients with systemic sclerosis have shown a mild to modest beneficial effect on skin disease with some noncontrolled trials also suggesting a potential beneficial effect in visceral disease.[93–95] In a preliminary 12-month study, IFN-γ1b in combination with prednisone demonstrated a substantial benefit in 18 patients with idiopathic pulmonary fibrosis who did not respond to glucocorticoids alone.[96] These results, however, will have to be confirmed in a larger study. In spite of its significant antifibrotic effects, thus far the data suggest that IFN-γ alone is not likely to have a major impact on fibrosing autoimmune diseases.

Vasculitis

The antiviral and antiproliferative activities of IFN-α have been well documented over the last two decades. Based on reports that IFN-α has a beneficial effect on patients with the hypereosinophilic syndrome, IFN-α was used with encouraging results in a small number of patients with Churg–Strauss vasculitis refractory to conventional therapy.[97] IFN-α alone or in combination with ribavirin has been used for the treatment of selected patients with moderate to severe cryoglobulinemic vasculitis related to hepatitis virus C infection.[98] IFN-α therapy has been associated with autoimmune thyroid disease or less commonly with polyarthritis in genetically susceptible individuals. In addition, its anti-angiogenic effects may exacerbate ischemia in patients with vasculitis.[99] Natural human IFN-α administered by the oral mucosal route for 12 weeks improved salivary output and decreased complaints of xerostomia in a randomized controlled trial involving 111 patients with primary Sjögren syndrome.[100]

Th2 cytokines

Chronic inflammatory arthritides such as rheumatoid arthritis and the spondyloarthropathies are characterized by synovial inflammation leading to erosion of calcified cartilage and subchondral bone. IL-1 and TNF-α are key mediators in the perpetuation of synovitis and cartilage and bone destruction. Other cytokines such as IL-6, IL-15, IL-17 and IL-18 probably play a less important role. These cytokines have also been shown to play a major role in inflammatory diseases of the bowel. Th2 cytokines such as IL-4 and IL-10 antagonize their pro-inflammatory effects and under certain circumstances even promote tissue repair, suggesting possible therapeutic roles in human disease.

Inflammatory bowel disease

Data in animals with genetic deletion of the IL-10 gene have unequivocally demonstrated the essential role of IL-10 in preventing exaggerated inflammatory responses to a variety of stimuli in various tissues. A double-blind, randomized, controlled study of 46 patients showed that a 1-week course of IL-10 resulted in complete remission in 50% of patients with Crohn's disease as compared to 23% in placebo-treated patients.[101] A more prolonged (28 days) subcutaneous administration of IL-10 was associated with modest clinical improvement in mild to moderate Crohn's disease but not in ulcerative colitis.

Inflammatory arthritides

Small studies in rheumatoid and psoriatic arthritis have failed to demonstrate a clinically significant response although individual joints may improve clinically, histologically, or by magnetic resonance imaging.[102] A modest beneficial effect has been consistently demonstrated in psoriatic skin.[102,103] Despite its major immunomodulatory and immunosuppressive effects, it is doubtful that IL-10 therapy is going to play an important role in the treatment of autoimmune inflammatory diseases.

Interleukin 11

In addition to its thrombocytopoietic effects, IL-11 has been shown to have anti-inflammatory and musculoskeletal protective effects. Phase I/II studies are in progress in patients with active Crohn's disease and rheumatoid arthritis, and early results suggest a potential benefit for patients with Crohn's disease.[104]

SUMMARY

It is clear that cytokine-based therapy has begun to make a mark on the clinical practice of medicine. It is still early in this approach

THERAPEUTIC PRINCIPLES

US Food and Drug Administration approved applications for cytokine therapy

- IFN-α
  - Hepatitis B
  - Hepatitis C
  - Condylomata acuminata
  - AIDS-associated Kaposi sarcoma
  - Hairy cell leukemia
  - Chronic myelogenous leukemia
  - Melanoma
  - Follicular lymphoma
- IFN-β
  - Multiple sclerosis
- IFN-γ
  - Chronic granulomatous disease
  - Osteopetrosis
- IL-2
  - Renal cell carcinoma
  - Melanoma
- IL-11
  - Chemotherapy-induced thrombocytopenia

to immunotherapy but there is good reason to be optimistic that successful applications will continue to expand. There is also reason to believe that combinations of selected cytokines may prove more useful than the current approach based on monotherapy.

REFERENCES

1. Malik AH, Lee WM. Chronic hepatitis B virus infection: treatment strategies for the next millennium. Ann Intern Med 2000;132:723.
2. Hoofnagle JH, Di Bisceglie AM. The treatment of chronic viral hepatitis. N Engl J Med 1997;336:347.
3. Wong DK, Cheung AM, O'Rourke K, Naylor CD, Detsky AS, Heathcote J. Effect of alpha-interferon treatment in patients with hepatitis B e antigen-positive chronic hepatitis B. A meta-analysis. Ann Intern Med 1993;119:312.
4. Niederau C, Heintges T, Lange S, et al. Long-term follow-up of HBeAg-positive patients treated with interferon alfa for chronic hepatitis B. N Engl J Med 1996;334:1422.
5. Liang TJ, Rehermann B, Seeff LB, Hoofnagle JH. Pathogenesis, natural history, treatment, and prevention of hepatitis C. Ann Intern Med 2000;132:296.
6. Davis GL. Current therapy for chronic hepatitis C. Gastroenterology 2000;118 (Suppl 1):S104.
7. Davis GL, Balart LA, Schiff ER, et al. Treatment of chronic hepatitis C with recombinant interferon alfa. A multicenter randomized, controlled trial. Hepatitis Interventional Therapy Group. N Engl J Med 1989;321:1501.
8. Di Bisceglie AM, Martin P, Kassianides C, et al. Recombinant interferon alfa therapy for chronic hepatitis C. A randomized, double-blind, placebo-controlled trial. N Engl J Med 1989;321:1506.
9. National Institutes of Health Consensus Development Conference Panel statement: management of hepatitis C. Hepatology 1997;26(Suppl 1):2S.
10. McHutchison JG, Gordon SC, Schiff ER, et al. Interferon alfa-2b alone or in combination with ribavirin as initial treatment for chronic hepatitis C. N Engl J Med 1998;339:1485.
11. Poynard T, Marcellin P, Lee SS, et al. Randomized trial of interferon α2b plus ribavirin for 48 weeks or for 24 weeks versus interferon α2b plus placebo for 48 weeks for treatment of chronic infection with hepatitis C virus. International Hepatitis Interventional Therapy Group. Lancet 1998;352:1426.
12. Davis GL, Esteban-Mur R, Rustgi V, et al. Interferon alfa-2b alone or in combination with ribavirin for the treatment of relapse of chronic hepatitis C. N Engl J Med 1998;339:1493.
13. Marcellin P, Boyer N, Gervais A, et al. Long-term histologic improvement and loss of detectable intrahepatic HCV RNA in patients with chronic hepatitis C and sustained response to interferon-alpha therapy. Ann Intern Med 1997;127:875.
14. Lau DTY, Kleiner DE, Ghany MG, Park Y, Schmid P, Hoofnagle JH. 10-Year follow-up after interferon-alpha therapy for chronic hepatitis C. Hepatology 1998; 28:1121.
15. Nelson DR, Lauwers GY, Lau JY, Davis GL. Interleukin 10 treatment reduces fibrosis in patients with chronic hepatitis C: a pilot trial of interferon nonresponders. Gastroenterology 2000;118:655.
16. Strander HA. Interferon in the treatment of human papilloma virus. Med Clin North Am 1986;Suppl:19.
17. Niimura M. Intralesional human fibroblast interferon in common warts. J Dermatol 1983;10:217.
18. Reichel RP, Fitz R, Neumann R, et al. Clinical study with recombinant interferon gamma versus interferon alpha-2c in patients with condylomata acuminata. Int J STD AIDS 1992;3:350.
19. Haglund S, Lundquist PG, Cantell K, Strander H. Interferon therapy in juvenile laryngeal papillomatosis. Arch Otolaryngol 1981;107:327.
20. Leventhal BG, Kashima HK, Weck PW, et al. Randomized surgical adjuvant trial of interferon alfa-n1 in recurrent papillomatosis. Arch Otolaryngol Head Neck Surg 1988;114:1163.
21. Leventhal BG, Kashima HK, Mounts P, et al. Long-term response of recurrent respiratory papillomatosis to treatment with lymphoblastoid interferon alfa-N1. N Engl J Med 1991;325:613.
22. Smith KL, Jacobson EL, Giordano M, et al. Restoration of immunity with interleukin-2 therapy. AIDS Reader 1999;9:56.
23. Kovacs JA, Baseler M, Dewar RJ, et al. Increases in CD4 T lymphocytes with intermittent courses of interleukin-2 in patients with human immunodeficiency virus infection. A preliminary study. N Engl J Med 1995;332:567.
24. Kovacs JA, Vogel S, Albert JM, et al. Controlled trial of interleukin-2 infusions in patients infected with the human immunodeficiency virus. N Engl J Med 1996;335:1350.
25. Davey RT Jr, Chaitt DG, Albert JM, et al. A randomized trial of high versus low-dose subcutaneous interleukin-2 outpatient therapy for early human immunodeficiency virus type 1 infection. J Infect Dis 1999;179:849.
26. Emery S, Capra WB, Cooper DA, et al. Pooled analysis of 3 randomized, controlled trials of interleukin-2 therapy in adult human immunodeficiency virus type 1 disease. J Infect Dis 2000;182:428.
27. Davey RT Jr, Murphy RL, Graziano FM, et al. Immunologic and virologic effects of subcutaneous interleukin 2 in combination with antiretroviral therapy: A randomized controlled trial. JAMA 2000;284:183.
28. Haas DW, Lavelle J, Nadler JP, et al. A randomized trial of interferon alpha therapy for HIV type 1 infection. AIDS Res Hum Retroviruses 2000;16:183.
29. Holland SM, Eisenstein EM, Kuhns DB, et al. Treatment of refractory disseminated nontuberculous mycobacterial infection with interferon gamma. A preliminary report. N Engl J Med 1994;330:1348.

30. Altare F, Jouanguy E, Lamhamedi S, Doffinger R, Fischer A, Casanova JL. Mendelian susceptibility to mycobacterial infection in man. Curr Opin Immunol 1998;10:413.
31. Altare F, Durandy A, Lammas D, et al. Impairment of mycobacterial immunity in human interleukin-12 receptor deficiency. Science 1998;280:1432.
32. Altare F, Lammas D, Revy P, et al. Inherited interleukin 12 deficiency in a child with bacille Calmette-Guerin and Salmonella enteritidis disseminated infection. J Clin Invest 1998;102:2035.
33. Doffinger R, Jouanguy E, Dupuis S, et al. Partial interferon-gamma receptor signaling chain deficiency in a patient with bacille Calmette-Guerin and Mycobacterium abscessus infection. J Infect Dis 2000;181:379.
34. Dorman SE, Holland SM. Mutation in the signal-transducing chain of the interferon-gamma receptor and susceptibility to mycobacterial infection. J Clin Invest 1998;101:2364.
35. Frucht DM, Holland SM. Defective monocyte costimulation for IFN-gamma production in familial disseminated Mycobacterium avium complex infection: abnormal IL-12 regulation. J Immunol 1996;157:411.
36. Jouanguy E, Dupuis S, Pallier A, et al. In a novel form of IFN-gamma receptor 1 deficiency, cell surface receptors fail to bind IFN-gamma. J Clin Invest 2000;105:1429.
37. Levin M, Newport M. Understanding the genetic basis of susceptibility to mycobacterial infection. Proc Assoc Am Physicians 1999;111:308.
38. Holland SM. Cytokine therapy of mycobacterial infections. Adv Intern Med 2000;45:431.
39. Chatte G, Panteix G, Perrin-Fayolle M, Pacheco Y. Aerosolized interferon gamma for Mycobacterium avium-complex lung disease. Am J Respir Crit Care Med 1995;152:1094.
40. Squires KE, Brown ST, Armstrong D, Murphy WF, Murray HW. Interferon-gamma treatment for Mycobacterium avium-intracellular complex bacillemia in patients with AIDS [Letter]. J Infect Dis 1992;166:686.
41. Johnson B, Bekker LG, Ress S, Kaplan G. Recombinant interleukin 2 adjunctive therapy in multidrug-resistant tuberculosis. Novartis Found Symp 1998;217:99.
42. Nathan CF, Kaplan G, Levis WR, et al. Local and systemic effects of intradermal recombinant interferon-gamma in patients with lepromatous leprosy. N Engl J Med 1986;315:6.
43. Sampaio EP, Moreira AL, Sarno EN, Malta AM, Kaplan G. Prolonged treatment with recombinant interferon gamma induces erythema nodosum leprosum in lepromatous leprosy patients. J Exp Med 1992;175:1729.
44. Villahermosa LG, Abalos RM, Walsh DS, Fajardo TT, Walsh GP. Recombinant interleukin-2 in lepromatous leprosy lesions: immunological and microbiological consequences. Clin Exp Dermatol 1997;22:134.
45. Kurkcuoglu N, Tandogdu R. Interferon gamma therapy for cutaneous leishmaniasis [Letter]. Arch Dermatol 1990;126:831.
46. Reed SG, Scott P. T-cell and cytokine responses in leishmaniasis. Curr Opin Immunol 1993;5:524.
47. Akuffo H, Kaplan G, Kiessling R, et al. Administration of recombinant interleukin-2 reduces the local parasite load of patients with disseminated cutaneous leishmaniasis. J Infect Dis 1990;161:775.
48. Chang Y, Cesarman E, Pessin MS, et al. Identification of herpesvirus-like DNA sequences in AIDS-associated Kaposi's sarcoma. Science 1994;266:1865.
49. Antman K, Chang Y. Kaposi's sarcoma. N Engl J Med 2000;342:1027.
50. Krown SE, Real FX, Cunningham-Rundles S, et al. Preliminary observations on the effect of recombinant leukocyte A interferon in homosexual men with Kaposi's sarcoma. N Engl J Med 1983;308:1071.
51. Mitsuyasu RT. Update on the pathogenesis and treatment of Kaposi sarcoma. Curr Opin Oncol 2000;12:174.
52. Quesada JR, Reuben J, Manning JT, Hersh EM, Gutterman JU. Alpha interferon for induction of remission in hairy-cell leukemia. N Engl J Med 1984;310:15.
53. Ratain MJ, Vardiman JW, Golomb HM. The role of interferon in the treatment of hairy cell leukemia. Semin Oncol 1986;13(Suppl 2):21.
54. Tallman MS, Peterson LC, Hakimian D, Gillis S, Polliack A. Treatment of hairy-cell leukemia: current views. Semin Hematol 1999;36:155.
55. Rai KR, Davey F, Peterson B, et al. Recombinant alpha-2b-interferon in therapy of previously untreated hairy cell leukemia: long-term follow-up results of study by Cancer and Leukemia Group B. Leukemia 1995;9:1116.
56. Capnist G, Federico M, Chisesi T, et al. Long term results of interferon treatment in hairy cell leukemia. Italian Cooperative Group of Hairy Cell Leukemia (ICGHCL). Leuk Lymphoma 1994;14:457.
57. Damasio EE, Clavio M, Masoudi B, et al. Alpha-interferon as induction and maintenance therapy in hairy cell leukemia: a long-term follow-up analysis. Eur J Haematol 2000;64:47.
58. Sawyers CL. Chronic myeloid leukemia. N Engl J Med 1999;340:1330.
59. Faderl S, Talpaz M, Estrov Z, Kantarjian HM. Chronic myelogenous leukemia: biology and therapy. Ann Intern Med 1999;131:207.
60. Talpaz M, McCredie KB, Mavligit GM, Gutterman JU. Leukocyte interferon-induced myeloid cytoreduction in chronic myelogenous leukemia. Blood 1983;62:689.
61. Talpaz M, Cortes J, O'Brien S, et al. Phase I study of polyethylene glycol (PEG) interferon alpha-2b (intron-A) in CML patients [Abstract]. Blood 1998;92(Suppl 1):151a.
62. Blade J, Esteve J. Viewpoint on the impact of interferon in the treatment of multiple myeloma: benefit for a small proportion of patients? Med Oncol 2000;17:77.
63. Wheatley K. Which myeloma patients benefit from interferon therapy? An overview of 24 randomized trials with 4000 patients. Br J Haematol 1998;102:140.
64. Peterson BA. Current treatment of follicular low-grade lymphomas. Semin Oncol 1999;26(Suppl 14):2.
65. Soubeyran P, Debled M, Tchen N, et al. Follicular lymphomas – a review of treatment modalities. Crit Rev Oncol Hematol 2000;35:13.
66. Haase-Statz S, Smalley RV. Role of interferon-alfa in NHL: still controversial? Oncology (Huntingt) 1999;13:1147.
67. Tepler I, Elias L, Smith JW II, et al. A randomized placebo-controlled trial of recombinant human interleukin-11 in cancer patients with severe thrombocytopenia due to chemotherapy. Blood 1996;87:3607.
68. Isaacs C, Robert NJ, Bailey FA, et al. Randomized placebo-controlled study of recombinant human interleukin-11 to prevent chemotherapy-induced thrombocytopenia in patients with breast cancer receiving dose-intensive cyclophosphamide and doxorubicin. J Clin Oncol 1997;15:3368.
69. Gallin JI. Interferon-gamma in the treatment of the chronic granulomatous diseases of childhood. Clin Immunol Immunopathol 1991;61:S100.
70. Gallin JI. Interferon-gamma in the management of chronic granulomatous disease. Rev Infect Dis 1991;13:973.
71. Gallin JI, Farber JM, Holland SM, Nutman TB. Interferon-gamma in the management of infectious diseases. [Clinical conference]. Ann Intern Med 1995;123:216.
72. Bemiller LS, Roberts DH, Starko KM, Curnutte JT. Safety and effectiveness of long-term interferon gamma therapy in patients with chronic granulomatous disease. Blood Cells Mol Dis 1995;21:239.
73. Key LL Jr, Ries WL, Rodriguiz RM, Hatcher HC. Recombinant human interferon gamma therapy for osteopetrosis. J Pediatr 1992;121:119.
74. Key LL Jr, Rodriguiz RM, Willi SM, et al. Long-term treatment of osteopetrosis with recombinant human interferon gamma. N Engl J Med 1995;332:1594.
75. Sneller MC, Strober W, Eisenstein E, Jaffe JS, Cunningham-Rundles C. NIH conference. New insights into common variable immunodeficiency. Ann Intern Med 1993;118:720.
76. Cunningham-Rundles C, Kazbay K, Hassett J, Zhou Z, Mayer L. Brief report: enhanced humoral immunity in common variable immunodeficiency after long-term treatment with polyethylene glycol-conjugated interleukin-2. N Engl J Med 1994; 331:918.
77. Rump JA, Jahreis A, Schlesier M, Stecher S, Peter HH. A double-blind, placebo-controlled, crossover therapy study with natural human IL-2 (nhuIL-2) in combination with regular intravenous gammaglobulin (IVIG) infusions in 10 patients with common variable immunodeficiency (CVID). Clin Exp Immunol 1997; 110:167.

78. Wills-Karp M. Immunologic basis of antigen-induced airway hyperresponsiveness. Annu Rev Immunol 1999;17:255.
79. Bini EJ, Weinshel EH. Severe exacerbation of asthma: a new side effect of interferon-alpha in patients with asthma and chronic hepatitis C. Mayo Clin Proc 1999;74:367.
80. Boguniewicz M, Schneider LC, Milgrom H, et al. Treatment of steroid-dependent asthma with recombinant interferon-gamma. Clin Exp Allergy 1993;23:785.
81. Boguniewicz M, Martin RJ, Martin D, et al. The effects of nebulized recombinant interferon-gamma in asthmatic airways. J Allergy Clin Immunol 1995;95:133.
82. Borish LC, Nelson HS, Lanz MJ, et al. Interleukin-4 receptor in moderate atopic asthma. A phase I/II randomized, placebo-controlled trial. Am J Respir Crit Care Med 1999;160:1816.
83. Leckie MJ, Ten Brincke A, Lordan J, et al. SB 240563, a humanized anti-IL-5 monoclonal antibody. Initial single dose safety and activity in patients with asthma. Am J Respir Crit Care Med 1999;159:A624.
84. Bryan S, O'Conner BJ, Matti S, et al. Effects of recombinant human interleukin-12 on eosinophils, airway hyperreactivity and the late asthmatic response. Lancet 2000;356:2149.
85. Gruschwitz MS, Peters KP, Heese A, Stosiek N, Koch HU, Hornstein OP. Effects of interferon-alpha-2b on the clinical course, inflammatory skin infiltrates and peripheral blood lymphocytes in patients with severe atopic eczema. Int Arch Allergy Immunol 1993;101:20.
86. Nielsen BW, Reimert CM, Hammer R, Schiotz PO, Thestrup-Pedersen K. Interferon therapy for atopic dermatitis reduces basophil histamine release, but does not reduce serum IgE or eosinophilic proteins. Allergy 1994;49:120.
87. Hanifin JM, Schneider LC, Leung DY, et al. Recombinant interferon gamma therapy for atopic dermatitis. J Am Acad Dermatol 1993;28:189.
88. Butterfield JH, Gleich GJ. Interferon-alpha treatment of six patients with the idiopathic hypereosinophilic syndrome. Ann Intern Med 1994;121:648.
89. Interferon beta-1b is effective in relapsing-remitting multiple sclerosis: I. Clinical results of a multicenter, randomized, double blind, placebo-controlled trial. The IFNB Multiple Sclerosis Study Group. Neurology 1993;43:655.
90. Jacobs LD, Cookfair DL, Rudick RA, et al. Intramuscular interferon beta-1a for disease progression in relapsing multiple sclerosis. The Multiple Sclerosis Collaborative Research Group. Ann Neurol 1996;39:285.
91. Randomized double-blinded placebo-controlled study of interferon beta-1a in relapsing/remitting multiple sclerosis. PRISMS (Prevention of Relapses and Disability by Interferon beta-1a Subcutaneously in Multiple Sclerosis) Study Group. Lancet 1998;352:1498.
92. Placebo-controlled multicentre randomized trial of interferon beta-1b in treatment of secondary progressive multiple sclerosis. European Study Group on Interferon beta-1b in secondary progressive MS. Lancet 1998;352:149.
93. Freundlich B, Jimenez SA, Steen VD, et al. Treatment of systemic sclerosis with recombinant interferon-gamma. A phase I/II clinical trial. Arthritis Rheum 1992; 35:1134.
94. Hunzelman N, Anders S, Fierbeck G, et al. Systemic scleroderma. Multicenter trial of 1 year of treatment with recombinant interferon gamma. Arch Dermatol 1997;133:609.
95. Grassegger A, Schuler G, Hessenberger G, et al. Interferon-gamma in the treatment of systemic sclerosis: a randomized controlled multicentre trial. Br J Dermatol 1998;139:639.
96. Ziesche R, Hofbauer E, Wittmann K, Petkov V, Block LH. A preliminary study of long-term treatment with interferon gamma-1b and low-dose prednisolone in patients with idiopathic pulmonary fibrosis. N Engl J Med 1999;341:1264.
97. Tatsis E, Schnabel A, Gross WL. Interferon-alpha treatment of four patients with the Churg–Strauss syndrome. Ann Intern Med 1998;129:370.
98. Lamprecht P, Gause A, Gross WL. Cryoglobulinemic vasculitis. Arthritis Rheum 1999;42:2507.
99. Cid MC, Hernandez-Rodriquez J, Robert J, et al. Interferon-alpha may exacerbate cryoglobulinemia-related ischemic manifestations: an adverse effect potentially related to its anti-angiogenic activity. Arthritis Rheum 1999;42:1051.
100. Ship JA, Fox PC, Michalek JE, Cummins MJ, Richards AB. Treatment of primary Sjogren's syndrome with low dose natural interferon-alpha administered by the oral mucosal route: a phase II clinical trial. IFN Protocol Study Group. J Interferon Cytokine Res 1999;19:943.
101. Van Deventer SJ, Elson CO, Fedorak RN. Multiple doses of intravenous interleukin 10 in steroid-refractory Crohn's disease. Gastroenterology 1997;113:383.
102. McInnes IB, Illei GG, Danning CL, et al. Interleukin-10 improves skin disease and modulates endothelial activation and leukocyte effector function in patients with psoriatic arthritis. Arthritis Rheum 1999;42:S377.
103. Asadullah K, Docke WD, Ebeling M, et al. Interleukin 10 treatment of psoriasis: clinical results of a phase 2 trial. Arch Dermatol 1999;135:187.
104. Sands BE, Bank S, Sninsky CA, et al. Preliminary evaluation of safety and activity of recombinant human interleukin 11 in patients with active Crohn's disease. Gastroenterology 1999;117:58.

Section 10 Prevention and Therapy of Immunologic Diseases
F Immune Modulation

Chapter 116 Cytokine Inhibitors and Receptor Antagonists

William P. Arend

Cytokines are mediators of cell–cell interactions and operate in a network of redundant and overlapping effects (Chapter 12). They serve important roles in normal physiology, for example in cell differentiation during embryogenesis and in host resistance to exogenous pathogens. A variety of natural mechanisms exist to regulate and control the effects of particular cytokines. Cytokines may lead to pathologic consequences in human autoimmune or chronic inflammatory diseases because of exaggerated production or inadequate inhibition. This chapter summarizes existing knowledge about approaches to modulation of the cytokine network, emphasizing, where possible, the results of clinical trials in human diseases.

INHIBITORS OF CYTOKINE PRODUCTION

Cytokines are produced during cell responses to a variety of stimuli, including bacterial products such as lipopolysaccharides (LPS), viral products, antigen–antibody complexes, complement fragments, and other cytokines themselves. Production of cytokines by lymphocytes may be inhibited by cyclosporin (CsA), largely accounting for the potent immunosuppressive effects of this compound. Other anti-inflammatory or immunosuppressive drugs, such as corticosteroids, may suppress cytokine production as one of their purported mechanisms of action.

IL-1 and tumor necrosis factor-α (TNF-α) may have potent pro-inflammatory effects in many human diseases, including asthma and rheumatoid arthritis. Agents that increase cellular cAMP levels and PGE_2 production may lead to a decrease in IL-1 and TNF-α synthesis and secretion through both transcriptional and post-transcriptional mechanisms. In addition, agents that inhibit IL-1β or TNF-α-processing enzymes comprise another potential mechanism of reducing the production of bioactive cytokines.

IL-6, in cooperation with other cytokines, has been shown to stimulate osteoclast function and bone resorption both in vitro and in vivo. The antiosteoporotic effects of estrogens may be mediated, at least in part, by inhibition of IL-6 production.[1] 17β-estradiol inhibits IL-1- and TNF-α-induced production of IL-6 from cultured osteoblasts and human primary bone cultures. Similar effects were observed with testosterone and progesterone, but at concentrations much higher than those of 17β-estradiol.

Some cytokines themselves block production of other cytokines. Both IL-4 and IL-10 are potent inhibitors of production of TNF-α, IL-1, IL-6, IL-8, and granulocyte-macrophage colony-stimulating factor (GM-CSF) production by monocytes and macrophages.[2,3] IL-4 also up-regulates production by macrophages of the specific IL-1 receptor antagonist, IL-1Ra.[4] Furthermore, IL-4 is very effective at suppressing streptococcal cell wall-induced arthritis in rats where IL-1Ra gene expression is enhanced in the synovial tissues. Initial studies employing therapeutic administration of IL-4 in human disease have exhibited considerable toxicity but clinical trials of IL-10 in rheumatoid arthritis are in progress.

> **KEY CONCEPTS**
>
> **Approaches to inhibition of cytokines**
> - Inhibitors of cytokine production
> - Opposing effects of cytokines
> - Antibodies to cytokines
> - Protein binding of cytokines
> - Regulation of receptor expression
> - Soluble cytokine receptors
> - Cytokine receptor antagonists

OPPOSING EFFECTS OF CYTOKINES

The stimulatory effects of a cytokine on a particular target cell may be specifically opposed by another cytokine. Although the opposing effects of cytokines have primarily been examined in vitro, many of these actions probably also occur in vivo. Thus, the balance between cytokines in the cell microenvironment is of prime importance in determining the phenotypic characteristics displayed by that cell.

An example of the opposing effects of cytokines can be seen in the fibroblast-like cell in the rheumatoid synovium.[5,6] The combination of IL-1, platelet-derived growth factor (PDGF), and fibroblast growth factor (FGF) differentiates synovial fibroblasts into a phenotype that rapidly proliferates and produces a high level of collagenase and a low level of collagen. The combination of PDGF and transforming growth factor-β (TGF-β), however, causes the synovial fibroblast to assume a more quiescent phenotype with production of a low level of collagenase and a high level of collagen. In addition, both TNF-α and IFN-γ oppose TGF-β-induced collagen and fibronectin synthesis by these cells. Macrophages are also influenced to exhibit different phenotypic characteristics by different cytokines: IL-1 and TNF-α induce collagenase production by these cells whereas both IL-4 and IFN-γ decrease this response.[7]

It should be emphasized that cells in vivo are bathed in a mixture of cytokines, which may have opposing effects. The nature and activation state of cytokine-producing cells present locally in tissues determine the cytokine mixture at an inflammatory site and hence their net biologic effect. Knowledge about opposing effects of cytokines has been applied in the treatment of scleroderma, where both IFN-γ and IFN-α have been evaluated as agents to reduce skin collagen. However, the results of clinical trials in scleroderma patients were disappointing as both forms of IFN failed to reduce the skin score. Furthermore, serious side-effects were observed, including a worsening in vasculopathy with IFN-γ treatment and a deterioration in lung function in scleroderma patients treated for 1 year with IFN-α.[8,9]

ANTIBODIES TO CYTOKINES

Antibodies to cytokines represent another mechanism to interfere with the effects of specific cytokines. Antibodies to certain cytokines may occur naturally or may develop in response to the therapeutic administration of some recombinant human cytokines. Additionally, monoclonal antibodies to a specific cytokine may be used therapeutically in an effort to inhibit the biologic effects of that cytokine (Table 116.1).

Naturally-occurring antibodies to cytokines

Naturally-occurring antibodies to IL-1α, IL-6, IFN-γ, and TNF-α have been described in human circulation. These autoantibodies may not necessarily inhibit the effects of a cytokine in vivo. For example, a high-affinity antibody to a cytokine, if directed against the receptor-binding epitope on the cytokine molecule, could block the interaction of that cytokine with specific cell-surface receptors. A lower-affinity antibody, however, or an antibody that did not recognize the receptor-binding region of a cytokine, actually might enhance the effects of a cytokine in vivo. This might occur if the antibody carried the cytokine to a tissue where the cytokine transferred to cell-surface receptors of high-avidity binding, leading to stimulation of that cell. Antibodies to cytokines also might prolong the life span of cytokines by preventing proteolytic degradation or glomerular filtration and excretion in the urine.

Naturally-occurring antibodies to IL-1α are present in low titer in approximately 25% of normal sera and occur in higher titer and more commonly in the sera of patients with rheumatoid arthritis, Graves' disease, or pernicious anemia.[10–12] Although these antibodies may block the receptor binding of IL-1α in vitro, it is possible that their major in vivo function is to act as a carrier for IL-1α in circulation. Anti-IL-6 antibodies are found in the sera of approximately 15% of normal blood donors and occur more commonly in the sera of patients with scleroderma.[13,14] The in vivo biologic consequences of these antibodies remain unknown.

Antibodies to cytokines
1. Naturally-occurring antibodies to cytokines a. To IL-1α, IL-6, IFN-γ, and TNF-α are present in the circulation of normal individuals b. May block or enhance biologic effects of the cytokine in vivo c. To IL-1α, are found more commonly and in higher titer in the sera of patients with rheumatoid arthritis, Graves' disease, or penicious anemia
2. Monoclonal antibodies to TNF-α a. Chimeric molecules, with the binding site murine and the remainder of the molecule human b. Effective in the treatment of steroid-resistant Crohn's disease, including patients with draining abdominal or peritoneal fistula c. Effective in the treatment of rheumatoid arthritis resistant to standard disease-modifying drugs when administered with methotrexate

Table 116.1 Antibodies to cytokines.

Monoclonal antibodies to TNF-α

Monoclonal antibodies to TNF-α have been evaluated for the treatment of Crohn's disease and rheumatoid arthritis. These antibodies are chimeric, the binding site being of murine origin and the remainder of the molecule human. Extensive data argue for the presence of a cytokine imbalance in the intestinal mucosa of patients with Crohn's disease and in the proliferative rheumatoid synovium. Furthermore, animal models of both of these human diseases have been successfully treated with anti-TNF reagents, leading to trials in patients.

Crohn's disease

In an initial open study, 10 patients with steroid-resistant Crohn's disease received a single infusion of a chimeric monoclonal antibody to TNF-α, called cA2, at 10 mg/kg.[15] Eight patients exhibited a dramatic improvement with normalization of Crohn's disease activity index scores and healing of ulcerations by colonoscopy within 4 weeks. The average duration of improvement was 4 months. The clinical efficacy of anti-TNF-α monoclonal antibody treatment in Crohn's disease was further established in a subsequent 12-week multicenter, double-blind, placebo-controlled trial.[16] All 108 patients had moderate to severe Crohn's disease that was resistant to standard therapy, and received a single infusion of either placebo or cA2 at 5 mg/kg or 10 mg/kg. At 4 weeks after treatment, 65% of the cA2-treated patients experienced a clinical response in comparison to 17% of the placebo group. A clinical remission was observed in 33% of the cA2-treated patients compared to 4% of the placebo group. Furthermore, at 12 weeks after the cA2 infusion, 41% of the treated patients and only 12% of the placebo group still manifested a clinical response. Of those Crohn's disease patients not responding to the initial treatment with the monoclonal antibody to TNF-α, the rates of response and remission to a second infusion were 34% and 17%, respectively, after 12 weeks. These observations suggested that a subgroup of patients with Crohn's disease were truly resistant to anti-TNF-α treatment.

The effects of anti-TNF-α monoclonal antibody treatment were next examined in Crohn's disease patients with draining abdominal or peritoneal fistulas.[17] Infusions of placebo or cA2 at 5 mg/kg or 10 mg/kg were administered at weeks 0, 2, and 6 in 94 adult patients with chronic unhealing fistulas of at least 3 months duration. The patients were seen in follow-up visits at 2, 6, 10, 14, and 18 weeks after the first infusion. A 50% or greater reduction in the number of draining fistulas from baseline at two or more consecutive visits was observed in 68% and 56%, respectively, of patients in the two cA2 treatment groups, compared to 26% of the patients who received placebo. In addition, closure of all fistulas occurred in 55% and 38%, respectively, of the Crohn's disease patients who received the two doses of the anti-TNF-α monoclonal antibody compared to 13% in the placebo group.

These results indicate that half or more of patients with Crohn's disease resistant to standard therapies exhibit dramatic improvements after a single treatment or multiple infusions with anti-TNF-α monoclonal antibodies. Clinical questions remaining include the long-term safety of TNF-α blockade and the optimal timing of repeat infusions. T cells are most important in this disease process, and these cells both express membrane-bound TNF-α and release free TNF-α from the cell surface through cleavage by a specific protease. The anti-TNF-α monoclonal antibody not only neutralizes soluble TNF-α, preventing its interaction with receptors on target cells, but the antibody also binds to the membrane form of this cytokine. The prolonged clinical response to a single infusion of cA2 in Crohn's disease suggests that antibody binding to membrane TNF-α may either kill cells by complement-mediated lysis or induce immunomodulatory consequences.[18] Finally, severe inflammation in the intestine has been observed in mice genetically deficient in production of either IL-10 or TGF-β. Additional cytokine approaches to treatment of inflammatory bowel disease may include the targeted administration of these cytokines by gene therapy.

Rheumatoid arthritis

TNF-α is produced in the inflamed synovial tissue of patients with rheumatoid arthritis, and anti-TNF-α treatments have successfully reduced both swelling and tissue destruction in animal models of inflammatory arthritis.[19] Anti-TNF-α monoclonal antibodies also have been successfully employed in the treatment of patients with rheumatoid arthritis. A randomized, double-blind, placebo-controlled trial of a single infusion of 1 or 10 mg/kg of the cA2 monoclonal antibody to TNF-α was carried out in 73 patients with active rheumatoid arthritis.[20] At 4 weeks after infusion of the high dose of cA2, when assessed by the Paulus criteria, 79% of patients exhibited a 20% response and 58% of patients had a 50% response. These results compared to 44% and 28% of patients from the low-dose group responding, and 8% of the placebo group. Although the responding patients relapsed after 2–4 months, equivalent clinical improvements resulted after subsequent repeat infusions of anti-TNF-α monoclonal antibodies.[21]

Multiple infusions of cA2 were then evaluated, either alone or combined with methotrexate, in a subsequent 26-week, double-blind, placebo-controlled trial in 101 patients with rheumatoid arthritis.[22] The patients were treated with infusions of cA2 at 1, 3, or 10 mg/kg, or with placebo, at weeks 0, 2, 6, 10, and 14, both with or without methotrexate 7.5 mg/week. Sixty per cent of patients receiving the anti-TNF-α monoclonal antibody at 3 or 10 mg/kg, with or without methotrexate, exhibited a 20% Paulus response with a median duration of 10.4 to >18.1 weeks. The more stringent 50% Paulus response was observed at 26 weeks in approximately 50% of the patients in the two higher dose cA2 groups who also received methotrexate, compared with approximately 20% of those who received cA2 alone. Patients who received repeat infusions of cA2 at the lowest dose, 1 mg/kg, without methotrexate failed to sustain a clinical response. However, low-dose cA2 in combination with methotrexate led to a Paulus response at both the 20% and 50% criteria levels in >60% of the patients, which was observed through 16 weeks but fell off to around 20% of patients at 26 weeks. Thus, repeat infusions of the anti-TNF-α monoclonal antibody yielded sustained responses in rheumatoid arthritis, and synergy was observed with methotrexate, possibly allowing lower doses of cA2 to be administered in combination therapy. For rheumatoid arthritis resistant to standard disease-modifying drugs, FDA approval has been granted for treatment with monoclonal antibodies to TNF-α only in combination with methotrexate, but not alone.

Safety of anti-TNF-α treatment

The safety of anti-TNF-α monoclonal antibody treatment also was assessed in the clinical trials in both diseases. In Crohn's disease with fistulas, patients receiving the higher dose of cA2 of 10 mg/kg exhibited more side-effects such as headache, abscess, upper respiratory infection, and fatigue.[17] There did not appear to be a dose-related incidence of adverse events in the rheumatoid arthritis trials, either without or with methotrexate, although similar side-effects as observed in Crohn's disease were described.[22] The incidence of infections requiring treatment with antibiotics in the 26-week trial in rheumatoid arthritis was 32% in the anti-TNF-α-treated patients in comparison to 21% in the patients who received methotrexate alone. These infections were primarily in upper respiratory or urinary tracts or cutaneous. More long-term experience with anti-TNF-α treatments will be necessary to ascertain whether serious infections or malignancies occur at higher rates.

PROTEIN BINDING OF CYTOKINES

Cytokine binding to proteins in vivo has been inferred from observing high molecular weight forms of some cytokines in serum or plasma. Both autoantibodies to cytokines and soluble cytokine receptors may comprise a large part of this binding activity. Two other human proteins, uromodulin and α_2-macroglobulin, also may bind cytokines in vivo, with mixed biologic consequences.

Uromodulin is an 85 kDa protein that is synthesized in the kidneys and may bind IL-1 and TNF-α locally in that organ.[23] This interaction could possibly inhibit the local effects of these two cytokines or retain them in the kidneys.

α_2-Macroglobulin is a large serum protein that binds many materials in the circulation and clears them by promoting uptake and degradation by phagocytic cells. The electrophoretic fast form of α_2-macroglobulin may bind to many cytokines, including IL-1, IL-2, IL-6, TNF-α, TGF-β, and PDGF.[24] This interaction may have a variety of consequences (Table 116.2). The interaction of IL-1β and IL-6 with α_2-macroglobulin may actually enhance the effects of these cytokines by retaining them in circulation and delivering them to tissues.[25] In contrast, TGF-β bound to α_2-macroglobulin is inhibited from interacting with cell-surface receptors for TGF-β but is rapidly cleared from circulation by the complex binding to hepatocyte receptors for α_2-macroglobulin.[26]

Consequences of α_2-macroglobulin binding of cytokines	
Immunoassays	Masking of antigenic epitopes on cytokines
Bioassays	Inhibition of stability or receptor binding of cytokines
In vivo effects	Inhibition of cytokine distribution, receptor binding, or degradation
Clearance	Cytokine clearance enhanced by α_2-macroglobulin binding to receptors on hepatocytes and macrophages

Table 116.2 Consequences of α_2-macroglobulin binding of cytokines.

REGULATION OF RECEPTOR EXPRESSION

The in vivo effects of many cytokines may be influenced by the relative levels of receptor expression on particular target cells. Depending on the presence of other cytokines or LPS in the cell microenvironment, the cell-surface receptors for TNF-α may either be up-regulated (by IL-1, IL-2, IL-4, IL-6, IFN-γ, or TNF-α itself), or down-regulated (by LPS). In a similar fashion, the expression of type I receptors for IL-1 may be enhanced on T cells by IL-2 and IL-4, on fibroblasts by PDGF and IL-1 itself, and on keratinocytes by IFN-γ. In contrast, type I IL-1 receptor expression on myeloid cells and articular chondrocytes is potently down-regulated by TGF-β.[27,28]

Expression of other cytokine receptors also is regulated by other cytokines or by cell differentiation. These largely in vitro observations have yet to be applied to the potential in vivo treatment of disease. However, the possibility exists that a particularly noxious or injurious effect of a cytokine in a disease process may be reduced by the administration of a therapeutic agent that decreases cell-surface receptor expression for that cytokine.

SOLUBLE CYTOKINE RECEPTORS

A potentially important mechanism for inhibition of cytokine effects is the presence of naturally-occurring soluble cytokine receptors which have been shown to exhibit a number of biologic activities. Some soluble cytokine receptors also have been developed by techniques of genetic engineering for application as therapeutic agents in human diseases.

Naturally-occurring soluble cytokine receptors

Receptors for numerous cytokines are normally found in circulation or in other body cavities. These are generated primarily by enzymatic cleavage of cell-surface receptors, but occasionally are separate gene products. The in vivo relevance of naturally-occurring soluble cytokine receptors remains unclear although they may inhibit cytokine effects by blocking binding to cell-surface receptors. In other instances, soluble cytokine receptors may enhance effects either by delivering cytokines to tissues or by interacting independently with cell-surface molecules responsible for inducing pathways of signal transduction (Table 116.3).

Two different receptors for TNF-α are present on the cell surface: 55 kDa or type I, and 75 kDa or type II. The extramembranous portions of both receptors also exist as soluble molecules and were originally described as TNF inhibitors in the urine of febrile patients, or of some normal individuals, and in the plasma of cancer patients. High concentrations of both types of soluble TNF receptors also have been described in the synovial fluids of patients with rheumatoid arthritis, in the supernatants of cultured alveolar macrophages, and in several biologic fluids from patients with inflammatory diseases. In addition, soluble TNF receptors may behave as acute-phase reactants, with plasma levels increasing as part of a general response to inflammation.[29] The biological relevance of naturally-occurring soluble TNF receptors in humans has not been established. However, in experimental models of disease in animals, soluble receptors may either enhance or inhibit the biologic effects of TNF-α, depending upon the relative concentrations of the cytokine and of the soluble receptors, and in what body space or compartment they are present.

Two different IL-1 receptors are present both on the plasma membrane and in soluble form, the latter as products of proteolysis from the cell surface (Fig. 116.1). Membrane-expressed type I IL-1 receptors possess a long cytoplasmic tail and are responsible for inducing intracellular responses. Type II IL-1 receptors on the cell surface exhibit a short cytoplasmic domain and fail to stimulate cells after ligand binding. The major biologic functions for type II IL-1 receptors appear to be as dummy receptors on the cell surface and as potential inhibitors of IL-1 activity in the soluble form. Soluble type II IL-1 receptors are present in normal plasma and in the synovial fluids of patients with rheumatoid arthritis; whether they inhibit IL-1 activity in vivo is not known.

Soluble IL-2 receptors are commonly present in the circulation and serve as a nonspecific indicator of autoimmune, infectious, inflammatory, or neoplastic diseases. These molecules bind IL-2 too weakly to inhibit function or to act as a carrier of this

Naturally-occurring soluble cytokine receptors	
Cytokine receptor	**Biologic effects of soluble receptors in vivo**
TNF-α	Possible inhibition or carrier
IL-1	Possible inhibition
IL-2	Marker of disease activity
IL-4	Possible carrier
IL-6	Stimulation of cell responses

Table 116.3 Naturally-occurring soluble cytokine receptors.

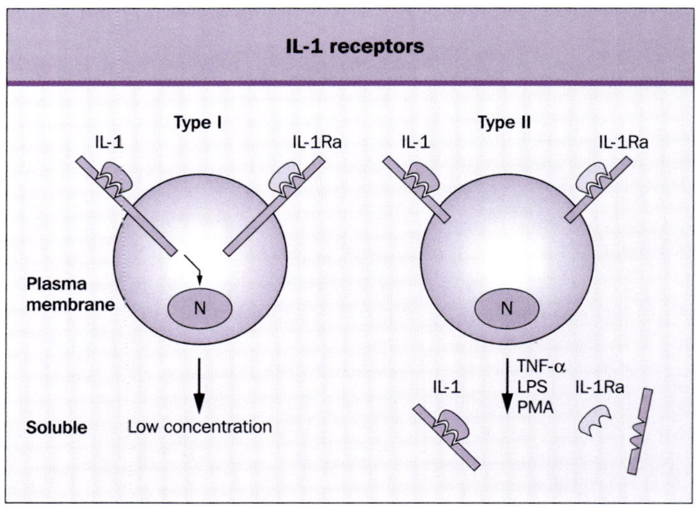

Figure 116.1 IL-1 receptors. Left. The type I IL-1 receptor has a long cytoplasmic tail and transduces intracellular responses after binding by IL-1α or IL-1β, but not by IL-1Ra. Soluble type I IL-1 receptors are found in low concentrations in plasma. Right. The type II IL-1 receptor has a short cytoplasmic tail and is not capable of generating intracellular responses. Treatment of type II IL-1 receptor-bearing cells, such as PMN, with TNF-α, bacterial LPS, or phorbol myristate acetate (PMA) leads to the proteolytic release of soluble type II IL-1 receptors which are present in high concentrations in plasma and synovial fluids. These soluble type II IL-1 receptors bind IL-1β avidly but bind IL-1Ra weakly.

cytokine. Measurement of serum levels of soluble IL-2 receptors may be clinically useful in the diagnosis and management of patients with certain T-cell malignancies or autoimmune diseases.

In contrast to the other soluble receptors discussed, soluble IL-4 receptors may be a product of an alternatively spliced RNA.[30] Although soluble IL-4 receptors inhibit many IL-4 effects in vitro, these naturally-occurring molecules may actually enhance IL-4 effects in vivo through acting as a carrier of this cytokine.[31] IL-4 bound to soluble receptors is protected from proteolytic degradation, and complexes of IL-4 and soluble receptors rapidly dissociate at 37°C.

The IL-6 receptor consists of two chains: an 89 kDa ligand binding unit (gp80) and a 130 kDa signal transducing unit (gp130). The extracellular portion of the gp130 chain is released from activated cells by proteolysis, generating a soluble IL-6 receptor that binds IL-6 with high affinity. Paradoxically, complexes of IL-6 and soluble IL-6 receptors actually stimulate cells by binding to the gp130 chain on the cell surface. Soluble IL-6 receptors are elevated in the circulation of patients with multiple myeloma and enhance the biologic responses of myeloma cells to IL-6. Thus, reducing the levels of circulating soluble IL-6 receptors in this disease may be a therapeutic goal.

Treatment of rheumatoid arthritis with soluble TNF receptors

A fusion protein was created consisting of two units of the extracellular portion of the human p75 TNF receptor coupled to the Fc portion of the human IgG_1 molecule (TNFR:Fc). This dimer bound soluble TNF-α with high affinity and inhibited in vitro biologic effects on target cells, leading to its evaluation as a therapeutic agent in patients with rheumatoid arthritis. In a multicenter, double-blind, placebo-controlled clinical trial in 180 patients with refractory rheumatoid arthritis, patients received twice-weekly subcutaneous injections of placebo or TNFR:Fc at 3 doses (0.25, 2, or 16 mg per square meter of body surface area).[32] An improvement of 20% or more in symptoms of active disease was observed in 75% of the high-dose group after 3 months of treatment compared with 14% of the placebo group. The TNFR:Fc was well tolerated with the only adverse events being mild injection site reactions and upper respiratory infections.

In a subsequent study of longer duration, 234 patients with active rheumatoid arthritis received twice-weekly injections of placebo or TNFR:Fc at 10 or 25 mg for 6 months.[33] Again, a dramatic clinical response was observed. At 6 months, 59% of the high-dose group exhibited a 20% response by the ACR criteria, with 40% demonstrating the more stringent 50% ACR response, in comparison to 11% and 5%, respectively, of the placebo group. In fact, a 70% ACR response (virtually no disease activity) was observed in 9% and 15% of patients who received the two doses of TNFR:Fc for 6 months compared to 1% in the placebo group. No difference in infections was observed between the three groups.

The soluble TNFR:Fc fusion protein was next examined in combination with methotrexate in patients with rheumatoid arthritis who exhibited persistent disease activity in spite of methotrexate therapy at a stable dose of 15–25 mg per week for at least 6 months.[34] Patients received 25 mg TNFR:Fc or placebo by twice-weekly injections, and continued to take their previous dose of methotrexate. The addition of the soluble TNFR:Fc fusion protein to methotrexate led to rapid and sustained clinical responses. The ACR 20%, 50%, and 70% criteria were met at 24 weeks by 71%, 39%, and 15%, respectively, of the patients receiving the soluble TNFR:Fc protein, compared to 27%, 3%, and 0%, respectively, of the placebo group. Again, injection site reactions were common in the patients receiving the fusion protein (42% vs. 7% in the placebo group), and no differences in rates of infections were observed between the three groups.

> **CLINICAL PEARLS**
>
> **Treatment of rheumatoid arthritis with soluble TNF receptor Fc fusion protein**
> - Two units of the extracellular portion of the human p75 TNF receptor were coupled to the Fc portion of the human IgG_1 molecule (TNFR:Fc).
> - Twice-weekly subcutaneous injections of TNFR:Fc alone were highly efficacious in the treatment of patients with refractory rheumatoid arthritis.
> - TNFR:Fc is also effective when used in combination with methotrexate in patients only partially responsive to the latter drug.
> - TNFR:Fc is also effective in juvenile rheumatoid arthritis, and possibly in other forms of inflammatory arthritis in adults.

In summary, soluble TNFR:Fc is a very effective treatment for rheumatoid arthritis resistant to the usual disease-modifying drugs. This therapeutic agent also is effective in patients with juvenile rheumatoid arthritis and is being examined in other forms of adult inflammatory arthritis. While soluble TNFR:Fc appears to be safe in the short term, more long-term experience will be necessary to observe whether any infectious or neoplastic complications will emerge. For rheumatoid arthritis resistant to other disease-modifying drugs, FDA approval has been granted for treatment with soluble TNFR:Fc either alone or in combination with methotrexate. However, within the first 6 months of availability of this agent, a number of deaths were reported from sepsis. A warning was issued by the manufacturer against use of TNF blockade in rheumatoid arthritis patients with acute or chronic infections. In fact, in a clinical trial with soluble p75 TNFR:Fc in patients with sepsis syndrome, overall mortality actually increased at 28 days in the higher-dose groups.[35]

Treatment of asthma with soluble IL-4 receptors

IL-4 is an important cytokine in mediating allergic inflammation and asthma through multiple mechanisms (Chapter 49). IL-4 promotes the differentiation of naive T cells into the Th2 phenotype, thus leading to the production of more IL-4 as well as IL-5, IL-9, and IL-13 (Chapter 15). In addition, IL-4 induces the switch to IgE production, up-regulates IgE receptor expression on a variety of cells, induces adhesion molecule expression on endothelial cells to enhance eosinophil migration into tissues, and up-regulates both mucin and 15-lipoxygenase production. The IL-4 receptor consists of a ligand-binding α-chain and a signal-transducing γ-chain also common to receptors for IL-2, IL-7, IL-9, and IL-15. Soluble IL-4 receptors have been produced by genetic engineering, consisting of the 54 kDa extracellular portion of the α-chain. Soluble IL-4 receptors, as well as anti-IL-4 antibodies, are effective in inhibiting IL-4 effects in vivo in mice and in vitro in human cell systems.

THERAPEUTIC PRINCIPLES

Treatment of asthma with soluble IL-4 receptors

- IL-4 is an important mediator of allergic inflammation and asthma:
  - — Promotes the differentiation of naive T cells into the Th2 phenotype.
  - — Induces the switch to IgE production and up-regulates IgG receptor expression.
  - — Enhances eosinophil migration into tissues through stimulating adhesion molecule expression on endothelial cells.
- A single dose of nebulized soluble IL-4 receptors is highly effective for up to 2 weeks in the treatment of patients with moderate atopic asthma requiring inhaled corticosteroids.

Soluble IL-4 receptors have recently been demonstrated to have therapeutic efficacy in asthma. In a double-blind, placebo-controlled trial, 25 patients with moderate atopic asthma requiring inhaled corticosteroids received either placebo or a single dose of nebulized IL-4R at 1500 μg or 500 μg.[36] The corticosteroids were stopped and the patients were followed through 15 days. The nebulized IL-4R had previously been shown to have an in vivo half-life of around 1 week. The patients receiving the high dose of IL-4R demonstrated clinical improvement in multiple parameters including FEV_1 on day 4, FEV_{25-75} on days 2 and 4, asthma symptom scores, and less β_2 agonist use, all in comparison with the low-dose or placebo groups. Most importantly, the patients did not worsen after discontinuing their corticosteroids, but their clinical course remained stable through 15 days after receiving a single dose of nebulized IL-4R. Although not studied, it was hypothesized that patients with nonallergic asthma as well as other atopic diseases such as allergic rhinitis and atopic dermatitis might also respond to the nebulized IL-4R.

CYTOKINE RECEPTOR ANTAGONISTS

Both TNF-α and IL-1 may be of central pathophysiologic importance in human autoimmune and chronic inflammatory diseases. These cytokines are primary products of monocytes and macrophages and can be produced by many other cells as well. TNF-α and IL-1 may be responsible for tissue destruction in many organs through inducing the production of matrix metalloproteinases (MMPs) by fibroblasts and other mesenchymal cells. The ubiquity of TNF-α and IL-1 production, and the pleiotropy of their effects, suggests that natural regulatory mechanisms must exist. The generation of soluble receptors for TNF-α and IL-1 may comprise such a mechanism.

The identification of a specific receptor antagonist for IL-1, termed IL-1Ra, represents the first description of a naturally-occurring receptor antagonist of any cytokine or hormone-like molecule. At least four different structural variants of IL-1Ra have been described to date, the first secreted and the rest intracellular isoforms. While the major function of secreted IL-1Ra (sIL-1Ra) may be to competitively inhibit the binding of IL-1 to plasma membrane receptors, intracellular IL-1Ra (icIL-1Ra) may exhibit additional effects inside cells. Recombinant IL-1Ra has successfully been applied as a therapeutic agent in rheumatoid arthritis.

CLINICAL PEARLS

IL-1 receptor antagonist in the treatment of rheumatoid arthritis

- A naturally-occurring competitive inhibitor of the binding of IL-1α and IL-1β to types I and II IL-1 receptors on target cells.
- One secreted and three or more intracellular isoforms may exist
- Requires 100-fold or greater excess amounts of IL-1Ra to inhibit IL-1 biologic responses in vitro or in vivo.
- The balance between endogenous IL-1Ra and IL-1 levels in a particular tissue may influence the relative propensity to develop an inflammatory disease.
- Is clinically effective in the treatment of rheumatoid arthritis when administered as daily subcutaneous injections.

Production and characteristics of IL-1Ra

Earlier studies on the identification of IL-1 inhibitory biologic activities in the supernatants of various cells, and the eventual purification and cloning of IL-1Ra, have been previously reviewed.[37] IL-1Ra appears to have evolved from a primordial form of IL-1, acquiring structural changes so that it binds to IL-1 receptors but fails to activate cells. Large amounts of IL-1Ra are necessary both in vitro and in vivo to inhibit the stimulatory effects of IL-1 (Fig. 116.2). This is because of the spare receptor effect whereby target cells are exquisitively sensitive to the occupancy of only a few type I IL-1 receptors per cells by IL-1α or β, and cells express a relatively large number of receptors. IL-1Ra binds strongly to both types I and II IL-1 receptors on cells, but interacts more avidly with soluble type I IL-1 receptor than with type II.[38] Thus, soluble type I IL-1 receptors actually may

Inhibition of IL-1 activation of cells

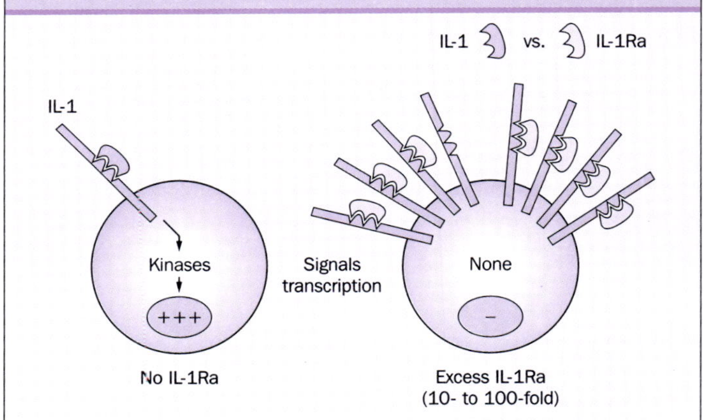

Figure 116.2 Inhibition of IL-1 activation of cells requires a great excess of IL-1Ra. Left. Occupancy of plasma membrane type I IL-Ra requires only a few molecules per cell of IL-1α or IL-1β to stimulate a full biologic response in a target cell. This is mediated by cytoplasmic kinases and enhanced transcription in the nucleus. Right. Because cells express relatively large numbers of type I IL-1 receptors, 10- to 100-fold excess amounts of IL-1Ra are necessary to block occupancy of only a few receptors by IL-1.

block the anti-inflammatory effects of IL-1Ra whereas soluble type II IL-1 receptors may be additive.

IL-1 and IL-1Ra are generally produced by the same cells but are differentially regulated. LPS induces the production of both molecules in monocytes, but adherent immune complexes or aggregated IgG stimulate primarily IL-1Ra production. The injection of small amounts of LPS into normal volunteers led to peak plasma levels of IL-1Ra that were 100-fold greater than IL-1β levels.[39] Furthermore, IL-4 or IL-10 enhance LPS-induced IL-1Ra production by monocytes and macrophages but inhibit IL-1 production. The relative concentrations of IL-1 vs. IL-1Ra in local tissues may be an important determinant of the net pro- or anti-inflammatory environment.

Role of endogenous IL-1Ra

The role in biology of IL-1Ra has recently been reviewed.[40] The tissue distribution of IL-1Ra in mice indicated that sIL-1Ra was found predominately in peripheral blood cells, lungs, spleen, and liver, while icIL-1Ra was present in large amounts in epithelial cells in the skin and gastrointestinal tract. Surprisingly, sIL-1Ra was produced by hepatic cells with the characteristics of an acute-phase protein both in vitro and in vivo, the first cytokine to exhibit this physiology.[41] Endogenous IL-1Ra is produced in numerous experimental animal models of disease, as well as in human autoimmune and chronic inflammatory diseases. The use of neutralizing antibodies to IL-1Ra demonstrated that endogenous IL-1Ra was an important natural anti-inflammatory protein in arthritis, colitis, and granulomatous pulmonary disease (reviewed in ref. 40).

The physiologic effects of endogenous IL-1Ra were further characterized by studies in transgenic B6CBAF1/J or gene-deleted C57BL/6J mice. Mice lacking all isoforms of IL-1Ra exhibited decreased body mass, did not reproduce well, were more susceptible to lethal endotoxemia, and were less susceptible to infection with *Listeria monocytogenes*, all in comparison to wild-type controls.[42] In contrast, mice overexpressing sIL-1Ra under control of the endogenous promoter were protected from the lethal effects of endotoxemia but were more susceptible to listeriosis. These observations were consistent with the known pathologic effects of unopposed IL-1 in endotoxemia and the protective role of IL-1 in host defense against organisms that multiply inside cells. Additional studies indicated that collagen-induced arthritis exhibited an earlier onset and was more severe in IL-1Ra gene-deleted mice, with the opposite pattern observed in IL-1Ra transgenic mice.[43]

The results of recent studies indicate that different phenotypes can be observed in IL-1Ra knockout mice depending on the strain studied. A chronic inflammatory arthritis resembling rheumatoid arthritis spontaneously developed in all IL-1Ra-deficient mice bred on a BALB/cA background but not on a C57BL/6J background.[44] In studies by other investigators, IL-1Ra-deficient mice bred on an outbred MF1 background spontaneously developed a lethal inflammatory arterial disease.[45] The results of these two studies indicate that the ratio of IL-1Ra to IL-1 may be an important influence on the development of inflammatory disease in the joints or vessel walls, depending on the interaction with products of other as yet unknown genes. Thus, endogenously-produced IL-1Ra may act a natural regulator of the pro-inflammatory effects of IL-1 in situations where other genes predisposing to early disease mechanisms may be operative.

Therapeutic use of IL-1Ra

Clinical trials with the administration of IL-1Ra have been carried out in sepsis syndrome and rheumatoid arthritis. Although the results of early studies indicated possible efficacy in a subset of patients with sepsis syndrome, subsequent clinical trials failed to reveal any benefit on mortality at 28 days. However, more positive effects have been observed in rheumatoid arthritis. In a preliminary study, 175 patients with active rheumatoid arthritis received subcutaneous injections of recombinant human IL-1Ra in 3 different doses in a varying schedule ranging from daily to once a week for 7 weeks.[46] By the end of the 3-week treatment phase, daily dosing appeared more effective than weekly dosing but the groups were too small to establish efficacy. The most frequent adverse reaction was inflammation at the injection site, observed in 62% of patients. In a subsequent, larger clinical trial, 472 patients were randomized into a 24-week, double-blind, placebo-controlled, multicenter study, receiving either placebo or a self-administered daily subcutaneous injection of IL-1Ra at 30, 75, or 150 mg.[47] At 24 weeks, 43% of the patients treated with the largest dose of IL-1Ra demonstrated a 20% response by the American College of Rheumatology criteria in comparison to 27% of patients with a 20% response in the placebo group. In addition, the rate of radiologic progression was significantly less in all patients who received IL-1Ra compared to placebo. Clinical trials in progress are examining the effect of IL-1Ra in rheumatoid arthritis over longer periods of time and when administered in combination with methotrexate.

SUMMARY AND CONCLUSIONS

This chapter has reviewed some of the mechanisms whereby cytokine effects are inhibited or blocked, illustrating that the cytokine network truly is self-regulating. Exaggerated effects of particular cytokines in disease processes may be due to unregulated production of pro-inflammatory cytokines, particularly IL-1 or TNF-α, or to inadequate production of anti-inflammatory cytokines such as IL-1Ra. In addition, cytokine effects may be regulated at the levels of production, protein binding, receptor expression, soluble receptor generation, or receptor binding. Successful clinical trials have been reported in patients with Crohn's disease infused with monoclonal antibodies to TNF-α, in patients with rheumatoid arthritis treated with monoclonal antibodies to TNF-α, soluble TNF

THERAPEUTIC PRINCIPLES

IL-1 and TNF-α in inflammatory diseases

- Both IL-1 and TNF-α may mediate acute inflammatory events in rheumatoid arthritis and other human infectious or autoimmune diseases.
- Either IL-1 or TNF-α may stimulate production of itself or of the other cytokine.
- Interfering with the effects of either cytokine by the following means is therapeutically beneficial in human disease:
  - — Monoclonal antibodies to TNF-α in Crohn's disease or rheumatoid arthritis.
  - — Soluble TNF receptors in rheumatoid arthritis.
  - — IL-1 receptor antagonist in rheumatoid arthritis.

receptors, or IL-1Ra, and in asthma patients receiving nebulized soluble IL-4 receptors. However, this area of clinical therapeutics is still in its infancy. Studies are in progress examining these or additional approaches to inhibition of cytokine production or effects in a variety of human autoimmune or inflammatory diseases.

REFERENCES

1. Girasole G, Jilks RL, Passeri G, et al. 17β-estradiol inhibits interleukin-6 production by bone marrow-derived stromal cells and osteoblasts in vitro: A potential mechanism for the antiosteoporotic effect of estrogens. J Clin Invest 1992;89:883.
2. Donnelly RP, Fenton MJ, Kaufman JD, et al. IL-1 expression in human monocytes is transcriptionally and posttranscriptionally regulated by IL-4. J Immunol 1991;146:3431.
3. De Waal Malefyt R, Abrams J, Bennett B, et al. Interleukin 10 (IL-10) inhibits cytokine synthesis by human monocytes: an autoregulatory role of IL-10 produced by monocytes. J Exp Med 1991;174:1209.
4. Fenton MJ, Buras JA, Donnelly RP. IL-4 regulates IL-1 and IL-1 receptor antagonist expression in human monocytes. J Immunol 1992;149:1283.
5. Lafyatis R, Remmers EF, Roberts AB, et al. Anchorage-independent growth of synoviocytes from arthritic and normal joints. Stimulation by exogenous platelet-derived growth factor and inhibition by transforming growth factor-beta and retinoids. J Clin Invest 1989;83:1267.
6. Sano H, Engleka K, Mathern P, et al. Coexpression of phosphotyrosine-containing proteins, platelet-derived growth factor-B, and fibroblast growth factor-1 *in situ* in synovial tissues of patients with rheumatoid arthritis and Lewis rats with adjuvant or streptococcal cell wall arthritis. J Clin Invest 1993;91:553.
7. Lacraz S, Nicod L, Galve-de-Rochemonteix B, et al. Suppression of metalloproteinase biosynthesis in human alveolar macrophages by interleukin-4. J Clin Invest 1992;90:382.
8. Polisson RP, Gilkeson GS, Pyun EH, et al. A multicenter trial of recombinant human interferon gamma in patients with systemic sclerosis: effects on cutaneous fibrosis and interleukin 2 receptor levels. J Rheumatol 1996;23:654.
9. Black CM, Silman AJ, Herrick AI, et al. Interferon-α does not improve outcome at one year in patients with diffuse cutaneous scleroderma. Results of a randomized, double-blind, placebo-controlled trial. Arthritis Rheum 1999;42:299.
10. Svenson M, Hansen MB, Bendtzen K. Distribution and characterization of autoantibodies to interleukin 1α in normal human sera. Scand J Immunol 1990;32:695.
11. Suzuki H, Kamimura J, Ayabe T, et al. Demonstration of neutralizing antibodies against IL-1α in sera from patients with rheumatoid arthritis. J Immunol 1990;145:2140.
12. Hansen MB, Svenson M, Bendtzen K. Human anti-interleukin-1α antibodies. Immunol Lett 1991;30:133.
13. Hansen MB, Svenson M, Diamant M, et al. High-affinity IgG autoantibodies to IL-6 in sera of normal individuals are competitive inhibitors of IL-6 in vitro. Cytokine 1993;5:72.
14. Takemura H, Suzuki H, Yoshizaki K, et al. Anti-interleukin-6 autoantibodies in rheumatic diseases. Arthritis Rheum 1992;35:940.
15. Van Dulleman HM, van Deventer SJH, Hommes DW, et al. Treatment of Crohn's disease with anti-tumor necrosis factor chimeric monoclonal antibody (cA2). Gastroenterol 1995;109:129.
16. Targan SR, Hanauer SB, van Deventer SJH, et al. A short-term study of chimeric monoclonal antibody cA2 to tumor necrosis factor α for Crohn's disease. N Engl J Med 1997;337:1029.
17. Present DH, Rutgeerts P, Targan S, et al. Infliximab for the treatment of fistulas in patients with Crohn's disease. N Engl J Med 1999;340:1398.
18. Garside P. Cytokines in experimental colitis. Clin Exp Immunol 1999;118:337.
19. Feldmann M, Elliott MJ, Woody JN, Maini RN. Anti-tumor necrosis factor-α therapy of rheumatoid arthritis. Adv Immunol 1997;64:283.
20. Elliott MJ, Maini RN, Feldmann M, et al. Randomised double-blind comparison of chimeric monoclonal antibody to tumour necrosis factor α (cA2) versus placebo in rheumatoid arthritis. Lancet 1994;344:1105.
21. Elliott MJ, Maini RN, Feldmann M, et al. Repeated therapy with monoclonal antibody to tumour necrosis factor α (cA2) in patients with rheumatoid arthritis. Lancet 1994;344:1125.
22. Maini RN, Breedveld FC, Kalden JR, et al. Therapeutic efficacy of multiple intravenous infusions of anti-tumor necrosis factor α monoclonal antibody combined with low-dose weekly methotrexate in rheumatoid arthritis. Arthritis Rheum 1998;41:1552.
23. Hession C, Decker JM, Sherblom AP, et al. Uromodulin (Tamm Horsfall glycoprotein): a renal ligand for lymphokines. Science 1987;237:1479.
24. James K. Interactions between cytokines and α_2-macroglobulin. Immunol Today 1990;11:163.
25. Borth W, Urbanski A, Prohaska R, et al. Binding of recombinant interleukin-1β to the third component of complement and α_2-macroglobulin after activation of serum by immune complexes. Blood 1990;75:2388.
26. LeMarre J, Hayes MA, Wollenberg GK, et al. An α_2-macroglobulin receptor-dependent mechanism for the plasma clearance of transforming growth factor-β in mice. J Clin Invest 1991;87:39.
27. Dubois CM, Ruscetti FW, Palaszynski EW, et al. Transforming growth factor β is a potent inhibitor of interleukin 1 (IL-1) receptor expression: proposed mechanism of inhibition of IL-1 action. J Exp Med 1990;172:737.
28. Redini F, Mauviel A, Pronost S, et al. Transforming growth factor β exerts opposite effects from interleukin-1β on cultured rabbit articular chondrocytes through reduction of interleukin-1 receptor expression. Arthritis Rheum 1993;36:44.
29. Chikanza IC, Roux-Lombard P, Dayer J-M, et al. Tumour necrosis factor soluble receptors behave as acute phase reactants following surgery in patients with rheumatoid arthritis, chronic osteomyelitis and osteoarthritis. Clin Exp Immunol 1993;92:19.
30. Mosley B, Beckmann MP, March CJ, et al. The murine interleukin-4 receptor: molecular cloning and characterization of secreted and membrane bound forms. Cell 1989;59:335.
31. Fernandez-Botran R, Vitetta ES. Evidence that natural murine soluble interleukin-4 receptors may act as a transport protein. J Exp Med 1991;174:673.
32. Moreland LW, Baumgartner SW, Schiff MH, et al. Treatment of rheumatoid arthritis with a recombinant human tumor necrosis factor receptor (p75)-Fc fusion protein. N Engl J Med 1997;337:141.
33. Moreland LW, Schiff MH, Baumgartner SW, et al. Etanercept therapy in rheumatoid arthritis. A randomized, controlled trial. Ann Int Med 1999;130:478.
34. Weinblatt ME, Kremer JM, Bankhurst AD, et al. A trial of etanercept, a recombinant tumor necrosis factor receptor: Fc fusion protein, in patients with rheumatoid arthritis receiving methotrexate. N Engl J Med 1999;340:253.
35. Fisher Jr CJ, Agosti JN, Opal SM, et al. Treatment of septic shock with the tumor necrosis factor receptor:Fc fusion protein. N Engl J Med 1996;334:1697.
36. Borish LC, Nelson HS, Lanz MJ, et al. Interleukin-4 receptor in moderate atopic asthma. Am J Respir Crit Care Med 1999;160:1816.
37. Arend WP. Interleukin-1 receptor antagonist. Adv Immunol 1993;54:167.
38. Arend WP, Malyak M, Smith MF Jr, et al. Binding of IL-1α, IL-1β, and IL-1 receptor antagonist by soluble IL-1 receptors and levels of soluble IL-1 receptors in synovial fluids. J Immunol 1994;153:4766.
39. Granowitz EV, Santos AA, Poutsiaka DD, et al. Production of interleukin-1 receptor antagonist during experimental endotoxemia. Lancet 1991;338:1423.
40. Arend WP, Malyak M, Guthridge CJ, Gabay G. Interleukin-1 receptor antagonist: role in biology. Annu Rev Immunol 1998;16:27.

41. Gabay C, Smith MF Jr, Eidlen D, Arend WP. Interleukin 1 receptor antagonist (IL-1Ra) is an acute phase protein. J Clin Invest 1997;99:2930.
42. Hirsch E, Irikura VM, Paul SM, Hirsh D. Functions of interleukin 1 receptor antagonist in gene knockout and overproducing mice. Proc Natl Acad Sci USA 1996;93:11008.
43. Ma Y, Thornton S, Boivin G, et al. Altered susceptibility to collagen-induced arthritis in transgenic mice with aberrant expression of interleukin-1 receptor antagonist. Arthritis Rheum 1998;41:1798.
44. Horai R, Saijo S, Hidetoshi H, et al. Development of chronic inflammatory arthropathy resembling rheumatoid arthritis in IL-1 receptor antagonist-deficient mice. J Exp Med 2000;191:313.
45. Nicklin MJH, Hughes DE, Barton JL, Ure JM, Duff GW. Arterial inflammation in mice lacking the IL-1 receptor antagonist gene. J Exp Med 2000;191:303.
46. Campion GV, Lebsack ME, Lookabough, Gordon G, Catalano M. Dose-range and dose-frequency study of recombinant human interleukin-1 receptor antagonist in patients with rheumatoid arthritis. Arthritis Rheum 1996;39:1092.
47. Bresnihan B, Alvaro-Gracia JM, Cobby M, et al. Treatment of rheumatoid arthritis with recombinant human interleukin-1 receptor antagonist. Arthritis Rheum 1998;41:2196.

Chapter 117 Monoclonal Antibodies and Soluble Protein Receptors

Ted R. Mikuls and Larry W. Moreland

INTRODUCTION

The immune system is composed of a complex array of cells and cell products which, in concert, direct host defense mechanisms to foreign antigens, protecting autologous cells from injury. Unfortunately, these defense mechanisms can, and often do, inflict serious harm on host tissues. 'Unchecked' inflammation, in response to either a foreign or auto-antigen, frequently leads to pathologic changes characteristic of disease (e.g. rheumatoid arthritis [RA]).

Traditional treatment approaches for diseases such as RA and systemic lupus erythematosus (SLE) have involved the use of potent immunosuppressive agents as a means of controlling inflammation. This approach has obvious limitations. In general, immunosuppressive regimens are associated with significant toxicity and, despite their potent effect at the cellular level, often lack significant clinical efficacy. Such limitations are apparent, for example, in the treatment of RA. Methotrexate (MTX), a potent immunosuppressant, is often considered the cornerstone of RA therapy, comparing favorably with other available disease-modifying antirheumatic drugs (DMARDs). Despite this fact, MTX, when used as a single agent, is rarely associated with disease remission and has a rate of continued use of approximately 65% at 5 years, an arguably low figure given the 'life span' of the disease.[1,2]

In recent years, there has been significant growth in our understanding of the molecular interactions that both promote and inhibit inflammation. T-cell activation has long been considered the seminal event in the development of immunity and has thus been implicated in the pathogenesis of several autoimmune diseases. At the center of T-cell activation is the specific interaction between the MHC antigen (Ag) complex and the T-cell receptor (TCR). It has become clear that T-cell activation requires a second (or co-stimulatory) signal. Several co-stimulatory, cell-surface receptors have been described, with particular attention given to the CD40/CD40 ligand (CD40L; CD154) and B7/CD28/CTLA4 interactions. T-cell activation leads to a cascade of events including T cell-dependent humoral immunity, activation of the antigen-presenting cell (APC), and the release of inflammatory mediators including cytokines and matrix metalloproteinases (MMPs). A corollary to the 'two-signal model' of T-cell activation is that MHC-Ag/TCR binding in the absence of co-stimulation may lead to antigen-specific T-cell apoptosis or anergy, a fact which has enormous therapeutic implications. The specificity of these molecules (cell-surface receptors, immunoglobulins, and cytokines) makes them ideal targets for directed therapeutic interventions, therapies that potentially lack the global immunosuppressive effects of many current treatment approaches.

AN OVERVIEW OF BIOLOGICAL AGENTS

Recent advances in biotechnology, particularly in the area of recombinant DNA technology, have made it possible to target these molecules specifically. Therapeutic applications of this technology are often referred to as 'biologicals' or 'biological agents'. Therapeutic approaches that have been tested in humans include the use of monoclonal antibodies (mAbs), soluble protein receptors, recombinant inhibitory cytokines, cytokine inhibitors, and metalloproteinase inhibitors (Fig. 117.1). In addition to being used as immunomodulators, mAbs may have other important applications, including the treatment of cancer and cardiovascular disease. In this chapter we will discuss the use of mAbs and soluble receptors (including fusion proteins) as potential therapeutic modalities.

The variable region on the mAb molecule allows for specific mAb–Ag interaction, an interaction that may be used to inhibit inflammation. MAb–Ag binding may lead to clearance of target molecules (via Fc–Fc receptor-mediated pathways); complement activation, and lysis of target cells; or competitive inhibition of normal molecular (ligand–receptor) interactions. Retreatment with murine mAbs is often limited by the formation of human anti-mouse antibodies (HAMAs). In an attempt to circumvent immunogenicity, chimeric constructs have been developed by fusing the constant region of human immunoglobulin (Ig) with

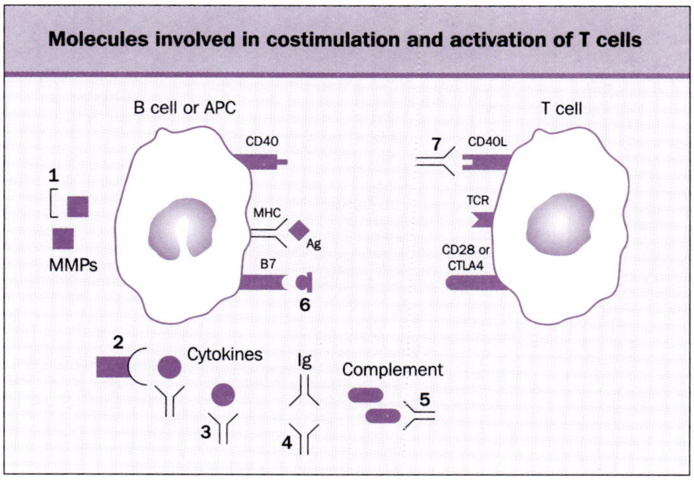

Figure 117.1 Molecules involved in co-stimulation and activation of T cells with subsequent release of cellular products. Biologicals targeting these molecules include: (1) metalloproteinase inhibitors; (2) soluble cytokine receptors; (3) anticytokine mAb; (4) anti-Ig mAb; (5) anticomplement mAb; (6) CTLA41g; (7) anti-CD40 mAb.

KEY CONCEPTS

The role of biological agents in immune diseases

- T-cell activation is considered a seminal event in the development of an immune response and is implicated in the pathogenesis of several autoimmune diseases.
- T-cell depletion has limited the use of biological agents targeting pan-T-cell antigens (i.e. anti-CD4 mAb).
- Current strategies have focused on the use of biological agents which:
  - target pro-inflammatory products of T-cell activation (i.e. cytokines and immunoglobulins)
  - inhibit co-stimulatory signaling between antigen-presenting cells and T cells.

the variable region from a murine Ig (Fig. 117.2). Although generally less antigenic than murine forms, chimeric mAbs have been associated with the development of human antichimeric antibodies (HACAs). Humanized mAbs, comprised of human variable and constant regions, have recently been developed and are under active investigation. Another limiting factor associated with the administration of anti-inflammatory mAbs has been the so-called 'cytokine release syndrome'.[3] Although relatively uncommon, this shock-like syndrome has been best described with OKT3 administration (an anti-T lymphocyte mAb) in renal transplant recipients and is thought to be mediated by cytokine release, complement activation, and neutrophil degranulation.

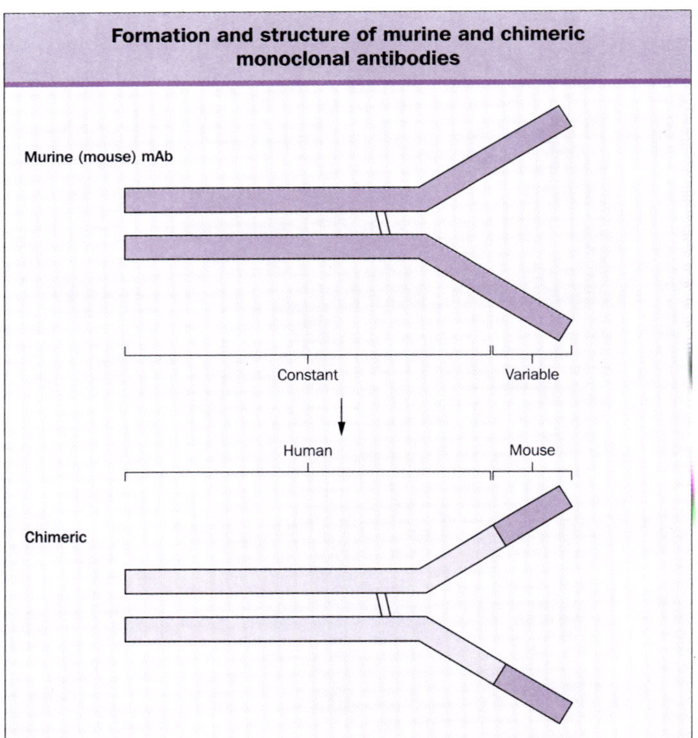

Figure 117.2 Formation and structure of murine (mouse) and chimeric monoclonal antibodies (mAbs). Chimeras are formed through the fusion of constant region of human immunoglobulin (Ig) with the variable region of murine Ig.

Soluble receptors (SRs) are composed of the extracellular domain of native transmembrane protein receptors and thus competitively inhibit the binding of complementary ligands with cell-surface receptors. Shed from the surface of cells, SRs (such as soluble tumor necrosis factor receptor [sTNFR]) may down-regulate the inflammatory cascade. As with mAbs, the use of recombinant SRs may be limited by their antigenicity as well as their relatively short serum half-lives. These problems have been abrogated by the development of fusion proteins, agents derived from linking SRs with conjugate proteins, most often Ig, a segment of Ig, or polyethylene glycol (PEG). Fusion of the SR with a conjugate protein may also increase the binding affinity of the SR for its complementary ligand.

AGENTS INHIBITING T-CELL CO-STIMULATION

MAbs and SRs that inhibit co-stimulatory signals have shown great promise in a variety of animal models of disease and in the process have provided much needed insight into the pathogenesis of these conditions. In contrast to anti-CD4 mAbs and mAbs targeting pan-T-cell markers, blockade of co-stimulation has not resulted in significant T-cell depletion or immunosuppression. B7 (CD80), a ligand expressed primarily on APCs, binds the T-cell receptor CD28 (Fig. 117.1). The resulting signal promotes T-cell activation, proliferation, and differentiation. Additionally, B7 binds CTLA4 (CD152), a receptor expressed almost exclusively on activated T cells. In contrast to the B7-CD28 signal, B7-CTLA4 signal is thought to be inhibitory, particularly since CTLA4 knockout mice have been shown to develop a fatal lymphoproliferative disorder.[4] CTLA4 has a higher binding affinity than CD28 for the B7 ligand. CTLA4Ig, a fusion protein composed of the extracellular domain of CTLA4 and the Fc portion of IgG_1, effectively inhibits B7–CD28 signaling, in contrast to CD28Ig which fails to inhibit this interaction.[5] Consequently, CTLA4Ig has been used in efforts to treat several diseases (psoriasis, RA, etc.), as a primary means of interrupting the B7–CD28 signal.

Similar to the B7–CD28 signal, CD40–CD40L interaction has been shown to play a pivotal role in T-cell activation. CD40L, also known as CD154 or gp39, is expressed on T cells. CD40, expressed primarily on B cells, has also been found on a host of other cells including dendritic cells, basal epithelial cells,[6] macrophages,[7] Langerhans cells,[8] endothelial cells,[9] and thymic epithelial cells.[10] Recently, CD40 expression has been described in synovial monocytes of RA patients,[11] in atheromatous plaques,[12] and in parenchymal and nonparenchymal kidney cells in patients with nephritis associated with SLE,[13] suggesting that the CD40–CD40L interaction plays a pivotal role in the pathogenesis of these disorders. The CD40–CD40L signal up-regulates B7 expression (providing positive feedback) and ultimately leads to activation of nuclear factor-κB (NF-κB). Nuclear translocation of NF-κB is necessary for T-cell growth, differentiation, and resistance to apoptosis as well as for effector functions of B cells and APCs.[14,15] Patients with genetic defects in the CD40L molecule (hyper-IgM syndrome) phenotypically display a lack of germinal centers and have severely impaired humoral immunity with deficient Ig class switching[16] (Chapter 34). MAbs targeting CD40L have been successful in inhibiting the CD40–CD40L signal.

CTLA4Ig[17] and anti-CD40L mAb[18] have both shown promise in murine models of organ transplantation. In these studies, co-stimulatory receptor blockade for 2 weeks following pancreatic

KEY CONCEPTS

The blockade of co-stimulatory signals

- In addition to the specific interaction of the MHC-antigen complex with the T-cell receptor, T-cell activation requires a 'second signal' (i.e. CD40/CD40 ligand and CD80 or 86/CD28 co-stimulation).
- MHC-antigen complex interaction with the T-cell receptor, in the absence of a co-stimulatory signal, may lead to antigen-specific T-cell anergy.
- Blockade of co-stimulation (with a combination of anti-CD40L mAb and CTLA4Ig) has proven successful in a primate model of allograft rejection.
- Co-stimulatory blockade may play a therapeutic role in a number of immune-mediated diseases including SLE, GVHD, multiple sclerosis, and psoriasis.
- In a phase I trial, CTLA4Ig administration was well tolerated and led to significant clinical improvement for patients with long-standing psoriasis.

islet cell transplantation (in diabetic mice) allowed for long-term graft function and diabetes-free survival. Furthermore, resection of the transplanted tissue led to disease recurrence. With re-transplantation from the original donor, the animal models again experienced permanent cure, while cells from a separate donor were promptly rejected. Inhibition of co-stimulatory signals not only prevented transplant rejection but also promoted tolerance to donor tissue.

Unfortunately, CTLA4Ig lacks efficacy in a primate model of organ transplantation.[19,20] In contrast, anti-CD40L, both alone and in combination with CTLA4Ig, has effectively inhibited rejection of renal allografts in rhesus monkeys.[19] In this study, animals given mismatched renal allografts were treated with the combination of anti-CD40L and CTLA4Ig for 28 days post transplantation. In contrast to control allografts (all of which were rejected within 8 days) animals receiving combination therapy maintained normal graft function for at least 6 months, suggesting that co-stimulatory blockade not only prevented rejection but also induced tolerance to donor antigen.

Co-stimulatory blockade has shown promise in several other models for disease. Anti-CD40L, for instance, has been effective in preventing the development of graft-versus-host disease (GVHD) in murine models.[21] Interestingly, GVHD can not be induced using T cells harvested from CD40L knockouts.[22] Both CTLA4Ig[23] and anti-CD40L[24] have also been effective in preventing the onset of collagen-induced arthritis and the development of anticollagen Abs. Atherosclerotic animal models given anti-CD40L mAb have shown reduced plaque formation, suggesting that inflammation, and specifically CD40–CD40L interactions, play an important role in the atherogenesis.[25] Anti-CD40L mAb[26] and CTLA4Ig[27] also blocked the development of experimental allergic encephalitis (EAE) in mice. Anti-CD40L mAb also ameliorates the course of disease when given subsequent to the development of EAE.[26] Activated CD40L$^+$ T cells residing next to CD40$^+$ cells have been found in lesions of patients with multiple sclerosis (MS), the human corollary to EAE.[26]

Both agents have been used successfully in animal models for SLE-associated glomerulonephritis.[28,29] Susceptible mice (NZB/W F1) showed decreased anti-DNA antibody production and prolonged survival even when CTLA4Ig was given after disease progression.[28] Brief blockade of the CD40–CD40L interaction with anti-CD40L mAb at disease onset produced an unexpected long-term benefit with a 60% reduction in the incidence of severe glomerulonephritis[30] compared to controls.

At the time of writing, only two human trials investigating the use of co-stimulatory blockade have been published. In a phase I, open-label, dose-escalating trial, CTLA4Ig was administered to patients with long-standing psoriasis.[31] Forty-six per cent of patients experienced at least 50% improvement (compared to 4% in the parallel control group). Response was dose-related, sustained benefit being seen in some cases. The agent was well tolerated without evidence of global immunosuppression or anti-CTLA4Ig antibody production.

In a more recent phase I trial, investigators examined the use of a humanized anti-CD40L mAb (IDEC-131) in patients with SLE.[32] Patients with symptomatic disease (n = 23) were given a single intravenous dose of IDEC-131. In this dose-escalation trial, anti-CD40L mAb administration was well tolerated and no major adverse effects were reported. Importantly, there was no anti-mAb antibody formation and no T-cell depletion. A multiple-dose phase II trial of IDEC-131 in SLE patients is currently underway. Human trials investigating the use of anti-CD40L mAb and CTLA4Ig in other diseases (e.g. RA) are ongoing. The role that these agents will play in the treatment of these conditions remains to be seen.

AGENTS TARGETING PRO-INFLAMMATORY CYTOKINES

Pathogenic production of pro-inflammatory cytokines has long been implicated in the pathogenesis of several autoimmune diseases. There is accumulating evidence, for instance, that IL-1 and TNF play important roles in the pathogenesis of RA,[33] inflammatory bowel disease (IBD),[34,35] and GVHD.[36,37] TNF has also been implicated in MS[38] and allograft rejection.[39,40] There are a number of other cytokines that may serve as potential targets for biologic interventions. IL-10, for instance, up-regulates autoantibody production and may be an appropriate target in patients with SLE. In this chapter we will discuss anti-TNF therapies as a paradigm for anticytokine modalities. The role of IL-1 in disease pathogenesis and IL-1 directed therapies are reviewed in more detail in Chapter 116.

TNF plays a pivotal role in the inflammatory cascade, stimulating the release of pro-inflammatory cytokines (including IL-1)[41] and matrix metalloproteinases (MMPs),[42] as well as inducing the expression of adhesion molecules.[43] Aberrant TNF production may, in part, be related to 'hyper-expression' of CD40L. CD40L$^+$ T cells can be found in excess in synovial tissue of patients with RA,[44] as well as in the intestinal mucosa of IBD patients.[45] Ligation of these cells with CD40 leads to significant TNF production in a dose-dependent fashion. Currently available biologicals that inhibit TNF include a chimeric anti-TNF mAb (infliximab), and a soluble TNF receptor (sTNFR) fusion protein (etanercept). Clinical trials evaluating infliximab and etanercept in autoimmune diseases are summarized in Table 117.1.

In 1998, the US Food and Drug Administration (FDA) approved etanercept (a sTNFR [p75]:Fc fusion protein), making it the first biological agent available for the treatment of RA.

Agent / Study population	Reference
Clinical trials on agents targeting TNF-α	
Infliximab	
CD	McCabe et al[52]
CD	van Dullemen et al[53]
CD	Targan et al[54]
CD (with fistulas)	Present et al[73]
CD	Baert et al[74]
RA	Elliott et al[55]
RA	Elliott et al[56]
RA	Elliott et al[75]
RA (in comb. with MTX)	Maini et al[57]
RA (in comb. with MTX)	Lipsky et al[76]
Psoriasis	Antoni et al[58]
Etanercept	
RA	Moreland et al[77]
RA	Moreland et al[46]
RA	Moreland et al[48]
RA	Moreland et al[51]
RA (in comb. with MTX)	Weinblatt et al[49]
RA (vs. MTX in early dis.)	Finck et al[50]
JRA	Lovell et al[60]
Psoriasis	Mease et al[59]

CD, Crohn's disease; RA, rheumatoid arthritis; MTX, methotrexate; JRA, juvenile rheumatoid arthritis.

Table 117.1 Summary of clinical trials on agents targeting tissue necrosis factor-alpha (TNF-α) including infliximab (anti-TNF mAb) and etanercept (sTNFR: Fc fusion protein).

More recently, the drug has gained approval for the treatment of juvenile rheumatoid arthritis (JRA). In a phase II trial,[46] 75% of RA patients receiving etanercept had 20% improvement as measured by American College of Rheumatology (ACR) criteria,[47] compared to 14% receiving placebo. Patients experienced a rapid decrease in both swollen and tender joint counts without significant dose-related toxicity.[46] A large multicenter phase III trial has confirmed both the efficacy and tolerability of etanercept in the treatment of RA.[48] At the end of 6 months, 59% of patients receiving etanercept (25 mg subcutaneously twice a week) met ACR criteria for 20% improvement. Injection site reactions were the only adverse event related to etanercept use.

In addition, etanercept has been shown to be safe and effective when used in combination with MTX for the treatment of patients with RA.[49] In a recent phase III trial, etanercept also compared favorably to MTX for the treatment of patients with early, active disease.[50] Patients receiving etanercept experienced more rapid clinical response and had fewer side-effects than patients taking MTX.

In long-term, open-label follow-up studies, etancercept has maintained its efficacy; minor injection site reactions remain the most frequently occurring adverse event.[51] Patients receiving etanercept are more prone to developing antinuclear antibodies (including antibodies to double-stranded DNA). Thus far, there have been no reports of lupus-like syndromes. Post-marketing reports of infections occurring in some patients warrant careful long-term follow-up and caution with the use of TNF inhibitors in patients with active infection. Continued long-term follow-up will be important in clarifying the significance of these findings.

Infliximab, a chimeric mAb, represents another means of inhibiting TNF. Intravenous infliximab has been approved by the FDA for the treatment of Crohn's disease and RA. The efficacy and safety of infliximab in the treatment of Crohn's disease have been clearly demonstrated in several studies.[52–54] In one study, infliximab use resulted in a 33% remission rate for patients with treatment-resistant Crohn's disease.[52]

Infliximab has been shown to be similarly efficacious for the treatment of RA. As with etanercept, infliximab displays a relatively rapid onset of action, giving it a clear advantage over standard disease-modifying agents which often take weeks to months to begin working. RA patients receiving infliximab in the initial phase I study[55] experienced a decrease in morning stiffness from a median duration of 180 minutes at study entry to 5 minutes at 6 weeks. In the same time period, infliximab administration was associated with a 73% reduction in pain scores. Swollen joint counts decreased from 18 to 5, and C-reactive protein levels fell from a median of 39.5 mg/dl to 8 mg/dl. Repeated dosing of infliximab has been complicated by HACA responses,[56] antibodies that could potentially limit the drug's long-term therapeutic effect. In a recent trial, HACA responses in RA patients were greatly diminished with the co-administration of MTX.[57] Patients receiving the combination of infliximab–MTX showed improvement in both the duration and magnitude of their clinical response.

Anti-TNF therapies hold promise for a number of other diseases. In a recent open-label trial of patients with refractory psoriatic arthritis, infliximab use was associated with substantial clinical and radiologic benefit.[58] The results from a double-blind, placebo-controlled trial of etanercept in patients with severe psoriatic arthritis and psoriasis are similarly encouraging.[59] Eighty-seven per cent of those receiving etanercept met criteria for improvement compared to only 23% of those receiving placebo. Etanercept has also proven to be effective and well tolerated in the treatment of JRA.[60] The median time to flare for JRA patients receiving etanercept was more than 116 days (less than one half had experienced flare by the trial's conclusion) compared to 28 days for those receiving placebo. Both infliximab and etanercept are being actively investigated for use in a variety of other diseases including MS, Wegener granulomatosis, GVHD, and Behçet's disease.

THERAPEUTIC PRINCIPLES

The inhibition of pro-inflammatory cytokines

- Etanercept, a soluble TNF receptor-Fc fusion protein, has FDA approval for the treatment of both rheumatoid arthritis and juvenile rheumatoid arthritis.
- Infliximab, a chimeric anti-TNF mAb, has FDA approval for the treatment of rheumatoid arthritis and Crohn's disease.
- In phase III clinical trials of rheumatoid arthritis, etanercept and infliximab have been well tolerated, displaying substantial disease-modifying properties.

AGENTS TARGETING IMMUNOGLOBULIN AND COMPLEMENT

Ig and complement also play crucial roles in inflammation and have become the target of novel therapeutic approaches in atopic asthma and SLE-associated glomerulonephritis. In atopic asthma patients, IgE binds to Fc receptors on inflammatory cells (mast cells and basophils) which are subsequently activated by cross-linking of the Fab of IgE with multivalent antigens. Activation of these cells leads to degranulation and release of mediators (e.g. histamine) which result in airway hyperresponsiveness. Parenteral administration of a humanized murine mAb (rhuMAb-E25) directed against the Fc-binding domain of IgE has been shown to suppress both the early- and late-phase responses to inhaled allergen in patients with asthma.[61] In a separate study, aerosolized delivery of anti-IgE (E25) failed to inhibit airway hyperresponsiveness in patients with asthma.[62] One patient receiving E25 developed anti-E25 antibodies, suggesting that the aerosolized route may also be more immunogenic than the parenteral route. A placebo-controlled clinical trial involving 317 patients with allergic asthma demonstrated that anti-E25 therapy administered over 20 weeks resulted in a marked decrease in serum IgE levels.[63] In addition, the asthma scores and steroid use in the treated patients decreased significantly compared to those of the placebo group, suggesting that this therapy may be useful in moderate to severe allergic asthmatics.[63]

Complement activation and decreased levels of serum complement (C3, C4, and CH50) are hallmarks of active SLE. Both the classical and alternative complement pathways are involved in active disease. Converging at C5, these pathways lead to the formation of the pro-inflammatory C5a molecule and the terminal membrane attack complex (C5b–C9). A mAb targeting C5 has been developed in an attempt to inhibit the formation of these pro-inflammatory molecules. In normal volunteers, administration of an anti-C5 mAb inhibited serum hemolytic complement activity for 12–24 hours in a dose-dependent fashion. A chimeric anti-C5 mAb (h5G1.1-mAb) has been tested in a phase I trial of patients with RA and has been shown to be well tolerated.[64] Patients given a single intravenous dose (8 mg/kg) of h5G1.1-mAb had a significant reduction in C-reactive protein levels compared to baseline and showed trends towards improved tender and swollen joint counts. The role that complement antagonists will play in the treatment of diseases such as RA and SLE awaits further study.

THE USE OF mAbs IN NONINFLAMMATORY CONDITIONS

The specificity of mAb binding makes these agents attractive for the treatment of many noninflammatory conditions. There is accumulating evidence, for instance, that mAbs may play an increasing role in the treatment of several malignancies. Three classes of cytotoxic mAbs have been described. The first two classes consist of unconjugated mAbs and mAbs conjugated to toxins or radioisotopes. The last class consists of a mAb acting as a carrier of a toxic gene. In general, the use of mAb–toxin conjugate proteins has been greatly hampered by significant dose-limiting toxicity including the relatively uniform development of a vascular leak syndrome.

In a phase II trial involving patients with relapsed low-grade and follicular nonHodgkin lymphoma (NHL), the administration of rituximab (an unconjugated anti-CD20 mAb) was associated with a 48% response rate.[65,66] Displaying little toxicity, rituximab is currently under active investigation for the treatment of other B-cell malignancies including chronic lymphocytic leukemia (CLL) and multiple myeloma (MM). Researchers are currently developing an anti-CD38 mAb that is to act as a carrier for a toxin gene. This DNA cargo may be internalized by $CD38^+$ (MM) cells via receptor-mediated endocytosis, resulting in the selective killing of MM cells.[67] Therapy directed at the alpha chain of the IL-2 receptor has been used clinically in the treatment of adult T-cell leukemia.[68,69] In addition, an alternative approach targeting the high-affinity IL-2 receptor using a fusion protein consisting of a portion of the diphtheria toxin protein and IL-2 is efficacious in the treatment of cutaneous T-cell lymphoma.[70] In 1999, the FDA approved the use of this fusion protein (DAB_{389}IL-2) for the treatment of persistent or recurrent cutaneous T-cell lymphoma if the cells are CD25 positive.

In addition to having an antitumor effect, mAbs may soon play a major role in the treatment of cardiovascular disease. CD40–CD40L signaling has been implicated in the development of atherosclerosis,[25] suggesting that blockade of this signal (with anti-CD40L mAb) may be of benefit. In addition to atherogenesis, platelet aggregation is regarded as a major culprit in the development of acute coronary syndromes, often complicating treatment interventions such as percutaneous transluminal angioplasty (PTCA).

Activation of the platelet glycoprotein (gp) receptor, IIb/IIIa, is recognized as the final common pathway in platelet aggregation and has thus become the target of biologic intervention. Abciximab, an anti-gpIIb/IIIa mAb, has been studied extensively in the treatment of acute coronary syndromes. In the EPIC trial (Evaluation of 7E3 for the Prevention of Ischemic Complications),[71] abciximab was given as an adjunct to PTCA for patients with unstable angina. Its use resulted in a more than 70% reduction in the 30-day incidence of death, acute myocardial infarction (MI), or urgent revascularization. Additionally, those receiving abciximab infusions had a 60% lower mortality at 3 years.[72] Currently, abciximab is used primarily as an adjunct to PTCA and other interventional procedures. The future role of this agent for the noninterventional medical management of acute coronary syndromes remains to be seen. Abciximab is currently being investigated for use in acute MI, administered in combination with low-dose thrombolytics.

THERAPEUTIC PRINCIPLES

The use of monoclonal antibodies in noninflammatory conditions

- mAbs targeting specific cell-surface antigens are under investigation in noninflammatory conditions including cardiovascular disease and neoplasia.
- The administration of rituximab (an unconjugated anti-CD20 mAb) has been associated with a 48% response rate in patients with relapsed low-grade follicular nonHodgkin lymphoma.
- Abciximab selectively binds the gpIIb/IIIa receptor, interfering with platelet aggregation, and has recently proven to be an important adjunctive therapy in patients with unstable angina undergoing percutaneous angioplasty.

CONCLUSIONS

Biological agents have given clinicians and patients alike a new, targeted approach in the treatment of several disorders. These agents, specifically mAbs and SRs, selectively bind target antigen and thus have obvious theoretical advantages over many standard treatment regimens. Importantly, selective molecular targeting has provided investigators with enormous insight into the pathogenesis of several poorly understood diseases including RA, SLE, GVHD, MS, and allograft rejection. In addition to an immunomodulating role, these agents may be used in traditionally noninflammatory disorders including CAD and cancer, diseases associated with significant morbidity and mortality.

With few exceptions, data supporting the use of biological agents in humans remain limited. Studies aimed at defining the role of these agents are underway. In addition to questions of safety and efficacy, these studies (and others sure to follow), will need to address several critical issues. For instance, given the agents' potential for antigenicity, re-treatment and long-term use may be difficult. A potential for untoward adverse events, including neoplasia and infection, will require rigorous and lengthy open-label follow-up. The use of biologicals as part of combination regimens, either with other biological agents or with standard modalities, will also require further study. In general, recombinant DNA technology involved in the production of biological agents is expensive, a cost that may seriously limit widespread acceptance of these drugs. Given concerns over cost and issues of antigenicity with retreatment, biologicals may soon play an increasing role as 'induction' therapies, given early on in the disease process, particularly considering the potency and relatively short onset of action of these agents. The precise role that biological agents play in the treatment armamentarium of physicians remains to be seen.

REFERENCES

1. Felson DT, Anderson JJ, Meenan RF. Use of short-term efficacy/toxicity tradeoffs to select second-line drugs in rheumatoid arthritis. A meta-analysis of published clinical trials. Arthritis Rheum 1992;35:1117.
2. Pincus T, Marcum SB, Callahan LF. Long-term drug therapy for rheumatoid arthritis in seven rheumatology private practices. II. Second-line drugs and prednisone. J Rheumatol 1992;19:1885.
3. Parlevliet KJ, Bemelman FJ, Yong SL, et al. Toxicty of OKT3 increases with dosage. A controlled study in renal transplant recipients. Transplant Intern 1995;8:141.
4. Tivol EA, Borriello F, Schweitzer AN, et al. Loss of CTLA-4 leads to massive lymphoproliferation and fatal multiorgan tissue destruction, revealing a critical negative regulatory role of CTLA-4. Immunity 1995;3:541.
5. Linsley PS, Wallace PM, Johnson J, et al. Immunosuppression in vivo by a soluble form of the CTLA-4 T cell activation molecule. Science 1992;257:792.
6. Clark EA. CD40: a cytokine receptor in search of a ligand. Tissue Antigens 1990;36:33.
7. Alderson MR, Armitage RJ, Tough TW, et al. CD40 expression by monocytes: regulation by cytokines and activation of monocytes by the ligand for CD40. J Exp Med 1993;178:669.
8. Caux C, Massacrier C, Vanbervliet B, et al. Activation of human dendritic cells through CD40 cross-linking. J Exp Med 1994;180:1263.
9. Karmann K, Hughes CW, Schechner J, et al. CD40 on human endothelial cells: inducibility by cytokines and functional regulation of adhesion molecule expression. Proc Natl Acad Sci USA 1995;92:4342.
10. Galy AHM, Spits H. CD40 is functionally expressed on human thymic epithelium. J Immunol 1992;149:775.
11. Sekine C, Yagita H, Miyasaka N, et al. Expression and function of CD40 on rheumatoid arthritis synovium. J Rheumatol 1998;25:1048.
12. Mach F, Schonbeck U, Sukhova GK, et al. Functional CD40 ligand is expressed on human vascular endothelial cells, smooth muscle cells, and macrophages: implications for CD40–CD40 ligand signaling in atherosclerosis. Proc Natl Acad Sci USA 1997;94:1931.
13. Yellin MJ, D'Agati V, Parkinson G, et al. Immunohistologic analysis of renal CD40 and CD40L expression in lupus nephritis and other glomerulonephritides. Arthritis Rheum 1997;40:124.
14. Rothe M, Sarma V, Dixit VM, et al. TRAF2-mediated activation of NF-kappa B by TNF receptor II and CD40. Science 1995;269:1424.
15. Cheng G, Baltimore D. TANK, a co-inducer with TRAF2 of TNF- and CD40L-mediated NF-kappaB activation. Genes Dev 1996;10:963.
16. Ramesh N, Geha RS, Notarangelo LD. CD40 ligand and the hyper-IgM syndrome. In: Ochs HD, Smith CIE, Puck JM (eds) Primary immunodeficiency diseases. New York, Oxford University Press, 1999, p 2331.
17. Lenschow DJ, Zeng Y, Thistlethwaite JR, et al. Long-term survival of xenogeneic pancreatic islet grafts induced by CTLA4Ig. Science 1992;257:789.
18. Parker DC, Greiner DL, Phillips NE, et al. Survival of mouse pancreatic islet allografts in recipients treated with allogenic small lymphocytes and antibody to CD40 ligand. Proc Natl Acad Sci USA 1995;92:9560.
19. Kirk AD, Harlan DM, Armstrong NN, et al. CTLA4-Ig and anti-CD40 ligand prevent renal allograft rejection in primates. Proc Natl Acad Sci USA 1997;94:8789.
20. Levisetti MG, Padrid PA, Szot GL, et al. Immunosuppressive effects of human CTLA4-Ig in a non-human primate model of allogeneic pancreatic islet transplanation. J Immunol 1997;159:5187.
21. Durie FH, Aruffo A, Ledbetter J, et al. Antibody to ligand of CD40, gp39, blocks the occurrence of the acute and chronic forms of graft-versus-host disease. J Clin Invest 1994;94:1333.
22. Buhlmann JE, Noelle RJ. Therapeutic potential for blockade of the CD40 ligand, gp39. J Clin Immunol 1996;16:83.
23. Knoerzer DB, Karr RW, Schwartz BD, et al. Collagen-induced arthritis in the BB rat: prevention of disease by treatment with CTLA-4-Ig. J Clin Invest 1995;96:987.
24. Durie FH, Fava RA, Foy TM, et al. Prevention of collagen-induced arthritis with an antibody to gp39, the ligand for CD40. Science 1993;261:1328.
25. Mach F, Schonbeck U, Sukhova GK, et al. Reduction of atherosclerosis in mice by inhibition of CD40 signalling. Nature 1998;394:200.
26. Gerritse K, Laman JD, Noelle RJ, et al. CD40–CD40 ligand interactions in experimental allergic encephalomyelitis and multiple sclerosis. Proc Natl Acad Sci USA 1996;93:2499.
27. Miller SD, Vanderlugt CL, Lenschow DJ, et al. Blockage of CD28/B7-1 interaction prevents epitope spreading and clinical relapse of murine EAE. Immunity 1995;3:739.
28. Finck BK, Linsley PS, Wofsy D. Treatment of murine lupus with CTLA4Ig. Science 1994;265:1225.
29. Early GC, Zhao W, Burns CM. Anti-CD40 ligand antibody treatment prevents the development of lupus-like nephritis in a subset of New Zealand black × New Zealand white mice. Response correlates with the absence of an anti-antibody response. J Immunol 1996;157:3159.
30. Mohan C, Shi Y, Laman JD, et al. Interaction between CD40 and its ligand gp39 in the development of murine lupus nephritis. J Immunol 1995;154:1470.
31. Abrams JR, Lebwohl MG, Guzzo CA, et al. CTLA4Ig-mediated blockade of T-cell costimulation in patients with psoriasis vulgaris. J Clin Invest 1999;103:1243.
32. Davis JC, Totoritis MC, Sklenar TA, et al. Results of a phase I, single-dose, dose-escalating trial of a humanized anti-CD40L monoclonal antibody (IDEC-131) in patients with systemic lupus erythematosus. [Abstract.] Arthritis Rheum 1999;42(suppl):s1264.
33. Koopman WJ, Moreland LW. Rheumatoid arthritis: anticytokine therapies on the horizon. Ann Intern Med 1998;128:231.

34. Derkx B, Taminiau J, Radema S, et al. Tumour-necrosis factor antibody treatment in Crohn's disease. [Letter.] Lancet 1992;42:173.
35. Ferpetti M, Casini-Raggi V, Pizarro TT, et al. Neutralization of endogenous IL-1 receptor antagonist exacerbates and prolongs inflammation in rabbit immune colitis. J Clin Invest 1994;94:449.
36. Herve P, Flesch M, Tiberghiem P, et al. Phase I–II trial of a monoclonal anti-tumor necrosis factor alpha antibody for the treatment of refractory severe acute graft-versus-host disease. Blood 1992;79:3362.
37. Autin JH, Weinstein HJ, Guinan EC, et al. Recombinant human interleukin-1 receptor antagonist in the treatment of steroid-resistant graft-versus-host disease. Blood 1994;84:1342.
38. Sharief MK, Phil M, Hentges R. Association between tumor necrosis factor alpha and disease progression in patients with multiple sclerosis. N Engl J Med 1991;325:467.
39. Bolling SF, Kunkel SL, Lin H. Prolongation of cardiac allograft survival in rats by anti-TNF and cyclosporine combination therapy. Transplant 1992;53:283.
40. Lin H, Chensue SW, Strieter RM, et al Antibodies against tumor necrosis factor prolong cardiac allograft survival in the rat. J Heart Lung Transplant 1992;11:330.
41. Brennan FM, Chantry D, Jackson A, et al. Inhibitory effect of TNF alpha antibodies on synovial cell interleukin-1 production in rheumatoid arthritis. Lancet 1989;2:244.
42. Shingu M, Nagai Y, Isayama T, et al. The effects of cytokines on metalloproteinase inhibitors (TIMP) and collagenase production by human chondrocytes and TIMP production by synovial cells and endothelial cells. Clin Exp Immunol 1993;94:145.
43. Moser RB, Schleiffenbaum B, Groscurth P, et al. Interleukin 1 and tumor necrosis factor stimulate human vascular endothelial cells to promote transendothelial neutrophil passage. J Clin Invest 1989;83:444.
44. Harigai M, Hara M, Nakazawa S, et al. Ligation of CD40 induced tumor necrosis factor alpha in rheumatoid arthritis: a novel mechanism of activation of synoviocytes. J Rheumatol 1999;26:1035.
45. Liu Z, Colpaert S, D'Haens GR, et al. Hyperexpression of CD40 ligand (CD154) in inflammatory bowel disease and its contribution to pathogenic cytokine production. J Immunol 1999;163:4049.
46. Moreland LW, Baumgartner SW, Schiff MH, et al. Treatment of rheumatoid arthritis with a recombinant human tumor necrosis factor receptor (p75)-Fc fusion protein. N Engl J Med 1997;337:141.
47. Felson DT, Anderson JJ, Boers M, et al. American College of Rheumatology preliminary definition of improvement in rheumatoid arthritis. Arthritis Rheum 1995; 38:727.
48. Moreland LW, Schiff MH, Baumgartner SW, et al. Etanercept therapy in rheumatoid arthritis. A randomized controlled trial. Ann Intern Med 1999;130:478.
49. Weinblatt ME, Kremer JM, Bankhurst AD, et al. A trial of etanercept, a recombinant tumor necrosis factor receptor: Fc fusion protein, in patients with rheumatoid arthritis receiving methotrexate. N Engl J Med 1999;340:253.
50. Finck B, Martin R, Fleischmann R, et al. A phase III trial of etanercept vs. methotrexate (MTX) in early rheumatoid arthritis. [Abstract.] Arthritis Rheum 1999;42(suppl):a280.
51. Moreland LM, Cohen SB, Baumgartner S, et al. Long-term use of etanercept in patients with DMARD-refractory rheumatoid arthritis. [Abstract.] Arthritis Rheum 1999;42(suppl):a1981.
52. McCabe RP, Woody J, van Deventer S, et al. A multicenter trial of cA2 anti-TNF chimeric monoclonal antibody in patients with active Crohn's disease. [Abstract.] Gastroenterology 1996;110 (suppl):a962.
53. van Dullemen HM, van Deventer SJH, Hommes DW, et al. Treatment of Crohn's disease with anti-tumor necrosis factor chimeric monoclonal antibody (cA2). Gastroenterology 1995;109:129.
54. Targan SR, Hanauer SB, van Deventer SJH, et al. A short-term study of chimeric monoclonal antibody cA2 to tumor necrosis factor (alpha) for Crohn's disease. N Engl J Med 1997;337:1029.
55. Elliott MJ, Maini RN, Feldmann M, et al. Treatment of rheumatoid arthritis with chimeric monoclonal antibodies to TNF-alpha. Arthritis Rheum 1993;21:318.
56. Elliott MJ, Maini RN, Feldmann M, et al. Repeated therapy with monoclonal antibody to tumour necrosis factor alpha (cA2) in patients with rheumatoid arthritis. Lancet 1994;344:1125.
57. Maini RN, Breedveld FC, Kalden JR, et al. Therapeutic efficacy of multiple intravenous infusions of anti-tumor necrosis factor α monoclonal antibody combined with low-dose weekly methotrexate in rheumatoid arthritis. Arthritis Rheum 1998;41:1552.
58. Antoni C, Dechant C, Lorenz H, et al. Successful treatment of severe psoriatic arthritis with infliximab. [Abstract.] Arthritis Rheum 1999;42(suppl):a1801.
59. Mease P, Goffe B, Metz J, et al. Enbrel® (etanercept) in patients with psoriatic arthritis and psoriasis. [Abstract.] Arthritis Rheum 1999;42(suppl):a1835.
60. Lovell DJ, Giannini EH, Lange M, et al. Safety and efficacy of Enbrel® (etanercept) in the extended treatment of polyarticular-course JRA. [Abstract.] Arthritis Rheum 1999;42(suppl):a279.
61. Frew AJ. Effects of anti-IgE in asthmatic subjects. Thorax 1998;53(suppl):s52.
62. Fahy JV, Cockcroft DW, Boulet LP, et al. Effect of aerosolized anti-IgE (E25) on airway responses to inhaled allergen in asthmatic subjects. Am J Respir Crit Care Med 1999;160:1023.
63. Migrom H, Fick R, Su JQ, et al. Treatment of allergic asthma with monoclonal anti-IgE antibody. N Engl J Med 1999;341:1966.
64. Jain RI, Moreland LW, Caldwell JR, et al. A single-dose, placebo controlled, double-blind, phase I study of the humanized anti-C5 antibody h5G1.1 in patients with rheumatoid arthritis. [Abstract.] Arthritis Rheum 1999;42(suppl):s42.
65. McLaughlin P, Grillo-Lopez AJ, Czuczman M, et al. IDEC-C2B8 (rituximab): clinical activity in clinically chemoresistant (CCRD) low-grade or follicular lymphoma (LG/F NHL) and in patients relapsing after anthracycline therapy (ANTHRA-RX) or ABMT. [Abstract.] Proc Am Soc Clin Oncol 1997;55(suppl):a16.
66. Maloney DG, Grillo-Lopez AJ, White CA, et al. IDEC-C2B8 (rituximab) anti-CD20 monoclonal antibody therapy in patients with relapsed low-grade non-Hodgkin's lymphoma. Blood 1997;90:2188.
67. Maloney DG, Donovan K, Hamblin TJ. Antibody therapy for treatment of multiple myeloma. Semin Hematol 1999;36(suppl):30.
68. Waldmann TA, White J, Goldman CK, et al. The interleukin-2 receptor: a target for monoclonal antibody therapy of human T-cell lymphotrophic virus 1-induced adult T-cell leukemia. Blood 1993;82:1701.
69. Waldmann TA, White JD, Carrasquillo JA, et al. Radioimmuno-therapy of IL-2Ra expressing adult T cell leukemia with Yttrium-90 labeled anti-Tac. Blood 1995;86:4063.
70. Duvic M, Cather J, Maize J, Frankel A. DAB_{389}IL-2 diphtheria fusion toxin produces clinical responses in tumor stage cutaneous T cell lymphoma. Am J Hematol 1998;58:87.
71. The EPIC investigators. Use of monoclonal antibody directed against the platelet glycoprotein IIb/IIIa receptor in high-risk coronary angioplasty. N Engl J Med 1994; 330:956.
72. Lincoff AM, Califf RM, Anderson K, et al. Evidence for prevention of death and myocardial infarction with platelet membrane glycoprotein IIb/IIIa receptor blockade by abciximab (c7E3 Fab) among patient with unstable angina undergoing percutaneous coronary revascularization. J Am Coll Cardiol 1997;30:149.
73. Present DH, Rutgeerts P, Targan S, et al. Infliximab for the treatment of fistulas in patients with Crohn's disease. N Engl J Med 1999;340:1398.
74. Baert FJ, D'Haens GR, Peeters M, et al. Tumor necrosis factor alpha antibody (infliximab) therapy profoundly down-regulates the inflammation in Crohn's iliocolitis. Gastroenterology 1999;116:22.
75. Elliott MJ, Maini RN, Feldmann M, et al. Randomized double-blind comparison of chimeric monoclonal antibody to tumor necrosis factor alpha (cA2) versus placebo in rheumatoid arthritis. Lancet 1994;344:1105.
76. Lipsky PE, St. Clair W, Kavanaugh A, et al. Long-term control of signs and symptoms of rheumatoid arthritis with chimeric monoclonal anti-TNF alpha antibody (infliximab) in patients with active disease on methotrexate. [Abstract.] Arthritis Rheum 1998;41(suppl):a364.
77. Moreland LW, Margolis GR, Heck LW, et al. Recombinant soluble tumor necrosis factor receptor (p80) fusion protein: toxicity and dose finding trial in refractory rheumatoid arthritis. J Rheumatol 1996;2:1849.

Chapter 118 Apheresis

Ellen F. Lazarus and Harvey G. Klein*

While the origins of therapeutic apheresis may be traced to the ancient practice of bloodletting, the first modern manual techniques for plasmapheresis were developed during the early days of artificial kidney research at the turn of the twentieth century.[1] The term *apheresis* derived from a Greek verb meaning 'to take away or withdraw', was coined to describe removal of one component of blood with return of the remaining components to the donor. Like phlebotomy, apheresis was used first to treat patients but later became more important for collecting blood components for transfusion. In addition to the emerging prominence of donor apheresis for the collection of plasma and cellular blood components, therapeutic apheresis, including derivative procedures using filters, columns, and even ultraviolet light, remains an important primary or adjuvant modality in the treatment of a wide variety of immunologic and nonimmunologic disorders. In the USA, more than 100 000 therapeutic apheresis procedures are performed each year for a wide variety of indications.[2]

PRINCIPLES OF APHERESIS

The principal objective of apheresis is efficient removal of some circulating blood component, either cells (cytapheresis) or some plasma solute (plasmapheresis). For most disorders, the treatment goal is to deplete the circulating cell or substance directly responsible for the disease process. Apheresis can also mobilize cells and plasma components from tissue depots. For example, lymphocytes can be mobilized from the spleen and lymph nodes of some patients with chronic lymphocytic leukemia, and low-density lipoproteins can be removed from tissue stores in patients with familial hyperlipoproteinemia. Apheresis can have other, less obvious effects. Lymphocyte depletion can modify immune responsiveness in some disease states, possibly by disturbing the control mechanisms of cellular immune regulation. Plasmapheresis enhances splenic clearance of immune complexes in certain autoimmune disorders.[3] When therapeutic effect is judged by clinical improvement rather than by efficiency of solute removal, apheresis is more often a helpful adjunct than a form of first-line therapy.

Several mathematical models formulated for different clinical conditions describe the kinetics of apheresis.[4,5] Removal of most blood components follows a logarithmic curve. The removal of 1.5–2 volumes will reduce an intravascular substance by about 60%, and processing larger volumes results in little additional gain. When the goal of plasmapheresis is to supply a deficient substance, for example plasma factors in the treatment of thrombotic thrombocytopenic purpura, replacement follows logarithmic kinetics similar to those developed for solute removal.

Specific cell removal with centrifugal automated cell separators depends on the number of cells available, the volume of blood processed, the efficiency of the particular instrument, and the separation characteristics of the different cells. Most commercially available instruments remove platelets and lymphocytes extremely efficiently. Granulocytes and monocytes cannot be cleanly separated from other cells by standard centrifugal apheresis equipment (Fig. 118.1). Optimal harvesting of these cells requires special

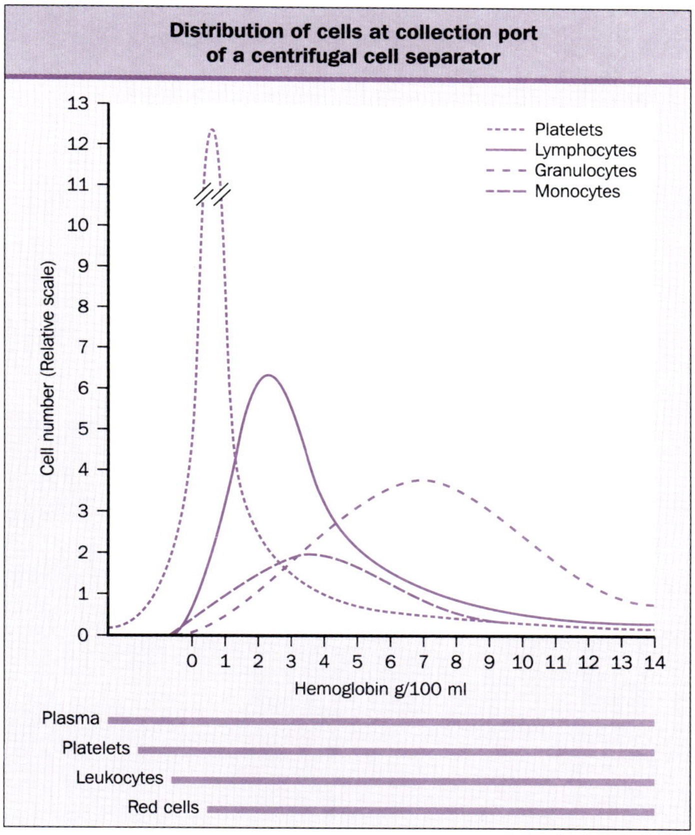

Figure 118.1 Schematic distribution of cells at the collection port of a centrifugal cell separator. The number and percentage of each cell type collected can be varied by adjusting the site of collection along the interface or by changing centrifugal force, blood flow rate, or rate of cell removal. (Reproduced with permission from Hoffman R (ed.) *Hematology: Basic Principles and Practice*, 3rd Edition. London, Churchill Livingstone, 1999.)

* The views of these authors represent scientific opinion and should not be construed as opinion or policy of the US Department of Health and Human Services, US Public Health Service, US Food and Drug Administration, or National Institutes of Health.

techniques such as stimulating the donor with corticosteroids or cytokines and adding sedimenting agents to enhance cell separation.

TECHNOLOGY AND TECHNIQUES

The plasmapheresis technique that originated in the animal laboratory required manual resuspension of red cells and posed a substantial risk of microbial contamination of the components being reinfused.[1] With the introduction of sterile, disposable, interconnected plastic blood bags, plasmapheresis became relatively safe and easy. However, manual apheresis proved too inefficient and labor-intensive for collecting large component volumes and raised concerns that the separated units of red blood cells might be reinfused accidentally into the wrong donor or patient. The introduction of automated on-line blood cell separators solved these problems.[6]

Automated apheresis instruments use microprocessor technology to draw and anticoagulate blood, separate components either by centrifugation or by filtration, collect the desired component and recombine the remaining components for return to the patient.[6] The equipment contains disposable plastic software in the blood path and uses anticoagulants containing citrate or combinations of citrate and heparin that do not result in clinical anticoagulation of the patient. Most instruments function well at blood flow rates of 30–80 ml/min and can operate from peripheral venous access or from a variety of multilumen central venous catheters.

Since the ideal method for treating disorders mediated by abnormal plasma components is to remove the offending substance selectively, a variety of on-line filtration and column adsorption techniques have been introduced or proposed. Ligands bound to a column matrix may be relatively nonspecific chemical sorbents such as charcoal or heparin, or specific ligands such as monoclonal antibodies and recombinant protein antigens. The two most successful clinical columns use staphylococcal protein A and dextran sulfate cellulose. Staphylococcal protein A has high affinity for the Fc portion of IgG_1, IgG_2, and IgG_4, and for immune complexes containing these IgG subclasses. The dextran sulfate cellulose columns selectively remove low-density lipoproteins and have proved effective in managing patients with homozygous hyperlipoproteinemia.

Manipulation of cellular components is also used as an apheresis technique to treat immunologic disorders. A procedure known as photopheresis involves on-line separation of leukocytes that are exposed to light-sensitizing agents and ultraviolet light before being returned to the patient. Commercial devices are available for performing this procedure.

THERAPEUTIC CYTAPHERESIS

Red cell exchange (erythrocytapheresis) is used most often to manage or prevent the acute vaso-occlusive complications of sickle cell disease such as acute chest syndrome, priapism, cerebrovascular accident, and intrahepatic cholestasis. Mechanical cell separators offer the advantages of speed and ease compared to manual exchange transfusion, and reduce the risks of rapid blood volume alteration and increased blood viscosity that may occur with simple transfusion. The rationale behind exchange transfusion involves improving tissue oxygenation and preventing microvascular sickling by diluting the patient's abnormal red cells, simultaneously correcting anemia and favorably altering whole blood viscosity and rheology. No clinical data support a single optimal level of hemoglobin A (HbA). For simple and exchange transfusions, raising the level of HbA to 70% while lowering the level of HbS to 30% is generally efficacious, although even higher levels of HbA may be required to treat an ongoing crisis.

Prophylactic exchange transfusion for sickle cell patients has also been used during pregnancy, before surgery, or for patients who have suffered a stroke. In a randomized study of sickle cell disease patients undergoing surgery, a conservative simple transfusion regimen (to increase the hemoglobin level to 10 g/dl) was as effective as an aggressive regimen (to lower the HbS level to less than 30%) with respect to perioperative nontransfusion-related complications. The patients in the aggressive regimen group received twice as many units of blood, had a proportionally increased RBC alloimunization rate, and experienced a greater number of hemolytic transfusion reactions.[7] The results of this and other studies suggest that if prophylactic preoperative exchange transfusion is used, it should be limited to those patients undergoing high-risk procedures in whom simple transfusion could not effectively raise the HbA level to at least 70%.

Transfusion prophylaxis is now clearly indicated for children with sickle cell anemia at high risk for stroke. A randomized controlled study demonstrated a 90% reduction in risk of stroke in children with sickle cell anemia and abnormal results on transcranial Doppler ultrasonography who were maintained at levels of HbA exceeding 30% by simple or exchange transfusion.[8] Long-term erythrocytapheresis may be preferable for patients at high risk for stroke who have developed iron overload to levels that are associated with organ damage.[9]

Red cell exchange transfusion, although relatively safe and convenient, carries all the complications of simple red cell transfusion. Patients are exposed to a large number of donors and are at small but significant risk of contracting hepatitis and other blood-borne infections. As many as one third of all patients develop red cell alloantibodies,[10] and life-threatening delayed hemolytic transfusion reactions have been reported. In addition, an immunohematologic study of multiply transfused sickle cell disease patients shows that 85% of heavily transfused patients are alloimmunized to HLA and/or platelet-specific antigens.[11] Most centers attempt to avoid inducing nonhemolytic transfusion reactions and HLA alloimmunization by using leukodepleted red cells. Extended red cell phenotyping at diagnosis and provision of phenotypically-matched blood, when practical, can reduce the risk of RBC alloimmunization and associated hemolytic transfusion reactions. Despite the removal of cells during exchange, patients remain in positive iron balance, although iron accumulation is slow and chelation is rarely required to prevent transfusional hemosiderosis.

Therapeutic leukapheresis has been used most successfully to help manage patients with acute or chronic leukemia and extremely high white blood cell (WBC) numbers (hyperleukocytosis). When the fractional volume of leukocytes (leukocrit) exceeds 20%, blood viscosity increases and leukocytes can interfere with pulmonary and cerebral blood flow and compete with tissue for oxygen in the microcirculation.[12] A single leukapheresis procedure generally reduces the WBC count by 20–50%. Leukapheresis is generally performed when the blast count is >100 000/mm^3 or when rapidly rising blast counts are >50 000/mm^3, especially when evidence of central nervous system or pulmonary symptoms appears. Chronic leukapheresis can provide acceptable control of the peripheral WBC count in clinical situations such as pregnancy, when cytotoxic

THERAPEUTIC PRINCIPLES

Common indications for therapeutic cytapheresis
- Red cell exchange
  - Sickle cell disease:
    acute complications
    prophylaxis for recurrent stroke
    frequent severe pain crises
  - Malaria with parasitemia >15%
- Leukapheresis
  - Leukemia with hyperleukocytosis syndrome
  - Cutaneous T-cell lymphoma (photopheresis)
  - Peripheral blood stem cell collection
- Plateletpheresis
  - Symptomatic thrombocytosis

agents may best be avoided, but cytoreduction alone does not appear to alter the course of the disease.

Lymphocyte depletion has been used therapeutically to modify patient immune responsiveness. Removal of large numbers of lymphocytes over a period of a few weeks can suppress peripheral lymphocyte counts in rheumatoid arthritis patients for up to 1 year and alter skin-test reactivity and lymphocyte mitogen responsiveness to a variety of stimulants.[13] Selected patients experience a modest but significant reduction in disease activity; however, the subset of patients who may derive substantial benefit from this therapy is difficult to identify.[14,15] Lymphocyte removal by apheresis has also been used to treat patients with multiple sclerosis; however, evidence of clinical efficacy is sparse and lymphocytapheresis is currently not recommended outside of clinical trials.[16]

Photopheresis is an automated extracorporeal photochemotherapy treatment that involves oral administration of a light-sensitizing agent, psoralen, followed by leukapheresis and ex vivo ultraviolet A irradiation of leukocytes. The treated cells are reinfused. This therapy has minimal toxicity and is highly effective in the treatment of patients with advanced cutaneous T-cell lymphoma. Additional disease states that may respond to photopheresis therapy include solid organ graft rejection and graft-versus-host disease following bone marrow transplantation.[17–19] While anecdotal reports of success are impressive, controlled trials of clinical efficacy of photopheresis in these settings are lacking. The mechanisms by which photopheresis effects tumor regression or allogeneic organ tolerance are unknown.

Therapeutic plateletpheresis is generally reserved for patients with myeloproliferative disorders and hemorrhage or thrombosis associated with an increase in circulating platelets. Many centers consider using plateletpheresis when the patient's peripheral platelet count is $>10^6/mm^3$, although no consistent relationship between the level of platelet elevation and the occurrence of symptoms has been found, and no generally accepted assay of platelet dysfunction predicts which patients are at risk. A single cytapheresis procedure can lower the platelet count by 30–50%. Attempts to maintain thrombocythemic patients at normal platelet counts by cytapheresis alone have not been successful; therefore, long-term chemotherapy should be instituted concurrently. Since most patients with thrombocytosis do not develop symptoms, prophylactic plateletpheresis is unwarranted, regardless of the platelet count.[20]

THERAPEUTIC PLASMAPHERESIS

In the 1960s, therapeutic plasmapheresis was initially applied to the management of diseases mediated by a pathogenic antibody, such as Waldenström's macroglobulinemia and hemolytic disease of the newborn in Rh-sensitized pregnant women. The growth of therapeutic plasmapheresis during the past 50 years owes as much to the development of new technology as to new insight into the pathophysiology of the diseases under treatment. The prevailing developmental strategy has been to complement plasmapheresis with more specific procedures to remove pathologic plasma constituents. An array of immunologic and physicochemical techniques, including cascade filtration, adsorption, immunoadsorption, cryoprecipitation, and photoinactivation, have been added to the plasmapheresis system for laboratory research and clinical applications.

Committees appointed by the American Society of Apheresis (ASFA), American Association of Blood Banks (AABB), and the American Academy of Neurology have published practice guidelines for using plasmapheresis in a wide variety of disease states.[21–23] ASFA and AABB have classified the indications for therapeutic apheresis into four categories based on the strength of the evidence of clinical efficacy for each disorder. Category I includes diseases for which therapeutic apheresis is standard and acceptable, either as a primary therapy or as first-line adjunct therapy. Category II includes diseases for which therapeutic apheresis is generally accepted but considered to be supportive or adjunctive to more definitive treatments. Category III includes diseases in which there is a suggestion of benefit, but for which existing evidence is insufficient to establish the efficacy of therapeutic apheresis or to determine the risk/benefit ratio. Category IV includes disorders for which controlled trials have not shown benefit or anecdotal reports have been discouraging. Common category I and II indications for therapeutic apheresis are listed in Table 118.1.

Metabolic diseases

Evidence that both cutaneous and vascular lesions regress in familial hypercholesterolemia as low-density lipoprotein levels are controlled by plasmapheresis has encouraged the use of several related procedures in patients with homozygous disease and in poorly controlled heterozygous patients. Low-density lipoprotein (LDL) apheresis is a procedure for specifically removing apolipoprotein B-containing lipoproteins from the blood by a variety of techniques including dextran sulfate cellulose adsorption, immunoadsorption, and heparin-induced extracorporeal precipitation. Short-term safety and efficacy have been demonstrated.[24] Continuing experience with this therapy will be required to prove long-term clinical benefit in patients with refractory hypercholesterolemia and coronary artery disease.

Plasmapheresis may be used in patients with other inherited metabolic disorders such as phytanic acid storage disease (Refsum's disease).[25] The frequency of exchange depends primarily on total body burden, rate of synthesis, and plasma concentration of the solute to be removed (Fig. 118.2).

Renal, autoimmune, and rheumatic disorders

Plasmapheresis appears to have at least a temporary adjunctive role in managing some disorders characterized by circulating autoantibodies. Early success was reported in patients with Goodpasture syndrome, a disorder characterized by specific pathogenic autoantibody directed against the renal glomerular and

Common indications for therapeutic plasmapheresis		
Disease	**Procedure**	**Indication category**
Metabolic		
Familial hypercholesterolemia	Selective adsorption	I
Phytanic acid storage disease	Plasma exchange	I
Autoimmune, renal, and rheumatic		
Cryoglobulinemia	Plasma exchange	II
Anti-glomerular basement membrane antibody disease	Plasma exchange	I
Rheumatoid arthritis	Immunoadsorption	II
	Lymphocyte-plasmapheresis	II
Hematological		
Thrombotic thrombocytopenic purpura	Plasma exchange	I
Post-transfusion purpura	Plasma exchange	I
Myeloma with hyperviscosity	Plasma exchange	II
Neurological		
Acute inflammatory demyelinating polyradiculoneuropathy	Plasma exchange	I
Chronic inflammatory demyelinating, polyradiculoneuropathy	Plasma exchange	I
Myasthenia gravis	Plasma exchange	I
Sydenham's chorea	Plasma exchange	II
PANDAS	Plasma exchange	II

Table 118.1 Common indications for therapeutic plasmapheresis. (Modified from McLeod BC. Introduction to the third special issue: clinical applications of therapeutic apheresis. *J Clin Apheresis* 2000;15:1. Reprinted by permission of Wiley-Liss, Inc., a subsidiary of John Wiley & Sons, Inc.)

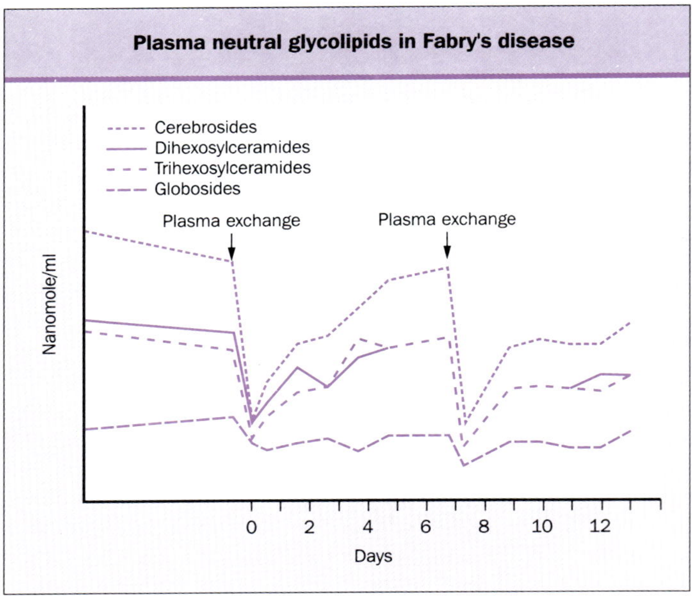

Figure 118.2 Plasma exchange to remove plasma neutral glycolipids in a patient with Fabry's disease. The plasma lipid recovery curve appears to be biphasic, reflecting initial re-equilibration from tissue stores and subsequent new synthesis of that glycolipid. (Reproduced with permission from Hoffman R (ed.) *Hematology: Basic Principles and Practice*, 3rd Edition. London, Churchill Livingstone, 1999.)

pulmonary alveolar basement membranes. Plasmapheresis has demonstrated similar success in a variety of disorders associated with specific autoantibodies, including myasthenia gravis, pemphigus, and Eaton–Lambert syndrome. Plasmapheresis can be used in addition to corticosteroids or cytotoxic agents in the treatment of life-threatening or organ-threatening symptoms in patients with cryoglobulinemia.[26] A recent randomized, double-blind, sham-controlled, multicenter trial has demonstrated efficacy of selective apheresis with the Prosorba® staphylococcal protein A column in rheumatoid arthritis patients with active disease who had failed to respond to treatment with methotrexate or at least two other second-line drugs.[27] In a continuation phase of this trial, 13 patients were re-treated with the Prosorba® column. A 78% response rate was obtained in patients who had previously responded to treatment (7/9); the response rate was 0% in the 4 patients who did not initially respond to immunoabsorption apheresis treatment.[28] The Food and Drug Administration has approved extended labeling for this immunoabsorption column to include treatment of moderate to severe rheumatoid arthritis. The decision to treat rheumatoid arthritis patients with therapeutic apheresis should be weighed against the disease status of the patient, the costs of the treatments, and the availability of potentially more effective disease-modifying anti-rheumatic drugs.

In other autoimmune disorders, such as immune thrombocytopenic purpura and immune inhibitors to coagulation proteins, plasmapheresis may be helpful during a catastrophic event. Plasmapheresis, often combined with glucocorricoid therapy, has been successful in the acute phase of these disorders and long-term remissions have been reported. Benefit in chronic disorders is less well established. Although therapeutic plasma exchange has been used in a variety of other immune disorders, such as systemic lupus erythematosus and systemic vasculitis, the benefits of this treatment remain unproven and these are generally considered to be category III or IV indications.[26]

Controversy surrounds the practice of combining cytotoxic drug therapy with plasmapheresis to prevent rapid resynthesis of antibody, so-called 'antibody rebound'. Although the rebound phenomenon is well established in animal models, investigational studies in healthy volunteers suggest that antibody rebound is not common. Controlled trials of plasmapheresis therapy that failed to demonstrate benefit in lupus nephritis and polymyositis have been criticized for not including a plasmapheresis-with-immunosuppression arm. Since many uncontrolled treatment protocols stipulate simultaneous use of immunosuppressive drugs and plasmapheresis, an apparent favorable outcome may result from the independent effects of the different treatments or some synergistic effect. The largest controlled trial of combined therapy for proliferative glomerulonephritis in SLE showed no benefit compared to controls.[29]

Neurological disorders

Controlled clinical trials of plasmapheresis have demonstrated efficacy in acute inflammatory demyelinating polyradiculopathy (Guillain–Barré syndrome) and chronic inflammatory demyelinating polyneuropathy (CIDP). However, intravenous immunoglobulin (IVIG) alone may be equally effective in the treatment of severe Guillain–Barré syndrome.[30] Two comparative trials of therapeutic apheresis versus IVIG in the treatment of CIDP also demonstrated equivalent efficacy as primary therapy in this disorder.[16]

Limited evidence from recent, small randomized trials suggests that other neurologic disorders mediated by pathogenic autoantibodies may respond to plasmapheresis, such as multiple sclerosis with acute fulminant CNS demyelination[31] and infection-triggered obsessive-compulsive disorder and tic disorders in childhood.[32] In the latter disorder, the offending antibody appears to be related to infection with the group A β-hemolytic streptococcus. While plasmapheresis has induced long-term remissions, re-infection with streptococcus has resulted in neurologic relapse.

Hematological diseases

Plasma exchange is the treatment of choice for thrombotic thrombocytopenic purpura (TTP), and this life-threatening disorder is one of the few indications for the use of fresh frozen plasma (FFP) as volume replacement fluid in therapeutic apheresis rather than crystalloid and/or colloid volume expanders. TTP is characterized by various combinations of the classic pentad of thrombocytopenia, microangiopathic hemolytic anemia, neurologic signs and symptoms, fever, and renal involvement. The pathogenesis of this disorder is better understood since the discovery, reported by Tsai et al[33] and Furlan et al[34] that a Ca^{2+}/Ba^{2+}-activated metalloproteinase that metabolizes large von Willebrand factor (vWf) multimers to smaller forms in normal plasma is reduced or absent in patients with chronic relapsing, acute idiopathic, and intermittently recurrent types of TTP. The vWf-cleaving proteinase is not produced or does not function properly in children with chronic relapsing TTP. These patients respond to FFP infusion alone, often remaining free of symptoms for several weeks. In contrast, an IgG inhibitory antibody most likely accounts for the decreased plasma vWf-cleaving proteinase activity in patients with acute idiopathic TTP. The presence of this autoantibody may explain why these patients require plasma exchange (for removal of the antibody) in addition to plasma infusion (to replace the inhibited vWf-cleaving proteinase).[35] Cryodepleted plasma, the plasma that remains after cryoprecipitate is prepared, is suggested by some authors to be as effective or possibly more effective than FFP in this setting.[36]

Post-transfusion purpura is a rare, serious complication of blood transfusion, usually affecting multiparous women or individuals with a history of prior transfusion, characterized by the precipitous onset of thrombocytopenia between 5 and 10 days after transfusion, occasionally complicated by intracranial hemorrhage or other bleeding problems. The disease is associated with the presence of antibodies in the plasma of affected patients directed against a platelet membrane antigen, usually HPA-1a; however, the mechanism of autologous platelet destruction has not been fully described. Although no controlled trials have been done to evaluate the role of therapeutic plasmapheresis in the treatment of this rare disorder, several reported cases show rapid resolution of thrombocytopenia and bleeding within 24–48 hours after the first procedure. IVIG has also been demonstrated to be effective in this disorder, and is now considered the first-line therapy in nonbleeding patients who do not require immediate resolution of thrombocytopenia, due to greater ease of administration and availability as compared to therapeutic plasmapheresis.[37]

Plasmapheresis has long been used to treat hyperviscosity syndrome due to Waldenström's macroglobulinemia and other malignant paraproteinemias. It is generally used as an adjunct to chemotherapy or other treatment to decrease paraprotein synthesis, although it may serve as primary therapy in some patients. Since the IgM proteins reside largely within the intravascular compartment, one or two procedures that remove one to one and a half plasma volumes each can return plasma viscosity to near normal levels.[38] For IgG or IgA paraproteinemias, more procedures may be necessary due to the large extravascular distribution of these immunoglobulins.

THERAPEUTIC PRINCIPLES

Immunologic diseases in which plasmapheresis is standard therapy

- Goodpasture syndrome
- Thrombotic thrombocytopenic purpura
- Post-transfusion purpura
- Guillain–Barré syndrome
- Chronic inflammatory demyelinating polyradiculopathy
- Myasthenia gravis

Replacement fluids for plasma exchange

The success of therapeutic apheresis procedures seldom depends on the composition of the replacement solution that is used, with the exception of thrombotic thrombocytopenic purpura. With therapeutic plasmapheresis for most other disorders, the primary function of the replacement solution is to maintain intravascular volume. Additional requirements include restoration of important plasma proteins, maintenance of colloid osmotic pressure, maintenance of electrolyte balance, and preservation of trace elements lost during a prolonged course of plasmapheresis procedures. In moderately well-nourished subjects, homeostatic mechanisms normally obviate the need for precise plasma replacement and 5% albumin or combinations of albumin and crystalloid are usually sufficient. Other patients should receive solutions prepared specifically to meet their individual requirements. Routine supplementation with calcium, potassium, or immunoglobulins is unnecessary. Concerns about use of human plasma-derived volume expanders and cost issues have led some centers to develop protocols for alternatives to albumin, such as hydroxyethyl starch, for full or partial volume replacement with plasma exchange.[39] These solutions are generally well tolerated. Since less than 500 ml volume is removed during most cell collection procedures and therapeutic cell depletions, no replacement beyond the anticoagulant and saline priming solution is required.

Complications of therapeutic apheresis

The current generation of blood cell separators is remarkably reliable and equipped with sensitive detection and alarm systems to alert the operator to potential problems. Automated apheresis is a minimal risk procedure for normal healthy donors. Adverse events occur more frequently and include more serious consequences in patients undergoing therapeutic apheresis, often due to problems associated with the underlying disease, vascular access, and exposure to allogeneic blood components. Even in the therapeutic setting, adverse events are relatively uncommon and are usually of mild to moderate severity. A recent survey of 18 apheresis centers reported an overall incidence of immediate adverse events of 4.75% (163/3429 therapeutic procedures), with only 26 events (0.76%) classified as severe. As would be expected, the incidence of adverse events in plasma exchange with plasma replacement was more than twice the rate in plasma exchange without plasma replacement (7.8% and 3.3%, respectively). There were 3 deaths reported in this survey; in each case, the physician supervising the procedure attributed the death to an underlying medical condition (extensive burn injuries in two patients and severe pericarditis in the third).[40] This finding is consistent with earlier reports, in which deaths were related to cardiac and respiratory causes in patients critically ill prior to apheresis, and the contributory role of the apheresis procedure was often questionable. The frequency of adverse reactions is strongly influenced by the experience of the operator and the nature of the patient population under treatment.[41] For example, in the recent multicenter survey, vasovagal events occurred more frequently in neurologic patients than in patients with other disorders, consistent with findings reported in previous studies.[40] A summary of the incidence of adverse events complicating therapeutic apheresis procedures, as reported in three recent studies, is presented in Table 118.2.

Expected and predictable effects of therapeutic apheresis include alterations in laboratory parameters due to removal and dilution by replacement fluids. A 5–20% decrease in hemoglobin/hematocrit, a 20–30% decrease in platelet count, and mild leukocytosis are commonly observed. Significant but transient abnormalities in coagulation tests will often occur after serial plasma exchange procedures, as well as clinically insignificant decreased levels of other plasma proteins.[5,44] The effect of a single blood volume plasma exchange on the intravascular levels of some blood constituents is summarized in Table 118.3.

The most common adverse effect of both donor and therapeutic apheresis is symptomatic hypocalcemia due to infusion of calcium-chelating citrate ions in the anticoagulant, and, if used as replacement fluid, anticoagulated donor plasma. This is usually manifested by mild perioral and/or acral paresthesia, requiring no intervention other than slowing the reinfusion rate. The benefit of small doses of oral calcium supplements in this setting is questionable, although the practice is widespread. Hyperventilation may exacerbate these symptoms. More severe citrate toxicity is very uncommon; signs may range from involuntary carpopedal spasm to frank tetany with spasm in other muscle groups, including life-threatening laryngospasm.[45] Controlled infusions of 10% calcium gluconate are effective in

Incidence (%) of selected adverse effects associated with therapeutic apheresis

	McLeod et al.[40a]	Mokrzycki & Kaplan[42b]	Couriel & Weinstein[43c]	Additional comments
Citrate reactions	1.5 (moderate–severe)	2.4 (paresthesias, muscle cramps, nausea)	8.9 (most mild, few with nausea or vomiting)	McLeod survey excluded transient paresthesias
Vaso-vagal (hypotension, syncope, seizure)	1.1	1.4	2.6	
Transfusion reactions	1.6	3.1	0.3	Usually urticaria associated with plasma replacement; 5 anaphylactoid reactions in a patient treated with FFP (Mokrzycki)
Access related	0.4	1.1	1.0	All of the severe complications and one of the fatalities in the Couriel study were related to use of central venous catheters
Severe cardiovascular events	0.1 (circulatory collapse and cardiac arrest)	0	0	
Severe respiratory events	0.3 (respiratory distress; one report of anaphylaxis)	0 (excluding the 5 anaphylactoid reactions, above)	0	
Death	0.1	0	0.5	All fatalities due to underlying disease or access-related (one report of arterial laceration in Couriel study)
Overall reaction rate (percentage of procedures)	4.75	9.7	17	

[a] The most numerous procedures were plasma exchange with albumin or saline replacement, or with allogeneic plasma replacement, and autologous PBSC collection; survey also included cytapheresis, column depletion, and photopheresis procedures.
[b] All procedures were performed with a membrane-based system (autopheresis C system modified for continuous flow).
[c] Most of the patients in this study (89%) were treated for neurologic disorders.

Table 118.2 Incidence (%) of selected adverse effects associated with therapeutic apheresis.

Constituent	Percentage decrease from baseline	Percentage recovery 48 hours after plasma exchange
Clotting factors	25–50	80–100
Fibrinogen	63	65
Immunoglobulins	63	~45
Paraproteins	30–60	Variable
Liver enzymes	55–60	100
Bilirubin	45	100
C3	63	60–100
Platelets	20–30	75–100

Changes in levels of blood constituents after one blood volume plasma exchange[a]

[a] Replacement fluid consisting of 4–5% albumin in 0.9% sodium chloride

Table 118.3 Changes in levels of blood constituents after one blood volume plasma exchange[a]. (Modified from Weinstein R. Basic principles of therapeutic blood exchange. In: McLeod BC (ed.) *Apheresis: principles and practice*. Bethesda, MD, AABB Press, 1997, p 264.)

the management of these complications. Acute severe hypocalcemia leading to fatal cardiac arrhythmia has been reported rarely in apheresis patients. Metabolism of citrate occurs predominantly in the liver and kidney, and patients with conditions affecting these organs are therefore at increased risk for severe citrate reactions. In addition, citrate toxicity has been reported due to mechanical dysfunction of the automated apheresis instrument.[46] A study of therapeutic plasma exchange procedures performed with and without 10% calcium gluconate infusion showed the effectiveness of continuous calcium infusion for the prevention of mild to moderate citrate toxicity;[47] however, careful monitoring is necessary to prevent inadvertent overdose if this procedure is adopted.

The most severe allergic complications occur when plasma is used as the replacement solution, and this risk increases with repeated exposure.[41] Allergic reactions to ethylene oxide, an agent used in the sterilization of plastic disposable equipment, have been reported.[48] Intravenous diphenhydramine is usually effective in managing these reactions; premedication with steroids and precautions against anaphylaxis may be necessary for sensitized individuals. Atypical (hypotension and flushing) and anaphylactic reactions have been reported in patients receiving ACE inhibitors undergoing different apheresis procedures; these medications should be discontinued for at least 24 hours prior to apheresis.[49] Although extremely rare, pyrogen reactions to human serum albumin during plasma exchange have been reported.[50] Serious complications indirectly associated with therapeutic apheresis include adverse consequences of vascular access, namely hemorrhage, pneumo or hemothorax, thrombosis, nerve damage, and infection. A retrospective review of 381 therapeutic plasma exchange procedures at one institution reported an approximately 1% incidence of severe complications, all of them related to central venous catheters[43] (Table 118.2).

PERIPHERAL BLOOD MONONUCLEAR CELL COLLECTION FOR TRANSPLANTATION AND OTHER CELL THERAPIES

Blood cell separators developed for hemapheresis are used increasingly for autologous and allogeneic peripheral blood stem cell (PBSC) collection and novel forms of cellular therapy. In the cell-processing laboratory, separation techniques have been developed for removing T lymphocytes, purging tumor cells, and selecting progenitor cells from autologous bone marrow harvests and PBSC collection products. Hematopoietic progenitor cells can be collected from peripheral blood and cryopreserved. The fresh or cryopreserved PBSC products are used to reconstitute hematopoietic and immunologic function in patients who receive myeloablative chemotherapy for a wide range of hematologic malignancies, nonmalignant hematologic disorders, and some solid tumors. Of particular interest for the immunologist is the use of T lymphocytes for immunotherapy. Lymphocyte concentrates prepared from leukocyte collections are used as immunotherapy for solid tumors, leukemic relapse after allogeneic hematopoietic stem/progenitor cell transplantation, and viral complications of bone marrow transplantation. Preliminary studies promise a role for both circulating hematopoietic progenitor cells and other mononuclear cells in the therapy of immunosuppressed patients and in gene therapy. The uses of peripheral blood mononuclear cells for adoptive immunotherapy and gene therapy are described in a number of recent reviews.[51–54]

Peripheral blood stem cell collection

Pluripotent hematopoietic progenitor cells, most likely including primordial hematopoietic stem cells capable of reconstituting the bone marrow and the immune system, have long been known to circulate in the peripheral blood. PBSC collections have several practical advantages compared to bone marrow harvests in that they: (1) eliminate risks associated with anesthesia, (2) permit collection of hematopoietic progenitor cells despite tumor involvement of the marrow or previous pelvic irradiation, (3) facilitate graft manipulations by obtaining greater numbers of $CD34^+$ cells, (4) permit repeated collection as necessary, and (5) can be safely performed on small children. Numerous studies show that PBSC transplantation consistently results in rapid hematopoietic recovery and durable engraftment in both autologous and allogeneic transplant settings. PBSCs are rapidly replacing bone marrow for transplantation after myeloablative therapy. Despite the 10-fold increase in the number of T lymphocytes in unmanipulated allogeneic PBSC collections, there does not appear to be an increase in the incidence or severity of acute GVHD, although the risk of chronic GVHD may be higher.[55]

Ordinarily, PBSCs circulate in extremely small numbers. The concentration of stem cells in the peripheral blood can be increased by the administration of cytokines such as granulocyte colony-stimulating factor (G-CSF) and granulocyte-macrophage CSF (GM-CSF), and by the administration of chemotherapy. $CD34^+$ hematopoietic stem cell levels in the peripheral blood generally rise 20–40-fold (from 1–2 cells/μl to 40–70 cells/μl) following G-CSF alone, and they may show an even greater increase (100–1000-fold) when chemotherapy rebound is enhanced by administration of G-CSF.[56] New cytokines in development or combinations of cytokines may further improve PBSC mobilization, resulting in reduced numbers and/or smaller volumes of leukapheresis procedures required to obtain adequate transplants. The appropriate mobilization strategy to use depends on the clinical situation. In the autologous transplant setting, the mobilization regimen may consist of chemotherapy with or without cytokine administration, depending on the patient's diagnosis and medical condition.

In vitro functional hematopoietic colony assays have been used to characterize and quantitate stem/progenitor cells collected by hemapheresis. Colony assays have limited clinical utility because they require 10–14 days to perform. Assays that use the CD34 antigen as a marker for primitive hematopoietic progenitor cells have the advantage of a relatively rapid turn-around time. Despite ongoing problems with inter- laboratory standardization, flow cytometric analysis of CD34 immunostained blood cells can be used effectively for 'real-time' decision-making about the timing and adequacy of PBSC collections. Recent and ongoing studies are evaluating a variety of approaches to achieve standardization and clinical utility of $CD34^+$ cell quantitation, including semi-automated flow cytometric analysis and microvolume fluorimetry.[57–60]

Although definition of a therapeutic dose remains controversial, most centers recommend a minimum of $2.0–5.0 \times 10^6$ $CD34^+$ cells/kg body weight. Within this range, recovery of neutrophil and platelet counts as early as 1–2 weeks post transplant is commonly observed. Greater numbers of $CD34^+$ cells confer a shorter time to hematopoietic recovery and concomitantly fewer blood component transfusions; however, significant improvement in transplant-related mortality or overall survival has yet to be demonstrated in this setting. Several clinical scale devices for positive selection of $CD34^+$ hematopoietic cells are available. $CD34^+$ selection by immune-affinity techniques ('positive selection') results in exclusion of unwanted cells, including occult malignant cells that do not express the CD34 antigen and T lymphocytes, without compromising the engraftment potential of the purified product. As yet no data confirm the clinical benefit of positive selection.

Several problems complicate the widespread use of PBSCs. For allogeneic donors, the discomfort of multiple-day cytokine administration may be a significant deterrent, and the long-term effects of exposure to these exogenous cytokines are unknown. Citrate toxicity is a frequent complication of PBSC collections that, though usually mild and transient, may be severe and even life-threatening in some individuals. Venous access requires large-bore multilumen catheters, and these appear particularly susceptible to clotting, especially when patients receive recombinant cytokine stimulation. Hemorrhage, especially in thrombocytopenic patients, is another potentially severe complication of central venous catheter placement. Patients who have received multiple prior cycles of chemotherapy occasionally fail to respond adequately to mobilization regimens, and even normal, healthy donors may fail to mobilize adequate numbers of peripheral hematopoietic stem/progenitor cells, for unknown reasons. Finally, PBSCs may be stored frozen in liquid nitrogen with the cryoprotectant dimethylsulfoxide. Rapid infusion of dimethylsulfoxide causes bradycardia, hypertension, fever, nausea, and vomiting. Toxicity is usually averted, however, by appropriate premedication and careful attention to infusion rates.

Immune reconstitution of patients undergoing hematopoietic stem/progenitor cell transplant may be prolonged and incomplete, especially in the setting of unrelated allogeneic donors. Donor mobilization using different cytokine cocktails and ex vivo manipulation of the PBSC graft show promise as strategies for improving the immune capability of transplanted patients.

REFERENCES

1. Abel J, Rowntree LG, Turner BB. Plasma removal with return of corpuscles (plasmaphaeresis). J Pharmacol Exp Ther 1914;5:625.
2. Rock G, Sutton DM. Apheresis: man versus machine. Transfusion 1997;37:993.
3. Lockwood CM, Worlledge S, Nicholas A, Cotton C, Peters DK. Reversal of impaired splenic function in patients with nephritis or vasculitis (or both) by plasma exchange. N Engl J Med 1979;300:524.
4. Collins JA. Problems associated with the massive transfusion of stored blood. Surgery 1974;75:274.
5. Weinstein R. Basic principles of therapeutic blood exchange. In: McLeod BC (ed.) Apheresis: principles and practice. Bethesda, MD, AABB Press, 1997, p 264.
6. Corbin F, Cullis HM, Freiriech E, et al. Development of apheresis instrumentation. In: McLeod BC, Price TH, Drew MJ (eds) Apheresis: principles and practice. Bethesda, MD, AABB Press, 1997, p 1.
7. Vichinsky EP, Haberkern CM, Neumayr L, et al. A comparison of conservative and aggressive transfusion regimens in the perioperative management of sickle cell disease. The Preoperative Transfusion in Sickle Cell Disease Study Group. N Engl J Med 1995;333:206.
8. Adams RJ, McKie VC, Hsu L, et al. Prevention of a first stroke by transfusions in children with sickle cell anemia and abnormal results on transcranial Doppler ultrasonography. N Engl J Med 1998;339:5.
9. Kim HC, Dugan NP, Silber JH, et al. Erythrocytapheresis therapy to reduce iron overload in chronically transfused patients with sickle cell disease. Blood 1994;83:1136.
10. Coles SM, Klein HG, Holland PV. Alloimmunization in two multitransfused patient populations. Transfusion 1981;21:462.
11. Friedman DF, Lukas MB, Jawad A, Larson PJ, Ohene-Frempong K, Manno CS. Alloimmunization to platelets in heavily transfused patients with sickle cell disease. Blood 1996;88:3216.
12. Lichtman MA, Rowe JM. Hyperleukocytic leukemias: rheological, clinical, and therapeutic considerations. Blood 1982;60:279.
13. Wright DG, Karsh J, Fauci AS, et al. Lymphocyte depletion and immunosuppression with repeated leukapheresis by continuous flow centrifugation. Blood 1981;58:451.
14. Wallace D, Goldfinger D, Lowe C, et al. A double-blind, controlled study of lymphoplasmapheresis versus sham apheresis in rheumatoid arthritis. N Engl J Med 1982;306:1406.
15. Karsh J, Klippel JH, Plotz PH, Decker JL, Wright DG, Flye MW. Lymphapheresis in rheumatoid arthritis. A randomized trial. Arthritis Rheum 1981;24:867.
16. Weinstein R. Therapeutic apheresis in neurological disorders. J Clin Apheresis 2000;15:74.
17. Dall'Amico R, Murer L, Montini G, et al. Successful treatment of recurrent rejection in renal transplant patients with photopheresis. J Am Soc Nephrol 1998;9:121.
18. Wolfe JT, Tomaszewski JE, Grossman RA, et al. Reversal of acute renal allograft rejection by extracorporeal photopheresis: a case presentation and review of the literature. J Clin Apheresis 1996;11:36.
19. Dall'Amico R, Rossetti F, Zulian F, et al. Photopheresis in paediatric patients with drug-resistant chronic graft-versus-host disease. Br J Haematol 1997;97:848.
20. Kessler CM, Klein HG, Havlik RJ. Uncontrolled thrombocytosis in chronic myeloproliferative disorders. Br J Haematol 1982;50:157.

21. Assessment of plasmapheresis. Report of the Therapeutics and Technology Assessment Subcommittee of the American Academy of Neurology. Neurology 1996;47:840.
22. Committee AAoBBH. Guidelines for therapeutic hemapheresis. Bethesda, MD, American Association of Blood Banks, 1995.
23. McLeod BC. Introduction to the third special issue: clinical applications of therapeutic apheresis. J Clin Apheresis 2000;15:1.
24. Gordon BR, Saal SD. Low-density lipoprotein apheresis using the Liposorber dextran sulfate cellulose system for patients with hypercholesterolemia refractory to medical therapy. J Clin Apheresis 1996;11:128.
25. Gibberd FB, Billimoria JD, Page NG, Retsas S. Heredopathia atactica polyneuritiformis (Refsum's disease) treated by diet and plasma-exchange. Lancet 1979;1:575.
26. Koo AP. Therapeutic apheresis in autoimmune and rheumatic diseases. J Clin Apheresis 2000;15:18.
27. Felson DT, LaValley MP, Baldassare AR, et al. The Prosorba column for treatment of refractory rheumatoid arthritis: a randomized, double-blind, sham-controlled trial. Arthritis Rheum 1999;42:2153.
28. Furst D, Felson D, Gendreau M. Patients with severe rheumatoid arthritis responding to treatment respond again on retreatment. Arthritis Rheum 1998;41:S316.
29. Wallace DJ, Goldfinger D, Pepkowitz SH, et al. Randomized controlled trial of pulse/synchronization cyclophosphamide/apheresis for proliferative lupus nephritis. J Clin Apheresis 1998;13:163.
30. Randomised trial of plasma exchange, intravenous immunoglobulin, and combined treatments in Guillain–Barré syndrome. Plasma Exchange/Sandoglobulin Guillain–Barré Syndrome Trial Group. Lancet 1997;349:225.
31. Weinshenker BG, O'Brien PC, Petterson TM, et al. A randomized trial of plasma exchange in acute central nervous system inflammatory demyelinating disease. Ann Neurol 1999;46:878.
32. Perlmutter SJ, Leitman SF, Garvey MA, et al. Therapeutic plasma exchange and intravenous immunoglobulin for obsessive-compulsive disorder and tic disorders in childhood. Lancet 1999;354:1153.
33. Tsai HM, Lian EC. Antibodies to von Willebrand factor-cleaving protease in acute thrombotic thrombocytopenic purpura N Engl J Med 1998;339:1585.
34. Furlan M, Robles R, Galbusera M, et al. von Willebrand factor-cleaving protease in thrombotic thrombocytopenic purpura and the hemolytic-uremic syndrome. N Engl J Med 1998;339:1578.
35. Moake JL. vWf and thrombotic thrombocytopenic purpura: Overview, workshop on von Willebrand factor and thrombotic thrombocytopenic purpura, National Institutes of Health, Bethesda, MD, July 31, 2000.
36. Rock G, Shumak KH, Sutton DM, Buskard NA, Nair RC. Cryosupernatant as replacement fluid for plasma exchange in thrombotic thrombocytopenic purpura. Members of the Canadian Apheresis Group. Br J Haematol 1996;94:383.
37. Grima KM. Therapeutic apheresis in hematological and oncological diseases. J Clin Apheresis 2000;15:28.
38. Drew MJ. Therapeutic plasma exchange in hematologic diseases and dysproteinemias. In: McLeod BC (ed.) Apheresis: principles and practice. Bethesda, MD, AABB Press, 1997, p 307.
39. Brecher ME, Owen HG, Bandarenko N. Alternatives to albumin: strach replacement for plasma exchange. J Clin Apheresis 1997;12:146.
40. McLeod BC, Sniecinski I, Ciavarella D, et al. Frequency of immediate adverse effects associated with therapeutic apheresis. Transfusion 1999;39:282.
41. Sutton DM, Nair RC, Rock G. Complications of plasma exchange. Transfusion 1989;29:124.
42. Mokrzycki MH, Kaplan AA. Therapeutic plasma exchange: complications and management. American Journal of Kidney Diseases 1994;23:817–827.
43. Couriel D, Weinstein R. Complications of therapeutic plasma exchange: a recent assessment. J Clin Apheresis 1994;9:1.
44. Wood L, Jacobs P. The effect of serial therapeutic plasmapheresis on platelet count, coagulation factors, plasma immunoglobulin, and complement levels. J Clin Apheresis 1986;3:124.
45. Strauss RG. Mechanisms of adverse effects during hemapheresis. J Clin Apheresis 1996;11:160.
46. Uhl L, Maillet S, King S, Kruskall MS. Unexpected citrate toxicity and severe hypocalcemia during apheresis. Transfusion 1997;37:1063.
47. Weinstein R. Prevention of citrate reactions during therapeutic plasma exchange by constant infusion of calcium gluconate with the return fluid. J Clin Apheresis 1996;11:204.
48. Leitman SF, Boltansky H, Alter HJ, Pearson FC, Kaliner MA. Allergic reactions in healthy plateletpheresis donors caused by sensitization to ethylene oxide gas. N Engl J Med 1986;315:1192.
49. Owen HG, Brecher ME. Atypical reactions associated with use of angiotensin-converting enzyme inhibitors and apheresis. Transfusion 1994;34:891.
50. Pool M, McLeod BC. Pyrogen reactions to human serum albumin during plasma exchange. J Clin Apheresis 1995;10:81.
51. Beutler E. Gene therapy. Biol Blood Marrow Transplant 1999;5:273.
52. Halene S, Kohn DB. Gene therapy using hematopoietic stem cells: sisyphus approaches the crest. Hum Gene Ther 2000;11:1259.
53. Hoffman DM, Gitlitz BJ, Belldegrun A, Figlin RA. Adoptive cellular therapy. Semin Oncol 2000;27:221.
54. Baron F, Beguin Y. Adoptive immunotherapy with donor lymphocyte infusions after allogeneic HPC transplantation. Transfusion 2000;40:468.
55. Storek J, Gooley T, Siadak M, et al. Allogeneic peripheral blood stem cell transplantation may be associated with a high risk of chronic graft-versus-host disease. Blood 1997;90:4705.
56. Leitman SF, Read EJ. Hematopoietic progenitor cells. Semin Hematol 1996;33:341.
57. Gutensohn K, Carrero I, Krueger W, et al. Semi-automated flow cytometric analysis of CD34-expressing hematopoietic cells in peripheral blood progenitor cell apheresis products. Transfusion 1999;39:1220.
58. Sutherland DR, Anderson L, Keeney M, Nayar R, Chin-Yee I. The ISHAGE guidelines for CD34+ cell determination by flow cytometry. International Society of Hematotherapy and Graft Engineering. J Hematother 1996;5:213.
59. Gratama JW, Braakman E, Kraan J, et al. Comparison of single and dual-platform assay formats for CD34+ haematopoietic progenitor cell enumeration. Clin Lab Haematol 1999;21:337.
60. Read EJ, Kunitake ST, Carter CS, Chau Q, Yu MY, Klein HG. Enumeration of CD34+ hematopoietic progenitor cells in peripheral blood and leukapheresis products by microvolume fluorimetry: a comparison with flow cytometry. J Hematother 1997;6:291.

Chapter 119

Experimental Immunotherapy of Autoimmune Disease

Lawrence Steinman and C. Garrison Fathman

This chapter focuses on selective and nonselective approaches to therapy of autoimmune disease, emphasizing studies in a prototypic model of T cell-mediated organ-specific autoimmune disease termed 'experimental autoimmune encephalomyelitis'. This disorder serves as an animal model for the human disease multiple sclerosis. Applications of experimental immune therapy to human diseases are also discussed.

EXPERIMENTAL AUTOIMMUNE ENCEPHALOMYELITIS: A PROTOTYPIC MODEL OF ORGAN-SPECIFIC AUTOIMMUNITY

Experimental autoimmune encephalomyelitis (EAE) is a useful model of acute demyelinating disease. Some forms of EAE reflect chronic demyelination with exacerbations and remissions characteristic of multiple sclerosis (MS). The chronic models of EAE reflect many of the pathophysiologic steps in MS. EAE reveals the role of certain adhesion molecules, the influence of T cells and antibodies reactive to components of the myelin sheath, the participation of metalloproteases in opening the blood–brain barrier, and the cytotoxic role of certain cytokines. EAE has been predictive for one of the three new therapies approved in the USA for treatment of MS; copaxone, a drug approved for use in relapsing remitting MS, was successful in treating various models of EAE. However, EAE has been a poor predictor of other immunotherapies. For example, the role of certain cytokines in EAE is contradictory to what is seen when tried experimentally in MS. Recognition of the discrepancies between MS and its experimental models is critical in attempting to design rational therapies for demyelinating disease. This also serves as a cautionary note in translating therapeutic approaches in experimental models to human disease in other autoimmune disorders.

Multiple sclerosis (MS) is an inflammatory demyelinating disease of central nervous system (CNS) white matter (Chapter 77). It is the major chronic disease of white matter, affecting approximately 350 000 individuals in North America, and about twice that number in Europe. MS is much less common in India and Asia, probably reflecting a genetic predisposition within a certain genotype encoded by the major histocompatibility complex (HLA) on chromosome 6 (Chapter 6). Individuals with a particular HLA type (HLA-DRB1*1501, formerly known as HLA-DR2), are three to four times more susceptible to MS than individuals who have a different HLA type at this locus. The incidence of MS in Northern Europe, where this allele is most common, is as high as 1 per 750 individuals. Females are affected twice as often as males.[1]

Approximately 85% of MS cases begin as relapsing-remitting disease, with episodes of neurologic impairment involving major white matter tracts impairing vision, other sensory modalities, motor performance, or coordination. Episodes of relapse and remission often evolve over many years to a more chronic form of disability without clearcut exacerbations. These clinical scenarios become important in the development of animal models of MS. The most useful animal models would develop acute attacks with specific neurologic deficits including paralysis. Then the animals would develop chronic neurologic disease, with relapsing episodes of paralysis followed by periods of clinical remission and ultimately permanent deficits. Many animal models of MS feature only acute attacks and recovery, a situation that is comparable to human syndromes of acute demyelinating disease, syndromes that are closely related to MS and may represent initial attacks of MS that are self-contained.

There are three acute demyelinating diseases – acute optic neuritis (AON), acute transverse myelopathy (ATM), and acute disseminated encephalomyelitis (ADE), affecting the central nervous system – that appear identical both clinically and pathologically to MS during exacerbations. Indeed, most relapses of chronic MS resemble these three acute conditions clinically and pathologically. There is no way to distinguish AON, ATM, and ADE from a first episode of MS, and in about 25% of cases these acute demyelinating syndromes culminate in recurrent episodes of inflammation involving the brain, optic nerve, or spinal cord. Upon the return of these syndromes, the illness is then called MS. The acute demyelinating attacks, lasting days to weeks, often occur following a viral infection. AON is manifest by a transient disturbance of vision, ATM is characterized by transient paralysis and sensory disturbances in the extremities, often with bowel and bladder dysfunction, and ADE is distinguished by various motor and sensory disturbances and occasionally by convulsions.

One of the first known examples of ADE occurred when 'paralytic accidents', referring to spinal cord inflammation leading to clinical paralysis, were noted after rabies immunization. This observation served as a basis for the development of models of acute experimental allergic encephalomyelitis.[2–4] The 'paralytic accidents' were due to an immune response directed at the brain tissue used for growing the attenuated rabies virus.

Once it was recognized that immunization with brain tissue could produce paralysis and demyelination in experimental animals, models of acute disseminated encephalomyelitis were developed in monkeys at the Rockefeller Institute by Rivers. Injection of a mixture of brain material with complete Freund's adjuvant, an emulsion made from killed *Mycobacterian tuberculosis*, permitted the development of highly reproducible models of acute paralysis and white matter inflammation.[4] The efforts of Rivers, Freund, and Kabat resulted in the establishment of animal models of experimentally induced autoimmunity in the nervous system, termed

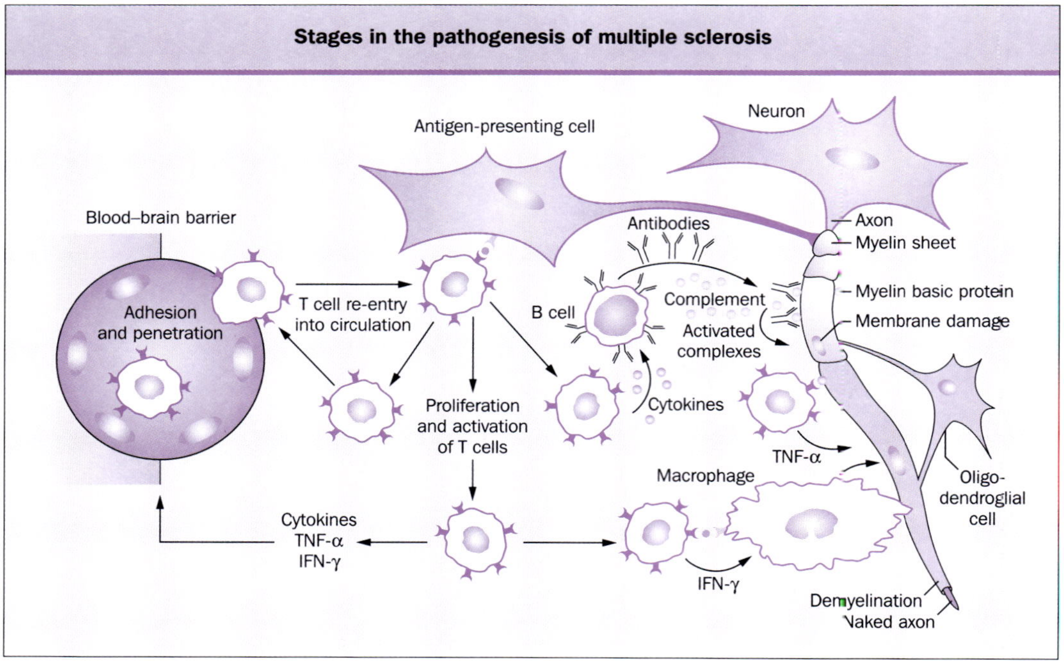

Figure 119.1 Stages in the pathogenesis of multiple sclerosis. (Redrawn from Steinman L. Multiple sclerosis: a coordinated immunological attack against myelin in the central nervous system. *Cell* 1996;85:299.)

'experimental allergic encephalomyelitis' (later to be interchanged with experimental autoimmune encephalomyelitis). In the basic protocol for inducing EAE, experimental animals are immunized with either foreign or self proteins from the white matter of the nervous system, usually myelin basic protein (MBP), proteolipid protein (PLP), or myelin oligodendroglial glycoprotein (MOG). The acute EAE models reflect many of the features of AON, ATM, and ADE. Unlike MS, these illnesses occur acutely and then resolve with varying degrees of residual disease in the optic nerves, spinal cord, or white matter of the brain. MS, in contrast to these acute diseases, is chronic, lasting a lifetime, and is commonly manifest by episodes of inflammation in the white matter, leading to permanent disabilities. With the development of models of relapsing EAE, investigators produced several animal models of MS that incorporate most of the features described below.

In MS, evidence points to an immune response against components of the myelin sheath. A widely accepted view of the process of demyelination identifies T cells, immunoglobulin and complement playing a central role in pathogenesis (Fig. 119.1). Adhesion molecules, cytokines, chemokines, HLA molecules and metalloproteases are critical participants in the development of the inflammatory response in brain. Initially, circulating autoreactive myelin-specific CD4 Th1 cells are activated in the periphery by nonself antigens, likely of microbial origin. CD8 T cells are also found in the CNS and are clonally restricted. However, the precise role of CD4 and CD8 T cells remains to be elucidated in MS.

The putative microbial components that activate the CD4 T cells must resemble CNS myelin proteins, and this resemblance between self and nonself molecules is called molecular mimicry[1,5] (Chapter 58) (Fig. 119.2). The circulating T cells that recognize molecules resembling myelin are captured on vascular endothelium in the brain, first by selectins and then by ligand–receptor interactions between integrin molecules. T cells then migrate through the endothelium in response to chemotactic signals. Once T cells are activated, they secrete metalloproteinases and

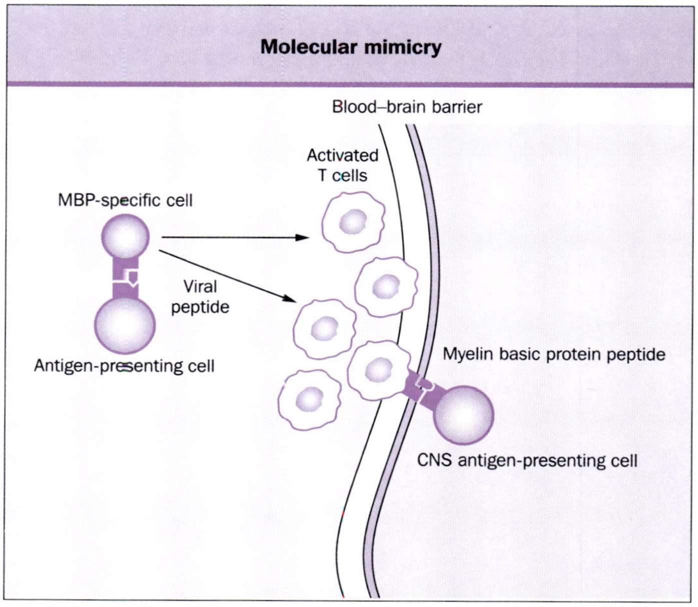

Figure 119.2 Molecular mimicry. Antibodies against human herpesvirus-6 n the blood of patients with multiple sclerosis (MS). (Redrawn from Steinman L, Oldstone MBA. More mayhem from molecular mimics. *Nature Medicine* 1997;12:1321.)

or other matrix-degrading enzymes, which facilitate their penetration through the basement lamina.

Microglial cells and astrocytes reactivate T cells locally in the CNS by presentation of myelin antigens complexed with MHC class II molecules. T cells stimulate macrophages by secretion of inflammatory cytokines, and macrophages in turn show increased phagocytic activity and release oxygen free radicals, nitric oxide metabolites, proteases, arachidonic acid derivatives, and complement components that damage myelin.

Comparisons between MS and EAE: presentation, genetics and pathology	MS	EAE
Clinical presentation		
Relapses and remissions	Present	Present
Paralysis	Present	Present
Ataxia	Present	Present
Visual impairment	Present	Present
Genetics		
MHC-linked susceptibility	Yes	Yes
Females more susceptible	Yes	Yes
Pathology in lesions		
T cells reactive to myelin	Present	Present
Antibodies to myelin	Present	Present
α4 integrin, complement	Present	Present
TNF-α, IFN-γ	Present	Present
Demyelination	Present	Present
Axonal dystrophy	Present	Present

Table 119.1 Comparisons between MS and EAE: presentation, genetics and pathology.

Autoantibodies against myelin antigens, such as myelin basic protein and myelin oligodendroglial glycoprotein, also have an important role in demyelination.[6–8] In addition to myelin damage in MS, there is clear evidence for axonal loss and dysfunction.[9] Many of the gene products involved in this immunopathogenic scenario of MS have been demonstrated at the sites of lesions by standard methods of immunohistochemistry, in situ hybridization, and reverse transcriptase-based PCR.

EAE reflects many of the features seen in MS (Table 119.1): females are twice as susceptible to MS as males and female mice also are overwhelmingly more susceptible to EAE induction. Susceptibility to EAE in mice is closely linked to loci in the major histocompatibility complex H-2, comparable with the HLA link in humans. T-cell and antibody responses to various myelin proteins, like MBP, MOG, and PLP can be detected in animals with EAE including cells found in the CSF. TCR rearrangements indicative of T-cell reactivity to myelin have been detected in demyelinating areas from brains of mice with EAE.[1] Similarly, antibody responses to MBP and to MOG can be detected at the site of vesiculating myelin in EAE brain.[7,8] Immunization with various myelin proteins in suitable adjuvants or with T-cell clones specific for certain peptides within these proteins can trigger chronic relapsing, demyelinating disease in rodents and non-human primates. In EAE, T-cell immune responses spread to different antigenic epitopes of a given myelin protein, and then spread to other myelin antigens, a phenomenon known as 'antigen spreading'. Immunization with microbial sequences resembling myelin antigens can either induce clinical paralysis and demyelination, or protect against disease in EAE.[5] This is often interpreted to mean that the microbe towards which the initial immune response is thought to have been directed actually triggered the disease.[6] Finally, in chronic relapsing EAE, there is also evidence for axonal pathology.[10]

KEY CONCEPTS

EAE: an animal model of the human disease MS
- Induced by immunizing with antigenic components of the myelin sheath.
- T cells, immunoglobulin, and complement are immunopathogenic.
- CD4+ T cells reactive to myelin antigens are found in the lesions.
- Susceptibility to EAE is greater in females and MHC linked.

THERAPY OF EAE AND MS

Inflammatory MS lesions have been demonstrated to include α4 integrin and matrix metalloproteases, CD4 T cells reactive to myelin proteins, and the cytokines IL-6, TNF-α and interferon gamma (IFN-γ). These have also been demonstrated in inflamed brain and spinal cord in EAE. Treatments with antibodies to α4 integrin,[11] to CD4 T cells reactive to myelin proteins,[12] and to the cytokines IL-6,[13] lymphotoxin, and TNF-α[14] have all reversed paralysis in various models of EAE (Table 119.2). Likewise, administration of small molecule metalloprotease inhibitors[15] and altered peptide ligands (APL) for T-cell receptors recognizing myelin antigens, has also reversed EAE.[5] This has led to clinical trials directed at α4 integrin, CD4, T cells reactive to myelin antigens, TNF-α, and IFN-γ. Many of these approaches are being tested in phase II clinical trials, where dose and timing of administration of the therapeutic agent are being ascertained. To date, the most promising therapeutic approach to come out of the EAE model is Copaxone. This synthetic polymer analog of myelin basic protein has been successful in reducing the relapse rate in MS in clinical trials, and is currently approved for treatment of MS.[16]

Nonspecific therapy of EAE: targeting cytokines, adhesion molecules, matrix metalloproteases

Beta interferon (IFN-β), approved for use in the USA and the EEU for treatment of relapsing MS, was originally tried as an antiviral compound for treatment of MS, a disease often linked to a viral etiology. After IFN-β was proved to be effective clinically in relapsing-remitting MS, it was shown that recombinant IFN-β could ameliorate EAE, though severe relapses were seen when IFN-β was discontinued.[17]

CD4 T-cell responses are divided into two categories (Chapter 16), based on the types of cytokines produced after stimulation: Th1 responses, commonly found in T cells from individuals with organ-specific autoimmune diseases like MS or rheumatoid arthritis, lead to production of IFN-γ and TNF-α; while Th2 responses,

Comparisons between MS and EAE: therapy	MS	EAE
Therapy		
IFN-γ, systemic	Worsens	Cures
anti-TNF-α, systemic	Worsens	Cures
IL-4 transduced T cells	Not done	Cures
TNF-α transduced T cells	Not done	Worsens
Copaxone	Improves	Cure
IFN-β	Improves	Improves
Altered peptide ligands	Improves	Cure
DNA vaccination	Not done	Cures

Table 119.2 Comparisons between MS and EAE: therapy.

commonly found in T cells from individuals with allergic conditions or parasitic infections, are characterized by the release of IL-4, IL-5, and IL-10. MS is considered a Th1-type autoimmune disease, as is EAE. However, EAE also can be induced with Th2-type T-cell clones,[18] demonstrating that other cytokines can assume critical functions in producing the phenotype characteristic of EAE. Although experimental autoimmune encephalomyelitis and experimental allergic encephalomyelitis are used interchangeably, perhaps it is more appropriate to refer to disease caused by Th1 clones as 'experimental autoimmune encephalomyelitis', while disease induced by Th2 clones could be referred to as 'experimental allergic encephalomyelitis'.

It is clear that two of the critical cytokines involved in the pathogenesis of MS are IFN-γ and TNF-α. A clinical trial was performed in the 1980s to test the efficacy of IFN-γ in MS. Results showed that IFN-γ exacerbated disease, and the trial was halted while in progress.[19] The results implied that IFN-γ is pathogenic in MS. Paradoxically, in EAE, systemic administration of IFN-γ protects against paralysis.[20]

Another cytokine believed to play a key role in MS is TNF-α. This is based on the observation that there is an increase in TNF-α in the cerebrospinal fluid preceding and during relapses of disease.[21] However, thus far in humans, treatments with monoclonal anti-TNF antibody and soluble TNF receptor have actually worsened MS.[22] The anti-TNF treatments that failed in MS have been successful in other diseases like rheumatoid arthritis and Crohn's disease, where TNF-α plays a critical role. Clinical trials with reagents that block TNF-α in the periphery have exacerbated MS, but therapeutic trials with phosphodiesterase inhibitors and other approaches like altered peptide ligands that can down-regulate TNF-α within the central nervous system have not been reported.

The discrepancies between the results with inhibition of TNF-α in EAE versus MS are quite perplexing. TNF-α and lymphotoxin are members of the TNF family of cytokines, and although they have different structures they both bind to the same receptors and produce similar biologic effects. Whether it is TNF-α or lymphotoxin that may be the key inflammatory mediator in EAE or MS is an open question. An attempt to resolve this issue has been addressed with mice in which TNF family members – either TNF-α, lymphotoxin, or both – are disrupted.

There is evidence that TNF-α, lymphotoxin, and members of the TNF receptor family may play a key role in the pathogenesis of oligodendroglial damage. TNF is elevated in relapses of MS and if has been demonstrated in MS lesions.[21,23] Myelin basic protein reactive T cells from MS patients expressing the disease-associated HLA-DRB1*15 allele produce increased levels of TNF-α.[24] Increased numbers of MBP-induced TNF-α and lymphotoxin mRNA-expressing mononuclear cells were also demonstrated in the blood and CSF of MS patients.[25] In vitro, TNF-α can damage myelin and injure oligodendrocytes in culture.[26] In various models of EAE, blockade of TNF-α with monoclonal antibodies or soluble TNF receptor constructs can prevent or reverse disease.[26] Therapy with altered peptide analogs of myelin basic protein which negatively regulate the expression of TNF-α reverses EAE, even after paralysis is apparent.[27] Negative regulation of TNF-α by IV phosphodiesterase inhibitors prevents and reverses EAE.[28,29] Astrocytes from strains of rats that are susceptible to EAE express higher levels of TNF-α than those from strains that are resistant to EAE.[30] Over-expression of TNF-α in the central nervous system in transgenic mice leads to spontaneous inflammatory demyelinating disease.[31]

Interestingly, however, in mice with the TNF-α and lymphotoxin genes deleted, full-blown inflammation can still develop in the CNS.[32] The mediators that can replace TNF-α when its gene is disabled should be identified because it may ensue that inhibiting TNF-α alone may allow another mediator to become up-regulated and replace it in the inflammatory cascade. Targeted gene deletion in mice of lymphotoxin alone, with TNF-α expression left intact, blocks the development of EAE.[14] However, Korner et al[33] showed that TNF, and not lymphotoxin, is essential for initial lymphocyte movement into the CNS. This indicates, at least in rodent models of demyelination, that lymphotoxin may play the decisive role in demyelination, rather than TNF-α. There is also evidence that at least under some circumstances TNF-α might have an anti-inflammatory role. Mice deficient in TNF-α develop a more severe form of EAE. The EAE in these TNF-α knockout mice can be reversed by administering TNF-α.[34] Nonetheless, the case for the pathogenic effect of TNF in MS and many of its animal models is strong and demands the question, how might TNF-α and lymphotoxin cause damage?

TNF receptor binding by TNF-α or lymphotoxin activates cellular mechanisms resulting in cell death. Fas/APO-1 (CD95) is a member of the TNF/nerve growth factor receptor family. Like TNF receptor activation, Fas/APO-1 activation also leads to cell death. Cell killing by T cells involves both the TNF receptor and Fas. Recently, it was shown that Fas ligation causes lysis of human oligodendroglial cells.[35] TNF also damages oligodendroglial cells in vitro. The cellular mechanisms leading to death from activation of the TNF receptor family are now being elucidated. In chronic MS, oligodendrocytes express Fas and TNF receptors, as well as the antiapoptotic molecule, bcl-2. However, oligodendroglial cells showed no evidence of apoptosis when DNA fragmentation was assayed.[36]

Thus, it is unclear from various EAE models whether TNF-α is a pathologic player, and should be inhibited, or whether it might indeed have protective effects. When myelin-specific T cells transduced with retroviruses carrying cytokines have been given to mice with EAE, IL-4 transduced T cells ameliorated EAE, while TNF-α transduced cells worsened disease. When targeting is more precise, using retrovirally transduced myelin-specific T cells that can home to the site of disease, a Th1 cytokine exacerbated and a Th2 cytokine ameliorated EAE.[37] The effects of cytokines and their inhibitors when given systemically, or when their genes have been disrupted globally, may be paradoxical, especially when interpreting results with potential therapeutics such as monoclonal antibodies or soluble recep-

THERAPEUTIC PRINCIPLES

Nonspecific strategies for immunotherapy of EAE/MS

- Therapy directed at cytokines, adhesion molecules, and matrix metalloproteases.
- IFN-γ therapy exacerbated MS.
- Anti-TNF therapy failed in MS.
- Inhibition of TNF-α by phosphodiesterase IV inhibitors prevents and reverses EAE.

tors that are unable to penetrate to the site of disease across the blood–brain barrier.

T-cell vaccination in EAE

Autoreactive T cells, attenuated by radiation, can be used as vaccines to prevent and treat the autoimmune diseases which in an unmodified state these same cells induce. The principle of T-cell vaccination is similar to traditional microbial vaccination against infectious agents. Pioneering work by Cohen and coworkers[38] demonstrated that T-cell vaccination is effective in preventing and treating many experimental autoimmune diseases, including EAE, experimental autoimmune uveitis, insulin-dependent diabetes mellitus in the NOD mouse, and adjuvant arthritis. The major target of the immune response in T-cell vaccination is the TCR hypervariable regions, including CDR3 or less variable CDR2, as predicted by their immunogenic property and sequence diversity.[39] Recent investigations involving immunization with various TCR peptides suggest that both the CDR2 and the CDR3 regions are likely to trigger the clonotypic interactions.[40,41] In experimental animals, a clonotypic regulatory T-cell response preventing EAE can be induced by immunizing rats with a synthetic peptide of the Vβ CDR2 region characteristic for encephalitogenic T cells. These anticlonotypic T cells are the major cellular component of the protective mechanism and are capable of conferring a specific protection to naive rats by adoptive transfer. Similarly, in humans, TCR peptides corresponding to both CDR2 and CDR3 regions are found to induce CD4 regulatory T cells in vitro.[42]

T-cell vaccination in MS

Zhang and coworkers conducted a phase I clinical trial in which patients with relapsing-remitting and chronic progressive MS were vaccinated with irradiated autologous MBP-reactive T cell clones.[43] Disease activity was monitored, including the frequency and severity of clinical exacerbation, neurological examination, and magnetic resonance imaging (MRI) of the brain lesions. Selected MBP-reactive T-cell clones (T-cell vaccines) were first activated in vitro and irradiated to render them incapable of proliferation. Each recipient received a total of three subcutaneous injections of 2–4 vaccine clones (15×10^6 cells for each clone) at 2–4-month intervals. The clinical trial revealed that the procedure used for vaccination trial was safe, technically feasible, and the autologous vaccine clones were well tolerated. After three vaccinations, no circulating MBP-reactive T cells were detected in the recipients, suggesting a depletion of the autoreactive T cells.

To investigate further whether depletion of MBP-reactive T cells in vaccinated patients correlated with clinical improvement, patients were monitored over a period of 2–3 years for various clinical parameters, including exacerbation rate, expanded disability status score (EDSS), and quantitative changes in brain lesions as detected by MRI. Each patient was paired with a control MS subject selected before vaccination. The 5 patients with relapsing-remitting MS exhibited a total of 3 exacerbations during 2–3 years after vaccination as compared to 16 relapses recorded during the 2-year period prior to vaccination.[44] In the 5 paired control MS subjects, the number of relapses was reduced from 12 to 9 during the same period of time. Consistent with the reduced rate of exacerbation in the vaccinated subjects, there was a net reduction of the end EDSS by 0.5–2.0 points in some patients. In contrast, EDSS recorded in paired control subjects showed a progressive increase over the same period of time, which reflects the natural course of the disease within this group of patients. In the 3 patients with chronic progressive MS, however, vaccination did not seem to alter the clinical course.

The semiquantitative analysis of the MRI scans revealed that in 5 out of 8 vaccinated patients, the total lesion score of the two MRI scans (taken shortly after vaccination and approximately 2 years after vaccination) did not differ significantly from respective baseline values, representing merely a 3.6% lesion increase.[44] In contrast, among the control subjects the brain lesions progressed over the same period of time. The total MRI lesion score of this group was increased by 39.5% in the scans taken at the end of the trial, as compared to the baseline scans. The stabilization of the brain lesions seen in some vaccinated patients may represent a significant improvement, considering that in the course of untreated MS, the lesions increase generally by at least 10% on a yearly basis similar to the control subjects seen in this phase I trial.

T-cell receptor peptide vaccination in EAE and MS

In 1989, Vandenbark, Offner and coworkers successfully prevented and treated EAE in Lewis rats using a synthetic peptide corresponding to the TCR CDR2 sequence of encephalitogenic MBP-reactive T cells.[45] They demonstrated that the protective effect could be conferred by anticlonotypic regulatory T cells induced by immunization with the TCR peptide. Howell and colleagues showed in an independent study that a synthetic peptide designed to correspond to the TCR CDR3 sequence of encephalitogenic T cells was also effective in treating EAE.[41] Thus, these studies suggested that vaccination with TCR peptides is effective in treating an autoimmune disease model through regulatory mechanisms by which myelin autoreactive T cells are suppressed.

Vandenbark and coworkers immunized MS patients with two synthetic TCR CDR2 peptides corresponding to TCR Vβ 5.2 and Vβ 6.1 in a clinical trial. Selection of these TCR peptides was based on the author's observation that both Vβ 5.2 and Vβ 6.1 were over-expressed by MBP-reactive T cells found in patients with MS.[46,47] In their clinical trials, patients received 4 weekly injections of the TCR peptides at varying dosage and received injections every 4 weeks thereafter. Vaccination with these two peptides induced specific T-cell responses and antibody reactivity in some patients (responders), which correlated inversely with the frequency of circulating MBP-reactive T cells.[48] The results of a double-blind, placebo-controlled clinical trial in 23 $DR2^+$ patients with MS revealed that this treatment was nontoxic and stabilized clinical progression in 6/23 MS patients who responded to vaccination.[49] The vaccination nonresponders underwent continuous clinical decline, and the frequency of their circulating MBP-reactive T cells remained unaltered during the course of the 1-year clinical trial. Interestingly, vaccination with the TCR peptides appeared to induce TCR peptide-specific T cells that preferentially produced IL-4 and IL-10 but not IFN-γ. TCR peptide-specific T cells induced by vaccination suppressed proliferation of MBP-reactive T cells and production of IFN-γ in vitro.

DNA vaccination in EAE

Instead of making vaccines composed of proteins or peptides, it is possible to construct a vaccine from the DNA encoding the

THERAPEUTIC PRINCIPLES

Antigen-specific therapy directed at EAE/MS

- T-cell vaccination using irradiated autologous MBP-reactive T-cell clones showed some efficacy in relapsing-remitting MS.
- Vaccination with synthetic TCR peptides (from MBP reactive T cells) showed some efficacy in MS and was effective in treating EAE.
- DNA vaccination using dominant TCR genes expressed in MS patient derived T cells is being evaluated.

intended antigen. The DNA in the vaccine is taken up by cells of the vaccinated subject, which then translate and transcribe the injected DNA and express the antigen encoded by it. The immune cells of the individual, in turn, mount an immune response to the antigen expressed by the transduced cells, giving rise to immunological memory. Upon a future exposure to the introduced antigen perhaps by an infectious agent, the immune system reacts in an enhanced manner and prevents the infection. This vaccination approach utilizes 'naked' DNA material (cloned in an expression vector) that encodes an antigen designed to induce both B-cell and T-cell responses to the antigen expressed by myocytes in the vicinity of the injection site.[50] Multiple injections of DNA encoding the variable region gene of the TCR commonly found on encephalitogenic T cells termed Vβ8.2, prevented EAE in mice.[39] Vaccination with the Vβ DNA from the TCR induced a shift in the pattern of cytokine produced by the encephalitogenic T cells. These encephalitogenic T cells no longer produced pro-inflammatory cytokines, IL-2 and IFN-γ after vaccination, and instead produced suppressive cytokines, including IL-4. Thus, the state of resistance to EAE induced by DNA vaccination is attributable to the shift of the Th1 'pro-inflammatory' cytokine pattern to the Th2 'suppressive' pattern. DNA immunization has now been extended to the treatment of EAE with DNA minigenes encoding myelin antigens.[51,52] This novel vaccination approach will be implemented for the treatment of MS. DNA vaccination to a dominant TCR V gene expressed on T cells, recognizing a critical myelin protein, might modulate the cytokine profile of myelin autoreactive T cells in the systemic circulation, and at the site of demyelinating lesions.

Altered peptide ligand therapy in EAE and MS

When a T-cell receptor encounters a variant of the antigen that it normally recognizes, an aberrant signal is induced within the cell. In the case of autoreactive T cells that normally produce pro-inflammatory cytokines the variant antigen may trigger suppressive cytokines. We have constructed altered peptide ligands for T cells recognizing fragments of myelin basic protein. These T cells induce paralysis and demyelination in experimental animals when triggered by the native myelin basic protein. However, when these T cells encounter altered peptide ligand, APL, they no longer produce the pathogenic cytokine IFN-γ and TNF-α, but rather produce IL-4 (Fig. 119.3). This can reverse EAE. Interestingly, the effect is 'trans-acting', in that paralytic disease induced with a specific myelin protein, such as proteolipid

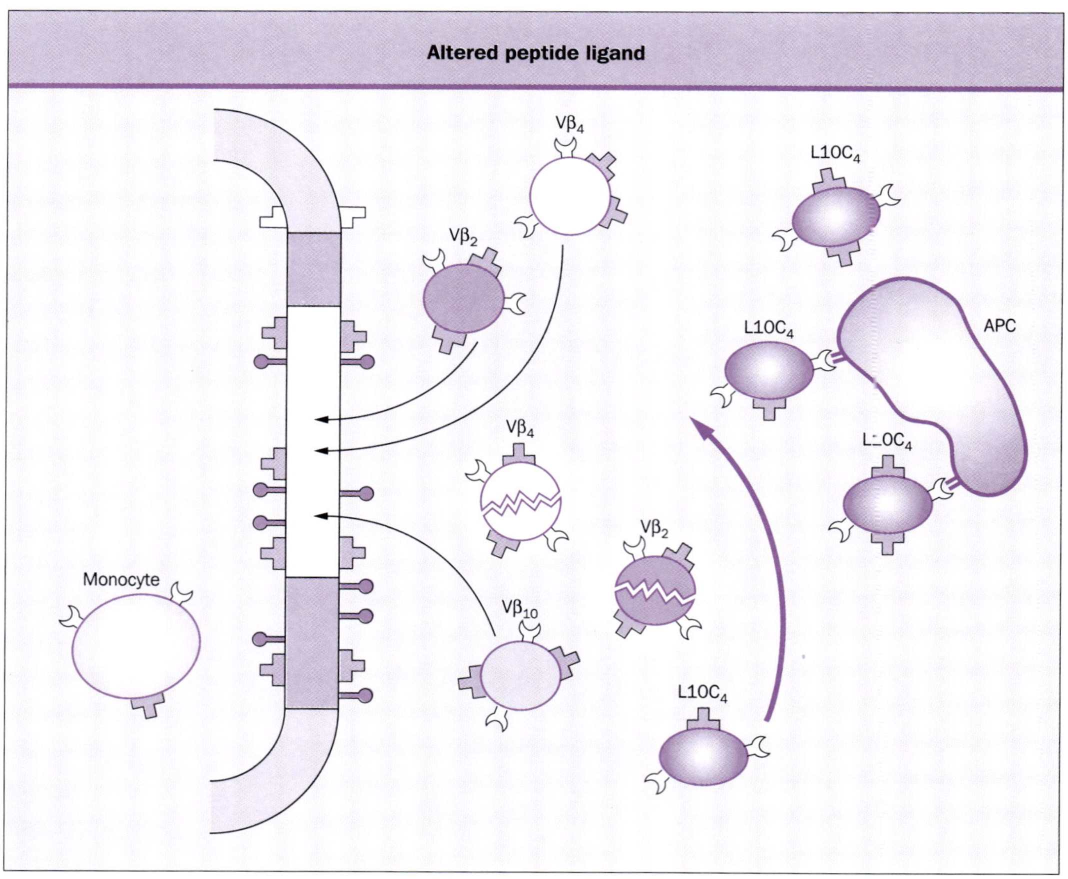

Figure 119.3 A rare T cell specific for the neuroantigen MBP in an inflammatory infiltrate, designated L10C4, is targeted by an altered peptide. Within 24 h there is an exodus of the entire nonspecific infiltrate. APC, antigen-presenting cell. (Redrawn from Steinman L. A few autoreactive cells in an autoimmune infiltrate control a vast population of nonspecific cells: a tale of smart bombs and the infantry. *Proc Natl Acad Sci USA* 1996;93:2553.)

protein, can be suppressed with an altered peptide ligand derived from an alternative myelin protein such a MBP. The trans-acting effect is mediated by IL-4, because antibodies to IL-4 can abrogate the suppression of disease.[1,27]

Hafler and coworkers showed that an altered MBP peptide could act as antagonist that blocked subsequent activation and induced a shift in cytokine production pattern.[53] After pretreatment with altered peptide, the autoreactive T-cell clones no longer produce TNF-α and IFN-γ but rather secrete TGF-β (an important suppressive cytokine). The in vivo effect of altered peptides of MBP has been demonstrated in experimental animals both to prevent and treat EAE. Karin and colleagues described that when the immunodominant MBP peptide (residues 87–99) was altered in that lysine (K) was replaced by alanine (A) at position 91, this mutant peptide lost ability to induce EAE and instead prevent and reverse ongoing EAE with clinical paralysis.[54] This altered MBP peptide (91K→A) suppressed EAE by inhibiting the production of TNF-α and IFN-γ.

Treatment of PLP-induced relapses of EAE has also been attenuated by the MBPp87–99.[55] Thus, APL therapy of EAE can have a trans-acting influence on immune responses to other myelin antigens. As the immune response spreads to various components of the supramolecular complex of myelin proteins, Th2 cytokines induced by administration of one myelin peptide may inhibit responses to other myelin antigens.[27,55,56] Thus, APL directed to one myelin antigen like MBP can inhibit immune responses to other myelin antigens.

These in vitro and in vivo studies suggest that alteration of a critical TCR contact residue of a pathogenic myelin peptide may modulate pathogenic autoreactive T cells, so that they deliver suppressive cytokines at the site of pathology. Thus, for its therapeutic application in MS, a myelin peptide derived either from MBP, MOG, or PLP must be altered at a specific position that renders myelin autoreactive T cells inactive and enables them to produce suppressive cytokines. Phase I and II trials with an altered peptide ligand for MBP have been completed in MS and are being evaluated.

The problem of epitope spreading and the outlook for antigen-specific therapy

The concept of epitope spreading described by Sercarz, Lehmann and colleagues for EAE delineates how antigen-specific autoimmune responses can spread to different epitopes on one protein, termed 'intramolecular epitope spreading'[57,58] or to other epitopes on other structural proteins, termed 'intermolecular epitope spreading'.[58] One decade ago there was enthusiasm that, at least for short periods in the pathogenesis of autoimmune disease, the immune response was highly restricted. There was hope that there might be an easy extrapolation to human diseases from experiments in rodents showing that 'cures' of clinical symptoms in models of autoimmune disease were possible after deletion of T cells bearing receptors with one T-cell V region product,[59,60] or immunization against that TCR V gene product.[41,45] The discovery of epitope spreading raised doubts that this simplistic approach targeting single TCR V genes, or even trying to tolerize to a single epitope on one autoantigen, would ever be clinically applicable once epitope spreading was underway. The evidence that epitope spreading occurs in human autoimmune diseases and in their animal counterparts is strong. However, we shall describe data from animal experiments that suggest that highly specific therapy of autoimmune disease remains a real possibility. Should our contention, that highly restricted approaches to the immunotherapy of autoimmune disease prove to be incorrect, we shall hedge our bet with a counterstrategy, DNA vaccination against multiple autoantigenic epitopes, an approach made possible by the ease of DNA immunization.[51,61]

THERAPEUTIC PRINCIPLES

Altered peptide ligand therapy of EAE/MS

- Altered MBP peptide ligand induces cytokine shifts to IL-4 and/or TGF-β production.
- Therapy with altered MBP peptide ligand (MBPp87–89, 91 K→A) reverses ongoing EAE.
- Altered peptide ligand is trans-acting in EAE, i.e. it blocks the response to other myelin epitopes.
- Phase I and II trials using altered peptide ligand have been undertaken in MS.

Success of highly selective immune therapy in EAE

Over the past decade, at least in animal models, highly selective therapies targeting either the T-cell receptor, or specific peptide epitopes of autoantigens, have proven successful in both the prevention and reversal of autoimmune disease. Many of these therapies that succeeded in EAE are now being tried in MS.[61] In 1988 and 1989, it was demonstrated that the T-cell response to pathogenic epitopes on myelin basic protein utilized a limited set of TCR V region genes.[47,59] Using this information EAE was either prevented or ongoing disease, including paralysis, was reversed with the administration of antibody to the TCR Vβ chain.[59] Disease reversal with the antibody to TCR Vβ8 was demonstrated even after paralysis was evident in PLSJ F1 mice immunized with whole MBP. Whole MBP contains multiple discrete epitopes of MBP that are capable of inducing EAE, including MBPp35–47 and MBPp89–101, which are recognized by TCR that do not use Vβ8. Therefore, at least in PLSJ F1 mice after the acute attack of EAE, there was evidence of a dominant autoimmune response, where the pathophysiology involved a very restricted attack against one epitope with T-cell receptors of limited diversity. This protection was checked for another 2 weeks after a single treatment with anti-Vβ8 antibody; whereas 12 of 19 mice were free of disease 72 hours after being treated during full-blown paralysis, after 2 weeks 14 of 19 mice remained free of disease. This indicates that although epitope spreading could occur, deletion of T cells expressing the dominant TCR Vβ8 chain resulted in stable disease suppression.[59]

The experiments using antibodies were followed by experiments showing that acute EAE in the Lewis rat could be prevented or reversed with immunization to Vβ8 peptides as previously noted.[39,45] At the same time it was shown that one could block EAE with altered peptide ligands that interfered with the pathogenic recognition of disease-inducing epitopes.[27,54,56,62,63] APL treatment altered the cytokine profiles of pathogenic T cells, and was able to reverse disease induced by antigens that contained multiple epitopes. T-cell infiltrates in EAE brain, known to be highly diverse, actually disappeared following the treatment of a paralyzed mouse with a single APL directed to one epitope.[27,56] The regression of the inflammatory infiltrate was mediated in part by the cytokine IL-4, as disease reversal was abrogated by anti-IL-4 treatment.[54] Finally, DNA vaccination to TCR gene products, and to specific myelin epitopes, was shown to prevent EAE.[39,51,52,61]

Epitope spreading in experimental and human autoimmune disease, focusing on EAE and MS

In EAE induced with an injection of an epitope of PLP, the immune reactivity of T cells can spread to other epitopes on PLP, and then on to other myelin antigens such as MBP and MOG. Tuohy and colleagues demonstrated that, during the course of EAE initiated by immunization to one epitope, both intramolecular and intermolecular epitope spreading allow the autoimmune response to evolve in an orderly manner to encompass detectable T-cell responses to other epitopes on the initiating antigen and to other myelin antigens.[64] Remarkably, the T-cell response to the initiating epitope was lost as disease progressed, a situation that is very different following immunization with a virus.[65]

In organ-specific autoimmune diseases such as MS, rheumatoid arthritis and insulin-dependent diabetes mellitus (IDDM), a vigorous debate remains as to what antigen triggered the initial autoimmune response. Further, there are arguments about what antigens dominate the diverse immune responses detected at the site of disease. Thus, in MS, where an apparent autoimmune T- and B-cell response occurs in the myelin sheath of the central nervous system, there are arguments whether the initial or dominant immune response might be directed at myelin basic protein (MBP),[1] myelin oligodendroglial glycoprotein (MOG),[66] proteolipid protein (PLP),[67] or various other myelin antigens.[68] In MS brain there is at least some evidence of clonally restricted T-cell responses to certain epitopes of MBP,[1,8,47] and that the antibody response in brain itself is highly restricted, with some overlap in the specificity of the T- and the B-cell response.[6–8] In IDDM, investigators debate whether the primary response is against glutamic acid decarboxylase,[69,70] insulin,[71] heat-shock protein 65,[72] or other islet cell antigens.

Tracking epitope spreading in human autoimmune disease is difficult, because it is hard to know exactly when disease was initiated. In fact it has been suggested that autoimmune diseases, such as MS and IDDM, are due to a clinical deficit that emerges years after the primary event. Tuohy and colleagues were able to follow, over a period of many years, the response of peripheral blood lymphocytes in patients with an isolated neurologic deficit, as it evolved into clinically definite MS.[64] As these patients progressed to MS, they lost reactivity to the myelin epitopes that were recognized during the initial immune response, and developed T-cell immune reactivity to other myelin epitopes, the converse of what was described as 'original antigenic sin'.[73] In this doctrine, the immune response to a subsequent exposure to a new strain of influenza virus boosts the response to the original strain of immunizing antigen. This doctrine pertains to both antibody and cytotoxic T-cell responses to viral antigens.[74] It is raised as a major problem for vaccine manufacturers who would like to immunize against viral variants.[75] This is a major challenge on a yearly basis for influenza vaccines, and a dramatic challenge for example in developing a vaccine to HIV, which is so variable. But examination of this doctrine reveals that quite the opposite seems to occur in autoimmunity! The immune response to the initiating self-antigen in autoimmunity disappears as disease enters the stage where clinical progression and then chronicity prevail (Fig. 119.4).[65]

In the face of epitope spreading there is evidence that targeted immune therapy might still work

If intramolecular and intermolecular epitope spreading are characteristic of the immune response in autoimmune disease, might this negate the possibility of antigen-specific immune therapy? As previously noted, data from Tuohy and colleagues,[64] and experiments by Acha-Orbea,[59] Brocke,[27] and Nicholson[76] indicate that

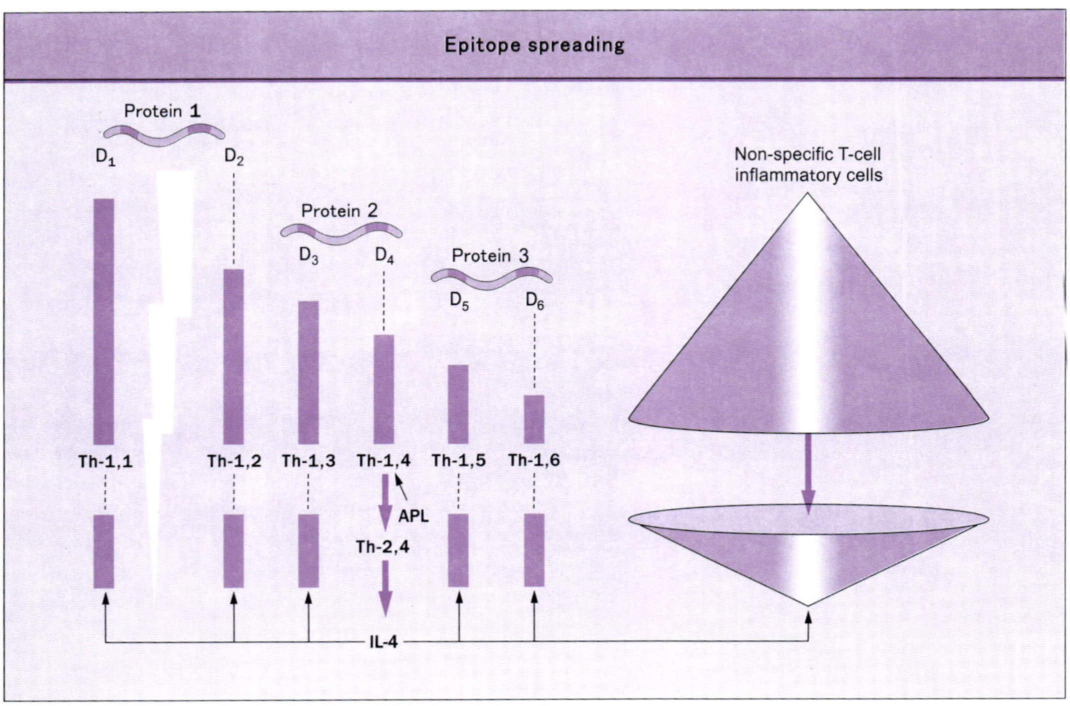

Figure 119.4 Mechanism for intramolecular and intermolecular epitope spreading in autoimmunity. (Redrawn from Steinman L. Absence of 'original antigenic sin' in autoimmunity provides an unforseen platform for immune therapy. *J Exp Med* 1999;189:1021.)

certain dominant immune responses prevail in chronic autoimmunity, and that control of these responses can culminate in amelioration of ongoing disease.[27,59] In the MS brain at autopsy for instance, T and B cells reactive to an epitope on MBP, p87–99, can be detected.[6–8,47] Indeed in MS, antibodies to MBPp87–99 can be seen at the site of disease, where vesiculated myelin is demonstrable by electron microscopy.[7] Tuohy et al showed that they could block relapses of EAE, after disease was initially induced with PLPp139–151, by administering MBPp87–99.[64] After mice were immunized with PLP, the immune response spread intramolecularly to other PLP epitopes, and then intermolecularly to other myelin antigens, including MBP. Epitope spreading was manifest clinically as relapsing paralysis. One of the antigens targeted by the immune response after intermolecular epitope spreading was MBPp87–99. Administration of this MBP fragment suppressed further episodes of paralysis. As previously noted, this trans-acting suppression may be mediated by cytokines such as IL-4, which are released after T cells encounter low-affinity MBP peptides or APL.[27] These results implied that if one can suppress an immune response to a critical immunogenic epitope that can be detected during chronic disease, then it may be possible to intervene and to treat autoimmunity, despite the fact that perhaps an alternate antigen or microbial mimic triggered the disease initially.

As previously discussed elsewhere,[65] the differences are stark between immunity to viral antigens, where 'original antigenic sin' provides a reasonable explanation for the persistence of responses to the first encounter with virus, and autoimmunity to self-antigens, where the initial immune response wanes over time. It is important to recognize some essential differences, however, between autoimmunity and immunity to microbes. In autoimmunity the antigen persists, though ancillary signals surrounding the self-constituent, such as cytokines, co-stimulatory molecules, and MHC, may vary over time, thus changing the 'antigenicity' of self. In immunity to microbes, the pathogen is either removed by the immune reaction, or immunity is subverted, resulting in persistence of the microbe, if the host survives. Elaborate microbial escape mechanisms include mutation of microbial genes and variations in microbial antigenicity, as well as the production of mediators with the properties of cytokines and chemokines that suppress immune attack. Often persistence involves microbial genes turning off critical genes in the host. Thus, 'original antigenic sin' may describe how certain immune responses to microbes remain dominant over time, a situation that occurs in autoimmunity. However, in autoimmunity the response to the inciting antigen fades, whereas in microbial immunity the initial response may dominate.

At present, the explanation of the persistence and dominance of the initial immune response to a virus can be explained with the concept of 'original antigenic sin'. Yet it is now clear that the very opposite of 'original antigenic sin' ensues as autoimmunity develops. What may confound immunization to viruses may be a potential blessing in the design of immune therapies to counter epitope spreading in autoimmune disease.

It may now be possible to tolerize directly to multiple epitopes by using DNA vaccines containing multiple myelin minigenes in MS, or multiple epitopes of various autoantigens in other autoimmune conditions. Whereas the economics of peptide-based therapy or monoclonal antibody therapy made such an approach prohibitively expensive, DNA vaccine technology will allow the constructions of plasmids with multiple epitopes, or TCR V regions, under the control of promoters that will enhance tolerization.[51,52,61]

CODA

Although EAE has many features that reflect what is known about the pathophysiology of MS, there also are many discrepancies between the pathology of EAE and MS. Therefore, extrapolations must be made with caution when predicting what might happen in MS, based on therapeutic results obtained in the EAE model. Results of ongoing clinical trials that include targeting $\alpha4$ integrin with humanized antibodies, metalloproteases with small molecule inhibitors, and T cells reactive to myelin antigens with humanized antibodies and altered peptide ligands, should allow us to judge the utility of EAE as a model to predict therapeutic efficacy for MS. So far, the development of the approved MS drug, Copaxone, based on its efficacy in EAE, and the success of IFN-β in treating EAE, must be balanced with the failures of anti-TNF-γ and IFN-γ in MS, after their successful use in various models of EAE. Thus, it is too early to judge whether amelioration of EAE will be a reliable predictor of success in treating MS.

A similar note of caution must be applied to experimental immunotherapy in other autoimmune disease models. However taken together these models have provided critical insights into the immunopathogenic basis of these diseases as well as identifying new approaches to their therapy.

REFERENCES

1. Steinman L. Multiple sclerosis: a coordinated immunological attack against myelin in the central nervous system. Cell 1996;85:299.
2. Stuart G, Krikorian KS. The neuro-paralytic accidents of anti-rabies treatment. Ann Trop Med Parasitol 1928;22:327.
3. Rivers TM, Schwentker FF. Encephalomyelitis accompanied by myelin destruction experimentally produced in monkeys. J Exp Med 1935;61:689.
4. Kabat EA, Wolf A, Bezer AL. The rapid production of acute disseminated encephalomyelitis in rhesus monkeys by injection of heterologous and homologous brain tissue with adjuvants. J Exp Med 1947;85:117.
5. Conlon P, Oksenberg JR, Zhang J, Steinman L. The immunobiology of multiple sclerosis: an autoimmune disease of the central nervous system. Neurobiol Dis 1999;6:149.
6. Wucherpfennig KW, Catz I, Hausmann S, Strominger JL, Steinman L, Warren KG. Recognition of the immunodominant myelin basic protein peptide by autoantibodies and HLA-DR2 restricted T cell clones from multiple sclerosis patients: Identity of key contact residues in the B-cell and T-cell epitopes. Clin Invest 1997;100:1114.
7. Genain CP, Cannella B, Hauser SL, Raine CS. Identification of autoantibodies associated with myelin damage in multiple sclerosis. Nat Med 1999;5:170.
8. Warren KG, Catz I, Steinman L. Fine specificity of the antibody response to myelin basic protein in the central nervous system in multiple sclerosis: The minimal B cell epitope and a model of its unique features. Proc Natl Acad Sci USA 1995;92:11061.
9. Trapp BD, Peterson J, Ransohoff RM, et al. Axonal transection in the lesions of MS. N Engl J Med 1998;228:278.

10. Raine CS, Cross AH. Axonal dystrophy as a consequence of long-term demyelination. Lab Invest 1988;60:714.
11. Yednock T, Cannon C, Fritz L, Sanchez-Madrid F, Steinman L, Karin N. Prevention of experimental autoimmune encephalomyelitis by antibodies against α4β1 integrin. Nature 1992;356:63.
12. Waldor MK, Hardy R, Herzenberg LA et al. Reversal of EAE with monoclonal antibody to a T cell subset marker (L3T4). Science 1985;227:415.
13. Gijbels K, Brocke S, Abrams J, Steinman L. Administration of neutralizing antibodies to interleukin-6 (IL-6) reduces experimental autoimmune encephalomyelitis and is associated with elevated levels of IL-6 bioactivity in central nervous system and circulation. Mol Med 1995;1(7):795.
14. Suen W, Bergman CM, Hjelmstrom P, Ruddle NH. A critical role for lymptoxin in EAE. J Exp Med 1997;186:1233.
15. Gijbels K, Galardy R, Steinman L. Reversal of EAE with a hydroxymate inhibitor of matrix metalloproteases. J Clin Invest 1994;94:2177.
16. Arnon R. The development of Cop-1 (Copaxone), an innovative drug for treatment of MS. Immunol Lett 1996;50:1.
17. Ruuls SR, de Labie MCDC, Wever K et al. The length of treatment determines whether IFN-β prevents or aggravates experimental autoimmune encephalomyelitis in Lewis rats. J Immunol 1996;157:5721.
18. Lafaille JJ, Keere FV, Hsu AL, Baron J, Hass W, Raine CS, Tonegawa S. Myelin basic protein T helper 2 cells cause experimental autoimmune encephalomyelitis in immunodeficient mice rather than protect them from disease. J Exp Med 1997;186:307.
19. Panitch HS, Hirsch RL, Schindler J, Johnson KP. Treatment of MS with gamma interferon: Exacerbations associated with activation of the immune system. Neurology 1987;37:1097.
20. Krakowski M, Owens T. Interferon-gamma confers resistance to EAE. Eur J Immunol 1996;26:1641.
21. Sharief MK, Hentges R. Association between TNFα and disease progression in patients with MS. N Engl J Med 1991;325:467.
22. van Oosten BW, Barkhof F, Truyen L, et al. Increased MRI activity and immune activation in two multiple sclerosis patients treated with the monoclonal anti-tumor necrosis factor antibody cA2. Neurology 1996;47:1531.
23. Hofman FM, Hinton DR, Johnson K, Merrill JE. TNF identified in MS brain. J Exp Med 1989;170:607.
24. Hermans G, Stinissen P, Hauben L, Van den Berg-Loonen E, Raus J, Zhang J. Cytokine profile of MBP-reactive T cells in MS and healthy individuals. Ann Neurol 1997;42:18.
25. Navikas V, He B, Link J et al. Augmented expression of TNFα and lymphotoxin in mononuclear cells in multiple sclerosis and optic neuritis. Brain 1996;119:213.
26. Selmaj KW, Raine CS. Tumor necrosis factor mediates myelin and oligodendrocyte damage in vitro. Ann Neurol 1988;23:339.
27. Brocke S, Gijbels K, Allegretta M, et al. Treatment of experimental encephalomyelitis with a peptide analogue of myelin basic protein. Nature 1996;379:343.
28. Sommer N, Löschmann PA, Northoff GH, et al. The antidepressant rolipram suppresses cytokine production and prevents autoimmune encephalomyelitis. Nat Med 1995;1:3,244.
29. Genain CP, Roberts T, Davis RL, et al. Prevention of autoimmune demyelination in non-human primates by a cAMP-specific phosphodiesterase inhibitor. Proc Natl Acad Sci USA 1995;92:8,3601.
30. Chung IY, Norris JG, Benveniste EN. Differential tumor necrosis factor α expression by astrocytes from EAE-susceptible and resistant rat strains. J Exp Med 1991;173:801.
31. Probert L, Akassoglou K, Pasparakis M, Kontogeorgos G, Kollias G. Spontaneous inflammatory demyelinating disease in transgenic mice showing central nervous system-specific expression of TNFα. Proc Natl Acad Sci USA 1995;92:11294.
32. Frei K, Eugster HP, Bopst M, Constantinuscu CS, Lavi E, Fonatana A. TNFα and lymphotoxin alpha are not required for induction of acute experimental autoimmune encephalomyelitis. J Exp Med 1997;185:2177.
33. Korner H, Riminton DS, Strickland DH, Lemckert FA, Pollard JD, Sedgwick JD. Critical points of TNF action in CNS autoimmune inflammation defined by gene targeting. J Exp Med 1997;186:1585.
34. Liu J, Marino MW, Wong G, et al. TNF is a potent anti-inflammatory cytokine in autoimmune mediated demyelination. Nat Med 1998;4:78.
35. D'Souza SD, Bonetti B, Balasingam V, et al. MS: Fas signaling in oligodendrocyte cell death. Exp Med 1996;184:2361.
36. Bonetti B, Raine CS. Multiple sclerosis: oligodendrocytes display cell death-related molecules in situ but do not undergo apoptosis. Ann Neurol 1997;42:74.
37. Dal Canto RA, Shaw MK, Nolan GP, Steinman L, Fathman CG. Local delivery of TNF by retrovirus-transduced T lymphocytes exacerbates experimental autoimmune encephalomyelitis. Clin Immunol 1999;90:10.
38. Lider O, Reshef T, Beraud E, et al. Anti-idiotypic network induced by T cell vaccination against experimental autoimmune encephalomyelitis. Science 1988;239:181.
39. Waisman A, Ruiz PJ, Hirschberg DL et al. Suppressive vaccination with DNA encoding a variable region gene of the T cell receptor prevents autoimmune encephalomyelitis and activates Th2 immunity. Nat Med 1996;2:899.
40. Vandenbark AA, Hashim GA, Offner H. Immunization with a synthetic T cell receptor V region peptide protects against experimental autoimmune encephalomyelitis. Nature 1989;341:541.
41. Howell MD, Winters ST, Olee T, et al. Vaccination against experimental allergic encephalomyelitis with T cell receptor peptides. Science 1989;246:668.
42. Saruham-Direskeneli G, Weber F, Meinl E, et al. Human T cell autoimmunity against MBP: CD4+ cells recognizing epitopes of the TCR beta chain from an MBP specific T cell clone. Eur J Immunol 1993;23:530.
43. Zhang J, Medaer R, Stinissen P, et al. MHC restricted clonotypic depletion of human myelin basic protein-reactive T cells by T cell vaccination. Science 1993;261:1451.
44. Medaer R, Stinissen P, Truyen L, et al. Depletion of myelin basic protein autoreactive T cells by T cell vaccination: Clinical trial in multiple sclerosis. Lancet 1995;346:807.
45. Vandenbark AA, Hashim G, Offner H. Immunization with a synthetic T cell receptor V-region peptide protects against experimental autoimmune encephalomyelitis. Nature 1989;341:541.
46. Kotzin B, Karuturi S, Chou YK, et al. Preferential TCR beta chain variable gene use in MBP-reactive T cell clones from patients with MS. Proc Natl Acad Sci USA 1991;88:9161.
47. Oksenberg JR, Panzara MA, Begovich AB, et al. Selection for T cell receptor Vβ-Dβ-Jβ gene rearrangements with specificity for a myelin basic protein peptide in brain lesions of multiple sclerosis. Nature 1993;362:68.
48. Chou YK, Morrison WJ, Weinberg AD, et al. Immunity to TCR peptides in multitude sclerosis. II. T-cell recognitia of Vβ5.2 and Vβ6.1 CDR2 peptides. J Immunol 1994;152:2520.
49. Vandenbark AA, Chou K, Whitham R, et al. Treatment of multiple sclerosis with T-cell receptor peptides: Results of a double-blind pilot trial. Nat Med 1996;10:1109.
50. Tang D, DeVit M, Johnston S. Genetic immunisation is a simple method to elicit an immune response. Nature 1993;356:152.
51. Lobell A, Weissert R, Storch MK, et al. Vaccination with DNA encoding an immunodominant myelin basic protein peptide targeted to Fc of immunoglobulin G suppresses experimental autoimmune encephalomyelitis. J Exp Med 1998;187:1543.
52. Ruiz P, Garren H, Ruiz I et al. Suppressive immunization with DNA encoding a self-peptide prevents autoimmune disease: modulation of T cell co-stimulation. J Immunol 1999;162:3336.
53. Windhagen A, Scholz C, Hollsberg P, et al. Modulation of cytokine patterns of human autoreactive T cell clones by a single amino acid substitution of their peptide ligand. Immunity 1995;2:373.
54. Karin N, Mitchell D, Ling N, Brocke S, Steinman L. Reversal of experimental autoimmune encephalomyelitis by a soluble variant of a myelin basic protein epitope: T cell receptor antagonism and reduction of interferon-γ and TNF-α production. J Exp Med 1994;180:2227.
55. Yu M, Johnson JM, Tuohy VK. A predictable sequential determinant spreading cascade invariably accompanies progression of EAE: A basis

for peptide-specific therapy after onset of clinical disease. J Exp Med 1996;183:1771.
56. Gaur A, Boehme SA, Chalmers D, et al. Amelioration of relapsing experimental autoimmune encephalomyelitis with altered myelin basic protein peptides involves different cellular mechanisms. J Neuroimmunol 1997;74:149.
57. Lehmann PV, Forsthuber T, Miller A, Sercarz EE. Spreading of T cell autoimmunity to cryptic determinants of an autoantigen. Nature 1992;358:155.
58. Steinman L, Conlon P. Viral damage and the breakdown of self-tolerance. Nat Med 1997;3:1085.
59. Acha-Orbea H, Mitchell DJ, Timmerman L, et al. Limited heterogeneity of T cell receptors from lymphocytes mediating autoimmune encephalomyelitis allows specific immune intervention. Cell 1988;54:263.
60. Urban JL, Kumar V, Kono DH, et al. Restricted use of T cell receptor V genes in murine autoimmune encephalomyelitis raises possibilities for antibody therapy. Cell 1988;54:577.
61. Steinman L. Assessment of the utility of animal models for multiple sclerosis and demyelinating disease in the design of rational therapy. Neuron 1999;24:511.
62. Karin N, Binah O, Grabie N, et al. Short peptide-based tolerogens without self-antigenic or pathogenic activity reverse autoimmune disease. J Immunol 1998;160:5188.
63. Vergelli M, Hemmer B, Utz U, et al. Differential activation of human autoreactive T cell clones by altered peptide ligands derived from myelin basic protein peptide (87–99). Eur J Immunol 1996;26:2624.
64. Tuohy VK, Yu M, Ling T, Kawczak JA, Kinkel RP. Spontaneous regression of primary autoreactivity during chronic progression of experimental autoimmune encephalomyelitis and multiple sclerosis. J Exp Med 1999;189:1033.
65. Steinman L. Absence of 'Original Antigenic Sin' in autoimmunity provides an unforseen platform for immune therapy. J Exp Med 1999;198(7):1021.
66. Kerlero de Rosbo N, Hofman M, Mandel I et al. Predominance of the autoimmune response to myelin oligodendrocyte glycoprotein (MOG) in multiple sclerosis: Reactivity to the extracellular domain of MOG is directed against three main regions. Eur J Immunol 1997;27:3059.
67. Zhang J, Markovic S, Lacet B, Raus J, Weiner HL, Hafler DA. Increased frequency of interleukin 2-responsive T cells specific for myelin basic protein and proteolipid protein in peripheral blood and cerebrospinal fluid of patients with multiple sclerosis. J Exp Med 1994;179:973.
68. Steinman L. Presenting an odd autoantigen. Nature 1995;375:739.
69. Baekkeskov S, Aanstoot HJ, Christgau S, et al. Identification of the 64K autoantigen in insulin dependent diabetes as the GABA-synthesizing enzyme glutamic acid decarboxylase. Nature 1990;347:151.
70. Atkinson MA, Bowman MA, Campbell L, Darrow BL, Kaufman DL, MacLaren NK. Cellular immunity to a determinant common to glutamic acid decarboxylase and Coxsackie virus in insulin dependent diabetes. J Clin Invest 1994;94:2125.
71. Castano L, Eisenbarth GS. Type-1 diabetes: A chronic autoimmune disease of human, mouse and rat. Ann Rev Immunol 1990;8:647.
72. Elias D, Reshef T, Birk O, van der Zee R, Walker MD, Cohen IR. Vaccination against autoimmune mouse diabetes with a T cell epitope of the human 65 kDa heat shock protein. Proc Natl Acad Sci USA 1991;88:3088.
73. de St Groth F, Webster R. Disquisitions on original antigenic sin. I. Evidence in man. J Exp Med 1966;124:331.
74. Klenerman P, Zinkernagel RM. Original antigenic sin impairs cytotoxic T lymphocyte responses to viruses bearing variant epitopes. Nature 1998;394:482.
75. McMichael A. The original sin of killer T cells. Nature 1998;394:421.
76. Nicholson LB, Murtaza A, Hafler BP, Sette A, Kuchroo VK. A T cell receptor antagonist peptide induces T cells that mediate bystander suppression and prevent autoimmune encephalomyelitis induced with multiple myelin antigens. Proc Natl Acad Sci USA 1998;94(17):9279.

Section 11 Diagnostic Immunology

Chapter 120

Assessment of Immunoglobulins and Antibodies

Russell Tomar and Henry A. Homburger

INTRODUCTION

One of the wonders of the immune system is its ability to form antibodies of essentially similar structure but with enormous diversity to react with 10^9 or more different antigenic sites. This diversity is based on a relatively small number of differentiating amino acids located primarily in the variable or hypervariable regions of the immunoglobulin molecule. The common as well as the variable components of immunoglobulins are more or less predetermined by one's genetic composition. More details about structural and functional genes are provided in Chapters 9 and 14.

Immunoglobulin diversity is necessary for antibody function but presents some unique problems for those needing to determine amount, type or activity. Most serum proteins are assessed indirectly by making antibodies to the desired substance. This antibody then becomes an intermediary to identify the serum protein. Finally, a 'marker' molecule, such as an immunofluorescent substance, an enzyme, a radioisotope etc., is attached to the identifying antibody. The specificity of the system depends largely on the uniformity of the antibody, and this depends very much on the uniformity of the original antigen. Immunoglobulins are diverse and not uniform, and so present challenges in the production of quality reagents.

The migration of immunoglobulins on electrophoresis is one piece of evidence for their diversity.[1,2] In the example of serum protein electrophoresis depicted in Figure 120.1, the stained protein bands representing albumin, α_1-, α_2- and β-globulins are easily demonstrated. Note that most of the protein bands, such as albumin, are sharply delineated, whereas the area representing the immunoglobulins, also known as the γ-globulins, is broad and diffuse. The apparent lack of resolution is due to the presence of many electrophoretically different immunoglobulins that migrate in the same general region. These small differences in the amino acid composition of immunoglobulins from healthy individuals provide the expected polyclonal display of γ-globulins. Subjects with 'normal' hypergammaglobulinemia and an M-protein are depicted in Figure 120.2. M-proteins are associated with malignancies and are discussed in detail in Chapter 99.

Each antibody-producing cell secretes an immunoglobulin that is more or less specific for that cell and its progeny. There are, however, a number of common regions in immunoglobulins that are sufficiently immunogenic to prepare antibodies to the different classes of immunoglobulins. This allows the laboratory to quantify immunoglobulins.

The common elements among immunoglobulins include their basic structure of two heavy and two light polypeptide chains. There are five different kinds of heavy chains, γ, α, μ, δ and ε, and two different kinds of light chains, κ and λ. Each set of heavy chains is chemically associated with a set of light chains, leading to the following possible formulae: γ2, κ2; γ2, λ2 (IgG); μ2, κ2; μ2, λ2 (IgM) and so forth. IgG, IgD and IgE antibodies are always found as monomeric units composed of two heavy and two light chains, whereas IgA and IgM are present in multmeric form.

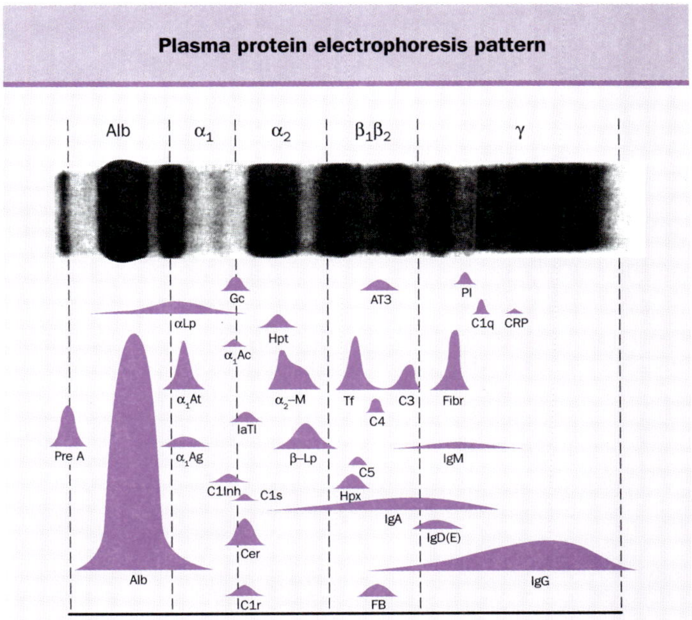

Figure 120.1 Plasma protein electrophoresis pattern in agarose gel is composed of five fractions, each composed of many individual species. Some of the major proteins are shown here in an artist's rendition for clarity. (Adapted from Laurell C B: Electrophoresis, specific protein assays, or both in measurement of plasma proteins? *Clin Chem* 1973;19:99.)

α_1Ac = α_1-antichymotrypsin
α_1Ag = α_1-acid glycoprotein
α_1At = α_1-antitrypsin
α_2-M = α_1-macroglobulin
α-LP = α-lipoprotein
Alb = Albumin
AT3 = Antithrombin III
β-Lp = β-lipoprotein
Complement components:
Clq, Clr, Cls, C3, C4,
C5 = As designated
Cllnh = Cl esterase inhibitor
Cer = Ceruloplasmin
CRP = C-reactive protein
Gc = Gc-globulin (vitamin D-binding protein)
FB = Factor B
Fibr = Fibrinogen
Hpt = Haptoglobin
Hpx = Hemopexin
Immunoglobulins:
IgA. IgD. IgE. IgG. IgM 6 = As designated
Pl = Plasminogen
Pre A = Prealbumin
Tf = Transferrin

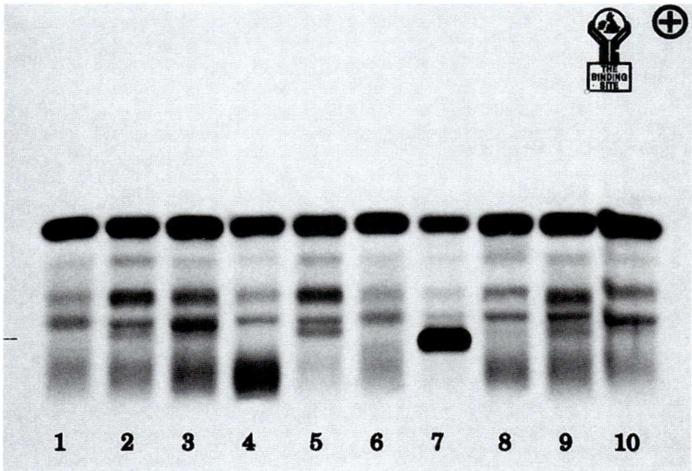

Figure 120.2 High-resolution protein electrophoresis of serum from 10 different subjects. The serum in lane 7 demonstrates an M-protein; the serum in lane 4 contains polyclonal hypergammaglobulinemia; the sample in lane 5 indicates probable hypogammaglobulinemia.

IgG is present in normal adult serum in concentrations of 800–1600 mg/dl. There are further amino acid differences that separate IgGs into four unique subclasses, distributed approximately as 66% IgG_1, 23% IgG_2, 7% IgG_3 and 4% IgG_4. IgA is present in serum at concentrations of about 40–220 mg/dl and is the principal immunoglobulin in secretory fluids. In secretions IgA exists as a dimer, which also contains a protein J chain and another peptide chain called the secretory component (SC). The latter is synthesized by mucosal epithelial cells and is joined to dimeric IgA during its movement through epithelial cells from the interstitial fluid to the luminal surface. Most IgM molecules are composed of five monomeric subunits linked by disulfide bonds and a J chain, to constitute a pentameric structure. Serum concentration of IgM ranges from about 120 to 400 mg/ml. IgD is a minor component in serum at about 3 mg/ml; in humans, and probably several other species, IgD is one of the principal immunoglobulins on the B-cell surface. IgE is the immunoglobulin present at the lowest concentration in serum, estimated at 17–450 ng/ml. IgE is the major immunoglobulin associated with immediate hypersensitivity reactions in humans. Immunoglobulin levels change with age, increasing during childhood as shown in Table 120.1. Levels may also vary by gender and race, although these differences are generally not clinically significant. The amino acids responsible for immunoglobulin classes or isotypes provide the structural backbone for the variable regions associated with antibody diversity. In addition, the common regions account for the different biological activities of the immunoglobulin classes and subclasses. It is the common regions, particularly those involved with class distinction, that allow for the immunoglobulin measurements in general clinical use. The changes often observed clinically in serum immunoglobulin levels include increased or decreased concentrations of one or more classes and excessive production of an M-protein. Determinations of the more variable function of antigen specificity are also in clinical use but require somewhat different methodological approaches. A more extensive discussion of immunoglobulins is presented by Ricardo and Tomar.[3]

Immunoglobulin levels			
	IgG	IgM	IgA
Cord blood	6.36–16.06	0.06–0.25	0.01–0.03
1 month	2.51–9.06	0.20–0.87	0.01–0.53
2 months	2.06–6.01	0.17–1.05	0.02–0.46
3 months	1.76–5.81	0.24–0.89	0.04–0.46
4 months	1.96–5.58	0.27–1.01	0.04–0.73
5 months	1.72–8.14	0.33–1.09	0.08–0.68
6 months	2.15–7.04	0.35–1.02	0.08–0.68
7–9 months	2.17–9.04	0.34–1.26	0.11–0.90
10–12 months	2.94–10.69	0.41–1.49	0.16–0.84
1 year	3.45–12.13	0.43–1.73	0.14–1.06
2 years	4.24–10.51	0.48–1.68	0.14–1.23
3 years	4.41–11.35	0.47–2.00	0.22–1.59
4–5 years	4.63–12.36	0.43–1.96	0.25–1.54
6–8 years	6.33–12.80	0.48–2.07	0.33–2.02
9–10 years	6.08–15.72	0.52–2.42	0.45–2.36
Adult	6.39–13.49	0.56–3.52	0.70–3.12

Reference ranges established by Beckman Laboratory using the Beckman nephelometer.

Table 120.1 Immunoglobulin levels (age-related reference ranges in g/l).

Laboratory testing for specific antibodies and autoantibodies is useful clinically to screen for disease, to establish specific diagnoses, and to monitor the clinical course of certain diseases. This is particularly true for diseases in which the antibody response is involved in pathogenesis, e.g. immediate hypersensitivity diseases, or where antibodies serve empirically as disease-specific markers or independent prognostic indicators.

METHODS FOR IMMUNOGLOBULIN DETERMINATION

Qualitative and semiquantitative methods

The following methods have two primary uses: to identify M-proteins and to rapidly estimate the quantity of γ-globulins. They provide only gross measures of the amounts of immunoglobulins and their classes. Study of body fluids other than serum generally require significant concentrating of the sample, in the range of 50–100-fold for urine.

Serum protein electrophoresis (SPEP)

Tiselius[4] described zonal electrophoresis in 1937. Because proteins display a net charge in an electrical field, under such conditions they will separate. Serum proteins are amphoteric and so their net charges are dependent on the pH of the buffer solution used. A protein in a buffer with a pH below the protein's iso-

CLINICAL PEARLS

Assessment of immunoglobulins

When to order a serum protein electrophoresis

- When there are signs and/or symptoms of diseases associated with M-proteins
- To follow the quantity of M-protein. Densitometry is usually more reliable than nephelometry to estimate the amount of M-protein.

When to order serum immunofixation

- To characterize the heavy and light chains of an M-protein, thereby confirming its presence
- To identify M-proteins that may be present in quantities below the ability of SPEP to detect. This should be reserved only for those instances where there is strong clinical indication of the presence of an M-protein

When to order quantitative immunoglobulins

- To evaluate possible immunoglobulin deficiency states, including those associated with an M-protein

electric point migrates towards the anode; conversely, in a buffer with a pH above its isoelectric point, it migrates towards the cathode. The size and shape of a protein molecule, the buffer's ionic strength, the frictional resistance of the supporting medium, the applied current, the temperature of the reaction and the duration of the charge all influence the quality and quantity of the separatory migration. Clinical laboratories most commonly use barbital buffers at pH 8.6, wherein γ-globulins have little charge and tend to be influenced by endosmosis as well as charge. In the past, paper and cellulose acetate were most commonly used as supporting media. The new standard is agarose, which offers less frictional resistance and clearer delineation of more discrete bands. Keren[5] summarizes methods to analyze monoclonal gammopathies as part of a multidisciplinary effort to develop clinical and laboratory guidelines.

Description of method

The sample – most commonly serum – is applied to a buffer-saturated support medium such as agarose, and placed on an electrophoretic apparatus that consists of buffer reservoirs and positive and negative electrodes. The application of electric current to the supporting medium separates the proteins according to their net charge at a standard pH 8.6. All major proteins except some immunoglobulin components migrate toward the anode. Following electrophoresis (usually based on a standardized time or by observation of a marker dye), the proteins are stained with a stain of choice, most commonly amido black or Coomassie blue. The strips containing the stained proteins are then visually reviewed and semiquantified with a densitometer.

Five zones are readily identified with cellulose acetate protein electrophoresis: (1) albumin; (2) α_1-globulin, consisting primarily of α_1-antitrypsin; (3) α_2-globulin containing haptoglobin and α_2-macroglobulin; (4) β-globulin, comprised of transferrin and complement components; and (5) the γ-globulins. As many as 12 discrete regions may be seen with high-resolution protein electrophoresis using agarose and controlled voltage and temperatures. These are shown in Figure 120.1, along with the serum proteins in each region. Other body fluids are commonly studied in the clinical laboratory, including urine for evidence of M-protein components, particularly light chains, and cerebrospinal fluid, particularly for oligoclonal immunoglobulins suggestive of certain disorders such as multiple sclerosis. The conditions under which these fluids are analyzed may differ from those used for serum, and attention should be paid to manufacturer instructions as well as literature citations.

Recommendations for use

Serum protein electrophoresis is used to look for the presence of monoclonal and/or polyclonal immunoglobulins. Hypogammaglobulinemia may be detected as well, but SPEP is not particularly sensitive and is not the preferred method unless other methods are not readily available. An M-protein should be further evaluated by other means and hypogammaglobulinemia should be confirmed by quantifying the major immunoglobulin classes. Densitometric analysis of stained proteins after SPEP is an excellent way of following therapy of diseases with M-proteins once the specific diagnosis has been established. This and other clinical points are described as part of clinical guidelines by Keren et al.[6]

Immunofixation electrophoresis (IFE)

Immunofixation (Fig. 120.3) has replaced immunoelectrophoresis (IEP) as the gold standard for establishing the presence of and characterizing an M-protein.[3] It is easier to perform, somewhat

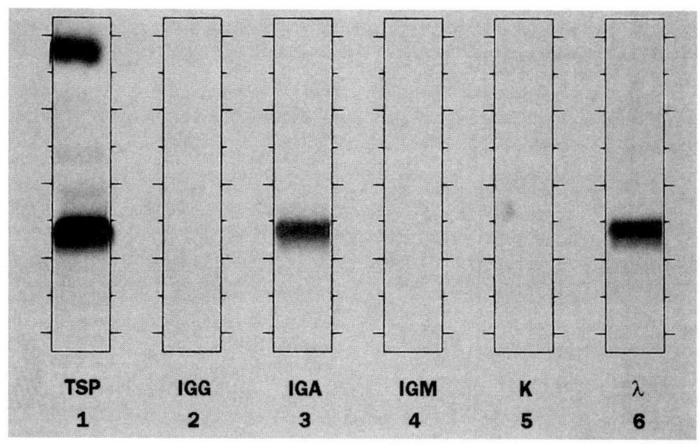

Figure 120.3 An immunofixation of serum from a patient with an IgA-λ M-protein. Lane 1 contains a serum protein electrophoresis. Lanes 2–6 represent serum samples from the same patient subjected to electrophoresis and then reacted with monospecific antisera to IgG, IgA, IgM, κ and λ.

KEY CONCEPTS

Qualitative/semiquantitative immunoglobulin testing

- Protein electrophoresis: evaluate for the presence of M-protein, monitor changes of M-protein
- Immunofixation electrophoresis (capillary electrophoresis, immunoelectrophoresis): characterize the heavy and light chains of M-protein, identify M-protein present in quantities below detection by protein electrophoresis

more sensitive, and easier to interpret than IEP. Alper and Johnson[7] described IFE in 1969, and it combines the resolution of zone electrophoresis with the specificity of an antigen–antibody precipitin reaction.

Description of method

The initial step in this procedure involves replicating lanes of high-resolution protein electrophoresis. After the proteins are separated, but before staining, the replicate electrophoretic strips are each incubated with a different specific antiserum, either in solution or with an antiserum-soaked membrane. Laboratories usually include antisera to IgG, IgA, IgM and κ and λ light chains, but leave one lane blank to look at an untreated (standard) SPEP. The quality of the antiserum is critical in that it must be specific for the intended target and of high titer. The protein band and its antiserum form a precipitate on the gel at the region of antibody–antigen equivalence, which is then washed to remove unreacted proteins. Following staining with amido black or Coomassie blue, the gel is reviewed manually. The location of the immunoprecipitate depends on the electrophoretic mobility of the specific protein.

Recommendation for use

Most laboratories use IFE after screening samples with SPEP and/or a quantitative immunoglobulin measurement. Although serum is the most common sample source, urine or cerebrospinal fluid may also be examined to search for and/or characterize M-proteins or their fragments. IFE has several advantages over IEP, including: (1) rapid turnaround time: IFE can be complete within 2 hours, whereas IEP requires overnight incubation; (2) increased sensitivity; (3) better resolution. This is particularly true of non-IgG M-proteins that might be lost in the 'umbrella' effect of IEPs; and (4) ease of interpretation compared to IEPs.

The disadvantages include the increased quality, quantity and hence cost of antisera required. Optimal resolution requires that the amounts of antisera be determined for each patient sample to avoid either excess dilution or excess antibody. In addition, because of the increased sensitivity of IFE, smaller bands are more frequently identified. These may be of uncertain clinical significance, leading to some difficulties in interpretation.

Capillary electrophoresis (CPE)

Capillary electrophoresis provides increased sensitivity, speed, and the potential for automation. Commercial instruments aimed at detecting M-proteins have entered the market and appear to be attractive to those laboratories with large sample numbers.

Description of method

Samples are aspirated from small wells into narrow-bore, negatively charged capillary tubes. An electrical current is applied and proteins migrate towards the cathode. The fractions are optically quantified at a wave length of 215 nm to produce a virtual electrophoretogram similar to those seen with traditional SPEP. There is no staining of the material and up to 40 samples per hour may be processed. CEP has been used to characterize M-proteins by a process called immunosubtraction. This requires the patient sample to be adsorbed with beads to which specific antisera, such as anti-IgM, anti-IgG, anti-IgA, anti-κ and anti-λ, are bound. After CEP of the adsorbed sample, an M-protein demonstrated before immunosubtraction would be expected to be absent when reacted with its class-specific antiserum.

Recommendation for use

CEP and immunosubtraction are relatively new and the advantages and disadvantages are not yet fully understood. Also, CEP is not yet accepted for urine or cerebrospinal fluid. Larger laboratories will be drawn to its automation capabilities, speed and potential cost savings. Clinicians may be drawn to its speed and potential improvement in sensitivity.[5]

Immunoelectrophoresis (IEP)

Grabar and Williams[8] described immunoelectrophoresis in 1953; this was later modified by Scheidegger.[9] IEP is a two-step procedure that combines the principles of zone electrophoresis with those of immunodiffusion and it is the older method used to identify M-proteins.

Description of method

The serum proteins are first separated by electrophoresis in a supporting medium such as agarose, commonly bound to a glass slide or plastic sheet. The separated proteins are reacted for up to 72 hours with specific antiserum placed in troughs running parallel to the electrophoretic migration. Antigen and antibody diffuse toward each other, forming elliptical precipitin arcs. The shape, position and size of each arc demonstrate the specific characteristics for each protein. Typically, γ-globulin from a healthy individual will form a balanced, evenly distributed smooth arc. Excess production of one type of immunoglobulin, i.e. an M-protein, leads to distortion by thickening or unbalancing the uniformity of the arc. The quality and quantity of antisera used are not as critical as in IFE.

Recommendations for use

Immunoelectrophoresis has been used extensively to study immunoglobulins in serum and other body fluids. Although largely supplanted by IFE, many laboratories throughout the world use IEP to search for and/or characterize M-proteins in the serum or urine. It is slower, somewhat less sensitive and more difficult to read than IFE. It may be less costly than IFE, particularly if the laboratory makes its own slides. The umbrella effect indicates that the most rapidly moving antigens in the greatest concentration, such as IgG and anti-IgG, may 'hide' other reactions, including M-proteins. Thus, IEP may be difficult to interpret and has less sensitivity for detecting M-proteins in smaller quantities, including IgA and at times IgM. Figure 120.4 illustrates the principle of IEP.

Quantitative methods

The immunoglobulin levels of a healthy population show significant variations due to age, gender, racial background, environmental factors and genetic makeup. Each locale must verify reference values by age, often by assessing a group of healthy individuals and comparing the results with data in the literature and/or supplied by the manufacturer.[10,11] Table 120.2 provides an example of some of these differences. Although there are international standards, variations in methods and techniques (as well as lack of interest in such standards) lead to great between site differences and imprecision.

Immunoglobulin levels outside of the reference range include low levels seen in hypogammaglobulinemia and increased levels associated with polyclonal hypergammaglobulinemia associated with chronic inflammation such as infections, autoimmune dis-

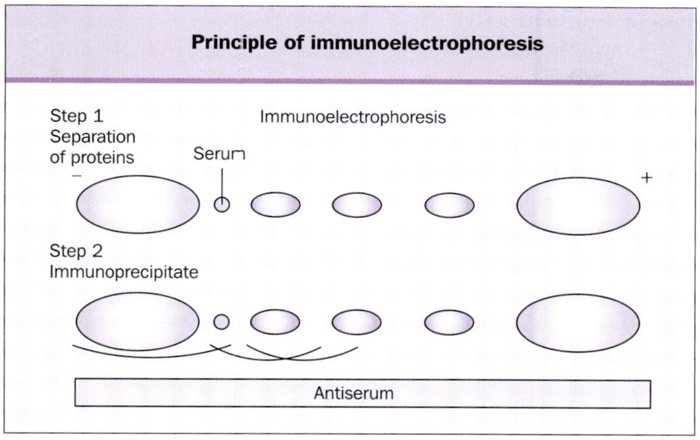

Figure 120.4 Principle of immunoelectrophoresis. In the first step, serum proteins are separated by electrophoresis. Antiserum is applied to the trough, and serum and antiserum diffuse into the agar. Precipitin arcs are formed for the individual serum proteins.

Serum IgG concentration in a biracial population

Sex	Age (years)	No. of samples tested	Whites Mean (±SE) (mg/ml)	No. of samples tested	Blacks Mean (±SE) (mg/ml)
	15–34	17	11.2 (7.3)	21	13.4 (6.5)
Men	35–54	17	10.8 (5.9)	19	13.5 (9.0)
	55–74	20	10.9 (7.4)	20	13.3 (5.8)
	15–34	19	10.6 (6.3)	18	15.6 (8.0)
Women	35–54	19	12.3 (3.4)	15	15.4 (6.4)
	55–74	20	10.9 (6.1)	16	14.2 (9.6)

Table 120.2 Serum IgG concentration in a biracial population. Adopted from Lichtman MA, Vaughan JH, Hames CG. The distribution of serum immunoglobulins, anti-gammaG globulins and antinuclear antibodies in White and Negro subjects in Evans County, Georgia. Arthritis Rheum 1967;10:204.

eases and chronic liver disease, or monoclonal hypergammaglobulinemia associated with multiple myeloma and Waldenström's macroglobulinemia. Immunoglobulins are commonly quantified to evaluate suspected immunoglobulin deficiency; monitor IgG replacement therapy; characterize monoclonal immunoglobulins in conjunction with other techniques (see above); and monitor the levels of the M-protein.

Radial immunodiffusion (RID)

RID is a precipitation method based on the principle that antigen and antibodies form precipitates in liquid or semifluid media. Under conditions of antibody excess, the quantity of the precipitate is directly related to the quantity of the antigen in the original mix. Ouchterlony[12] had demonstrated that precipitins would form in agar, and later agarose, in a manner that was related to the relative quantities of each. Mancini[13] and later Fahey and McKelvey[14] added antibody to the medium and then antigen to wells cut into the medium. The amount of precipitin, generally measured in distance migrated from the antigen well, is mathematically related to the quantity of antigen added to the well. Mancini allowed the reaction to go to completion, i.e. until all migration stopped. Fahey and McKelvey took measurements after designated intervals. Both related the diameter of the precipitin circles to simultaneously run controls. RID has been and is being used to measure many antigen–antibody combinations. Other precipitation methods used to look for specific antibodies will be discussed later.

Description of method

A predetermined dilution of specific antiserum is mixed with agar or agarose and allowed to gel, usually in a Petri dish or a glass slide. A series of small wells are cut in the agar to be filled with samples containing antigen. As the antigen diffuses into the agar it forms a precipitate with the antibodies contained in the gel. Once antigen–antibody equivalence is reached, an opaque precipitation ring develops around the antigen well, the diameter of which is proportional to the concentration of the antigen in solution placed in the well. The diameter may be measured either at the endpoint, when the antigen has completely reacted with the antibody (typically 48–72 hours), or after a fixed diffusion time, usually 24 hours. The concentration of the unknown sample is estimated by measuring the diameter of the ring produced by the sample and plotting this on a concentration–diameter curve established with standards containing known amounts of the antigen. The lower limit of this method's sensitivity is approximately 0.3–0.5 mg/dl. Within limitations, the ring diameter for a given antigen concentration can be increased by decreasing the antiserum concentration in the gel.

Recommendation for use

Radial immunodiffusion is used to measure the concentration of many proteins, including serum immunoglobulins and IgG subclasses. The method is simple to perform and requires very little equipment. Its major limitations include the duration of time required, the relative imprecision of the assay, with its coefficient of variation often greater than 10%, its relative insensitivity and inapplicability for materials in low concentrations, and its dependence on not only antigen quantity but also antigen shape. There are a few situations in which RID can lead to erroneous estimates of immunoglobulin concentrations. IgM is usually a large molecule with a sedimentation coefficient of 19S. However, in some instances IgM may be found in a monomeric, 7S form, including Waldenström's macroglobulinemia and ataxia–telangiectasia. As the RID standards are 19S, the more rapidly migrating 7S IgM will form a larger ring of precipitation and thus give an erroneous overestimate of serum IgM.

The opposite situation occurs when high concentrations of 7S (IgG) rheumatoid factor are present in the sample. Rheumatoid factor is usually a 19S IgM antibody directed against the Fc portion of IgG. At times, 7S IgG antibodies will be directed towards the Fc portion of other IgG molecules. In this case the IgG, instead of diffusing freely through the agar–antibody medium, interacts and forms complexes with the IgG antibody in the medium, thereby retarding migration, reducing the ring size and underestimating the concentration of serum IgG.

A third situation in which spurious results may arise occurs when testing for IgA levels in patients with IgA deficiency. These patients not uncommonly have antibodies against cow and goat protein. Because the antibody in the agar–antibody mixture is frequently produced in goats, the patient's serum may react with goat specific proteins in the antiserum to form a precipitin ring, giving a false positive response for IgA in an IgA-deficient subject.

KEY CONCEPTS

Quantitative immunoglobulin testing
- Assess immunoglobulin class or subclass levels, monitor changes in monoclonal immunoglobulin: radial immunodiffusion, nephelometry, electroimmunodiffusion
- Assess specific antibody levels: immunoassay

Nephelometry

Although radial immunodiffusion was previously the standard technique for immunoglobulin quantitation, it has now been replaced by automated nephelometry. This modification of the precipitin reaction depends on the light-scattering of immune complexes in solution. The amount of scattered light produced by soluble immune complexes is then measured in a photoelectric cell as optical density. As antigen concentration increases, the scattered light increases. In contrast to the standard precipitin reaction, which requires the concentrations of antigen and antibody to be at equivalence, nephelometry operates best with antibody excess.

Description of the method

A standard curve is developed by reacting increasing concentrations of the antigen of interest with a constant (and large) quantity of specific antiserum. Increasing amounts of immune complexes scatter more light, and so the intensity of scattered light is directly related to the antigen concentration. Antigen can be measured accurately in the antibody excess portion of the precipitin curve and, to maintain this relationship, increased antigen concentration requires additional dilutions of the sample.

End-point (or fixed-time) nephelometry represents a method in which the maximum scattered light is measured after the antigen–antibody reaction has reached equilibrium, or after a fixed reaction time. The antigen concentration in the unknown sample is calculated from a response curve produced with reference standards containing known amounts of the antigen tested under the same conditions.

Rate nephelometry is an alternative method in which the peak rate of immune complex formation is measured. As soluble immune complexes are formed during an antigen–antibody reaction, the quantity of scattered light over time may be plotted as a sigmoid curve. The upper inflection point in the curve represents the peak rate of immune complex formation and is directly proportional to the antigen concentration. The antigen concentration of an unknown sample is calculated by comparing the sample's peak rate of light scatter against an established reference curve. Rate nephelometry is the most commonly used automated method for protein determination in the United States. Available instruments provide an automated platform with barcoding and computer controls to provide rapid and reproducible results with relatively high throughout. The coefficients of variation for most systems used in clinical laboratories are within 5%.

Recommendations for use

Over 87% of laboratories that take proficiency testing programs from the College of American Pathologists use nephelometry to measure immunoglobulins. Less than 2% use RID. Some disadvantages of nephelometry include its increased start-up and running costs, although these may be more than compensated for by the savings in personnel. Other potential problems include antisera specificity, i.e. poor reactivity of the commercial antisera with unusual M-proteins; dilutional issues with M-proteins, leading to quantitative confusion; and temperature maintenance problems with cryoglobulins. In general, densitometric readout of SPEPs is a better way to follow the quantity of M-proteins during therapy and the course of the disease. Finally, other particles or discoloration in serum due to increased lipids or bilirubin may increase background light scatter and make interpretation difficult or impossible.

Electroimmunodiffusion (EID)

Laurell[15] developed electroimmunodiffusion (EID) to quantify specific proteins in solution. The technique differs from radial immunodiffusion in its use of an electric field to induce migration of the protein under study into the antibody-containing gel. Antigen–antibody complexes form a visible precipitate in the form of a cone or 'rocket'. The length of the cone is proportional to the amount of antigen in the sample.

Description of method

In this method the samples and standards are placed in wells cut in the antiserum-containing agar or agarose and the plate is electrophoresed until migration is complete. The antigen–antibody complex forms precipitin cones of a height proportional to the amount of antigen. A standard curve is constructed and the concentration of the unknown samples extrapolated from the curve. The sensitivity of the test is in the order of 0.1–0.5 mg/dl. Because of its costs and relative imprecision, this method has been replaced by nephelometry and ELISA.

Radioimmunoassay (RIA)

Yalow and Berson[16] developed the radioimmunoassay (RIA) to measure insulin in human plasma. The assay is based on binding the substance of interest by a radiolabeled specific antibody, or inhibition of binding by a radiolabeled antigen. RIA is uncommon in clinical laboratories today but its principles serve as benchmarks for most subsequent assays with similar sensitivity.

Description of method

Initially, most RIAs were competitive assays in which the concentration of the unknown antigen was incubated with known quantities of specific antibody and radiolabeled antigen. Simultaneously, a standard curve was developed with a fixed amount of the antibody and increasing quantities of radiolabeled antigen. The degree of inhibition by the unknown provided an indirect measure of its concentration. In current practice the antigen–antibody complexes are separated from the unbound radiolabeled antigen and 'bound' and 'free' and/or 'total' radioactivity determined. High concentrations of antigen in the test sample may nonspecifically interfere with the specific reaction.

A noncompetitive RIA binds specific antibody to a solid phase, usually a polystyrene tube or plate, to 'capture' the antigen of interest. The test serum is exposed to the antibody bound to the solid phase, allowing serum antigens to react with the specific antibody. The excess serum is washed away and a second radiolabeled antibody, directed against the antigen, is added. Excess (unbound) labeled antibody is washed away, and the level of radioactivity is directly related to the antigen concentration in the sample. Unknowns are compared to a standard curve generated with reference serum having known concentrations of antigen. Noncompetitive methods have largely replaced the more cumbersome competitive systems.

Recommendations for use

RIA demonstrates excellent sensitivity and precision and may be used to measure a variety of antigens, antibodies, drugs, hormones and related materials in human body fluids. Proteins present in serum in very low concentrations, such as IgE and IgG_4, can also be effectively measured by this technique. However, there are major disadvantages, including high cost, short reagent half-life, difficulty with disposal of radiolabeled reagents, and potential safety issues related to radionuclides.

Enzyme-linked immunosorbent assay (ELISA)

Engvall and Pearlman[17] decribed the enzyme-linked immunosorbent assay (ELISA), which is based on similar principles to radioimmunoassay, except that an enzyme replaces the radioactive label on the antibody or antigen. The 'readout' is dependent on the enzyme acting upon a chromogenic substrate. Competitive and noncompetitive assays can be set up using methods analogous to those for RIA.

Description of method

There are many variations of the ELISA methods.[18] In one common procedure that measures antibodies to a specific antigen, plastic microtiter wells are coated with the target antigen. This is followed by incubation with serum that putatively contains the antibody of interest. After washing, the plates are reacted with an enzyme-labeled antibody such as anti-IgG. Following washing, a selected substrate is added, the enzyme–substrate reaction is allowed to proceed, and the resultant color is spectrophotometrically determined. The intensity of the color is directly related to the concentration of the specific antibody and is determined by comparison with a standard curve. ELISA is a sensitive method that can measure proteins in nanogram quantities, eliminates the need for radioactive materials, and uses reagents that have a long shelf life.

Recommendations for use

The sensitivity of an ELISA is comparable to that of a radioimmunoassay. One potential disadvantage is the relatively large size of an enzyme label that theoretically could interfere with the antigen–antibody reaction. A second potential problem is the possible carcinogenicity of some of the substrates. None the less, clinical laboratories regularly use ELISAs to measure IgE and to look for and quantify specific antibodies, as discussed later in this chapter. The relative sensitivities of several different assays are listed in Table 120.3.

KEY CONCEPTS

Immunoassay

- Competitive inhibition: labeled antigen binding to specific antibody
- Noncompetitive: solid-phase bound reactants (antigen or antibody)
- Assay named based on detection system: radioimmunoassay (RIA), enzyme-linked immunosorbent assay (ELISA), fluorescence immunoassay (FIA)

Comparative sensitivity of assays

Method	Estimated sensitivity
Double immunodiffusion	>0.1 μg/ml
Immunofluorescence	<0.1 μg/ml
Enzyme-linked assays	1–10 ng/ml
Immunofixation	5–10 μg/ml of M-protein
Electroimmunodiffusion	1–5 μg/ml
Agglutination	0.02–1.0 μg
Hemagglutination	0.001 μg
Complement fixation	0.05 μg

Table 120.3 Comparative sensitivity of assays. In general, the more sensitive an assay the less specific it becomes. Many assays in clinical use were validated using older, less sensitive procedures. One should not assume the same specificity when the test is done using the newer, more sensitive procedure. Adapted from Nakamura RM, Tucker ES, Carlson IH. Immunoassays in the clinical laboratory. In: Henry JB (ed) *Clinical diagnosis and management by laboratory methods*, 18th edn. Philadelphia, WB Saunders, 1991

IMMUNOASSAYS FOR SPECIFIC ANTIGENS

A universal feature of immunoassay methods for specific antibodies is the use of antigens as reagents in the analytical systems. The nature of the reagent antigen defines the specificity of the antibodies that are detected and measured.[19,20] Reagent antigens can be crude preparations that contain the antigens of clinical interest, or highly purified or recombinant molecules.

Reagent antigens of clinical interest are often highly complex molecules, usually proteins or glycoproteins, bearing several different sites (epitopes) that react with antibodies in patients' specimens. The clinical applications of tests for specific antibodies often are directly related to the nature of the reagent antigens. Tests that employ crude or complex antigen preparations, e.g. whole cells or tissue substrates in the test for antinuclear antibodies, are useful primarily as screening tests, whereas tests that employ highly purified or recombinant antigens, e.g. tests for antibodies to some microbial antigens or extractable nuclear antigens, may detect antibodies that are disease-specific markers.[21]

The nature of the reagent antigen also influences the precision and accuracy of tests used to quantify the level or concentration of specific antibodies. Quantification performed using crude antigen as a reagent tends to be semiquantitative and imprecise, with the result expressed as a titer (i.e. the reciprocal of the dilution of test specimen used in the assay). In contrast, highly purified antigen may be used to prepare a pure preparation of specific antibodies by affinity chromatography, which enables calibration of the test system either in mass units (e.g. micrograms of antibody protein per milliliter) or in arbitrary quantitative units.[22]

The antigens of interest in clinical immunology belong to several different chemical classes, including proteins and glycoproteins, lipids, nucleic acids, carbohydrates and haptens.[23] The principal analytic methods discussed below are adaptable for use with proteins, glycoproteins and nucleic acid antigens.

Measurement methods for specific antibodies

Precipitation methods

Precipitation methods have been used in clinical immunology laboratories for decades to detect both antigens and specific antibodies. They are based on the antigen–antibody precipitin reaction originally described by Heidelberger and Kendall.[24] In this reaction, a multivalent antigen reacts with antibodies in a fluid or semisolid matrix such as an agar gel to form an insoluble lattice of antigen–antibody complexes. The presence of a precipitin indicates the presence of specific antibodies to one or more of the antigens in the sample. Precipitation occurs over a range of concentrations of antigens and antibodies called the equivalence point (Fig. 120.5). If the concentration of either reactant is too great, precipitation does not occur and only soluble complexes are formed.

A modification of the basic immunoprecipitation technique, called **double immunodiffusion**, is most commonly used to detect specific antibodies.[12] In this adaptation, an aqueous solution of reagent antigen is placed in the center well of an agar slide and positive control sera and specimens to be tested for the presence of specific antibodies are pipetted into wells that surround the center well. After 24–48 hours of incubation, which permits diffusion of the antigen and antibodies throughout the gel, precipitin lines form that can be detected visually. The antibody specificity in the test specimen is evaluated by examining the pattern of convergence between the unknown precipitin and the control having an antibody of known specificity. The possible reactions include identity (fusion), partial identity (one spur) and nonidentity (two spurs) (Fig. 120.6).

The double-immunodiffusion method is simple to perform and requires no special equipment. However, the technique is qualitative and only sensitive to concentrations of antibodies greater than approximately 0.1 μg/ml. The relative lack of sensitivity of this method limits its application in the laboratory to situations in which patients' sera contain relatively high concentrations of specific antibodies.[25] The results of double-immunodiffusion tests are also subject to errors of interpretation. False negative results may occur if the concentration of antigen is not carefully adjusted to produce a zone of equivalence with the concentration of antibodies usually encountered in patients' specimens. In addition, multiple precipitin lines of unknown specificity may be seen with clinical specimens, and these precipitins can obscure the identification of specific antibodies of clinical interest. The double-immunodiffusion method cannot be used to detect antibodies to haptens and monovalent antigens, which fail to form an insoluble lattice with specific antibodies.[13]

Counterimmunoelectrophoresis (CIEP) is a modification of the basic immunoprecipitation technique that uses electrophoresis to enhance the rate of migration of antigen and antibodies in a gel matrix.[26] By adjusting the pH of the electrophoresis buffer solution, antigen and specific antibodies are made to migrate in opposite directions toward the center of the slide, where immunoprecipitation can occur (Fig. 120.7). CIEP is a somewhat more sensitive technique than conventional double immunodiffusion, but it is technically demanding and has limited application in the clinical laboratory for detecting most specific antibodies.

Precipitin reaction

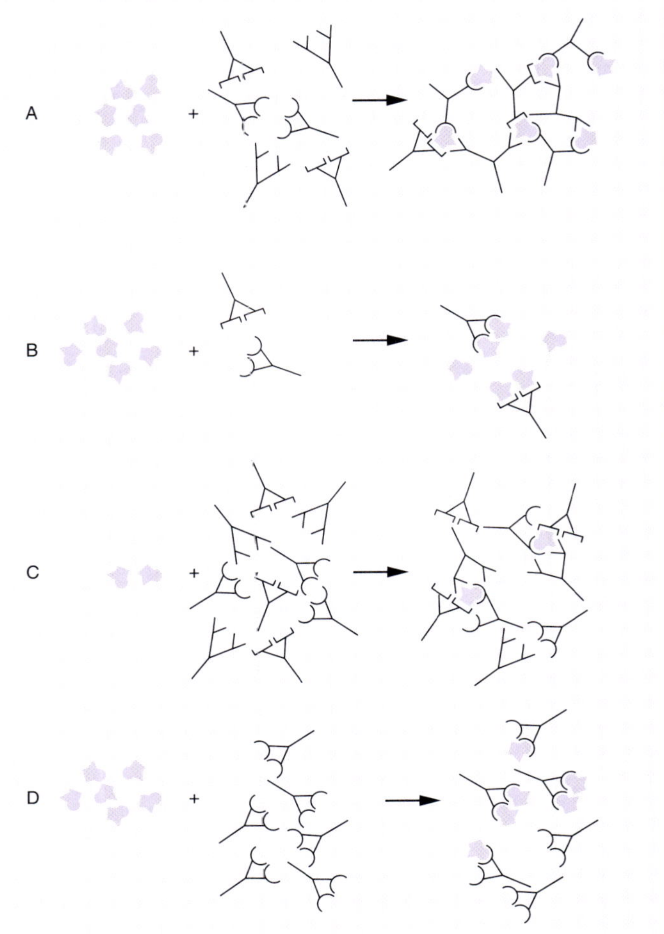

Figure 120.5 Precipitin reaction. Antigen molecules are represented as having three different antigenic sites (epitopes) on their surface. Three different types of antibodies are illustrated, each having binding regions for one of the three types of antigenic sites. (**A**) Near the equivalence point, lattice formation occurs and a precipitate forms. (**B**) In the presence of excess antigen the concentration of antibody is insufficient for cross-linking. Lattice formation does not occur and complexes are soluble. (**C**) In the presence of excess antibody lattice formation does not occur and complexes are soluble. (**D**) In the presence of a monoclonal antibody each antigen molecule is bound at a single site. No cross-linking can occur and complexes remain soluble.

KEY CONCEPTS

Specific antibody testing

Semiquantitative: double immunodiffusion, counterimmunoelectrophoresis, agglutination, indirect immunofluorescence, immunoblot

Quantitative: immunoassay

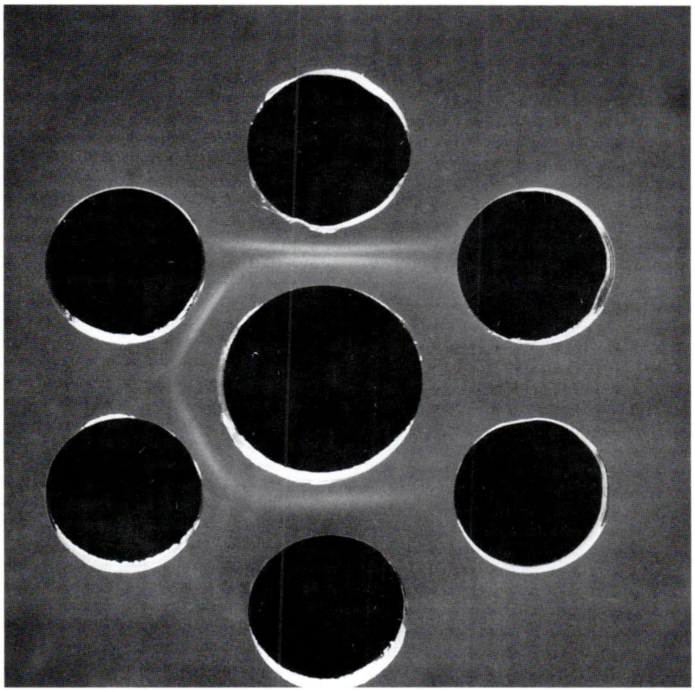

Figure 120.6 Double immunodiffusion for autoantibodies to extractable nuclear antigens U_1RNP and Sm. The center well was loaded with U_1RNP/Sm antigen. Outside wells were loaded with control sera or patients' sera as follows (counterclockwise from top well): anti-U_1RNP and anti-Sm control, patient 1 in duplicate; anti-U_1RNP control, patient 2 in duplicate. Precipitin formed with serum from patient 1 shows line of identity (fusion of precipitins) with anti-U_1RNP control sera.

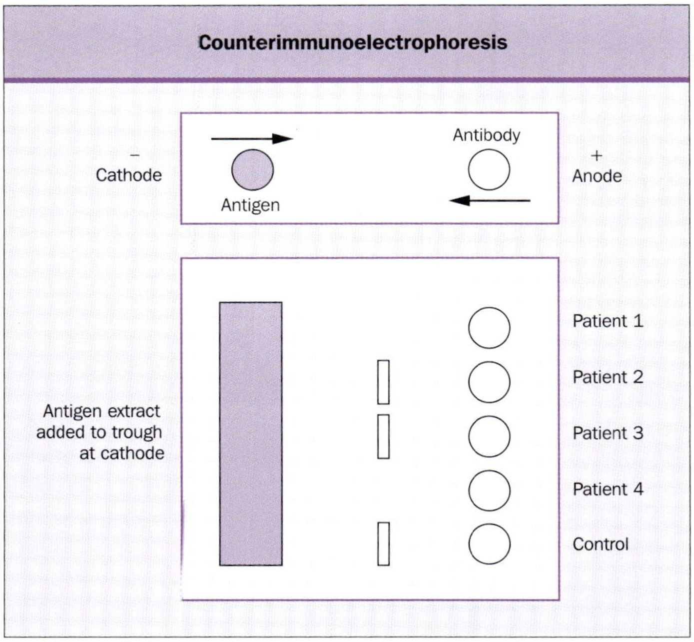

Figure 120.7 Counterimmunoelectrophoresis. Antigen and antibody migrate toward the center of an agar slide. Precipitins that form in the same position as the control indicate the presence of antibodies of the same specificity.

Agglutination

Agglutination is the aggregation or clumping of visible but discrete particles in an antigen–antibody reaction to form a larger mass. The fundamental immunologic principle of agglutination reactions is the same as previously described for precipitin reactions. Initially, antigen–antibody recognition occurs, followed by binding, and then by visible aggregation of antigen particles. On occasion agglutination is incomplete because the necessary antibody bridging of adjacent antigen particles fails to occur.

Agglutination assays for specific antibodies can be performed using insoluble native antigens such as bacterial cells, antigen-coated particles such as latex beads, or red blood cells to which antigens have been attached by chemical coupling. Agglutination assays require a stable particle on which antigen is accessible for binding, and a reaction solution of proper ionic strength and viscosity to prevent incomplete agglutination.[27] Most of the commercially available agglutination tests that are designed to detect antibodies specify the use of serum (not plasma) or cerebrospinal fluid.[28] The sensitivity and specificity of these tests are determined by the purity of the antigens coupled to insoluble particles.

In general, the advantages of agglutination methods are their ease of performance; speed of performance, usually requiring less than 10 minutes; high degree of analytic sensitivity (comparable to immunometric methods, discussed later); and the enormous variety of antibodies that can be detected. In addition, with the exception of cold agglutinins, the tests are usually not affected by temperature. One of the major disadvantages of agglutination methods is that the reactions are only semiquantitative. For example, although qualitative test results are highly reproducible, for most test systems the quantitative results are only accurate to a fourfold difference in antibody titer.[27] The other important disadvantage of agglutination methods is the occurrence of the prozone phenomenon, in which agglutination is inhibited by extreme antibody excess as a result of poor lattice formation and steric hindrance.[29]

Agglutination techniques are used routinely in the diagnosis of infectious diseases, in transfusion medicine for typing of blood cells, and in commercial assays for the detection of autoantibodies in patients with autoimmune diseases. Numerous agglutination-based diagnostic tests are available because of the ease with which the test reagents can be developed. For example, some red blood cells, bacteria and fungi can be agglutinated directly by serum antibodies. Indirect agglutination tests are also available in which a vast repertoire of soluble antigens can be passively adsorbed or chemically coupled to red blood cells or inert particles (e.g. latex beads).[29]

Direct agglutination

Direct agglutination, as the name implies, is the aggregation of particles brought about by the interaction of specific antibodies with particulate antigens. To agglutinate an antigen all that is required is a reaction solution of the proper ionic strength and an antibody with two or more receptors that cross-link adjacent antigen particles (Fig. 120.8). IgM antibodies are more efficient than IgG antibodies in agglutination reactions. IgM antibodies usually aggregate particulate antigens based on the size of the antibody molecule, whereas IgG antibodies may require the addition of substances such as bovine serum albumin or dextran to alter the viscosity and charge of the reaction solution before agglutination can occur.[27,29] In some direct agglutination tests, red blood cells or bacteria are treated with enzymes such as papain or

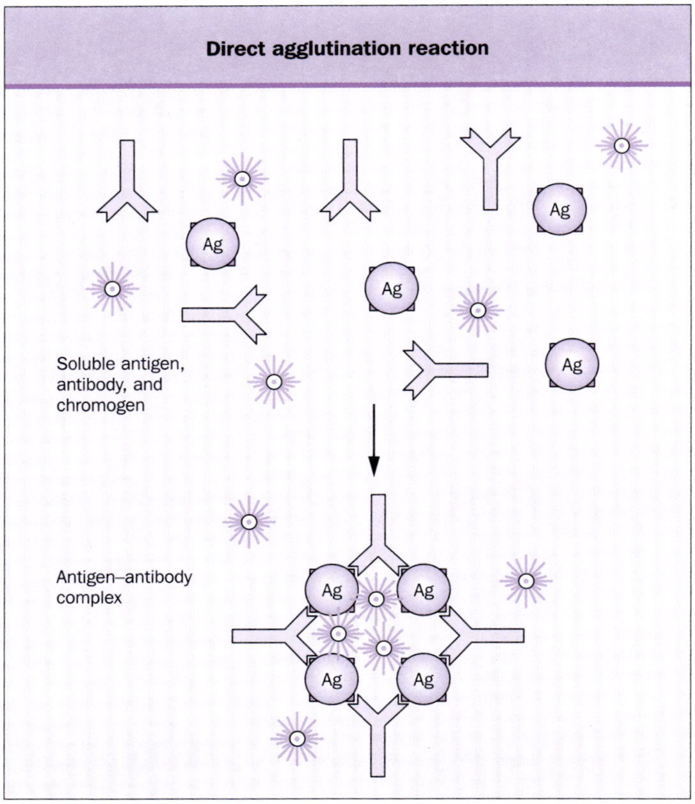

Figure 120.8 Direct agglutination reaction. Particulate antigen reacts with specific antibodies to form an insoluble matte. Chromogen particles are trapped in the matte, indicating that the reaction has taken place.

DNase to increase the exposure of surface antigens, remove blocking structures, or in some way alter the configuration of external membrane components to enhance the agglutination reaction.[27] In the direct agglutination tests, if the techniques are highly standardized then the only reagents necessary are positive and negative controls for qualitative tests, a serum that can be diluted for quantitative tests, some measurement of antigen concentration (such as a McFarland standard for opacity), and a control for nonspecific agglutination.

The most common use of the direct agglutination test procedure is in blood banking, in particular for ABO typing of eythrocytes.[30] Direct agglutination tests are also widely used for serotyping of bacteria, e.g. *Campylobacter* and other enteric pathogens involved in outbreaks of foodborne human gastroenteritis, and in the diagnosis of brucellosis and leptospirosis.[28]

Indirect agglutination

By far the most widely used of the agglutination methods are the indirect assays.[31] A number of baterial antigens, viruses, endo- and exotoxins and ovalbumin adsorb directly on to red cells, but for most applications agents such as tannic acid, bisdiazobenzidine and glutaraldehyde are used to couple antigens to red blood cells.[29] In addition to red blood cells, bentonite, a form of siliceous earth, and latex are used as carriers for protein or polysaccharide antigens. Latex is the most commonly used carrier and is an aggregate of polystyrene molecules held together by van der Waal's attractive forces. The functional groups on the latex spheres originate from the compound used as the initiator of polymerization. Thus some proteins bind directly to these functional groups, whereas others are covalently coupled using carbiodimides or other suitable reagents.[32]

Latex agglutination (LA) tests are commonly used in the diagnosis of bacterial, fungal, rickettsial and parasitic diseases, but are infrequently used in the diagnosis of viral diseases. Currently, LA tests are available only for specific antibodies to rubella, HIV, group C rotaviruses, and for Epstein–Barr virus screening.[33,34] LA methods are also used to detect autoantibodies to purified nuclear antigens and rheumatoid factor.

Indirect hemagglutination (IHA) uses antigens coupled to erythrocytes to test for the presence of specific antibodies. IHA tests have been developed for detecting specific antibodies to parasites, including protozoan, trematode, cestode and nematode species.[35] IHA is also used in the confirmation of syphilis, in the diagnosis of herpes simplex virus infection, and as a test for penicilloyl antibodies of the IgM and IgG isotypes in patients with immune-mediated drug reactions.[36]

A third form of agglutination test is the **antibody-mediated incomplete agglutination** reaction. The direct antiglobulin test used in the diagnosis of autoimmune and drug-induced immune hemolytic anemia and to determine antibody directed to Rh antigens on erythrocytes is a form of the original Coombs' test. In this technique, antiglobulin antibodies produced in a heterologous species are added to detect subagglutinating or nonagglutinating amounts of antierythrocyte antibodies.[29] The direct Coombs' test detects specific antibodies or other serum proteins that bind to a patient's erythrocytes. The indirect Coombs' test is a two-stage reaction in which first the patient's serum is incubated with commercially available red blood cells, and then the antiglobulin serum is added.[29] Still another variation on the Coombs' test uses enzyme-treated erythrocytes to increase assay sensitivity.[37]

Finally, **flocculation**, a term used mainly in syphilis serology, describes the reaction of a microscopically visible particle (antigen) with an invisible substance (antibody) to form aggregates that can either be seen microscopically, as in the Venereal Disease Research Laboratory (VDRL) slide test, or visualized by the addition of a particle such as charcoal, which becomes entrapped in the antigen–antibody lattice, as in the rapid plasma reagin (RPR) card test for syphilis. In these tests the antigen–antibody reaction particles stay suspended, rather than settling in a clump or forming a matte pattern.

Indirect immunofluorescence

Indirect immunofluorescence (IF) is the technique most commonly used in clinical laboratories to screen for specific antibodies that react with cellular antigens. IF is more sensitive than double immunodiffusion and faster to perform. The increased sensitivity of IF enables the detection of human antibodies in concentrations less than 0.1 μg/ml.[38,39] The technique is semiquantitative, with results expressed in titers, and is readily adaptable to the detection and measurement of many clinically important specific antibodies.[21]

IF tests are performed by incubating patients' diluted sera with thin sections of animal or human tissues or cultured cells that have been fixed chemically to allow intracellular penetration of specific antibodies. After the incubation, unbound antibodies and serum proteins are washed off the slide and a second-stage antibody, e.g. fluorochrome-conjugated antihuman immunoglobulin, is added to the substrate tissue. This reagent antibody binds to any specific antibodies that have been captured by antigens in the substrate. Depending upon the specific test application, a fluorochrome-labeled antihuman immunoglobulin reagent can be chosen that reacts with any or all of the prevalent isotypes of human immunoglobulin, including IgG, IgM and IgA. Bound antihuman immunoglobulin antibody is visualized using a fluorescent microscope. Incident light at a wavelength optimal to excite the fluorochrome is directed at the substrate slide, and light emitted by the fluorochrome is isolated by appropriate filters and transmitted to the microscope objective, where it can be visualized. The presence of specific antibodies is indicated by fluorescence of the tissue or cells on the substrate slide.

The accurate performance of IF testing for specific antibodies requires careful attention to quality control of the test specimen, substrate slides, and fluorochrome-conjugated antihuman immunoglobulin antiserum.[40] Sera from fasting patients are optimal for testing, as lipemic or hemolyzed sera may produce increased background fluorescence. In addition, each test set-up must include known negative and positive control sera. Long-term quality control requires comparison testing of successive lots of substrate slides with known negative and positive control sera to ensure that there is minimal nonspecific binding of human immunoglobulins in the negative sera and comparable binding of specific antibodies, defined by similar end-point titers (plus or minus one dilution) for the positive control sera. Successive lots of antihuman immunoglobulin antisera are also compared to ensure reproducibility of the analytical system. These reagents are characterized in terms of their antibody to total protein content, fluorochrome to protein ratio (typically in the range of 3 molecules of fluorochrome per molecule of protein), and the dilution of reagent antiserum that yields maximal specific to nonspecific fluorescence, as demonstrated with well-characterized positive and negative control sera.[41,42] In most IF assays it is also desirable periodically to test a weakly reactive (positive) control serum to ensure that there has been no loss of analytic sensitivity from storage of the substrate slides or fluorochrome-conjugated antiserum.

The IF technique is widely used to screen for autoantibodies, antibodies associated with immune-mediated inflammatory diseases, and antibodies to some bacteria and spirochetes in infectious diseases.

Immunoblotting (Western blots)

Immunoblotting, also called Western blotting, is a method used to identify specific antigens in complex mixtures and is a modification of the various EIA techniques. The proteins are initially separated by molecular weight using sodium dodecylsulfate polyacrylamide gel electrophoresis (SDS-PAGE). The separated proteins are transferred (blotted) and immobilized on to a semipermeable solid medium, such as nitrocellulose. Antibody to one or more of the separated proteins is incubated with the immobilized proteins. This method can also be applied to the study of antibodies, as is the detection of antibodies to HIV polypeptides.

Description of method

Immunoblotting consists of several steps: (1) electrophoretic separation of proteins by molecular weight on SDS-PAGE; (2) transfer of the separated proteins from the polyacrylamide gel to a nitrocellulose or similar support; (3) identification of the specific antigens by reacting the immobilized antigens with antibody putatively against the antigens of interest. The antibody may be directly labeled with enzyme or radioisotope, or unlabeled when an enzyme or radionuclide-labeled second antibody directed against the first is used. The reactive proteins appear as dark bands on a whitish or gray background. Molecular weight standards are run to permit the estimation of molecular weights of the separated proteins. The number and intensity of the bands depends on the concentration and number of antigens in the test material. The sensitivity of the test is partly related to the specific antibody titer, as well as to the amplification system in use. Picogram quantities of polypeptide can be detected.

Western blotting is the gold standard for confirming the presence of antibody to HIV. In this procedure, HIV antigens are separated by SDS-PAGE, the polypeptides immunobilized on a solid medium, and patient serum, thought to have antibodies to HIV, incubated with the membrane. A second antibody, labeled with enzyme, is added, followed by substrate. Positive and negative controls are also run simultaneously. Most laboratories have adopted the guidelines recommended by the Association of State and Territorial Public Health Laboratory Directors and the Centers for Disease Control and Prevention.[43,44] This approach involves reporting the results as positive, indeterminate or negative. A positive test result is defined by the presence of any two of the following bands: p24, gp41 or gp 120/160. An indeterminate result is the presence of no more than one of these three bands, with or without other nondiagnostic bands. A negative result is the absence of bands or the absence of any of the three diagnostic bands. Figure 120.9 demonstrates a serum positive for antibodies to HIV-1 by Western blot.

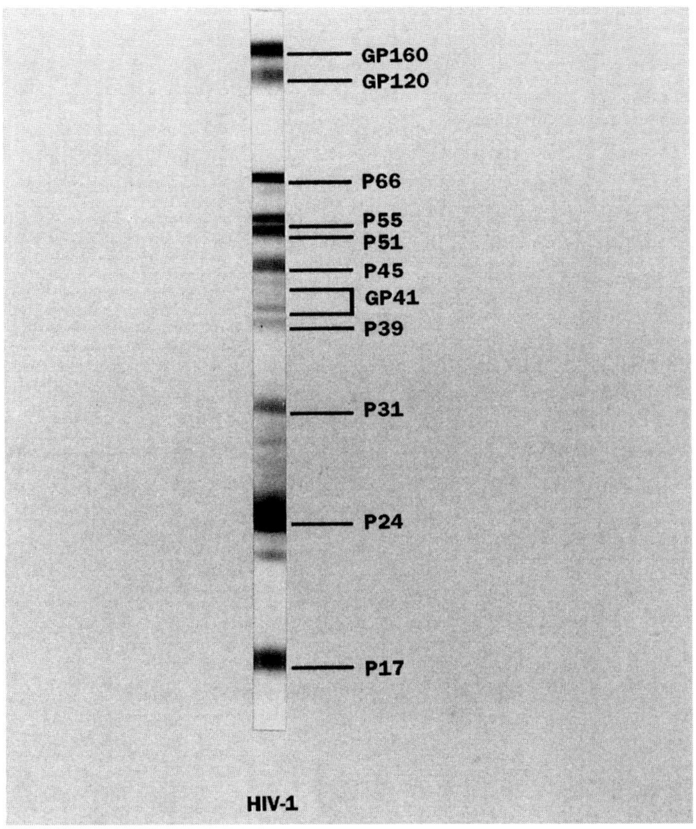

Figure 120.9 Western blot analysis for antibodies to HIV proteins. A positive test is defined by the presence of any two of the following bands: P24 (core protein), GP41 and GP120/160 (envelope proteins).

Immunometric methods

Immunometric methods are EIA variants that are widely used and versatile analytical systems for the detection and measurement of specific antibodies. These methods, also called sandwich immunoassays, make use of a solid-phase conjugate of reagent antigen (the immunosorbent) to capture specific antibodies from patients' specimens. Specific antibodies bound to the immunosorbent in the first stage of the assay are detected in the second stage by incubating with a polyclonal or monoclonal antihuman immunoglobulin antibody that has been labeled with an enzyme, radionuclide or luminescent molecule.[45] In the final stage of the assay, the amount of labeled second-stage antibody that has been bound to the immunosorbent is determined by measuring a colored or fluorescent product generated by the enzyme label (Fig. 120.10) or by counting radioactivity.

Immunometric methods offer several advantages that account for their popularity. A variety of methods have been developed to couple antigens covalently or noncovalently to the solid-phase immunosorbent, and each of the principal chemical classes of antigen mentioned previously, including some haptens, has been adapted to immunometric methods.[45,46] Antigen immunosorbents can be prepared from crude antigen mixtures for use in screening tests, or from highly purified antigens for use in the measurement of marker antibodies or quantitative assays. Immunometric methods are very sensitive compared to precipitin or agglutination techniques. Analytical sensitivity is in the range of 1–10 ng of antibody protein per milliliter, which is adequate for the measurement of specific antibodies of all human isotypes and subclasses, including IgE and IgG. subclasses. The increased analytical sensitivity of immunometric assays is largely a result of amplification of the signal produced by the binding of labeled second-stage anti-immunoglobulin antibody. As noted above, the second-stage antibody is typically labeled with an enzyme or radionuclide. Commonly used enzyme labels such as alkaline phosphatase generate many moles of measurable product for each mole of second-stage antibody bound to the immunosorbent, and radionuclides emit measurable radiation that can be counted to a predetermined end-point of total counts. The analytic sensitivity of immunometric methods is limited primarily by the ratio of specific to nonspecific binding of immunoglobulin in the first stage of the assay.[45] Immunosorbents with low levels of nonspecific binding afford maximum analytical sensitivity.

The most common immunometric assay for specific antibodies is the enzyme immunoassay (EIA). In this an antigen is adsorbed noncovalently to the wells of a polystyrene microtiter plate. Different types of plastic plates have been developed to maximize the adsorption of different chemical classes of antigen, including proteins and glycoproteins, phospholipids and nucleic acids, as well as to minimize nonspecific binding of immunoglobulins. EIA may be used to detect specific antibodies qualitatively or to make semiquantitative measurements of specific antibodies by use of a standard curve calibrated in units. For qualitative applications, the absorbance in wells incubated with diluted patients' serum is compared to a negative (nonimmune) control serum pool. Positive results are indicated by absorbances significantly greater than the negative control pool, typically at least twice the negative control (background) level. For more quantitative applications, the absorbance in wells that contain diluted patients' serum is compared to a standard curve (Fig. 120.11). In either application, positive and negative control sera must be run with each plate to ensure that all steps in the procedure have been performed properly. There are also limitations on the accuracy and precision of semiquantitative tests performed by EIA. EIA methods are inherently quite variable, and successive tests on the same serum often yield results that vary by as much as 15–20%.[45,46] In addition, the standard curve of absorbance versus antibody level is usually nonlinear (Fig. 120.11). Consequently, even though results are often reported on a continuous scale in units, it is best to regard them as semiquantitative. Results are often interpreted as falling within ranges, e.g. negative, borderline, weakly positive and strongly positive, with each category defined by a range of values expressed in units.

As noted above, the EIA method is performed in microtiter plates in which the antigen is adsorbed noncovalently to the plastic plate. In other applications of the basic immunometric method, antigen is coupled covalently to a solid phase, such as a paper disk or a suspension of particles, to prepare the immunosorbent. This is particularly common with allergen immunosorbents used to test

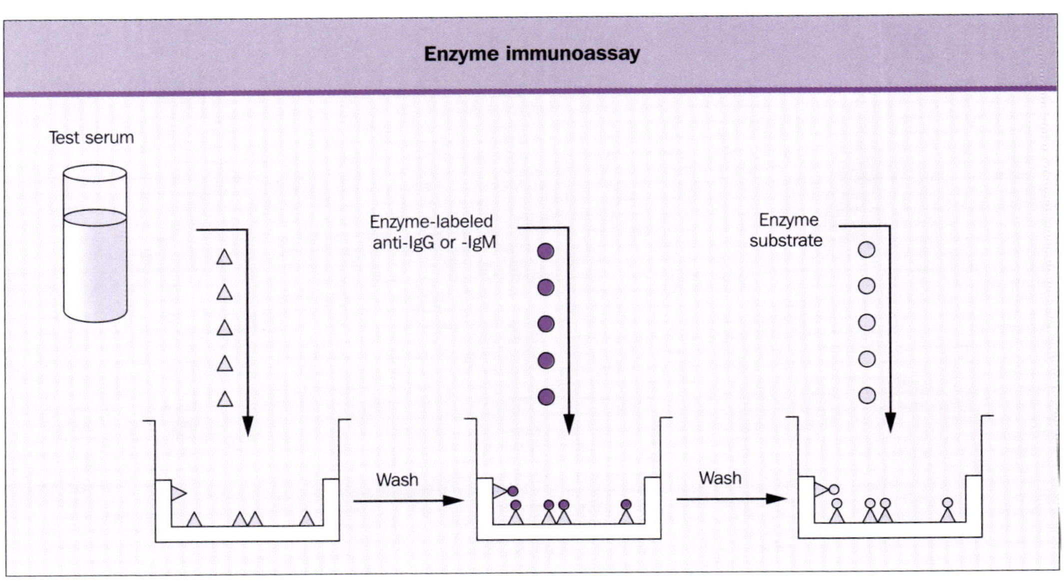

Figure 120.10 Enzyme immunoassay. See text for explanation.

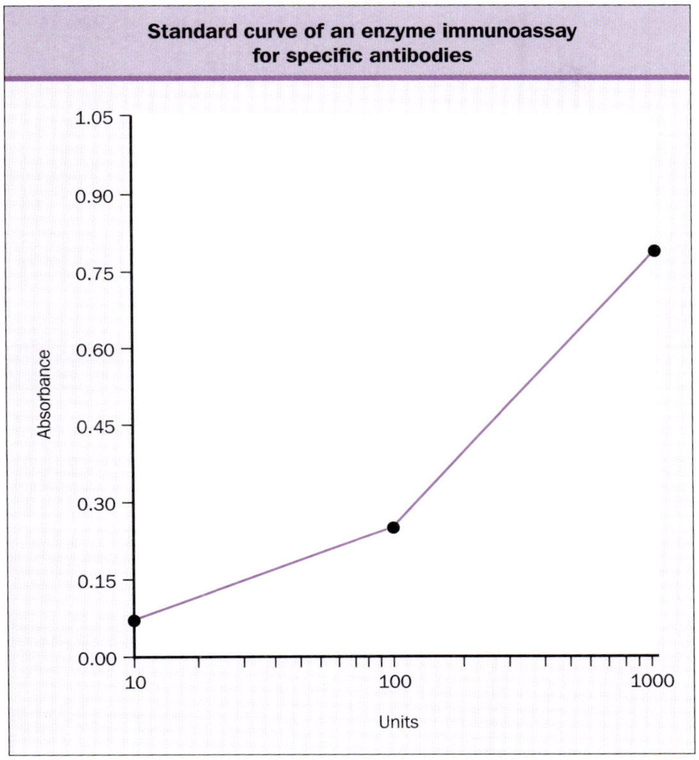

Figure 120.11 Standard curve of an enzyme immunoassay for specific antibodies. The standard curve is calibrated in arbitrary units and is nonlinear. Results <10 are negative, 10–99, weakly positive, and ≥ 100 strongly positive.

for specific IgE antibodies. The principal advantages of covalent coupling are that the antigen immunosorbents are stable indefinitely, and successive lots of immunosorbent can be characterized in terms of the amount of antigen coupled per gram of solid phase and the capacity to bind antibodies from well-characterized positive control pools.[47] Regardless of the method used to prepare the immunosorbent, however, the same limitations regarding accuracy and precision of testing noted earlier apply.

ASSESSMENT OF LABORATORY PERFORMANCE

Because of the wide variety of analytic methods available to perform laboratory tests for specific antibodies, clinicians need a resource with which to judge the performance (sensitivity and specificity) of the methods that they have access to in their own practices. Much information can be found from the results of federally mandated laboratory proficiency testing programs. The US Clinical Laboratory Improvement Amendment of 1988 established a single set of federal standards that applies to laboratories that test human specimens, and periodic proficiency testing is part of this program of standards.[48] Data from large interlaboratory proficiency testing programs often include results from hundreds of different laboratories. These data are useful to indicate the level of performance for each laboratory compared to the entire group of peer laboratories that use the same analytic methods.

REFERENCES

1. Laurell CB. Electrophoresis, specific protein assays, or both in measurement of plasma proteins? Clin Chem 1973;19:99.
2. McPherson RA. Specific proteins. In: Henry JB (ed) Clinical diagnosis and management by laboratory methods, 18th edn. Philadelphia, WB Saunders, 1991.
3. Ricardo MJ, Tomar RH. Humoral immunity: antibodies and immunoglobulins. In: Henry JB (ed) Clinical diagnosis and management by laboratory methods, 18th edn. Philadelphia, WB Saunders, 1991.
4. Tiselius A. A new apparatus for electrophoretic analysis of colloid mixtures. Trans Faraday Soc 1937;33:534.
5. Keren DF. Procedures for the evaluation of monoclonal immunoglobulins. Arch Pathol Lab Med 1999;123:126.
6. Keren DF, Alexanian R, Goeken JA, Gorevic PD, Kyle RA, Tomar RH. Guidelines for clinical and laboratory evaluation of patients with monoclonal gammopathies. Arch Pathol Lab Med 1999;123:106.
7. Alper CA, Johnson AM. Immmunofixation electrophoresis: a technique for study of protein polymorphism. Vox Sang 1969;17:445.
8. Grabar, P, Williams CA. Méthode permettant l'étude conjuguce des propriétés électrophoriques et immunochimiques d'un mélange de protéines, application au sérum sanguin. Biochim Biophys Acta 1953;10:1934.
9. Scheidegger JJ. Une microméthode de l'immunoélectrophorèse. Int Arch Allergy 1955;7:102.
10. Lichtman MA, Vaughan JH, Hames CG. The distribution of serum immunoglobulins, anti-gammaG globulins and antinuclear antibodies in White and Negro subjects in Evans County, Georgia. Arthritis Rheum 1967;10:204.
11. Bawa N, Tomar RH. Laboratory evaluation of immunoglobulin function and humoral immunity. In: Henry JB (ed) Clinical diagnosis and management by laboratory methods, 19th edn. Philadelphia, WB Saunders, 1996.
12. Ouchterlony O, Nilsson LA. Immunodiffusion and immunoelectrophoresis. In: Wier DN (ed) Handbook of experimental immunology, Vol 32, St Louis, Blackwell, 1986.
13. Mancini G, Carbonara AO, Heremans JF. Immunochemical quantitation of antigens by single radial immunodiffusion. Immunochemistry 1965;2:235.
14. Fahey JL, McKelvey EM. Quantitative determination of serum immunoglobulins in antibody agar plates. J Immunol 1965;94:84.
15. Laurell CB. Quantitative estimation of proteins by electrophoresis in agarose gel containing antibodies. Ann Biochem 1966;15:45.
16. Yalow RS, Berson BA. Immunoglobulin specificity of human insulin: application to immunoassay on insulin. J Clin Invest 1961;40:2190.
17. Engvall E, Perlman P. Enzyme-linked immunoabsorbent assay (ELISA): quantitative assay of immunoglobulin G. Immunochemistry 1971;8:871.
18. Nakamura RM, Tucker ES, Carlson IH. Immunoassays in the clinical laboratory. In: Henry JB (ed) Clinical diagnosis and management by laboratory methods, 18th edn. Philadelphia, WB Saunders, 1991.
19. Benjamin DC, Berzofsky JA, East IJ, et al. The antigenic structure of proteins: a reprisal. Annu Rev Immunol 1984;2:67.
20. Sela M. Antigenicity: some molecular aspects. Science 1969;166:1365.
21. Tan EM. Antinuclear antibodies: diagnostic markers for autoimmune diseases and probes for cell biology. Adv Immunol 1989;44:93.
22. Van Norstrand MD, Malinchoc M, Lindor KD, et al. Quantitative measurement of autoantibodies to recombinant mitochondrial antigens in patients with primary biliary cirrhosis: relationship of levels of autoantibodies to disease progression. Hepatology 1997;25(1):6.
23. Goodman JW. Antigen determinants and antibody combining sites. In: Sela M (ed) The antigens, Vol 3. New York, Academic Press, 1975.

24. Heidelberger M, Kendall FE. A quantitative study of the precipitin reaction between type III pneumococcus polysaccharide and purified homologous antibody. J Exp Med 1929;50:809.
25. Wilson MR, Saunders RD. Immunodiffusion assays for antibodies to small nuclear ribonucleoproteins and other cellular antigens. In: Rose NR, deMacario EC, Fahey JL, et al. (eds) Manual of clinical laboratory immunology, 4th edn. Washington DC, American Society for Microbiology, 1992.
26. Feldkamp CS, Carey JL. Standardization of immunoassay methodologies. In: Rose NR, de Marcario EC, Folds JD, et al. (eds) Manual of clinical laboratory immunology, 5th edn. Washington DC, ASM Press, 1997, p 1168.
27. Kasahara Y. Agglutination immunoassays. In: Rose NR, de Marcario EC, Folds JD, et al. (eds) Manual of clinical laboratory immunology, 5th edn. Washington DC, ASM Press, 1997, p 7.
28. Tinghitella TJ. Antibody detection for the diagnosis of infectious disease. In: Tilton RC, Balows A, Hohnadel DC, et al. (eds) Clinical laboratory medicine. St Louis, Mosby-Year Book, 1992.
29. Stites DP. Clinical laboratory methods for detection of antigens and antibodies. In: Sites DP, Stobo JD, Fundenberg HH, et al. (eds) Basic and clinical immunology, 5th edn. Los Altos CA, Lange Medical, 1984.
30. Johnson CL. Blood group antigens and antibodies. In: Tilton RC, Balows A, Hohnadel DC, et al. (eds) Clinical laboratory medicine, St Louis, Mosby-Yearbook, 1992.
31. Pope V, Larsen SA, Schriefer M. Immunologic methods for diagnosis of spirochetal diseases. In: Rose NR, de Marcario EC, Folds JD, et al. (eds) Manual of clinical laboratory immunology, 5th edn. Washington DC, ASM Press, 1997, p 510.
32. Hirayama C, Ihara H, Shibata M, et al. Polypeptide artificial carrier particles for use in passive agglutination imunoassay. Polymer J 1991;23:161.
33. Kuzuya M, Fujii R, Hamano M, et al. Rapid detection of human group C rotaviruses by reverse passive hemagglutination and latex agglutination tests using monoclonal antibodies. J Clin Microbiol 1993;31:1308.
34. Farhat SE, Finn S, Chua R, et al. Rapid detection of infectious mononucleosis-associated heterophile antibodies by a novel immunochromatographic assay and a latex agglutination test. J Clin Microbiol 1993;31:1597.
35. Wilson M, Schantz PM, Tsang VCW. Clinical immunoparasitology. In: Rose NR, de Marcario EC, Folds JD, et al. (eds) Manual of clinical laboratory immunology, 5th edn. Washington DC, ASM Press, 1997, p 575.
36. Adkinson NF Jr. Tests for immunological reactions to drugs and occupational allergens. In: Rose NR, de Marcario EC, Folds JD, et al. (eds) Manual of clinical laboratory immunology, 5th edn. Washington DC, ASM Press, 1997, p 893.
37. Petz LD. Autoimmune hemolytic anemias. In: Rose NR, de Marcario EC, Folds JD, et al. (eds) Manual of clinical laboratory immunology, 5th edn. Washington DC, ASM Press, 1997, p 1018.
38. Nakamura RM, Tan EM. Recent advances in laboratory tests and the significance of autoantibodies to nuclear antigens in systemic-rheumatic diseases. Clin Lab Med 1986;6:41.
39. Molden DP, Nakamura RM, Tan EM. Standardization of the immunofluorescence test for autoantibody to nuclear antigens (ANA): use of reference sera of defined antibody specificity. Am J Clin Pathol 1984;82:57.
40. Quality assurance for the indirect immunofluorescence test for autoantibodies to nuclear antigen (IF-ANA): approved guideline. NCCLS I/LA2-A, Vol 16(11), December 1996.
41. Tan EM, Fritzler MJ, McDougal JS, et al. Reference sera for antinuclear antibodies. Antibodies to native DNA, Sm, nuclear RNP, and SS-B/La. Arthritis Rheum 1982;25:1271.
42. McDougal JS, Kennedy S, McDuffie FC. Standards and quality assurance for immunologic tests. Standards and reference materials for autoantibodies to nuclear antigens. In: Rippey JH, Nakamura RM (eds) Diagnostic immunology: technology assessment and quality assurance. Skokie IL, College of American Pathologists, 1983.
43. Centers for Disease Control Update. Serologic testing for antibody to human immunodeficiency virus. MMWR 1988;36:833.
44. Centers for Disease Control. Interpretation and use of the Western blot assay for serodiagnosis of human immunodeficiency virus type 1 infections. MMWR 1989;38(Suppl 7):1.
45. Carpenter AB. Enzyme-linked immunoassays. In: Rose NR, de Marcario EC, Folds JD, et al. (eds) Manual of clinical laboratory immunology, 5th edn. Washington DC, ASM Press, 1997, p 20.
46. Gosling JP. A decade of development of immunoassay methodology. Clin Chem 1990;36:1408.
47. Wide L, Bennich H, Johansson SGO. Diagnosis of allergy by an in vitro test for allergen antibodies. Lancet 1967;2:1105.
48. Federal Register 1992;57(40) Washington DC, United States Government Printing Office, pp 7139, 7245.

Chapter 121

Flow Cytometry

Thomas A. Fleisher, Jack J.H. Bleesing and Gerald Marti

INTRODUCTION

Flow cytometry provides a platform for rapid, multiparameter analysis of single cells in suspension. This is commonly applied for the identification of human lymphocyte subsets, a method referred to as immunophenotyping that has seen increasing applications over the past 15 years as a result of at least four developments. First, insights into the differentiation and function of human lymphocytes have opened new avenues for clinical investigation. Second, the number of monoclonal antibodies specific for lymphocyte surface antigens has expanded, providing a wide array of immunophenotyping reagents. Third, instrument operation and data analysis have become less complex and developments in fluorochrome chemistry have facilitated multicolor analysis. Finally, the need for absolute CD4 T-cell counts as part of disease assessment and follow-up for patients infected with the human immunodeficiency virus (HIV) introduced a definitive clinical need for this technology. In addition to the applications in HIV infection, immunophenotyping has become a routine approach for the evaluation of lymphoproliferative disorders and has been applied in the study of immunodeficiency disorders and immune-mediated diseases.

Flow cytometry can also be used for the evaluation of intracellular parameters, including the identification of changes linked to cellular activation or programmed cell death and the detection of specific intracellular proteins. This technique also can be applied to evaluate cell cycle status (i.e. G_0-G_1, S, G_2-M) based on DNA staining, a technique that is commonly performed to characterize certain tumors. Finally, a new flow-based method using tetramer technology has great promise in the characterization of antigen-specific T cells associated with normal immune responses following immunization and in association with disease states.

This chapter focuses on the underlying concepts of flow cytometry, including basic instrument mechanics and principles of data management. Immunophenotyping-related issues, including optimal lymphocyte gating and directed use of test reagents, are also reviewed. In addition, a brief overview of intracellular probes, cell cycle analysis, tetramer technology and nonlymphocyte-directed applications is given. These discussions are aimed at identifying the utility as well as the limitations of flow cytometry.

INSTRUMENTATION

The basic components of a flow cytometer are shown in Figure 121.1: they include the illumination source, optical bench, fluidic system, electronics and computer.[1–3] Illumination in a standard, single-beam clinical instrument is generated by a monochromatic light source using an air-cooled argon ion laser (488 nm wavelength). The point where the light illuminates the cell (particle) is referred to as the interrogation (analysis) point. In clinical instruments this intersection typically occurs within a quartz flow cell, whereas in cell sorters the beam intersects the cells flowing as a jet stream in air. The optical bench contains lenses that focus the illumination beam into a specific shape, with defined size at the interrogation point to ensure a consistent area of illumination. Light (both nonfluorescent and fluorescent signals) generated from each illuminated cell is collected and measured. These light signals are optically coupled with a detection system consisting of sets of filters linked to photodetectors. The filters are designed and strategically located to separate the desired light signals and direct them to each individual photodetector. Filters for the nonfluorescent signals correspond to the emission signal wavelength (e.g. blue), whereas those for the fluorescence channels are chosen to correspond with the emission signals of specific fluorochromes (e.g. green, orange or red; see Fluorochrome section). The photodetectors consist of photomultiplier tubes for the fluorescence and side (90°) scatter signals and a photodiode for the forward (low-angle) scatter signal. The light signals produced from each cell are converted into digital

Simplified design of a flow cytometer

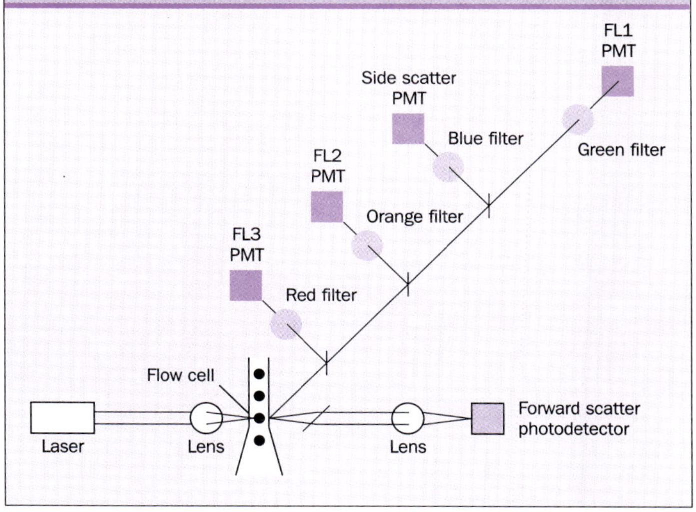

Figure 121.1 Simplified design of a flow cytometer with one illumination source (laser) set up to collect five parameters. These include the two nonfluorescent parameters (blue light) forward and side scatter, as well as three fluorescent parameters, green (FITC), orange (PE) and red (PerCP) light.

signals that can be interpreted using either linear or log amplification. Highly sensitive solid-state detectors are likely to replace photomultiplier tubes to provide more linear amplification.

The fluidic system consists of sheath fluid that moves the sample stream and thus provides the flow in a flow cytometer. Cells (particles) in suspension are injected into the moving sheath fluid, establishing a hydrodynamically focused single-file flow of cells through the interrogation point. This process maintains the cell stream in a constant, central location within the column of sheath fluid by controlling the sample delivery rate and the sheath fluid velocity.[4] Because the location and shape of the incident light beam is fixed, this process of centrally fixing the cell stream ensures that all cells are illuminated by the same area of the light beam, exposing each to the same excitation energy and reducing signal variation. Thus, the difference in magnitude of the emission signal generated by each cell reflects differences between the cells, and is not confounded by cell movement within the excitation beam. The use of hydrodynamic focusing has the additional advantage of producing little or no change in cell shape, although it may have an effect on cell orientation. The lack of alteration in cell shape provides a mechanism for distinguishing 'architectural' differences between specific leukocyte types (see Gating section).[5,6]

The choice and arrangement of the filters allows for the simultaneous evaluation of multiple colors (parameters) on each cell even if one color is substantially brighter than the others. Thus, a flow cytometer provides a platform to assess multiple parameters as discrete pieces of information on many cells in short periods of time, typically collecting data on 1000–2000 cells per second.

The internal electronics in the flow cytometer provide the system for converting analog light signals (photoelectrons) received at the photodetectors into digital signals for acquisition and storage in a computer. The intensity of these converted signals is measured on a relative scale that is generally set in either 256 or 1024 equal increments (referred to as channels). A specialized analysis program is used and typically the results generated are depicted graphically as a single-parameter histogram displaying specific light (fluorescence) intensity (x-axis) versus cell number (y-axis) (Fig. 121.2). Two-color (parameter) studies can be evaluated with a pair of histograms (one for each color) or with a single plot displaying both parameters. The latter include dot, contour or isometric plots that simultaneously display both parameters versus cell frequency (Fig. 121.3).

The correlated multiparameter data for each cell are frequently stored in the computer using a format known as list mode storage, which enables the retrieval of all collected data. Specialized computer software enables data analysis, which in immunophenotyping studies is typically based on the presence or absence of specific antibody binding. Cell cycle analysis evaluates fluorescence intensity as a measure of cellular DNA content, based on the intercalation or binding of a DNA-specific dye. Most programs enable the operator to evaluate the number of events, percentage of events, mean and/or median channel fluorescence, and selected statistical measures for each identified cell population/subpopulation. The mean or median channel fluorescence is a measure of fluorescence intensity and can be used to determine the number of antigen molecules per cell.[7]

The evaluation of clinical flow data in immunophenotyping usually involves setting criteria for distinguishing lymphocyte subpopulations. Establishing the boundaries of the negative or nonstained cells is one approach. This is a very common technique used in clinical laboratories that provides relatively con-

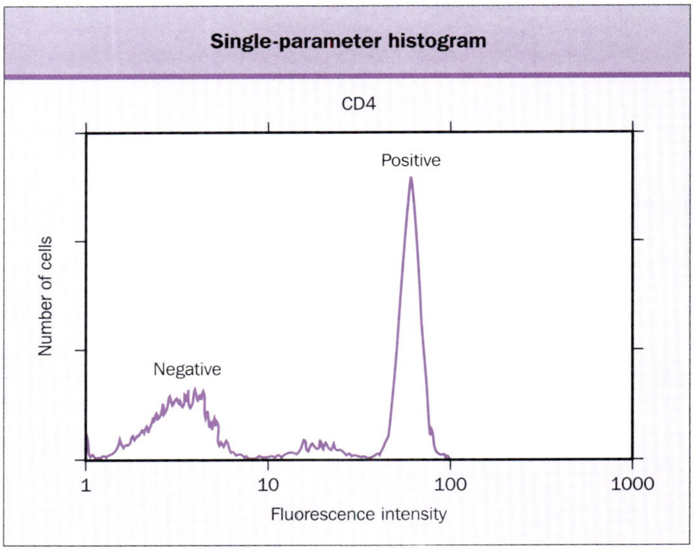

Figure 121.2 Single-parameter histogram demonstrating the negative cell subpopulation (autofluorescence and nonspecific antibody binding) and a positive cell subpopulation. Integrating the area under each curve would provide the numbers and percentage of cells present in each respective subpopulation. The very small subpopulation defined between the negative and positive peaks represents low-density CD4 expression found on the few monocytes contained within the lymphocyte gate.

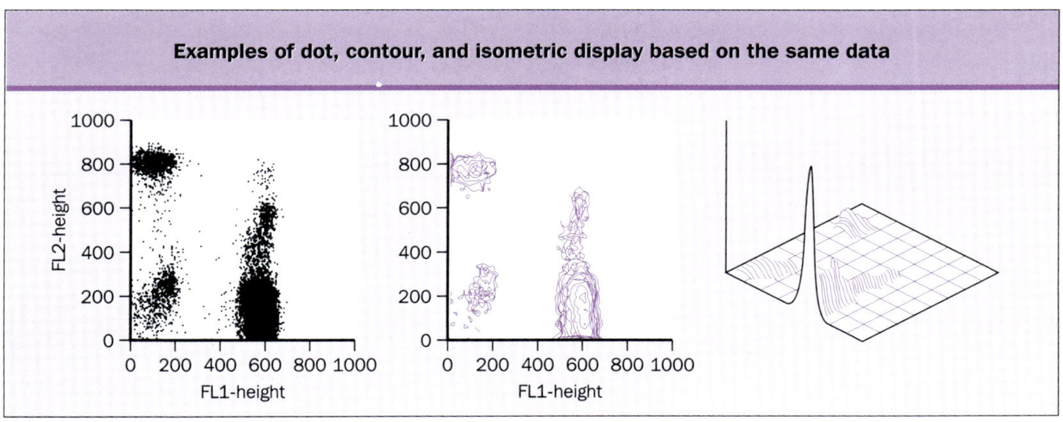

Figure 121.3 Examples of dot, contour and isometric displays based on the same two-color data. All three techniques enable simultaneous evaluation of both parameters.

sistent criteria for negative versus positive discrimination. When dealing with DNA staining, a consistent cellular source of DNA (e.g. chicken erythrocytes) is used as an internal reference for evaluating DNA content and evaluating the cell cycle distribution.

FLUORESCENCE REAGENTS

The standard indicator system in flow cytometry is based on one or more fluorochromes, dyes that absorb and emit light of defined wavelengths.[8,9] The energy lost during the return of excited electrons to their ground state yields emitted light with a longer wavelength (lower energy) than the excitation wavelength. Fluorochromes are usually directly conjugated (linked) to monoclonal antibodies, enabling direct staining. Alternatively, indirect staining can be done using an unlabeled primary monoclonal antibody followed by washing and the addition of a fluorochrome-conjugated antibody reactive with the first antibody (e.g. goat antimurine immunoglobulin). The direct method is technically easier and more readily adaptable to multicolor studies, but the indirect method may be more sensitive. Currently there are a number of fluorochromes available for use and at least three specific fluorochromes are commonly used for immunophenotyping with a single argon-laser (488 nm – blue) excitation beam. These are fluorescein isothiocyanate (FITC), phycoerythrin (PE) and peridin chlorophyll protein (PerCP), which emit green, orange and red light, respectively. In addition, an alternative third color (red) has been developed based on energy transfer using one fluorochrome (e.g. PE) to provide the excitation energy for a second fluorochrome (e.g. a cyanine dye such as Cy5) that is the source of emitted light. Most clinical instruments collect five parameters from each cell, the three fluorescence signals (green, orange, red) and the two nonfluorescence signals (forward and side scatter). Four-color studies can be accomplished with a combination of tandem conjugated reagents, and instruments with additional light sources are available for six- (or more) color analysis. The instrument-linked computer can acquire any combination of parameters on a large number of cells – typically 10 000 or more – for display and analysis. The number of events (cells) analyzed varies and must be increased when evaluating very small subpopulations of cells, in order to acquire statistically relevant data.

Studies of intracellular parameters require specific fluorescent probes that can be loaded into the cells. Intracellular protein evaluation requires cell fixation and permeabilization in order to allow monoclonal reagents access to the cell interior. Activation-induced changes involve probes that include calcium-sensitive dyes (e.g. fluo-3), glutathione-sensitive dyes (e.g. monochlorbimane) and H_2O_2-responsive dyes (e.g. dihydrorhodamine 123).[10,11] Assessment of DNA content can be performed with dyes that intercalate double-stranded DNA and RNA including propidium iodide and ethidium bromide.[12,13] In addition there are ultraviolet-excited DNA dyes that are highly specific for DNA, including Hoechst 33258 and 4,6-diamidino-2-phenylindole (DAPI); acridine orange is used for simultaneous staining of DNA/RNA.

IMMUNOPHENOTYPING

Gating

The proper assessment of a cell mixture often requires initial identification of lineage-specific cells, an approach referred to as gating. In practical terms, gating for immunophenotyping maximizes lymphocyte and minimizes nonlymphocyte inclusion in the evaluation. This is a particularly important process in analyzing whole blood samples, as lymphocytes normally represent a minority leukocyte population in adult peripheral blood. Directing the study to lymphocytes enables the generation of accurate statistics regarding subpopulations as well as eliminating any contributions from contaminating cells. The latter issue is particularly problematic when multiple lineages express the same surface antigens (e.g. CD4 is found on lymphocytes and monocytes). In addition, nonspecific binding of monoclonal reagents through the Fcγ receptor, as well as the presence of cytophilic human immunoglobulin on monocytes, can also affect the results. Gating techniques can also be used to confine the evaluation to other cell types, such as monocytes or granulocytes.

Traditional gating involves the use of the two standard nonfluorescent parameters, forward angle (low angle) and side (90°) light scatter (Fig. 121.4A).[5,6] Forward scatter is a reflection of cellular cross-sectional area (with a relationship to cell size) and refractile index, whereas side scatter is an indication of the cellular granularity and surface irregularity. The combination of these two nonfluorescent parameters provides a convenient means of distinguishing between a mixture of lymphocytes, monocytes and granulocytes (in the absence of red blood cells and platelets). With the light scatter-based distinction, lymphocytes have the lowest forward and side scatter, monocytes have higher forward and side scatter, and granulocytes have very high side scatter (Fig. 121.4A). This method is effective in distinguishing a relatively pure population of lymphocytes under most circumstances. However, the presence of nucleated red cells, large platelets or other particulate debris can produce contaminating events (cells) within the 'lymphocyte gate'. Furthermore, malignant lymphoid cells may not fit into the previously outlined standard light scatter patterns.

A method to confirm the integrity of the scatter-based lymphocyte gate has been devised using two directly conjugated monoclonal reagents, CD45 and CD14.[14] These 'gating reagents' provide a three-part differential. Lymphocytes have the highest level of CD45 binding but are negative for CD14; granulocytes have a lower level of CD45 binding and an intermediate level of CD14 expression; and monocytes have high levels of both CD45 and CD14 expression. Importantly, nonleukocytes, including erythrocytes and platelets, are negative using both reagents. In addition, malignant leukocytes that have characteristics of very early precursor cells are often CD45 and CD14 negative. Gating reagents provide a reliable means of checking the scatter-based lymphocyte gate for the frequency of nonlymphocytes within the gate and the extent of lymphocyte exclusion from the gate (Fig. 121.4B). Guidelines for an acceptable degree of contamination within the lymphocyte gate, as well as the level of lymphocyte exclusion, are contained within the US National Committee

KEY CONCEPTS

Gating
- Method to define cell population of interest
- Typically performed using forward and side scatter
- Should be confirmed with gating (monoclonal) reagents

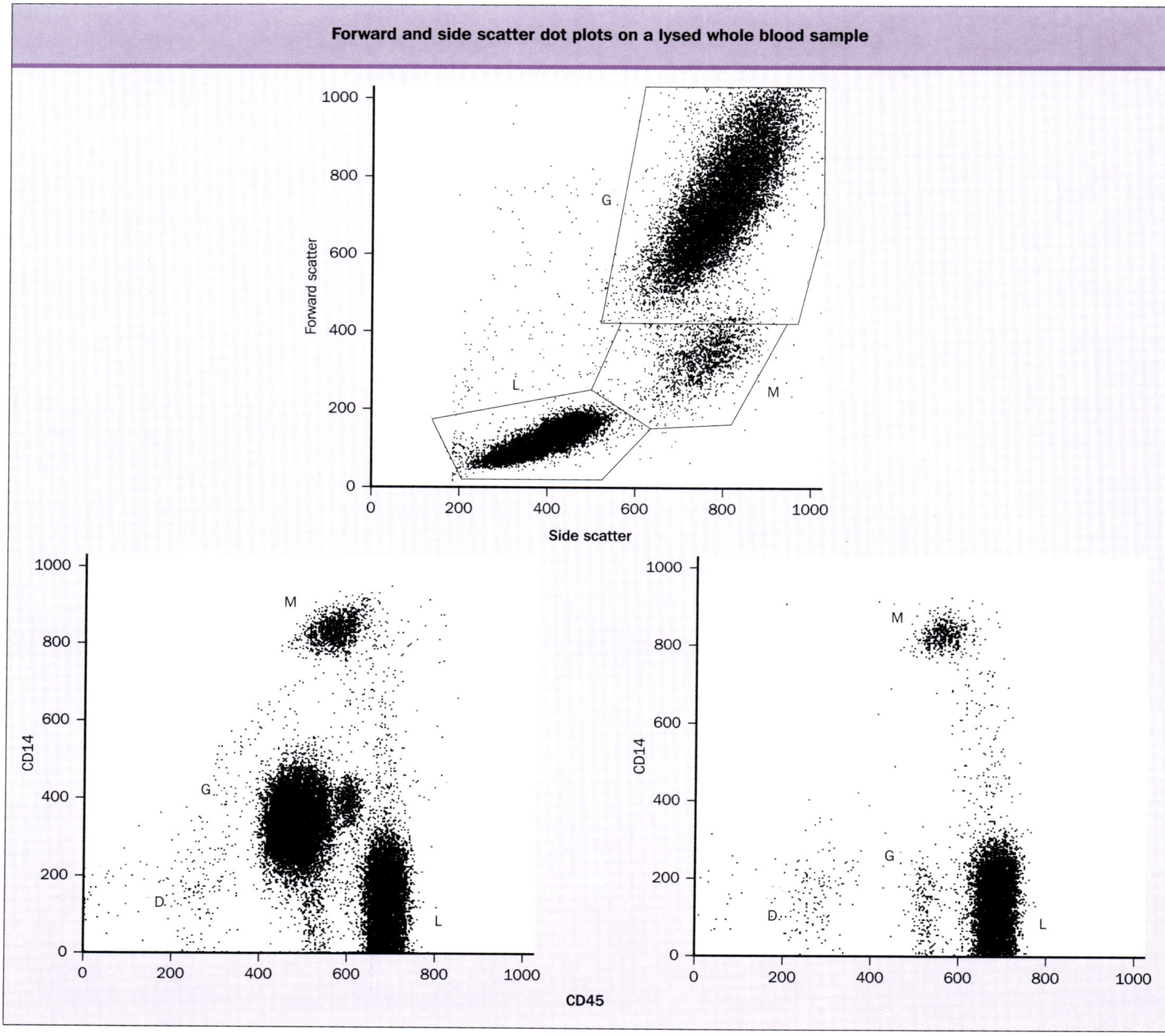

Figure 121.4 Top panel: forward and side scatter dot plots on a lysed whole blood sample, demonstrating the basic three-part leukocyte differential with lymphocytes (L), monocytes (M) and granulocytes (G). **Lower panel**: Dot plot with CD45/CD14 gating reagents showing the fluorescence distribution of all cells (left) and the fluorescence pattern of the scatter-based lymphocyte gate (right). The cellular elements identified include lymphocytes (L), monocytes (M) and granulocytes (G), as well as a small number of nonlysed red blood cells and/or debris (D).

for Clinical Laboratory Standards (NCCLS) guideline for lymphocyte immunophenotyping.[15] Each laboratory must establish its own guidelines and act accordingly when the data do not conform to these standards.

Data presentation

The usual approach for presenting one-color data is the single-parameter histogram (Fig. 121.2), a graphic presentation of cell number on the *y*-axis versus fluorescence (light) intensity on the *x*-axis. Integration of curve areas provides data on the number of cells defined within the confines of the fluorescence intensity selected. Often there are two distinct distributions, with one identifying cells that were not bound by the monoclonal reagent and the second representing cells bound by the antibody. Negative cells produces low-level fluorescence that results from cellular autofluorescence, together with any nonspecific binding of the monoclonal reagent. The level of this signal varies between different cell types. Interpretation of two cell populations (i.e. negative and positive) is simplified when the two distributions demonstrate distinct baseline separation, but the evaluation of two overlapping distributions is more difficult.

Multicolor data can be evaluated using a series of single-parameter histograms that consider each parameter independently. However, it is more informative to present two parameters

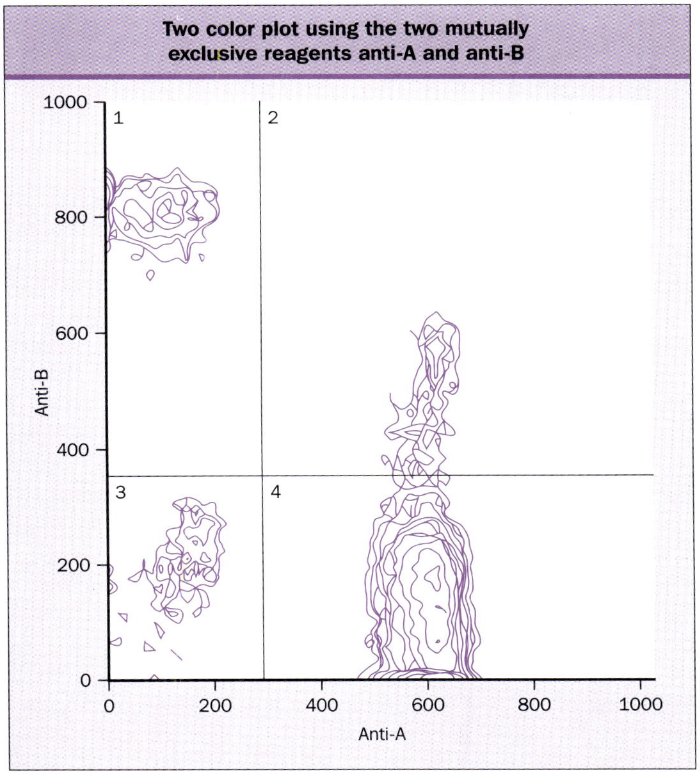

Figure 121.5 Two-color contour plot using the two mutually exclusive reagents anti-A and anti-B. Cells that express antigen A or antigen B mutually exclusively are found in quadrants 1 and 4 (A+B– or A–B+), and those that express both are located in quadrant 2 (A+B+); those that express neither are found in quadrant 3 (A–B–).

simultaneously using a correlated display (Fig. 121.5), and two-color displays are recommended for clinical flow cytometry whenever possible.[15,16] This approach enables the characterization of four different phenotypes: A+/B–, A–/B+, A+/B+, A–/B– (using the two model reagents anti-A and anti-B). When three reagents are used simultaneously, eight different immunophenotypes can be identified; the simultaneous use of *n* monoclonal reagents could identify 2^n subpopulations. The multicolor approach can provide a means to further resolve subpopulations, and has been particularly useful in the evaluation of cellular differentiation and activation as well as clarifying overlapping cell subpopulations.

A commonly used convention to identify positive cells is based on establishing a marker (discriminator) at the fluorescence histogram channel number that includes 98% or 99% of the negative cells. As previously noted, negative cells refers to cellular autofluorescence plus nonspecific binding. The latter is based on the fluorescence resulting from cells incubated with directly conjugated control monoclonal antibodies of the appropriate class or subclass (e.g. IgG_1, IgG_{2a}, IgG_{2b} or IgM) that are not specifically reactive with human lymphocyte surface antigens. The negative cell discrimination can be relatively simple to apply unless there is significant overlap between two populations, in which case this approach underestimates the frequency of positive cells.

The level of fluorescence produced by different fluorochromes varies: the brightest of the three standard immunophenotyping dyes is phycoerythrin. This observation has been used to demonstrate that varying the fluorochrome can alter the resolution of antigens expressed at low concentrations.[17] As a general rule, phycoerythrin is the best for direct staining studies evaluating 'dim' positive markers.

KEY CONCEPTS

Data presentation
- Fluorescence intensity is plotted versus cell number
- Can present data on more than one parameter on each cell
- Multicolor data presentation may increase cell subpopulation resolution

It should also be noted that the fluorescence signals emitted by different fluorochromes are not completely separated by the filters. The correction of this overlap is accomplished by electronic subtraction of the overlapping signal, a process referred to as electronic compensation. The overlap is particularly significant when using FITC and PE in combination, because FITC produces orange light in addition to its primary green signal. Compensation involves subtraction of the orange signal produced by FITC from the orange signal produced by PE. The availability of tandem conjugates adds another level of complexity, as does four-color flow cytometry, particularly when performed with a single light source. Overlap between fluorochrome combinations must be compensated, and proper compensation is absolutely critical for multicolor flow cytometry; a general approach to this was published recently.[18]

The fluorescence intensity of histogram patterns can be compared between different cell preparations when the same reagent and experimental set-up are used. This enables semiquantitative comparison of the antigen density between the various cells studied. However, fluorescence data obtained using different reagents generally are not comparable, because of the variability based on differences in antibody affinity and fluorochrome-to-protein ratio.

Quality control is a critical component of clinical flow cytometry to ensure optimal results.[19] This includes monitoring instrument set-up and performance, as well as optimizing sample preparation and reagents and standardizing controls and data interpretation. Quantitative flow cytometry based on fluorescence standard curve provides quantitative data in units referred to as molecular equivalents of soluble fluorochrome (MESF). When properly constructed standard curves are used, quantitative data for different reagents can be generated and compared.[7,20] Finally, participation in interlaboratory proficiency testing surveys, such as the triannual samples provided by the College of American Pathologists (CAP), is an important additional measure to monitor laboratory performance.

Methods

Whole-blood lysis represents the most common technique used for sample preparation in the flow cytometry laboratory.[15,20,21] This method consists of mixing a fixed volume of anticoagulated whole blood (or bone marrow) with one or more directly conjugated monoclonal antibodies, followed by incubation at a designated temperature and time. Next the red blood cells are lysed, the sample is washed and then run into the flow cytometer, usually following fixation in paraformaldehyde to reduce the infectious risk. The nonlysed cells remaining include all peripheral blood leukocytes, as well as any nonlysed red cells, platelets and debris. The heterogeneity of the sample necessitates careful lymphocyte gating in order to generate accurate immunophenotyping data. The advantages of the whole-blood lysis method include fewer preparation steps, less sample handling, and a lower likelihood of differential lymphocyte loss. This last point can occur when density gradient techniques are used to prepare mononuclear cells for analysis. For example, there is a variable but significant loss of T-cell subsets and B cells during the separation (ref. 20; personal observation). Alternative sources of cells (e.g. bronchial alveolar lavage fluid, fine-needle aspirates) can also be evaluated with flow cytometry.[22] Patient studies must be determined with the same methods and reagents as used in the determination of the control ranges to ensure comparability.

The application of control ranges must take into account the fact that significant changes take place in lymphocyte distribution during childhood, as well as among the very elderly.[23–28] There are also immunophenotypic differences induced by drugs, including tobacco products, such that information on current medications should be obtained whenever possible.[23,24,29] Other factors can also have an impact on lymphocyte distribution, including race, sex, diurnal variation and recent viral infection.[23,24,30]

The choice of immunophenoptyping reagents depends on the cells being studied and the question being asked. However, regardless of the specific set-up, the inclusion of a tube with the gating reagents (CD45 and CD14) to confirm the integrity of the standard lymphocyte gate is recommended.[13] In addition, control reagents should be included to establish the fluorescence intensity of negative cells. Additional important controls include a pan-T cell, B cell, and NK cell marker for every sample (Table 121.1). This provides a very valuable internal control, based on the principle that the whole is the sum of its parts. Thus, the total percentage of lymphocytes in the gate, as determined by the gating reagents, should approximately equal the sum of the percentages for T cells, B cells, and NK cells. A technical or biological explanation must be identified when this relationship does not hold. Biological explanations for a significant difference would include the presence of immature or malignant cells that were not identified by the reagents chosen. In addition, if the gating reagents (CD45/CD14) had not been included, contaminating cells (e.g., myeloid precursors, nucleated red blood cells, large platelets) with forward- and side-scatter characteristics similar to those of lymphocytes could not be ruled out. Potential technical problems include reagent or fluorochrome degradation, failure to add a reagent, and a host of others. Evidence for any major technical error should result in repeating the study.

Additional data that can be used for controls depend on the set-up. For example, the availability of multiple antibodies that identify a similar cell subpopulation is a useful check (e.g. total T cells by comparing CD3 and CD5 or CD2; total B cells by comparing CD19 and CD20). In addition, the determination of subsets within a lymphocyte subpopulation is another mechanism to validate results (e.g. the number of $CD4^+$ and $CD8^+$ cells should be approximately equal to the number of $CD3^+$ cells unless there is a significant number of double-negative T cells). Finally, the use of specific reagents in more than one tube enables comparison between the repeat values as a measure of consistency. The application of these various internal checks should be performed by the flow operator as a simple means of checking the validity of the data. Insights regarding unusual biological findings may also be uncovered through this type of evaluation (e.g. the presence of an increased population of $CD4^+/CD8^+$ double-negative T cells).[31]

The challenge in performing immunophenotyping is to accurately identify cells with specific surface characteristics (antigens). As previously noted, the capacity to discriminate specific cell subpopulations is often enhanced through the directed use of antibody combinations. The typical data generated consist of the percentage of negative versus positive cells when using one reagent, and multiple subpopulations when using more than one reagent. Regardless of the experimental design, it is important to consider not only the percentage but also the absolute number of cells within each subpopulation. This is most commonly obtained by multiplying the relevant percentage from the flow cytometer by the absolute lymphocyte count obtained using a white blood count and differential. For example, when assaying for CD4 T-cell counts, the percentage of $CD4^+$ cells is multiplied by the peripheral absolute lymphocyte count to yield the absolute CD4 count. A potential problem with this approach is the requirement for two separate procedures (i.e. dual platforms) to generate the final result. This introduces the possibility of additive error, based on the inherent errors of the two different methods, and has fueled a search for approaches to perform both tasks by flow cytometry (i.e. a single platform). One alternative involves the inclusion of a fixed number of fluorescent beads (in a defined volume) in each tube as a reference standard to generate absolute numbers without requiring additional data. Regardless of the approach, the reporting of both percentages and absolute numbers is necessary when immunophenotyping peripheral lymphocytes.

The objective of evaluating malignant cells is often to characterize the lineage and differentiation level of the abnormal cells, rather than quantifying subpopulations.[32] The pattern of reactivity combined with fluorescence intensity is often useful in identifying leukemic patterns whereas the absolute number of cells may not be required. However, flow cytometric detection and quantification of rare abnormal cells can be useful in evaluating minimal residual disease in lymphoproliferative disorders.

Lymphocyte surface antigens for immunophenotyping

T cell
Pan-T cell: CD3, CD2, CD7, CD5
Major T-cell subset: CD4, CD8
Surface antigens associated with function: CD28, CD38, CD45RA, CD45RO, CD62L
Activation antigens: CD25, CD40L, CD69, CD71, HLA-DR
B cell
Pan-B cell: CD19, CD20, surface immunoglobulin
Major B-cell subset: CD5, CD21
Surface antigens associated with function: CD27
Activation antigens: CD23, CD25
NK cell
Pan-NK cell: CD16, CD56
NK subset: CD2, CD8, CD57

Table 121.1 Selected lymphocyte surface antigens for immunophenotyping.

Immunophenotyping studies

The majority of immunophenotyping studies are directed at quantifying a specific cell subpopulation, evaluating for the pres-

> **CLINICAL RELEVANCE**
>
> **Immunophenotyping studies**
> - Can be used to identify cell subsets, establish lineage, stage of cell differentiation, state of cell activation, and assess for clonality
> - Lymphocyte results should be checked by T cells + B cells + NK cells = 100%
> - Are not the equivalent of lymphocyte function studies

ence or absence of a particular surface antigen, identifying the differentiation level of specific cells, determining cell lineage, establishing monoclonality, or examining for evidence of cell activation.

Quantification of a particular cell subpopulation can be readily accomplished with flow cytometry. The evaluation of absolute CD4 T-cell counts has formed the basis for monitoring patients infected with HIV.[33,34] The quantitation of $CD34^+$ hematopoietic stem cells in donor peripheral blood or bone marrow is used in many cellular reconstitution protocols.[35] Subpopulation characterization can also be useful in the evaluation of patients with clinical history and laboratory findings suggestive of immune deficiency. It is very important to recognize that immunophenotyping identifies the presence or absence of cells: it does not provide data regarding the function of those cells. This point is clearly illustrated by the finding of normal B-cell numbers in most patients with common variable immune deficiency, but absent B cells in patients with X-linked agammaglobulinemia, despite the fact that both patient groups fail to produce immunoglobulins.[36,37] These examples point out that immunophenotyping by flow cytometry is valuable for identifying specific cells, but assessment of relevant cell function requires additional testing.

Flow cytometry can be used to test for the presence or absence of a specific surface antigen. An example of this type of application is in the evaluation of a patient with a history of recurrent skin infections, delayed wound healing and persistent granulocytosis that is suggestive of leukocyte adhesion deficiency.[38] This disorder results from a defect in the gene encoding CD18, preventing the expression of three different heterodimeric adhesion molecules each containing CD18 (Chapter 37). This disorder can usually be diagnosed by studying granulocytes and lymphocytes for the expression of the three different CD11 isoforms, as well as CD18. In certain patients who demonstrate antigen expression but at low levels, it may be necessary to confirm the diagnosis by demonstrating a failure of adhesion molecule up-regulation following cell activation.

The directed use of the large array of monoclonal reagents can help address questions regarding the level of cell differentiation. Antibodies that are specific to precursors represent one approach, and would include the thymocyte marker CD1, or the pre-B-cell marker CD10 (CALLA). However, many surface antigens found on immature cells also are expressed on mature cells. Examples of these include CD2 and CD7 found on thymocytes and circulating T cells, or CD19 and HLA-DR found on pre-B as well as B cells. Thus the pattern of surface antigen expression can also help distinguish the level of differentiation. The best approach to determine the developmental level of a particular cell population or subpopulation is to evaluate using a combination of reagents that span the natural history of the cell lineage.

The previous approach represents the basic principle for testing in leukemia and lymphomas. It must be recognized that malignant cells can have altered forward and side-scatter characteristics, as well as diminished or no CD45 expression.[32] Thus, under these circumstances the conventional approaches to gating may have to be modified. The application of immunophenotyping can complement the morphologic and cytochemical methods, enabling the optimal classification and therapeutic approach. The standard approach may include determining whether specific antigens are present as well as the level of expression. Malignant cells may express antigens associated with different lineages, such that antibody panels used in these studies must also be directed at identifying the cell lineage. Lineage-directed studies can provide insight into shared expression of specific antigens.

Issues of monoclonality can be dealt with using flow cytometry when analyzing B cells, and in some circumstances when studying T cells. Normally B cells are a heterogeneous mixture of mutually exclusive κ or λ light-chain-positive cells. The distribution of light-chain expression can be evaluated for clonal excess using a method called the Komogorov–Smirnov D value comparison.[39,40] Light-chain clonal excess will usually be accompanied by an excess in B cells expressing one particular heavy chain (α, γ, μ or ε). The capacity to evaluate T-cell monoclonality by flow cytometry is more restricted owing to limited reagent availability. The approach consists of using T-cell antigen receptor α- or β-variable chain-specific reagents looking for evidence of clonal excess. This test is useful when positive but less so when negative, as monoclonal reagents do not identify the entire repertoire of T-cell antigen receptors.

The state of lymphoid activation can be addressed by evaluating for the presence of surface antigens that either are found only on activated cells or are up-regulated following activation. These include receptors for specific growth factors (e.g. IL-2 receptor α chain, CD25), receptors for critical elements required for cell growth (e.g. transferrin receptor, CD71), ligands that are critical for cell–cell communication following activation (CD40 ligand on T cells), and surface antigens that are up-regulated as a result of activation (e.g. adhesion molecules, HLA-DR, CD69). Such studies must take into account the temporal relationship of the various surface antigens in association with cell activation. In addition, chronic in vivo activation may impart a different pattern from that found with in vitro studies.

INTRACELLULAR EVALUATION

Cellular activation

Ligand binding and transmembrane signal transduction resulting in cellular activation can be evaluated using flow cytometry. Changes in intracellular ionic calcium concentration (Ca^{2+}) are frequently used to monitor cell activation after ligand binding. These changes are associated with the activation of phospholipase C and protein kinase C. In general, three reagents have been used to measure Ca^{2+}: quin 2, indo-1, and fluo-3. Quin 2 has a low excitation coefficient and is not useful for flow cytometry; indo-1 requires ultraviolet excitation; and fluo-3 can be excited by 488 nm but does not permit radiometric analysis. Nevertheless, because of its ease of use fluo-3 is currently the most widely used probe for intracytoplasmic Ca^{2+} evaluation by flow cytometry. Strict attention must be paid to loading conditions, the presence or absence of free Ca^{2+} in the media, experimental temperature,

CLINICAL RELEVANCE

Intracellular flow cytometry
- Activation-directed studies:
  - Calcium flux
  - Intracellular messenger phosphorylation
  - Oxidative burst: neutrophils
- Intracellular cytokine studies:
  - Clarify the Th1/Th2 status of an immune response
  - Can be assessed in an in vitro antigen specific response
  - Can be combined with cell surface studies

baseline measurements and calibration. This approach can be combined with cell surface marker or cell cycle evaluation.[10]

In addition to Ca^{2+} measurements, intracellular pH changes related to cellular activation can be evaluated. The most useful probe for pH is SNARF-1.[10] This can be excited at 488 nm and allows for ratiometric analysis with detection at 575 and 640 nm.

Glutathione (glutamylcysteinylglycine, GSH) is an important antioxidant generated during cell activation that can be measured by flow cytometry.[10] The fluorescent probe monochlorobimane is most commonly used for this measurement, but it is complicated by the need to determine GSH by an independent method such as HPLC.

Additional approaches to evaluate cellular activation include assessment of intranuclear markers (Ki-67, PCNA) as well as surface proteins that are up-regulated following cellular activation (e.g. CD69, CD25, CD71).[41] Actual cell division can be evaluated using lipophilic membrane dyes (e.g. PKH26) that lose 50% of their fluorescence with each round of cell division.[42] This approach also can be used to label target cells in cell-based cytotoxicity assays.[43] Flow cytometry has proved very useful for the evaluation of programmed cell death (apoptosis). This often involves the assessment of changes in the cell membrane (annexin V binding) that appear early following the induction of apoptotic pathways.[44]

Recently, an activation signal-specific application of flow cytometry has been reported. In this method, detection of phosphorylated STAT-1 was performed following interferon-γ stimulation of monocytes. The approach was found to be more sensitive than immunoblotting and may be generally applicable for the detection of proteins altered by cell activation, depending on the availability of reagents specific for the activation-altered protein.[45]

The assessment of oxidative burst following cell stimulation plays a central role in neutrophil functional evaluation. This can be most readily assessed by flow cytometry using the hydrogen peroxide-sensitive dye dihydrorhodamine 123. The procedure involves loading the dye into the cells, stimulating with phorbol myristate acetate (PMA), and evaluating for fluorescence by flow cytometry.[11] This test has proved to be extremely accurate in diagnosing patients with chronic granulomatous disease (CGD) and carriers of X-linked CGD.[46] A major advantage of this method is its sensitivity, which allows the detection of one normal cell in a population of 1000 abnormal cells. This makes assessment of oxidative burst a useful tool in following allogeneic granulocyte survival after transfusion into patients with CGD, as well as in evaluating the effectiveness of allogeneic stem cell transplantation and gene therapy in CGD.

Intracellular cytokine detection

After the introduction of a system for fixation and permeabilization of cells that preserved cell morphology and intracellular antigenicity, it became possible to analyze cytokine-producing cells at the single-cell level by flow cytometry.[47,48] This provides a platform for multiparameter analysis, which allows for the simultaneous detection of two or more intracellular cytokines in combination with cell surface markers, or other intracellular markers. Important aspects of intracellular cytokine detection include lymphocyte activation, the use of a protein transport inhibitor during activation, the use of proper controls and the choice of antibodies. As there is little or no spontaneous cytokine production in resting lymphocytes, intracellular cytokine detection requires activation. Initial experience was based on supraphysiological stimulation by PMA and ionomycin, but antigen-specific activation systems have also proved to be feasible. It should be emphasized that, regardless of the activation method, the duration of activation is an important variable, as individual cells reach maximum cytokine production at different times. In addition, different cytokines have different optimal periods of activation. It is recommended to establish a proper kinetic profile, depending on the biological system or clinical condition being studied.[47]

To increase the amount of intracellular cytokines, inhibitors of intracellular protein transport, such as monensin or brefeldin, are commonly used and lead to the accumulation of proteins within the cell. Nonspecific binding of the antibody reagents is an issue, as permeabilization allows access not only to the cytokine of interest, but also to other proteins present in much greater quantities than on the cell surface. In addition, fixation further increases nonspecific binding. Subclass-matched controls may be insufficient and the use of both a negative control sample, which contains an excess of unlabeled or 'cold' anticytokine antibody, and a subclass-matched control sample provides the optimal control. When the conjugated anticytokine is added to the negative control sample it can only bind to other proteins in a nonspecific manner, thereby providing a measure to discriminate between specific and nonspecific binding.[47] The use of directly conjugated anticytokine antibodies not only simplifies the staining procedure, but also provides a better distinction between specific and nonspecific binding than do unlabeled antibodies. Because the fixation agent may change the native state of certain epitopes, it is also important to use antibodies that recognize antigens after fixation.

One of the main applications of intracellular cytokine detection by flow cytometry has been the study and refinement of the Th1/Th2 paradigm.[49] It has recently become clear that the regulated secretion of cytokines can be used to study the response of individual T cells to polyclonal stimuli and specific antigens. A recently described method for measuring antigen-specific T-cell cytokine expression, after a short culture in whole blood, offers a useful alternative to the tetramer-based approach discussed later in the chapter (Fig 121.6).[50]

Cell cycle analysis

In addition to surface immunophenotyping and cytoplasmic characterization, flow cytometry is also used in cell cycle analysis. Propidium iodide (PI) is the most commonly used fluorochrome, owing to its optimal linear DNA-binding capacity in a variety of different cell types. Thus, a single-parameter histogram of DNA

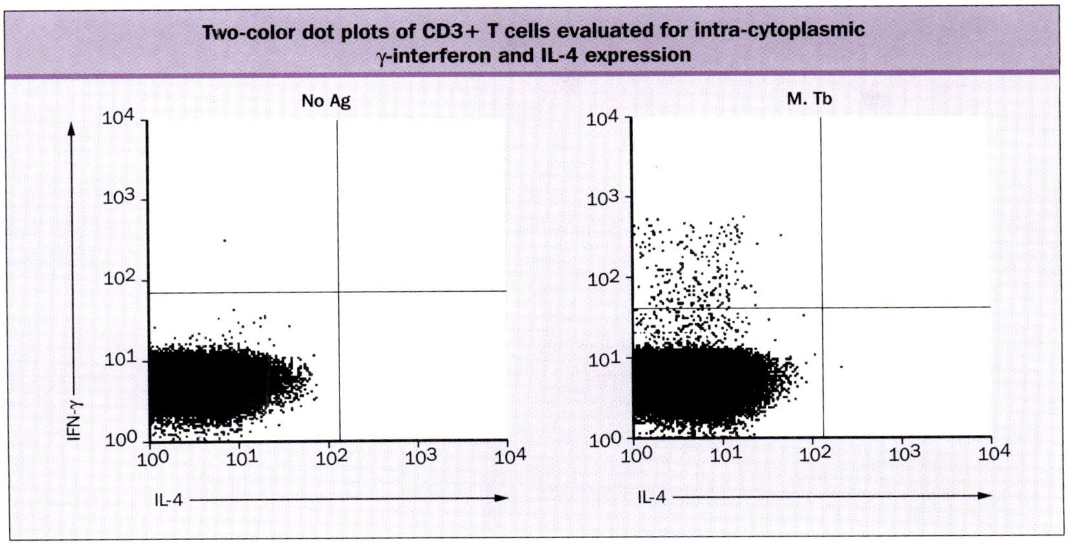

Figure 121.6 Two-color dot plots of CD3⁺ T cells evaluated for intracytoplasmic interferon-γ and IL-4 expression. The donor had a positive skin test to PPD and demonstated a Th1 pattern of cytokine expression (interferon-γ) in response to *Mycobacterium tuberculosis* antigen, with an absence of a Th2 cytokine pattern (IL-4). (Courtesy of Calman Prussin.)

content using PI readily permits the determination of cell cycle compartments, expressed as the percentage of cells in G_0–G_1, S and G_2-M. In addition to these conventional parameters, the presence or absence of aneuploidy can be determined by inspection of the G_0–G_1 peak and/or use of a DNA index (ratio of abnormal DNA content to a diploid DNA standard). Also, elevation in the S and/or G_2-M phase can be detected. The optimal display of these data uses a combination of side scatter versus DNA content. Recently it has been noted that cells observed on the histogram in the area below the level of G_0–G_1 may be undergoing apoptosis.[51] Additional flow-cytometric approaches to evaluate this process are being studied.[52,53]

It should be noted that several different computer algorithms have been developed to determine the relative proportion of each cell cycle compartment, and the selection of a software program is not a trivial process. The major instrument manufacturers supply cell cycle analysis programs, and there are also third-party programs available. Generally the optimal program should be capable of modeling two or more aneuploid populations, subtracting debris (particularly if formalin-fixed paraffin-embedded archival material is used) and accurately estimating S-phase cells.[12,54] The combination of a surface marker and cell cycle has been very useful in differentiating normal cell populations from tumor cell populations.[55] One example is the use of either anti-κ, anti-λ or B-cell reagents to separate the aneuploid B-cell clone from the remaining normal, reactive B cells in a lymphoid cell mixture. Another uses cytokeratin as a marker to distinguish between the tumor cells and the inflammatory cells that are present.[56]

The other major event that has occurred in cell cycle analysis has been the development of technology using the incorporation of bromodeoxyuridine.[13,57] This thymidine analog is used to directly determine the percentage of S-phase cells. Also, when used in kinetic studies it permits a determination of the individual times for the components of the cell cycle and a determination of the growth fraction. Finally, recent developments have resulted in the availability of two anticyclin reagents to evaluate cell cycle transition points in malignant cells.[58,59]

PEPTIDE–MHC TETRAMERS

In contrast to B cells, direct visualization of antigen-specific T cells in vivo has, until recently, been unsuccessful. In 1996, Altman et al. introduced a novel flow-cytometry-based methodology that enables the direct visualization and quantification of antigen-specific T cells.[60] By generating soluble peptide–MHC multimers, such that multiple TCRs are engaged at the same time, the avidity of these multimeric ligands for the peptide-specific TCR is greatly increased. The methodology involves engineering a biotinylation recognition sequence on to the COOH terminus of the extracellular domain of one chain of the MHC molecule which, after combining with a specific antigenic peptide, is bound by avidin or streptavidin. As both avidin and streptavidin have four biotin-binding sites, the result is a tetrameric peptide–MHC complex that serves as a ligand for T cells specific for both the peptide and MHC. Flow-cytometric detection is achieved by labeling streptavidin with a fluorochrome. The major pitfall to this approach is the need to know the antigen-derived peptide and its HLA-restrictions, as well as the HLA type of each subject studied. Since the initial report, an increasing number of tetramer-based studies have appeared. Most have focused on the MHC class I-mediated

CLINICAL RELEVANCE

Cell cycle analysis
- Useful to screen percentage of S phase and aneuploidy
- Applied primarily in malignant cell evaluation
- Can be combined with cell surface studies

KEY CONCEPTS

Peptide–MHC tetramers
- Useful to assess the number of antigen-specific T cells
- Can be directed at both $CD4^+$ and $CD8^+$ T cells
- Requires information about the antigenic peptide and HLA (MHC) restriction

immune response, in both mice and humans, to a variety of infectious agents, including HIV, Epstein–Barr virus (EBV) and others.[60–62] Since the initial description with class I-restricted recognition, detection of antigen-specific CD4 T cells with tetramers of soluble MHC class II molecules and covalently linked peptide has also been reported.[63]

In addition to demonstrating the feasibility of this approach, the published studies have provided several new insights into the MHC class I-mediated immune response (Chapter 17). For example, it has become clear that the extent of the MHC class I-mediated cellular response is much greater than previously estimated. Furthermore, the extensive proliferation of CD8 T cells during an acute infection is not the result of bystander activation, but represents an expansion of antigen-specific CD8 T cells. One possible explanation is that, in contrast to previously used techniques such as the limiting dilution assay, tetramer-based assays do not depend on in-vitro cell division and survival. Peptide–MHC tetramer assays have also shown promise in the study of the kinetics of primary and secondary immune responses, as well as in a better understanding of concepts such as immunodominance and clonal exhaustion.[62,64]

An obviously attractive aspect of this technology is that tetramer staining can be combined with a variety of cell surface and intracellular phenotypic and functional markers. Already there are indications that the phenotype of antigen-specific T cells varies between individuals and between different phases of the immune response. In addition, tetramer-positive T cells can be sorted for further analysis, such as cytotoxicity assays or in vitro expansion.[64] The tetramer-based technology has not only proved useful for the study of the immune response to infectious agents, it has also been applied to the study of oral tolerance, autoimmune conditions and tumor immunology.[65–67] It is likely that this highly sensitive and specific technology will find many more applications and will lead to new discoveries and a reassessment of certain existing concepts.

CONCLUSION

Immunophenotyping by flow cytometry has become readily available in larger clinical laboratories. The application of this technology has moved forward in parallel to significant improvements in instrumentation and the expansion in the availability of reagents. The latter have defined a large array of lymphocyte surface molecules, but the function of some of these has yet to be delineated.

Properly performed, flow cytometry can provide rapid and accurate lymphocyte subpopulation identification. The primary clinical indications of immunophenotyping remain quantifying CD4 T-cell counts in HIV infection, lineage assignment in leukemias and lymphomas, and assessing $CD34^+$ stem cells for transplantation. Additional uses include characterizing immune deficiency disorders, evaluating immune-mediated inflammatory diseases, and assessing patients following organ transplantation. The real utility of these newer applications remains to be fully clarified and, in most settings, immunophenotyping does not represent a diagnostic procedure but rather plays a part in the evaluation and understanding of complex disorders and the longitudinal evaluation of immunomodulatory therapy.

It is critical to recognize that immunophenotyping is a means of identifying cells, but it is not directed at cell function. The expansion of flow-cytometric techniques to evaluate intracellular characteristics and the evolution of MHC–tetramer technology is moving this platform into the cell function arena. These newer approaches are expanding the utility of flow cytometry as a valuable tool for the characterization of immune function and responses.

REFERENCES

1. Wood JCS. Clinical flow cytometry instruments. In: Bauer KD, Duque RE, Shankey TV (eds) Clinical flow cytometry, principles and application. Baltimore, Williams & Wilkins, 1993.
2. Shapiro HM. How a flow cytometer works. In: Shapiro HM (ed) Practical flow cytometry, 2nd edn. New York, Alan R. Liss, 1998.
3. Givan AL. Instrumentation beyond the black box. In: Givan AL (ed) Flow cytometry, first principles. New York, Wiley Liss, 1992.
4. Kachel V, Fellner-Feldegg H, Menke E. Hydrodynamic properties of flow cytometry instruments. In: Melamed MR, Lindmo T, Mendelsohn ML (eds) Flow cytometry and sorting. New York, Wiley Liss, 1990.
5. Salzman GC, Crowell JM, Martin JC, et al. Cell classification by laser light scattering identification and separation of unstained leukocytes. Acta Cytol 1975;19:374.
6. Thompson JM, Gralow JR, Levy R, Miller RA. The optimal application of forward and ninety-degree light scatter in flow cytometry for the gating of mononuclear cells. Cytometry 1985;6:401.
7. Vogt RF, Marti GE, Schwartz. Quantitative calibration of fluorochrome intensity for clinical and research applications of leukocyte immunophenotyping by flow cytometry. In: Tyrer HW (ed) Critical issues in biotechnology and bioengineering, Vol 1. Norwood NJ, Ablex Publishing, 1995.
8. Waggoner A, Ernst LA. Fluorescence reagents for flow cytometry. In: Bauer KD, Duque RE, Shankey TV (eds) Clinical flow cytometry, principles and application. Baltimore, Williams & Wilkins, 1993.
9. Shapiro HM. Parameters and probes. In: Shapiro HM (ed) Practical flow cytometry, 2nd edn. New York, Alan R. Liss, 1998.
10. Rabinovitsch PS, June CH, Kavanagh TJ. Measurements of cell physiology: ionized calcium, pH and glutathione. In: Bauer KD, Duque RE, Shankey TV (eds) Clinical flow cytometry: principles and application. Baltimore, Williams & Wilkins, 1993.
11. Vowells SJ, Sekhsaria S, Malech HL, Shalit M, Fleisher TA. Flow cytometric analysis of granulocyte respiratory burst: a comparison study of fluorescent probes. J Immunol Meth 1995;178:89.
12. Braylan RC, Benson NA, Nourse V, et al. Correlated analysis of cellular DNA, membrane antigens and light scatter of human lymphoid cells. Cytometry 1982;2:337.
13. Darzynkiewicz Z, Traganos F, Kimmel M. Assay of cell kinetics by multivariate flow cytometry using the principle of strathmokinesis. In: Gray JW, Darzynkiewicz Z (eds) Techniques in cell cycle analysis. Clifton NJ, Humana Press, 1987.
14. Loken MR, Brosnan JM, Bach BA, Ault KA. Establishing optimal lymphocyte gates for immunophenotyping for flow cytometry. Cytometry 1990;11:453.
15. National Committee for Clinical Laboratory Standards. Clinical applications of flow cytometry: quality assurance and immunophenotyping of peripheral blood lymphocytes. NCCLS Document H42, Villanova PA, 1992.
16. Thorthwaite JT, Seckinger D, Sugarbaker EV, et al. Dual immunofluorescent analysis of human peripheral blood lymphocytes. Am J Clin Pathol 1984;82:48.

17. Jackson AL, Matsumoto H, Janszen M, et al. Restricted expression of p55 interleukin 2 receptor (CD25) on normal T cells. Clin Immunol Immunopathol 1990;54:126.
18. Stewart CC, Stewart SJ. Four color compensation. Cytometry 1999;38:161.
19. Owens MA, Loken MR. Quality control of flow cytometer and reagents. In: Owens MA, Loken MR (eds) Flow cytometry principles for clinical laboratory practice. New York, Wiley Liss, 1995.
20. Schwartz A, Marti GE, Poon R, Gratama JW, Fernandez-Repollet E. Standardizing flow cytometry: a classification system of fluorescence standards used for flow cytometry. Cytometry 1998;33:106.
21. Renzi P, Ginns LC. Analysis of T cell subsets in normal adults: comparison of whole blood lysis technique to Ficoll–Hypaque separation by flow cytometry. J Immunol Meth 1987;98:53.
22. Yamada M, Tamura N, Shirai T, Kira S. Flow cytometric analysis of lymphocyte subsets in the bronchoalveolar lavage fluid and peripheral blood of healthy volunteers. Scand J Immunol 1986;24:559.
23. Burton RC, Ferguson P, Gray M, et al. Effects of age, gender, and cigarette smoking on human immunoregulatory T-cell subsets: establishment of normal ranges and comparison with patients with cancer and multiple sclerosis. Diagn Immunol 1983;1:216.
24. Tollerud DJ, Clark JW, Brown LM, et al. The influence of age, race, and gender on peripheral blood mononuclear-cell subsets in healthy nonsmokers. J Clin Immunol 1989;9:214.
25. Denny T, Yogev R, Gelman R, et al. Lymphocyte subsets in healthy children during the first 5 years of life. JAMA 1992;267:1484.
26. Kotylo PS, Fineberg NA, Freeman KS, et al. Reference ranges for lymphocyte subsets in pediatric patients. Am J Clin Pathol 1993;100:111.
27. Reichert T, DeBruyere M, Deneys V, et al. Lymphocyte subset ranges in adult Caucasians. Clin Immunol Immunopathol 1991;60:190.
28. Wiener D, Shah S, Malone J, et al. Multiparameter analysis of peripheral blood in the normal pediatric population by flow cytometry. J Clin Lab Anal 1990;4:175.
29. Tollerud DJ, Clark JW, Brown LM, et al. The effects of smoking on T cell subsets. A population based survey of healthy Caucasians. Am Rev Respir Dis 1989;139:1446.
30. Levi FA, Canon C, Touitou Y, et al. Circadian rhythms in circulating T lymphocyte subtypes and plasma testosterone, total and free cortisol in five healthy men. Clin Exp Immunol 1988;71:329.
31. Sneller MC, Straus SE, Jaffe ES, et al. A novel lymphoproliferative/autoimmune syndrome resembling murine lpr/gld disease. J Clin Invest 1992;90:334.
32. Banks PM. Immunophenotypic markers useful in diagnosing and classification of hematopoietic neoplasms. In: Knowles DM (ed) Neoplastic hematopathology. Baltimore, Williams & Wilkins, 1992.
33. Philips AN, Lee CA, Elford J, et al. Serial CD4 lymphocyte counts and development of AIDS. Lancet 1991;337:389.
34. Yarchoan R, Venzon DJ, Pluda JM, et al. CD4 count and the risk for death in patients infected with HIV receiving antiretroviral therapy. Ann Intern Med 1991;115:184.
35. Sekhsaria S, Fleisher TA, Vowells SJ, et al. G-CSF recruitment of $CD34^+$ progenitors impaired mobilization in chronic granulomatous disease and ADA deficient patients. Blood 1996;88:1104.
36. Wright JJ, Wagner DK, Blaese RM, et al. Characterization of common variable immunodeficiency: characterization of patients with distinctive immunophenotypic and clinical features. Blood 1990;76:2046.
37. Anker R, Conley ME, Pollok BA. Clonal diversity in the B cell repertoire of patients with X-linked agammaglobulinemia. J Exp Med 1989;169:2109.
38. Schmalsteig FC. Leukocyte adherence defect. Pediatr Infect Dis J 1988;7:867.
39. Berliner N, Ault KA, Martin P, Weinberg DS. Detection of clonal excess in lymphoproliferative disease by κ/λ analysis: correlation with immunoglobulin gene rearrangement. Blood 1986;67:80.
40. Young IT. Proof without prejudice. Use of the Kogomorov–Smirnov test for the analysis of histograms from flow systems and other sources. J Histochem Cytochem 1977;25:935.
41. Mardiney MMIII, Brown MR, Fleisher TA. Measurement of CD69 expression: a rapid and efficient means to assess mitogen or antigen induced proliferative capacity in normals. Cytometry 1996;26:305.
42. Allsopp CE, Nicholls SJ, Langhorne J. A flow cytometric method to assess antigen-specific proliferative response of different subpopulations of fresh and cryopreserved human peripheral blood mononuclear cells. J Immunol Meth 1998;214:175.
43. Slezak SE, Horan PK. Cell-mediated cytotoxicity. A highly sensitive and informative flow cytometric assay. J Immunol Meth 1989;117:205.
44. Shounan Y, Feng X, O'Connell PJ. Apoptosis detection by annexin V binding: a novel method for quantitation of cell-mediated cytotoxicity. J Immunol Meth 1998;217:61.
45. Fleisher TA, Dorman SE, Anderson JA, Vail M, Brown MR, Holland SM. Detection of intracellular phosphorylated STAT-1 by flow cytometry. Clin Immunol 1999;90:425.
46. Vowells SJ, Fleisher TA, Sekhsaria S, Alling DW, Maguire TE, Malech HL. Genotype dependent variability in flow cytometric evaluation of reduced nicotinamide adenine dinucleotide phosphate oxidase function in patients with chronic granulomatous disease. J Pediatr 1996;128:104.
47. Prussin C. Cytokine flow cytometry: understanding cytokine biology at the single-cell level. J Clin Immunol 1997;17:195.
48. Carrock Sewell WA, North ME, Webster DB, Farrant J. Determination of intracellular cytokines by flow cytometry following whole-blood culture. J Immunol Meth 1997;209:67.
49. Rostaing LM, Tkaczuk J, Durand M, et al. Kinetics of intracytoplasmic Th1 and Th2 cytokine production assessed by flow cytometry following in vitro activation of peripheral blood mononuclear cells. Cytometry 1999;35:318.
50. Suni MA, Picker LJ, Maino VC. Detection of antigen-specific T cell cytokine expression in whole blood by flow cytometry. J Immunol Meth 1998;212:89.
51. Hotz MA, Gong J, Tragonos F, et al. Flow cytometric detection of apoptosis: comparison of assays of *in situ* DNA degradation and chromatin changes. Cytometry 1994;15:232.
52. Gorczyca W, Turziak T, Kram A, et al. Detection of apoptosis-associated DNA strand breaks in fine needle aspiration biopsies by *in situ* end labeling of fragmented DNA. Cytometry 1994;16:169.
53. Gong J, Tragonos F, Darzynkiewicz Z. A selective procedure for DNA extraction from apoptotic cells applicable for gel electrophoresis and flow cytometry. Ann Biochem 1994;218:1.
54. Wheeless LL, Coon JS, Cox C, et al. Precision of DNA flow cytometry in inter-institutional analyses. Cytometry 1991;12:405.
55. Shankey TV, Rabinovitch PS, Bagwell B, et al. Guidelines for implementation of clinical DNA cytometry. Cytometry 1993;14:472.
56. Zarbo RJ, Visscher DW, Crissman JD. Two-color multiparametric method for flow cytometric DNA analysis of carcinomas using staining for cytokeratin and leukocyte-common antigen. Anal Quant Cytol Histol 1989;11:391.
57. Gray JW, Dolbeare F, Pallavicinic M, et al. Flow cytokinetics. In: Gray JW, Darzynkiewicz Z (eds) Techniques in cell cycle analysis. Clifton NJ, Humana Press, 1987.
58. Gong J, Tragonos F, Darzynkiewicz Z. Simultaneous analysis of cell cycle kinetics at two different DNA ploidy levels based on DNA content and cyclin B measurements. Cancer Res 1993;53:5096.
59. Gong J, Tragonos F, Darzynkiewicz Z. Expression of cyclins B and E in individual MOLT-4 cells and in stimulated human lymphocytes during their progression through the cell cycle. Int Oncol 1993;3:1037.
60. Altman JD, Moss PAH, Goulder PJR, et al. Phenotypic analysis of antigen-specific T lymphocytes. Science 1996;274:94.
61. McMichael AJ, O'Callaghan CA. A new look on T cells. J Exp Med 1998;187:1367.
62. Murali-Krishna K, Altman JD, Suresh M, et al. Counting antigen-specific CD8 T cells: a reevaluation of bystander activation during viral infection. Immunity 1998;8:177.
63. Crawford F, Kozono H, White J, Marrack P, Kappler J. Detection of antigen-specific T cells with multivalent soluble class II MHC covalent peptide complexes. Immunity 1998;8:675.

64. Kuroda MJ, Schmitz JE, Barouch DH, et al. Analysis of gag-specific cytotoxic T lymphocytes in simian immunodeficiency virus-infected rhesus monkeys by cell staining with a tetrameric major histocompatibility complex class I-peptide complex. J Exp Med 1998;187:1373.
65. Gütgemann I, Fahrer AM, Altman JD, Davis MM, Chien Y-H. Induction of rapid T cell activation and tolerance by systemic presentation of an orally administered antigen. Immunity 1998;8:667.
66. Ogg GS, Dunbar PR, Romero P, Chen J, Cerundolo V. High frequency of skin-homing melanocyte-specific cytotoxic T lymphocytes in autoimmune vitiligo. J Exp Med 1998;188:1203.
67. Lee PP, Yee C, Savage PA, et al. Characterization of circulating T cells specific for tumor-associated antigens in melanoma patients. Nature Med 1999;5:677.

Chapter 122 Assessment of Lymphocyte and Monocyte Function

Anna Nowak-Wegrzyn and Howard M. Lederman

INTRODUCTION

Lymphocytes and monocytes can be evaluated by assessing their numbers and functional activity. Enumeration of lymphocytes and monocytes provides a first estimate of their status because severe deficiencies in the numbers of these cells are generally associated with impaired function, and increased numbers may indicate pathologic processes such as infection, inflammation or malignancy. However, cell function does not always correlate with cell number. Some patients may have reduced numbers of cells that function normally, whereas others have normal numbers of cells with impaired function. In practice, tests of cell number and function are usually necessary when evaluating a patient suspected of being immunodeficient.

The functions of lymphocytes and monocytes can be evaluated separately or in concert with other cells. In general, testing in vitro offers the opportunity to investigate specific abilities of cells in a controlled environment, whereas testing in vivo may be more reflective of cooperation between different components. These two approaches therefore complement each other.

This chapter focuses on those methods that are generally available at commercial laboratories and for which normative data are available. As our understanding of lymphocyte and monocyte biology advances, there is an increasing number of assays that can be performed in individual circumstances and at selected research laboratories. As appropriate, these assays are noted but not covered in detail.

ASSESSMENT OF B LYMPHOCYTE FUNCTION

The laboratory analysis of B-cell function focuses on the measurement of immunoglobulins and antibodies, as these are the unique protein products of differentiated B lymphocytes. However, it is important to remember that the function of B lymphocytes is dependent on the accessory function of T lymphocytes and antigen-presenting cells. Defects in any of these cells or their soluble products can result in abnormal antibody production. Quantification of serum IgG, IgA and IgM concentrations, along with measurement of specific antibody responses to immunization or natural infection, will identify the great majority of patients with abnormal humoral immunity, although they may not fully identify the underlying pathophysiology. Enumeration of B cells and measurement of IgG subclass concentrations is useful in selected patients.

Measurement of IgG, IgM and IgA

Measurement of serum immunoglobulins IgG, IgM and IgA is a useful screening test of humoral immunity because most patients with humoral immunodeficiencies will have decreased serum immunoglobulins. Immunoglobulin concentrations are commonly measured by either rate nephelometry or radial immunodiffusion (RID). Rate nephelometry is fast, accurate for immunoglobulin concentrations greater than 0.1 g/l, and can be performed in serum, urine and cerebrospinal fluid. RID is slower but less expensive. Low-level kits can detect as little as 0.01 g/l and are useful in evaluating hypogammaglobulinemic patients. RID may yield misleading results if abnormally large molecules (macroglobulinemia) or partially degraded immunoglobulin molecules (as may be found in urine) are present.[1] Serum immunoglobulin concentrations must be interpreted by comparison with normal ranges for age. IgG and IgM concentrations approach adult values by about 6 years of age; IgA concentrations increase until puberty.[2]

Low imunoglobulin concentrations can be found in patients with decreased production (i.e. primary immunodeficiency, immunosuppressive therapy) and in patients with increased protein losses (i.e proteinuria, protein-losing enteropathy, severe burns). Usually, the history and physical examination provide clues to the presence of syndromes leading to excess loss. Measurement of serum albumin concentration can be helpful: patients with decreased immunoglobulin production usually have normal albumin concentrations, whereas increased protein loss generally results in low concentrations of both albumin and immunoglobulins. One exception is the patient with hypogammaglobulinemia and secondary intestinal disease (infection or inflammation), who may develop decreased albumin as a consequence of diarrhea.

A finding of normal or elevated serum immunoglobulin levels in a patient with a history of recurrent infections should prompt an evaluation for IgG subclass deficiency, specific antibody deficiency, viral infection (HIV, EBV), lymphoreticular malignancy and gammopathy.

Measurement of IgG subclasses

Rare patients with increased susceptibility to infection have normal or borderline total serum IgG levels but low levels of one or more IgG subclasses and/or inadequate specific antibody responses.[3]

The quantification of IgG subclasses requires the use of subclass-specific monoclonal antibodies in either an immunoassay or by nephelometry. Measurements of IgG subclasses are complicated by the cross-reactivity of some anti-subclass antisera and the fact that some of the subclasses are normally present in low concentrations. A rough assessment of the accuracy of IgG subclass measurement is made by comparison with total serum IgG level; the sum of all IgG subclasses should approximately equal the total serum IgG level. IgG subclass concentrations vary with age and do not follow a normal distribution within the population. For example, the normal reference range for IgG_4 includes 0 g/l at some ages. The interpretation of IgG subclass deficiency in the absence of specific antibody deficiency must be made with great caution. It is controversial whether IgG subclass measurements in the absence of antibody measurements are ever useful.

Measurement of secretory IgA

Secretory IgA deficiency almost always occurs concomitantly with selective serum IgA deficiency. In secretions, IgA exists as a dimer that contains a J chain and secretory component. The latter is synthesized by mucosal epithelial cells and covalently binds to dimeric IgA as it passes through mucosal epithelial cells. For patients with symptoms of defective mucosal immunity but normal levels of serum IgA, measurements of secretory IgA can be made in saliva, tears, nasal fluid or gastric secretions.[4] These measurements are hampered by low concentration and difficulty in obtaining samples, and are therefore of limited value in clinical practice.

Measurement of IgE

Abnormalities of IgE, both high and low, are common in incomplete antibody-deficiency syndromes. IgE levels may be moderately elevated in Wiscott–Aldrich syndrome, DiGeorge anomaly, Nezelof syndrome; severely elevated in hyper-IgE syndrome; and reduced or absent in ataxia–telangiectasia. High IgE levels may be found in patients with parasitic infection or atopic disorders. Even though specific IgE may be absent in subjects without atopy, the finding of measurable specific IgE levels in a patient undergoing an evaluation for immunodeficiency can provide indirect evidence for a preserved mechanism of isotype switching, which requires the cooperation of B and T lymphocytes.

Measurement of IgD

Determination of IgD level usually is not indicated in the evaluation of suspected antibody deficiency. However, it is helpful for the evaluation of suspected hyper-IgD syndrome, a rare problem characterized by periodic fever, lymphadenitis and arthritis.[5] Serum IgD levels in this disorder are typically >150 IU/ml or >20 mg/dl as measured by radial immunodiffusion, radioimmunoassay or enzyme-linked immunosorbent assay.

Evaluation of hypergammaglobulinemia/ dysgammaglobulinemia

Some patients have elevated serum immunoglobulin levels. Causes of hypergammaglobulinemia include monoclonal gammopathy of undetermined significance (MGUS), multiple myeloma, Waldenström's macroglobulinemia, amyloidosis, chronic lymphocytic leukemia, collagen vascular disease, and a variety of chronic viral infections such as HIV, HBV and EBV. These may lead to poly-, oligo- or monoclonal expansion of B-cell populations, with resulting gammopathy. Serum protein electrophoresis (SPEP) is a useful screening test for the presence of monoclonal proteins. Immunofixation electrophoresis (IFE) should be carried out to confirm the presence of a monoclonal protein and to determine its immunoglobulin heavy- and light-chain components.[6]

Natural antibody levels

Natural antibodies are those present without deliberate antigenic challenge. Isohemagglutinins are natural IgM antibodies to polysaccharide blood group antigens A and/or B if the antigens are not on the patient's red cells.[7] Individuals with blood type AB do not form isohemagglutinins, and children under 1 year of age generally do not either. Other natural antibodies include heterophile antibodies (antibodies to sheep erythrocytes) and antibodies to streptolysin O, *Escherichia coli* and endotoxin. Nearly all normal individuals have antibodies at titers of at least 1:10 to some or all of these antigens because of their widespread distribution in food, inhaled particles and the respiratory flora.

Specific antibody concentration

Specific antibody concentrations should always be used to assess the significance of low or borderline-low immunoglobulin class or subclass levels in patients with recurrent infections. Specific antibody function is also an excellent measure of the return of immune function after bone marrow transplantation or immunosuppressive chemotherapy.

The results of the antibody measurements need to be interpreted in the context of the patient's age and previous exposure, either by natural infection or by immunization. In the first months of life the measurement of IgG antibodies is likely to reflect transplacentally transferred maternal antibodies, in addition to the infant's own response to immunization or infection. In this setting, measurements of IgM or IgA antibodies are more informative because they indicate the host response. Although the random measurement of antibody concentration may be a useful screening test, it is often more informative to measure antibodies prior to and after immunization. In general, responses are considered normal if antibody levels equal or exceed values known to be required for protection, or if there is a fourfold or greater rise in antibody level after immunization. In some situations high preimmunization antibody concentration due to recent infection or transplacental transfer of maternal antibody can diminish the magnitude of the increase. Antibody concentrations are usually measured in serum, which is stable for several months when separated and stored at –70°C.

KEY CONCEPTS

Evaluation of B-lymphocyte function

- Measurement of serum IgG, IgM, and IgA is a useful screening test.
- Immunoglobulin measurements should be interpreted in the context of age, susceptibility to infections and antibody responses.
- Specific antibody responses to T-dependent (protein) and T-independent (bacterial polysaccharide) antigens are useful in evaluating for suspected immunodeficiency or the return of immune function after bone marrow transplantation or immunosuppressive therapy.
- Enumeration of B lymphocytes is helpful in further characterization of an immune defect and/or the maturity of B lymphocytes.
- In vitro studies of B lymphocyte function evaluate B-lymphocyte proliferation, secretion of antibody and isotype switching.

Vaccines used in evaluation of immunodeficiency	
Vaccine	**Criteria for response**
T-dependent	Evaluation 2–3 weeks after immunization
Diphtheria toxoid	Protective level >0.01 IU/ml; usual response after primary immunization >1.0 IU/ml
Tetanus toxoid	Protective level >0.01 IU/ml; usual response after primary immunization >1.0 IU/ml
Hemophilus influenzae type b conjugate	Protective level >0.15 μg/ml; usual response after primary immunization >1.0 μg/ml
T-independent	Evaluation 3–4 weeks after immunization
Pneumococcal polysaccharide	Protective level estimated to be 0.15 μg/ml; usual response to immunization ≥ 0.8 μg/ml for majority of vaccine serotypes

Live viral vaccines such as oral polio, mumps/measles/rubella and varicella should never be used in the evaluation of suspected immunodeficiency because they may cause disseminated, potentially fatal infection in an immunocompromised host.

Table 122.1 Vaccines commonly used in the evaluation of suspected immunodeficiency.

The majority of vaccines are T dependent, that is, they can activate B cells only in the presence of T cells (Table 122.1). The evaluation of antibody responses to tetanus toxoid, diphtheria toxoid or *Haemophilus influenzae* type b (HiB) conjugate vaccines is the most useful method for assessing the response to T-dependent antigens. These vaccines are administered early in life as part of the routine childhood immunization schedule, they induce strong antibody responses in the majority of vaccinated subjects, and they have excellent safety profiles. There is no contraindication to their use even in severely immunocompromised patients, as none are a live vaccine and thus, cannot transmit disease. There are standardized laboratory methods available for the measurement of specific antibodies that provide quantitative results interpretable in the context of well-characterized normative data.

There are several methods for the determination of circulating diphtheria toxin antibodies. Only protective toxin-neutralizing antibodies inhibit diphtheria toxin activity in animals or in cell culture, whereas neutralizing and nonneutralizing antibodies can be detected by in vitro methods. In vivo toxin neutralization assays compare the dose of diphtheria toxin antibodies necessary to protect a rabbit or guinea pig against the erythrogenic effect with the dose of a standard preparation of diphtheria antitoxin.[8] In vitro assays are based on the capability of serum containing antidiphtheria toxin antibodies to neutralize the cytopathic effect of the toxin on the tissue culture system. Both of these neutralization assays are considered to be gold standards. Alternative methods for the measurement of antidiphtheria antibodies include ELISA and passive hemagglutination assays. Both are quantitative and reproducible, and so are useful for measuring response to immunization. However, because the ELISA and passive hemagglutination assays detect both neutralizing and nonneutralizing antibodies, the results are less accurate for predicting protection. Commercial ELISA assays can detect IgG anti-diphtheria toxin antibodies but correlate poorly with toxin neutralization assays, particularly for sera containing less than 0.1 IU/ml of diphtheria toxin antibodies. Passive hemagglutination assays are performed using turkey, chicken, horse or sheep erythrocytes, sensitized by diphtheria toxin. These assays also lack sensitivity for sera containing less than 0.1 IU of diphtheria toxin antibodies. For all assays, international reference standards for diphtheria toxin antibodies are available. Primary immunizations in infancy induce protective levels of diphtheria toxin antibodies (≥ 0.01 IU/ml) in over 97% of infants. Ten days after booster vaccination there is typically a 5–10-fold increase in the levels of antibodies. Levels of 0.01–0.09 IU/ml represent some degree of protection, 0.1 IU/ml reflects full protection, and levels greater than 1.0 IU/ml provide long-term protection.

Similar to the methods for diphtheria anti-toxin antibodies, the most reliable method for determining tetanus anti-toxin levels is a mouse neutralization assay. ELISA and hemagglutination assays may be used, with the same caveats discussed above.[9] Interpretation is identical to that of anti-diphtheria toxin results.

HIB conjugate vaccine induces anti-PRP (capsular polyribositol phosphate) antibodies, which may be measured by either radioantigen-binding assays or ELISA. These assays are commercially available and accurate. Based upon epidemiologic studies, an antibody level of 0.15 μg/ml is protective, and post-immunization responses of ≥ 1 μg/ml are considered indicative of long-term immunity.[10]

Live viral vaccines (e.g. oral polio, mumps/measles/rubella and varicella) should never be used for the evaluation of suspected immunodeficiency because they may cause disseminated infection in an immunocompromised host.

It is also important to measure antibody responses to T-independent antigens, such as pneumococcal and meningococcal polysaccharide vaccines, that activate B cells even in the absence of T cells. There is little or no response to T-independent antigens in individuals less than 2 years of age, and the usual adult magnitude of response is not achieved in individuals under 5 years of age. Lack of response to polysaccharide antigens is correlated with a deficiency of IgG_2 and IgG_4 in some patient populations.[11] A variety of assays may be used to measure pneumococcal antibodies. In the older radioimmunoassay (RIA) method, serum is incubated with radiolabeled capsular polysaccharide, and antigen–antibody complexes are precipitated with ammonium sulfate and separated by centrifugation. The radioactivity of the resulting pellet is measured and results are reported in nanograms of antibody nitrogen/ml.[12] The protective antibody level is 200–300 ng of antibody nitrogen/ml; normal healthy adults usually develop >800 ng antibody nitrogen/ml 3–4 weeks after immunization.[13] The major limitation of this method is that it measures antibodies to type-specific polysaccharides as well as antibodies to cell-wall C-polysaccharide, although the latter does not confer protection. Newer ELISA assays incorporate a preabsorption step with C-polysaccharide and then measure type-specific IgG antibodies in comparison to a Food and Drug Administration reference serum.[14] One limitation of these assays is the lack of information about IgM antibodies that may play a role in protection. The protective antibody level is estimated to be 0.15 μg/ml.[15]

Response to bacteriophage φX174 and keyhole-limpet hemocyanin

The evaluation of ability to form antibody in patients on γ-globulin replacement therapy requires special consideration because these individuals are passively receiving antibodies to many common vaccine antigens. Neoantigens such as bacteriophage φX174[16] or keyhole-limpet hemocyanin (KLH)[17] are useful for this purpose as there is no natural exposure to them. Both vaccines have been used safely in immunocompromised hosts. IgM and secondary IgG responses can be measured by ELISA; in the case of φX174, clearance of bacteriophage from blood can also be measured.

Quantification of B lymphocytes

B cells comprise 10–20% of the total lymphocytes circulating in peripheral blood, and are usually measured by flow cytometry using an antibody to cell surface antigens. Because B-cell surface antigens appear and disappear in an orderly sequence as they differentiate, flow cytometry can also yield information about the maturity of B lymphocytes. Pre-B cells can be identified in the bone marrow and peripheral blood as cells containing cytoplasmic μ chains without surface immunoglobulin and by the presence of specific surface markers (e.g. CD10). Mature B lymphocytes express specific markers, including CD19, CD20 and CD21, as well as surface IgM and IgD. If a delay between sample collection and processing is anticipated, it is imperative that a normal control specimen be obtained simultaneously and sent to the laboratory for parallel analysis. Although not used as a primary mode of diagnosis, immunohistochemical staining for B lymphocytes in relevant biopsy specimens (e.g. rectal mucosa, duodenum, bronchi) may be helpful in establishing or supporting the diagnosis of immunodeficiency.

In vitro assessment of B-lymphocyte function

In vitro studies of B-cell immune function are used primarily in the research setting to identify cellular defects causing impaired antibody synthesis. These tests evaluate B-cell proliferation, secretion of antibody and isotype switching. In addition, the ability of T cells to provide help for B-cell differentiation can be assessed.

Purified B cells are placed in tissue culture and stimulated with mitogens (e.g. formalin-fixed *Staphylococcus aureus* Cowan strain, SAC), antibodies directed against surface molecules (e.g. anti-IgM antibody) and/or cytokines. The rate of cell proliferation can be assessed by measuring ^{3}H-thymidine incorporation in stimulated and resting cells. The same stimuli (often used in combination, such as SAC plus IL-2) can also induce the secretion of immunoglobulin, and the concentrations of individual immunoglobulin isotypes in the culture supernatant can be measured by ELISA (Fig. 122.1).

Cell-mixing experiments allow for evaluation of the helper T-lymphocyte function to support antibody synthesis. Activated T cells (after stimulation with mitogen or anti-CD3 antibody) are

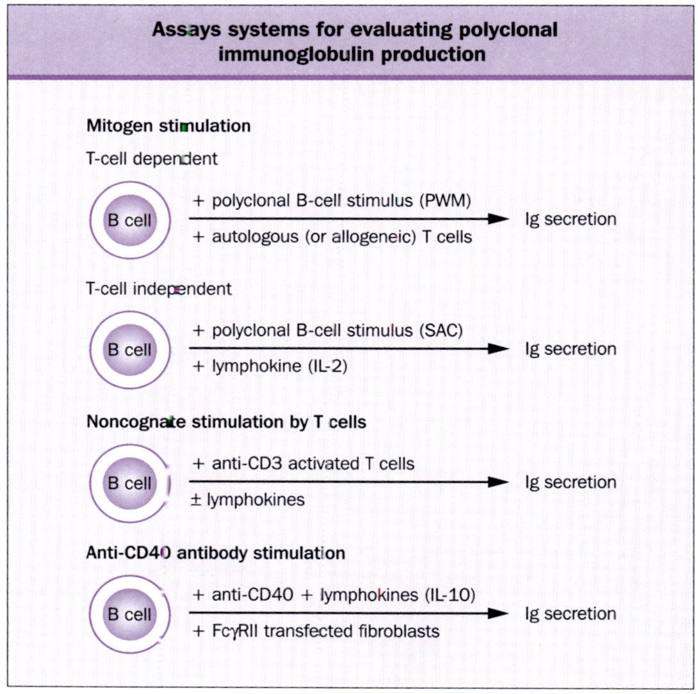

Fig. 122.1 Assay systems for evaluating polyclonal immunoglobulin production. The mitogen stimulation assays are technically the simplest to perform and can be designed to evaluate immunoglobulin production in a T cell-dependent and T cell-independent assay system. The noncognate activation by T cells is particularly useful to evaluate T helper cell function for immunoglobulin production. The anti-CD40 stimulation model enables evaluation of (T cell signal-dependent) isotype switch and allows viable B cells to be maintained in culture for up to several weeks.

mixed with purified B cells. B lymphocytes proliferate and secrete IgG, IgA and IgM when cultured in the presence of T lymphocytes and pokeweed mitogen. B lymphocytes, cultured in the presence of anti-CD40 or soluble CD40 ligand, secrete IgG almost exclusively; they secrete IgM and IgA if exposed to IL-10; and they secrete IgE if exposed to IL-4.[18] Measurement of B-cell proliferation and immunoglobulin secretion in response to a variety of stimuli and in the presence or absence of T lymphocytes may help to distinguish between intrinsic defects in B lymphocytes and defective helper T-lymphocyte function.

Identification of gene defects

The gene defects responsible for many primary immunodeficiency diseases have been identified (Chapters 34, 35) and molecular genetic techniques offer an exciting opportunity to confirm specific diagnoses. Identification of a mutation may allow genetic counseling for prenatal diagnosis, carrier detection and risk of recurrence. Increased precision in diagnosis will undoubtedly also lead to better delineation of the clinical expression of primary immunodeficiency diseases. The principles of mutation analysis are described in Chapter 125 and the importance of this diagnostic approach is illustrated by the following case.

A 16 month-old boy with a history of recurrent upper and lower respiratory infections was evaluated for immunodeficiency. Serum IgG, IgA or IgM were undetectable by nephelometry and he had less than 1% B lymphocytes in peripheral blood. A presumptive diagnosis of X-linked agammaglobulinemia was made on the basis of severe panhypogammaglobulinemia and the absence of peripheral blood B lymphocytes in a young male child. Several years later, the gene for X-LA was identified, the patient's blood was submitted for mutational analysis but no mutations were identified. Additional phenotypic studies revealed a normal number of pro-B cells but no pre-B cells. Further molecular analysis identified a homozygous splice mutation in the BLNK gene that encodes a cytoplasmic adapter protein essential for signal transduction after antigen cross-links immunoglobulin on the B lymphocyte surface.[19] The BLNK gene is not on the X chromosome, and the patient was given accurate information about the autosomal recessive nature of the mutation and the very low risk of clinical disease for his immediate offspring.

ANALYSIS OF T LYMPHOCYTES AND CELL-MEDIATED IMMUNITY

T lymphocytes have a central role in many phases of the immune response. They are the effector cells of cell-mediated immunity and they secrete cytokines that regulate every aspect of humoral and cell-mediated immune responses. There are two general approaches to the evaluation of T cells: measurement of number and measurement of function. Each has limitations. Numbers of total T lymphocytes ($CD3^+$) and individual T lymphocyte subsets ($CD4^+$, $CD8^+$) are easily measured by flow cytometry (Chapter 121). However, although the quantification of T-lymphocyte populations provides valuable information, cell surface markers do not always correlate with cellular function. For example, CD4 'helper' T lymphocytes are functionally diverse. Some CD4 cells secrete cytokines (e.g. IL-4 and IL-6) that drive B-cell proliferation and differentiation to immunoglobulin-secreting plasma cells; some CD4 cells secrete cytokines (e.g. IL-10) that suppress immunoglobulin synthesis; and some CD4 cells secrete cytokines (IL-2, interferon-γ) that stimulate the proliferation and function of CD8 cytotoxic T lymphocytes and natural killer cells. As a result, in most cases assessment of T lymphocytes requires the measurement of T-cell number *and* T-cell function. Standard laboratory methods for assessing T-lymphocyte function include measurement of in vitro lymphoproliferative (LPA) responses to mitogens and antigens as well as in vitro cytotoxic function. These tests are limited by the requirement for specialized laboratories, the need to rapidly deliver viable cells to those laboratories, and the wide variation observed among normal individuals. One other method, measurement of delayed-type hypersensitivity responses, requires no laboratory facilities but has not been well standardized.

Delayed-type hypersensitivity skin tests

Delayed-type hypersensitivity (DTH) skin tests may be used as a screen for T-lymphocyte function and as a means of detecting prior exposure or immunity to specific pathogens (e.g. *Mycobacterium tuberculosis*). Reagents are widely available and the tests are easily applied by the clinician. Recall antigen extracts are injected intradermally or pressed into the skin epicutaneously with a pronged applicator. Erythema and induration are recorded 24 and 48 hours later, and are the result of the accumulation of Langerhans cells, CD4 lymphocytes and macrophages, and the release of vasoactive mediators, with subsequent leakage of serum proteins into the tissue. If properly performed, DTH skin test results correlate well with other measures of T-cell function.[20]

The clinical significance of DTH skin testing is strongly dependent upon antigen potency and standardization, the number of skin tests performed and injection technique. Results obtained using poorly standardized or outdated extracts, or those not intended for DTH testing, may be inconclusive or misleading. In general, because the positive response rate of even the best recall antigens is only 60–70% in normal populations, multiple skin tests should be used in evaluating T-cell function.[21,22] Only a few reagents have been standardized and licensed for DTH skin testing. These include candida, tetanus toxoid, mumps, tuberculin, coccidioidin and histoplasmin. The choice of reagent is made depending partly on the history of prior exposure by immunization (e.g. tetanus, mumps) or environment (e.g. candida, tuberculin). For the purposes of evaluating immune function, the former are often the most useful as the exposure can be controlled and the subject can be immunized as necessary prior to testing (Table 122.2). Candida is useful because of ubiquitous exposure, but coccidioidin and histoplasmin are restricted to endemic regions of infection, and only a small percentage of the US population has been sensitized to tuberculin. Intradermal injection of antigen is preferred because of its more reliable delivery. The amount of antigen delivered by epicutaneous application is affected by the nature of the subject's skin and the application technique, and for these reasons epicutaneous application should be avoided. Dinitrochlorobenzene (DNCB), a powerful primary sensitizer, can be used without previous sensitization; however,

Reagents for delayed-hypersensitivity tests

Antigen	Source	Concentration for test
Candida albicans	Candin® ALK Laboratories	Calibrated by manufacturer by testing in normal adults; use undiluted
Mumps	MSTA® Connaught	40 CFU/ml
Tetanus toxoid	Tetanus toxoid[a] USP (fluid), Connaught	0.8 Lfu/ml, dilute tetanus toxoid USP 1:10 in 0.03% sterile human albumin in 0.9% NaCl with phenol
Tuberculin, purified protein derivative	Tubersol®,[b] Connaught	50 Tu/ml

[a] Tetanus toxoid USP (fluid) is not the same product as tetanus toxoid adsorbed for immunization.
[b] Should not be administered to individuals with previous positive tuberculin skin test.

Table 122.2 Useful reagents for delayed-type hypersensitivity tests.

KEY CONCEPTS

Evaluation of T-lymphocyte function

- Quantification of T cells and T-cell subsets is useful, but does not always predict function.
- Delayed-type hypersensitivity skin tests evaluate in vivo T-cell function but have a significant rate of false negative results.
- In vitro tests of T lymphocyte function require specialized laboratory facilities.
- Lymphoproliferative assays are best used as qualitative measures of T-lymphocyte function, i.e. function absent or present.

CLINICAL PEARLS

Causes of cutaneous anergy

- T-cell dysfunction
  - HIV infection
  - Primary immunodeficiency
  - Secondary immunodeficiency
- Infections
  - Fever
  - Leukocytosis
- Malnutrition
- Atopic dermatitis
- Malignancy
- Immunosuppressive therapy
  - Corticosteroids
- Age
  - Infancy
  - Advanced age
- Collagen vascular disease
- Other
  - Uremia
  - Anemia
  - Sarcoidosis

this substance has generally fallen into disfavor because severe cutaneous reactions may occur. Finally, under investigational protocols, keyhole-limpet hemocyanin (KLH) has been used as an antigen to which most subjects have had no previous exposure. In fact, DTH, antibody and lymphoproliferative responses can each be measured after primary and booster immunizations with KLH.

DTH skin tests are best used as a qualitative measure of T-cell function. Quantitative measurements are possible, but because they require flawlessly reproducible technique and cumbersome scoring systems they are not clinically useful. It should also be emphasized that DTH reagents may induce non-T-cell-dependent inflammation, such as immediate hypersensitivity or arthus reactions, but these are usually distinguished from delayed-type skin responses by their early onset and relatively brief duration. If necessary, a punch biopsy specimen can be obtained for pathologic examination to confirm the presence of a DTH response.

Anergy – defined as the lack of response to multiple recall antigens – is associated with a wide range of clinical disorders.[23] One of the limitations of DTH skin testing is the high percentage of false negative results among those patients likely to be evaluated, including infants and hospitalized patients with chronic illnesses. For example, the majority of immunologically normal infants under the age of 12 months will not react to candida or tetanus antigens, either because of lack of prior exposure to those specific antigens or because of immunologic immaturity.[24] Thus, positive delayed-type hypersensitivity reactions should be considered indicative of grossly intact cell-mediated immunity, but a negative test should not, by itself, be considered diagnostic of cell-mediated immune dysfunction.

Quantification of T cells

T-cell quantification is useful for the management of HIV-infected patients and for evaluating patients with suspected immunodeficiency. The method of choice for enumerating lymphocyte populations in peripheral blood is flow cytometry. This technique, described in detail in Chapter 121, involves incubating blood cells with fluorochrome-conjugated monoclonal antibodies directed against lineage-specific cell surface proteins. The fluorescence of individual cells is quantified from which the percentage of lymphocytes bearing the specific cell surface protein in question can be reported. Flow cytometry can be adapted to quantify virtually any cell surface antigen for which there is a monoclonal antibody. By staining cells with several antibodies, each conjugated to a different fluorochrome, functional properties of individual cells may be inferred. For example, this technique can identify naive ($CD45RA^+$) and memory ($CD45RO^+$), or resting ($HLA\text{-}DR^-$) and activated ($HLA\text{-}DR^+$) subsets of $CD4^+$ or $CD8^+$ T lymphocytes. Analysis of lymphocyte subsets is best interpreted in terms of absolute numbers of cells, although most laboratories express data in the form of ratios or percentages.

In vitro assessment of T-cell function

In vitro studies of T-cell function are labor intensive and difficult to standardize, but are useful in the evaluation of selected patients. For example, in young children with a high incidence of anergy to DTH skin tests, proliferation assays are indicated as a functional screen for primary T-cell abnormalities. In addition, T-cell proliferation and cytotoxicity assays can be used to further investigate those anergic patients with clinical evidence of T-cell dysfunction.

T-cell proliferation is required for many aspects of the normal immune response. Proliferation is triggered by activation of the T-cell antigen receptor by a foreign peptide bound to a major histocompatibility complex (MHC) Class I or Class II molecule on the surface of an antigen-presenting cell. The T-cell receptor transduces signals to the nucleus, which causes coordinate gene transcription, cytokine secretion and cell division. The proliferative activity of T cells can be examined by activating peripheral blood lymphocytes with recall antigens such as tetanus toxoid or candida, mitogens such as phytohemagglutinin or concanavalin A, monoclonal antibodies to the T-cell receptor CD3, or irradiated allogeneic lymphocytes.[25] After an incubation period of 3–7 days, depending on the stimulus, cell proliferation is quantified by measuring the incorporation of ^3H-thymidine into DNA. Normal values of T-cell proliferation have a wide distribution, and laboratory-specific normal data must be used in interpreting test results. Generally, these tests are best used as qualitative measures of T lymphocyte function (i.e. function absent or present) because of the wide variation in results among normal subjects, and even among blood samples collected from a single individual on different days or different times of the same day. Results of replicate cultures may be reported as median counts per minute (cpm) or median stimulation index (SI), which is the ratio of cpm in antigen- or mitogen-stimulated cultures divided by the cpm in unstimulated cultures. The SI may be the best method for comparing results among subjects in multicenter trials, with positive results defined as SI > 5.0 for antigen responses and SI >10.0 for mitogen responses. The specific cut-off for SI depends on the type and concentration of antigen and the cell density in culture. The disadvantage of using SI to establish positive or negative results is that for weak responses the SI is very strongly dependent upon the absolute cpm in unstimulated cultures. Small variations in this number may lead to wide variations in SI. As a rule, both cpm and SI should be used to interpret results.

A critical issue in the performance and interpretation of T-lymphocyte function by LPA is the condition of the blood sample.[26] In many cases blood must be transported to a laboratory at a distant site and cells may be subjected to very high or very low ambient temperatures during transit. To minimize this problem, cells should be shipped in well insulated containers and minimum/maximum thermometers should be included. If a delay between sample collection and performance of the assay, or distant transport, is anticipated it is imperative that a blood specimen from a normal individual be included as a control. Even with all of these factors controlled, overnight delay in processing specimens can lead to loss of positive responses.

T-cell cytotoxicity assay

The ability of T cells to kill allogeneic targets is evaluated with an in vitro chromium release assay.[27] T cells from the test subject are sensitized by a 7-day incubation with irradiated (and thus unable to replicate) cells from an unrelated donor. Target cells are prepared from a second aliquot of donor cells by labelling with ^{51}Cr. The sensitized T cells from the test subject are then incubated with the prepared target cells in varying effector to target cell ratios. The cytolytic function of the test cells correlates with the amount of ^{51}Cr that is released into the medium via cell lysis. The percentage of lysis depends upon a number of variables, including the number of target cells. Normal values must be provided by the laboratory performing the test. If target cells express HLA Class I molecules in common with the effector cells, the assay system can also be used to detect cytotoxicity specific for viral antigens expressed by virus-infected target cells (Fig. 122.2).

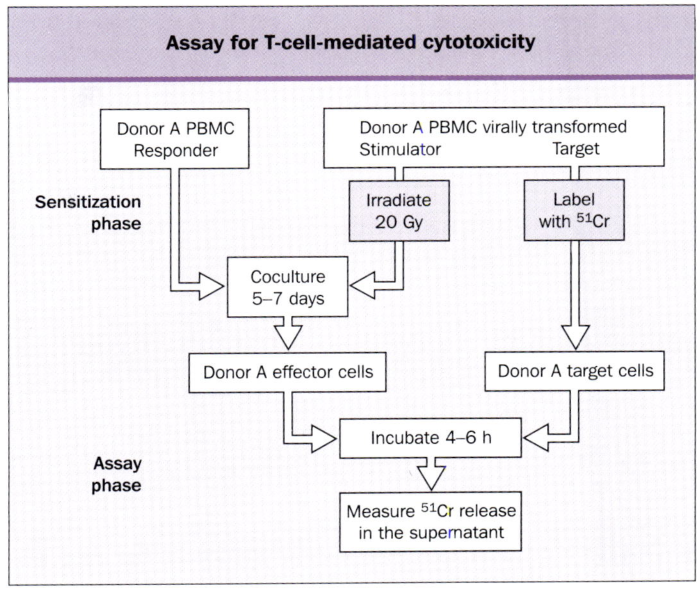

Fig. 122.2 Assay for T cell-mediated cytotoxicity with virally modified (infected) targets demonstrating the sensitization step using irradiated, virally modified stimulator cells in coculture with the responder cells for 5 to 7 days. This procedure is followed by the assay phase with the use of the effector cells generated during the sensitization step. These cells are incubated for 4 to 6 hours with ^{51}Cr-labeled target (virally transformed) cells, and then ^{51}Cr released into the supernatant is measured. This assay typically tests CD8 T cell-mediated cytotoxicity, in which case the effector cells and the stimulator/target cells must share MHC Class I molecules. The test can also be performed with the same allogeneic cells for stimulator and target cells.

Cytokine assays

Many aspects of the immune response are initiated or regulated by networks of cytokines. As our understanding of these relationships expands, it is inevitable that some instances of immune system dysfunction will be linked to defects in cytokine production or receptor function. Examples that have already been reported include the association of IL-2 deficiency with some cases of severe combined immunodeficiency,[28] and the paracrine stimulation of myeloma tumor cells by IL-6.[29] Soluble IL-2 receptor levels in peripheral blood have been used as markers of inflammation in patients with chronic inflammatory diseases such as rheumatoid arthritis. Although none of these have yet attained routine clinical use, it is likely that the measurement of cytokine levels will have a role in patient diagnosis and/or management within the next few years.

Cytokine levels in body fluids such as serum or cerebrospinal fluid can be quantified in some circumstances. However, it is often more useful to stimulate T lymphocytes or mixed populations of mononuclear cells from peripheral blood (B lymphocytes, T lymphocytes and monocytes) with antigens or mitogens, as described for lymphocyte proliferation assays. Culture supernatants are collected at various times after stimulation and cytokine concentrations are measured as the assay output, instead of or in addition to measuring lymphocyte proliferation. Cytokines are most often quantified by the use of monoclonal antibodies in a sandwich enzyme-linked immunosorbent assay.[30]

Measurement of cytokine secretion into culture supernatants provides a measure of the relative magnitude of lymphocyte responses to various stimuli, but it does not provide information on the number or percentage of responding cells. These data can be obtained by using flow cytometry to detect cells containing intracellular cytokines, cells in the G2/S/M phases of the cell cycle, or cells expressing surface activation molecules such as HLA-DR and the high-affinity IL-2 receptor (CD25) (Chapter 121). Alternatively, individual cytokine-secreting lymphocytes can be detected by ELISPOT assay. Nitrocellulose-backed microtiter plates are coated with monoclonal antibody to the cytokine of interest. Serially diluted single-cell suspensions are added to wells and incubated for 6–24 hours. Cells are then removed by washing, and localized spots of secreted cytokine are detected by adding an enzyme-labeled second anti-cytokine antibody followed by substrate then detecting color in the areas of the antibody–cytokine complex.[31]

ASSESSMENT OF NATURAL KILLER CELL FUNCTION

Natural killer cells are large granular lymphocytes that are defined by their cytotoxic capabilities. Unlike CD8 T cells, they do not display clonally specific antigen receptors, although their cytolytic activity is down-regulated by binding to Class I MHC molecules (Chapter 18).[3] These cells may be important for host defense against intracellular pathogens and tumor cells, and may have a role in promoting hematopoiesis. NK-cell number can be estimated by counting cells ($CD3^-$) that bear both CD56 (NKH1) and CD16 (low-affinity IgG receptor) surface proteins. NK-cell activity is usually measured in the laboratory with a chromium release assay that utilizes a particular tumor cell line (K-562) as the target.[33,34] Using antibody-coated target cells the assay can also be adapted to determine antibody-dependent cellular cytotoxicity (ADCC) based on the expression of Fcγ receptors by NK cells (Fig. 122.3). NK cells may be pretreated with IL-2 or interferon to boost cytolytic activity. There is a wide variation in the NK-cell activity of normal subjects, and interpretation must be based upon normative data from the laboratory.

NK cytotoxicity and ADCC

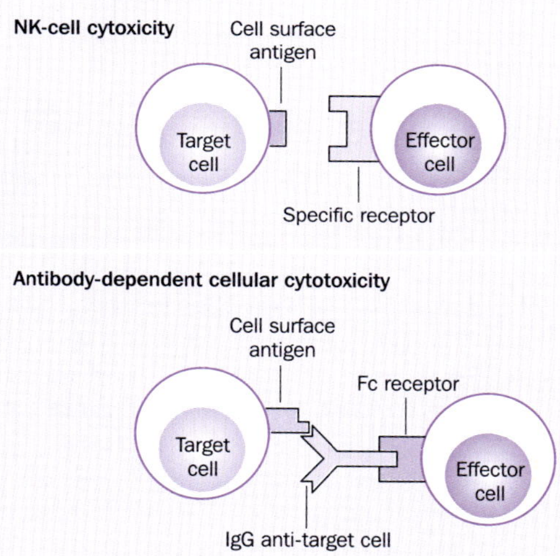

Procedure

- Targets for NK cells are selected cell lines (K562), for ADCC are IgG coated cell lines (P815), for cytokine-enhanced cytotoxicity are usually cell lines (targets for IL-2 induced LAK cells include fresh tumor cells as well as cell lines)
- Cytokine-enhanced killing requires either direct addition (IFN) to assay or effector cell preincubation (IL-2)
- Incubate effector cells with ^{51}Cr-labeled target cells for 4–6 hours
- Measure ^{51}Cr release into the supernatant

Fig. 122.3 NK cytotoxicity and ADCC. The NK effector cell binds directly to the appropriate target cell without prior sensitization and mediates target cell lysis. ADCC depends on immunoglobulin bound to the target cell surface to act as a 'bridge' between the target cell and the effector cell via an Fc receptor on the cytotoxic cell.

ASSESSMENT OF MONOCYTE FUNCTION

Monocytes have numerous functions in the immune response, many of which overlap with the functions of other cell types. Monocytes are phagocytic cells, although their microbicidal capacity is somewhat less than that of neutrophils. Monocytes can process and present antigen, as well as secrete cytokines, prostaglandins, complement components and other mediators of inflammation. Cells of the macrophage lineage are essential for bone and tissue remodeling during growth and development. Absolute monocyte deficiency is thought to be incompatible with life.

Monocyte functions shared with other phagocytic cells, especially neutrophils, include chemotaxis, phagocytosis and intracellular killing. These are usually evaluated in conjunction with the function of neutrophils, because of the difficulty in isolating sufficient numbers of monocytes. Furthermore, no abnormalities of these functions have been described that selectively affect monocytes but not neutrophils.

Functions of monocytes not shared by neutrophils include antigen processing and presentation, and cytokine production. However, many of these are also subserved by other cell types. For example, dendritic cells and B lymphocytes are also highly effective for antigen processing and presentation; complement components are also secreted by hepatocytes; cytokines IL-6, IL-10 and TNF-α are also secreted by T lymphocytes; and IL-12 is also produced by B lymphocytes. One of the unique products of monocytes is neopterin.

Monocyte enrichment/purification

Circulating monocytes in the blood make up 3–8% of the total leukocytes or about 300–600 cells/mm.[3] There are several techniques for isolating highly enriched monocyte populations.[35] They can be isolated from whole blood by density gradient centrifugation in slightly hyperosmotic solutions, because monocytes have a lower buoyant density than other leukocytes. This isolation method does not perturb monocyte function, and the cell yield is >60% with purity >90%. Other methods purify monocytes by positive selection with monocyte-specific cell surface antigens. For example, this can be accomplished by using magnetic beads coated with monoclonal antibody against the CD14 membrane antigen. During a short incubation period, monocytes bind to the anti-CD14-coated magnetic beads, and complexes of beads and monocytes can be isolated using a magnet. The same monoclonal antibody can be used to sort cells by flow cytometry. Both methods select populations of high purity, but yield may vary and be low. More importantly, positive selection methods carry the risk that binding a cell surface receptor will alter cell function. In fact, CD14 is the receptor for bacterial lipopolysaccharide and cross-linking CD14 can activate the cell, inducing oxidative metabolism and cytokine secretion. Monocytes can be purified by negative selection techniques, in which magnetic beads are coated with antibodies against all leukocytes except monocytes, or by similar flow cytometry-based techniques. In these methods there is no concern that monocytes can be activated by the selection process. However, the purity of the final product depends on whether the antibody cocktail contains a sufficient variety of antibodies to remove all other cell populations, and is thus usually less than that of positively selected cells.

Antigen processing and presentation

Monocytes function as antigen-processing cells by ingesting foreign particles, degrading proteins and presenting antigenic peptides via constitutively expressed cell surface Class I and II MHC molecules. Monocytes generally do not express high levels of Class II MHC molecules unless they are activated by interferon-γ and, to a lesser extent, by GM-CSF, IL-4 or IL-13. In contrast, IL-10 decreases Class II MHC expression. Class I and Class II MHC molecules on the monocyte surface can be measured by flow cytometry. There are diseases in which Class I or Class II MHC antigens are not expressed on leukocytes (bare lymphocyte syndrome). However, the lack of histocompatibility antigen expression is not an exclusive property of the monocyte, and these diseases can be diagnosed by testing the more abundant lymphocyte populations in peripheral blood.

Research protocols are available to assess antigen processing and presentation Freshly purified monocytes can be incubated with antigen, excess antigen can be removed by washing, and the 'antigen-pulsed' monocytes can be then added to the purified HLA-matched T lymphocytes or T-lymphocyte cell lines. The adequacy of antigen presentation is assessed by quantifying IL-2 production and/or the proliferation of antigen-specific T cells.[36] Presentation of antigen via Class I MHC can be assessed by infecting the monocytes with a relevant virus or transfecting an antigen into the monocytes. These 'endogenous' antigens are then presented on cell surface MHC-I molecules. The peptide-bearing monocytes are labeled with ^{51}Cr and then used as targets for antigen-specific cytotoxic CD8 T-cell clones, in which case the assay measures the cytotoxicity of the ^{51}Cr-labeled monocytes. These tests are not available in commercial laboratories.

Cytokine and neopterin production

Activated monocytes secrete a variety of cytokines. Cytokine production can be assessed by adding microbial antigens such as candida or tuberculin to mixed populations of T lymphocytes and monocytes. Antigen-specific T lymphocytes secrete cytokines (e.g. IFN-γ) that activate monocytes to produce cytokines. Alternatively, bacterial lipopolysaccharide directly actives monocytes. In either case, monocyte-derived cytokines (IL-1, IL-6, IL-8, IL-12, IL-18, GM-CSF, TNF-α, TGF-β) released into culture supernatants can be measured by ELISA. One clinical application of cytokine induction assays is the measurement of monocyte function in HIV infection:[37] TNF-α production has been most useful for this purpose. Other monocyte-derived cytokines of clinical interest include IL-8, a chemotactic factor for neutrophils and lymphocytes that has been implicated in the pathogenesis of the adult respiratory distress syndrome, and IL-18, a cytokine that stimulates IFN-γ production by T lymphocytes.[38,39] Recently, deficiencies of IL-12 production and in the expression of the IFN-γ receptor on monocytes have been identified in individuals with disseminated bacille Calmette–Guérin (BCG) and disseminated *Mycobacterium avium* infections.[40–43]

Neopterin is one of the unique products of monocytes. Neopterin is derived from guanosine triphosphate within the biosynthetic pathway of tetrahydrobiopterin, an essential cofactor for tyrosine and tryptophan hydroxylation that plays an important role in the biosynthesis of catecholamines and serotonin.[44] In monocytes, large amounts of neopterin are accumulated at the expense of biopterin derivatives owing to a constitutive deficiency of pyruvoyltetrahydropterin synthase. The exact role of neopterin in the immune system remains obscure, but it is released from monocytes after in vitro incubation with IFN-γ. Commercial assays are available for measuring neopterin in serum, urine and cerebrospinal fluid. Neopterin levels are elevated in patients with viral, bacterial or protozoal infections, rheumatoid arthritis, systemic lupus erythematosus, acute graft-versus-host disease, AIDS and certain malignancies. In infections, neopterin levels precede the occurrence of detectable antibodies to the pathogen. As it is a unique product of monocytes, neopterin concentrations in body fluids can be regarded as an indirect estimate of monocyte activation.[45]

> **KEY CONCEPTS**
>
> **Evaluation of monocyte function**
>
> - Monocyte chemotaxis, phagocytosis and intracellular killing are usually evaluated in conjunction with the function of neutrophils.
> - Antigen processing and presentation by monocytes can be assessed.
> - Induced cytokine assays quantitate secretion of cytokines by monocytes after activation with IFN-γ. Relevant cytokines include: IL-1, IL-6, IL-8, IL-12, IL-18, TNF-α, GM-CSF, TGF-β.
> - Neopterin, a unique product of activated monocytes, can be measured as an indirect estimate of monocyte activation.

Chemotaxis and adherence

Chemotaxis, or directed cellular motion, occurs when monocyte surface receptors bind any of a number of stimuli, including complement components (C3a and C5a), leukotriene B_4, IL-8, and a variety of bacterial products. Following activation, mechanical cytoskeletal changes propel the cell toward the source of the stimulus. Impaired chemotaxis may be associated with the absence of chemoattractant substances or corresponding receptors, defects in cell adhesion molecules, cytoskeletal abnormalities or extrinsic inhibitors.[46]

Functional assays of monocyte chemotaxis or adherence can be performed in vitro or in vivo, but are difficult to interpret because of the inherent variability of these tests and the lack of well-standardized normative data. Monocyte chemotaxis can be assessed in vitro with a chemotactic chamber (Boyden technique) or the double microfilter radioimmunoassay using ^{51}Cr-labeled cells. Isolated monocytes are placed in the upper chamber, separated by a Millipore filter from a chemotactic stimulus placed in the lower chamber. The usual chemotactic stimuli are human serum to which endotoxin, zymosan, antigen–anti-body complexes have been added to cause the release of C3a and C5a, or the bacterial peptide f-met-leu-phe. The number of cells migrating toward the chemotactic stimulus is assessed by microscopy of the lower side of the filter. Some laboratories perform an agarose well test, which may be more reproducible.[47] Three wells are cut in the gel, one for the cell suspension, one for a chemoattractant and one for a buffer control. After incubation, the distance of directed cellular migration toward the chemoattractant and control wells is measured and compared with data from simultaneous normal controls. The Rebuck skin window is an in vivo procedure to assess the morphology and motility of cells in the inflammatory response. The skin is abraded superficially with a scalpel blade over an area of 4 mm^2, a cover slip is placed over the site, and then changed at 30-minute intervals for 24 hours. The number of leukocytes migrating and adhering to the cover slip is counted. An initial influx of polymorphonuclear cells occurs within 2 hours, and monocytes migrate within 12 hours.[48] Monocyte chemotactic defects have been observed in normal neonates, Wiskott–Aldrich syndrome and Chediak– Higashi syndrome (Chapter 37).

Phagocytosis

Phagocytosis and the associated oxidative burst are essential for the destruction of pathogenic microorganisms by monocytes. Defects in monocyte phagocytosis are usually secondary to infection, drugs, alcohol, and systemic diseases such as systemic lupus erythematosus and monocytic leukemia. Primary defects of phagocytic uptake are rare. Patients with leukocyte adhesion deficiency type I and with actin dysfunction syndrome show defects in particulate-mediated phagocytosis. More commonly, phagocytic defects are the result of opsonic defects rather than intrinsic abnormalities of the leukocytes.

Phagocytic assays measure the ability of monocytes and/or neutrophils to recognize and ingest particles or microbial agents. Particles that are coated (opsonized) with antibody and/or complement are engulfed with much greater avidity than uncoated particles because phagocytes have receptors for the Fc portion of IgG and for C3b. Latex-coated particles, as well as antibody and/or complement-coated microbial targets, are traditionally used to test phagocytosis. In these assays monocytes or neutrophils are incubated with their targets under conditions that promote their interaction (e.g. gentle rotation). After incubation, targets not associated with phagocytic cells are removed by washing. If radiolabeled targets are used, phagocytosis may be assessed by measuring the radioactivity associated with phagocytic cells (the assumption is that targets that adhere to phagocytic cells have been or will be phagocytosed) and expressing the result as percentage radioactivity ingested.[49] One can visually count the percentage of cells with ingested targets and express the result as a phagocytic index (percentage of phagocytes with ingested particles).[50] The phagocytic index can also be calculated by using fluorescein-labeled targets and detecting phagocytes with or without ingested targets in a flow cytometer.[51] Phagocytic assays are used predominantly in research: there are no standardized methods of performing them and no available reference values except those established for specific methods in individual laboratories.

Tests for monocyte/neutrophil phagocytic and microbicidal activity

Activated monocytes produce a number of oxidative microbicidal compounds through the activation of the enzyme NADPH oxidase.[52] Other antimicrobial compounds, such as lysozyme and proteolytic enzymes are preformed in the granules and released on phagocytosis of particles.[53] Deficiencies of several of these substances have been linked to decreased microbial killing and clinical immunodeficiency.

The respiratory burst, generated by a group of proteins collectively known as NADPH oxidase, can be readily measured in the laboratory using the NBT (nitroblue tetrazolium) test.[54] A fresh sample of monocytes is incubated with yellow NBT and then activated with either latex particles or phorbol ester (PMA). Monocytes with a normal respiratory burst will reduce NBT to formazan, a blue product that precipitates within cells and can be detected by light microscopy. This test can be performed with a few drops of blood on a microscope slide.[55] It is essential that fresh blood specimens from normal controls are processed with each test, because monocytes are labile and oxidative activity deteriorates rapidly after blood is collected from the patient. NADPH oxidase activity can also be estimated by measuring the spontaneous release of light (chemiluminescence). This light is produced by oxygen metabolites produced by the respiratory burst in activated phagocytes.[56] Oxidative burst may also be assessed by flow cytometry using cells loaded with a hydrogen peroxide-sensitive dye, dihydrorhodamine. This test may be used to follow allogeneic granulocyte survival after transfusion or allogeneic stem cell transplantation. It it also sensitive and accurate in diagnosing patients with chronic granulomatous disease (CGD) and carriers of X-linked CGD (Chapter 121).

Measurement of specific granule components may be warranted in patients with decreased monocyte function in whom other screening tests are not diagnostic. Leukocyte glucose-6-phosphate dehydrogenase deficiency has been associated with decreased leukocyte microbicidal activity[57] and this enzyme is readily measured in the clinical laboratory. Special staining techniques for lactoferrin, vitamin B_{12}-binding proteins and myeloperoxidase can also be performed in some laboratories. Chediak–Higashi syndrome, a disease in which monocytes have a defect in migration, chemotaxis and intracellular killing, is associated with striking giant granules in peripheral leukocytes and blood marrow.

The ability of cells to phagocytose and kill microorganisms can be assessed by mixing fixed ratios of white blood cells and viable bacteria. At various times thereafter aliquots of the cell suspension are removed and viable bacteria are quantified by culture.[58] These tests are best performed in a research laboratory, and always require the simultaneous testing of neutrophils from a normal individual as a control.

REFERENCES

1. Check IJ, Papadea C. Immunoglobulin quantitation. In: Rose NR, Conway de Macario E, Folds JD, Lane HC, Nakamura RM (ed) Manual of Clinical Laboratory Immunology, 5th edn. Washington DC, ASM Press, 1997.
2. Jolliff CR, Cost KM, Stivrins PC, et al. Reference intervals for serum IgG, IgA, IgM, C3 and C4 as determined by rate nephelometry. Clin Chem 1982;28:126.
3. Oxelius V. Chronic infections in a family with hereditary deficiency of IgG2 and IgG4. Clin Exp Immunol 1974;17:19.
4. South MA, Warwick WJ, Wollheim FA, et al. The IgA system. III. IgA levels in the serum and saliva of pediatric patients – evidence for a local immunological system. J Pediatr 1967;71:645.
5. Drenth JPH, Haagsman CJ, vander Meer JWH, et al. Hyperimmunoglobulinemia D and periodic fever syndrome: the clinical spectrum in a series of 50 patients. Medicine 1994;73:133.
6. Ledue TB, Garfin DE. Immunofixation and immunoblotting. In: Rose NR, Conway de Macario E, Folds JD, Lane HC, Nakamura RM (eds)

Manual of Clinical Laboratory Immunology, 5th edn. Washington DC, ASM Press. 1997.
7. Auf de Maur C, Hodel M, Nydegger UE, et al. Age dependency of ABO histo-blood group antibodies: reexamination of an old dogma. Transfusion 1993;33:915.
8. Efstratiou A, Maple PA. WHO Manual for the laboratory diagnosis of diphtheria. No. ICP-EPI 038(C). Geneva, World Health Organization, 1994.
9. Melville-Smith ME, Seagrott VA. Watkins JT. A comparison of enzyme-linked immunosorbent assay (ELISA) with the toxin neutralization test in mice as a method for the estimation of tetanus anti-toxin in human sera. J Biol Standards 1983;11:137.
10. Peltola H, Käeyhty H, Sivonen A, et al. *Haemophilus influenzae* type b capsular polysaccharide vaccine in children: a double-blind field study of 100,000 vaccines in children 3 months to 5 years of age in Finland. Pediatrics 1977;60:730.
11. Umetsu DT, Ambrosino DM, Quinti I, et al. Recurrent sinopulmonary infections and impaired antibody responses to bacterial capsular polysaccharide antigen in children with selective IgG-subclass deficiency. N Engl J Med 1985;313:1247.
12. Schiffman G, Douglas RM, Bonner MJ, et al. A radioimmunoassay for immunologic phenomena in pneumococcal disease and for the antibody response to pneumococcal vaccines – I. Methods for the radioimmunoassay of anticapsular antibodies and comparison with other techniques. J Immunol Meth 1980;33:133.
13. Landesman SH, Schiffman G. Assessment of the antibody response to pneumococcal vaccine in high risk populations. Rev Infect Dis 1981;35S:184.
14. Koskela M. Serum antibodies to pneumococcal C polysaccharide in children: response to acute pneumococcal otitis media and vaccination. Pediatr Infect Dis J 1987;6:519.
15. Rennels MB, Edwards KM, Keyserling HL, et al. Safety and immunogenicity of heptavalent pneumococcal vaccine conjugated to CRM_{197} in United States infants. Pediatrics 1998;101:604.
16. Pyun KH, Ochs HD, Wedgewood RD, et al. Human antibody responses to bacteriophage φX-174: sequential induction of IgM and IgG subclass antibody. Clin Immunol Immunopathol 1989;152:5957.
17. Curtis JE, Hersh EM, Harris JE, et al. The human primary immune response to keyhole limpet haemocyanin: interrelationships of delayed hypersensitivity. Clin Exp Immunol 1970;6:473.
18. Nonoyama S, Farrington M, Ishida H, et al. Activated B cells from patients with common variable immunodeficiency proliferate and synthesize immunoglobulin. J Clin Invest 1993;92:1282.
19. Minegishi Y, Rohrer J, Coustan-Smith E, et al. An essential role for BLNK in human B cell development. Science 1999;286:1954.
20. Gordon EH, Krouse HA, Kinney JL, et al. Delayed cutaneous hypersensitivity in normals: choice of antigens and comparison to in vitro assays of cell-mediated immunity. J Allergy Clin Immunol 1983;72:487.
21. Palmer DL, Reed WP. Delayed hypersensitivity skin testing. I. Response rates in a hospitalized population. J Infect Dis 1974;130:132.
22. Grossman J, Baum J, Gluckman J, et al. The effect of aging and acute illness on delayed hypersensitivity. J Allergy Clin Immunol 1975;55:268.
23. Palmer DL, Reed WP. Delayed hypersensitivity skin testing. II. Clinical correlates and anergy. J Infect Dis 1974;130:138.
24. Kniker WT, Anderson CT, McBryde JL, et al. Multitest CMI for standardized measurement of delayed cutaneous hypersensitivity and cell-mediated immunity. Normal values and proposed scoring system for healthy adults in the USA. Ann Allergy 1984;52:75.
25. James SP. Measurement of proliferative responses of cultured lymphocytes. In: Coligan JE, Kruisbeck AM, Margulies DH, Shevach EM, Strober W (eds) Current Protocols in Immunology. John Wiley & Sons, New York, 1994;pp 7.10.1–7.10.10
26. Weinberg A, Betensky RA, Zhang L, Ray G. Effects of shipment, storage, anticoagulant, and cell separation on lymphocyte proliferation assays for human immunodeficiency virus-infected patients. Clin Diagn Lab Immunol 1998;5:804.
27. Carpenter CB. Lymphocyte-mediated cytotoxicity. In: Rose NR, Friedman H, Fahey JL (eds) Manual of Clinical Laboratory Immunology, 3rd edn. Washington DC, ASM Press, 1986.
28. Weinberg K, Parkman R. Severe combined immunodeficiency due to a specific defect in the production of interleukin-2. N Engl J Med 1990;322:1718.
29. Portier M, Rajzbaum G, Zhang XG, et al. In vivo interleukin 6 gene expression in the tumoral environment in multiple myeloma. Eur J Immunol 1991;21:1759.
30. Aziz N, Nishanian P, Mitsuyasu R, Detels R, Fahey JL. Variables that affect assays for plasma cytokines and soluble activation markers. Clin Diagn Lab Immunol 1999;1:89–95.
31. Czerkinsky C, Andersson G, Ekre HP, et al: Reverse ELISPOT assay for clonal analysis of cytokine production. I. Enumeration of gamma-interferon-secreting cells. J Immunol Meth 1988;110:29.
32. Bakker AB, Wu J, Phillips JH, Lanier LL. NK cell activation: distinct stimulatory pathways counterbalancing inhibitory signals. Hum Immunol 2000;1:18–27.
33. Ortaldo JR, Bonnard GD, Herberman RB. Cytotoxic reactivity of human lymphocytes cultured in vitro. J Immunol 1977;119:1351.
34. Komiyama A, Kawai H, Yabuhara A, et al. Natural killer cell immunodeficiency in siblings: defective killing in the absence of natural killer cytotoxic factor activity in natural killer and lymphokine-activated killer cytotoxicities. Pediatrics 1990;85:323.
35. Wahl LM, Smith PD. Isolation of monocyte/macrophage populations. In: Coligan JE, Kruisbeck AM, Margulies DH, Shevach EM, Strober W (eds) Current protocols in immunology. John Wiley & Sons, New York, 1995, p 7.6.1.
36. Harding CV. Techniques for studying phagocytic processing of bacteria for Class I or II MHC-restricted antigen recognition by T lymphocytes. Meth Cell Biol 1994;45:307.
37. Wallis RS, Lederman HM, Sprintzler J, et al. Measurement of induced cytokines in AIDS clinical trials using whole blood: a preliminary report. Clin Diagn Lab Immunol 1998;5:556.
38. Baggiolini M, Dewald B, Moser B. Interleukin-8 and related chemotactic cytokines-CXC and CC chemokines. Adv Immunol 1994;55:97.
39. Dinarello CA. Interleukin-18. Methods 1999;19:121.
40. Altare F, Lammas D, Revy P, et al. Inherited interleukin 12 deficiency in a child with bacille Calmette–Guérin and *Salmonella enteritidis* disseminated infection. J Clin Invest 1998;102:2035.
41. Fruch DM, Holland SM. Defective monocyte costimulation for IFN-γ production in familial disseminated *Mycobacterium avium* complex infection. J Immunol 1996;157:411.
42. Casanova JL, Ochs H. Interferon-gamma receptor deficiency: an expanding clinical phenotype? J Pediatr 1999;35:543.
43. Dorman SE, Holland SM. Mutation in the signal transducing chain of the interferon gamma receptor and susceptibility to mycobacterial infection. J Clin Invest 1998;101:2364.
44. Nichol CA, Smith GK, Duch DS. Biosynthesis and metabolism of tetrahydrobiopterin and molybdopterin. Annu Rev Biochem 1985;54:729.
45. Wachter H, Fuchs D, Hausen A, et al. Neopterin as a marker for activation of cellular immunity: immunologic basis and clinical application. Adv Clin Chem 1989;27:81.
46. Yang KD, Hill HR. Neutrophil function disorders: pathophysiology, prevention, and therapy. J Pediatr 1991;119:343.
47. Nelson RD, Quie PQ, Simmons RL. Chemotaxis under agarose: a new and simple method for measuring chemotaxis and spontaneous migration of human polymorphonuclear leukocytes and monocytes. J Immunol 1975;115:1650.
48. Rebuck JW, Crowley JH. A method of studying leukocytic functions in vivo. Ann NY Acad Sci 1955;59:757.
49. Cates KL, Marsh KH, Granoff DM. Serum opsonic activity after immunization of adults with *Haemophilus influenzae* type b–diphtheria toxoid conjugate vaccine. Infect Immun 1985;48:183.
50. Winkelstein JA, Drachman RH. Deficiency of pneumococcal serum opsinizing activity in sickle-cell disease. N Engl J Med 1968;279:459.
51. Bassoe CF, Bjerknes R. Phagocytosis by human leukocytes, phagosomal pH and degradation of seven species of bacteria measured by flow cytometry. J Med Microbiol 1985;19:115.
52. Segal AW. The electron transport chain of the microbicidal oxidase of phagocytic cells and its involvement in the molecular pathology of chronic granulomatous disease. J Clin Invest 1989;83:1785.

53. Falloon J, Gallin JI. Neutrophil granules in health and disease. J Allergy Clin Immunol 1986;77:653.
54. Baehner RL, Nathan DG. Quantitative nitroblue tetrazolium test in chronic granulomatous disease. N Engl J Med 1968;278:971.
55. Repine JE, Rasmussen B, White JG. An improved nitroblue tetrazolium test using phorbol myristate acetate-coated coverslips. Am Soc Clin Pathol 1978;71:582.
56. Stephens P, Winston DJ, Van Dyke K. In vitro circulation of opsonic and granulocyte function by luminol-dependent chemiluminescence: utility in patients with severe neutropenia and cellular deficiency states. Infect Immun 1978;22:41.
57. Cooper MR, DeChatelet LR, McCall CE. Complete deficiency of leukocyte glucose-6-phosphate dehydrogenase with defective bacteriocidal activity. J Clin Invest 1972;51:769.
58. Clawson CC, Repine JE. Quantitation of maximal bactericidal capability in human neutrophils. J Lab Clin Med 1986;88:316.

Chapter 123

Assessment of Neutrophil Function

Douglas B. Kuhns

INTRODUCTION

Neutrophils, also known as polymorphonuclear neutrophils (because of their multilobed nucleus) or granulocytes (because of their array of cytoplasmic granules) are major contributors to host defense against invading microorganisms, particularly bacteria and fungi. They are bone marrow-derived, terminally differentiated cells that are no longer capable of cellular division. Neutrophils have a short life span in the circulation ($t_{1/2}$ = 6–8 hours), but probably live an additional 1 or 2 days in the surrounding tissue.[1] Despite this short half-life, neutrophils in the blood are normally maintained between 3000 and 6000 cells/mm^3 and represent from 30 to 50% of the leukocytes found circulating in the peripheral blood (Chapter 22).

Neutrophils have a characteristic and unique morphology. Human neutrophils have a diameter of 10–15 μm and a volume of 346 μm^3. The cytoplasm represents 63% of the cell, the nucleus 21%, the granules 15%, and the mitochondria less than 1%.[2] The nucleus of the mature neutrophil is segmented into three to five lobes. Although the significance of this segmentation is not currently understood, it has been shown that the chromosomes are randomly distributed between the lobes.[3] Neutrophils have large cytoplasmic granules that are heterogeneous in size and shape and contain numerous proteins synthesized during specific stages of neutrophil maturation. It is the large content of myeloperoxidase in the azurophilic granules that gives pus its greenish color. With relatively few mitochondria, neutrophils derive much of their energy from glycolysis, using ample glycogen stores.

There are four pools of neutrophils *in vivo*: the bone marrow pool (~90% of the total), the circulating pool (~3% of the total), the marginated pool (~4% of the total) adherent to the endothelium, and the remainder located in the tissues as exudative or extravasated neutrophils.[4] Neutrophils are produced in the bone marrow and released into the blood and tissues. About 55–60% of the bone marrow is dedicated to the production of neutrophils.[5] Once in the circulation, neutrophils do not return to the marrow. However, circulating cells can exchange with the marginated pool. Elevation of systemic epinephrine stimulates the release of neutrophils from the marginated pool and a doubling of the number of neutrophils in the peripheral circulation.[6] The administration of glucocorticoids results in the mobilization of neutrophils from the bone marrow reserve.[7] The administration of endotoxin can cause a decrease in the number of circulating neutrophils within 30–90 minutes, presumably due to increased margination of neutrophils to the endothelium.[8] Subsequently there is a pronounced neutrophilia at 3–5 hours that is probably due to G-CSF-induced release of neutrophils from the bone marrow stores.[9]

In the peripheral circulation, neutrophils roll along the vascular endothelium, transiently attaching to and detaching from it. This low-affinity adhesion is mediated by the adhesive glycoproteins known as selectins.[10,11] These are lectin-binding proteins expressed on the surface of both neutrophils and vascular endothelial cells. L-selectin (CD62L) is expressed on the surface of neutrophils[12,13] and E-selectin (CD62E) is expressed on the surface of endothelial cells.[14] As the rolling neutrophils near the focus of infection they respond to chemoattractants, e.g. C5a, interleukin-8 (IL-8), platelet-activating factor, leukotrienes, and bacterial formylated peptides generated at the infectious focus, with functional activation of the β_2-integrins.[15] The β_2-integrins are heterodimeric glycoproteins with differing α subunits (CD11a or LFA-1, CD11b or MAC-1, and CD11c or gp150) and a common β_2 subunit (CD18). They are adherence receptors that recognize extracellular matrix proteins and complement factors (CD11b/CD18 = complement receptor type 3 and CD11c/CD18 = complement receptor type 4). Activation of the integrins induces tighter adherence of the neutrophils to vascular endothelial cells and a cessation of rolling. In addition, the neutrophils undergo a dramatic shape change, from the normal spheroid shape with relatively smooth membrane to a flattened triangular shape with ruffled lamellipodia.[16] Homophilic interactions of platelet/endothelial cell adhesion molecule (PECAM or CD31), a member of the immunoglobulin superfamily that is expressed on the surface of neutrophils and at the lateral cell–cell junction of endothelial cells, direct the neutrophil to the cell junction.[17] Neutrophils then detach from the endothelium and migrate through a gap in the vascular endothelium created by the contraction of juxtaposed vascular endothelial cells. Once the neutrophil has migrated out of the lumen of the vasculature and into the extravascular space, it migrates along chemotactic gradients to the focus of the infection.

In the tissue, neutrophils initiate their primary function, the ingestion and killing of bacteria. Phagocytosis requires two distinct stages: adhesion (attachment) and internalization. Neutrophils do not express specific receptors for each specific microorganism. Instead, microorganisms become coated or opsonized with specific immunoglobulins and complement fragments such as C3b and iC3b. Neutrophils recognize these targets using Fc receptors and adhesion molecules, including the β_2-integrins such as CD11b/CD18. Treatment of neutrophils with the chemotactic peptide formyl-methionyl-leucyl-phenylalanine (fMLF), bacterial lipopolysaccharide (LPS) or cytokines (IL-1, GM-CSF etc.) results in increased expression of neutrophil surface receptors (Fc receptors CD11b/CD18, and CD11c/CD18). These receptors act alone or synergistically to enhance the adhesion of neutrophils to antibody- and complement (C3b and iC3b)-coated microorganisms, resulting in increased phagocytosis, respiratory burst activity and degranulation. Zippering of the receptor–ligand interactions promotes the extension of pseudopods around the organism. As the extending pseudopods meet, the membranes fuse, enveloping the microorganism and resulting in the formation of the phagosome.[18] Defects in any quantitative and qualitative aspects of ligand–receptor interaction can impair phagocytic efficiency.

The neutrophil has an extensive array of storage granules that can be defined by the biosynthesis of particular granule proteins at the given stage of neutrophil maturation.[19] Granules are classified into four distinct populations, azurophilic, specific, gelatinase and secretory. Azurophilic granules contain myeloperoxidase, lysozyme, defensins, proteases and the acid hydrolases. Specific granules contain lactoferrin, lysozyme and vitamin B_{12}-binding protein; they also serve as storage pools for CD11b/CD18 and cytochrome b_{558} of the O_2^--generating enzyme NADPH oxidase. The gelatinase granules are a subset of the specific granules that have a high content of gelatinase. The secretory granules are highly mobilizable intracellular vesicles that contain alkaline phosphatase and other surface antigens.

As the phagosome forms, the azurophilic granules fuse with the phagosomal membrane and release their complement of acid hydrolases, defensins and myeloperoxidase, enzymes that can potentiate the digestive and microbcidal activities of the neutrophil, resulting in the formation of the phagolysosome. The secretion of specific and secretory granules is thought to release mediators of inflammation (such as lactoferrin) and mediate the translocation of additional receptors (CD11b/CD18, fMLF receptors and laminin receptors as well as cytochrome b_{558} of the NADPH oxidase) to the plasma membrane. Translocation of these receptors modulates neutrophil adhesion, movement, phagocytosis and respiratory burst activity. Factors that affect signal transduction, metabolic activity, microfilament rearrangement and microtubule assembly regulate the degranulation process.

Accompanying the fusion of the granule to the phagolysosome is the assembly of the multicomponent O_2^- generating enzyme NADPH oxidase, an enzyme complex consisting of at least two cytosolic components,[20] $p47^{phox}$, $p67^{phox}$, and two membrane components,[21,22] $p22^{phox}$ and the cytochrome b_{558}, $gp91^{phox}$. This enzyme reduces molecular O_2 to O_2^- utilizing NADPH generated by the oxidation of glucose through the pentose pathway. O_2^- dismutases either spontaneously, or through the action of superoxide dismutase, to form H_2O_2. In the presence of metal such as Fe^{2+}, H_2O_2 and O_2^- can react to form the highly reactive hydroxyl radical, $OH^{\bullet}$. Alternatively, the azurophilic granule constituent myeloperoxidase catalyzes the formation of hypochlorous acid from H_2O_2 and Cl^-. The combination of reactive oxygen intermediates (ROI), antimicrobial peptides and the degradative lysosomal enzymes results in the ultimate destruction of the microorganism. Excess production of ROI species and the release of lysosomal enzymes can lead to tissue damage and inflammation.

Neutrophils display a diverse array of cellular functions. Abnormalities in these can severely compromise host defense, leading to recurrent bacterial and fungal infections. To localize specific deficiencies of neutrophil function, assays have been developed that mimic these functions both in vivo and in vitro. Often, a preliminary screening of several neutrophil functions is performed to localize deficits and then more vigorous testing of specific function is performed. Assays to assess neutrophil function should address several limitations: the number of cells required for the assay, the type of cell preparation needed (isolated neutrophils versus whole blood), the overall incubation time for the assay, the complexity of the assay and the rapidity of data collection. These issues become more critical if several functional assays are planned concurrently. Because neutrophils cannot be stored or frozen, control neutrophils from a normal volunteer are usually assayed in parallel to validate the results. This generally doubles the number of assays to be performed. In addition, isolation of neutrophils can take 1–2 hours, limiting the time available for functional assays. Fluorescent probes have increased the sensitivity of many of the assays and eliminated the need for radioactive probes. The use of multiwell plates and multiwell plate readers has reduced the number of cells required and has facilitated the collection of data.

KEY CONCEPTS

Generation of reactive oxygen intermediates

The stepwise reduction of O_2 leads to reactive oxygen intermediates and finally to H_2O.

$$\underset{\text{Oxygen}}{O_2} + e^- \rightarrow \underset{\text{Superoxide anion}}{O_2^-} + 2H^+ + e^- \rightarrow \underset{\text{Hydrogen peroxide}}{H_2O_2} + e^- \rightarrow$$

$$\underset{\text{Hydroxyl radical}}{OH^{\bullet}} + OH^- + e^- \rightarrow \underset{\text{Water}}{H_2O} + \tfrac{1}{2}O_2$$

KEY CONCEPTS

Assays of neutrophil function

Because of the time required to isolate neutrophils and their short life span, functional assays should be designed with minimal complexity and rapid data collection

MICROSCOPIC EXAMINATION OF NEUTROPHILS

Clinical indications and implications

A microscopic examination of neutrophils in a peripheral blood smear with a differential stain is useful in the diagnosis of several neutrophil defects. Neutrophils from patients with Chediak–Higashi syndrome exhibit abnormally large, cytoplasmic granules that result from the fusion of azurophilic granules early in neutrophil maturation. Neutrophils from patients with specific granule deficiency are characterized by decreased granularity in the cytoplasm. Specific granule deficiency has recently been shown to be a result of a defect in the CCAAT/enhancer binding protein-ε (CEBP-ε), a member of the leucine zipper family of transcription factors.[23]

Principle and interpretation of laboratory assessment
Blood smears are stained with Wright–Giemsa differential stain or a histochemical stain for myeloperoxidase, such as benzidine dihydrochloride.[24]

ISOLATION OF NEUTROPHILS

Clinical indications and implications
Assays that avoid neutrophil isolation are preferred because of the artifactual preactivation of neutrophils during isolation.[25] However, most assays require isolated neutrophils to eliminate any possible contributions of other leukocytes and blood components. In general, blood should be drawn using either citrate or heparin (10 units/ml) as the anticoagulant and maintained at 20–25°C in polypropylene containers. Most isolation protocols require 1–2 hours to obtain purified neutrophils.

Principle and interpretation of laboratory assessment
Most neutrophil isolation protocols use differences in the cell density as a basis for the separation. The relative densities of blood cells are as follows: erythrocytes > neutrophils and eosinophils > monocytes, lymphocytes and basophils > platelets. Ficoll–Hypaque is a solution of sodium diatrizoate (a dense iodinated molecule) and Ficoll (a polysaccharide) with a density (1.083 g/ml) that falls between that of neutrophils and that of the mononuclear cells. To isolate neutrophils,[26] whole blood is diluted with saline and underlaid with Ficoll–Hypaque. The cells are centrifuged for 30 minutes at 500 *g*. The less dense monocytes, lymphocytes, basophils and platelets remain at the upper interface of the Ficoll–Hypaque, and the denser erythrocytes and neutrophils pass through it and pellet at the bottom. The mononuclear cells are carefully harvested and the remaining Ficoll–Hypaque aspirated. The erythrocyte/neutrophil pellet is resuspended with saline and mixed with 3% dextran. Dextran promotes the formation of rouleaux by the erythrocytes, causing them to sediment rapidly at 1 *g*. The neutrophil-enriched supernatant fluid is harvested from the bulk of the erythrocytes. Contaminating erythrocytes are removed by hypotonic lysis using 0.2% saline. The isotonicity is quickly restored with an equal volume of 1.6% saline. A second hypotonic lysis removes many of the red cell ghosts. In general, $1–2 \times 10^6$ neutrophils can be isolated per milliliter of whole blood from a normal subject with a normal white blood cell count.

A second neutrophil isolation protocol that uses a discontinuous gradient of plasma/Percoll has often been used to minimize the exposure of neutrophils to trace contamination by bacterial lipopolysaccharide (LPS) and reduce neutrophil preactivation.[27] Neutrophils prepared by the plasma/Percoll isolation protocol exhibit reduced fMLF-stimulated O_2^- production. However, treatment of the neutrophils with LPS (10 μg/ml) in the presence of 1% serum (as a source of LPS-binding protein) results in priming of the neutrophils and enhanced O_2^- production after stimulation with fMLF.

NEUTROPHIL ADHERENCE

Clinical indications and implications
The adherence of neutrophils to the endothelium is a prerequisite step to the migration of neutrophils into the tissues. Neutrophils isolated from patients with leukocyte adhesion deficiency type 1 (LAD-1) who lack the common β_2-integrin subunit, CD18, exhibit abnormal adherence to endothelium,[28] and are therefore unable to migrate efficiently into the surrounding tissues, often resulting in marked granulocytosis.[29] Leukocyte adhesion deficiency type 2 (LAD-2) is a milder form of the disease in which patients exhibit a defect in fucose metabolism and glycoprotein biosynthesis.[30] Neutrophils from patients with LAD-2 exhibit abnormal expression of the glycoprotein, L-selectin, and fail to roll along the endothelium. However, they do exhibit normal β_2-mediated adherence.

Principle and interpretation of laboratory assessment
The adhesive function of phagocytes is commonly assessed by the passage of 1 ml of whole blood through a column filled with nylon fiber. Adherence is measured as the difference in the absolute neutrophil count of the precolumn sample and of the sample after passage through the column.

Alternatively, isolated neutrophils can be induced to adhere to plastic using a 96-well plate, either uncoated or pre-coated with fetal bovine serum or a specific extracellular matrix protein such as fibrinogen or fibronectin. Endothelial cell monolayers harvested from human umbilical veins can serve as a more physiological substrate for the measurement of cell adhesion. Isolated neutrophils are preloaded with the cell-permeant acetoxy methyl ester derivative of the fluorescent dye, calcein. Nonspecific esterases in the cytosol cleave the acetoxy methyl ester moiety, trapping the fluorescent probe in the cytosol. The labeled neutrophils are added to each well and incubated in the absence or presence of phorbol myristate acetate (PMA) to promote adherence through activation of the integrins. At the end of the incubation, the wells are washed three times to remove nonadherent cells. The fluorescence of each well is determined with a fluorescent plate reader and compared to the fluorescence of a control well with a known number of fluorescent cells. As shown in the left panel of Figure 123.1, under control conditions less than 10% of the neutrophils adhere to plastic or to plastic coated with fetal bovine serum. Slightly more neutrophil adherence is observed in wells coated with fibrinogen. Treatment of normal neutrophils with PMA for 30 minutes results in the adherence of more than 90% of the neutrophils under all conditions. This adherence assay is valuable in the diagnosis of patients with leukocyte adhesion deficiency. As shown in the right panel of Figure 123.1, neutrophils isolated from patients with LAD-1 generally exhibit less than 5% adherence under control conditions, and do not increase adherence after treatment with PMA, in striking contrast to the neutrophils obtained from normals.

NEUTROPHIL CHEMOTAXIS

Clinical indications and implications
Neutrophil migration is a prerequisite for neutrophil accumulation at sites of inflammation. Patients with leukocyte chemotactic defects usually show recurrent skin abscesses and occasional life-threatening invasive infections.

Principle and interpretation of laboratory assessment
The assessment of neutrophil chemotaxis in vivo can be evaluated using skin windows. Skin blisters are gently raised on the volar surface of the forearm using a vacuum pump and an eight-well blister device, with little hemorrhage or vascular damage. The roof of the blister is removed and the exposed skin lesion is

Adherence of neutrophils to plastic: normal vs leukocyte adhesion deficiency

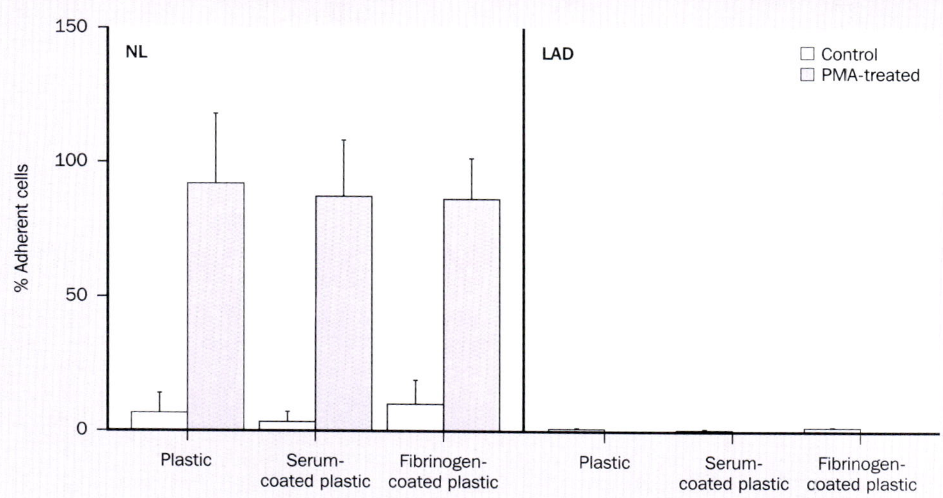

Figure 123.1 Adherence of neutrophils to plastic: normal *vs.* leukocyte adhesion deficiency. Neutrophils (1 X 10^7/ml HBSS without divalent cations) were pre-loaded with calcien-AM (5 μg/ml) for 15 minutes at 37°C. The cells were washed twice and resuspended in HBSS/HEPES with 2% BSA at a cell concentration of 2 X 10^6/ml. The wells of a 96-well plate were coated for 1 hour at 37°C with 32 μl of either buffer alone, fetal bovine serum, or fibrinogen (2.5 mg/ml). The wells were washed three times and then cells were added to each well (160 μl/ml, 3.2 X 10^5/well). Affter a 10 minute preincubation at 37°C, PMA (100 ng/ml) was added and the plate was incubated for 30 minutes at 37°C. The wells were then washed three times with HBSS/ HEPES to remove nonadherent neutrophils. The percentage of adherent cells was determined by the ratio of the flourescence of the well compared to the flourescence of a known standard well. The panel (NL) on the left represents the data (mean ± S.D) from 22 normal subjects and the panel on the right represents the data from 3 patients with leukocyte adhesion deficiency.

bathed with autologous serum using a skin window chamber. Over 24 hours, exudative neutrophils accumulate in the autologous serum bathing the skin lesion. The skin chamber provides a mechanism for characterizing the immune cells, as well as soluble immune mediators, that accumulate in the autologous serum during the evolution of the inflammatory response.[31]

Chemotaxis in vitro is generally measured using a modified Boyden chamber. This includes three components: a lower (chemo-attractant) chamber, a nitrocellulose or polycarbonate filter layer, and an upper cell chamber. The lower compartments of the chamber are filled with a chemoattractant such as fMLF (10^{-8} M) or IL-8 (10 ng/ml). Recently, a rapid fluorescence-based measurement of neutrophil chemotaxis has been described that uses a new 96-well disposable chemotaxis chamber[32] and can be read in a fluorescence plate reader. The lower chamber containing the chemoattractant is separated from the cellular compartment by a filter. However, instead of a top chamber, the filter has a hydrophobic mask that creates surface tension in the cell suspension, keeping it in a position directly above the chemoattractant chamber. In this assay, neutrophils labeled with the fluorescent dye calcein-AM are placed on top of the filter. The chemotaxis chamber is incubated for up to 60 minutes at 37°C. The nonmigrating neutrophils on the top of the filter are rinsed off with buffer and then the plate is read in a fluorescence plate reader. The number of migrating neutrophils can be determined by comparing the fluorescence to a standard well with a known number of fluorescent neutrophils. Fewer than 5×10^6 fluorescent-neutrophils are needed to determine neutrophil chemotaxis using several doses of the chemoattractants fMLF, IL-8, C5a, and leukotriene B_4. The advantages of this new assay are the high sensitivity, the rapid acquisition and analysis of data, and the reduced labor involved in loading the upper chamber and acquiring the data. The 96-well format also allows for multiple comparisons to be made under identical conditions.

EXPRESSION OF SURFACE ANTIGENS

Clinical indications and implications

The expression of neutrophil membrane antigens is altered in vivo during exudation[33] or after challenge with intravenous endotoxin.[9] Flow-cytometric analysis of adhesion molecules on the neutrophil cell surface can indirectly reflect neutrophil adhesion function. Patients with leukocyte adhesion deficiency type I exhibit a deficit in the expression of the common β_2-integrin CD18, resulting in deficiency in CD11a, CD11b, CD11c, and CD18.[34]

Principles and interpretation of laboratory assessment

The expression of cell surface antigens is determined on neutrophils stained with directly labeled monoclonal antibodies and analyzed by flow cytometry. Neutrophils stained with nonspecific isotype antibodies are used to determine the nonspecific background staining. To determine the expression of circulating neutrophils and avoid artifacts induced by neutrophil isolation, an aliquot of whole blood can be stained with the appropriate antibody prior to lysis of the erythrocytes. During flow-cytometric analysis, the neutrophils are easily differentiated using their forward light scatter and right-angle light scatter. As very little blood is needed (100 μl) for each antigen, the neutrophils can be stained with a panel of antibodies to many relevant surface antigens, so that a more complete representation of surface antigen

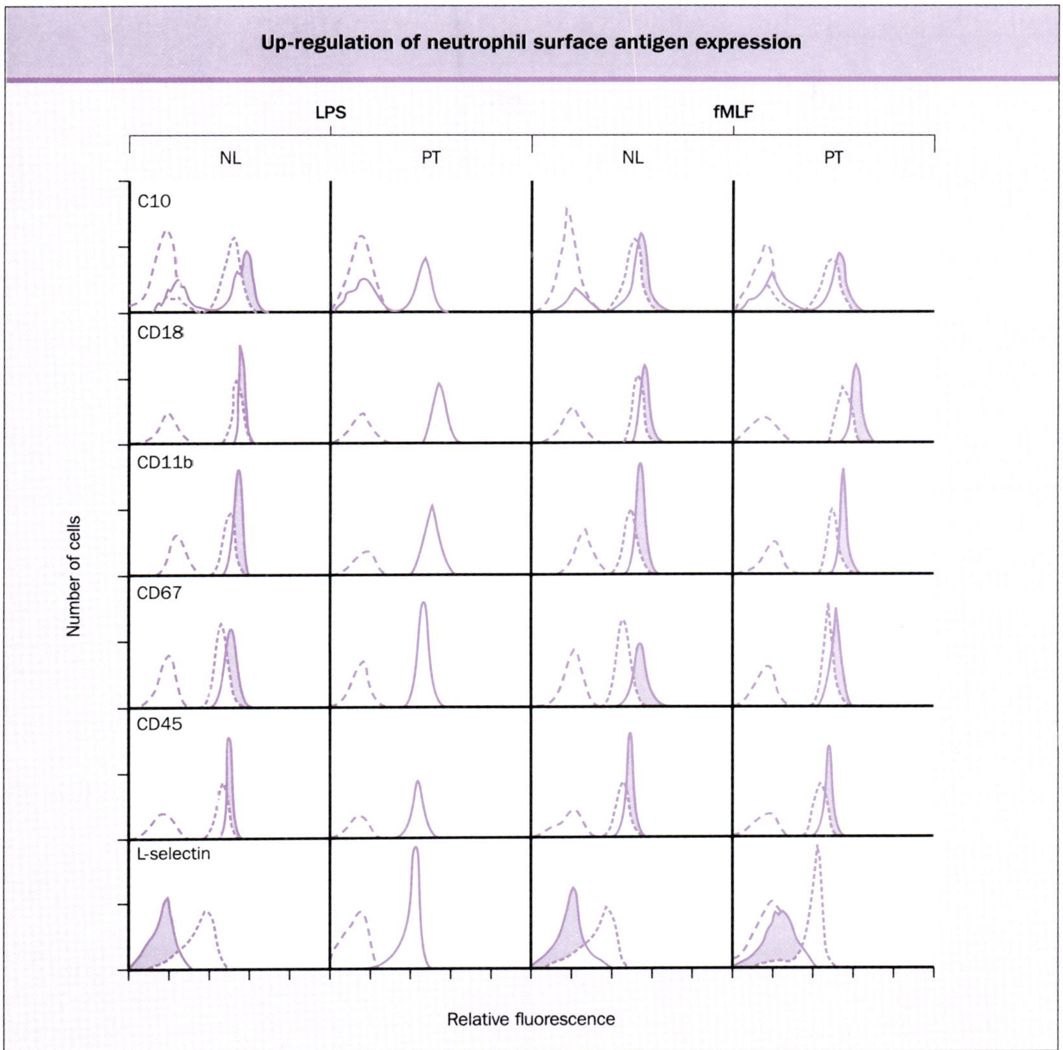

Figure 123.2 Up-regulation of neutrophil surface antigen expression Neutrophils (2.5×10^6/ml HBSS+10% AB sera) were treated with either LPS (100 ng/ml) or fMLF (0.1 μM) for 30 minutes at 37°C. The cells were washed and stained with C10 (an antibody that demonstrates neutrophil heterogeneity), CD18, CD11b (antibodies to β_2 integrins), CD67 (a specific granule marker), CD45 (the common leukocyte antigen) and L-selectin. The dotted lines represent the isotype control, dashed lines represent control neutrophils, and solid lines represent stimulated cells. Differences between control and stimulated cells have been shaded. (From Kuhns DB, Long Priel DA, Gallin JI. Endotoxin and IL-1 hyporesponsiveness in a patient with recurrent bacterial infections. J Immunol 1997;158:3959 with permission.)

expression on neutrophils can be obtained. The panel should include the β_2-integrins (CD11a, CD11b, CD11c, and CD18), selectins (CD62L), Fcγ receptors I, II, and III (CD64, CD32 and CD16), leukosialin (CD43), the common leukocyte antigen (CD45), and markers for the specific granules (CD67) and azurophilic granules (CD63). During exudation, the expression of CD11b, CD18, and CD45 is increased over that observed in peripheral neutrophils, but the expression of CD43 (leukosialin) and CD62L is markedly reduced.[33]

The expression of surface antigens can also be used to assess the responsiveness of neutrophils to particular ligands,[35] such as fMLF and LPS, as shown in Figure 123.2. Isolated neutrophils are incubated for 30 minutes at 37°C in the absence or presence of ligand. The neutrophils are then stained with antibody to a specific surface antigen and analyzed for alteration in expression, either up-regulation because of translocation of latent antigen to the plasma membrane, or down-regulation due to shedding of antigen. These studies can also be performed to assess latent intracellular pools of specific antigens. In moderate leukocyte adhesion deficiency, there is a reduced basal expression of the β_2-integrins, and stimulation fails to cause any further up-regulation of the surface expression of membrane antigens.[29]

PHAGOCYTOSIS

Clinical indications and implications

The recognition and ingestion of bacteria and fungi is an important initial step in the microbicidal response of neutrophils.

Principles and interpretation of laboratory assessment

To assess phagocytosis, neutrophils are incubated in the presence of human serum with various target particles, including latex-coated beads, zymosan, and heat-killed bacteria. Phagocytosis of the target particles can be analyzed either with direct visualization using a light microscope or by quantification based on fluorescence. Phagocytosis of fluorescent bacteria can be quantified with a flow cytometer to estimate phagocytosis at the single-cell level, or with a fluorescence plate reader to estimate overall phagocytosis. In analyzing phagocytosis, it is important to differentiate noningested particles attached to the cell surface from particles that have been internalized. This obstacle can be overcome with the use of fluorescent-labeled bacteria. Certain dyes quench the fluorescence of any extracellular bacteria so that only internalized bacteria are included in the analysis, e.g. trypan blue quenches fluorescein.

NEUTROPHIL DEGRANULATION

Clinical indications and implications

The proteases, acid hydrolases and inflammatory mediators released from storage granules in the neutrophils can mediate bacterial killing, tissue damage, healing and immune regulation. Lactoferrin that is released from specific granules can chelate iron, resulting in a bactericidal or bacteriostatic effect. Elevation of plasma lactoferrin is an indication of intravascular activation and degranulation of neutrophils.[9]

Principle and interpretation of laboratory assessment

Stimulation of neutrophils with various secretagogues can result in the release of granular enzymes into the extracellular fluid. Treatment of the neutrophils with cytochalasin b (5 µg/ml) disrupts microfilament assembly and facilitates the release of both specific and azurophilic enzymes. Because the stimulation of neutrophil degranulation is often accompanied by O_2^- generation and oxidative inactivation of enzymes, both the cell supernatant fluid and the cell pellet should be analyzed to determine the percentage of enzyme released. To differentiate degranulation from cell lysis, the release of the cytosolic enzyme, lactate dehydrogenase, should be monitored simultaneously.

The release of azurophilic granules can be assessed by determination of β-glucuronidase activity. Supernatant fluids or cell extracts obtained from stimulated neutrophils are incubated with 4-methylumbelliferyl-β-D-glucuronide in a 96-well plate. The reaction is stopped with the addition of ammonium hydroxide/glycine buffer, pH 10. The results are determined on a fluorescence plate reader and compared to a standard curve of 4-methylumbelliferone. Methylumbelliferone-derived substrates are also available for other acid hydrolases, phosphatases and lysozyme. Several different enzymes can be analyzed on the same plate and compared to the same standard curve. Alternatively, the release of azurophilic enzymes can be monitored with the marker enzyme myeloperoxidase using commercially available enzyme-linked immunoassays. CD63 is also found in the membrane of azurophilic granules and migrates to the neutrophil surface after stimulation with fMLF in the presence of cytochalasin b.[25]

The release of specific granules can be assessed by determination of vitamin B_{12}-binding protein or lactoferrin. To measure vitamin B_{12}-binding protein, supernatant fluids or cell extracts obtained from stimulated neutrophils are incubated with ^{57}Co-labeled vitamin B_{12}. Charcoal is added to absorb excess vitamin B_{12} and total vitamin B_{12} activity is determined from the remaining protein-bound vitamin B_{12} and the specific activity of the radioligand.[36] Lactoferrin is determined by enzyme-linked immunoassay using rabbit anti-human lactoferrin antibody.[37] The carcinoembryonic antigen CD66b (formerly CD67) is found on the neutrophil surface and the specific granules, and its expression on the surface of the neutrophils is increased after stimulation with fMLF and LPS.[35]

The secretory granules usually contain proteins that are translocated into the membrane from cytosol during degranulation. Detection of the constituents of secretory granules can be assessed by flow-cytometric analysis of the change in expression of surface proteins such as adhesion molecules, and cytochrome b_{558} of the NADPH oxidase.

GENERATION OF REACTIVE OXYGEN INTERMEDIATES

Clinical indications and implications

The release of reactive oxygen intermediates (ROI) such as O_2^- and H_2O_2 is an important component of neutrophil bactericidal machinery. Neutrophils isolated from patients with chronic granulomatous disease (CGD) have a defect in the NADPH oxidase and are unable to generate ROI, resulting in an oxygen-dependent bactericidal defect (Chapter 37). Microorganisms causing infections in patients with CGD are usually catalase positive, such as *Staphylococcus aureus* and *Escherichia coli*, but not catalase-negative bacteria such as streptococci, because the CGD neutrophil can utilize the H_2O_2 generated by the catalase-negative bacterium during the killing process. NADPH, the source of reducing potential utilized by the oxidase, is provided by metabolism of glucose through the pentose phosphate pathway.

Principles and interpretation of laboratory assessments

The production of superoxide (O_2) can be detected using the reduction of cytochrome c. Because O_2^- causes a one-to-one stoichiometric reduction of ferricytochrome c to ferrocytochrome c, the resultant increase in the absorption spectrum at 550 nM can be used to quantity the production of O_2^-. Superoxide dismutase is added to an identical tube to control for the nonspecific reduction of cytochrome c. However, as cytochrome is not permeable to the cells, the detection of O_2^- is limited to that released into the extracellular milieu. Neutrophils isolated from normal volunteers produce 0.42 ± 0.67 nmol/10^6 neutrophils/10 minutes under resting conditions. Treatment of normal neutrophils with PMA results in 35.92 ± 11.92 nmol/10^6 neutrophils/10 minutes (Fig. 123.3). An estimate of normal O_2^- production over 60 minutes can be obtained by reducing the number of neutrophils in the assay to 2×10^5. Neutrophils isolated from patients with chronic granulomatous disease fail to produce O_2^- in response to PMA in 10 minutes. However, some patients with autosomal forms of CGD have low, but detectable O_2^- production in 60 minutes. Neutrophils isolated from X-linked heterozygous carriers of CGD can yield a full spectrum of O_2^- production, whereas neutrophils from autosomal recessive carriers of CGD generally yield a normal response. Although the detection of O_2^- by reduction of cytochrome c is useful in the diagnosis of patients with CGD, it cannot be used in the diagnosis of carriers because of the wide spectrum of responses.

KEY CONCEPTS

Common assays of neutrophil function

- Adherence to plastic or endothelial cells
- Chemotaxis in a Boyden chamber or multiwell chamber
- CD11a,b,c; CD18; CD62L; CD16; CD32; CD64; CD43 expression by flow cytometry
- Phagocytosis of latex beads, zymosan or heat-killed bacteria
- Generation of reactive oxygen intermediates by reduction of ferricytochrome c, reduction of NBT or by DHR fluorescence
- Bactericidal activity against *Staphylococcus aureus*
- Generation of nitric oxide

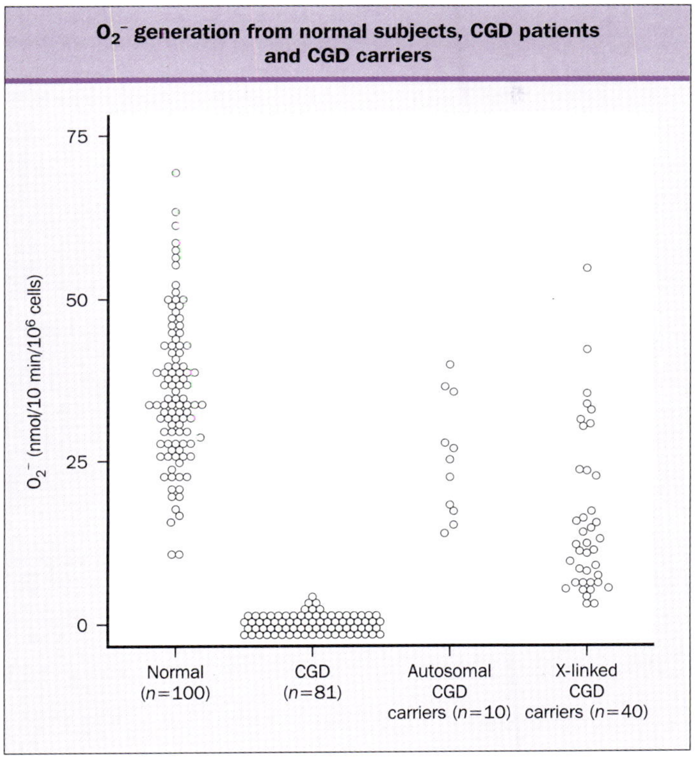

Figure 123.3 O_2^- Generation from normal subjects, CGD patients and CGD carriers. Neutrophils (1×10^6/ml HBSS) were incubated in the presence of 150 μM cytochrome c in the presence of PMA (100 ng/ml) for 10 minutes at 37°C. The reaction was terminated by centrifugation at 4°C. Reduction of cytochrome c was monitored at an analytical wavelength of 550 nm. O_2^- generation was calculated using a μmolar extinction coefficient of 0.0211. An identical tube containing superoxide dismutase (100 μg/ml) served as a blank.

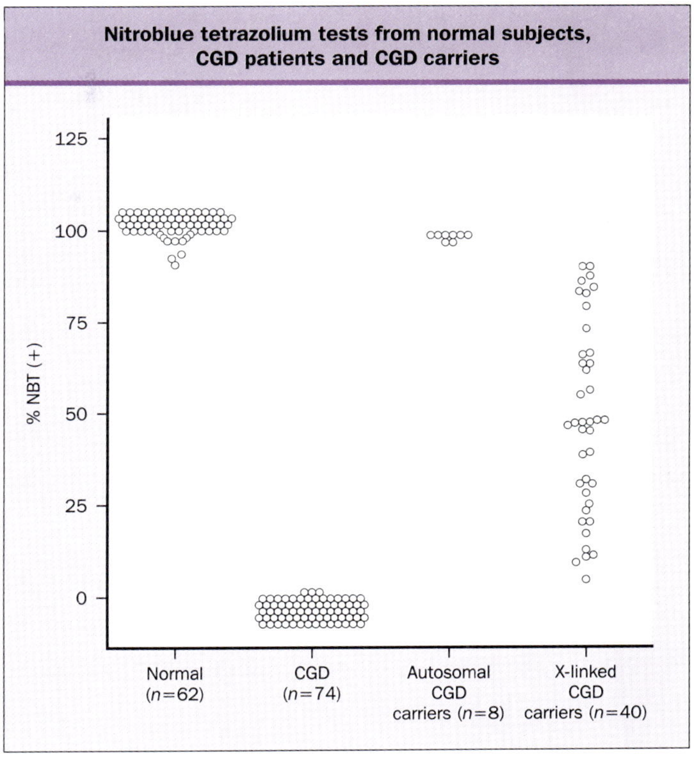

Figure 123.4 Nitroblue tetrazolum tests from normal subjects, CGD patients and CGD carriers. Neutrophils (1×10^6/ml HBSS) were incubated in the presence of nitroblue tetrazolium (1 mg/ml) and PMA (100 ng/ml) for 30 minutes at 37°C in a slide chamber. The slide was washed twice with HBSS and counterstained with safranin O. Two hundred cells were manually counted using a microscope and scored as the percent NBT (+).

In addition, the extracellular release of H_2O_2 can be measured in a horseradish peroxidase-induced phenol red oxidation assay. PMN suspensions in the presence of horseradish peroxidase and phenol red are exposed to either PMA or buffer alone. An increase in absorbance is measured at 600 nm by PMA stimulated normal neutrophils.

The nitroblue tetrazolium (NBT) test is a qualitative assay of O_2^- production. Either whole blood or isolated neutrophils are mixed with NBT in a chamber slide and stimulated with PMA for 15–30 minutes at 37°C. The neutrophils are allowed to settle on the slide, which is then air-dried, fixed with methanol, counterstained with 0.1% safranin and examined under a microscope. The NBT test yields a visual record of the reduction of the nitroblue tetrazolium dye to the insoluble blue-black deposits of formazan. Normal neutrophils, but not neutrophils from CGD patients, reduce the yellow dye to black-brown-blue aggregates in the cells (Fig. 123.4). Because of the random inactivation of the X chromosome, X-linked carriers of CGD exhibit both NBT (+) and NBT (–) neutrophils. The percentage of NBT (+) neutrophils in X-linked carriers of CGD ranges from 5 to 95%. The drawback of the NBT test is the labor-intensive enumeration of sufficient neutrophils to obtain an accurate reflection of the percentage of positive cells. The NBT can be used to diagnose X-linked carriers of CGD, but cannot differentiate autosomal carriers from normal subjects.

An alternative to the NBT is a flow-cytometric assay using dihydrorhodamine-1,2,3 (DHR).[38] Neutrophils are loaded with the non-fluorescent dye and then stimulated with PMA for 15 minutes at 37°C. The H_2O_2 produced oxidizes the dye and results in increased fluorescence, detectable with a flow cytometer. Catalase is added to prevent cell-to-cell diffusion of H_2O_2. Because dye is localized to the cytoplasm and catalase is present in the extracellular fluid, the dihydrorhodamine-1,2,3 assay detects the intracellular production of reactive oxygen metabolites. Stimulation of normal neutrophils (A) with PMA results in a two-log shift in the fluorescence intensity (Fig. 123.5). Neutrophils from an X-linked carrier of CGD (B) exhibit mosaicism, with a negatively stained population and a brightly stained positive population. Neutrophils from patients with X-linked CGD who lack gp91^{phox} (C) express little increase in fluorescence, whereas those from patients with a deficiency in p47^{phox} exhibit a slight increase in fluorescence. The major advantages of the dihydrorhodamine-1,2,3 assay are the sensitivity, the signal-to-noise ratio, and the ease of counting a large number of cells.

BACTERICIDAL ACTIVITY

Clinical indications and implications

Assessment of bactericidal activity is a general test that encompasses a broad spectrum of neutrophil function. To show normal

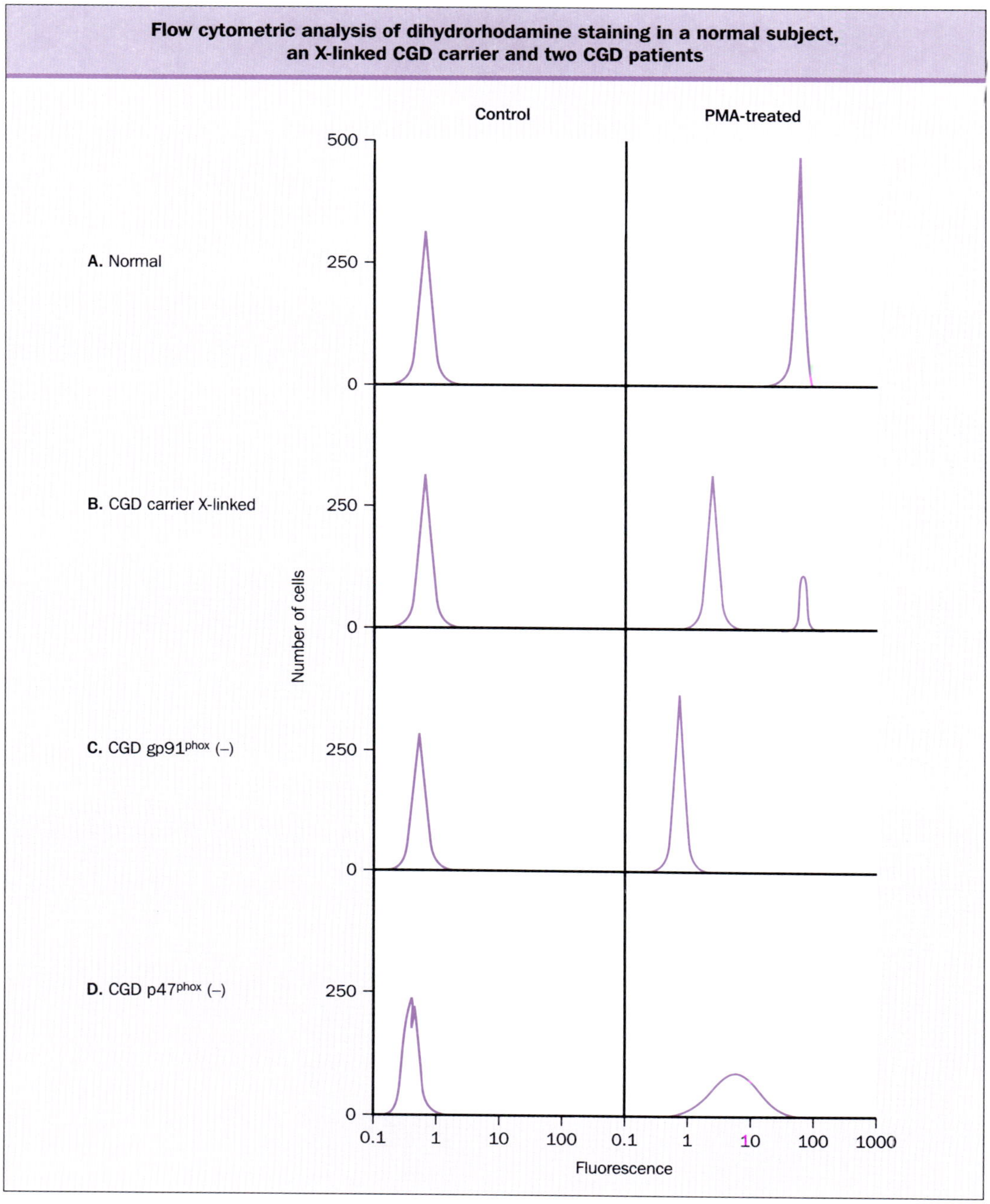

Figure 123.5 Flow cytometric analysis of dihydrorhodamine staining in a normal subject, an X-linked CGD carrier and two CGD patients. Whole blood (1.2 milliliter collected with EDTA as anticoagulant) was lysed using ammonium chloride-potassium bicarbonate solution. The remaining leukocytes were resuspended in HBSS and incubated with dihydrorhodamine 1,2,3 (100 μM) for 5 minutes at 37°C. The cells were then incubated an additional 15 minutes at 37°C either with buffer (control) or PMA (400 ng/ml). The cells were immediately analyzed by flow cytometric analysis. Neutrophils were differentiated by forward light scattering and right angle light scattering. The analyses presented represent 5000 events within the gated area.

bactericidal activity the neutrophil must be able to recognize and ingest bacteria, and then activate a potent microbicidal response that may include both oxidative and nonoxidative mechanisms.

Principles and interpretation of laboratory assessment

Challenging neutrophils with viable bacteria at a fixed bacteria: neutrophil ratio is a useful assay to assess the ability of neutrophils to recognize, ingest and kill bacteria (typically *Staphylococcus aureus*, substrain 502A). The bacteria are suspended in trypticase soy broth and grown in a shaker water bath at 37°C, monitoring the $OD_{650\ nm}$ until the bacteria are in log phase. In order to add a known number of bacteria, preliminary studies should be performed to determine the number of viable bacteria (i.e. colonies) versus the $OD_{650\ nm}$. An $OD_{650\ nm}$ of 0.200 yields approximately 0.8–1 × 10^8 bacteria/ml.

Because neutrophils do not directly recognize bacteria but instead recognize the opsonins (immunoglobulins, complement C3b and iC3b), the assay requires the presence of serum to provide opsonins for its opsonic activity. A pool of freshly frozen AB sera from at least 10 donors yields the best results. Commercially available pools of AB have proved less satisfactory, presumably because of decreased complement and opsonic activity during processing. Neutrophils in the presence of human serum and viable bacteria are incubated at 37°C for 90–120 minutes on an end-over-end rotator. Control reactions, such as bacteria alone and bacteria with serum alone, are included in the study to exclude the possibilities of serum bactericidal activity or poor bacterial viability. At indicated times, an aliquot of the neutrophil suspension is lysed in distilled water to release viable bacteria. A fraction of the lysate is added to a 22 mm Petri dish, mixed with melted trypticase soy agar, and then allowed to solidify. The plates are incubated for 48 hours at 37°C, and colony formation is enumerated by either manual counting or image analysis. The data are presented as percent killing of the original bacterial challenge. At a low (fewer than four bacteria per neutrophil) multiplicity of infection (MOI), neutrophils kill >90% of the bacteria (Fig. 123.6). However, increasing the MOI – i.e., increasing the bacterial challenge – reduces the efficiency of bacterial killing. The multiplicity of killing reaches a plateau at 10–15 bacteria. Challenge of neutrophils with a low MOI can be useful in identifying patients with a marked defect in the ability to kill, whereas challenge with a higher MOI can be useful in identifying those with more subtle defects.

Effect of multiplicity of infection on neutrophil staphylocidal activity

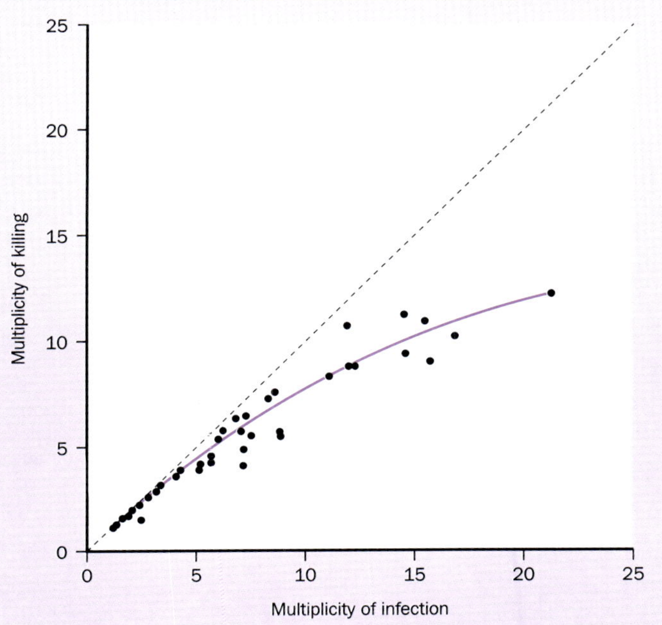

Figure 123.6 Effect of multiplicity of infection on neutrophil staphylocidal activity. Neutrophils (5 X 10^6/ml of HBSS with 10% AB sera) were challenged with increasing multiplicity of infection using *Staphylococcus aureus*, substrain 502A. After incubation for 90 minutes at 37°C, the number of remaining viable bacteria was determinated by colony counting. Each data point represents the mean of triplicate determinations. The multiplicity of killing was calculated as the difference between the multiplicity of infection and the multiplicity of surviving bacteria. The dotted diagonal line represents the theoretical 100% multiplicity of killing.

GENERATION OF REACTIVE NITROGEN INTERMEDIATES

Clinical indications and implications

The release of nitric oxide (NO) and other reactive nitrogen intermediates from phagocytes[39,40] has been implicated in bacterial killing and tumor cytotoxicity.

Principles and interpretation of laboratory assessments

Because of its short half-life and reactivity, direct measurement of NO is difficult. However, its release can be monitored using one of its stable end-products, nitrite (NO_2), which reacts with the colorimetric Griess reagent to form a purple azo dye.[41] However, in many biological fluids, particularly plasma and serum, the stable end-product of NO release is primarily nitrate (NO_3^-), which cannot be detected with the Griess reagent. Treatment of samples with nitrate reductase results in the enzymatic conversion of NO_3^- to NO_2^-.[42] Alternatively, deproteinated plasma samples can be added to a 96-well filter plate containing cadmium powder, which catalyzes the conversion of NO_3^- to NO_2^-. The sample is then drawn through the filter with a vacuum manifold and collected in a separate 96-well plate. Griess reagent is added to detect the NO_2^- and the absorbance is determined on a 96-well plate reader. With this protocol, the level of NO_3^- + NO_2^- in normal human plasma is 45.9 μM (range 27.6–88.9 μM, n=12).

ACKNOWLEDGMENT

This project has been funded in whole or in part with Federal funds from the National Cancer Institute, National Institutes of Health, under Contract No. NO-CO-56000. The content of this publication does not necessarily reflect the views or policies of the Department of Health and Human Services, nor does mention of trade name, commercial products, or organization imply endorsement by the U.S. Government.

REFERENCES

1. Bainton DF. The cells of inflammation: a general view. In: Weissman G (ed). The cell biology of inflammation, 2nd edn. New York, Elsevier/North-Holland, 1980.
2. Hallett MB. The significance of stimulus–response coupling in the neutrophil for physiology and pathology. In: Hallett MB (ed) The neutrophil: cellular biochemistry and physiology. Boca Raton, CRC Press, 1989.
3. Campbell MS, Lovell MA, Gorbsky GJ. Stability of nuclear segments in human neutrophils and evidence for the role of microfilaments or microtubules in their genesis during differentiation of HL60 myelocytes. J Leuk Biol 1995;58:659.
4. Athens JW, Raabs SO, Haab OP et al. Leukokinetic studies. IV. The total blood, circulating and marginal pool and the granulocyte turnover rate in normal subjects. J Clin Invest 1961;40:989.
5. Bainton DF Developmental biology of neutrophils and eosinophils. In: Gallin JI, Snyderman R (eds) Inflammation: basic principles and correlates, 3rd edn. Philadelphia, Lippincott Williams & Wilkins, 1999.
6. Joyce RA, Boggs DF, Haiba U, Srodes CH. Marginal neutrophil pool size in normal subjects and neutropenic patients as measured by epinephrine infusion. J Lab Clin Med 1976;88:614.
7. Dale DC, Fauci AS, Guerry D, Wolff SM. Comparison of agents producing a neutrophilic leukocytosis in man. J Clin Invest 1975;56:808.
8. Wolff SM, Rubenstein M, Mulholland JH, Ailing DW. Comparison of hematologic and febrile response to endotoxin in man. Blood 1965;26:190.
9. Kuhns DB, Alvord WG, Gallin JI. Increased circulating cytokines, cytokine antagonists, and E-selectin after intravenous administration of endotoxin in humans. J Infect Dis 1995;171:145.

10. Springer TA. Adhesion receptors of the immune system. Nature 1990;346:425.
11. Long MW. Blood cell cytoadhesion molecules. J Exp Med 1992;20:288.
12. Tedder TF, Matsuyama T, Rothstein DM, Schlossman SF, Morimoto C. Human antigen-specific memory T cells express the homing receptor necessary for lymphocyte recirculation. Eur J Immunol 1990;20:1351.
13. Griffin JD, Spertini O, Ernst TJ, et al. Granulocyte–macrophage colony-stimulating factor and other cytokines regulate surface expression of the leukocyte adhesion molecule-1 on human neutrophils, monocytes and their precursors. J Immunol 1990;145:576.
14. Bevilacqua MP, Pober JS, Mendrick DL, Cotran RS, Gimbrone MA Jr. Identification of an inducible endothelial–leukocyte adhesion molecule. Proc Natl Acad Sci USA 1987;84:9238.
15. Kishimoto TK, Baldwin ET, Anderson DC. The role of β_2 integrins in inflammation. In: Gallin JI, Synderman R (eds) Inflammation: basic principles and correlates, 3rd edn. Philadelphia, Lippincott Williams & Wilkins, 1999.
16. Gallin JI, Rosenthal AS. The regulatory role of divalent cations in human granulocyte chemotaxis. Evidence for an association between calcium exchanges and microtubule assembly. J Cell Biol 1974;62:594.
17. Vaporciyan AA, Delisser HM, Yan H-C, et al. Involvement of platelet–endothelial cell adhesion molecule-1 in neutrophils recruitment in vivo. Science 1993;262:1580.
18. Shaw DR, Griffin FM Jr. Phagocytosis requires repeated triggering of macrophage phagocytic receptors during particle ingestion. Nature 1981;289:409.
19. Borregaard N, Cowland BJ. Granules of the human neutrophilic polymorphonuclear leukocyte. Blood 1997;89:3503.
20. Volpp BD, Nauseef WM, Clark RA. Two cytosolic neutrophil oxidase absent in autosomal recessive chronic granulomatous disease. Science 1988;242:1295.
21. Parkos CA, Dinauer MC, Walker LE, Allen RA, Jesitis AJ, Orkin SH. Primary structure and unique expression of the 22-kilodalton light chain of human neutrophil cytochrome b. Proc Natl Acad Sci USA 1988;85:3319.
22. Segal AW, Cross AF, Garcia RC. Absence of cytochrome b-245 in chronic granulomatous disease: a multicenter European evaluation of its incidence and relevance. N Engl J Med 1983;308:245.
23. Lekström-Himes JA, Dorman SE, Kopar P, Holland SM, Gallin JI. Neutrophil specific granule deficiency results from a novel mutation with loss of function of the transcription factor CCAAT/enhancer binding protein epsilon. J Exp Med 1999;189:1847.
24. Kaplow LS. Simplified myeloperoxidase stain using benzidine dihydrochloride. Blood 1965;26:215.
25. Kuijpers TW, Tool ATJ, van der Schoot CE, et al. Membrane surface antigen expression on neutrophils: a reappraisal of the use of surface markers for neutrophil activation. Blood 1991;78:1105.
26. Boyum A. Isolation of mononuclear cells and granulocytes from human peripheral blood. Scand J Clin Lab Invest 1968;21:77.
27. Haslett C, Guthrie LA, Kopaniak MM, Johnston RB Jr, Henson PM. Modulation of multiple neutrophil functions by preparative methods or trace concentrations of bacterial lipopolysaccharide. Am J Pathol 1985;119:101.
28. Buescher EB, Gaither T, Nath J, Gallin JI. Abnormal adherence-related functions of neutrophils, monocytes, and Epstein–Barr virus-transformed B cells in a patient with C3bi receptor deficiency. Blood 1985;65:1382.
29. Anderson DC, Schmalsteig FC, Finegold MJ et al. The severe and moderate phenotypes of inheritable Mac-1, LFA-1 deficiency: their quantitative definition and relation to leukocyte dysfunction and clinical features. J Infect Dis 1985;152:668.
30. Etzioni A, Frydmann M, Pollack S et al. Recurrent severe infections caused by a novel leukocyte adhesion deficiency. N Engl J Med 1992;327:1789.
31. Kuhns DB, DeCarlo E, Hawk DM, Gallin JI. Dynamics of the cellular and humoral components of the inflammatory response in skin blisters in humans. J Clin Invest 1992;89:1734.
32. Frevert CW, Wong VA, Goodman RB, Goodwin R, Martin TR. Rapid fluorescence-based measurement of neutrophil migration in vitro. J Immunol Meth 1998;213:41.
33. Kuhns DB, Long Priel DA, Gallin JI. Loss of L-selectin on human neutrophils following exudation *in vivo*. Cell Immunol 1995;164:306.
34. Anderson DC, Springer TA. Leukocyte adhesion deficiency: and inherited defect in the Mac-1, LFA-1, and p150, 95 glycoproteins. Annu Rev Med 1987;38:175.
35. Kuhns DB, Long Priel DA, Gallin JI. Endotoxin and IL-1 hyporesponsiveness in a patient with recurrent bacterial infections. J Immunol 1997 158:3959.
36. Gottlieb C, Lau K-S, Wasserman LR, et al. Rapid charcoal assay for intrinsic factor (IF), gastric juice unsaturated B12 binding capacity, antibody to IF, and serum unsaturated B12 binding capacity. Blood 1965;25:875.
37. Hetherington SV, Spitznagel JK, Quie PG. An enzyme-linked immunoassay (ELISA) for measurement of lactoferrin. J Immunol Meth 1983;65:183.
38. Emmendörfer A, Hecht M, Lohmann-Matthes ML, Roesler J. A fast and easy method to determine the production of reactive oxygen intermediates by human and murine phagocytes using dihydrorhodamine-1,2,3. J Immunol Meth 1990;131:269.
39. Schmidt HHHW, Seifert R, Bohme E. Formation and release of nitric oxide from human neutrophils and HL-60 cells induced by a chemotactic peptide, platelet activating factor and leukotriene B4. FEBS Lett 1989;244:357.
40. Green LC, Ruiz de Luzuriaga K, Wagner DA, et al. Nitrate biosynthesis in man. Proc Natl Acad Sci USA 1981;78:7764.
41. Green LC, Wagner DA, Glogowski J, et al. Analysis of nitrate, nitrite, and [^{15}N]nitrate in biologoical fluids. Anal Biochem 1982;126:131.
42. Gilliam MB, Sherman MP, Griscavage JM, Ignarro LJ. A spectrophotometric assay for nitrate using NADPH oxidation by *Aspergillus* nitrate reductase. Anal Biochem 1993;212:359.

Section 11 Diagnostic Immunology

Chapter 124 Assessment of Human Allergic Diseases

Robert G. Hamilton

Allergies comprise a spectrum of IgE-mediated immediate-type hypersensitivity reactions that manifest as skin reactions (urticaria, dermatitis), respiratory reactions (asthma or rhinitis), gastrointestinal symptoms and, in their most extreme condition, anaphylactic shock. Reactions such as these are generally precipitated by exposure of a genetically predisposed and sensitized individual to a variety of substances that are ubiquitous in the environment and which are usually tolerated well by most healthy individuals. This chapter reviews the principles and methods used in the diagnosis and management of individuals with allergic disease. It focuses on in vivo and in vitro methods for the detection and quantification of total serum IgE and allergen-specific IgE. Other analytes used in the work-up and management of the allergic patient are discussed, including mast cell tryptase, eosinophil cationic protein, precipitating IgG antibodies, and the environmental assessment of aeroallergens in indoor environments.

BIOLOGICAL PROPERTIES OF IgE

In 1921 Prausnitz and Kustner (PK) reported that an intradermal injection of serum from an allergic individual into the skin of an unsensitized (nonallergic) individual, followed 24 hours later by injection of specific antigen into the same skin site, induced local itching and swelling that was surrounded by a zone of erythema.[1] This passively transferred allergic or *PK reaction* reached a maximum within 10 minutes, persisted for about 20 minutes, and gradually disappeared. The antibody mediating this reaction was shown to be thermolabile, losing its sensitizing activity after heating serum at 56°C for several hours. In 1967 this antibody was identified as a fifth human immunoglobulin isotype and designated IgE.[2,3] Table 124.1 contrasts the established properties of IgE (reaginic) antibodies with those documented for IgG antibodies that have been implicated in the modulation of the human allergic reaction (see also Chapter 14).

Serum IgE concentrations are the lowest of the five human immunoglobulin isotypes (0–0.0001 g/l, 0.004% of the total adult serum immunoglobulin).[4] Approximately 50% of IgE is localized in the extravascular space. Its short biological half-life in peripheral blood of 1–5 days is due primarily to a relatively high fractional catabolic rate (37% intravascular pool catabolized/day). IgE does not pass the placenta or activate the classic complement pathway. Its reaginic (mast-cell sensitizing) activity is dependent upon its ability to bind to the α chain of the high affinity IgE Fc-ε receptor (FcεRI) that resides on the membrane surface of basophils and mast cells.

CLINICAL RELEVANCE OF TOTAL SERUM IgE AND IgE ANTIBODY

The human 'allergic' state involves two discrete phases: a sensitizing event and a subsequent challenge.[5] A foreign substance (allergen) initially enters the blood (e.g. Hymenoptera venoms, drugs), respiratory tract (e.g. pollens, spores, dust mite fecal particles, natural rubber latex allergen on glove cornstarch powder), or gastrointestinal system (e.g. foods). Macrophages and T-cell lymphocytes interact with the allergen and present it to B-cell lymphocytes, which differentiate into plasma cells. In genetically predisposed individuals some activated plasma cells produce IgE antibodies that bind to IgE Fc receptors on the surface of mast cells in the connective tissue of the skin, respiratory and digestive tracts, and around blood vessels and basophils in the blood. These events comprise the *sensitization phase*.

Upon a subsequent allergen exposure (*challenge*) of the sensitized individual, allergen cross-links IgE molecules attached to basophil and/or mast-cell surface receptors, causing degranulation and the release of chemical mediators: histamine, slow-reacting substance of anaphylaxis, neutrophil chemotactic factor of anaphylaxis, platelet-activating factor, kinin-producing enzymes (kallikrein) and, in the case of mast cells, prostaglandin D_2 (Chapter 45). Moreover, the activation process causes the release of mast-cell proteases such as the serine esterase, tryptase, which itself has become a serological marker of the mast-cell degranulation process.[6] All these events may ultimately lead to an immediate-type hypersensitivity response that manifests as a spectrum of reactions, ranging from localized swelling and erythema in the skin (wheal and flare) to more systemic bronchoconstriction, urticaria (hives), angioedema, and, in severe cases, anaphylaxis and death. During the evaluation of an individual suspected of having an allergic disease, IgE is the primary analyte that is monitored in tissue by in vivo provocation methods (e.g. skin testing) or measured in serum by in vitro assays.

Total serum IgE

The concentration of IgE in the serum is highly age dependent.[4] Cord serum IgE concentrations are low, usually <2 kU/l (<4.8 μg/l), because IgE does not readily cross the placenta. Serum IgE levels progressively increase in healthy children up to the age of 10–15 years. The rate of this rise towards adult levels is slower than that of IgG but comparable to the observed rise of IgA. Atopic infants have an earlier and steeper rise in serum IgE levels during their early years compared to age-matched nonatopic controls.[7] Total serum IgE gradually declines in an age-dependent manner from the second to the eighth decades of life.

Table 124.1 Properties of IgE and IgG antibodies.

Properties of IgE and IgG antibodies

Property	IgE	IgG_1	IgG_2	IgG_3	IgG_4
Heavy (H) chain class	ε	γ^1	γ^2	γ^3	γ^4
H-chain molecular weight (kDa)	70	50	50	60	50
H-chain carbohydrate (av %)	18	3–4	3–4	3–4	3–4
H-chain number oligosaccharides	5	1	1	1	1
Light-chain type	κ and λ	κ and λ	κ and λ	κ and λ	κ and λ
Averaged Ig light chain K/L ratio		2.4	1.1	1.4	8.0
Molecular weight of secreted form (kDa)	190	150	150	160	150
H-chain domain number	5	4	4	4	4
Hinge (amino acids)	none	15	12	62	12
Interchain disulfide bonds per monomer	NA	2	4	11	2
pI range mean (SD)	NA	8.6 (0.4)	7.4 (0.6)	8.3 (0.7)	7.2 (0.8)
Tailpiece	No	No	No	No	No
Allotypes	Em1	G1m: a(1), x(2), f(3), z(17)	G2m: n(23)	G3m: b1(5), c3(6), b5(10), b0(11) b3(13), b4(14) s(15), t(16), g1(21), c5(24), u(26), v(27), g5(28)	G4m Gm4a(i) Gm4b(i)
Distribution: % intravascular	50	45	45	45	45
Biological half-life (days)	1–5	21–24	21–24	7–8	21–24
Fractional catabolic rate (percent intravascular pool catabolized per day)	71	7	7	17	7
Synthetic rate (mg/kg/day)	0.002	33	33	33	33
Percent total immunoglobulin in adult serum	0.004	45–53	11–15	0.03–0.06	0.015–0.045
Approximate adult range: age 16–60 in serum g/l	0–0.0001 non-atopics	5–12	2–6	0.5–1	0.2–1
Functional valency	2	2	2	2	1–2
Transplacental transfer	0	++	+	++	++
Binding to phagocytic cells		++	+	+−	±
Binding to basophils and mast cells	+++	?	?	?	?
Complement activation classical pathway	0 + Alter path	++	+	+++	0

NA = not available.

A patient's serum IgE level should be compared with reference intervals established with sera from an age-stratified, healthy skin test-negative (nonatopic) population such as the one reported by Barbee et al.[7] After age 14, serum IgE levels > 333 kU/l (>800 μg/l) are considered abnormally elevated and strongly associated with atopic disorders such as allergic rhinitis, extrinsic asthma and atopic dermatitis. Extreme elevations in serum IgE are commonly observed in parasite infections and are necessary for the diagnosis of the hyper-IgE syndrome. Normal or low total IgE levels in some individuals with asthma suggest that IgE-mediated mechanisms play only a minor or insignificant role in the pathogenesis of their condition. Low total serum IgE levels can thus support the diagnosis of nonallergic (intrinsic) asthma and help to exclude bronchopulmonary aspergillosis. The reported overlap between IgE levels in atopic and nonatopic populations, however, is considerable.[7–12] Thus although an elevated serum IgE can be useful in confirming the clinical diagnosis of allergic respiratory or skin diseases, a low or normal value does not eliminate the possibility of IgE-mediated mechanism. This fact is illustrated by the observation that a group of adults with allergic asthma had a mean serum IgE level of 1589 ng/ml (range 55–12 750 ng/ml), with only about half of them having IgE concentrations >800 ng/ml. In contrast, approximately 90% of patients with atopic dermatitis had elevated total serum IgE levels (mean 978 kU/l, range 1.3–65 208 kU/l, where 1 IU = 2.4 ng/ml). Parasitic infections, selected immunodeficiency states, cancer (Hodgkin's disease, bronchial carcinoma), rheumatoid arthritis, liver disease and atopic dermatitis (eczema) are several other disease states that have been associated with a dysregulation of total serum IgE levels.[13–18] The total serum IgE must therefore be interpreted carefully within the relevant clinical context for each patient.

Allergen-specific IgE

In contrast to total serum IgE, the presence of allergen-specific IgE antibody on basophils or skin mast cells or in the serum is highly predictive of an individual's propensity to exhibit an allergic response upon re-exposure to that allergen. Before its identification as a novel immunoglobulin in 1967, IgE was only detectable with in vivo bioassays (skin test, bronchial or nasal provocation tests). Purification of IgE myeloma protein and the subsequent production of antisera specific for IgE led to the development of the first in vitro assays (radioallergosorbent test or RAST) for the detection of allergen-specific IgE antibody in serum.[19] Since then, many commercial variants based on the original noncompetitive solid-phase radioallergosorbent test design have been developed (Table 124.2). Several of these assays have not obtained FDA clearance and are thus marketed only outside the USA.

A number of studies have compared the diagnostic sensitivity and specificity of in vivo and in vitro assays in the diagnosis of human allergic disease. Such intermethod comparisons have shown that IgE antibody results generated by serological (immuno) assay usually agreed well with leukocyte and mast-cell histamine release assays,[20–22] and provocation tests such as the skin test and inhalation provocation test.[20,23,24]

The more sensitive the patient, the better the correlation between methods. Two groups directly examined the diagnostic sensitivity, specificity and efficiency of three IgE antibody assay formats from one commercial manufacturer using three common aeroallergen specificities (cat dander, short ragweed and *Alternaria*).[25,26] These three formats were selected because they represented the evolution in assay designs from the original paper disk RAST (Phadebas RAST or PhRAST) to the modified RAST (MRAST) that used a two-point calibration curve, to the most modern CAP system employing an allergosorbent with a higher binding capacity and a more quantitative calibration system. The investigators used the manufacturer's defined positive thresholds and a skin-prick test (PST) as the reference method for defining the presence or absence of allergic disease. The sensitivity (number of positive in vitro assay results among subjects with a positive PST/total number of subjects with a positive PST) ranged from 44% (PhRAST, *Alternaria*) to 100% (MRAST, cat). The sensitivity of three assays was highly dependent on the allergen specificity and the assay format (allergosorbent, label, and method of calibration). The specificity (number of negative in vitro assay results among subjects with a negative PST/total number of subjects with a negative PST) was high in most cases (range 83% MRAST to 100% CAP/PhRAST). The efficiency of these methods (percentage of patients correctly classified as diseased and nondiseased using the PST as the reference method) ranged from 76% (PhRAST) to 91% (CAP). Both groups of investigators agreed that of these three assay methods, the CAP system, with its enhanced allergosorbent and improved calibration system, represented an advance in technology that achieved increased sensitivity while maintaining assay specificity. Further optimization of the 0.35 kIUa/l positive threshold in the CAP has been suggested by receiver–operator curve analysis depicting the relationship between increasing specificity and decreasing sensitivity of an assay, compared to skin test results, as the positive threshold decision criterion is made increasingly strict.[26]

Even when the same allergen is used in the different in vivo and in vitro assays, from 10% to 25% of the patients with a positive in vivo provocation test have no detectable specific IgE in their serum as measured by in vitro methods.[25,26] In a study to evaluate these mismatches, van der Zee et al[27] conducted 660 paired skin test and RAST measurements to grass pollen, house dust mite and cat dander. Out of 1980 skin test/RAST combinations using the same allergen source there were 140 discrepancies, with >90% of these being positive skin reactions without detectable allergen-specific IgE antibodies in serum (negative RAST). The authors confirmed more than 80% of these discordant results with a repeat RAST and skin test, and then performed basophil histamine release studies as an independent measure of IgE antibody. Histamine was released from washed leukocytes of 82% of 28 RAST-negative–skin-test-positive patients using the relevant extract. These results support the concept that optimally performed serological immunoassays are inherently less sensitive than bioassays such as the skin test when the same allergen source is used in both.[27,28] Differences in the results obtained with provocation and serological tests can generally be traced to either the heterogeneity of the allergen preparation used and/or the inherent sensitivity of the assays.

The clinical importance of these differences in diagnostic sensitivity between skin test and serologic analysis may be less important for patients with allergies to inhaled (pollen, dust mite and epidermal) allergens than in those facing life-threatening anaphylactic reactions caused by Hymenoptera stings, drug administration or occupational natural rubber latex allergen exposure. In these latter cases, skin tests are preferable to in vitro immunoassay analyses for the detection of allergen-specific IgE antibodies.[29] Immunoassay analyses of IgE antibody in serum may, however, be helpful in certain cases where the patient has taken antihistamines, β-receptor stimulants or high-dose steroids which can reduce the provocation test's measured response in children, pregnant women and elderly patients, in whom skin testing may not be well tolerated; and when dealing with allergens (e.g. foods, molds) where commercial extracts can be highly variable or labile.[30]

Table 124.2 Commercially available allergen-specific IgE antibody immunoassays.

Commercially available allergen-specific IgE antibody immunoassays

Manufacturer	Assay name	Chemistry	Allergen reagent[b]	Interpolated units
Abbott[a]	MATRIX	SP-NC	NiC-paper	SIgE/ml
AlerCHEK[a]	EIA	SP-NC	Paper disk	Positive/negative
Bio Whittaker	FAST PLUS	SP-NC	Plastic well	IU/ml
Chiron Diagnostic Corporation[a]	Magic Lite	SP-NC	Paramagnetic particles	IU/ml
Diagnostic Products Corporation	AlaSTAT standard and extended	FP-NC	Soluble polymer	IU/ml
Hycor HY-TEC	EIA	SP-NC	Paper disk	IU/ml
Hycor (Ventrex)	Modified EAST/RAST	SP-NC	Paper disk	Adjusted counts
MAST Immunosystems	MAST (LUM)	SP-NC	Cellulose threads	LU
MAST Immunosystems	MAST (CLA)	SP-NC	Cellulose threads	mV
Pharmacia UpJohn	Phadebas RAST	SP-NC	Paper disk	PRU/ml
Pharmacia UpJohn	Modified RAST	SP-NC	Paper disk	Normalized counts
Pharmacia UpJohn	CAP System	SP-NC	Sponge	kIUA/l
Pharmacia UpJohn	CAP System (ASM)	SP-NC	Sponge	% Reference
Sanofi Diagnostics/Pasteur	RAST/EAST	SP-NC	Paper disk	AU/ml
Sanofi Diagnostics/Pasteur	modified RAST/EAST	SP-NC	Paper disk	Normalized counts
Quidel	Allergen Screen	SP-NC	Dipstick	Positive/negative
THABEST IgE	EAST	SP-NC	Paper disk	SIE units

AU/ml, allergy units per ml;
ASM, Alternate Scoring Method;
CLA, chemiluminescent assay;
EAST, enzyme-allergosorbent test;
EIA, enzyme immunoassay;
FAST, fluorescent allergosorbent test;
FP, fluid-phase immunoassay;
IU/ml, arbitrary international units per ml (not recognized as truly international units);
kUA/l, kilo units (allergen-specific) per liter (based on total IgE heterologous reference curve);
LU/(LUM), luminescence units (luminometer);
MAST, multiple antigen simultaneous test;
NC, noncompetitive binding immunoassay;
Nic, nitrocellulose;
PRU/ml, arbitrary Phadebas RAST Units per ml;
RAST, radioallergosorbent test;
sIgE/ml, specific IgE units per ml (based on allergen-specific IgE homologous reference curve);
SIE units, specific IgE units;
SP, solid-phase immunoassay.
[a]These immunoassays are not actively used in North America.
[b]Solid phase to which the allergen has been insolubilized.

DIAGNOSTIC METHODS

A combination of in vivo provocation and in vitro laboratory tests is used to support the clinical diagnosis of allergic disease. The actual tests selected will ultimately depend upon the nature of the disease process under investigation (e.g. extrinsic asthma, urticaria/angioedema, rhinitis/sinusitis or anaphylaxis).

Initial clinical laboratory tests

Following a medical history and physical examination, the patient who is suspected of having allergic disease may undergo several blood tests. A complete blood count and/or a total blood eosinophil count, if performed, should be obtained before any systemic corticosteroids or epinephrine are administered. Normal whole blood eosinophil levels range from 0 to 500 cells/50 mm^3. Children generally have higher normal levels (mean 240 cells/mm^3, 95% confidence limit = 0–740 cells/mm^3), with peak levels occurring at 4–8 years of age. Most laboratories consider a differential white blood cell count with an eosinophil level greater than 5–10% of the total white cell count to be abnormal. Blood, sputum and nasal secretion eosinophilia is characteristic of asthma, whether or not allergy is present. In a bronchitic sputum specimen neutrophils predominate. A neutrophilic nasal discharge is characteristic of sinusitis. Other laboratory tests that may be ordered include pulmonary function tests and a chest X-ray or sinus CT scan, as indicated.

In vivo provocation testing

Both the skin test and nasal/bronchial provocation tests are useful diagnostic tools for the confirmation of immediate-type hypersensitivity reactions associated with allergic disease, and in the identification of the offending allergens in the work-up for avoidance therapy.

Skin tests

Guerin and Watson[31] described a three-phase response in the skin that occurs during an immediate-type skin test reaction following the administration of a stimulus (allergen or histamine-positive control) into the skin. First, a bluish-white area appears that involves the constriction of capillaries and which typically disappears within minutes. Second, an erythemic peripheral halo or flare appears as a result of arteriole dilatation. Finally, a circular urticarial papule or wheal is observed, as a result of extravasation of plasma into the skin, which is generally maximal by 15–20 minutes. The immediate wheal and flare reaction can be followed by a late-phase reaction in 5–6 hours that appears as a poorly defined edema-like reaction and usually disappears by 24 hours. The administration of an allergen extract can be accomplished by either a prick/puncture or intradermal injection.[32]

Puncture skin testing involves placing a drop of allergen extract on the skin of the forearm or back and the introduction of allergen into the epidermis with a needle puncture. A variety of single-point, multipoint and bifurcated needles have been used.[33] After the prick or puncture, the excess allergen is removed by blotting with tissue paper or gauze. An immediate reaction (wheal and erythema) is read at 15–20 minutes as it reaches its maximum size. Care is taken to space individual tests at a sufficient distance from each other so as not to produce overlapping erythema. Because of the direct skin irritation, bleeding can produce false positive results with some crude allergen extracts.

The intradermal skin (ID) test is 1000–10 000 times more sensitive by concentration than is the puncture test. A 0.01–0.05 ml volume (optimally 0.02 ml) of diluted allergen extract in a 0.5–1.0 ml syringe is injected intracutaneously through a 26–27 gauge needle. An 0.02 ml injection will initially produce a superficial 2–3 mm diameter bleb. Like the puncture test the ID skin test is read at 15–20 minutes, when the reaction is maximal. Dilutions of extract of more than 1:1000 w/v are commonly used to minimize false positive irritation and the potential for systemic reactions. Subcutaneous administration of the allergen can lead to a false negative result. The volume of allergen extract that is injected only slightly influences the size of the wheal and flare reaction, whereas the concentration is the most important determinant of final ID skin test results. Intradermal testing allows an investigator to perform a skin test titration to determine quantitatively the patient's skin sensitivity. For serial titration the same volume (e.g. 0.02 ml) of 3–10-fold serial dilutions of allergen extract is injected into different sites in the skin and the concentration of allergen required to produce a wheal or erythema of a defined mean diameter (e.g. 8 mm wheal) is interpolated. The higher the concentration of allergen required to induce the defined wheal or erythema size, the less sensitive the patient is to that allergen preparation.

KEY CONCEPTS

IgE (reaginic) antibody detection

- Allergen-specific IgE can be detected in skin test by a puncture or intradermal administration of allergen or in the serum by laboratory-based immunoassays.
- In general, the intradermal skin test is more sensitive than a puncture skin test, which is roughly comparable to the best in vitro methods for IgE antibody detection in serum.
- Because the results of in vitro tests for IgE antibody vary considerably between methods, proficiency testing surveys are essential to evaluate performance.
- Double-blind placebo-controlled food challenge is the gold standard for definitive diagnosis of food allergies.

Figure 124.1 shows the relationship that we have observed between the *Dermatophagoides pteronyssinus* (*Dpt*, dust mite)

Relationship between the IgE anti-*D. pteronyssinus* (*Dpt*) in the skin and serum

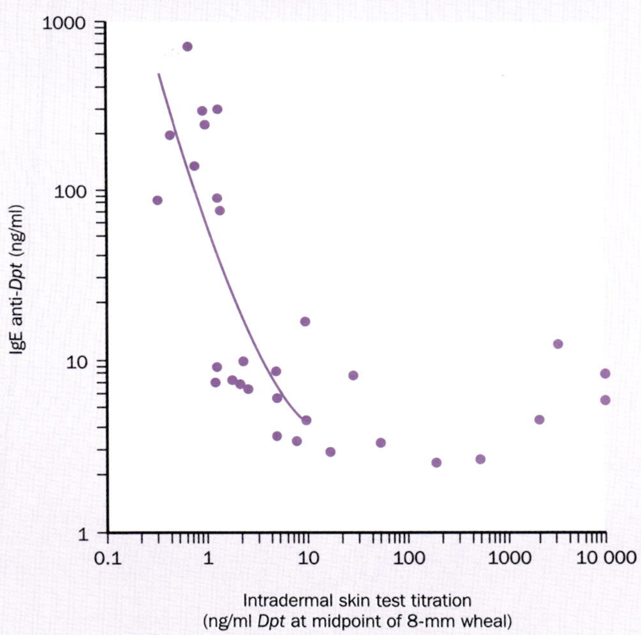

Figure 124.1 Relationship between the IgE anti-*D. pteronyssinus* (*Dpt*) in the skin (*x*-axis, intradermal skin test titration; ng/ml of *Dpt* required to produce an 8 mm wheal) and serum (*y*-axis, ng/ml of IgE anti-*Dpt* as measured by RAST; sensitivity = 2 ng/ml). These results were obtained by testing the skin and serum of 30 dust mite-allergic individuals with varying degrees of clinical sensitivity using the same *Dpt* extract in both the RAST and the ID skin test titration study. A lower 'titer' of antigen required to induce an 8 mm wheal (e.g., higher degree of skin sensitivity) was strongly correlated ($r = 0.77$; $P < 0.001$) with a higher serum IgE antibody level in individuals with the higher level of skin sensitivity (<10 ng/ml midpoint). Less sensitive patients (titers > 10 ng/ml *Dpt*) had lower levels of serum antibody (2–15 ng/ml), which did not relate well with skin sensitivity.

specific IgE antibody in sera from 30 dust mite-allergic subjects, as measured by a radioallergosorbent test in ng/ml, the lower the ID skin test midpoint *Dpt* allergen extract titer required to produce an 8 mm wheal in the same individuals. Using the same *Dpt* extract in both tests, a higher degree of skin sensitivity (i.e. lower titer of antigen required to induce an 8 mm wheal) was strongly correlated ($r = 0.77$, $P < 0.001$) with higher serum IgE antibody levels in those with the higher levels of skin sensitivity (<10 ng/ml midpoint). Figure 124.2 shows the strong correlation in wheal size that is observed in the same *Dpt*-allergic patients receiving the same dust mite extract in a single puncture skin test and a midpoint intradermal skin test titration.

Both the puncture and the ID skin test procedures produce a maximal wheal and flare size by 15–20 minutes, which is measured with a millimeter ruler or caliper. The maximal diameter and the midpoint perpendicular diameter are then averaged to generate an index. A permanent record of the skin reaction can be made by applying adhesive cellulose tape over the wheal and flare skin area, which has previously been outlined with a felt-tip or ballpoint pen. Using a single concentration of allergen, the ID skin test may be graded based on one of several reported systems[32] (Table 124.3). Alternatively, a midpoint titer may be interpolated from a skin test titration including serial three or 10-fold dilutions of the allergen extract. Some investigators prefer to use the erythema (flare) size rather than the wheal size obtained during titration studies because the slope of the flare's regression line with dose is steeper.[34] The strong relationship between the size of the intradermal erythema and wheal that we have observed with the mean of 304 duplicate skin tests is shown in Figure 124.3. This relationship is useful to know because in many dark-skinned subjects the erythema is difficult or impossible to assess.

Skin testing grading system

Grade or Class	Wheal size (mm)	Erythema size (mm)
0	No discernible wheal	
1+	≤ $\frac{1}{2}$ × histamine wheal	
2+	> $\frac{1}{2}$ × histamine and < 1 × histamine wheal	
3+	= size of histamine wheal ± 1 mm	
4+	> 1 × histamine wheal and < 2 × histamine wheal	
5+	> 2 × histamine wheal	
Alternative skin test grading system for intradermal skin testing only involving interpretation of wheal and erythema responses[b]		
0	<5	<5
+/–	5–10	5–10
1+	5–10	11–20
2+	5–10	21–30
3+	10–15	31–40
4+	> 15 with pseudopods	41–50

[a]Prick/puncture histamine (3–10 mg/ml); ID histamine (100 μg/ml).

Table 124.3 Grading system for puncture and intradermal skin testing using histamine as a reference[a]. [b]Modified from Norman PS In: Middleton E, Ellis EF, Reed CE (eds) *Allergy: principles and practice*, 2nd edn. St. Louis, CV Mosby, 1982.

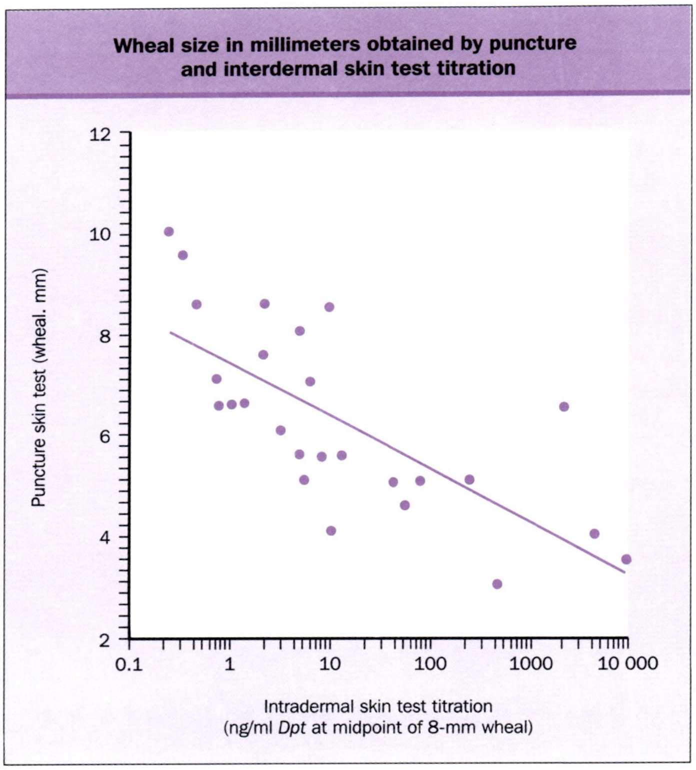

Figure 124.2 The wheal size in millimeters at a single dose of *Dpt* allergen administered in a puncture skin test in compared to the titer or ng/ml of the same *Dpt* allergen obtained in an ID skin test titration on the same 26 dust mite-allergic patients to produce an 8 mm wheal. These data indicate that the wheal size obtained with a single allergen dose by the less labor-intensive puncture skin test is as predictive ($r = 0.72$, $P < 0.001$) of the relative patient sensitivity as the more technically complex intradermal skin test titration study, which involves the administration of seven increasing concentrations of the same allergen into different skin sites.

Bronchial and nasal provocation tests

Bronchial and nasal provocation challenges are performed primarily as a research procedure to identify a relationship between an inhaled substance and a change in the patient's bronchial or nasal physiology. Bronchoprovocation studies with methacholine can also be useful in the diagnosis of difficult cases of asthma. The bronchoprovocation procedure involves the administration of either methacholine or histamine via a calibrated nebulizer, starting at doses of 0.05–0.1 mg/ml and doubling the concentration up to 10–25 mg/ml. Alternatively, allergen extracts can be administered in increasing doses. Pulmonary function is monitored after each dose. A positive response is usually defined as the concentration of agonist that results in a drop in the forced expiratory volume per second (FEV-1) of 20% or more from the baseline (which must be >70% of that predicted for valid interpretation). More extensive details regarding the methods and interpretation of bronchial challenges are presented elsewhere.[35]

Nasal provocation in its simplest form involves the controlled administration of buffer (human serum albumin–saline) or increasing concentrations of allergen into a washed nasal passage. The symptoms (e.g. number of sneezes) induced and/or mast cell mediators released into nasal lavage fluids (e.g. TAME esterase and histamine) after each concentration of allergen indicates the relative level of sensitivity to that allergen. Nasal airway resistance

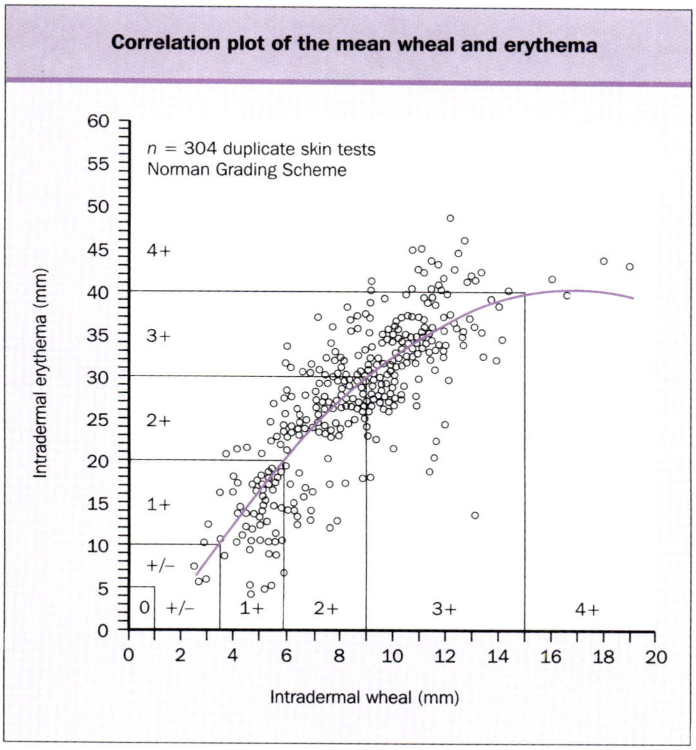

Figure 124.3 Correlation plot of the mean wheal (*x*-axis) and erythema (*y*-axis) in millimeters for the mean of 304 duplicate intradermal skin tests to dust mite (*D. pteronyssinus*) obtained in a population of dust mite-sensitive individuals. The relationship is highly correlated ($r = 0.82$, $P < 0.001$) in grades 0–3+, indicating that either can be used to judge the degree of intradermal skin sensitivity. In highly allergic individuals (>35 mm erythema), however, the slope declines dramatically, indicating that wheal size may be more discriminating than erythema.

is a less satisfactory end-point because of high intrinsic variations. Details of the procedure and applications can be found elsewhere.[36]

A hooded exposure chamber has been described for simultaneous nasal and bronchial challenges as a diagnostic procedure for assessing occupationally induced latex allergy.[37] The challenge involves bathing the subject's conjunctiva and upper and lower airways with air alone, placebo (untreated) cornstarch, and then graded concentrations of latex cornstarch, each for 3-minute intervals separated by 15 minutes. Following each challenge the peak expiratory flow rates (PEFR) and chest and rhinoconjunctival symptoms scores are monitored. Every 18 minutes this procedure is repeated with a different particle type or concentration until either symptoms are observed or the highest dose of cornstarch allergen has been administered. Symptoms reported by the subject are recorded using a validated symptom score instrument.[38] The challenge is considered positive if one of three conditions are met: the PEFR decreases by ≥ 15%; a PEFR drop occurs of at least 10% with a symptom score of ≥ 3; or a symptom score of ≥ 6 is obtained. The particle size distribution is monitored for consistency on a laser particle counter. This procedure has been particularly useful in problematic diagnostic cases involving a discordant clinical history and latex skin test and/or serological test result.

Double-blind placebo-controlled food challenge

Food-induced gastrointestinal reactions (e.g. nausea, colic, vomiting and diarrhea) may occur within minutes to hours following the consumption of food allergens by a sensitized individual.[39] Commonly eaten foods that are known to contain potent allergens include cow milk (caseins, β-lactoglobulin, α-lactalbumin), chicken egg white (ovalbumin, ovomucoid, ovotransferrin), cereal grains (wheat, rye, barley, oats), legumes (peanut, soybean, white bean), fish and seafood (shrimp, crabs, lobsters, oysters). Diagnosis of a food allergy begins with a medical history, which includes an assessment of diet diaries and elimination diets as necessary. Skin tests and serological tests for IgE antibody to extracted food allergens and open food challenges with fresh and cooked foods may also be used to identify suspect foods. No evidence is available to indicate that food-specific IgG or IgG4 antibody levels have any diagnostic value. The double-blind placebo-controlled food challenge (DBPCFC) is considered the definitive diagnostic test for food allergy.[40,41] This normally begins with strict elimination of the suspect foods for 7–14 days before the challenge. An equal number of randomly alternating food allergen and placebo challenges, starting with 125–500 mg of lyophilized food, are then administered to the patient in a fasting state, doubling the dose every 15–60 minutes. Clinical reactivity can be ruled out once 10 g of lyophilized food blinded in liquid or capsules is tolerated.[39] Negative DBPCFCs must then be confirmed with an open feeding challenge under observation to rule out possible false negative challenges. An extensive discussion of the DBPCFC and variables influencing its outcome is presented elsewhere.[39–41]

In 1997, sera from 300 children and adolescents who had been previously evaluated by a skin test and DBPCFC were analyzed in the CAP system for food-specific IgE antibody.[42] In this group, allergy to egg, milk, peanut and soy accounted for 87% of the confirmed allergic reactions. The investigators were able to determine a diagnostic level of IgE antibody for egg (6 kIUa/l), milk (32 kIUa/l), peanut (15 kIUa/l) and fish (20 kUa/l), above which they could predict clinical reactivity in this group with more than 95% certainty. They concluded that by measuring the concentration of food-specific IgE antibody with the CAP system, it was possible to identify a subset of children who were highly likely (>95%) to experience a clinical reaction to egg, milk, peanut or fish. Quantitative serological measurements for food-specific IgE antibody may therefore be able to eliminate the need for time-consuming DBPCFCs in a significant number of children who are suspected of having food allergy.

CLINICAL LABORATORY (IN VITRO) TESTING

Most diagnostic allergy laboratories offer a variety of serological tests that can be useful in the diagnosis of allergic disease. Analytes commonly measured in these laboratories include the total serum IgE, allergen-specific IgE, Hymenoptera venom-specific IgG, the venom-RAST inhibition test and mast cell tryptase. Basophil histamine release (BHR), although rarely offered as a clinical test because of the requirement for fresh blood, is a useful investigational method that will also be reviewed in this section.

Total serum IgE

Of the diagnostic allergy tests that are performed in the clinical laboratory, total serum IgE is currently the only analyte regulated under the Clinical Laboratory Improvement Act (CLIA) of 1988. There are currently 33 different commercial assays licensed in the United States to measure the total level of IgE in serum (see College of American Pathologists [CAP] proficiency survey).[43] Of these, nine are most extensively used by clinical laboratories. These assays are almost exclusively two-site, noncompetitive immunometric assays in which a solid-phase anti-IgE is used in molar excess to capture IgE from a small aliquot of serum. Following a buffer wash to remove unbound serum proteins, a different antihuman IgE labeled with a radionuclide, enzyme or fluorophor is added in molar excess to detect bound IgE. The removal of unbound detection antibody is followed by the development and quantification of the response signal. The quantity of the final assay response signal (counts per minute bound, optical density, fluorescence signal units) measured is proportional to the amount of human IgE bound in the middle of the sandwich between the capture and the detection antibodies. The minimum detectable concentration of most commercial assays is in the range of 0.5–1 μg/l (1 kIU/l is equivalent to 2.4 μg/l of IgE). The intermethod agreement of the different commercial IgE assays can be regarded as excellent (e.g. intermethod CVs typically <10% for serum IgE levels ≥ 30 kIU/l).[43] This good performance is due in part to the availability of a World Health Organization IgE International Reference Preparation (WHO 75/502). For researchers interested in performing their own total serum IgE assays, details of a model polyclonal antibody-based immunoradiometric assay (IRMA) and monoclonal antibody-based immunoenzymetric assay (IEMA) for total serum IgE are presented elsewhere.[44] Nonatopic age-adjusted reference intervals for total serum IgE must be used for normative interpretation.[4]

Allergen-specific IgE

Specific IgE antibody is not on the list of regulated analytes as defined by Federal CLIA-88 statutes. As such, clinical laboratories performing specific IgE measurements in serum need to use an FDA-approved procedure/kit, but they are not currently subject to rigorous scrutiny by regulators in terms of performance on external proficiency testing programs. There are currently 11 manufacturers of commercial IgE antibody assays (Table 124.2). Some of these offer several versions of their assay using similar reagents and formats, but may have different schemes for computing and reporting of the final results. The majority of the assays used in diagnostic allergy laboratories use an immunometric (labeled-antibody) assay design that is traceable back to the first IgE antibody assay reported by Wide et al in 1967.[19] This assay, which was called the radioallergosorbent test or RAST, employed three primary reagents: an allergosorbent or allergen of interest insolubilized on a solid support (e.g. cellulose paper disk); a labeled antihuman IgE detection reagent; and the patient's serum (source of human IgE antibody). An alternative assay format (e.g. AlaSTAT) uses labeled allergens that initially interact with IgE antibody in a rapid solution phase chemistry. This reaction is followed by binding of the allergen–antibody complex to a solid phase and the detection of bound IgE with a labeled antihuman IgE. In all of these assays the solid-phase supports, reagents, buffers, incubation times and temperatures, sample volumes, assay kinetics and computation methods (data reduction schemes and units) vary substantially.

The most highly variable component of the IgE antibody assay is the allergen-containing reagent. The National Committee on Clinical Laboratory Standards (NCCLS) has established a guideline that defines the characteristics of immunologic assays for human IgE antibodies to specific allergens.[45] The guideline provides a nomenclature scheme for allergens and procedures for qualifying the allergen-containing reagents used in IgE antibody assays. There are a reported 300–400 allergens of clinical interest. Some of these share structurally similar or cross-reactive epitopes, and others possess entirely unique IgE antibody-binding determinants. Allergens as a whole have been conveniently grouped into extracts of weed pollen, grass pollen, tree pollen, animal epidermals, molds, house dust mites, parasites/insects, occupational allergens, drugs, venoms and foods. Among different species of a genus, such as ragweed (e.g. Canyon, Desert, Giant, Short, Silver, Southern, Western), there is extensive allergenic cross-reactivity. Extensive allergenic cross-reactivity has also been documented within a particular pollen group, such as the grasses (June, Brome, Timothy, Perennial Rye, Fescue, Orchard, Red Top, Salt, Sweet Vernal, Velvet). In contrast, certain grass pollens, such as those produced by Bermuda Grass, Johnson Grass and cultivated corn, oat and wheat, are minimally cross-reactive (allergenically distinct). Variations in the allergenic content of source materials, the extraction process from the raw source material, allergen-reagent manufacturing methods, differential binding to various allergosorbent supports, instability during storage, heterogeneity of internal reference allergen standards, and differences in characterization procedures (antisera, assays) make the production of reproducible allergens for in vitro use a challenge. Table 124.4 lists the most commonly requested allergen specificities that are available as diagnostic products. Of these groups, the foods have experienced the largest increase in availability of new allergen specificities. Most of these are available from at least one manufacturer as a Food and Drug Administration-approved reagent, which means that the allergosorbent or labeled allergen has been through a systematic evaluation process using serum from clinical history- and skin test-positive patients.

The second attribute that varies widely among commercially available IgE antibody assays is the unitage that provides an estimate of IgE antibody content in a serum. There is no industry-wide IgE antibody reference sera with precalibrated amounts of antibody. From a practical point of view this would be difficult to accomplish for all the clinically important allergen specificities, as each would require its own calibrated serum pool. Serum from at least 10 individuals allergic to each clinically relevant allergen specificity would have to be identified. For most allergens of interest the primary allergens have not even been identified. It is therefore not possible for manufacturers of IgE antibody assays to cross-calibrate their assay's results to a common reference preparation so that the mass estimates of IgE antibody generated by the different assays can be directly compared. Primary reference sera, if available, could be calibrated using a laboratory procedure called depletion analysis or, if the allergens' specificities are known, other calibration schemes.[46]

The presence of IgE antibody in a patient's serum can generally be reliably determined using the manufacturer's-derived positive threshold. These semiquantitative results are reported as positive/negative, or in arbitrary classes (e.g. 0–VI, 0–6). Some manufacturers, however, have adopted a more quantitative calibration scheme. One such employs a total serum IgE ('hetero-

Selected allergen specificities		
Weeds	**Epidermals**	**Foods**
Common ragweed (short)	Cat dander	Egg white
Western ragweed	Dog epithelium	Milk
Giant ragweed (tall)	Horse dander	Codfish
False ragweed	Cow dander	Barley
Wormwood (sagebrush)	Dog dander	Oat
Mugwort (sagebrush)	Guineapig epithelium	Corn
Oxeye daisy	Pigeon droppings	Rice
Dandelion	Goose feathers	Sesame seed
English plantain	Mouse epithelium	Pea
Lamb's quarters	Mouse urine proteins	Peanut
Russian thistle	Rat epithelium	Soybean
Goldenrod	Rat urine proteins	White bean
Cocklebur	Rat serum proteins	Hazel nut
Rough pigweed	Mouse serum proteins	Brazil nut
Scale	Budgerigar droppings	Almond
Rough marsh elder	Budgerigar feathers	Crab
Firebrush (Kochia)	Budgerigar serum	Shrimp
Sheep sorrel	Duck feathers	Tomato
		Pork
Grasses	**Molds**	Orange
Sweet vernal	*Penicillium notatum*	Potato
Bermuda	*Cladosporium herbarum*	Coconut
Orchard	*Aspergillus fumigatus*	Tuna
Meadow fescue	*Candida albicans*	Salmon
Timothy	*Alternaria tenuis*	Strawberry
Common reed grass	*Botrytis cinerea*	Baker's yeast
June Grass–Kentucky blue	*Helminthosporium halodes*	Garlic
Red top (Bent)	*Fusarium moniliforme*	Apple
Johnson grass	*Stemphylium botryosum*	Egg yolk
Brome	*Rhizopus nigricans*	Chicken meat
Cultivated rye	*Aureobasidium pullulans*	α-Lactalbumin
Velvet	*Phoma betae*	β-Lactoglobulin
Wheat pollen	*Epicoccum purpurascens*	Casein
Meadow foxtail	*Trichoderma viride*	Gluten
Canary (Reed)		Lobster
	House dust mites	Cheese (Cheddar)
Trees	*Dermatophagoides*	Cheese, mold type
Maple (Box elder)	*pteronyssinus*	Kiwi fruit
Alder	*Dermatophagoides farinae*	Celery
Birch		Parsley
Hazel nut	**House dust**	Melons
Beech	House dust – Greer	Lamb
Mountain cedar	House dust – Hollister Stier	Mustard
Oak		Malt
Elm	**Insects**	Mango
Olive	Cockroach	Cacao
Walnut	Mosquito	
Sycamore		**Drugs**
Willow	**Occupational**	Penicilloyl G/V
White pine	Wild silk	Beef/pork insulin
Eucalyptus	Silk	Human insulin
Acacia	Isocyanate TDI	Protamine
Mesquite	Isocyanate MDI	Vancomycin
Melaleuca	Isocyanate HDI	
Pecan	Ethylene oxide	**Venoms**
Italian cypress	Phtallic anhydride	White-faced hornet
Cottonwood	Formaldehyde	Yellowjacket
White ash	Natural rubber latex	*Polistes* paper wasp
	Cotton seed	Yellow hornet
	Sunflower seed	Honey bee
	Trimellitic anhydride	Bumble bee
	Natural rubber latex	Imported fire ant

Table 124.4 Selected allergen specificitie.

logous') calibration curve[46] from which allergen-specific IgE antibody results are interpolated. Using this procedure, quantitative estimates of IgE antibody are assigned in kIU/l or μg/l that is traceable to the WHO IgE antibody reference serum. This heterologous interpolation approach has become the next best strategy to actually having a calibrated IgE antibody reference serum for each allergen specificity, which at present is unrealistic.

Some investigators have proposed that IgE antibody to 10–15 aeroallergens may account for most of the aeroallergen-related disease in western Europe and North America. Although the particular 10–15 allergen specificities may vary for children and adults, or for individuals in Europe, Asia and North America, it has been possible to develop a multiallergen IgE antibody screening test that is highly predictive of the results obtained by a panel of skin tests or in vitro IgE antibody tests. In these assays, the 10–15 most common allergens are insolubilized on a single solid phase (e.g. Phadiatop) or in individual locations on one solid support (e.g. Matrix). In an alternative test, several food allergens of most relevance to pediatric allergy patients may also be attached to the same solid phase (Chapter 52). These screening assays are most useful in confirming the absence of significant atopic disease in individuals who are suspected of having an intrinsic or non-IgE-mediated disease process. The negative predictive value of this single test is much higher than total serum IgE in identifying nonatopic individuals. Such a test can minimize the need for multiple in vivo or in vitro allergen-specific IgE measurements in patients with a low clinical probability of atopic disease. The use of such screening tests in unselected populations is likely to generate many false positive results, however, as IgE antibody responses are much more frequent than is symptomatic disease.

Competitive RAST inhibition assay

The soluble allergen, competitive inhibition format of the radioallergosorbent test, or its nonisotopic counterparts, has been widely used by researchers, allergen manufacturers and regulators to determine the relative potency of allergen extracts.[47] One practical research application of the RAST inhibition assay has been as a tool for monitoring the concentration of latex allergen released from latex gloves, condoms and other latex-containing consumer products that have been undergoing manufacturing process changes to reduce allergen content.

In the diagnostic allergy laboratory the RAST inhibition assay has been used to confirm an IgE antibody assay's minimum detectable dose (sensitivity) and nonspecific binding, and to document the allergen specificity of IgE antibody binding as a part of a quality control program. The one clinical application of the RAST inhibition assay has been as an adjunct to define the appropriate therapeutic composition of venoms for insect sting-allergic patients who have multiple potentially cross-reactive sensitivities and have elected to receive immunotherapy[48] (Chapter 47). The primary indication for this test is a strong skin reactivity or a high level of serum IgE antibody to yellowjacket venom (YJV), and a weak skin reactivity or low level of serum IgE antibody specific for *Polistes* wasp venom (PWV). The structural similarity between vespid and *Polistes* wasp phospholipase A1/B (*Ves g* I; *Pol a* I) and Hyaluronidase (*Ves g* II; *Pol a* II) frequently produces IgE antibody cross-reactivity. We have evaluated the sera of 305 Hymenoptera venom-allergic patients who had >2 ng/ml of IgE antibody to YJV and PWV. The clinical question for these patients was whether PWV should be included in their venom immunotherapy together with yellowjacket or mixed vespid venom. Using this procedure, the venom RAST inhibition assay

CLINICAL PEARLS

Clinical utility of Hymenoptera venom RAST inhibition test
- Useful in identifying venom cross-reactive IgE antibodies and selecting appropriate venoms for immunotherapy.
- One-third of venom-allergic patients with concomitant yellowjacket venom (YJV) and *Polistes* wasp venom (PWV) sensitivity can be treated with YJV alone or mixed vespid venoms, owing to >95% cross-reactive IgE anti-PWV with soluble YJV.

identified one-third (36.4%) of subjects with a primary YJV sensitivity who were candidates for exclusion of PWV from their immunotherapy regimen because their IgE anti-PWV was >95% cross-inhibitible with soluble YJV.[48]

Allergen-specific IgG

Allergen injections during immunotherapy are known to enhance the production of specific IgG 'blocking' antibodies (Table 124.1).[49] Quantitative measurements of total IgG antibodies or IgG subclass antibodies in studies of allergic rhinitis do not generally correlate with control of clinical symptoms in individual patients. However, clinically successful immunotherapy is almost always accompanied by high serum levels of allergen-specific IgG.[50] In contrast, the presence or levels of IgG antibodies specific for food antigens have shown no correlation with the results of positive double-blind placebo-controlled food challenges.

Allergen-specific IgG antibody measurements may be helpful in determining optimal therapy in patients with Hymenoptera venom sensitivity. In a prospective study, Hymenoptera venom-specific IgG antibodies were monitored in the serum of 109 venom-allergic patients to examine whether IgG antibody levels could predict the risk of a systemic reaction after a sting challenge in patients receiving venom immunotherapy.[51] Of the 211 venom sting challenges performed in this group over a 4-year period, systemic symptoms occurred in 16% of those with less than 3 μg/ml of venom-specific IgG antibody, and in only 1.6% of those with venom IgG levels greater than 3 μg/ml. The highest rate of allergic reactions (26%) occurred in patients who had both a venom-specific IgG antibody level less than 3 μg/ml and fewer than 4 years of venom immunotherapy.[51] Therefore, quantitative venom-specific IgG antibody levels appear to be of value in individualizing the dose and frequency of injections while maximizing the protective effects. The clinical utility of the IgG antibody measurement may be restricted to the first 4 years of venom immunotherapy.

CLINICAL PEARLS

IgG antibody measurements
- Clinically successful aeroallergen immunotherapy is almost always accompanied by high serum levels of allergen-specific IgG.
- Quantitative venom-specific IgG antibody levels can be of value in individualizing venom doses and frequencies for patients on immunotherapy for up to 4 years.
- Food-specific IgG and IgG4 assay results do not correlate with the results of double-blind placebo-controlled food challenges.

Mast-cell tryptase

Two types of mast cells have been identified in skin, respiratory and digestive tract connective tissues based on the types of neutral proteases present in their secretory granules. One group contains only tryptase, whereas the other contains both tryptase and chymase.[52] Upon activation of the mast cells these proteases are released in parallel with prestored histamine and newly generated vasoactive mediators.

Mast-cell tryptase (MW 134 kDa) is a serine esterase with four subunits, each with an enzymatically active site. In mast cells, from 10 to 35 pg of tryptase per cell is reportedly stored attached to heparin. When dissociated from heparin, it rapidly degrades into its monomers and loses enzymatic activity. As basophils are a rather insignificant source of tryptase release, tryptase in serum has been proposed as a marker of mast-cell activation. Levels of immunoreactive tryptase in the serum (plasma) of healthy adults are less than 5 μg/l (most <2.5 μg/l). Elevated levels of tryptase (>10 μg/l as measured by immunoassay) can be detected in serum from 1 to 4 hours after the onset of systemic anaphylaxis with hypotension.[6,53] In some cases tryptase may reach levels as high as 1 mg/l. Recommended times for serum collection for a serum tryptase is 30 minutes to 4 hours after the onset of an acute event. Although postmortem specimens are often difficult to analyze for tryptase because of gross hemolysis, levels above 10 μg/l in these specimens may also be considered abnormal. Elevated tryptase can be detected usually within 15–30 minutes of an allergen challenge, and it declines with an approximate half-life of 2 hours. This contrasts with histamine, which peaks more quickly – within 5–10 minutes after an event – and may return to baseline levels in less than 1 hour. Tryptase has also been detected in bronchoalveolar lavage fluid, nasal lavage fluid, tears and skin chamber fluid, but there are currently no clinical indications for such measurements.

Basophil histamine release

The potent vasoactive mediator histamine is stored in cytoplasmic granules of basophilic leukocytes and mast cells and released along with other mediators of inflammation in response to both immunologic and nonimmunologic stimuli.[49,54] The basophil histamine release (BHR) assay has been particularly useful as quantitative assay of allergen potency, and as a research model for the study of triggering mechanisms of mediator release from basophils. In its most basic form,[54] peripheral blood leukocytes are isolated from a donor and incubated with varying concentrations (e.g. 3–10-fold dilutions) of allergen extract or antihuman IgE as a positive control. Histamine release is complete within 30 minutes, and then histamine in the supernatant is measured by enzymatic, radiometric or spectrophotofluorometric techniques. The donor BHR dose–response curve is characteristically bell-shaped with a linear ascending portion, maximum or peak at the optimal cross-linking allergen dose, and a descending portion at higher than optimal allergen concentrations. The concentration of allergen required to induce 50% histamine release defines the relative sensitivity of the patient's basophils for a given allergen extract. The BHR assay can also be performed using anticoagulated whole blood. Details of the BHR assay are given elsewhere.[54,55]

Patient sensitivity for a given allergen can be determined with a positive BHR test. BHR test results are highly correlated with those determined by skin testing[56] and bronchoprovocation.[57] Although the BHR test has been most widely used in research laboratories owing to its expense and the need for fresh blood, it can be successfully applied to the clinical diagnosis of allergy in selected cases, as the results obtained parallel those of other IgE antibody tests. BHR has also been a useful tool for clarifying discrepancies between skin test and serological IgE antibody test results.[27]

PROFICIENCY SURVEY FOR TOTAL AND ALLERGEN-SPECIFIC IgE ANTIBODY ASSAYS

The College of American Pathologists (CAP) conducts the only independent diagnostic allergy laboratory proficiency survey in the United States.[58] It is designed to fulfill the proficiency testing requirements for regulated analytes such as total serum IgE, which is considered a highly complex test as specified by US Public Law 100–578, the Clinical Laboratory Improvement Amendments of 1988 (CLIA-88). Every 17 weeks (three cycles per year), five challenge sera are sent to each laboratory to be analyzed for both total serum IgE and IgE antibody to five allergen specificities. Two additional wildcard serum specimens are sent throughout the year to evaluate the ability of laboratories to accurately measure specific IgE antibody to a number of less common allergen specificities, such as natural rubber latex (an occupational allergen), Hymenoptera venoms and unusual foods (kiwi, avocado). Each challenge specimen is unique, and therefore, the survey routinely assesses interlaboratory (intramethod) variation. Split serum samples are occasionally sent to assess intralaboratory variation.

Data from the 15 yearly total serum IgE challenges are reported in the participants' summaries as the mean, standard deviation, coefficient of variation, median, low value and high values for each assay method. A pass/fail designation for total serum IgE is returned to the participating laboratory and state licensing agencies because it is regulated by CLIA-88. Those laboratories that generate total serum IgE measurements outside their peer group mean $\pm$ 3 SD are classified 'out of control'. Except for the occasional nonatopic serum, interlaboratory/intramethod and intermethod coefficients of variation for total serum IgE are routinely $\leq$ 15%.

Allergen-specific IgE is not a CLIA-88-regulated analyte. Moreover, allergen-specific IgE results are reported by different assays in nonequivalent arbitrary units or classes (Table 124.2). There are some assays that also report out quantitative kIU/l results, and these are also tabulated in the participants' summary.[59] Specific IgE survey results are currently evaluated based only on the qualitative class assignment for peer laboratories that use the same assay method. Without a uniform calibration scheme the relative level of IgE antibody, as indicated by the class with the different methods, cannot be directly compared. Even within a given method, care must be exercised when extrapolating the performance data of a particular allergen specificity to overall assay performance. An assay that performs well in detecting specific IgE to one particular allergen specificity may not perform equally well in detecting IgE antibodies to other allergen specificities. Overall method performance is highly dependent on the quality of the allergen-containing reagent used in the assay. A more extensive discussion of the strengths and limitations of the SE external proficiency survey is presented elsewhere.[43,58]

OTHER SERUM ANALYTES

Several other analytes may be measured in the diagnostic allergy laboratory to support the differential diagnosis of allergies, asthma or hypersensitivity pneumonitis, and to aid in the management of asthmatic patients. These include eosinophil cationic protein, human IgG-precipitating antibodies specific for antigens in organic dusts, and cotinine.

Eosinophil cationic protein (ECP)

ECP is a basic protein that can be detected in the granules of the eosinophil in different forms, with molecular weights ranging from 18.5 to 22 kDa.[60] Elevated levels of ECP have been detected in the serum, sputum and nasal secretions of individuals undergoing a late-phase allergic reaction (usually 6–24 hours after exposure), when an eosinophil influx is predominant at the reactive site.[61,62] Levels of immunoreactive ECP detected in the serum of 100 healthy subjects ranged from 2.3 to 16 μg/l (95% range, geometric mean of 6 μg/l). ECP measurements have had limited clinical utility as an analyte for monitoring patients with extrinsic asthma and other allergic diseases where eosinophils may play a role in tissue damage.

Precipitating IgG antibodies (precipitins)

Hypersensitivity pneumonitis (HP), also known as extrinsic allergic alveolitis, is a hypersensitivity reaction to antigenic organic dusts (e.g. molds, bird droppings) involving the lung interstitium and terminal bronchioles[63] (Chapter 84). Hours after a heavy antigenic exposure an acute form of hypersensitivity pneumonitis can occur, with chills, fever, malaise, cough and shortness of breath. Whereas histology of the lung lesions indicates a cell-mediated pathology, most patients with hypersensitivity pneumonitis have high levels of IgG antibody to the offending antigen in their serum. The double diffusion method (Ouchterlony) of measuring precipitating antibodies by diffusing antigen (extract) and antibody (control or patient's serum) towards each other in agarose gel has been used to identify the presence of specific precipitating antibodies in the serum of HP patients. Precipitating antibodies or precipitins can be detected in the serum of nearly all ill patients, but also in the serum of as many as 50% of asymptomatic individuals who have been exposed to the relevant organic dusts.[64] Immunoassays for IgG antibody to the appropriate organic dust antigens may be less useful clinically because they are too sensitive. They typically detect IgG antibody in the sera of a much higher number of patients than do the immunodiffusion methods. Precipitin assays are currently available with specificities for the thermophilic actinomyces (*M. faeni*, *T. vulgaris* and *T. candidus*), aspergillus (*A. fumigatus*, *A. niger*, *A. flavus*), pigeon serum, *Aureobasidum pullulans*, and fecal particles from parakeets and a variety of exotic household birds (Cockatiel, Amazon).

Cotinine

Passive or second-hand smoke exposure is considered a trigger for asthma in some children. Because parental self-reports of smoking status are not always reliable and custody cases often need definitive measures of passive smoke exposure, a number of biochemical markers (thiocyanate, nicotine, cotinine and carbon monoxide) in the plasma, saliva and urine have been used to validate claims of parental nonsmoking.[65] Analysis of nicotine by gas chromatography or immunoassay is specific to tobacco, but its biological half-life is short. In contrast, cotinine, the major metabolite of nicotine, has a longer half-life and has become the marker of choice for monitoring passive smoke exposure. The rate of cotinine clearance in urine from nonsmokers (27.3±1.9 h) is significantly longer than that of smokers (15.4±1.2 h).[66] A diagnostic sensitivity of 97–99% and specificity 81–83% for cotinine in plasma, saliva and urine using 13.7, 14.2 and 49.7 ng/ml as their respective positive cut-off values[65] indicates that cotinine can serve as an effective marker of passive nicotine exposure regardless of the biological specimen that is collected.

ASSESSMENT OF ENVIRONMENTAL AEROALLERGENS

IgE-mediated diseases are currently managed using a combination of three approaches: pharmacotherapy of symptoms, allergen-specific immunotherapy, and allergen avoidance. Of these, avoidance or the separation of the allergen and the patient is potentially the least expensive, best tolerated and most effective approach for reducing allergy symptoms and minimizing increased sensitization. The level of aeroallergens in the indoor and outdoor environments can be highly relevant for the clinical management of allergic patients.

Indoor environments

The indoor home environment has become an important target for allergen control. Of the many known allergen specificities, aeroallergens produced by dust mites (*Dermatophagoides farinae, D. pteronyssinus*), fur-bearing pets (cats, dogs) and rodents (mice, rats), indoor insects (cockroach) and a limited number of common molds (*Penicillium, Aspergillus, Alternaria* and *Cladosporium*) are known to produce the majority of indoor allergic diseases.[67] A number of diagnostic allergy laboratories have the capability to evaluate dust specimens collected by allergic patients from carpeted areas of their homes, workplaces and schools. They can use one of several inexpensive dust collectors that fit on to most standard household vacuum cleaners. Once sent to the laboratory, the crude dust specimen is processed to generate extracted soluble proteins. These are then evaluated by a panel of monoclonal antibody-based immunoenzymetric assays to quantify indicator indoor aeroallergens: *Der f* 1 and *Der p* 1 (25 kDa allergens excreted into fecal particles by dust mites [*D. farinae, D. pteronyssinus*]), *Fel d* 1 (35 kDa allergen excreted by the sweat glands of the domestic cat [*Felis domesticus*]), *Bla g* 1/*Bla g* 2 (25–36 kDa allergens produced by the German cockroach [*Blatella germanica*]), *Mus m* 1 (19 kDa allergen excreted into urine by the mouse [*Mus musculus*]) and *Rat n* 1 (17 kDa allergen excreted in urine by the rat [*Rattus norvegicus*]). A viable mold spore analysis can also be performed on 5 mg of fine dust in a microbiological culture plate containing Sabouraud's dextrose agar.[67]

Each of these allergens may be considered an 'indicator' molecule because it allows the homeowner to track the relative levels of their associated allergen source(s) by room throughout the house. Figure 124.4 shows a representative distribution of *D. farinae* (*Der f* 1) and *D. pteronyssinus* (*Der p* 1) group 1 allergen levels as measured by enzyme immunoassay in 647 and 741 fine dust specimens, respectively, from across the United States. Levels of *Der p* 1 and/or *Der f* 1 allergen >2000 ng/g of fine dust have been associated with an increased risk of allergic symptoms in sensitized individuals, whereas levels >10 000 ng/g of fine dust have been associated with an increased risk of sensitization. For cat, *Fel d* 1 levels >8000 ng/g of fine dust have been proposed as a threshold for sensitization. Any cockroach allergen detected in an environment (>0.5 unit/g fine dust) identifies an indoor area that places cockroach-allergic individuals at some risk for symptoms and sensitization. Finally, viable mold spore levels above 25 000 colonies/g of fine dust place the home above

Distribution of *D. farinae* (*Der f* 1) and *D. pteronyssinus* (*Der p* 1) group 1 allergen levels in American homes

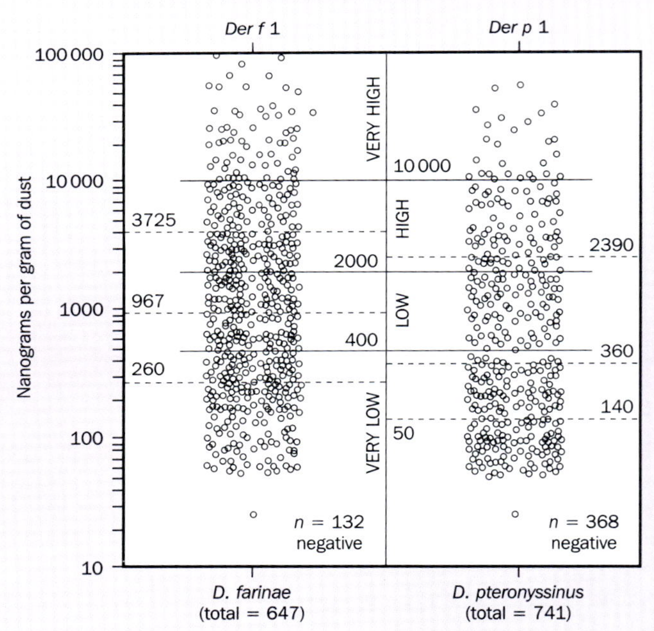

Figure 124.4 Distribution of *D. farinae* (*Der f.* 1) and *D. pteronyssinus* (*Der p.* 1) group 1 allergen levels as measured by monoclonal antibody based-enzyme immunoassay in 647 and 741 fine dust specimens, respectively, from across the United States. Results are reported in nanograms of allergen per gram of fine dust. The allergen levels are divided into quartiles, with the levels of demarcation noted by dashed lines. Proposed risk levels are also noted at 400, 2000 and 10 000 ng/g by solid lines. (From Hamilton RG, Chapman MD, Platts-Mills TAE, Adkinson NF Jr. *Immunol Allergy Pract* 1992;14:9.

CLINICAL PEARLS

Indoor aeroallergen analyses

- Predominant indoor aeroallergens include dust mites, cockroaches, epidermal allergens (cat, dog, mouse, rat) and a limited number of molds.
- Quantitative analysis of house dust samples enables allergic subjects to assess the individual risk for symptoms and/or sensitization in a particular home and to monitor the effects of environmental control.

the 75th percentile for homes monitored across the United States. In cases where these proposed threshold levels are exceeded, the allergic individual is encouraged to take action to reduce the allergen levels. A detailed discussion of strategies for doing this is beyond the scope of this chapter, but can be found elsewhere.[67,68] Repeat household dust allergen measurements following an intervention allows monitoring and documentation of allergen reduction.

Outdoor environments

In most major cities across the United States an aerobiology station has been established to perform a daily evaluation of the outdoor air for pollen and mold spore levels. This information is transmitted to local weather stations and newspapers for public use. An aerobiology network has been established by the American Academy of Allergy, Asthma and Immunology to certify participating laboratories and monitor their performance. This network also collates and disseminates pollen and mold data across the nation throughout the allergy season. The station coordinator oversees pollen/mold collectors that are mounted on a platform or rooftop, typically one story off the ground (e.g. 13 feet), ideally in an open space distant from trees. The device currently used by most sites is the rotorod, which is a rotating arm cascade impactor that contains a pair of 1.59 mm wide plastic rods which extend during rotation on a central arm at a defined time interval (e.g. 10–60 s every 10 min).[69] Pollen and mold spore levels are reported in grains or spores per cubic meter of air sampled for the previous 24-hour period. The duration of rotation can be adjusted to minimize the risk of the rod becoming overloaded during periods of high pollen and mold density, as such overloading can lead to gross inaccuracies. The efficiency of particle collection on the rod decreases with particle size (e.g. 7 μm particle with 10% efficiency to 25 μm with 100% efficiency).[70] Fungal spores are relatively small: they vary in size from 1 μm to more than 100 μm, with many spores in the range of 7–12 μm. Pollen grains are larger, with diameters of 20–70 μm. Other devices for spore collection include inertial samplers such as suction impactors. These devices have a higher efficiency for small particle collection and collect longitudinal samples over a 24 hour or 5-day period. Despite the greater cost, many stations are gradually adopting the suction impactor collectors in their routine daily pollen and mold spore counting to enhance the efficiency of collection.

REFERENCES

1. Prausnitz C, Kustner H. Studine uber die Ueberemfindlichkeil. Zentrabl Bakteriol Mikrobiol Hyg 1921;86:160.
2. Ishizaka K, Ishizaka T. Physiochemical properties of reaginic antibody. I. Association of reaginic activity with an immunoglobulin other than gamma A or gamma G globulin. J Allergy 1967;37:169.
3. Johansson SGO. Raised levels of a new immunoglobulin class (IgND) in asthma. Lancet 1967;2:951.
4. Hamilton RG. Human immunoglobulins. In: Leffell MS, Rose N (eds.) Handbook of human immunology. Boca Raton, CRC Press, 1998.
5. Frick OL. Immediate hypersensitivity. In: Stites DP, Stobo JD, Fudenburg HH, Wells JW (eds) Basic and clinical immunology. Los Altos, CA, Lange Medical Publications, 1992; p 250.
6. Schartz LB, Yunginger JW, Miller J, et al. Time course of appearance and disappearance of human mast cell tryptase in the circulation after anaphylaxis. J Clin Invest 1989;83:1551.
7. Barbee RA, Halomen M, Lebowitz M, et al. Distribution of IgE in a community population sample: correlations with age, sex and allergen skin test reactivity. J Allergy Clin Immunol 1981;68:106.
8. Kjellman M, Johannson SGO, Roth A. Serum IgE levels in healthy children quantified by a sandwich technique (PRIST). Clin Allergy 1976;6:51.
9. Wittig HJ, Belloit J, DeFillippi I, et al. Age-related serum IgE levels in healthy subjects and in patients with allergic disease. J Allergy Clin Immunol 1980;66:305.
10. Saarinen UM, Juntunen K, Kajosarri J, et al. Serum immunoglobulin E in atopic and non-atopic children aged 6 months to 5 years. Acta Paediatr Scand 1982;71:489.
11. Dati F, Ringel KP. Reference values for serum IgE in healthy non-atopic children and adults. Clin Chem 1982;28:1556.
12. Nye L., Merritt TG, Landon J, et al. A detailed investigation of circulating IgE levels in a normal population. Clin Allergy 1973;1:13.
13. Wuthrich B. Serum IgE in atopic dermatitis. Clin Allergy 1978;8:241.
14. Grennan DM, Palmer DG. Serum IgE concentration in rheumatoid arthritis: lack of correlation with gold toxicity. Br Med J 1979;8:1477.
15. Buckley RH, Becker WG. Abnormalities in the regulation of human IgE synthesis. Immunol Rev 1978;41:388.
16. Amlot PL, Green LA. Atopy and immunoglobulin E concentrations in Hodgkin's disease and other lymphomas. Br Med J 1978;1:327.
17. Halligran R, Arrendal H, Hiesche P. Elevated immunoglobulin E in bronchial carcinoma: its relation to the histology and prognosis of the cancer. J Allergy Clin Immunol 1981;67:398.
18. Levo Y, Shalalit N. Serum IgE levels in patients with liver disease. Ann Allergy 1981;47:456.
19. Wide L, Bennich H, Johansson SGO. Diagnosis by an *in vitro* test for allergen specific antibodies. Lancet 1967;2:1105.
20. Norman PS, Lichtenstein LM, Ishizaka K. Diagnostic tests in ragweed hay fever. A comparison of direct skin tests, IgE antibody measurements and basophil histamine release. J Allergy Clin Immunol 1973;52:210.
21. Foucard T. Immunochemical and biological determination of reagins. A comparison between the radioallergosorbent test (RAST) and the test for histamine release from passively sensitized chopped human lung (CHLT). Int Arch Allergy Appl Immunol 1972;42:711.
22. Hoffman DR. Comparison of methods of performing the radioallergosorbent test: Phadebas, Fadal Nalebuff and Hoffman protocols. Ann Allergy 1980;45:343.
23. Hogarth-Scott RS, McNichol RN, Williams HE, et al. Diagnosis of allergy *in vitro*: a comparison between skin sensitivity testing and serum levels of specific IgE antibody in children. Med Aus 1973;1:1293.
24. Berg T, Bennich H, Johansson SGO. *In vitro* diagnosis of atopic allergy. I. A comparison between provocation tests and the radioallergosorbent test. Int Arch Allergy Appl Immunol 1971;40:770.
25. Kelso JM, Sodhi N, Gosselin VA, et al. Diagnostic performance characteristics of the standard Phadebas RAST, modified RAST and Pharmacia CP system versus skin testing. Ann Allergy 1991;67:511.
26. Williams PB, Dolen WK, Koepke JW, et al. Comparison of skin testing and three *in vitro* assays for specific IgE in the clinical evaluation of immediate hypersensitivity. Ann Allergy 1992;68:35.
27. Van der Zee JS, De Groot H, van Swieten P, et al. Discrepancies between skin test and IgE antibody assays: studies of histamine release, complement activation *in vitro* and occurrence of allergen-specific IgG. J Allergy Clin Immunol 1988;82:270.
28. Bernstein IL. Proceedings of the task force on guidelines for standardizing old and new technologies used for the diagnosis and treatment of allergic diseases. J Allergy Clin Immunol 1988;82:487.
29. Hamilton RG, Adkinson NF Jr, Multi-Center Latex Task Force. Diagnosis of natural rubber latex allergy: multi-center latex skin testing efficacy study. J Allergy Clin Immunol 1998;102:482.
30. Hamilton RG, Biagini RE, Krieg EF, Multi-Center Latex Task Force. Diagnostic performance of FDA-cleared serological assays for natural rubber latex specific IgE antibody. J Allergy Clin Immunol 1999;103:925.

31. Guerin B, Watson RD. Skin tests. Clin Rev Allergy 1988;6:211.
32. Norman PS. Skin testing. In: Middleton E, Ellis EF, Reed CE (eds) Allergy: Principles and practice, 2nd edn. Mosby, St. Louis, 1982, p 295.
33. Nelson HS, Lahr J, Buchmeier A, McCormick D. Evaluation of devices for skin prick testing. J Allergy Clin Immunol 1998;101:153.
34. Turkeltaub PC, Rastogi SC, Baer H, et al. A standardized quantitative skin test assay of allergen potency and stability. Studies on the allergen dose–response curve and effect of wheal, erythema and patient selection on assay results. J Allergy Clin Immunol 1982;70:343.
35. Chai H. Bronchial challenges. Clin Rev Allergy 1988;6:231.
36. Naclerio RM, Norman PS, Fish JE. In vivo methods for study of allergy: mucosal tests techniques and interpretation. In: Middleton E, Reed CE, Ellis EF, Adkinson NF Jr, Yunginger JW (eds) Allergy: principles and practice, 3rd edn. St. Louis, Mosby, 1988, p 437.
37. Kurtz KM, Hamilton RG, Adkinson NF Jr. Role and application of provocation in the diagnosis of occupational latex allergy. Ann Allergy Asthma Immunol 1999;83:634.
38. Pipkorn U, Granerus G, Proud D. The effect of a histamine synthesis inhibitor on the immediate nasal allergic reaction. Allergy 1987;42:496.
39. Sampson HA. Adverse reactions to foods. In: Middleton E, Reed CE, Ellis EF, Adkinson NF Jr, Yunginger JW, Busse WW (eds) Allergy: principles and practice, 4th edn. St. Louis, Mosby, 1993, p 1661.
40. May CD. Objective clinical and laboratory studies of immediate-hypersensitivity reactions to foods in asthmatic children. J Allergy Clin Immunol 1976;58:500.
41. Bock SA, Sampson HA, Atkins FM, et al. Double-blind placebo controlled food challenge as an office procedure: a manual. J Allergy Clin Immunol 1988;82:986.
42. Sampson HA, Ho DG. Relationship between food-specific IgE concentrations and the risk of positive food challenges in children and adolescents. J Allergy Clin Immunol 1997;100:444.
43. Diagnostic Allergy [SE] Survey, College of American Pathologists (CAP), 325 Waukegan Road, Northfield, IL 60093–2750, 1999, p 1–7.
44. Hamilton RG, Adkinson NF Jr. Immunological tests for diagnosis and management of human allergic disease: total and allergen-specific IgE and allergen-specific IgG. In: Rose NR, De Macario EC, Folds JD, Lane HC, Nakamura RM (eds) Manual of clinical laboratory immunology, 5th edn. Washington DC, American Society for Microbiology, 1997, p 881.
45. National Committee on Clinical Laboratory Standards (Matsson PNJ, Hamilton RG, eds) Evaluation methods and analytical performance characteristics of immunological assays for human IgE antibody of defined allergen specificities: approved guideline 1/LA20-A, 1997.
46. Hamilton RG, Butler JE. Quantitation of specific antibodies: methods of expression, standards solid phase considerations and specific applications. In: Butler JE (ed) Immunochemistry of solid phase immunoassays. Boca Raton, FL, CRC Press, 1991, Chapter 9.
47. Yunginger JW, Adolphson CR. Standardization of allergens. In: Rose NR, De Macario EC, Fahey JL, Friedman H, Penn GM (eds) Manual of clinical laboratory immunology, 4th edn. Washington DC, American Society for Microbiology, 1992, p 678.
48. Hamilton RG, Wisenauer JA, Golden DB, Valentine MD, Adkinson NF Jr. Selection of Hymenoptera venoms for immunotherapy based on patient's IgE antibody crossreactivity. J Allergy Clin Immunol 1993;92:651.
49. Lichtenstein LM, Holtzman NA, Burnett LS. A quantitative *in vitro* study of the chromatographic distribution and immunoglobulin characteristics of human blocking antibody. J Immunol 1968;101:317.
50. Lichtenstein LM, Norman PS, Winkenwerder WL. A single year of immunotherapy of ragweed hay fever: immunologic and clinical studies. Ann Intern Med 1971;75:663.
51. Golden DBK, Lawrence ID, Hamilton RG, Kagey Sobotka A, Valentine MD, Lichtenstein LM. Clinical correlation of the venom-specific IgG antibody level during maintenance venom immunotherapy. J Allergy Clin Immunol 1992;90:386.
52. Craig CS, Schwartz LB. Tryptase and chymase: markers of distinct types of human mast cells. Immunol Res 1989;8:130.
53. Miller JS, Schwartz LB. Tryptase levels as an indication of mast cell activation in a patient with Hymenoptera anaphylaxis and mastocytosis. N Engl J Med 1987;316:1622.
54. Lichtenstein LM, Osler AG. Studies on the mechanisms of hypersensitivity phenomenon. IX. Histamine release from human leukocytes by ragweed pollen. J Exp Med 1964;120:507.
55. MacGlashan DW Jr, Schleimer RP, Lichtenstein LM. Qualitative differences between dimeric and trimeric stimulation of human basophils. J Immunol 1983;130:4.
56. Siraganian RP. Automated histamine analysis for *in vitro* allergy testing. II. Correlation of skin test results with *in vitro* whole blood histamine release in 82 patients. J Allergy Clin Immunol 1977;59:214.
57. Wegner F, Hockamp R, Rutschke A, Becker B, Reinhardt D. Superiority of the histamine release test above case history, prick test and radioallergosorbent test in predicting bronchial reactivity to the house dust mite in asthmatic children. Klin Wochenschr 1983;61:43.
58. Fifield R, Hamilton RG. Inter-laboratory 'external' quality assessment programs for the diagnostic allergy laboratory. J Clin Immunoassay 1993;16:144.
59. Hamilton RG, Adkinson NF Jr. Clinical laboratory methods for the assessment and management of human allergic diseases. Clin Lab Med 1986;6:117.
60. Gleich GJ, Loegering DA. Immunobiology of eosinophils. Annu Rev Immunol 1984;2:429.
61. Hallgren R, Bigelle A, Veuge P. Eosinophil cationic protein in inflammatory effusions as evidence of eosinophil involvement. Ann Rheum Dis 1984;43:556.
62. Dahl R, Venge P, Fredens K. The eosinophil. In: Barnes PJ, Rodger I, Thompson N (eds) Asthma: basic mechanisms and clinical management. London, Academic Press, 1988.
63. Pepys J. Hypersensitivity diseases of the lungs due to fungi and organic dusts. Monogr Allergy 1972;4:69.
64. Fink JN. Hypersensitivity pneumonitis. In: Middleton E, Reed CE, Ellis EF, Adkinson NF Jr, Yunginger JW (eds). Allergy: principles and practice, 3rd edn. St. Louis, Mosby, 1988, p 1237.
65. Jarvis MJ, Tunstall-Pedoe H, Feyerabend C, Vesley C, Saloojee Y. Comparisons of tests used to distinguish smokers from non-smokers. Am J Public Health 1987;77:1435.
66. Haley NJ, Sepkovic DW, Hoffmann D. Elimination of cotenine from body fluids: disposition in smokers and non-smokers. Am J Public Health 1989;79:1046.
67. Hamilton RG, Chapman MD, Platts-Mills TAE, Adkinson NF Jr. House dust aeroallergen measurements in clinical practice: a guide to allergen free home and work environments. Immunol Allergy Practice 1992;14:9.
68. Wood RA, Eggleston PA, Lind P, et al. Antigenic analysis of household dust samples. Am Rev Respir Dis 1988;137:358.
69. Solomon WR. Techniques of air sampling. In: Sheldon JM, Lovell RM, Mathews KP (eds). Manual of clinical allergy, 2nd edn. Philadelphia, WB Saunders, 1967.
70. Edmonds RL. Collection efficiency of rotorod samplers for sampling fungus spores in the atmosphere. Plant Disease Reporter 1972;56:704.

Chapter 125 Molecular Methods

John W. Belmont

Molecular analysis of nucleic acids provides broad tools for the clinical laboratory. The purpose of this chapter is to review the basic principles that underlie clinical molecular genetic testing, to review the range of methods that can be employed, and to suggest a multidisciplinary approach for implementation in immunological disorders.

BASIC PRINCIPLES

Genome structure and gene expression

The human genome is thought to contain 30 000–40 000 genes[1–3] distributed on 23 pairs of chromosomes (http://www.ncbi.nlm.nih.gov/genemap/; http://www.ncbi.nlm.nih.gov/UniGene/). The total length of one copy of the genome is $\sim 3 \times 10^9$ nucleotide bases. The protein coding segments (exons) are split by noncoding DNA sequences (introns). Some of the noncoding DNA contains regulatory elements that direct the expression of the genes, control chromatin conformation, act as origins for DNA replication, and produce the large-scale chromosome structure. About 40% of the total DNA is accounted for by families of repeated sequences. These repeat elements are generally silent but may become involved in mutational mechanisms of deletion and insertion. Each cell expresses only a subset of the entire gene repertoire, but previous views of gene expression are being rapidly modified by growing experience with gene expression microarrays.[4,5] 'Housekeeping' genes are expressed in almost all tissues and cell types, where they perform basic metabolic and structural functions. Other genes are under very specific control and their expression is restricted to one or a few cell types. Differential gene expression specifies the unique functions of cells, e.g. globin in erythrocytes, immunoglobulin in B cells, and T-cell receptor in T cells. Genes that coordinate the expression of groups of tissue-specific genes primarily encode transcription factors that regulate the rate of mRNA transcription on their target genes. A few of these apparently act as 'master' genes during particular developmental processes or in specific cell lineages. Some of these master genes may be involved in leukemias and lymphomas. So far, immune deficiency genes appear to be in the category of genes that perform cell type-specific functions or that control cell growth[6].

Polymorphic variation and linkage

A genetic map relates one gene to another based on how often they are inherited together. The maternal and paternal copies of the genome are nonidentical at many nucleotide positions. The differences are called *polymorphisms* and, when comparing two arbitrary chromosomes, they occur in $\sim 1/1000$ nucleotides.[7] Polymorphisms arise over time in a group of individuals because of mutation in the DNA. Some polymorphisms involve simple sequence repeats so that there is variation in the number of repeat units. These are called short tandem repeats (STR) and form the basis of the most widely applied genetic marker maps (described later in this chapter). In contrast to STRs, the most common polymorphisms involve a change in a single nucleotide position. Large databases of single nucleotide polymorphisms (SNPs – pronounced 'snips') are being accumulated (http://www.ncbi.nlm.nih.gov/SNP/). It is thought that there could be $1\text{–}3 \times 10^6$ SNPs available across the human genome. Many STR and SNP polymorphisms are found in noncoding DNA, presumably because these segments are not subject to 'purifying' negative selection in evolution. Functionally significant polymorphisms occur in protein coding sequences and in regulatory noncoding DNA sequences at frequencies that can vary widely between loci.

The composition of genes and their alleles in an individual is called the *genotype*. The individual's genotype interacts with the environment both in development and in maturity to create the *phenotype*. Some components of the phenotype, like skin rash, can be relatively simple, while other phenotypes may be based on complex laboratory evaluation (e.g. in T-cell proliferation). A key distinction should be drawn between discrete traits and those that are represented by a quantitative continuum. Many laboratory values, which are essentially quantitative, can be reduced to discrete traits by assigning them to 'normal' or 'abnormal' status. Polymorphisms presumably account for the majority of variation that is observed at the phenotype level between healthy individuals and between populations. Common polymorphisms are usually considered to have minor allele frequencies of at least 5%. This is an arbitrary cutoff and there are actually many more low-frequency alleles in most DNA segments examined to date; more rare polymorphisms are generally uncovered as more individuals are surveyed. Some of these polymorphisms are population-specific and there is a general correlation of allele frequency with the age of polymorphism, i.e. the older the polymorphism the greater the allele frequency and the greater the likelihood that it will be observed in all ethnic groups. Polymorphisms are the key to tracking the inheritance of whole segments of adjacent DNA and are thus used to follow disease genes in families.

During the formation of the haploid germ cells – ova and sperm – one member (homolog) of each parental chromosome pair is segregated to one of two daughter nuclei (first meiotic division, Fig. 125.1). Because each chromosome is essentially independent of the others, genes on different chromosomes are independently segregated and unlinked. During meiosis, *recombination* between homologous chromosomes leads to further mixing of the two parental genomes. Each chromosome may cross

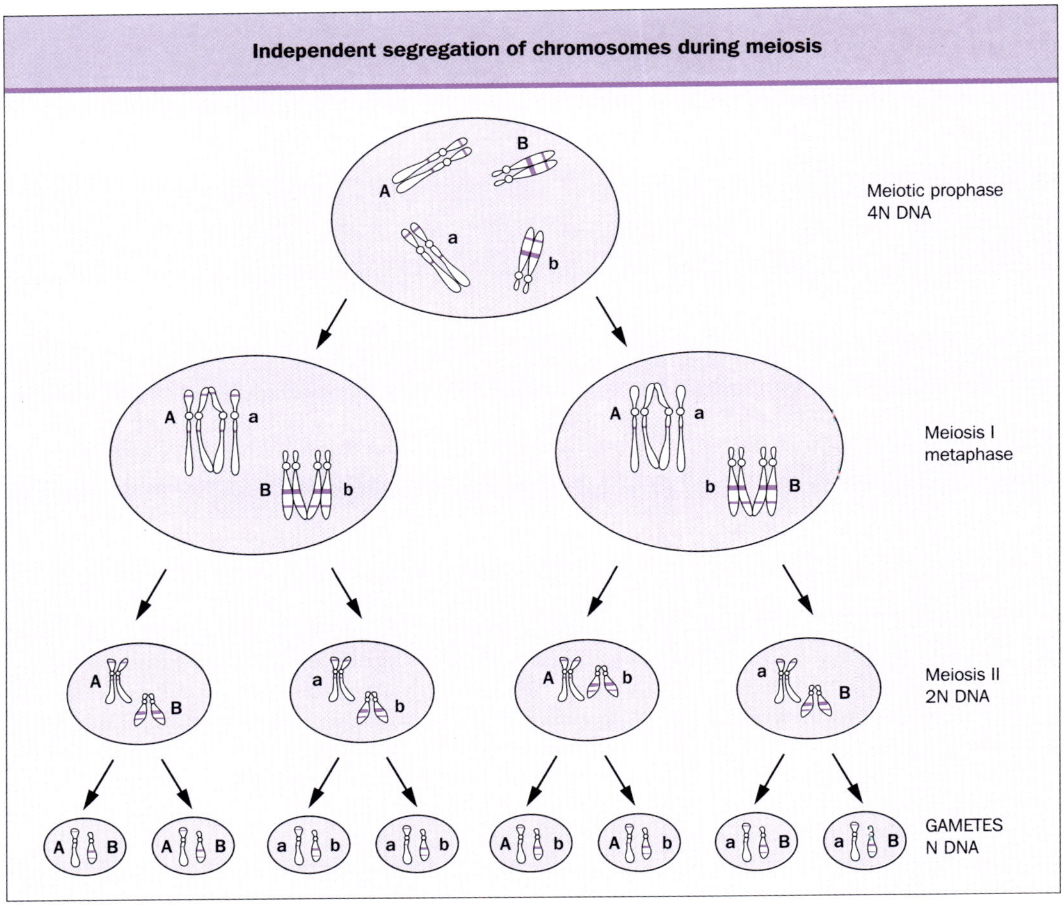

Figure 125.1 Independent segregation of chromosomes during meiosis. The diploid adult cells give rise to all combinations of parental chromosomes. Genes on different chromosomes are unlinked. Detection of this phenomenon depends on distinguishing allelic polymorphisms, i.e. A or a, B or b.

over an average of 2–3 segments at meiosis. If several genes or markers are on the same chromosome then the phase in which they start may favor one allele association over another (Fig. 125.2). If the genes are far apart on a chromosome then it is likely that at least one crossover point will come between them during meiosis. If the genes are close to one another they will tend to segregate together. If they are very close they will essentially always segregate together. Since the physical distance between two genes determines whether they will be inherited as a block during meiosis, a statistical relationship can be developed that indicates how likely two segments are to be co-inherited. *Linkage* between two loci can be quantified as the recombination fraction – θ. Linkage is present if the fraction of recombination is less than 0.5 (i.e. a 50:50 chance of co-inheritance). θ is often expressed in centimorgans (cM) so that if two loci are 1 cM apart then there is a 1% chance of recombination at meiosis. 1 cM is equivalent to approximately 1 million base pairs of DNA. However, the recombination fraction between two loci can be affected by factors other than physical distance, e.g. the presence of repeat sequences that may favor recombination or proximity to the centromere that may suppress recombination.

Genes can be mapped in relation to one another by a linkage map. Genes that are physically close can be shown to be predominantly co-inherited. The usual way to express this relationship is with the LOD score – log of the odds of linkage – that compares the chance of two gene segments to be co-inherited with the situation in which they are unlinked. Conventionally, if the LOD is >3.0 (or 1000:1 in favor of the genes being linked) the results are considered significant. One major achievement of the human genome project has been to develop dense linkage maps for humans.[8,9] The use of marker loci that show a high degree of polymorphism is particularly useful for this.

Linkage mapping played a large role in the identification of the X-linked immune deficiency genes (Chapters 34–37). Linkage has been much less useful for the identification of autosomal recessive genes responsible for rare immune deficiencies because average family sizes are not large enough to be used by themselves. Another difficulty is that similar diseases (phenotypes) can be caused by mutation in more than one gene locus (locus heterogeneity). Linkage testing, however, can be a very powerful method for individual family studies once a disease gene has been identified. DNA can be examined directly without the need to identify the specific disease mutation or to test the mutant

KEY CONCEPTS

Human genomics

- The human genome encompasses approximately 35 000 genes, but each cell expresses only a subset of those genes.
- Genetic and physical maps of the genome are essential to molecular diagnosis of immune system diseases.
- Genetic maps depend on the co-inheritance of DNA segments – linkage – to derive gene order on individual chromosomes.
- Physical maps of the genome describe the exact gene locations on a chromosome. The genome DNA sequence is the finest scale physical map of the genome.

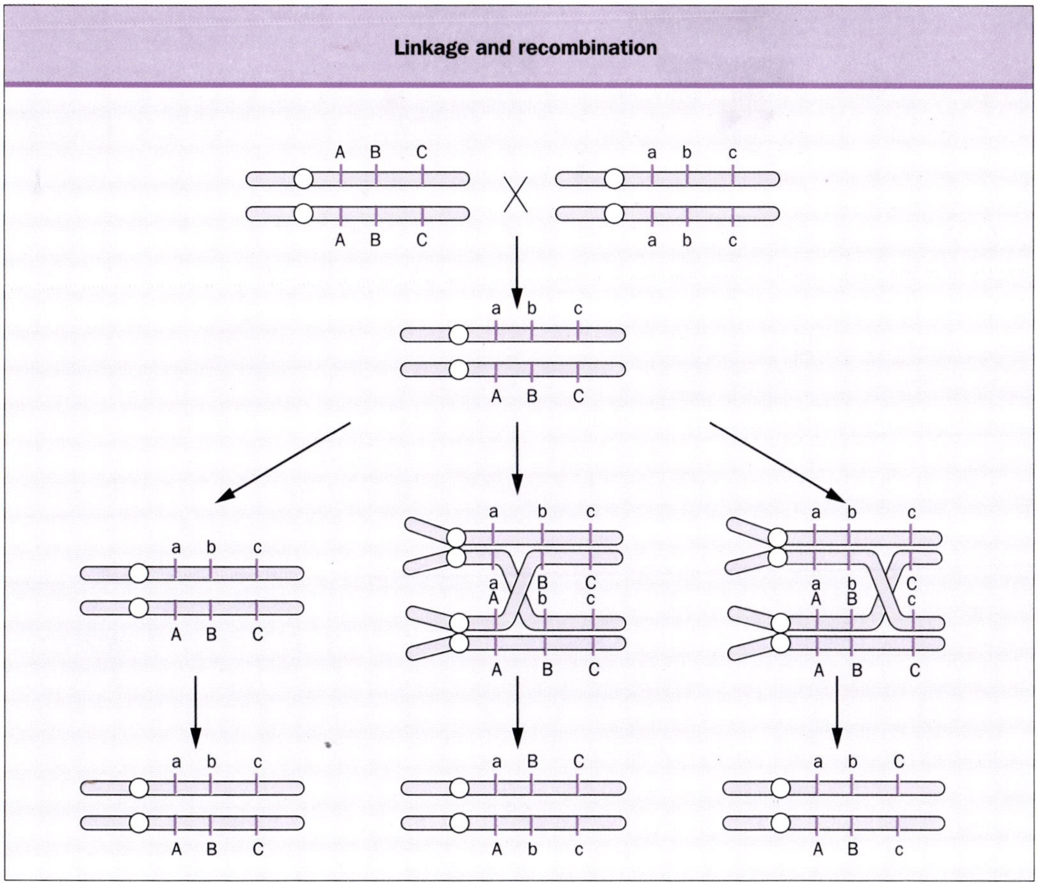

Figure 125.2 Linkage and recombination. Genes that are physically close to one another on a chromosome tend to be inherited as a block. The farther apart they are, the more likely it is that a recombination will take place during meiosis. DNA markers, like microsatellites, are used to distinguish the two parental alleles. Blocks of co-inherited genes create a *haplotype* that is stably inherited within families. A new haplotype is created by recombination.

gene product. Many of the markers used for clinical analysis in primary immune deficiencies are either contained within the disease gene or are physically close and thus show no recombination ($\theta = 0$). Although these markers are preferred, highly accurate diagnoses can be made with markers that are farther away. This is accomplished by testing markers that flank each side of the disease gene.

Physical maps and molecular cytogenetics

Genetic or linkage maps can be contrasted with the physical gene map. Physical maps are different from the genetic map in that they describe how genes are arranged in the DNA on a scale as large as a whole chromosome and as fine as a single nucleotide. At the most coarse level of the physical map, genes are placed in chromosome segments corresponding to the Giemsa stain banding pattern of metaphase chromosomes. The availability of the draft human DNA sequence has provided a nearly complete fine-scale physical map of the human genome (http://www.ncbi.nlm.nih.gov/genome/guide/). Although the draft sequence leaves uncertainty about the order of DNA elements over intervals of about 1000–15 000 nucleotides, the larger-scale order is very precisely known. This physical map is encompassed in a set of bacterial artificial chromosome (BAC) clones that have DNA inserts of approximately 90 000–250 000 nucleotides. These clones partially overlap one another creating a 'golden path' (http://genome.ucsc.edu/goldenPath/hgTracks.html) of coverage across most of the genome (Fig. 125.3). These clones have formed the scaffold for the public genome sequencing project. BAC clones now provide extremely useful reagents for both research and clinical purposes.

A very important way to localize genes after they have been cloned is to hybridize them directly to a chromosome spread. The technique, called fluorescence in situ hybridization (FISH), allows detection and electronic enhancement of signals from the chromosome spread to directly localize genes.[10] FISH is used for cytogenetic examination of tumors, leukemias, and lymphomas. In the DiGeorge syndrome, characteristic deletions of chromosomes 22q11 or 10p13 can only be detected with FISH (Chapter 40). BAC clones are exceptionally convenient as probes because their order is generally known and their size is technically advantageous for signal intensity.

Mutation

Mutations may involve small or large deletions, insertions, inversions, or duplications. Mutations occurring outside coding sequences of genes or that do not change the protein encoded by the gene may have no phenotypic effect at all. They become one of the huge pool of neutral polymorphisms in the genome. Single base changes in a triplet amino acid codon, on the other hand, often disturb the normal function of proteins. These are described as missense (i.e. causing an amino acid substitution), nonsense (i.e. terminating translation), or frameshift (changing the reading frame, usually leading to translation termination within a few codons). Mutations affecting regulatory or splice signal sequences in RNA can also be deleterious. A primary mechanism of mutation is misincorporation of nucleotides during DNA replication by DNA polymerase. A second important mechanism occurs at CpG dinucleotides.[11] The cytosine is often methylated and chemical deamination of the methylated cytosine gives the base thymidine. At the next round of replication the CG may be changed to TG or CA depending on

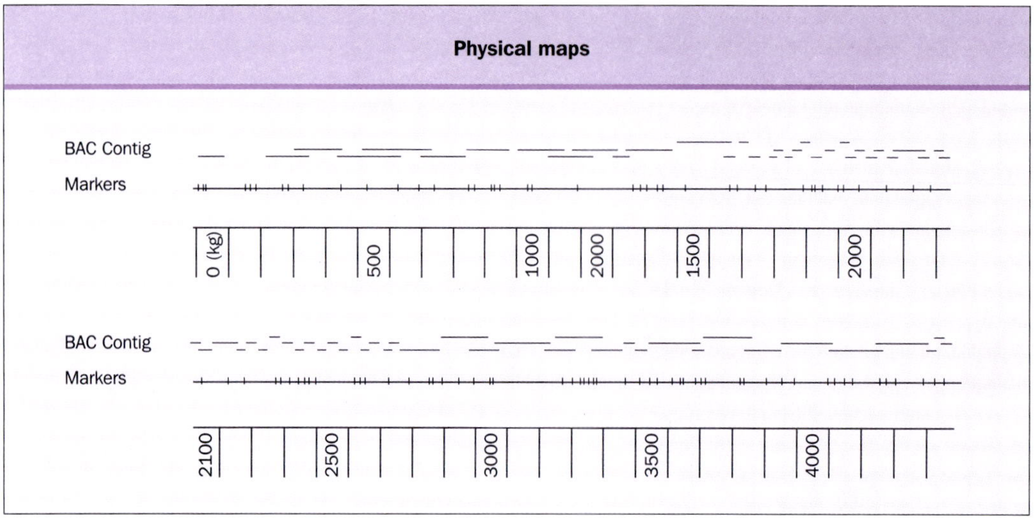

Figure 125.3 Physical maps. A contig of bacterial artificial chromosome (BAC) clones forms an overlapping path of coverage over millions of base pairs. These BACs and some smaller clones have been used to produce libraries for sequencing the genome and are coupled in the public databases to the genomic sequence.

which DNA strand was altered. CG is found in the amino acid codons of Arg, Ser, Pro, Thr, and Ala. These amino acids are frequently involved in coding sequence mutations. Finally, an entirely different and novel mechanism for mutation is expansion of unstable triplet repeat segments.[12] So far, no disorder that affects the immune system has been associated with this mechanism. As outlined below, mutation screening will have a continuing and expanding role in clinical molecular testing.

Heritable mutations may arise in either the male or female germline but the sex-related frequency is influenced by the mutational mechanism. Chromosomal nondisjunction, for example, occurs predominantly during female meiosis and has a strong maternal age effect. The fact that spermatogonial proliferation occurs throughout life and involves many more cell replications than oogenesis increases the single base mutation frequency in the paternal germline. A 20-fold risk for point mutations and a 11-fold risk of mutations at CpG dinucleotides occurring in the male germline has been observed in the factor IX gene.[13–15]

Clinicians must cope with both locus and allele *heterogeneity*. Locus heterogeneity means that the same or a similar phenotype results from mutation in one of several different genes. For example, severe combined immune deficiency (SCID) may result from mutation in the adenosine deaminase, interleukin-2 receptor γ chain genes, etc. Allelic heterogeneity, on the other hand, means that the disease is caused by different mutations in the same gene. For severe X-linked disorders, allele heterogeneity is typically high because in the past most affected individuals did not live to reproduce and because the diseases arise by repeated new mutations. At autosomal loci some mutations occurred in the distant past or have a high frequency in a particular population. In the heterozygous state, recessive mutations may be weakly deleterious, neutral, or actually confer a small advantage. In cystic fibrosis[16] and Tay–Sachs disease,[17] for example, a few mutations account for a large percentage of the abnormal alleles. The heterozygote frequency in those disorders may be increased by relative resistance to *Salmonella*/cholera[18] and tuberculosis,[19] respectively. Because the mutant alleles are common, it is possible to test affected individuals and potential carriers directly for those mutations. Certain important HLA alleles that increase the risk of autoimmune disease may owe their prevalence to either founder effects or selective advantage in the period when infectious burden was high and life span short. In contrast, none of the immune deficiencies (with the possible exception of the SCID seen in Native Americans of the Southwest[20]) result from common mutations that would permit efficient screening. In the autosomal recessive immune deficiencies most patients have two different mutations (*compound heterozygosity*) at the disease locus unless there is parental consanguinity.

KEY CONCEPTS

Mutation

- Mutation can occur by deletion, insertion, or duplication of short or long DNA segments.
- Single-base mutations can be caused by replication errors or by chemical deamination of methyl-cytosine.
- Single-base mutations can affect protein coding sequence, regulatory sequences, or the RNA splice signals within a gene.
- The parental origin of mutations (maternal or paternal) affects which mutational mechanisms were most likely responsible.
- A disease can be caused by mutations in several alternative genes (locus heterogeneity).
- Most primary immune deficiency disease occurs because of different kinds of mutations in particular genes (allelic heterogeneity).

X chromosome inactivation

Disturbances in the pattern of X inactivation are interesting phenomena in women who are carriers of X-linked immune deficiencies. At the level of an individual cell only a single X chromosome is active. Since either the maternal or paternal X chromosome is expressed exclusively, women are *mosaic* for X chromosome gene expression. Measurement of X chromosome activity in the blood cells of normal women shows that on average the contribution of maternal and paternal X chromosomes is approximately 50%. Extreme skewing of X inactivation often results from abnormal proliferation of blood cells. X inactivation analysis can be used to demonstrate clonal growth of premalignant (e.g. myelodysplasia) and malignant cells. In three classic X-linked immune deficiencies (severe combined immune deficiency, agammaglobulinemia, and Wiskott–Aldrich syndrome) one of the X chromosomes bears a mutation that affects the growth or survival of cells expressing that mutant allele. As a consequence, the affected stem cell and its daughters have a selective disadvantage in growth. In a female carrying mutations at the X-linked severe combined immune deficiency (XSCID MIM #300400), agammaglobulinemia (XLA MIM *300300), or Wiskott–Aldrich (WAS MIM *301000) loci, cell competition and compensation mechanisms lead to decreased contribution of cells expressing the mutant allele among affected cells. In XLA, the B-cell lineage shows selective use of the nonmutant active X.[21] In XSCID, skewing of X inactivation is observed in B cells, T cells, and NK cells.[22,23] In WAS, some degree of skewing of X inactivation can be observed in all hematopoietic lineages but is most prominent and consistent in the T cells.[24] Historically, skewed X inactivation was very helpful in linkage mapping of these conditions. As a clinical test, X inactivation now has reduced importance compared to direct mutation analyses. There may be some role for X inactivation assays to clarify carrier status when mutation analysis is incomplete or unsuccessful.

DESCRIPTION AND PRINCIPLES OF DNA DIAGNOSTIC TECHNIQUES

The overriding theme of all DNA diagnostic techniques is the specific detection of one or a few segments of DNA in the complex mixture of sequences encompassing the genome. There are four key techniques in gene diagnosis: restriction enzyme digestion, DNA:DNA hybridization, polymerase chain reaction, and DNA sequencing. In addition to these four core laboratory techniques one should now add computer-based data management or *bioinformatics* as a necessary diagnostic laboratory discipline.

Southern and Northern blotting

Southern analysis was one of the first techniques to find wide clinical application. For the first time it was possible to examine qualitatively an individual gene from many patients and their families. In a Southern blot,[25] genomic DNA is digested with a restriction enzyme that cuts at a short specific (4–8 base pairs) segment of DNA (Fig. 125.4). The very long pieces of chromosomal DNA are cleaved into much smaller units that range from a few hundred to tens of thousands of base pairs. The digested genomic DNA is separated on the basis of fragment length on an agarose gel. Because genomic DNA is very complex, the digested DNA looks like a random smear, but because cleavage by the restriction enzyme is sequence specific, the pattern of digestion is very reproducible. The separated DNA is transferred and fixed to a filter membrane and then incubated with a labeled and denatured DNA probe. The probe is most commonly labeled with ^{32}P, but non-radioactive probes, particularly those using chemiluminescence technology, rival the sensitivity achieved with radiolabeling. When

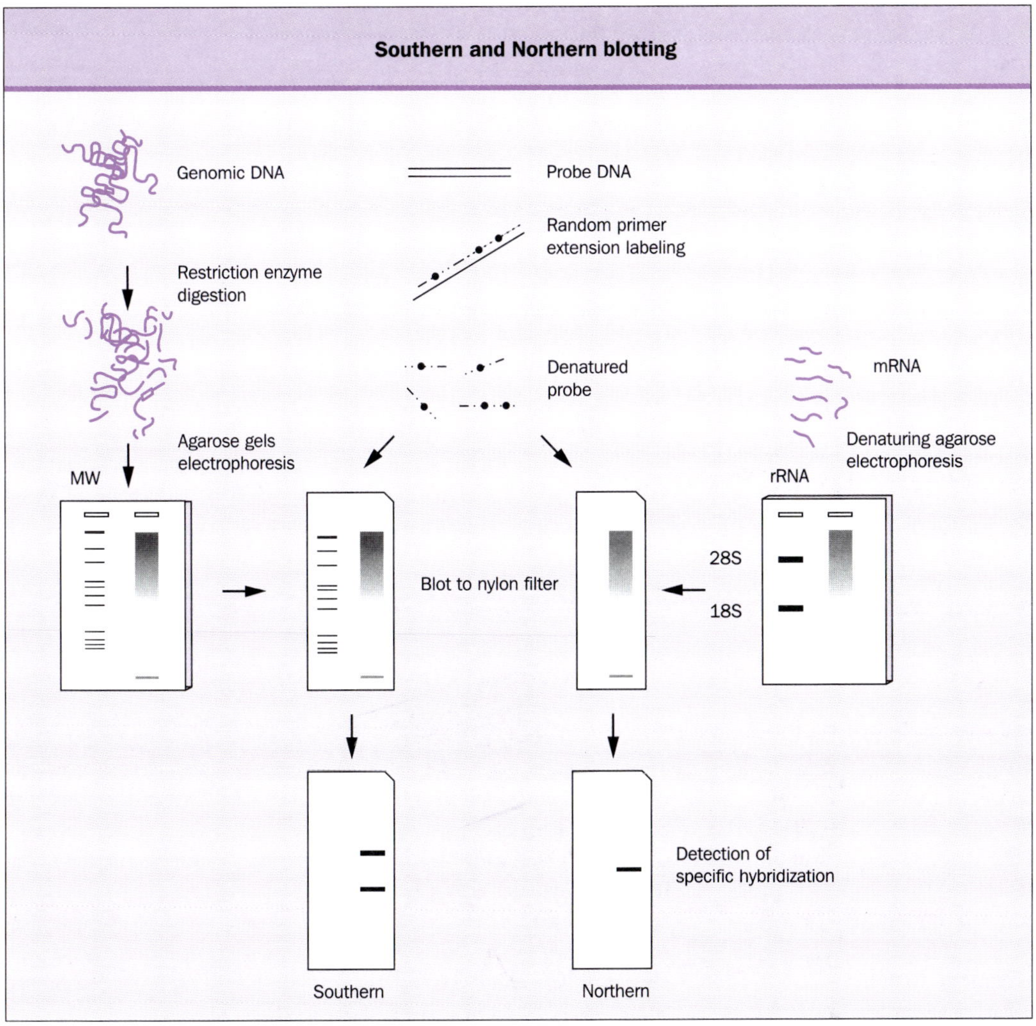

Figure 125.4 Southern and Northern blotting. Probe DNA is usually produced by incorporation of ^{32}P-dCTP into newly synthesized DNA. See text for further explanation.

the probe DNA finds a complementary sequence on the filter, it hybridizes. The hybrids are stable to washing while nonspecifically bound probe is washed away. The filter is then analyzed by autoradiography or a phosphor imaging device. Northern analysis is very similar but instead of using enzyme-digested genomic DNA one probes RNA. Whole RNA or affinity-purified mRNA can be used. The RNA is separated under denaturing conditions to avoid the self-hybridization (secondary structure) that might affect migration in the gel.

Southern analysis continues to be useful in analysis of the immunoglobulin and T-cell receptor loci in leukemias and lymphomas. The main utility of Southern analysis is that it can scan many thousands of base pairs of DNA. It is likely to remain a preferred method in clinical applications in which the complexity or primary sequence of the locus makes DNA amplification difficult.

X-chromosome inactivation

To measure X inactivation one must distinguish the two chromosomes and determine whether the products of those chromosomes are equally active. Various assays have been used but the human androgen receptor locus (HAR) is most widely applied.[26] HAR contains a highly polymorphic (90% heterozygosity) trinucleotide repeat in the first exon. This repeat is within ~100 bp of two Hpa II restriction enzyme sites that are methylated on the inactive X chromosome but unmethylated on the active X. In the normal situation, some DNA from both alleles is active and some is inactive. Therefore, the PCR products from Hpa II-cut DNA reflect the presence of both allele templates. If one allele is exclusively active its potential to be a template is destroyed by Hpa II digestion and it will disappear from the PCR products. X-inactivation studies have a limited role in carrier detection within XLA, XSCID, and WAS pedigrees and nuclear families, but may occasionally be helpful if direct mutation detection is unsuccessful.

Fluorescence in situ hybridization (FISH)

FISH provides a significant advance over older techniques that used radioactive labels for probing genes directly on chromosome spreads.[27] In its simplest form a cloned gene segment is labeled with biotin or digoxygenin tagged nucleotides. These are detected with secondary antibodies and high-sensitivity immunofluorescence techniques. The probe is hybridized to chromosomes from cells that are prepared to allow visualization of early metaphase (condensed) chromosomes. A locus appears as two pairs of dots corresponding to the sister chromatids from the two chromosomal homologs. Cells that are in interphase (when the DNA is largely unfolded in the nucleus) can also be probed. In the interphase cell, two single signals are observed corresponding to the two chromosomes. FISH plays an important role in detecting known common rearrangements such as the deletions observed in DiGeorge syndrome[28] or the translocation of *BCR-ABL* in chronic myelogenous leukemia.[29] FISH studies on interphase cells are used as a very rapid test for common chromosomal disorders such as trisomy 18 and trisomy 13.[30] Recent advances in FISH technology have emphasized its capability for multiple parallel assays. One new approach to the study of children with birth defects is subtelomeric FISH in which probes have been defined for the subtelomeric region of all the autosomes.[31] This approach allows for single-step assessment for submicroscopic deletions and rearrangement that have previously escaped detection. A related method is called spectral karyotyping in which chromosome painting probes are each labeled with a different 'color'. This method has shown great promise as a research tool in neoplastic disease.[32,33]

PCR and microsatellites

DNA amplification using the polymerase chain reaction (PCR) was a watershed advance in detection of specific nucleic acid sequences.[34] PCR depends on the ability of two short synthetic oligonucleotides to find the DNA that closely matches each one (Fig. 125.5). A thermostable enzyme is added that can synthesize new DNA using each oligonucleotide as a primer, resulting in a doubling of the segment between the primers. The presence of the complementary oligonucleotide allows a second strand of complementary DNA to be synthesized. This constitutes one cycle of PCR. When this cycle is repeated, the segment of DNA inbetween the oligonucleotides is geometrically increased. RNA can also be amplified by first synthesizing complementary DNA (cDNA) using viral reverse transcriptase (RT-PCR). The amount of product then becomes great enough to detect, either by hybridization or by direct visualization on an ethidium bromide-stained gel. PCR can theoretically detect a single molecule of DNA or RNA. Thus, small cell or tissue samples can be analyzed very rapidly. One variation is to label one of the oligonucleotides, either with a radioactive molecule like ^{32}P or with a fluorescent tag. PCR provides the starting point for linkage assays, mutation analysis, and DNA sequencing. RT-PCR is finding use in the quantitation of mRNA from blood cells, e.g. in measuring cytokine transcription from activated T and B cells.

Segments of DNA that are polymorphic can be readily detected by PCR. A class of polymorphism that is easily distinguished by PCR is called a microsatellite. These short tandem repeats (STR) are principally dinucleotide, trinucleotide, and tetranucleotide elements that vary in the number of repeat subunits between individuals[35] STRs have much higher mutation rates[36,37] than single nucleotide positions (~1000-fold greater). This instability creates extensive families of alleles. In general, the longer the uninterrupted repeat segments, the greater the chance that the element will be polymorphic. At many of these loci the heterozygosity is 70–90%. Polymorphic short tandem repeats are distributed in the genome approximately every 40 000 bases. It has been possible to identify them either close to or within most genes of medical interest. Their high degree of heterozygosity and the ease of the assay, have made microsatellites an important tool for clinical linkage testing.

DNA sequencing

The direct determination of a DNA sequence[38] is fundamental to mutation identification (Fig. 125.6). The most commonly used method depends on termination of DNA synthesis by chemically modified nucleotides (dideoxy-NTPs). A single-stranded DNA template is hybridized to a primer that can recognize a short known segment of DNA. Often this primer segment is simply part of the bacterial cloning vector. The single-stranded DNA is obtained from bacterial plasmid/phage vectors or it may be produced by DNA amplification. The primer acts as a starting point for DNA synthesis by a bacterial DNA polymerase that is added to the reaction. If the reaction were allowed to go to completion, the polymerase would synthesize a new complementary DNA strand on the single-stranded template and then fall off the end. In DNA sequencing, four separate reactions are set up, each

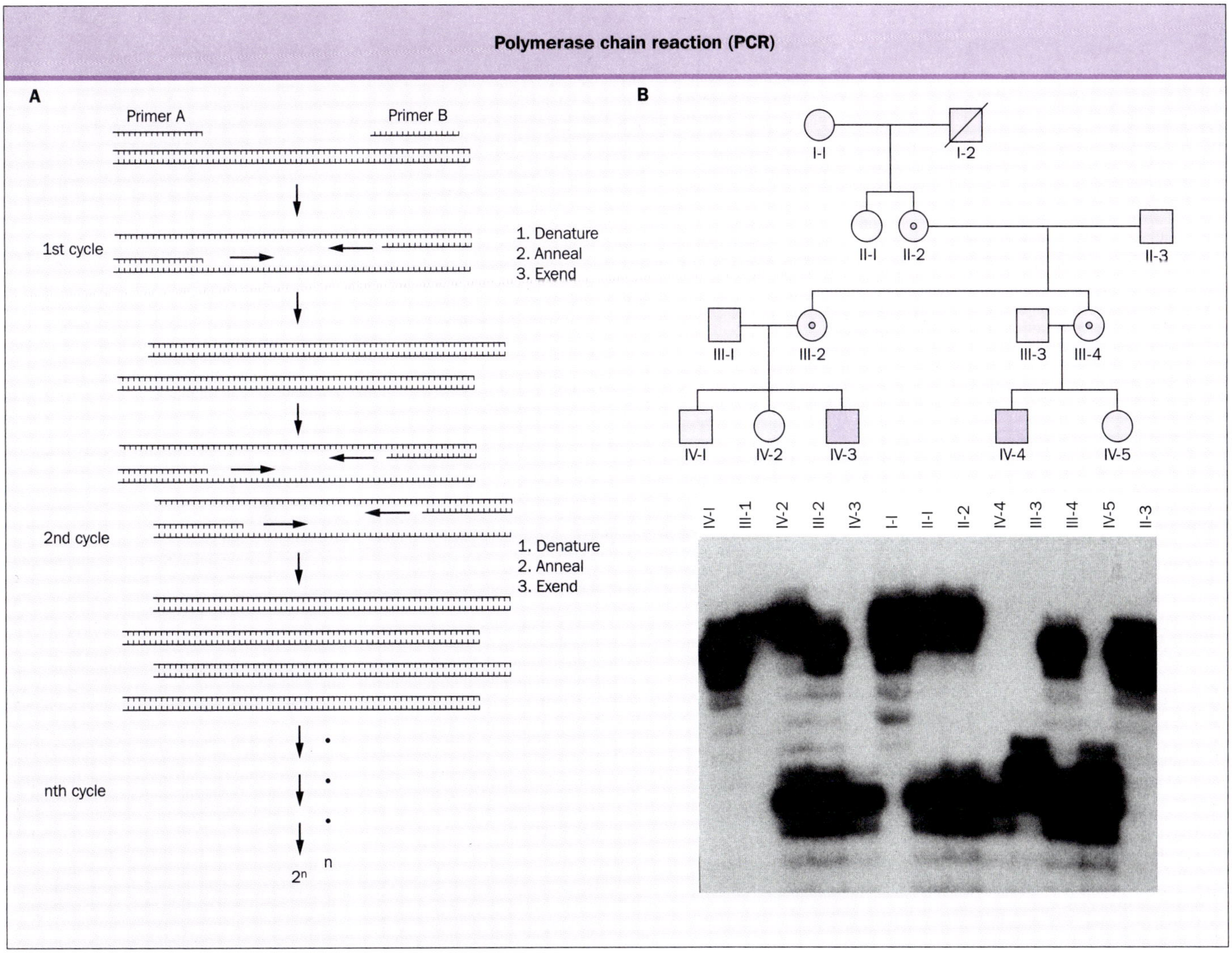

Figure 125.5 Polymerase chain reaction. (**A**) Primers that hybridize to the target sequence are used to initiate multiple cycles of synthesis, melting, annealing, and synthesis. In practice, the potential geometric increase in DNA tapers off as reaction components become limiting. (**B**) PCR flanking a triplet $(AAT)_n$ repeat segment at DXS101 allows detection of allelic differences. This polymorphism is tightly linked to the XLA locus and can be used to track inheritance of the disease in a family.

'spiked' with one of the four possible dideoxy nucleotides (ddATP, ddTTP, ddCTP, or ddGTP). As synthesis proceeds, some of the strands incorporate a dideoxy nucleotide and no further extension can take place. In each reaction a family of molecules is synthesized whose unit lengths are determined by whether the reaction had been terminated by incorporation of a specific nucleotide at a given position. Either the primer or the nucleotides may be labeled. The reaction products are separated on a denaturing polyacrylamide gel. In the past, the sequencing primers were end-labeled with ^{32}P and the pattern of band lengths was visualized by autoradiography with each nucleotide reaction in a single lane of a large gel. Automated techniques for DNA sequencing using laser scanning of fluorophore or infrared-labeled reactions have largely replaced ^{32}P. By the use of four different fluorescent labels the reaction products can be analyzed in a single lane of the gel. Two classes of chemistries are popular: 'dye primer', in which the primers of each reaction are tagged with different fluorophores, and 'dye terminator', in which the dideoxynucleotides are themselves labeled with fluorophores. Unequal signal intensities, variable signals within reactions, and gel migration differences between reactions due to the mass properties of the fluorophores presented significant limitations for the early automated sequencing chemistries. Recent advances in both dye primer[39] and dye terminator chemistry[40] have greatly improved the accuracy of quantitation and base calling. Automated techniques for template preparation and robot-assisted reaction chemistry are becoming more common. The original instrumentation for automated fluorescent sequencing used large polyacrylamide gels, but the most recent generation of instruments exploits large renewable capillary electrophoresis arrays. These instruments (PE Biosystems 3700 and Molecular Dynamics MegaBACE) have been crucial to the rapid production of the draft human genome sequence, and newer generation instruments can be expected to have further increased throughput and reduced cost.

Mutation scanning and detection

Individual mutation analysis has become the principal focus of diagnostic molecular biology. Improvements are continuing to

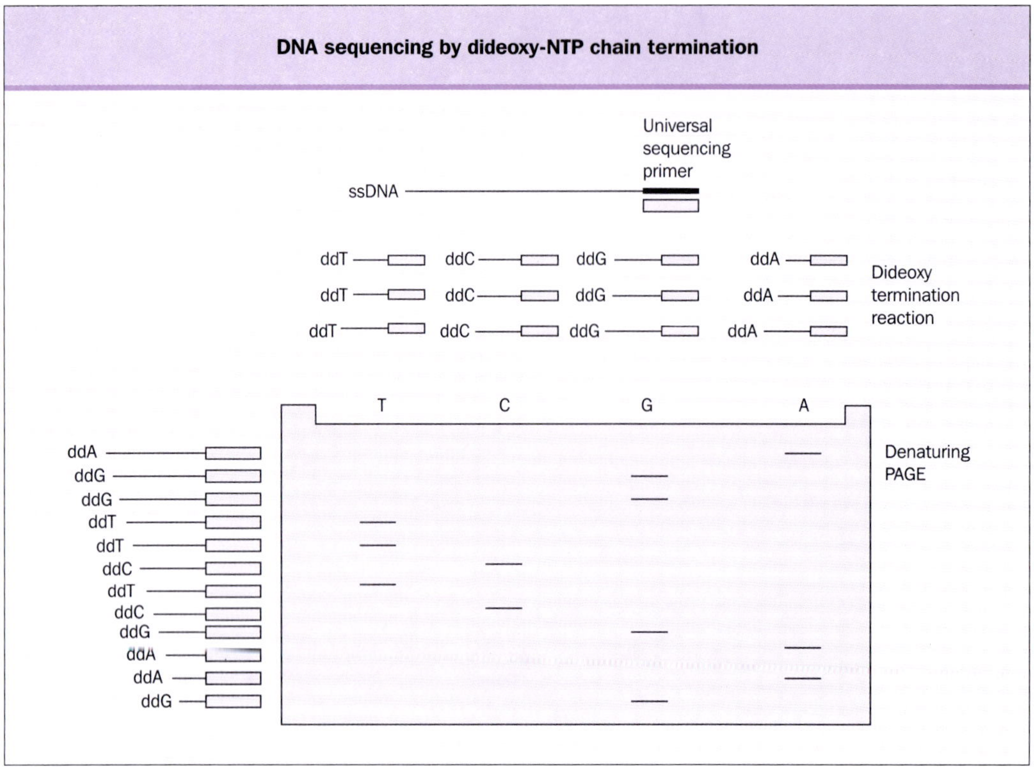

Figure 125.6 DNA sequencing by dideoxy-NTP chain termination. Copying of the DNA by the polymerase is terminated at specific positions when a ddNTP is incorporated. The ddNTP is added mixed with dNTPs so that, in each reaction, only some new strands terminate while others continue through to the next complementary nucleotide. The sequencing products can be visualized by autoradiography or by laser scanning in an automated sequencer.

allow for faster, less expensive, and more extensive screening of individual patient samples. Ideally, mutation analysis begins with some knowledge of the mutational spectrum at a particular locus. Some mutations recur commonly because of the large-scale genomic structure around a disease gene. Examples of this are the common inversions of the factor VIII locus[41] and the common deletions seen in the spinal muscular atrophy locus,[42] both of which involve recombination between repeated elements. Common mutations, such as the ΔF508 in cystic fibrosis[43,44] and the N370S in Gaucher's disease,[45] illustrate simple mutations that have high allele frequency due to population effects. Certain nucleotide positions may have a greater rate of mutation and these may explain recurrent, albeit rare, mutations in some genes. Beyond these common mutations, the mutational spectrum at these loci and most others is very diverse. Mutations 'private' to particular families are routinely observed. Clinical mutation analysis, therefore, must deal with known common mutations, identify family-specific mutations, and flexibly genotype at-risk individuals once a familial mutation is found.

KEY CONCEPTS

Molecular methods

- Most DNA diagnostics rely on DNA hybridization restriction enzyme digestion, polymerase chain reaction (PCR), and/or DNA sequencing.
- Southern blots directly detect a DNA segment within the complex mixture of the entire genome.
- PCR allows an exponential amplification of a DNA segment from the genome, allowing multiple analytical procedures on the single pure sequence.
- There are numerous methods for mutation detection in amplified DNA, but the analysis of heteroduplexes by DHPLC is one of the simplest and most sensitive.
- Bioinformatics is an emerging discipline relevant to molecular diagnosis. Integration of bioinformatics techniques plays a necessary role in data acquisition and interpretation.

Detection of an unknown mutation

Several methods have been described that can be used for the detection of single-base substitutions in DNA.[46,47] Different circumstances govern whether it is more desirable to study cDNA synthesized from mRNA or to use genomic DNA for analysis. These factors include the accessibility of the cell type that normally expresses the gene, the level of mRNA expression, and the size of the gene. If genomic DNA is used, then the structure of the gene must be known in order to design PCR primer sets that allow amplification of each exon. Amplification from mRNA allows examination of the coding sequence in the most efficient units. The availability of the draft human genome sequence makes determination of gene structure and amplimer design for genomic DNA much simpler than ever before. Amplification from genomic DNA will, therefore, be the most commonly used method. There are several factors that make genomic DNA a preferred template for mutation analysis: (1) the chemical stability of DNA is greater than that of RNA; (2) genomic DNA is readily obtained from any tissue or cell source, particularly small samples of peripheral blood; (3) some mutations cause mRNA instability leading to amplification failure of the mutated transcript. It should be noted that any mutation that directly affects amplification, such as deletion or mutation in the amplimer sequence itself, can produce misleading results. It is always desirable to have parental specimens available to serve as reference for proving biallelic inheritance in the affected offspring.

In general, there are four classes of methods used for mutation detection: (1) mutation site cleavage; (2) conformation alteration; (3) denaturing electrophoresis or chromatography; and (4) direct mutation site detection. Cleavage methods must differentially attack variant versus wild-type sequences.[48] Most often this is achieved by hybridizing the test sequence to a standard wild-type probe. Initial efforts to detect single-base mutations relied on the mismatch of the mutant DNA with normal DNA. In one variation, RNAse A detected single-base mismatch bulges in RNA:RNA hybrids.[49,50] The sensitivity is about 60% when one strand is interrogated and can be increased by the addition of RNAse 1 or RNAse T1 as alternative enzymes for mismatch hybrid cleavage. Enzymatic detection of DNA mismatches with T4 endonuclease VII (T4E7) has also been reported.[51–53] This method is somewhat simpler than the RNAse protocol and does not require specific template preparation steps. In the base excision and sequence scanning[54] (BESS) uracil glycosylase is used to cleave T positions in which uracil has been partially substituted. The result is much like a T lane in a sequence reaction. Chemical modification is another cleavage-based approach to mutation detection. Chemical base modification allows specific cleavage of single-base mismatch bulges in DNA hybrids.[55,56] Amplified DNA is probed with a labeled normal DNA and then treated with a chemical such as osmium tetroxide. The mismatched base is chemically modified and is then sensitive to cleavage by piperidine. The main advantage of cleavage methods is that relatively long DNA segments of 800–1000 nucleotides can be reliably analyzed. However, the required multistep procedures often do not compare favorably with direct DNA sequencing in either cost or complexity. The RNAse, T4E7, and BESS T methods are all available as commercial kits, but compared to other screening techniques they have not been used very widely.

Mismatch cleavage techniques are rather demanding and most investigators have shifted instead to simpler strategies. In single-strand confirmational polymorphism (SSCP),[57,58] the amplified DNA PCR product is denatured and then separated on a native acrylamide gel. (Fig. 125.7A). Single-stranded DNA assumes some secondary structure due to internal base pairing, and each strand has a unique mobility based on size and shape. Under appropriate conditions, using short segments of DNA, single-base differences can be seen to alter the mobility in the acrylamide gel of one or both of the complementary DNA strands. Using 150–200 nucleotide-long PCR products, 70–95% of mutations can be detected with this method. A method that combines a single Sanger dideoxy sequencing reaction with an SSCP-like analysis on a nondenaturing gel is 'dideoxy fingerprinting'– ddF – and by creating families of fragments it can achieve somewhat higher sensitivity than SSCP over longer DNA fragments.[59,60]

A similar method is called heteroduplex analysis.[61] This method depends on the hybridization of complementary strands of mutant and normal (wild-type) alleles. This creates a mixture of heteroduplexes and homoduplexes with three resulting types of DNA hybrids: mutant/mutant, normal/normal, and the heterodimer that contains one mutant and one normal DNA strand. The mismatch configuration of this heterodimer means that it tends to migrate slightly differently in an agarose or acrylamide gel and can thus be detected. In both SSCP or heteroduplex scanning the PCR products can be detected by incorporation of ^{32}P-labeled

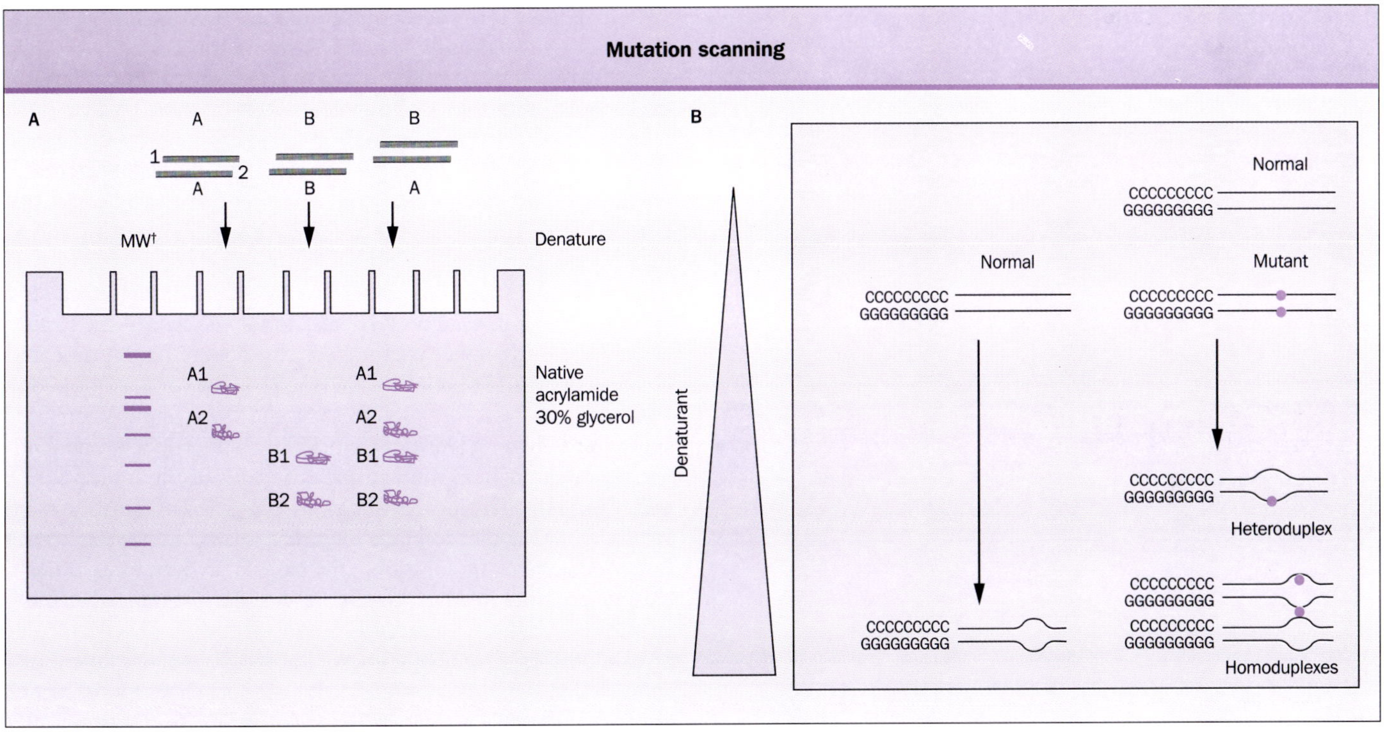

Figure 125.7 Mutation scanning. (**A**) Single-strand conformation (SSC). After PCR of either RNA or genomic DNA the products are denatured and then separated in a native acrylamide gel. Subtle differences in the folding of single-strand molecules, including single-nucleotide changes, lead to distinctive migration in the gel. (**B**) Denaturing gradient gel electrophoresis (DGGE). After PCR with primers that introduce a 'G-C clamp' sequence, the products are separated in gel containing a gradient of denaturant. As the double-stranded DNA migrates through the gradient it reaches a point where a discrete domain begins to unwind. The DNA then abruptly stops migrating in the gel. Single-nucleotide differences can be detected by the position at which the DNA reaches its stopping point. A heterozygous individual's DNA will form heteroduplexes during the last round of PCR. Heteroduplexes may have very distinctive migration in the gel because of increased instability at the mismatched bases.

nucleotides or using ethidium staining. Another method is called denaturing gradient gel electrophoresis (DGGE).[62] Here one uses PCR primers that have a 30–50 bp segment of G homopolymer on one end (Fig. 125.7B). After amplification with this primer the double-stranded DNA product has a G-C tail. This 'G-C clamp' is more stable to denaturing conditions than the remaining portion of the DNA so that it provides a stable domain that is the last to melt as the DNA unwinds. The PCR product is electrophoresed at ~60°C through a gel that contains a gradient of urea. As the DNA reaches conditions when partial melting first begins, it stops migrating through the gel. DNA segments with even single-base differences can show easily distinguishable gel migration patterns. Denaturing high performance liquid chromatography[63–65] (DHPLC) is the latest entry in heteroduplex analysis, incorporating rapid and robust separation and detection technologies for heteroduplex detection (Fig. 125.8A). This method directly detects single-nucleotide and insertion/deletion variation in crude PCR products. DHPLC uses a polystyrene-divinylbenzene copolymer matrix in a temperature-controlled column chromatography format. A linear gradient of acetonitrile at regulated temperatures allows separation of DNA from the column matrix based on fragment size and the presence of unstable heteroduplex structures. Under partially denaturing temperatures, the heteroduplexes elute from the column earlier than the homoduplexes because of their reduced melting temperature. Optimization involving more than three temperatures is not usually required because mutations are detectable over a broad range of column temperatures. If melting domains within a fragment differ by more than 10°C, however, runs at different temperatures may be required to screen both domains adequately (Fig. 125.8B).

Denaturing high-performance liquid chromatography

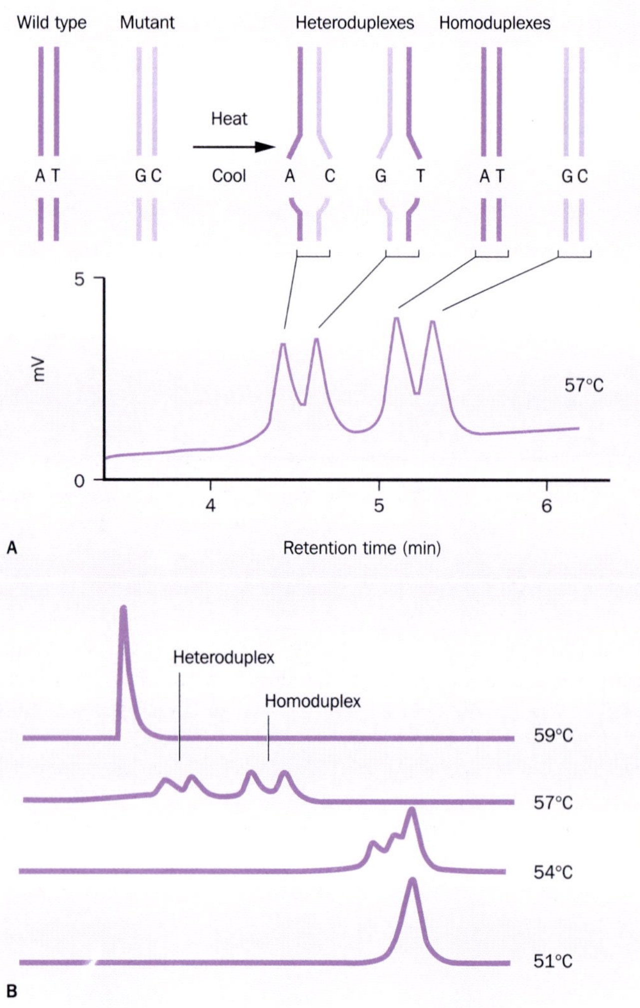

Figure 125.8 Denaturing high-performance liquid chromatography (DHPLC). (**A**) DNA heteroduplexes are separated from homoduplexes by their characteristic melting profile in a temperature-controlled acetonitrile gradient. (**B**) Resolution of the heteroduplexes from homoduplexes is temperature dependent.

An individual bearing compound heterozygous mutations at an autosomal locus will produce both heteroduplex and homoduplex PCR products and these can be detected with high sensitivity in a DHPLC system. An individual bearing a homozygous mutation at an autosomal locus or a hemizygous mutation at an X-linked locus will produce only homoduplexes. Depending on the nature of the mutation, the mutant homoduplexes may not be reliably distinguished from wild-type sequence based only on their elution profile on the column. Intentional introduction of wild-type DNA or PCR products as a secondary procedure can then be employed.

Detection of a known mutation

Once a mutation has been identified in a patient, the entire family can be tested. A typical method is called allele-specific oligonucleotide hybridization (ASO; Fig. 125.9).[66] This method and the related one called reverse dot blot hybridization are extremely useful for detecting common mutations in a population or for single family testing. As more mutations have been identified in genes commonly associated with human disease, other techniques that lend themselves to automation have been developed. The simplest of these is called oligonucleotide ligation assay[67] (OLA). In this procedure, pairs of specific oligonucleotides are designed to match exactly the wild-type and variant sequence. After a denaturing step, the temperature is reduced to one at which the oligos may hybridize with the single-strand template. Thermal-stable ligase is used to ligate the two oligos and the cycle is repeated. One popular method is to capture the ligated oligos in an ELISA so that the ligated products can be detected by conventional antibody and enzyme processes and quantified in a standard 96 well format plate reader. 'Molecular beacons' are specialized oligonucleotides that contain a fluorophore and a fluorescence-quencher group at opposite ends of the molecule[68–70] (Fig. 125.10). The probe oligos are designed to form a stem structure with an intervening loop that is complementary to the target sequence. In solution, the molecular beacon assumes a hairpin structure in which the fluorescence emission is quenched. In the presence of a perfectly matched target, the molecular beacon unfolds, placing the fluorophore and quencher far enough apart so that the fluorophore is no longer quenched. Fluorescence emission increases during PCR amplification. To determine if a known mutation is present, specific probe oligos are designed to be exact matches for the wild-type and mutant DNA sequences. Different fluorophores with minimally overlapping emission spectra are used for each probe oligo and their differential hybridization is monitored at each cycle of amplification. Specialized instrumentation is used to monitor single reactions or reactions in a 96 well format during the PCR amplification

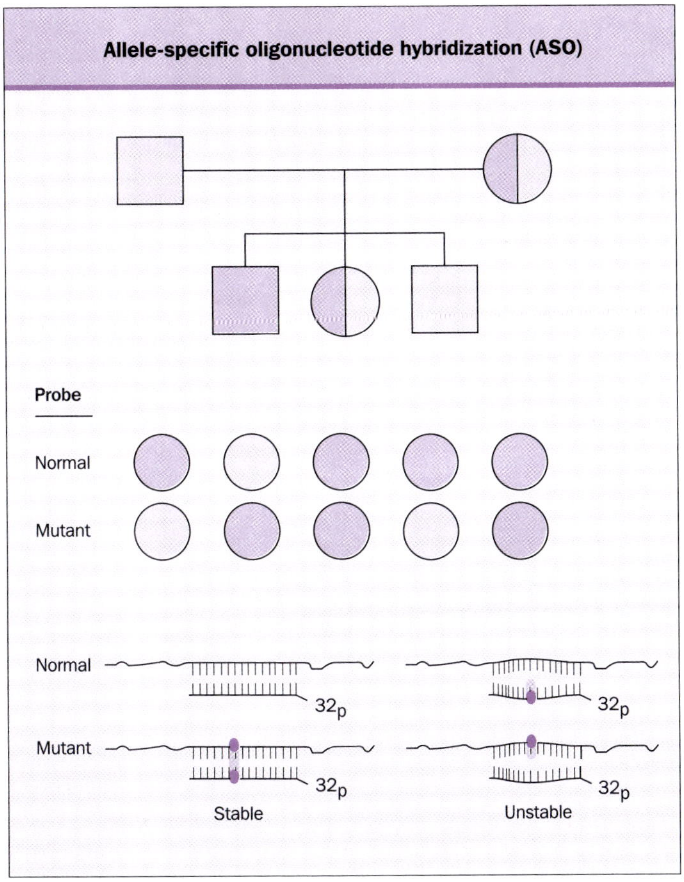

Figure 125.9 Allele-specific oligonucleotide hybridization (ASO). ASO is used to detect known mutations. PCR products from each individual in the pedigree are spotted on to a nylon filter. The filter is then probed with labeled oligonucleotides representing either the wild-type or mutant sequence. The filter is then washed under conditions that are close to the melting temperature. The imprecise base pairing between the normal or mutant probes and the PCR products leads to instability and the probe washes away. The resulting specific patterns allow determination of genotype.

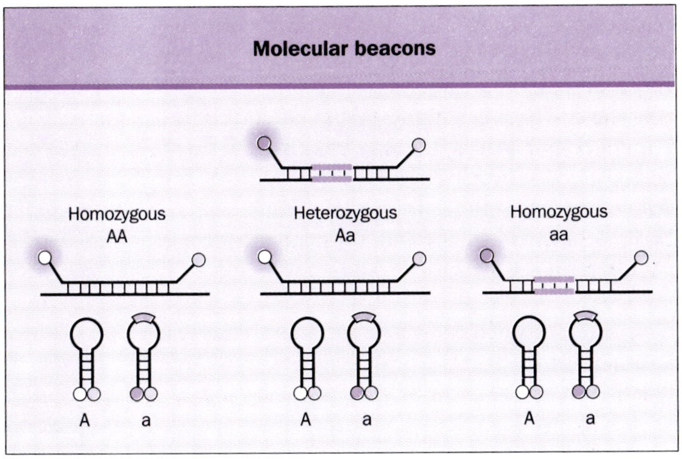

Figure 125.10 Molecular beacons. Fluorophore-tagged oligonucleotides specific for the wild-type and mutant allele are hybridized during a PCR reaction to the DNA amplimers. The opening of the oligo hairpin allows the fluorophore to emit light at its characteristic wavelength and the result is quantitatively detected as the PCR reaction progresses.

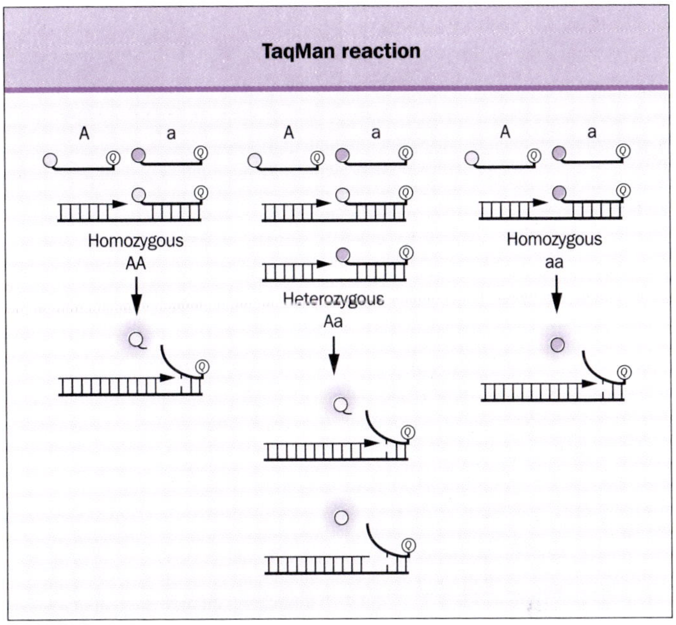

Figure 125.11 TaqMan reaction. Allele-specific fluorophore-tagged oligonucleotides are hybridized to single-strand DNA produced during a PCR reaction. Strand displacement leads to cleavage of the fluorophore and release from quenching. The intensity and wavelength of the emitted light is monitored during the course of the PCR.

process. Another technique, the TaqMan reaction[71–74] (Fig. 125.11), uses the same kind of instrumentation to monitor the PCR reaction in real time, but employs a slightly different approach to allele recognition. In the TaqMan method, the fluorophore is attached to the 5′ end of the probe and a quencher to the 3′ end. The 3′ end is modified so that it cannot be used as a primer for polymerase extension. In its native state this oligo is quenched. The TaqMan probe hybridizes to the target sequence as it is produced in the PCR reaction. As the Taq polymerase extends on the template, the probe oligo is displaced and the 5′ end becomes a substrate for the exonuclease activity of the polymerase. Cleavage of the 5′ base from the oligo releases the fluorophore and the quenching is relieved. The increase in fluorescence emission as the PCR reaction proceeds is monitored in the instrument. Allele-specific genotyping for mutant or wild-type forms is again accomplished by design of specific probe oligos for each sequence. These will compete with one another and the fluorescence emission will correspond to the oligo that exactly matches the target sequence. Both molecular beacons and TaqMan reactions are robust and, because they occur in solution without need for electrophoretic fragment separation, they lend themselves to scale-up automation. Limitations include the need for very precise probe design (which may require several rounds of optimization), the cost of custom fluorophore-tagged oligos, and the requirement for at least four oligos for each reaction.

Microarrays

Ordered arrays of DNA oligonucleotides could potentially have a revolutionary impact on mutation screening and diagnosis. Array 'printing' allows many thousands of DNAs or oligonucleotides to be spotted on activated glass surfaces.[75,76] An alternative approach is direct synthesis of oligonucleotides on the surface using photoactive chemistry and masking templates.[77–79] This process is very similar, in principle, to the fabrication of microelectronics devices and so has given these arrays the nickname of 'gene chips'. In its simplest form, DNA 'targets' derived from the patient or tissue source are amplified and labeled with fluorophores and are used to determine complementary binding by massively parallel hybridization to the probes fixed on the array. Such arrays are extraordinarily useful tools for monitoring gene expression at thousands of loci in a single assay.[80,81] This approach could interrogate an entire known sequence by hybridizations to a single array that covers each nucleotide site in stepwise fashion. In this way, the array would be used as a highly parallel ASO assay. Microarrays have been used both to assay for known mutations and polymorphisms and for the primary screening process – a kind of sequencing by hybridization.[82–84] There are several limitations to this approach relating to the specificity of the hybridization, i.e. it is difficult to obtain conditions of specific and sensitive hybridization across many thousands of unique sites. This has stimulated interest in alternative detection chemistries that depend on primer extension or ligation to detect sequence variants[85,86] (Fig. 125.12). Primer extension on the surface of the gene chip can be thought of as a form of 'minisequencing'. The incorporation of a single labeled nucleotide at the primer allows specific interrogation of the template sequence adjacent to the primer. The most serious limitation of both hybridization and minisequencing methods is the preliminary step of preparing the template DNA for analysis. Nonamplified genomic DNA is too complex (i.e. the concentration of any particular sequence is too low) to be analyzed directly. Robust amplification schemes that allow parallel amplification of hundreds of segments simultaneously are required. Future developments will likely require at least a 10-fold increase in the number of positions that can be amplified to produce the template targets for microarray analysis. Two variants of microarray technology are of current interest. In one system, specifically 'colored' microspheres are used as the surface for oligonucleotide attachment.[87,88] Hybridization is detected using fluorophore-tagged probe DNA in a flow cytometry instrument. In principle, this could allow highly parallel analyses of multiple alleles and positions. Another alternative is single-nucleotide primer extension followed by array printing on a specialized matrix. The resulting microarrays are then analyzed by matrix-assisted laser-desorption time-of-flight (MALDI-TOF) mass spectroscopy.[89,90] The individual analyses are extraordinarily fast and the genotyping is precise because of the single-atom specificity of the mass spectroscopy. It is unclear which of these systems will have the most utility, but each has great promise.

Microarray for genotyping

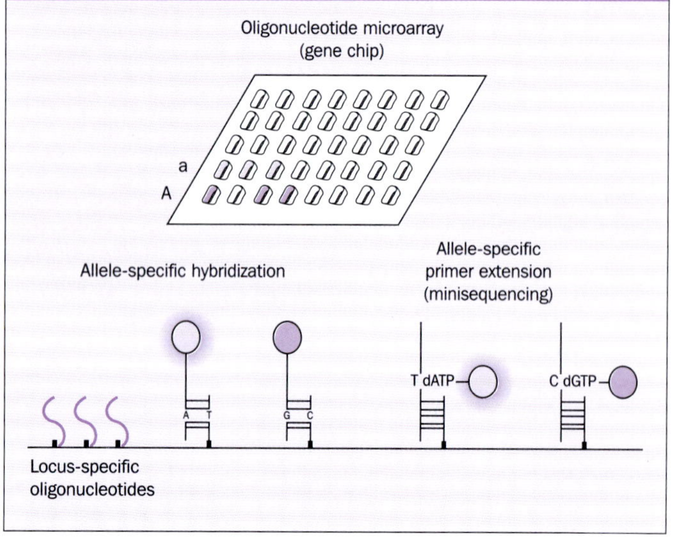

Figure 125.12 Microarray for genotyping. Oligonucleotides are printed or synthesized on a glass surface. Allele-specific hybridization is detected by the position in the array. An alternative (and perhaps more robust) chemistry is single-nucleotide extension, a form of 'minisequencing'.

Bioinformatics

Bioinformatics has emerged as a fundamental discipline in molecular biology as enormous DNA and protein sequence databases, linkage maps, physical maps, and other integrated data sets have been generated by individual labs and the human genome project. The growing number of genetic loci that are already known to be important in immunological disease renders it critical that both research and diagnostic laboratories make maximal use of automated processes in sample archiving, data acquisition, data analysis, and reporting.

Internal databases and data acquisition

Laboratory information management (LIM) systems are widespread and each laboratory must deal with the generic operational problems of sample accession, tracking, and reporting. DNA diagnostic laboratories have several unique problems and resources that deserve comment. Indefinite long-term sample archiving or 'DNA banking' is an important option given the rapid progress being made in the genetic contribution to many diseases. In this way, sample material may be reanalyzed as testing methods advance. Relational databases (usually implemented on Oracle or SQL servers) should integrate sample accession, physical archive, quality control, and genotype information. Automated data acquisition is an important component of DNA sequencing and fluorescent-tagged STR genotyping. Instrument-specific and secondary base-calling programs are necessary for data interpretation. Currently, the programs PHRED[91,92] and POLYPHRED[93] (http://genome.washington.edu/) set the standard by incorporating automated analysis of data quality. Use of internal size standards and other quality control measures are required for the accurate fragment length determination that is so critical to STR genotyping. Automated procedures for data file export to analytical software and data archiving on indelible media are also important issues. The number of patient-specific data records and the complexity of relationships within family-based testing make it difficult for manual processes to achieve the required reliability.

Data interpretation and public sequence databases

Computer-based methods for genotype and DNA sequence data interpretation are necessary for efficiency and cost-effectiveness. It should be noted that the estimation of genetic risks based on genotype data requires a knowledge of specialized statistical procedures whose description is beyond the scope of this chapter.[94] Incorporation of linkage data with pedigree structure information and ancillary biochemical or immunological testing should use a Bayesian approach in which *prior* probabilities (pedigree, lab testing, etc.) are integrated with the *conditional* probabilities

Chapter 127 Immunohematology

Linda M. Griffith and Harvey G. Klein

INTRODUCTION

The practice of transfusion medicine is based on the knowledge of blood groups acquired from serologic studies in the early 1900s to the present. Landsteiner's original observation of red cell agglutination provided the basis for serologic investigation that made practical transfusion therapy possible. More recent contributions from biochemistry and molecular biology have increased our knowledge of red cell antigen systems. Storage methods for whole blood and plasma, developed as recently as the 1940s, made transfusion routinely available for patient care. Other notable advances included practical methods for the separation of whole blood into components, including red cells, platelets and plasma, the collection of selected components, testing for infectious disease and criteria for quality assurance.

Today, serologic and other immunohematologic methods continue to define our understanding of compatibility. Serologic methods for the investigation of individual patient sera remain essential for the selection of a compatible transfusion. The transfusion history of a patient, expressed as antibodies formed in response to foreign antigens, is reflected in the recipient serum. The antigen phenotype of a cellular component, rather than the genotype of the donor, is more important for predicting compatibility. Phenotypic analysis of a cellular component for matching with the patient may be critical for the management of a challenging clinical case. This chapter reviews the major antigen systems and serology for red cells, platelets and granulocytes – the immunohematology that constitutes the scientific basis for medical transfusion practice.

TRANSFUSION AND COMPATIBILITY TESTING

Although blood transfusion traces its beginnings to William Harvey's discovery of the circulation of blood in 1628, immunohematology dates to Landsteiner's observation in 1901 that sera from certain subjects agglutinate the red blood cells of other subjects.[1] Landsteiner described isoagglutination, blood groups, and the potential significance for blood transfusion. A decade then passed before laboratory tests for blood groups were performed for clinical purposes, and before cross-matching of donor and recipient was introduced. Epstein and Ottenberg, in 1908,[2] first suggested that blood groups were inherited. Landsteiner's technique of using 5% saline cell suspensions at room temperature or in the cold favored the detection of direct agglutinating IgM antibodies, especially the reciprocal antibodies of the ABO blood group system.

Early blood group serology was further advanced by two techniques: (1) injecting human red blood cells into animals and absorbing the species antibodies from the immune sera that resulted with other human red cells. The blood groups M, N and P were described in this way by Landsteiner and Levine in 1927;[3] (2) investigation of clinical hemolytic transfusion reactions and hemolytic disease of the newborn (erythroblastosis fetalis).[4] The agglutinins or red cell antibodies detected in these studies were indirect agglutinins, but these so-called 'incomplete' or indirect IgG antibodies could be induced to agglutinate red cells by heating the mixture on a slide, by suspension in albumin, or by treating the target red cells with enzymes. Such crude physical and chemical methods of enhancing antigen–antibody interaction, for example by reducing the negative charge on the red cell or by exposing membrane epitopes, are still used today. Red cell serology entered a period of intense activity in 1945, with the description of the direct antihuman globulin test (DAT) or Coombs' test. The addition of serum from a rabbit sensitized against human globulin produced agglutination of red blood cells coated with IgG antibody.[5] Modifications of the DAT permitted screening of sera from transfused patients, the definition of additional blood groups, and pretransfusion cross-matching.

Blood groups

Over 25 genetically determined human blood group systems have been described. An international nomenclature has been devised and is maintained by the International Society of Blood Transfusion (ISBT) Working Party on Terminology for Red Cell Surface Antigens.[6] There are also a number of rare red cell antigens, called 'private' antigens, and numerous 'public' antigens, serologic determinants found on almost all red cells tested. Red cell antigens are epitopes located on the proteins and lipids of the red cell membrane that are capable of eliciting antibody production.

Traditionally red cell antigens were defined by serologic investigations, and over 250 blood groups antigens have been characterized. Reagent polyclonal human antisera obtained from multiply transfused patients and multiparous females were used in those studies. Now, biochemical and molecular biologic investigations have provided a structural basis for understanding red cell membrane composition. Many antigens have been discovered to be related to one another, owing to polymorphisms of a parent molecule, and thus comprise a blood group system. Biosynthetic pathways have been deciphered for several blood group antigen systems. The chromosome locations of the genes that define most blood group antigen systems have been identified and the involved genes have been cloned and sequenced.[7,8]

Antigenic determinants of the red cell membrane are located on a wide variety of biochemical structures. For example, ABO antigens are located on certain carbohydrate chains that are attached to either membrane lipids or several integral membrane proteins. Lewis antigens are glycosphingolipids that circulate in plasma and attach to the red cell surface. The Rh antigens are integral to the membrane, and may be complexes of lipid and protein. Members of the MNS antigen system are membrane-spanning glycoproteins known as the glycophorins. Other less familiar antigens, such as Cromer, are located on glycosylphosphatidylinositol (GPI)-linked proteins, which are extensions of the membrane. Most blood group antigens are specific to the red cell. However, the A, B and H antigens, among others, are expressed on many different human tissues. The functions of many red cell antigens have now been defined and include transport, adhesion and regulation of complement. Several red cell antigens have been associated with specific diseases. The Cromer blood group system is located on decay-accelerating factor, which is affected in paroxysmal nocturnal hemoglobinuria (PNH), and Duffy antigens act as receptors for certain malarial parasites. Especially informative are 'null' phenotypes that result in hematologic abnormality. For example, the absence of Kell precursor substance is associated with the McLeod syndrome of red cells; also, certain Rh null individuals may develop compensated hemolytic anemia.

Several important blood group systems have carbohydrate determinants (Table 127.1). The ABO system – the most important blood group for transfusion – as well as the Lewis, P, and I systems, has similar biosynthetic pathways in which genes code for glycosyl transferases, attaching specific sugars to common precursor structures.[9] The oligosaccharide chains that determine the ABO type of red cells are carried predominantly on the red cell protein bands 3 (the anion exchanger AE1) and 4.5 (the glucose transporter). Also, glycosphingolipids carrying these oligosaccharides are adsorbed to the red cell from plasma. The immunospecific epitope usually consists of only a few sugar molecules on the membrane structure, and alteration of a single immunodominant sugar is sufficient to elicit a different antibody. Subjects who lack the A or B antigen develop the corresponding 'naturally occurring' IgM antibody within a few months of birth, possibly as a result of exposure to environmental agents such as bacteria that possess these common antigens. Polysaccharide antigens usually elicit formation of IgM antibodies; however, notable exceptions include the clinically important IgG anti-A,B responsible for one form of hemolytic disease of the newborn and the IgG anti-P (Donath–Landsteiner antibody) responsible for paroxysmal cold hemoglobinuria (PCH). ABO blood typing requires both 'forward' red cell grouping with reagent anti-A and anti-B and 'reverse' serum grouping using the subject's serum and reagent red cells.

Safe transfusion practice prohibits infusing A, B or AB blood to patients whose red cells lack the corresponding antigens, because the recipient's plasma contains anti-A and/or anti-B isohemagglutinins. Most fatal hemolytic transfusion reactions result from patient and donor sample errors that end in ABO-incompatible transfusions.[10,11] Although group O red cells may be given to patients of groups A, B or AB when type-specific blood is not available, plasma from some group O individuals contains a potent hemolytic antibody. Therefore, group O whole blood should not be given to recipients other than group O, except in an emergency.

Protein blood group systems such as Rh, Kell, Kidd and Duffy are structurally quite diverse, but as a group generally elicit IgG antibodies after the primary immune response is stimulated by transfusion or pregnancy (Table 127.1). These IgG antibodies, when present in a recipient, are likely to cause hemolysis of incompatible transfused red cells. Clinically, the Rh system is second in importance only to the ABO system. Antibodies to Rh constitute about half of all alloantibodies made by recipients of ABO type-specific component transfusions. The system is complex and consists of two polypeptides, RhD and RhCE.[12] Red cells are typed for transfusion as either Rh positive or Rh negative, based on the presence or absence of the RhD polypeptide antigen, using RhD antisera. Eighty-five per cent of Caucasian blood donors test positive for RhD. Individuals either possess or

Table 127.1 Selected red cell antigen systems.

Selected red cell antigen systems			
System or collection	**Symbol**	**Associated antigens**	**Membrane component**
Polysaccharide blood groups			
ABO	ABO	A, B, AB, O	Anion exchanger (AE-1), protein 4.5, lipids
Lewis	LE	Le^a, Le^b	Type 2 oligosaccharides
Hh	H	H	AE1, protein 4.5, lipids
Ii	I	I, i	AE1, protein 4.5, lipids
P	P1	P_i	Glycolipid
Protein blood groups			
Rh	RH	D, CE, Ce, cE, ce, C^w	Rh proteins
MNS	MNS	M, N, S, s, U	M, N: glycophorin A S, s: glycophorin B
Lutheran	LU	Lu^a, Lu^b	Lutheran glycoprotein
Kell	KEL	K, k, Kp^a, Kp^b, Js^a, Js^b	Kell protein
Duffy	FY	Fy^a, Fy^b, Fy^3	Chemokine receptor
Kidd	JK	Jk^a, Jk^b, Jk^3	Urea transporter
Xg	XG	Xg^a	Xg glycoprotein
Cromer	CROM	Cr^a, Tc^a, Tc^b, Tc^c	Decay accelerating factor (CD55) (GPI linked)
Chido/Rogers	CH/RG	Ch^1, Ch^2, Rg^1, Rg^2	C4 complement (adsorbed from plasma)
Cartwright	YT	Yt^a, Yt^b	Acetylcholinesterase (GPI-linked)
Landsteiner-Weiner	LW	LW^a, LW^{ab}, LW^b	LW glycoprotein

KEY CONCEPTS

Blood groups

- Subjects who lack the polysaccharide blood group antigens A and B demonstrate the corresponding naturally occurring antibodies. These antibodies are responsible for most fatal transfusion reactions.
- Of the more than 40 different alleles and variants of the Rh system, RhD is the most important and determines 'Rh' positivity.
- Alloimmunization occurs in about 1% of transfused patients. A minority of the alloantibodies are clinically significant.

entirely lack RhD polypeptide: there is no antithetical Rhd polypeptide. This, then, explains the extreme antigenicity of RhD when transfused to individuals lacking that antigen on their red cells. The *Rh*C and *RhE* genes are closely linked and the antigens expressed on a single combined polypeptide, RhCE. There are two alleles for each antigen, *Rh*C and *Rhc*, and *RhE* and *Rhe*. Possible polypeptides thus include RhCe, RhcE, RhCE and Rhce. Antibodies to these other Rh antigens are also clinically important. More than 40 different variant Rh alleles, many the result of crossover events during meiosis, have been recognized serologically.

Immunogenicity of red blood cell antigens

With more than 250 blood group antigens identified by the ISBT study group, it is fortunate that blood transfusion does not require phenotypically identical cells. Relatively few blood group antigens are clinically important, and transfusion recipients do not always form antibodies to antigens they lack. Alloimmunization depends on several factors, including the immune responsiveness of the recipient (an inherited characteristic that may be modified by disease or treatment), the immunogenicity of the particular antigen, the dose and schedule of antigen exposure, and the likelihood that a recipient who lacks a specific antigen will be exposed to that antigen, a function of the ethnic diversity of the particular population. Interaction of these factors makes it difficult to predict any individual patient's response to transfusion. For the most potent immunogen, RhD, as little as 0.1 ml blood is sufficient to elicit an antibody response.[13] However, some apparently normal subjects fail to respond to repeated stimulation, and patients with leukemia and certain solid tumors develop anti-RhD far less frequently than expected.[14] Because alloimmunization can occur only when a subject lacks the sensitizing antigen, the risk of alloimmunization decreases as the prevalence of antigen increases in a population, and estimates of relative risk of immunization have been calculated.[15] One reason proposed for the high rate of alloimmunization observed among transfused patients with sickle cell disease is the disparity in antigens between Caucasian blood donors and African-American recipients.[16]

TECHNIQUES FOR DETERMINING COMPATIBILITY

Serologic compatibility testing for the purposes of red blood cell transfusion relies primarily on in vitro RBC agglutination and hemolysis as a detection system. Historically, compatibility testing was introduced to predict and avoid potential immunologic destruction of the transfused red cells and the severe, occasionally fatal, consequences to the recipient. Preventing alloimmunization to red cells is of lesser importance except for response to RhD in negative recipients, particularly women of childbearing age. Detailed descriptions of the pretransfusion testing process can be found elsewhere.[17]

Serologic compatibility testing involves three complementary strategies:

1. RBC phenotyping and antigen matching, done primarily for the ABO system to prevent reactions resulting from naturally occurring antibodies, and for the RhD antigen to avoid alloimmunization. Routine extended phenotyping and matching is unnecessary and impractical. However, for particular situations, such as repeated transfusions of patients with sickle cell disease, the approach has some advocates.
2. Antibody screening and identification. The recipient's serum is screened for preformed alloantibodies using a limited panel of cells of known phenotype. The panel includes clinically significant antigens, such that antibodies would cause hemolytic transfusion reactions. If alloantibodies are detected, they are identified by additional panel testing and antigen-negative blood is provided.
3. Serologic crossmatching. The recipient's serum is incubated with donor cells, both as a final check of ABO compatibility and as a screen for any preformed antibodies directed toward antigens not present on the original screening cells. This combination of testing dramatically reduces the risk of hemolytic transfusion reactions. Immediate hemolysis can be life-threatening; delayed hemolysis with fever and jaundice, and decreased red cell survival manifested by mild anemia are other sequelae of an incompatible transfusion. Unfortunately, previously formed antibodies do not always persist at detectable levels in the serum, and negative serology does not guarantee compatibility. As a general rule, antigen-negative blood must be provided for patients who have a documented history of clinically significant red cell alloantibodies, even if their serum does not currently contain detectable levels of that antibody.

KEY CONCEPTS

Serologic testing

- Serologic compatibility relies primarily on tests with hemagglutination end-points.
- Compatibility testing employs limited red cell phenotyping, serum screening for antibodies, and specific donor–recipient cross-matching.
- A history of a clinically significant alloantibody requires the provision of antigen-negative blood, as alloantibody reactivity may decline to undetectable levels.
- Serologic compatibility does not exclude clinically important hemolytic reactions. In vivo red cell survival studies may be necessary to determine compatibility.

Testing techniques

The presence or absence of antigens on red cells, and the identification of antibodies to red cells in patient sera, continue to be determined in hospital blood banks and reference laboratories today by labor-intensive serologic methods (Fig. 127.1). Serology is also the basis for most additional testing that may be required to solve specific clinical problems. In the serologic tube agglutination test, red cell agglutinates (clumps of cells) are visualized and the extent of agglutination is assessed empirically.

Technical judgement is required both to optimize the serologic tube test and to select a testing strategy for challenging individual patient specimens. For particulate red cell antigen–antibody complexes, as with soluble antigen–antibody systems, the accuracy and reproducibility of testing depend on optimizing the assay. The formation of agglutinates may be enhanced by techniques that optimize antigen–antibody reaction. Variables include temperature, ionic strength, pH, incubation time, and ratio of antigen to antibody. When red cell membrane antigens are exposed to pentameric IgM antibody, multiple adjacent cells may be bound together. IgM antibodies generally react more avidly at lower temperatures, possibly owing to conformational changes in the red cell membrane. Low pH enhances the reaction of some IgM antibodies, for example against the M antigen of the MNS system. The normal negative charge of sialic acid residues on the red cell surface (ζ potential) tends to keep cells apart, and so neutralization of the charge will enhance test sensitivity. Ordinarily bivalent IgG molecules cannot bridge the 240 Å distance between cells. Thus, detection of IgG antibodies may require additional enhancement. Centrifugation, the addition of positively charged molecules such as albumin or polybrene, removing the negative charge of the red cells by mild enzyme treatment, and additional cross-bridging by the use of a secondary antihuman globulin (AHG) antibody all enhance the agglutination reaction. The desired end result is the reproducible formation of clumps or 'agglutinates' visible to the eye or other detection system.

Commercial typing reagents are either high-titered polyclonal human alloantibodies prepared from the plasma of sensitized donors, or monoclonal antibodies. Monoclonal reagents currently available include antibodies reactive with the ABO, Rh, MN, Lewis and Kidd blood group systems, and some components of complement. Plant lectins are occasionally useful for some identifications. For example, *Dolichos biflorus* lectin, when diluted properly, reacts with only the A_1 subtype of the ABO system.

Arguably the most important test in diagnostic red cell immunohematology is the antihuman globulin (AHG) test, or Coombs' test. The AHG test detects antibodies that coat the surface of the cell (sensitize the cell) but do not completely span the 240 Å distance between cells, as is necessary for direct agglutination. Cells sensitized by primary antibody, usually IgG, are then detected by the addition of a secondary AHG reagent, which forms a bridge between coated red cells and results in agglutination. Two kinds of AHG test are important for transfusion medicine.

1. The direct antihuman globulin test (DAT, direct Coombs' test) is used to ask what antibodies are attached to the patient's own red cells. The patient's red cells are collected and washed, and then incubated with AHG reagent. A positive DAT identifies red cells that were coated with antibody or complement in vivo. These antibodies may be eluted from the patient's red cells and studied separately to determine their antigen specificity. The DAT is important in the diagnosis of autoimmune hemolytic anemia, hemolytic disease of the newborn, drug-induced immune hemolysis, and hemolytic transfusion reactions.

2. The indirect antihuman globulin test (IAT, indirect Coombs' test) is used to ask what antibodies are present in the patient's serum. The serum is collected and incubated with reagent red cells. The reagent red cells, with patient antibody now attached in vitro, are washed before the addition of AHG reagent. The IAT is used to assess circulating patient antibody in serum antibody detection and identification tests, and in cross-matching for transfusion. The IAT is also used for red cell phenotyping, with known reagent antibody added to the patient or component red cells to be phenotyped. Clinically significant antibodies are usually of the IgG isotype, and so commercial polyspecific AHG reagents are designed to be sensitive to a wide variety of IgG antibodies. Polyspecific AHG reagents generally also react with the C3d component of complement, and often with the C3b, C4b and C4d components as well. These reagents are not designed to detect IgA or IgM specifically, although some reagents react with the common light chains of these immunoglobulins.

Agglutination may be described by the strength of the interaction, and the quantity of antibody present. Several visual grading systems have been devised to score the strength or affinity/avidity of the agglutination reaction. Strength of reaction is one important factor used to distinguish multiple antibodies from one another when present in a single serum sample.[18] The

Eight-cell panel for determining specificity of antibodies to red blood cells

Cell	Rh–hr	Rhesus					Kell		Duffy		Kidd		MNS				Lewis		P	Serum results		
		D	C	E	c	e	K	k	Fy^a	Fy^b	Jk^a	Jk^b	M	N	S	s	Le^a	Le^b	P_1	RT	37	IgG
1	R_1R_2	+	+	0	0	+	0	+	+	0	+	0	+	0	+	0	0	+	+	0	0	0
2	R_2R_2	+	0	+	+	0	0	+	0	+	+	+	0	+	0	+	+	0	0	0	0	0
3	R_0r	+	0	0	+	+	0	+	0	0	+	0	0	+	0	+	0	0	+	0	0	0
4	r'r	0	+	0	+	+	+	+	+	+	0	+	+	+	+	+	0	+	0	0	w+	2+
5	r''r	0	0	+	+	+	0	+	0	+	+	0	+	0	+	+	0	+	+	0	0	0
6	rr	0	0	0	+	+	+	+	+	+	+	+	+	+	0	+	+	0	+	0	w+	2+
7	rr	0	0	0	+	+	0	+	0	+	0	+	+	0	+	0	0	+	0	0	0	0
8	rr	0	0	0	+	+	+	0	+	+	0	+	0	+	0	+	0	+	+	0	1+	3+

Figure 127.1 Eight-cell panel for determining specificity of antibodies to red cells. Cells 4, 6 and 8, which carry the K (Kell) antigen, are nonreactive at room temperature (RT), react weakly at 37°C and more strongly by the indirect antiglobulin test (IgG). Cell 8, which reacts most strongly, is homozygous for K since it lacks k. (Courtesy of Jo Lynn Procter.)

KEY CONCEPTS

Direct antiglobulin test and indirect antiglobulin test

- The direct antiglobulin test (DAT) is used to determine whether patient red cells have been coated in vivo with immunoglobulin, complement, or both.
  - The DAT is an important part of the evaluation of hemolytic events, including autoimmune hemolytic anemia, hemolytic transfusion reactions and hemolytic disease of the newborn.
  - A positive DAT may result from autoantibodies to red cell antigens, alloantibodies to recently transfused red cells, or drug effects.
  - Maternal antibodies of IgG isotype may cross the placenta to coat fetal red cells.
  - A positive DAT does not necessarily equate with hemolysis or shortened red cell survival.
- The indirect antiglobulin test (IAT) is used to determine which antibodies are in patient serum.
  - The IAT most often detects serum alloantibodies from prior transfusion or pregnancy.
  - Red cell alloantibodies are difficult to detect when patients have autoantibody in their serum; adsorption and elution studies can detect hidden alloantibodies and improve transfusion safety.
  - Antigen-negative red cells must be provided for transfusion when a patient has a history of alloantibody formation, even when no antibody is detected by IAT.
  - The rate of alloimmunization is 1% per unit of red cells transfused.

quantity of antibody can be determined by titration, or serial dilutions, against an antigen-positive cell using the presence or absence of agglutination as an end-point. Estimates relating the amount of antibody bound to a cell or present in serum to the strength of agglutination are crude at best, and do not predict clinical outcome.

Recent alternatives to standard tube assays include column agglutination and automated solid-phase technology. Column agglutination, also known as gel agglutination testing, has been widely adopted for some routine serology in blood banks.[19] Gel agglutination requires relatively less experience for performance and accurate interpretation than does tube agglutination. It is based on controlled centrifugation of red cells through dextran acrylamide gel contained in microtubes: During centrifugation, agglutinated red cells are trapped within the gel and unagglutinated red cells pellet at the bottom of the tube. Semiautomated solid-phase technology is available for large-scale ABO and RhD typing of donor red cells and is used in most collection centers. The test method is known as solid-phase red-cell adherence (SPRCA). In the direct test, as would be used in forward typing, reagent antibody is attached to a microplate well and donor red cells are added. If the red cells express the corresponding antibody they adhere to the sides of the well, but if negative they settle to the bottom. In the indirect test, as would be used in reverse typing, microplate wells coated with reagent red cells are reacted with donor serum. Unbound serum is washed away, and then indicator red cells coated with antihuman globulin are added. Additional methods, including affinity column technology, are available and useful in investigational and research settings.

In vivo compatibility

When a patient has multiple alloantibodies, selection of the 'least incompatible' red cells for transfusion can be accomplished by using either an in vitro serologic strategy known as differential agglutination, or in vivo red cell survival studies. Differential agglutination was initially developed as an in vitro technique for investigation of the life span of circulating red blood cells.[20] Later the test was adapted to assess transfusion compatibility. Differential agglutination methods have the disadvantages of being labor intensive, limited by the required differences in red cell antigens, and dependent upon the experience of the technician quantifying the agglutination reactions. Further, variables including temperature, antibody titer and strength of the agglutination reaction in vitro do not necessarily correlate with clinical hemolysis. Therefore, radiolabeled or biotinylated in vivo red cell survival studies are now more commonly used as an 'in vivo cross-match' for the patient who is incompatible with available donor units based on serologic testing, or when the survival of transfused red cells appears shortened in the absence of serologically demonstrable antibody. In general, 75% 1-hour survival of ^{51}Cr-labeled red cells predicts acceptable transfusion safety and efficacy.[21] The older in vivo crossmatching technique using clinical evidence of hemolysis, such as the appearance of plasma free hemoglobin or decrease in haptoglobin, has essentially been abandoned.

HEMOLYTIC REACTIONS

Hemolytic transfusion reactions

Immune hemolysis can occur intravascularly or extravascularly (Chapter 72). Intravascular immune hemolysis involves antibody-mediated complement activation, red cell membrane lysis, and the release of free hemoglobin into the plasma. The free hemoglobin is bound by albumin, haptoglobin and hemopexin, or is excreted unbound in the urine. The most common symptoms are fever, chest pain, nausea, flushing and dyspnea. Common signs include hypotension, hemoglobinuria, generalized bleeding and oliguria. Fatal hemolytic transfusion reactions are most commonly immediate, intravascular, and related to incompatibilities in the ABO system (74% of all immediate fatal reactions reported to the US FDA during a 10-year period[11]). Fatalities are most often the result of shock, disseminated intravascular coagulation, and renal failure mediated by antigen–antibody-induced immune hemolysis, complement activation and cytokine release.

Extravascular hemolysis results when immune-sensitized erythrocytes, usually coated with IgG and/or complement components, are removed by reticuloendothelial macrophages via their Fc and/or C3b receptors. Extravascular hemolysis is characterized by hyperbilirubinemia, an elevated serum lactic acid dehydrogenase (LDH) level, and a falling hematocrit. In some cases alloantibody may be detectable on transfused red cells by the DAT in the absence of clinical or laboratory evidence of hemolysis. Such cells are said to be 'sensitized' ('coated') and such alloantibodies are considered clinically insignificant, despite causing decreased survival of affected red cells. Extravascular hemolysis can be immediate and severe, but is more often delayed for days to weeks and insidious in onset. About one-third of these reactions are asymptomatic and unexpected. The frequency, estimated at between

CLINICAL PEARLS

Transfusion reactions

- Intravascular hemolysis, usually related to antibodies to the ABO system, is frequently acute and fulminant and may be complicated by shock, renal failure and disseminated intravascular coagulation (DIC).
- Most alloantibodies do not fix complement and do mediate extravascular hemolysis, usually insidious and often unrecognized. Fever, mild jaundice, mild anemia and a positive DAT may be present.
- Poor platelet increments following platelet transfusions may indicate developing alloantibodies to the HLA system or, less frequently, platelet-specific alloantibodies.
- Rh immunoglobulin injections can prevent primary immunization of Rh-negative patients who receive blood components with Rh-positive red cells.

1:500 and 1:6000 units transfused, is probably an underestimate.[22] Commonly implicated alloantibodies are those to the Rh, Kell, Kidd, Duffy and MNS systems. The triad of fever, anemia and a history of blood transfusion should alert the clinician to the possibility of delayed hemolysis. Immune-mediated hemolytic transfusion reactions are more common in women because of prior sensitization to red blood cell antigens during pregnancy, and increase in frequency with age, reflecting the higher likelihood of prior sensitization to red cell antigens.

Most hemolytic reactions result from the transfusion of red cells to a sensitized recipient, although infusions of plasma-containing components with a high-titer alloantibody can hemolyze the recipient's red cells. Routine screening of donor sera for alloantibodies has made such reactions uncommon. Even less common is hemolysis related to an incompatibility between two transfused units of blood – 'interunit incompatibility'.

Laboratory diagnosis of a hemolytic transfusion reaction should include examination of pre- and post-transfusion specimens for the presence of alloantibody and change in the status of the DAT, as well as visual inspection of the post-transfusion plasma and urine for evidence of hemolysis. The complete blood count may reveal a less than expected rise in hemoglobin, and a blood smear may show spherocytes and polychromasia. Hyperbilirubinemia and elevated LDH usually accompany delayed reactions. When immune hemolysis is suspected, the alloantibody must be sought and identified. Occasionally the DAT and alloantibody cannot be detected even by sensitive techniques, but serial red cell phenotyping indicates loss of red cells with a particular antigen. Repeated specimens should be assayed weeks and even months after the suspected transfusion episode. The frequency of alloimmunization in different series is variable and depends on the level of suspicion, the system of detection, and the nature and length of the patient follow-up. Alloimmunization probably occurs with about 1% of units transfused.[23]

One unusual form of delayed hemolysis results after solid organ or bone marrow transplantation as a result of antibodies produced by 'passenger' B lymphocytes from the graft. ABO-mismatched bone marrow transplants can be associated with significant immunohematologic consequences, depending on whether the mismatch is major or minor, and whether the transplant is myeloablative or nonmyeloablative. For nonmyeloablative transplants, relatively stable chimeric marrow and immune systems are created in the recipient. Further investigation will be required for an understanding of hemolysis and other immunohematologic consequences of the chimeric state.[24,25]

Hemolytic disease of the newborn

Diamond et al[26] linked four clinical disorders of the newborn – hydrops fetalis, icterus gravis neonatorum, congenital anemia and erythroblastosis fetalis – as manifestations of a single disease. The illness described, now known as hemolytic disease of the newborn (HDN), results from sensitization of the mother to fetal red blood cell antigens (Chapter 72). Stimulation occurs from the transplacental passage of fetal cells possessing an antigen that the mother lacks. This induces maternal IgG antibody, which crosses the placenta and binds to fetal blood cells and other tissues. HDN does not occur commonly with the first pregnancy.

Although many red cell antigens can cause maternal sensitization and HDN, the most important remains RhD because of its frequent association with clinical disease and because of the severity of the illness. RhD is expressed on fetal red cells by the 4th week of gestation, so that sensitization may occur early in the first trimester. As little as 0.25 ml of fetal blood can sensitize the mother. However, about one-third of susceptible women fail to be immunized, despite significant fetomaternal hemorrhage, an observation that may be related to the mother's genetic makeup. Concurrent ABO incompatibilities, if present, may destroy fetal cells in the maternal circulation before sensitization can occur. Finally, pregnancy has been postulated to have a protective effect against sensitization.[27] The risk of fetomaternal hemorrhage is greatest at the time of delivery. First-trimester spontaneous abortion, amniocentesis and abdominal trauma all increase the risk of sensitization earlier in pregnancy. Approximately 8% of susceptible women develop anti-RhD after the first pregnancy with an RhD-positive fetus. Fetal cells in the maternal circulation can be detected by the erythrocyte rosetting assay, and semiquantitative detection is possible using the Kleihauer–Betke acid elution test or an enzyme-linked antiglobulin test.[28]

At the first prenatal evaluation, obstetric patients should be typed for ABO and Rh status and screened for preformed antibodies. Therapies directed toward decreasing the risk or severity of HDN in sensitized women have not proved effective. However, careful fetal monitoring with ultrasound, amniocentesis and percutaneous umbilical cord blood sampling can predict the need for fetal transfusion and early delivery. When infants present with unexplained jaundice, anemia, hydrops or a positive DAT, HDN caused by antibodies other than anti-RhD should be suspected. If the infant is group A or B and the mother is group O, ABO-related HDN is possible, a disease at least as common as Rh disease but far less severe. For diagnosis, antiglobulin testing should be performed and the antibody should be eluted from neonatal red cells and identified.

The prevention of primary sensitization to RhD antigen is now possible by administering Rh immune globulin (RhIg) to susceptible pregnant women during periods of risk of sensitization. RhIg prophylaxis is administered routinely at week 28 of pregnancy and within 72 hours of delivery. RhIg may also be used for RhD-negative recipients of RhD-positive blood components. Although it is obvious that circulating RhD-positive red cells are coated by the RhIg injection, the mechanism by which this injection prevents isoimmunization remains unclear.[29]

Red cell reactive autoantibodies

The first reports that patients may make antibodies directed against their own blood cells were by Donath and Landsteiner almost a century ago. The postulated causes of autoimmune cell destruction include cross-reacting antibodies, alterations to self-antigens (as may happen with drugs), revealed cryptantigens, and immune complexes fixed to 'innocent bystander' blood cells. In addition, the self-antigen may be normal but abnormal antibody production may occur. Examples include the production of anti-i due to Epstein–Barr virus (EBV) stimulation of B lymphocytes in infectious mononucleosis; the production of anti-I in mycoplasma pneumonia, and the loss of T-cell regulation in AIDS and some lymphoproliferative disorders, with ensuing autoantibody production. Some individuals also produce 'aberrant' autoantibody concomitant with the production of 'appropriate' alloantibody.[40] This phenomenon is illustrated by the appearance of autoantibodies in some cases of hemolytic transfusion reactions. Also, patients such as those with sickle cell anemia, who require frequent transfusion, may make autoantibodies in the setting of active production of multiple alloantibodies.

When a patient is discovered to have a positive DAT, further laboratory investigation and correlation with clinical information will help determine the clinical relevance of this observation. A positive DAT can be due to the presence of autoantibodies, alloantibodies, or both. An isolated DAT does not necessarily imply hemolysis. Other laboratory tests will help determine whether compensated hemolysis or hemolytic anemia is associated with the DAT. Some laboratories go to great lengths to characterize an isolated DAT. However, when autoantibody can be eluted from the red cells but alloantibodies are not present in the serum, and the patient has not been recently transfused, further serologic evaluation of the antibody is rarely rewarding.

Warm reactive autoantibodies and warm autoimmune hemolytic anemia

The clinical syndromes resulting from autoimmune hemolysis are directly related to the mechanism of red blood cell lysis and to the isotype and thermal amplitude of the autoantibody. Most warm-reacting antibodies (30°C or higher in vitro) are IgG, most commonly IgG_1 and IgG_3.[31] Warm-reacting IgM and IgA antibodies are unusual and their clinical significance, when found together with IgG, is unclear. Most warm-reacting antibodies are directed against protein antigens, including those that have blood group specificity, for example Rh, K, Jka and Ge. Among these, antigens of the Rh system are implicated most frequently in warm autoimmune hemolytic anemia. However, autoantibody specificity is not usually helpful for diagnosis or for selecting blood for transfusion. Red blood cells coated with IgG are removed relatively efficiently by specific macrophage receptors, primarily in the spleen.[32]

IgG-mediated warm-reacting autoimmune hemolytic anemias comprise about 70% of all autoimmune hemolytic anemia. Slightly more women than men are affected.[33] The degree of anemia is variable and the onset may be gradual. Mild jaundice and hepatosplenomegaly may be appreciated. No cause or association is determined for about half of all cases. Of the others, viral infections in childhood, medications, connective tissue disorders, lymphoproliferative disease and inherited immune deficiency states are among the most common associations.[34]

CLINICAL PEARLS

Autoimmune hemolysis

- Most cases of autoimmune hemolytic anemia result from warm-reacting IgG autoantibodies of broad specificity.
- Lymphoproliferative disorders, connective tissue disorders, medications and childhood viral infections are most frequently associated with warm autoimmune hemolysis.
- Cold autoantibodies that react in vitro at temperatures below 30°C are common but rarely clinically significant.
- Different mechanisms of drug-induced immune hemolysis may require specialized laboratory testing, including drug coating of reagent cells, drug addition to serum samples, or elution of antibody from affected cells and incubation with drug-coated reagent cells.

Cold reactive autoantibodies and cold agglutinin disease (cold agglutinin syndrome)

Cold-reacting antibodies are generally directed at polysaccharide antigens and are usually IgM antibodies. Cold autoantibodies react optimally at 0–5°C, but often have a broad thermal amplitude. Hemolysis and in vivo agglutination are usually confined to antibodies that react at 30°C or higher.

Cold autoantibodies, also known as cold agglutinins, may accompany viral infections, mycoplasma pneumonia or lymphoid malignancies (Chapter 72). They are frequently IgM antibodies directed against the I, i and Pr antigens. Cold agglutinins fix complement to the red cell surface during the passage of blood through the cooler extremities. Sensitized red cells are subsequently removed from circulation by C3b receptors located on macrophages of the liver and spleen. Patients with clinically significant cold-reacting autoantibodies may exhibit chronic anemia, episodes of acute hemolysis, or a syndrome characterized by painful acrocyanosis of the ears, nose and distal digits, referred to as cold hemagglutinin disease (CHD). Cold IgM autoantibodies may make both direct and reverse grouping for ABO difficult to perform and interpret. Prewarmed blood samples and reagents are often necessary to assure accurate testing when cold agglutinins are present.

The Donath–Landsteiner antibody is a rare, biphasic cold-reacting IgG antibody that is usually directed against the polysaccharide P antigen. It is associated with childhood viral infections such as measles and mumps, and with infection by *Treponema pallidum*. Cold-reacting anti-P antibodies fix complement to the red cell surface as blood passes through the vasculature of the cooler extremities.[35] Red cells sensitized by complement are subsequently hemolyzed by activation of the complement cascade upon return to the warmer central circulation of the patient. Acute attacks of intravascular hemolysis and hemoglobinuria may occur upon exposure to cold temperatures, and are referred to as paroxysmal cold hemoglobinuria (PCH).

DRUGS AND IMMUNOHEMATOLOGY

A variety of drugs may elicit the formation of antibodies directed against the drug itself or against antigens on the blood cell surface.

The most carefully studied examples of drug-related immune cytopenia involve the red cell. Drug-induced immune neutropenia and thrombocytopenia (for example 'quinine purpura') are also well established. Drug-induced red cell antibodies may produce an isolated positive DAT with no other sequelae, or may result in severe hemolytic anemia. When a patient presents with hemolysis and a positive DAT, it is important to include drug etiology in the differential diagnosis (Chapter 72).

PLATELETS

Platelets display a relatively unique set of glycoprotein antigens that occur predominantly on platelets and megakaryocytes, but are not restricted to them (Table 127.2). Most platelet-specific antigens occur in biallelic systems present as platelet glycoproteins, and have been studied at the molecular level.[36] The functions of several platelet glycoproteins have been determined. For example, glycoprotein Ia/IIa is important for platelet binding to exposed collagen, and this interaction is further strengthened by interaction of platelet glycoprotein Ib/IX with von Willebrand factor deposited on damaged endothelium. Platelet aggregation is also critical for hemostasis, and is mediated by the interaction of fibrinogen with platelet glycoprotein IIb/IIIa. Other antigens found on platelets include the red cell alloantigens ABH, Lewis, Ii and P. ABH antigens occur as intrinsic glycoprotein and absorbed glycosphingolipid antigens. Lewis antigens occur only on glycosphingolipids adsorbed from plasma. These antigens are less dense on platelets than on red cells. HLA Class I antigens, including HLA-A and HLA-B antigens, are intrinsic membrane constituents strongly expressed on platelets as well as other cell types, including lymphocytes and neutrophils.

Individuals can become refractory to repeated platelet transfusion, primarily due to antibodies to nonself HLA Class I antigens. Antibodies are developed in response to white cells present in transfused platelet and red cell units, or to fetal blood that enters the maternal circulation during pregnancy. Antibodies to foreign HLA-A and HLA-B Class I antigens then interact with transfused platelets having those specificities. Antibodies to platelet-specific antigens may also occur for about 10% of HLA-alloimmunized patients, and may be important in specific clinical conditions. Evaluation of a suspected case of HLA alloimmunization may include antigen phenotyping of the intended recipient and/or characterization of antibodies in serum from that individual, so that a donor lacking those specificities can be selected (Fig. 127.2 and Chapter 126).

When patients transfused with cellular blood components become alloimmunized to platelets, HLA antibodies can appear as soon as 10 days after transfusion.[37] The multicenter randomized blinded Trial to Reduce Alloimmunization to Platelets (TRAP) demonstrated that either leukocyte reduction by filtration or inactivation by ultraviolet B (UVB) irradiation was effective in reducing HLA antibody generation from 45% to 17–21%, independent of the number of donor exposures.[38] Platelet refractoriness was reduced from 13% to 3–5%. Antibodies to platelet-specific glycoproteins developed in 6–11% of all patients.

Selected platelet antigen systems

System	Glycoprotein location	Antigens	Original name
HPA-1	GPIIIa	HPA-1a HPA-1b	Zw^a, Pl^{A1} Zw^b, Pl^{A2}
HPA-2	GPIb	HPA-2a HPA-2b	Ko^b, Sib^b Ko^a, Sib^a
HPA-3	GPIIb	HPA-3a HPA-3b	Bak^a, Lek^a Bak^b, Lek^b
HPA-4	GPIIIa	HPA-4a HPA-4b	Pen^a, Yuk^b Pen^b, Yuk^a
HPA-5	GPIa	HPA-5a HPA-5b	Br^b, Zav^b Br^a, Zav^a, Hc^a
HPA-6	GPIIIa	HPA-6a HPA-6b	Ca^b Ca^a
HPA-7	GPIIIa	HPA-7a HPA-7b	Mo^b Mo^a
HPA-8	GPIIIa	HPA-8a HPA-8b	Sr^b Sr^a

Table 127.2 Selected platelet antigen systems.

HLA antibody screen

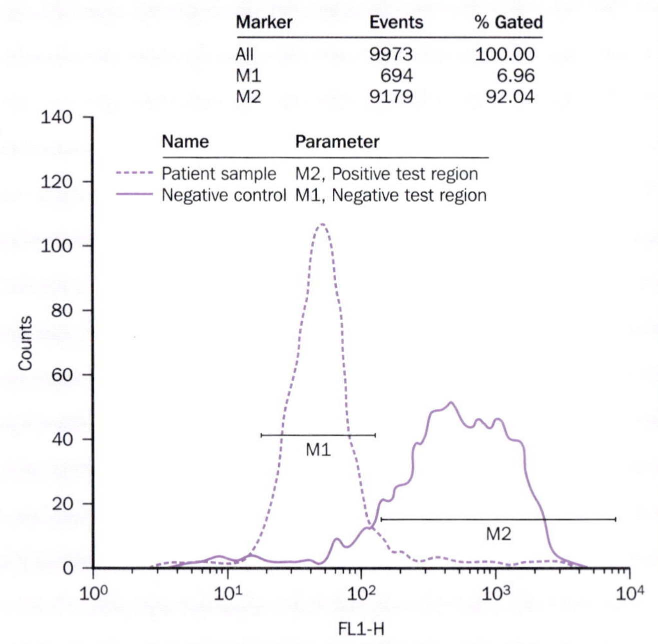

Figure 127.2 HLA antibody screen. Histograms are overlaid for HLA Class I microbead reactions with patient serum containing 92% panel reactive antibody (PRA) and negative serum. A pool of 30 different microbeads coated with purified HLA Class I antigens, including all common as well as many rare Class I antigens, is reacted with either patient serum or negative control serum. Unreacted serum antibodies are removed by washing. Bound anti-HLA antibodies are quantitated by reaction with fluorescent-labeled anti-human IgG and flow cytometric analysis. M1 is the negative region defined by reaction of control serum with Class I beads. M2 is the positive test region occupied by Class I beads coated with patient anti-HLA antibodies. For the patient specimen 9973 Class I beads are assessed, of which 9179 or 92.04% have bound anti-HLA antibodies. The patient is therefore said to have 92% PRA. (Courtesy of Melissa Schepperly and Toni Simonis.)

Considerations in the selection of a platelet component for transfusion include ABO type (although the role of A and B antigens in platelet transfusion incompatibility is debated) and HLA type, if the patient is known to be alloimmunized. For highly alloimmunized patients, or if HLA-matched platelets are not available, platelets tested for compatibility by cross-matching provide a therapeutic option.[39]

The biochemistry of platelet antigens and the quantification and characterization of antiplatelet antibodies have contributed to our understanding of the pathophysiology of various thrombocytopenic conditions. Thrombocytopenia associated with platelet alloantibodies and autoantibodies find parallels with several of the immune-mediated anemias.[40] Autoimmune thrombocytopenia associated with infections, lymphoproliferative disorders and drugs, as well as neonatal alloimune thrombocytopenia and post-transfusion purpura, is discussed in Chapter 74.

GRANULOCYTES

Granulocyte serology and antigen systems are far less well understood than those of red blood cells and platelets. Methods for detecting granulocyte antibodies are discussed in Chapter 73. Significant progress has been made in the methods for collection and transfusion of granulocytes. It is now possible to prepare therapeutic quantities of viable neutrophils, with post-transfusion increments approaching near physiologic range. Our knowledge of granulocyte serology, although rudimentary, has contributed to our understanding of clinical responses to granulocyte transfusion for life-threatening fungal and bacterial infections in neutropenic patients. Granulocytes possess a number of neutrophil-specific antigen systems, as well as HLA antigens (Table 127.3). The major red cell antigens are not found on granulocytes. Many granulocyte-specific antigens were identified during the investigation of alloimmune neonatal neutropenia (ANN), other autoimmune neutropenias, or transfusion reactions (Fig. 127.3).[41]

Neutrophils can now be collected for therapeutic transfusion to neutropenic patients with life-threatening infections.[42] When donors are stimulated with growth factors such as G-CSF, with or without steroids, post-transfusion increments in patients approach the physiologic range for circulating granulocytes. Limiting factors for granulocyte transfusion include HLA alloimmunization, pulmonary toxicity and chill–fever reactions. The majority of transfused patients rapidly develop anti-HLA antibodies.[43] Many alloimmunized patients suffer severe chill–fever reactions or pulmonary toxicity with subsequent transfusions. Trafficking studies with radiolabeled neutrophils have demonstrated reduced recovery, half-life and migration in the presence of leukoagglutinating antibodies.[44] HLA antibodies appear to be the major culprits in these immune-mediated reactions. The role of neutrophil-specific antibodies is less clear. In practice it is convenient to screen potential granulocyte recipients for HLA antibodies. Alloimmunized patients are then transfused with only HLA-matched compatible components, or not at all. Although it is difficult to prove a correlation of pulmonary toxicity with the presence of HLA antibodies, that trend is apparent. It is likely that either HLA antibodies, or neutrophil-specific antibodies for which HLA antibodies are a surrogate marker, are the culprit for pulmonary toxicity, which is the major limitation for granulocyte transfusion. In very ill patients hemodynamic instability has also been observed, the physiologic basis for which is poorly understood. Unfortunately, screening and compatibility testing with a single assay is unlikely to predict the tolerance and efficacy of granulocyte transfusions. Now that it is possible to obtain therapeutic doses of granulocytes, clinical trials are needed to prove efficacy and develop guidelines for the transfusion of this component.

Neutrophil antigen systems

System	Antigens	Location
NA	NA1, NA2	FcγRIIIb (CD16)
NB	NB1	58–64 kDa glycoprotein
NC	NC1	FcγRIIIb (CD16)
5	5a, 5b	Unknown
9	9a, 9b	Unknown
Unnamed	Mart, Ond	αL (CD11a) αM (CD11b)
Unnamed	LAN, SH	FcγRIIIb (CD16)

Table 127.3 Neutrophil antigen systems.

NA antigen phenotyping of granulocytes

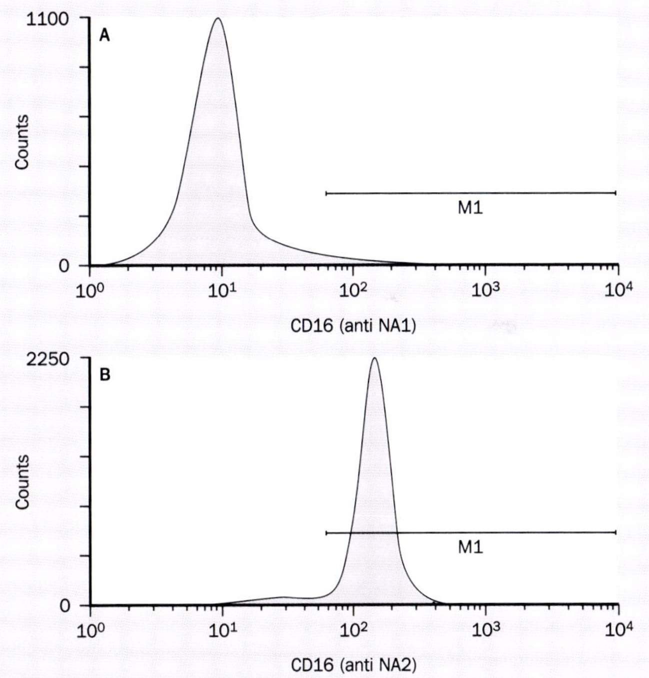

Figure 127.3 NA antigen phenotyping of granulocytes. Donor granulocytes are typed using murine monoclonal antibodies to CD16 specific for either the NA1 or NA2 epitope. Whole blood is incubated with fluorescent-labeled monoclonal antibodies. Fluorescence intensity of granulocytes is quantitated by flow cytometry following lysis of red cells. M1 is the positive test region. (**A**) Anti-CD16 having NA1 specificity is incubated with donor cells. Only 1.58% of cells are stained. (**B**) Anti-CD16 specific for NA2 is incubated with donor cells. 95.8% of granulocytes are positive for NA2. Therefore, these donor granulocytes express the NA2 epitope of CD16 and are negative for the NA1 epitode. (Courtesy of Kazuhiko Matsuo and David Stroncek.)

REFERENCES

1. Landsteiner K. Über Agglutinationserscheinungen normalen menschlichen Blutes. Wien Klin Wochenschr 1901;49:1132.
2. Epstein AA, Ottenberg R. Simple method of performing serum reactions. Proc NY Pathol Soc 1908;8:117.
3. Landsteiner K, Levine P. On the inheritance of agglutinogens of human blood demonstrable by immune agglutinins. J Exp Med 1928;48:731.
4. Levine P, Burnham L, Katzin EM, et al. The role of isoimmunization in the pathogenesis of erythroblastosis fetalis. Am J Obstet Gynecol 1941;42:925.
5. Coombs RRA, Mourant AE, Race RR. A new test for the detection of weak and 'incomplete' Rh agglutinins. Br J Exp Pathol 1945;26:255.
6. Daniels G. Terminology for red cell antigens – 1999 update. Immunohematology 1999;15:95.
7. Reid ME. Molecular basis for blood groups and function of carrier proteins. In: Silberstein LE (ed) Molecular and functional aspects of blood group antigens. Bethesda, MD, American Association of Blood Banks, 1995, p. 75.
8. Telen MJ. Erythrocyte blood group antigens: polymorphisms of functionally important molecules. Semin Hematol 1996;33:302.
9. Yamamoto F, Clausen F, White T, et al. Molecular genetic basis of the histo-blood group ABO system. Nature 1990;345:229.
10. Honig CL, Bove JR. Transfusion associated fatalities: review of Bureau of Biologics reports 1976–1978. Transfusion 1980;20:653.
11. Sazama K. Reports of 355 transfusion associated deaths: 1976 through 1985. Transfusion 1990;30:583.
12. Avent AD, Reid ME. The Rh blood group system: a review. Blood 2000;95:375.
13. Woodrow JC, Finn R. Transplacental hemorrhage. Br J Haematol 1966;18:357.
14. Lichtiger B, Surgeon J, Rhorer S. Rh-incompatible platelet transfusion therapy in cancer patients. Vox Sang 1983;45:139.
15. Giblett ER. A critique of the theoretical hazard of inter- vs. intraracial transfusion. Transfusion 1961;1:233.
16. Sosler SD, Jilly BJ, Saporito C, et al. A simple, practical model for reducing alloimmunization in patients with sickle cell disease. Am J Hematol 1993;43:103.
17. Vengelen-Tyler V (ed): Pretransfusion testing. In: Technical manual. 13th edn. Bethesda, MD, American Association of Blood Banks, 1999, p. 375.
18. Marsh ML. Scoring of hemagglutination reactions. Transfusion 1972;12:352.
19. Langston MM, Procter JL, Cipolone KM, Stroncek DF. Evaluation of the gel system for ABO grouping and D typing. Transfusion 1999;39:300.
20. Ashby W. The determination of the length of life of transfused blood-corpuscles in man. J Exp Med 1919;29:267.
21. International Committee for Standardization in Haematology. Recommended method for radioisotope red-cell survival studies. Br J Haematol 1980;45:659.
22. Pineda AA, Brzica SM, Taswell HF. Hemolytic transfusion reaction. Recent experience in a large blood bank. Mayo Clin Proc 1978;53:378.
23. Lostumbo MM, Holland PV, Schmidt PJ. Isoimmunization after multiple transfusions. N Engl J Med 1966;275:141.
24. Petz LD. Hemolysis associated with transplantation. Transfusion 1998;38:224.
25. Gajewski JL, Petz LD, Calhoun L, et al. Hemolysis of transfused group O red blood cells in minor ABO-incompatible unrelated-donor bone marrow transplants in patients receiving cyclosporine without post-transplant methotrexate. Blood 1992;79:3076.
26. Diamond LK, Blackfan KD, Baty JM. Erythroblastosis fetalis and its association with universal edema of the fetus, icterus gravis neonatorum, and anemia of the newborn. J Pediatr 1932;1:269.
27. Keith L, Danis RP, Berger GS. Clinical experience with the prevention of Rh isoimmunization – a historical comparative analysis. Am J Reprod Immunol Microbiol 1984;5:84.
28. Ness PM, Riley JZ. The detection of feto-maternal hemorrhage by enzyme-linked antiglobulin test (ELAT). In: Frigoletto FD, Jewett JF, Konugres AA (eds). Rh hemolytic disease – new strategy for eradication. Boston, GK Hall, 1982.
29. Pollack W, Gorman JG, Freda VJ. Rh immune suppression: past, present, and future. In: Frigoletto FD, Jewett JF, Konugres AA (eds) Rh hemolytic disease – new strategy for eradication. Boston, GK Hall, 1982.
30. Mohn JF, Lambert RM, Bowman HS, et al. Experimental production in man of autoantibodies with Rh specificity. Ann NY Acad Sci 1965;124:477.
31. Engelfriet CP, von dem Borne AEGK, Beckers DO, et al. Autoimmune hemolytic anemia – serological and immunological characteristics of the autoantibodies: mechanisms of cell destruction. Semin Hematol 1974;7:328.
32. Schreiber AD, Frank MM. Role of antibody and complement in the immune clearance and destruction of erythrocytes. I. In vivo effects of IgG and IgM complement fixing sites. J Clin Invest 1973;51:575.
33. Chaplin H Jr. Clinical usefulness of specific antiglobulin reagents in autoimmune hemolytic anemia. Prog Hematol 1973;8:25.
34. Pirofsky B. Autoimmunization and the autoimmune hemolytic anemias. Baltimore, Williams & Wilkins, 1969.
35. Berger M, Gaither TA, Frank MM. Complement receptors. Clin Immunol Rev 1981–1982;1:471.
36. Kickler T. Platelet immunology. In: Anderson KC, Ness PM (eds). Scientific basis of transfusion medicine. Philadelphia PA, W.B. Saunders, 2000, p. 227.
37. Howard JE, Perkins HA. The natural history of alloimmunization to platelets. Transfusion 1978;18:496.
38. The Trial to Reduce Alloimmunization to Platelets Study Group. Leukocyte reduction and ultraviolet B irradiation of platelets to prevent alloimmunization and refractoriness to platelet transfusions. N Engl J Med 1997;337:1861.
39. Gelb AB, Leavitt AD. Crossmatch-compatible platelets improve corrected count increments in patients who are refractory to randomly selected platelets. Transfusion 1997; 37:624.
40. von dem Borne AEG Jr, Kuijpers RWAM, Goldschmeding R. Platelet antigens in alloimmune thrombocytopenia, In: Nance SJ (ed) Clinical and basic science aspects of immunohematology. Arlington VA, American Association of Blood Banks, 1991.
41. Shastri KA, Logue GI. Autoimmune neutropenia. Blood 1993;8:1984.
42. Klein HG, Strauss RG, Schiffer CA. Granulocyte transfusion therapy. Semin Hematol 1996;33:359.
43. Stroncek DF, Leonard K, Eiber G, Malech HL, Gallin JI, Leitman SF. Alloimmunization after granulocyte transfusions. Transfusion 1996;36:1009.
44. McCullough JJ, Weiblen BJ, Clay ME, et al. Effect of leukocyte antibodies on the fate, in vivo, of indium-111-labelled granulocytes. Blood 1981;58:164.

Appendices

SELECTED CD MOLECULES AND THEIR CHARACTERISTICS

CD molecule	Predominant distribution	Identity/function
CD1a–e	Thymocytes, subset of lymphocytes, antigen-presenting cells	MHC Class 1-like molecules; presentation of non-peptide antigens to T cells; thymic T cell development
CD2	T cells	Binds to LFA-3; receptor for CD48; T cell activation; adhesion
CD3	T cells	T cell signaling complex; associated with T cell receptor (TCR)
CD4	T cell subset	TCR co-receptor; interacts with MHC Class II molecules on antigen presenting cells; identifies T cells with helper function; signal transduction
CD5	Most T cells, thymocytes, B cell subset	Binds to CD72; regulation of cell proliferation/activation; identifies B-1 B cell subset
CD6	Thymocytes, T cells, B cell subset	Binds CD166 (ALCAM); adhesion; mediates binding of developing thymocytes with thymic epithelial cells; thymic development; T cell activation
CD7	Pluripotent hematopoietic cells, thymocytes, T cells	T cell and NK cell development
CD8	T cell subset	TCR co-receptor; interacts with MHC Class I molecules on antigen presenting cells; identifies T cells with cytotoxic function
CD10	B cells	Neutral endopeptidase; enkephalinase; B cell development; common acute lymphoblastic leukemia antigen (CALLA)
CD11a	Leukocytes	α chain of LFA-1; pairs with CD18; interacts with ICAM; adhesion and cellular migration
CD11b	Monocytes, granulocytes, NK cells	α chain of complement receptor 3 (CR3); pairs with CD18; adhesion molecule
CD11c	Monocytes, granulocytes, NK cells	α chain of complement receptor 4 (CR4); pairs with CD18; adhesion molecule
CD14	Granulocytes, monocytes/macrophages	Receptor for LPS/LPB complex; myeloid differentiation antigen; cell activation
CD16a,b	NK cells, monocytes/macrophages, neutrophils	FcγRIIIA and FcγRIIIB (low affinity IgG receptors-type III); phagocytosis; ADCC
CD18	Leukocytes	β chain of β2 integrin molecules, including LFA-1, CR3, and CR4; pairs with CD11a, b, and c
CD19	B cells	BCR co-receptor; signal transduction; complexes with CD21
CD20	B cells	Role in B cell activation/differentiation
CD21	B cells; follicular dendritic cells	Complement receptor type 2 (CR2): C3d receptor; B cell co-receptor subunit; EBV receptor
CD22	B cells	Associates with BCR; signaling; regulation of B cell activation; adhesion
CD23	B cells, macrophages, eosinophils, platelets, follicular dendritic cells	FcεRII; (Low affinity IgE receptor)
CD24	Leukocytes	Heat stable antigen; co-stimulation; adhesion
CD25	Activated T cells and B cells	α chain of IL-2 receptor, low affinity IL-2 binding; signaling for cell proliferation/differentiation

CD molecule	Predominant distribution	Identity/function
CD26	Activated T cells and B cells; macrophages	Dipeptidyl peptidase; role in extracellular adhesion; cell activation
CD27	T cells; B cell subset	Co-stimulation; T cell proliferation
CD28	T cells	Binds B7-1 (CD80) and B7-2 (CD86); T cell co-stimulation; signal transduction
CD29	Leukocytes	Integrin β1 chain; pairs with CD49a-CD49f to form VLA-1-VLA-6 integrins, respectively; adhesion; signal transduction; development
CD30	Activated B cells and T cells	Binds to CD153; T cell activation/regulation/differentiation
CD31	Monocytes, granulocytes, platelets, endothelial cells, B cells	PECAM-1; Binds to CD38; adhesion; signal transduction
CD32	B cells, monocytes/macrophages, granulocytes, eosinophils	FcγRII (low affinity IgG receptor-type II) phagocytosis; ADCC; B cell regulation
CD34	Hematopoietic progenitor cells; capillary endothelium	Mucosialin; binds to CD62L; adhesion
CD35	Leukocytes; erythrocytes	Complement receptor 1 (CR1); C3b and C4b receptor; phagocytosis
CD36	Monocytes/macrophages; endothelium; platelets	Binds oxidized LDL; scavenger receptor; binds apoptic cells; adhesion and endocytic receptor; GPIIIb; platelet adhesion and aggregation
CD38	NK cells; T cell and B cell subsets; monocytes	Binds CD31; cyclase; hydrolase; cell activation
CD40	B cells; antigen-presenting cells	Binds CD154 (CD40 ligand); B cell proliferation differentiation, and survival; T cell co-stimulation
CD41	Megakaryocytes/platelets	Glycoprotein IIb; α IIb integrin chain; binds fibronectin, fibrinogen, von-Willebrand factor, thrombospondin; extracellular adhesion; platelet aggregation
CD43	Leukocytes (except resting B cells)	Leukocyte sialoglycoprotein; may bind CD54; signal transduction; adhesion; anti-adhesion
CD44	Leukocytes; memory T cells; erythrocytes	Binds hyaluronan, collagen, fibronectin, laminin, osteopontin; extra- and intercellular adhesion; T cell co-stimulation; leukocyte homing
CD45	Leukocytes (pan-leukocyte marker)	Protein tyrosine phosphatase; cell differentiation; lymphocyte signal transduction and activation
CD45RA	Naive T cell marker (in conjunction with low CD62L); B cells, monocytes	CD45 isoform
CD45RB	B and T cell subsets, monocytes/macrophages, granulocytes	CD45 isoform
CD45RO	Memory T cell marker; B cells, monocytes/macrophages	CD45 isoform
CD46	Hematopoietic cells	Membrane cofactor protein (MCP); binds to C3b and C4b and regulates complement pathway
CD47R	Leukocytes; endothelium	Integrin-associated protein (IAP); leukocyte migration, extravasation and activation
CD48	Leukocytes (not neutrophils)	Binds CD2; adhesion; co-stimulation
CD49a-f	Various distributions	Integrin α1-6 chain; binds to CD29 to form VLA-1 to VLA-6; binds extracellular matrix components such as fibronectin, laminin, collagen (CD49D binds VCAM-1, fibronectin, MadCAM-1, invasin); lymphocyte homing; extracellular adhesion; embryonic development
CD50	Thymocytes, B cells, T cells, monocytes, granulocytes	ICAM-3; adhesion
CD51	Platelets/megakaryocytes, granulocytes, monocytes, T cells	Integrin α chain; associates with CD61; binds vitronectin, fibronectin, fibrinogen; extracellular adhesion; T cell co-stimulation; epithelial inflammatory response
CD54	Broad distribution; increased on activated leukocytes	ICAM-1; binds LFA-1; adhesion; leukocyte transendothelial migration, rhinovirus receptor
CD55	Hematopoietic cells and some non-hematopoietic cells	Decay accelerating factor (DAF); binds complement fragment C3b; regulation of complement activation
CD56	NK cells	NKH-1; adhesion
CD57	NK cells, T cell subset, B cells, monocytes	Oligosaccharide expressed on cell surface glycoproteins

CD molecule	Predominant distribution	Identity/function
CD58	Hematopoietic cells and nonhematopoietic cells	LFA-3; binds CD2; adhesion; lymphocyte co-activation
CD59	Hematopoietic cells and non-hematopoietic cells	Binds complement components C8 and C9 and regulates assembly of complement membrane attack complex
CD61	Platelets/ megakaryocytes, macrophages	Integrin β3 subunit; associates with CD41 or CD51
CD62E	Endothelium	ELAM-1 or E-selection; binds sialyl-lewis X; adhesion; mediates rolling interaction of neutrophils on endothelium and neutrophil extravasation
CD62L	B cells, T cells, monocytes, NK cells	LECAM-1, LAM-1 (or L-selectin); binds CD34 and GlyCAM; adhesion; mediates rolling interactions with endothelium and call extravasation
CD62P	Platelets/megakaryocytes, endothelium	P-selectin; binds sialyl-Lewis X; mediates interaction of platelets with neutrophils and monocytes; mediates rolling interaction of neutrophils with endothelium
CD64	Monocytes/macrophages	FcγR1 (High affinity IgG receptor)
CD68	Monocytes/macrophages	Macrosialin; early activation antigen; role in phagocytic activity
CD69	Activated T cells, B cells, macrophages, NK cells	Early activation antigen; costimulation
CD70	Activated B and T cells; macrophages	Binds to CD27; costimulation
CD71	Activated leukocytes	Transferrin receptor; cell activation
CD72	B cells	Ligand for CD5; B cell activation and differentiation; costimulation
CD73	B and T cell subsets	Ecto-5' nucleotidase; allows nucleoside uptake
CD74	MHC Class II expressing cells	MHC Class II associated invariant chain; involved in antigen processing and peptide presentation in antigen-presenting cells
CD77	Germinal center B cells	
CD79a,b	B cells	Igα, Igβ; components of BCR complex that mediate signal transduction
CD80	Monocytes/macrophages, dendritic cells, activated B cells	B7-1; ligand for CD28 and CTLA-4; T cell interaction with antigen-presenting cells; co-stimulation
CD81	Lymphocytes	Associates with CD19 and CD21 to form B cell co-receptor complex; costimulation; adhesion
CD86	Monocytes, activated B cells	B7-2; ligand for CD28 and CTLA-4; T cell interaction with antigen-presenting cells; co-stimulation
CD87	Granulocytes; monocytes/macrophages, activated T cells	Urokinase plasminogen activator receptor
CD88	Granulocytes, macrophages, mast cells	Complement component fragment C5a receptor
CD89	Monocytes/macrophages, granulocytes, B and T cell subsets	FcαR (IgA receptor)
CD91	Monocytes	α2 macroglobulin receptor
CD94	NK cells, NK cells	Inhibits killing
CD95	Broad distribution	Fas or Apo-1; induces apoptosis after being bound by Fas ligand
CD102	Resting lymphocytes, monocytes, endothelial cells	ICAM-2; binds LFA-1 (CD11a/CD18); adhesion; T cell costimulation
CD103	Intraepithelial lymphocytes, T cell subset	αE integrin; T cell development and co-stimulation
CD104	Epithelial cells, Schwann cells	β4 integrin; epidermal adhesion to basement membrane
CD105	Endothelial cells, bone marrow cell subset, activated macrophages	Endoglin; adhesion
CD106	Endothelial cells	VCAM-1; ligand for VLA-4; lymphocyte adhesion; embryonic development
CD107a,b	Epithelial cells, subsets of monocytes, granulocytes, and lymphocytes	LAMP-1 and LAMP-2; adhesion

CD molecule	Predominant distribution	Identity/function
CD110	Hematopoietic stem cells, megakaryocytes, platelets	Thrombopoietin receptor; megakaryocyte proliferation and differentiation
CD114	Granulocytes	G-CSF receptor; regulates granulopoiesis
CD115	Monocytes/macrophages	M-CSF receptor; cell differentiation
CD116	Monocytes, neutrophils, eosinophils	GM-CSF α chain receptor; cell differentiation
CD117	Hematopoietic progenitors	c-kit; stem cell factor (SCF) receptor; hematopoietic cell differentiation
CD118	Broad distribution	Type 1 interferon (interferon α/β) receptor
CD119	Broad distribution	Interferon γ receptor
CD120a	Hematopoietic cells, nonhematopoietic cells, myeloid cells	TNF receptor-type 1; signal transduction; apoptosis
CD120b	Hematopoietic cells, nonhematopoietic cells, myeloid cells	TNF receptor-type II; signal transduction, apoptosis
CD121a	Thymocytes, T cell subset, fibroblasts, epithelial cells, and brain cells	IL-1 receptor-type I; signal transduction
CD121b	T cell subset, mycloid cell subsets	IL-1 receptor-type II
CD122	NK cells, T cell and B cell subset	IL-2 and IL-15 receptor β chain; signal transduction; regulation of lymphocyte development, differentiation, activation and proliferation
CD123	Bone marrow stem cells, granulocytes, monocytes, megakaryocytes	IL-3 receptor α chain; cell development and differentation
CD124	Mature B and T cells, hematopoietic precursor cells	IL-4 receptor; signal transduction; lymphocyte development, activation, differentiation and proliferation
CD125	Eosinophils, basophils, B cell subset	IL-5 receptor; eosinophil and B cell growth and differentiation
CD126	Activated B cells, plasma cells, T cells, granulocytes, monocytes/macrophages; also expressed on epithelial cells, fibroblasts, hepatocytes, and neural cells	IL-6 receptor α chain; regulation of B cell and T cell differentiation and function; hematopoiesis
CD127	Bone marrow lymphoid precursors, pro-B cells, T cell precursors, T cell subset, monocytes	IL-7 receptor α chain; signal transduction; B and T cell proliferation and differentiation
CD128	Neutrophils, basophils, T cell subset	IL-8 receptor; neutrophil activation and migration
CD129	T cells	IL-9 receptor α chain; T cell proliferation
CD130	Broad distribution	IL-6 receptor β chain (with CD126); signal transduction
CD131	Lymphocytes, granulocytes, monocytes	IL-3, IL-5 and GM-CSF receptor; common β chain; signal transduction; see CD123 and CD125
CD132	Lymphocytes	Common γ chain of high affinity receptor for IL-2 (with CD25 and CD122), IL-4 (with CD124), IL-7 (with CD127), IL-9 (with CD129), and IL15 (with CD122) receptors; signal transduction
CD134	Activated T cells	OX-40 antigen of TNFR superfamily (binds OX-40 ligand); T cell–B cell interaction and T cell costimulation
CD135	Lymphoid and myeloid cell progenitor subsets	Flt3 ligand receptor; development of mycloid and lymphoid progenitors
CD137	Activated T cells	4-1BB; binds 4-1BB ligand and extracellular matrix components; T cell–B cell interaction and T cell costimulation; extracellular adhesion; signal transduction
CD138	B cell subset, plasma cells	Syndecan-1; binds interstitial matrix proteins; B cell–matrix interactions
CD140a,b	Endothelial cells	PDGF receptor α and β chain; embryonic development; signal transduction; chemotaxis
CD141	Endothelium	Thrombomodulin (binds thrombin); regulates coagulation
CD142	Endothelium	Tissue factor; binds plasma factors VII/VIIa; hemostasis, coagulation, and angiogenesis
CD143	Endothelium	Angiotensin-converting enzyme (ACE); binds angiotensin 1; regulates blood pressure

CD molecule	Predominant distribution	Identity/function
CD144	Endothelium	VE-cadherin; cell–cell adhesion; maintenance of endothelium integrity
CD150	T and B cell subsets	Surface lymphocyte activation marker (SLAM); B cell–T cell interaction; costimulation
CD151	Not defined	PETA-3; regulates platelet aggregation and mediator release
CD152	Activated T cells	CTLA-4; binds B7-1 (CD80) and B7-2 (CD86); T cell costimulation–negative signal
CD153	T cells	CD30 ligand; T cell activation, differentiation, and regulation
CD154	Activated T cells	CD40 ligand; T cell costimulation
CD156a	Leukocytes, B cells	Transmembrane glycoprotein; disintegrin and metalloproteinase domain (ADAM) family member; leukocyte adhesion and protease function; infiltration of myelomonocytic cells
CD156b	Broad distribution	TNF-α converting enzyme (TACE); disintegrin and metalloproteinase domain (ADAM) family member; cleaves TNF and transforming growth factor-α from cell surface, thereby releasing soluble form
CD158	NK cells	Killer cell immunoglobulin (Ig)-like receptors (KIR); family of molecules that inhibit NK cytotoxic activity
CD159a	NK cells	NKG2a (killer cell lectin-like receptor)
CD161	NK cells	Natural killer cell receptor-P1; target cell recognition; NK cell activation
CD162	Granulocyte and T cell subsets	P-selectin glycoprotein ligand-1 (PSGL-1); adhesion
CD166	Activated T cells, B cells	ALCAM; binds CD6; T cell activation; thymocyte development
CD167a	Epithelial cells	Discoidin domain receptor 1 (DDD1); tyrosine kinase receptor; binds to collagen; cell–cell contact and adhesion
CD178	Activated T cells; various tissue cells	Fas ligand (ligand for CD95); binding to Fas triggers apoptosis
CD179a	Pro B and pre B cells	VpreB; forms surrogate light chain with CD179b; early B cell differentiation
CD179b	Pro B and pre B cells	Lambda 5; forms surrogate light chain with CD179a; early B cell differentiation
CD180	B cells	RP105; toll-like receptor family; regulates B cell recognition and signaling of LPS
CD183	Effector/memory T cells	CXCR3 receptor for interferon-inducible chemokines IP10, Mig, and I-TAC; chemotactic migration of effector T cells into areas of inflammation
CD184	Leukocytes; hematopoietic progenitors	CXCR4 receptor for chemokines such as stromal cell derived factor-1 (SDF-1) (fusin); chemotaxis; HIV-1 co-receptor
CD195	Broad distribution; myeloid cells, lymphocytes, T lymphocytes, neurons, epithelium, endothelium	CCR5 receptor for chemokines such as macrophage inflammatory proteins, MIP-1α and MIP-1β, and RANTES; chemotaxis; HIV-1 coreceptor
CDw197	Lymphoid tissues, B cells, T cell subset	CCR7 chemokine receptor; chemotaxis; T cell homing and migration
CD201	Endothelial cells	Protein C receptor; coagulation
CD204	Myeloid cells, monocytes/macrophages	Macrophage scavenger receptor-1 (MSR1); mediates binding, internalization and processing of various negatively charged macromolecules
CD206	Dendritic cells, macrophages, myeloid cells, endothelial cells	Mannose receptor, C-type 1; binds microorganisms; phagocytosis
CD207	Dendritic cells, Langerhans cells	Langerin; mannose receptor; phagocytosis and internalization of antigen for processing
CDw210	Broad distribution	Il-10 receptor α and β chain;
CD212	T cells, NK cells	IL-12 receptor β-1 chain;
CD213a1,a2	Lymphocytes, bronchial epithelial and smooth muscle cells	IL-13 receptor α1 and α2 chains
CDw217	Activated T cell subset	IL-17; cytotoxic T-lymphocyte-associated serine esterase 8; stimulates cell activation; induces osteoclast differentiation factor (ODF)
CD220	Broad distribution	Insulin receptor; stimulates glucose uptake

CD molecule	Predominant distribution	Identity/function
CD221	Broad distribution	Insulin-like growth factor 1 receptor; cell signaling; activation, and differentiation
CD222	Broad distribution	Mannose-6-phosphate receptor; insulin-like growth factor-2 receptor
CD226	NK cells, platelets, monocytes, T cell subset	Platelet and T cell activation antigen 1 (PTA1); adhesion
CD233–242	Erythrocytes	Various erythrocyte membrane antigens, including blood group associated glycoproteins
CD246	T cells	TCR or CD3 zeta chain; associated with TCR and CD3; couples TCR recognition with T cell signaling

Abbreviations

ADCC, antibody dependent cellular cytotoxicity;
ALCAM, activated leukocyte cell adhesion molecule;
BCR, B cell receptor for antigen;
EBV, Epstein–Barr virus;
ELAM, endothelial leukocyte adhesion molecule;
G-CSF, granulocyte colony stimulating factor;
GM-CSF, granulocyte macrophage colony stimulating factor;
ICAM, intercellular adhesion molecule;
LAM, leukocyte adhesion molecule;
LAMP, latent membrane protein;
LDL, low density lipoproteins;
LECAM, lymphocyte endothelial cell adhesion molecule;
LFA, lymphocyte function antigen;
LPB, lipopolysaccharide binding protein;
LPS, lipopolysaccharide;
M-CSF, macrophage colony stimulating factor;
MHC, major histocompatibility complex;
NK cells, natural killer cells;
PDGF, platelet-derived growth factor;
PECAM, platelet endothelial cell adhesion molecule;
PETA, platelet-endothelial cell tetraspan antigen;
TCR, T cell receptor for antigen;
TNF, tumor necrosis factor;
TNFR, tumor necrosis factor receptor;
VCAM, vascular cellular adhesion molecule;
VLA, very late antigen.

This list was adapted from the results of the 7th International Workshop on Human Leukocyte Differentiation Antigens (HLDA7) held in Harrogate, UK in June, 2000 (see http://gryphon.jr2.ox.ac.uk).

LABORATORY REFERENCE VALUES

Serum immunoglobulin levels

Age	IgG gm/L	IgM gm/L	IgA gm/L
Cord blood	6.36–16.06	0.06–0.25	0.01–0.03
1 month	2.51–9.06	0.20–0.87	0.01–0.53
2 months	2.06–6.01	0.17–1.05	0.02–0.46
3 months	1.76–5.81	0.24–0.89	0.04–0.46
4 months	1.96–5.58	0.27–1.01	0.04–0.73
5 months	1.72–8.14	0.33–1.09	0.08–0.68
6 months	2.15–7.04	0.35–1.02	0.08–0.68
7–9 months	2.17–9.04	0.34–1.26	0.11–0.90
10–12 months	2.94–10.69	0.41–1.49	0.16–0.84
1 year	3.45–12.13	0.43–1.73	0.14–1.06
2 years	4.24–10.51	0.48–1.68	0.14–1.23
3 years	4.41–11.35	0.47–2.00	0.22–1.59
4–5 years	4.63–12.36	0.43–1.96	0.25–1.54
6–8 years	6.33–12.80	0.48–2.07	0.33–2.02
9–10 years	6.08–15.72	0.52–2.42	0.45–2.36
Adult	6.39–13.49	0.56–3.52	0.70–3.12

Data generated by Beckman Labs using a Beckman rate nephelometer (see Chapter 120)

Total serum IgE (IU/ml)

Age	Gender	Geometric mean	Upper 95% confidence limit
6–14 years	M	42.7	527
	F	43.3	344
15–24 years	M	33.6	447
	F	18.6	262
25–34 years	M	16.8	275
	F	16.6	216
35–44 years	M	21.7	242
	F	19.3	206
45–54 years	M	19.2	254
	F	13.3	177
55–64 years	M	21.3	354
	F	11.7	148
65–74 years	M	21.2	248
	F	11.5	122
>75 years	M	18.4	219
	F	9.2	124
6–75 years	all M	22.9	317
	all F	14.7	189

Data generated using prick skin test negative (i.e. house dust mite, Bermuda grass, tree mix, weed mix, mold mix) individuals by Barbee RA, et al. J Allergy Clin Immunol 68:106, 1981 (with permission).

Lymphocyte immunophenotype: adult reference range (95% confidence interval)

Surface antigens	Percent positive	Cells/mm³
T cells		
CD3	61–84%	832–2028
CD5	60–82%	828–1994
CD2	74–89%	992–2079
CD3/CD4	32–58%	474–1405
CD3/CD8	11–36%	188–720
CD4/CD45RO	12–29%	196–522
CD4/CD45RA	3.5–22.5%	57–481
CD8/CD45RO	2–9.5%	33–192
CD8/CD45RA	3.5–22%	53–413
CD8/CD28	7.5–30%	145–583
CD8/CD57	2.5–23.5	39–417
CD3/HLA–DR	≤ 15.1%	≤ 291
CD3/CD25	≤ 37.4%	≤ 756
B cells		
CD19	5.5–16%	94–378
CD20	5–16%	88–330
CD20/CD5	1.5–10%	24–220
NK cells		
$CD3^-/CD16^-CD56^+$	6.5–29.5%	120–490
Lymphocytes	17–41%	1173–2640

Data gererated in the Flow Cytometry Section, Immunology Service, DLM, CC, NIH, Bethesda, MD. The 95% confidence interval for the WBC is 4300–9200/mm³.

Age–dependent lymphocyte immunophenotype reference range (95% confidence interval)						
	T-cell surface antigens					
	CD3		CD3/CD4		CD3/CD8	
Age	Percent Positive	Cells/mm³	Percent positive	Cells/mm³	Percent Positive	Cells/mm³
Neonate	28–76	600–5000	17–52	400–3500	10–41	200–1900
1 wk–2 mo	60–85	2300–7000	41–68	1700–5300	9–23	400–1700
2–5 mo	48–75	2300–6500	33–58	1500–5000	11–25	500–1600
5–9 mo	50–77	2400–6900	33–58	1400–5100	13–26	600–2200
9–15 mo	54–76	1600–6700	31–54	1000–4600	12–28	400–2100
15–24 mo	39–73	1400–8000	25–50	900–5500	11–32	400–2300
2–5 yr	43–76	900–4500	23–48	500–2400	14–33	300–1600
5–10 yr	55–78	700–4200	27–53	300–2000	19–34	300–1800
10–16 yr	52–78	800–3500	25–48	400–2100	9–35	200–1200
Adult	55–83	700–2100	28–57	300–1400	10–39	200–900

	B-cell and NK-cell surface antigens			
Age	CD19		$CD3^-/CD16–56^+$	
	Percent positive	Cells/mm³	Percent positive	Cells/mm³
Neonate	5–22	40–1100	6–58	100–1900
1 wk–2 mo	4–26	600–1900	3–23	200–1400
2–5 mo	14–39	600–3000	2–14	100–1300
5–9 mo	13–35	700–2500	2–13	100–1000
9–15 mo	15–39	600–2700	3–17	200–1200
15–24 mo	17–41	600–3100	3–16	100–1400
2–5 yr	14–44	200–2100	4–23	100–1000
5–10 yr	10–31	200–1600	4–26	90–900
10–16 yr	8–24	200–600	6–27	70–1200
Adult	6–19	100–500	7–31	90–600

Data generated by Comans-Bitter WM, et al. J Pediatr 130:388, 1997 (with permission).

Lymphocyte proliferation (95% confidence interval)	
	Counts per minute
Mitogens	
Unstimulated	0–8,707
PHA 10 ug/ml	79,067–197,169
ConA 50 ug/ml	49,591–189,654
PWM 100 ng/ml	36,957–158–404
Antigens	
Tetanus toxoid (40ng/ml)	2,013–23,173
Candida (1:2000 wt:vol)	1,620–9,908

Data generated by the Allergy Immunology Department, Texas Children's Hospital, Baylor College of Medicine, Houston, TX

NEUTROPHIL OXIDATIVE BURST

NBT test > 95% granulocytes positive (stained) following PMA stimulation

DHR assay: adult control stimulation index* = 123–273

$$\text{* equals: } \frac{\text{mean channel fluorescence of PMA stimulated cells}}{\text{mean channel fluorescence of unstimulated cells}}$$

Data generated in the Flow Cytometry Section, Immunology Service, DLM, CC, NIH, Bethesda, MD.

CHEMOKINES

Class	Systemic name	Chemokine		Receptor(s)	Receptor(s) expressed on
	CXCL1	GRO-α, MGSA	Growth-related oncogene-α	CXCR2 DARC	N, M, T, NK Erythrocytes
	CXCL2	GRO-β MIP-2α	Growth-related oncogene-β	CXCR2	N, M, T, NK
	CXCL3	GRO-γ MIP-2β	Growth-related oncogene- γ	CXCR2	N, M, T, NK
	CXCL4	PF4	Platelet factor 4		
	CXCL5	ENA-78	Epithelial cell derived neutrophil attractant-78	CXCR2	N, M, T, NK
	CXCL6	GCP-2	Granulocyte chemoattractant protein-2	CXCR1, CXCR2	N, M, T, NK, Ba
CXC (α)	CXCL7	NAP-2	Neutrophil activating peptide-2	CXCR2	N, M, T, NK
	CXCL8	IL-8	Interleukin-8	CXCR1, CXCR2 DARC	N, M, T, NK, Ba Erythrocytes
	CXCL9	MIG	Monokine-induced by interferon g	CXCR3	T, NK, B
	CXCL10	IP-10	Interferon g-inducible protein-10	CXCR3	T, NK, B
	CXCL11	I-TACK	Interferon inducible T cell a chemoattractant	CXCR3	T, NK, B
	CXCL12	PBSF SDF-1	Pre-B-cell growth-stimulating factor Stromal cell-derived factor 1	CXCR4	T,B,M,DC
	CXCL13	BCA-1 BLC	B cell-attracting chemokine-1 B-lymphocyte chemoattractant	CXCR5	B,T
	CXCL14	BRAK bolekine	Chemokine isolated from breast and kidney tissue		
	CCL1	I-309	Inducible 309	CCR8	T, M
	CCL2	MCP-1	Monocyte chemoattractant protein-1	CCR2, CCR5 DARC	M, T, NK, DC, Ba Erythrocytes
	CCL3	MIP-1α	Macrophage inflammatory protein 1a	CCR1, CCR5	N, M, T, NK, DC, Eo, Ba
	CCL4	MIP-1β	Macrophage inflammatory protein 1b	CCR5, CCR8	M, T, DC
	CCL5	RANTES	Regulated on activation of normal T cells expressed & secreted	CCR1, CCR3, CCR5 DARC	N, M, T, NK, DC, Eo, Ba Erythrocytes
	CCL7	MCP-3	Monocyte chemoattractant protein-3	CCR1, CCR2, CCR3, CCR5	N, M, T, NK, DC, Eo, Ba
	CCL8	MCP-2	Monocyte chemoattractant protein-2	CCR2, CCR3, CCR5	M, T, NK, DC, Ba, Eo
	CCL11	Eotaxin-1		CCR3, CCR5	Ba, Eo, T, M, DC
	CCL13	MCP-4 CKβ-10	Monocyte chemoattractant protein-4 Chemokineβ-10	CCR2, CCR3, CCR5	M, T, NK, DC, Ba, Eo
	CCL14	MCIF CKβ-1 HCC-1 NCC-2	Macrophage colony inhibitory factor Chemokineβ-1 Hemofiltrate CC chemokine-1 Novel CC chemokine-2		
	CCL15	LKN-1 MIP-5 HCC-2 MIP-1δ	Leukotactin Macrophage inflammatory protein-5 Hemofiltrate CC chemokine-2 Macrophage inflammatory protein Iδ	CCR1, CCR3	N, M, T, NK, DC, Eo, Ba
	CCL16	LEC NCC-4 HCC-4	Liver-expressed chemokine Novel CC chemokine-4 Hemofiltrate CC chemokine-4		
CC (β)	CCL17	TARC	Thymus and activation-regulated chemokine	CCR4, CCR8, DARC	T, M, NK, DC, Ba Erythrocytes
	CCL18	PARC DC-CK1 MIP-4 AMAC-1 CKβ-7	Pulmonary and activation-regulated chemokine Dendritic cells chemokine-1 Macrophage inflammatory protein-4 Alternative macrophage activation-associated CC chemokine Chemokineβ-7		
	CCL19	ELC MIP-3β CKβ-11 Exodus-3	EBV-Induced gene 1 -ligand chemokine Macrophage inflammatory protein-3β Chemokineβ-11	CCR7	T, M, DC, B
	CCL20	LARC MIP-3α Exodus	Liver & activation-regulated chemokine Macrophage inflammatory protein-3α	CCR6	T, DC, B

Class	Systemic name	Chemokine		Receptor(s)	Receptor(s) expressed on
	CCL2I	SLC CKβ-9 Exodus 2 6Ckine	Secondary lymphoid tissue chemokine Chemokineβ-9	CCR7	T, M, DC, B
	CCL22	MDC STCP-1	Macrophage derived chemokine Stimulated T-cell chemoattractant protein-1	CCR4	T, NK, DC, Ba
	CCL23	MPIF-1 CKβ-8	Myeloid progenitor inhibitory factor-1 Chemokineβ-6	CCR1	N, M, T, NK, DC, Eo, Ba
	CCL24	MPIF-2 CKβ-6 Eotaxin-2	Myeloid progenitor inhibitory factor-2 Chemokineβ-8	CCR3	Ba, Eo, T
	CCL25	TECK	Thymus-expressed chemokine	CCR9	T
	CCL26	Eotaxin-3		CCR3	Ba, Eo, T
	CCL27	CTACK	Cutaneous T cell-attracting chemokine	CCR10	K, T
XC (γ)	XCL1	Lymphotactin ATAC SCM-1α	 Activation-induced, T cell-derived, and chemokine-related Single cysteine motif-1α	XCR1	M, T
	XCL2	SCM-1 β	Single cysteine motif-1β		
CX_3C (δ)	CX_3CL1	Fractalkine		CX_3CR1	M, NK, T

Abbreviations for cells: B, B cells; Ba, Basophils; DC, Dendritic cells; Eo, Eosinophils;M, Macrophages/Monocytes; N, Neutrophils; NK, Natural Killer cells ; T, T cells.

CYTOKINES

Cytokine	Abbreviation	Receptor family	Signaling	Source	Target	Action	Knockout phenotype
Cardiotrophin-1	CT-1	Type I (hematopoietin) gp130-utilizing	Jak1, Stat3	myocardial cells	myocardium	growth	
Ciliary Neurotrophic Factor	CNTF	Type I (hematopoietin) gp130-utilizing	Jak1, Stat3	Schwann cells, astrocytes	neuronal cells	survival	Progressive atrophy and loss of motor neurons
Colony Stimulating Factor, Granulocyte	G-CSF	Type I (hematopoietin) homodimeric	Jak2, Stat3	many tissues, macrophages, endothelium, fibroblasts	committed progenitors	differentiation, activates mature granulocytes	neutropenia
Colony Stimulating Factor, Granulocyte-Macrophage	GM-CSF	Type I (hematopoietin) β_c utilizing	Jak2, Stat5	T cell, Macrophages, endothelium, fibroblasts	immature and committed myelo-monocytic progenitors, mature macrophages and granulocytes, dendritic cells	growth, differentiation, survival, activation	pulmonary alveolar proteinosis
Colony Stimulating Factor, Macrophage	CSF-1 or M-CSF	Type I (hematopoietin)	Ras/Raf/MAPK	macrophages, endothelium, fibroblasts, other cells	committed myelomonocytic progenitors	differentiation, proliferation, survival	monocytopenia, osteopetrosis, female infertility
Erythropoietin	Epo	Type I (hematopoietin) homodimeric	Jak2, Stat5	kidney, liver	erythroid precursors	erythroid differentiation	embryonic lethal, severe anemia
FLT-3/FLK-2 Ligand	FL	Type I (hematopoietin)	Ras/Raf/MAPK	diverse tissues	myeloid cells, especially dendritic cells	proliferation, differentiation	Reduced repopulating hematopoietic stem cells, reduced B cell precursors
Growth Hormone	GH	Type I (hematopoietin) homodimeric	Jak2, Stat5b	pituitary and placental GH genes (2)	diverse tissues	Growth, adipocyte differentiation, induces IGF-1	Dwarfism*
Interferon-α/β	IFNα/β	Type I (hematopoietin)	Jak1, Tyk2, Stat1, Stat2	macrophages, fibroblasts, other	all NK cells	antiviral, antiproliferative, increased MHC Class I activation	susceptibility to viral infections
Interferon-γ	IFNγ	Type I (hematopoietin)	Jak1, Jak2, Stat1	Th1 T cells, NK cells	macrophages, endothelium, NK cells	activation, increased MHC Class II expression, increased antigen presentation	susceptibility to bacterial infections
Interleukin-1α/β	IL-1 α/β	IL-1/TLR	IRAK, MyD88, TRAF6, NF-κB	many cells, especiallly macrophages	CNS, endothelial cells, liver, thymocytes, macrophages	fever, anorexia, activation, acute phase reactants, costimulation, activation, cytokine secretion	
Interleukin-2	IL-2	Type I (hematopoietin) γ_c utilizing	Jak1, Jak3, Stat5	T cells	T, B, NK cells, macrophages	proliferation, cytotoxicity, IFNγ secretion, antibody production	lymphoproliferation*
Interleukin-3	IL-3	Type I (hematopoietin) β_c utilizing	Jak2, Stat5	T cells	immature hematopoietic progenitors of multiple lineage	growth, differentiation, survival	no defects in basal hematopoiesis
Interleukin-4	IL-4	Type I (hematopoietin) γ_c utilizing	Jak1, Jak3, Stat6	Th2 T cells, mast cells	T cell, B cell, macrophage	proliferation,Th2 differentiation, IgG4 and IgE production, Inhibition of cell-mediated immunity	Defective Th2 differentiation and IgE production, decreased allergic responses

Interleukin-5	IL-5	Type I (hematopoietin) β_c utilizing	Jak2, Stat5	Th2 T cells	eosinophil, B cell	proliferation, activation	Decreased eosinophilia, defective CD5+ B1 B cell development
Interleukin-6	IL-6	Type I (hematopoietin) gp130-utilizing	Jak1, Stat3	macrophage, fibroblasts, endothelium, epithelium, T cells, other stromal cells	liver, B cell, T-cell, thymocytes, myeloid cells, osteoclasts	acute phase reactants, proliferation, differentiation, costimulation, proliferation	Reduced Ig, esp IgA, T lymphopenia, impaired acute phase response
Interleukin-7	IL-7	Type I (hematopoietin) γ_c utilizing	Jak1, Jak3, Stat5	bone marrow, thymic stromal cells, spleen	thymocytes, T cells, B cells	growth, differentiation, survival	SCID
Interleukein-8	IL-8	See Chemokines					
Interleukin-9	IL-9	Type I (hematopoietin) γ_c utilizing	Jak1, Jak3, Stat5	Th2 T cells	T cells, mast cell precursors	proliferation	
Interleukin-10	IL-10	Type I (hematopoietin)	Jak1, Tyk2, Stat3	Th2 T cells, others	macrophages	decreased MHC Class II expression, decreased antigen presentation	exaggerated inflammatory response and autoimmune disease
Interleukin-11	IL-11	Type I (hematopoietin) gp130-utilizing	Jak1, Stat3	stromal cells	hematopoietic stem cells	proliferation	
Interleukin-12	IL-12	Type I (hematopoietin) heterodimeric	Jak2, Tyk2, Stat4	macrophages, B cells	T cells, NK cells	Th1 differentiation, proliferation, cytotoxicity	Defective Th1 differentiation, susceptibility to bacterial infections
Interleukin-13	IL-13	Type I (hematopoietin) heterodimeric	Jak1, Tyk2, Stat6	activated T cells	B cells, macrophages	costimulator of proliferation, IgE, increased CD23, and Class II, inhibits cytokine secretion and cell-mediated immunity	Defective Th2 responses and IgE production, decreased allergic responses
Interleukin-15	IL-15	Type I (hematopoietin) γ_c utilizing	Jak1, Jak3, Stat5	many cells	T-cells, especially memory cells, NK cells	proliferation, survival	absence of NK and memory cells
Interleukin-16	IL-16	CD4		lymphocytes, eosinophils, mast cells, lung epithelium, fibroblasts	CD4 T cells	recruitment and activation of CD4 T cells	
Interleukin-17	IL-17	IL-17R		T cells	many cells	induces cytokine production, I-CAM1 surface expression, T cell proliferation, neutrophil maturation	
Interleukin-18	IL-18	IL-1/TLR	IRAK, MyD88, TRAF6, NF-κB	macrophages	T cells, NK cells	proinflammatory, enhances Th1 responses, enhances NK cell cytotoxicity	enhancement of allergen-induced eosinophilia
Leptin		Type I (hematopoietin) homodimeric	Jak2/Stat3	adipocytes	hyothalamus, thyroid	Satiety, controls metabolic rate	obesity
Leukemia Inhibitory Factor	LIF	Type I (hematopoietin) gp130-utilizing	Jak1, Stat3	uterus, macrophage, fibroblasts, endothelium, epithelium, T cells	embryonic stem cells, neurons, hematopoietic cells	survival	Decreased hematopoietic progenitors, defective blastocyst implantation

continued

CYTOKINES (*contd.*)

Cytokine	Abbreviation	Receptor family	Signaling	Source	Target	Action	Knockout phenotype
Lymphotoxin-α	LTα	TNF		activated T cells and B cells	many cells	cytolysis, lymph node architecture, activation	aberrant lymph node structure
Oncostatin M	OSM	Type I (hematopoietin) gp130-utilizing	Jak1, Stat3	macrophage, fibroblasts, endothelium, epithelium, T cells, others	myeloid cells, liver, embryonic stem cells	differentiation, acute phase induction	
Prolactin	Prl	Type I (hematopoietin) homodimeric	Jak2, Stat5a	pituitary and uterine Prl genes (2)	mammary epithelium	growth, differentiation	infertility, lactation defects
Stem cell factor	SCF, c-kit ligand	Receptor Tyrosine Kinases	Ras/Raf/ MAPK	bone marrow stromal cells	pluripotent stem cell	activation, growth	defective hematopoietic stem cell proliferation, melanocyte production and germ cell development
Thrombopioietin	Tpo	Type I (hematopoietin) homodimeric	Jak2, Stat5	liver, kidney	committed stem cells and megakaryocytes	platelet	Severe thrombocytopenia
Transforming Growth Factor-β 1, 2, 3	TGFβ 1, 2, 3	TGF-β Receptor serine kinase family	SMADs, SARA, FAST-1, TAK1	T cells, macrophages, other cells	T cell, macrophages, other cells	inhibits growth and activation	
Tumor Necrosis Factor-α	TNFα	TNF	TRAFs, TRADD, FADD, Caspases,	macrophages, T cells	neutrophils, macrophages, endothelium, CNS, muscle, fat	adhesion, activation, adhesion, cytokines, coagulation, fever,	Fever deregulation

Index

References for tables and figures are indicated by **bold text**.